CPR FOR ADULTS OR CHILDREN OVER 8 YEARS OLD

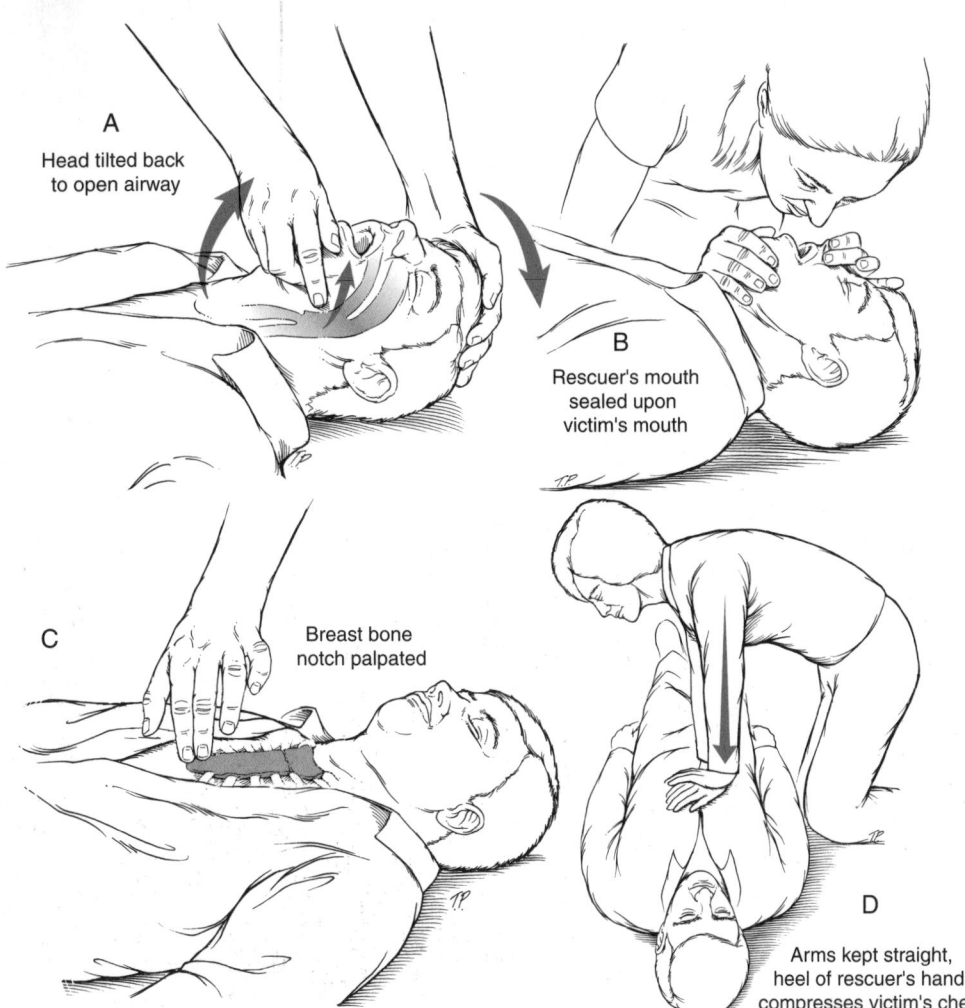

A
Head tilted back
to open airway

B
Rescuer's mouth
sealed upon
victim's mouth

C
Breast bone
notch palpated

D
Arms kept straight,
heel of rescuer's hand
compresses victim's chest

(A) Position the victim on his back. Lift the chin and tilt back the head to open the airway. (B) Kneel next to the victim, pinch his nose shut, and forcibly exhale two times into his mouth without allowing an air gap between your mouth and his. (C) Place two fingers of your left hand above the breast-bone notch. (D) Perform chest compressions by placing the heel of your hand 1 to 1½ inches above the base of the victim's breast; use your other hand to provide support, while with both hands you compress the chest 1½ to 2 inches 15 times rapidly, alternating the chest compressions with giving two breaths. Keep your arms straight. Do 80 to 100 compressions a minute (see page 362).

CPR FOR INFANTS

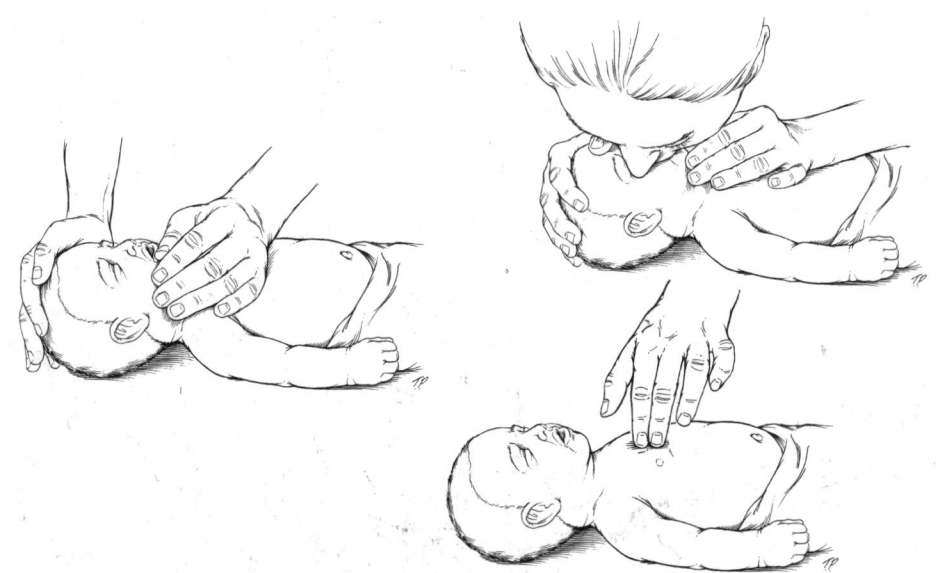

Resuscitating an infant is similar to resuscitating an adult, but compress the infant's chest only 1 inch and only with the middle fingers of the hand; perform only five compressions before cycling back to the breathing (two breaths after five compressions). Do 100 compressions a minute. For children between the ages of 1 and 8 years old, follow these directions but use the heel of the hand for compression and perform one breath after five compressions, except for the initial two breaths. Do 80 to 100 compressions a minute (see page 363).

JOHNS HOPKINS
Family Health Book

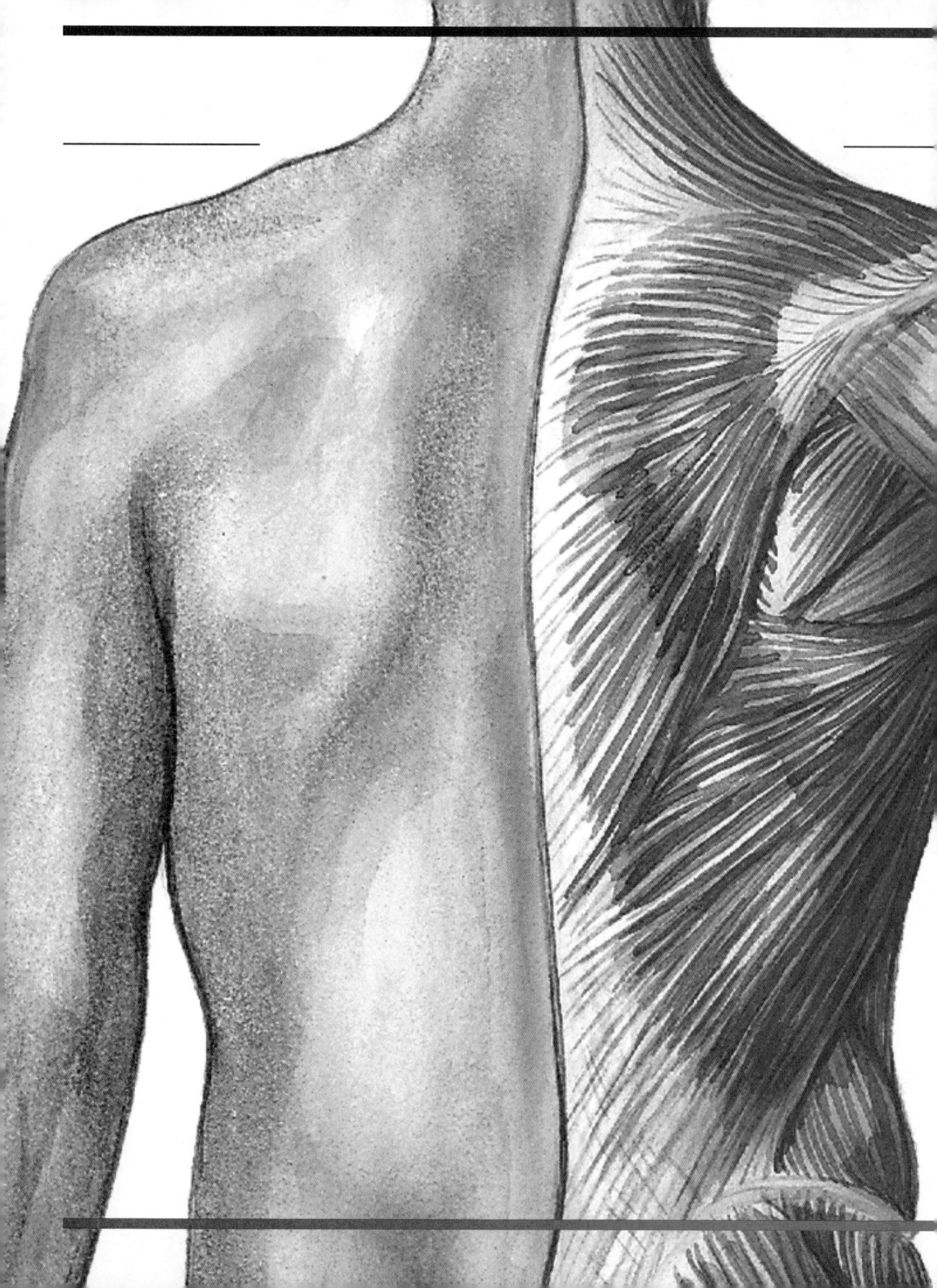

JOHNS HOPKINS

Family Health Book

EDITOR-IN-CHIEF

Michael J. Klag, M.D., M.P.H.

ASSOCIATE EDITORS

Robert S. Lawrence, M.D.

Ada R. Davis, Ph.D.

John K. Niparko, M.D.

ILLUSTRATIONS

Art as Applied to Medicine,
The Johns Hopkins University

Timothy H. Phelps, M.S., F.A.M.I., C.M.I.

David A. Rini, M.F.A., C.M.I.

Corinne Sandone, M.A.

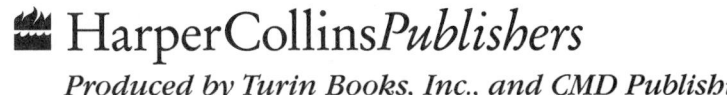

HarperCollins*Publishers*

Produced by Turin Books, Inc., and CMD Publishing

The Johns Hopkins Family Health Book is designed to give you information on various medical conditions, medications, and procedures for your personal knowledge and to help you be a more informed consumer of medical and health services. It is not intended to be complete or exhaustive, nor is it a substitute for the advice of your physician. You should seek medical care promptly for any specific medical problem you or your family members may have.

You can learn more about Johns Hopkins on the World Wide Web at http:// hopkins.med.jhu.edu/. For assistance in arranging a visit to the Johns Hopkins Medical Institutions—from scheduling appointments to receiving guidance on hotels and transportation—please call Johns Hopkins USA at 1-800-507-9952 (or locally, at 410-614-USA1). Client services coordinators are available Monday through Friday from 8:30 a.m. until 5:00 p.m. (Eastern).

Address correspondence related to this book to:

Editor, Johns Hopkins Family Health Book
c/o Office of Consumer Health Information
1830 E. Monument Street Suite 2-200
Baltimore MD 21205

JOHNS HOPKINS FAMILY HEALTH BOOK. Copyright ©1999 by The Johns Hopkins University. All rights reserved. Printed in the United States of America. No part of this book may be used or reproduced in any manner whatsoever without written permission except in the case of brief quotations embodied in critical articles and reviews. For information address HarperCollins Publishers, Inc., 10 East 53rd Street, New York, NY 10022.

HarperCollins books may be purchased for educational, business, or sales promotional use. For information please write: Special Markets Department, HarperCollins Publishers, Inc., 10 East 53rd Street, New York, NY 10022.

FIRST EDITION

Designed by Jeannette Jacobs

Library of Congress Cataloging-in-Publication Data
Johns Hopkins family health book/ by Johns Hopkins University.
        p.   cm.
    Includes index.
    ISBN 0-06-270149-5
    1. Medicine, Popular.   I. Johns Hopkins University.
    RC81.J64 1999   98-38133
    616—dc21   CIP

99 00 01 02 03 CMD XWC 10 9 8 7 6 5 4 3 2 1

Acknowledgments for color insert photographs

The photographs on page C-48 were provided courtesy of the Library of the Horticultural Society of New York.

The photographs of osteoarthritis, page C-42, butterfly rash of lupus,* page C-27, gout, page C-42, and Raynaud's phenomenon, page C-27 were reprinted from the *Clinical Slide Collection on Rheumatic Diseases,* copyright 1997. Used with permission from the American College of Rheumatology. *Identity masked electronically.

The photographs of mastitis, page C-27, stye, page C-46, rubeola, page C-31, rubella,* page C-31, mumps,* page C-30, and strep throat, page C-40 were reprinted from the slide collection *Infectious Diseases*, copyright 1981, RECOM Publishers, D-Fritzlar, Germany. *Identities masked electronically.

The photograph of milia on page C-33 is reprinted from *Atlas of Pediatric Dermatology*, edited by Bernard A. Cohen, M.D., copyright 1993, used with permission of Mosby International Limited.

The color blind tests used on page C-46 were provided courtesy of the Good-Lite Company, Forest Park, IL.

A *Letter* from the *Editor*

All of us at Johns Hopkins receive telephone calls from families and friends whenever they develop a health problem. We provide input on the next step in pinning down the cause of symptoms, talk about the implications of new diagnoses, and help our callers to negotiate our complicated health care system.

Our purpose in writing this book is to give you a similar resource for health information. To do this, we have drawn on the faculty of our Schools of Medicine, Hygiene and Public Health, and Nursing. Although we have assembled an encyclopedic compendium of information, there is no substitute for a therapeutic encounter with a concerned and competent health care professional. We hope, instead, to supplement and facilitate these interactions. All providers recognize that persons leave their office not only with new information but also with many questions. This book is equivalent to that telephone call to "your friend the doctor" who helps you to answer such questions.

The philosophy of the editors is to follow the principles of evidence-based medicine whenever possible. The implications of this approach are that we have used recommendations for use of screening tests and disease treatment from organizations such as the U.S. Preventive Health Services Task Force that weigh the evidence from clinical trials and other research. Many "alternative medicine" treatments have not been subjected to such evaluation and, thus, do not find a place in this book.

A few items to orient you as you use this book. We have chosen to use the term "doctor" as a generic term for all health care professionals. This choice was made for the sake of simplicity. We recognize, however, that excellent health care is provided by nurse practitioners, nurse clinicians, physician assistants, optometrists, podiatrists, physical therapists, occupational therapists, and a host of other professionals. Where appropriate we describe the role of these health care providers.

The book is organized into 5 main sections: Staying Healthy, Health Over the Life Course, First Aid and Emergency Care, Body Systems and Disorders, and Becoming a Partner in Your Health Care. The Body Systems and Disorders section loosely follows a head-to-toe organization. Entries about diseases and conditions follow a template. First, we describe symptoms associated with the disease. Second, the signs that the doctor observes on physical examination in persons with the condition, as well as laboratory findings, are listed. Third, we describe the pathophysiology of the condition in "What is It?" Fourth, we give an overview of available treatment for the condition. When applicable, we have also added a section on prevention of the condition.

The *Johns Hopkins Family Health Book* represents a colossal effort. We hope that it is so polished that you don't see the sweat, but sweat there was, and we would like to acknowledge the contributions of those who made this book possible. My associate editors, Ada Davis, Bob Lawrence, and John Niparko, dedicated an enormous amount of time and talent to oversee this book from start to finish. The more than 110 Hopkins faculty who were involved demonstrated unceasing commitment to producing the most accurate and highest quality information, as well as exceptional patience with our impositions on their busy schedules. Tim Phelps, David Rini, and Cory Sandone of the Johns Hopkins Department of Art as Applied to Medicine proved to us repeatedly that a well-drawn picture is worth a thousand words. Michael Linkinhoker and Bradley Powell provided superb assistance in preparing art for production. Chris Becker and Mary Capotosto in the Johns Hopkins Office of Consumer Health Information moved mountains of paper and coordinated a myriad of communications with aplomb. Molly Mullen brought a fresh and expert viewpoint to review of page proofs.

Adrian Zackheim and Linda Cunningham at HarperCollins and Scott Sherman, assistant dean of the Johns Hopkins School of Medicine, were present at the creation and provided leadership and support throughout the long gestation of this volume. Channa Taub of Turin Books provided invaluable assistance in the creation and editing of this book. Patty Leasure at HarperCollins guided us through the publishing process and Tricia Medved stepped in to bring the book down the home stretch. Assistants Rob Amell and Greg Chaput kept things running smoothly. Jennifer Mitchell, Donna Balopole, and the wonderful staff at CMD did a superb job of integrating all of the work into the volume you are holding.

Lastly, the editorial board owes a great deal to Ron Sauder, Director of the Office of Consumer Health Information. He went above and beyond the call of duty at every step of the process.

Read in good health!

Michael J. Klag, MD, MPH

The *Editors*

Editor-in-Chief

Michael J. Klag, M.D., M.P.H., is David M. Levine Professor of Medicine, and Director, Division of General Internal Medicine at The Johns Hopkins University School of Medicine. He is also the Associate Director for General Medicine of the Department of Medicine. Dr. Klag holds joint appointments in the Departments of Epidemiology and Health Policy and Management at The Johns Hopkins University School of Hygiene and Public Health. Dr. Klag received his M.D. degree at the University of Pennsylvania School of Medicine in 1978 and his Master of Public Health degree at The Johns Hopkins University School of Hygiene and Public Health in 1987. Dr. Klag practices general internal medicine at Johns Hopkins and is a fellow of the American College of Physicians. He has published in many medical journals, serves on the editorial board of the *American Journal of Medicine*, and is an editorial consultant to numerous other journals.

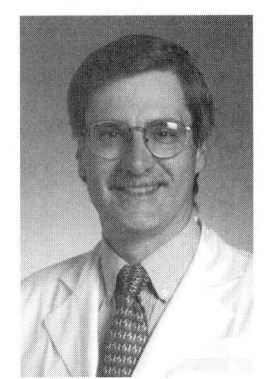

Associate Editors

Robert S. Lawrence, M.D., is Associate Dean for Professional Education and Programs and Professor of Health Policy and Management at The Johns Hopkins University School of Hygiene and Public Health and Professor of Medicine at The Johns Hopkins University School of Medicine. He received his M.D. degree at Harvard Medical School and is a Master of the American College of Physicians and a Fellow of the American College of Preventive Medicine. He currently serves as a consultant to the Task Force on Community Preventive Services at the Centers for Disease Control and Prevention.

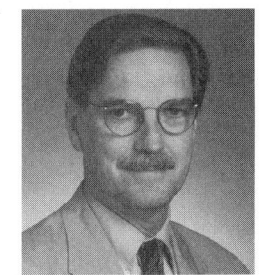

Ada Romaine Davis, Ph.D., is Associate Professor and Director of Baccalaureate Programs at The Johns Hopkins University School of Nursing. She graduated from Kings County Hospital School of Nursing, earned degrees at the University of Maryland, and is certified as an Adult Nurse Practitioner and as an Editor in the Life Sciences. She is a member of the New York Academy of Sciences and is included in *Marquis' Who's Who Among American Educators.*

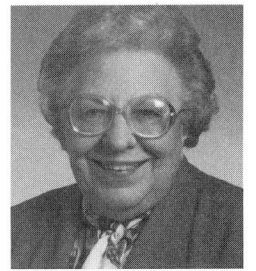

John Kim Niparko, M.D., is Professor and Director of the Division of Otology, Neurology, and Skull Base Surgery in the Department of Otolaryngology—Head and Neck Surgery, at The Johns Hopkins University School of Medicine. He is a graduate of the University of Michigan, where he earned his M.D. with Distinction. He has been named one of the "Best Doctors in America" and is currently Assistant Editor of the *Archives of Otolaryngology—Head and Neck Surgery.*

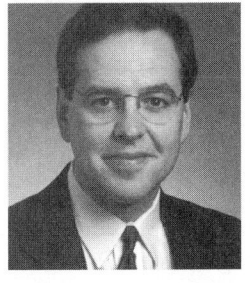

List of Editors and Contributors

Bernard Guyer, M.D., M.P.H. *Professor and Chair, Maternal and Child Health*

Henry R. Halperin, M.D. *Associate Professor of Medicine*

Ada Hamosh, M.D., M.P.H. *Assistant Professor of Pediatrics*

Jennifer A. Haythornthwaite, Ph.D. *Associate Professor of Medical Psychology and Psychiatry*

Kathy J. Helzlsouer, M.D. M.H.S. *Associate Professor of Epidemiology and Oncology*

Barbara Howard, M.D. *Assistant Professor of Pediatrics*

Orest Hurko, M.D. *Associate Professor of Neurology, Medicine, Neurological Surgery, and Pediatrics; Clinical Director, Greenberg Center for Skeletal Dysplasia*

Alain Joffe, M.D. *Associate Professor of Pediatrics; Director, Adolescent Medicine*

Constance J. Johnson, M.D. *Associate Professor of Neurology; Director, Neurovascular Center, Johns Hopkins Bayview Medical Center*

Paramjit Kaur Joshi, M.D. *Associate Professor of Psychiatry; Assistant Professor of Pediatrics*

Michael J. Kaminsky, M.D. *Associate Professor of Psychiatry; Clinical Director, Psychiatry*

Jean S. Kan, M.D. *Helen B. Taussig Professor of Pediatric Cardiology*

Adam S. Kibel, M.D. *Instructor in Urology*

Alan M. Lake, M.D. *Associate Professor of Pediatrics*

Michael A. Levine, M.D. *Professor of Pediatrics, Medicine, and Pathology; Director, Division of Pediatric Endocrinology*

Horace K. Liang, M.D. *Assistant Professor and Residency Director, Emergency Medicine*

Paul S. Lietman, M.D., Ph.D. *Wellcome Professor of Clinical Pharmacology; Professor of Medicine, Pediatrics, Pharmacology and Molecular Sciences; Director, Division of Clinical Pharmacology; Director of Research for Johns Hopkins Singapore*

Donlin M. Long, M.D., Ph.D. *Professor and Director, Neurosurgery*

Ellen J. MacKenzie, Ph.D. *Professor of Health Policy and Management; Director, Center for Injury Research and Policy; Senior Associate Dean, Academic Affairs, School of Hygiene and Public Health*

Warren R. Maley, M.D. *Assistant Professor of Surgery*

Carole Marcus, M.D. *Associate Professor of Pediatrics; Medical Director, Pediatric Sleep Lab*

Simeon Margolis, M.D., Ph.D. *Professor of Medicine, Endocrinology Division; Professor of Biological Chemistry*

Edward G. MacFarland, M.D. *Associate Professor of Orthopaedic Surgery; Director, Sports Medicine and Shoulder Surgery*

Victor A. McKusick, M.D. *University Professor of Medical Genetics*

Patrick A. Murphy, M.D. *Professor of Medicine and Molecular Biology and Genetics*

Susanne Ogaitis, M.S.P.H. *Assistant Director for External Affairs; Center for Injury Research and Policy*

Jean Ogborn, M.D. *Assistant Professor of Pediatrics; Assistant Director, Pediatric Emergency Medicine*

Bruce A. Perler, M.D. *Professor of Surgery; Director, Vascular Surgery Fellowship and Vascular Noninvasive Laboratory*

Deborah Persaud, M.D. *Assistant Professor of Pediatrics*

Timothy H. Phelps, M.S., F.A.M.I., C.M.I. *Associate Professor, Art as Applied to Medicine*

Leslie Plotnick, M.D. *Associate Professor of Pediatrics*

Martin Pomper, M.D., Ph.D. *Assistant Professor of Radiology*

Eva Pressman, M.D. *Assistant Professor of Gynecology and Obstetrics*

David A. Rini, M.F.A., C.M.I *Assistant Professor, Art as Applied to Medicine*

Leon A. Rosenberg, Ph.D. *Joint Appointment, Psychiatry and Pediatrics; Professor, School of Continuing Studies*

Roberto Salvatori, M.D. *Instructor in Medicine and Endocrinology*

Jonathan Samet, M.D., M.S. *Professor and Chair, Epidemiology*

Corinne Sandone, M.A. *Assistant Professor, Art as Applied to Medicine*

Brian S. Schwartz, M.D., M.S. *Associate Professor of Environmental Health Sciences; Director, Division of Occupational and Environmental Health*

William W. Scott, Jr., M.D. *Associate Professor of Radiology and Orthopaedic Surgery; Director, Orthopaedic Radiology*

Henry M. Seidel, M.D. *Professor Emeritus, Pediatrics*

Bruce K. Shapiro, M.D. *Associate Professor of Pediatrics; Vice President, Kennedy Krieger Institute*

Phillip R. Slavney, M.D. *Eugene Meyer III Professor of Psychiatry and Medicine*

Philip L. Smith, M.D. *Professor of Medicine; Instructor in Anesthesiology*

Paul D. Sponseller, M.D. *Associate Professor of Orthopaedic Surgery; Head, Division of Pediatric Orthopaedics*

Kerry J. Stewart, Ed.D. *Associate Professor of Medicine*

Craig A. Vander Kolk, M.D. *Associate Professor of Plastic Surgery; Assistant Professor of Pediatrics*

Judith W. Vogelhut, B.S., C.P.N.P., I.B.C.L.C. *Nurse Coordinator, Pediatrics, Breast Feeding Center*

Allen Walker, M.D. *Assistant Professor of Pediatrics; Director, Pediatric Emergency Medicine*

Patrick C. Walsh, M.D. *David Hall McConnell Professor and Director, Urology*

David B. Weishampel, Ph.D. *Professor of Cell Biology and Anatomy*

S. Elizabeth Whitmore, M.D. *Assistant Professor of Dermatology*

Fredrick M. Wigley, M.D. *Professor of Medicine; Director, Molecular and Clinical Rheumatology*

Modena Wilson, M.D., M.P.H. *Professor of Pediatrics; Director, General Pediatrics and Adolescent Medicine*

Robert A. Wise, M.D. *Professor of Medicine*

Robert J. Wityk, M.D. *Assistant Professor of Neurology and Medicine*

CONSULTING EDITORS

Ayse Ali Atasoylu, M.D. *Fellow, General Internal Medicine*

Diane M. Becker, Sc.D. *Associate Professor, Medicine; Director, Center for Health Promotion; Joint Appointment, Health Policy and Management*

Jeanne Marie Clark, M.D., M.P.H. *Fellow, General Internal Medicine*

Thomas Philip Erlinger, M.D. *Fellow, General Internal Medicine*

John A. Flynn, M.D. *Assistant Professor, Internal Medicine and Rheumatology; Clinical Director, General Internal Medicine*

Todd William Gress, M.D. *Fellow, General Internal Medicine*

Cary Philip Gross, M.D. *Fellow, Robert Wood Johnson Clinical Scholar Program and General Internal Medicine*

David Morgan Huchton, M.D. *Fellow and Resident, Otolaryngology-Head and Neck Surgery*

George R. Huggins, M.D. *Deputy Chairman, Clinical Affairs; Chairman, Gynecology/Obstetrics, JHBMC*

Brian S. Kuszyk, M.D. *Fellow, Resident, Radiology and Radiographical Science*

Julie R. Lange, M.D. *Assistant Professor, Surgery*

Daniel J. Lee, M.D. *Fellow, Johns Hopkins Hospital; Assistant Resident, Department of Otolaryngology-Head and Neck Surgery*

Terrence P. O'Brien, M.D. *Assistant Professor, Ophthalmology; Director, Refractive Eye Surgery; Director, Ocular Infectious Diseases*

Kimberly Peairs, M.D. *Assistant Professor, General Internal Medicine*

Christopher Sciamanna, M.D. *Fellow, General Internal Medicine*

Jodi Segal, M.D. *Fellow, General Internal Medicine*

Stephen D. Sisson, M.D. *Assistant Professor, Medicine*

John Song, M.D. *Fellow, General Internal Medicine*

Francisco A. Tausk, M.D. *Assistant Professor of Dermatology*

Michael Weiner, M.D. *Fellow, General Internal Medicine*

Albert W. Wu, M.D., M.P.H. *Associate Professor, Health Policy and Management; Joint Appointment, Internal Medicine*

* Unless otherwise noted all positions listed above are at The Johns Hopkins University Schools of Medicine, Nursing, and Public Health.

PUBLISHING & PRODUCTION ACKNOWLEDGMENTS

The Johns Hopkins University and Health System Office of Consumer Health Information

Scott Sherman, *Assistant Dean*
W. Ronald Sauder, *Director*
Molly L. Mullen, *Editor*
Mary Capotosto, *Publications Coordinator*

HarperCollins*Publishers*, Inc.
Patricia Leasure, *Executive Editor*
Tricia Medved, *Editor*
Jeannette Jacobs, *Graphic Designer*

Turin Books, Inc
Channa Taub, *Editorial Director*

CMD Publishing, *a division of Current Medical Directions, Inc.*
Jennifer Mitchell, *Vice President, Publishing*
Sarah Butterworth, *Vice President, Marketing and Development*
Donna Balopole, *Production Director*
Linda Fetters, *Indexer*

Hermitage Publishing Services, *Page Composition*

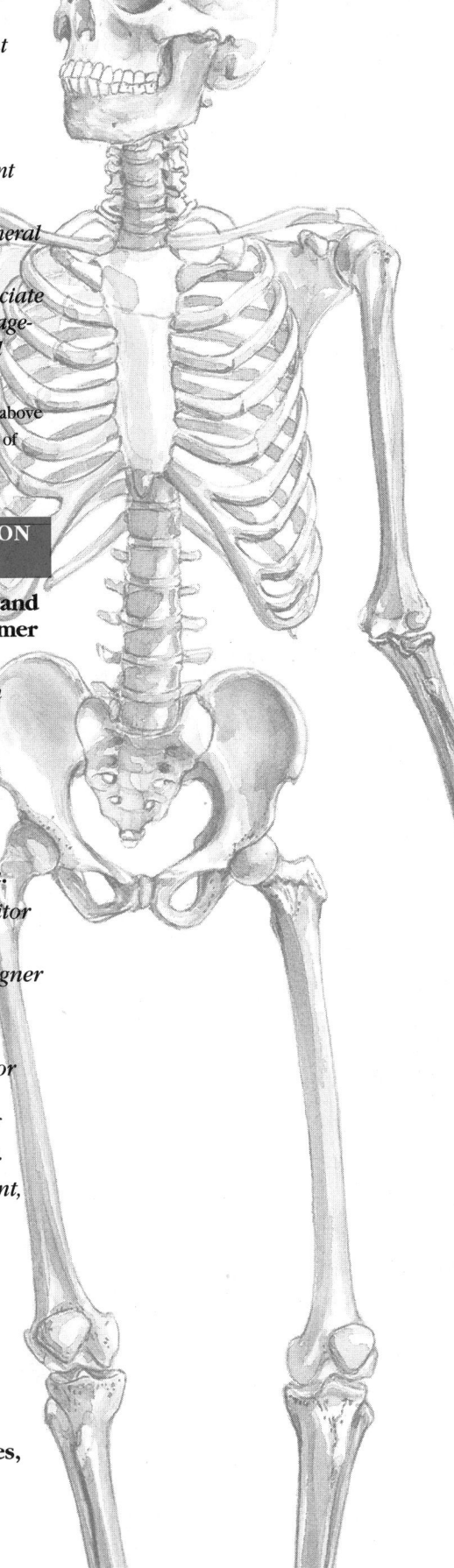

CONTENTS

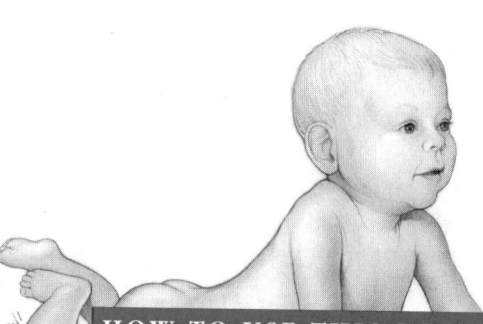

HOW TO USE THIS BOOK   xiv

Read this section first to learn how the book is organized and to find out where to look for the information you need, whether you are trying to interpret your symptoms, wish to know more about a medication that you are taking, or are looking for general health and nutrition facts.

PART 1. STAYING HEALTHY   1

Eating right and exercising are crucial to preventing disease and maintaining a desirable weight. But staying healthy also means making your home safe and understanding the devastating effects of smoking and substance abuse. This section discusses the basic components of a healthy diet and shows you how to design a personalized exercise program for everyone in your family. You will also learn how to childproof your home and evaluate it for dangerous toxins such as radon or lead, how to recognize if you or someone you know has a problem with drugs or alcohol, and what techniques are effective for quitting smoking.

PART 2. HEALTH OVER THE LIFE COURSE   109

Each stage of life has a special set of health concerns. This section explains what to expect during a pregnancy and how to care properly for an infant. As your child grows, you will need to know how to interpret common symptoms such as a fever or stomach ache and to be able to recognize problems in speech or vision that could impede your child's development. In adulthood the focus turns to setting life goals and building lasting relationships. The chapter on seniors dispels myths about aging and provides advice on staying physically and mentally fit and overcoming age-related health problems related to vision and hearing.

PART 3. FIRST AID AND EMERGENCY CARE   349

Knowing the basics of first aid is vital to your family's health. Not only does it give you the power to quickly soothe the pain of everyday cuts and bruises, but in the case of a sudden injury or illness it can mean the difference between life and death. This chapter will show you how to build a proper first-aid kit and give you the tools to evaluate health emergencies. Learn how to address everyday sprains and strains, what to do in the event of a severe asthma attack or febrile seizure in your child, and the warning signs of a heart attack or stroke.

PART 4. BODY SYSTEMS AND DISORDERS   417

Knowing how to interpret your symptoms is the first step in recognizing a potential health problem. These chapters discuss the functions of various body systems and describe the most common or serious health problems related to them. You will learn what your symptoms mean, what signs the doctor looks for and the tests used during diagnosis, how a problem develops, and what can be done to treat or prevent it. Each chapter also discusses self-care measures and advises you on when your doctor should be called.

PART 5. BECOMING A PARTNER IN YOUR HEALTH CARE   1381

Taking charge of your health means being an informed patient and forming a partnership with your doctor. Knowing how to find the right doctor or health care plan for you and your family and understanding your rights as a patient are important parts of that process. This section also prepares you for what to expect before and during surgery and explains how to get the most out of your medications while minimizing side effects. The last chapter offers advice to families on how to come to terms with the death of a loved one and how to cope when someone close to you is seriously ill.

PART 6. APPENDICES   1501

INDEX   1603

*C*olor Atlas of Anatomy, Disorders, and Diseases follows page 1276

How *to* Use *this* Book

Structure of the Book

When it comes to your health, you want answers fast. A comprehensive source of information for the entire family, *Johns Hopkins Family Health Book* is organized

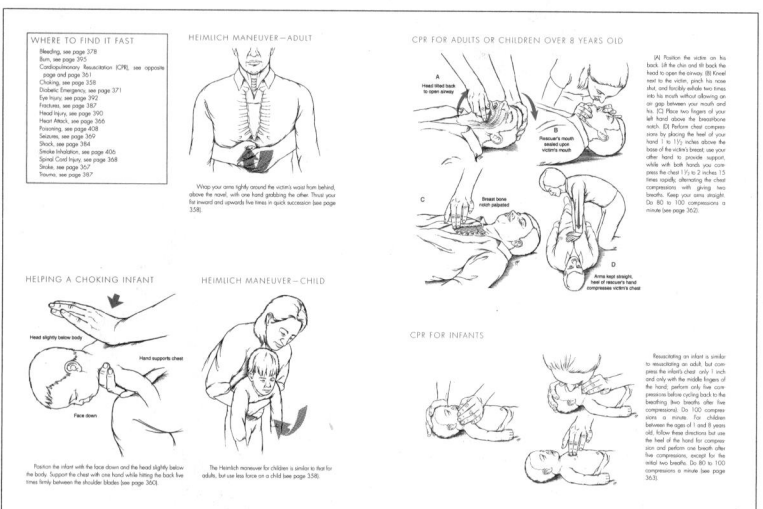

for easy use. It is divided into six main sections and a comprehensive index. The first four sections are devoted to different areas of your physical and mental well-being. Part 5 describes the rapidly changing face of modern health care, and Part 6 contains helpful appendices including a glossary of common medical terms and a medication directory. A thorough index, which includes symptoms highlighted in color, enables you to find any topic quickly.

A unique feature of this book is its three-tiered emergency reference system:

1. When seconds to minutes count in a life-threatening emergency, such as choking and major blood loss, turn at once to the first aid section shown on the pages inside the front and back covers; these illustrated pages provide quick access to emergency techniques for choking, bleeding, and stroke along with listings of both stroke and heart attack signs. A Where to Find It Fast index directs you to first aid techniques within the text.

2. When you have a few more minutes to administer first aid, turn to Chapter 13, First Aid and Emergency Care, for detailed coverage of many emergencies; this chapter can be quickly found by looking for the text pages that are edged in red ink.

3. Before emergencies even occur or after they are stabilized, in-depth information on many diseases and disorders can be found in the chapters in Part 4: Body Systems and Disorders.

The following is a description of each section of the book; for an overview of any individual chapter, you can turn to the detailed table of contents at the start of the chapter.

Part 1. Staying Healthy

Proper diet and regular exercise form the foundation of healthy living. This section explains how a balanced approach to your nutritional needs can be accomplished without giving up the joy of eating. You

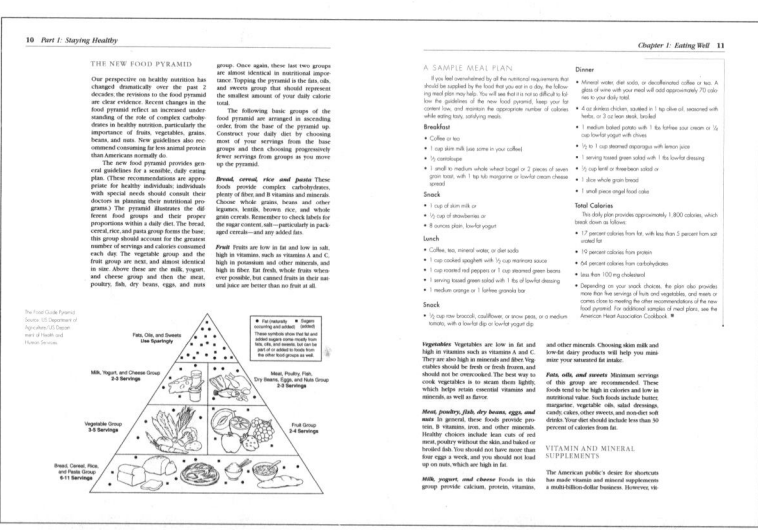

will also learn how eating right and staying fit can help you maintain a healthy weight and prevent disease while avoiding the perils of dangerous dieting and unhealthy eating habits. This section also contains advice for staying safe and preventing injury inside and outside the home and includes information on fire safety, childproofing your house, avoiding environmental toxins, and the potentially dangerous consequences of sun exposure. Chapter 4 explains why it is crucial to stop smoking and surveys the latest smoking cessation techniques. This section concludes with a chapter on the devastating effects of alcohol and drug addiction and includes information on how to recognize if you or someone you know has a substance abuse problem and where to turn for help.

Part 2. Health Over the Life Course

This section contains a wealth of information for every member of your family, from the youngest to the oldest. It is your guide to growth and development, to learning, living and changing together as a family, and to aging. After a chapter on the role of genetics and the importance of understanding hereditary medical conditions, this sections proceeds step by step from birth to the senior years. It explains the best way to plan for and manage a pregnancy and discusses the developmental stages vital to your child's growth. This section also contains advice for parents and teens on the challenges posed by the adolescent years, from simple growing pains to issues of health and sexuality. The chapter on adulthood discusses the importance of setting career goals and

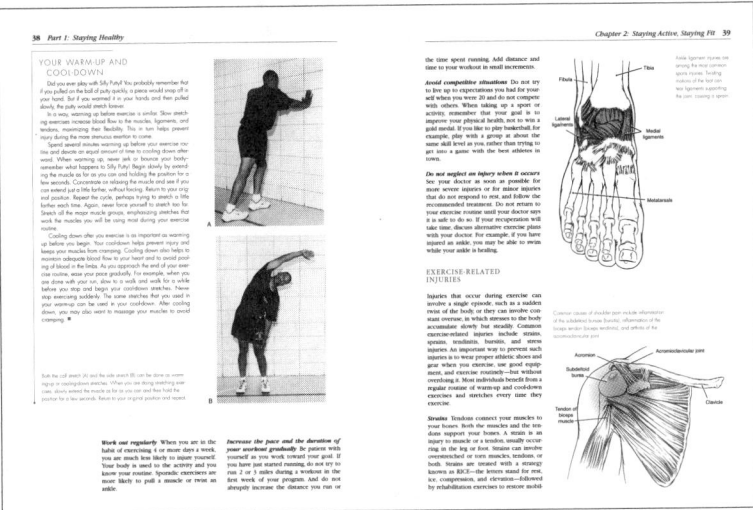

building solid relationships while coping with the inevitable stresses of modern life. The final chapter distinguishes fact from myth in the aging process and discusses health concerns of seniors, such as osteoporosis and the disorders that cause dementia; it also includes information on identifying and correcting vision and hearing problems.

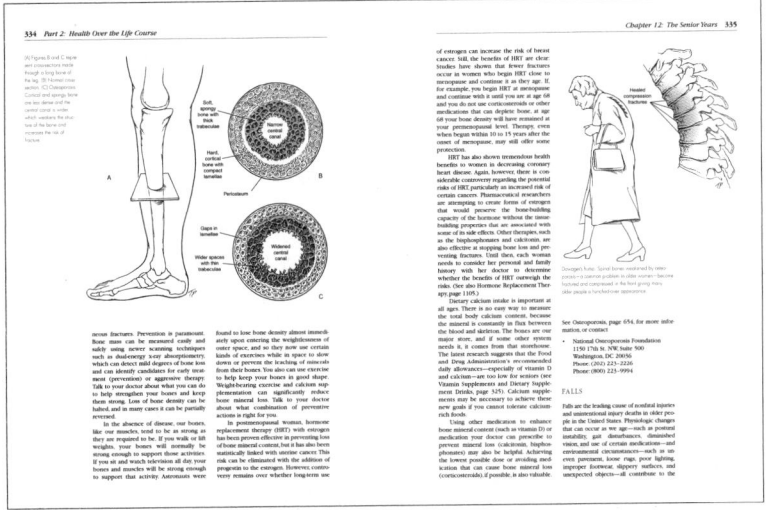

Part 3. First Aid and Emergency Care

Knowing how to respond properly to a medical emergency such as a heart attack or stroke can often mean the difference between life and death. First aid is also important in helping to reduce the severity of an injury and to speed healing, as well as to soothe the pain of everyday cuts and bruises. This easy-to-find chapter explains how to evaluate and address a broad range of injuries and medical emergencies, from a nuisance nosebleed to life-threatening trauma. For even faster reference, first aid procedures for major life-threatening situations where response time is limited are printed inside the front and back covers of the book.

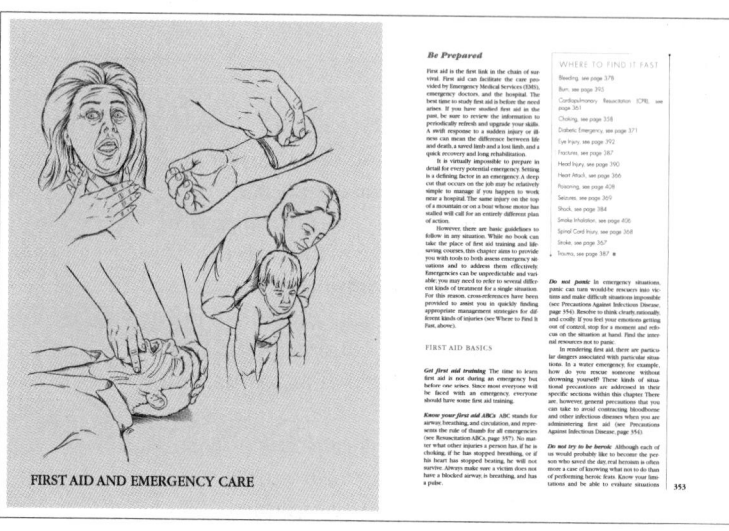

FIRST AID AND EMERGENCY CARE

Part 4. Body Systems and Disorders

While this book is not a substitute for professional medical care, understanding how to interpret your symptoms and knowing what to expect during a doctor's examination are an important part of being an informed patient. The 17 chapters in this section explain the most common or serious medical conditions

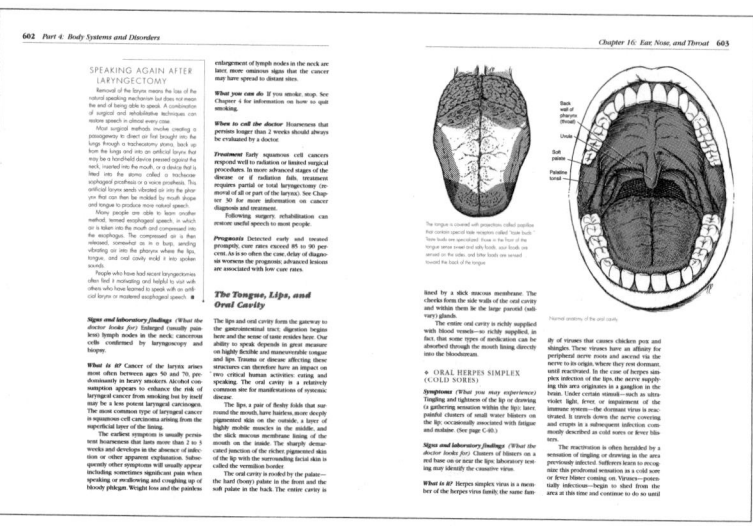

affecting various systems of the body and include the latest research from experts at Johns Hopkins. The discussion of each condition begins with a list of symptoms (which are what you may experience) and signs (what the doctor looks for during an examination) and demystifies the tests used during diagnosis.

Symptoms and signs are listed in order of how commonly they occur, with more frequent symptoms and signs listed first. In addition, since some symptoms and signs occur individually during illness while others appear as a group, this is distinguished in the text. When symptoms occur separately from each other, you may experience one of them and not the others; this type of listing is separated by semi-colons—for example, "headache; runny nose; fever." Listings of symptoms that usually occur together are separated by commas—for example, "headache, runny nose, and fever." This distinction applies to the sections on both the symptoms and the signs and laboratory findings of disease entries.

Part 4 of the book also discusses how diseases develop and who is usually affected and describes when it is appropriate to use self-care measures such as over-the-counter medications. It also explains what you can do to prevent a condition from developing in the first place and compares the success rates of various treatment options. Diseases and disorders that are described in greater detail with subheadings such as signs, symptoms and laboratory findings, and treatment are indicated with a ❖ icon.

This section of the book also includes a 48-page color insert; the first half of the insert features original color drawings of major body systems and parts; the second half consists of color photographs of a variety of diseases and disorders, including dermatologic and ophthalmic problems.

Part 5. Becoming a Partner in Your Health Care

Because informed patients usually receive the highest level of care, the chapters in this section aim at making the rapidly changing world of modern health care easier to understand. This section is your source for information on health care plans, choosing the best doctor for you and your family, and preparing for surgery. It also explains how medications get approved by the Food and Drug Administration (FDA) and provides general tips for using your medications safely. The chapter on home care and long-term care discusses the role of caregivers and explains what to look for in a nursing home or other facility. The last chapter offers advice to families on coping with the death or illness of a loved one.

Part 6. Appendices

The Medication Directory contained in this section is particularly useful if you want to know more about your medications. It provides key information on over 80 commonly prescribed drugs. You will learn how your medication works and what it is typically used for. It explains which side effects are of no concern and which are cause to

glossary (an extensive list of commonly used medical terms with easy-to-understand explanations), a listing of the normal values for many commonly prescribed laboratory tests, normal growth charts for children, and reproductions of forms known as advance directives (such as a living will,

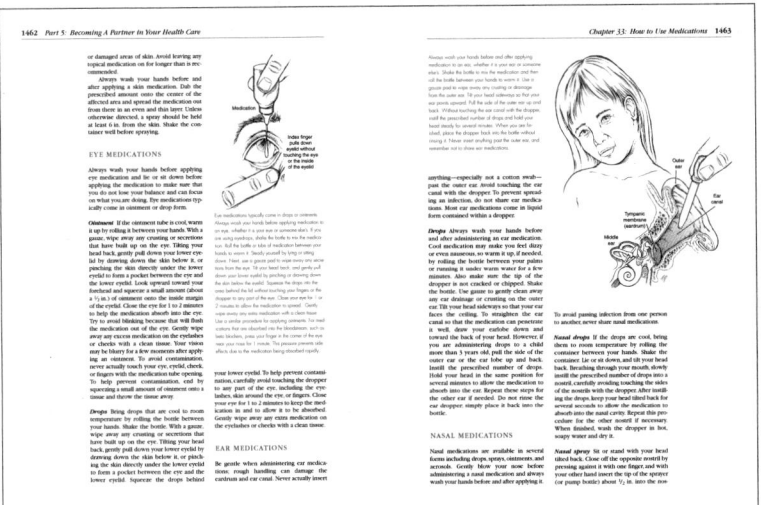

appointment of a health care agent, and health care instructions) that will enable you—in advance of an incapacitating accident or illness—to make health care decisions and/or to name someone to make those decisions on your behalf.

The Index

The detailed index at the end of the book is a dual-function index and makes it easy for you to access topics within the text. Diseases, disorders, and syndromes, symptoms, parts of the body, and types of tests are all included as main entries in the index and boldface numerals are used to indicate any primary discussions. Symptom main entries are highlighted in color so that they can be noted quickly, and illustrations in the text are indicated with italic page numbers.

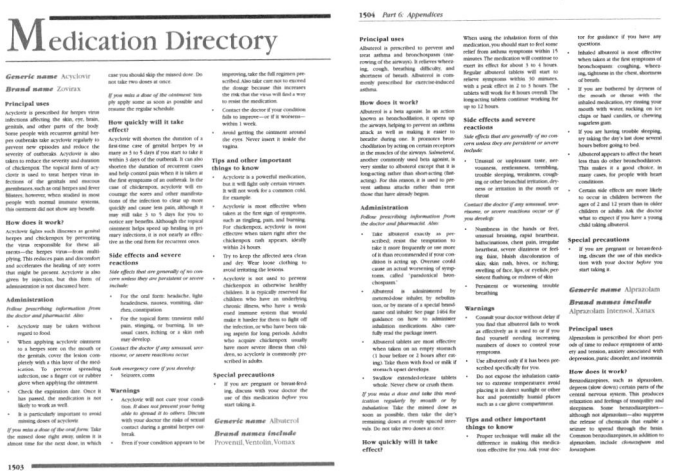

call a doctor. It also contains warnings about which medications should not be combined and discusses the effect that your medication may have on an existing medical condition. Part 6 also contains a

JOHNS HOPKINS
Family Health Book

PART ONE
Staying Healthy

Eating Well

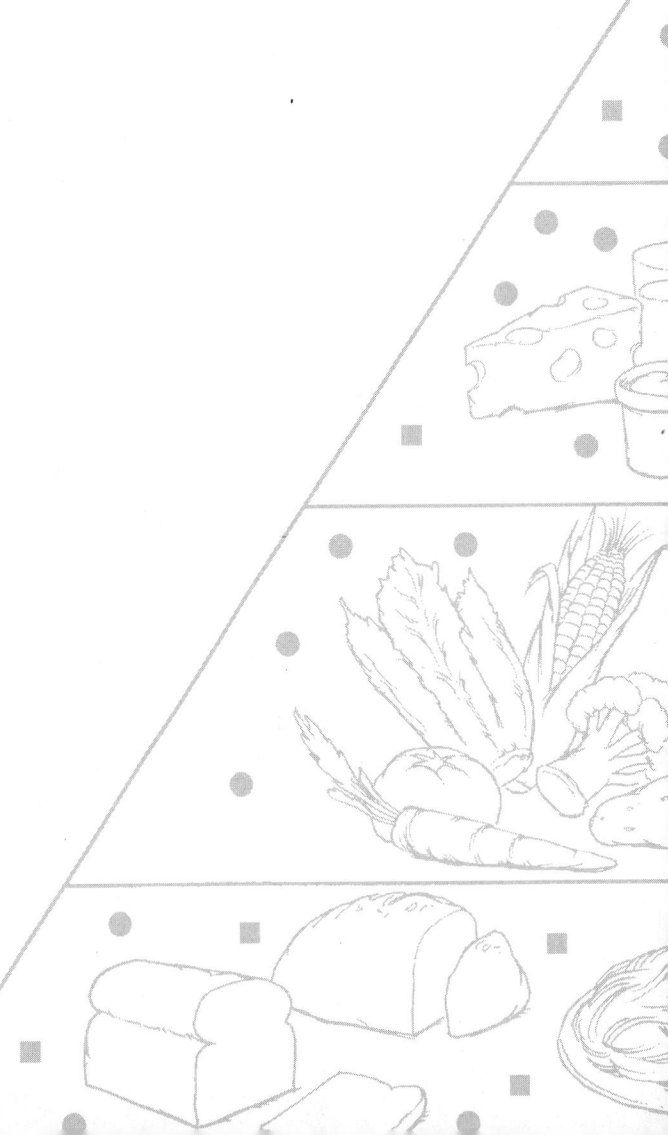

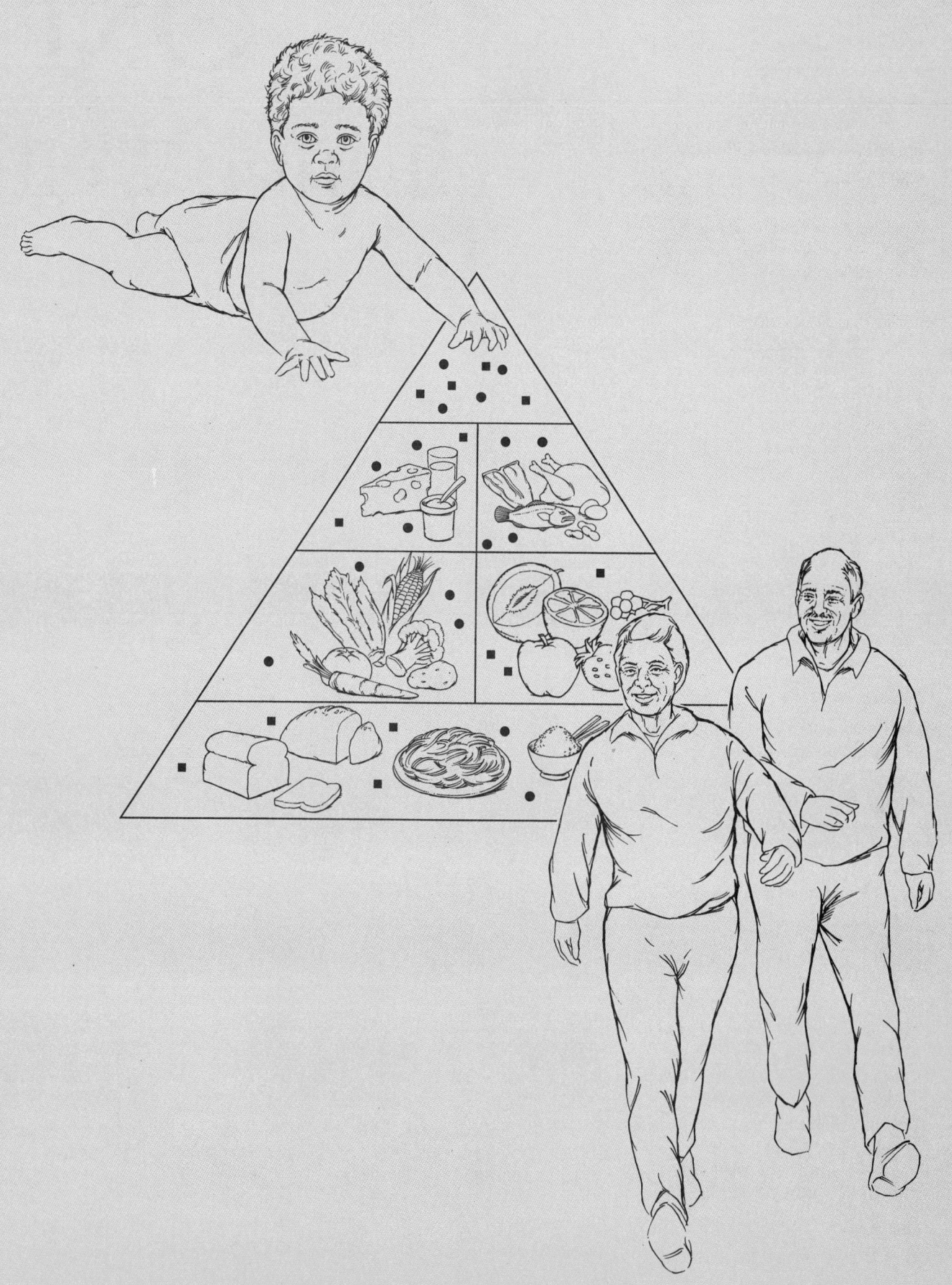

EATING WELL

Nutrition and Good Health

Americans are preoccupied with both food and dieting, and these two preoccupations are often at odds. What we need is a balanced approach to nutritional needs and gastronomical pleasures so that food becomes a healthy and joyful part of daily life.

The word *diet*, originally from the Greek for "a way of life," has become synonymous with suffering for many Americans. But whether we refer to what we eat as our diet, our daily fare, or our nutritional program, the only way to solve the riddle of maintaining a desirable weight and meeting our nutritional needs is to eat a variety of healthy foods in moderation every day.

How we view food and diet has changed dramatically in this century. Less than 100 years ago, malnutrition was a major medical problem in the United States. Many people did not get the proper nutrients from food and suffered from scurvy, goiter, rickets, and stunted growth. Minor illnesses would often lead to death in people weakened by malnutrition.

In the affluent period following World War II, food was enjoyed as one of the rewards of prosperity. The American diet became richer in calories and fat, and included meals such as eggs and bacon, and steak and potatoes. Fast food and manufactured snack foods became plentiful; at the same time technological advances in the workplace and at home made life more sedentary. As a result, most Americans began to put on extra pounds. Today, even though many families live below the poverty line, obesity in children and adults is our biggest nutritional problem, and a contributing factor in a host of chronic medical conditions.

We may not be what we eat, but our health irrevocably depends on what we eat. A healthy, balanced diet is truly the staff of life. All the pills in the world do not have the power that fresh vegetables and fruits, lean proteins, and the right amount of essential fatty acids and complex carbohydrates have for ensuring good health. This chapter provides the information you need to construct a diet that is an essential part of your overall program of good health.

CHILDREN AND NUTRITION

The nutritional needs of children are different from those of adults. Be careful to take the special needs of growing children into account as you create a nutritional plan for the improved health of your entire family.

There is almost universal agreement that children under the age of two should not be put on a fat-restricted diet. At this age, the fat a child consumes is essential to growth and development. When your child reaches age two, you may want to talk with your pediatrician about beginning to substitute 1 or 2 percent milk for whole milk and increasing your child's consumption of low-fat foods.

As your child grows, the best way to ensure that he is getting the necessary nutrients without becoming overweight is to help him establish healthy eating habits. This includes having healthy snacks in the house, including fresh fruit, whole wheat crackers and bread, and low-fat alternatives to snack foods. If your child is overweight, speak with your doctor about ways of changing eating habits gradually and subtly. Never force an overweight child to lose weight; such a plan is neither healthy nor effective. Instead, implement lifestyle changes that will allow your child to "grow" into his weight. Exercise should be encouraged and noneducational TV viewing should probably be limited. Keep high-calorie snacks out of the house and do not use food as a reward. For further information on nutrition in children, see Chapter 9. ∎

WHAT IS A HEALTHFUL DIET?

Although nutritional requirements vary depending on age, physique, gender, and individual health profile, all of us need varying amounts of the basic components of a healthy diet: protein, fat, carbohydrate, vitamins, minerals, and water. Only the three macronutrients—protein, carbohydrate, and fat—provide the calories that the body needs for energy. However, the micronutrients—vitamins and minerals—are just as essential for growth, development, and overall good health. Although fiber is not a nutrient, it is important for good health and disease prevention. Water is essential for sustaining life.

Protein After water, protein is the most plentiful substance in the body. It is essential for growth and repair of body tissues, including internal organs, blood, muscles, and skin, as well as for the formation of antibodies, hormones, and enzymes. Protein is a source of energy and heat, as well as an important component in the elimination of waste. Proteins are composed of amino acids; 22 amino acids are known to be vital for health. Of these 22, 14 are synthesized by the adult body. The remaining 8, called the essential amino acids, can only be obtained from the food we eat.

Fruits, vegetables, nuts, beans, and other foods contain some protein; however, meat, eggs, and cheese and other foods from animal sources contain complete proteins, which means they provide adequate amounts of all eight essential amino acids. Your daily diet must include enough protein to replenish the body's supply of essential amino acids because the body cannot synthesize them. If you do not eat foods from animal sources, you will need to eat a variety of plant protein sources in combination to ensure that you obtain sufficient amounts of all the essential amino acids.

How much protein people need to consume on a daily basis varies. Some research has indicated that Americans consume too much protein. However, recent emphasis on consuming more complex carbohydrates, or "carbo-loading," for better athletic performance, and on the health benefits of a vegetarian diet has caused many Americans to consume smaller and smaller amounts of complete protein. As you construct your nutrition plan, remember that adequate daily amounts of complete protein are essential for your health. The US Senate Select Committee on Nutrition and Human Needs recommends that approximately 12 percent of your total daily calories come from protein. This means that normal, healthy adults should consume roughly 40 to 70 g of protein every day.

Fat A certain amount of fat is necessary in a healthy diet. Babies and young children especially need adequate fat in their diet for proper brain development. Unfortunately, most Americans consume too much fat, making fat 40 percent or more of their caloric intake, rather than the recommended 30 to 35 percent. Too much fat, particularly saturated fat, may lead to heart disease and obesity, and put you at greater risk for other diseases and chronic conditions.

Fat is a substance made up of fatty acids or lipids. Depending upon their chemical structure, fatty acids are saturated, monosaturated, or polyunsaturated. The more hydrogen a fatty acid contains, the more saturated the fat is. Saturated fats are the "fattest" fats—and are the fats that may hurt your health.

There are two polyunsaturated fatty acids that are called essential fatty acids because the body cannot manufacture them; they must be obtained through diet. Essential fatty acids are necessary for healthy growth and metabolism. Although Americans consume far too much saturated fat, some studies show that as many as 10 percent of Americans may be deficient in the essential fatty acids. Essential fatty acids are obtained from sunflower seeds, walnuts, green leafy vegetables, and canola, soybean, and walnut oils.

Dietary fat helps to transport the fat-soluble vitamins A, D, E, and K, so that they can be absorbed and utilized. Cells use fat to aid in a great number of body functions, including membrane formation, nerve-impulse conduction, hormone production, metabolic function, brain function, immune function, reproductive function, and skin and hair health.

Problems with fat arise when 10 percent or more of your daily calorie consumption comes from saturated fat. Saturated fats are found in meats, dairy products, butter, and oils high in saturated fats, such as coconut oil, palm oil, corn oil, and cottonseed oil (see Common Foods and Cooking Ingredients High in Saturated Fats, this page).

COMMON FOODS AND COOKING INGREDIENTS HIGH IN SATURATED FATS

In a healthy nutrition plan for adults, the following foods and cooking ingredients should be avoided entirely or used only sparingly.

- Butter
- Coconut oil
- Palm oil
- Cocoa butter
- Lard ■

CUTTING DOWN ON FAT

Cutting down on the amount of fat you consume is easier than you think. Keep in mind that you are only cutting down and not eliminating fat from your diet. Concentrate on controlling the amount of saturated fat you consume. Remember that children need more fat than adults; you should not attempt to limit your children's fat intake in the same way that you do your own (see Children and Nutrition, page 5).

When grocery shopping, read the labels. Products containing more than 30 percent fat should be eaten infrequently. Use whole milk sparingly, as a treat in coffee, for example. For general consumption, try to replace whole milk with low-fat (1 or 2 percent) or skim milk. Buy only lean meat. For cooking and salads, choose oils that are good sources of monounsaturated fat such as olive oil and canola oil.

In planning dinner menus, substitute fish and chicken for red meat in main dishes whenever possible. When you do serve red meat, trim off all the excess fat before cooking. Use low-fat methods of cooking, such as broiling, roasting, or baking, rather than frying. Always use an oil low in saturated fat for sautéing. Replace high-fat ingredients in your favorite recipes with low-fat alternatives. For example, use a fat-free sour cream substitute, yogurt, or cottage cheese, instead of real sour cream. Choose a low-fat dressing for salads or make your own low-fat dressing. For snacks, eat fruits and vegetables, rather than fatty snacks such as potato chips, chocolate bars, or cookies. When it is time for dessert, serve fruit.

When you go out to dinner, your goal should be to have fun without losing sight of all your new-found good eating habits. Here are some easy-to-follow tips:

- Ask for sauces and dressings on the side.

- Choose a salad instead of an appetizer.

- Choose a main course that is steamed.

- Ask the waiter how individual dishes are prepared.

- Choose a fruit or sorbet for dessert. ∎

Fatty acids also affect blood cholesterol and triglyceride levels—triglycerides are the principal blood lipids (fats). Saturated fat tends to raise the total blood cholesterol level and should be avoided. Although saturated fat has few redeeming features, unsaturated fats are important components of healthy nutrition. Monounsaturated fat can raise levels of high-density lipoprotein (HDL), or "good" cholesterol, without significantly raising overall cholesterol levels. Polyunsaturated fat can lower overall cholesterol levels, but at the expense of HDL levels. For more information, see Cholesterol and Dietary Fats, page 793 and Understanding Your Lipid Profile, page 794.

Fat is higher in calories than any other calorie source. There are 9 calories per gram of fat, compared to 4 calories per gram of carbohydrate or protein. This means that even if you consume smaller amounts of fat than carbohydrate or protein, you may actually be consuming more calories. If you are overweight, restricting your intake of fat should help reduce your daily total of calories and help you lose weight.

Carbohydrates Carbohydrates provide fuel for the body in the form of glucose, which is used to produce energy for every cell in the body. Carbohydrates also assist in the metabolism of other nutrients.

There are two kinds of carbohydrates, simple and complex. Complex carbohydrates are starches; they are found in legumes, nuts, vegetables, and whole grains. Simple carbohydrates are sugars; they are found in refined sugars and fruits. Simple carbohydrates are often viewed as the "bad" carbohydrates. However, this label applies only to refined sugars found in candies and snacks, rather than to fruits, which supply other important nutrients along with simple sugars.

Complex carbohydrates are digested more slowly than simple carbohydrates and provide a steady source of energy. They do not give the burst of energy associated with sugars, sometimes called a "sugar rush." The American Heart Association recommends that Americans cut back on refined sugars and increase the amount of complex carbohydrates to approximately 55 percent of the total amount of calories consumed in a day.

Fiber Fiber comes from the cell walls of plants. All fibers help slow the absorption of glucose into the body and aid digestion. They may help prevent colon cancer. Fiber is classified as a carbohydrate and supplies no vitamins, minerals, or calories. Fiber plays an important role in proper digestion without increasing your caloric intake. People in developing countries where fiber consumption is five to six times that of Americans rarely have constipation, which is a problem which afflicts approximately 100 million Americans. Gastrointestinal tract and digestive disorders plague almost

HIGH FIBER FOODS

	SERVING SIZE	TOTAL FIBER (g)	SOLUBLE FIBER (g)	INSOLUBLE FIBER (g)
Breads, Cereals, and Pasta				
Rye bread	1 slice	2.7	0.8	1.9
Whole-grain bread	1 slice	2.9	0.1	2.8
Brown rice	½ cup, cooked	1.3	1.3	0.0
Bran, 100% cereal	½ cup	10.0	0.3	9.7
Oats, whole	½ cup, cooked	1.6	0.5	1.1
Fruits				
Apple	1 small	3.9	2.3	1.6
Apricots	2 medium	1.3	0.9	0.4
Banana	1 small	1.3	0.6	0.7
Blackberries	½ cup	3.7	0.7	3.0
Grapefruit	½ fruit	1.3	0.90	0.4
Peach	1 medium	1.0	0.5	0.5
Pear	1 small	2.5	0.6	1.9
Pineapple	½ cup	0.8	0.2	0.6
Plums	2 medium	2.3	1.3	1.0
Strawberries	¾ cup	2.4	0.9	1.5
Tangerine	1 medium	1.8	1.4	0.4
Legumes				
Kidney beans	½ cup, cooked	4.5	0.5	4.0
Lima beans	½ cup, cooked	1.4	0.2	1.2
Pinto beans	½ cup, cooked	2.9	2.2	0.7
White beans	½ cup, cooked	4.2	0.4	3.8
Vegetables				
Broccoli	½ cup, cooked	2.6	1.6	1.0
Lettuce	½ cup, raw	0.5	0.2	0.3
Parsnips	½ cup, cooked	4.4	0.4	4.0
Peas	½ cup, cooked	5.2	2.0	3.2
Potatoes	1 small	3.8	2.2	1.6
Summer squash	½ cup, cooked	2.3	1.1	1.2
Zucchini	½ cup, cooked	2.5	1.1	1.4

Source: US Department of Agriculture database.

half of all Americans. These disorders may be relieved or eliminated by adequate fiber in the diet.

There are two types of fiber, water-soluble and water-insoluble. Water-insoluble fibers include cellulose, lignin, and hemicelluloses; they are found in wheat bran, whole grains, and vegetables. Although these fibers do not dissolve in water, they absorb water, which makes it easier for the intestines to eliminate waste products. Pectins, gums, and mucilages are all water-soluble fibers. Pectins are found in apples, citrus fruits, legumes, and certain vegetables. Gums and mucilages are found in legumes and oats. Pectins and gums slow sugar absorption, which can be helpful to people with diabetes. Water-soluble fibers may also help to lower low-density lipoprotein (LDL) cholesterol, or "bad" cholesterol, although this effect is still being debated.

The National Cancer Institute recommends that an individual consume between 20 and 35 g of fiber a day. Consumption of fiber in the average American diet amounts to about 10 g a day. Good sources of water-insoluble fiber include all-bran cereal, shredded wheat, asparagus, brussels sprouts, and green beans. Good sources of water-soluble fiber include oat bran, dried split peas, dried white beans, strawberries, apples, and bananas. It is best to try to get your fiber from foods, rather than supplements. If you are not used to a fiber-rich diet, increase the amount of fiber in your diet gradually.

Vitamins Vitamins are small, complex, organic (carbon-containing) chemicals that assist in the body's chemical reactions. Vitamins are often referred to as the spark plugs of the cells because they work as catalysts, triggering cellular metabolic reactions. The deficiency of any one vitamin will cause signs and symptoms of disease associated with that particular vitamin deficiency. In general, vitamins cannot be synthesized by the body. They must be obtained from the foods you eat or from supplements. There is no single food that contains all the vitamins.

There are 13 essential vitamins. These are divided into two categories, the water-soluble vitamins, such as vitamin C and all the B vitamins, and the fat-soluble vitamins, A, D, E, and K. The fat-soluble vitamins are more easily stored by the body than the water-soluble vitamins. Vitamins A and D are stored by the liver for up to 6 months and can be toxic when taken in large amounts. Because of the body's ability to store fat-soluble vitamins, taking excessive amounts of any of the fat-soluble vitamins may result in unpleasant symptoms or toxicity. Because the body cannot store the water-soluble vitamins in large amounts, you need to consume them every day. Taking large doses of water-soluble vitamins may not be dangerous to your health, but it may be a waste of money because once the saturation level, or threshold, is reached any excess is eliminated in the urine. See Dietary Guidelines: USRDAs, RDIs, and RDAs, page 16.

Minerals Minerals are inorganic substances. The body needs some minerals, such as calcium, potassium, iron, phosphorus, and magnesium, in relatively large amounts. Others, called trace minerals, are necessary for good health in much smaller amounts. They include zinc, iodine, copper, selenium, and manganese.

Taking isolated mineral supplements is usually not recommended, although taking supplemental calcium is recommended for women and some men to prevent osteoporosis. Taking excessive amounts of individual minerals can be dangerous to your health and may cause bloating, weight gain, headaches, hypertension, kidney disease, and depression.

Water Although water has no food value, the body cannot survive without it. Water is the most plentiful substance in the body. It accounts for 55 to 65 percent of body weight in adults and an even higher percentage in infants, yet when we think about nutrition, we tend to forget that water is an essential nutrient and that our health depends on it. A person can live without food for weeks; without water, a person will die in only a few days.

Water is important in the regulation of body temperature, the conduction of nerve impulses, digestion and elimination, and the maintenance of the immune system. Water carries nutrients, hormones, and antibodies to and from cells.

Because your body can store only small amounts of water, it is important to keep replenishing your body's water supply. Water is essential in keeping the brain adequately hydrated. It takes only a one percent fluid loss for the body to begin to become dehydrated. If you are of average weight and height and in good health, you lose approximately 2 cups of water a day simply by breathing, 2 more cups through perspiration, and approximately 6 cups through bowel movements and urination.

Everyone should drink at least eight 8-oz glasses of water a day. Although most of us know that we should drink plenty of water, few of us actually make the effort to drink the recommended eight glasses a day. Most of us drink only when we are thirsty, even though drinking plenty of water is one of the best and easiest ways to help maintain a healthy body. If you have trouble drinking 8 oz of water at a time, try drinking smaller glasses of water more frequently. If you exercise or work manually you should increase your water consumption. You should also drink more water in hot climates or if anything, such as diarrhea or fever, has increased your body's water loss. While there is water in everything that you drink, you should not substitute coffee or soda for water. Caffeinated beverages act as diuretics and may increase your need for water, rather than replenish your body's water supply.

Caffeine is a drug that stimulates your central nervous system and can make you feel as if you have more energy. Although the effects of caffeine vary from individual to individual, usually one to two cups of coffee is sufficient to provide a stimulant effect. Caffeine also increases the amount of blood flow to the kidneys which, in turn, increases the production of urine. Thus, caffeine acts as a diuretic. It cannot be counted toward your daily intake of eight glasses of water or other liquids. In fact, if you drink coffee regularly, you should drink more water during the day.

Small amounts of caffeine, such as those in soft drinks or in two cups of coffee a day, are not considered harmful to your overall health or detrimental to a healthy nutrition plan. Large quantities of caffeine, however, may lead to restlessness and trembling, insomnia, and gastrointestinal problems including diarrhea. Try to cut back if you drink more than three cups of coffee or five to six cups of tea a day. (Tea has substantially less caffeine than coffee and is considered to have some health benefits.) Caffeine can be addictive; decrease your caffeine intake gradually to avoid the headaches that can result from suddenly giving it up.

THE NEW FOOD PYRAMID

Our perspective on healthy nutrition has changed dramatically over the past 2 decades; the revisions to the food pyramid are clear evidence. Recent changes in the food pyramid reflect an increased understanding of the role of complex carbohydrates in healthy nutrition, particularly the importance of fruits, vegetables, grains, beans, and nuts. New guidelines also recommend consuming far less animal protein than Americans normally do.

The new food pyramid provides general guidelines for a sensible, daily eating plan. (These recommendations are appropriate for healthy individuals; individuals with special needs should consult their doctors in planning their nutritional programs.) The pyramid illustrates the different food groups and their proper proportions within a daily diet. The bread, cereal, rice, and pasta group forms the base; this group should account for the greatest number of servings and calories consumed each day. The vegetable group and the fruit group are next, and almost identical in size. Above these are the milk, yogurt, and cheese group and then the meat, poultry, fish, dry beans, eggs, and nuts

group. Once again, these last two groups are almost identical in nutritional importance. Topping the pyramid is the fats, oils, and sweets group that should represent the smallest amount of your daily calorie total.

The following basic groups of the food pyramid are arranged in ascending order, from the base of the pyramid up. Construct your daily diet by choosing most of your servings from the base groups and then choosing progressively fewer servings from groups as you move up the pyramid.

Bread, cereal, rice and pasta These foods provide complex carbohydrates, plenty of fiber, and B vitamins and minerals. Choose whole grains, beans and other legumes, lentils, brown rice, and whole grain cereals. Remember to check labels for the sugar content, salt—particularly in packaged cereals—and any added fats.

Fruit Fruits are low in fat and low in salt, high in vitamins, such as vitamins A and C, high in potassium and other minerals, and high in fiber. Eat fresh, whole fruits whenever possible, but canned fruits in their natural juice are better than no fruit at all.

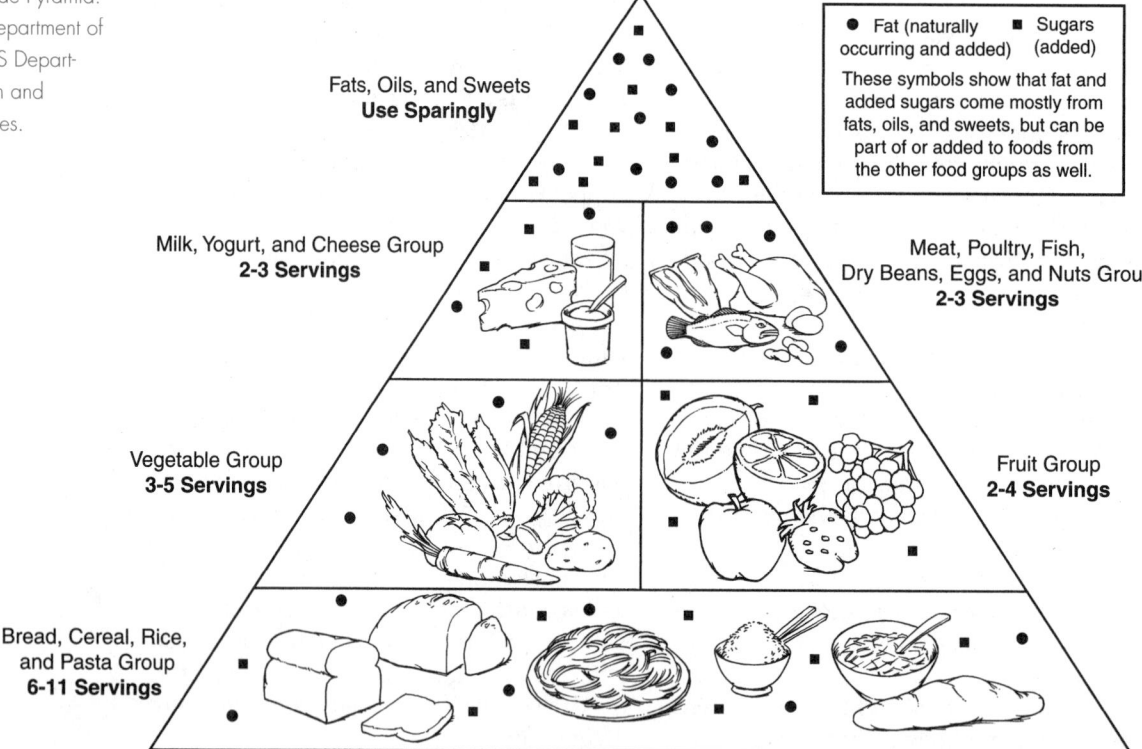

The Food Guide Pyramid. Source: US Department of Agriculture/US Department of Health and Human Services.

Fats, Oils, and Sweets
Use Sparingly

● Fat (naturally occurring and added)   ■ Sugars (added)

These symbols show that fat and added sugars come mostly from fats, oils, and sweets, but can be part of or added to foods from the other food groups as well.

Milk, Yogurt, and Cheese Group
2-3 Servings

Meat, Poultry, Fish, Dry Beans, Eggs, and Nuts Group
2-3 Servings

Vegetable Group
3-5 Servings

Fruit Group
2-4 Servings

Bread, Cereal, Rice, and Pasta Group
6-11 Servings

A SAMPLE MEAL PLAN

If you feel overwhelmed by all the nutritional requirements that should be supplied by the food that you eat in a day, the following meal plan may help. You will see that it is not so difficult to follow the guidelines of the new food pyramid, keep your fat content low, and maintain the appropriate number of calories while eating tasty, satisfying meals.

Breakfast

- Coffee or tea
- 1 cup skim milk (use some in your coffee)
- $\frac{1}{2}$ cantaloupe
- 1 small to medium whole wheat bagel or 2 pieces of seven grain toast, with 1 tsp tub margarine or low-fat cream cheese spread

Snack

- 1 cup of skim milk *or*
- $\frac{1}{2}$ cup of strawberries *or*
- 8 ounces plain, low-fat yogurt

Lunch

- Coffee, tea, mineral water, or diet soda
- 1 cup cooked spaghetti with $\frac{1}{2}$ cup marinara sauce
- 1 cup roasted red peppers or 1 cup steamed green beans
- 1 serving tossed green salad with 1 tbs of low-fat dressing
- 1 medium orange or 1 fat-free granola bar

Snack

- $\frac{1}{2}$ cup raw broccoli, cauliflower, or snow peas, or a medium tomato, with a low-fat dip or low-fat yogurt dip

Dinner

- Mineral water, diet soda, or decaffeinated coffee or tea. A glass of wine with your meal will add approximately 70 calories to your daily total.
- 4 oz skinless chicken, sautéed in 1 tsp olive oil, seasoned with herbs, or 3 oz lean steak, broiled
- 1 medium baked potato with 1 tbs fat-free sour cream or $\frac{1}{4}$ cup low-fat yogurt with chives
- $\frac{1}{2}$ to 1 cup steamed asparagus with lemon juice
- 1 serving tossed green salad with 1 tbs low-fat dressing
- $\frac{1}{2}$ cup lentil or three-bean salad *or*
- 1 slice whole grain bread
- 1 small piece angel food cake

Total Calories

This daily plan provides approximately 1,800 calories, which break down as follows:

- 17 percent calories from fat, with less than 5 percent from saturated fat
- 19 percent calories from protein
- 64 percent calories from carbohydrates
- Less than 100 mg cholesterol
- Depending on your snack choices, the plan also provides more than five servings of fruits and vegetables, and meets or comes close to meeting the other recommendations of the new food pyramid. For additional samples of meal plans, see the *American Heart Association Cookbook*. ■

Vegetables Vegetables are low in fat and high in vitamins such as vitamins A and C. They are also high in minerals and fiber. Vegetables should be fresh or fresh frozen, and should not be overcooked. The best way to cook vegetables is to steam them lightly, which helps retain essential vitamins and minerals, as well as flavor.

Meat, poultry, fish, dry beans, eggs, and nuts In general, these foods provide protein, B vitamins, iron, and other minerals. Healthy choices include lean cuts of red meat, poultry without the skin, and baked or broiled fish. You should not have more than four eggs a week, and you should not load up on nuts, which are high in fat.

Milk, yogurt, and cheese Foods in this group provide calcium, protein, vitamins, and other minerals. Choosing skim milk and low-fat dairy products will help you minimize your saturated fat intake.

Fats, oils, and sweets Minimum servings of this group are recommended. These foods tend to be high in calories and low in nutritional value. Such foods include butter, margarine, vegetable oils, salad dressings, candy, cakes, other sweets, and non-diet soft drinks. Your diet should include less than 30 percent of calories from fat.

VITAMIN AND MINERAL SUPPLEMENTS

The American public's desire for shortcuts has made vitamin and mineral supplements a multi-billion-dollar business. However, vitamin and mineral supplements are no substitute for good nutrition and should only be used in addition to a healthy eating plan.

Taken sensibly and in moderation, however, supplements can play an important, supportive role in ensuring a healthy nutrition plan. Seniors, who often consume fewer calories than they did in middle-adulthood, may not be getting the vitamins they need from their daily food and should talk to their doctors about taking a supplement (see The Nutritional Needs of Seniors, page 26). Vitamin supplements are also appropriate for children and pregnant or lactating women, who should discuss taking a supplement with their doctors. When choosing a vitamin and/or mineral supplement, be careful not to get one that contains megadoses of vitamins and minerals. If you are a reasonably healthy adult, amounts equal to, or slightly above, the recommended dietary allowance (RDA) for each nutrient should be adequate (see Dietary Guidelines: USRDAs, RDIs, and RDAs, page 16). A supplement should provide 100 percent, or close to 100 percent, of the RDA for each vitamin and mineral listed, rather than 100 percent of two or three vitamins and 20 or 30 percent of others. Avoid supplements that provide many times the RDA of any nutrients; the safety of taking megadoses of vitamins and minerals has not been established. Women of childbearing age should be particularly careful in their selection.

If you eat a variety of foods in sufficient quantities you are likely to get all the vitamins and minerals that you need. If you can afford it, most experts would agree that taking a daily multivitamin or mineral supplement can help ensure that you are getting the vitamins and minerals that you need to stay healthy. There is debate about the value of taking supplements containing relatively higher amounts of one or more nutrients. Provided below is information on three supplements and the pros and cons of taking them.

Ensuring an adequate intake of folic acid prior to conception and during early pregnancy reduces the risk of neural tube defects, including anencephaly and spina bifida, congenital defects in which either the brain or spinal cord is not fully formed. Although the RDA for folic acid is 0.18 mg, the American Academy of Pediatrics and the Centers for Disease Control and Prevention (CDC) recommend that all women of child-bearing age should be getting 0.4 mg of folic acid daily to protect the health of their fetus should they become pregnant. If you wait until you realize you are pregnant to be concerned about your folic acid intake, it may be too late. Certain women should be particularly concerned about getting enough folate (a more general term for the vitamin that includes folic acid), such as women with a family history of neural tube defects. It is possible to consume 0.4 mg of folate from the foods that you eat; good sources of folate are orange juice, breakfast cereals, and greens such as spinach, collards, and chard. However, to be certain that you are getting an adequate amount of folic acid, you may want to take a multivitamin supplement that contains 0.4 mg of folic acid.

Women over age 25 should take calcium supplements. Many experts also agree that higher intakes than the RDA of 800 mg —between 1,000 mg and 1,200 mg a day— provide further protection against osteoporosis, particularly during the postmenopausal years.

Antioxidants are more controversial. An antioxidant is a chemical or substance that inhibits the oxidation of another substance to which it is added. Oxidation causes metal to rust or food to turn brown or rancid. When you squeeze lemon juice on a slice of avocado, you are preventing oxidation. Free radicals are by-products of the oxidation process. Recently, there has been intense interest in the role of antioxidants in destroying free radicals in the body. Some scientists believe that free radicals may hasten the aging process and may also contribute to the development of cancer, and that a diet rich in antioxidants may prevent or decrease the severity of many chronic diseases, including cancer. Antioxidants may also contribute to keeping HDL levels high and LDL levels low, because LDL is the oxidized form of HDL. However, there is much debate on the subject. No study has shown a direct link between a diet rich in antioxidants and the prevention of cancer. In fact, in a recent study of long-term, male smokers in Finland, the group taking antioxidants had a slightly higher death rate.

Natural antioxidants include vitamin E, vitamin C, carotenoids (some of which the body converts into vitamin A), and selenium. Until further long-term studies of antioxidants are performed, there is likely

WHAT VITAMINS DO FOR YOUR BODY

VITAMIN	SIGNIFICANT SOURCES	PHYSIOLOGIC BENEFITS	DEFICIENCY SYMPTOMS	OVER-CONSUMPTION SYMPTOMS
Vitamin A	Butter, whole milk, cheese made from whole milk, eggs, liver, dark green and deep yellow vegetables, peaches, carrots, cherries, papaya, mangoes	Beneficial to vision and reproduction. Also assists in growth of mucous membranes, bones, skin, and hair	Night blindness, weight loss, impaired growth in children. More severely, drying of the cornea and blindness	Dryness of the mucous membranes, nausea, double vision, headaches, enlargement of the liver and spleen, and birth defects
Vitamin D	Salt-water fish, fish-liver oils, liver, egg yolks. Exposure to sunlight, which changes the cholesterol in the skin to vitamin D	Assists in the absorption of calcium, which is beneficial to teeth and bones	Rickets in children and osteomalacia in adults	Nausea, weight loss, constipation. More severely, mental retardation and kidney and heart damage
Vitamin E	Whole grain cereals, vegetable oil, cheese, shellfish, liver, milk, broccoli, cabbage	Acts as an antioxidant. Slows the development of cataracts. Beneficial to reproduction and red blood cells	Appetite loss, reproductive problems, and stunted growth	At very high doses, headaches, fatigue, and muscular weakness
Vitamin K	Green leafy vegetables, cauliflower, eggs, and dairy products. Also produced by bacteria in the intestine	Proper clotting of blood	Increased tendency to bleed and abnormal blood clotting	Menadione, a form of vitamin K, may cause anemia and infantile jaundice in high doses
Vitamin C (ascorbic acid)	Oranges, orange juice, other citrus fruits and fruit juices, potatoes cooked in the skin, tomatoes, strawberries, collard greens, lima beans, green leafy vegetables, broccoli	Assists in the healing of wounds, resistance to infection, assists in the absorption of iron, acts as an antioxidant, assists in the formation of collagen. May reduce the risk of some cancers and cataracts	Fatigue, increased risk of infection, appetite loss, muscular weakness. More severely, scurvy, poor wound healing, bleeding gums, bone pain, and psychological changes	Diarrhea
Thiamin (vitamin B_1)	Whole grain cereals, seafood, legumes, ham, kidney, liver, raisins, soybeans, nuts, seeds	Beneficial to growth, digestion, metabolism of carbohydrates, nervous system, and heart	Fatigue, constipation, weight loss, muscular weakness. More severely, beriberi: edema, heart failure, and psychological symptoms from confusion to psychosis	None
Riboflavin (vitamin B_2)	Beef, ham, kidney, liver, chicken, raw eggs, dark green and leafy vegetables, whole grain cereal	Beneficial to respiration, vision, skin, nails, hair, lips, tongue, and the metabolism of protein, carbohydrates, and fats	Sore throat, cracks at the corner of the mouth, rash, swollen tongue, chapped lips, and psychological problems	None
Niacin (vitamin B_3)	Chicken, turkey, ham, rabbit, liver, kidney, yeast, tuna, whole grain cereals, nuts	Necessary in the digestion of food. May be used to lower cholesterol when taken in large doses under medical supervision	Weight loss, nausea, headache. More severely, skin rash, sore tongue, diarrhea, nervousness, and psychological changes	Heart arrhythmias, ulcers, high blood pressure and uric acid, flushing, and liver problems

WHAT VITAMINS DO FOR YOUR BODY (continued)

VITAMIN	SIGNIFICANT SOURCES	PHYSIOLOGICAL BENEFITS	DEFICIENCY SYMPTOMS	OVER-CONSUMPTION SYMPTOMS
Folic Acid (folate)	Orange juice, liver, chicken, legumes, yeast, dark green and leafy vegetables, wheat germ, bran	Assists in the synthesis of nucleic acids and amino acids, formation of red blood cells. May help reduce the risk of neural-tube birth defects when taken in early pregnancy	Weight loss, diarrhea, anemia, and bleeding gums	Convulsions in epileptics and may obscure certain forms of anemia
Vitamin B_6	Kidney, liver, salmon, tuna, chicken, wheat germ, whole grain cereal, yeast, dark green and leafy vegetables, potatoes, prunes, bananas	Beneficial to the metabolism of protein and carbohydrates, important in red blood cell formation and nerve functions	Itchy and scaly skin, confusion, depression, inflammation of the mouth, and infantile convulsions	Destruction of sensory nerves
Biotin	Beef, chicken, lamb, pork, veal, kidney, liver, egg yolk, fish, rolled oats, brown rice, nuts, seeds, legumes, yeast. Also made by intestinal bacteria	Assists in the metabolism of protein and carbohydrates, and the synthesis of fats	Nausea, appetite loss, depression, hair loss, and dry, scaly skin	None
Vitamin B_{12}	Beef, kidney, liver, poultry, herring, sardines, shellfish, cheese, eggs, milk. Significant amounts are not found in plant foods	Necessary for red blood cell formation, beneficial to growth, digestion, and the metabolism of protein, carbohydrates, and fats	Sore tongue, anemia, and neurological symptoms	None
Pantothenic Acid	Kidney, liver, whole grain cereals, peas, soybeans, lobster, eggs, seeds, vegetables	Beneficial in the metabolism of carbohydrates and fats and in the production of various hormones and neurotransmitters	Listlessness, fatigue, and burning-feet syndrome. Deficiency is rare because of wide distribution in foods.	Virtually non-toxic, diarrhea only at high doses

to be disagreement on whether supplements containing antioxidants are helpful or harmful.

FOODS RICH IN CALCIUM

The RDA for calcium in adolescents and young adults is 1,200 mg a day; for both men and women age 25 and over it is 800 mg. Many Americans consume far less calcium than the RDA. Women, in particular, tend to avoid foods high in calcium such as dairy products, because they are afraid of their high calorie and high-fat content. Many other Americans avoid these foods because they do not tolerate the lactose in dairy products. However, many foods contain calcium and can be substituted for dairy products. New low-fat dairy products contain as much or more calcium than the high-fat products. For example, skim milk contains more calcium than whole milk on a per-calorie basis. Orange juice with added calcium or a calcium supplement may also be used to ensure enough calcium in the diet of all Americans, from pre-teens and teens to adults and seniors. Although 800 mg is the present RDA for most adults, many doctors recommend that pregnant or nursing women, postmenopausal women, and seniors get 1,000 to 1,200 mg of calcium a day. It is important not to use "natural" calcium supplements because they are not absorbed.

A list of calcium-rich foods that will help you get as much calcium as possible from your food choices is shown in the table on this page.

One of the reasons that calcium is so crucial to a woman's diet is to guard against osteoporosis. Osteoporosis is a debilitating disease that affects many women during their postmenopausal years. Most experts agree that prevention of osteoporosis depends on getting as much calcium as possible into your bones while they are still forming, a process that begins in the womb and is largely completed by age 30. When women reach menopause, the decrease in estrogen causes them to lose minerals such as calcium from their bones. If your bones lose a lot of calcium or do not have much to start with, osteoporosis may result and the risk of bone fracture goes up. There is some debate about whether high calcium intake can help you after you reach menopause. Foods can provide you with the 1,000 to 1,300 mg of calcium you are likely to need each day; good sources include milk, yogurt, cheese, and fish with bones, such as salmon and sardines. Other less well-known sources include calcium-fortified orange juice, corn tortillas, tofu, soybean flour, and cashews. Depending on whether you like (or tolerate) dairy products, and whether or not you have a family history of osteoporosis, you may decide that taking a calcium supplement makes good sense.

MAKING HEALTHY CHOICES FOR YOU AND YOUR FAMILY

When it comes to nutrition and maintaining your ideal weight, there is no quick fix or magic bullet. The only real dietary revolution is to admit, finally, that there is no substitute for a well-balanced diet and to resolve to make moderate eating habits a life-long goal. By following the recommendations contained in the new food pyramid, you can find a balanced nutrition plan that works for you.

A varied, well-balanced diet not only will help you maintain your overall health and protect against disease, but also will give you more energy and make you feel better. Once you begin to feel the positive effects of healthy eating habits, you will be further motivated to continue your efforts.

CALCIUM-RICH FOODS

FOOD	AMOUNT	CALCIUM (mg)
Dairy products		
Whole milk	1 cup	290
2% milk	1 cup	297
Skim milk	1 cup	302
Buttermilk	1 cup	285
Yogurt, plain low-fat	8 oz	415
Cheddar cheese	1 oz	206
Swiss cheese	1 oz	272
American cheese	1 oz	174
Cottage cheese	½ cup	62
Soybean products		
Soy milk, calcium fortified	8 oz	200–300
Tofu, soft	4 oz	50
Tofu, hard, with calcium	4 oz	160–230
Grains		
Biscuit, homemade from mix	1	34–58
Cereal, processed	½ cup cooked	49
Waffle, frozen	1	85
Fruits and vegetables		
Broccoli	½ cup cooked	88
Cabbage	½ cup cooked	44
Beet greens	½ cup cooked	99
Collards	½ cup cooked	152
Dandelion greens	½ cup cooked	140
Kale	½ cup cooked	89
Rhubarb	½ cup cooked	174
Mustard greens	½ cup cooked	138
Spinach	½ cup cooked	83
Swiss chard	½ cup cooked	73
Turnip greens	½ cup cooked	138
Leeks	1–2 medium	26

The US Department of Health and Human Services and the US Department of Agriculture have established dietary guidelines for everyone over age two. These guidelines, which are consistent with the food pyramid, will help you maintain a desirable weight for your height and age, improve your overall health, and lower your risk for certain diseases, such as high blood pressure, heart disease, stroke, diabetes, and possibly some forms of cancer. There are a few key points to follow:

• Eat a wide variety of foods.

• Increase the amount of fruits, vegetables, and grains that you eat.

- Choose a diet low in fat, particularly saturated and polyunsaturated fat.
- Choose a low-sodium diet.
- Use sugar in moderation, if at all.
- Maintain a desirable weight.
- Drink alcohol only in moderation.

In addition, it is recommended that women and adolescent girls choose a nutrition plan that is rich in calcium, folate, and iron. Most women of child-bearing age obtain only about half the calcium they need from the foods they eat and should consider taking a calcium supplement.

The amount of calories that you should consume daily depends on your level of physical activity, sex, and age. In general, children, teenage girls, active women, and sedentary men need approximately 2,200 calories a day, while sedentary women and older people in general need about 1,600 calories a day. Teenage boys, active men, and very active women need about 2,800 calories a day. If you are unsure about your caloric needs, talk to your doctor.

Do not be discouraged if the habits of a lifetime do not change overnight. Changes made in small increments are far more likely to be long-lasting than any revolutionary, overnight changes. Gradual adjustments in food choices, the size of meals, and the amount of daily physical activity are far more likely to be permanent. Over time, the rewards of improved health and increased energy will help you to stick to your new routine.

DIETARY GUIDELINES: USRDAs, RDIs, AND RDAs

The US recommended daily allowances (USRDAs) were developed by the Food and Drug Administration (FDA) in 1968 to be used on food labels. However, the Nutrition Labeling and Education act, passed in 1990 and implemented in 1994, has rendered the USRDA obsolete. They have been replaced by RDIs (reference daily intakes). For now USRDA and RDI values are identical and may be used interchangeably, although this will probably change in the future. The name change was made to avoid confusion between the USRDAs, which are set by the FDA, and recommended dietary allowances (RDAs), which are determined by the National Research Council of the National Academy of Sciences.

RDAs provide one of the standards used to determine the daily values as listed on the new food labels. For the first time, RDAs provide recommended daily intakes for cholesterol, fat, carbohydrate, fiber, sodium, and potassium, in addition to other vitamins and minerals. RDAs refer to the amounts of essential nutrients needed on a daily basis to prevent nutritional deficiencies in nearly all healthy individuals.

RDAs are listed on labels of vitamin and mineral supplements and packaged foods. Vitamin and mineral labels must include listings for the seven essential vitamins and minerals. Manufacturers may elect not to list the USRDAs for the other essential nutrients. The transition to RDIs, also referred to as dietary reference intakes (DRIs), will take approximately 4 years. For the moment, the most consistent recommendations are the RDAs. The RDAs for vitamins, minerals, and the other essential nutrients are shown on the left.

RDAs

	MALES		FEMALES	
	AGE 25–50	OVER 50	AGE 25–50	OVER 50
Fat-Soluble Vitamins				
Vitamin A (mg)	1,000	1,000	800	800
Vitamin D (mg)	5	5	5	5
Vitamin E (mg)	10	10	8	8
Vitamin K (mg)	80	80	65	65
Water-Soluble Vitamins				
Vitamin C (mg)	60	60	60	60
Thiamin (mg)	1.5	1.2	1.1	1.0
Riboflavin (mg)	1.7	1.4	1.3	1.2
Niacin (mg)	19	15	15	13
Vitamin B_6 (mg)	2.0	2.0	1.6	1.6
Folate (mcg)	200	200	400	180
Vitamin B_{12} (mg)	2.0	2.0	2.0	2.0
Minerals				
Calcium (mg)	800	800	800	800
Phosphorus (mg)	800	800	800	800
Magnesium (mg)	350	350	280	280
Iron (mg)	10	10	10	30
Zinc (mg)	15	15	12	15
Iodine (mcg)	150	150	150	175
Selenium (mcg)	70	70	55	65

READING THE LABELS

Until recently, food labels were often difficult to understand; however, the FDA has now implemented guidelines to make label reading less confusing and more useful to the consumer. Not only can you ascertain the nutrient content of a particular product, but the labels can also guide you as to the portion size you should be eating to obtain nutritional benefits and avoid consuming too many calories or too much fat. To put the new labeling guidelines to good use, you need to know how to read the label.

Portion, or serving, sizes are provided in familiar household measurements or units, as well as in grams. Next, the "Amount Per Serving" section of the label gives you the number of calories in each portion and the number of calories from fat. Comparing your usual portion size with the recommended portion will help you avoid excess calories. Below, the total calorie count of a serving is broken down into amounts of fat; cholesterol; sodium; carbohydrate, including sub-listings for dietary fiber and sugars; and protein. This allows you to structure your daily calorie intake in terms of percentages of protein, carbohydrate, and fat. Beneath these readings, the vitamin and mineral content is listed, including percentages of the daily requirement of each vitamin and mineral obtained from one portion. Then the composition of the food is described in terms of total fat, saturated fat, and other components.

The new labeling laws guard against claims that a product is lower in fat than it really is by instituting uniform portion sizes based on normal servings of a particular food. A label can no longer state that one piece of a high-fat snack food is a por-

NUTRITION FACTS LABEL

Most food packages contain a nutrition label similar to this one that contains important information for comparing food for purchase or for planning a diet. The information presented on this label reflects the Food and Drug Administration's rules for food labeling published in 1992 and 1993.

Serving Size Serving sizes on the new food labels are meant to reflect the amount people actually eat and are expressed in common household and metric measures.

Nutrients This section describes the amount of each major nutrient found in one serving. Each label must include information on total fat, saturated fat, cholesterol, sodium, total carbohydrate, dietary fiber, sugars, protein, vitamin A, vitamin C, calcium, and iron. These nutrients were chosen because they reflect today's health concerns and are listed in order of importance to current dietary recommendations.

Calories per Serving The number of total calories and calories from fat appear on each label. It may be helpful to estimate the percentage of calories from fat in each serving by dividing the calories from fat by the total calories. Many health organizations recommend no more than 30 percent of calories from fat.

Daily Values Daily values represents the percentage of a day's requirement of a nutrient that is provided by one serving. Percentages are based on a 2,000 calorie diet and need to be adjusted if you consume much more or less each day.

Calories per Gram The number of calories in 1 g of each major energy-producing nutrient are listed here.

Nutrition facts label (see text for explanation). Source: Food and Drug Administration, 1994.

Nutrition Facts

Serving Size 14 crackers (31g)
Serving Per Container About 7

Amount Per Serving

Calories 120   Calories from Fat 35

	% Daily Value*
Total Fat 4g	6%
Saturated Fat 0.5g	3%
Polyunsaturated Fat 0.5g	
Monounsaturated Fat 1.5g	
Cholesterol 0mg	0%
Sodium 310mg	13%
Total Carbohydrate 19g	6%
Dietary Fiber Less than 1g	4%
Sugars 2g	
Protein 2g	

Vitamin A 0%	•	Vitamin C 0%
Calcium 4%	•	Iron 6%

* Percent Daily Values are based on a 2,000 calorie diet. Your daily values may be higher or lower depending on your calorie needs:

		Calories:	2,000	2,500
Total Fat	Less than		65g	80g
Sat Fat	Less than		20g	25g
Cholesterol	Less than		300mg	300mg
Sodium	Less than		2,400mg	2,400mg
Total Carbohydrate			300g	375g
Dietary Fiber			25g	30g

Calories per gram:
Fat 9 • Carbohydrate 4 • Protein 4

WHAT IS A PORTION?

Determining the appropriate portion size of specific foods can be confusing, but the new food labeling system can help. At the top of the label, you will see the portion size described in several ways. While some measurements such as grams or ounces, may be difficult to translate into a serving size, at least one description will be in familiar household measurements, such as tablespoons or number of pieces. A portion of fruits and vegetables should generally be ½ cup or more. Portion sizes for meats, poultry, and fish should be approximately 3 oz, or about the size of the palm of your hand if your hands are of average size. Portion sizes for beans, legumes, and other complex carbohydrates should vary from ½ to 1 cup. When calculating portion sizes for sweets, the general rule is to choose less, rather than more, although this can be the hardest rule of all to follow. ■

tion size when people realistically consume a portion of a dozen pieces. In addition, the new guidelines make it more difficult to make false claims about products. Claims of health benefits can only be made if an established nutrient-disease connection has been well documented. Restrictions on nutrient descriptions have also been implemented. Because the rules for claiming that a product is low in sodium or low in fat are stricter, such claims can now be trusted.

BEWARE OF RESTAURANT PORTIONS

FOOD	USDA SERVING	AVERAGE RESTAURANT SERVING
Bagel	2 oz	4–5 oz
Chips	2 oz	3 oz or more
French fries	3 oz	6–8 oz
Ice cream	½ cup	1 cup or more
Pasta	1 cup	3 cups
Meat	3 oz	6–16 oz
Salad dressings	2 tbs	4 tbs or more
Sandwich	4 oz	9–12 oz
Pizza slice	5 oz	9 oz or more

Portion sizes vary widely in restaurants. The wide variety of portion sizes served in restaurants helps to explain why many Americans underestimate portion size of foods they eat by as much as 50 percent. The above table can help you avoid overeating the next time you eat out.

You may read various descriptions of nutrient content on new food labels, including terms such as "fat-free" or "light." Until the recent restructuring of food labeling, such claims could be misleading; now, if you read such terms on a label you can trust the labeling. These terms can only be used if the food meets strict requirements. The following criteria for terms commonly used on labels have been defined by the American Heart Association.

Cholesterol-free Cholesterol-free foods have no more than 2 mg of cholesterol and no more than 2 g of fat per serving.

Fat-free A fat-free food has no more than 0.5 g of fat per serving.

Low-fat A low-fat food has no more than 3 g of fat per serving.

Extra lean Extra lean foods have no more than 5 g of fat per serving. No more than 2 g are from saturated fat and there are no more than 95 mg of cholesterol per serving.

Lean A lean product has no more than 10 g of fat per serving. No more than 4 g come from saturated fat and there are no more than 95 mg of cholesterol per serving.

Light (lite) A food that is considered "light" must meet one of several criteria. It must either be ⅓ lower in calories, or be ½ lower in fat as compared to the higher calorie, higher fat equivalent, or it must be ½ lower in sodium as compared to the higher sodium equivalent. Be aware that a light food does not have to meet all three criteria; check the label.

Reduced-sodium Foods that are listed as reduced-sodium foods have at least ¼ less sodium per serving than similar, high-sodium equivalents.

The Health Risks of Obesity

The most common and costly nutritional problem in the United States is obesity. Approximately 55 percent of Americans can be categorized as obese or overweight, according to standards recently set by the

DETERMINING IF YOU ARE OVERWEIGHT

Whether or not you are overweight or obese can be determined by calculating your body mass index (BMI), which is your weight in kilograms divided by the square of your height in meters. According to new standards set by the National Heart, Lung, and Blood Institute, a BMI of 18.5 to 24.9 means that you are normal weight, a BMI of 25.0 to 29.9 is defined as overweight, and obesity is indicated by a BMI of 30.0 or more. You can use the chart on the right to calculate your BMI, and you can also calculate your BMI on the Internet at http://www. nhlbisupport.com/bmi/

Whether this weight or BMI is healthy for you is as individual as most other aspects of health. For example, if you have a family history of diabetes you should not be content with a weight that is in the high end of the normal range. To help prevent diabetes, you should strive for a weight in the low to mid-normal range, because any more weight increases the risk of diabetes. If you were slender and fit in college but now weigh 20 percent more than you did then, you are probably overweight and should consider a new fitness and nutrition program, even if your weight falls within the average range. Remember, average does not necessarily imply optimal health. If you are an athlete who lifts weights and has higher than average muscle mass, your BMI may be more than the average but you may not be overweight. On the other hand, if you are small-boned with a small frame and your weight places you in the high range of average BMI, you may still be overweight. The best way to determine if you are overweight is to discuss what you should weigh with your doctor.

Finally, if the weight you have gained is mainly at your waist, you may be at higher risk for heart disease and should consider losing weight, whether or not your weight is normal. ■

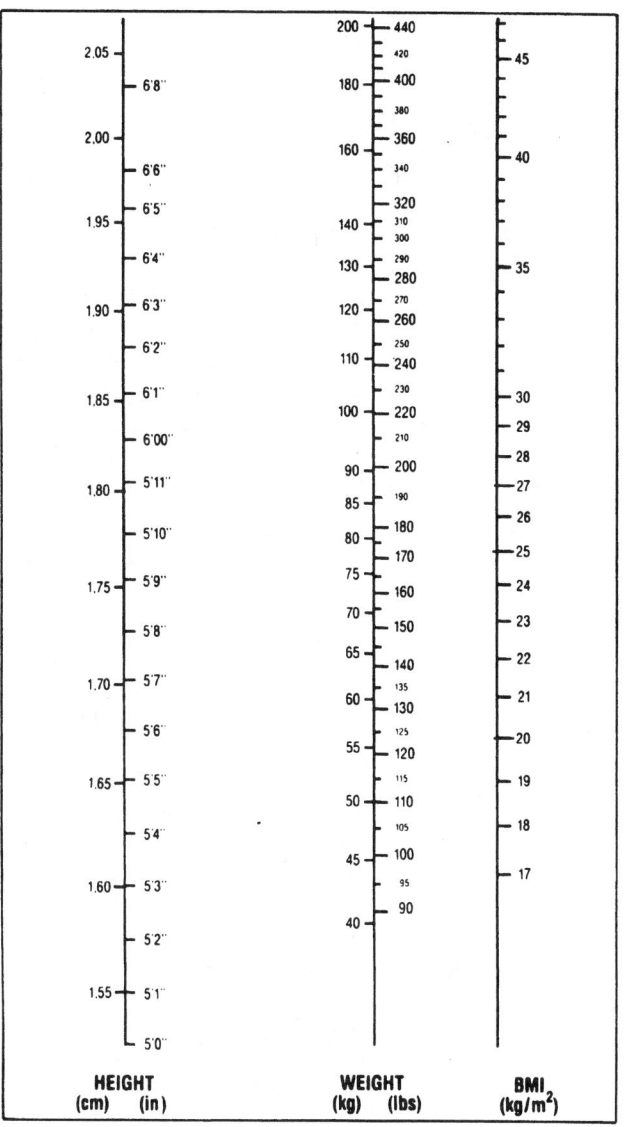

Body Mass Index (BMI). Obesity (overweight) is defined by the BMI because taller persons also weigh more. To calculate your BMI, take a ruler or straight edge and make a line connecting your height and your weight. The point where the line crosses the third bar is your BMI. Obesity is currently defined as a BMI of 30 or above. Source: Adapted from Health Canada's 1988 nomogram contained in *Canadian Guidelines for Healthy Weights*. With permission of the Minister of Public Works and Government Services Canada, 1998.

National Heart, Lung, and Blood Institute. Technically, obesity is defined as an excess of body fat: in men when fat accounts for 25 percent of total body weight and in women when fat accounts for 30 percent of body weight. However, because body fat can be difficult to measure, an excess of body weight is commonly used to determine obesity. People are considered medically obese when their body weight is 20 percent or more above the desirable weight for their height, sex, and body build.

Obesity is a major health risk. Obesity increases your risk for hypertension (high blood pressure) and forms of heart disease, stroke, type 2 diabetes mellitus, and certain types of cancer. It may also increase your risk of complications during or after surgery, especially surgery performed under general anesthesia, as well as lengthen your recovery time after illness or surgery. In women, obesity may complicate pregnancy and can lead to early menopause. Obesity is also associated with an increased risk for varicose veins, sleep apnea, and gallstones. While the risk of osteoarthritis is not increased, the pain and disability associated with existing osteoarthritis is worsened by obesity. In addition, obesity may be responsible for low self-esteem and may lead to depression. When body weight is more than 30 percent above the desirable body weight, obesity is associated with a decrease in longevity. About the only health risk that is lower in obese individuals is the risk of osteoporosis and hip fractures, probably because excess weight stimulates bone-strengthening hormonal factors.

If you are obese, the most important step that you can take to improve your overall health and lower your risk of disease is to achieve and maintain weight loss.

A WEIGHT LOSS PROGRAM

Losing weight and keeping it off requires a permanent shift in lifestyle. Chronic dieting and fad diets not only do not work, they may contribute to the problem. The fundamental problem is that most Americans consume too many calories, particularly with high-fat and high-sugar foods, and persist in leading sedentary lives. Your game plan for weight loss should combine an increase in the amount of energy you spend with a decrease in the calories you consume on a daily basis. It is a fundamental change that must be made gradually and maintained over time.

As many as 95 percent of the participants in research studies involving dieting regain the weight that they worked so hard to lose. If you are overweight and have tried dieting time and again to no avail, you are not alone. You may need to change your strategy. Most successful and permanent weight-loss involves shifting your priority from finding a diet that might work tem-porarily, to changing your lifestyle to include healthier foods and more physical activity. Rather than seeing food as the enemy, you need to make healthy foods your ally. You need not starve to lose weight and keep it off, you simply need to change the foods that you eat. As you increase the amount of fresh fruits and vegetables and grains and other complex carbohydrates in your diet, begin to cut down on the amount of fatty foods, particularly foods high in saturated fat. (It should be noted that this weight loss program is not appropriate for children or adolescents, whose nutritional needs are different from adults. See Children and Nutrition, page 5, as well as Chapter 9.)

When designing your weight loss plan, it is as important to choose foods that you enjoy eating as it is to choose healthy foods. If you plan a meal that is unappetizing to you, you are much more likely to compensate with a dessert or snack on foods that will undo all your good work. It is also important to eat enough of the foods you choose so that you are not hungry and tempted to snack on junk food. Remember when creating your meal plans that quick fixes from simple carbohydrates (sugar), low-fiber foods like white bread, and high-fat snack foods like potato chips are digested quickly and are less filling than high-bulk, low-fat foods. Quick fixes soon leave you hungry for more. Complete proteins—dairy products, lean meats, poultry, and fish—and complex carbohydrates—whole grain breads, lentils, grains, beans, and other legumes—are digested more slowly, keep you satisfied longer, and give you the energy you need. You should concentrate on including a substantial amount of complex carbohydrates, 55 percent of your caloric intake, and a sufficient amount of protein, about 20 percent of your caloric intake, in your diet.

Although eating a diet that is low in fat is essential to any weight loss program, it is still important that you restrict your daily calorie intake and increase your level of physical activity. If you think of food as fuel, you need to consume less and burn more to lose weight successfully.

A pound of excess weight is equivalent to approximately 3,500 calories. While most new and habitual dieters want immediate and noticeable results, the most successful weight loss program is one in which you lose weight slowly but steadily by building

CALORIE VALUES

Not all of the nutrients that provide energy are created equal. Some foods, such as sugar and alcohol, provide only empty calories. Fiber, on the other hand, provides no nutrients or calories but contributes to health. The following is a list of the calorie content of the various food components we consume.

- 1 g of fat: 9 calories

- 1 g of protein: 4 calories

- 1 g of carbohydrate: 4 calories

- 1 g of alcohol: 7 calories

- 1 g of fiber: 0 calories

These values provide an additional tool in making wise choices about the foods you eat. Choosing foods rich in protein and complex carbohydrate and low in fat can help keep your calorie consumption down while providing you with the nutrition you need. ■

up a daily calorie deficit. The daily calorie deficit refers to the difference between your daily intake and expenditure of calories. A reasonable calorie deficit is 500 calories a day, or if you are extremely overweight, 1,000 calories a day. The greater your calorie deficit, the faster your weight loss. However, when you eat less than 1,000 calories a day, you are likely to become so hungry that you end up overeating and undermining the progress you have made.

Some fad diets claim that you can lose a pound a day, which works out to a calorie deficit of approximately 3,500 a day. Such goals and claims are far-fetched. While you might see significant weight loss during the first week of a fad diet, it is almost always due to water loss and not fat loss. Fat loss is essential to true weight loss. With your calorie deficit between 500 and 1,000 calories a day, you will lose between 1 and 2 lbs a week on average. It is important to keep in mind that your goal is a calorie deficit, not a recommended calorie intake, of 500 to 1,000 calories a day. Your goal should be moderate and steady weight loss, which is the best way to ensure that you will continue to lose weight and will keep lost weight off.

Many experts suggest that you keep a diary of what you eat, at least for the first few days of your new nutritional plan. This may be helpful for two reasons. Seeing exactly what you eat and when may help you make changes based on an awareness of the times of day that you eat the most and the reasons why you do. A diary may also be helpful because knowing that you will write down what you eat can encourage you to choose to skip food that you do not really need.

Last, but not least, increase the amount of physical activity in your daily life. Physical activity burns fat and improves muscle tone, helping you lose inches as well as pounds. For more information on increasing your activity level safely and effectively, see Chapter 2.

As we age we tend to need fewer calories to maintain our ideal weight. To avoid the arduous task of trying to take off excess weight once you have already put it on, it is important to begin to eat smaller portions and to monitor your calories as early as in your 30s. The earlier you get started eating a healthy diet, the fewer weight problems you are likely to have later on.

Many people, particularly as they get older, tend to think of losing weight as an impossible task. Losing weight is always difficult, and it may indeed become harder to do so as you age. Like any major lifestyle change, losing weight demands serious effort and perseverance. You must keep the rewards of losing weight constantly in sight to motivate you to work steadily toward your goal. Try not to worry or get discouraged if you hit a plateau. Steady effort is the best insurance that you will reach your goal.

Sometimes people find it impossible to lose weight on their own, particularly those who are very obese. A morbidly obese person is someone who weighs over 100 lbs

DIET AIDS

Obesity is a very difficult problem to solve and a difficult condition to treat. Controlling obesity depends on making nutritional and lifestyle changes, and in some cases medication may be useful initially to help reduce weight and motivate the patient. Some experts believe that if medication proves helpful, it should be continued indefinitely to help maintain weight loss.

Some of these medications are available over-the-counter, others must be prescribed by a doctor. The medications that are prescribed fall into two classes. Vasoactive amine medications curb appetite. Serotonergic medications provide the brain with more serotonin, which may help to quiet brain centers that control appetite and help increase the sense of satisfaction.

The combination of these two classes of medication has given rise to the controversial, widely publicized, and recently withdrawn "fen-phen" therapy for obesity.

Both drugs had been on the market individually for years, and each drug had been approved individually by the FDA; however, the two-drug combination had not been approved. Their combined use received a great deal of attention after a 4-year study that had demonstrated their success in promoting weight control with few side effects or complications. More recent reports of dangerous side effects and possible complications due to this drug combination—including a high rate of valvular heart disease, leading to open-heart surgery in some cases—resulted in the FDA recommendation that fenfluramine (Pondimin or Redux) be withdrawn from the market. Phentermine was not withdrawn and is still presented to aid weight loss. Although medications should be prescribed only for people who are clinically obese and under the supervision of a doctor, millions of prescriptions have been written in the United States solely for the purpose of cosmetic weight loss.

Weight loss medication is approved only for those for whom weight is a health hazard. If you are only 10 to 20 lbs overweight, such drug therapy is not appropriate. It is important to realize that in controlled trials the use of medication to control appetite results in only about $1/4$ lb of additional weight loss a week as compared to placebo. Even when appropriately prescribed, medication should only be a part of a comprehensive approach to weight loss and weight maintenance. Without substantive changes in eating habits and lifestyle any effect medication may have on your weight will be lost once the therapy ends. ■

more than the average weight for his height and build. Until recently, surgery for morbidly obese people had been considered largely ineffective. But new research has indicated that surgery for obesity, or bariatric surgery, is often successful in patients who cannot lose weight by traditional methods. Bariatric surgery, however, is still considered a last resort; all options should be thoroughly explored before undergoing surgery (see When You Can't Do It Alone, below).

MAINTENANCE: KEEPING THE WEIGHT OFF

Losing the weight you need to lose is only the first step in weight control. Maintaining that weight loss is the crucial next step and the step so many dieters are unable to take. To maintain your ideal weight, you need to maintain all your new, healthy eating and exercise habits. Think of staying fit as a lifelong project. You can help yourself stay motivated by reminding yourself that you have not just been on a diet, you have fundamentally changed your life for the better.

Once you have established the number of calories that you should consume daily to maintain your new weight, the best insurance for weight maintenance is to keep up your new level of physical activity. Exercise is not the most effective way to lose weight initially, but it is an excellent way to maintain lower weight once weight loss has been accomplished. If you return to a sedentary lifestyle, you will burn fewer calories; any calories that are not burned will become that excess weight you just worked so hard to lose.

If you lost weight with the help of a formal weight loss program, stay in touch with friends you made in the program. Sharing a common goal with others can help you stay motivated. Exercising with a friend and socializing with friends who are physically active will help you stay active and keep the weight off.

Do not weigh yourself every day; weight fluctuates with water retention and you may be needlessly disheartened. You should, however, weigh yourself once a week. If you find that you are slowly but steadily gaining weight, reevaluate your eating habits, calorie and fat intake, and level of physical activity, before the progress you have made is undermined.

WHEN YOU CAN'T DO IT ALONE

If you find that you cannot make the lifestyle changes that you need to make in order to lose weight and keep it off, there are ways to get help. If you have failed at dieting, do not buy any over-the-counter diet pills or other diet drugs that promise weight loss. These aids are as suspect as fad diets; they do not work in the long run.

If you have failed at dieting, admit that you have a problem. Talk to your doctor. Unless you are very obese, medical intervention will probably not be necessary. There are some weight loss programs that are recommended by doctors for effective weight loss. They include Take Off Pounds Sensibly (TOPS) and Weight Watchers. With your doctor's approval, you might consider joining one of these groups. These programs work because they address lifestyle changes. They teach you to choose different foods and to judge portion sizes. The plans also offer ways to increase your daily physical activity and make exercise a part of your life. In addition, there are meetings that you can attend to check your progress and receive support when the going gets rough. Most importantly, these programs focus on long-term goals. Check listings in your area for local chapters, and remember to make sure that you have found an accredited

FAD DIETS

When many of us contemplate losing weight, we often look for a shortcut first. Unfortunately, there are no shortcuts and there is no substitute for a healthy, lifelong eating plan. Every year, hundreds of fad diets are advertised, prompting millions of Americans to resolve, once again, to try a new way to lose weight. But fad diets do not work. You may suffer through hunger pangs for 2 weeks and drop 10 lbs, but as soon as you return to your former lifestyle, you will almost certainly put the weight back on. In addition, some studies have shown that "yo-yo" dieting may cause additional increases in weight when you do gain weight back, as well as possible increases in health risks.

The propaganda around fad diets suggests that weight loss depends on magical solutions. The truth is that most fad diets are based on false or misleading claims, and some may actually be harmful. These claims also mislead the consumer by suggesting that something other than a permanent modification in food-related behaviors will solve the problem of keeping weight off. The only diet that works is one that results in overall and long-term changes in eating habits and lifestyle. ■

branch of the national organization. Many university or teaching hospitals also have weight loss clinics or obesity centers that offer programs.

Nutrition and Disease Prevention

Staying active and eating well are two of the most important components of disease prevention. A healthy diet that is low in fat, provides the nutrients you need, and is rich in complex carbohydrates and fiber can lower your risk of heart disease, type 2 diabetes, osteoporosis, and some forms of cancer. Good nutrition also protects against many diseases that do not have a direct link to dietary habits; eating wholesome foods every day helps ensure that your body has the nutrients to support all its systems, including the immune system, the first line of defense in fighting disease.

THE HEALTHY HEART DIET

Nutrition plays a major role in fighting heart disease. The link between diet, hypertension, and other forms of coronary heart disease is well documented. Your daily choice of what you eat and drink plays a major role in your risk for heart disease, which is the leading cause of death in the United States. The American Heart Association recommends that all Americans eat a diet low in fat, particularly saturated fat, and low in cholesterol.

When your cholesterol level is elevated for a long period of time, plaque develops in your arteries and causes atherosclerosis, or hardening of the arteries. Atherosclerosis impedes blood flow to and from the heart, and increases the risk of a heart attack. A diet low in fat and cholesterol can help prevent atherosclerosis. The American Heart Association also recommends a low-sodium diet to lower the risk of hypertension, which can lead to cardiovascular disease and stroke (see below).

In general, a healthy-heart diet should include no more than 30 percent of calories from fat. Less than 10 percent of calories should come from saturated fat, and no more than 10 percent should come from polyunsaturated fats. Monounsaturated fats, found in olive oil, canola oil, peanut oil, many nut oils, peanut butter, and avocados, should account for most of your calories from fat. You should not consume more than 300 mg of cholesterol a day and no more than 2,400 mg (2.4 g) of sodium. In addition, you should eat a varied diet to ensure proper vit-

Fatty deposits (atherosclerotic plaques) in the arteries can obstruct the flow of blood in the heart, brain, or elsewhere. A clot may form over the plaque and completely block flow, leading to damage to the organ that the blood vessel supplies with blood. In the heart this can cause a heart attack (myocardial infarction) and in the brain this can cause a stroke. Diets high in saturated fat and cholesterol can lead to atherosclerosis (hardening of the arteries) and the diseases associated with it.

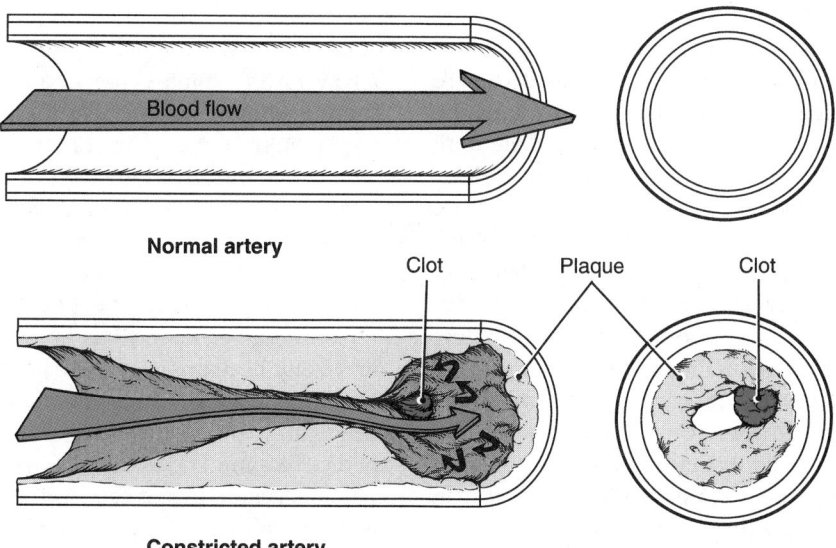

Normal artery

Clot   Plaque   Clot

Constricted artery

SODIUM CONTENT IN CONDIMENTS AND SEASONINGS

FOOD ITEM	AMOUNT	SODIUM (mg)
A-1 sauce	1 tbs	275
Baking powder	1 tsp	339
Baking soda	1 tsp	821
Barbecue sauce	1 tbs	130
Bleu cheese dressing	1 tbs	153
Chili	1 tbs	227
Chili powder	1 tsp	26
Garlic salt	1 tsp	1,850
Horseradish, prepared	1 tbs	198
French dressing	1 tbs	214
Italian dressing	1 tbs	116
Ketchup	1 tbs	156
Mayonnaise	1 tbs	78
Meat tenderizer	1 tsp	1,750
Monosodium glutamate (MSG)	1 tsp	492
Mustard, prepared	1 tsp	65
Olives, green	4	323
Olives, black	3	96
Onion salt	1 tsp	1,620
Pickle, dill	1	928
Pickle, sweet	1	128
Relish, sweet	1 tbs	124
Russian dressing	1 tbs	133
Soy sauce	1 tbs	1,029
Tabasco sauce	1 tsp	24
Tartar sauce	1 tbs	182
Teriyaki sauce	1 tbs	690
Thousand Island dressing	1 tbs	109
Worcestershire sauce	1 tbs	206

amins and nutrients. If you drink alcohol, drink less than two drinks a day. If you smoke, give it up (see Chapter 4). If you are overweight, you will also need to limit the amount of calories you consume daily until you have lost the desired amount of weight; do this under your doctor's supervision. Finally, to ensure the health of your heart, you will also need to make physical activity a part of your daily life (see Chapter 2). Consult your doctor before beginning any new exercise regimen. Taking the dietary precautions necessary to ensure a healthy heart will also help protect you against other diseases, such as diabetes. For more information on a heart-friendly diet, see Lifestyle Changes for a Healthy Heart, page 797.

REDUCING SODIUM IN YOUR DIET

New guidelines recommend that you limit your sodium intake to no more than 2,400 mg a day. If you suffer from heart disease or have had a heart attack, you should limit your daily sodium intake to less than 2,000 mg. A low-salt diet is not harmful and can help prevent hypertension and heart disease. Your body actually needs much less than 2,400 mg of sodium each day. For more information, see Chapter 20.

However, few Americans adhere to the recommended guidelines. The average American consumes 4,000 mg or more of sodium each day; it is estimated that the average American consumes 15 lbs of salt a year. After sugar, salt is the leading food additive in the United States. Salt is not good for your health because excess sodium causes your body to retain fluid and can lead to hypertension.

To reduce the sodium in your diet, avoid processed and canned foods with added sodium. Read the new food labels carefully for sodium content and avoid those foods high in sodium, which include most cheeses, condiments and seasonings (see this page). When cooking, flavor your dishes with spices rather than salt. At the table, use a salt substitute sparingly. Salt substitutes contain potassium chloride and should only be used with the approval of your doctor (see About Salt Substitutes, page 803).

IS THERE A CANCER PREVENTION DIET?

What you eat will not prevent all cancers, but it may lower your risk for certain cancers. There is some evidence that a high-fat diet may be linked to a higher risk for certain cancers, including cancer of the colon, uterus, breast, and prostate. Additionally, obesity increases the risk for certain cancers, including cancer of the colon, uterus, ovary, pancreas, prostate, and breast in older women.

Although research has yet to prove a direct link between diet and cancer prevention, the National Cancer Institute and the American Cancer Society have agreed on dietary recommendations to help lower the risk of certain types of cancer. These recommendations include the following:

- Eat a varied, well-balanced diet, concentrating on including at least five portions of fresh fruits and vegetables in your diet every day. Do not overcook vegetables because it diminishes their nutritional value. Steaming vegetables is the healthiest way of cooking, as it allows retention of the most vitamins and minerals.

- Eat foods that are high in fiber. Foods high in fiber include grains, whole grain breads, lentils, and legumes.

- Cut down on the amount of saturated and polyunsaturated fat in your diet.

- Concentrate on including foods in your diet that are high in vitamins C and A. Foods that are high in vitamin C include oranges, grapefruits, strawberries, green peppers, red peppers, and broccoli. Foods that are high in vitamin A include yellow vegetables such as squash, deep green vegetables such as spinach, and sweet potatoes, carrots, apricots, and peaches. Studies have shown that vitamin C may act as an antioxidant and reduce the production of some carcinogenic compounds. Vitamin A may lower your risk of certain cancers, including cancer of the larynx, pharynx, and lung.

- Eat cruciferous vegetables such as broccoli, cauliflower, cabbage, brussels sprouts, kale, and Swiss chard. Some research shows that cruciferous vegetables may lower the risk of colon, stomach, and lung cancers.

- Cut back on the amount of smoked and salt-cured foods.

- Cut back on the amount of processed foods and foods containing nitrites.

- Limit the amount of alcohol you consume to no more than two drinks a day.

- Make physical activity a daily part of your life.

CONTROLLING TYPE 2 DIABETES MELLITUS THROUGH DIET

More than 10 million Americans have type 2 diabetes mellitus (formerly called non-insulin-dependent diabetes mellitus), and the number is rising. Over 80 percent of people with diabetes are overweight. Diet is crucial in controlling type 2 diabetes because bringing weight and blood sugar levels close to normal ranges helps prevent many of the long-term complications of the disease.

If you are overweight, the first step to controlling your diabetes is to control your weight. By losing weight, you will lower your insulin resistance, which allows your body to begin to control blood glucose levels. Your diet will be basically the same as the healthy heart diet and the diet that lowers the risk of certain cancers, but you will need to pay special attention to your calorie intake in order to reach your desired weight. You will also have to carefully restrict the sweets in your diet. Consult your doctor before beginning any weight loss program.

The American Diabetes Association recommends cutting about 500 calories from your daily total during the initial weight loss period, while maintaining a nutritionally balanced diet. Limit the fat in your diet to less than 30 percent of your overall calories, with less than 10 percent of calories coming from saturated fats. Approximately 50 percent of calories should come from complex carbohydrates, including fresh vegetables, grains, lentils, beans and other legumes, and whole grain breads. Include fruit, but limit fruit juices because of their sugar content. By concentrating on obtaining 50 percent of your calories from complex carbohydrates, you will likely lower the amount of calories you consume, since many of these are foods low in calories. You will also increase the natural fiber content in your diet, which will aid digestion. Some studies even show that fiber may aid in controlling blood glucose levels. Protein should comprise between 12 and 20 percent of your diet.

In addition to changing how much you eat and the types of foods that you eat, modifying your meal pattern is also important. Smaller, more frequent meals or small meals combined with high-protein or complex carbohydrate snacks throughout the day limit the amount of glucose the body has to metabolize at any given time, which helps regulate blood glucose levels.

Finally, increasing your level of physical activity is almost as important as your diet in managing diabetes. Before beginning an exercise plan, however, consult your doctor, especially if you have experienced any side effects relating to your diabetes, such as poor circulation. For more information on diabetes, see Diabetes Mellitus Type 2, page 1179.

MANAGING LACTOSE INTOLERANCE

Lactose is the principal sugar found in milk. Lactose must be broken down into the simple sugars glucose and galactose before it can be used by the body. This process occurs with the aid of the intestinal enzyme, lactase.

When lactase is in short supply or not present at all, lactose intolerance occurs. It is estimated that about 70 percent of adults worldwide experience some degree of lactose intolerance. Lactose intolerance may develop at any age, but the age at which it occurs is often related to ethnic background. Asians, blacks, and Hispanics tend to develop lactose intolerance at about age 5, while whites often develop it around age 60 or 70. When lactase is not present, lactose remains in the small intestine, where it causes gas and bloating. As bacteria triggers fermentation of the undigested sugar, cramping and diarrhea occur. Lactose intolerance is different from a milk allergy. Milk allergies occur in only 1 percent of adults and are accompanied by symptoms such as a runny nose, diarrhea, vomiting, hives, and even asthma. Lactose intolerance and milk allergy can only be determined by your doctor.

A lactose-restricted diet can help manage lactose intolerance. On such a diet, high-lactose dairy products such as milk, cream, ice cream, and fresh cheeses, are eliminated or replaced with more easily digested dairy products such as yogurt and hard cheeses. Yogurt that contains live and active cultures can often be tolerated because the bacterial cultures contained in the yogurt digest some lactose. No dairy product should be eaten on an empty stomach; instead, it should be combined with other foods at meals. Drinking lactose-reduced or lactose-free milk is also recommended. A lactase supplement, such as Lactaid, may be used. People who are lactose intolerant are also likely to need a calcium supplement (see Calcium-Rich Foods, page 15).

Many people with a lactose deficiency may be able to consume moderate amounts of milk and other dairy products without experiencing symptoms of lactose intolerance. Research has also shown that people with lactose deficiency who consume moderate amounts of lactose on a regular basis may adapt and eventually experience no symptoms.

LACTOSE CONTENT OF COMMON FOODS

FOOD ITEM	LACTOSE (g)/ 100 g of food
American cheese	5
Brie	0–2
Butter and margarine	1
Buttermilk	5
Cheddar cheese	0–2
Condensed or evaporated milk	11
Cottage cheese	3
Cow's milk (whole, low-fat, or skim)	5
Cream cheese	2
Feta cheese	4
Half-and-half	4
Ice cream	3–8
Ice milk	8
Light cream	4
Mozzarella	0.3
Muenster cheese	1
Parmesan	0–3
Ricotta	3
Roquefort	2
Swiss cheese	1–2
Yogurt	2–6

NUTRITIONAL NEEDS OF SENIORS

Although the nutritional requirements of seniors have been the focus of much research, there is no evidence that the nutritional needs of older people change. In fact, the USRDAs are essentially the same for seniors as for younger adults. However, seniors need fewer calories per day. It can be a challenge to get sufficient nutrients while consuming fewer calories, which is all the more reason for seniors to choose their food with care and make proper nutrition a priority.

Although undernutrition is a problem for many seniors, so is weight gain. It is easy to put on unwanted extra pounds as activity levels decrease with age, therefore it is important that seniors also watch their weight.

If you are older and in good health, following the healthy heart diet will give you the nutrients you need, help you maintain a desirable weight, and protect against disease (see page 23). To prevent osteoporosis, older individuals should make sure to include plenty of calcium in their diet and perhaps also take a daily calcium supplement (see page 14).

As you plan your diet, keep in mind that changes occur as you age that affect digestion and absorption of nutrients. If it is difficult for you to prepare properly nutritious meals, contact local agencies that may be able to help you maintain an adequate diet with meal delivery (see Avoiding Undernutrition, page 323).

Older people who suffer from a chronic disease often find it difficult to follow a healthy nutrition plan because of lack of appetite or interest. The following tips may help you get the nutrients you need and maintain your weight.

- Vary the foods you eat. Eating a variety of foods can help you maintain your appetite and your interest in eating.

- As long as you are not suffering from heart disease, maintain an adequate fat intake by including olive oil and other oils, nuts, and even a small amount of butter in your diet. Consuming a moderate amount of fat will ensure that you consume enough calories every day. Fat also adds flavor to food, which can help restore a flagging appetite.

- Keep a record of what you eat during the day, trying to concentrate on getting enough fruits, vegetables, and complex carbohydrates such as beans, lentils, and grains. If you see from your notes that you are not eating as well as you should be, consult your doctor.

- Weigh yourself once a week. If your weight drops and you are not trying to lose weight, see your doctor.

- Talk to your doctor about how medications that you may be taking affect your nutritional needs.

- When family or friends ask if they can do anything for you, suggest that they bring you a healthy, home-cooked meal and healthy, ready-to-eat snacks.

Although a nutritional supplement cannot cancel the effects of poor eating habits, it can protect you from some vitamin and mineral deficiencies. All seniors should consider taking a multiple vitamin and mineral supplement that provides the RDA of essential vitamins and minerals (see Vitamin Supplements and Dietary Supplement Drinks, page 325).

Food Safety

Just as it is important to make healthy choices in terms of what we eat, it is also important to prepare food in a healthy manner to avoid infection and spoilage.

Food poisoning occurs when you eat contaminated food. Contamination occurs when proper hygiene is not maintained during food preparation. The best safeguards against food contamination are a clean kitchen, proper food storage and refrigeration, proper hygiene during preparation, and thoroughly cooked foods. See Avoiding Food Contamination, page 28.

Common symptoms of gastrointestinal infection caused by food poisoning include nausea, stomach ache, vomiting, and diarrhea. Cases of food poisoning may range from mild to severe. Most cases of food poisoning last only a few hours, although food poisoning caused by contaminated cream or mayonnaise may last 12 hours or more. For most individuals, food poisoning is unpleasant and debilitating, but it lasts no more than 24 to 36 hours. However, for children, the elderly, and individuals with compromised immune systems, the health risks of food poisoning are far greater.

A common cause of food poisoning is the bacteria *Staphylococcus aureus*, or staph. A staph infection may be caused by spoiled mayonnaise or cream, or the bacteria may have spread from the hands of a person preparing food. Staph infection lasts about 12 hours and is rarely serious. *Salmonella* bacteria, found most frequently in meat, poultry, and eggs, are responsible for a common form of food poisoning that can be lethal. Symptoms include fever and gastrointestinal discomfort; they usually appear the day after eating contaminated food, although symptoms may appear up to 48 hours after eating contaminated food.

Eating fish contaminated with ciguatoxin may also cause food poisoning. Ciguatoxin poisoning occurs mainly in tropical areas. Symptoms include nausea or vomiting, general gastrointestinal discomfort, rash, achiness, tingling of the mouth and tongue, and numbness in the hands and feet. Symptoms may last a month or more. Sushi, which is made of raw fish, may also cause abdominal pain and vomiting. The source of this infection is a parasite found in the crustaceans on which fish feed. Hepatitis A can be caused by eating raw shellfish. Remember that when you eat sushi or raw shellfish, you do so at your own risk.

Diarrhea may also be caused by *Clostridium perfringens*. This infection may occur when cooked meat is left out of the refrigerator for too long. Symptoms occur about a day after eating contaminated food and last about a day. Another form of diarrhea, traveler's diarrhea, may be caused by *Escherichia coli* bacteria. *E. coli* is common in the water supplies of many countries, and is sometimes found even in US water systems. *E. coli* may also be present in meat that has not been fully cooked. Diarrhea from an *E. coli* infection can be severe and may last for several days.

Modern canning techniques have made botulism a very rare form of food poisoning nowadays; however, when it occurs, it can be lethal. Botulism is caused by *Clostridium botulinum*, which can grow in the absence of oxygen. Check all cans before opening them to see if they are swollen or dented or if the button on the top of the can has popped, all of which are signs of a possible risk of botulism.

For more information on food poisoning, traveler's diarrhea, and other infections caused by contaminated food and water, see Foodborne and Waterborne Infections, page 869.

should also be served well done. Many recipes provide cooking times that leave meat and fish undercooked and unsafe to eat; adjust times so that meat or fish is thoroughly cooked. Many restaurants serve fish rare to almost raw. Remember to request your fish well done. Serving rare meat and fish might be considered sophisticated, but there is nothing sophisticated about a case of food poisoning (see page 61). To prevent foods from becoming contaminated by bacteria, take the following precautions:

- Wash your hands with warm, soapy water before beginning any food preparation; wash them again after you have finished.

- Clean all kitchen equipment including your cutting board and any utensils before and after preparing food. Use hot soapy water.

- Designate one cutting board for meat and poultry only.

- Disinfect cutting boards using a solution of 2 tsp of household bleach in 1 qt of hot water. Wash the board thoroughly after disinfecting.

- Replace cutting boards periodically.

- Thaw meat and poultry in the refrigerator or microwave, not at room temperature.

- Do not use cracked eggs.

- Clean all foods thoroughly.

- Refrigerate leftovers immediately.

- Do not keep leftovers more than a day or two.

- Do not eat raw fish or meat, uncooked marinades, or undercooked eggs.

- Throw away moldy foods, except cheese. Cheese may be eaten as long as the moldy patches are thoroughly cut away.

AVOIDING FOOD CONTAMINATION

Meat, poultry, and eggs present the greatest risk of contamination. To lower the risk of food poisoning, these foods must be thoroughly cleaned under hygienic conditions and thoroughly cooked. Meat should be cooked until it is well done. If it is pink inside, it is not safe to eat. Fish and chicken

ORGANIC FOODS

Many people are now choosing to eat organic foods whenever possible to ensure that their diet is not contaminated with pesticides and other toxins. Organic fruits and vegetables are foods that are grown in soil that has been kept pesticide-free for 3 years. Livestock that is given only organic feed and no hormone or vitamin supplements provide organic beef and poultry.

The United States Department of Agriculture and the FDA set acceptable pesticide levels for all food. By these standards the pesticide levels in the food supply are safe. However, these levels are established by assessing the average amount of fresh produce that Americans eat and then calculating the amount of pesticides contained in this average amount. At present, there is some debate over the amount of fruits and vegetables that Americans consume. The FDA assessment of this amount is considered very conservative according to many nutritionists and some food-safety advocacy groups. According to the National Resources Council, safe pesticide levels as determined by the FDA represent a diet that includes only small amounts of fruits and vegetables. Fruits and vegetables actually constitute a far greater portion of the daily diet of many people. There is some legitimate concern, therefore, that pesticide levels in foods may be too high, or, at least, that safe pesticide levels have yet to be adequately established.

Organic foods offer an alternative for those who are concerned about the pesticide level in their food. But organic products can have drawbacks. Always check to make sure that organic milk has been pasteurized. Milk that has not been pasteurized may be more dangerous to your health than a small residue of pesticide. You should only buy organic foods from a reputable merchant. Farms and companies that produce organic foods vary in quality and in the definition of organic that they use. And simply because foods are labeled organic, do not neglect to follow basic food-handling precautions, such as washing fruits and vegetables and handling meat and poultry properly.

ALCOHOL AND NUTRITION

Alcohol affects the entire body; abuse of alcohol can damage every organ in the body, from the skin to the heart and brain.

Alcoholism is associated with nutritional deficiencies and prolonged alcoholism may lead to malnutrition and disease. Excessive alcohol consumption over a long period of time often leads to gastric bleeding. In addition, it may damage the pancreas and cause pancreatitis, which can be fatal. Alcohol-related malabsorption may lead to vitamin deficiencies. People who consume large amounts of alcohol may not eat properly; they tend to replace calories from food with calories from alcohol, which may lead to the development of vitamin deficiencies, particularly of the B vitamins.

Prolonged abuse of alcohol also causes liver damage. Approximately one in five long-term heavy drinkers will develop cirrhosis of the liver. Protein metabolized by a damaged or cirrhotic liver is broken down into ammonia and other compounds; eventually, toxins accumulate, which can lead to unconsciousness and brain damage. If you are a heavy drinker and find you cannot cut back on your own, you should seek help. For more information on stopping alcohol abuse, see Chapter 5.

Two

Staying Active, Staying Fit

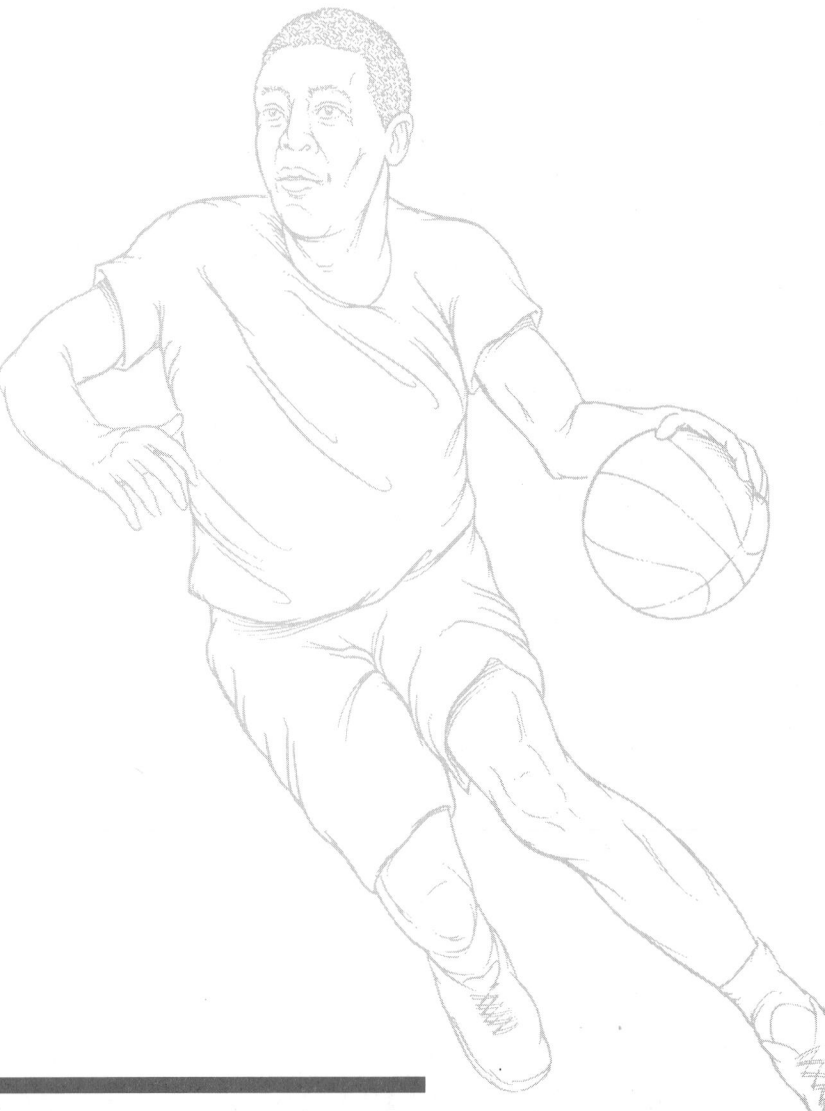

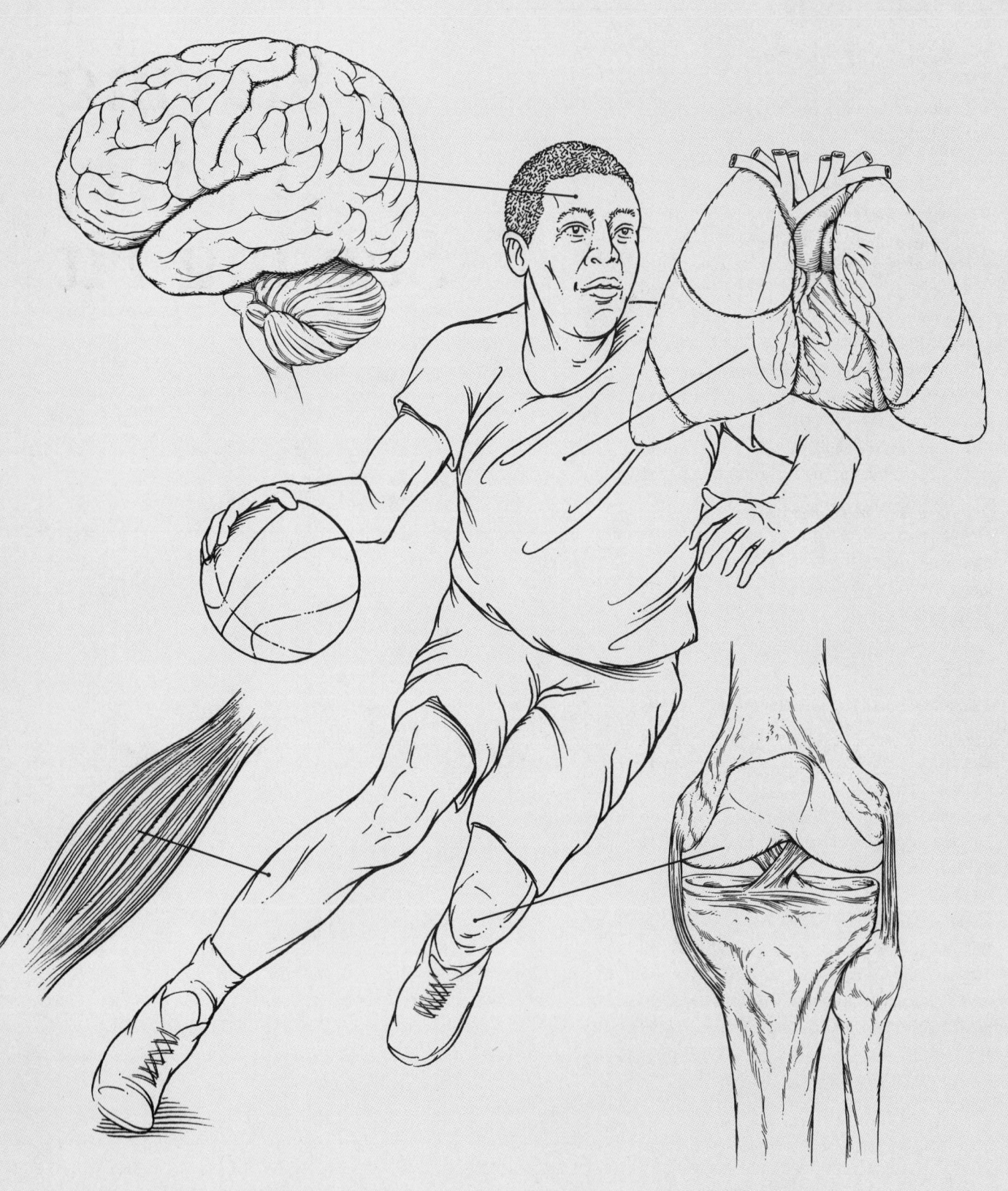

STAYING ACTIVE, STAYING FIT

The Benefits of Physical Activity

Twentieth-century advances in technology have played a greater and greater role in easing the physical demands of our daily lives; the resulting dependence on technology has made us increasingly sedentary. Few Americans walk to work or to the grocery store. We use the remote to change the television channel, the electric can opener to open a can. Our lives are filled with shortcuts that may improve many aspects of how we live but that can also undermine our good health, which depends on leading a physically active life.

Physical activity is vital to good health, and yet in our sedentary culture many of us make exercise our lowest priority, after work, family, and of course, eating. Instead of making physical activity an indispensable part of our daily routine, we tend to treat exercise as something we will do when we someday have the time. We tell ourselves we will work out on the weekend or, even worse, get back to exercising when we get that promotion or when the children are older. But without physical activity, the body cannot stay fit. And the longer you go without exercising, the harder it will be for your body to do what you ask it to do.

The number of Americans who are physically inactive is alarming. According to the 1996 Surgeon General's Report, approximately 25 percent of adult Americans do not engage in any physical activity. More than 60 percent of Americans are not physically active for 20 minutes at a time, three times a week, which is the minimal physical activity level recommended for fitness of the heart and blood vessels, or cardiovascular fitness. In addition, approximately 14 percent of children do not engage in any vigorous or even moderate physical activity. And physical inactivity is more prevalent in women and girls, blacks, and Hispanics.

The health and fitness benefits of physical activity cannot be overstated: Exercise is essential for maintaining cardiovascular fitness, muscle strength, stamina, balance, and joint flexibility. Strength-developing exercise improves overall musculoskeletal health, and stretching maintains flexibility. Physical activity also increases energy level, improves mood, and diminishes anxiety and stress. Exercise can be beneficial in avoiding weight gain and in helping replace fat with muscle.

Moderate exercise performed consistently can prevent or control heart disease and diabetes. Higher levels of physical activity are linked with increased levels of high density lipoprotein (HDL), the "good" cholesterol in the blood. If you are a smoker, increasing your level of physical activity may motivate you to cut down on your smoking. Women who exercise may lessen the debilitating effects of osteoporosis, or avoid the disease altogether. Physical activity is also one of the best means we have of ensuring that we age well and enjoy life more fully. Exercise can even increase life expectancy.

While the connection between physical activity and overall good health has been known throughout history, in recent decades cardiovascular fitness has taken center stage. Many experts recommended moderate to intense exercise primarily as a way to improve cardiorespiratory health. Such activity, which increases endurance and improves the way the body makes use of oxygen, is known as aerobic exercise. But focusing on aerobic exercise can cause people to ignore other, equally important forms of activity, such as resistance exercise to improve muscle strength and endurance, and other exercises to promote flexibility, dexterity, and balance. The 1996 Surgeon General's Report recommends moderate levels of a variety of these activities to promote general health. If you have been inactive, it is recommended that you begin to increase your level of activity gradually, eventually aiming for regular activity for 30 minutes on all or most days of the week. For maximal health benefits, aerobic activity should be combined with periods of weight-resistance activity (see Combined Exercise for General Health, page 34).

LEADING A PHYSICALLY ACTIVE DAILY LIFE

No one is too young or too old to exercise. Exercise can be a family activity, or it can be something you enjoy alone. And any exercise or physical activity is better than none. You will be surprised how much you can increase your level of physical activity simply by making conscious choices about how you perform everyday tasks. The American Heart Association states that nearly

COMBINED EXERCISE FOR GENERAL HEALTH

To be complete, an exercise program must include different but complementary types of activity: aerobic exercise, resistance exercise, and flexibility training.

"Aerobic" means "oxygen-using." Aerobic exercise increases your body's demand for oxygen, and raises your heart rate. Regular aerobic exercise increases the efficiency with which your body uses oxygen, strengthening your heart, increasing your endurance, enhancing your immune system, and maintaining your overall health. Besides increasing cardiovascular health, calorie-burning aerobic exercise is instrumental in any weight-loss program.

After 2 or 3 minutes the ability to sustain exercise is dependent on the ability to take in oxygen from the air we breathe. For this reason, aerobic exercise increases the rate and depth of your breathing and the heart rate increases in order to deliver oxygen to the muscles. It also causes your body to become warmer and eventually causes you to perspire in order to get rid of excess heat. To achieve full benefits, aerobic exercise must last at least 20 continuous minutes and must be performed at least three or four times a week. Examples of aerobic activity include walking, jogging, bicycling, iceskating, in-line skating, aerobic dancing, and swimming.

In addition to aerobic exercise, resistance exercise is also important. Resistance exercises strengthen the body and tone the muscles. The name refers to the fact that to increase muscle mass and strength, you must increase the amount of resistance the muscle encounters as it moves. Resistance exercise involves slow movement of specific muscle groups. Other names for resistance exercise are weight-training exercise and muscle strengthening or conditioning.

A set of weight-training exercises, such as arm curls or bench presses, usually does not last the 2 or 3 minutes necessary to begin increasing heart rate and the sustained demand for oxygen. Most weight-training exercises are considered anaerobic because they do not require a steady source of oxygen to complete the task, the way running a mile does. However, resistance exercises may improve metabolism by increasing lean muscle, which is the body's calorie-burning engine, and by burning blood glucose at a faster rate than aerobic exercise. Resistance exercise does not raise your heart rate significantly, but it can raise your blood pressure to very high levels when performing the exercise. People with high blood pressure or other risk factors should consult a physician before starting a vigorous resistance exercise program.

Besides improving muscle strength, resistance exercise slows down the loss of bone and muscle mass that normally occurs as we age. It is particularly helpful in addressing age-related changes in body composition. Resistance exercise also improves balance, which can help you avoid falls and reduce your risk of bone fractures.

Weight-lifting, isometric exercises, sit-ups and push-ups, and exercising with various resistance enhancers such as rubber tubing are all examples of resistance exercise. Daily activities such as shoveling snow or lifting and carrying heavy packages can technically be defined as resistance exercise, but such activities are usually not performed with enough regularity to constitute complete exercise.

Flexibility is also important. A complete exercise routine includes stretching. Particularly as we age, flexibility is important for performing everyday tasks efficiently and for preventing falls.

The benefits of exercise depend on the intensity, duration, and frequency with which it is performed. By definition, exercise requires a higher level of intensity than normal activity. For example, walking is good exercise if done briskly, but simply strolling along a sidewalk will not significantly improve cardiovascular strength.

As discussed above, exercise must last a certain amount of time to be effective and the duration or intensity of your exercise routine should increase over time, up to a certain point. During the first weeks and months of running or jogging, work to increase the distance you cover or the speed at which you cover the same distance.

Frequency is probably the most important element in any successful exercise program. Exercising one day a week is not enough to provide maximal health benefits. Moreover, exercising only occasionally may actually increase your risk of injury. To improve your level of physical fitness, you need to perform your exercise routine or engage in some sustained physical activity for 20 to 30 minutes on most days (four or more) of the week. No matter how complete your exercise routine may be, it is of little good to your overall health if you do not do it regularly. ■

everyone can become moderately fit and reduce the risk of cardiovascular disease simply by increasing the level of physical activity in their daily life, and by maintaining that level of activity.

Success in establishing exercise as a part of your life depends on changing your attitude toward it. If the thought of exercise seems daunting, remember that to get yourself started, you do not necessarily have to "work out," you just have to move.

The easiest way to become more active is to examine your daily routine and see where you might add a physical component to your activities. For example, if you work on the fifth floor of an office building, try taking the stairs instead of the elevator. If you become winded after one or two flights, try walking a few flights and taking the elevator the rest of the way. Gradually, work up to walking the entire way. If you drive to work even though the distance is only a mile or two, try walking or bicycling. If you take the bus to work, get off the bus 10 blocks from your office and walk the rest of the way. Instead of driving when you do errands, walk or bicycle. When you go to the shopping mall, park your car a distance from your favorite store and walk to the mall. In stores, take the stairs instead of the escalator.

Even doing chores around the house can increase your level of physical activity. According to the Surgeon General, 30 minutes of gardening or 45 minutes washing and waxing a car can help (see What Is a Moderate Amount of Physical Activity? page 36). Instead of hiring a cleaning person, clean the house yourself. Recent research shows that housecleaning—mopping, vacuuming, dusting, and polishing—is a valuable form of physical activity. If you use a portable phone, pace while you make your phone calls instead of sitting in a chair. If you have stairs in your house, walk them more often. Take the dogs for long, brisk walks. If you like to garden, work in the garden using hand tools. Weed the garden and rake the leaves yourself. Mow the lawn with a hand mower, not a power mower. These are just a few suggestions of how to increase your level of daily physical activity without changing your life. Once you change your attitude toward exercise and increase your level of activity, you have taken the first step toward becoming a more physically active person.

Many see exercise as another chore instead of as something intimately connected to enjoyment of life. Still others who have been sedentary for a long time have ready excuses for remaining so. If you have back problems or suffer from arthritis or any other chronic pain, you may think exercise would be too painful—and use this as an excuse to remain inactive. The fact is that for many health conditions staying inactive will not relieve your pain and it can even worsen your condition. Physical activity is important for everyone, including those with chronic conditions or physical disabilities. Remaining inactive and not using the muscles that you can may aggravate existing problems and possibly create new problems.

In most cases, the benefits of an intelligently planned exercise regimen far outweigh any risks involved in exercise; still, to minimize the risk of injury you need to make sure you are exercising safely and responsibly. As in all areas of life, moderation is the key to exercising safely. Americans, however, tend to have some difficulty embracing the concept of moderation. We tend to think more is better. Particularly when we know something is good for us, we think we can't get enough. This pioneer spirit coupled with the increasing popularity of many sports, exercise programs, and exercise fads has contributed to the rise of injuries related to sports and to overuse of the body.

Exercise is most worthwhile when it is done safely and when it is accompanied by the proper warm-up and cool-down techniques. Middle-aged and older adults, and younger persons at increased risk for heart disease, should not commence a vigorous exercise routine without consulting a doctor. If you have been sedentary for a long time or have a history of heart disease or any other illness, your doctor will probably recommend an exercise stress test before you begin to exercise (see Getting a Safe Start, page 37).

The most important step in making exercise a part of your life is to choose goals that are realistic and manageable. For example, if you have never been cross-country skiing before, do not attempt a 10-mile ski over rough terrain your first day on the trails. Whatever activity you choose, start gradually and remember that any progress is progress. Once you have established a certain exercise as a part of your routine you can build up to a more strenuous level, but make sure exercise is a positive habit and part of your life before you challenge yourself further.

Try to think of exercising as something pleasurable—a reward, not a punishment. If you choose a form of exercise that you dislike but that you think will be "good for you," you probably will not stick with it. Choose an activity that you enjoy. If you enjoy swimming, make swimming your activity of choice. If you like to walk, take a 30-minute walk every day. If you find walking alone gets boring, find a walking buddy, or listen to music or a book on tape while you are walking. You need not condemn yourself to a dreary routine of calisthenics and running on a treadmill. A long walk is not only beneficial aerobic exercise, it can be a pleasure as well. Using free weights or machines can also be an enjoyable substitute for calisthenics. The more you enjoy

WHAT IS A MODERATE AMOUNT OF PHYSICAL ACTIVITY?

To achieve a moderate amount of physical activity, select activities that you enjoy and that fit into your daily life. A "moderate" amount of physical activity uses approximately 150 calories of energy a day, or 1,000 calories a week. Amount of activity is a function of the combination of duration, intensity, and frequency. The same amount of activity is obtained in longer sessions of moderately intense activities such as brisk walking, or in shorter sessions of strenuous activities such as running. The following list arranges equivalent amounts of different activities in an ascending order of strenuousness. Less vigorous activities requiring more time are at the top and more vigorous activities requiring less time are at the bottom.

- Washing and waxing a car for 45 to 60 minutes
- Washing windows or floors for 45 to 60 minutes
- Playing volleyball for 45 minutes
- Playing touch football for 30 to 45 minutes
- Gardening for 30 to 45 minutes
- Wheeling self in wheelchair for 30 to 40 minutes
- Walking 1¾ miles in 35 minutes (20-minute/mile)

- Basketball (shooting baskets) for 30 minutes
- Bicycling 5 miles in 30 minutes
- Dancing fast (social dancing) for 30 minutes
- Pushing a stroller 1½ miles in 30 minutes
- Raking leaves for 30 minutes
- Walking 2 miles in 30 minutes (15-minute/mile)
- Water aerobics for 30 minutes
- Swimming laps for 20 minutes
- Wheelchair basketball for 20 minutes
- Basketball (playing a game) for 20 minutes
- Bicycling 4 miles in 15 minutes
- Jumping rope for 15 minutes
- Running 1½ miles in 15 minutes (10-minute/mile)
- Shoveling show for 15 minutes
- Stairwalking for 15 minutes

Source: Physical Activity and Health: A Report of the Surgeon General, 1996. ■

SAFETY TIPS

Exercise-related injuries are all too common. It is important to exercise safely, especially as we grow older and become at greater risk for injury. The following tips can help.

- When exercising, you should feel that you are working somewhat hard, but not *too* hard. You should not feel that you are straining.
- Warm up before you work out and cool down afterwards.
- Pay attention to your body. If you experience serious muscle fatigue, stop and rest.
- Pace yourself. Do not overexert yourself at the beginning of your exercise session.
- Breathe deeply and regularly. Avoid holding your breath during exertion; this robs your body of the oxygen it needs during exercise.

- Stop for water breaks every 20 minutes or as often as you need.
- If you experience any of the following symptoms, stop exercising immediately.
  - Dizziness
  - Blurred vision
  - Heart palpitations
  - Chest pain or pressure
  - Neck pain
  - Pain running down your left arm
  - Faintness
  - Nausea
  - Breathlessness ■

THE FOUR S's

The American Heart Association suggests that you maximize your safety while exercising by paying attention to The Four S's.

Stretch Before exercising, warm up by stretching. Concentrate on those muscles and tendons that will be used in your exercise program. For example, if you plan to run, stretch the muscles in your calves, thighs, and ankles. If you plan to lift weights, stretch your arms, shoulders, back, and neck.

Surface The harder the surface, the greater the stress on your muscles and bones. Grass or dirt is better for running than concrete and a surface with "give" is best for aerobic dance.

Shoes No matter what the activity, the proper shoe can protect you from injury.

Style Your form is also important in protecting you from injury. Whatever your exercise of choice, learning how to exercise properly will help prevent injury. ■

your chosen activities, the more likely you are to keep exercising and to reap the benefits of becoming fit. If you need further motivation to make exercise a priority, consider how much easier your daily life will be when you are in good shape. Every physical activity—bending to pick something up, climbing the stairs, running to catch a train—is easier when you are physically fit.

Getting a Safe Start

Anyone who wants to increase their level of physical activity should do so slowly and carefully. Most people can increase their level of physical activity safely, as long as they do it sensibly.

CONSULTING YOUR DOCTOR

The American College of Sports Medicine has established guidelines to help people decide whether they should undergo a medical examination and a clinical exercise test before starting an exercise program. Generally, medical consultation is not necessary for men age 40 or younger and women age 50 or younger, who have no known medical risks or conditions. These individuals can begin a moderate or even a vigorous exercise program at any time. Healthy men over age 40 and women over age 50 should speak with their doctors before starting a vigorous program, but can usually begin to exercise at a moderate level without medical advice.

AVOIDING INJURY

The most common injuries that occur while exercising result from excessive demands placed on muscles, bones, and other tissues. You can minimize your risk for exercise-related injury by approaching your fitness goals realistically, by taking precautions when you exercise, and by doing your workout, if not daily, at least every other day.

Having risk factors for coronary artery disease changes the picture. These risk factors include age, 45 and over for men, 55 and over for women; a family history of heart disease; cigarette use; high cholesterol level; diabetes; and a sedentary lifestyle. People who have two or more risk factors may begin moderate exercise without a doctor's approval if they are not having symptoms, but they should speak with a doctor before engaging in more vigorous exercise. People who have two or more risk factors and who are experiencing symptoms should also see their doctor first, as should all people with any known cardiac, pulmonary, or metabolic disease before beginning a moderate exercise program.

If you are just beginning an exercise program, start slowly and build up your routine gradually. Allow yourself a couple of weeks or a month to reach the goal you have set for an adequate workout. For example, if you have been inactive and choose running as your exercise, begin by incorporating three 30-minute workouts into your weekly schedule. During each workout, alternate running 10 minutes and walking 10 minutes. If you become breathless, slow down and take walking breaks more frequently.

If you were an athlete when you were young and decide to return to a favorite sport at the age of 40, do not begin by trying to impress your friends with feats you have not performed in 20 years. Trying to show off or compete above your present competence level makes you a prime candidate for injury. Start getting back in shape gradually and do not expect to perform at the same level as when you were younger.

The following common sense guidelines will help minimize your risk of injury.

Consult your doctor If you have multiple risk factors and/or symptoms of coronary artery disease, or known cardiac, pulmonary, or metabolic disease, talk to your doctor before beginning an exercise routine or taking up a sport (see Consulting Your Doctor, above).

Warm up before exercising and cool down afterwards Stretching exercises increase blood flow to your muscles and lower muscle tension, minimizing the risk of injury during your workout. Stretching after your workout allows your muscles a chance to cool down, helping you avoid muscle pulls and strains (see Your Warm-Up and Cool-Down, page 38).

Choose a sport or activity that is right for you For example, if you have problems with your knees, swimming would be a better choice than running.

YOUR WARM-UP AND COOL-DOWN

Did you ever play with Silly Putty? You probably remember that if you pulled on the ball of putty quickly, a piece would snap off in your hand. But if you warmed it in your hands and then pulled slowly, the putty would stretch forever.

In a way, warming up before exercise is similar. Slow stretching exercises increase blood flow to the muscles, ligaments, and tendons, maximizing their flexibility. This in turn helps prevent injury during the more strenuous exertion to come.

Spend several minutes warming up before your exercise routine and devote an equal amount of time to cooling down afterward. When warming up, never jerk or bounce your body—remember what happens to Silly Putty! Begin slowly by extending the muscle as far as you can and holding the position for a few seconds. Concentrate on relaxing the muscle and see if you can extend just a little farther, without forcing. Return to your original position. Repeat the cycle, perhaps trying to stretch a little farther each time. Again, never force yourself to stretch too far. Stretch all the major muscle groups, emphasizing stretches that work the muscles you will be using most during your exercise routine.

Cooling down after you exercise is as important as warming up before you begin. Your cool-down helps prevent injury and keeps your muscles from cramping. Cooling down also helps to maintain adequate blood flow to your heart and to avoid pooling of blood in the limbs. As you approach the end of your exercise routine, ease your pace gradually. For example, when you are done with your run, slow to a walk and walk for a while before you stop and begin your cool-down stretches. Never stop exercising suddenly. The same stretches that you used in your warm-up can be used in your cool-down. After cooling down, you may also want to massage your muscles to avoid cramping. ■

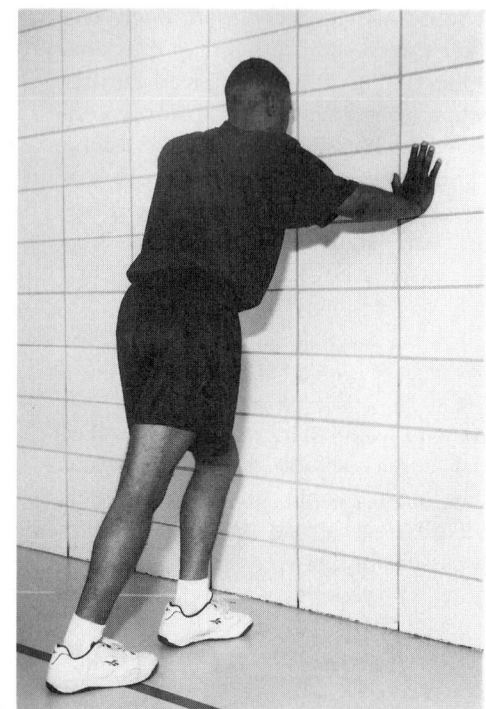

A

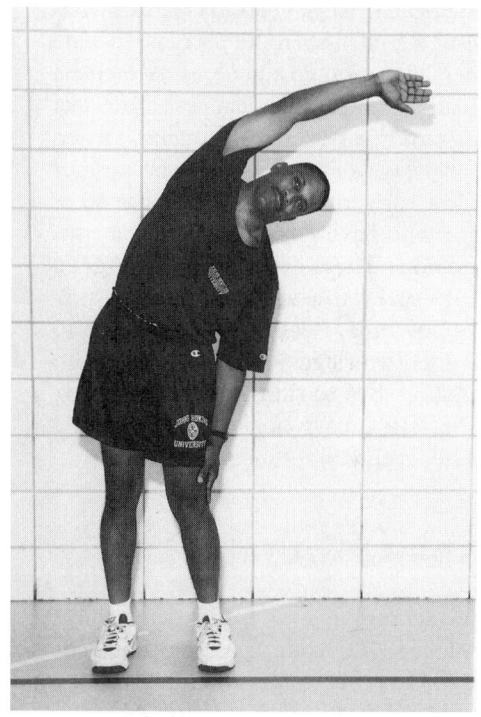

B

Both the calf stretch (A) and the side stretch (B) can be done as warming-up or cooling-down stretches. When you are doing stretching exercises, slowly extend the muscle as far as you can and then hold the position for a few seconds. Return to your original position and repeat.

Work out regularly When you are in the habit of exercising 4 or more days a week, you are much less likely to injure yourself. Your body is used to the activity and you know your routine. Sporadic exercisers are more likely to pull a muscle or twist an ankle.

Increase the pace and the duration of your workout gradually Be patient with yourself as you work toward your goal. If you have just started running, do not try to run 2 or 3 miles during a workout in the first week of your program. And do not abruptly increase the distance you run or the time spent running. Add distance and time to your workout in small increments.

Avoid competitive situations Do not try to live up to expectations you had for yourself when you were 20 and do not compete with others. When taking up a sport or activity, remember that your goal is to improve your physical health, not to win a gold medal. If you like to play basketball, for example, play with a group at about the same skill level as you, rather than trying to get into a game with the best athletes in town.

Do not neglect an injury when it occurs See your doctor as soon as possible for more severe injuries or for minor injuries that do not respond to rest, and follow the recommended treatment. Do not return to your exercise routine until your doctor says it is safe to do so. If your recuperation will take time, discuss alternative exercise plans with your doctor. For example, if you have injured an ankle, you may be able to swim while your ankle is healing.

EXERCISE-RELATED INJURIES

Injuries that occur during exercise can involve a single episode, such as a sudden twist of the body, or they can involve constant overuse, in which stresses to the body accumulate slowly but steadily. Common exercise-related injuries include strains, sprains, tendinitis, bursitis, and stress injuries. An important way to prevent such injuries is to wear proper athletic shoes and gear when you exercise, use good equipment, and exercise routinely—but without overdoing it. Most individuals benefit from a regular routine of warm-up and cool-down exercises and stretches every time they exercise.

Strains Tendons connect your muscles to your bones. Both the muscles and the tendons support your bones. A strain is an injury to muscle or a tendon, usually occurring in the leg or foot. Strains can involve overstretched or torn muscles, tendons, or both. Strains are treated with a strategy known as RICE—the letters stand for rest, ice, compression, and elevation—followed by rehabilitation exercises to restore mobil-

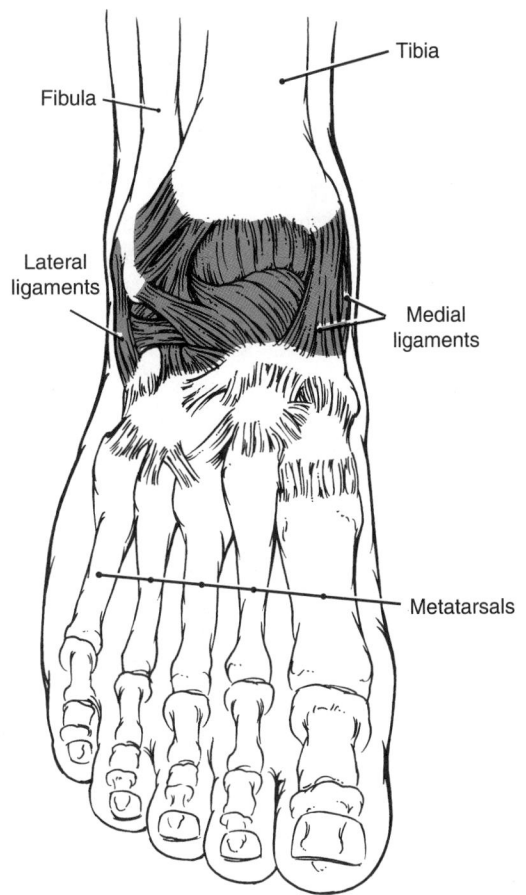

Ankle ligament injuries are among the most common sports injuries. Twisting motions of the foot can tear ligaments supporting the joint, causing a sprain.

Common causes of shoulder pain include inflammation of the subdeltoid bursae (bursitis), inflammation of the biceps tendon (biceps tendinitis), and arthritis of the acromioclavicular joint.

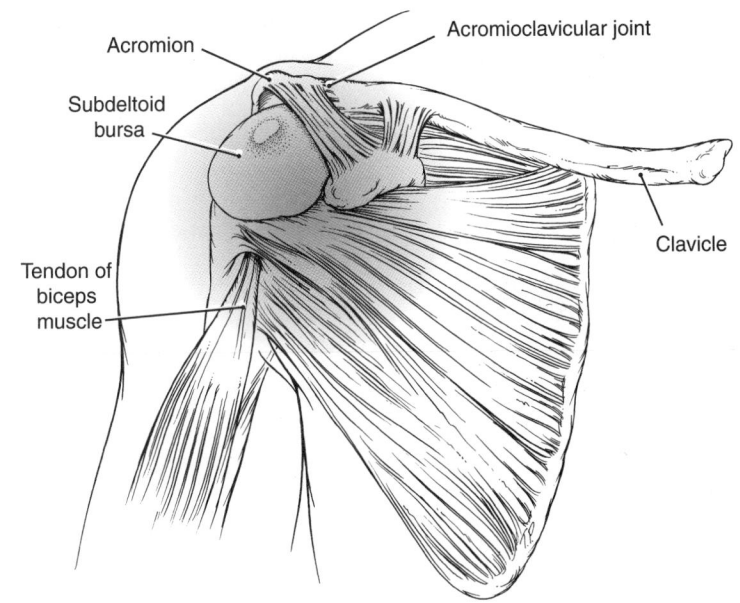

CARING FOR YOUR BACK

The stresses and strains of life affect the whole body, but one of the most vulnerable areas is the back. To protect your back, practice good posture, holding your shoulders back and your chin level, pulling in both your stomach and buttocks. Do not bend at the waist when lifting heavy objects; squat and let your knees—not your back—do the work. When exercising, avoid sudden, jerking motions and stressful twists and turns. Also avoid sleeping on your back or stomach and make sure the mattress you sleep on is very firm.

Both flexion (bending) exercises and extension (straightening) exercises can strengthen your back and protect it from injury. The following exercises should be done at least three times a week to be effective. If you have never done these exercises before, begin by repeating each exercise two or three times and work up to 10 repetitions in 1 to 2 weeks. If you have any discomfort or pain in your back, stop the exercise and see your doctor. If you have had a back injury or have a history of back problems, consider consulting your doctor before beginning any exercise routine.

Flexion Exercises

1. Lie on your back with your knees bent. Flatten your lower back against the floor by contracting your stomach muscles and rolling your pelvis up toward your stomach. Hold for a count of five and release.

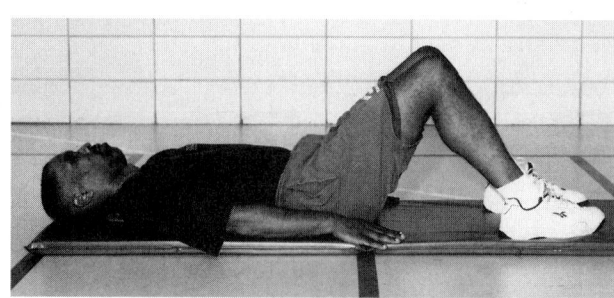

2. Lie on your back with your legs extended. Lift one knee to your chest and hold it there with your arms while flexing your foot toward your head. Count to five and release. Repeat the exercise with the other leg.

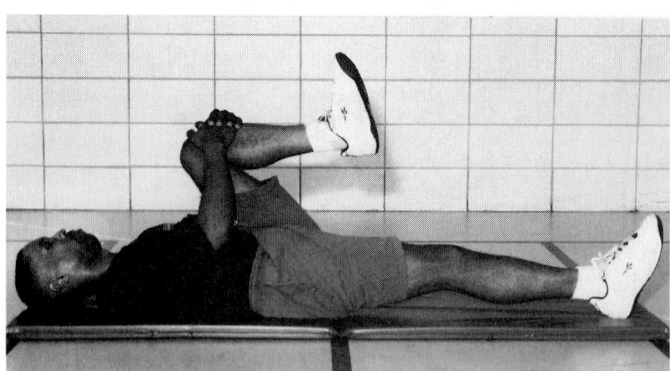

3. Lie on your back with your knees bent. Grasp your hands behind your head and lift your head from the floor, pulling your shoulders up to approximately a 45-degree angle. Hold for a count of five and release.

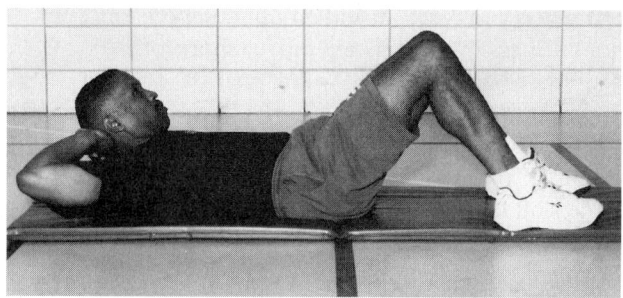

4. Do exercise no. 1 in a standing position with your back against the wall and your feet a few inches from the wall.

Extension Exercises

1. Lie on your stomach with your hands at your sides, palms up, and tighten your buttocks. Count to five and release.

2. In the same starting position, raise your head and chest while arching your upper back, squeezing your shoulders together and up toward your back. Hold for a count of five and release.

3. In the same starting position, slowly raise one leg into the air as far as you can to a count of five and then slowly lower it to a count of five. Repeat with the other leg.

4. Repeat exercise no. 3, raising both legs together to a count of five; then lower both legs together to a count of five.

Pelvic Stretch

Lie flat on your back. Pull your knees up until your legs form a triangle with your feet flat on the floor. With your back flat, swivel your pelvis and legs to the right so that your knees touch the floor. Hold for a count of five. Swivel back to center. Then swivel your pelvis and legs to the left so that your knees touch the floor. Count to five and return to center. Repeat the stretch three times. Gradually work up to 10 stretches. ∎

ity. In cases of severe strain, surgery may be necessary.

Sprains Ligaments support the joints of your body, connecting one bone to another. If ligaments become stretched or torn, usually as a result of a twist or a fall, a sprain can occur. Ankles, knees, and wrists are especially vulnerable to sprains. Sprains are treated the same way as strains, using the RICE strategy. Torn ligaments may require surgery.

Tendinitis Inflammation—pain, irritation, and swelling—often results when body tissue suffers an injury. Inflammation arising in a tendon or in the connective tissue covering the tendon is called tendinitis. Tendinitis usually results from a series of small repeated stresses that eventually aggravate the tendon until it becomes inflamed. Tennis players, swimmers, golfers, and baseball players are prone to tendinitis in the shoulder or arm; runners, soccer players, basketball players, and people who do aerobic dance are prone to tendinitis in the leg or the foot. Treatment for tendinitis involves rest to relieve the stress on the tendon, and possibly the use of anti-inflammatory drugs. Continued stress on an inflamed tendon may cause the tissue to rupture, which will require surgery.

Bursitis A bursa is a sac filled with fluid located between a bone and a tendon or muscle. Its function is to allow the tendon to slide over the bone smoothly. Bursitis—a swollen or irritated bursa—results from repeated small stresses and overuse. The condition, which often occurs in conjunction with tendinitis, is treated with rest and anti-inflammatory drugs. Aggravating the condition by trying to maintain your exercise routine will only make it worse.

Stress fractures If a bone is repeatedly stressed during overuse, tiny breaks can occur. These breaks, called stress fractures, develop most often in the legs and feet, particularly in people who run on hard pavement.

If you work out regularly, pay close attention to your body's warning signs. Fatigue, tightness in a muscle, or pain may mean you are trying too hard. Stress injuries may also occur because of poor balance or lack of flexibility. Often such injuries develop

CLIMATE, ALTITUDE, AND EXERCISE

The environment in which you live will affect the duration and intensity of your exercise routine, as well as what you wear while exercising. Use common sense in tailoring your workout to changing environmental factors. For example, you can expect to be winded sooner when running at a higher altitude than when running at sea level, and you should adjust accordingly. If you go from Miami, which is at sea level, to Denver, the Mile-High City, reduce the duration and intensity of your usual exercise routine for a few days until you have adjusted to the higher altitude.

If you live in a climate where winter temperatures are very cold, consider a winter exercise program that can be done at home or at a gym. If you are a runner, you may want to do your running on a treadmill during the coldest months of the year. If you love to run outdoors even in the cold, dress accordingly and expose as little skin as possible to reduce the risk of frostbite. A face mask and scarf will help protect against frostbite. In cold weather, make sure you breathe through your nose because your nostrils warm the air before it reaches your lungs. It is a good idea to dress in layers, which provide added warmth and can be removed as you warm up. A layer of polar fleece or a windbreaker further protects from the cold and wind. When snow or ice are present, your risk of falling is greater; you may want to forgo your run or exercise indoors.

In hot weather, plan to exercise in the early morning or early evening, when temperatures are cooler, or do your workout in an air-conditioned facility. In warmer weather, make sure to drink plenty of water before and after you exercise. Stop frequently to drink water when exercising for a prolonged period of time; carry a water bottle if necessary. If you exercise aerobically for an hour and have been sweating heavily, you may require a sports drink, such as Gatorade, to replenish fluids, salts, and important minerals, and to prevent muscle cramps. In hot weather your body sends blood to the skin to help keep it cool, so there is less blood available to the muscles. Consider adjusting your routine to avoid overexertion. In hot climates, wear loose-fitting clothing made of natural fibers that breathe. For safety precautions for avoiding heat stroke, see Under the Sun, page 69. ■

at the site of a previous injury. To minimize the risk, your program should include exercises that improve flexibility, such as stretches or yoga. If you have had a stress injury before, be particularly aware of any signs of stress in that area. For more information on the types of injuries described above, see Chapter 17.

Staying Active to Prevent Disease

Physical activity contributes to good health in innumerable ways. This section reviews the specific benefits of physical activity in preventing or relieving cardiovascular disease, osteoporosis, and age-related health problems.

CARDIOVASCULAR FITNESS

One of the most important risk factors for heart disease is physical inactivity, but fortunately this is a risk factor that you have the power to change. By exercising, you can also control a number of other risk factors for coronary artery disease. Moderate exercise, such as a half-hour walk three to four times a week, can reduce blood pressure; lower triglyceride levels; increase high-density lipoprotein (HDL), or "good" cholesterol, levels; and help control weight. Moderate exercise performed three or four times a week increases your heart's ability to pump blood and decreases the rate at which it beats at rest and at any given level of exercise. For more information on risk factors for cardiovascular disease and lifestyle changes that can prevent it, see Chapter 20.

Under medical supervision, an exercise program can help you recuperate from a heart attack faster and more completely. Carefully prescribed aerobic exercise may also be beneficial if you suffer from chest pains due to angina pectoris. Research has demonstrated that regular exercise can lower mortality in cardiac patients by as much as 25 percent.

Before you begin to exercise, you should be examined by your doctor if you have multiple risk factors or suffer from symptoms of heart disease, or have had a major heart attack. In some cases, your doctor may want you to undergo an exercise stress test before you begin to exercise. If you suffer from poorly controlled angina, uncontrolled hypertension (high blood pressure), congenital heart disease, complex arrhythmias, or another severe heart condition, your doctor may ask you to refrain from exercising until your condition improves after medical or surgical treatment.

An exercise program is most likely to benefit your cardiovascular fitness if you do it regularly. Once you stop, deterioration in cardiovascular conditioning occurs in only a few weeks. If your motivation is flagging and you feel like quitting, remember that it may take weeks or months to regain the conditioning benefits your exercise program has given you.

PREVENTING OSTEOPOROSIS

Like most tissues of the body, the bones constantly regenerate themselves. This process, called remodeling, keeps the bones strong. As we age, however, new bone is formed more slowly. The bones become thinner and weaker. This loss of normal bone density may eventually result in osteoporosis. While older men are also at risk for osteoporosis, the disease is far more common in women. Some degree of osteoporosis is present in one out of every four women over age 45 and nine out of ten women over age 75. Doctors agree that regular exercise—weight-bearing aerobic exercise and weight training—is one of the few effective methods available for preventing osteoporosis or for treating existing osteoporosis. They also agree that leading a sedentary life increases the risk of osteoporosis later in life.

It is never too late to begin weight-bearing exercise to lessen the effects of osteo-

---

LOWERING YOUR STRESS LEVEL

Research shows that regular aerobic exercise can lower your level of stress. Whether you choose to walk, run, ride a bicycle, skate, or engage in any form of aerobics, regular exercise can help you keep the stress in your life under control.

In addition, simple breathing exercises during the day can help control your stress level. Here are some tips.

Practice Breathing Continually When we are under stress, we have an unconscious tendency to hold our breath or at least to breathe less often. To counteract this tendency, during the day, at the office or at home, practice breathing in and out rhythmically and continually, without speeding up or slowing down. Feel your breath as you breathe in and out. Draw each breath deeply into year lower lungs and diaphragm, expanding your ribcage as you breathe in.

Slow Down Your Breathing Take time during the day to breathe more slowly. Breathe in while counting to five, hold your breath for a count of five, then breathe out. Repeat the exercise five times.

Diaphragmatic Breathing Diaphragmatic breathing—deep, abdominal breathing—may be used anywhere, at any time, to reduce stress immediately. To master the technique, sit erect in a chair and close your eyes. Place one hand on your chest and the other on your abdomen. Count slowly to four as you inhale, pausing briefly at the top of the breath. Then exhale to a count of six. Be aware of your hands as you breathe. Try to increase the motion of the hand on the abdomen while minimizing the motion of the hand on the chest. The lower hand should rise as you inhale and sink as you exhale. ■

EXERCISE AND WEIGHT LOSS

One-half of all adult Americans are overweight. While many people successfully lose weight, most gain it back, often because they return to old eating habits and because they are not physically active. For sedentary people, keeping weight off is an enormous struggle. In contrast, the best predictor of success in losing weight and keeping it off is physical activity.

There are two chief components to effective weight loss: taking in fewer calories and increasing the rate at which your body burns calories. When your body burns more energy than it takes in you create a calorie deficit. As a result, your body starts burning excess fat stored in the cells. This, in turn, leads to weight loss.

Regular exercise is an invaluable part of any complete weight loss program and it is essential in keeping weight off once you have lost it. Exercise not only builds muscles and contributes to cardiovascular health, it also burns calories, creating a greater calorie deficit. The more you exercise, the more calories you burn, and the faster you can lose weight.

Although less widely known, an important factor in weight loss is the change in basal metabolism, your body's metabolic rate, caused by calorie restriction. When you take in fewer calories, your basal metabolism decreases, which means that your body slows down to adjust to the reduced intake of calories. Over time, it becomes harder and harder to lose weight and keep it off. For this reason, calorie restriction by itself is not enough for effective weight control. However, exercise increases your metabolic rate. Thus, calorie restriction and exercise go hand in hand to produce effective, long-term weight loss.

If you have been inactive for a long period of time and you are obese, you should consult your physician before you begin exercising. Your doctor will probably give you an exercise stress test to determine the health of your heart and the activity level appropriate for you. If you are very obese, even walking a quarter of a mile or raising your hands 10 times above your head may be strenuous at first. Start slowly and add to your routine gradually. ■

porosis and reduce the risk of fracture. A woman of 40 who incorporates weight-bearing exercise in her life today can help prevent osteoporosis later in life. Even a woman of 70 with osteoporosis can slow further bone loss by beginning a regular, weight-bearing exercise routine.

Examples of weight-bearing exercises are walking (including walking on a treadmill), jumping rope, jogging, or using motorized stairs. While non-weight-bearing exercise, such as swimming, is an excellent workout for the heart, it is less effective in preventing bone loss, although recent research shows that even swimming can help prevent osteoporosis. Weight-training exercise is also an excellent way to prevent or control osteoporosis.

AGING AND FITNESS

There's some truth to the old cliché, "It's better to wear out than to rust out." The body is built for physical activity. When we do not use our bodies, our muscles atrophy and our stamina and flexibility diminish. We become less agile. The chores of daily life become harder to execute, requiring dependence on others, and we increase the likelihood of injuring ourselves while performing routine tasks. Without exercise, the aging process can be that much more difficult.

Physical activity helps you enjoy life more, increases your confidence as you grow older, and results in less dependence on others. It also lowers your risk of injury by improving flexibility and balance. Best of all, remaining physically active can lengthen your life. Life expectancy is higher for those who are even moderately active and rises even higher for those who are very active. Increased longevity with a greater ability to enjoy life should be motivation enough to stay fit as we grow older.

Start putting your body to work and you will be surprised to discover that the flexibility and strength you thought were lost forever can be regained at least partially. You will also experience improved general health and fitness. In its way, staying physically active is as important an investment in your future as saving for retirement. Just as you would not think twice about contributing to your pension fund, you should begin investing in physical activity today to ensure a happy, healthy, and independent life in later years.

Your Personal Exercise Plan

In developing your personal exercise plan, your goal should be to select a variety of activities that you like and that fulfill your body's various needs. Remember that neither aerobic exercise (walking, running, swimming) nor resistance exercise (weight lifting and weight training) alone will be enough to ensure your cardiovascular fitness, stamina, strength, and flexibility. A combination of activities is necessary for overall health (see Combined Exercise for General Health, page 34). In choosing an exercise program, it is important to consider not only what you wish to achieve from your program, but also your age and overall physical condition and health.

As you plan, think of what you enjoy doing most. If you like to be outdoors when you exercise, choose a sport or activity that you can do outdoors, but make provisions for a rainy day by having an alternate activity that you can do indoors. If you prefer exercising indoors, you can join a gym or exercise at home. It is estimated that about 60 to 80 percent of all Americans who exercise do so at home. Exercising at home may involve a routine as simple as a combination of yoga positions and jumping rope, or a more complex exercise routine that involves use of home exercise machines. Exercise videos that include both weight training and aerobic routines are good options for home exercise.

The intensity, frequency, and duration of your exercise program determine health and fitness benefits. Intensity refers to how hard you are working while you are exercising. Walking briskly, for example, provides more aerobic benefits than walking at a slow pace. One of the best ways to measure the intensity, and thus the effectiveness, of your exercise routine is by determining your target heart rate (see Finding Your Target Heart rate, this page). The American Heart Association recommends staying in your target-heart-rate zone (THRZ) for approximately 20 minutes, three times a week, while the American College of Sports Medicine recommends sessions of "continuous aerobic activity" in the THRZ that last from 15 to 60 minutes, three to five times a week. Whichever approach you adopt, be careful not to overdo it. Most exercise-related injuries occur because people push themselves too hard.

Remember the importance of warming up before you exercise and cooling down afterward (see Your Warm-Up and Cool-Down, page 38). In addition, drink plenty of water before and after you exercise to replenish lost body fluids. During exercise, stop to drink water every 20 to 30 minutes, especially if the air temperature is warm. Increase the duration and the intensity of the exercise gradually to prevent injury and overuse of muscles and tissues. If you become an avid exerciser, consider cross-training—alternating your activities so that you are exercising different muscles more strenuously on different days. Cross-training also helps prevent boredom and reduces

FINDING YOUR TARGET HEART RATE

Aerobic exercise makes your heart beat faster, which results in more oxygen-carrying blood being pumped to the muscles. When not exercising, however, the healthy heart beats slowly, because each beat pumps more blood per beat. One of the first signs of improved conditioning and fitness is a lower resting heart rate. An unconditioned person's heart may beat over 90 times a minute; someone who is in shape can pump the same total amount of blood each minute at a rate of 60 or less beats a minute. In a 24 hour period, an unconditioned person's heart may beat 40,000 times more than a conditioned person's heart. A heart working so hard is less desirable for cardiovascular health.

To lower your resting heart rate and gain the other benefits of aerobic conditioning, you have to determine your target heart rate zone (THRZ) and maintain a pace that keeps your exercising heart rate at that level for your entire aerobic session. During your workout, you can take your pulse to ensure that you are maintaining your THRZ.

Experts vary on what the recommended THRZ should be. The American Heart Association considers 60 to 75 percent of your maximal heart rate to be your THRZ, while the American College of Sports Medicine recommends a THRZ of 60 to 90 percent of your maximal heart rate. Beginning exercisers are generally advised to stay in the low range; as fitness improves, your THRZ can increase.

Here is an example of how to calculate your target heart rate. Assume that your goal is 70 percent of your maximal heart rate. Subtract your age from 220, then calculate 70 percent of the remainder. Thus, if you are 50 years old, your THRZ would be 119 beats per minute (220 − 50 = 170; 70% of 170 = 119). If you are older or have led a sedentary lifestyle, your physician may recommend a lower THRZ of 50 percent instead of 65 or 70 percent. Once you have determined your THRZ, pace yourself to maintain this heart rate during the main portion of your workout, until you begin your cool-down.

Taking Your Pulse During and after your aerobic exercise routine, you will need to take your pulse to ensure that you have reached your THRZ. You should take your resting pulse before you begin your routine, again after you finish your warm-up stretches, and once more immediately after you finish your workout.

- To find your pulse, press your index and middle fingers together and place them on your inner wrist below your thumb.

- Count the number of beats in 15 seconds.

- Multiply by four to obtain total beats per minute. ■

the risk of injury. You might choose to walk 3 days a week and swim twice a week, or you might choose to take an aerobic dance class twice a week and go roller-skating three times a week. In addition to aerobic exercise, your exercise routine should include resistance exercise for overall conditioning. A well-rounded exercise program includes activities that build cardiovascular endurance as well as activities that improve flexibility, strength, and conditioning.

The following are some of the most popular outdoor and indoor exercise choices. Other sports and activities—such as tennis, golf, soccer, and basketball—can also help you stay fit. Keep in mind, however, that unless you participate in brisk games several times a week, you should regard sports activities as only one part of your exercise routine, rather than the whole show. Playing golf, tennis, or basketball once a week is fine when incorporated as part of a varied program that gets you moving three or more times a week.

WALKING

Walking is now the most popular sport in America. About 40 million Americans walk to keep fit, and the number is growing. If you choose walking, take into account any physical or health limitations, remember to warm up and cool down, and build your program gradually. In fact, if you have been sedentary for a long time, walking is the perfect way to slowly and gently increase your level of physical activity (see A Sample Exercise Plan, page 50).

Whether you are young or old, in perfect shape or overweight, athletic or not, walking is an activity that you can usually fit into your schedule with little trouble. Walking does not take a lot of preparation beforehand, nor does it require any special attire except for a sturdy, well-fitting pair of good sneakers or walking shoes. Since walking is a low-impact exercise, the risk of injury is low. And walking is free.

You can walk to work. You can walk around the block. You can walk down a country road. You can walk when you are on vacation to explore a new city or a new country. If it is raining you can walk in a shopping mall. If you walk for health, however, resist the temptation to stop intermittently to admire the scenery or do your errands. Walking in fits and starts provides little or no aerobic benefit.

To make walking a worthwhile aerobic activity, you need to walk long enough and fast enough. If you choose walking as your activity, plan on spending more time exercising per week than you would if you chose a higher-intensity aerobic activity, such as running or bicycling. If walking is your sole form of aerobic activity, the Institute for Aerobic Research suggests a goal of walking about 3 miles in 45 minutes, at least four or five times a week. Once you are able to walk 4 miles comfortably without stopping, consider longer treks or hikes, pick up your pace, or carry hand weights while you walk to increase the intensity of your workout.

Good posture is important. Poor posture can shorten your stride, strain your back, disturb your balance, and tire you early. When you walk, keep your neck and shoulders relaxed and hold your head up high. Bring your foot down lightly to the ground, heel first. Then roll your weight forward across the sole of your foot and push off gently with your toes. Your feet should point straight ahead and you should avoid hyperextending, or locking, your knee. As one leg advances, the opposite arm should advance.

Good walking shoes are essential for comfort and safety while walking. Your walking shoe should have a padded insole, midsole, and heel, with a good arch. You should be able to wiggle your toes in the shoe. The sole should be firm and thick to protect your foot on concrete or rocky terrain. The upper part of the shoe can be canvas, leather, or nylon; it should be properly ventilated so that perspiration can escape.

SWIMMING

Swimming is the second most popular sport in America after walking. Gliding through the water can be soothing as well as invigorating. Properly performed, swimming gives your entire body a good workout. The buoyancy of the water allows you to exercise without placing weight-bearing stress on your body, which can prevent stress-related injuries to muscles, bones, and joints. If you have injured yourself in another sport or activity, swimming is an excellent aerobic alternative while you are recuperating. Swimming is also an excellent choice if you are older and taking up exercise after a period of being sedentary because the risk of injury is low and because swimming can help relieve pain and stiffness due to arthritis or lower back problems.

Your target heart rate is about 10 to 13 beats lower for swimming than it is for other aerobic activities. Because you are horizontal in the water when swimming, your heart has an easier time pumping blood with each beat. As a result, it is impossible to generate the same increase in heart rate as with other aerobic activities, unless you are swimming at an Olympic pace! When you measure your pulse after swimming, do not worry if it is less elevated than it is during another aerobic activity (see Finding Your Target Heart Rate, page 44).

If you already know how to swim, you probably will not need lessons. However, if you are a beginning swimmer or have not been swimming for a number of years, taking a few lessons or swimming with a coach for a couple of sessions will help you develop an efficient, energy-saving stroke. The crawl, or freestyle, is considered the best aerobic swimming stroke because it conserves energy and maximizes aerobic benefits. The backstroke, breaststroke, or sidestroke may be used for short break periods during a 30-minute workout. If you have a history of back problems, you may want to use a snorkel to ensure that you keep your lower back flat while you swim.

RUNNING OR JOGGING

Jogging is defined as moving slower than 9 minutes per mile; running involves faster speeds. Although the jogging craze may have peaked in the 1980s, running is still a very popular sport in America. Some people simply love to run. Others choose running because they can gain aerobic benefits faster than walking. If you use proper technique and wear proper running shoes, running is one of the fastest ways to get a full aerobic workout, as well as to lose weight. Both jogging and running confer aerobic benefits, although for maximum aerobic benefit you need to spend more time jogging at your target heart than running.

Be aware, however, that nearly 75 percent of all sports injuries are caused by running. Choosing the right surface and

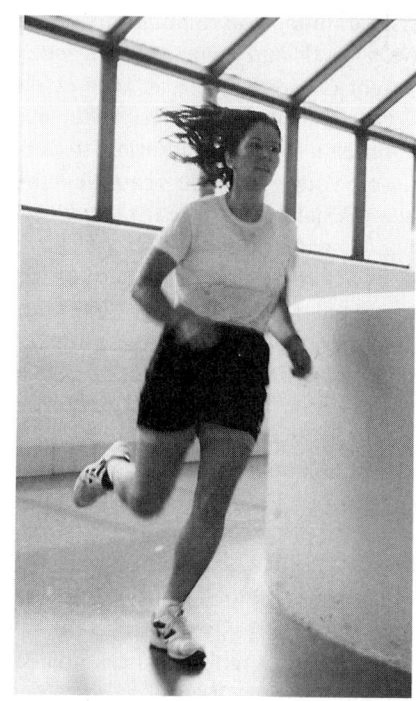

Jogging on an indoor track.

the right running shoe is essential in minimizing your risk of injury. A smooth, flat surface can help you maintain a steady stride at your target heart rate. Running on hard surfaces such as concrete, asphalt, and blacktop greatly increases your risk of injury. The best surface for running is a synthetic indoor or outdoor track. A grassy field, dirt road, or outdoor cinder track are also good. If you run on a road, wear bright-colored clothing so that you will be easily seen. If you run outdoors, remember that poor weather conditions increase your risk of injury. When roads are icy or slippery try to do your running on an indoor track or treadmill.

Running on hard surfaces puts tremendous stress on your muscles, bones, and joints. Wherever you run, wear good running shoes to ensure adequate shock absorption and to prevent strains, sprains, tissue tears, and stress fractures. Women should buy running shoes made specifically for women, because the shape of a woman's foot is significantly different from that of a man's. Children should also wear quality running shoes, even if they are likely to outgrow the shoe before they wear it out. Studies show that when running, children strike the ground with a force approximately three-and-a-half times greater than their body weight. In contrast, adults create an average impact of about two-and-a-half times their body weight. Well-fitting, thick, cotton socks are important for the comfort of your feet and for added shock absorption. Lace your running shoes tightly enough to keep the foot from sliding inside the shoe.

In running, your posture and stride are important. Your back should be flat, your pelvis vertical, and your chest slightly elevated. Your neck should be elongated and your shoulders relaxed. If you run on a banked track or road that is not level, remember to alternate the side of the road on which you train. Running on only one side of an incline causes your body to compensate for the incline and can lead to stress and injuries. When running, land evenly on your heel, roll your weight forward onto the ball of the foot, and push off with the toes. Every stage of your running stride should be smoothly executed, and the opposite arm should move forward at the same speed as the foot. Practicing good posture and running technique will help you minimize your risk of injury.

Long-term problems associated with running can be minimized by cross-training with another sport. Try not to run every day. Swimming or bicycling are excellent alternate aerobic-exercise choices for runners.

AEROBIC DANCE

For those who find it difficult to motivate themselves to exercise, aerobic dance can be a good way to get moving. Many fans of aerobic dance find that the variety of creative steps keeps boredom at a minimum while maximizing the opportunity for a good workout.

Most gyms offer classes in aerobic dance and there are many aerobic dance studios across the country. While aerobic dance is an excellent form of aerobic activity, the injury rate among both instructors and students is very high. The most common reasons for injury are improper footwear, improper floors, overly strenuous or complicated high-impact routines, and overtraining.

As is true of running and walking, the proper shoe can make the difference between safety and injury during aerobic dancing. Most major athletic shoe companies now design shoes specifically geared to the needs of aerobic dancers. Your shoe should adequately absorb shock and minimize the twisting of the foot. Heel, arch, and ankle support are critical to a safe workout. Because many movements in aerobic dance require landing squarely and with considerable force on the ball of the foot, your shoes should provide additional padding in that area.

Synthetic floors that come in interlocking pieces are now available for any size room; these floors are the most common choice for aerobic dance studios. Concrete or other hard surfaces are inappropriate. Thick carpet should also be avoided because it can create undue stress on your ankles and cause you to slip during side-to-side motions. High-density industrial carpet or wood floors are better choices.

Choose a routine that is compatible with your individual ability. Practice aerobic dance only with a certified aerobic dance instructor; check the instructors' credentials before joining a gym or aerobic dance studio. Warm up and cool down before and after your workout.

EXERCISE MACHINES

Using a variety of exercise machines can give you an excellent indoor aerobic workout. Many people prefer using machines, whether at home or at a gym, because they are convenient and because the ability to work out does not depend on good weather. Among the most popular exercise machines are cross-country ski machines, stationary bicycles, rowing machines, treadmills, and motorized stairs. Belonging to a gym gives you the option of varying your routine by using different machines. If you are purchasing one of these machines for your home, remember that quality varies widely. Research a machine before buying. Selecting a quality brand will lower your risk of stress-related injury and provide you with a more satisfying workout.

Jumping rope is an efficient and cost-effective form of indoor aerobic activity that does not involve machinery. A jump rope costs little and is extremely portable. Even in a small apartment, simply rearranging the furniture will probably give you enough space to jump rope in place.

BICYCLING

Many people find riding a bicycle more fun and less monotonous than walking, running, or swimming. Cycling allows you to travel greater distances, explore new places, and combine exercise with sightseeing. However, to gain the aerobic benefits of cycling, you need to pedal rhythmically and maintain a constant speed of approximately 15 miles an hour. Cycling at speeds of less than 10 miles an hour provides less aerobic benefit.

Choosing the right bicycle is essential if you plan to bicycle regularly. Since a bicycle is an expensive investment, it is best to borrow or rent one initially and take your time determining which size and model are right for you. Touring, recreational-sport, and mountain bikes are all possibilities. Before choosing a bike, test-ride a number of different models.

There are four important considerations in choosing a bicycle. First, determine which riding position is best for you. Until recently there were two basic choices: upright or bent over in a racer's crouch. Now a third option, the recumbent pose, is available. Recumbent bicycles allow you to lean back, as if sitting in a reclining chair,

An in-line skater wearing proper safety equipment: wrist guards, knee and elbow pads, and a helmet.

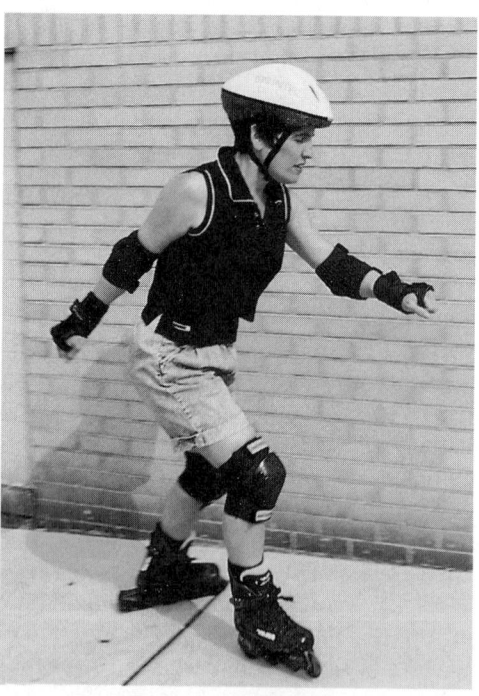

while you pedal. These models can be expensive. Next, make sure that the frame size is proportional to your height and leg length. If the bicycle frame is too large or too small, you will probably experience tension and pain while you ride. Third, consider the number of gears that you will need. Shifting from one gear to another will allow you to pedal at a steady pace while going up and down hills. Finally, select a tire width: thin, medium, or wide. Wide tires give the softest, most comfortable ride, whereas thin tires give speed.

If you are a beginner or have not cycled for a while, consider working with a trainer or coach before going on long solo rides. For beginners, the most important things to learn are how to get on and off the bike and how to stop smoothly and safely. Your first rides should take place on flat terrain. Adjust the seat and handlebars so that your leg is fully extended at the bottom point of the circle when you pedal. Ride bending forward from the hips, not the waist, with your back straight and your neck and shoulders relaxed. As you grip the handlebars, bend your elbows slightly for better leverage.

Safety in bicycling is of supreme importance. Do not try maneuvering a bike in traffic until you are a confident bicyclist. Remember that poor weather conditions, rough terrain, or bad equipment increase the risk of being thrown off a bike or getting into an accident. Reflective rear-view mirrors should be mounted on the handlebars of your bicycle for added visibility. Most serious injuries that occur usually involve the head. All cyclists should wear a fitted, protective, hard-shell helmet that meets or surpasses the standards set by the American National Standards Institute (ANSI). In many states, use of such helmets is the law for riders of any age.

ICE SKATING AND IN-LINE SKATING

Skating can be one of the most enjoyable ways of getting your aerobic exercise. In recent years old-fashioned roller-skating using heavy skates with several pairs of wheels has been supplanted by several variations of the sport. Roller-skiing involves short skis with rollers attached to the base and in-line skating simulates ice skating by using molded, hockey skate uppers attached to a single row of roller wheels that resembles the blade of an ice skate. The American Heart Association has endorsed both in-line skating (roller-blading) and ice-skating as safe and effective aerobic exercise options for cardiorespiratory fitness. Recent research confirms that skating is as effective as running or cycling for increasing aerobic fitness, reducing stress, and burning fat. In-line skating at a speed of 10 miles an hour is equivalent to jogging at 5 miles an hour. Skating also provides unique exercise benefits. It tones the buttocks and outer thighs, and provides excellent exercise for the pelvis and legs. It is also one of the few activities that exercises the backs of the thighs.

Whatever form of skating you choose, equipment is important. Ice skates and in-line skates can be expensive, so you may want to rent before you buy. Choose a sturdy boot that is high enough to support your ankle but that does not cover the calf. The tongue of the boot should be well padded and there should be cushioned support for the toes, arch, and heel. Your blades or rollers should be well made of high-quality material and you should have the blades of your ice skates sharpened periodically. In-line skaters should wear wrist guards, knee and elbow pads, and a helmet. Ice-skating and in-line skating may be done on indoor or outdoor rinks. In-line skating may also be done in an empty parking lot, on pathways, or on roads where skating is permitted. If you are a beginner at either sport, taking a few lessons will help you learn the right stroking technique, how to turn, and how to stop, and lower your risk of injury.

WEIGHT TRAINING

Strength and endurance training is as important as aerobic exercise for your overall health. Muscle strength and endurance increase when muscles are forced to adapt to an imposed demand. Progressive resistance exercise, or PRE, is the best way to increase muscle strength and endurance. In PRE, a specific level of resistance is introduced into an exercise and then increased incrementally over a period of weeks and months. This resistance may come from body weight, rubber tubing, free weights, or weight machines.

Weight training is becoming an increasingly popular choice among people of all ages for intensifying muscle strength and endurance, and improving or maintaining body composition. The two types of weights used in a weight-training program are free weights and weight machines.

Free weights include dumbbells, which are weights held in one hand, and barbells, which are weights that require a two-handed grip. Both dumbbells and barbells are inexpensive and easy to use and store at home. Before purchasing free weights, consult a qualified instructor to decide what amount of weight is right for you and to develop an appropriate routine. You may want to invest in a good pair of training gloves for better grip. Although many people wear training belts for back protection, a recent study showed that such belts do not provide much extra support.

Weight-training machines are a major feature of most gyms and fitness centers, but they also can be purchased for the home and many inexpensive models are now available. If you opt to use machines in your weight-training routine, try working out at a gym with a trainer before making the decision to buy a machine for home use.

A weight-training routine consists of both repetitions and sets. A repetition is one complete cycle of a particular weight-lifting exercise. For example, one repetition of a biceps curl begins with your arm straight down by your side, palm facing out, gripping your weight or pressing against the machine. Bending your elbow, you lift the weight to shoulder height. The repetition ends as you lower the weight back to thigh level. Beginners should try between 5 to 10 repetitions of an exercise to build muscle strength. Work up to 15 or more repetitions for areas dense in muscle fibers, such as the forearms and calves, to increase endurance.

A set is the number of repetitions that you do in sequence. Beginners should try to complete one or two sets of each strength and endurance exercise. If you choose to do two sets of an exercise back-to-back, rest 5 to 10 seconds after the first set and then repeat for the second set; or you can do one set of each of the exercises in your routine and then go on to the second set for each exercise.

Your muscles need to rest between sessions of weight training. Most experts agree

A SAMPLE EXERCISE PLAN

Whatever exercise you choose, consider your age and level of conditioning before you start. Contrary to what you might think, even walking as a form of exercise takes a certain amount of endurance and conditioning at the beginning. Here is a plan to get you off to a safe start. You should do your routine at least every other day. Do warm-up exercises before you begin and cool-down exercises when you are done.

- Week 1: Walk slowly for 5 minutes. Then walk briskly for 5 minutes. Finish by walking slowly for 5 minutes—for a total of 15 minutes.

- Week 2: Walk slowly for 5 minutes. Then walk briskly for 7 minutes. Finish by walking slowly for 5 minutes—for a total of 17 minutes.

For the first 6 weeks of the plan, add to your brisk-walking time in 2-minute intervals. For the second 6 weeks of the plan, add to your brisk-walking time in 3-minute intervals. By the twelfth week of the plan, you should be able to walk 30 minutes briskly and 40 minutes altogether without stopping. If you feel pain or undue strain, or if you are obese and feel winded, stop and rest. To increase the intensity of your workout, carry light hand weights, which will raise your heart rate and burn more calories. Start with ½-lb or 1-lb hand or wrist weights and gradually increase to 3 lbs in each hand. Move your arms back and forth naturally, gripping the weights gently. If you have heart disease, high blood pressure, or injuries such as a strain or tendinitis, do not use hand weights. ■

that intensively exercised muscles need a rest of 48 hours. To ensure your muscles get adequate rest, you may want to split your weight-training routine, exercising the upper body one day and the lower body the next.

To ensure safety, choose weight or resistance levels that you can manage easily. The number of repetitions and sets is more important in building muscle strength and endurance than the amount of weight that you use. When trying new routines it is helpful, though by no means essential, to

have someone act as a spotter until you feel comfortable with the exercises. Always remember to warm up before your routine and cool down afterwards.

YOGA

Yoga is good for the body and the mind. Practicing even just a few of the yoga postures two or three times a week can increase flexibility, improve balance, help you breathe more deeply, and lower your stress level. While yoga is not considered an aerobic exercise, it can ease tension and calm your mind while working your muscles and joints. Once you have learned the postures with the help of a qualified instructor, you can do yoga at home without expensive equipment.

Many gyms and fitness centers offer yoga classes and many metropolitan areas have yoga centers that offer classes and one-on-one instruction. Books and videotapes are available that teach basic yoga poses that you can practice at home. A tape may be easier for beginners than a book. If you decide yoga is the right physical activity for you, remember to supplement your yoga routines with at least 20 minutes of aerobic exercise three times a week.

STAYING MOTIVATED

For most of us, taking care of ourselves can pose a real challenge. Staying motivated is difficult. Here are some suggestions to help you plan, and maintain, a good exercise routine.

- Don't make excuses. The two biggest excuses for avoiding exercise are "I don't have time" and "I don't have any place to exercise." If you have time to read this, you have the time to exercise. And you don't need a gym or a track. You can increase your activity level enough to gain aerobic benefits simply by walking to work or jogging in place.

- Set realistic goals. One sure way to fail is to expect feats from yourself that are impossible to attain. Experts agree that any physical activity is better than none. Set small goals when you start out, and you will be less likely to get discouraged.

- Stick to your workout schedule, unless you are sick. If you start letting other events interfere with exercise, you will skip sessions more frequently.

- Exercise with a friend, if possible. The buddy system is one sure way to keep motivated. Usually, when one friend's inspiration lags, the other's remains strong, and vice versa. Having company when you are working out can help the time go faster. The buddy system works even if all you do is accompany each other to the gym and then go your separate ways.

- Think long term. Do not expect your physical condition to change overnight, or even in a month. When you start exercising, think of it as starting a life-long habit, whose benefits you will reap every day for the rest of your life.

- Stay active while traveling. Do not give up your hard-won progress when you go away on vacation. You may want to take a break from the routine you do at home, but try to stay active in other ways. For example, if you work out in a gym at home and you go to a beach resort for vacation, walk on the beach and swim instead of using the machines in the hotel.

- Reward yourself. Each time you reach a goal, whether it is simply sticking to your routine for a month, increasing the distance you can run, or the amount of weight-lifting sets you can complete, give yourself a reward.

THREE

Everyday Safety

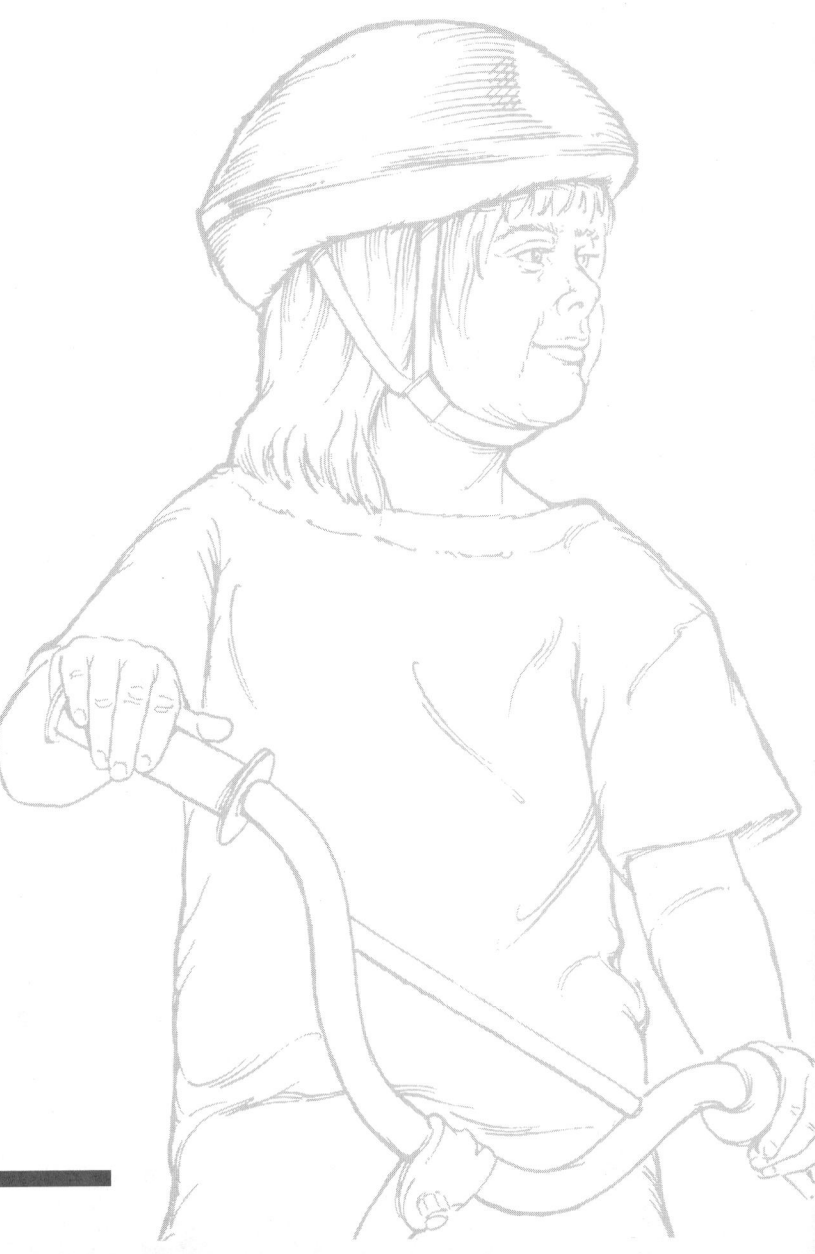

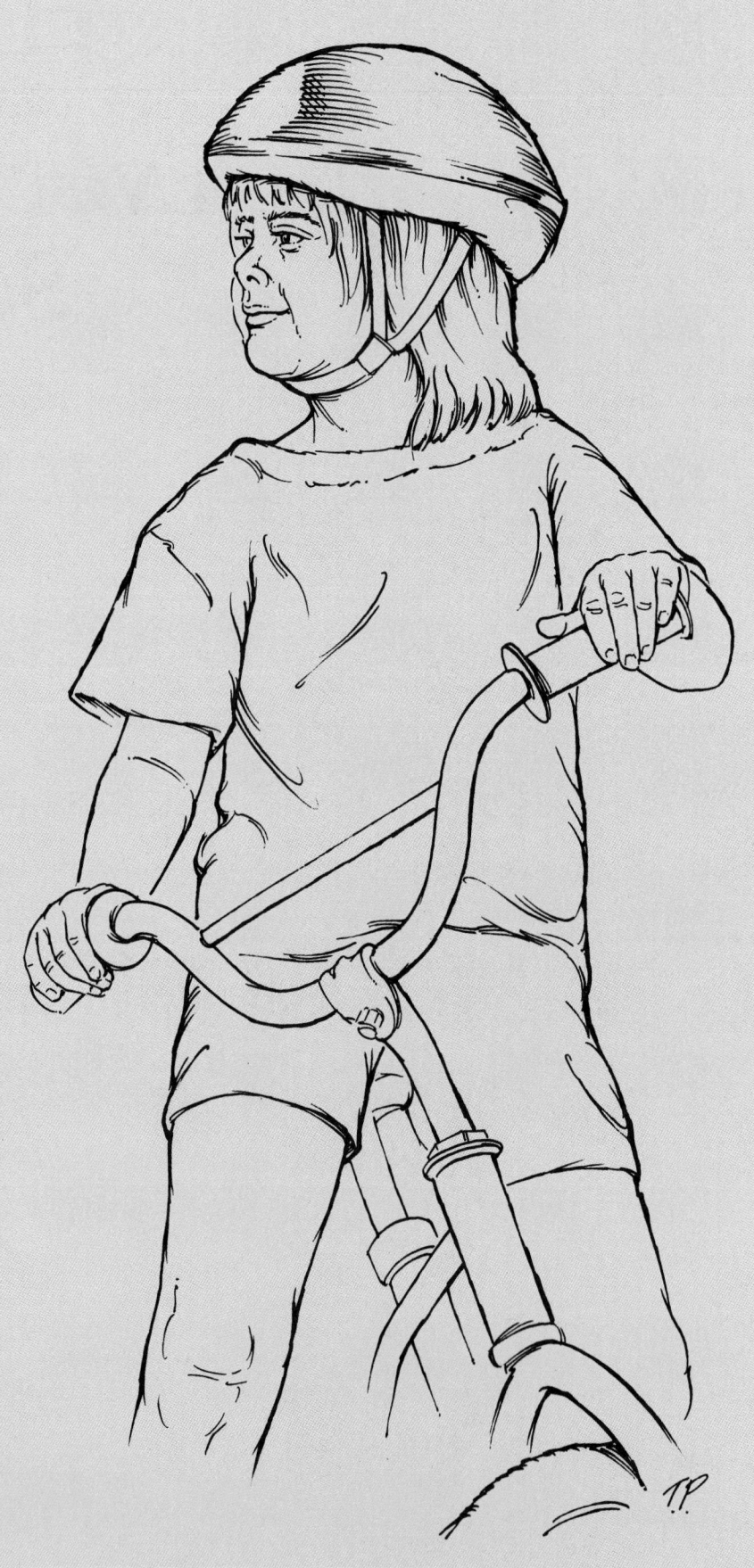

EVERYDAY SAFETY

Staying Safe

Safety is a state of mind—a healthy state of mind. Protecting yourself and your family from life's preventable injuries and tragedies is within your power. You can help keep your family and home safe by recognizing and eliminating safety hazards and planning how you will respond to emergency situations. The pay-off in good health is significant. Hospital emergency room statistics are a tally of preventable injuries, big and small. Injuries are the leading cause of death for children and young adults, and the fourth leading cause of death for all age groups. Most injuries can be prevented, or their consequences minimized, with a bit of forethought and planning.

Although there are many home safety products on the market, safety does not have to be an expensive proposition. Smoke detectors, which cost about $10, are one of the most inexpensive investments you can make in your family's safety. In the long run, safety pays off financially. Injuries cost money and time, in addition to causing pain and suffering. Some safety improvements will earn you rebates on your car or home-owners' insurance. Many safety improvements are completely free: a rearrangement of furniture or rugs that prevents a serious fall; a fire drill with your children that gives you peace of mind. The success of your safety efforts is measured in injuries that do not happen, and your family's good health.

Safe at Home

Keeping yourself and your family safe at home need not be expensive or intrusive. Simple common sense measures can help prevent injuries, accidents, and fires.

THE SAFE-HOME TOUR

Once or twice a year make a safety tour of your house to catch problems before they turn into safety hazards. For the extra precautions you should take when there are children living in your house, see Child-Proofing Your Home, page 59.

Attics, crawl spaces, and storage areas

- Be aware that storage areas that are accessed only occasionally often harbor potential hazards.

PUTTING RISK IN PERSPECTIVE

Risks to health and safety are usually discussed in relative terms and stated as odds or percentages. We often hear that a given activity carries a "1 in 50,000 chance of dying" or a "40 percent chance of living longer." Most of us lack the skill to process this kind information as we make decisions about daily behavior. In addition, we tend to overestimate risks that are out of our control, such as terrorist attacks or natural disasters, and underestimate the risks of the things we do every day.

To put some of these things in perspective, death or injury from driving or riding in an automobile is one of the greatest risks Americans face on a daily basis. Yet many of us are far more fearful about air travel, which poses a much smaller threat to life. About 110 people die every day—40,000 people each year—in automobile accidents. That is equivalent to 130 jumbo jets crashing each year. If a plane crashed every three days, would we continue to fly? So why do so many of us neglect the simple safety measure of wearing a seat belt, which can reduce the risk of dying in an accident by more than 40 percent?

With all the recent news-making weather catastrophes, we tend to overestimate risks from floods, hurricanes, tornadoes, or earthquakes. However, the risk of heart attack—often controllable through lifestyle and dietary changes—is about 1 chance in 2,800, whereas the risk of dying in a tornado—largely uncontrollable—is about 1 chance in 56,000. A few dozen people have died from eating foods contaminated with the new strain of E. coli bacteria, so we are careful to cook our ground beef until it is well done. But even though 500,000 people die each year from smoking-related illnesses, smokers continue to light up.

This chapter cannot and does not try to weigh out every risk or give the odds of dangers on every event or behavior. It does try to make you aware of the most common hazards so that you can eliminate existing dangers and anticipate new ones, as well as prepare for what you cannot control by planning for emergencies. ■

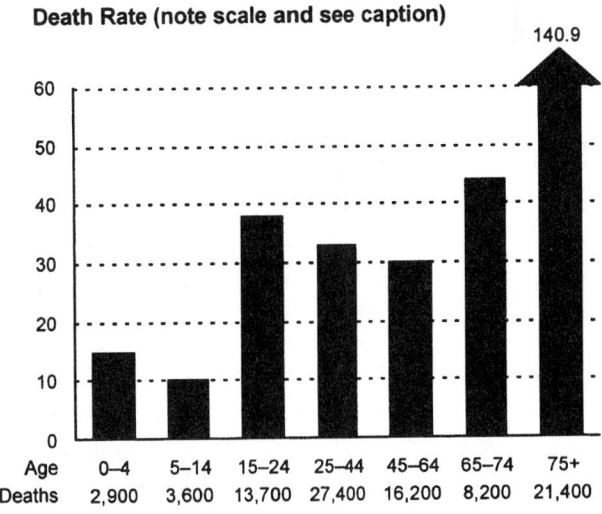

Death Rate (note scale and see caption)

Age	0–4	5–14	15–24	25–44	45–64	65–74	75+
Deaths	2,900	3,600	13,700	27,400	16,200	8,200	21,400

Deaths due to unintentional injuries in 1996. The term "unintentional" covers most deaths from injury and poisoning. Excluded are homicides (including legal intervention), suicides, deaths for which none of these categories can be determined, and war deaths. The rate in the above graph is based on deaths per 100,000 population in each age group. The total number of deaths from unintentional injury was 93,400, a rate of 35.2 deaths per 100,000 population. Source: National Safety Council, Accident Facts 1997 Edition, Itasca, IL; used with permission.

FIRE SAFETY CHECKLIST

- Make sure you have at least one smoke detector installed on every level of your home and near the bedroom area.

- Test the smoke detector monthly and vacuum the grill work periodically.

- Replace the smoke detector batteries twice a year. An easy way to remember this task is to change smoke detector batteries when you change your clocks in the spring and fall.

- Keep multipurpose (ABC) fire extinguishers in your kitchen, your basement or utility area, your garage, and your car. Home fire extinguishers are rated as "A" for wood, paper, or trash fires; "B" for flammable liquids and grease fires; and "C" for electrical fires.

- Post the fire response number and your home's address and location prominently near every phone.

- Have an escape plan for yourself and your family. Be sure that all windows and doors on the escape route can be easily opened from the inside. Make sure everyone, even small children, knows how to get out and where to meet outside to be sure that everyone got out safely.

- Make sure that children understand that they cannot hide from fire and that they must not return to the house for pets or special toys. Teach them to "Stop, Drop, and Roll" if their clothing catches fire and to stay close to the floor if there is smoke.

- Have at least two ways to get out of each area of your house in case fire is blocking one exit.

- Be sure there are safe ways to escape second-story or basement bedrooms.

- If you live in an apartment building, memorize the number of doors from your own to the safety exit. Stay off the elevators in the event of a fire.

- Keep matches and cigarette lighters where children can never get them. Never use a cigarette lighter to entertain a small child or allow a child to play with lighters or matches, even under supervision.

- Never smoke in bed and never allow anyone to smoke in bed in your home.

- Use extreme caution if you smoke in an upholstered chair or couch.

- Check for unextinguished smoking materials after guests leave. Do not empty ash trays into waste baskets or trash until the next morning; leave them in the sink overnight.

- If you are buying new furniture or bedding, check for and select fire-retardant upholstery and mattresses.

- Keep ashtrays and smoking materials away from bedding, curtains, and upholstered furniture.

- Check electrical cords for fraying; never run electrical cords under rugs or across a floor area.

- Do not overload electrical outlets or extension cords.

- Replace any appliances, switches, or cords that feel hot to the touch.

- Make sure that space heaters, wood stoves, and furnaces are properly installed, vented, and maintained. Keep them at least 3 ft from walls, furniture, curtains, rugs, or anything flammable. Do not use kerosene space heaters. Electric space heaters should be the type that switch off automatically if they are tipped over. Fireplaces, chimneys, and vents should be inspected at least once a year, and cleaned and repaired promptly if necessary. ■

- A smoke detector is an inexpensive safety investment for storage spaces. Battery-operated smoke detectors do not always perform well in unheated areas. Get one that runs on regular house current if your storage area gets cold in the winter. A smoke detector should be placed in each space or room that is enclosed by walls.

- Repair damaged wiring or insulation.

- Store items well away from heat ducts, chimneys, and exposed wiring. Stack boxes and containers carefully so they do not topple over.

- Keep rodent poisons and traps where children and pets cannot get at them.

Bedrooms

- Make sure heavy furniture, especially chests of drawers, cannot tip over even when the drawers are extended. Secure them to the wall with angle brackets if necessary.

- Electric blankets present several risks for electric shock and fire and should be unplugged when not in use. Replace electric blankets and mattress pads if they have frayed wiring. To avoid damage to the wiring, make sure that electric blankets are never tucked in.

- Do not keep any medication in your bedside table if you have children living at home or visiting. If you take a medication with a potential for dangerous overdose, such as sleeping aids or pain medication, keep it where you must be awake and alert to take a second dose.

- Consider installing a phone within reach of the bed. Have bedside lamp switches within easy reach. If you wear glasses keep them close at hand as well.

- Keep a small flashlight near your bedside for emergencies.

- If you use a humidifier or vaporizer, clean it regularly according to the manufacturer's instructions to prevent bacterial or mold contamination. Consider replacing an older humidifier, which can spread molds and mineral dust, with a newer model.

Stairways and halls

- Scatter rugs can be a tripping hazard. If you must use them, make sure they have non-slip pads underneath.

- Frayed carpeting can be hazardous throughout the house, but is particularly dangerous on steps, where tripping can lead to serious falls. Make sure all carpeting on stairs is well secured and replace any carpeting that has tears or holes.

Bathroom

- Use a non-slip tub mat or stick-on appliqués in your tub or shower if it does not have a non-skid surface.

- Keep electrical appliances, such as hair dryers, curlers, curling irons, and shavers well away from sinks and tubs, and unplugged when not in use. Never use electrical appliances when your hands are wet or if the bathroom floor is wet from a bath or shower.

- Have a ground fault circuit interrupt (GFCI) outlet installed in your bathroom. GFCI outlets have a shock-protection device that detects a short circuit and shuts off the electricity. Remember not to turn on light switches or appliances when your hands are wet.

- Keep medications, vitamin and mineral supplements, and personal care products out of the reach of your own or visiting children. Do a quick check on the contents of the medicine cabinet and discard items whose expiration dates have passed.

- Do not mix bathroom cleansers containing chlorine with cleansers containing ammonia. Fumes produced by the

resulting chemical reaction may be dangerous.

- Set your hot water thermostat between 120 and 125°F. Higher temperatures may lead to scalding injuries.

Living room

- Make sure your television stand is stable and will not tip over. Check bookcases to be sure they cannot topple over; secure them to the wall with angle brackets if necessary.

- Do not run electrical cords or extension cords either under rugs, where they can be a fire hazard, or across floors, where they can be tripped over.

- Do not overload extension cords or electrical outlets. Older homes, in particular, are often "underwired," though they may have plenty of wall outlets. Check the electrical capacity of your home to be sure it can handle your electrical load safely.

- Avoid playing excessively loud music, which can lead to hearing loss.

Kitchen

- Keep knives stored safely where small children cannot reach them. Always use food grinders and processors with their safety guards in place.

- Check the exhaust vent over the kitchen range to make sure it is clean and free of grease build-up that can catch fire.

- Consider putting a non-slip mat in front of the kitchen sink to prevent slippery floors.

- Get in the habit of leaving infrequently used kitchen appliances unplugged to reduce the risk of fire. Make sure that all appliances have three-pronged, grounded plugs. Have a GFCI installed in any outlets near the kitchen sink.

- If you use a gas range, make sure that there is no gas odor and that the pilot lights and burners are burning cleanly.

Basement

- Keep freezers locked. Secure the doors of infrequently used refrigerators, storage lockers, or other places where children could get trapped. Immediately

A SAFER HOME FOR THE ELDERLY

We may not want to admit it, but our physical capabilities do change as we get older. A household arrangement that was once navigated with ease can turn into an obstacle course when our eyesight fails or our knees become less steady. Since older people are more vulnerable to falls, burns, and other accidents, and have more difficulty recovering from an accident, prevention is important for better overall health and greater independence.

Preventing Falls

Failing eyesight; diminished strength, endurance, and flexibility; and drowsiness caused by medication or interrupted sleep all make the elderly especially at risk for injury from falls. For older people, falls can have consequences far beyond a bump on the knee. A broken hip or ankle can bring on a series of medical problems requiring extended hospital and nursing home stays. Falls are the most common cause of fatal injuries in older people. Falls that do not result in injury can still have serious consequences because the person who has fallen cannot get up and call for help. If you live alone, plan regular check-ins from family or friends. Locate telephones where they can be reached from the floor and in the bathroom. A portable phone or a portable electronic alert system could be a lifesaver.

Some simple preventive measures can substantially reduce the risk of falling. First, increase the lighting in stairways, hallways, and in the bathroom. Cataracts, a common eye condition in older people, can reduce the amount of light the eye perceives, so more light often is needed. Cataracts may also make you more vulnerable to glaring light, so do not overdo it. Just be sure not to create a fire hazard by using a higher wattage light bulb than your fixtures allow.

Several thousand older people end up in emergency rooms every year because they have tripped on throw rugs or runners. Remove rugs and runners that are worn or frayed or that tend to slide or bunch up. Use double-sided tape under rugs to secure them to the floor. You can also purchase special rubber matting that can be cut to fit under your rugs. The slip-resistant backing on many rugs will wear off with repeated washings; replace old rugs or secure them with tape. Check stair treads, and replace worn or loose treads or carpet.

Make sure that beds, chairs, and bathroom fixtures are at the right height; adapt them if they require too much up or down motion to get into or out of easily. A sturdy step stool is a must for reaching high objects. Install grab bars in the bath or shower and next to the toilet. If the toilet is too low for comfortable use, purchase a seat-height extender.

Be wary of making extensive changes all at once. As we age, memory is our best friend and our worst enemy. Rearranging the furniture to make things easier may trip up unwary feet that tread a familiar path from years of habit.

Preventing Burns and Scalds

Our skin thins with age, so older people are much more vulnerable to scalds and burns. This, and decreased mobility, combine to make fire a particular risk for the elderly. Smoking brings additional risks, causing the greatest number of fatal fires for the elderly. Older people who smoke should be encouraged to quit and should never smoke in bed or when drowsy. Many fire-related deaths are caused by smoke and toxic fumes created by smoking materials smoldering in upholstered furniture or mattresses. Use extra care in keeping ashtrays and smoking materials away from curtains, papers, and other flammable materials.

More than 70 percent of deaths from clothing fires are to people over age 65. Be careful of stray ashes from smoking materials. Roll long sleeves back when cooking; avoid cooking or tending fireplaces or wood stoves in loose or highly flammable clothing. If clothing does catch fire, remember to "Stop, Drop, and Roll" to extinguish the flames. To avoid hot spills in the kitchen, turn pot handles toward the rear of the stove.

Use electric blankets with care. Never fall asleep with a heating pad; heating pads may cause burns with prolonged use, even at their lowest settings. To prevent scalding, set water heater temperatures at 120°F or "low," and always touch-test the water before entering a bath or shower. If the water temperature in the shower fluctuates, have a plumber install a special balancing valve that will even out extremes in temperature. ■

remove the door of an emptied refrigerator.

- **Make sure your furnace, hot water heater, and clothes dryer are properly vented and that the vents are free of leaves, lint, and other debris.**

- **Use only the right size fuses and circuit breakers. Never substitute a larger fuse or a penny for the proper fuse. If you have continual problems with blown fuses or tripped breakers, track down the short circuit or overload before it causes a fire.**

Garage

- **Never leave a car or any other engine running in an attached garage. If your garage is attached to living areas, install a carbon monoxide detector in the living space.**

- **Do not store gasoline, power tools, paints, or chemicals where children can find them. Be sure that gasoline and fuels are stored in tightly capped, approved containers and that they are well away from furnaces or gas water heaters or dryers.**

- Unplug electrical power tools when they are not in use.

- Make sure that overhead garage-door openers are working properly and are programmed to reopen when something blocks the path of closure.

Around the house

- Make sure that entrances are well lit and stairs have handrails.

- Keep walkways, decks, porches, and stairways free of obstacles. If water, ice, or sand make walkways slippery, think about making minor structural changes, such as adding roof gutters, floor grates, or non-slip surfaces.

- Take a look up to check for areas where falling ice, roof tiles, or other airborne hazards might create a problem.

- Check the electrical entrance to the house and entrances for cable and phone services to make sure they are in good condition and clear of shrubbery and tree branches.

- Carbon monoxide monitors should be installed near wood stoves and gas furnaces.

CHILD-PROOFING YOUR HOME

Making sure that your home is a safe environment for your growing child requires your forethought. Child-proofing is not a one-time-only event, but an ongoing process. Try to stay two steps ahead of ever more active and curious youngsters.

Keep infants out of harm's reach by providing a secure environment. Make sure that furnishings and equipment are sturdy and safe (see page 60). Keep your infant's sleep and play areas free of strangulation or suffocation hazards. Blind or drapery cords should be hooked out of reach of children and should not form a continuous loop. Plastic bags, pillows, and even extra fluffy comforters may cause suffocation; keep them out of infants' cribs, bedrooms, and play areas. Make sure crib bumper pads are securely fastened and cannot entangle a sleeping infant. The spaces between crib slats should be narrow enough to make strangulation impossible. Mobiles should be securely fastened to the ceiling or a crib

arm. They should not have any small parts that could choke a baby or long strings that could entangle a baby. Do not use crib gyms that extend across the crib. Infants' clothing should be non-flammable and free of stray threads that might wind around a tiny finger or toe. Remove cords for tying hoods closed and any long ribbons and trims that might choke or entangle a baby.

Before your child starts to crawl, get down to the child's level and have a look at household furnishings that might present a hazard. Electrical outlets should be plugged with outlet covers and electrical cords secured against curious fingers. Never leave a young child unattended in a room where a fire is lit. Look at coffee tables and book cases, and make sure they will not topple over when your little one uses them for chin-ups. Pad the sharp corners and edges of coffee tables and other furnishings. Part of the child-proofing process includes protecting your possessions from your children. Move precious possessions to a high closet shelf. Many common household plants are poisonous; if any of yours are on the list on page 410, discard them.

Depending on the contents, kitchen and bathroom cabinets and drawers may need child-proof latches. Never transfer a poison to a different container, particularly to one that might appeal to a child, such as a soda bottle. Most children learn to open "child-proof" latches eventually, so remove all cleansers and poisons from under the bathroom and kitchen sinks. Store them well out of reach in a place that locks or latches. This month's crawling baby will be climbing soon enough, so you might as well find a safe and permanent storage place for hazardous household cleansers, preferably one with a lock.

If your kitchen range has front controls, you may want to install special knob covers that will keep toddlers from turning on the burners. Get in the habit of keeping hot cups of coffee or tea, alcoholic drinks, and sharp knives well away from a baby's or toddler's long reach. Remember, too, to keep the cupboard doors and the dishwasher door latched. Get in the habit of keeping pot handles turned toward the back of the stove. Never cook with a child in your arms or in an infant carrier; they could get badly burned. Make sure that toddlers cannot get into the trash, pet food dishes, or spoiled food scraps.

EVALUATING CHILDREN'S TOYS AND FURNISHINGS FOR SAFETY

Whether you are buying new furnishings for your baby or using hand-me-downs from a friend, you need to evaluate all of your baby items for safety. Even though there are some mandatory and some voluntary standards, you cannot assume that all baby products are universally and uniformly safe. Here are a few things to look for.

Toys Toys marked "Not for children under 3" are so labeled because they have small parts that might be a choking hazard. Respect these age limits. You should always check toys thoroughly before you let your child play with them. Make sure the toy has no small, loose parts and that wheels, button eyes, and other small parts are securely fastened. Look for cords or strings longer than 7 in. and loops or openings more than 14 in. around, which might be strangulation hazards. Look for any sharp edges. Check wooden toys for splinters. Toy-chest lids should stay open automatically when lifted up so that the lid cannot fall shut on a child. Toy chests should also have vent holes so that a child will be able to breathe if she should get trapped inside.

Cribs and Beds All recently manufactured cribs meet a safety standard that reduces the potential for entrapment injuries. If you are using an older crib, measure the distance between the slats to make sure they are no more than 2⅜ in. apart. If they are, discard the crib and get a new one; it is not safe for your baby. Make sure that the mattress fits snugly against the sides of the crib and does not pull away from the corner posts. The corner post should not be more than 1/16 in. higher than the end panels, so that a baby cannot catch her clothing and strangle. Make sure the design does not include open work or cutout areas on the headboard or footboard where a baby's head could be entrapped. The crib's hardware and latches should be complete and working properly. And finally, make sure that the wood is smooth, not splintered, and that the paint is lead free.

When babies are old enough to stand up in their cribs, lower the crib mattress so they cannot fall out or climb out. Remove anything in the crib that they could use to climb up and over the rail.

Bunk bed mattresses and box springs should have adequate support so they cannot collapse. Make sure the railing of the top bunk will prevent a child from falling and that the gaps between mattresses and bunk bed guardrails are less than 3½ in. so that children cannot get trapped. Children under age 6 should not use a top bunk.

Strollers Strollers should have a wide base to prevent tipping. The shopping basket should be low over the front or back wheels so that the stroller will be stable even with an extra load. Safety belts and harnesses are a must. Make sure the brakes lock the wheels securely. Folding strollers should have an effective locking device so that the stroller cannot fold up with the baby in the seat. Make sure that the frame will not pinch little fingers.

Playpens Wooden play pens are not widely used anymore. If you are using one make sure that the slats are less than 2⅜ in. apart, as you would for a crib. Mesh play pens should have small perforations; the mesh should be intact with no tears or holes. Make sure the covering of the top rail is intact. Never leave a baby in a mesh play pen with the side down. Even a tiny infant can get trapped between the mesh and the mattress and suffocate.

Walkers More than 27,000 children are injured each year in walker-related accidents, the most serious involving falls down stairways. The American Academy of Pediatrics recommends that parents not use walkers for their children. A better choice is one of the bouncing seats that are stable and secure, and still entertaining. Walkers allow babies who could not move under their own power to get around very quickly and reach things they would not get to otherwise.

It is strongly recommended that you never put your child in a walker. If you insist on using a walker even though they are a proven hazard, please observe the following precautions that will lessen but not eliminate the risks to your baby. Make sure that doors to stairways are closed at all times; keep babies in walkers out of the kitchen where hot oven doors and cooking activities are a great risk. A walker should have a wide wheel base to prevent tipping. The coil springs should have covers over them to keep fingers from getting pinched. You should not use a walker that has an X-frame that could pinch or even amputate your baby's fingers. Make sure that the seat is securely attached to the frame. ■

In the bathroom use a bath sponge, nonslip mat, or bath seat to keep your child safer in the tub, but *never* leave a baby or toddler unattended or alone with a sibling in a tub of water, even for a minute. Lower your water heater thermostat to 120°F and touch test the water temperature before placing a child in the tub. Always run a little cold water into the baby's bath last, to cool the faucets to the touch. You may want to have a plumber install anti-scald valves on the tub faucet and showerhead. Put personal care products and appliances out of reach. Consider installing a lock on your medicine cabinet. Only purchase medications and vitamin supplements in child-proof containers. Many medications that seem benign to adults can be toxic to children—acetaminophen and iron supplements are two examples—so use care with every substance. Keep ipecac syrup in your first aid kit and the poison control center phone number posted on every phone. Do not, however, ever give ipecac syrup to induce vomiting unless instructed by a health care professional; it can exacerbate some poisonings.

Small children can drown in very shallow water. Consider any amount of water that could cover a child's nose and mouth to be a potential hazard—this includes toilets, scrub buckets, and aquariums, as well as the more obvious hazards of bathtubs, wading and swimming pools, garden pools, and hot tubs.

Put gates at the top and bottom of every stairway; keep doors to stairways latched. Window screens are meant to keep bugs from coming in a window not to keep children from falling out. Install bars or other window guards, particularly on upper-story windows.

One of the greatest child-proofing challenges is keeping the house free of choking hazards. Jewelry, coins, paper clips, staples, erasers, safety pins, broken or deflated balloons, button batteries, and nails and other small hardware items are just a few of the things little children will find and put in their mouths. If you have older children, their toys will inevitably have some small parts that are hazardous to younger siblings. Read the manufacturers' warning labels and follow them. Enlist an older child's cooperation in keeping small toys picked up and designate an area where they can safely play with "big kids' toys."

Edible choking hazards include hot dogs—the primary cause of choking in children—grapes, raisins, raw carrots, hard candies, popcorn, and nuts. Keep babies away from these foods completely. Even when a child has a full set of teeth and can chew food thoroughly, foods that are very dense, round, or solid may still be choking hazards. Cut hot dogs lengthwise and crosswise into small pieces that cannot lodge in the throat. Carrots can be shredded or parboiled; grapes can be cut in half. Do not allow children to play games with food or run or play with food in their mouths.

Children, even babies and toddlers, will imitate adults, so never take medication in front of children. In addition to keeping cigarette lighters and matches out of the reach of children, make sure to put cigarettes away too; many children have eaten tobacco products. Keep alcoholic beverages on a high shelf or in a locked cabinet. Remind visitors to keep purses and luggage securely closed to little fingers.

Children can get trapped in large appliances. Remove doors before storing appliances like refrigerators or freezers.

Take a careful look at outdoor play areas. Make sure none of your shrubs or

THE CHILDREN'S SAFETY CENTER

Many injuries to young children occur in the place parents believe their children are most safe—at home. The Children's Safety Center at Johns Hopkins offers families individualized services and safety counseling to help achieve home safety. For free home-safety educational materials and counseling by an experienced health educator, call (410) 614-5587 between 10 AM and 4 PM EST, weekdays. ∎

ornamental plants is poisonous. Providing children with a fenced play area is a good way to keep them in and other hazards, such as stray pets, out. If you live near a busy street or a large body of water, a fenced play area can give you greater peace of mind, although close supervision of small children is always necessary. Since children may wander, swimming pools, fountains, or hot tubs in neighbors' yards are also a hazard to your child; a fenced play area can help keep your child at home and in view.

Child-proofing can reduce hazards, but it cannot take the place of good supervision. Many injuries and poisonings occur when parents are momentarily distracted by a phone call or someone at the door. A portable telephone can free you up to keep an eye on the children, and a baby monitor can help you keep tabs on napping or playing children even when you are not in the room with them.

The real key to successful child-proofing is creating an environment where your child is free to explore without injuring herself and without worrying you. With time and plenty of good-humored preemptive and preventive effort, your children will learn to respect the limits you set.

SAFE IN THE KITCHEN

The kitchen is the heart of a home, and probably the most dangerous room in the house. If you want to make your kitchen a safer place, evaluate your kitchen for fire safety, safe food handling, and safe use of kitchen equipment.

In addition to the fire safety tips discussed above, take a second look at your cooking appliances and the cooking area to eliminate fire hazards. Move flammable pot holders, cooking oils, and drippings containers away from your kitchen range. Keep a container of salt or baking soda near the kitchen range to extinguish small cooking fires. You can also extinguish grease fires by covering the cooking pan with a tight lid. Never put water on a grease fire. Keep a multipurpose fire extinguisher near the kitchen. Make sure that toaster, coffee pots, and other small appliances will not ignite nearby objects.

No cooks want to poison their guests, but poor food handling practices can do just that. Increasingly virulent strains of bacteria that thrive within improperly prepared food products make it more important than ever to develop good kitchen habits. Poultry and meat products require special care; juices from the raw meat can contaminate knives, cutting boards, and other foods. If you are planning on chopping or cutting up both vegetables and meat, cut up the vegetables first, then the meat. Next wash the cutting board and the knives thoroughly in hot soapy water and air dry or pat dry with paper towels. Wash your hands with warm water and soap for at least 20 seconds. Partisans of wood and plastic cutting boards have been making conflicting claims about which remain safer from contamination. The jury is still out, but so far plastic cutting boards, which can be washed more thoroughly, seem to have the more valid claims. Sanitize both wood and plastic cutting boards periodically by washing with a solution of 2 tsp liquid chlorine bleach in 1 qt of water. Replace either type of cutting board when worn; deep grooves are hard to clean and may harbor bacteria.

Foods should be cooked thoroughly. Undercooked eggs, poultry, and meat may all cause food-borne illness. Ground beef should be cooked to an internal temperature of 160°F, pork to 170°F, and poultry to 180°F. Eggs should be heated to 140°F for at least 3½ minutes. Do not serve food containing raw eggs, such as traditional eggnogs; or raw meat, such as steak tartare. Raw fish and shellfish may also present hazards and should not be eaten by pregnant women, children, the elderly, or infirm individuals. Be sure to wash vegetables and fruits thoroughly to remove bacteria and pesticide residue.

Keep hot food hot and cold food cold. Extended warming of food may just breed bacteria if the food is not heated through to a high enough temperature. Refrigerate foods promptly. Foods containing eggs and dairy products will spoil if they sit out at room temperature. Picnics and outdoor meals present additional challenges because hot summer days may speed spoilage.

If you do any home canning, freezing, or preserving, get the latest guidelines on good practices from your local Cooperative Extension Service office and follow them to the letter. Not only will you get better results, but your efforts will result in a safer product.

Microwave oven doors and seals should be kept in good condition. Use a grounded, three-prong plug and locate the microwave well away from the kitchen sink. Follow the manufacturer's instructions for use. Never put metal objects, metal or foil pans, or aluminum foil in a microwave. Some glass containers may explode; be sure that containers are labeled "microwave safe." If you use paper plates or towels in microwave cooking, do not over do the cooking time or power because you could set the paper on fire. Microwaves do not always heat food evenly; part of the food may feel cool and other parts may be dangerously hot. This is especially dangerous with baby bottles. Never warm baby bottles in a microwave oven. Test other foods carefully before you serve them.

Your kitchen can present risks for falls, burns and scalds, and injuries from knives and other sharp objects. Wipe up spills as they happen to prevent slips and falls on wet floors. Do not reach over steaming pots or add water to a pot that has boiled dry. Always remember to keep pot handles turned away from the range or the flow of kitchen traffic. Hot grease causes terrible burns, so be especially careful of frying pans and oven broiler pans. Food grinders, processors, blenders, graters, and disposal systems may be dangerous. Follow the manufacturer's instructions and use the safety features. Unplug all appliances when you are not using them and before you clean them. In addition to the hazard of mixing chlorine- and ammonia-containing cleansers together, handle all kitchen cleaning products with care and read their caution labels. Automatic dishwasher detergent can cause caustic burns to eyes and skin, to the lungs if inhaled, and to the gastrointestinal tract if swallowed.

GUN SAFETY

Guns in the home pose an unreasonable danger to those who live there. Studies have shown that keeping a gun in the house is related to increased homicides and suicides among the residents of that house. The best advice is not to have a gun in your house.

If you do keep a gun in the home, it is very important that you follow a few simple rules. Always keep guns locked and unloaded. Store ammunition separately, and keep it locked as well. Children should never have access to a gun.

If you shoot guns recreationally, be sure to use protective devices over your ears to prevent hearing loss. If you are exposed to high noise levels during your workday, participating in noisy recreational activities like shooting puts you at greatly increased risk for hearing loss.

INVISIBLE DANGERS: RADON, CARBON MONOXIDE, AND LEAD

Though we might prefer not to worry about what we cannot see, the dangers of radon, carbon monoxide, and lead are a real concern.

Radon Radon is a colorless, odorless, and completely imperceptible radioactive gas that escapes from soil and bedrock. It enters homes through basement foundations and floor drains, through water supplies, and through some natural gas supplies. Radon causes no immediate irritation or symptoms and there are no early signs of exposure. Unfortunately, even though radon seems benign in the short run, it has the long-term effect of increasing the risk of lung cancer. Radon exposure is particularly dangerous for smokers, who are already at 10 to 20 times higher risk for lung cancer than nonsmokers. Risks of radon exposure in children are not known, but it is a concern because children often spend more time at home and indoors, and have a greater number of years of potential exposure.

Radon gas is created by the decay of naturally occurring radioactive radium, a

FIREWORKS

Fireworks are beautiful, exciting, fun—and extremely dangerous. In fact, many states have laws limiting their use to public displays licensed by fire departments or local governments.

All fireworks have an explosive charge and some kind of fuse to light the charge. Both can be very unpredictable. Many people are injured when they try to light one or re-light an unexploded charge. Fireworks cause thousands of serious injuries every year, including many eye injuries that result in permanent blindness. Fireworks may also cause acoustic trauma leading to hearing loss.

The safest approach to fireworks is from a distance. Children love fireworks but, unfortunately, they are the ones who are often injured. Try to limit your family's firework exposure to public displays. If you cannot resist, follow these safety tips.

- Do not allow anyone but a sober adult to handle fireworks. Even sparklers carry substantial risks for burns in children.

- Always read the safety instructions.

- Do not allow children or anyone else to throw fireworks at other people or pets.

- Keep a bucket of water nearby to put out any sparks or grass fires. Never use fireworks during a drought. Brush fires spread quickly in dry conditions; you will be in trouble with the law on top of everything else.

- Never try to re-light a dud. Douse it with a bucket of water.

- Never put fireworks in another container to explode; the resulting shrapnel may cause serious injury or death. ■

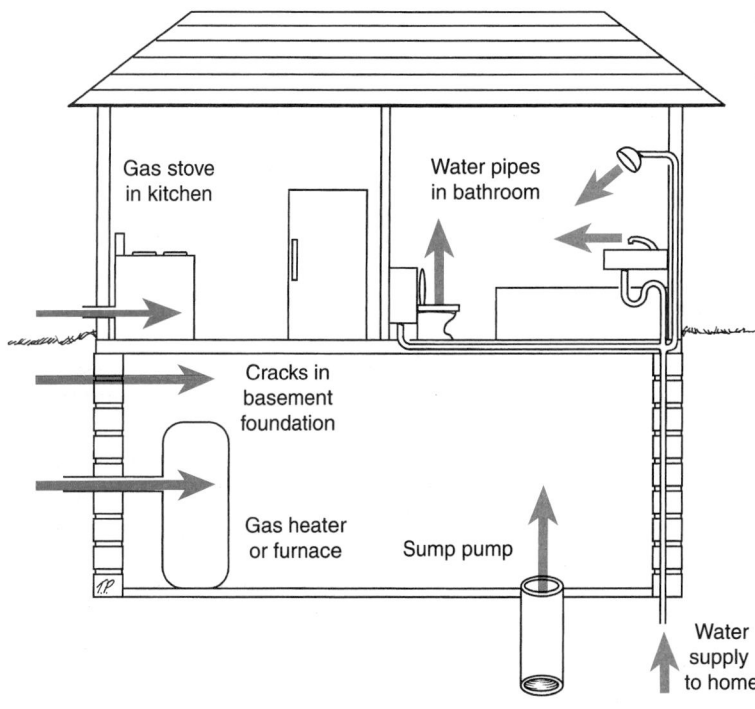

Entry points for radon into the home.

common component of soil and bedrock. The US Environmental Protection Agency estimates that about 10 percent of American homes have radon concentrations above the limits that the agency considers acceptable. Some areas of the country have geologic formations that are more prone to radon release than others, but nearly every state has areas where radon is a problem. Even within one neighborhood, some homes will have radon problems and some will not. The only way to know whether you have radon in your home is to test for it, and many states now require a radon test whenever real estate is sold.

Home kits to test for radon are available in many hardware and home building supply stores. Home test kits typically require the test unit to remain in a closed basement or lowest level of the house for a specified period of time. The test kit is then returned to a laboratory for evaluation. Other radon monitoring systems are available either for home or professional use. If your home is heated with natural gas or gets its water from a groundwater source in a radon area (municipal water supplies do not usually pose a radon problem), you may want to measure radon concentrations in the upper levels of your home because radon is released from the water when you use the shower, wash the dishes, or run the water for any reason. Read test kit instructions carefully and seek advice from your state's Department of Environmental Protection before you proceed.

If you do find unacceptable levels of radon in your home, radon abatement measures can restore your home's healthful air quality. Some common measures involve sealing basement floors and venting the basement or crawl space area. Most states offer guidance in addressing radon problems.

Carbon monoxide Carbon monoxide is also a colorless, odorless, and imperceptible gas. Unlike radon, however, carbon monoxide constitutes an immediate danger that will kill you in high enough concentrations. Carbon monoxide is produced by the incomplete combustion of fuels in stoves, grills, furnaces, gas-fired water heaters or clothes dryers, and gasoline engines.

The symptoms of carbon monoxide poisoning are slow to build and often mimic flu-like illness. Common symptoms include headaches, dizziness, weakness, drowsiness, nausea, vomiting, confusion, and disorientation. When carbon monoxide reaches very high levels, it causes loss of consciousness and death.

Following the safety measures described in this chapter will help keep you safe from carbon monoxide poisoning. Furnaces and other heating appliances, and gas dryers and water heaters should be properly installed and vented. Have a technician check them every year. If you ever feel that they are not operating properly, have them serviced right away. Always keep vents and chimneys clear. Never use a charcoal or gas grill in an enclosed space. Dozens of people die every year because they have attempted to run a charcoal grill inside the house or garage.

Internal combustion engines in cars and power equipment are another source of carbon monoxide fumes. Never leave a car or other power equipment running in an attached garage because fumes may travel unannounced into the living areas of the house. Make sure that your car's exhaust system is operating properly. If you must keep the car idling outside, leave one or more of the car windows cracked open. Never leave children in a car while it is running. Not only might they try to operate the car, but children, who are much more vulnerable to carbon monoxide, may succumb quickly if fumes get into the car. If you must keep the car idling in winter weather, be sure that the exhaust pipe is free of snow.

Carbon monoxide monitors are now available for home use and cost from $30 to $80 for most models. They should be installed on the ceiling in a hallway near the bedroom area of the house and in garages attached to living areas. Carbon monoxide detectors sound an alarm before carbon monoxide levels reach the danger point.

Lead Childhood lead poisoning is one of this country's most serious preventable health problems in children. Many American children have hazardous levels of lead in their bodies. Children with high levels of lead may suffer from nervous system damage, hearing problems, headaches, slowed growth, and behavioral and learning problems, including hyperactivity. Lead is dangerous to adults, too. Long-term exposure may cause muscle and joint pain, high blood pressure, nervous system disorders, and problems with digestion, reproduction, memory, and concentration.

Now that leaded gasoline has been largely phased out, the greatest source of lead exposure is the lead paint that was used in the interior of older homes. Pottery and dishes made with lead glazes also pose risks, as does soil contaminated by peeling or chipping exterior paint. Lead was widely used in paints until 1978, and lead solder was used in plumbing until the 1980s. Homes built before these years are likely to have a problem with either lead paint or lead in the water.

If you think your home has lead paint or lead in the plumbing, there are simple steps you can take to reduce your children's risk.

- Have your children tested for lead, even if they seem healthy.

- Check your home for lead hazards. Home test kits are available, although the results are not always accurate. State health departments can offer advice and test your water for lead.

- Clean floors, window sills, and other surfaces regularly with a damp cloth and an all-purpose cleaner to remove dust that may contain lead. Rinse the cleaning sponge thoroughly after every use and do not use it for other purposes.

- Wipe the soil off your shoes before entering the house.

- Wash your children's hands, bottles, pacifiers, and toys frequently.

- Do not serve food on imported or handmade pottery because the glazes often contain lead. Crystal decanters may carry a similar risk.

- Feed your children a healthy diet high in calcium. Good nutrition reduces lead absorption.

If you do have lead paint in your home, do not try to remove it yourself. Get professional help from a contractor specializing in lead paint removal. Contact your state's department of public health for a list of resources. Improper paint removal may make the problem worse. Do not sand, scrape, or use chemical paint removers on lead paint. Paint-removing appliances that use heat, either propane or electricity, are especially dangerous because they vaporize the lead and release the fumes into the air.

Until you can get professional help, clean frequently, keep paint chips swept up, and dispose of them carefully.

Safe on the Road

Americans are increasingly on the move; it seems as if we are always on our way to somewhere. Accidents do not stop at our front door, and neither does the need for safety consciousness.

SAFE IN THE CAR

If you want to do the one thing that will best improve your safety and long-term health: use your seatbelt! Many states have laws requiring seat belt use, but even if the law does not require it, buckle up every time and do not start the car until all of your passengers are buckled up as well. Automobile accidents are the leading cause of injury and death in healthy individuals, taking the lives of nearly 45,000 Americans each year.

The safest place for children of any age is in the back seat. If you have a car with a passenger-side air bag, *never* place a rear-facing safety seat in the front seat. The force of the inflating air bag will hit the back of the safety seat behind the child's head causing brain and spinal cord injuries, or death. It is best to not place any children, smaller adults (generally 5 ft tall and under), or fragile elderly persons in a front seat where there is an air bag; however, if there are no other suitable seating positions, a few precautions can decrease the risk of injury. Slide the vehicle seat back as far as possible, and make sure that the person is secured properly in a seat belt or forward-facing child safety seat. A car can be retrofitted with an on/off switch to deactivate the passenger-side air bag; you might want to consider this modification if you anticipate having children or shorter adults as frequent passengers. Remember, too, that the bed of a pick-up truck is never a safe place for passengers, whatever their age.

Keep your vehicle's windows clear of anything that will obscure your view. Loose papers can blow around in the wind and be a dangerous distraction. Sudden stops can turn ice scrapers, books, and toys into dangerous flying objects. Do not pile up your

USING CHILD SAFETY SEATS

Car crashes are the leading cause of death and injury for children. If you are concerned about your children's safety, the most important thing you can do is make sure they ride properly buckled up. Infants and small children should always ride in approved child safety seats. Laws requiring child restraints vary by state, but most require children under age 4 or 5 to be in an approved safety seat appropriate for their age and weight.

The safest place for a child of any age is in the car's back seat and the safest place for a child safety seat is in the center position of the back seat. Some rear seats have a small hump in the center that makes a car seat unstable. In that case, install the seat on the side. *Never put a rear-facing safety seat in a front seat where there is a passenger-side airbag. Properly secure all children in the back seat.* Airbags inflate at a high speed; infants and older children not buckled up properly have been killed or seriously injured by the impact. Previously, people put infants in rear-facing seats up front where they could be monitored; however, this is extremely hazardous in cars with passenger-side air bags. You may want to have an on-off switch installed that deactivates the passenger-side air bag.

The car seat you select must fit your baby's size and weight and must fit properly in your car. Check the label to be certain it meets current federal safety standards.

Child safety seats come in three types. Infant seats are safe for children under 20 lbs and less than 1 year of age and are used in a rear-facing position. Premature infants should not be placed in regular infant seats until they weigh at least 6 lbs; check with your doctor about safely transporting a premature baby. Toddler car seats hold children from 20 to 40 lbs and are used in a front-facing position. Many car seats, called convertible seats, convert from rear-facing to front-facing for use by both infants and toddlers. Many booster seats are made to be used with lap/shoulder belts. If only a lap seat belt is available, be sure to use a booster seat or travel vest approved for use in lap-belt-only cars.

Many hospitals and public health agencies have car seat rental or loan programs. If you decide to buy or use a second-hand car seat, make sure that it was made after January 1, 1981. Be certain it is free of cracks and that all parts are operating properly. Check with the manufacturer to make sure the seat has not been recalled for safety problems. If a car seat has been in an accident, it is no longer safe to use. Discard it and get a new one.

Child safety seats come with a number of features; some will fit in your car better than others. Try before you buy. The seat must be stable and work with the seats and seat belts in your car. If you are going to be using the seat in a second car, check it in both. The seat belts of some cars will not hold a child safety seat properly; you will need to have the seat belt modified. Other seat belts require the use of a locking clip. If the seat is not secured properly, your child will not be protected. Read the section in your car owner's manual on "Child Restraints." You can also call the safety seat manufacturer's toll-free customer service line or your car dealership's service department. ∎

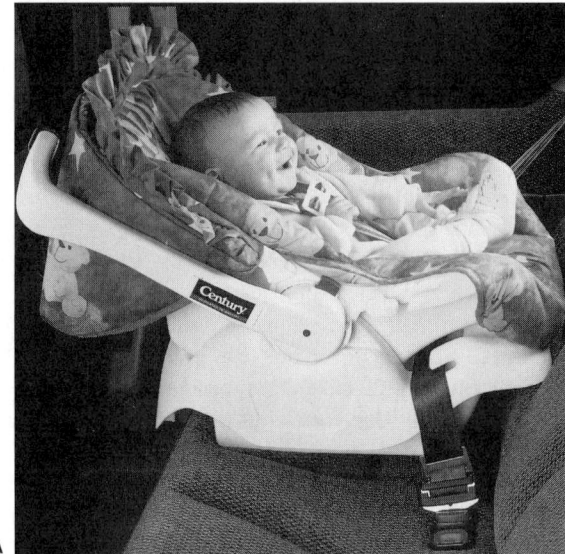

A

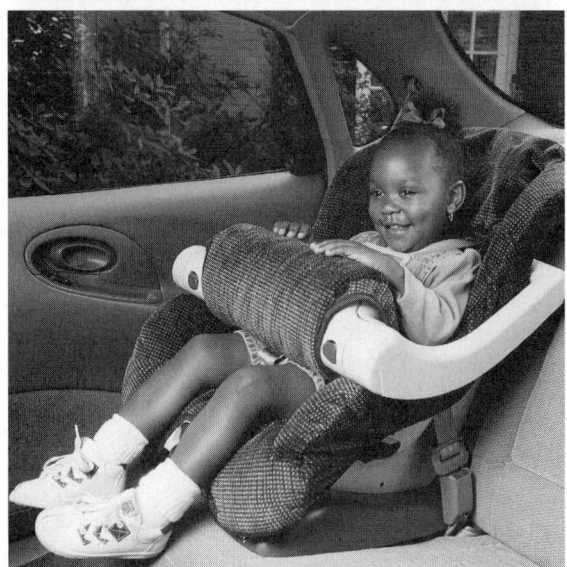

B

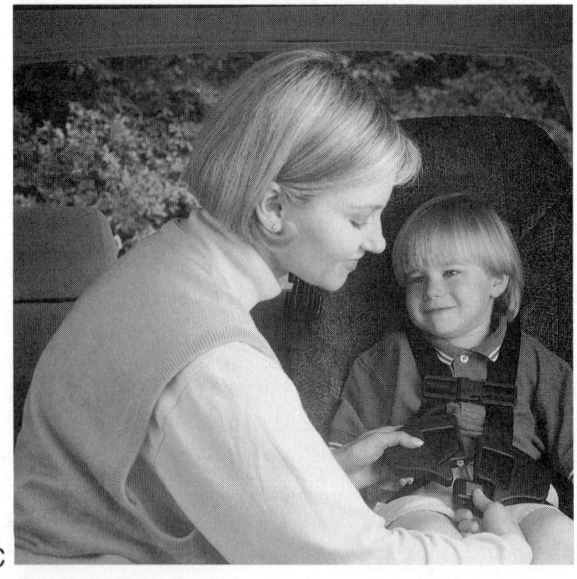

C

Child safety seats are to be used only in the rear seat of the automobile. (A) Children under 1 year of age and who weigh less than 20 lbs must be placed in a rear-facing car seat such as an infant seat or a "convertible" seat used rear-facing. (B) Toddlers weighing between 20 and 40 lbs should be placed in forward-facing seats with built-in harness straps. (C) Some booster seats can be used with a harness until 40 lbs, after which the harness system is removed and the adult lap and shoulder belt restrain the child and the seat until about 65 lbs. (Courtesy Century Products, Macedonia, OH; used with permission.)

cargo to the point where your rear or side vision is obstructed. Make sure all cargo is properly secured. Keep your defrosters and windshield wipers and washers working well so that you will have good visibility at all times.

Do not exceed posted speed limits—speed limits save lives. Drive defensively. The best drivers stay alert to road conditions and watch what other drivers are up to. Signal your own intentions clearly but never assume another driver sees you or your signal. Always give yourself plenty of time and room to react to other vehicles. Changing road and weather conditions warrant changes in your driving. Do not be afraid to slow down in rain, fog, snow, or ice. If other drivers want to go faster than you think is prudent, find a safe place to pull over and let them pass.

Do not drive when you have been drinking or using any drugs, even over-the-counter medications, that might make you drowsy or impair your judgment. Even small amounts of alcohol slow your reaction time. If you expect to be drinking, make alternate arrangements for getting home. If you are fatigued, *do not drive*. Even the best driver becomes a menace dozing at the wheel.

Cross railroad crossings carefully. Never race a train to the crossing or go around railroad crossing gates.

Teenage drivers are at high risk for accidents. Make sure young drivers in your family have adequate instruction and practice in safe, defensive driving before you let them on the road. Establish firm ground rules about when and where they may drive and how many passengers they may have along. Make it clear that under no circumstances may they drive after drinking or using drugs. Make arrangements for them to be picked up after events that might include drinking. If you have input into choosing the car your teenage drives, remember that bigger cars are safer in collisions. Many of the small sport utility vehicles popular with young drivers are unstable and prone to rollovers.

SAFE ON WHEELS

Motorcycles, mini-bikes, all-terrain vehicles, and snowmobiles share some similar risks. You should be sure to wear a helmet whenever you ride on any such vehicle, even if it is not required by law. Children should not be allowed to operate any motorized vehicle, even off the road; they do not have the strength, coordination, maturity, or judgment necessary for safe operation. It is also not safe for children to ride on open vehicles, even with an adult driving. These vehicles can reach very high speeds but offer no protection in a crash and little protection from falls off the vehicle.

Motorcycles are covered by state motor vehicle regulations and almost all states require the use of approved helmets and eye protection. Even if you ride in a state that does not, you should still wear a helmet all of the time. Eye protection and protective clothing are also essential for safety.

Some states regulate the off-road use of motorized vehicles, such as all-terrain vehicles and snowmobiles. Look for an operator's safety class in your area or ask the dealer where classes are offered. Assess the potential safety problems of the equipment before you buy. Three-wheeled all-terrain vehicles have been implicated in fatalities and serious injuries, and should not be used.

BIKING AND SKATING SAFETY

Think helmets when you think about safety for bicycles, skateboards, and in-line skates. Every bike rider, child or adult, should wear an approved, appropriately sized bike helmet every time they ride, whether on the street or not. If you enjoy skateboards or in-line skates, a helmet is also a necessary part of your equipment. Approved helmets carry a Snell or ANSI sticker, which indicates that the helmet meets certain safety standards. Helmets prevent head injuries from falls and collisions, which are the cause of the vast majority of fatalities and serious injuries from these sports. The protection helmets provide to the skull, forehead, eyes, ears, nose, and cheeks is profound. Over 70 percent of injuries to these areas are preventable. In addition to helmets, skateboarders and in-line skaters should also use wrist guards and elbow and knee pads.

Bicycles are considered to be vehicles and are subject to the same rules of the road as cars and trucks. Bike riders should always ride with, not against, traffic and use the approved hand signals to indicate turns and stops. Stop at stop signs and lights. Before turning check for traffic behind you and on both sides. Being predictable keeps you safer; do not dart in and out of traffic or from between parked cars. When biking in wet conditions, watch out for wet debris that may cause skidding, and remember that your brakes may not respond as well as they do in dry conditions. When riding at night, use reflectors and lights and wear reflective clothing to ensure your visibility. Be sure to practice defensive riding. Watch out for the drivers around you and do not assume that they see you or know what you are about to do.

Keep your children safe by limiting their bike riding, skateboarding, or in-line skating to daylight hours and safe areas. Bike riding should be limited to bike paths and quiet streets. Even quiet streets are not safe for skating sports, so help your children find safe places to skate where they will not create a hazard to other pedestrians. Make sure your children know the basic rules of the road and how to watch out for other vehicles before they venture out. Be sure bicycles and other equipment fit the child and have an age-appropriate design; for example, young children usually cannot manage hand brakes safely. To be sure the bike fits, have your child stand with feet flat on the ground straddling the center bar; there should be at least 1 in. clearance.

PEDESTRIAN SAFETY

Children need to be taught, and adults reminded, about the basic rules of pedestrian safety. Always use sidewalks if available; if you must walk on the road or in the street, walk on the left, facing traffic. If you find yourself out after dark, try to find a light-colored article of clothing to wear as an outer garment. Wear reflective clothing if you walk or jog after dark. Purchase children's outerwear with reflective patches. If you are out during times of decreased visibility, give drivers extra time to see you and respond. Heavy rain, fog, or high snow banks make it hard to see pedestrians and hard to stop quickly.

Cross at crosswalks, read the traffic lights, and watch for turning cars and cars that do not stop. Teach your children how to look for oncoming traffic—look left,

right, then left again. Do not cross the street between parked cars, and teach your children not to do it either. If your children walk to school, plan their route for safety and walk it with them a few times. Keep in mind that children under age 12 may judge speed and distance poorly; make sure they never cross alone at difficult intersections.

Safe Outdoors

Outdoor recreation brings balance to our lives and gives us a chance to exercise, get some fresh air, and have fun. A little thought given to safety will prevent injuries and accidents while we enjoy the outdoors.

PLAY IT SAFE

Playing hard does not mean you cannot play safe. Before you head to the backyard, the playground, or the trails, think a bit about safety.

Playground equipment, whether it is in your own backyard or in a public park, should be safe and in good repair. Falls account for approximately 75 percent of all injuries related to playground equipment. Therefore, the surface under and around playground equipment is the most critical safety factor on a playground. Hard, paved surfaces, such as concrete and asphalt, are dangerous, as are hard-packed earth, soil, and grass. Loose-fill surfaces, such as sand, pea gravel, mulch, and hardwood chips should be at least 9 to 12 in. deep to provide adequate protection. Acceptable synthetic surfaces include rubber tile and pour-in-place systems.

Make sure playground equipment is securely anchored so it will not tip over. Strangulation hazards on playground equipment include vertical posts, gaps, openings between $3\frac{1}{2}$ and 9 in. that can trap a child's head, and open connecting links, such as S-hooks, that can catch a child's clothing. Swings on S-hooks can swing right out of the hook; swing chains can pinch fingers. Swing seats should be made of lightweight materials such as rubber, canvas, or plastic to reduce injuries from impact. Adequate guardrails and protective barriers on equipment can prevent falls. You should also inspect equipment for sharp edges, protrusions, pinch points, and hot surfaces. Many public playgrounds do not yet meet all of these standards; you may need to talk with the school or recreation department about making your neighborhood playgrounds safer. In the meantime try to keep your children off the equipment. Do not let children play on equipment that is not appropriate for their size, age, and skill level.

Always check games and other outdoor toys for safety and limit their use to appropriate ages. Some games, such as croquet, are best for older children. High-powered water guns, lawn darts, and BB guns, which can be deadly, are unsafe for any age. The chalk markings used for many field sports contain lime, which may cause skin irritations or even caustic burns. Avoid contact with the chalk markings on the ground and keep well away when they are being applied to a field.

Children should never play on or near railroad tracks. Teach them not to walk on tracks or climb on railroad cars.

Before you venture out for a hike, plan ahead for safety. If you are headed for unfamiliar territory, take a map and check it carefully. Talk to park personnel or rangers about unusual trail or weather conditions, insects, poisonous snakes or plants, or animal hazards. Weather can change quickly, so keep an eye on the sky for signs of fast-moving storms. Always take along a lightweight, preferably waterproof jacket, even if the day is fine. Take along insect repellents if ticks, chiggers or mosquitoes are a problem, but use them only according to the label instructions. Treat all snakes as if they were poisonous. Do not approach or pick up any wild animal, even if it looks sick or injured. Know what poison ivy and oak and sumac look like and teach everyone in your party to avoid them. (See Bites and Stings, page 397; Severe Contact Dermatitis/Poison Ivy, Oak, and Sumac, page 407; Animal-Borne Infections, page 886; Plant Dermatoses, Poison Ivy, Oak, and Sumac, page 1335; and Insect Sting Allergic Reactions, page 1339).

Dress for hiking in sturdy comfortable shoes with non-slip soles and as heavy a sock as you can comfortably wear with your shoes. Blisters can make even a short hike a miserable experience, and the wrong footgear may cause a turned ankle, a fall, or worse. Dress in layers, with lighter clothing underneath, that you can add and remove as the day warms and cools. If you hike to higher or lower terrain, the temperature and

---

TEN ESSENTIALS FOR HIKING AND CAMPING

1. Map of the area

2. Extra food

3. Extra water or water purification supplies

4. Extra clothing

5. Sunscreen and sunglasses

6. Insect repellent

7. Waterproof matches and fire starter

8. Flashlight

9. Knife

10. First aid kit ■

---

the weather may be quite different at your destination.

Always pack a few extra high-energy snacks beyond what you need for your lunch, just in case you are gone longer than you expect. In addition to a jacket, also pack a hat for protection against the sun or cold, sunscreen, sunglasses, insect repellent, a small first aid kit, waterproof matches and fire starter, a flashlight, a pocket knife, and plenty of water. Trailside water supplies are often not safe for drinking. (See Ten Essentials for Hiking and Camping, above.)

UNDER THE SUN

Exposure to the sun has a direct relationship to incidence of skin cancer. You can greatly reduce your risk—and keep your skin looking younger—by covering up and using sunscreen. Wear a hat and long sleeves when you are in the sun. Wear sunglasses to decrease the risk of cataract formation. Protect exposed areas with a sunscreen product that is appropriate for your skin type and the time you will be exposed. Although people with fair complexions are at greater risk for skin cancer and need to take more precautions and use stronger sunscreens, no one is free of risk.

Excessive exposure to hot, humid weather can lead to heat exhaustion and heat stroke. These are medical emergencies that require immediate care (see Environmental Emergencies, page 402). The very young and the very old are particularly susceptible; to minimize the risk of heat stress, they should drink plenty of fluids and seek shelter from the heat. In the hottest weather, athletes and outdoor enthusiasts must moderate their activity, increase their fluid intake, and cool down frequently with cool water. In very hot weather, keep in mind that your fluid intake must go beyond just quenching your thirst. If you drink only when you are thirsty, you will not adequately replace fluids lost through perspiration.

POOL AND WATER SAFETY

Safety around the water starts with knowing how to swim. Call your local Red Cross, YMCA or YWCA, or recreation department for times and places of water safety and swimming classes. Formal swimming lessons are generally not recommended for children younger than 5 years old, and definitely not recommended for children younger than 2 years old. Even children who know how to swim and understand water safety rules must always be carefully supervised around the water. Familiarity with cardiopulmonary resuscitation (CPR) techniques can be life saving at poolside (see Cardiopulmonary Resuscitation, page 361 and Near-Drowning, page 405).

If you have your own swimming pool, it must be completely fenced on all four sides; there should be no direct access from within the house. Fences should be at least 6 ft high. Gates should be self-closing with the latch near the top. Be sure there are no openings around the gate or under the fence that children could wriggle through. Establish firm ground rules about pool and poolside behavior: no horseplay, no glass bottles or drinking glasses, and no swimming after drinking alcohol. Keep safety equipment, such as a pole and a life preserver on a rope, readily accessible near the pool. Never let children swim or play near the water without adult supervision. If possible, keep a portable phone near the pool. It can save precious minutes in an emergency and will reduce the chance that you will be called away from supervising your children if the phone rings. CPR training is a must for all pool owners.

Even backyard wading pools may present hazards for little children. Never let your children play unattended in or near a wading pool. Get in the habit of emptying the pool after every use. Not only will you eliminate a drowning hazard, but water-filled pools attract stray and wild animals, which is a concern in areas where rabies is becoming epidemic in the animal population. Keep in mind that large buckets, pails, or even aquariums can pose drowning hazards for small children.

Flotation devices for children who do not yet swim are a mixed blessing. Those that are unstable are downright dangerous. Flotation devices and toys may allow children to get into deeper water than they can safely manage; they should be watched especially closely when using them. Flotation toys are no substitute for close supervision and will not prevent drowning.

Older children should be taught the dangers of swimming or rafting in deep or fast-moving rivers or creeks. They should also be warned never to walk out on ice-covered lakes.

Safe boating requires a knowledge of your boat and equipment, attention to the weather, and adherence to boating safety rules. Many boating accidents involve alcohol. Never operate a boat if you are under the influence of alcohol or drugs. Insist that everyone wear their life jacket and make sure your boat is equipped with the right sizes and types for your passengers. Do not exceed your boat's weight and passenger limits.

Water sports, such as water skiing and personal watercraft (jet-skis), present further hazards from impact injuries, entanglement, collisions with other craft, and drowning. Follow the safety rules for the sport, always wear an approved flotation device, and be alert to other water traffic. Mixing alcohol and water sports is a recipe for disaster.

WEATHERING THE STORMS

Many people underestimate the power and force of nature, probably more so now that many of us earn our livings away from the land and spend most of our time inside buildings. Take a hint from the loggers, farmers, and fishermen: thunder, lightning, hail, blizzards, and heavy winds should be taken seriously.

If you are outdoors in threatening weather, try to find safe shelter immediately.

"Safe" is a relative term that depends on what is available and what kind of storm is approaching. Many storms have combinations of two or three hazards, so your plans should cover all the bases.

Lightning is best survived in your car unless it has a convertible top, because the tires provide good insulation against the electrical charge. Your car is good shelter in a storm as long as you are clear of potentially falling trees and not parked in a flash flood zone. If you cannot get to shelter in a lightning storm, find a low-lying area and crouch in it. Do not seek shelter under a tree. Lightning strikes the highest point around and the area under a tree struck by lightning will be electrically charged. Water is a very good conductor of electricity, so avoid puddles or ditches with standing water if you can. Do not seek shelter in any kind of metal building or storage shed. If you are in the water or in a boat, get to shore immediately and take shelter.

High winds are dangerous in themselves and can escalate into tornadoes or twisters. Seek shelter inside if a tornado is threatening. A car might protect you in a heavy wind, but automobiles and mobile homes are not good places to ride out a tornado. If you can, seek shelter in a basement or at least in a well-reinforced interior room away from any windows.

If power lines are down, stay away. If you are in your car with downed power lines on or near it, stay there. Do not try to get out. The tires are providing you with protective insulation, which you lose when you try to get out. Never touch a power line even if it looks dead.

Severe weather—hurricanes, floods, and tornadoes—and natural disasters such as earthquakes and forest fires have been a staple of the evening news for the last few years. It is certainly not necessary to worry excessively about natural disasters. We cannot control them and the chances of experiencing even one major storm or earthquake are still very small, no matter where you live. Still, a little forethought and planning never hurt and could go a long way toward assuring your comfort and well-being under difficult circumstances.

Almost all natural events create similar problems; only the geography and a few details differ. Preparing your house and your car with a few basic supplies can help you weather the storms comfortably and safely.

EMERGENCY SUPPLIES FOR HOME AND CAR

Home

- Flashlight and extra batteries, and candles and matches

- Bottled water, ideally 3 gallons per person

- Food that can be consumed without cooking, plus a mechanical can opener. Have a 3-day supply of food for each person.

- Sterno and matches for boiling water, and small pot or kettle.

- Three-day supply of medications and any special supplies that you may need, such as ready-to-use baby formula and diapers.

- If feasible, a safe source of auxiliary heat, such as a vented heater or wood and kindling for a fireplace. Never use a gas or charcoal grill.

- First aid kit

- Transistor radio and extra batteries

Car

- Flashlight and extra batteries, and matches

- Bottled water

- High-energy snacks such as chocolate bars, granola bars, cheese crackers, or peanut butter crackers

- "Space Blanket" or regular blanket for warmth or shelter from the sun.

- Shovel and bag of kitty litter for winter travel, extra coolant for travel in hot weather

- Sturdy shoes or boots and an extra jacket, hat, and gloves for winter travel

- First aid kit

- Flares ■

LAWN, GARDEN, AND FARM CHEMICALS AND EQUIPMENT

It takes a lot of work to keep a lawn and yard in shape. The amount of equipment and chemicals that we use in the process is growing by the year. Lawn mowers and tractors, trimmers, hedge shears, tillers, leaf blowers, chain saws, and snow blowers are great tools, but they can be dangerous if they are not properly used and maintained.

Do not wear loose clothing, long sleeves, scarves, or jewelry that might get caught in equipment. Tie back long hair. Never reach into or under equipment unless the engine is completely turned off—and not just stalled. Safety switches, guards, and other devices are there for a reason; do not bypass them. Do not mow the lawn barefoot or in sandals or smooth-soled shoes; one slip on the damp grass and you could be headed for severe injury. Before you mow, check the yard for stray toys, sticks, and small stones. Make sure no children are in the vicinity when you are mowing. Debris and innocent objects turn into dangerous shrapnel when thrown by a mower blade.

Do not let children use lawn mowers or other power equipment until they are big enough to handle such equipment safely and mature enough to handle it responsibly. You are the best judge of when your child has the ability to be mindful of the consequences of their actions and exercise good judgment. Most children do not reach this point until the teen years. While it is important that children share in family chores, they should not be put in danger.

FARM SAFETY

Whether farming is your hobby or business, make safety your business on the farm. Although farm life can look idyllic, farming is one of the most hazardous occupations. Because farming is often a family affair, children are too often the victims of farm accidents. Some common sense measures can help protect every one on the farm, young or old.

Getting crops in and out can be a stressful task, especially when the weather is not cooperating. Do not work with hazardous equipment when you are overtired. Non-farm workers have shift limits on hazardous equipment; set limits on your own and your family's work times.

Keep children safe on the farm and do not let children under age 18 operate hazardous equipment. Do not let children under age 14 operate farm equipment at all. Do not let anyone operate your equipment until they have completed safety training. Keep youngsters out of work areas, where their lack of maturity and judgment makes them inadvertent hazards themselves. Be sure not to let children work beyond their level of ability or stamina.

Your local Cooperative Extension Service office has information on farm safety and may sponsor farm safety workshops for the whole family. ■

Carrying children, or anyone else, as passengers on riding mowers, tractors, or other farm equipment is extremely dangerous. Deaths and amputations are not uncommon. Always use ear protectors when operating noisy equipment; lawn mowers, leaf blowers, and chain saws are among the kinds of equipment most hazardous to your hearing. Respirators that provide protection from airborne particles are essential when handling fertilizers, powdered pesticides, and animal feeds. Surgical-type dust masks will provide no protection against these hazards and should never be substituted for respirators. It is important to wear protective clothing, gloves, and masks when handling pesticides and herbicides because many of these chemicals are very well absorbed through the skin. Remember to launder chemical-soaked clothing separately from the regular family wash and run an empty wash cycle afterwards to clean the washing machine.

Treat your power equipment with respect. Maintain machinery in good repair, paying special attention to protective shields and safety features. Do not disable any safety feature. Use the seatbelts on ride-on equipment. When equipment is parked, lock the brakes and take the keys. Always leave a tractor's power takeoff (PTO) in neutral and leave front-end loader buckets and similar equipment in the down position.

Store lawn, garden, and farm chemicals in a locked cabinet or shed. Read the manufacturer's instructions carefully before you use them and follow the cautions to the letter. If protective masks or clothing are required, never use the product without them. Home gardening and lawn products may contain powerful pesticides and herbicides, as do commercial farm products. Do not allow your children to use them or to be in the area when you are applying them. Keep your children off the lawns for a few days after pesticide or herbicide has been applied.

Safe at Work

Although occupational injuries have dropped dramatically, too many people are still injured needlessly at work. Workplace safety depends on a partnership between the employer and the employee. It is the employer's responsibility to provide a safe work environment, proper equipment, and training. It is up to the employee to use that training to work safely without endangering herself or others.

ERGONOMICS AT WORK

Ergonomics is a scientific discipline devoted to the study of human work. Ergonomics analyzes the relationships among people at work, the implements they use, and the physical and psychological demands of the work environments. Employers and employees can use the principles of ergonomics to make work safer and more efficient. Repetitive strain injury (RSI), including carpal tunnel syndrome and tendonitis, is the fastest growing type of occupational injury, even exceeding back injuries in many instances. RSI is caused by repetitive motions, forceful motions, awkward postures, or application of direct pressure to body areas not meant to withstand them. People who commonly suffer from RSIs are cashiers, computer operators, assembly-line workers, meat packers, and food service workers. RSI causes inflammation and pain, and can be permanently disabling if it is not dealt with properly.

Often simple adjustments to work areas or to the way a task is performed reduce physical stress and risk for RSI. Most companies have consultants available to analyze work stations and task performance. Sometimes workers can modify their own work habits by changing how they do a task or by taking more frequent breaks. Do not use splints, braces, or other orthopedic aids without medical supervision. They can cause more harm than good if they are not correctly prescribed and adjusted.

Back injuries are a common workplace injury in many different occupations. Lifting and twisting with a heavy object in your arms is particularly risky. Proper lifting requires bending at the knees and lifting with a straight back. If you must lift heavy objects, follow proper back mechanics. If your job requires regular heavy lifting, start a conditioning program to build your back, arm, stomach, and thigh muscles.

WORKPLACE HEALTH AND SAFETY

During the past two decades, workplace injuries have decreased dramatically. The Occupational Safety and Health Administration (OSHA) has gotten a great deal of negative press on issues of over-regulation, but its efforts have paid off in reduced injuries and fatalities. Many companies have found that increased attention to worker safety pays off with a cleaner work environment, less waste, less lost time, and better productivity. Employees should do their part by using the safety equipment provided and pointing out safety hazards to supervisors and management. Nevertheless, on average in the United States 17 people die each day due to work-related causes.

Noise in the workplace may cause long-term hearing loss and creates a further safety hazard when verbal instructions and warning devices cannot be heard. Noise exposure is cumulative. If your noise exposure on the job is high, take steps to keep it low at other times. Avoid recreational activities with high noise levels, such as listening to loud music or shooting guns. Do not wear a personal stereo to drown out workplace noise; it can increase both your hearing loss and your vulnerability. Noise abatement is one strategy to reduce the hazard, but you should still wear effective ear protection that is rated for the noise level at your workplace. Also be sure to wear adequate ear protection during activities outside of work that have a high noise level.

Eye injuries from foreign objects and chemicals are another hazard. Health care workers need to protect their eyes from body fluids. Safety glasses or prescription eyewear made with safety glass are adequate in many cases. Some workplaces require wraparound glasses that also protect the eyes from the side.

Chemicals, dust, gases, fumes, and smoke are all hazards when inhaled. Learn to identify the hazards in your workplace and the proper way of working with or around each one. Seek health and safety training from your employer. Obtain the Material Safety Data Sheets from your employer and read about the chemicals that you use. Depending on the materials being used, protective equipment should include respirators, dust masks, and even air-supplied hoods. Some work may require pro-

ELECTROMAGNETIC FIELDS: WHAT ARE THE RISKS?

The hazard of electromagnetic radiation is a controversial issue in workplace and home safety. Electromagnetic fields (EMFs) are created by electric appliances such as computer monitors, television sets, cellular phones, electric motors, hair dryers, and nondigital electric clocks. Other sources of EMFs include high-tension power lines, microwaves, and radar. The scientific community is divided over whether or not EMFs present health hazards, and if so, what kinds. Some studies have linked the use of police radar to an unusual form of cancer. High-tension power lines have been linked to clusters of child leukemia cases. Another study found clusters of miscarriages in women who worked at computer terminals.

None of these studies are conclusive, and another recent study has found no health risks from EMFs. The issue is further complicated by difficulties in agreeing on how to measure EMFs. Some industries have decided not to wait the years it will take for science to catch up with current health concerns. Many computer monitor manufacturers have voluntarily adopted Swedish standards to cut down on EMF emissions from their computer displays.

While science debates, you can protect yourself from these potential, but unproven hazards by limiting your exposure as much as you can. EMFs drop exponentially with distance. The further you sit away from a computer monitor, television, or electric clock, the less radiation will reach you. Keep your appliances in good repair; microwave ovens and computer monitors often have shielding inside the cases. If you work near large electric motors or any equipment that uses microwave technology, keep your distance. ■

tective clothing as well. If you work with or around chemicals and are not supplied with uniforms, make sure your clothing is not laundered with the rest of the family wash.

Secondhand cigarette smoke is another workplace hazard. If your workplace allows smoking, try to get your employer to consider making it smoke-free.

Travel Safe

Many of the same safety measures that you take at home will serve you well when you travel. When you stay in a hotel, always review the location of fire exits, stairways, and fire equipment. Memorize the way to the fire exit, in case you have to find it with smoke obscuring your view. Make a plan for two ways to get out in case one of the exits from your floor is blocked by fire. Keep your room key and any personal necessities right next to your bed and have a robe and slippers handy in case you have to make a quick exit. You may also want to pack a small flashlight when you travel.

Air and rail travel are far safer than driving to work or even crossing a busy street, but we often fear them more because air and rail accidents are so widely reported. You can take certain personal safety and health measures when you fly. Always wear your seat belt when you are in your seat, stay away from alcoholic beverages, and wear comfortable shoes and comfortable, nonflammable clothing that covers as much of your body as possible. Listen carefully to the safety briefings before the flight and follow instructions about stowing your carry-on luggage. Request a seat close to an exit. Count the number of rows to the nearest exit, in case you have to reach it in smoky conditions.

You may want to use a child safety seat if you are traveling with a child under 2 years old. While so few infants die in air crashes that child seats are not required for air travel, young children are much safer during turbulence when secured in a safety seat. The airlines do require that the safety seat be approved for use on airplanes, however, so check with your airline first. If you do use a child safety seat, airlines require that you pay for that seat at the full adult fare. If you are flying and then renting a car or using a relative's car, make sure that your child safety seat is compatible with all the different vehicles. Car rental agencies usually rent child safety seats at a small additional charge.

IMMUNIZATIONS FOR INTERNATIONAL TRAVEL

Before you leave on a trip outside the country, you need to make sure that you have the appropriate immunizations to cover both the disease risks and the government requirements of the areas where you will be traveling. Each country has its own immunization requirements, which can change depending on local disease outbreaks. You can find out what is needed through your doctor, a travel health clinic, or directly from the Centers for Disease Control and Prevention (CDC). You can contact the CDC through their International Travel Voice Information System at (404) 332-4555 or FAX Information Service at (404) 332-4565. The CDC also maintains up-to-date travel information on the Internet that includes information on a range of travel-related health risks in addition to immunization requirements, at http://www.cdc.gov/ travel. For more information on specific diseases, see appropriate entries in the chapters in Part 4: Body Systems and Disorders.

The World Health Organization has adopted International Health Regulations that govern the process by which countries require specific vaccinations. The regulations recommend official International Certificates of Immunization for specific diseases which some countries may require. Knowing your itinerary is important because some required immunizations are determined by where you have been and for how long. Although the international regulations are widely used, border guards in some countries have been known to require documentation for specific immunizations that their governments do not officially require. It is important to be aware of the potential for these situations before you leave.

Deciding which immunizations to get is a matter for careful discussion with your doctor. Some required immunizations may be contraindicated for you if you have certain medical conditions; others immunizations may not be required, but would be helpful in keeping you healthy on your trip. Mild reactions to immunizations are not uncommon. You might experience local pain, tenderness, muscle stiffness at the site of injections, mild headache, malaise, or a low-grade fever. Call your doctor if any mild symptom lasts more than two days or if you experience more severe symptoms such as hives, cramps, or abdominal pain.

Be sure to allow enough time before your departure to research and receive the necessary immunizations. Some immunizations require a series of injections over a period of time, or take time to build their protective effect; others interact and cannot be given at the same time.

Travel immunizations and children Sorting out immunization schedules for children who will be traveling can be a bit complicated. Discuss the subject with your child's pediatrician or a specialist in travel health. Some standard immunizations for children should be given on an accelerated schedule if you plan to travel. The CDC has recommendations for accelerating immunization schedules for children specific to different ages. Infants still have maternal immunities for some diseases and cannot be given vaccines for others.

PREVENTING TRAVELER'S DIARRHEA

Traveler's diarrhea, contracted from contaminated food or water, is a miserable and not infrequent experience—definitely not one to write home about. You can prevent it and reduce your risk of cholera, typhoid, and hepatitis A by following simple rules about eating and drinking while traveling (see Chapter 21).

FOUR

Smoking and How to Stop

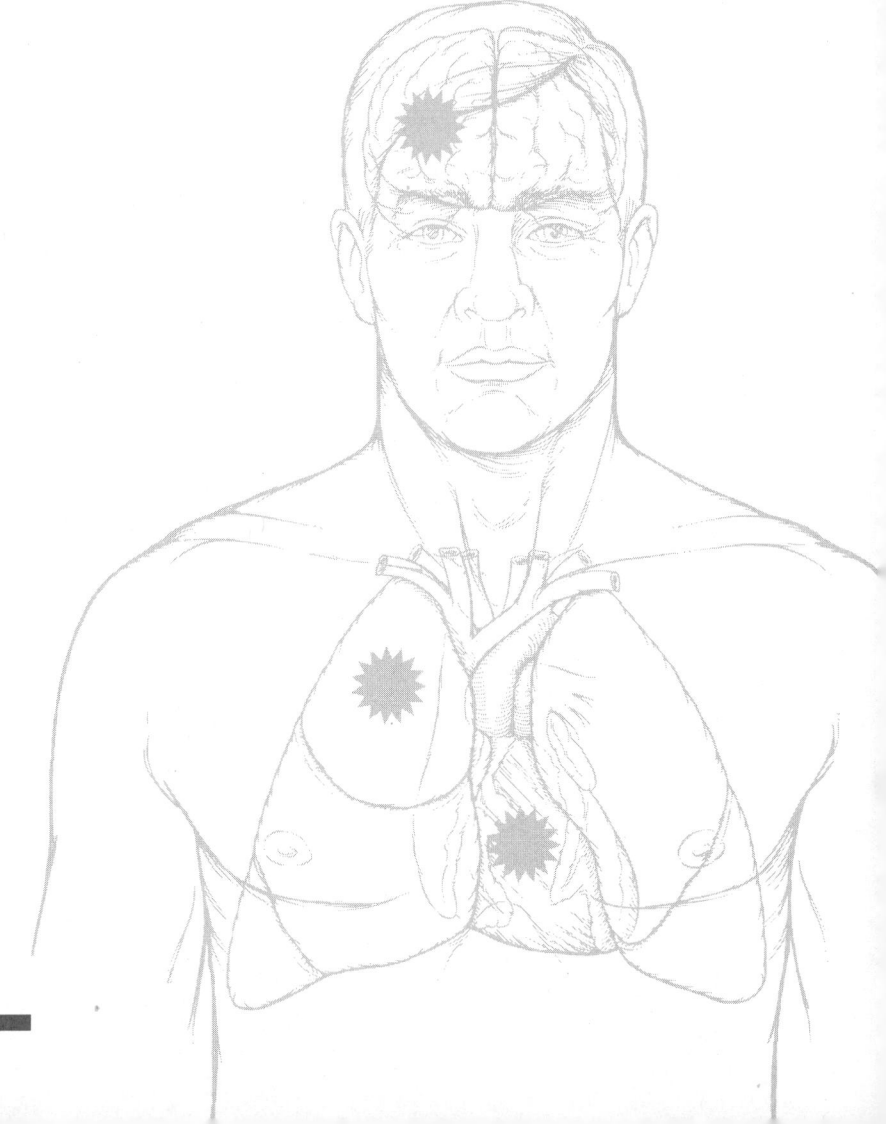

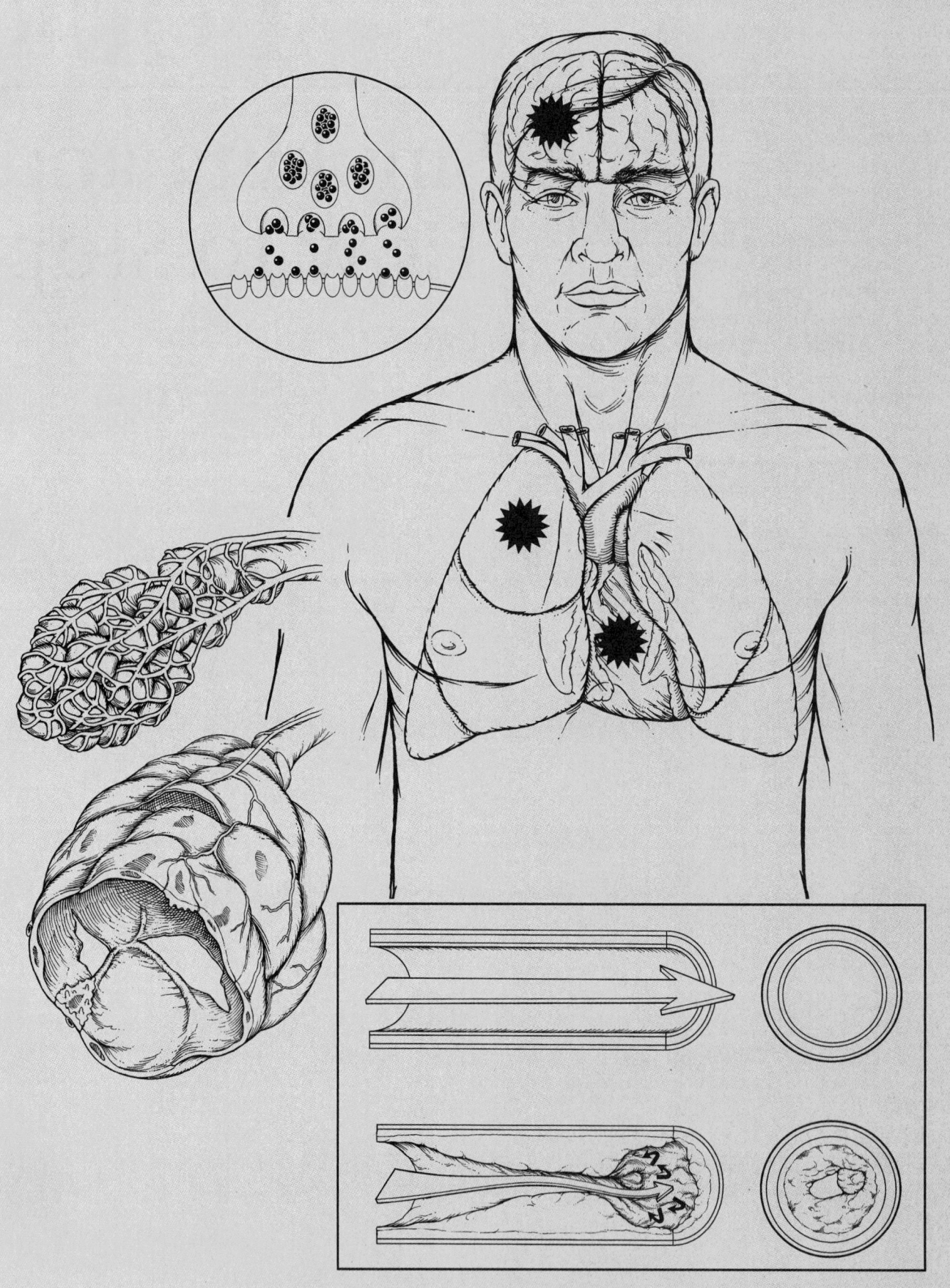

SMOKING AND HOW TO STOP

Kicking the Habit

This is a small chapter in a large book. But if you smoke and you are concerned about your health and the health of your family, this is the most important chapter in the book. The single most important thing you can do for your own health and the health of those around you is to stop smoking.

The problem for most tobacco users is not what action to take, but how to take it. As anyone who has tried to stop smoking will attest, kicking the habit is one of the hardest things you can do. But it can be done and is done every day. There are nearly as many people in the United States today who identify themselves as former smokers as there are people who smoke and the number of former smokers increases daily.

If you have tried to stop smoking on your own in the past and have met with limited success—a few days, weeks, or months without tobacco—you should not look at it as failure. You have greatly increased your odds of stopping the next time you try.

Most smokers, even in light of the truly adverse health consequences, find that smoking genuinely gives them pleasure. It is also genuinely hard to stop smoking. Nicotine is addicting and the craving for a cigarette can persist, even years after a smoker has stopped. Smokers are hesitant to go through the trauma of giving it up, saying, "You have to die of something." Invariably, smokers say this when they are still relatively healthy; they live to regret it when they find themselves bound to an oxygen tank, undergoing chemotherapy, or having open heart surgery at age 50.

THE PRIMARY HEALTH RISKS OF SMOKING

One in six deaths in the United States is tobacco-related. Tobacco use impairs the immune system, making users more susceptible to colds, flu, and every other non-tobacco-related illness.

If a single virus caused all the deaths, all the birth defects, and all the health care costs that tobacco does, governments all over the planet would move to find the virus, then find a vaccination or a cure. But tobacco is an important cash crop. Through huge campaign contributions and other outlays of money, the tobacco industry influences our government. Tobacco is the single most preventable cause of death in America, yet our government subsidizes its cultivation.

Cancer Tobacco smoke contains many powerful carcinogens (cancer-causing substances). Not only does tobacco smoke cause lung cancer and many other cancers of the mouth and throat, it also can cause cancer of the esophagus, stomach, bladder, kidneys, and pancreas. Tobacco smoke has been shown to cause cancers not only in smokers but in nonsmokers who are exposed to their smoke. Even smokeless tobacco products can cause cancer of the tongue, gums, throat, stomach, and esophagus.

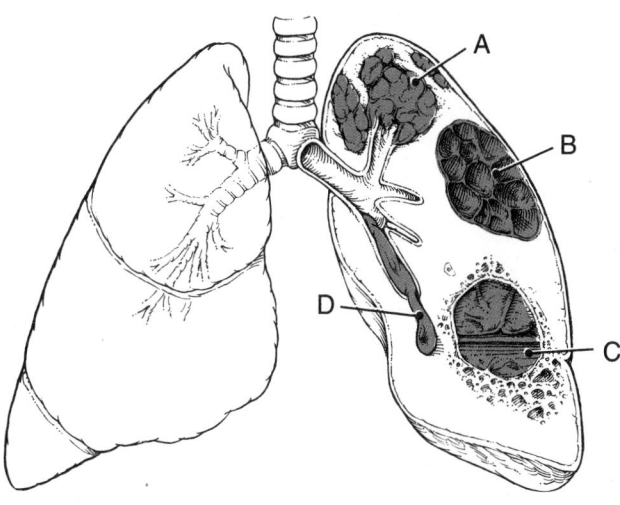

Smokers are at increased risk of lung cancer, lung abscess, emphysema, and chronic bronchitis. (A) Lung cancer is one of the most deadly cancers, since it has often spread beyond the lungs by the time it is discovered. (B) Smokers are more likely to develop pneumonia, which can lead to a lung abscess if untreated. (C) Emphysema is the result of damage to the small air sacs (alveoli) that allow oxygen to pass into the body. For that reason, people with severe emphysema often need to wear supplemental oxygen. (D) People with chronic bronchitis frequently cough up phlegm (sputum) and wheeze often.

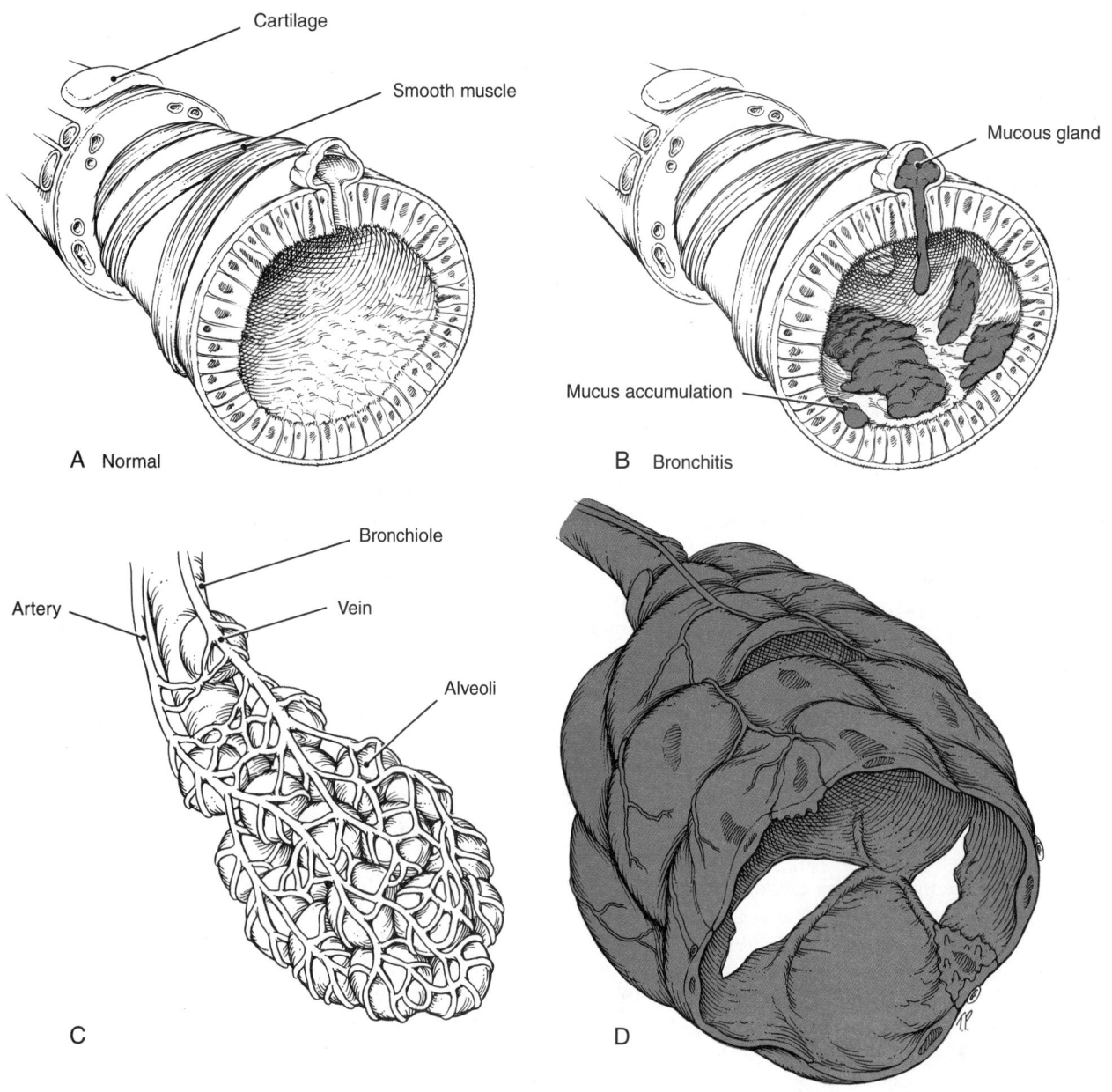

Cartilage

Smooth muscle

A   Normal

Mucous gland

Mucus accumulation

B   Bronchitis

Bronchiole

Artery

Vein

Alveoli

C

D

Smoking often causes bronchitis (B) and emphysema (D). Compared to the normal airway (A), smoking irritates and narrows the airways and increases production of mucus by the mucous glands. Compared to the normal air sacs (alveoli) (C), years of smoking can destroy the walls separating the alveoli, which makes them useless for transporting oxygen from the lungs to the body. These changes often lead to excessive coughing, mucus production, and difficulty breathing.

Other lung disease Smoking causes chronic obstructive pulmonary disease, or emphysema, an incurable though preventable lung disease characterized by shortness of breath, coughing, and a serious impairment of the ability of the lungs to work. Smoking worsens asthma, which is a chronic and potentially fatal disease that causes inflammation of the bronchial tubes, resulting in wheezing and shortness of breath. Smokers are also more prone to pneumonia.

Cardiovascular disease Although people most readily associate smoking with lung cancer and emphysema, more people die from cardiovascular (heart and blood vessel) conditions caused by smoking. In addition to nicotine, tobacco smoke contains thousands of other compounds, many of them acutely poisonous; carbon monox-

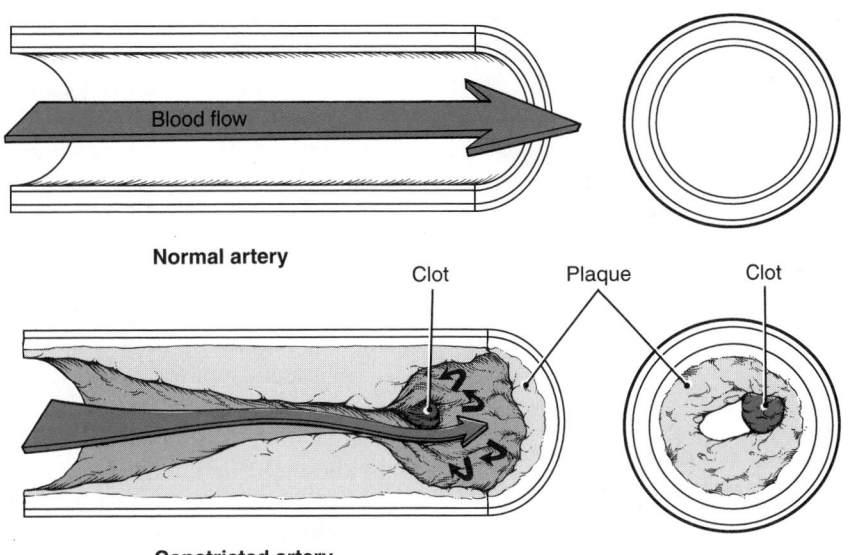

Normal artery

Clot Plaque Clot

Constricted artery

Atherosclerosis. Tobacco smoking accelerates the process of atherosclerosis, or hardening of the arteries, which is the deposition of fatty material in the walls of arteries that forms plaques. Growth of the plaque or blood clot formation over the plaque can obstruct blood flow and damage the organ that the artery supplies with blood.

ide is present in tobacco smoke in high concentrations. Carbon monoxide has a doubly poisonous effect when combined with nicotine. When you inhale cigarette smoke, carbon monoxide replaces the oxygen that should be in your red blood cells. Nicotine is a stimulant and causes the heart to work harder, but the oxygen the heart needs to do this extra work has been replaced by carbon monoxide, which forces the heart to work even harder for oxygen. Atherosclerosis (hardening of the arteries) and stroke are also caused by tobacco smoke.

The dangers of secondhand smoke

More people are thought to die annually from exposure to secondhand tobacco smoke than from AIDS. Although it is difficult to quantify the impact of exposure to

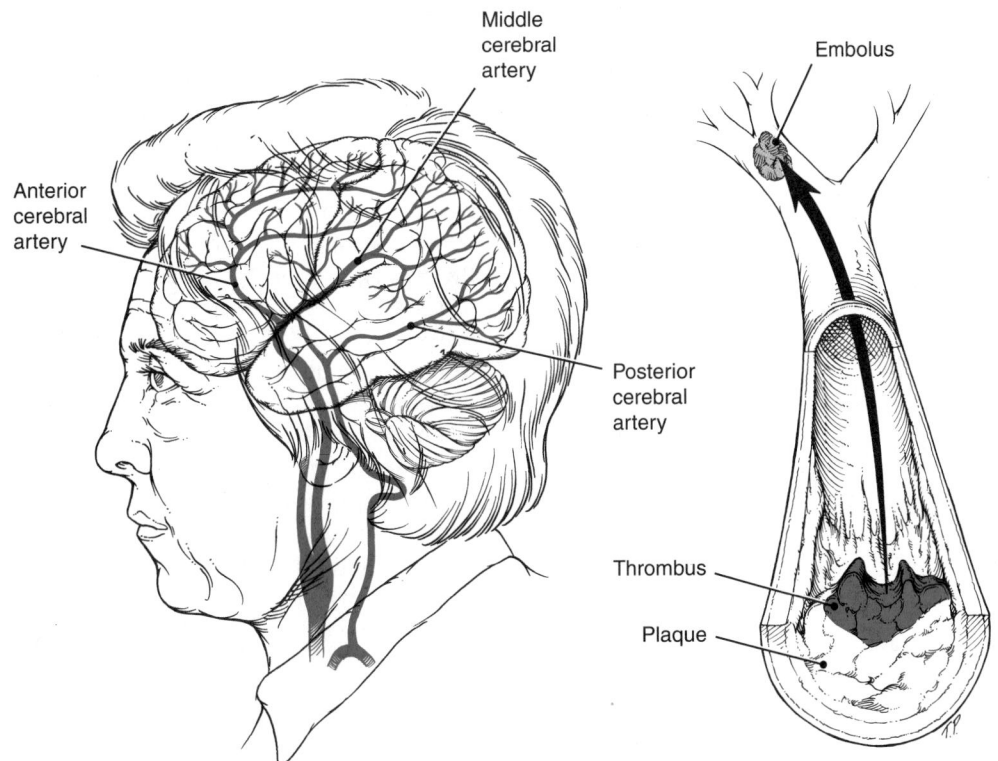

Middle cerebral artery

Anterior cerebral artery

Posterior cerebral artery

Embolus

Thrombus

Plaque

Atherosclerosis in the brain. Blockage of an artery in the brain (cerebral artery) typically results in a stroke. Plaque formation causes narrowing of a cerebral artery, which can be completely obstructed by a blood clot (thrombus), or part of the plaque can break off (embolus) and block blood flow further into the brain. Blockage of blood flow from a thrombus or embolus is called a stroke. The risk of heart attack and stroke falls significantly after a person stops smoking.

secondhand smoke precisely, studies done on children whose mothers were very light smokers demonstrate that even the blood of these children showed significantly higher markers for the presence of nicotine than that of children whose parents did not

WHAT IS NICOTINE?

Nicotine—the active, addictive ingredient in tobacco—is, in large doses, a fatal poison that is used as an agricultural insecticide.

In smaller doses nicotine is a stimulant of the central nervous system (CNS) and acts in a manner similar to amphetamines and cocaine. Nicotine stimulates production of dopamine, the neurotransmitter most closely associated with excitement and arousal.

Nicotine affects what is known as the autonomic nervous system, or that part of the nervous system that controls the functions we do not have to think about consciously, such as breath, heartbeat, and digestion. Within seconds of inhaling, the smoker will experience a quickening of the heartbeat, a constriction of the blood vessels, and the euphoric state characteristic of stimulants. First-time smokers may experience nausea or diarrhea, transitory effects that are replaced quickly by the high of nicotine.

Studies show that nicotine has "good" effects. It has been shown to improve concentration, relieve boredom and anxiety, and reduce the tendency toward aggression and irritation. It may also increase alertness. These effects may in part account for the difficulty many have in stopping. But all these positive effects can be obtained elsewhere, without the cost to health. ■

Tobacco has powerful effects on the brain that are mediated through its effects on dopamine in the junctions between nerve cells. (A) In a nonsmoker, dopamine crosses the nerve junction (synaptic cleft) and activates a receptor on the other side. Some of the dopamine does not make it all the way across the cleft and is broken down in the junction by enzymes. (B) In a smoker, more receptors are activated on the opposite side of the junction because much more dopamine travels down the nerve fiber and less is broken down in the junction. The end result is an increase in the amount of dopamine in the brain. When a smoker stops smoking, dopamine levels fall and trigger the symptoms of withdrawal.

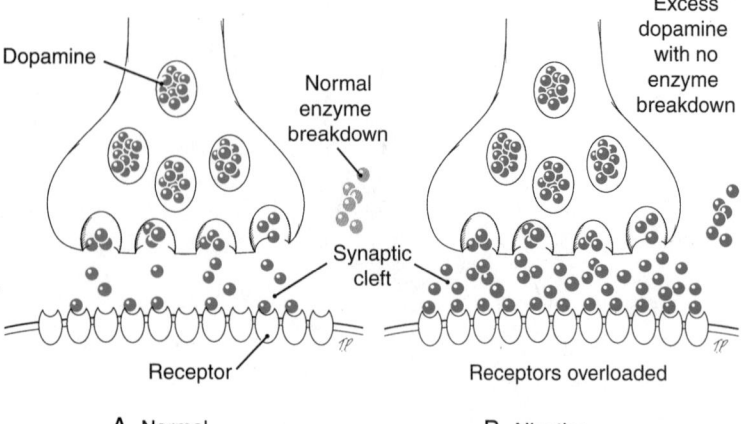

smoke. In households where both parents smoke, the risk is multiplied. Children who are continually exposed to cigarette smoke in early life are at higher risk for chronic bronchitis, asthma, and pneumonia, all of which are potentially fatal. In certain jurisdictions in the United States, the presence of smokers in a household has sufficed as justification for changing custody arrangements from the smoking parent to the nonsmoking parent.

While most of the smoke that cigarette, pipe, and cigar smokers expose themselves to is filtered, or not even inhaled, the sidestream smoke that nonsmokers are exposed to comes primarily from the burning end of the cigarette, cigar, or pipe, with no benefit of filtration. Therefore sidestream smoke has a much higher, undiluted concentration of "tar," nicotine, and all the other gases that make up tobacco smoke. People with respiratory problems or heart conditions should be particularly careful to limit their exposure to sidestream smoke.

DO "LIGHT" CIGARETTES REDUCE THE RISKS OF SMOKING?

Many people believe that smoking "light" cigarettes reduces the chance of getting cancer or heart disease. The predominance of light cigarettes on the market reflects this belief—6 out of 10 packs of cigarettes sold are low tar and nicotine brands. However, research indicates that there is little difference in the risks associated with regular cigarettes and the light varieties. Government procedures for testing the tar and nicotine content of cigarettes, which are overseen by the Federal Trade Commission, but performed by the tobacco companies themselves, have not changed since 1967. This is true even though the manner in which cigarettes are designed and manufactured has changed considerably since the 1960s.

If you smoked a light cigarette exactly the same way a smoking machine does, you would probably get the same amounts of tar and nicotine as the machine measures. However, the machine, unlike the smoker, has no blood level of nicotine that it must reach in order to feel satisfied. Studies show that smokers, consciously or unconsciously, adjust the way that they smoke or the amount that they smoke in order to maintain levels of nicotine in their blood. Light cigarettes frequently have pinholes punched in the filter. When the machine smokes the cigarette, air is brought in with the smoke, diluting it. People often compensate for the diluted smoke by covering the pinholes with their fingers or lips, or by drawing more deeply or frequently on the cigarette. In some cases, smoking light cigarettes may actually cause the smoker to inhale more tar and nicotine.

STEPS TOWARD STOPPING

You will need some time to prepare yourself mentally for the psychological and physical jolt that stopping can bring. There are many different approaches that you can take, but set out with a plan.

- Talk to your doctor about nicotine-replacement therapy and see if it is right for you (see below). If stopping smoking has proven too emotionally difficult for you in the past, ask your doctor if there is some other medical therapy that might be helpful to you, such as antidepressants (see Smoking and Depression, page 85). Your doctor may know of a support group program that you might enter and should also be able to give you advice on diet and exercise.

- Talk to your employer, religious leader, or one of the community organizations that sponsor smoking cessation programs. For addresses of organizations, see Tobacco Cessation Help, page 84.

- Consider alternative methods such as hypnosis or acupuncture. Although there is little scientific evidence to support their use, some former smokers have had success with these methods.

- If you are not the type to join groups and think the only way for you is to stop cold turkey, construct a plan (see page 84). Remember many people have successfully stopped smoking on their own.

NICOTINE REPLACEMENT THERAPY

Nicotine replacement therapy is designed to help smokers stop smoking by tapering off nicotine gradually, usually over a three-

WHAT IS "TAR"?

The "tar" in cigarette smoke is not actually tar but a sticky, tar-like residue of up to 4,000 compounds that make up tobacco smoke. Lung tissue is lined with a layer of mucus that rests on fine, protective hairs called cilia. The cilia beat in a sweeping motion, which protects the fragile lungs much the same way that eyelashes protect the eyes. The cilia stop incoming particles or microorganisms from embedding themselves in the lungs and then sweep them out.

The gases in cigarette smoke interfere with the cilia. Inhaled cigarette smoke coats the lungs with tarry residue and exposes the cilia to more particles than they can handle. With the cilia unable to clean the lungs, lung tissue gets gummed with tar. The many potent carcinogens (cancer-causing substances) in the tar remain in the lungs and are replenished each time a smoker lights up. Our bodies are exposed to carcinogens every day; generally defenses such as the cilia and the immune system round up these carcinogens and send them packing. Tobacco smoke, however, suppresses the immune system as well as disables the cilia, causing prolonged exposure to carcinogens. ■

month period, using nicotine gum (Nicorette) or the transdermal nicotine patch ("the patch"). Instead of going cold turkey, you stop smoking and exchange your cigarettes for either the gum or the patch to soften the impact of stopping. While the gum and the patch are less harmful than cigarettes, nicotine is still a poison and in these forms may still cause many of the complications that smokeless tobacco causes.

The patch delivers nicotine directly through the skin. For some people, the patch is more effective than gum because it is available in different strengths. You apply a patch to a bare, unobtrusive area of skin. The nicotine in the patch is delivered into the bloodstream through the capillaries at the surface of the skin. The patch keeps blood levels of nicotine constant throughout the day, so you should never have a craving. The patch may cause insomnia, in which case it can be removed at night and replaced in the morning.

The latest development in nicotine replacement therapy is nicotine nasal spray, which has been shown to be as effective as

TOBACCO CESSATION HELP

- Nicotine Anonymous World Services
  P.O. Box 591777
  San Francisco, CA 94159-1777
  Phone: (415) 750-0328

- The Phoenix Institute
  3459 East Livingston Ave.
  Columbus, OH 43227
  Phone: (800) 346-6356
  http://www.PhoenixInst.com
  e-mail: GeorgeL@PhoenixInst.com

- American Cancer Society
  1599 Clifton Rd., N.E.
  Atlanta, GA 30329
  Phone: (800) ACS-2345
  http://www.cancer.org

- American Heart Association
  1280 Parker Rd.
  Denver, CO 80231
  Phone: (800) AHA-USA1

- American Lung Association
  1740 Broadway
  New York, NY 10019-4274
  Phone: (212) 315-8700

- National Cancer Institute
  9000 Rockville Pike
  Building 31, 4A-18
  Bethesda, MD 20892
  Phone: (800) 4CANCER

- National Heart, Lung, and Blood Institute
  Information Center
  P.O. Box 30105
  Bethesda, MD 20824-0105
  Phone: (301) 951-3260

- Quitnet
  http://www.quitnet.org

- Office on Smoking and Health
  4770 Buford Highway, N.E.
  Mail Stop K-50
  Atlanta, GA 30341-3724
  Phone: (800) CDC-1331

- US Department of Veterans Affairs
  Veterans Health Services and Research
  Administration
  302 West Washington St., Room E-12
  Indianapolis, IN 46204-2738
  Phone: (317) 232-3910 ■

the gum and the patch. Because the nasal spray may cause sinus irritation, it is not recommended for people who have asthma, allergies, or any other sinus condition.

TIPS ON STOPPING COLD TURKEY

- Select a day for stopping. Choose a date no more than 2 months away. Think of it as the first day of the rest of your life. You might select a date of particular importance: your birthday, your child's birthday, your wedding anniversary.

- Mark your date on every calendar you come in contact with. Ask your friends and even your boss to mark it on their calendars. Tell friends, co-workers, everyone you can think of, that your day is coming.

- Some smoking cessation programs advocate keeping a little journal with you and taking a moment to write down the date, time of day, and reason every time you light up. If possible, jot down a few notes after smoking and analyze what a given cigarette has done for you. This will show you your pattern of smoking and will provide you with a written record of when and why you smoke, making it simpler to avoid the smoking cues. For example, if you smoke after a meal you can devise a strategy to sidestep that cue, such as popping a piece of sugar-free gum in your mouth.

- Before your stopping day arrives, try different methods of preparing for it. Try going smoke free for a single day prior to your stopping date. This will prove to you that no single day without tobacco is intolerable. Or you could try tapering off before your day arrives. Structure the tapering-off around the amount of time you go without a cigarette, rather than the number of cigarettes you smoke. For example, most smokers love the morning's first cigarette best. Your body has been deprived of nicotine for 8 hours; those first few puffs give you the biggest high of the day. Delay your first cigarette for 2 hours every day for a week. The following week, delay it 3 hours, and so on, as you work your way up to your stopping date.

- Before going cold turkey, some people force themselves to smoke as much as they possibly can right up until going to bed on their last smoking day. The idea is to make oneself literally sick of smoking.

- The night before your stopping day, soak all the cigarettes you have around the house in water and then toss them in the garbage. Get rid of matches, lighters, and ashtrays.

- Some people take the money they would have spent on cigarettes and save it for a special treat. Try to give yourself a concrete reminder of the rewards you are gaining by not smoking.

AVOIDING A RELAPSE

One of the most important things you can do after you have stopped is find ways to occupy yourself during moments when you might previously have lit up. Try candies, gum, or drinking water. Or try exercises every time you feel a desire for a cigarette. You'll be breathing better; doing a few toe-touches or pushups every time you want a cigarette will let you feel your improved breathing, which will remind you of your improved health.

Try to avoid drinking alcohol for the first several weeks or months after you stop smoking. Drinking and smoking go hand in hand. Drinking lowers inhibitions and makes it easier to say, "One cigarette can't hurt," which will lead to another and another. In the beginning, limit your participation in social situations that might cue smoking, and only return to them slowly and carefully. Avoid smoke-filled rooms. Eventually, you will wonder how you could ever have tolerated being around smokers.

Although most former smokers report having gone through withdrawal alone, support groups can be effective in helping you withstand your cravings. They can also build self-esteem, especially as you help others in the same way as you have been helped.

If you do relapse, do not worry. If you stayed smoke-free for a week, the cigarettes you did not smoke saved you as much as $15. And since you did not smoke those cigarettes, there is that much less tar in your lungs. You have also proven to yourself that you can stop.

Most smokers do not stop on the first try. In fact, for many people it takes four or five attempts. Even nicotine replacement therapy has a success rate of only about 28 percent. But if 100 people go on a nicotine replacement regimen and only 28 succeed

ONCE A SMOKER, ALWAYS A SMOKER?

It is useful to borrow from the Alcoholics Anonymous model: once an alcoholic, always an alcoholic. Once a smoker, always a smoker. Relapse is possible at any time. Some smokers have stopped for years only to begin again after some emotional cue. Relapse is prevented only through constant vigilance. The addict who can "just have one" and not become a full-blown addict again is rare.

No single day without smoking is intolerable. Take it one day at a time. ■

in stopping, that does not mean that the remaining 72 will never stop. It only means they did not stop that time. All of them wanted to stop or they would not have been in the program.

Knowing that most former smokers had limited success their first time out should help you. You have tried. Your attempt probably gave you insights into the difficulty of stopping. Why did you go back to smoking? Did you have a drink and decide one cigarette would not hurt? How can you alter your approach to smoking cessation in order to make it completely successful next time?

Smoking and Depression

Research indicates a correlation between depression and smoking; smokers are more likely to experience depression. Nicotine affects the same parts of the nervous system that are involved in clinical depression as well as obsessive-compulsive behaviors and eating disorders. Some smokers may use the stimulant effect of cigarettes to lift them out of depression. Because of this, people with depression may have more difficulty stopping smoking.

Some people with depression in smoking cessation programs have become nearly suicidal without nicotine. Trials are now under way in order to establish whether some of the new serotonin-enhancing anti-depression drugs such as sertraline (Zoloft) and fluoxetine (Prozac) are effective in making stopping easier for smokers who also suffer from depression. Bupropion (Zyban) is another antidepressant, unrelated to sertraline and fluoxetine, that has also been proven to be as effective as nicotine replacement products in helping people stop smoking.

Some doctors have begun to view nicotine replacement as a long-term therapy for people with depression who stop smoking, instead of one that lasts only for a matter of months. Although nicotine is a poison and is harmful in any form, it is considerably less harmful when delivered through gum, the patch, or nasal spray instead of in cigarette smoke.

IF YOU CANNOT STOP SMOKING NOW

There are steps you can take to guard your health even if you cannot or will not stop smoking. Make extra efforts regarding physical fitness, nutrition, and medical checkups as precautionary measures.

Exercise

The first step you can take toward improving your health and lowering your risks for heart and lung disease is to exercise regularly. Regular exercise will help you cut back on your smoking, make you feel better, and improve your overall cardiovascular health.

Talk to your physician and set up a regular exercise program—it could be as simple as a brisk, daily 30-minute walk.

Diet

If you are like many smokers, your diet is not particularly good. Because nicotine is an appetite suppressant you probably skip meals. An important step you can take toward improved health is to make sure you eat a balanced diet (see Chapter 1). Speak with your doctor about taking a vitamin supplement.

Calcium

For many years now we have been aware of the difficulties older women face with osteoporosis (see Osteoporosis, pages 331 and 654). This disintegration of the skeleton is much more serious in smokers than nonsmokers. Smokers use up more calcium daily than nonsmokers and therefore need to replenish it more frequently. Calcium supplements can be effective, although direct dietary sources such as milk and other dairy products are better.

Overall Health Maintenance

It is particularly important that smokers see their doctors for annual checkups to keep tabs on risk factors for cardiovascular problems and cancer. Your doctor should monitor your cholesterol levels, along with your blood pressure and other indicators for diseases of the blood vessels such as atherosclerosis. You should also have tests that would indicate the presence of cancers. Many cancers are curable if discovered and treated early. Regular eye exams for cataracts are also important if you smoke. ∎

Weight Gain

For many people, a significant roadblock to stopping smoking is potential weight gain. Statistically speaking, you are likely to gain some weight when you stop smoking. Do not let your vanity get the better of you. Smoking is far more harmful to your health than a slight weight gain.

The myth may once have been that smokers were people with oral fixations who simply replaced cigarettes with food when they stopped smoking. However, research shows that smoking makes people metabolize food differently. A smoker eating exactly the same diet as a nonsmoker will burn approximately 200 more calories than the nonsmoker. Not only is nicotine an appetite suppressant, it is also a metabolic poison that helps burn calories. If nicotine addiction did not kill you in the process, it would be a weight-loss wonder drug. However, it will kill you. You need to take a healthier approach than smoking to control your weight.

There are several steps that you can take to keep yourself from a precipitous weight gain when you stop smoking:

- Do not add to your stress by fretting over your weight. Tackle one issue at a time. Give yourself at least a week after stopping smoking before you embark on any kind of serious diet. An initial failure to keep your weight down might provoke an emotional low, which could lead quickly to a relapse.

- Exercise is a valuable way to keep weight down and spirits up. The runner's high you have heard about is real. Many people who once were addicted to nicotine now find themselves committed to athletics. If you have led a sedentary lifestyle and smoked heavily, however, do not start a strenuous exercise program without consulting your doctor.

- Drink plenty of water. Water can give you a feeling of fullness that will take the edge off hunger pangs and will also help clean out your system.

- If you feel a need for sweets, try sugarless gum or candy.

- If you need something to do with your hands, try keeping celery or carrot sticks cut into cigarette-sized pieces on hand. Carry them with you.

For Parents of Teenage Smokers

Probably one of the most disheartening discoveries parents can make is to find that their child has taken up smoking. A teenager who takes up smoking may want to differentiate himself from you, to try to prove that he is more of an adult than he really is, and more in control of his life than you might let him be. So what is the proper way to react when you discover that your teenager has been smoking?

Many parents' first reaction is anger, followed by a desire to take some kind of punitive action. This kind of reaction may stop some children from smoking, but for many adolescents this will only fuel their desire to smoke. Before taking action, take the time to analyze why your child has taken up smoking. It is likely that your child is using cigarettes in an effort to deal with some perceived inadequacy.

Rational explanation is not likely to penetrate your teenager's protective armor. Anger and threats will probably only set you at odds with your child; an adversarial relationship will benefit neither of you. You may feel that punishment is necessary. If you do, make certain that the punishment is within a framework of a larger plan that includes your involvement, such as arranging counseling with a social worker or someone from your church or temple. Most importantly, talk to your child. Remember that peer pressure is complex. Often a strong desire to belong puts children under pressure to conform to their peers. Peer groups are also powerful because they seem to offer a readily adoptable identity to teenagers concerned with finding their identities.

Find out if your child is using smoking to compensate for feelings of inadequacy and try to identify the roots of these feelings. Perhaps he is feeling overwhelmed by the pressures of school or of looming college admissions, and smoking seems to relieve the anxiety. Perhaps he feels socially awkward, even outcast. Perhaps your child sees cigarettes as a way to gain control over obesity. Keep in mind that the parts of the CNS that nicotine interferes with appear to be those that are also associated with depression, eating disorders, and obsessive-compulsive behaviors (see Smoking and Depression, page 85).

THE COSTS OF TOBACCO

- Percentage of minors who are successful in purchasing tobacco products: 67

- Estimated number of smokers in the United States: 52,000,000

- Number of packs of cigarettes smoked daily in the United States: 75,000,000

- Price of a pound of tobacco leaf, in dollars: 1

- Approximate number of cigarettes that can be made from a pound of tobacco: 600

- Number of cigarettes in a pack of cigarettes: 20

- Average cost of a pack of cigarettes, in dollars: 2.2

- Amount the tobacco industry spends annually on promotion, in dollars: 6,000,000,000

- Estimated annual health care expenditure in the United States on tobacco-related illness, in dollars: 5,000,000,000

- Number of days it takes to become addicted to nicotine: 7

- Approximate number of deaths annually in the United States from tobacco-related illness: 500,000

- Estimated number of deaths annually from secondhand smoke: 37,000

- Approximate percentage of people who take up smoking after age 25: 0

- Maximum number of years of education the average smoker has completed: 12

- Age at which many small children are able to recognize "Joe Camel" as a smoking-related icon: 3

- Age at which most teenagers begin experimenting with tobacco: 14.5

- Age by which teenage smokers have become regular users: 18

- Estimated number of young Americans who take up smoking daily: 3,000

- Rank of heart disease in killing smokers: 1

- Approximate number of years after stopping smoking until a former smoker's risk for heart disease returns to normal: 3 ■

The most important thing you can do is to get some kind of counseling for your child to discover what kind of inadequacy your child feels, so that you can look for other ways to address it. If your child feels weak or bullied, perhaps courses in karate or weight training may help build self-esteem. If your child feels out of control and is developing an eating problem or depression, he should have professional help.

If you smoke yourself, the problem is multiplied. You might take your child with you to your doctor, who could explain the kinds of deleterious effects smoking has on the body. Better still, resolve to help your child by helping yourself—the two of you can go through a smoking cessation program together.

Do not lose hope if your child continues to smoke despite all your efforts. Many a 17-year-old who will not listen to reason turns into a sensible 21-year-old who successfully kicks the habit.

TARGETING CHILDREN

The best customer is a life-long customer. Although it claims otherwise, the tobacco industry aims to start smokers young. People who do not begin smoking while they are children or adolescents are unlikely to start later in life.

Eighty percent of smokers tried tobacco before their eighteenth birthday. Teenage smokers, on average, begin experimenting with tobacco between ages 14 and 15 and become regular smokers by the time they are 18. It is estimated that teenagers consume more than half a billion packs of cigarettes a year, as well as more than 25 million containers of smokeless tobacco.

Children are more susceptible to the messages paid for by the billions that the tobacco industry spends on advertising each year. They include not only magazine ads and billboards, but also giveaway merchandise such as T-shirts, hats, and tote bags, all with logos that appeal to fashion-conscious adolescents. Tobacco companies sponsor sporting and musical events, many of which are televised. This allows the tobacco industry to get around the ban on television advertising, while forging an association between a cigarette brand and activities that teenagers admire. All of these ads and promotions sell lifestyle more than the product itself; the implied message is that to enjoy the lifestyle, all you have to do is smoke the brand. To adolescents and children who want to differentiate themselves from their parents, who are subject to peer pressure, and who are trying to appear more adult, the models offered by tobacco advertising are powerful magnets.

Children tend to view themselves as immortal; to them cigarettes seem harmless enough. They also see lots of people around who smoke but who appear quite healthy. Most children—like nearly everyone who starts smoking—do not see themselves as beginning a long-term addiction. It is only when they try to stop that they realize that they are hooked.

Alcohol and Substance Abuse

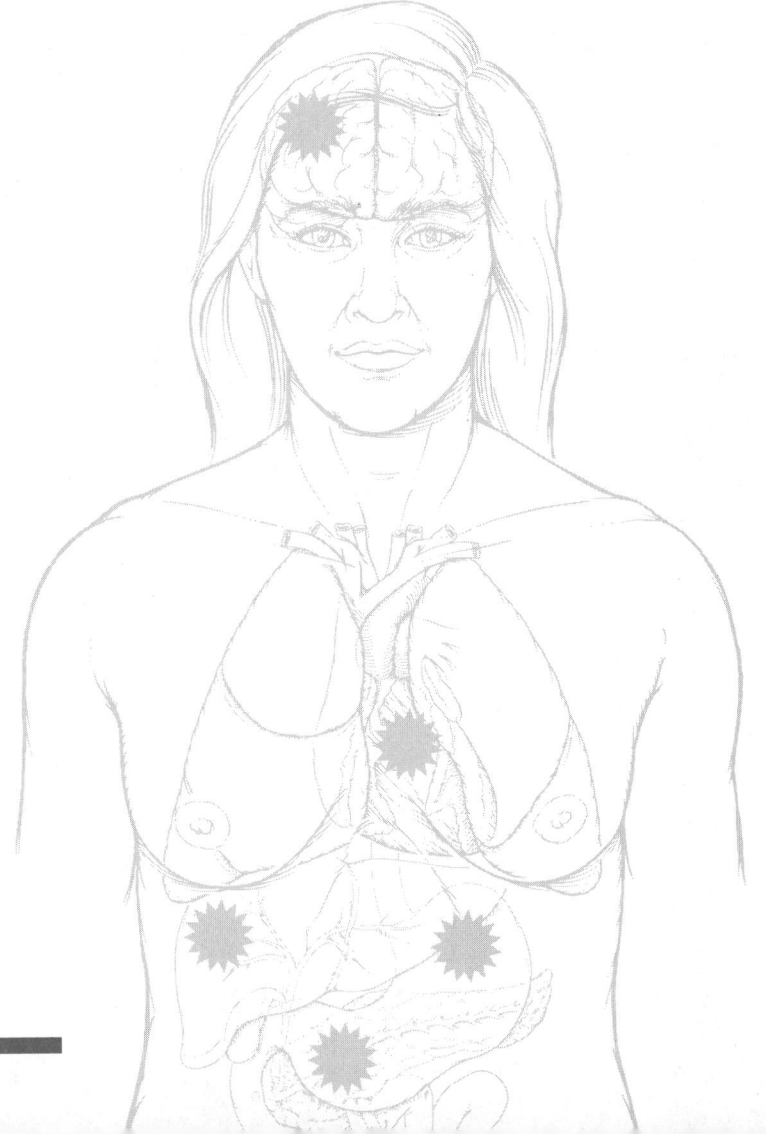

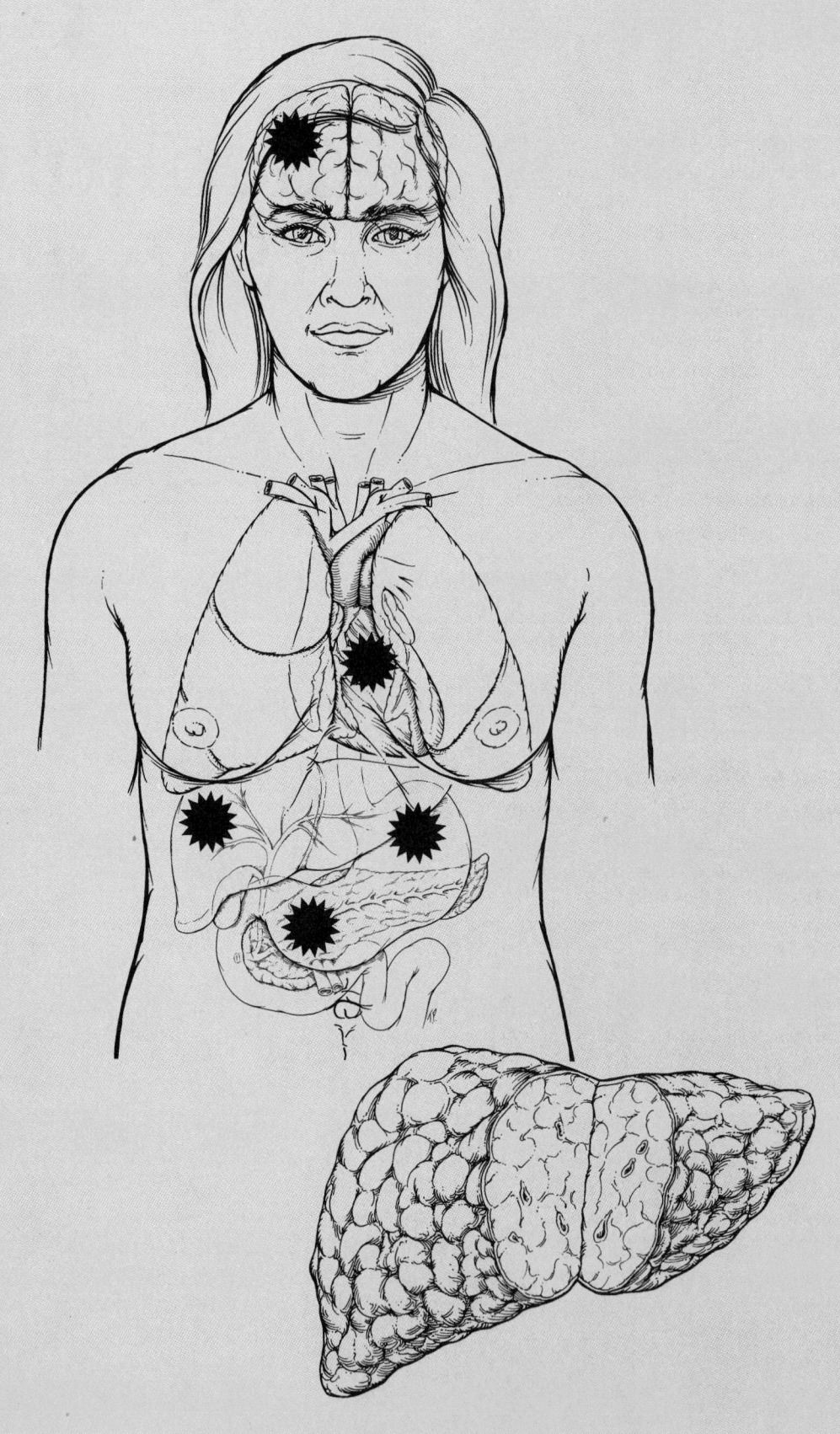

ALCOHOL AND SUBSTANCE ABUSE

Is There a Problem?

If you are worried that someone you love has a problem with alcohol or other drugs, they may well have one. If you are worried that your own alcohol or other drug usage has escalated to a problem level, it is quite possible that it has. The hallmark of problem use of alcohol or any other drug is an awareness that the drug is affecting the quality of the user's life or the quality of life of the user's family.

Problem use of alcohol or other drugs does not necessarily mean addiction or dependence. A person with an alcohol problem may not wake up every morning needing a drink. A person with a drug problem may go to work without getting high. But research has demonstrated that *any* use of psychoactive drugs has the potential to cause damage; psychoactive refers to the ability of a chemical to change a person's state of mind rapidly—to euphoria, excitability, depression, or another mood.

How can you tell if use of alcohol or another drug is problem usage? This chapter will help you determine when there is a problem and offer guidelines on how to resolve it. For the purposes of this discussion we will use alcoholism throughout the chapter to refer to the harmful use of alcohol—the most commonly abused drug. Our comments, however, are also applicable to the harmful use of other substances.

WHAT IS MODERATE ALCOHOL USE?

Moderate, or safe, drinking is not easy to define, but it should not be confused with social drinking. Social drinking is that which is acceptable in the particular group in which it occurs. Social drinking at a church dinner is considerably different from social drinking at a fraternity keg party. Moderate drinking is drinking that does not generally cause problems, either for the drinker or for society—the drinker's family, friends, as well as others who may be tangentially involved, such as other drivers on the road.

It is difficult to specify precisely how much alcohol can be safely consumed because a given dose of alcohol will affect different people differently. However, numerical definitions of moderate drinking do exist. Guidelines put forth jointly by the US Department of Agriculture and the US Department of Health and Human Services define moderate drinking as no more than one drink a day for most women and no more than two drinks a day for most men. A standard drink is generally considered to be 12 oz of beer, 5 oz of wine, or 1.5 oz of 80-proof distilled spirits. Each of these drinks contains roughly the same amount of absolute alcohol, approximately 0.5 oz or 12 g.

The difference between acceptable amounts of alcohol for men and women reflects research findings that women become more intoxicated than men at equivalent doses of alcohol. This results, in part, from an enzyme in stomach tissue that breaks down alcohol before it can reach the bloodstream and cause intoxication. The enzyme is present in both males and females but it is four times more active in males. In addition, women have proportionately more fat and less body water than men. Because alcohol is dissolved in water in cells throughout the body, a given dose of alcohol becomes more highly concentrated in relation to the total body water of a woman than of a man. Since the proportion of body water decreases with age, a limit of one drink a day for seniors is recommended. Recent studies have reported an increase in alcoholism in the elderly. If you are over age 65 and find it difficult to limit yourself to one drink a day, consult your doctor, who may be able to help you before a serious problem with alcohol develops. Your doctor can also address any underlying problems such as depression that may be contributing factors to the urge to drink.

The guidelines for moderate alcohol use exclude the following persons who should not consume alcoholic beverages at all: women who are pregnant or trying to conceive, men who are trying to become fathers, people who plan to drive or engage in other activities that require attention or skill, people taking medication including over-the-counter (OTC) medications, recovering alcoholics, and people under the age 21. Alcohol use should also be avoided by people with certain medical conditions such as peptic ulcer. Drinking should be avoided completely by people who have been diagnosed with alcoholism.

WHAT IS ALCOHOLISM?

Once viewed as a sign of weak character, alcoholism is now known to be a disease,

WARNING: COMBINING ALCOHOL AND MEDICATIONS

The combination of alcohol with many prescription and OTC medications can be fatal. This warning is directed not only to alcohol abusers, but also to those who drink alcohol in moderation. Alcohol in any amount has the potential for dangerous interaction with many medications.

Drugs that depress the central nervous system—opioids, sedatives, and hypnotics—can combine with alcohol to create other compounds that multiply the effect of both drugs. The result is an increased likelihood of overdose, as well as automobile and household accidents.

OTC medications can have potentially fatal interactions with alcohol. One of the most dangerous and too often ignored is the interaction between alcohol and OTC pain relievers. Drinking alcohol regularly even at modest levels can activate certain enzymes that break acetaminophen into chemicals that are potentially damaging to the liver, even if the acetaminophen is taken at recommended dosages. The amount of alcohol that it takes to cause this reaction varies from person to person. To be safe, anyone who has more than two alcoholic drinks a day should not use acetaminophen.

Alcohol can also interact with:

- Antihistamines, exaggerating any drowsiness the medications can cause
- Nonsteroidal anti-inflammatory drugs (NSAIDs) such as ibuprophen and similar OTC pain relievers
- Sedatives and hypnotics (sleeping pills)
- Cardiovascular medication
- Antiulcer medication
- Antiseizure medication
- Antipsychotic medication
- Antidiabetic medication
- Antidepressants

There are nearly 3,000 prescription medications available, and millions of different individuals taking millions of potential combinations of them. If you have any questions about the medications you are taking and the likelihood that they might interact with alcohol, or with one another, consult with your doctor or your pharmacist. They should be aware of all the drugs you are taking, OTC as well as prescription, and will be able to assess the potential interactions. Be especially careful if you are a senior, because many drug-drug and alcohol-drug interactions are more extreme in older adults. If you see more than one doctor, make sure each knows all the medications you take. Also listen to your pharmacist. Most prescription drugs that may have hazardous interactions with alcohol are packaged at the pharmacy with clear warning labels. Do not ignore these warnings. Whenever you are in doubt, consult your doctor. ■

ALCOHOL AND DRUG ABUSE IN THE UNITED STATES

In a national household survey in 1993, 14 percent of adults ages 18 to 25 and 3 percent of adults over age 35 reported using illicit drugs within the last month. Occasional use of marijuana accounts for a large proportion of reported drug use, but many drug users use other illicit drugs including cocaine, heroin, phencyclidine (PCP or angel dust), methaqualone (Quaaludes), and hallucinogens; legal drugs not prescribed by a doctor including amphetamines, benzodiazepines, barbiturates, and anabolic steroids; or inhalants including amyl nitrate, butyl nitrate, gasoline, nitrous oxide, glue, and other solvents. An estimated 5 million Americans smoke marijuana at least once a week, almost half a million use cocaine weekly, and over half a million have used heroin or other injectable drugs in the past year. Some researchers estimate that up to half a million Americans are addicted to heroin and 1 to 1.6 million currently use drugs intravenously. Drug use is more common among men, the unemployed, adults who have not completed high school, and urban residents.

Heavy drinking, or more than 5 drinks a day, 5 days a week, is reported by 10 percent of adult men and 2 percent of women. The discrepancy may be slightly misleading, because alcohol is metabolized differently in men and women (see What is Moderate Alcohol Use?, page 91). On average, 5 drinks for a man are equivalent to 10 drinks for a woman.

In large community surveys that used detailed interviews, the prevalence of alcohol abuse and dependence in 1992 broke down as follows.

Men

Ages 18 to 29	17 to 24 percent
Ages 30 to 44	11 to 14 percent
Ages 45 to 64	6 to 8 percent
Over age 65	1 to 3 percent

Women

Ages 18 to 29	4 to 10 percent
Ages 30 to 44	2 to 4 percent
Ages 45 to 64	1 to 2 percent
Over age 65	less than 1 percent

The statistics above indicate that problem usage is frequently outgrown. What seemed like a good idea in high school or college—getting stoned, drinking to blackout levels, using hallucinogens—can seem childish and foolish to an adult with substantial responsibilities at work and at home. But if you take any 10 individuals from the ages 18 to 25 who occasionally engage in excessive drinking or drugging, it is impossible to predict who will or will not outgrow the behavior, or who might be at risk for such behavior later in life.

As statistics demonstrate, heavy drinking is not the norm in the general population. Less than one in four Americans has trouble controlling the use of alcohol. If you notice that you are still using alcohol or other drugs the way you did in your younger years while all your former party-mates have settled down to moderation or abstinence, you should contact your doctor to discuss your usage and whether treatment is warranted. ■

one of the single most destructive diseases in the world. Alcoholism costs billions of dollars annually in medical expense, countless lost hours in work time, and innumerable lives lost due to complications, automobile accidents, and suicide. It cuts across all social classes, afflicting the wealthy and the poor.

Many people mistakenly believe that dependence under any circumstance equals addiction. This is not the case. Terminally ill cancer patients, for example, may need morphine regularly to cope with physical pain, but this does not make them morphine addicts. People with epilepsy often depend on powerful barbiturates to control potential seizures; however, they are not addicted. Addiction involves both physical and emotional dependence that causes serious disruption in other aspects of a person's life.

The conventional view for decades was that alcoholism is an addiction to, or physical dependence on, alcohol; however, scientific viewpoints on problem usage of alcohol or other drugs have been evolving in recent years. Although alcoholism has traditionally been viewed as a disease of addiction, there is a growing recognition that addiction represents only the extreme end of problem alcohol or other drug use. For many people with alcoholism, actual physiological dependence is only a late stage of the disease and is preceded by many years of problem use. Many problem drinkers have medical or social problems attributable to alcohol without typical signs of full-blown addiction; others are at risk for future problems due to hazardous drinking, whether it takes the form of chronic consumption or frequent binges.

EVALUATING THE PROBLEM

One of the first and most important steps in treating the disease of alcoholism is admitting that there could be a problem. It is essential that you understand that alcoholism, or other drug abuse, is a disease. It is not your fault that you have the disease, but it is your responsibility to seek treatment for it.

Alcoholism is highly treatable. Your chances for recovery and for turning your life around are excellent, regardless of whether you are engaged in hazardous use or are fully dependent and experience withdrawal symptoms if you try to stop. Make an appointment to see your doctor. If you speak openly and honestly, your doctor can help you determine if you have a problem with alcohol and if necessary offer suggestions for treatment.

You should also regularly assess your patterns of alcohol consumption yourself. Frankly consider how much you have been drinking and if you have been drinking more lately. Stop and think if your drinking has hurt yourself or others. Ask yourself why you drink. With regular, honest self-screening, you may discover signs that your alcohol use is potentially dangerous. Just as you would for a suspicious lump on your body, you should contact your doctor and discover if the warning sign is cause for further testing or treatment. The Alcohol Use Disorders Identification Test (AUDIT) was designed to help doctors detect problem use of alcohol or other drugs, but you can use it yourself to gauge whether your own drinking or drug use is dangerous (see page 94).

Often problem drinking can be precipitated by a major life crisis—a divorce,

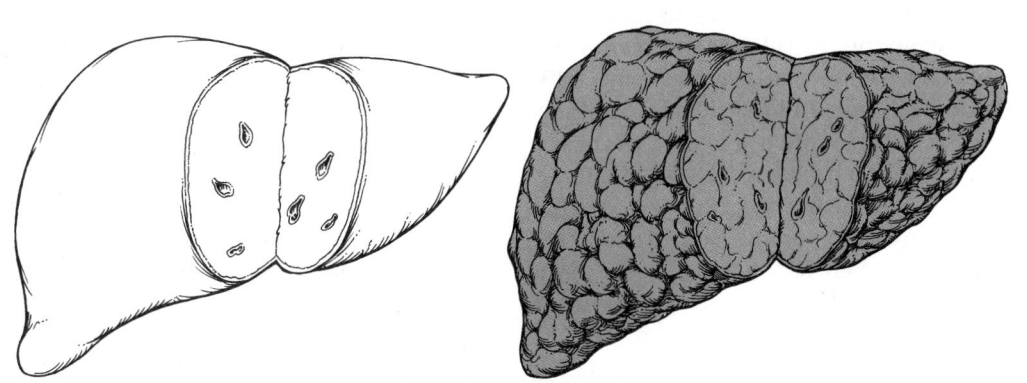

Chronic damage of liver cells, usually from drinking alcohol. leads to scarring, dysfunction, and eventually failure of the liver.

AUDIT: ALCOHOL USE DISORDERS IDENTIFICATION TEST

POINTS PER ANSWER	0	1	2	3	4
How often do you have a drink containing alcohol?	Never	Monthly or less	2–4 times a month	2–3 times a week	4 or more times a week
How many drinks do you have on typical day of drinking?	None	1–2	3–4	5–6	7–9
How often do you have 6 or more drinks on one occasion?	Never	Less than monthly	Monthly	Weekly	Daily or almost daily
How often during the last year have you found that you were unable to stop drinking once you had started?	Never	Less than monthly	Monthly	Weekly	Daily or almost daily
How often during the last year have you failed to do what was normally expected of you because of drinking?	Never	Less than monthly	Monthly	Weekly	Daily or almost daily
How often during the last year have you needed a first drink in the morning to get yourself going after a heavy drinking session?	Never	Less than monthly	Monthly	Weekly	Daily or almost daily
How often during the last year have you had a feeling of guilt or remorse after drinking?	Never	Less than monthly	Monthly	Weekly	Daily or almost daily
How often during the last year have you been unable to remember what happened the night before because you had been drinking?	Never	Less than monthly	Monthly	Weekly	Daily or almost daily
Have you or someone else been injured as a result of your drinking?	Never		Yes, but not in the last year		Yes, during the last year
Has a relative, doctor, or other health care provider been concerned about your drinking or suggested you cut down?	Never		Yes, but not in the last year		Yes, during, the last year

A score of higher than 8 out of the possible 40 points suggests the presence of problem drinking and indicates the need for more in-depth assessment. A score higher than 10 is an even greater indicator that problem drinking exists.

the death of a loved one, or the diagnosis of disease. Problem drinking can build from responsible, moderate usage that grows to harmful levels when a person's life is disrupted by difficult changes. A person can go for virtually the entirety of her adult life having one glass of wine with dinner and then find that retirement, loneliness, or some other emotional change can lead her to problem drinking. Similarly, a college student may initially use an amphetamine to stay up late to study for exams and then fall into using the drug when she goes out dancing, wants to lose a few pounds, or feels a little down. Neither of these people has necessarily become addicted, but clearly their use is becoming a problem and could easily become dependence. However, the danger is that both would deny the possibility of a problem. Denial is a complex process that contributes both to the escalation to problem use and to the continuance of addiction.

DENIAL AND MOTIVATION

Denial pushes the user of alcohol down the slippery slope of abuse; motivation is the equipment with which he climbs back up to reclaim life. Denial is measured by how much a person is willing to ignore their desire for a drink and the problems that substance use is causing in their lives. Motivation is measured by how much a person wants to retake her life, work, and family.

Denial is a complex mechanism. Perhaps one of the reasons alcoholism has been judged on moral grounds is the confounding power of denial, which can manifest in a person almost like a second personality. In a sense, alcohol acts like an invading, self-perpetuating organism. In order to maintain its hold on its "host," it fools a person into believing that there is no alcohol problem, despite considerable evidence to the contrary, including diminishing work performance, scrapes with the law, and blackouts. There are as many manifestations of denial as there are people with alcoholism. People make irrational excuses for their behavior: I am not an alcoholic because I do not drink in the morning; I am not an alcoholic because I drink alcohol-free beer every other day; because I have never passed out; because I never drink directly from the bottle; because I drink the same amount as anyone. These excuses are themselves a signal of serious disease. Denial can also work to compound alcohol abuse with other problems. People who abuse alcohol are more likely to smoke cigarettes, use other drugs, and have a poor diet than those who do not. People who abuse alcohol are 35 times more likely to use cocaine, 17 times more likely to use sedatives, 13 times more likely to use opioids, 12 times more likely to use hallucinogens, 11 times more likely to use stimulants, and 6 times more likely to use marijuana and related drugs. Surveys show that at least 90 percent of people with alcoholism are nicotine dependent.

Denial is also present in the co-alcoholic or codependent relationship. Out of a misplaced sense of love or loyalty, a spouse or child will minimize or completely deny that their loved one has a problem, or that the loved one's disease is creating problems for others. Often, doctor and family must work to break down denial by confronting the person with alcoholism with the reality and the gravity of the situation. Sometimes a formal intervention can accomplish this (see page 103). Research shows that motivation is crucial to successful treatment, even if the motivation comes from an external source rather than an inner desire to overcome the disease. The threat of losing one's family, going to jail, or losing a job can be a significant motivating factor for many people. Many employers have found it to their benefit to install employee help programs; for every dollar spent on treatment and prevention in employee assistance programs, it is estimated that employers save $4 to $7.

Although the threat of loss may motivate some people to seek treatment, it will not necessarily do so for everyone. "Hitting bottom" is sometimes the only way to break down persistent denial. Of course, hitting bottom means different things to different people. One individual may hit bottom when she wrecks the family car; another may be homeless, begging and stealing in order to buy a bottle, and still not have hit bottom.

Group therapy, such as that offered in treatment facilities and Alcoholics Anonymous (AA) meetings, is perhaps the most powerful tool in breaking down denial and strengthening motivation to get and stay sober. Most of these groups are conducted by recovering alcoholics who have been through the process of denial themselves and are particularly well equipped to spot denial in others and help them overcome it. Denial is also a fundamental reason why recovery is an ongoing, lifelong process. Even recovering alcoholics who have been sober for years can fall into patterns of diseased thinking—"Just one drink can't hurt"—which can lead to relapse.

Motivation begins with recognizing that there might be a problem and continues with finding the will to seek treatment and to make treatment work. Often, motivation grows as a person sees the benefits and rewards of sobriety and aspires toward them instead of falling back into the diseased thinking of denial. Motivation ebbs and flows like any other state of mind; sometimes it is buoyed by hope and enthusiasm, sometimes it sinks under hopelessness. People with alcoholism should be aware that these ups and downs are part of the nature of recovery.

Research has shown that even with the most minimal resources, people who are highly motivated are more often able to succeed in attaining and maintaining sobriety. In the elderly, normal mechanisms for coping may have become so completely disrupted by the loss of loved ones, particularly a spouse or child, or by the depression that can sometimes accompany retirement, or even by the aging process itself, that treatment for alcoholism can be more difficult because of a lack of motivation. Building motivation for the elderly may require assistance from family members or another social network, such as the person's church or temple.

PREVENTION

Prevention has been shown to be one of the most effective means of reducing rates of problem or addictive usage of alcohol or other drugs.

From 1979 until 1992, alcohol and other drug use declined significantly in the general US population, despite the boom in cocaine and crack cocaine use in the 1980s. For the last several years, sales of hard liquor have declined and beer sales have remained level at best. Wine sales have also been flat. This is true not only in the United States but also in much of Europe.

Thanks to the efforts of numerous organizations—some governmental, but many private with an emotional stake in the issue, such as Mothers Against Drunk Driving (MADD) and Students Against Drunk Driving (SADD)—the consumption of alcohol, marijuana, cocaine, and heroin, and the deaths linked to them, declined steadily. There are probably also significant demographic and social trends that contributed to this decline, including the aging of the baby boom generation and the increased concern of that generation with its overall health and well-being.

Prevention comes in many forms, and quite simple ones can be very effective, such as the designated driver rule. Many school districts have created programs that minimize situations in which alcohol and other drug use can occur. The "all-night prom" is one example: A high school holds an all-night, drug- and alcohol-free party after the prom, which discourages students from wandering off in their cars to hangouts, hotels, or beaches. These efforts at prevention cost minimal amounts of money, but save countless lives.

It is important to note that during the period of the 1980s and early 1990s, core use of drugs—that is, use by the regularly using segment of the population—showed little change. This indicates that prevention efforts have their most significant effect on casual or experimental users, or those who are not yet users. The numbers suggest that prevention really does work. But prevention must be an ongoing battle in a war that is never over. Currently, alcohol, marijuana, and other drug use has begun to rise. In 1993, hospitals throughout the United States reported an all-time high in drug-related emergency room visits, which is considered an important indicator of drug use in the community. The government has recently reported a 141-percent rise in marijuana use among young people. A recent study showed that between the years 1992 and 1995, overall teenage drug use more than doubled. When teenagers do not view the use of alcohol or other drugs as dangerous to their health—and many foolishly do not—their use increases substantially. These increases are not limited to the United States, but are occurring in Canada and Europe as well. Efforts at prevention need to be redoubled; it must be realized that cuts in programs to prevent alcohol and other drug abuse in the end result in increased expense.

The Disease Model of Addiction

Alcoholism in particular and addiction in general have been thought of as a disease by some in the medical profession for more than a century. In 1935 AA was founded by two alcoholics, one a stockbroker, the other a doctor, in the belief that alcoholism could be treated as an illness.

In 1956 the American Medical Association officially designated alcoholism a disease. By coming up with specific diagnostic criteria—those signs and symptoms that constitute alcoholism—medical professionals have been able to more effectively plan, monitor, and evaluate treatment. Over the years, treating alcoholism as a disease has led to considerable success in helping alcoholics stay sober. Yet none of the available treatment programs can promise to cure every case. Currently it is believed that 70 percent or more of alcoholics can be treated effectively with lasting success.

Despite the fact that the medical profession has treated alcoholism and addiction as a disease for nearly half a century, many people still view alcohol and other drug addic-

THE DOPAMINE CONNECTION

Dopamine is a neurotransmitter, a chemical the brain uses to communicate. All of the communication between the brain and body, and within the brain itself, takes place via a system called neurotransmission. The central (brain) and peripheral (body) nervous systems consist of vast networks of nerve fibers. These nerve fibers are made up of individual nerve cells, or neurons. Thoughts and sensations are transmitted from neuron to neuron along these fibers by means of chemical neurotransmitters. The neurotransmitters carry the signal over the synapse, or the gap that separates individual neurons from one another. When a signal is sent—and signals flow constantly—the neuron floods the synapse with the neurotransmitter particular to a given sensation or command. At this writing, there are some 60 known neurotransmitters at work in the human body. Each neuron is equipped with receptors that will accept particular neurotransmitters and no others. In the use of psychoactive drugs, what seems to happen is that the drug "impersonates" a neurotransmitter, and overwhelms it.

Dopamine, serotonin, and norepinephrine are the three neurotransmitters most closely linked to mood, memory, and habit. Medications that affect serotonin levels make up the largest number of antidepressants on the market today. Norepinephrine is involved in many of the same responses as dopamine, such as the "fight-or-flight" response, but it is dopamine that has recently been most closely scrutinized in addiction research. Dopamine is involved in the basic biological process of pain avoidance and pleasure pursuit.

Cocaine and other stimulants, which attach almost exclusively to dopamine receptors, apparently either deplete dopamine or exhaust the body's normal response to dopamine when the user is not using the drugs. This effect is known as down-regulation of dopamine production and receptors. Recent research has shown that cocaine taken intravenously increases the dopamine avail-

able to the body, although it is not yet completely clear that such an increase affects the user's high. In the wake of the euphoria of cocaine or another central nervous system stimulant, the body is left struggling to make up for the wild "spending spree" of neurotransmitters during the euphoric period. This effect may help explain why 90 percent of people with alcoholism are nicotine-dependent, and why people with alcoholism are many times more likely to use cocaine, sedatives, opioids, hallucinogens, stimulants, and marijuana than other people.

Substance abuse promises intense euphoria, which is often followed by an intense low. The most difficult aspect of treating and preventing addiction is the variation in how people react to the pains and pleasures of intoxication. Some people find that the hangover that can follow alcohol use or the low that can follow sustained cocaine use is not worth the transient euphoria the drugs produce. Others will find those episodes of physical and psychic pain a small price to pay for the euphoria that the drug provides. Drugs that provide initial euphoria with almost no pain, such as crack cocaine, are likely to be the most addictive.

Medicine has long sought methods of pain relief that are not psychoactive. It was hoped that the development of heroin might end addiction because it would require such a tiny dose. It did not end addiction. Heroin, once the hero of pain relief, is now classified as a schedule-I drug in the United States, that is, it is deemed too dangerous to be medically useful. At this point, it is hard to imagine a pain-killing medication that does not interact with the emotional pleasure centers in the brain. This may be because new discoveries indicate that dopamine and other neurotransmitters govern emotional state and physical pain simultaneously; consequently, the two may be inextricably linked. Researchers may soon be able to design medications that block the psychoactive properties of pain relievers by preventing them from interacting with neurotransmitters. ■

tion as a problem of character rather than a biological dysfunction. How can something that represents a choice—such as taking a drink—be considered a sign of disease? In fact, part of the disease of addiction is that the addict loses the ability to choose, which is often difficult for someone who has never lost control to understand. Given that alcoholism is a disease, is it contagious? Can you catch alcoholism the way you can catch a cold? Is it genetically passed on or does it depend on environmental factors, like skin cancer does? Can you get addiction from repeated exposure? Actually, as research progresses more and more specialists agree that alcoholism may be at least in part contagious, genetically linked, and environmentally determined.

Addiction is not contagious in the true sense of the word. But psychology plays an

important role in addiction. Particularly with adolescents and young adults who are susceptible to peer pressure, exposure to alcohol or other casual drug use in others can lead an individual to decide that alcohol or other drug use is acceptable and appropriate.

The genetic component to addiction is still under debate. In the 1970s studies documented that alcoholism runs in families. The question still remains whether alcoholism runs in families because children learn to become alcoholics from their home environments; because children inherit genes that create an underlying predisposition for addiction; or both. Various genes hypothesized to be linked to alcoholism have been examined, but none has yet passed a rigorous test for linkage. Genes might play a direct role in the development of alcoholism, such as in affecting the body's metabolism of alcohol, or they might play a less direct role, such as influencing personality in a way that makes an individual vulnerable to alcoholism. The best research available on the issue are Danish cross-adoptive studies that examined siblings adopted into different families. Boys had a higher likelihood of involvement in AA if their biological father was an alcoholic than boys who were raised by an alcoholic, adoptive father but whose biological father was not an alcoholic.

The environmental element of addiction is its social aspect. A person's emotional health—and propensity toward addiction—is often directly related to factors such as stress, self-esteem, employment, childhood victimization from either physical or sexual abuse, and a sense of either hopefulness or hopelessness. Social drinking, for example, does not necessarily mean moderate drinking. It means drinking in a manner consistent with a particular social setting. If everyone is drinking to the point of unconsciousness at a particular social occasion, drinking to the point of unconsciousness would constitute social drinking in that particular setting.

Although there is as yet no way of predicting who will be struck by the disease of alcoholism, researchers continue to explore the various social, genetic, and biologic mechanisms that may contribute to alcoholism and addiction. Promising research into neurotransmitters and the biochemistry of the brain will likely provide more useful medication to treat the disease of alcoholism.

❖ PROBLEM USE OF ALCOHOL OR OTHER DRUGS

Symptoms *(What you may experience)*
At least one or more of the following:

- Failure to fulfill obligations at work, school, or home, which can range from coming to work or class with a hangover that makes it difficult to complete expected tasks, to spending the night in a bar instead of returning home to deal with an important responsibility such as child care

- Drinking or drug use in situations in which it is physically hazardous; for example, driving a car, boat, or motorcycle after drinking or using drugs, or riding with others who have been drinking or using drugs

- Recurring legal problems related to alcohol or drug use, such as arrests for possession or driving under the influence

- Continued alcohol or drug use despite the knowledge of resulting social, occupational, psychological, or physical problems, including drinking despite a driving while under the influence (DWI) citation, drinking while taking medication that interacts with alcohol, staying out all night "partying" and going in to work without having slept, or going to work or school while under the influence of alcohol or other drugs

- Focusing on the desire for alcohol or drugs to the exclusion of other activities; for example, needing a drink after work before doing anything else

- Losing control of drinking; for example, intending to have "just one" but drinking or drugging all night

Signs *(What the doctor looks for)* A person who has a problem with alcohol or other drugs may have increased physical problems, including stomach problems, hypertension (high blood pressure), heart irregularities, weight loss, poor diet, anxiety or panic attacks, insomnia, and other problems. A young, otherwise healthy person who occasionally abuses alcohol, cocaine, or marijuana, may not show any outward symptoms. In many cases, especially involving adolescents, the doctor may need to talk to other family members in order to establish patterns of problem usage.

A doctor will seek information regarding alcohol or other drug use by asking questions about how much a person drinks, when she drinks, and if she uses other drugs. The answers may lead the doctor to suspect a problem, which would prompt the doctor to ask further questions. If the disease has not yet progressed to the stage of dependency, a doctor will probably not be able to detect problem usage without the cooperation of the patient. Although interviews with doctors can sometimes feel like interrogations, it is important to remember that your doctor is trying to make an

TREATMENT RESOURCES

- Adcare Hospital Helpline
  Phone: (800) ALCOHOL (252–6465)
  24-hour toll-free referrals

- Alcoholics Anonymous (AA)
  Web site: http://www.alcoholics-anonymous.org
  Information on AA, including on-line meetings

- Al-Anon
  Phone: (800) 367–9996
  AA's sister organization for families of people with alcoholism

- American Council on Alcoholism
  Phone: (800) 527–5344
  Toll-free referrals; counseling for people with alcoholism and their families

- Center for Substance Abuse Treatment
  Phone: (800) 662–4357 – English
  Phone: (800) 622–9832 – Spanish

- Cocaine Anonymous (CA)
  Web site: http://www.ca.org

- Narcotics Anonymous (NA)
  Web site: http://www.na.org

- National Alliance of Methadone Advocates
  Web site: http://www.methadone.org/nama1.html

- National Clearinghouse for Alcohol and Drug Information
  Phone: (800) 729–6686
  Web site: http://www.health.org
  Toll-free referrals; information with a focus on prevention and health-related issues

- National Council on Alcoholism and Drug Dependence
  Phone: (800) 622–2255
  Toll-free referrals

- Web of Addictions
  Web site: http://www.well.com/user/woa
  Information on alcohol and other drug abuse, with links to other web sites ∎

honest appraisal of a potential problem in order to recommend treatment. You are partners, not adversaries.

What is it? Abuse of alcohol or another drug is an early stage of the disease of addiction. Although it may not necessarily lead to full-blown addiction, it can easily progress to dependence.

What you can do Stop. The only truly reliable cure for alcoholism or other drug abuse is abstinence. If your problem usage has not escalated to the later stages of addiction, you may be able to stop with minimal assistance. Stopping on your own, however, can be difficult and lonely, and is often unsuccessful. In most cases seeking help is advisable. Talk to your doctor or contact one of the organizations that help people with alcoholism and other addictions (see above).

When to call the doctor If you suspect that you or a loved one might have a problem, you should contact your doctor. It is vital to get an objective professional opinion. Although the AUDIT questions (see page 94) can help you determine if a problem exists, they are no substitute for a medical opinion. If you suspect that your use of alcohol or other drugs has slipped, even slightly, into the problem area, talk to your doctor. If you are concerned about a friend

or family member, discuss the behavior that concerns you with a doctor. It may turn out that you need not worry, but recognizing that there might be a problem is one of the most important elements of successful treatment, and successful treatment can significantly reduce the likelihood of abuse becoming full-blown dependence. As with all disease, the earlier the diagnosis, the better the prognosis.

Treatment Although there is evidence to indicate that some people can curtail or cut off problem alcohol or other drug use on their own, the most effective treatment involves structured support. Whether through the looser structures of AA, Narcotics Anonymous (NA), Cocaine Anonymous (CA), or similar 12-step programs, or through tightly structured residential programs, most people need help in developing coping mechanisms, living with others soberly, and making amends to those they may have hurt because of their alcoholism (see Treatment for Alcoholism, page 102).

Prognosis Alcoholism is a highly treatable illness. When a person is motivated, and supported by family, co-workers, health care professionals, and others, there is a very high recovery rate. Relapse is frequent during the early phase of treatment and may even be a fundamental part of the recovery process.

❖ ADDICTION TO ALCOHOL OR OTHER DRUGS

Symptoms *(What you may experience)*

- Diminished effects of the drug and consequent need for increased amounts to achieve the same effect

- Preoccupation with the drug including how to obtain it and when to be able to use it

- Wernicke-Korsakoff syndrome symptoms (includes amnesia and confusion)

- Blackouts, which are not loss of consciousness but loss of memory such as the failure to recall the "good time" of the previous night

- Unexplained seizures

- Stomach or intestinal problems including bloody vomit due to gastrointestinal bleeding

- Ill effects from interactions with medications (see page 92)

- Fainting or passing out

- Lowered resistance to infection

- Night sweats

- Depression

- Suicidal thoughts or attempts

- Hypertension

Signs *(**What the doctor looks for**)* Signs of all but the most advanced alcoholism are quite subtle. A doctor will look for the odor of alcohol on the breath, or the odor of breath mints or cigarettes. The doctor will look for physical manifestations of long-term alcohol or other drug use such as signs of liver disease, which include puffiness of the face, small testicles, and small or thin arms and legs in relation to the body; inflammation of the liver; hypertension; heart arrhythmias; gynecomastia (breast growth in men); and cuts or bruises that cannot be readily explained. A person who is a problem user of alcohol or other drugs will often demonstrate an increase in minor trauma including bumps, bruises, cuts, and scrapes, which may come from carelessness or even from fighting. A doctor will often look for confirmation of excessive alcohol or other drug use in blood tests.

If there is reason to suspect addiction, a doctor will ask about drinking or drug use.

As with many other diseases, talking may be the best diagnostic tool. Answers themselves may be symptomatic. A person with alcoholism will respond in ways that are characteristically different from a person without the disease. Because denial is such a potent force—the single most difficult hurdle to overcome in treatment—a doctor may want to talk to the spouse or other loved ones in order to make an objective determination. Doctors who specialize in alcohol or other drug addiction understand how to break down denial and get to the truth of a diagnosis of addiction.

What is it? Addiction differs from dependence, which does not exhibit most of the symptoms of advanced alcoholism listed previously. Addiction to alcohol or another drug occurs when the body has become so accustomed to the presence of a mood-altering substance that the disruption it causes to the body and brain becomes a person's normal state. A person with alcoholism, therefore, needs the drug just to feel normal. In addition, addiction is progressive, which means that a person with the disease needs greater and greater amounts to obtain the same effect.

Most drugs that are commonly abused target a single neurotransmitter (see The Dopamine Connection, page 97) but alcohol cuts a wide swath through the central nervous system, affecting many of the neurotransmitters involved with mood and emotion. This "taking over" of the brain's inner workings can lead to powerful urges that a person with alcoholism simply cannot control, and which she then attempts to cover up with denial (see page 94).

Addiction usually follows a predictable pattern. For whatever reason, a person experiments with a drug. Most people who experiment soon give up the drug and go on with their lives. Some abuse the drug for a while, then leave it alone. Still others—the smallest percentage of people who experiment—continue using the drug. To these people, the drug appeals to a complex combination of social, genetic, and psychological factors within them and they move to the maintenance phase of addiction. In this middle stage people use regularly and may experience effects such as reduced stress, merriment, or the sense of being superhuman as very strong reinforcements to their drug use. But soon they reach the tolerance stage when the body becomes accustomed to having a particular amount of the drug in its system. At the tolerance stage people must use more in order to achieve the same pleasurable effect. Often the pleasurable effect disappears, but the memory of the pleasurable effect is so strong that people continue using larger amounts until finally they are using amounts that would kill a nonuser, even though they may never experience the high that they first fell in love with. Depending on the drug, the transition from maintenance to tolerance may be either slow or very rapid. Certain drugs, such as crack cocaine, have such powerful reinforcement mechanisms that addiction can occur quite rapidly. Alcohol, on the other hand, has significant downsides, such as making a person hungover and sick, which make it less rapidly addictive.

In full-blown addiction, the sudden absence of the drug may cause a violent physical or emotional reaction known as withdrawal. In the case of alcoholism, this can lead to hallucination, nearly suicidal depression, and even fatal seizures (see Delirium Tremens, above). Usually, the state of withdrawal is essentially the opposite of the action of the drug. People who are withdrawing from cocaine or amphetamines may become massively depressed. Those withdrawing from sedating drugs, such as alcohol or benzodiazepines (Valium or Librium), may become highly agitated.

What you can do Stop. Get help.

Try to assess your alcohol or other drug use by honestly answering the AUDIT questions (see page 94). If you have any reason to suspect that you might have a problem or the beginnings of a problem, seek help from your doctor. If you do not have a regular primary care physician, seek a referral, which you can do through many avenues. You can consult the employee handbook or guide to medical benefits at your workplace to discover what, if any, resources are available to you through work. You can contact AA or a similar organization (see page 99). Your clergyman also may be able to refer you to a self-help group.

When to call the doctor Call your doctor if you suspect you have a problem with addiction or the beginnings of a problem, or if you suspect that a loved one has a problem or the beginnings of a problem. Call as soon

DELIRIUM TREMENS

Delirium tremens, or the DTs, is an extreme reaction to alcohol withdrawal that occurs in persons who have stopped drinking after having become tolerant of high amounts of alcohol on a daily basis. Although delirium tremens is most commonly associated with alcohol, withdrawal from other drugs can produce similar effects on long-term, high-dose users. The effects of withdrawal may last as long as a month or even continue in one form or another for several months; these cases require clinically supervised detoxification. Episodes can be very violent, even fatal. Symptoms of delirium tremens are both physical and psychological and usually consist of exhausting physical tremors and hallucinations, often of bugs or other creatures crawling on the skin. The hallucinations may render the patient delirious and incoherent. Proper nutrition, medication, and supervision are necessary to bring a person through the phase of delirium. ∎

as you develop a suspicion. Delay can only make the problem worse and treatment more difficult. A loved one who is in crisis may be ready to accept a recommendation to change.

Treatment Treatment can range from intensive inpatient therapy including detoxification, to unsupervised attendance of AA meetings (see Treatment for Alcoholism, page 102).

Prognosis With sustained treatment of at least 2 years, good motivation, and strong support, the prognosis for recovery is excellent.

❖ CO-ALCOHOL DEPENDENCE

Symptoms *(What you may experience)*

- Psychological distress manifested in symptoms such as anxiety, aggression, anorexia nervosa, bulimia, depression, insomnia, hyperactivity, and suicidal tendency
- Psychosomatic illness (ailments that have no biological basis and clear up after the co-alcoholism clears up)
- Family violence or neglect
- Alcoholism or other drug abuse

Signs *(What the doctor looks for)* Unless a person discusses the problems caused by a family member's alcoholism with a doctor, co-alcoholism may only be diagnosed after an emergency room visit or a police intervention following an episode of domestic violence. A doctor may also discover co-alcoholism when another illness fails to respond to conventional treatment, or when a family member is diagnosed with alcoholism.

What is it? Co-alcoholism is a mirror of alcoholism. Like alcoholism, co-alcoholism is a progressive, chronic disease that without treatment can kill the co-alcoholic. Co-alcoholism is similar to post-traumatic stress disorder, or what was once called shell shock. Co-alcoholism is a protective behavior that a person initially develops as a survival mechanism, and leads to denial that can be as strong in the person who suffers from co-alcoholism as in the person with alcoholism. It can include secretive behavior that is protective of the person with alcoholism, and denial of the disease or the existence of a problem. It is also characterized by a psychological numbing that removes a person from natural emotional reactions, which then resurface like nightmares and leave a person feeling anxiously alert, guilty, and traumatized.

What you can do If you are concerned that a loved one has alcoholism or another drug dependency and you find that it is affecting your own health, you should understand that you can get help even if your loved one will not. You can, on your own, begin to take control of your life and stop your own suffering. Consult your doctor and find out about outpatient treatment programs such as Al-Anon or Alateen. These programs offer guidance, support, and information about getting well.

When to call the doctor Call your doctor if you suspect that someone you love has a problem with addiction. You may not even realize that you yourself are affected beyond just worrying about your loved one. Because co-alcoholism is a survival mechanism, you may be blind to the extent to which the behavior of your loved one is affecting your health. What may have become normal for you would be a virtually intolerable state for someone else. If you have been forced to lie for your loved one or otherwise enabled his or her behavior, if you have experienced either verbal or physical abuse, if you have explained away bruises received in abuse as the result of falling down stairs or walking into doors, if you have been humiliated by your loved one's behavior, or if you have experienced aches and pains or have become depressed and despairing as a result of the behavior of your loved one, get help.

Treatment The most effective treatment known is group therapy, usually in the form of Al-Anon, Nar-Anon, Alateen, or Alatot. These organizations work on the same principles as AA. For additional information on the various therapies available to help you deal with the many emotional difficulties that can result from being co-dependent, see Chapter 27.

Prognosis With sustained treatment, the prognosis is excellent for recovery of full health, although this does not mean that the family situation will necessarily be repaired. In some cases, breaking the cycle of co-dependence can help motivate the addicted individual to seek help. But equally often, it may be necessary to come to peace with the fact that the family member may never stop abusing alcohol or drugs. In some instances this may mean the end of a marriage, in others it may mean coming to terms with the shortcomings of a parent.

Treatment for Alcoholism

If you do not or your loved one does not believe there is a problem, then it is difficult to initiate treatment. All treatment is based on motivation. Successful treatment is problematic at best unless the addicted individual has a clear desire to make treatment work. Denial is the most difficult hurdle to overcome in this process. Denial can prevent a person from seeing both the valuable things to be lost by not engaging in treatment and the valuable things to be gained by adhering to treatment (see page 94). Once denial has been overcome, treatment for alcoholism can be quite effective. Over time it can lead to a reversal of many of the complications of drinking or other drug use. With the assistance of a doctor and a good recovery program, there is an approximate 70 percent rate of recovery. The success rate of spontaneous, or self-driven, recovery, is only about 4 to 25 percent.

INTERVENTION

The active intervention is a group confrontation that is planned. Because people with alcoholism are so steeped in denial, a one-on-one confrontation with a spouse or friend will often only provoke more guilt in the person with alcoholism and then increased denial because of the guilt. In an intervention family, friends, colleagues, and others connected with the situation team up to compel the person with alcoholism to listen to overwhelming evidence of her disease. Although the intent is not to hurt, interventions can be painful events for the person with alcoholism as well as loved ones.

Substance abuse counselors are often trained as intervention specialists. Any time a family or group of friends considers an intervention, an intervention specialist should be consulted. Participants may understandably be angry or even hateful, and may in the heat of the moment get carried away and try to humiliate the person with alcoholism. This is dangerous and counterproductive. A poorly executed intervention can be worse than no intervention at all and rather than get a person to admit the disease, it can lead to suicide or a worsening of the alcohol or other drug abuse.

An intervention specialist will help select appropriate participants and will train them in how to keep focused on the subject of the intervention. The counselor will help participants enumerate specific examples of how the person with alcoholism has let them down, or hurt or humiliated them. The counselor will also work with participants to anticipate potential objections to treatment, real as well as imagined. In the intervention itself, the counselor acts as referee, keeping the person with alcoholism from deflecting or denying evidence of the disease and keeping the participants on the subject. The intended outcome of a planned intervention is to get the person with alcoholism to agree to a specific treatment program.

After the intervention participants, particularly those who instigated the process, may feel let down or guilty. They may feel that they have betrayed someone they love. This is a natural reaction to a painful situation that exposes rather than hides wounds. Even though it may be quite painful, confronting addiction is a necessary part of the process of healing. ■

The object of treatment is recovery, or sustained periods of abstinence that will eventually lead to progressively longer, if not permanent, periods of total abstinence. Recovery is an ongoing process that will last the lifetime of the person with alcoholism. Built into the definition of recovery is the likelihood of relapse or near-relapse. Professionals in the treatment of alcoholism never refer to sober alcoholics as "former" alcoholics, but always as "recovering" alcoholics. The distinction is crucial. A person cannot quit an addiction the way one quits a job, certain of never going back. A person with alcoholism can only stop. An addict is always an addict. The disease may remain in remission, but the danger that it might return is always present.

Moderation Management (MM) is a recent movement that maintains that moderation and not abstinence should be the ultimate goal of treatment for people with alcoholism. MM is winning hopeful adherents, but its success rate is still quite dubious. Most professionals believe that in practice moderation has not been shown to be effective at all and that it can actually be deadly. While certain individuals may outgrow problem usage of alcohol or another drug, there is always the potential for problem usage to return later in life. The only truly effective treatment for alcoholism is therefore total and sustained abstinence.

How can total and sustained abstinence be achieved? Many people with alcoholism find this long-term goal to be completely unrealistic when they first confront sobriety. Going without a drink forever is a goal too unreachable even to attempt. This is what makes the AA slogan "One day at a time" so profound to the alcoholic, even though it might seem completely self-evident and even silly to someone without alcoholism. The goal of recovery is not a lifetime of sobriety, but the short-term goal of a single day of sobriety.

Most often, treatment for problem alcohol or other drug use is precipitated by an intervening circumstance. This could be a passive intervention such as an arrest for driving under the influence or a sense of hitting bottom after marital, financial, or other difficulties. Or it could be deliberate, such as a planned intervention, in which family and friends sit a person down in a controlled setting and confront her with the irrefutable evidence of her addiction. The intervention includes an enumeration of all the ways in which the disease has caused shortcomings in the person's relationships, life, and responsibilities. This technique was inadvertently invented by a husband who was worn out by his wife's illness. Together with the rest of the family, he confronted her with how it had affected them all. Intervention has been found to be tremendously useful when carried out in a loving and supportive manner under the guidance of an intervention specialist (see above).

DETOX AND INPATIENT TREATMENT

Some researchers maintain that as many as half of people with alcohol or other drug addiction need to be hospitalized at the beginning of treatment. People who have not progressed to full-blown addiction may not need such close scrutiny and can recover using appropriate levels of outpatient care alone (see page 106). Adolescents, particularly when parents have no control over them, may need the strict supervision of hospitalization even if their disease has not progressed to full-blown addiction.

Detoxification, or detox ("drying out"), often begins with admission to a hospital or the detox unit of a treatment center. Detox is the process of removing the substance of abuse from the body, or detoxifying the system. If the patient cooperates, detox from alcohol can be done safely and without severe withdrawal symptoms. Detoxification can be done at home in some circumstances, but under no circumstances should it be done without close medical supervision (see Delirium Tremens, page 101). If your insurance will not cover inpatient detox, consult your doctor about undergoing detox at home. In some cases, medication is necessary, but most specialists agree that detoxification without medication goes more quickly, which means that the process of recovery can begin that much sooner.

Withdrawal levels differ from person to person, depending upon the duration of the addiction and the level of tolerance that was achieved. People who had been taking doses of alcohol or other drugs that would have killed nonusers may experience severe withdrawal symptoms, while others may experience only mild effects. Physical withdrawal lasts only a few days or at most a few weeks; however, emotional withdrawal may last a lifetime for some people, ebbing and flowing over the years. In others, personal growth through self-empowerment can minimize or eliminate emotional withdrawal.

After detoxification, psychiatric or physical ailments may appear that the alcoholism or dependence on another drug had concealed. This effect is known as comorbidity. The other ailment may be directly caused by alcoholism, such as liver disease, or it may be unrelated. If depression persists after stopping alcohol, treatment for depression will make relapse less likely.

If your medical insurance or place of employment covers inpatient treatment, or if you can afford it, then it may be wise to take advantage of this option. Inpatient treatment is particularly recommended for adolescents and people who have been abusing alcohol or another drug since adolescence (see If You Suspect Your Child Is Using Alcohol or Other Drugs, page 105). The time is spent, usually 2 to 6 weeks, in a crash course in sobriety and includes intensive group therapy combined with living with other recovering addicts—all at different stages of recovery—as well as a complete physical workup, examination for co-morbid conditions, and an intensive nutritional regimen, which can all be powerful tools for breaking down denial and helping rebuild a new physical, mental, and spiritual outlook on life. Inpatient programs teach sobriety coping mechanisms, as well as strategies for dealing with cravings and for avoiding relapse. Even if a person has not gone into treatment willingly but has been forced, as happens with adolescents and people mandated by the courts or the social service system, inpatient treatment can effectively begin to motivate a person to reclaim her life.

For some people with alcoholism, particularly those in the later stages of the disease, inpatient treatment should be followed by an outpatient treatment program.

If you have no strong network of sober, non-codependent friends or loved ones, inpatient treatment can remove you from diseased surroundings and help you reorient your thinking. It can also give codependent loved ones important time to sort out their lives and seek support.

If you or your loved one have attempted suicide or had suicidal thoughts, inpatient treatment can also be crucial to ensuring safety. Deep depression sometimes accompanies withdrawal, and feelings of hopelessness and helplessness can be easier to overcome in an inpatient setting. If you have a co-morbid condition, recovery at an inpatient facility can include medical treatment of that condition.

As an inpatient, you or your loved one will learn about AA, CA, NA, or other appropriate organizations; attend intensive group therapy sessions; and begin to assess, with the help of counselors, the state of your life.

IF YOU SUSPECT YOUR CHILD IS USING ALCOHOL OR OTHER DRUGS

As a parent, it is your responsibility not to facilitate alcohol or other substance abuse in your children. If you are aware that your child uses alcohol or other drugs, drinks to the point of getting a hangover, or gets into legal trouble due to drinking or other drugs, you need to be proactive and take steps to address the problem. To ignore a child's abuse of alcohol or other substances is essentially to condone it.

Letting your child know how you feel about the possibility of her drinking or using drugs can prevent your child's condition from worsening. Intervention often leads to a positive outcome. Steps may include—but are not limited to—speaking openly with your child about abuse of alcohol or other drugs, buying a urine-testing kit to determine abuse, or more intense measures such as setting up treatment for substance abuse. Regardless of the degree of abuse, playing an active role can help give your child a life free from alcohol or other drug abuse and addiction. It is important to do something to help your child before it's too late.

The first thing to do is watch out for the warning signs of adolescent drug abuse, as outlined by the National Institute on Alcoholism and Alcohol Abuse:

- Physical signs including persistent fatigue, repeated health complaints, red and dull eyes, and a steady cough

- Emotional signs including personality change, sudden mood change, irresponsible behavior, low self-esteem, depression, and a general lack of interest

- School-related signs including a drop in grades, many absences, and discipline problems

- Social signs including new friends who are less interested in standard home and school activities, scrapes with the law, and changes to less conventional styles in dress and music

Do not try to make a diagnosis on your own. Try to talk openly with your child about use and abuse of alcohol and other drugs, and make sure she knows that you care and are watching her behavior. You should consult your child's doctor in order to rule out other causes for these symptoms. Depression, for example, is common in adolescents; when undiagnosed it can mean serious trouble for your family. You should also alert your child's doctor to the possibility of drug abuse. A doctor's advice or warnings may have an effect on your child that your own advice or warnings may not.

If use of alcohol or other drugs has become a large enough part of your child's life for you to begin to notice, then likely the drug use has become abuse. Many parents are tempted to ignore what their children are going through and call it only a phase, but it is important to remember that ignoring an adolescent's problem enables the young person to continue the behav-

ior. It is also important to remember that abuse and addiction can tear families apart. Examine your own lifestyle. What are your drinking or drug habits? What is your attitude about drinking? Are you having emotional or financial difficulties that make it hard to give your child the attention she needs?

Contact a therapist or counselor who specializes in adolescent addiction. Discuss your concerns with the counselor and find out what resources are available in your area. You need not limit your contact to one counselor. Interview a few. Chances are that you will be working with this specialist for some time; find someone with whom you can connect and who can connect with your child, someone who you feel can be objective and nonjudgmental. Discuss the level of the problem. Is your child disappearing for days at a time, or is the problem restricted to a decline in the quality of her school work? Find out what kind of treatment is appropriate.

The next step is intervention (see page 103). Intervention with an adolescent can be both easier and more difficult than intervention with an adult. It can be more difficult because adolescents are often rebellious. Add to their rebelliousness the denial and secrecy involved in addiction, and intervention can face serious obstacles. But because adolescents are minors, you can send your child to a treatment facility to receive help even without her consent, which you could not do were she an adult.

Chances are good that your child wants to be caught, but that is not all she wants. Your child may want the guidance of an adult, which should be provided by a counselor in whom she can confide. It is up to you to find good counseling including individual counseling for your child and family counseling. It is difficult for a counselor to evaluate an adolescent without information about the dynamics of the family. These sessions may be grueling. They may take you out of work and be expensive if your insurance does not pay for them. In the end, however, the emotional and financial toll will be considerably less than if you do not intervene. Most counselors will ask parents who are themselves drinkers or drug users to rid the home of all such substances.

Some adolescents will need inpatient treatment. Some will have more than one problem—an emerging co-morbid problem, such as severe depression in conjunction with substance abuse. Some adolescents may only need outpatient treatment and strict guidance.

Whatever the case, all adolescents require strict but predictable and sensible discipline from their parents. Many experts on adolescent difficulties recommend drawing up a contract between you and your child. This way, a child's responsibilities and rights are spelled out in black and white, as well as what your child can expect of you. Your counselor should have examples of such contracts that can be tailored to your family's particular situation.

With a stable home environment, conscientious care, a stable routine, established goals, predictable rules, and judicious limits on freedoms, treatment can help your child mature into a responsible, sober adult. ■

You will be guided to set short-term life and treatment goals. It is also an important time for your family to share in counseling and learn about behaviors that they may have developed in order to cope, such as enabling. Groups like Alanon, Alateen, and Alatot exist to help family members of people with alcoholism.

OUTPATIENT TREATMENT, AA, AND GROUP THERAPY

Outpatient treatment is the first type of treatment many people with alcoholism attempt. It may be the only treatment necessary, although for many, it will be continuous, at least in the form of ongoing attendance of AA meetings. It is the most affordable, most available, and the least intrusive kind of treatment. You can continue to work and to live at home while you begin to rebuild your emotional, spiritual, and physical life. For outpatient treatment to succeed, however, it must be intensive and thorough, and should be monitored by your doctor with regular follow-up over an extended period of time.

Outpatient therapy makes up the largest portion of all treatment for alcoholism and has many levels of intensity. The most intensive is close to inpatient treatment; a person would go to treatment early in the morning and stay until evening, essentially only coming home to sleep. At the other end of the spectrum, a person might attend only occasional AA, CA, or NA meetings, or other group therapy sessions, which may be all that is needed. Many recovering alcoholics, however, attend AA meetings on a weekly, even daily, basis, for decades. For many, AA becomes an extended family.

Group therapy has proven to be the most effective route to successful recovery, perhaps because people who have been dependent upon alcohol or other drugs themselves are well-equipped to spot the signs of denial in others and the diseased thinking that can lead up to relapse. Groups of people in recovery also help one another deal with feelings of guilt or shame, and with the experience of recurring cravings. Various types of group therapy should be employed including professionally mediated counseling involving the family, and AA or other group-encounter meetings. These kinds of therapy can help firmly break

down denial and offer a supportive way out of the cycle of guilt and shame. The group is also there to offer invaluable support in the event, or likelihood, of relapse. Many substance abuse specialists consider the group setting to be the single most important aspect of treatment.

If you were to pick up the telephone right now, you could probably find an AA meeting in your area in the very near future, perhaps even tonight. You might even be offered a ride to it. Members of AA believe that regular attendance at meetings is fundamental to recovery; some attend a one-hour meeting on a daily basis. You can even attend an AA meeting on-line (see Treatment Resources, page 99). If you are not comfortable with the spiritual aspect of AA, consult your doctor about other possibilities for group therapy.

In some cases, alcohol or other drugs played such a large role in the user's life that personal relationships change quite profoundly when their use ceases. Families may require counseling in order to establish healthy relationships, perhaps for the first time. In addition, alcoholism in its active state may have covered up other social and psychological problems; indeed, these problems may have been contributing factors to the progression of the addiction. If a full recovery from alcoholism is to be achieved, individual or family counseling may be necessary to deal with both old trauma and new changes (see Chapter 27 for more information on the kinds of therapies available). Despite the pain and hard work involved, the most positive prognosis for recovery from alcoholism is the new potential for personal growth, maturity, integrity, and freedom.

MEDICATIONS FOR TREATMENT

There are two prescription medications that can help in recovery; however, they cannot take the place of motivation. Medication is most effective in people who are highly motivated.

Disulfiram (Antabuse) is a drug that changes the way ethyl alcohol (the active ingredient in alcoholic drink) is metabolized in the body. Disulfiram has been used for more than 40 years and is considered quite safe although it has certain hazards

AA: THE 12-STEP MODEL FOR SOBRIETY

Begun in the 1930s, Alcoholics Anonymous (AA) now has as many as 100,000 offshoots worldwide, including Narcotics Anonymous (NA), and Cocaine Anonymous (CA), and even Debtors Anonymous (DA), plus a host of other 12-step programs. There are also some very valuable related groups that assist the families of people with alcoholism, such as Alanon, Alateen, and Nar-Anon.

AA is a self-sustaining, not-for-profit organization that runs on $1 donations from its members to pay for coffee and keep the lights on. To avoid conflicts of interest, AA purposely does not rely on money from other organizations.

The AA model is one of the most important tools available for treatment of alcohol and other drug abuse, and can be used in conjunction with other forms of therapy. AA relies on a series of assisted steps to sobriety. In the words of AA, the program operates when a recovering alcoholic passes along the story of her own problem drinking, describes the sobriety she has found in AA, and invites the newcomer to join the informal fellowship.

When you begin AA, CA, or NA you are newly sober. With the assistance of a sponsor who is also in recovery, you begin to learn how to maintain your sobriety one day at a time. Over time, you change your life and your thinking. On a purely biological level, you return your brain and body to as close a semblance of the pre-addiction chemical equilibrium as is possible. In many cases, much of the damage done can be undone. In certain cases, however, damage may be irreversible.

If you can follow the 12 steps, you are encouraged to do so. If you feel uncomfortable doing so, you are not forced. But you will be asked to keep your mind open, attend meetings regularly, stay sober, read AA literature, and listen as other people in recovery describe their personal experiences in maintaining sobriety.

Each meeting lasts an hour, and begins with a recitation of the 12 steps and 12 traditions, and ends with a recitation of the Lord's Prayer. In between, people get up, introduce themselves by first name only, and tell their stories. Meetings can be lively, with those attending listening for signs of denial, relapse, or lack of sincerity.

You can call your sponsor day or night if you need a shoulder to lean on. You are encouraged not to take on any romantic relationships during the first year of sobriety, nor to make any other serious, life-affecting decisions, because your decision-making capacity may still be impaired by the disease. You are also encouraged not to use any other substances, even to the point of refusing pain medication, recognizing that addiction to one drug is the same disease as addiction to another and that relapse could and often does result from any contact with a drug. All are encouraged to continue to attend meetings for the entirety of their lives and many do. Indeed, in the initial period, successful participation in AA may require a substantial investment of time—as many as 90 meetings in 90 days. Most feel that the time investment is worthwhile. Many feel they owe their lives to the brother- and sisterhood of their 12-step program. ▶

when combined with alcohol. The medication works through what is known as the alcohol-disulfiram reaction; essentially, it makes you sick if you drink. If your doctor prescribes it for you, you must be alcohol-free and must avoid products such as OTC cold medicines and mouthwashes that could contain alcohol. If you are at a party where alcohol is being consumed, you should maintain a careful watch over your glass, as even the slightest amount of alcohol will make you very sick. Symptoms include feelings of panic, flushing, sweating, and an overall sense of discomfort including headache and possibly breathing difficulties. Symptoms last for about 30 minutes and may also include vomiting and chest pains. Although it is rare, people who have heart or respiratory difficulties can die from the reaction. Disulfiram can be a significant aid to recovering alcoholics, because the very real nature of the reaction frees them from a certain amount of choice: they understand that they cannot drink and so simply avoid it.

Naltrexone is a recently approved drug that can be useful not only for people addicted to alcohol but also to opioids. Alcohol and opioids attach to the receptors for the neurotransmitter endorphin, which is the body's natural painkiller, thought to be the source of the well-known "runner's high." Naltrexone blocks the ability of alcohol or opioids to attach to the receptor, which in turn prevents the experience of a high even if a person drinks or uses drugs. Naltrexone is safe and effective. In the future researchers may come up with an extended-release form of the medication—an implant—that could be useful in people who have difficulty maintaining their sobriety.

For many years methadone, a synthetic opiate that is as addictive but not as pleasurable as morphine or heroin, has been used with measured success in the treatment of heroin, morphine, or other opiate addiction. Replacement methadone therapy (methadone maintenance) has helped some people become drug-free, but in most

◆ The 12 Steps

1. We admitted we were powerless over alcohol—that our lives had become unmanageable.

2. Came to believe that a Power greater than ourselves could restore us to sanity.

3. Made a decision to turn our will and our lives over to the care of God as we understood Him.

4. Made a searching and fearless moral inventory of ourselves.

5. Admitted to God, to ourselves, and to another human being the exact nature of our wrongs.

6. Were entirely ready to have God remove all these defects of character.

7. Humbly asked Him to remove our shortcomings.

8. Made a list of all persons we had harmed, and became willing to make amends to them all.

9. Made direct amends to such people wherever possible, except when to do so would injure them or others.

10. Continued to take personal inventory and when we were wrong promptly admitted it.

11. Sought through prayer and meditation to improve our conscious contact with God as we understood Him, praying only for knowledge of His will for us and the power to carry that out.

12. Having had a spiritual awakening as the result of these steps, we tried to carry this message to alcoholics and to practice these principles in all our affairs.

The 12 Traditions

1. Our common welfare should come first; personal recovery depends on AA unity.

2. For our group purpose there is but one ultimate authority—a loving God as He may express Himself in our group conscience. Our leaders are but trusted servants; they do not govern.

3. The only requirement for AA membership is a desire to stop drinking.

4. Each group should be autonomous except in matters affecting other groups or AA as a whole.

5. Each group has but one primary purpose—to carry its message to the alcoholic who still suffers.

6. An AA group ought never endorse, finance, or lend the AA name to any related facility or outside enterprise, lest problems of money, property, and prestige divert us from our primary purpose.

7. Every AA group ought to be fully self-supporting, declining outside contributions.

8. AA should remain forever nonprofessional, but our service centers may employ special workers.

9. AA, as such, ought never to be organized; but we may create service boards or committees directly responsible to those they serve.

10. AA has no opinion on outside issues; hence the AA name ought never be drawn into public controversy.

11. Our public relations policy is based on attraction rather than promotion; we need always maintain personal anonymity at the level of press, radio, and films.

12. Anonymity is the spiritual foundation of our traditions, ever reminding us to place principles before personalities.

(Courtesy of Alcoholics Anonymous; used with permission.) ■

cases it simply reduces problems related to opiate-addiction rather than ending addiction itself. By offering an oral substitute for heroin or morphine, specialists attempt to give people who are either unwilling or unable to get clean an alternative to progressively escalating addiction. Methadone replacement therapy may help people with addiction remove themselves from some of the psychological cues of their addiction, particularly the use of hypodermic syringes, and may help lessen the spread of blood-borne diseases such as acquired immonodeficiency syndrome (AIDS) and hepatitis. It may also help reduce crime associated with addiction, although it has been shown to be less effective than detoxification and sobriety. For those people who do not have the motivation to recover from addiction, methadone maintenance may offer an alternative to crime and incarceration.

PART TWO
Health Over *the* Life Course

Family History, Genetics, and Your Health

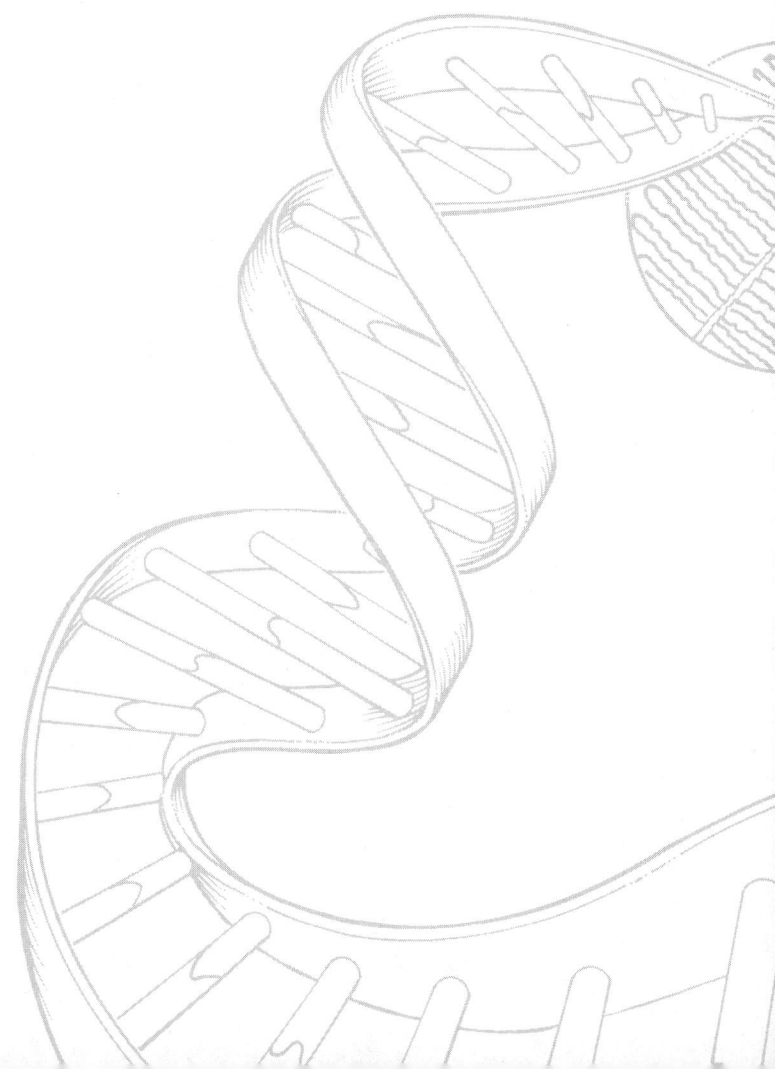

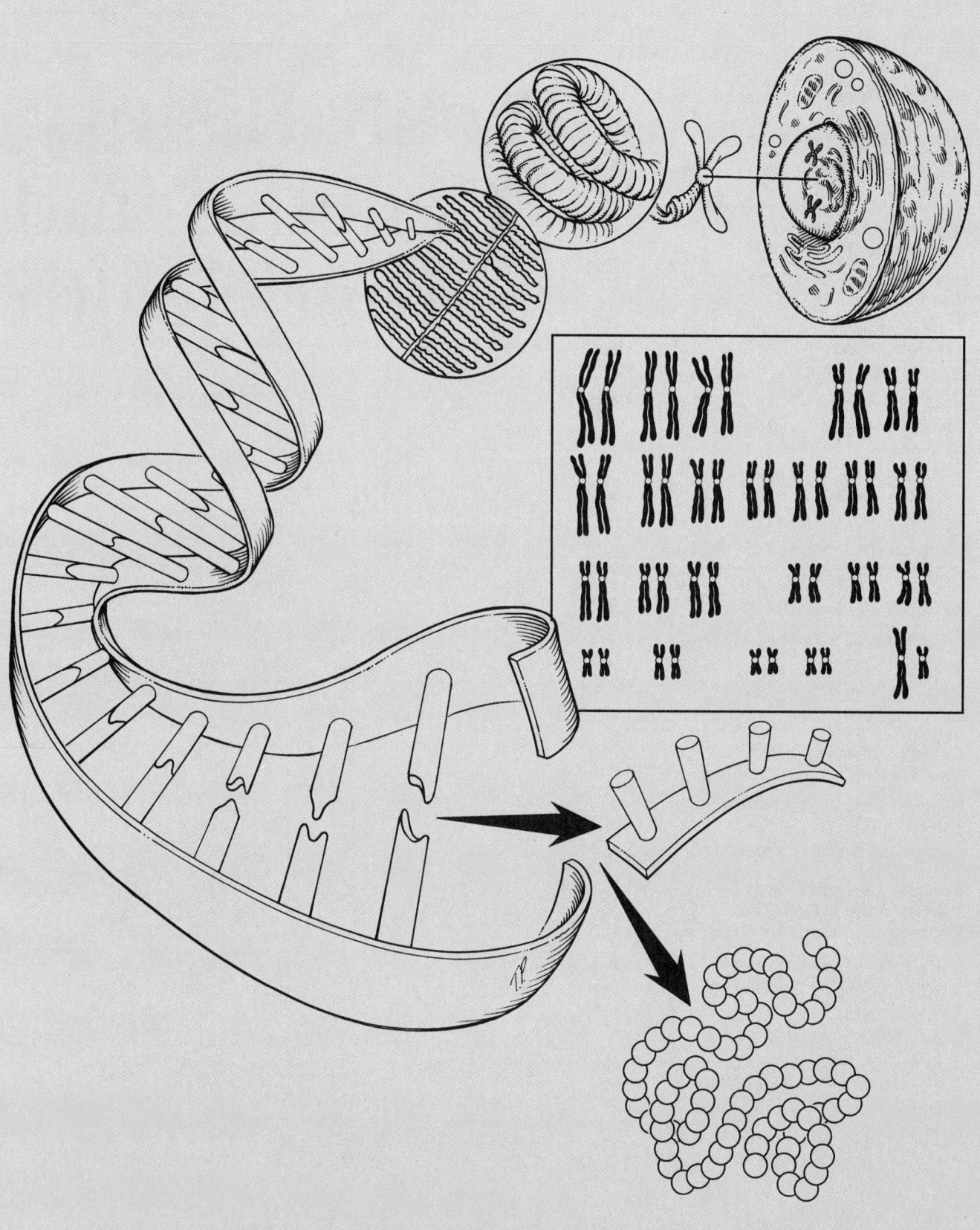

SIX

FAMILY HISTORY, GENETICS, AND YOUR HEALTH

Genetic Research

Imagine looking for a needle in a haystack, except that you are looking for a particular needle not in stacks of hay, but in stacks of needles—23 pairs of stacks, in fact. An impossible task? But imagine that the needle (or needles, in this case) may actually be the key that unlocks the mysteries of countless diseases, from cancer and obesity to birth defects and chronic disease. In a sense, this is what genetic research is and what genetic researchers do.

Genetic research is perhaps the single most exciting area of biomedical research today, and although it is still in many respects in its infancy, it has already provided us with an astonishing font of knowledge. In the words of Johns Hopkins professor Dr. Bert Vogelstein, "what we're doing now would have seemed like science fiction" only a few years earlier. Genetic research has told us not only about what causes particular genetically linked disorders, such as Marfan syndrome or cystic fibrosis, but has also provided a tremendous wealth of insight and knowledge into how our genes affect our health, particularly our susceptibility to chronic diseases such as cancer, cardiovascular disease, arthritis, and many others.

As they search through the haystacks of the human genome (and the genomes of other life forms that inhabit our planet), genetic researchers are almost daily disproving many of the myths of what genes do and discovering things that, in the words of Johns Hopkins researcher and professor Dr. Jef Boeke, "no one else in the world ever knew before." This knowledge has begun to have, and will continue to have, a profound impact on our health. Although any genetic researcher will be quick to point out that genes do not necessarily equal destiny, they most certainly do *affect* destiny. And the more we understand about our individual family history and our individual genetic makeup, the more we will be able to take control of our health.

Genetic Inheritance

A multitude of factors can affect health, but perhaps none is as important as the unique genetic blueprint we receive from our parents at conception. Much of what we inherit is beyond our capacity to change—we cannot change our eye color, for example. But much of our genetic inheritance is a fortune we can build upon or squander. Height, for example, is determined by the genes, yet a malnourished child will not achieve the full height "written" in his genes. Similarly, the predisposition to disease is sometimes set in stone—if you inherit a particular genetic defect, you will inevitably develop a certain disorder. For people with these disorders, hope may lie with the work of genetic researchers, who may uncover the gene responsible and eventually develop a treatment or cure. But more commonly, a genetic predisposition to disease is something that can be influenced by the lifestyle choices you make. Indeed, with a basic understanding of how genetics works, and by understanding the factors that influence genetic expression, we can directly affect and lower our risk of developing many diseases.

We begin as a single, unique cell, the zygote, that is created from the union of our parents' germ cells—the sperm and egg—and the genetic material combined in that single cell goes on to govern the creation of all of the nearly 10 trillion cells that make up an adult human.

Our genes, in turn, work with one another not only to create us but to continue creating and renewing us as life goes on. While there are certain cells that replicate themselves only very slowly, if at all, once we are grown, such as the lenses of the eyes and the nerves, there are many more cells that replicate constantly. Those parts of the body that are in constant contact with the environment (such as the skin and digestive tract), those that are involved with reproduction (such as the ovaries and testes), and the organs that manufacture the enzymes and hormones that we need to keep metabolism going (such as the liver, pancreas, and kidneys), must constantly renew and replenish themselves. It is the genetic material within the cells that provides these parts of the body with the information and the ability to function and to maintain themselves, and how well they do so is partly governed by genetic makeup itself, but it is more profoundly affected by environment—the foods you eat, the exercise you enjoy, the air you breathe, and the emotional and physical stresses to which you are subjected.

THE BUILDING BLOCKS OF LIFE

In humans (and in most other forms of life), the basic building block of life is deoxyribonucleic acid (DNA). DNA is a miracle of elegance that contains all of the information it takes to make us. Bound together on the famous double helix of DNA, which resembles a spiral-shaped ladder, are coding triplets, sequences of three chemicals known as nucleotides: adenine (A), cytosine (C), guanine (G), and thymine (T). These four different types of nucleotides are combined in various groups of three to code the details of the genetic information. Generally speaking, the more complex a creature is, the more DNA it has.

DNA makes life possible because it is able to copy, or replicate, itself. When DNA replicates, the double helix splits apart into two separate strands and as it splits, an enzyme makes a mirror image copy of each strand. This process results in two identical copies of the original DNA. The genetic code contained in DNA tells the body's machinery how to build proteins; this code is translated by ribonucleic acid (RNA). Messenger RNA reads the code from DNA through a process called transcription. Outside of the cell's nucleus another form of RNA, transfer RNA, carries single amino acids to messenger RNA. The amino acids, the building blocks of proteins, are then joined together in the correct sequence, as determined by messenger RNA, to form proteins.

If DNA is the basic code of life, then an individual gene is the basic string of code, which is long enough to instruct the creation of a particular protein necessary for the normal development and function of the body. From each parent we get a set of genes that govern each trait. In this case a trait is more than just hair or eye or skin color but rather all of the things that go into making up a body. So from each parent we get genes that control how, for example, our blood vessels are made and shaped.

A gene by itself is not especially useful; it is the interplay of genes that makes us who we are. Genes themselves, researchers have discovered, actually make up less than 10 percent of our genome, which is the sum of all of our genetic material. The larger percentage of the genome is made up of some materials whose functions are understood and some whose functions are yet to be clearly delineated. Some of these materials are tools that our cells used at the beginning of life to spur our rapid growth and create our different parts. In the adult, this material is "shut down," but still exists in the genome.

All of our cells contain the entirety of our genetic material, and all of our cells know what to do, when to do it, and, as importantly, when to stop doing it. Consider how it is that your liver is where it belongs, rather than where your big toe is. Consider also that if, for example, your skin cells did not die and get sloughed off when they were replaced, there would be the potential for truly monstrous results. Apoptosis, or programmed cell death, is an important genetic function governed by specific genes.

Chromosomes are the trees on which the genes are stored. The basic design of the human body is to have a total of 46 chromosomes that are arranged into 23 pairs, half of which are acquired from each parent at conception. There are 22 pairs of autosomes (non-sex chromosomes) and one pair of sex chromosomes. Traits that are carried on the X chromosome are described as X-linked and all others are described as autosomal. Some genetic disorders, most notably Down syndrome, are the result of an extra chromosome (pair 21 has a third chromosome). Other genetic disorders can result from the lack of a chromosome.

Except for the sex chromosomes, each of the other 22 pairs of chromosomes is what is known as homologous, that is, each of the chromosomes in the pair are identical, and carry the same genes for the same functions in the same locations. Each gene that resides in one of these homologous locations (or loci) is termed an allele, and each of us has two alleles for every type of gene. When these two alleles are the same (each, for example, coding for brown eyes), that gene is termed homozygous. When the two alleles are different—one, for example, coding for brown eyes, the other for blue—that gene is termed heterozygous.

The zygote (the cell resulting from the union of sperm and egg), which begins to divide almost immediately, contains all of the genetic information it needs in order to construct a fully formed human being. The only requirement is a favorable environment and sufficient energy and nutrition.

Understanding Your Family History and Its Role in Disease Prevention

In some respects, our genes are a hand of cards we are dealt and must play. There are some genes your parents may have passed on to you, or that you may pass on to your children, that make some conditions inevitable. There are also unique mutations that can take place at the union of sperm and egg. But inevitable conditions appear to make up the smallest proportion of genetically related diseases. The largest number of genetically related disorders are what is known as multifactorial, or determined by more than one gene as well as interaction with the environment—the air we breathe, the food we eat, the exercise we enjoy (see page 121). In many respects, once we are conceived, environment can play as crucial a role in our health as our genes themselves. Looked at from another perspective, it can be said that environment plays an even more important role, given that environment is something we can manipulate to a significant degree. Indeed, this is why good prenatal care and the health of the mother during pregnancy can lead to avoidance of some birth defects and greater overall health for the child.

As the study of genetics has progressed, we have begun to understand more and more that our environment in combination with our genes often holds the key to long-term good health. As we have begun to live longer, defeat infectious illness, and reduce accidental deaths by improved safety, many of our health concerns have shifted to the diseases that were once thought to be the result of aging. Conditions such as diabetes, arthritis, cardiovascular disease, and cancer are indeed more common as we age, but research has increasingly shown that they are not an inevitable part of aging. Many factors play a role in these diseases, not only our genetic heritage but also our lifestyle choices and environments. Research shows that they are anything but inevitable. If we understand our genetic heritage and its risks, we may be able to alter our environments and lifestyles to reduce our risk of these health problems and live longer and healthier lives.

The aim of this chapter is to help you understand how your family history affects your predisposition towards certain diseases, explain some of the many exciting things happening in genetic research today, and give you some insight into how you can use that knowledge to improve your health.

HOW DOES HEREDITY INFLUENCE HEALTH?

Heredity encompasses not only the unique set of traits we inherit from our parents, it also encompasses traits that are common to our species. We get many diseases simply because we are humans, and we do not get others because our species is not susceptible to them.

Most researchers believe that we all arose from the same genome, then scattered, in discrete populations, to the various ends of the earth. That part of the human genome that has been mapped would seem to bear this out. Each of our discrete populations took certain characteristics with them and these characteristics evolved over the millennia to adapt to their particular environments. Still, we all share certain basic genetic tendencies, and as such are all more or less susceptible to particular genetically related disorders.

Our ethnic heritages also play a role in our heredity. Each ethnic heritage brings with it certain genetic risks and benefits. Jewish people of eastern European descent (Ashkenazim), for example, are about 100 times more likely to conceive a child with Tay-Sachs disease than any other population. Similarly, the vast majority of individuals with the blood disease known as sickle cell anemia (believed to be a protective mechanism against the ravages of malaria) are of African descent (see Chapter 22 for more information on sickle cell anemia).

Gender too affects our genetic inheritance. There are certain genes that are expressed in women but not in men, and vice versa, and there are certain genetic disorders that can be seen in both men and women.

Finally, our families reflect most closely our genetic heritage. But even in the same family, there is variation in genetic expression; for example, two brothers may share only some of half of their genes in common; the other half may vary considerably. Con-

THE HUMAN GENOME AND THE HUMAN GENOME PROJECT

Our individual genome is the sum of our genetic material. The human genome is the genetic material of one individual. Despite our vast individual differences we are, at the genetic level, remarkably similar. Whether we are blue-, green-, or brown-eyed, the genes that code for eye color—and all of our other traits—reside in the same places on the same chromosomes.

With this knowledge, a number of different researchers from different backgrounds—and unaware of each other's similar ideas—began, in the early 1980s, to believe that a complete sequencing of our genetic structure could be an inestimable boon to research. Some researchers theorized that it might even offer potential solutions to otherwise intractable problems, such as cancer and birth defects. If the gene (or genes) that may be involved in a particular illness were identified, its location determined, and the protein it produces understood, all sorts of doors for treatment might be opened: turning off or turning on the gene; developing gene-specific medication or genetic vaccines; or even replacing a defective gene.

In the mid-1980s, Dr. Robert Sinsheimer, at that time the Chancellor of the University of California, Santa Cruz, met with a group of prominent researchers in order to try to initiate a program that would sequence the human genome. His effort failed to attract adequate funding. At about the same time, Nobel Prize-winning molecular biologist Dr. Renato Dulbecco gave the idea an early public airing in *Science* magazine. But it was not until Charles DeLisi at the US Department of Energy's Office of Health and Environmental Research came up with a similar idea as a result of his work with inherited mutations that someone was able to invest the notion with sufficient institutional savvy and clout. By the late 1980s, the Department of Energy and the National Institutes of Health were working together, as their agreement put it, "to coordinate research and technical activities related to the human genome."

In a nutshell, the very ambitious goal of the Human Genome Project (HGP) is to create what might be called a reference map of the human genome. The mission the HGP has set for itself is "to determine the complete sequence of human DNA." In executing this vast undertaking, the HGP would also sequence the genetic makeup of a selection of other organisms that researchers often turn to as models of genetic behavior. In the end, researchers hope to be able to say with confidence which genes reside where on which chromosomes, and what they control. Because genes make up only about 10 percent of the genome, another facet of the project is to map the other genetic material and determine its function. Indeed, certain genetic material known as polymorphisms that were thought to be little more than inconsequential variation, have, under the

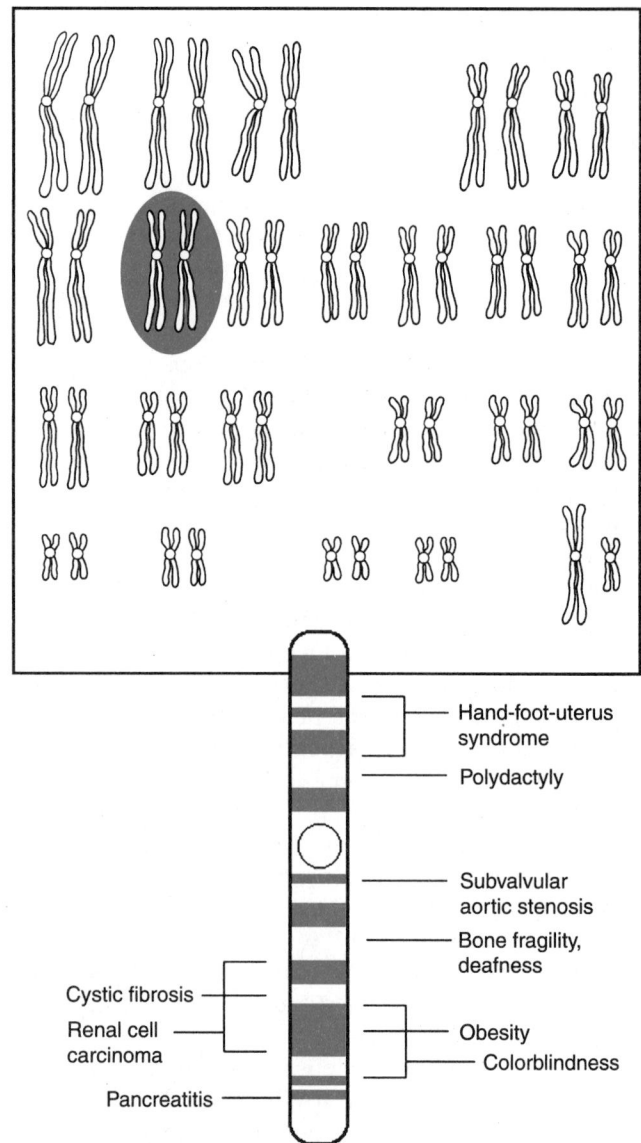

Gene map. Chromosomes of DNA typically contain a short arm (known as p) and a long arm (known as q), and each contains many genes. Abnormal genes can lead to a wide variety of diseases. Sample maps of chromosomes 6 through 12 are shown, along with the locations along the chromosomes where abnormalities in genes can lead to specific diseases. The locations are numbered in great detail for easy and consistent reference.

watchful eyes of Johns Hopkins researchers Dr. Bert Vogelstein, Dr. Kenneth Kinzler, and others, recently been shown to play a significant role in colon cancer.

Although the HGP has already taken several years, it is currently ahead of schedule. It is expected to take many more ▶

sider the example of twins. If two people are genetically identical, why do they not fall prey to the same illnesses? Think the same thoughts? Have the same tastes? Some of the most interesting studies in genetics have been done on identical twins, following both those twins who grew up together and those who were separated at birth. Astonishing differences and similarities can be manifest: one may be schizophrenic, the

▶ years—if it finally proves possible. In the end, it should give researchers (and has done so already) an astonishing array of tools, some of them potentially dangerous.

Indeed, part of the HGP is known as ELSI, an acronym for the ethical, social, and legal implications of genetic research. Nearly anyone who has heard of genetic research understands at some level that this research seeks to understand the very fiber of our being, thus leaving open the possibility of science fiction becoming science fact. While the technology to justify such worry exists mostly in the future, there are numerous instances where our burgeoning knowledge of genetics opens numerous questions (see page 129).

In terms of individual health and preventive medicine, the sought-after map of the human genome will give researchers a much better idea of which conditions are truly genetic and which are not, which are triggered by environmental factors, and perhaps how to defeat such environmental triggers. There will no doubt be many surprises.

Currently, the largest repository of information is the Online Mendelian Inheritance in Man (OMIM) database at Johns Hopkins University. The findings of researchers are posted in this database as they are made. The database is available to researchers throughout the world who are looking for specific information (see page 121).

For more information on the HGP, see the National Institutes of Health's World Wide Web pages devoted to the National Human Genome Research Institute at http://www.nhgri.nih.gov/hgp/ ■

other not; one may become alcoholic, the other not; one may be gay, the other not. Clearly—since twins are presumed to be genetically identical—environment must play a role from the very beginning of their lives.

CLONING AND TWINS

We human beings have been manipulating the genetic material of other species for millennia, and the results of those experiments are all around us. From the spots on a Dalmatian to the disease resistance of hybrid tomatoes to the docility and meatiness of domestic cattle, we have been trying to improve on "God's handiwork" since time began. Even studies of human mating behavior have shown that we select a mate not merely for love but for particular genetic traits we want to emphasize in our offspring.

But with the recent news that man has at last succeeded in cloning animals comes a wave of concern over the moral, ethical, and philosophical implications of such advanced manipulation.

In science fiction novels, cloning has been taken to varying extremes—castes of workers as identical as ants; chimerical combinations of species; and duplicates of evil geniuses who are in training to take over the world. These occasionally frightening, occasionally humorous fantasies on tapping into genetics' unmapped possibilities reflect, as art should, our collective fears and dreams. But in dreams, as the poet Delmore Schwartz said, begin responsibilities.

Cloning is the sexless reproduction of life using genetic material of a single, already existing parent, as opposed to sexual reproduction, which utilizes all new genetic material combined sexually from two parents. In the case of Dolly, the cloned Scottish sheep, genetic material was extracted from a single living cell in a 6-year-old adult ewe's udder and implanted in an already fertilized egg cell, thus replacing the new genetic material in the egg. The egg then was implanted in another, surrogate mother ewe and brought to term in an otherwise normal pregnancy. Dolly was the result.

Although the process sounds on paper perfectly logical and straightforward, it is in fact not simple at all, and the success that is Dolly resulted only after hundreds of failures. While Dolly is a genuine clone, the technology by which she was produced is still very much experimental, and in order to validate scientifically the technique that led to her birth, other laboratories must duplicate the method with similar results.

Despite being 6 years younger—and being created from 6-year-old genetic material—Dolly would seem to be the twin of the elder ewe. Yet this is something that the researchers do not yet know. What Dolly is not and never will be is the *same* ewe. No life is ever truly identical to any other life.

Despite countless science fiction scenarios that have depicted clones as identical to their genetic sources—sharing the same thoughts and fears, the same desires and skills—this is the stuff of fiction and fantasy and not reality.

We have had genetically identical humans (and animals) for eons—twins—but even identical twins are identical only at the zygote stage. In a sense, we cannot know beyond any doubt—because we do not yet have the technology to analyze the entirety of any single human's genome—that identical twins are indeed identical, gene for gene.

In any case, one twin has never been a replacement for the other. If indeed it becomes possible to clone humans, any human born from such a process would be as separate and distinct an individual as any identical twin is, with all the differences that twins have, but as importantly, with all the spiritual, ethical, and legal rights and protections of any other individual human. So cloning cannot duplicate us, offer us a new body to take over when our old one wears out, or offer us replacement parts.

Dr. Victor McKusick of Johns Hopkins is one of the foremost experts on genetics in the world and is himself a twin. Is his brother, Vincent McKusick, also a leading geneticist?

Though Vincent McKusick is similar in build and height to his brother and was genetically identical at conception, he is, as we might expect, a completely different man. Indeed, the "identical" brother is the recently retired chief justice of the Supreme Court of Maine. McKusick the geneticist suggests that personality is far more malleable by environment than physical characteristics. Research into the workings of the brain show that personality is subject to physical change by education, accident, and experience—factors that explain why complete strangers sometimes seem to have more in common with us than members of our own families. Genes may be replicable, but individual experience seldom is. Likewise, physical characteristics are also influenced by chance in development. The DNA fingerprint is absolutely identical in identical twins but the dermatoglyphic fingerprints are distinctive in every person because of chance events that influence development of the finger pads early in utero. Similarly, in the brain, the migrating neurons may take slightly different pathways in monozygotic twins.

Cloning, while it does have considerable possibilities in the field of medical research, could not, for example, recreate Albert Einstein, if somehow live tissue from Einstein still existed. Research indicates that what made Einstein Einstein was experience and environment as well as genetics.

MENDELIAN INHERITANCE

Gregor Mendel, a 19th-century Austrian monk, is regarded as the father of the modern study of genetics because he defined the mechanics by which traits are passed from parent to child. The mechanics of this transfer of traits we refer to now as Mendelian inheritance. It was Mendel who first arrived at the conclusion that our genes are paired in the somatic or ordinary cells of the body, but are segregated, or occur singly, in our germ cells, or sex cells (eggs or sperm).

Mendel performed his research on pea plants, but from these experiments much was learned about the genetic transmission of particular traits in humans. Mendel learned, for example, about dominant and recessive genes—a principle that is important in understanding how parents can pass on a disease they do not have to their children.

One of the easiest ways of illustrating the principle of dominant versus recessive is by looking at how eye color is passed from parents to child. Let us say, for example, that the gene for brown eyes is B (dominant) and the gene for blue eyes is b (recessive). The genes of brown-eyed parents can be either BB or Bb. In the latter case, the dominant trait—brown eyes—will be expressed, even though the parent also carries a recessive gene for blue eyes. The parent will never have blue eyes, but he may pass on that recessive gene to his child if he has a child with someone else who is either Bb (brown-eyed, but carrying a recessive gene) or bb (blue-eyed). Thus, two brown-eyed parents, each of whom carries a recessive gene (Bb), can have a blue-eyed child. But as a rule, two blue-eyed parents (bb) never have a brown-eyed child (although there are exceptions to the rule).

The child who has the BB or the bb genetic makeup is known as homozygous, and has identical genes in the same gene pair. The child who has the Bb trait is called heterozygous, and has different genes in the same gene pair. Since brown eye color is the dominant trait, that child will always exhibit the phenotype or expressed trait, of brown eyes, but may still carry the recessive gene for blue eyes. His genotype is Bb.

This kind of inheritance, known as autosomal dominant or autosomal recessive, works the same way for genetically deter-

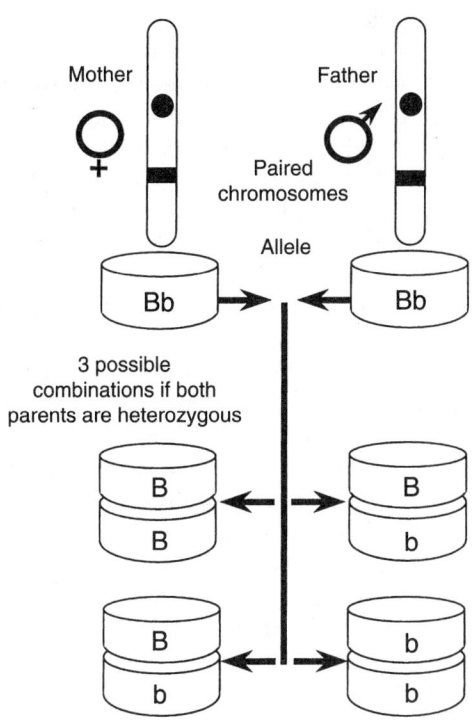

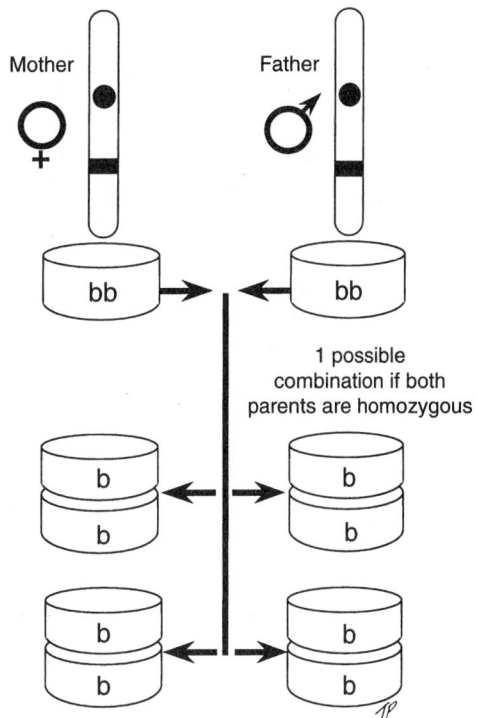

Patterns of autosomal inheritance. Alleles are alternative forms of genes on part of a DNA chromosome. Because most chromosomes are paired, genes are generally represented by two alleles. (A) A person with brown eyes may have a combination of alleles (Bb) or two identical alleles (BB, not shown). Each brown-eyed parent with the combination (Bb) could donate either type of allele (B or b) to a child, so a child whose parents both have Bb alleles could have brown eyes (BB or Bb) or blue eyes (bb). (B) A person with blue eyes has two identical alleles (bb). Each blue-eyed parent donates one of his or her b alleles to a child, so a child whose parents both have blue eyes also has blue eyes ("bb").

mined disorders as it does for eye color. (Autosomes are the nonsex chromosomes.)

Autosomal dominant inheritance occurs when a single gene with the trait (Bb) produces a person affected with a genetically determined disorder. In autosomal dominant conditions, every affected person usually has an affected parent except where the condition arises from a new mutation. For example, in achondroplasia, a form of dwarfism, 80 percent or more of cases do not have an affected parent. Most autosomal dominant disorders are rare and therefore, most affected persons have only a single copy of the disorder gene (Bb); that is, they are heterozygous. When persons with a dominant trait for a disorder have children with persons who do not carry the trait (bb), on the average, one-half of their children will be affected and half will not. Those children who are born with the B trait—if they have children with an unaffected person—have the same likelihood (50 percent) of passing along the trait. Those children born without the dominant (B) trait will not carry the gene and will not pass it along to their children.

Autosomal recessive inheritance is generally characterized in this way: if two unaffected but heterozygous people (Bb) have children, each of their children can be BB, Bb, bB, or bb, that is, there is a one-in-four chance that a child will be born homozygous for the recessive trait (bb) and express it; a one-in-two chance a child will be, like the parents, heterozygous for the recessive trait (Bb or bB) and not express it; and a one-in-four chance a child will be homozygous (BB) for the dominant trait. Only the fourth child (BB) would have no chance of passing on the trait to his own children.

Thus if both parents are carriers of a recessive gene for cystic fibrosis, for example, neither parent would have the disease, but there is a one-in-four chance any of their children might inherit the recessive gene from both parents and thereby develop the disease.

Other kinds of Mendelian inheritance in man include X-linked recessive inheri-

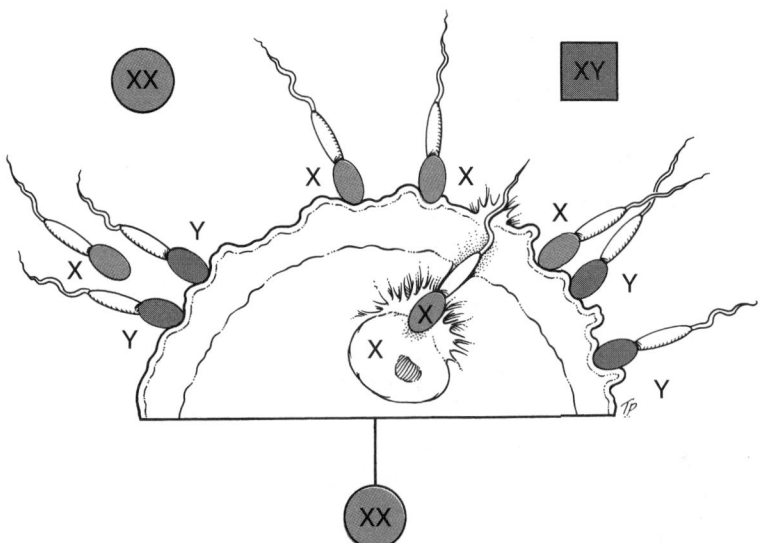

Sex chromosomes unite when a man's sperm penetrates a woman's egg. Women (XX) donate an X chromosome to their children. Men (XY) can donate either an X or a Y chromosome. Thus a child's sex is determined by which of the father's chromosomes is donated through the sperm. A girl receives an X chromosome from her father whereas a boy receives a Y chromosome from his father.

tance. In understanding sex-linked disorders, it is important to keep in mind that males are XY and females are XX as far as their sex chromosomes are concerned. A female child receives an X chromosome from each parent; a male receives an X chromosome from his mother and a Y chromosome from his father.

X-linked inheritance is so called because the responsible gene is carried on the X chromosome rather than on one of the autosomes. An example of X-linked recessive inheritance, in which nearly all those affected are male, is hemophilia (see Chapter 22 for more information on hemophilia). The trait is passed along by a heterozygous mother to half her offspring (statistically speaking), although only the males (who are hemizygous—having only one X chromosome) will express it. Since the trait is linked to the X sex chromosome, which always comes from the mother, an affected male cannot pass the disorder to his sons, although he passes the carrier gene to all his daughters.

Although these laws of inheritance follow mathematical principles, there are other genetic factors, many of which are not clearly understood, that blur the neat patterns of these equations. Thus brown eyes are dominant and blue recessive, but some children have hazel, green, or gray eyes. This has to do with something scientists call the penetrance or expressivity of genes. A gene may be recessive, for example, yet still make its presence felt. This characteristic applies to the inheritance of disorders as well, which is why children in the same family inheriting the same genetic defect can, depending on the rest of their genetic makeup, express the disease in varying ways. In one child, the disease may be extremely severe; in the other, although the genetic defect exists, the disease itself may be virtually undetectable.

Another of Mendel's genetic laws is that of independent assortment, which asserts that the genes for particular traits are transmitted from one generation to another independent of genes for other traits. The reason for independent assortment is that genes are located on different chromosomes. If a parent is a carrier of blue eye color (Bb) and also a carrier of the cystic fibrosis gene, there is no relationship between whether the eye gene for blue eyes and the gene for cystic fibrosis are transmitted to the child. The reason for independent assortment of genes for different traits is the location of the genes on different chromosomes. Even genes on the same chromosome will assort independently if they are sufficiently far apart that crossing over occurs between the genes during formation of the eyes and sperm. The genes that govern eye color, for example, do not group with the gene for cystic fibrosis. If a man with brown eyes who is a carrier of blue eye color and a carrier of cystic fibrosis has children with a woman who has similar genetic makeup, there is no relationship between whether the eye gene for blue eyes and the gene for cystic fibrosis are transmitted to their children. Children who have brown eyes and children who have blue eyes are equally likely to inherit the cystic fibrosis gene.

One relatively recent discovery that has changed our understanding of the Mendelian laws of dominance and recessivity is imprinting. With certain traits it appears that certain genes or groups of genes have been imprinted, or are chemically different depending on their origin, so that the same trait is expressed differently depending on whether it comes from the father or the mother.

Imprinting was discovered during the gene-mapping process when it was found that two distinctly different genetic diseases, each assumed to be caused by a different gene or set of genes, turned out to be caused by exactly the same gene. The only difference at the genetic level is apparently that the expressing gene came from the father or the mother. At the metabolic level the difference is two completely different diseases.

WHAT DOES MENDELIAN INHERITANCE MEAN FOR YOU?

When your doctor or a genetic counselor helps you assess your genetic risk for a particular condition, he can look at your genetic pedigree, at the suspected disorder (and how it is transmitted), and help determine either how likely you are to carry the trait and pass it along to your children, or how likely you (or your children) are to express the disorder if it is something that appears later in life. But the doctor's counsel is limited somewhat by the inevitability of genetic laws. You may be advised, for example, what your chances are of having a child with a particular disorder, and you can choose not to have children or, in some cases, to test the fetus in utero, but you cannot prevent or remedy the genetic defect should it occur. In some cases of late onset disease, however, you can prevent the disease from occurring by removing the organ at risk—the colon, for example, can be removed if you discover that you have inherited the genetic disorder called familial adenomatous polyposis (FAP) that inevitably leads to colon cancer.

Much more complex is multifactorial inheritance. Here there is no clear-cut cause-and-effect relationship between genetic mutation and disease, and there is much you can do to protect yourself from many diseases for which you may be at risk. Take, for example, a pale-skinned person who is more prone to skin cancer. By avoiding excessive exposure to sunlight, he can greatly reduce his risk for skin cancer. If he spends long hours in the sun and gets repeated bad sunburns, skin cancer will be an ongoing concern for most of his later

ONLINE MENDELIAN INHERITANCE IN MAN (OMIM)

The Online Mendelian Inheritance in Man (OMIM) Website is the brainchild of Dr. Victor McKusick, a genetics expert at Johns Hopkins. OMIM is the online version of his encyclopedic work *Mendelian Inheritance In Man*, published first in book form in 1966. OMIM is the single largest database of information on genetic disorders and the genes that underlie them. The information is updated daily. Geneticists, researchers, doctors, and genetic counselors, as well as ordinary citizens, rely on it for the latest information. Authored by Dr. McKusick and his colleagues and maintained by the National Center for Biotechnology Information, OMIM can be viewed by anyone with access to a computer and the World Wide Web at: http://www.ncbi.nlm.nih.gov/omim ∎

life. By maintaining careful vigilance over changes in the skin (such as new moles and discolorations), however, he can work with his doctor to stop skin cancer as soon as it happens and before it has a chance to spread.

GENETICALLY DETERMINED DISORDERS

The human genome is incredibly complex, and virtually everyone has some genetic abnormalities. Mutations and degradations to the genetic code occur almost all the time, but most mutations are insignificant; indeed, the cells have protective mechanisms that assist in rooting out and destroying mutated cells. In most cases, we are unaware of the abnormal genes within our own bodies. Carriers of a recessive gene for Tay-Sachs disease, for example, would have no way of knowing that they carried a defective gene unless they were tested for it or, in uniting with another Tay-Sachs carrier, had a child with Tay-Sachs. And many genetic abnormalities, such as those that cause near-sightedness, are so common or treatable that they are considered within the norm by most of us.

Genetic abnormalities or mutations can occur in a variety of ways. A defective gene can be passed from parent to child, or spontaneous mutations can occur at the moment of conception. These are mutations or abnormalities of the germ cells, or the genetic material supplied by the sperm and the egg.

Mutations can occur as single-gene mutations, in which a single gene accounts for a recognizable pattern of disorder, or as chromosomal abnormalities. Examples of some of the most serious single-gene mutations are Tay-Sachs disease, cystic fibrosis, FAP, and hemophilia. Because these disorders are due to only a single gene, they have been relatively easy to map and to develop tests for. Chromosomal aberrations or abnormalities can occur if there are too many chromosomes (Down syndrome, for example, is the result of an extra chromosome in pair 21), or if there is a defect or abnormality in one of the chromosomes or, possibly, if there is only a single chromosome where there should be a pair (Turner syndrome, for example, results when a girl is born with only a single sex chromosome). Although these single-gene and chromosomal mutations are present at birth, the disorder they cause may have an onset early in life (even in the womb) or much later. Though genetic abnormalities cannot be altered or repaired given our present medical knowledge, some of the disorders they cause can be effectively treated, but for others there is no treatment.

While there is much that is black-and-white about single-gene and chromosomal abnormalities—if you have this particular defect, you will inevitably suffer this particular disorder—there is much that is gray in these areas, too. A child can be severely affected by Down syndrome, for example, or mildly affected by Down syndrome, though the chromosomal error is the same. Our genetic makeup appears to have many checks and balances that affect the penetrance or expressivity of a genetic disorder. Children within a single family may each inherit the same genetic defect, yet depending on the rest of their genetic makeup the disorder may express itself severely or virtually invisibly.

This is even more true of genetic abnormalities or mutations that occur in the somatic cells (the cells of the body). These mutations, which are far more common, are not present at birth but rather occur sometime during the life span. In many cases, these mutations are caused by environmental insults, such as the ultraviolet rays of the sun that cause skin cancer. Mutations of the somatic cells are not inherited, but the propensity to develop these mutations may be inherited in the same way that fair skin is passed from parent to child. Genetic mutation of our bodies' cells may be extremely detrimental to our health (causing cancer, for example) or may have no effect on our health whatsoever because of the body's protective mechanisms. Even more importantly, genetic mutations are often within our power to prevent by making lifestyle and environment alterations.

Polygenic or multifactorial conditions are dependent not on a single gene but on the interaction of several genes, as well as the interaction of the environment. In many cases, genetic abnormalities do not cause the disease so much as they increase the propensity to develop the disease. While particular genes involved in various conditions (such as breast or colon cancer) may be identified, the presence of these genes does not inevitably lead to the disorder. Many factors are responsible for these disorders to be expressed, and if all the factors are not present, the disorder may not occur. Recent studies on the breast cancer genes, for example, have shown that many genes appear to play a role and that the presence of a defective gene increases one's risk but does not guarantee that cancer will occur.

LOCATING THE GENES RESPONSIBLE FOR GENETIC DISORDERS

Many important genetic diseases have been mapped to specific chromosome locations, and it often seems that new ones are being located weekly. The enormous amount of media attention these discoveries receive often leaves the reading public with the impression that a cure lies just around the corner. Identifying genetic markers is, however, only one step on the long and winding road that can lead to treatment and possibly cure.

The following are some important genetic diseases that have been mapped to specific chromosome locations:

- Huntington's disease
- Cystic fibrosis
- Hemophilia A
- Marfan syndrome
- Sickle cell anemia

- Beta-thalassemia
- Alpha-thalassemia
- Fragile X syndrome
- Phenylketonuria
- Duchenne's muscular dystrophy
- Retinoblastoma
- Familial hypercholesterolemia
- Polycystic kidney disease
- Gaucher's disease
- Hemochromatosis
- G6PD deficiency
- Tay-Sachs disease
- Neurofibromatosis type 1 and 2
- Familial polyposis coli

For the diseases noted above, cloning of the identified genes has been accomplished, either partially or completely, but there are other diseases, such as cleft palate, for which locations have been mapped but the genes not yet cloned. For some diseases, such as familial breast cancer, familial Alzheimer's disease, and prostate cancer, genetic markers have been mapped and the genes themselves cloned, but these particular genes are responsible for only a small number of the cases of the disease. Indeed, these genes may not actually cause the disorder, but rather may increase one's risk of acquiring the disorder. The cloning of a gene is an important step on the path toward possible gene therapy. By cloning the gene, researchers can then reproduce it synthetically in order to create enough of it to use experimentally. One of the ways genetic researchers look for genetic markers is by studying certain populations that arose from a relatively contained group of common ancestors: the Amish, Ashkenazi Jews, South African Afrikaners, French Canadians, Finns, and certain others are favorites of researchers because of their relatively homogeneous gene pool. If one of the founders of the population had by chance a mutation that is responsible for a disorder, that single heritable mutation is much easier to trace than it would be in the general population.

But just because a population is easy to study does not mean that it is more likely to suffer from particular disorders. Consider the front-page news of the discovery by Johns Hopkins researchers of the first known gene related to familial colorectal

cancer, or FCC. Although it was suspected that certain types of colorectal cancer ran in families, and FCC is believed to account for an estimated 15 to 50 percent of all colorectal cancers, its genetic basis remained something of a mystery until this particular mutation was discovered in a single patient of Ashkenazi Jewish descent (Ashkenazim, or Jews of European descent, account for about 95 percent of all American Jews). Researchers, believing that the many common genetic traits of this group might provide insights into the causes of FCC, went on to study 766 Ashkenazim. The researchers found the mutation in over 6 percent of those studied. The Johns Hopkins team then studied blood and tissue samples of 211 Ashkenazi Jewish colon cancer patients. They found that one in six of those patients who developed colorectal cancer before age 66, and one in eight of those who developed colorectal cancer at any age, had the mutation. Moreover, the mutation was found in nearly one-third of Ashkenazi patients with a family history of colorectal cancer.

But after the headlines appeared when the FCC study was reported, many people mistakenly deduced from it that colon cancer was more common in Jews than in others, or even—wildly—that all Jews had the mutation or that all who had the mutation would contract the disorder. This is clearly not the case.

While the study and the simple test the researchers devised to detect the mutation are specific to the Ashkenazi Jewish population, the investigators say it provides important clues about FCC among the general population as well. This is also true of studies of the breast cancer genes in the same population. Kenneth Kinzler, PhD, associate professor of oncology and codirector of the FCC study, noted that "Studying specific populations makes the discovery of genetic mutations easier. These findings then serve as a paradigm for the general population."

More than 130,000 cases of colon cancer are diagnosed in the United States each year. At least 15 percent to as many as half of these cases are thought to have a hereditary component. FCC is the most common hereditary form. FAP and hereditary non-polyposis colon cancer, two other inherited syndromes well defined by Hopkins researchers in prior studies, account for another 3 to 5 percent of colon cancers. The remaining cases occur sporadically, with no as-yet apparent inherited genetic link, among the general population.

Mormons, because of the meticulous genealogic records of their population, are also a favorite for genetic study. It was in a group of largely Mormon women in Utah that the BRCA1 gene, which has been linked with breast cancer, was first isolated.

But again that does not mean that only Mormon women have the mutation—indeed it exists throughout the population. Researchers were able to take those records and work backwards to a result that could then be applied to the population as a whole.

The list above is by no means a comprehensive list of all the genes linked to various disorders that have been discovered. Any list made today would be outdated tomorrow. See page 121 for further information on genes that have been linked to disease.

For questions and answers about a new gene test for colon cancer among the Ashkenazi Jewish population, call the Johns Hopkins Hereditary Colorectal Cancer Program at (410) 955-4041.

Genetics and Health Care

When you first visit a doctor you may be asked to arrive at your appointment early, and before you see the doctor you are usually handed a clipboard with a stack of papers to fill out. Some of these forms are for insurance purposes, but most of the others relate to your medical history, what medications you may be using—both prescription and over-the-counter—and also to your family history and your genetic background.

If you see a cardiologist, for example, you will likely be asked about the incidence of cardiovascular disease in your family, as well as other related conditions—did anyone have a stroke? Heart attack? Is there diabetes in your family? If you see a gastroenterologist, you may be asked about incidence of bowel cancer, inflammatory bowel disease, and so on, in your family. If you are being screened for breast cancer, you may be asked whether there is any history of breast cancer in your family. The more you know about your family history, the more you will be able to assist your doctor in your

health care (see page 126 for more information on gathering and representing these data.)

The goal of these screening questions is to concentrate health efforts in protecting you from diseases for which you are at the greatest risk. In the United States, for example, all adults are at risk for cardiovascular disease, statistically speaking, because it is the number one cause of death. Adults who have a family history of cardiovascular disease are at even greater risk. Fortunately, there are many things we can do to reduce our risk of cardiovascular disease such as exercising more, eating a heart-healthy diet, and not smoking (see Chapter 1 and Chapter 2).

For people with a family history of a particular cancer, there are a variety of precautionary measures to take. One is more frequent screening for cancer, because early diagnosis and treatment are two of the most effective weapons against cancer. Another is to reduce environmental triggers—avoiding the sun's ultraviolet rays or the harmful chemicals in tobacco will greatly reduce the risk of skin or lung cancer, for example. For some people who are at very high risk for a particular cancer, more aggressive preventive measures might be considered. Prophylactic removal of the colon or the breast, for example, might be a preventive measure for those people whose family history marks them as almost certain targets of these cancers.

GENE THERAPY

Although limited gene therapy has been employed in a medical setting for a few years now, most such treatments remain theoretical and are as much guesswork as science. Yet gene therapy is by no means science fiction.

What is gene therapy and what can it accomplish?

A gene, you may recall, works with other genes to code for a protein, or to cause a particular protein to be made. While we know proteins most prominently as the stuff of which our muscles and other tissues are made, proteins have a multiplicity of other functions—everything from neural transmission to immune function and beyond. A defective gene, then, may cause the manufacture of nothing at all, or of a defective protein that has implications throughout the body.

The idea behind gene therapy seems relatively simple: replace a defective gene with a good one. The illustration to the right gives an example of one method of gene therapy. Actually doing so is a good deal more difficult. In a human being, it is estimated that there are about 10 trillion cells—an astonishing number when you consider that each cell has an entire copy of a person's genetic material in it.

Therefore, replacing a defective gene is a very complicated process because each of our body's cells has a copy of the defective gene. In order to fix the defective gene, a significant number of cells would, in theory, have to be invaded and their genetic material replaced. How do we accomplish this?

There would seem to be a number of different possibilities. Experiments have used different methods to insert new genes into the cells of research animals with differing levels of success. In some cases the genomes of these animals have actually incorporated the genes and passed them along to their offspring.

In the early 1980s researchers at the University of Pennsylvania performed experimental gene therapy on families of mice with a malfunctioning growth gene by injecting into the eggs of parent mice a growth hormone gene from rats. Only about 1 percent of these experiments worked—from most standpoints, not a very high success rate—but that they were successful at all is astonishing. In those mice in which the therapy worked, "cured" mice grew normally. More importantly, the genetic defect appeared to have been erased from the mice's genome so that these new, normal mice did not pass along the defect to their offspring. There was of course no effect on the parent mice. Although this sort of treatment is exponentially more complex in human beings—not only from a medical but also from an ethical point of view—the experiments do offer some hope that workable therapies can be developed.

Another, different kind of gene therapy that is possible is the bone marrow transplant, which aims to transplant certain kinds of marrow cells as well as the genetic material within them that enables them to regenerate. Consider the example of severe

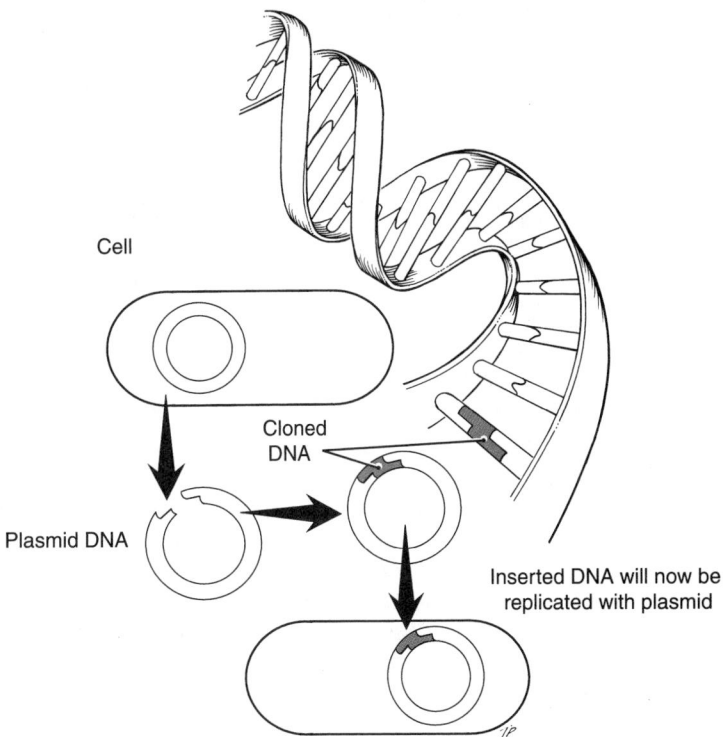

Cell

Cloned DNA

Plasmid DNA

Inserted DNA will now be replicated with plasmid

Cloning using plasmids. Plasmids are circular DNA molecules that exist in nature and can replicate independently. Additional DNA fragments can be joined to a plasmid and will then be replicated many times.

combined immune deficiency syndrome, the "bubble boy" disease (see Chapter 22). In this disorder about 25 percent of sufferers are unable to create a particular enzyme because of a genetic defect. The absence of this enzyme impairs the body's ability to produce the immune system's all-important killer T cells. This lack leaves the person with severe combined immune deficiency syndrome unable to ward off the diseases a normal immune system would regularly prevent or defeat. T cells are generated by a very small number of marrow cells that exist in every normal immune system, and although they make up only a tiny fraction of the actual marrow, they are remarkably prolific. Sometimes cells with this ability (and the genetic material that enables them to reproduce themselves) can be transferred to other people. You may know that with bone marrow transplants, marrow donors must be a close match to the recipient. This means that the genetic material supplied by the donor must be similar enough to that of the recipient that the transplant will take, or that the transplanted cells will enter the recipient's body and work the way they do in the

CONSTRUCTING A FAMILY GENETIC TREE

In largely homogenous societies where there has not been as much ethnic mixing as there has in the United States, people may have a much more complete idea of what genetic diseases they or their children could be prone to. But in the genetic mixture that exists in the melting pot of the United States, heritages may be so diverse and families so far-flung that we may be completely unaware of the susceptibilities and predispositions that are in our genes.

As more and more information about genes becomes available, a considerable part of preventive medicine is likely to be devoted to understanding the genetic variables in our past and using them to our health advantage. In an ideal setting, every doctor would have a genetic pedigree of his patients that he could use to rule out specific disorders or to get clues as to how to treat them. He could spot trends and recommend genetic testing or recommend particular diet or lifestyle changes that would be beneficial. In an era where medical records are more accessible than financial histories, having a genetic pedigree on file can be a double-edged sword. But knowing your own family history still has considerable value. The question is, how do you put it together?

A family pedigree is very much like a family tree of the sort you would use to map your family's social history. If you have a personal computer, software packages are available that can help you map both your family's social and medical history. In the case of a family or genetic pedigree, the tree describes the patterns of inheritance of particular genetic traits and the incidence of particular disorders in the family. A family tree can give you wonderful insight into who your forebears were—lawyers, bankers, inventors, kings, queens, or knaves. Similarly, a genetic pedigree can give you and your doctor wonderful information that can help you prevent disease.

In order to establish your genetic pedigree, it is best to go back as far as you can, past your parents to your grandparents, great grandparents, and even great-great-grandparents. This can represent a substantial amount of history, but collecting it can be a fascinating and rewarding experience. You will want to collect the following two pieces of information about each family member that you research (and as many others as possible).

- Cause of death. This can be done by obtaining a death certificate from the municipality in which the person died if no one in your family can recall the cause of death.

- Any chronic disorders such as heart disease, alcoholism, or diabetes—in short, anything at all you can find about their medical history.

Constructing a Family Genetic Pedigree

Here are the figures used in a family genetic pedigree to describe the members of the family, their position in the family, and so on.

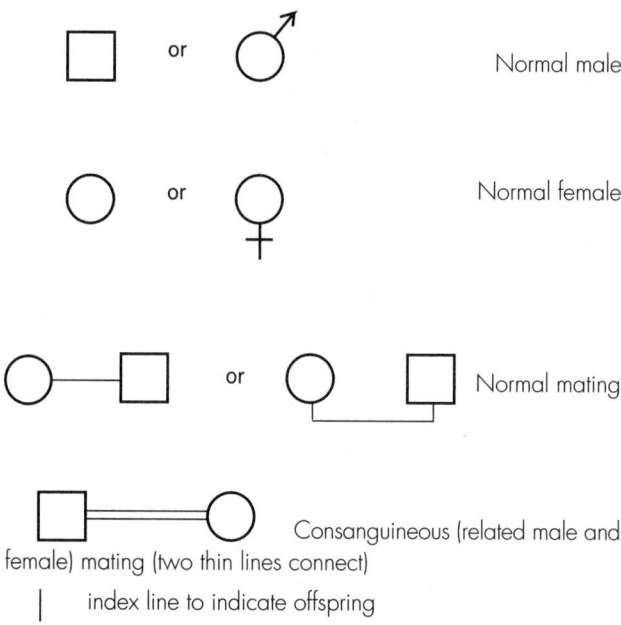

Normal male

Normal female

Normal mating

Consanguineous (related male and female) mating (two thin lines connect)

index line to indicate offspring

A fully darkened circle or square indicates a person homozygous for a particular trait or disease.

A darkened figure indicates a person affected with a particular trait or disease (see page 118).

The symbols can also be divided as many as four times in order to describe the varying ways people may manifest a particular syndrome.

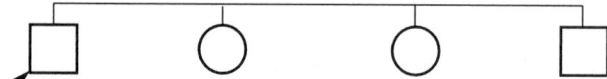

Brothers and sisters (or siblings) of particular parents; arrow indicates the proband, or the person whose pedigree is described by the diagram (see below).

Siblings whose inheritance of a trait or syndrome is unknown or unimportant can, for preservation of space, be described by a square or circle with the number of brothers or sisters in it.

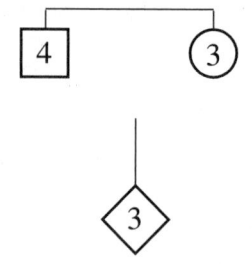

If the gender of the siblings is unknown, they can be indicated by a diamond. Multiple siblings of unknown gender can be described by a diamond with the number of siblings in it.

Abortions or miscarriages are described by a small darkened circle.

Identical, or monozygotic, twins are described by a pair of circles or squares, connected to the parents by single, angled index lines and to one another by a straight index line. Fraternal, or dizygotic, twins are described by a pair of circles or squares, ▶

or a circle and a square, without being connected to each other by a straight index line. If it is uncertain whether the twins

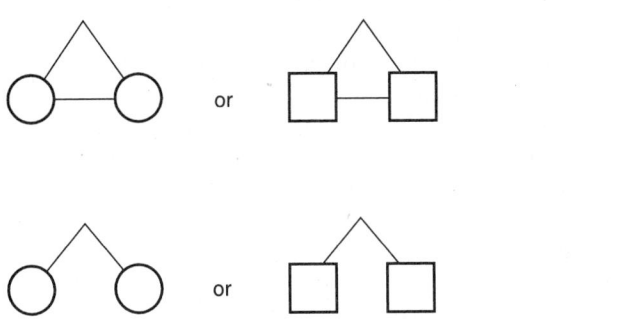

were mono- or dizygotic, a question mark is entered between the twin sibs.

A diagonal line through the circle or square or a windowpane shape in the middle of the circle or square is used to designate a deceased member of the family.

Each generation of the family is designated with a roman numeral. If you were beginning with your father's family, for example, and began with his parents, the first line of the chart would be designated I and would include his grandmother and grandfather. The second line—your parents—would be II, and your line—the person whose history is being described is called the index case, the proband, or the propositus (male), and proposita (female)—is III.

Putting it Together: The Smith Family

Below is a family pedigree for the fictitious Smith family, some members of which have the autosomal dominant disorder known as familial adenomatous polyposis (FAP) a single-gene disorder that causes the individual to grow polyps in the colon, or large intestine, beginning around the age of 11 years. The growths increase as the years go on, leading almost certainly to colon cancer, unless prophylactic treatment is begun. The disease is transmitted vertically, that is, from parent to child, with a 50 percent risk that the child of an affected parent will have the disease.

1. Stan Smith has FAP. His wife, Brenda, is unaffected. They have three children, Stan, Jr., Jennifer, and Laura. All were at 50 percent risk of developing FAP. Stan, Jr., and Laura are affected.

2. Stan, Jr., and his wife, Elizabeth, have two children. Although both children had a 50 percent chance of inheriting FAP, neither did. Neither will pass the gene along to their children.

3. Jennifer and her husband, Mark, have two children. Since Jennifer is unaffected there was no risk of FAP to her children.

4. Laura and her husband, John, have three children. All the children had a 50 percent chance of inheriting FAP; two are affected.

In some cases, when working up a family pedigree, you may want to make more than one if you are tracking the presence of more than one condition. Still, individual symbols can be divided to indicate as many as four traits. There are computer programs available that can allow you to include a variety of information for each member of your family. ■

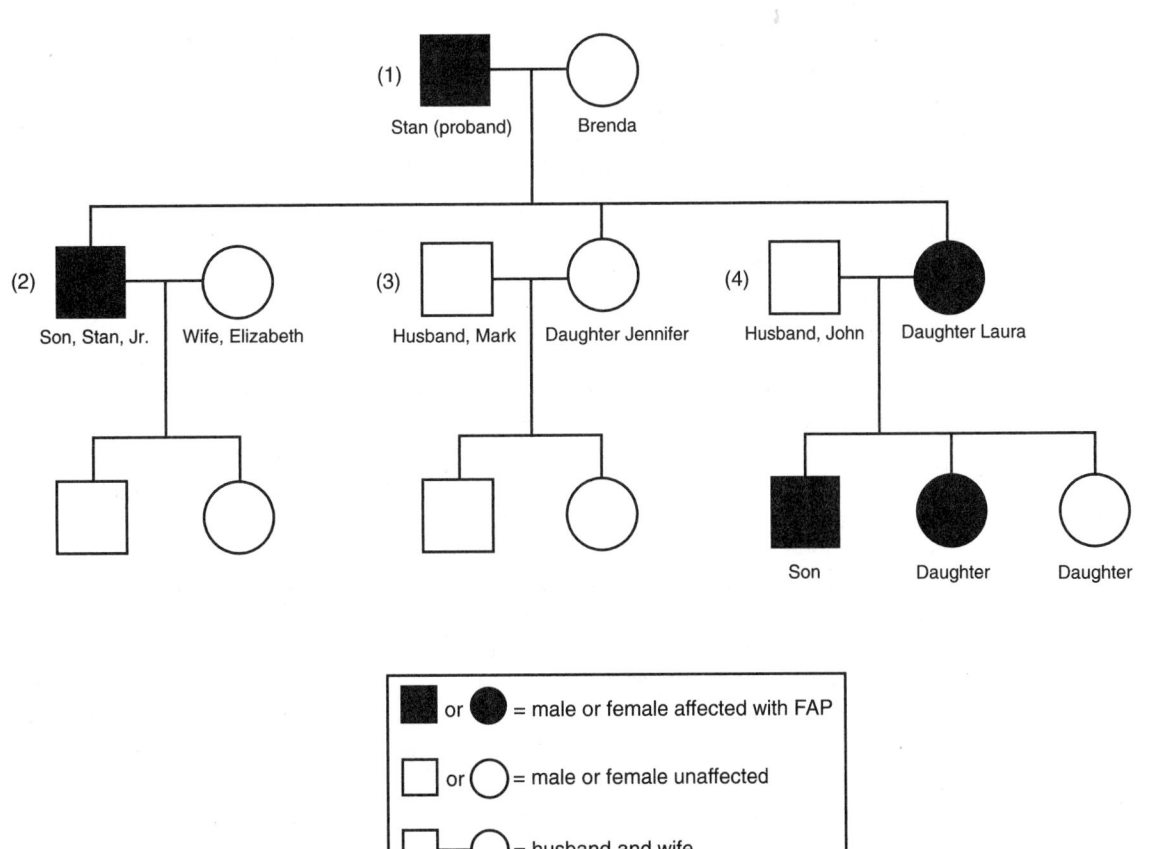

donor without being rejected. People who have severe combined immune deficiency syndrome may have healthy siblings from whom they can obtain such a bone marrow transplant.

In a successful treatment of this type (which is by no means guaranteed because of the small numbers of these cells), the person can actually be cured. In this case, the faulty gene is not replaced throughout the body, but cells with healthy genetic material capable of reproducing themselves are introduced and are able to replicate themselves sufficiently to bolster the immune system to normal capacity. But the therapy, as it stands today, fails more often than it succeeds. This is because the cells in question represent such a small fraction of the marrow cells. If the transplanted marrow contains none of them, it will not work. If the genetic material is not closely enough matched, then the transplanted cells will be immunologically rejected.

There are still other experimental techniques in the experimental stages that may allow for yet other kinds of genetic therapy.

Curiously, perhaps the most popular tools for genetic therapy researchers are retroviruses, or the class of virus to which the virus that causes acquired immunodeficiency syndrome (AIDS) belongs. Retroviruses gain their name from their ability to reverse some of the genetic replication process and insert genetic material into cells. If researchers can succeed in infecting a sufficient number of genetically defective cells with healthy genes, cures for many diseases may be possible. It may be possible to use lymphocytes, or white blood cells, the agents-at-large of the immune system, to "piggyback" genetic material around the body. In this case, disabled viruses with new genetic material are attached to the cells and inserted all around the body. The viruses make their way into the cells and leave the good genetic material.

To fight kidney cancer, for example, researchers have developed and begun testing a genetically engineered cancer vaccine that contains an immune system activating gene. A retrovirus carries a potent immune system activating gene into the cancer cells; the gene supercharges the immune system, causing it to seek and destroy cancer cells. Similar vaccines are being tested for use in prostate and pancreatic cancers; results have been promising although use of these vaccines outside of small human trials is still years away.

Viruses, of course, even disabled ones, have the potential to be dangerous. Could a disabled virus that is clever enough to insinuate itself into cells also find a way to re-enable itself once in the body? One of the difficulties of AIDS research has been the virus's ability to adapt to its surroundings and change its genetic shape. How will foreign particles such as viruses react with the immune system? Is there not the potential to make matters even worse?

With each potential solution comes an increased number of questions, all of which need to be answered before gene therapy can be as regular a part of our medical arsenal as antibiotics and vaccinations. In theory it should be possible to replace individual defective genes; in some rare cases it has been done. But at the moment, the tools we have are blunt and they make the research process a little like driving a nail with dynamite: one blast in hundreds may drive the nail in exactly right.

So while there is considerable hope for the future, genetic therapy is not yet a standard tool for doctors.

ONCOGENES: SWITCHED-ON CANCER GENES

One of the most fascinating aspects of our bodies' genetic code is that the genetic material in our cells not only knows when to turn itself on but when to turn itself off. From the undifferentiated cell created by the union of our parents' germ cells, our bodies create the 10 trillion highly differentiated and specialized cells of the adult. All of these cells have genetic information built into them that not only spurs particularized growth but also includes the information to stop growth when it is appropriate to do so. There is also information to trigger apoptosis, when it is time for one cell to move aside and make room for its daughter cells.

The genes that promote growth have become known as proto-oncogenes. Accompanying them in the genome are genes known as suppressor genes that are programmed to halt growth. Most—in fact, nearly all—of the time, they do their jobs perfectly well. Some of the first research in this area was conducted at the Johns Hopkins Oncology Center, although major credit goes to Princeton for developments in this area. The p53 tumor suppressor gene is the most commonly mutated gene in human cancer. When the gene is mutated, its growth-halting programming can be damaged, thus allowing mutated cells to grow unabated. While our cells are equipped with considerable defense and repair mechanisms, occasionally one of these proto-oncogenes becomes mutated and turns on growth when it should not. Or one of the suppressor genes, such as p53, fails and cannot adequately control growth, which allows a tumor to grow.

Research into the p53 gene has led to the development of screening tests for certain types of colon cancer, and has helped lay the groundwork for similar discoveries in other types of cancer, such as the BRCA1 gene that has been implicated in breast cancer.

Genetic Counseling and Testing

Because of a growth in understanding over the last several years of how the human genome works and the increase in the sophistication of technology for analyzing genes and identifying their locations on chromosomes, there are now hundreds of genetic disorders for which people can be tested.

Most gene testing is as simple a procedure as having blood drawn—so simple that too often people are not even aware they are being tested for a genetic disorder. It is in the lab where the sophisticated procedures take place. Lab technicians remove your white blood cells, and then they remove the genetic material in them. The genetic material (DNA) is then broken down and analyzed for a particular defective gene or set of genes.

Despite the ease with which genetic material can be removed and sent to the lab, these tests are not at all like having your family doctor take a throat culture to see if you have a strep infection. Indeed, some of these tests have so many potential ramifications and variables that genetic counseling has rapidly become a necessary component of all such testing. If you are to be tested, you need to understand not only the medical implications of both positive and nega-

tive results, but the potential emotional and financial implications of the results.

In the past, when genetic tests were few, genetic counseling was something nearly every doctor could do in the office. But with the proliferation of genetic tests, the issue has become considerably more complex. Genetic counseling is only about 20 to 25 years old as a specialty, and there are about 1,500 genetic counselors in the United States. Recent studies have shown that if you are deciding to have genetic testing performed, proper counseling by an experienced counselor can prove invaluable in helping you make the decision that is right for you (see page 132).

PRENATAL GENETIC COUNSELING AND TESTING

Prenatal testing is the most well-known type of genetic testing. When a couple is deciding to conceive, they may be referred by their doctor to a genetic counselor because of the possibility that one or both families may carry a particular genetic disorder. Much counseling on routine matters is still performed by obstetricians in the office (those matters related, for example, to the age of the parents), but recent research has shown that assistance from an experienced counselor can, for those choosing to have genetic testing performed, prove invaluable in making informed, sensible decisions based on the latest information available.

Preconception genetic testing involves taking samples of both prospective parents' blood and analyzing its DNA content for abnormal genes. This is usually performed on couples who are at a high risk for a particular genetic defect, either because there is a family history of a disease (such as cystic fibrosis) or because they are part of a group at high risk for a particular disease (such as Jews of Eastern European descent, who are at high risk of being Tay-Sachs carriers).

Prenatal genetic testing is performed while the fetus is in utero. Again, this is usually performed when there is a family history of a particular disease or when parents are part of a group at high risk for a particular disease, such as women over age 35, who are at high risk for conceiving babies with Down syndrome. Prenatal genetic testing is most commonly performed using one of three methods:

- Amniocentesis, in which amniotic fluid is drawn from the womb during pregnancy

- Chorionic villus sampling, which is similar to amniocentesis, but performed earlier in the pregnancy

- Percutaneous umbilical blood sampling, in which fetal blood is removed from the umbilicus via a needle inserted into the mother's abdomen

Each of these methods is low risk and designed to give the doctor or counselor what is known as a karyotype of the fetus, or what is essentially a portrait of the fetus's chromosomes. This allows the counselor or doctor to look for known abnormalities. For more information on these prenatal screening tests, as well as postnatal screening tests for genetic abnormalities, such as phenylketonuria, see Chapter 7.

HOW DOES GENETIC COUNSELING WORK?

A genetic counselor will explain to prospective parents the mechanics of genetic inheritance. He will explain how testing works and what the tests can show and what they cannot show (some tests are quite accurate, while others can miss the trait).

Once testing has been performed—whether on the parents before conception or on the fetus in utero—the counselor will receive the results and can then present the potentialities. Most often the news is good—neither of the parents carries the trait, or only one does, and the trait, although it may be carried by offspring, will not express. If both parents happen to carry the trait, or if one parent carries a dominant trait that expresses later in life, the counselor will explain what having the trait means and how the parents might choose to work with it. This information would include everything from considering adoption rather than conception to terminating a pregnancy if the fetus, after conception, tests homozygous for the genetic disorder. If the parents decide they want to assume the risk then the counselor would explain how the disease works and what the likely outcome would be.

For example, for some diseases, such as Tay-Sachs disease, the testing is quite reliable, and the baby's outcome—an early death—inevitable. For others, such as cystic fibrosis, the testing is not so certain. About 4 percent of the white population in the United States carries the recessive trait, and about 70 to 85 percent of carriers can be identified. Once conception takes place, further genetic testing on the fetus can be performed and will demonstrate whether the fetus is homozygous for the trait. A child with cystic fibrosis may die quite young but can sometimes survive into young adulthood. While a counselor cannot tell a couple what they should do, he can guide the couple through the potential outcomes, discuss treatment options, and may make referrals to psychologists or to clergy in order to help prospective parents make such difficult and weighty decisions.

Genetic Counseling of Adults with a Family History of a Genetic Disease

Genetic counseling of healthy adults (or young adults) who have a high hereditary risk factor for a particular disorder that is expressed later in life is a relatively new but growing branch of genetic counseling. The disorders being tested for are often single-gene disorders, but they can also be multifactorial, and testing is almost always sought on the basis of family history. It is in these sorts of tests where counseling can be of greatest value. Many of the disorders that can be found through testing cannot as yet be treated, so counseling before testing is essential to making an informed decision on whether to have the test at all. While a negative test result can allow a person to breathe easier and go on with life, a positive result can seem like a death sentence and can lead to anxiety and depression. A genetic counselor can help a potential carrier of the trait consider all of the potential ramifications of a positive test result, including the possibility of loss of medical insurance for a preexisting condition or even the possibility of employment discrimination, and can help the person make a rational decision about the wisdom of testing.

Too often, according to many genetic counselors, testing is performed before counseling is done, and the counselor has to play catch-up. Ideally, anyone who is recommended to have genetic testing ought to see a genetic counselor before the testing is performed so that the nature of the test and the nature of the results are explained and all the implications are made clear. According to a recent study by Johns Hopkins researchers, the nature and implications of genetic testing are too often inadequately addressed before testing is performed (see page 132).

WHAT A GENETIC COUNSELOR WILL NEED

When you see a genetic counselor about the possibility of family-linked disease, the counselor will want as much of your family medical history as possible, going back at least four generations. He will want as thorough a medical history as you can obtain of your parents, their siblings, their parents, grandparents, and great-grandparents. In some cases, the only information available to you may be the cause of death, but that is important for a counselor to have in order to assess your risk and the necessity of any tests. He will also need as much information as possible about all your other first-degree relatives (brothers and sisters) and their incidence of disease. Some of this information you will know, but some will require research (see page 126).

WHAT CAN GENETIC TESTING AND COUNSELING DO FOR YOU?

Because a genetic counselor is specifically educated to address particular types of

GENETIC TESTING AND INSURANCE COVERAGE

Companies that provide health coverage want very much to know the results of genetic testing: a subscriber with a positive test could end up being quite costly to the insurer down the road. There is still very little legal precedent in this area. Some argue that discrimination based on a genetic test is against the law. But insurance companies have already argued with some success that a genetic predisposition toward breast, prostate, or some other cancer makes it a preexisting condition and therefore one that is not covered under the insurance.

A genetic test has the potential to be life changing. Many genetic counselors recommend that before someone undergoes testing he should beef up his insurance and make sure he has adequate health and life insurance that will cover him even if a genetic defect is discovered. But the issue is still thorny—some people have had themselves tested under a false identity so that test results would not get back to their insurance carrier. Too often, say genetic counselors, people are referred to them only after a positive result and come to counseling without having had adequate education on the process.

The issue of insurance coverage for genetic conditions will not be settled soon. No doubt more genetic assays will come on the market and more people will be denied insurance coverage for their illnesses. The responsibilities of both parties will probably only be resolved after considerable debate, but clearly the technology we have at the moment has outpaced our ability to use it in the most responsible fashion.

Should You Have Genetic Testing?

This is a question all individuals will have to answer for them-

selves, with a thorough understanding of the potential health benefits as well as the limitations, and also the potential for discrimination.

If you are tested for a genetic mutation or defect, it is possible to do so without your insurer's knowledge if you pay for the test out of your own pocket. Not disclosing a preexisting condition to your insurer, however, can be grounds for cancellation of the entire policy. If you have the test done under your own name, the results will still be in your medical records, and should you ever change your health or life insurance plans, any prospective insurer will gain access to those records. Anonymous testing is possible, but it carries the same risk of cancellation of your coverage. It is wise to consult a genetic counselor before undergoing this type of genetic testing so that you will be aware of all the potential risks, benefits, and ramifications.

Genetic testing should be an asset to your doctor and your health, but it is not yet so simple an equation. Geneticists and researchers have formed a coalition, as part of the Human Genome Project, to look into the repercussions of genetic testing (see page 116). Known as ELSI (an acronym for ethical, legal, and societal implications), the coalition is attempting to institute uniform procedures and protocols for genetic testing and influence legislation related to the ethical, legal, and social implications of genetic testing.

Recently legislation was proposed that would make a person's genetic pedigree irrelevant in obtaining health insurance. It is a positive step, but far from becoming the law of the land. ■

GENETIC DISEASE SUPPORT GROUPS

- The Alliance of Genetic Support Groups
  A nonprofit organization providing information for individuals and families who have genetic disorders. They can be reached on the World Wide Web at http://www.medhelp.org/geneticalliance/

- American Cancer Society
  Phone: (800) ACS–2345
  Web site: http://www.cancer.org

- American Self-Help Clearinghouse
  Northwest Covenant Med Center
  25 Pocono Rd.
  Denville, NJ 07834–2995
  Contact person: Edward J. Madara, Executive Director
  Phone: (201) 625–9565
  Fax: (201) 625–8848
  TDD number: (201) 625–9053
  Web site: http://www.cmhc.com/selfhelp

- The American Society of Human Genetics
  9650 Rockville Pike
  Bethesda, MD 20814–3998
  Phone: (301) 571–1825
  Web site: http://www.faseb.org/genetics/ashg/ashgmenu.htm

- Directory of National Genetic Voluntary Organizations
  This is a Web site that offers hypertext links to many of the hundreds of support organizations that exist to help individuals and families with genetic disorders, which include conditions as diverse as breast cancer, hypercholesterolemia, and Shprintzen's syndrome.
  Web site: http://medhlp.netusa.net/agsg/agsgsup.htm

- The Joseph and Rose Kennedy Institute of Ethics
  This teaching and research center offers moral and ethical perspectives on the ethics of genetic research and links to other sites where information may be obtained.
  Web site:http://guweb.georgetown.edu/kennedy/

- March of Dimes
  National Office
  1275 Mamaroneck Ave.
  White Plains, NY 10605
  Web site: http://www.modimes.org/ ■

genetic tests, he may be able to inform you more thoroughly than your doctor about the implications of the tests you are considering. First of all, a genetic counselor may help you decide if the test is even necessary. If the test is necessary, the genetic counselor will make certain that you understand what a positive result means and does not mean, and what a negative result means and does not mean. In some cases, a negative result does not rule out the potential for illness completely, so you need to be aware of this. Additionally, a counselor will educate you about the potential ramifications of a positive result on the test not only in terms of what it indicates about your likelihood of disease, but also what it can mean in terms of social factors, such as your emotional response and the economic realities. If you test positive for a cancer gene, your insurance company may consider any cancer arising out of that genetic mutation to be a preexisting condition and therefore one that is not covered under your insurance (see page 131). The genetic counselor may also refer you to psychological counseling, or to support groups and organizations dedicated to research on particular genetic and birth defects.

THE IMPORTANCE OF PROPER GENETIC COUNSELING

A recent study by Johns Hopkins researchers demonstrates that many doctors may not yet be equipped to supply their patients with the information about genetic testing that they would like.

Dr. Francis Giardiello, associate professor of medicine at Johns Hopkins, was the lead author of a recent nationwide study reported in the *New England Journal of Medicine* that looked into whether people received adequate genetic counseling or gave written, informed consent to having genetic tests. The study found results that are quite disturbing.

Nearly a third of the doctors surveyed did not know the limitations of the particular genetic test, did not fully understand how to interpret the test, and did not know how to counsel their patients adequately. Some people did not even know they were being tested. Dr. Giardiello reported that "Before genetic testing for cancer susceptibility became available commercially, the tests were offered in a research environment and delivered according to controlled protocols." While it is relatively easy to ensure that such protocols are followed in the research environment, such controls are not so easily established and maintained in the average doctor's office.

The "inadequacies in the genetic testing process" that Dr. Giardiello and his colleagues demonstrated had as much to do with a negative result as a positive one. The genetic test examined in the study was for a mutation of the adenomatous polyposis coli

(APC) gene, a tumor suppressor gene found by Johns Hopkins researchers in 1991 to be linked to colon cancer. A positive test for an APC gene mutation indicates that an affected individual has an inherited genetic mutation called familial adenomatous polyposis, or FAP, in which hundreds of polyps can form in the large intestine. Nearly all patients with FAP go on to develop colorectal cancer later in life if prophylactic surgery (surgery that prevents the spread of the disease) to remove the colon is not performed at some point.

A positive test result should indicate to the patient and the doctor that the patient's colon needs to be kept under surveillance and eventually removed. But, as the researchers pointed out, a negative test result does not necessarily mean that the patient's colon can be treated as normal and mostly ignored. According to the study, the test can identify an APC gene mutation in affected members of families only about 80 percent of the time. If the person being tested has a parent, brother, or sister with FAP, the detection level rises close to 100 percent. If a doctor has sufficient reason to suspect FAP but the test is negative, the disease may still be possible and some level of surveillance may still be warranted.

The study reported these worrisome results: less than 20 percent of people being tested were given genetic counseling before the test; only slightly more than 15 percent gave informed consent before the testing was performed; and in nearly a third of the cases the doctor ordering the test misinterpreted the results.

Most geneticists who are involved in working with families or individuals whose family histories reveal a predisposition for certain diseases feel strongly that before any genetic screening is performed, genetic counseling should occur. Counseling of individuals and family members provides them with information about the complexity of the necessary decision making and the many personal and ethical issues and concerns surrounding genetic testing. The more clearly the individual or family understands and appreciates the ways in which genes affect our bodies and interact with lifestyle behaviors, the better able they will be to make sound decisions regarding genetic testing for themselves and the better they will understand the ramifications of having such genetic screening performed. An example is that of the tumor suppressor gene p53 which, if mutated, results in the chaotic proliferation of cells of certain types of familial colon cancer and other cancers.

Questions to be answered in this and other instances include: Would the individual benefit from knowing that his genetic makeup shows a defective or mutated gene? Or would such knowledge cause months or years of needless worry in the event that no tumor developed? Would this knowledge increase the likelihood of participation in regular or more frequent exams to ensure early detection and treatment of colon cancer? Many of the answers would probably be maybe yes, maybe no. The many pros and cons inherent in these situations need to be discussed thoroughly between the genetic counselor and the individual or family to arrive at a decision that is best for everyone concerned.

For more information on genetic counseling, you can contact:

National Society of Genetic Counselors
233 Canterbury Dr.
Wallingford, PA 19086
Phone: (610) 872-7608

Pregnancy and Childbirth

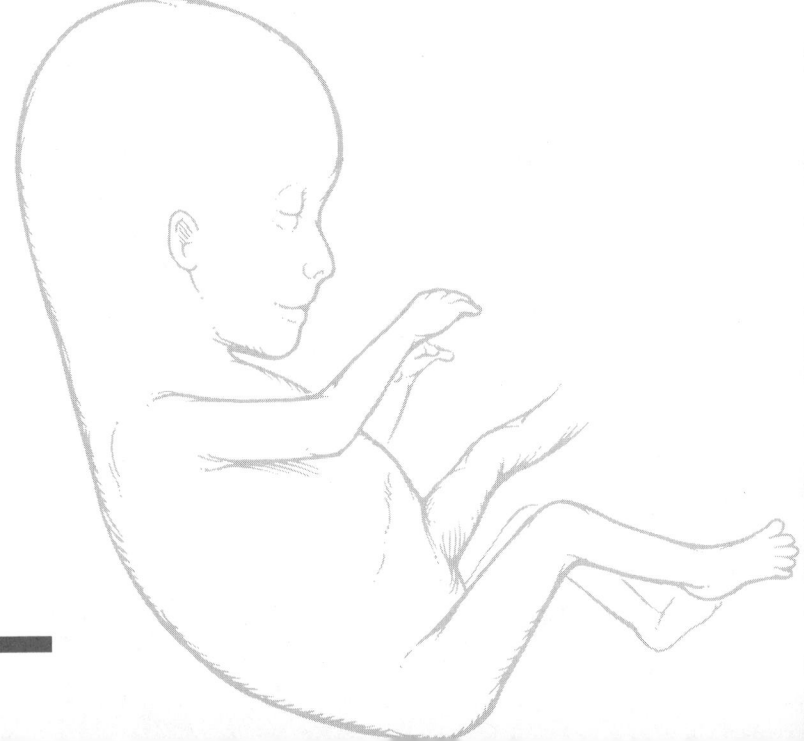

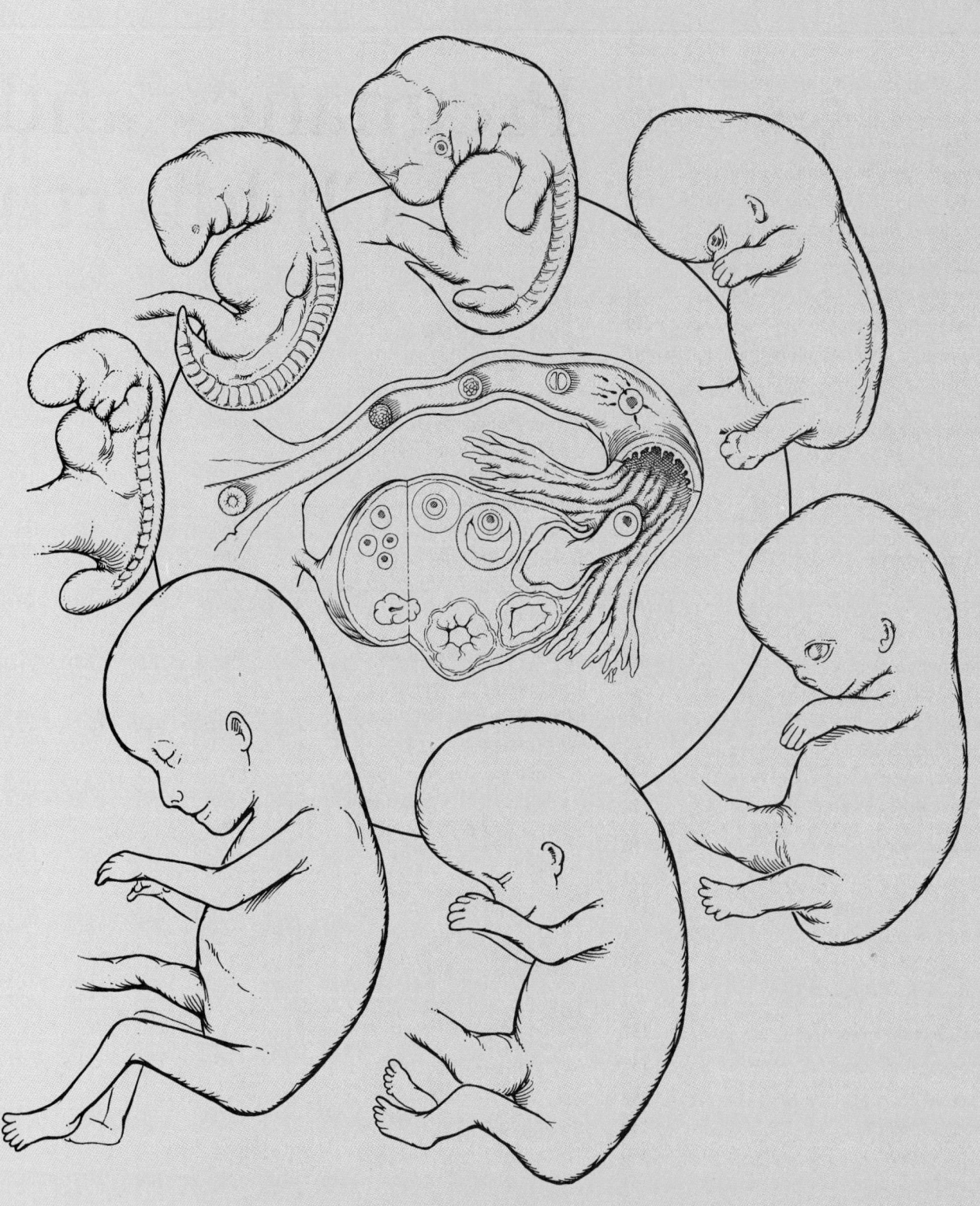

PREGNANCY AND CHILDBIRTH

The decision to have a baby is usually a joyful one. In the vast majority of cases, the pregnancy is uneventful, labor and delivery are uncomplicated, and a healthy baby is born. Nevertheless, an uneventful pregnancy and normal birth cannot be taken for granted. Becoming pregnant and having a baby are natural—but the more you prepare for your pregnancy and the better care you take of yourself and the baby growing inside you, the greater your chances of having a healthy pregnancy and a healthy, normal baby.

This chapter is dedicated to mapping the course of pregnancy and delivery—including the special issues and problems that may occur—and to helping you have the healthiest pregnancy possible. Through prenatal care, you can work with your health care provider to avoid the problems that can be avoided and to cope successfully with those problems you may have to face in order to achieve the desired outcome—a healthy baby and a healthy mother.

Planning Ahead for Pregnancy

There are measures every couple can take to establish the best possible chances for becoming pregnant and for the birth of a healthy child. Preconceptional care—the care of a woman planning for pregnancy—involves ascertaining in advance any conditions or problems the woman might be at risk for, identifying any special needs she might have, and ensuring that she is as healthy as possible *before* she gets pregnant. Such care is important, because the organs of the fetus begin to form as early as day 17 of the pregnancy—before most women are aware that they have conceived.

If you or your partner smoke and you are contemplating trying to become pregnant, the first thing you should do is quit smoking. Having such a positive goal to focus on—the birth of a healthy baby—may give you both the motivation you've needed all along to do something you know will be good for your own health and that is now essential for the health of your baby. If you are trying to get pregnant, you should also avoid alcohol. Your partner should limit his alcohol intake to one or two drinks per day,

because alcohol may inhibit fertility as well as cause birth defects. Marijuana also inhibits fertility and should be avoided, as should all other illegal drugs. Any prescription drugs that you may be taking should be discussed with your doctor prior to your trying to conceive.

Women who are considering getting pregnant should eat a healthy diet rich in calcium and B vitamins and avoid excessive amounts of caffeine, which strips nutrients from the body and may also inhibit fertility (see A Recommended Diet, page 138). If you are planning for pregnancy, you will also want to discuss your plans with your health care provider and ask for a prenatal vitamin supplement. It is usually recommended that

CONFIRMING A PREGNANCY

A missed period is the simplest and most convincing sign of pregnancy in the woman with regular menstrual periods. If you are trying to get pregnant and you miss a period, you should see your doctor for a pregnancy test. Other early signs of pregnancy, which you may or may not experience, include

- Nausea and vomiting

- Tender breasts

- Needing to urinate frequently

- Aching and heaviness in the pelvic area

- Implantation bleeding (slight vaginal bleeding that occurs approximately 7 days after conception)

There are many home test kits available that promise to tell you if you are pregnant by the first day of a missed period. These tests, which are more reliable than they used to be, work by detecting the presence of the hormone human chorionic gonadotropin (HCG) in your urine. If you get a positive result from a home kit, you are most likely pregnant and should see your doctor. A negative result may not be accurate, however. So if you experience symptoms of pregnancy, consult your doctor so that more accurate testing can be done. The lab urine HCG test is 95 percent accurate 3 weeks after conception; the blood serum test is 95 percent accurate 8 to 10 days after conception and 100 percent accurate 6 weeks after. ■

137

A RECOMMENDED DIET

Women often assume that they are supposed to eat more while they are pregnant. The truth is, what they need to do is eat nutrient-dense foods that supply more nutrients per calories consumed. This means you should minimize your intake of "empty" calories. Concentrate on getting most of your calories from fruits and vegetables, meat, fish, chicken, dairy products, legumes, beans, and other complex carbohydrates. Avoid desserts, candies, and other sweets, which provide very few nutrients. The key to a healthy pregnancy diet is improving the intake of nutrients, rather than solely increasing the number of calories.

If you are of average size and weight, you should consume approximately 2,200 to 2,400 calories a day while you are pregnant. If you exercise regularly during pregnancy, you should consume more calories than an inactive pregnant woman, though the exact number of calories depends on the extent of your exercise routine. Your health care provider can advise you as to how many additional calories you should consume.

For the health of your baby and yourself, it is important that you include the following important elements in your pregnancy diet.

Calcium A growing fetus depends on calcium for the formation of bones and teeth. More than 30,000 mg of calcium are utilized during a pregnancy, mostly in the development of the fetal skeleton. The greatest amount of calcium is needed in the last trimester. Increasing your calcium intake strengthens your baby's bones and your own. Calcium deficiency is also associated with preeclampsia and eclampsia.

Dairy products such as milk, cheese, and yogurt are rich in calcium. Four servings a day of dairy products are recommended for pregnant women. A cup of skim milk (skim milk has more calcium than whole milk), a cup of yogurt, or an ounce of cheese constitutes a serving. For women who are lactose intolerant, calcium supplements may be necessary.

Protein Protein helps your body do its own repair work during this taxing time, and it is important for the healthy development of your baby. Foods rich in protein include fish, poultry, meat, eggs, and milk. Beans and peas (kidney and navy beans, lentils, split peas), nuts, peanut butter, and tofu also contain adequate amounts of protein. Two to four servings a day are recommended.

Vitamins Although you should get most of the vitamins you need from the food you eat, prenatal vitamin supplements are recommended for all pregnant women. During pregnancy the B vitamins (particularly folic acid), vitamin C, and vitamin A are particularly important for fetal growth and development. Vitamin C is found in fresh fruits and vegetables, such as oranges and orange juice, grapefruit and grapefruit juice, strawberries, cantaloupe, mangos, broccoli, Brussels sprouts, raw cabbage, spinach, tomatoes, and tomato juice. Vitamin A is found in asparagus, broccoli, Brussels sprouts, chard, spinach and other dark green leafy vegetables, carrots, winter squash, sweet potatoes, apricots and cantaloupe. Good sources of folic acid are oranges and orange juice, cantaloupe, and green leafy vegetables.

Minerals Minerals are also important in a healthy pregnancy. The minerals you need are provided by a healthy diet and are also included in your prenatal vitamins. Some women do require iron supplements during pregnancy. However, you should not take an iron supplement unless your doctor recommends it; too much iron can be harmful to your health and can worsen constipation.

Liquids It is extremely important to drink plenty of liquids while you are pregnant. If you are experiencing morning sickness, try peppermint or chamomile tea or another herbal tea that is easy on the stomach. Water, fruit juices, milk, soup, and broth are also good choices. Decaffeinated teas and coffees are fine, but caffeine should be avoided. ■

WEIGHT GAIN RECOMMENDATIONS

For pregnant women of average weight, a gain of between 25 and 35 pounds is recommended. For underweight women, 28 to 40 pounds is recommended, and overweight women should gain no more than 25 pounds. If you were overweight when you became pregnant, ask your doctor to help you plan a diet that will give you the nutrients you and your fetus need without adding unnecessary pounds.

Approximately 20 pounds of the weight gained during pregnancy is due to your baby's weight and the necessary changes your body goes through to accommodate pregnancy. During a normal pregnancy, the weight of your uterus increases by about 2 pounds or more, as does the weight of your breasts. In addition, the extra blood your body supplies to nourish the fetus weighs about 3½ pounds. The placenta and membranes account for about 1½ pounds. The amniotic fluid weighs about 2 pounds. At birth, the average baby weighs between 7 and 7½ pounds.

During your pregnancy, it is best to gain weight gradually. Some women feel they should begin to gain weight immediately upon hearing that they are pregnant. It is best to curb this impulse, because the bulk of your weight gain should occur toward the end of your second trimester and into your third trimester. In your first trimester, your best strategy will be increasing your calorie intake moderately, concentrating on getting proper nutrients and vitamins, and drinking plenty of fluids. ■

INTRAUTERINE GROWTH RETARDATION

During your pregnancy, you are the sole source of all nutrients your fetus needs for healthy growth and development. If the supply of these nutrients is limited for any reason, the fetus suffers and fetal growth may be affected. When a fetus is deprived of nutrients, the newborn baby may suffer from a condition called intrauterine growth retardation (IUGR). Babies with IUGR often have problems after birth.

An infant who is born below the tenth percentile in weight is considered to be growth-restricted. This situation occurs when the fetus does not receive adequate nourishment from the mother via the placenta. Infants born below the tenth percentile do not have adequate body fat to maintain a normal temperature or blood sugar level. Such an infant may grow slowly throughout early childhood. IUGR may also lead to delayed intellectual development.

Smoking, drinking too much alcohol, and taking illegal drugs can slow the growth of the fetus. Eating a poor diet or dieting in order to avoid putting on weight also puts your baby at risk for IUGR. If you are very underweight when you begin your pregnancy, you'll need to improve your diet to avoid putting your baby at higher risk for IUGR. Exercising strenuously throughout your pregnancy may also deplete nutrient stores and deprive the fetus of necessary calories. If you are having trouble giving up drugs or alcohol or maintaining an adequate pregnancy diet, talk to your doctor about getting help. In many cases, IUGR can be prevented by making appropriate changes in your lifestyle and by getting the help you need to give up bad habits early on in your pregnancy.

Often, however, IUGR may be caused by pregnancy-related conditions and is not related to lifestyle choices at all. Such conditions include abnormalities of the umbilical cord or placenta, malformations or infections of the fetus, and the presence of more than one fetus. In such a case, if a sonogram confirms that the fetus is failing to grow at a normal rate and your pregnancy is far enough along that the fetus is viable, immediate delivery may be recommended to prevent further malnutrition. ■

women planning to conceive take sufficient amounts of folic acid, a B vitamin that is essential to the early development of the fetus. Taking at least 400 mcg of folic acid a day has been found to reduce the risk of neural tube defects (congenital malformations of the spine or skull), the most common of which is spina bifida. This can be done through diet, as many foods are now fortified with folic acid, or by taking a supplement.

CHOOSING A HEALTH CARE PROVIDER

Though the majority of women choose medical doctors (obstetrician/gynecologists [OB/GYNs] or family doctors) to guide them through their pregnancy, labor, and delivery, an increasing number are turning to certified nurse-midwives. How should you make the decision about who's right for you? It is very important that you find someone you feel comfortable with; look for someone whose personal style and training match your needs and expectations. It may be useful to interview a number of practitioners before making a final decision.

Obstetricians are highly trained specialists who are capable of handling nearly any complication; if yours is a high-risk pregnancy, an obstetrician will be best suited to work with you. A family doctor has more broad-based training and will view your pregnancy in the context of your well-being and that of your family. Certified nurse-midwives are trained to view childbearing as a natural process; they usually can spend more time with a woman and tend to be more flexible in approach than many doctors. They care for women with low-risk pregnancies. If you are interested in working with a midwife, be sure that your insurance will cover midwifery care.

Prenatal Visits: Working with Your Health Care Provider

The greatest gift you can give your newborn is to take care of yourself and your pregnancy by receiving prenatal care.

If your pregnancy is not complicated, your prenatal visits to your health provider will take place approximately once a month for the first 6 months of your pregnancy, and then every 2 to 3 weeks until the last month, when they will occur weekly.

Your first prenatal visit will probably be longer than the others. Your health care provider will review your health history and perform a medical examination that will include height, weight, and blood pressure measurements, as well as a series of tests, including:

EXERCISING SAFELY DURING PREGNANCY

Pregnancy is not the time to start a rigorous exercise routine—but it is also not the time to *stop* exercising. If you have not yet conceived, beginning an exercise regimen that you can carry through your pregnancy should be an important part of your pre-conception plan. While no studies have shown that exercise has an impact on fetal development, exercise can help you develop strength and endurance—both of which aid in making pregnancy, labor, and delivery go more smoothly.

When you are pregnant, hormonal changes can make you more vulnerable to injury. Your joints are particularly vulnerable because the connective tissues that hold them together stretch more easily. Games such as tennis or squash should be avoided, because the sudden changes in direction you make when running for a ball may damage your already vulnerable joints. Deep bending and any other movements that may tax your joints should also be avoided. After approximately the fourth month of pregnancy, you should also avoid doing any exercises lying on your back, a position which may decrease blood flow to your baby.

Swimming, walking, and low-impact aerobics are excellent forms of exercise while you are pregnant. High-impact aerobics should be avoided. So should strenuous or dangerous sports, such as mountain climbing, scuba diving, horseback riding, water skiing, and downhill skiing.

The ideal exercise class for you to take is one taught by a trained professional and designed to fit the needs of pregnant women. Such a class will not only help you get the exercise you need—and get it safely—but it will also give you much needed support from other pregnant women who share your concerns.

Here are some exercises and stretches you may find helpful during pregnancy.

Abdominal Curl-Up During pregnancy, your abdominal muscles will be stretched by your growing uterus. Abdominal strengthening exercises can help during this process and after the baby is born, when you are wondering where your flat stomach has gone. The curl-up is a modified sit-up done with knees bent and the back pressed flat against the floor. To make sure you exercise all your abdominal muscles, you should do your curl-ups both straight and diagonally (elbow points to opposite knee as you lift up).

Pelvic Tilt Pelvic tilts help strengthen the lower part of the abdominal wall. With your knees bent and feet flat on the floor, pull in your abdominal muscles while squeezing your buttocks tightly together and rotating your pelvis so that the small of your

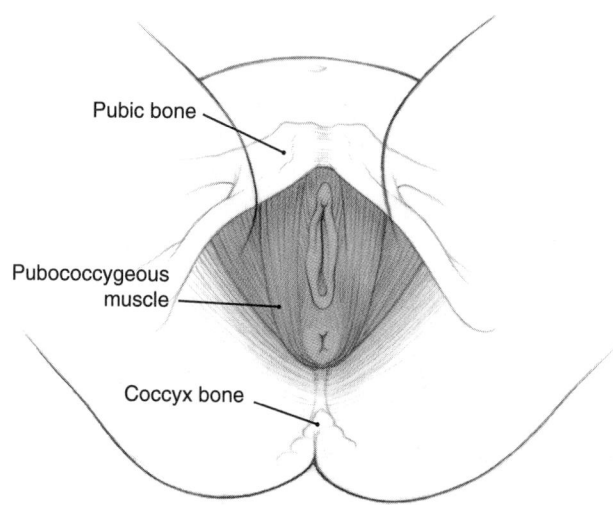

The pubococcygeus muscle connects the pubic bone to the coccyx. Exercising it daily during pregnancy can help facilitate the second stage of labor.

back presses against the floor. Slide your heels along the floor until your legs are fully extended while maintaining the pelvic tilt. Then straighten your legs and lift them to a 90-degree angle above your waist, while maintaining the pelvic tilt. Finally, lower your legs until you feel that your abdominal muscles are maximally stressed. This usually occurs at a 45-degree angle. For more information on the above exercises, see the illustrations in Chapter 2.

Pelvic Floor Exercises (Kegel Exercises) The muscles that comprise the pelvic floor are extremely important during pregnancy and help facilitate the second stage of labor. Most women are unaware of the pubococcygeus muscle, which connects the coccyx to the pubic bone; consequently, they do not exercise it or the other muscles of the pelvic floor. You can locate the pubococcygeus muscle by urinating and stopping the flow in midstream—the muscle you use to stop the flow is your pubococcygeus muscle. Or you can ask your doctor to help you locate it during your initial prenatal examination. Once you have identified the muscle, begin to exercise it by tightening the vaginal and anal sphincters. These contractions should be done slowly, in a group of three or four, with a rest afterwards. They can be done anywhere throughout the day; during the course of a day you should do a total of about 50. Perform these exercises, which are known as Kegel exercises, throughout your pregnancy and after the baby is born. ■

- Blood tests to check your blood type and Rh factor and establish if you have anemia, hepatitis B virus, certain sexually transmitted diseases (STDs), and immunity to rubella (German measles)

- A pelvic exam to determine the size of your uterus and the configuration of your pelvis

- A urine test for glucose (which may indicate the presence of diabetes), protein (which may reflect changes in the kidneys), and signs of infection

- A Papanicalaou (Pap) smear to monitor changes in your cervix, if you have not had one recently.

TWINS AND OTHER MULTIPLE PREGNANCIES

One to 2 percent of pregnancies in the United States result in multiple births. The introduction of fertility drugs has caused a rise in this number, because fertility drugs stimulate multiple ovulations to help a woman increase her chances of becoming pregnant. Naturally occurring multiple births seem to run in families.

Twins are the most common form of multiple birth. Two types of twins are possible—identical and fraternal. If two separate eggs are fertilized, fraternal twins result. If a single fertilized egg divides into two fetuses, identical twins result. Naturally occurring fraternal twins are the most common form of multiple births. The frequency of fraternal twins depends on a number of factors and also varies among ethnic groups. White women have a one in 100 chance of giving birth to fraternal twins; black women, one in 79. Regardless of ethnic background, identical twins occur in one out of 250 births.

Three or more fetuses may be produced in a single pregnancy, although this situation occurs far less frequently than twins. For example, triplets occur naturally in only one out of every 10,000 births, though fertility drugs have increased the occurrence of triplets overall.

In all multiple births, the risk increases for certain problems for both the mother and the fetuses. The risks to the mother include preeclampsia, gestational diabetes, anemia, hydramnios (too much amniotic fluid), and hemorrhage at delivery. In general, babies who are twins are more than twice as likely to have birth defects, though advances in coping with premature births have made it possible for most twins to thrive. Preterm labor and delivery are more common in cases of multiple pregnancy. Early diagnosis is the most important factor in preventing complications in any multiple birth. Here are some signs that may alert you and your doctor to the possibility of a multiple birth:

- A genetic history of twins

- The use of fertility drugs or in vitro fertilization

- A larger-than-expected uterus for the number of weeks of your pregnancy

- The detection of more than one heartbeat

If you are carrying more than one fetus, you will need to schedule more frequent prenatal visits so that your doctor may monitor you more closely to detect and prevent complications. ∎

If you are 35 or over, or if you have a familial history that may include genetic abnormalities or other risk factors, you will want to discuss with your doctor what prenatal tests you would like to have (see Prenatal Tests and Diagnoses, page 148).

Most subsequent prenatal visits are brief, unless there are complications in your pregnancy. Each routine prenatal visit will include the following procedures:

- A urine sample to check for glucose and protein

- Checking blood pressure to make sure it remains within the normal range

- A weight measurement to ascertain that you are gaining enough, but not too much, weight

- After 12 weeks, monitoring the heartbeat of the fetus

- Measuring the size of the uterus and position of the fetus

THE RISKS OF PREGNANCY AFTER AGE 35

A woman over the age of 35 who becomes pregnant is likely to have a normal pregnancy and give birth to a normal baby. But she should be aware of certain higher risks that she faces.

The best insurance that your needs as an older mother will be met to your satisfaction is to choose an OB/GYN who has expertise in the older mother and high-risk pregnancies. A doctor who has a specialty in working with older mothers will be in the best position to guide you through your pregnancy and advise you should difficulties arise.

Conditions for which pregnant women over age 35 are at greater risk include hypertension, preeclampsia and eclampsia (see pages 160 and 161), and gestational diabetes (see page 155). The chances of having a baby with Down syndrome increase steadily with age: Down syndrome occurs in one out of 200 children born to women over age 35, while only one in 1,400 children born to women in their 20s will have it. In addition, women who conceive after the age of 35 are at greater risk for miscarriage (see page 150), stillbirth, and intrauterine growth restriction (see page 139). The risk of placenta previa (see page 160) is also higher over the age of 35, and labor and delivery tend to be slightly longer in the older mother.

THE RISKS OF TOBACCO, ALCOHOL, AND OTHER DRUGS

Any woman who smokes, drinks alcohol, or takes illegal drugs during pregnancy is putting her pregnancy at risk and jeopardizing the chances for the birth of a healthy baby. If you think you may have a problem with tobacco, alcohol, or drugs, you should deal with it before trying to get pregnant.

Smoking The most obvious effect of tobacco on newborns is low birth weight. Women who smoke more than a pack of cigarettes a day give birth more frequently to lower-birthweight babies, who are at greater risk for infection and illnesses. Women who smoke are also at greater risk for miscarriage, placental abruption or separation, and fetal death.

Alcohol Excessive consumption of alcohol during pregnancy retards fetal growth and may also lead to fetal death or to fetal alcohol syndrome. Features of this syndrome include growth restriction, brain and spinal cord abnormalities, and characteristic facial changes. In addition, approximately 33 percent of babies whose mothers drank heavily during pregnancy have some form of congenital abnormality, as compared to only 5 percent of babies whose mothers did not drink. Most doctors agree that it is better to abstain from alcohol altogether during pregnancy, because it is impossible to calculate what is a safe amount of alcohol to drink.

Illegal drugs Illegal drugs, such as amphetamines, cocaine, crack cocaine, and heroin, pose serious risks in pregnancy. About half of the babies born to addicted mothers are born addicted themselves and with other chronic health problems. In addition, babies born to mothers who use drugs are two to six times as likely to be born prematurely or to suffer growth restriction. If you use drugs, your pregnancy is also much more likely to become complicated by hypertension (high blood pressure) and hemorrhage (bleeding).

MEDICATIONS DURING PREGNANCY

When you are pregnant, it is best to assume that any drug you take, even an over-the-counter medication such as aspirin, will affect your baby, too. Therefore, during pregnancy it is best to avoid taking any drugs—including aspirin and acetaminophen (Tylenol)—unless you have an existing condition, such as epilepsy, diabetes, or hypertension, that makes taking medication necessary. If you have such a condition, your health care provider will suggest a medication for you to take during your pregnancy that is least likely to hurt the fetus. Sometimes women develop urinary tract infections during pregnancy; if this happens, an antibiotic should be prescribed, because the risk of the infection to the mother and fetus is greater than the risk of the antibiotic. In addition, if a woman runs a high fever during a bout with the flu, acetaminophen may be recommended to bring down the fever, because a high fever may be dangerous to the fetus. As with all medications, it is important not to exceed the recommended dose.

The most dangerous time to take medication is in the first trimester of pregnancy, when the greatest amount of fetal development occurs and when the fetus is most vulnerable. Any medication you take should be considered a risk and should be discussed with your health care provider. The following is a partial list of drugs that may be dangerous to the fetus if taken during pregnancy.

- *Isotretinoin (Accutane).* This acne medication may cause severe central nervous system, facial, and ear abnormalities as well as heart disease.

- *Coumarin derivatives (dicumarol, warfarin [Coumadin]).* These anticoagulants are used by some patients with heart disease and may cause mental retardation, blindness, skeletal abnormalities, deafness, heart disease, and stillbirth.

- *Phenytoin (Dilantin).* This antiseizure medication is used by patients with seizure disorders. It may cause facial and limb abnormalities, growth restriction, heart defects, and tumors.

- *Streptomycin.* This antibiotic may cause deafness.

- *Tetracycline.* This antibiotic may cause bone abnormalities and discoloration of teeth.

- *ACE inhibitors (captopril).* These medications used to treat hypertension (high blood pressure) can cause injury or death to the fetus when taken during the second and third trimester of pregnancy.

This is only a partial list of medications that may endanger your pregnancy. When you decide to become pregnant it is a good idea to talk with your health care provider about all drugs, vitamins, and alternative or homeopathic medicines that you might be using, whether or not you think they are significant.

INFECTIOUS DISEASES DURING PREGNANCY

There are certain infectious diseases that can damage the health of the fetus. The best known of these is German measles (rubella). Rubella is a mild disease when contracted in childhood but, if contracted during the first 16 weeks of pregnancy, can severely damage the fetus. If you are already pregnant and were never infected with or immunized against rubella, you should avoid any contact with anyone who may have the disease, and you should be immunized after giving birth.

Influenza (the flu) may also be harmful to the fetus. In fact, a high temperature from any cause can be fatal to the fetus or bring on premature labor. If you are pregnant and have a fever of 101°F or more, consult your health care provider.

Some studies have shown a link between bacterial infections in the mother and premature birth. In the event of infection, be sure to consult your health care provider.

The following is a partial list of other infections that may be a problem in pregnancy (see Chapter 21 for more detailed information).

AIDS Acquired immunodeficiency syndrome (AIDS) is a fatal disease. A woman may be infected by having intercourse with an infected partner, sharing a needle when taking intravenous drugs, or by blood transfusion. Approximately 25 percent of babies born to women who are infected with the human immunodeficiency virus (HIV), which causes AIDS, are HIV-positive. Transmission of HIV to the fetus is markedly decreased (to 8 percent) if the mother takes the antiviral drug zidovudine (Retrovir; known as AZT) during pregnancy. The newborn baby must receive the medication for 6 weeks postpartum. If you are infected with HIV, you should not breastfeed if your baby does not have HIV; the virus can be transmitted to the baby through your breast milk.

Chlamydia infection *Chlamydia trachomatis* is a sexually transmitted bacterium that may cause conjunctivitis (pinkeye) and pneumonia in newborns. Infants with this condition are treated with antibiotics.

Gonorrhea Gonorrhea is a sexually transmitted disease that can infect your baby's eyes. You should be tested for gonorrhea before or during your pregnancy. If you test positive for gonorrhea, you should be treated with antibiotics.

Group B streptococcus (GBS) This bacterium is part of normal vaginal flora and may be transmitted from mother to child during childbirth. Approximately 5 to 30 percent of women have this strain of bacteria in their vagina and/or rectum, but only one or two out of every 100 babies whose mothers are affected develop infection. GBS is relatively harmless to the mother—although it is associated with an increased risk of fever after delivery—but it can be life-threatening to the newborn.

A baby who is infected will show symptoms within 24 hours of birth (early onset) or from 1 week to 3 months (late onset) with an average of 24 days. The predominant problem is meningitis (infection of the coverings of the brain), which must be treated immediately with antibiotics. Infection of the newborn can be prevented if the mother at risk is treated with antibiotics during labor. Risk factors include a woman's water breaking more than 18 hours before the baby is delivered, fever during labor, and preterm delivery. If the mother previously gave birth to an infected baby, this is also considered a risk factor. Neonatal sepsis (blood poisoning) occurs in 4 of every 1,000 live births. The mortality rate for babies born with neonatal sepsis can be up to 50 percent in premature infants and up to 25 percent in full-term babies. In the long term, neonatal sepsis may lead to mental retardation and severe disabilities. A newly developed vaccine for pregnant women that would also provide newborns with protection against GBS is being tested, but it is not yet available.

Hepatitis B Hepatitis B virus can infect the liver and is transmitted in the same ways as HIV. Hepatitis B can cross the placenta to the fetus or be transmitted to your baby after birth through contact with you. The risk of premature birth is higher if you have hepatitis B, which may also cause liver failure or lead to liver cancer. If you are diagnosed with hepatitis B, your baby should be given an injection of antibodies after birth. You should not breast-feed if you are infected with the virus. Hepatitis B vaccine is now recommended for all newborns as well as all adults with risk factors for hepatitis B such as contact with body fluids of an infected person or intravenous drug use.

Herpes simplex virus If you have genital herpes, you will be examined when you are in labor to see if you have active herpes lesions. If so, your health care provider will recommend a cesarean section to avoid exposing the baby to the virus during vaginal birth (see Cesarean Section, page 168). Genital herpes can cause severe complications for the newborn. Antiviral medication may be useful in pregnancy, so consult your health care provider.

Syphilis It is usually required by state law that all pregnant women be tested for the STI syphilis. Testing is usually done during your first prenatal visit and again in the third trimester. In the event that you test positive for syphilis, it can be treated immediately with penicillin. Congenital syphilis can cause growth restriction, premature labor, and stillbirth, as well as abnormalities of the bones, teeth, and hearing.

Urinary tract infections Acute cystitis occurs in approximately 1 percent of pregnancies and is one of the most common complications of pregnancy. These infections are treated with antibiotics. Untreated urinary tract infections have been associated with preterm labor.

Toxoplasmosis Toxoplasmosis can be contracted by respiratory contact with infected cat feces or by eating undercooked meat or fish. If you are pregnant and have a cat that goes outside, you should avoid changing the litter box. It is estimated that toxoplasmosis is acquired in utero by one in every 800 to 1,400 babies born throughout the world. Of those infected, most have minor symptoms.

Fifth disease/parvovirus infection Parvovirus B19 causes a systemic viral infection that usually occurs in epidemics. The symp-toms of the infection, which is also called fifth disease, include malaise, headache, rash, and a slight (if any) fever. Fetal loss and a serious condition called fetal hydrops (excessive swelling due to the effect of the virus on red blood cells) have been reported in pregnant women. In children, a red "slapped cheeks" appearance is typical, as is a rash on the trunk. The symptoms of parvovirus B19 infection are similar to those of scarlet fever, but without a high fever. The prognosis for recovery from parvovirus B19 infection is excellent.

A HEALTHY PREGNANCY AND CHRONIC HEALTH PROBLEMS

With proper medical attention and state-of-the-art prenatal care, many women with chronic diseases are able to manage pregnancy with few, if any, problems and give birth to a healthy baby. In most cases of chronic hypertension and diabetes, women are still able to conceive and to carry the pregnancy to term.

Asthma Five percent of women of reproductive age are affected by asthma. Asthma is a chronic respiratory condition, and it is difficult to predict how pregnancy will affect the problem. For some women, attacks worsen, while for others, the condition remains stable or even improves. While asthma may make you more prone to respiratory infection during pregnancy, most asthmatic women can carry a pregnancy safely to term. Virtually all medications used for the treatment of asthma are safe during pregnancy, but special care should be taken when steroids are used.

Heart problems A pregnant woman's heart works especially hard. If you have a preexisting heart condition, the added strain of your pregnancy on your heart may cause heart failure. However, this situation is rare, and if you are in good shape and are otherwise healthy, your pregnancy will probably be normal and your baby will most likely be healthy. During your pregnancy, your health care provider will monitor you for excessive weight gain, fluid retention, and anemia (low red blood cell count), all of which can be dangerous for a pregnant woman with heart problems. If you were born with your heart condition, you may undergo a special ultrasound examination during your pregnancy to look at the fetal heart.

Hypertension Hypertension is a common and often dangerous medical problem during pregnancy. Some women have chronic hypertension, while others develop hypertension during pregnancy. In both cases, the risk to the fetus is significant. The rate of fetal death is higher, and babies of hypertensive mothers tend to be smaller than average.

There are drugs that can be used to control hypertension; however, several antihypertensive agents, especially ACE inhibitors, can have adverse effects and should be avoided. ACE inhibitors are medications used to treat hypertension but should be discontinued during pregnancy as they can cause injury to the fetus if taken during the second and third trimesters. Women who have hypertension before getting pregnant should discuss their medications with their doctors and make necessary changes prior to conceiving.

Diabetes If you have diabetes and are contemplating becoming pregnant, you should discuss the implications of pregnancy on your health and the health of the fetus. The risk of congenital abnormalities in the fetus is three times higher if the mother has diabetes. Studies indicate that tight control of blood glucose levels just prior to conception and during pregnancy reduces this risk significantly. During the time you are trying to conceive you can maintain this control by adhering to a diabetic diet and by monitoring your blood glucose levels several times a day.

If you have diabetes and you become pregnant, you should be under the care of a high-risk obstetrician (a specialist in maternal-fetal medicine) or an experienced endocrinologist (a specialist in the treatment of disorders of the glands). To protect both your health and the health of the fetus, your pregnancy will be monitored more closely than the pregnancies of women who do not have diabetes. Women who have vascular complications related to diabetes will need to be monitored particularly closely.

The cesarean section rate for women with diabetes is as high as 50 percent and may be due to many factors (large babies, abnormal fetal heart rate patterns, preeclampsia). In many cases, however, vaginal delivery is completely safe. During labor and delivery, blood glucose levels may require control with a glucose and insulin infusion. There is an increased risk of dystocia (failure to progress in labor) and physical injury to babies born to women with diabetes, even in the delivery of normal size babies. Therefore, the second stage of labor should be closely monitored by an obstetrician who specializes in the care of women with diabetes. After delivery, your insulin requirements will need to be adjusted.

Seizure disorders In very rare cases, the medication you may be taking to control a seizure disorder may cause birth defects, or contribute to a low-birth-weight infant or to infant death. Prior to becoming pregnant, you should discuss your medication with a doctor who has experience in caring for pregnant women with seizure disorders and who can guide you in making the safest medication choice possible. Higher doses of folic acid may be recommended in some cases. The risk to the mother and fetus from recurrent seizures is much greater than the risks associated with medications taken to control them.

The First Trimester

A normal pregnancy lasts 40 weeks counting from the first day of your last period, or 38 weeks counting from the day of conception. A baby is considered full-term if it is born anywhere from 3 weeks before the due date to 2 weeks after it. Only 5 percent of babies actually arrive on the due date.

While the 40 weeks of pregnancy are divided into three trimesters, this division is fairly arbitrary. In terms of the fetus's development, the number of weeks completed is more significant. For the pregnant woman, however, each trimester carries with it a variety of developments and concerns, and we address those throughout this chapter.

NORMAL CHANGES AND EVENTS

At the very beginning of a pregnancy, some women notice physical changes almost immediately, while others do not realize they are pregnant until a pregnancy test confirms the pregnancy. When your pregnancy is confirmed, any discomfort you may be feeling will probably seem minor compared to your good news. The more you do to stay

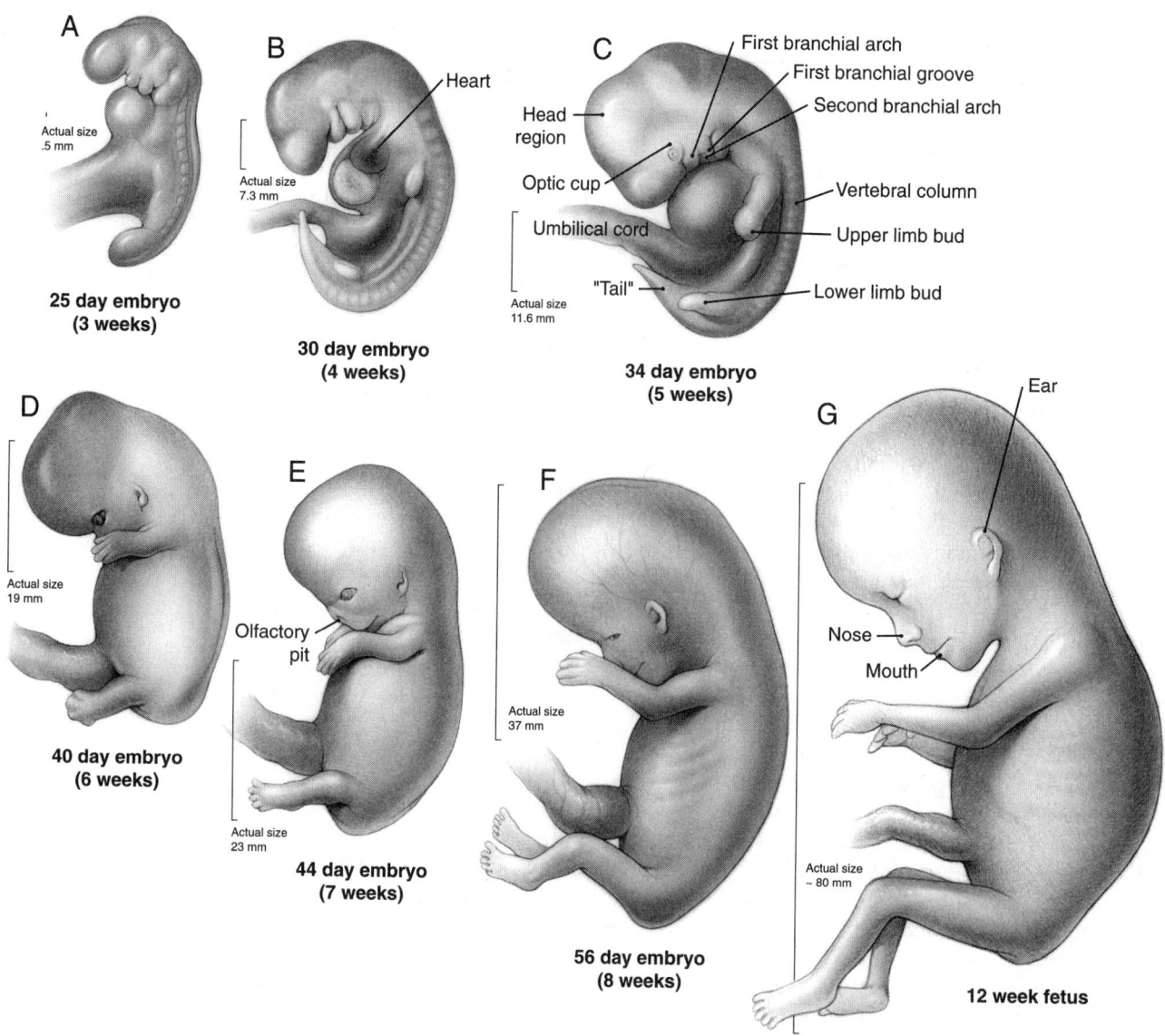

A

Actual size
.5 mm

**25 day embryo
(3 weeks)**

B

Heart

Actual size
7.3 mm

**30 day embryo
(4 weeks)**

C

First branchial arch
First branchial groove
Second branchial arch

Head
region

Optic cup

Vertebral column

Umbilical cord

Upper limb bud

"Tail"

Lower limb bud

Actual size
11.6 mm

**34 day embryo
(5 weeks)**

D

Actual size
19 mm

**40 day embryo
(6 weeks)**

E

Olfactory
pit

Actual size
23 mm

**44 day embryo
(7 weeks)**

F

Actual size
37 mm

**56 day embryo
(8 weeks)**

G

Ear

Nose

Mouth

Actual size
~ 80 mm

12 week fetus

Fetal development in the first trimester of pregnancy. (A) By three weeks, the vertebral column begins to form, and head and tail regions appear. Branchial arches will develop into parts of the ear and neck. (B) By 4 weeks, limb buds start to appear, and the heart is developing. (C) At about 5 weeks, limb buds elongate and olfactory and optic systems are developing. (D) At 6 weeks, the brain is developing, and the upper limbs and face become more distinct. (E) Nose and mouth are more developed by 7 weeks. (F) At 8 weeks, the head is less flexed. (G) By 12 weeks, the neck has elongated, further facial development occurs, and limbs are changing positions. By this time in pregnancy, the critical structures have formed.

healthy and nurture your pregnancy during the first trimester, the better your chances of having a normal pregnancy and a healthy baby. While this may not be the time to announce your good news to the world, it is the time to invest in your future and your baby's future by taking excellent care of yourself. This includes getting the rest you need, eating a healthy diet (see A Recommended Diet and Weight Gain Recommendations, page 138), taking prenatal vitamins, being conscientious about your prenatal visits, and establishing an exercise routine that is appropriate for pregnancy (see Exercising Safely During Pregnancy, page 140).

Your body undergoes major physical changes during the 40 weeks of pregnancy. Inevitably, most pregnant women experience some discomfort during part or all of their pregnancy. Changes that you may expect during this first trimester include the following:

Breast changes For many women, one of the first signs of pregnancy is an increasing tenderness of the breasts. Your breasts will continue to grow throughout your pregnancy in preparation for breast-feeding. The nipples, as well as the skin surrounding the nipples, may become darker, and the veins in your breasts may become more prominent. Your bra size may also increase, or even double, during pregnancy. Wearing a comfortable cotton bra with wide shoulder straps and good support may help ease any discomfort.

Skin changes Most skin changes occur later on in pregnancy. But almost immediately, many women notice a darkening of the nipple and the areola (the area around the nipple).

Increased frequency of urination One of the most common and earliest signs of pregnancy is increased frequency of urination. The need to urinate frequently is common throughout pregnancy, but if you find you need to urinate constantly or have any discomfort with urination, check with your doctor to make sure you do not have an infection.

Flatulence Increased flatulence may occur throughout pregnancy. If you find that you suffer more frequently from flatulence, avoid gas-producing foods such as beans, cabbage, fried foods, and onions.

Nausea Nausea, or morning sickness, may occur as early as the fourth or fifth week of pregnancy. While some women experience nausea in the morning (hence, the name), nausea can occur at any time of the day or night. Most women find that nausea disappears by the second trimester, but some women experience nausea throughout their pregnancies.

Rhinitis Rhinitis or "pregnant nose" may occur at any time during pregnancy, but it tends to worsen later in pregnancy. Rhinitis is caused by the swelling of the mucous membranes in the nose and throat, due to increased estrogen levels. If rhinitis becomes a chronic irritation, your doctor may consider appropriate medication.

Sexual changes As long as your pregnancy is normal, your sex life will be normal, too—that means what is normal for you and your partner. Some women experience increased sexual desire during pregnancy, while others find that the effect of pregnancy is just the opposite. Most changes in your sex life will occur in the later stages of pregnancy as your shape changes and your begin to experience more of the symptoms that may make sexual intercourse more uncomfortable, and therefore less desirable (see The Third Trimester, Normal Changes and Events, page 157).

If you are experiencing a difficult pregnancy or if there are known risk factors in your medical history, your doctor may tell you to limit your sexual relations. Your doctor will restrict intercourse if you have any unexplained bleeding, if you have a history of miscarriage, and, later in pregnancy, if placenta previa is known to exist.

Tiredness Many women experience extreme fatigue during the first 2 months of pregnancy and then again in the last trimester.

MORNING SICKNESS

Approximately 50 percent of pregnant women experience some form of morning sickness or nausea, which may or may not include vomiting. Morning sickness can begin as early as 2 weeks after conception. It usually ends sometime during the third month, often abruptly, but in rare cases it continues throughout the pregnancy. Despite its name, morning sickness can occur at any time of day or night.

Although the cause of morning sickness is unknown, hormonal changes are suspected of playing a role. A cure has proven equally elusive: although there are medications that can safely treat morning sickness, none should be taken routinely. There are, however, ways to relieve the symptoms, and you might try some of the following suggestions:

- An empty stomach will only increase your nausea. Try eating small meals throughout the day. Eat before you feel hungry.

- Avoid fried, spicy, or greasy food. Dry crackers relieve nausea for some women.

- Drink plenty of fluids. This is easier said than done if liquids make you feel queasy, but it is important to replace fluids if you are vomiting.

- Do not mix food and activity; do not rush through a meal, particularly in the morning.

- Wearing special wristbands designed for motion sickness may also help lessen symptoms.

Many women with morning sickness worry that their inability to hold down food can harm the developing fetus. This is rarely a problem, however. If your morning sickness is chronic and severe, your doctor may administer nutrition intravenously to ensure your well-being and that of your baby. ■

During the first weeks of pregnancy, your body is undergoing tremendous metabolic changes, which can account for your feelings of exhaustion. If you cannot find the time to nap during the day, try going to bed earlier and finding time for a short rest during the day.

PRENATAL TESTS AND DIAGNOSES

Many tests are available today to help a doctor monitor your health and that of your fetus with minimal risk to your pregnancy.

Ultrasound The most commonly used noninvasive test is an ultrasound exam, also called a sonogram, which may be used very early in the pregnancy to determine the location, size, and number of fetuses. Using ultrasound, a fetal sac may be visible as early as 6 weeks. Dating a pregnancy using ultrasound is most accurate before the 20th week.

Amniocentesis Amniocentesis is an invasive test that can be used to diagnose many conditions. It is most commonly used to determine whether you are carrying a fetus

with a chromosomal abnormality such as Down syndrome (mental retardation with some physical defects; see The Risks of Pregnancy After Age 35, page 141).

Amniocentesis is generally performed between the 15th and 18th weeks of pregnancy, early in the second trimester. The test is recommended for women who are 35 or older, who have a family history of genetic abnormalities, or who have previously given birth to an abnormal child. At present it is the most thorough prenatal test available.

The procedure usually takes only a few minutes. First, the doctor observes an ultrasound image of the fetus to avoid injuring it with the needle. Then, the doctor inserts a long, thin needle through your abdomen into the amniotic sac. A small amount of amniotic fluid is drawn into the needle and the needle is removed. Some women experience painful uterine contractions while the needle is in place. The fluid is sent to a laboratory for analysis. These tests take 7 to 14 days, because the cells from the amniotic fluid must be grown in a culture medium to be studied for chromosomal distribution. Amniocentesis can be used to diagnose certain single-gene disorders, neurologic defects, kidney diseases, and metabolic disorders as well as chromosomal abnormalities. Amniocentesis can also reveal the sex of the baby.

Chorionic villi sampling CVS, as it is often called, is an alternative to amniocentesis. The test can detect chromosomal and other genetic abnormalities and can be performed earlier in the pregnancy than amniocentesis (10 to 12 weeks). This is before most pregnant women have shared their news with others and when termination of a pregnancy is a less arduous procedure and recovery is easier.

Chorionic villi are the branching structures that form the placenta. CVS involves sampling the villi by inserting a catheter through the cervix. When the placenta is on the front wall or top of the uterus, a needle may be inserted through the abdomen, as with amniocentesis.

CVS provides the same information as amniocentesis regarding chromosomal abnormalities, except for neural tube defects. The test is therefore followed by alpha-fetoprotein analysis a few weeks later in the pregnancy (see page 149). The risk of mis-

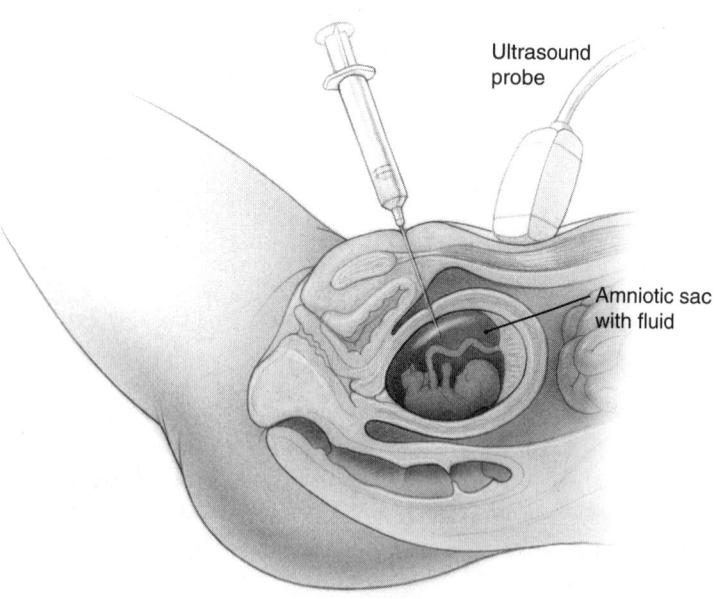

Amniocentesis can detect some fetal abnormalities. A thin needle is inserted through the abdomen into the amniotic sac to remove fluid for laboratory testing. Pictures of the area are obtained by an ultrasound device during the procedure.

Ultrasound probe

Amniotic sac with fluid

carriage with CVS is slightly greater than with amniocentesis, but the risk has diminished as the procedure has been refined. Results of a CVS are available within 10 to 14 days of the test.

Alpha-fetoprotein analysis/triple screen

Maternal alpha-fetoprotein analysis is a blood test that can be instrumental in detecting defects in the nervous system. This test is performed on maternal blood and presents virtually no risk to the mother or the fetus; therefore, most doctors offer it to all pregnant women when they are in the 16th week of pregnancy. This test is not diagnostic; it simply indicates risk.

Alpha-fetoprotein is produced by every fetus. In normal pregnancies, only a small amount crosses the placenta into the mother's blood. But in cases where a defect in the fetal skin is present, much larger amounts of alpha-fetoprotein are found in the mother's blood. Neural tube defects, such as spina bifida, are rare, occurring in approximately 1 to 2 births out of 1,000. High alpha-fetoprotein levels occur much more often (in about 50 out of 1,000 pregnant women), but in many cases the level indicates that twins are being carried or that the fetus is older than was previously thought. When a high level of the protein is found, ultrasound is performed. If ultrasound fails to detect an abnormality, amniocentesis may be performed. Abnormally low levels of alpha-fetoprotein in maternal blood are associated with chromosomal abnormalities of the fetus. When the alpha-fetoprotein test is combined with two other tests (tests for the hormones human chorionic gonadotropin [HCG] and estriol—the triple screen), an adjusted risk of chromosomal abnormality can be determined and amniocentesis can be offered for diagnosis.

Fetal blood sampling

Percutaneous fetal blood sampling involves taking fetal blood from the umbilical cord or intrahepatic vein to test for certain disorders. This test is performed in the late second or third trimester and can be used to diagnose chromosomal abnormalities, hemophilia and other blood protein deficits, sickle-cell anemia, thalassemia (Cooley's anemia), and thrombocytopenia (low number of platelets). It can also detect antibodies to such infectious agents as cytomegalovirus and *Toxoplasma*.

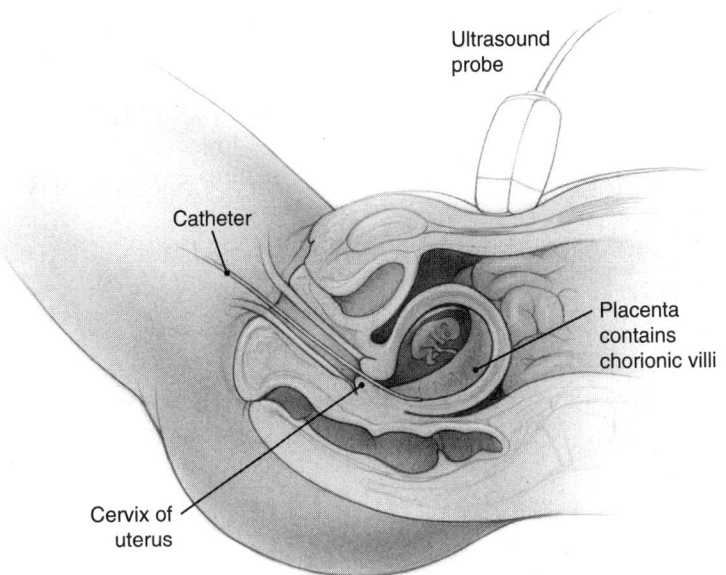

Chorionic villous sampling (CVS) can be performed earlier than amniocentesis. A catheter or needle is inserted into the uterus to obtain the sample from the placenta.

RHESUS INCOMPATIBILITY

Rhesus isoimmunization or incompatibility can occur when a woman who is Rh negative is carrying a fetus that is Rh positive. This can occur when the father of the child is Rh positive. When the blood of a fetus that is Rh positive mixes with the blood of a mother who is Rh negative, the mother's blood may develop antibodies that will then attack the fetus's red blood cells. Isoimmunization usually doesn't happen in first pregnancies; however, if you have miscarried or had an abortion previously and are Rh negative, you may already be sensitized, which means you have already developed antibodies. In the past, isoimmunization was a major cause of fetal and newborn mortality. However, the discovery and utilization of anti-D immune globulin (RhoGAM) has been one of the major advancements in obstetrics in recent decades. Now all pregnant women are tested to see if they are Rh negative. If a pregnant woman is Rh negative, the father's blood will also be tested. If his blood is Rh positive, the pregnant woman will be given a shot of Rh immune globulin when she is 28 weeks pregnant to prevent isoimmunization should any fetal blood leak into her bloodstream. All women who are pregnant—or who are planning on becoming pregnant—should be routinely screened for rhesus and antibody status. Rh immune globulin should be given earlier in pregnancy to Rh-negative mothers with possible Rh-positive fetuses when amniocentesis, CVS, or other procedures are performed, or if bleeding occurs.

ECTOPIC PREGNANCY

An ectopic pregnancy occurs when an egg is fertilized but implants *outside* of the uterine cavity. This is a rare event: less than 1 percent of all pregnancies are ectopic. The most common location for an ectopic pregnancy is the fallopian tube, although 5 percent of ectopic pregnancies occur in the abdomen, cervix, or ovary. When an egg implants in the fallopian tube, the tube eventually ruptures because it cannot expand to accommodate the growing embryo. Diagnosis of an ectopic pregnancy before the tube ruptures is difficult, but this is the only way to avoid a medical emergency.

Because a ruptured ectopic pregnancy can be extremely dangerous, it is important

In an ectopic pregnancy, a fertilized egg implants outside the uterine cavity, which prevents normal fetal development. Ectopic pregnancy sometimes leads to medical emergencies, such as the rupture of a fallopian tube. The inset shows an enlarged fallopian tube due to ectopic pregnancy.

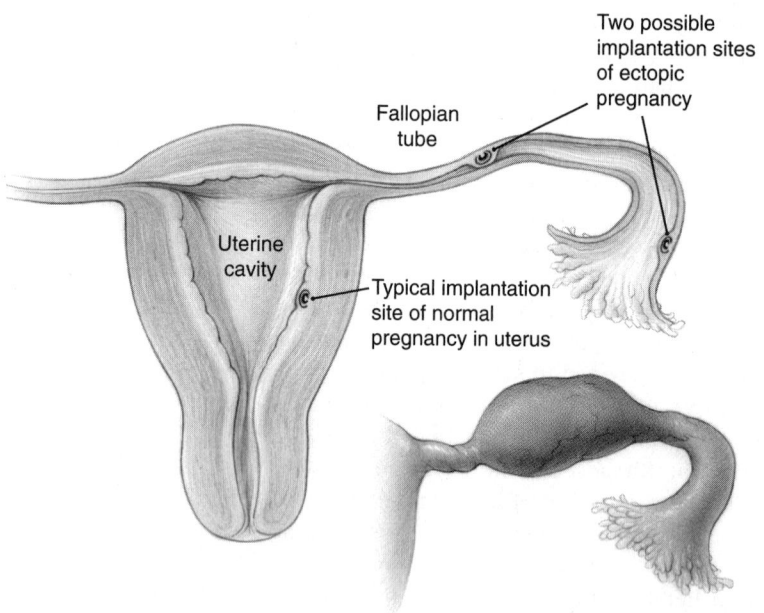

Fallopian tube

Two possible implantation sites of ectopic pregnancy

Uterine cavity

Typical implantation site of normal pregnancy in uterus

to be aware of the signs and symptoms of such a pregnancy. The following are abnormal changes after a missed period, which may indicate an ectopic pregnancy:

- Bleeding or spotting
- Fainting and weakness
- General pain in the abdomen, or pain localized on either side of the abdomen. The pain may be experienced as cramping, stabbing, or tearing pain and may occur with bleeding. Pain may also be experienced during intercourse.

If you experience any of these symptoms, you should notify your doctor immediately. The sooner an ectopic pregnancy is diagnosed, the better the chances of saving the fallopian tube. Ectopic or tubal pregnancies are diagnosed by testing levels of pregnancy hormones and progesterone and with the use of sonograms (ultrasound examination). When an ectopic pregnancy is diagnosed early, the medication methotrexate may be recommended to destroy the pregnancy. Laparoscopic surgery can also be used to remove the embryo. If a rupture occurs, more complicated abdominal surgery is often necessary—including removal of the damaged fallopian tube in some cases.

MISCARRIAGE (SPONTANEOUS ABORTION)

Spontaneous abortion, or miscarriage, occurs in 30 to 40 percent of all pregnancies and occurs before the 20th week of pregnancy. While this number sounds high, many of these miscarriages occur so early in the pregnancy that the women are not even aware of having miscarried, and a spontaneous abortion is interpreted as a "heavy" or "late" period.

Heavy bleeding during pregnancy, with or without the presence of clots or tissue, is a sign of impending miscarriage. Lower abdominal pain, cramping, and watery discharge (from the amniotic sac) are also common signs of miscarriage. Miscarriage may occur so rapidly that it is impossible for a woman to reach the doctor's office or the hospital in time. If you miscarry at home, you should try to place fetal tissue, which will appear as a red-gray mass or clot, in a clean container. This will allow a pathologist to examine it and confirm the miscarriage. If a miscarriage occurs at home, you will also be examined afterwards to make sure all of the fetal tissue has been expelled. You may be given a blood test to determine the level of HCG present, which might indicate that some products of conception remain in the uterus. When only part of the tissue is expelled, the miscarriage is referred to as "incomplete." Incomplete miscarriages are more common after the eighth week of pregnancy, when the placenta becomes more strongly attached. In such situations, the doctor will perform a dilation and curettage (D&C) to scrape the inside of the uterus. This minor surgery is usually performed in the doctor's office but sedation and hospitalization may sometimes be necessary.

Women who miscarry in the second trimester may find that their breasts become engorged with milk a few days later. Such engorgement may cause physical discomfort, but generally diminishes within a day or two. If this occurs, do not expel milk to relieve your discomfort, as this will only encourage your body to produce more milk. If you do experience pain, aspirin, acetaminophen, or ibuprofen may be taken and cold compresses applied to your breasts.

In many cases, after a woman has physically recovered from a miscarriage, the emotional consequences linger and may be, in fact, more severe. You may find that your health care provider focuses on your physical problems to the exclusion of your emotional experience of the miscarriage. Many women experience bereavement and need to mourn the loss of a pregnancy. Miscarriage has emotional as well as physical consequences for all women, and you should ask for help if you are having trouble with your emotional recovery.

Causes of miscarriage The causes of miscarriage vary and are often unclear. Present research indicates that low levels of the hormone progesterone may be a cause of pregnancy loss in the first 20 weeks of gestation, though there is no confirming research that administration of progesterone prevents miscarriage. In high-risk pregnancies where miscarriage is an especially great risk, bed rest or hospitalization may be recom-

mended. Clinical trials are under way using immunotherapy—the maternal injection of paternal lymphocytes—to prevent miscarriage, but such treatment has not yet been proven conclusively and is not available to the general public.

Almost all couples who experience miscarriage wish to know why it happened, and are frustrated when it is impossible for the doctor to give them a specific answer. This is particularly distressing when couples are planning to conceive again and want to do everything they can to avoid a subsequent miscarriage. There are, however, certain factors that often cause miscarriages. The most common cause of a miscarriage is abnormal development of the embryo, fetus, or placenta. Fifty to 60 percent of early miscarriages are attributed to chromosomal abnormalities; the earlier the miscarriage, the more likely that chromosomal abnormalities were the cause. In most of these cases, the problem is unlikely to repeat itself, and future pregnancies are not at risk.

Abnormalities of the uterus Variations in the shape or size of the uterus or the presence of fibroid tumors (benign growths) in the uterus can cause miscarriage. Though she does have a greater risk of miscarriage, a woman with an abnormal uterus or fibroid tumors may have no problem carrying a pregnancy to term. If, however, a misshapen uterus or a fibroid tumor that does not allow room for the fetus to grow causes a miscarriage, such problems may be corrected with surgery, greatly increasing the chances for a successful pregnancy.

Incompetent cervix Incompetent cervix, a condition in which the cervix (the neck of the uterus) fails to remain closed for the

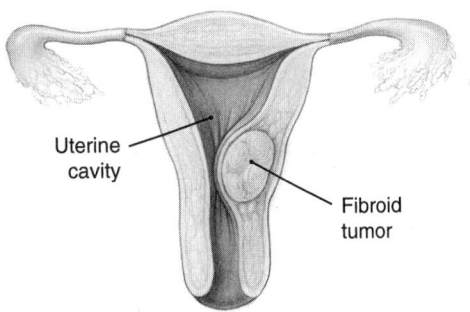

Uterine cavity

Fibroid tumor

Fibroid tumor of the uterus. These benign growths of the uterus can impair fetal growth and cause miscarriages, depending on their location. Surgery can sometimes correct the problem.

duration of a pregnancy, is another structural abnormality that is associated with an increased risk of miscarriage. A woman with an incompetent cervix may do well during the first trimester of pregnancy, but the cervix tends to dilate prematurely as the fetus increases in size and weight during the second trimester. If the condition is diagnosed early, before the second trimester, the situation can be treated by encircling the cervix with a ring stitch or by placing a band around it to keep it closed (see cervical cerclage, pages 154 and 155). These devices are removed when the pregnancy has reached term and it is time for labor.

Disorders of the endocrine system   In rare cases, thyroid dysfunction or another disorder of the endocrine system may increase a woman's risk of miscarriage.

Other factors   Other factors that may contribute to an increased risk of miscarriage include:

- Exposure to the hormone diethylstilbestrol (DES) in utero
- Maternal disease such as sickle cell anemia or lupus erythematosus
- Maternal age
- Use of drugs, alcohol, tobacco, or caffeine
- Malnutrition
- Trauma
- Genetic abnormality

TERMINATION OF PREGNANCY

While prenatal testing makes it possible to reassure most expectant mothers that they are carrying a healthy baby, it forces others to make painful choices. Personal and religious beliefs influence the decision to undertake prenatal testing, and they certainly play a large part in decisions that have to be made if the results of the testing reveal genetic abnormalities in the fetus.

Before the 24th week of pregnancy, the options for aborting a fetus include vacuum suction, D&C, and induction of labor. In a vacuum suction abortion, a tube attached to a suction device is inserted through the cervix into the uterus. Vacuum suction and D&Cs are performed under local anesthesia, often with intravenous (IV) sedation. After 16 to 18 weeks of pregnancy, termination may be performed by induction of labor. Medication is administered through the vagina or by an IV tube, leading to expulsion of the fetus in 12 to 24 hours. This method of abortion allows for autopsy of the fetus, the findings of which may be important for planning future pregnancies.

In some states, certain state laws affect the decision to abort after the 12th week of pregnancy. If you are considering abortion in the second trimester, you will want to obtain information on the laws in your state before making your choice.

Aborting a fetus for medical reasons is an emotional as well as physical trauma. Coping with your feelings of ambivalence and loss is an important part of your recovery. Accepting that conflicting emotional responses are part of the recovery process and giving yourself time to grieve can help. If you find that you are having difficulty coping with the experience, you may want to consult a psychotherapist.

The Second Trimester

NORMAL CHANGES AND EVENTS

By the second trimester, which includes the fourth, fifth, and sixth months of pregnancy, the fear of miscarriage has probably subsided for most women. And, just as you have adjusted emotionally to the pregnancy, your body has adjusted physically, as well. Many women in the second trimester experience a lessening of fatigue and, sometimes, even an extra boost of energy that allows them to accomplish what they want to accomplish before the baby comes. Many women also note that they feel increasingly forgetful and absentminded. By the second trimester, nausea has disappeared, or at least decreased, for most women, but occasional headaches, dizziness, or faintness may have been added to the list of complaints. Women also report a white, nonirritating vaginal discharge called leukorrhea.

Sometime during the second trimester, you will begin to feel your baby kicking and moving around. Some pregnant women worry if they do not feel their baby kick during the fourth month, but this should not be cause for concern. Though the fetus begins to move as early as the seventh week of pregnancy, the first sign of life, or "quickening," usually becomes evident anywhere between the 16th and 22nd weeks of pregnancy. While most mothers experience fetal movement as one of the greatest joys of pregnancy, it may also become a continuing cause of anxiety. At times, you may feel your baby move all day long, while at other times you may not notice any movement. This is normal. When you are busy and moving around a great deal, your baby will tend to be lulled by the rocking motion of your movements, and you may also tend to be less aware of each individual kick. This is why most women notice the greatest movement in the evening or early morning, when they are at rest and paying attention, and when the fetus is suddenly deprived of the gentle rocking motion provided when you are walking and moving around.

The following are some common issues and concerns that arise during the second trimester.

Backache Backache is one of the most common problems of pregnancy; it is caused by changes in posture required by the growing fetus. Backache is most common in the second and third trimester. Women who have had back problems before are especially prone to back pain during pregnancy. Your health care provider may be able to recommend exercises you can safely do to strengthen your back muscles, which will help relieve back pain.

Bleeding gums As pregnancy progresses, many women experience swollen or bleeding gums. You may notice your toothbrush is pink when you brush your teeth, and that your bleeding gums become progressively worse. Most women find that these symptoms disappear once the baby is delivered.

Braxton-Hicks contractions Braxton-Hicks contractions are sometimes referred to as practice contractions, as the uterus begins to flex in preparation for childbirth. Not all women experience them, but they can begin sometime after the 20th week of pregnancy and continue through the third trimester. During a Braxton-Hicks contrac-

tion, the uterus hardens for about a minute and then returns to normal. Such contractions are generally not painful, and are felt earlier and more often by women who have already delivered a child.

Breathing problems As the fetus grows, the pressure of the uterus on the bottom of your rib cage may cause you to feel short of breath or to experience the sensation of being unable to breathe. In fact, the lungs do not have as much room to expand and take in air as the fetus becomes larger. Many women find this problem to be particularly difficult at night. Sleeping propped up by pillows may help to ease your discomfort.

Gastrointestinal problems Most women find that nausea, or morning sickness, has subsided by the second trimester, but that heartburn has arrived to take its place. Heartburn is a common complaint during both the second and third trimester; as the fetus grows, it often presses on other organs, including the stomach, making digestion difficult. Most women find that eating smaller meals and snacks throughout the day helps to relieve heartburn.

Gas and constipation are also common complaints throughout pregnancy, particularly in the later months. Drinking plenty of water may help relieve constipation. Unfortunately, some foods that help alleviate constipation also produce gas. Your choices will depend on which problem bothers you more.

Muscle and leg cramps As pregnancy progresses, some women complain of cramping in the muscles, particularly in the legs. You may avoid, or at least lessen, cramping by pointing your toes up toward your head while stretching your legs.

Numbness or tingling of the extremities Numbness or tingling in your hands and feet is normal, particularly during the last two trimesters of pregnancy. However, if numbness persists, you should check with your doctor to make sure you are not suffering from another condition—for example, carpal tunnel syndrome (see Chapter 17 for more information).

Rhinitis As pregnancy progresses, many women complain of "pregnant nose," or rhinitis, which is caused by a swelling of the mucous membranes in the nose and throat. As with many of the symptoms of pregnancy, rhinitis is attributable to the increased production of estrogen. If you find this condition to be particularly irritating, your doctor can prescribe medication that will not harm the fetus.

Skin changes Skin changes occur throughout pregnancy, but they are more noticeable in the second and third trimesters. During the later trimesters, about half of all pregnant women notice slightly depressed, pinkish or reddish lines or markings on the skin of the abdomen. Called striae gravidarum, and more commonly known as stretch marks, they may also appear on the breasts, thighs, and lower back. After delivery, they will shrink and change to a silvery color, but they never disappear.

Also, it is common for brown patches to appear on the face or neck during pregnancy. These are referred to as chloasma, and usually disappear soon after the birth of the baby. In some women, particularly those with dark hair and complexions, the skin of the abdomen may become pigmented from the breastbone to the pubic bone and a dark line, known as a linea nigra, may form straight down the belly. This is caused by an increase in melanocyte-stimulating hormone, and the line usually disappears several months after the baby is born.

Redness of the palms may also occur later in pregnancy. This temporary redness is due to changes in estrogen levels. Many women, particularly Caucasian women, may also develop tiny red spots on the face, neck, chest, or upper arms. These are called spider hemangiomas and are also attributed to changes in estrogen levels. They generally disappear after delivery.

Swelling/Edema Almost all women experience some degree of edema—swelling due to excessive accumulation of fluid in the tissues—in their limbs during the second and third trimesters of pregnancy. Swelling of the feet, ankles, and hands is most common; your face may also become puffy. Minor swelling is normal; it is caused by the increased weight of the uterus, which may slow down blood and fluid circulation, particularly in the lower limbs. Edema can be relieved by elevating your legs, avoiding standing for long periods, and wearing support hose. Drinking eight glasses of water a

day is also important. If you are concerned with the degree of swelling you are experiencing—if, for example, when you press your finger into the swelling it leaves a temporary depression (known as pitting edema)—you should consult your doctor to eliminate the possibility of preeclampsia (see page 160).

Varicose veins Varicose veins may appear or worsen in the second and third trimesters of pregnancy, particularly in the ankles, calves, or thighs, and sometimes in the vulva. Poor circulation in the legs will make them worse, so avoid standing still for long periods of time. Try to lie down and elevate your legs whenever possible. Many women find that support hose offer some relief.

MEDICAL PROBLEMS

The second trimester is usually one in which the expectant mother feels a resurgence of energy and the joy of feeling her baby kick for the first time. But in some cases, problems do occur. The following are the most common conditions that pregnant women may face in their second trimester.

❖ INCOMPETENT CERVIX

During pregnancy the cervix has a vital function to perform—to retain the fetus, placenta, and amniotic fluid as the fetus matures in the uterus. If the cervix cannot perform this function, miscarriage or premature delivery will occur, usually during the second trimester or very early in the third trimester.

In some cases, a congenital or traumatically acquired weakness of the cervix may make this job impossible. Multiple pregnancies may also inhibit the function of the cervix. If your doctor suspects that your cervix may be "incompetent" because it has already begun to dilate early in your pregnancy, she will want to perform a cervical cerclage, a surgery that stitches together the cervical ring to prevent the expulsion of the fetus. This surgery has been found to be effective in preventing miscarriage or premature birth in approximately 90 percent of such cases. When your pregnancy has reached full term, the stitches will be cut in preparation for delivery. (See pages 151, 152, and 155.)

❖ GESTATIONAL DIABETES

Symptoms *(What you may experience)*
Excessive thirst; excessive urination. (If you are receiving adequate prenatal care, however, you may not experience any symptoms before you are diagnosed, since your doctor will check your urine for glucose and protein at each prenatal checkup.)

Signs and laboratory findings *(What the doctor looks for)* Your doctor will check your blood glucose levels with a blood test and recommend a glucose tolerance test. The American College of Obstetricians and Gynecologists recommends the 1-hour glucose tolerance test for most pregnant women.

What is it? Three to 5 percent of all pregnant women are diagnosed with gestational diabetes, and it is one of the more common conditions that develops during the pregnancies of older women. Gestational diabetes occurs because the hormones produced during pregnancy to help preserve the pregnancy may also inhibit the production of insulin. This contra-insulin effect usually begins at 20 to 24 weeks into the pregnancy.

If you are diagnosed with gestational diabetes, this does not necessarily mean that you or your baby will have diabetes after your baby is born. However, a woman who has had gestational diabetes has a higher risk of developing diabetes later in life. Gestational diabetes is generally not responsible for birth defects, which usually are caused during the first trimester. Babies born to women with gestational diabetes may be very large, because the fetus converts the extra glucose that crosses the placenta into fat. If your health care provider suspects that you are carrying an abnormally large baby, a cesarean section may be recommended.

If the baby is very large and vaginal delivery is attempted, shoulder dystocia may result. This is a situation in which the baby's head is delivered, but the shoulders become stuck. It is always an emergency. If your doctor thinks your baby will be larger than average, the risk of shoulder dystocia is eliminated by cesarean delivery. Approximately 30 percent of women with abnormal glucose levels give birth to larger-than-average babies.

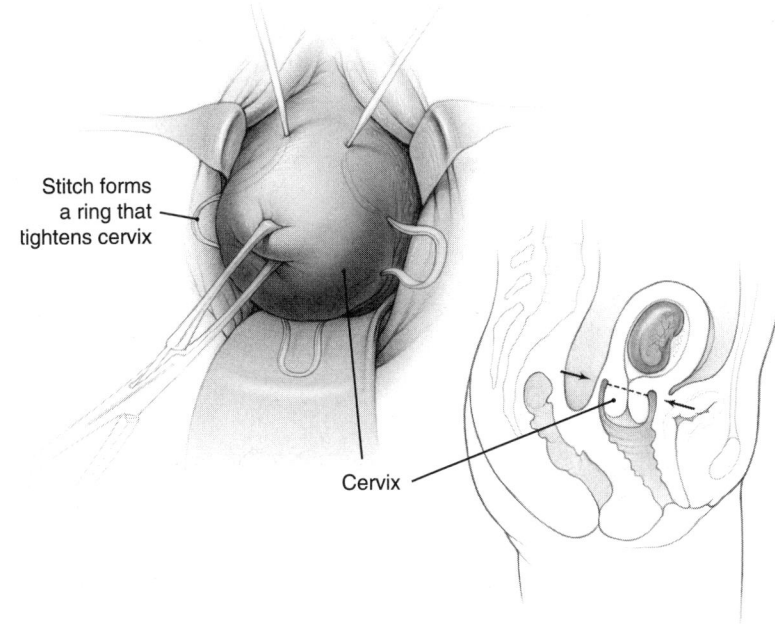

Stitch forms a ring that tightens cervix

Cervix

To prevent miscarriage or premature birth, a woman with a weak cervix may need to undergo cerclage during pregnancy. The cervical ring is stitched together to prevent expulsion of the fetus. The stitches are later cut to prepare for delivery.

What you can do In many cases, when gestational diabetes is not severe, the condition can be controlled with dietary changes alone. If you are diagnosed with gestational diabetes, your doctor will recommend that you see a nutritional counselor who will help you fashion a diet low in carbohydrates and fats to lower your blood glucose levels. That means that you will have to cut down on potatoes, foods made from white and processed flours such as bread and pasta, and refined sugars (sweets of all kinds, fruit juices, etc.). You should adhere to this diet strictly and remember that any cravings you may indulge with foods that are not on your list of healthy choices may worsen your condition and adversely affect the health of your baby. You should also drink plenty of water (at least eight glasses a day) if you have no heart problems.

Treatment Maintaining control of your blood glucose levels is the key to preventing complications in cases of gestational diabetes. Toward this goal, your health care provider will schedule you for more prenatal visits in order to monitor your condition closely. If your condition is severe enough, your doctor will probably prescribe small doses of insulin. This hormone replacement therapy to control your blood glucose levels will probably only last for the duration of your pregnancy, as long as your blood glucose levels return to normal after the baby is born. In addition, your doctor may request that you purchase a glucometer in order to monitor your own blood glucose level more closely (see Chapter 26).

Prognosis Excellent, as long as you are committed to maintaining tight control of your blood glucose levels.

❖ HYDRAMNIOS

Symptoms *(What you may experience)* Shortness of breath; indigestion or nausea. Your abdomen may become distended or you may experience abdominal pain. Premature labor may also occur.

Signs and laboratory findings *(What the doctor looks for)* If your doctor suspects hydramnios, she will want you to have an immediate ultrasound examination to determine the severity of the condition.

What is it? Hydramnios is a condition in which there is an excessive amount of amniotic fluid. The condition is usually harmless, but it becomes serious in one out of 1,000 pregnancies. Complications usually occur in women with diabetes that has not been well controlled and in women carrying twins or multiple fetuses. Severe hydramnios is a sign of some abnormality in the pregnancy. It is associated with birth defects including malformations of the gastrointestinal tract and central nervous system. Normally, in the second trimester, the fetus begins to urinate and to swallow amniotic fluid, regulating the amount of fluid in the process. Certain birth defects can lead to hydramnios by preventing the fetus from swallowing fluid or by causing excessive urination.

Treatment If the condition is not severe, no treatment will be prescribed. If hydramnios begins to interfere with breathing, amniotic fluid may be removed through amniocentesis. While this may relieve pain, it must be done repeatedly and increases the risk for premature labor. You may also

be hospitalized and given medications to inhibit uterine contractions in an effort to avoid premature labor.

Prognosis Depends on the cause and degree of severity.

❖ PREMATURE (PRETERM) LABOR

Symptoms *(What you may experience)* Abdominal cramping, sometimes accompanied by diarrhea; a dull lower backache; regular abdominal contractions; increased vaginal discharge. Fluid rushing from your vagina that may be watery or bloody (your "water breaking") may also accompany or precede preterm labor.

Signs and laboratory findings *(What the doctor looks for)* If your cervix has begun to efface or dilate, preterm labor will be diagnosed. Your doctor should give you a pelvic exam to ascertain that your water has broken.

What is it? Preterm labor is physiologically similar to labor at term, but it occurs too early (before the 36th week of pregnancy). Preterm labor is a major cause of infant death and physical complications for the infant after birth, including respiratory and developmental problems. In many instances, preterm, premature babies need special medical assistance simply to breathe, stay warm, and eat. Eight to 10 percent of babies born in the United States are born preterm. Ongoing medical problems are most common in babies born before the 32nd week of pregnancy.

In many cases, it is impossible to determine the cause of preterm labor, but the following may be possible causes: intrauterine infection, incompetent cervix (see page 154), placenta previa (see page 160), preeclampsia and eclampsia (see pages 160 and 161), rupture of membranes (see page 162), death of the fetus (see page 162), multiple fetuses, history of premature labors, smoking, maternal disease, and hemorrhage. Women over 40 and teenagers are also at increased risk, as are women who receive little or no prenatal care.

What you can do Find out if you have any risk factors for preterm labor. These include the following:

- A history of preterm birth or preterm labor
- Being pregnant with twins or multiple fetuses
- Abnormalities of the cervix (such as incompetent cervix)
- Being exposed in utero to DES
- Bleeding in the second trimester of pregnancy
- Placenta previa
- Gestational diabetes
- Hypertension

If you find you are at risk for preterm labor, you should take special care of yourself during pregnancy. You should avoid lifting heavy objects and avoid strenuous activity during pregnancy. You should also avoid extensive traveling. Your doctor will probably want you to come for more frequent prenatal visits. In some cases, your doctor may ask you to abstain from or restrict sexual activity or to monitor yourself for contractions after intercourse. Your partner should use a condom during intercourse so that you minimize the risk of infection and avoid exposure to seminal fluid, which may increase contractions. If you have experienced preterm labor before, bed rest may be prescribed.

When to call the doctor If you experience regular contractions (like menstrual cramps), changing vaginal discharge, sudden increase in lower back discomfort, or vaginal bleeding, you may be in premature labor. Do not wait for further confirmation—consider the situation an emergency and contact your doctor immediately.

Treatment The treatment for this condition will vary according to the age of the fetus.

There is no definite treatment to stop labor, though promising results have been noted with magnesium and ritodrine (Yutopar). If you are admitted to the hospital because labor may have begun early, medications may be used to prevent uterine contractions and stop your labor, as long as the labor is detected in the earliest stages and you and your baby are not at risk for infection. These medications may lower your blood pressure or raise your heart rate. They may also raise blood glucose levels, especially in women with diabetes. These medications also cross the placenta and

have relatively the same side effects on the fetus as on the mother. Their use must be carefully monitored and has yet to be correlated with a definitive improvement in the outcome of preterm labor.

Recently, a device that monitors uterine contractions at home was approved by the Food and Drug Administration (FDA) for use by women who have had a previous birth due to premature labor. This monitoring device is used in conjunction with daily contact with your doctor or an obstetric nurse. Some believe it may help to detect preterm labor earlier, thus improving the effectiveness of therapies that prevent uterine contractions and that prolong the pregnancy. However, the device has not been shown to improve the outcome of premature labor over frequent medical contact and may increase the frequency of hospital admissions and the use of medications.

Advances in the care of premature infants have made it possible to save many. Unfortunately, most babies born before the third trimester still do not survive. If you are at risk for preterm labor, you should work with your doctor to minimize that risk and try to ensure a healthy pregnancy. Your doctor may prescribe a course of corticosteroid medication to lower the risk of complications in the newborn.

The Third Trimester

NORMAL CHANGES AND EVENTS

By now you are probably used to feeling your baby kick and move inside you. Except when the kicks keep them up at night, most pregnant women find feeling their baby moving around one of the most pleasurable experiences of pregnancy, as they begin to get to know the baby by the way he or she moves and kicks inside. The third trimester is the time to prepare for childbirth by enrolling in a class where you can prepare for labor and practice breathing techniques and other methods of easing your delivery. It is also the time to begin to ready your home for the arrival of a new baby.

During the third and last trimester many women report an increasing boredom with the pregnancy and, at the same time, increased apprehension about the birth and health of the baby. During the third trimester, fetal activity continues and is often perceived as rolling rather than the kicking of the late second trimester. Most pregnant women continue to suffer from one or more of the common complaints, but have generally become so used to them that they notice them less. Common complaints during the third trimester include heartburn and constipation, achiness in the lower abdomen, an itchy abdomen, an increase in whitish vaginal discharge (leukorrhea), headaches, leg cramps, backache, hemorrhoids, increased problems with varicose veins in the legs, and continued nasal congestion. It is best not to use over-the-counter medications to relieve congestion; discuss this issue with your health care provider. In addition, many women begin to experience increased difficulty sleeping, breathlessness, Braxton-Hicks contractions, and leaking colostrum (pre-milk) from the breasts.

During the ninth month of pregnancy, or from the 36th week on, you should have weekly checkups with your doctor or nurse-midwife, which may include internal examination of the cervix for effacement and dilation, especially in the last 2 weeks. You will also receive instructions from your doctor regarding when to call if you think you are in labor.

You will find that during the final weeks of pregnancy, any change in symptoms or how you are feeling will raise the question "Is it time?" Most women experience at least a few false alarms during this time; this is normal. Two to four weeks before delivery, you may experience a release of pressure and a decrease in abdominal discomfort that is called lightening or dropping. This sensation means that engagement, where the fetus's head enters the pelvic cavity, has occurred. This descent of the fetus into the pelvic cavity often makes it a little easier for pregnant women to breathe and to sleep at night. If you have had children before, lightening rarely occurs until you go into labor. A sign that labor may be imminent is the passage of what is called a bloody show. This is a mucus-like discharge, tinged pinkish or brownish with blood. It is usually a sign that your cervix is effaced or in the process of dilating, which often, but not always, means that labor is about to begin. As with all aspects of pregnancy, what is normal varies from woman to woman. Once you have noted a bloody show, your labor may begin in hours, or it may be days away. If the discharge becomes bright red, notify your doctor immediately.

The following are the most common complaints of women during the third trimester.

Bleeding gums (see The Second Trimester, page 152)

Braxton-Hicks contractions If you haven't already experienced Braxton-Hicks contractions (uterine contractions not associated with cramps or labor), you may find that you are beginning to experience them now. If you have felt them before, you may find that they are more frequent and more intense in the third trimester.

Breast changes In addition to the increased fullness of your breasts, toward the end of your pregnancy you may notice a watery, yellowish fluid leaking from your nipples. This liquid is called colostrum and nourishes your baby during the first few days of life with protective antibodies that fight infection.

Breathing problems If you experienced shortness of breath during the second trimester, you will probably continue to experience difficulty breathing during the last trimester of pregnancy. As the fetus continues to grow, your lungs have less and less space to expand. Many women complain that shortness of breath makes sleeping difficult at night. Extra pillows may help alleviate the problem, and you may find that your discomfort eases after the fetus drops and the head engages for delivery.

Gastrointestinal problems For some women, gastrointestinal problems persist in the third trimester and many women have increasing difficulty with constipation. This is often due to the pressure of the fetus on the abdominal organs or to hormonal changes caused by pregnancy that slow the digestion of food. Drinking enough fluids (at least 8 glasses of water a day), eating a diet rich in fruits and vegetables, and maintaining your exercise program will help.

Hemorrhoids Hemorrhoids may occur or worsen during the later stages of pregnancy, due to the pressure of the fetus on the mother's organs. Before taking any hemorrhoid medication, you should consult your doctor. Minimizing constipation—by following the same health practices mentioned under Gastrointestinal problems—will also help.

Pelvic discomfort Many women complain of increased pelvic and buttock discomfort during the third trimester. This can be compounded by a feeling of increased heaviness and lethargy.

Sexual changes During pregnancy, some women find that their sexual desire increases, while others find that it decreases. While many women continue to enjoy sex throughout their pregnancy, almost all pregnant women find that sexual activity naturally decreases sometime during the third trimester. This can occur because many women experience a lessening of sexual desire. A number of factors may interfere with sexual desire, including physical discomfort, fears of harming the baby, feeling less desirable, and changes in vaginal secretions. Leakage of colostrum may be heightened during sexual stimulation; this may be disconcerting during foreplay, though it is nothing to worry about. Due to the increased blood flow to the vaginal area because of hormonal changes, some women also experience increased engorgement of the genitals after orgasm, and an uncomfortable fullness may persist.

Changes in your partner's responsiveness will also be a factor; some men draw closer to their partners during pregnancy and some become more distant. Some couples fear that sexual relations can harm the fetus, but in normal pregnancies and when both partners are healthy, this should not be a concern. Should there be a complication in your pregnancy, your doctor or midwife may request that you abstain from sex. For example, if you have a history of preterm labor or placenta previa (see page 160), or if your membranes have ruptured, your doctor will request that you abstain from sex.

Skin changes During the third trimester, the skin changes you have already noticed will persist. In addition, you may find that your abdomen feels itchy and that your navel has begun to protrude (see The Second Trimester, Normal Changes and Events, page 152).

Sleeping problems In the third trimester, you may find you have trouble sleeping as your weight and the size of the baby increase. As delivery approaches, sleep may become particularly difficult, due to breathing problems and the impossibility of finding a comfortable position. Extra pillows and lying on one side, with one leg crooked above the other and a pillow between your knees, may help. Taking warm (not hot) baths, drinking hot milk, and practicing relaxation techniques may also help. You should do everything you can to get the sleep you need *before* you give birth to prepare for labor and for the many sleepless nights you may face after the baby is born.

Swelling During the third trimester, swelling of the ankles and feet is usually normal. If you are concerned, see your doctor to eliminate the possibility of preeclampsia (see page 160). Swelling of the hands and face should be brought to the attention of your health care provider.

Varicose veins Varicose veins may worsen during the third trimester. Now it is even more important to keep your legs elevated whenever possible and to make sure you don't spend too much time standing in place.

MEDICAL PROBLEMS

While most pregnancies proceed smoothly toward the delivery date, there are certain problems that may often occur during the final trimester of pregnancy.

❖ ANTEPARTUM HEMORRHAGE

Antepartum hemorrhage refers to bleeding that occurs in the second half of pregnancy. While such bleeding is no longer a common cause of death in the industrialized world, it can still be fatal if it is not addressed immediately. Causes of antepartum hemorrhage include placenta previa (see page 160), cervical damage, and separation of the placenta from the uterine wall.

Light to heavy vaginal bleeding in the second half of pregnancy can be caused by many different conditions and is sometimes accompanied by abdominal pain. In many cases, bleeding is mild and will cease on its own without treatment. If you do have bleeding during the second half of your pregnancy, your doctor or health care provider will want to monitor you more closely throughout the rest of pregnancy, perhaps seeing you about once a week. If bleeding persists or becomes heavy, you may be hospitalized for observation. Your doctor may recommend immediate delivery of the baby by cesarean section. In all cases, antepartum hemorrhage should be considered a serious symptom of a pregnancy that may be in jeopardy.

❖ PLACENTA PREVIA

Symptoms *(What you may experience)* Painless vaginal bleeding (almost all cases of placenta previa have no symptoms in the first trimester).

Signs and laboratory findings *(What the doctor looks for)* If you have had vaginal bleeding, ultrasound will be performed to check the location of the placenta. This may include a vaginal ultrasound.

What is it? Placenta previa is a condition that occurs in a small percentage of pregnancies in which the placenta is situated low in the uterus, either completely or partially covering the cervix. The major cause of the complication is hemorrhage in the last trimester of pregnancy, causing a major risk to the life of both mother and child.

Most cases of placenta previa can now be diagnosed with ultrasound during the second trimester of pregnancy; more than 90 percent of the cases diagnosed during the second trimester correct themselves, so that the placenta becomes normally situated later in the pregnancy. (Approximately 5 to 6 percent of placentas are found to be low-lying during the second trimester.)

When to call the doctor If you experience any vaginal bleeding, contact your doctor, who will probably schedule you immediately for an ultrasound exam to evaluate your condition.

Treatment If a woman is asymptomatic (that is, has no bleeding) but ultrasound shows that the placenta is located completely over the cervix after 32 weeks of pregnancy, cesarean section is the only safe method of delivery. If there is any bleeding and you are in the late third trimester, your doctor may recommend that you have a

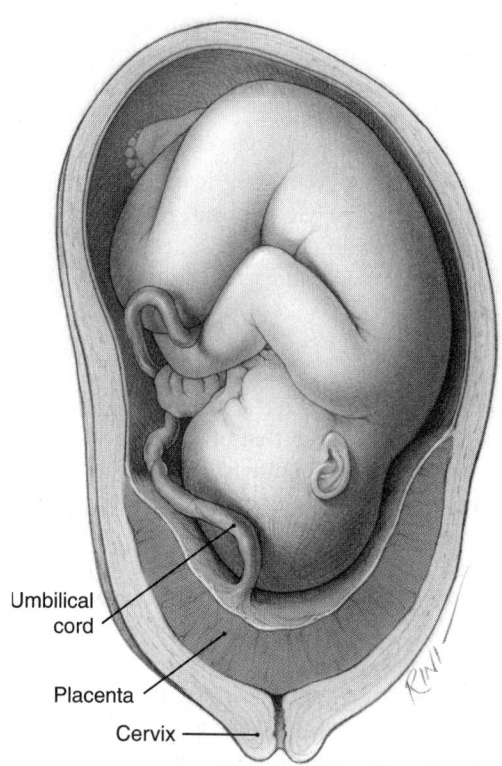

Umbilical cord

Placenta

Cervix

In placenta previa, the placenta blocks the cervical opening, and vaginal bleeding can occur. If the placenta does not become normally situated later in pregnancy, a cesarean section is required for a safe delivery.

cesarean section right away to prevent any complications to you or your baby from further bleeding from the placenta. The cesarean section should be performed immediately to avoid hemorrhage and damage to both mother and child. If hemorrhaging occurs and is severe, blood transfusions may be necessary.

Prognosis Good, as long as the condition is diagnosed early.

❖ PREECLAMPSIA

Symptoms *(What you may experience)* Edema (marked swelling of the hands, feet, and face due to excessive water retention); rapid weight gain (2 to 3 pounds a week); headache; epigastric pain (in the upper-middle region of the abdomen); seeing spots in front of your eyes.

Signs and laboratory findings *(What the doctor looks for)* Hypertension; pitting edema (when the swelling is pressed with a finger a temporary depression remains); proteinuria (protein in the urine).

What is it? Preeclampsia usually develops late in pregnancy and is defined as pregnancy-induced hypertension. The condition may be mild or severe. Fortunately, advances in diagnostic techniques and treatment for mother and fetus have minimized the risk of this condition, unless eclampsia ensues.

Treatment The best way to ensure early diagnosis and treatment of preeclampsia is to see your doctor or health care provider for your regular prenatal checkups. If you notice any signs that might indicate preeclampsia in your third trimester, such as swelling or puffiness (as listed above), see your doctor immediately. Because of the risk of preeclampsia, during your last 4 to 6 weeks of pregnancy, your doctor will want to see you once a week.

In all cases of preeclampsia, the goal of treatment is to keep blood pressure below dangerous levels (160/110 mmHg), to prevent damage to the mother's organ systems, and to deliver a healthy baby.

Treatment for preeclampsia varies depending on the severity of the hypertension and the stage of gestation at which it is diagnosed. Bed rest may be recommended if the preeclampsia is mild. A doctor may prescribe antihypertensive agents (blood pressure-lowering drugs) such as hydralazine (Apresoline). You may be instructed to report to a local hospital for a test of fetal well-being, such as a non-stress test (NST), to monitor the fetus's heart rate and assess its health.

When preeclampsia is more severe, hospitalization may be necessary. In a hospital setting, it is easier to monitor the pregnant woman's blood pressure, conduct regular or non-stress tests to monitor the condition of the fetus, and treat any emergencies. An ultrasound examination is performed to determine whether the fetus is continuing to grow and develop normally. Sometimes immediate delivery is the best treatment, particularly when the results of careful fetal assessment indicate that the fetus is in jeopardy.

Prognosis Excellent, as long as the diagnosis is made early. See your doctor regularly for prenatal checkups.

❖ ECLAMPSIA

If preeclampsia is not diagnosed early and controlled, a more serious condition called eclampsia may develop. Eclampsia is one of the most dangerous conditions possible in pregnancy. A woman with eclampsia may suffer severe convulsions, followed by coma. Eclampsia may be fatal to both the mother and the baby and must be treated as an emergency.

Symptoms *(What you may experience)* Blurred vision; convulsions; unconsciousness.

Signs and laboratory findings *(What the doctor looks for)* If you are still conscious and have complained of blurred vision, your doctor will check your blood pressure and check for protein in the urine.

What is it? Eclampsia is severe, pregnancy-induced hypertension resulting in seizures. It can be extremely dangerous to both the mother and the fetus and is sometimes fatal.

What you can do The best thing you can do is to try to prevent eclampsia. If you have been diagnosed with preeclampsia, take this diagnosis seriously: drink plenty of fluids and be vigilant about taking your antihypertensive medications if they have been prescribed. Do not be cavalier about this diagnosis. All women should strive for a healthy pregnancy, but in your case maintaining a healthy pregnancy is absolutely necessary to protect yourself and your baby. It can be difficult to be diligent, because patients with preeclampsia frequently feel fine—but it is most important that you take this situation very seriously.

Treatment You and the baby will be given intensive care, and critical decisions will be made regarding urgent need for delivery. The best treatment for eclampsia is immediate delivery of the baby.

Prognosis Once your baby is delivered, the prognosis is usually good for a complete recovery, with special care. Before your next pregnancy, you should be carefully evaluated for chronic vascular disease. Even if all is normal, you should still be followed closely.

❖ PREMATURE RUPTURE OF MEMBRANES

Symptoms *(What you may experience)* A trickle or gush of liquid from your vagina that does not stop.

Signs and laboratory findings *(What the doctor looks for)* A vaginal exam to determine that your membranes have ruptured.

What is it? The membranes surrounding the fetus usually rupture just as labor is about to begin or during labor. However, in some cases the membranes rupture early, before it is time for your labor to begin. If this happens, there is a risk that labor will also begin soon afterwards and that you will, therefore, deliver your baby preterm. Once the amniotic sac ruptures, the baby is at risk for infection.

When to call the doctor This situation should be considered an emergency if you are more than 3 weeks ahead of your due date. You should contact your doctor and go to the hospital for assessment. Your doctor may give you antibiotics during labor to lower the risk of infection in the newborn.

Treatment If your membranes have ruptured early, you should be hospitalized. Amniotic fluid collected from your vagina will be tested to assess the development of your baby's lungs. If the lungs are mature,

labor will be induced in order to avoid the risk of infection to the baby that can occur once the membranes rupture. If the lungs are not mature, your doctor may try to postpone labor with the use of drugs. If this choice is made, you will remain hospitalized so that the fetus may be monitored closely for infection.

Prognosis Good, when the condition is recognized and you and your newborn baby receive immediate attention.

INTRAUTERINE DEATH

Perhaps the most terrible burden a pregnant woman might bear is to be informed that the child she is carrying has died in utero (in the uterus).

If such a diagnosis has been determined via ultrasound evaluation, you should not feel rushed to decide whether to induce labor right away or to let nature take its course. Do not let yourself feel pressured by your doctor or by well-meaning family members who may wish to help relieve your suffering. Although you and they may feel that a quick delivery would be the best choice, it is not always the safest plan. Proceeding slowly—not rushing to deliver the stillborn baby—may make future pregnancies less risky.

If, however, labor does not begin within 6 weeks of the diagnosis of intrauterine death, you will be given drugs to induce labor. Ask for bereavement counseling if you think it would help.

Unless there were additional complications in your pregnancy, the outlook for future pregnancies is considered to be the same as for earlier ones.

POSTMATURITY (PROLONGED PREGNANCY)

Postmaturity refers to pregnancies that last 42 weeks or more, or are "post-term." The risks involved in post-term pregnancy include an approximately twofold increase in infant death due to asphyxia (lack of oxygen) and congenital malformations. There is also a higher chance of having an abnormally large baby (macrosomia).

FALSE LABOR

A week or two before your true labor begins, you may notice what feels like one or more series of uterine contractions. These contractions will feel like a dull ache or a tightening of the abdominal muscles with accompanying pressure in the pelvic area or lower back. It can be difficult to distinguish between the intermittent contractions of false labor and the early stages of real labor.

False labor, or prodromal labor contractions, is characterized by irregular, intermittent contractions that usually disappear if you walk around or lie down. False labor may be caused by fatigue and is often experienced in the evening. In general, the best distinguishing factor between true labor and false labor is that true labor pains are regular and persistent and will increase in frequency, strength, and duration, while false labor contractions will not. True labor contractions radiate from back to front, while false labor contractions are located in the abdomen and stop and start irregularly. If you are in the early stages of true labor, you may pass your mucous plug or notice a bloody "show." Also, your water may break. ■

If your pregnancy continues for 42 weeks or more, your doctor may suggest inducing labor. Prostaglandins (medications that increase uterine contractions) may be used to enhance the probability of a successful induction. If your labor does not progress, a cesarean section will be recommended.

Labor and Delivery

As your due date approaches and you become more and more sensitive to the slightest sensations in your uterus, you will probably ask yourself more than once, "Is this the beginning of labor?" Then, finally, you will say to yourself, without a doubt, "I'm in labor."

In the weeks prior to your due date, you may feel intermittent contractions characterized by a dull ache in the lower pelvic region, pressure in the lower back, or a sensation of tightening in the abdominal wall. You may also feel the baby drop down into the pelvic area—or at least you will be aware that your baby has shifted inside you—possibly relieving pressure and allowing you to, literally, breathe more easily. This phenomenon is called engagement or dropping, and the decrease in discomfort it produces is called lightening, a term many mothers find apt because of the physical sensation involved.

During the last weeks of your pregnancy you may find also that the mucous plug of the cervix, which protects the baby from vaginal germs, may dislodge. You can tell when this has occurred because your vaginal discharge will be heavier and pinkish in color. This discharge is referred to as bloody show.

The rupture of the membranes—also referred to as the water breaking or breaking of the bag of waters—usually occurs during labor. For about 20 percent of women it happens before labor, often during engagement. While rupture of the membranes may cause a gush of clear fluid, a slow trickle may also result. It may be hard for a woman to be sure of the source of this trickle; continued leakage means loss of amniotic fluid, not a urine flow. If you think your membranes have ruptured, you should call your doctor. Once this occurs, the fetus is susceptible to infection. If there is a greenish tinge to the discharge, you should tell your doctor as well, as this may indicate the presence of meconium (the fetus's stool), a sign that the fetus may be in distress. In any case, once your water has broken, your doctor will probably advise you to go to the hospital.

Successful labor and delivery depend on the position of the fetus, the dimensions of the pelvic passage, the contractions of the uterus, and the pushing by the mother to help the baby out.

Approximately 96 percent of babies settle into the uterus in the vertex or head-first position. In a small percentage of births, the baby is in the breech or feet-first position. Even more rarely, a baby may settle across the uterus (see Abnormal Fetal Positions, page 164). If the physician is unable to coax the baby into the head-first position, surgical (cesarean) delivery is sometimes necessary.

Most pelvic passages are wide enough to accommodate delivery. In the rare cases that the pelvic passage is too narrow, a cesarean delivery is required.

Finally, the baby is pushed out by the contractions of the uterus. True labor commences when all the muscles of the uterus begin to contract in concert, as if they were one big muscle. The interval between contractions decreases so that they are about 2 to 3 minutes apart as the birth of the baby becomes imminent.

THE STAGES OF LABOR

While labor is a continuous process, it is divided into three distinct stages.

First stage: Onset of contractions to full dilation of cervix The first stage of labor prepares the way for your baby's birth. During your pregnancy your cervix gets progressively softer and spongier in preparation for labor. As term approaches, the cervix begins to shorten in a process called effacement. The cervix is approximately an inch and a half long before effacement; afterward, it is so thin that it almost disappears. Additionally, pressure from the baby's head and the contractions of the uterus gradually force the cervix to dilate, creating a wider and wider opening. Full dilation is considered 10 centimeters.

The first stage of labor can have two phases. In the first phase, contractions are approximately 3 to 10 minutes apart. This phase lasts from the onset of dilation to 3 to

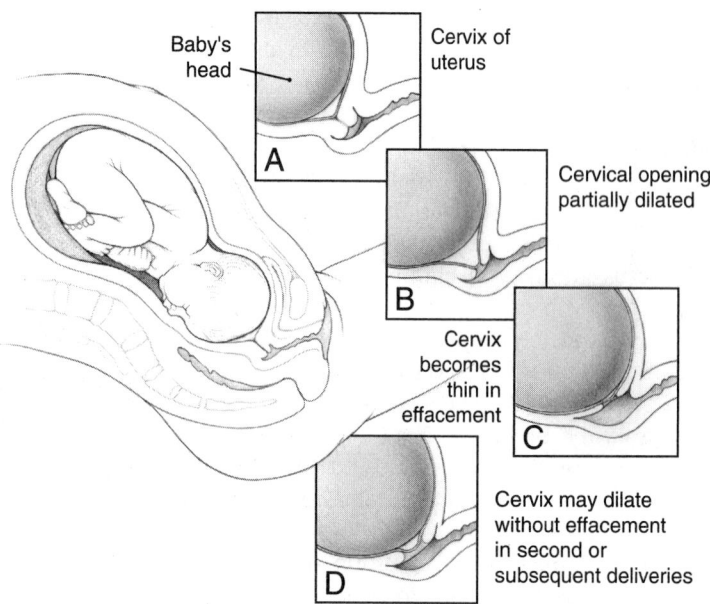

Baby's head

Cervix of uterus

A

Cervical opening partially dilated

B

Cervix becomes thin in effacement

C

Cervix may dilate without effacement in second or subsequent deliveries

D

Cervical dilation and effacement during labor. During labor, the cervix becomes softer and often becomes shortened (effacement). (A) Partial effacement occurs as the baby's head pushes against the cervix. (B) The cervical opening begins to enlarge (dilate) to allow the baby to be pushed out. (C) As the fetal head descends, the cervix will completely efface. (D) In second or subsequent deliveries, the cervix may become dilated prior to effacement.

5 centimeters' dilation and may continue for up to 24 hours in a first pregnancy. The second phase of the first stage of labor lasts from 3 to 5 centimeters to the full dilatation of the cervix. Contractions are approximately 2 to 5 minutes apart, and this phase may continue for up to 8 hours in a first pregnancy.

Unfortunately, it is impossible to predict how long or how difficult the first stage of labor may be. Some women dilate relatively quickly, and their contractions during this time are tolerable. Other women experience quite painful contractions, yet dilation occurs very slowly, leaving the laboring woman exhausted. This varies from woman to woman, but it may also vary from pregnancy to pregnancy in the same woman. In any case, once you are fully dilated, your body is prepared for the actual birth of your baby.

Second stage: Full dilation of cervix until delivery of the baby During the second stage of labor, uterine contractions are stronger; they now come every 2 to 3 min-

ABNORMAL FETAL POSITIONS

By the last month of pregnancy, most babies have settled into the head-down (vertex) presentation. Of those that do not, the majority (roughly 3 percent of term pregnancies) will be in a breech presentation when labor begins. In the breech position, the infant's buttocks are positioned closest to the cervix, so the buttocks or the feet will emerge first. More rarely, the baby may be in transverse position (lying on its side). Most breech and transverse babies are born healthy, though they are at higher risk for some problems than babies delivered head first. If a baby's position is not head down toward the end of the third trimester, your doctor may try to turn the baby manually before your labor

begins. This procedure is called external cephalic version. While cesarean section was once recommended in most breech births, it is now chiefly recommended in emergencies or if the baby is footling breech (in which one or both of the baby's feet are positioned below the buttocks). ■

Fetal positions. (A) Usually, the baby's head is closest to the cervix, so the head emerges first. Some babies, however, have higher risks of complications during labor if they assume less common positions in the uterus. (B) In the breech position, the infant's buttocks are closest to the cervix. (C) Rarely, the baby is in transverse position (on its side).

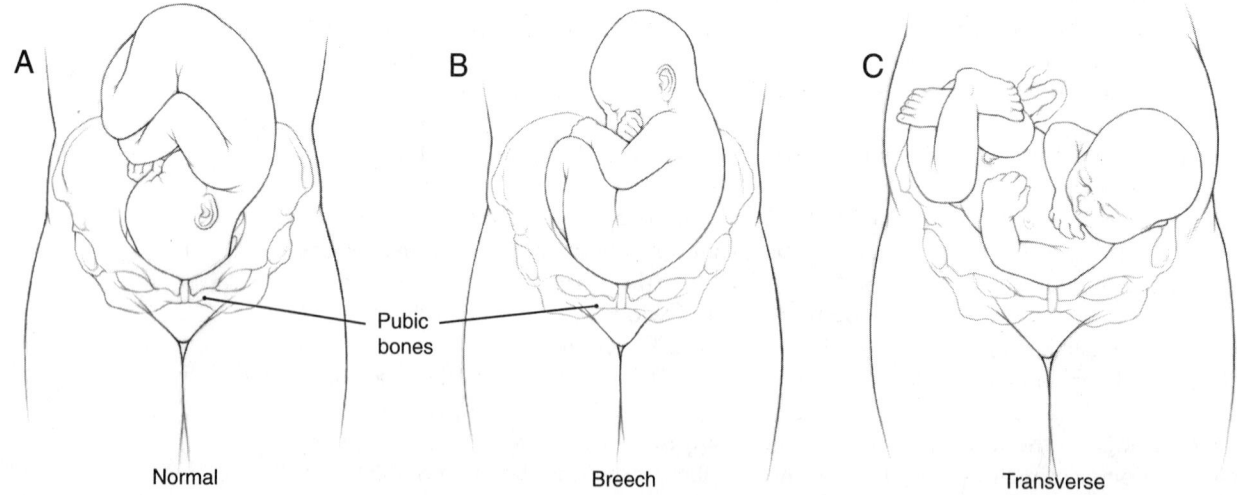

A

B

Pubic bones

C

Normal

Breech

Transverse

PAIN MANAGEMENT

The discomfort of labor can be managed in two ways. You and your partner may practice what is referred to as natural (or psychoprophylactic) childbirth. The most common form of natural childbirth is the Lamaze method, which involves breathing techniques and other strategies that may relieve the discomfort of labor and facilitate the birth process. The other method of pain management is through the use of analgesics and anesthetics considered safe for delivery. It is wise to be informed about the alternatives, so that you and your doctor can make the right decision as labor proceeds.

The analgesics used to relieve pain during labor and delivery include butorphanol (Stadol) and meperidine (Demerol). Butorphanol and meperidine are both narcotics, but butorphanol also has some antinarcotic properties, which make it better for short-term use. Narcotics decrease pain; but they may also depress breathing in the newborn and therefore cannot be given close to delivery. Tranquilizers may also be used during labor to calm the mother and decrease nausea and vomiting.

Three forms of anesthesia may be used during labor and delivery: epidural, spinal, and general.

Epidural Anesthesia Epidural, or caudal anesthesia, is the most popular choice of anesthesia because it offers relief during labor, the dosage can be regulated, and it allows the mother to be awake for the birth of her baby. An epidural has minimal side effects. It can be administered as early as the first stage of labor,

but it may make it difficult for you to push as labor progresses.

An epidural is administered while you are lying on your side or sitting on the edge of the bed. Your back is washed with an antiseptic soap, and the skin around the area will be numbed with a local anesthetic. It is important to remain still while the epidural is being administered. After the needle is inserted into the epidural space in the casing of the spinal cord, a catheter is left in place so that small, continuous doses may be given without an additional needle stick. The drug takes about 10 to 20 minutes to take effect. The procedure is usually not painful.

Spinal Anesthesia A spinal block involves the injection of a drug directly into the spinal canal. Two different types of medications can be used: narcotics or local anesthetics. A spinal block with local anesthetics is generally used only for cesarean delivery. It allows the mother to be awake and alert for the birth of her baby, but the numbness may last from 6 to 8 hours after delivery and it may cause headaches in the first days following delivery. A spinal injection of narcotics can be used to control the pain of labor. It may be done during the placement of an epidural or by itself. The advantage of spinal narcotics is that they offer more complete pain relief and no decrease in muscle strength. The disadvantage is that the effects last only 2 to 3 hours.

General Anesthesia General anesthesia involves the administration of drugs, via injection or inhalation, that cause numbness quickly and that will put you to sleep for the duration of the birth. General anesthesia was once a very popular choice, even for mothers who were not undergoing a cesarean delivery. However, it is now used only in emergency cesarean deliveries, some multiple births, cases of retained placenta, and in certain breech births. General anesthesia carries a risk of aspiration of stomach acids into the lungs. This is a potentially deadly complication and is more likely to occur in pregnant patients. ■

Epidural and spinal anesthesia. These blocks are commonly used in childbirth because they allow the mother to be awake for the birth of her baby and because they relieve the pain of labor. Both techniques allow for temporary pain blockage below the level of the chest. The techniques differ by the depth of the needle when the pain medication is infused (spinal anesthesia is injected deeper), although both are performed below where the spinal cord ends to avoid damaging the cord.

PROCEDURES YOU MAY ENCOUNTER DURING LABOR AND DELIVERY

The course of labor and delivery varies widely from pregnancy to pregnancy. During this time, which may be as short as a few hours or as long as a few days, you may find yourself unexpectedly facing certain tests or procedures. The following are some procedures commonly carried out during normal labor and delivery; being prepared for them may help you avoid undue anxiety and concern.

Induction of labor

In certain cases, labor may have to be artificially induced. Medical reasons for induction of labor include diabetes, preeclampsia, and eclampsia (see pages 160 and 161), premature rupture of membranes (see page 162), Rh disease (see page 149), postmaturity (see page 162), and high blood pressure. Generally, labor is induced by injecting the synthetic hormone oxytocin (Pitocin) into the mother to bring on uterine contractions. Oxytocin can also be given to speed up labor already in process. Contractions induced by oxytocin tend to be more intense and more frequent.

Fetal Monitoring

Electronic fetal monitoring allows your doctor to record your baby's heartbeat during labor. If you have had any complications in your pregnancy, this technique may also be used before labor begins to monitor your baby.

In many hospitals, electronic fetal monitoring has become almost routine. When active labor begins, transducers are placed on the mother's abdomen to monitor uterine contractions and the fetal heart rate. If the amniotic membranes have already ruptured, internal monitoring may be used. In this procedure, an electrode will be inserted through your vagina and attached to the baby's scalp. Your contractions and your baby's response to these contractions can then be monitored. During uterine contractions, the baby's blood supply is temporarily reduced. If an infant's health has been compromised by complications in a pregnancy, a dangerous level of stress may be placed on the baby during contractions. Even in some normal pregnancies, the stress level may become elevated. If a baby's heart rate indicates continued distress, your doctor may recommend an immediate cesarean delivery.

Fetal Scalp Blood Sampling

If your doctor suspects that the fetus is in continued distress, an additional test, called fetal scalp blood sampling, may be performed to help confirm the diagnosis. During this test, a small instrument is inserted through the partially dilated cervix to obtain a blood sample from the scalp of the baby. The acid-base balance of the fetus is then measured in what is called a pH test. If the test registers a trend toward an acid pH, fetal distress is confirmed. Such confirmation indicates the need for an immediate delivery, usually by cesarean section.

Episiotomy

An episiotomy is a small incision made in the area between the vagina and the rectum. This cut is made immediately after ▶

utes and last approximately 60 to 90 seconds. As the baby descends, you will begin pushing to help the process along. The more you can push in conjunction with your contractions, the more you facilitate the birth of your baby. The second stage of labor can last several minutes (for women who have delivered a child before) or up to 3 hours (for first babies). At this time, the doctor may cut an episiotomy—a small incision in the vaginal opening to make more room for the baby's head.

The baby's head is said to have crowned when it can be seen at the opening of the vagina. It will then emerge slowly. The rest of the baby's body follows more rapidly. At the moment your baby is born, you will probably be experiencing physical exhaustion and elation at the same time. You will hear your baby's first cries and hold your baby for the first time. As overwhelming as this moment may be, your work is not yet done.

Third stage: Delivery of the placenta

Once the baby has been born, the uterus begins to shrink, getting smaller and thicker and reducing the size of the area to which the placenta had been attached. Finally, the placenta detaches and is pushed out of the vagina. After delivery of the placenta, the uterus contracts even further, which prevents excessive bleeding. Normally, this stage of labor takes only 5 to 10 minutes. See Retained Placenta, page 168, for more information about what occurs should the placenta not be delivered within 30 minutes.

While you are expelling the placenta, a doctor will be examining the newborn and and evaluating its health. Most hospitals use the Apgar score, whereby the newborn is evaluated on the basis of five signs—**a**ppearance (color), **p**ulse (heartbeat), **g**rimace (reflex), **a**ctivity (muscle tone), and **r**espiration (breathing)—and given a score from zero to two for each one. Thus, the total score can be from zero to 10. The assessment is performed 1 minute after birth and again at 5 minutes. While Apgar scores were developed to assist in the

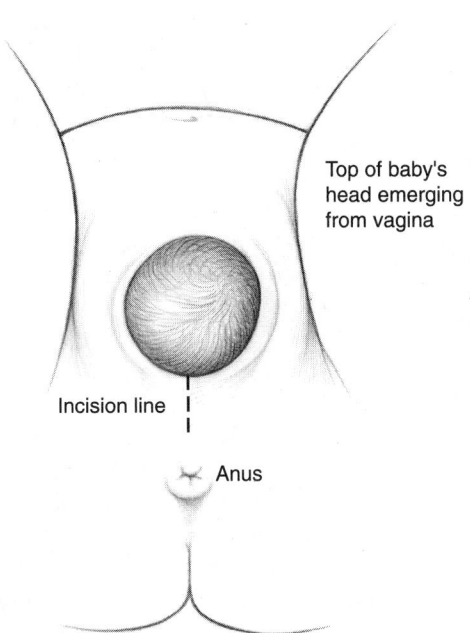

Top of baby's head emerging from vagina

Incision line

Anus

An episiotomy may facilitate the second stage of labor. Before the baby's head emerges, an anesthetic is injected between the vagina and the anus. An incision is then made to widen the opening for the baby, and the incision is stitched after delivery.

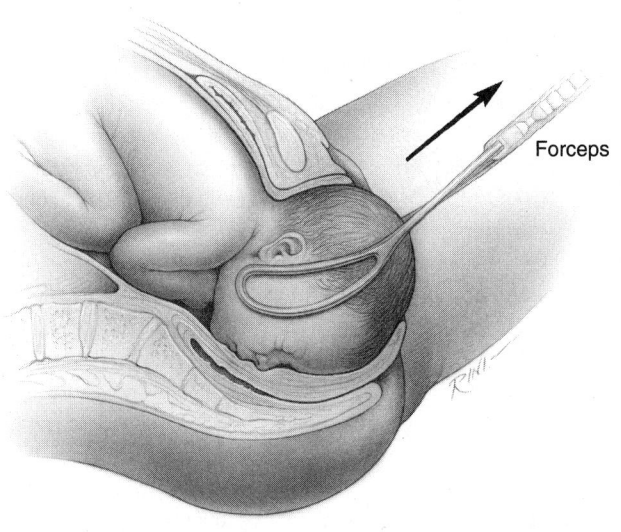

Forceps

Forceps (tong-like instruments) may be needed to assist delivery. When the cervix is completely dilated, forceps help to grip the baby's head gently and guide it through the pelvis.

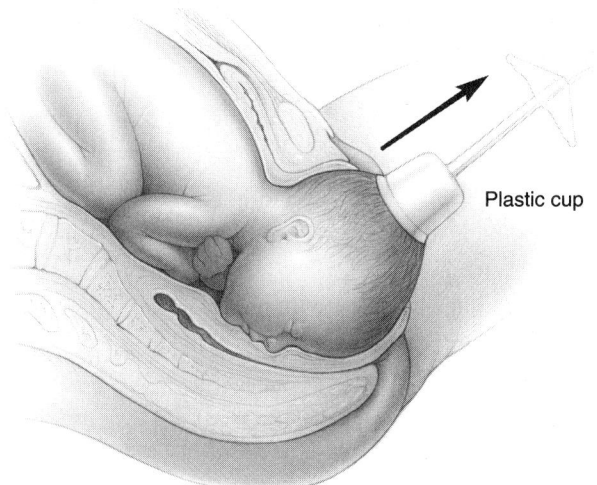

Plastic cup

Vacuum is an alternative device to assist delivery. Suction applied to a plastic cup over the baby's head can help to pull the baby down the birth canal. Temporary bruising may occur on the baby's head.

▶ the head has crowned during delivery in order to facilitate a rapid delivery and prevent tearing of the vulva or the vagina. Just before the emergence of the baby's head, a local anesthetic is injected between the vagina and the rectum, and the incision is made. The incision is then stitched up after delivery. This procedure is performed in somewhere between 50 and 90 percent of first-time mothers. Between 25 and 35 percent of women who have previously had a child will have an episiotomy. If you do not wish to have an episiotomy, be sure to discuss your wishes with your doctor before you go into labor. Though an episotomy can be avoided in some cases, it may be necessary if the baby is not tolerating the second stage of labor.

Forceps or Vacuum Extraction

In some cases vaginal deliveries must be aided by forceps or vacuum extraction. The use of forceps or vacuum extraction may be needed when the baby is too large to move through the birth canal unaided, when there is oxygen deprivation or other signs of fetal distress, or when the mother is too exhausted to push. Forceps are metal instruments that look like tongs. In the past, doctors used them to reach high into the birth canal, which necessitated a great deal of force and often bruised the baby. At present, however, forceps are used only when the cervix is completely dilated and the baby's head is within 2 inches of the mouth of the vagina.

Vacuum extraction was developed to replace forceps delivery and is preferred by some health care providers. In vacuum extraction, a plastic cup is fitted over the baby's head. A pump then gently attaches the cup to the baby's head, and the doctor can use it to pull the baby down the birth canal and out the vagina. As with a forceps delivery, there may still be slight swelling or bruising to the baby's head, but the bruises usually disappear within a few days. ■

PROLONGED LABOR

Prolonged labor is generally described as labor lasting 20 hours or more in a first birth and 14 hours or more in subsequent ones. Prolonged labor can be disheartening and exhausting, and lack of sleep and dehydration may add to your distress. Many women also become frustrated during prolonged labor because they feel the situation is somehow a reflection upon themselves; if they could only try harder, they feel, perhaps the situation would be different. But it is important to remember that even though you may be doing everything right, prolonged labor may still occur.

Failure to progress in labor is defined either by an overall measurement of time elapsed or by measuring the cervical dilation rate per hour during the time you have been in active labor. If the cause of prolonged labor is ineffective uterine contractions, an intravenous infusion of a synthetic hormone called oxytocin (Pitocin) may be used to stimulate contractions. In most cases, inducing contractions in this manner is successful. When it is not, a cesarean section may be necessary. Another form of inducing labor is by amniotomy (cutting the membranes), but this technique necessitates a firm commitment to immediate (within 24 hours) delivery to avoid infection.

Sometimes, the reason for prolonged labor is the inability of the fetus to pass through the pelvis (cephalopelvic disproportion or CPD). A diagnosis of CPD may be confirmed if uterine contractions of adequate intensity are ensured and labor still fails to progress; in this case, a cesarean section will be recommended. ∎

RETAINED PLACENTA

The placenta is normally expelled about 5 to 10 minutes after birth. This process is sometimes facilitated by placing the newborn at the mother's nipple. The sucking process helps trigger uterine contractions that expel the placenta. Expulsion of the placenta may also be facilitated by the administration of oxytocin, by cutting the umbilical cord immediately after birth, and by applying traction to the cord to help the placenta separate from the uterine wall.

If the placenta is not naturally expelled 30 minutes after birth, it is considered to be retained and must be removed manually. A retained placenta generally has not separated from the uterine wall. This procedure may be more difficult after oxytocin has been administered, since the uterus will be more firmly contracted. Once the placenta is removed it will be inspected. If a piece of the placenta is missing, the uterus will be explored manually. If any of the placenta remains in the uterus, it can cause serious infection. ∎

resuscitation of newborns, if the score remains below 5 at 5 minutes of life, the chance of neurologic impairment of the baby is greater. The Apgar score is not a specific indication of asphyxia, but an assessment of the infant's transition to life outside the womb.

CESAREAN SECTION

A cesarean section (also called C-section) refers to the delivery of the baby via one incision in the mother's abdominal wall and then another in the uterine wall. While the idea of delivering a baby through an incision in the abdominal wall is represented in Greek mythology and in cave paintings in Africa, the first cesarean sections in which both mother and child survived were not performed until the mid-1800s. However, the surgery did not become common practice until well into the 20th century. Now, most hospitals report birth rates for cesarean sections of between 20 and 25 percent.

In the 1970s, the rate of cesarean deliveries increased threefold in the United States. It should be noted that the increase in cesarean deliveries has been accompanied by a decrease in both infant and mother mortality. But while cesarean delivery may prevent complications for mother and child, its growing rate raises concerns that some cesarean deliveries are unnecessary.

The number of births by cesarean section is now decreasing. In many cases, a cesarean delivery is the right choice to protect the health of both the baby and the mother. Being an informed patient can help you and your partner make the right decision with your doctor, should a choice need to be made.

There are many situations in which a cesarean delivery is safest for the baby and mother. Here are some of the more common ones.

Active herpes virus If you have genital herpes and the virus has been active within 4 weeks of your due date, your doctor will schedule you for a cesarean section. A baby born vaginally during an outbreak of herpes can suffer severe consequences, including brain damage.

Placenta previa When the placenta covers, or partially covers, the cervical opening (placenta previa), vaginal delivery would lead to extensive hemorrhage and possibly fetal death.

Abruption Abruption refers to the sudden, premature separation of the placenta from the uterine wall. This interferes with the baby's oxygen supply and is a medical and surgical emergency.

Cephalopelvic disproportion (CPD) CPD occurs when the baby's head is too large to pass safely through the mother's pelvis during delivery.

Macrosomia Macrosomia refers to a baby who weighs more than 10 lbs at birth. These very large babies are especially common among women who have uncontrolled gestational diabetes. If a sonogram determines that your baby is likely to be significantly larger than average and if you still have 2 weeks until your due date, a cesarean section may be recommended.

Preeclampsia and eclampsia If preeclampsia has been diagnosed, your doctor will monitor your situation carefully. She may recommend a cesarean section if labor is not progressing or if the fetal heart pattern is worrisome.

Prolapsed cord The umbilical cord is called prolapsed if it moves down into the cervix or vagina, becoming stuck between the cervix and the baby. If blood flow to the baby is impaired, an emergency cesarean may be necessary.

Postmature fetus A fetus is considered postmature if it is 2 weeks overdue. In that case, macrosomia may result. If your baby is overdue, your doctor will discuss the possibility of inducing labor or performing a cesarean section (see Postmaturity, page 162).

Multiple Births A woman who is expecting twins has about a 5 percent greater chance of having a cesarean delivery. If a woman is carrying three or more babies, cesarean section is almost always recommended (see Twins and Other Multiple Pregnancies, page 141).

Before the surgery a urinary catheter will be inserted into the bladder to prevent damage to it. An intravenous (IV) catheter will be inserted to permit fluids to be given during the surgery. Your abdomen will be washed and any excessive body hair may be clipped. If the situation is an emergency, you may be given general anesthesia, which means you will be asleep throughout the surgery. If it is not an emergency, you may be consulted regarding anesthesia. If you want to be awake for the birth of the baby, you have a choice between spinal block or epidural anesthesia (see page 165). A spinal block offers the assurance of complete numbness, but it takes longer to wear off. An epidural may not leave you completely numb to all pain, but it will wear off more quickly. Epidurals are often chosen by doctors because their dosage can be regulated during surgery. In many hospitals, your partner is allowed to accompany you to the delivery room and be present during the surgery and the delivery of your baby.

In a cesarean section, the abdominal wall is first incised, and the uterus is then opened to remove the baby. Various locations are used for both the abdominal and the uterine incisions. (A) Vertical abdominal incision. (B) Transverse abdominal incision. (C) Classic uterine incision. (D) Low vertical uterine incision. (E) Low transverse uterine incision.

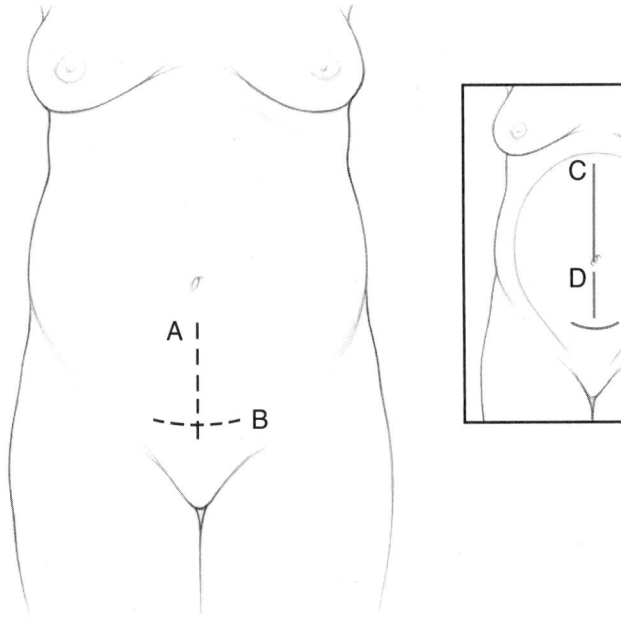

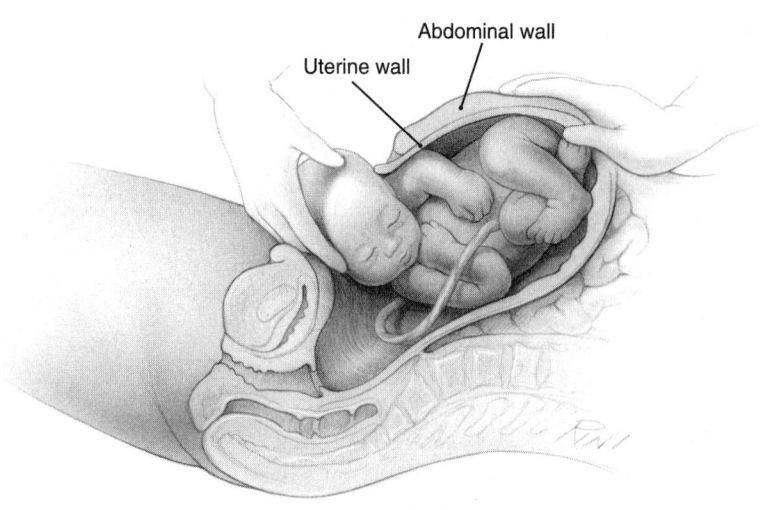

Abdominal wall
Uterine wall

Cesarean birth. After the abdominal incision is made, the uterus is cut and the baby is carefully removed.

The doctor will first make an incision through the wall of the abdomen. In most cases, a transverse or horizontal incision is now used, just above the pubic hairline. This is also referred to as a bikini incision. In some situations, the doctor may make a vertical, or midline, incision from the navel to the public bone. Once the abdomen has been opened, another incision, usually transverse, is made in the wall of the uterus in order to deliver the baby. It is important for you to know the type of incision used on the uterus (transverse or vertical), as this is one of the factors that will affect your ability to give birth vaginally in the future.

When the baby has been delivered and the placenta has been removed, first the uterus is closed with internal sutures, and then the abdomen is closed with sutures or metal clips. After a dressing is applied, you

VAGINAL BIRTH AFTER CESAREAN

The myth of "once a cesarean, always a cesarean" has been shaken in the last decade. Today many women are able to experience a successful vaginal delivery after a previous cesarean section. If you have delivered by cesarean section in the past and are pregnant again, talk with your doctor about the possibility of vaginal birth after cesarean (VBAC).

There are many reasons why you may wish to consider VBAC:

- *Birth experience.* With a vaginal delivery you can probably participate more in the delivery of your baby and you may be surrounded by the people whom you choose to be present in the delivery room, which may not be the case for a cesarean section.

- *Easier recovery.* A cesarean section usually takes longer to heal. If you have a vaginal delivery you will most likely be discharged from the hospital more quickly than you will if have a cesarean section and you will also be able to resume normal activities such as driving or exercise much sooner.

- *Lower risk profile.* The risk of complications for the mother is much lower with a vaginal delivery than a cesarean section because a cesarean section is, in fact, major surgery.

There are several medical factors that must be assessed when considering a vaginal versus cesarean delivery in any woman. For those who have already had cesarean sections, an important factor to determine is the type of incision that was used. There are three types of incisions:

- Transverse incision, made horizontally across the lower part of the uterus

- Low vertical incision, made vertically in the lower part of the uterus

- High vertical (classical) incision, made vertically in the upper part of the uterus Your external scar bears no relation to the type of incision that was made in your uterus, so your doctor will need to check your medical records for this information.

If you had a transverse incision there is less risk of complications during vaginal delivery. The risks are not well defined with a low vertical incision; you will need to evaluate your options with your doctor. If you had a high vertical incision the risks of vaginal delivery are significantly greater and VBAC is not recommended.

Your desires must be considered along with your doctor's medical opinion before a final decision is made. If you do not wish to attempt a vaginal delivery it is your right to insist upon a cesarean section. However, if you are a good candidate for VBAC the benefits will in most cases outweigh the risks.

Once you have decided on a vaginal delivery, certain measures will be taken during labor and delivery to minimize the risks that exist with VBAC. You will probably require extra support and encouragement during labor. Talk with your doctor about the best way to meet your needs. You may wish to attend a childbirth class with your partner or, if your doctor agrees, enlist the support of a doula (person who provides support to new mothers both during delivery and recovery afterwards). Your doctor may recommend or even require that you give birth in a hospital setting so that emergency equipment is readily available should a problem arise; however, some women do choose to deliver in birthing centers or at home. Prepare yourself by discussing with your doctor procedures that may be used during labor. It is also important to discuss the possibility that you may encounter difficulty at the same point in labor that led to your previous cesarean section so that you and your doctor will have an understanding regarding how to approach the situation should it arise again. ■

will be able to hold your baby and to try to nurse it. Early contact with your baby is very important and is certainly one good reason to remain awake during your cesarean section.

After surgery you will be taken to the recovery room. In recovery, your blood pressure and respiration will be checked regularly, and you will be monitored for any excessive vaginal bleeding.

The sooner you begin to get up and walk around after a cesarean delivery, the sooner you will recover. While you do not want to tax yourself unnecessarily, you should try to get out of bed within 12 to 24 hours with the help of a nurse or your partner as soon as you feel ready. You will probably be in pain or at least feel discomfort for several days after the operation. If your doctor has not already prescribed a pain reliever, you should ask her for one that you can take while nursing.

Until recently, most women stayed in the hospital for at least 5 days after a C-section. In recent years, that stay has grown shorter. Consult with your doctor and your health insurance provider to learn what is anticipated in your situation and how much of that stay will be covered by your health care plan.

Most women rapidly regain normal body functions after a cesarean section. After 4 to 6 weeks, you should be able to resume a full range of normal activities. Having a C-section should not interfere with breast-feeding, and it does not rule out a normal vaginal delivery in future pregnancies if the incision on the uterus is transverse.

❖ POSTPARTUM HEMORRHAGE

Symptoms *(What you may experience)* Continued heavy bleeding after delivery.

Signs and laboratory findings *(What the doctor looks for)* Your vaginal bleeding will be monitored closely after delivery. If the bleeding is too rapid (more than 1 pad per hour), if you pass large clots (larger than a golf ball), if you become light-headed, if your blood pressure drops, or if your pulse increases, you will be examined to find the source of bleeding.

What is it? The most common form of obstetrical hemorrhage is postpartum hemorrhage, which refers to heavy vaginal bleeding after delivery is completed. It is usually caused by the failure of the uterus to contract successfully when the placenta separates from the uterus (uterine atony). In some cases, the bleeding is heavy, while in others there is only a steady seepage. Sometimes the blood may collect in the uterus and not pass through the vagina. In this case, the uterus becomes distended. If not treated immediately, postpartum hemorrhage can be very serious, sometimes necessitating a hysterectomy.

Treatment Postpartum hemorrhage is treated most often with prostaglandins or the hormone oxytocin (Pitocin). These drugs are administered to make the uterus contract, which will stop the hemorrhaging. Prostaglandins are injected into the wall of the uterus. If this treatment is not successful, a surgical procedure called a bilateral hypogastric artery ligation, which involves tying off the blood vessels to stop the bleeding, may be performed to avoid a hysterectomy. Selective arterial embolization (a procedure that blocks off the bleeding artery) may be an option in medical centers that have an interventional radiologist on staff, but only if the bleeding is not life threatening. In the event that these procedures are not successful, a hysterectomy may be necessary.

After the Baby Is Born

The birth of your baby will transform your life in many ways, one of which becomes immediately obvious: suddenly, you are not the focus of the doctors', nurses', and your partner's attention; the newborn baby is. At first this will be a relief, but once you head home with your new baby, you'll have to make certain you get the rest and care *you* need to maintain your own health so that you can care for your baby.

POSTPARTUM CONCERNS

No aspect of childbirth is as neglected as the period directly following the birth of the child. While a great deal of attention is paid to preparing for birth, very little is given to the mother's recovery after birth.

Many new mothers are unprepared for the potential stresses of this period. From caring for your episiotomy to postpartum depression, there may be much to contend with, in addition to the rigors of caring for the newborn.

Here are some of the issues and concerns a new mother may face directly after childbirth:

- Uterine cramping. Some women experience uterine cramps as the uterus returns to its normal size and shape. These cramps usually last for about a week and may be more intense if this is not your first baby. Though these contractions may be painful, they are a healthy and necessary part of your recovery.

- Episiotomy. Recovering from an episiotomy can be very painful. Cold, wet compresses immediately following delivery may lessen the discomfort; you can continue to use them when you come home from the hospital. You may also want to take frequent warm baths to ease pain, aid healing, and help keep the area clean. A spray bottle filled with water can also be helpful in cleansing the perineum after delivery. All stitches used for episiotomy repairs will dissolve on their own.

- Hemorrhoids. During pregnancy, labor, and delivery, hemorrhoids may appear or worsen. Cold witch hazel compresses may help relieve discomfort, as may hemorrhoid creams or gels. Sitz baths may also be helpful, and so may sitting on specially designed pillows. Your hemorrhoids will gradually decrease in size and may eventually disappear.

- Breast engorgement. Two to four days after delivery, your breasts may become engorged, and you may feel fullness or discomfort. Applying ice packs helps to relieve discomfort; however, this will decrease milk production, so avoid using ice packs if you are nursing. Applying a wet, warm cloth to the breast will help relieve discomfort for nursing mothers. If you are not nursing, you should not pump or stimulate your breasts as this will simply cause greater milk production. Medications to prevent milk production are not recom-

mended because of possible serious side effects such as stroke.

In the past, women stayed in the hospital for several days following a normal delivery. In recent years, that stay has shrunk to 24 to 48 hours, depending upon the legal requirements of the state you live in and the amount of time your health care plan will cover. Many women feel that they will recuperate better at home and want to leave the hospital as quickly as possible. Others feel that it will be stressful and physically taxing to return home so quickly. Discuss the alternatives with your health care provider. If you do return home quickly, it is important to limit what you do, so that your body will not be overtaxed.

In the weeks after delivery, you should monitor your health for any abnormal changes. If you experience any of the following, you should contact your doctor.

- Fever
- Persistent pain in the area between the vulva and anus
- Nausea and vomiting
- Painful urination
- Bleeding that is heavier than your normal period
- Hot, tender breasts

Your doctor will want to see you about 4 to 6 weeks after your delivery to monitor your recovery and overall health. It is important that you keep this appointment and not neglect your own needs after the baby is born.

WELL-BABY CARE

While in the hospital, the baby is examined either by the hospital pediatrician or by a pediatrician you have chosen yourself. You will be asked to decide this before your baby is born. Because many insurance companies do not cover well-baby care, you would do well to check with yours to see what charges they will cover for a healthy newborn's stay in the hospital.

Once you return home from the hospital, your pediatrician will want to see your newborn in 1 to 2 weeks. Your baby's heartbeat and respiration will be checked, as well as weight gain and the healing of the navel—the space where the umbilical cord was formerly attached. If your baby is a boy and he has been circumcised, the circumcision will also be checked. In the first year of life, your pediatrician will want to see the baby every 2 to 3 months. During the first 2 years of life, your baby should receive a series of standard shots for immunization against childhood diseases.

In the first weeks of your baby's life, your pediatrician's help can be indispensable. She will alert you to any birthmarks or rashes your baby might have, listen to your concerns about colic, sleep, feedings, and other issues—and help you learn when to worry and when not to worry. See Chapter 8 for more information on well-baby care and other concerns about your newborn's health.

BREAST-FEEDING

To breast-feed or bottle-feed? It's a matter of personal choice.

It is now widely acknowledged, however, that "breast is best." Breast milk has properties that even the best formulas cannot provide:

- Breast-fed babies tend to get sick less often, because their mother's immunities are transferred through the milk. They also have a lower incidence of ear infections and allergies.

- Breast milk is a complete food, providing your baby with protein, carbohydrates, fat, and all the nutrients a baby needs; however, your pediatrician may need to prescribe a supplement for iron, vitamin D, and fluoride in some cases. Breast milk changes as the baby grows, offering a combination of ingredients that is perfectly suited to the baby's needs.

- Breast milk helps protect against infection in the digestive tract.

- Breast milk is more digestible than formulas based on cow's milk or soy milk.

- Breast milk is relatively low in cost (the mother just needs to increase her caloric intake) and requires no bottles, nipples, or other paraphernalia. It is always available, it is always at the right temperature, and it will not spoil unless it is expressed and not refrigerated.

- Babies are rarely allergic to breast milk.

- Breast-fed babies do not typically become constipated and are less likely to get diaper rash. Bowel movements of breast-fed babies are less offensive-smelling than those of bottle-fed babies.

- Breast-fed babies are not likely to be overfed, as may occur with bottle-feeding.

- There are advantages to the mother's health from breast-feeding: the uterus shrinks faster and breast-feeding mothers have a reduced risk of early breast cancer, ovarian cancer, and postmenopausal hip fractures.

- Breast-feeding helps build the mother-child bond.

While the advantages of breast-feeding (or nursing) are clear, some women choose not to nurse for a variety of reasons. One important benefit to bottle-feeding is that it allows the father to participate in feeding the baby. Some women also choose to bottle-feed because they feel that bottle-feeding is less disruptive to a couple's sex life; lactation hormones can keep the vagina relatively dry (though vaginal lubricants can help with this problem), and some couples find leaky breasts less than seductive (although the larger breast size of the nursing mother may be a positive factor for some couples). Other reasons mothers choose to bottle-feed include not having to worry about what they eat or drink, a desire for a freer daily schedule, and having a demanding job outside of the home that may make breast-feeding complicated. Additionally, some women choose not to breast-feed because they sense they are too impatient for a task they envision as time-consuming, they are squeamish about such close physical contact, they belong to a community or a culture that is not supportive of breast-feeding, or they feel uncomfortable about nursing in front of other people or in public. It is important for a mother who plans to bottle-feed to try to nurse her baby for at least a few days or weeks. Colostrum (pre-milk), which the baby receives only during the first days of nursing, is especially rich in many valuable substances not found in formulas.

Unfortunately, there are some women who want to breast-feed and cannot for medical reasons, such as a serious infection, debilitating illness (heart problems, severe anemia, or kidney impairment), or because they are taking medications that may pass into the breast milk. A few infants may be unable to nurse because of lactose intolerance or other medical issues. Premature birth and an undeveloped "sucking reflex" may prevent nursing initially, but mothers may pump and store milk until their infants are ready to nurse.

Whatever your reasons for choosing breast or bottle, feeling comfortable with the decision you make will make it the right one for you and your baby.

Once breast-feeding is established, it feels like the most natural and loving bond between mother and child. But getting there can be a trying experience for the exhausted new mother. Most women find that breast-feeding goes relatively smoothly from the beginning, but sometimes babies do have trouble latching on at first. The more often you try to nurse the baby, the better the chances that the baby will "get the hang of it" and your new role as a nursing mother will proceed smoothly. If problems continue, you should consult your doctor, the baby's pediatrician, or a lactation consultant. Many hospitals offer programs to help nursing mothers, or you can contact your local chapter of the La Leche League for support and information.

Make sure you are in a comfortable position when you nurse your baby. Start by supporting your breast with the hand that is not holding your baby, and brushing the baby's lips with the nipple until they open. Try not to put the nipple into the baby's mouth. Let your baby latch on and make sure the areola (dark area around the nipple), as well as the nipple, is in the baby's mouth. Also, check that your breast is not blocking the baby's nose. A steady, rhythmic motion visible in the cheeks will assure you that the baby is suckling. When you want to change breasts, or if the baby has finished but is still holding onto the nipple, break the suction by gently inserting your finger into the corner of your baby's mouth. Never pull the nipple out abruptly, as you might injure the nipple.

Many new mothers worry about their milk supply, but they should be assured that most nursing mothers produce enough milk to meet the newborn baby's needs. Breast milk is produced according to the law of supply and demand: If the baby nurses regularly, your breasts will be stimulated to make enough milk to keep up. If you or your doctor have any concern regarding your milk supply, you can usually build it up by nursing as often as possible for 48 hours. (If your baby is not hungry enough to nurse every 2 or 3 hours, you can pump milk from your breasts with a breast pump.) At first, however, mothers often experience the opposite problem—engorgement—which results in swollen and painful breasts. To relieve engorgement, nurse more often for shorter periods or use a breast pump to relieve your swollen breasts. And be sure to wear a supportive nursing bra, even at night. (Nursing bras and pads are also invaluable in absorbing the milk that may leak from your breasts at inopportune times.) After a short time, your body's milk supply and your baby's demands will start to synchronize.

The frequency of feedings will vary from newborn to newborn, but newborn babies demand and need to eat every 2 to 3 hours. If your baby does not demand to nurse at least six times a day during the first month of life, you can try offering the breast more often than your baby demands. Some babies may be less efficient at making their needs known than others. Breast-fed babies tend to gain weight more slowly than formula-fed babies. This is fine, as long as the weight gain is adequate. The health benefits breast milk confers outweigh the extra ounces formula may provide. Remember to nurse the baby from each breast at each feeding, if possible, by switching to the other breast halfway into the feeding. This will help you avoid sore or engorged breasts and will also help to make sure that the milk supply in each breast is adequate. You should start the next breast-feeding session with the breast you ended on during the previous nursing session or with the breast that feels heavier.

Many breast-feeding mothers choose at some time to express and store breast milk. Milk can be refrigerated for up to 48 hours or frozen for up to 6 months.

As a nursing mother, you have special nutritional needs. Be sure to maintain the healthy eating habits you adopted during pregnancy to ensure adequate milk produc-

PROBLEMS WITH YOUR BREASTS

The most common problems women encounter while breast-feeding are engorgement, cracked nipples, blocked milk ducts, and infectious mastitis.

Engorgement

If milk is not removed as it is formed in the breast, engorgement results. This may occur when feedings are limited or short. If your baby is feeding regularly and your breasts still feel engorged, you should pump milk from your breasts with a manual or electric breast pump, both of which can be purchased in most drugstores. If needed, a larger, more efficient electric breast pump can be rented for a reasonable monthly rate from many drugstores and hospitals. Do not worry about having enough milk for your baby. Pumping your breasts may even increase your milk production, and you can freeze the expressed milk in a sterile bottle or plastic bag for later use. Be prepared for it to take some time for your milk supply to synchronize with your baby's needs. This will occur naturally as you and your baby adjust to one another.

Cracked Nipples

If you do not dry your nipples sufficiently after nursing, they may become reddened, cracked, and sore. To prevent your nipples from becoming cracked, let them air-dry after nursing before putting on your bra and clothing, and wear a loose-fitting, cotton nursing bra. If you do develop cracked nipples, your doctor can prescribe a soothing cream or ointment.

Blocked Milk Ducts

Sometimes engorgement can lead to a blocked milk duct. A blocked duct occurs when milk collects in a duct and pressure rises. It may feel like a tiny, hard lump in your breast. If you feel such a lump, contact your doctor. If the pressure is not relieved, an inflammatory reaction can occur.

Infectious Mastitis

If an area of your breast becomes red, swollen, warm, and painful, and your pulse rises and you become feverish, you may have infectious mastitis. You should contact your doctor immediately. While mastitis is not always infectious, it is usually treated with antibiotics to avoid further complications (see Mastitis, Chapter 19). It is recommended that you continue nursing

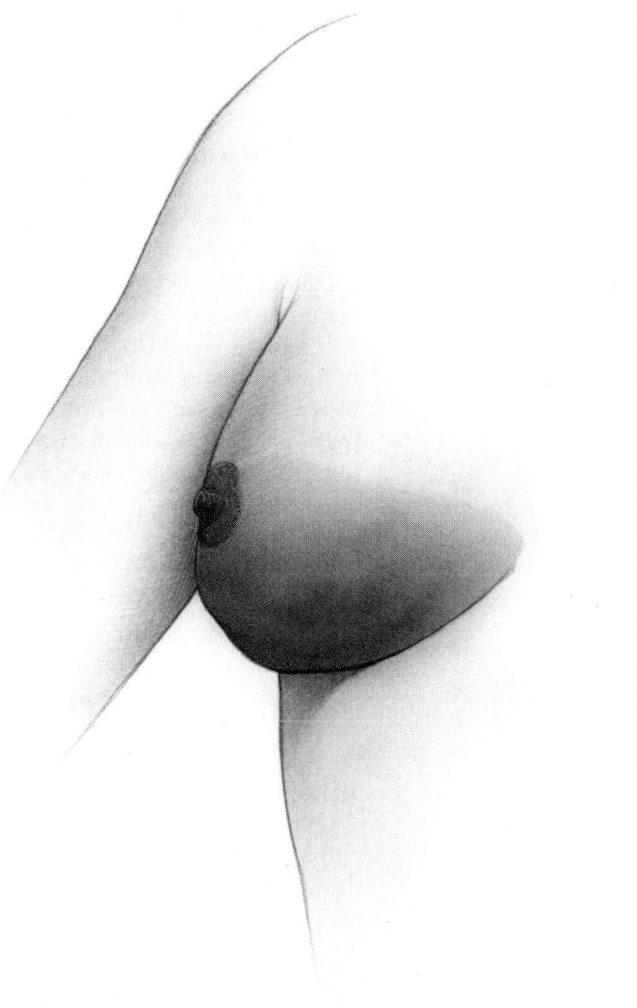

Infectious mastitis. A red, swollen, warm, painful breast can indicate this inflammatory condition. Antibiotics are sometimes needed for treatment. Continued nursing is usually encouraged to prevent engorgement.

your baby, if you can, to prevent engorgement. The antibiotics your doctor prescribes to treat the infection will not harm your baby. ■

tion and nutritional health for yourself and your baby.

A nursing mother requires about an additional 600 calories a day. These additional calories should be consumed to ensure an adequate intake of calcium (for the mother's needs) from milk and other dairy products, and the other nutrients discussed in A Recommended Diet, page 138.

Drinking plenty of fluids is just as important to adequate milk production as is a healthy diet. The best choice of beverages to meet this requirement is water. If you are a nursing mother, you should drink a minimum of eight glasses of water a day while nursing and more than that if you are thirsty.

IF YOU HAD GESTATIONAL DIABETES

While women with gestational diabetes are generally told that "everything will go back to normal" once the baby is born, more than 50 percent of women who have had gestational diabetes end up developing diabetes within the next 10 years. This sobering fact should motivate you to watch your diet and exercise regimen closely following pregnancy.

You should also make sure that you have annual checkups and talk to your doctor about your blood glucose levels. If they are consistently on the high end of normal, you should be particularly careful about monitoring your diet, and you should discuss with your doctor other measures you may take to prevent diabetes. (For more information on diabetes, see Chapter 26.)

POSTPARTUM DEPRESSION

Many women experience postpartum depression—a lingering unhappiness after childbirth, which may vary in degree from a mild sadness to an extremely serious condition that warrants immediate medical attention.

Usually, the main causes are lack of psychological and social support, as well as rapid changes in hormone levels. But confusion regarding how we define and treat serious postpartum depression may also cause women to suffer needlessly and to endanger their own and their children's welfare because their conditions were not taken seriously.

Almost all new mothers experience a normal letdown once their babies are born. After the expectation and excitement of pregnancy, the rigors of caring for a newborn can be a rude awakening. Excitement is replaced by exhaustion. Despite reading and preparing ahead of time, few mothers are prepared for the relentless demands of a newborn baby or the 24-hour nature of the job.

One way to minimize postpartum depression is to prepare ahead of time for the possibility of a letdown after birth. Discuss your fears regarding caring for a newborn with friends and family and ask other mothers for practical advice on the daily life of a new mother. In addition, be ready to shift your priorities to accommodate your new baby. Don't expect to resume an intense business or social schedule immediately, and don't make unrealistic demands on yourself, such as keeping an immaculate house or making a seven-course meal for guests. Your life has changed, and accepting just how much it has changed is the first step in this period of adjustment.

In addition, the most practical way to avoid exacerbating postpartum depression is to plan strategically with your partner and other family members to ensure that you get enough rest. You will be up a lot at night, even if you are not breast-feeding. Try to nap or at least rest when your baby does. You should be as dedicated to getting the rest you need as you are to tending to your baby.

Also, don't be afraid to ask for help. When a new baby has arrived, so do many guests. Ask them to help out with shopping, housework, and errands. And make sure you are eating well. Hunger can contribute to feelings of depression.

Extremely serious cases of postpartum depression require medical intervention. If you feel you are suffering from a severe case of depression that no amount of rest or support seems to alleviate, don't be deterred by well-meaning family and friends who insist your "blues" will pass. You should consult your doctor immediately. Sometimes, antidepressant medication will be prescribed by your doctor, who may also recommend counseling. If you are breast-feeding you should discuss the risk of side effects before taking any medication. It may be possible for you to continue breast-feeding while taking medication, but you should discuss this with your doctor.

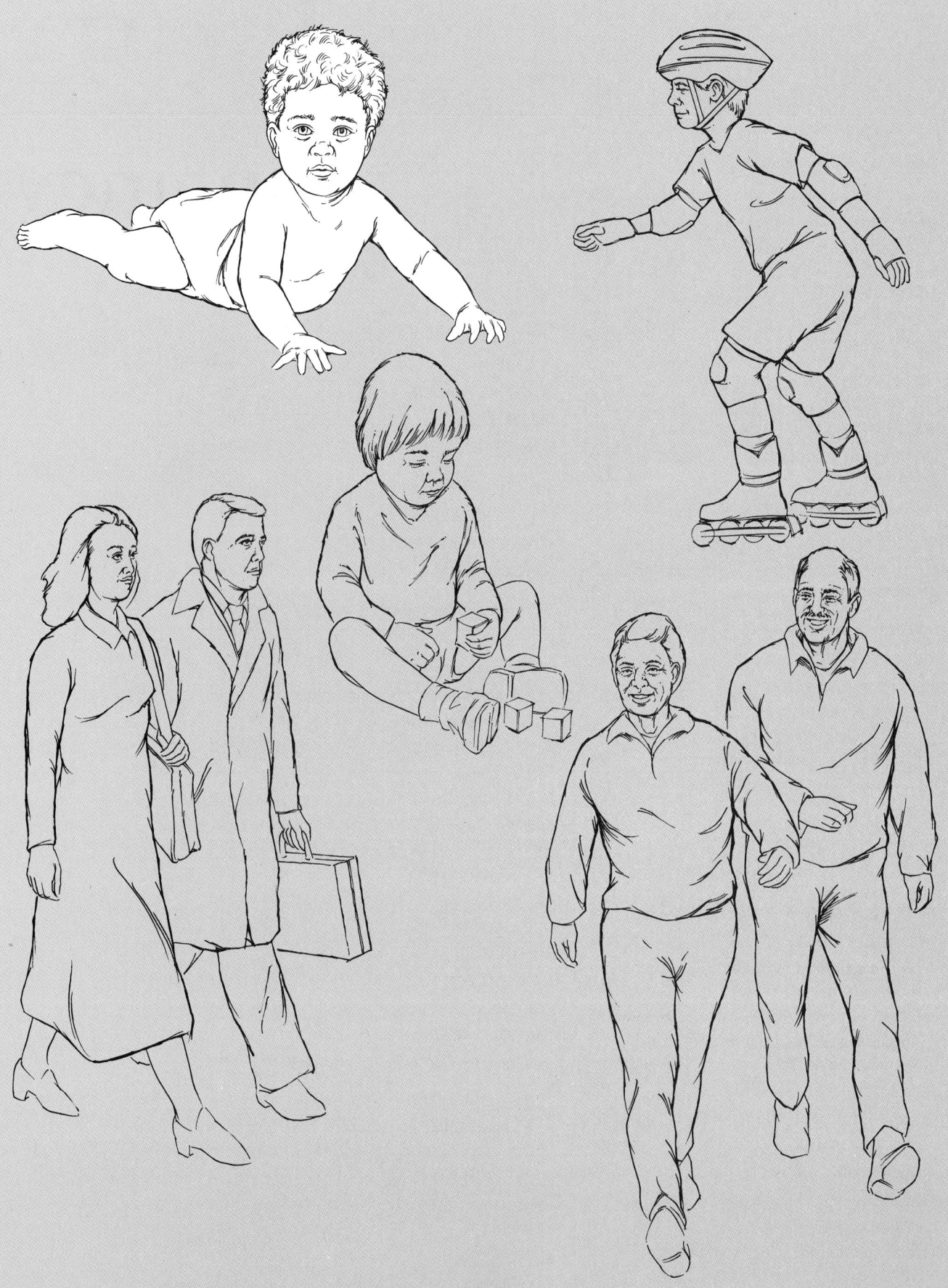

INFANCY

Your Newborn Baby

Nothing is as exciting as meeting and holding your new baby for the first time. After 9 months of waiting, the much loved and eagerly awaited new member of your family has arrived. From the first moments of life, your baby's new and various needs will take precedence over your own, because your newborn is dependent upon you for everything. And though your newborn will sleep from 14 to 18 hours a day, you'll be amazed how his needs will keep you busy most of the day and much of the night. During this time, it is best to simplify your life as much as possible. Your first priority is caring for your baby. Your second priority is getting the rest you need to care for your baby well. One of the best pieces of advice new mothers receive is to nap when the baby naps, for rare is the newborn that sleeps through the night. Expect your sleep to be interrupted and to be sleeping less than you would like. If you have trouble falling asleep when your baby is napping, try resting and relaxing. By all means, try not to use these precious moments of quiet to return calls or catch up on housework. And when friends and family visit and ask if they can help, let them. In other words, let other things wait, if possible, and devote your time to getting to know your baby. This is not an indulgence, it is a necessity for your baby's healthy development. Remember, you are investing in a lifelong relationship.

WHAT YOUR NEWBORN WILL LOOK LIKE

Most new parents find that their beloved newborn does not look quite like the bundle of angelic beauty they may have anticipated. At birth, the head of the newborn is about one quarter of the total length and will seem large in comparison to the rest of the body. Newborn babies generally seem very skinny. Their legs are spindly. Their bellies may appear swollen, and unless your baby was delivered by cesarean section, the head may be bruised and appear misshapen. Labor takes its toll on the newborn as well as the mother, and a baby delivered vaginally may have bloodshot or swollen eyes because of the pressure of delivery. In addition, the nose may be flattened, the chin asymmetric, and the head almost pointy. Some babies are born bald, while others are born with a full head of hair that may be matted down like a cap or standing straight up, giving the baby a startled expression. When all of these aspects are considered, most newborns appear more comic than beautiful.

The skin of the newborn is often pinkish, and usually thin and transparent enough to allow the blood vessels to be visible. Often, newborn babies, particularly those born prematurely, may be covered, particularly on the shoulders, forehead, and cheeks, with soft, downy hair, called lanugo. Lanugo generally disappears within the first weeks of life.

One of the great guessing games new parents indulge in involves eye color. Your baby's eyes will not resolve themselves into their permanent color until between the third and sixth months of life. Most darker skinned babies with dark eyes are born with the eye color they will have throughout life. White babies, however, may be born with eyes whose color changes during the first year. Because pigmentation of the iris often continues to increase through the first year of life, the actual color and depth of color of your baby's eyes may not be clearly determined until your baby is about 1 year old.

The evidence of birth may not be what the first-time parent may be expecting, but in less than a minute, the new parent adjusts, and in a matter of days or weeks, the evidence of birth disappears, leaving your newborn more beautiful than ever.

THE NORMAL NEWBORN

Full-term babies include all babies born between the 38th and 42nd week after the mother's last menstrual period. Most full-term newborns weigh between 5 lb, 5 oz and 10 lb, and they are usually between 18 and 22 in. long. Your newborn will lose from 6 to 10 percent of his birth weight in the first days after birth, due to fluid loss and relatively small feedings. An initial weight loss is natural, and your healthy baby will soon regain this weight.

During the first month of life, your baby will probably gain about 2 lb (see Nutrition, page 200). Newborns are hungry at erratic hours throughout the day and night. After 1 week of life, most newborns eat every 2 to 5 hours. At this point, it is important to let your baby establish his own feeding schedule by letting your baby eat whenever he

INITIAL ROUTINE TESTS

There are several tests your baby may have in the delivery room or newborn nursery. Of these, the Apgar score is the most common. It is a score assigned at 5 and 10 minutes after birth that depicts how well your baby seems to be dealing with extrauterine life. Depending on the laws of your state, your baby will also be tested for certain metabolic disorders (such as galactosemia, phenylketonuria, and hypothyroidism) that are best diagnosed and treated as soon as possible after birth to prevent or lessen permanent damage.

The Apgar Score Most infants score between 7 and 9 and require no treatment after birth except to have the mucus suctioned from the nose to clear the airway. Babies that score between 0 and 4 at 1 minute after birth require immediate medical treatment.

	SCORE		
	0	**1**	**2**
Heart rate	Absent	<100	>100
Respiratory effort	Absent, irregular	Slow, crying	Good
Muscle tone	Limp	Some flexion of extremities	Active motion
Reflex irritability (nose suction)	No response	Grimace	Cough or sneeze
Color	Blue, pale	Extremities blue	Completely pink

The Apgar score is assessed at 1 and 5 minutes. For neonatal distress, assessment is repeated at 10 and 20 minutes.

Source: Johnson KB: The Harriet Lane Handbook. A Manual for Pediatric House Officers. 13th Ed. Mosby-Year Book, St. Louis, 1993, as adapted from Apgar V: Anesth Analg 32:260, 1953; used with permission.

Phenylketonuria Phenylketonuria (PKU) is an inherited disorder that involves an enzyme deficiency affecting the ability to break down the amino acid phenylalanine present in most foods, including regular formula and breast milk. One of every 10,000 babies has PKU. If untreated, it can cause severe brain damage. All states now require that all newborns be tested for PKU. The test is simple, requiring only a few drops of your baby's blood. The test is usually performed when your baby is at least 3 days old, because the accuracy of the test depends on your baby having consumed a good amount of protein. Because most newborns and their mothers have been released from the hospital by this time, a trip back to the hospital or to your doctor may be necessary.

Congenital Hypothyroidism This deficiency affecting the production of thyroid hormone occurs in about 1 of every 4,000 babies born and is twice as likely to occur in girls. Because initial symptoms are rare and early treatment can greatly benefit those who have the disorder, almost all newborns are tested immediately for hypothyroidism. For more information on hypothyroidism, see Chapter 26.

Galactosemia Galactosemia is a very rare, inherited disorder that affects only 1 in approximately 45,000 newborns. It is a serious disease that involves an enzyme deficiency that inhibits the ability to metabolize galactose, which is present in milk as well as some other foods. Lethargy, severe diarrhea, persistent jaundice, and difficulty feeding can all be signs of galactosemia. Most states now require a test for galactosemia as part of the newborn hereditary metabolic screen. ■

seems hungry. Over the first month, the number of times your baby eats in a 24-hour period may diminish from seven or eight to five or six. Length of feedings may also vary during these early days of life. A breast-fed baby may want to nurse as long as 40 minutes or as short as 10 minutes at each feeding. After 1 month of life, your baby's eating habits may still not be fully established, but they will probably be more regular. During the first 2 weeks of life, your baby will be consuming approximately 16 to 18 oz of breast milk or formula per day. By 1 month, your baby may be consuming as much as 25 oz of milk or formula per day. If your baby is growing at the normal rate, you will know that the amount of milk or formula that he is taking is the correct amount.

Your newborn generally has his first bowel movement during the first 24 hours of life. Do not be startled if this stool is tarry and greenish or black. It is composed of residual amniotic fluid and intestinal secretions and is called a meconium stool. By the third or fourth day, meconium stools are replaced by transitional stools, as your baby begins to consume milk. At 1 week, your baby will probably be passing three to five stools a day or more. However, if your baby goes a day without passing a stool, do not worry, as long as he is feeding well.

The stool of a breast-fed baby is loose and odorless. The stool of a formula-fed baby tends to be more pasty, or thicker, and has a slight fecal smell. After a month of life, most babies have settled into having three or four bowel movements a day. These usually occur after feedings. Some breast-fed babies may have a bowel movement only once a day or every other day after the first few weeks. This is normal and nothing to worry about. If you notice any sudden changes in your newborn's bowel movements, call your doctor.

At birth, your baby's cry is his major form of expression, though newborns may also express themselves through gurgling or throaty sounds. As with other aspects of a newborn's development and personality, how frequently and intensely your baby cries is as individual as your baby is. Almost immediately, you will be able to recognize your baby's cry. Very soon, you will also be able to decipher what it is your baby needs when he is crying.

Often, both newborn boys and girls may have swollen breasts or genitals because of the surge of female hormones from the placenta immediately preceding birth. Sometimes you can even see a milky discharge from the breasts. If your baby is a girl, you may also notice a vaginal discharge, which is sometimes bloody. This is normal.

Your newborn will emulate the fetal position directly after birth. When placed on his stomach, the baby can roll his head to the side. When held on your shoulder, he can lift his head. The newborn's fists are clenched. If you pull your newborn into a sitting position by his arms, the newborn's head will loll forward or backward. By 1 month, the newborn's head will still roll forward or backward when not supported. If you pry his fingers open, the month-old baby can grasp the handle of a rattle but will drop it immediately. Your newborn baby can hear and distinguish volume. He can also see and can focus on and follow objects approximately 8 to 12 in. in front of his face.

For the first weeks of life, your newborn may sleep from 14 to 18 hours in a 24-hour period. When putting your baby down to sleep, always place him on his back, not on his side and especially not on his stomach (see Sudden Infant Death Syndrome, page 190).

Newborns tend to be alert for about 30 minutes every 4-hour period. The newborn may sleep seven or eight times during the day and evening. After about 1 month, most babies taper off to three or four naps a day and a nighttime block of sleep of about 5 or 6 hours. As most new parents know, however, the sleeping patterns of newborns are highly variable and hardly ever convenient. As your baby grows older, sleeping through the night becomes a possibility for both your baby and you.

Early Concerns

This section covers some common conditions that occur in healthy newborns. These conditions may be apparent at birth or may develop in the days following birth when you and your baby may be still in the hospital or already at home.

BIRTHMARKS

Birthmarks are very common and may appear at birth or soon after birth. Some birthmarks may grow before they fade. There are many kinds of birthmarks. Most are harmless and require no treatment. The following is a list of the most common ones.

Strawberry hemangioma This is strawberry red in color, soft, and raised. It may be as small as your baby's fingernail or as large as an adult hand. (See page C-33.) Hemangiomas are benign tumors comprised of blood vessels. They may appear anywhere on the body, though strawberry hemangiomas are found most often on the face, back, chest, or scalp. They usually appear during the first 2 months of life and are more common in girls. Strawberry hemangiomas tend to grow rapidly for 1 to 3 months. They stop growing between 6 and 12 months and usually begin to go away after a child's first birthday, fading to a pearly gray and eventually disappearing in most cases. They can remain at a fixed size for a period of months or years, however. Approximately 50 percent of these birthmarks disappear before the child is 5 years old, 70 percent by 7 years, and 90 percent before the child is 9 years old. Unless rare complications develop, treatment is generally not recommended, because it can lead to scarring. As difficult as it may be to adhere to watchful waiting, in most cases it is the best choice for your child, unless the birthmark interferes with a function, such as vision.

Sometimes a hemangioma develops deeper in the skin as a spongy lump with normal-colored or purplish overlying skin. The natural history of these hemangiomas is similar to strawberry marks. Watchful waiting is also the best treatment in most cases.

Port-wine stain, or nevus flammeus This purple-red birthmark may appear anywhere on the body. About half of these birth-marks appear on the face. They are red or purple marks composed of blood capillaries. Although the size varies, most are small. In rare cases, port-wine stains cover up to half of the body. A port-wine stain is composed of mature, dilated blood vessels and is present at birth. This birthmark is considered permanent. For the last 10 years, yellow lasers have been used safely and effectively to treat port-wine stains. Because the risk of scarring is negligible and younger children have a better response, treatment should begin as early in infancy as possible. (See page C-33.)

Salmon patches, or nevus simplex These may also be referred to as stork's bites. They appear as salmon-colored patches, particularly on the neck, eyelids, forehead, and around the mouth and nose. Salmon patches appear on 50 to 70 percent of healthy newborns. During the first 2 years of life, they begin to fade, and in most cases they are hidden by normal hair and skin pigment. Thus, they cause less concern than other birthmarks.

Mongolian spots Occurring most often on black infants, mongolian spots are second to salmon patches as a cause of birthmarks. They are blue to blue-black in appearance and occur most frequently on the back and buttocks, although they may be found anywhere on the body. Mongolian spots usually disappear with age, although some remain into adulthood.

Milia These look just like whiteheads and may be present on a newborn's face at birth or appear in the first few months of life. These miniature cysts disappear without treatment, and you should refrain from trying to squeeze them or treat them in any other manner. (See page C-33.)

Purpura This is not a birthmark but rather a purple-colored rash caused by blood vessel hemorrhage. It may appear on the skin or inside the mouth. Purpuric lesions may be associated with a number of infections and disorders or can even be the result of a trauma to the skin. The underlying cause of the discoloration may be serious, and you should contact your doctor immediately to rule out the possibility of a disease such as meningitis, which requires emergency treatment.

CAPUT SUCCEDANEUM

Caput succedaneum is the swelling of the scalp tissue that sometimes occurs at birth as powerful muscles push the baby through the relatively narrow opening at the end of the uterus. After a few days, this soft swelling disappears and the baby's head appears normal. Caput succedaneum can sometimes be difficult to distinguish from cephalohematoma (see page 186). If the baby's face led the way through the birth canal, it may be swollen.

CRADLE CAP

Cradle cap, or seborrheic dermatitis, is a common skin condition that may occur at any age. However, it is most common in newborns and often lasts through the first several months of life. It is characterized by dry, scaly skin that may appear in patches or all over the scalp, and it may extend down the forehead to the eyebrows and ears. Skin creases under the arms, neck, and diaper area may be affected. These patches may be crusty and yellowish and can give the scalp the appearance of being dirty, but cradle cap is not a result of poor hygiene. The cause of cradle cap is not fully understood, but it may be related to the baby's hormones or a yeast that commonly inhabits the scalp and skin. (See page C-32.)

Caput succedaneum. The baby's scalp tissue sometimes swells as the baby travels through the birth canal during delivery. The swelling generally disappears after a few days.

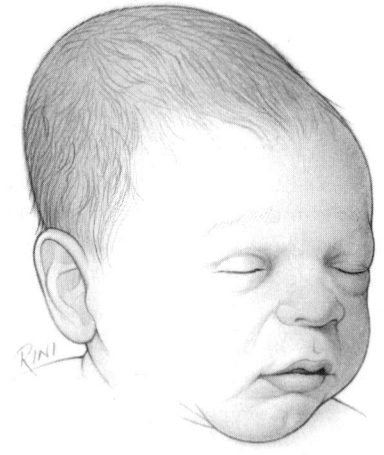

CIRCUMCISION

Circumcision refers to cutting away the foreskin that covers the glans (tip) of the penis. Circumcision has been practiced as a religious or cultural rite in the Jewish, Moslem, and other faiths and among African tribes for thousands of years. It became a common procedure in the United States early in this century, because it was believed that it made cleanliness easier and helped prevent penile infection and cancer. Many doctors today believe there is no medical reason to perform circumcision. Rather, the decision is one to be made by the parents for religious, cultural, or personal reasons. Because there is disagreement about the medical reasons for circumcision, you may want to discuss circumcision with your doctor before making your decision.

Although circumcision can be performed at any time, the procedure is usually done soon after birth. Doctors have believed that for newborns the pain is not severe and lasts for a short time only; but more and more hospitals are appropriately using local anesthesia for the procedure. When the circumcision is performed in a hospital by a doctor or by an experienced religious person, the chances of complications, such as infection or hemorrhage are minimal, although there rarely may be damage to the penis severe enough to require corrective surgery.

It takes about 10 days to 2 weeks for a circumcision to heal. In the days following your baby's circumcision, diapers should be changed frequently to protect the penis from infection. Cover the exposed raw glans with petroleum jelly at each diaper change for at least 3 days following circumcision. The penis should be

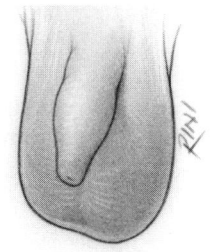

Uncircumcised penis

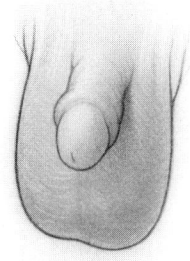

Circumcised penis

In a circumcision procedure, which usually occurs soon after birth, the foreskin covering the tip of a boy's penis is cut away. Although the procedure is frequently performed, whether it is medically desirable is not clear. Local anesthesia can be used to minimize pain.

washed with soap and water daily. Superficial bleeding and redness are normal, but if you notice anything unusual about your baby's penis—swelling, a foul smell, severe redness, or discharge—you should call your doctor immediately.

If you choose not to have your baby circumcised, you should be particularly attentive to hygiene. Be certain to clean only what you can see. Do not retract the foreskin at any time. It usually takes about 3 or 4 years for the foreskin to be easily retractable. Never force it. ■

Cradle cap generally disappears without treatment within the first few months of life. Your doctor may recommend washing the scalp daily with an antiseborrheic shampoo. You may want to massage the dry patches with oil and also scrub them gently with a soft toothbrush. Do not scrub too hard or too frequently; you will only irritate your baby's skin.

EPSTEIN'S PEARLS

If you see little white bumps on your baby's gums and are concerned your baby may be sprouting teeth too early, you can probably relax. In most cases, these bumps are only tiny, keratin-filled cysts, called Epstein's pearls. Some babies develop tiny, yellowish patches on the roof of the mouth. These cysts or patches are common and harmless and will disappear on their own without medical treatment. Epstein's pearls may be mistaken for natal teeth.

EARLY TEETH

Rarely, a baby is born with one or two primary (baby) teeth, called natal teeth, already in place, or sometimes primary teeth erupt within 30 days after birth and are called neonatal teeth. If natal teeth are extremely loose, they are sometimes removed to avoid the possibility of the newborn swallowing and choking on them; otherwise, they should be allowed to remain. If early teeth are removed to prevent choking, a dentist should see your baby for regular checkups. The permanent teeth will come in when your child is approximately 6 or 7 years old.

ERYTHEMA TOXICUM

Approximately 50 percent of babies born at term develop erythema toxicum 1 to 3 days after birth. This common rash appears less frequently among premature infants. The rash may appear on your baby's face, back, chest, or limbs. It is characterized by red, blotchy areas that may contain white centers or pimply areas or pustules. But perhaps what is most characteristic about erythema toxicum is its ephemeral nature; it can come and go within minutes. This rash is benign and disappears without treatment.

INNOCENT HEART MURMUR

Most parents react to the diagnosis of a heart murmur with fear. The heart is a most vital organ, and no parent wants to consider the possibility of a defect in how the heart works, particularly this early in life. If your doctor detects a heart murmur when your baby is in the hospital or in the first months after birth, it means the doctor has examined the heart and heard extra heart sounds. Usually, the doctor can tell if the sounds mean that there is a problem with the heart simply by the loudness, location, and type of sound.

Very few heart murmurs signal a heart abnormality, but some do. Your doctor may want to continue to listen to your baby's heart murmur over a period of time, have special tests done, or have you visit a pediatric cardiologist to decide whether or not medical and surgical treatment will be necessary (see Congenital Heart Defects, page 224).

Innocent, or functional, heart murmurs are frequently found in newborns and even in older children and do not indicate a congenital heart defect or other abnormality. Murmurs often disappear with time. If your baby has a functional heart murmur, no restrictions on activity are needed; his heart is perfectly normal.

JAUNDICE

Jaundice is one of the most common conditions in newborns and in most cases seems more serious to new parents than it actually turns out to be. Characterized by yellowing of the skin and whites of the eyes, jaundice is a condition that generally begins to appear on the second or third day of a baby's life and may last for a week or more. If your baby is premature, it may appear earlier and last longer. With mothers and babies now being discharged so soon after birth, jaundice may not become apparent until after discharge. You should contact your doctor if you notice signs of jaundice once you are at home with your baby.

Jaundice occurs when bilirubin is produced in newborns in greater quantities than their very immature livers can safely excrete. Bilirubin, which is yellowish in color, is produced when red blood cells are broken down and the oxygen-carrying pigment, called hemoglobin, is freed. When more bilirubin is produced than can be processed by the newborn's immature liver and eliminated, bilirubin levels in the blood increase, causing the yellowish or jaundiced appearance of the skin. This is called physiologic jaundice and at usual levels is common and not dangerous.

If physiologic jaundice is diagnosed in your newborn before you and your baby leave the hospital, in rare cases, your doctor may want to keep your baby in the hospital for observation. It is more likely that your doctor will have you return the next day for another test. Your baby's bilirubin level will be checked periodically through blood tests and will usually diminish over a day or two. Usually, physiologic jaundice requires no further treatment. Severe cases are treated with phototherapy. Phototherapy is conducted with a lamp called a bili-light or with a bili-blanket. Your baby is naked during the treatment so as much skin as possible is exposed to the light. His eyes are covered to protect them from the ultraviolet rays, and extra feedings may be encouraged because of the excess water loss that can occur through the skin.

In rare cases, bilirubin levels are too high or jaundice develops too quickly or too late to be physiologic. In these situations, special blood tests will be done to determine the cause, which may be infection, congenital liver or blood problems or related to breast-feeding. Knowing the cause will help your baby's doctor determine how to handle the condition.

THRUSH

Sometime during the first few weeks of life, you may notice a fuzzy, white coating on your newborn's tongue or inside of his cheeks. If you brush away the coating, the skin below may appear red or raw. These are symptoms of thrush (oral candidiasis). Thrush is a yeast infection a healthy newborn can contract during or after the birth process. If you think your baby may have thrush, you should let your doctor know. An antifungal agent, nystatin, will be prescribed to put in your baby's mouth. Thrush can be irritating and interfere with your baby's feedings, but it is not serious in a baby with a normal immune system. (See page C-40.)

UMBILICAL HERNIA

Normally, the opening in the abdominal wall where blood vessels extend into the umbilical cord during pregnancy closes completely after birth. When it does not, the navel (or belly button) may look huge, and a loop of the infant's intestine may protrude into it at times. This is called an umbilical hernia. Umbilical hernias are more common in black babies than white babies, and they usually disappear without intervention. Small openings will close, and the protrusion will disappear within the first months of life. Larger openings may take several years to resolve.

In the past, belly bands and other manners of binding the abdomen were recommended. These methods of treatment are not only ineffectual and outmoded, they

may also irritate your baby's skin, an additional problem a new parent doesn't need.

The surgical procedure to correct umbilical hernias is not complicated, but, because umbilical hernias almost always resolve themselves, many doctors recommend postponing consideration of surgical correction until your child is at least 6 or 7 years old. An umbilical hernia becomes an emergency only if the intestine gets stuck in it, which happens rarely. Get medical attention if

- The lump suddenly becomes much larger.
- The lump that protrudes when the baby is crying does not get soft when crying stops.
- The lump cannot be pushed in and remains hard to the touch.
- The lump or the area around the lump is tender, red, or sore.
- *Or* your baby is vomiting continuously.

Umbilical hernias should not be confused with a navel that protrudes before the stump of the cord drops off or a normal-sized navel that extends outward after the cord drops off, commonly known as an "outie."

Special Concerns

Most babies are born within 2 weeks of the projected due date after a normal pregnancy, labor, and delivery. Some healthy

If the abdominal wall does not close completely after birth, the navel may protrude. This protrusion is called an umbilical hernia. These hernias usually disappear after months to years without complications or intervention. Surgery may be necessary if a large hernia persists or complications develop.

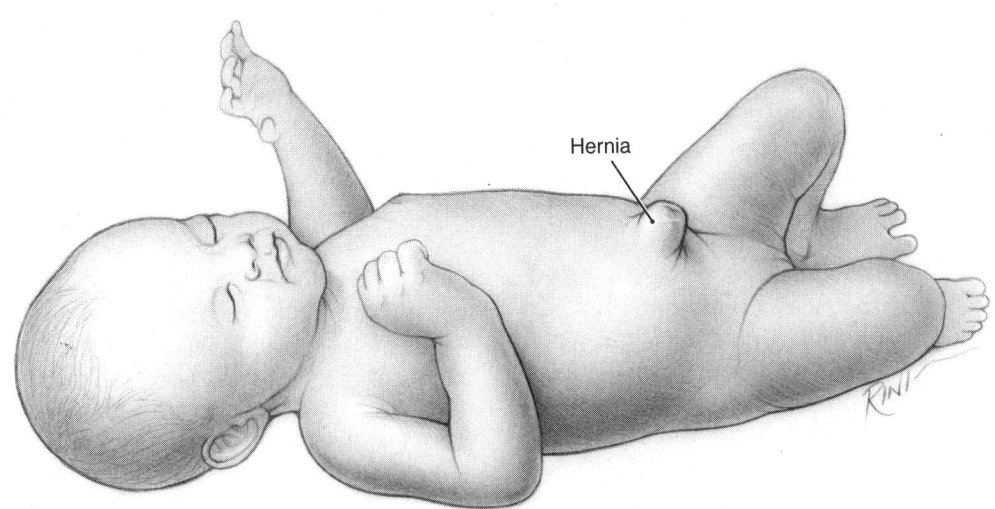

Hernia

babies, however, face early challenges for a variety of reasons, including a difficult birth process, premature birth, and low birth weight. Some of the problems these babies may face are covered in this section.

A DIFFICULT BIRTH

In most cases, childbirth is painful, but the labor and delivery are normal. However, between 6 and 8 of each 1,000 newborns suffer an injury during the birth process. These injuries almost always occur despite the best obstetric care and may occur because the uterus is a powerful muscle pushing the baby through a tight space. There is a lot of pressure on the baby. Conditions that raise the small risk of birth injury include breech birth, an abnormally large fetus, a difficult or prolonged labor, a rapid delivery, or a small pelvis. The use of forceps may sometimes cause a birth injury (see Procedures You May Encounter During Labor and Delivery, page 166). The most common birth injuries follow.

Lacerations Sometimes during a cesarean delivery, the baby's skin may be cut with the scalpel as it enters the uterus. These lacerations are most common on the baby's scalp, buttocks, or thighs and are usually minor. They are treated with bandaging or stitches and usually heal well.

Cephalohematoma Cephalohematoma occurs when, due to the pressure of labor, blood collects under the outside covering of the skull bone, creating a firm swelling. A minor skull fracture sometimes occurs along with this swelling. Cephalohematoma may be related to a forceps- or vacuum-assisted delivery, and treatment is rarely necessary. The blood usually disappears within 2 weeks to 3 months. The presence of a cephalohematoma may put the infant at risk for elevated bilirubin levels (see Jaundice, page 184).

Brachial plexus injury Stretching of the nerves of the neck can lead to brachial plexus injury. This is most common when the baby's shoulder is caught behind the pubic bone during delivery (shoulder dystocia). Brachial plexus injury can involve the nerves leading to the upper arm, the lower arm, or both. Most cases resolve with time, but occasionally there is permanent weakness. Treatment of brachial plexus injury involves physical therapy of the involved arm.

Facial nerve palsy When there is pressure on the facial nerve as the infant descends through the pelvis, facial nerve palsy may result. It may also be caused by pressure from a forceps delivery. Facial nerve palsy is a form of paralysis that may affect the entire injured side of your baby's face. The eye on the injured side may not close completely, and the corner of the mouth may droop. Recovery from this injury depends on how badly the nerve is damaged. Recovery is often rapid and complete.

Fractured collar bone Injury to the collar bone, or clavicle, is the most common bone injury during birth, though it often goes unrecognized initially. If the collar bone has been fractured, your baby may be unable to move the arm on the injured side. Your baby may also cry when moved. Some fractures need no treatment except gentle care when handling the baby. With more serious fractures, the arm and shoulder may need to be immobilized for the baby's comfort and to aid healing. The collar bone will heal in 7 to 10 days.

PREMATURITY AND ITS CHALLENGES

Babies born at an estimated gestational age of less than 37 weeks are considered premature; every year, over 200,000 babies are born prematurely in the United States. Many premature babies are also low-birth-weight babies, that is, babies who weigh less than 2,500 g (5 lb, 8 oz). Some premature babies are only a little shy of the 2,500 g mark and are able to catch up quickly and go home from the hospital only a few days later. Others, however, may be so small at birth that they fit in the palm of an adult hand. These babies require months of intensive medical treatment before they can be allowed to go home. Some small babies are not premature; they just did not grow well in the uterus. They are called small for gestational age (SGA). Some premature babies are also SGA. Some special concerns of prematurity do not apply to full-term babies who are SGA, whose organs may be mature. On the other hand, the cause of the poor growth

COMMON HEALTH PROBLEMS IN LOW-BIRTH-WEIGHT BABIES

Low-birth-weight babies weigh less than 2,500 g (5 lb, 8 oz). Low-birth-weight babies are usually but not always the result of premature birth. Premature babies are born at an estimated gestational age of less than 37 weeks. Common problems of low-birth-weight babies include the following:

Jaundice

Low-birth-weight babies develop jaundice more frequently than do full-term babies (see Jaundice, page 184).

Necrotizing Enterocolitis This bowel disease involves damage to the intestinal tissue. It is the most common gastrointestinal emergency in infants and is usually diagnosed within the first 20 days of life. The symptoms include vomiting, blood in the stool, and a swollen belly, as well as lethargy and respiratory failure. A baby suffering from this bowel disease will usually be put on intravenous feedings and antibiotic therapy. Further treatment, including surgery, will depend on the severity of the symptoms and the progress of the disease.

Apnea Apnea refers to periods when breathing ceases. Though any newborn may have short periods of apnea, premature and low-birth-weight babies are more likely to experience periods of breathing cessation. Apnea of prematurity is diagnosed if a newborn experiences periods of breathing cessation longer than 15 seconds in duration. When breathing ceases for a prolonged period, it is associated with bradycardia, a slow heart rate. If apnea has been observed in your baby, further testing will be done to determine whether or not your baby's breathing should be monitored with a machine.

Bronchopulmonary Dysplasia Bronchopulmonary Dysplasia (BPD) is a form of chronic lung disease particularly common in low-birth-weight babies. This condition is a result of immature lungs, the treatments (oxygen and mechanical ventilation) needed to sustain breathing and gas exchange, and other, unknown factors. Babies with BPD gain weight slowly and may also be subject to apnea of prematurity. Precautions must be taken to prevent respiratory infection, which can lead to respiratory failure. Some babies with BPD still require oxygen or medication when they are sent home from the hospital. In most cases, the condition is outgrown as the lungs reach full maturity.

Hypoglycemia The consequences of hypoglycemia, or low blood sugar, can be severe in low-birth-weight infants. If left untreated, hypoglycemia can cause seizures, brain damage, or both. Fortunately, hypoglycemia is screened routinely during the first 24 to 48 hours of life and longer in sick newborns.

Retinopathy of Prematurity Retinopathy of prematurity (ROP), also formerly referred to as retrolental fibroplasia, is an eye disorder seen in premature infants. Of the 40,000 premature infants born in the United States each year, only about 5 percent develop ROP. Many factors contribute to ROP, but the most important factor is immaturity. The smaller the baby, the higher the risk. ROP afflicts four of five babies weighing less than 750 g (about 1 lb, 10 oz) at birth; only 3 in 100 babies weighing 1,500 to 1,750 g (3 lb, 5 oz to 3 lb, 14 oz); and is rare in infants weighing over 2,000 g. ROP can lead to scarring and/or distortion of the retina, an increased risk of myopia or nearsightedness, amblyopia, or wandering eye, and blindness. A baby with ROP is treated by a pediatric ophthalmologist. Laser surgery may be performed to destroy excess growth of blood vessels in the eye in an attempt to avert blindness (see Blindness or Visual Loss, page 218, for more information.)

Intraventricular Hemorrhage The germinal matrix (an area in the developing brain from which nerve cells migrate to the cortex), filled with veins, arteries, and capillaries, is present in the immature brain of a fetus but disappears at about the 38th week of pregnancy. Premature babies are at increased risk for brain hemorrhage because of the fragility of this network of vessels. A minority of preterm infants suffer intraventricular hemorrhage during the first 72 hours of life. Babies who suffer severe hemorrhages are at greater risk for hydrocephalus and neurodevelopmental disabilities including cerebral palsy, mental retardation, and learning disabilities.

Patent Ductus Arteriosus The patent (open) ductus arteriosus (a fetal blood vessel near the heart) is a normal and essential structure in the fetus. Just after birth, however, the ductus arteriosus is supposed to close. In 15 to 35 percent of very low-birth-weight babies, this duct does not close quickly enough on its own. In most cases, there are no symptoms except sometimes shortness of breath, but if untreated, persistent patent ductus arteriosus can lead to heart failure. Treatment with indomethacin, an antiprostaglandin drug, is generally successful in closing the duct. In certain cases, surgery may be necessary. (See Patent Ductus Arteriosus, page 225, for more information.) ∎

before birth may have important implications after birth as well.

If you are the parent of a premature baby, the most important thing to remember is that prematurity is a temporary condition. Focusing on doing all you can to help your baby grow and thrive can help you through this difficult time. When a preterm infant is born, many parents are struck by the fragility of their infant. Preterm infants look thin and may be covered with a fine layer of hair, called lanugo. Their ears may seem odd because the cartilage that gives them shape has yet to develop. Sexual organs may not be fully developed. The cries of preterm infants may sound weaker than the lusty cries of full-term babies. Premature babies are easily stressed by cold temperatures. Fortunately, in recent years, tremendous strides have been made in caring for babies born prematurely. And in many cases, when your premature baby reaches 40 weeks, the gestational age at which he should have been born, except for a relatively long and narrow head, your baby will look very much like other infants. In many cases, his development will catch up with his age in the first year or two of life.

THE NEONATAL INTENSIVE CARE UNIT

If your baby is born prematurely, he will probably spend the first few days, weeks, or even months after birth in the neonatal intensive care unit (NICU) or the intermediate care nursery. The NICU is a highly technical environment that can seem frightening and intimidating at first. The babies are on special warming tables or in isolettes—a see-through, fully enclosed bassinet formerly called an incubator—to help them maintain body temperature. You should be prepared to see a number of tubes and wires connecting tiny infants to intravenous (IV) bottles, machines monitoring heart and respiratory rate, and ventilators, which deliver oxygen and help the babies breathe. Most of this equipment makes noises from time to time, signaling the nurses to check it or the baby. Even though your baby's first "home" is very unlike your family's home, you can become involved in the care of your baby almost from the beginning. Spending time with your baby, and touching him and talking to him, holding and feeding him when he is ready, and talking with the doctors and nurses caring for your child will help ease your fear and will be beneficial to your baby as well.

Family-centered care is endorsed by NICUs, and a variety of support systems are available to parents. Although rooming-in with your baby (sleeping at your baby's bedside) is not possible in the NICU environment, most permit 24-hour-a-day visitation by parents and grandparents. Breast-feeding is encouraged, and lactation specialists are available to mothers. Pumping your breasts to keep up your milk supply and to provide your baby with breast milk until he can nurse is something that only a mother can do. Most NICUs have social workers or case managers available to each family to assist with insurance issues, transportation and lodging needs, and referral to community resources for premature babies.

Your baby will probably have a primary nurse who is involved in coordinating care and can be an invaluable resource to you. Along with the pediatricians, your primary nurse will keep you up-to-date about your baby's progress and will let you know what to expect next. The primary nurse can also offer suggestions about how to personalize your child's care and can recommend developmentally appropriate stimulation and infant comfort measures. As your baby progresses, your primary nurse can help you become more comfortable with the daily care of your infant including feeding, burping, bathing, and changing diapers.

As your baby gets stronger, he will probably be transferred to an intermediate care nursery or step-down unit. This occurs when your baby still needs to be in the hospital but no longer requires intensive care. You can look at this as your baby's first graduation. This is also a sign that your baby is nearing hospital discharge, and so it becomes important to have everything ready at home. The hospital nursing staff may provide a series of parent classes on well-baby care, infant car seat use, and infant cardiopulmonary resuscitation. Any special needs your child may have will be reviewed with you before discharge, and the nursery staff will make sure that you have the appropriate equipment and/or medication that your baby will need.

Identifying a primary care doctor to care for your baby after hospital discharge is a key component of the transition from hospital to home. Choosing a doctor, if you do not already have one, should be done as early in the hospitalization as possible. This will give the NICU doctors the opportunity to keep your doctor informed about your baby's progress before discharge.

Premature birth and hospitalization of an infant are always stressful for families, and a prolonged NICU hospitalization will have ups and downs. Parents commonly have feelings of guilt, secretly blaming themselves for their baby's problems, or feelings of loss over the perfect or more "normal" baby they imagined. They may feel inept around the experienced NICU nurses and powerless in the hospital environment. Seek out parent groups to share your feelings, and take advantage of the support of the hospital staff and members of your community.

RESPIRATORY DISTRESS SYNDROME

Low-birth-weight babies and babies who are born preterm sometimes suffer from what is known as respiratory distress syndrome (RDS) because their lungs are not fully developed or do not function well enough for them to get enough oxygen into and carbon dioxide out of the blood.

RDS, also called hyaline membrane disease, is a major cause of death for premature newborns. The more premature the baby, the more likely is RDS and the more severe it may be. RDS is rare in full-term infants. A newborn with RDS has inadequate amounts of certain lipoproteins, called surfactants, that help prevent the collapse of the small air sacs in the lungs when the newborn breathes. Recently, tremendous progress has been made in the prevention and treatment of RDS by blowing artificial surfactant into the lungs of premature newborns to provide the missing agent until they become mature enough to make it themselves. RDS generally improves after 5 to 7 days. However, residual damage to immature lungs can cause chronic lung disease.

RDS is usually recognized soon after birth because a baby with RDS has trouble breathing. Blood tests and an x-ray of the lungs are used to confirm the diagnosis. The level of intervention is determined by the severity of the respiratory distress. Most babies with RDS need extra oxygen. Sometimes the baby is assisted with a technique called continuous positive airway pressure (CPAP), which blows oxygenated air into the baby's nose under pressure to help open the air sacs in the lung. Sometimes a ventilator is needed to breathe for the baby completely for a while. Because the premature baby's lungs are delicate and may be injured by the oxygen and the pressure from the ventilator, the goal is to provide adequate support as gently as possible. The baby is likely to be fed intravenously or through a feeding tube to the stomach until his breathing improves.

PNEUMOTHORAX

Pneumothorax occurs when small ruptures in the air sacs of a newborn's lungs allow air to escape into the space between pleurae, the delicate membranes that enclose the

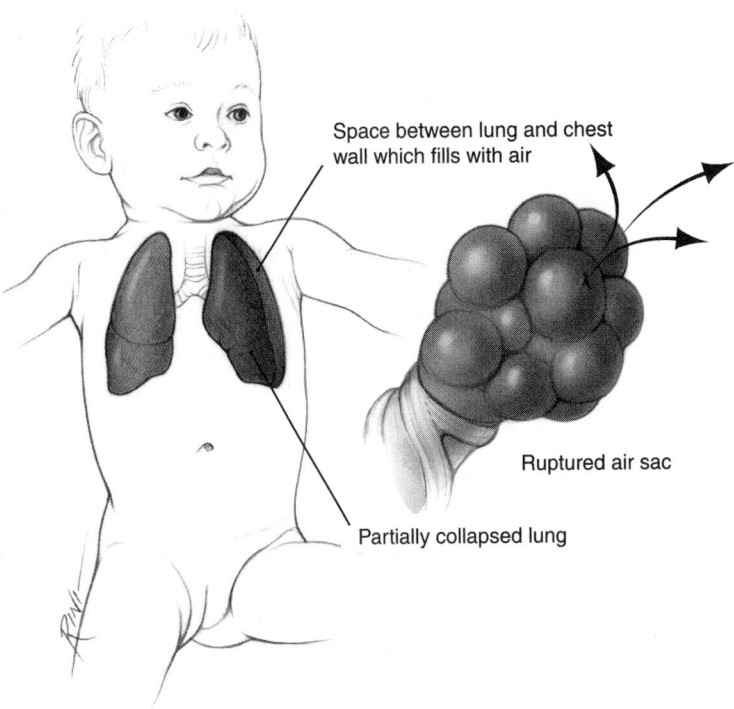

Space between lung and chest wall which fills with air

Ruptured air sac

Partially collapsed lung

Pneumothorax. If air sacs in a lung rupture, air can leak from inside the lung to the space between the lung and the chest wall, causing the lung to collapse partially. This can lead to sudden shortness of breath and sometimes requires a tube to be inserted through the chest wall to remove the air collection.

lungs and line the inside of the chest wall. This may result in the partial collapse of a lung. When a pneumothorax occurs in a newborn, it is usually in a baby with RDS (see above) whose breathing is being assisted. The pressure needed to push air into the baby's lungs may be forceful enough to rupture air sacs.

Pneumothorax can cause sudden deterioration in an infant with severe lung disease. An x-ray may be taken to confirm the diagnosis. If a significant amount of air has entered the pleural space, a tube will be inserted through the chest wall to drain out the misplaced air and allow the lung to reexpand.

TRANSIENT TACHYPNEA

Some full-term infants may suffer from transient tachypnea (also called retained fetal lung fluid): rapid shallow breathing that is believed to result from a delay in the reabsorption of fetal pulmonary fluid. This condition occurs more commonly in infants delivered by cesarean section, perhaps because the compression of the baby's chest during vaginal delivery assists in the clearing of fluid in the lungs. Some infants with transient tachypnea may need to breathe extra oxygen for a short time. Antibiotics may be given if a diagnosis of pneumonia cannot be ruled out. If the newborn is breathing too rapidly to be fed orally, intravenous feedings or feedings through a tube inserted through the nose or mouth into the stomach may be necessary. Most infants with transient tachypnea recover within 3 days with no ill effects.

SUDDEN INFANT DEATH SYNDROME

Sudden infant death syndrome (SIDS), also known as crib death, is the term used to name the sudden death, usually during sleep, of an otherwise healthy infant. All new parents worry about their newborn all the time, including when their baby is sleeping. Your baby may keep you up for nights on end crying, and then the one night he is sleeping peacefully, you may find yourself up every 15 minutes checking to make sure your baby is breathing. All new parents have heard about crib death and know that sometimes, and for no explicable reason, newborns do not wake up, which makes every parent worry even more when their baby is sleeping. The medical profession has not been able to adequately explain the causes of SIDS.

SIDS is the major cause of death for infants between the ages of 1 week and 1 year (most deaths from SIDS occur in the first 6 months), and SIDS is responsible for the deaths of over 5,000 babies in the United States every year. The chances of SIDS striking are between 1 and 2 in 1,000.

Recent research has indicated that there are two very important things that parents can do to help prevent SIDS. When you place your baby down to sleep, lay the baby on his back rather than on his stomach or side. Since this recommendation has been made to parents regularly by their pediatricians, the rate of SIDS has declined. The second most important risk factor and one that you can control is exposure to smoke. Infants exposed to cigarette smoke before or after birth have a greater risk of SIDS.

Also at higher risk for SIDS are low-birth-weight babies, premature babies, the babies of women who take illegal drugs, babies who have had a sibling who has died of SIDS, and babies who have stopped breathing and had to be revived. It should be noted that babies who are not in any of these categories may still die of SIDS.

When SIDS strikes The parent who goes to wake a baby up in the morning and finds the child has died is not only grief stricken but desperate to find a reason for this sudden death. Parents tend to blame themselves, thinking if they had only done something differently, this would not have happened. But in most cases, self-recrimination is unfounded. The cause or causes of SIDS are unknown. When infants are placed on their backs during sleep instead of their stomachs, the number of deaths related to SIDS falls dramatically. The most widely accepted theory suggests that SIDS results when infants sleeping on their stomachs are accidentally asphyxiated. This theory is corroborated by studies showing that certain types of bedding materials are associated with an increased rate of SIDS.

For more information about SIDS, call the national SIDS Alliance at (800) 221-SIDS, or visit The SIDS Network on the World Wide Web (http://sids-network.org).

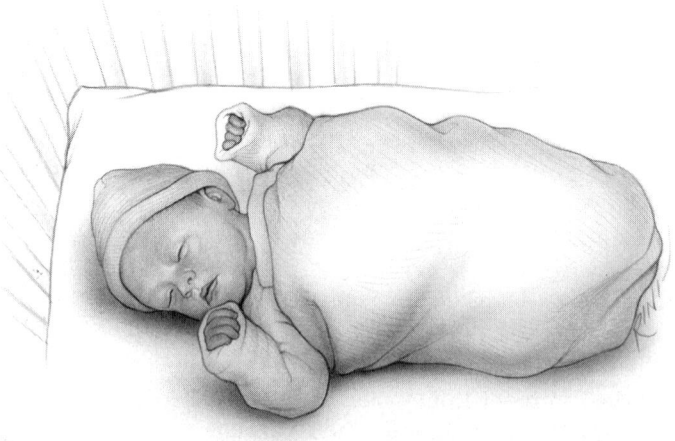

Recent research shows that babies who sleep on their backs have a lower risk of sudden infant death syndrome (SIDS) than babies who sleep in other positions.

Caring for Your Infant

The first months of your baby's life are likely to be both exciting and exhausting. The life of the entire family is changed by the addition of a new baby in the house. Your baby will make enormous strides in growth and development and require enormous amounts of energy and care from his parents. Be patient with yourself as a parent, with each other, and with your newborn as he adjusts to life outside the womb and begins to grow and develop quickly and in remarkable ways. Your most important responsibilities as parents are to keep your baby safe and well, and to love your baby, as you form a bond of attachment for life.

WELL-BABY CARE

For most new parents, your baby's doctor will be someone you turn to frequently—an invaluable source of information, advice, and reassurance. Your doctor will offer you experienced guidance through these early years, if you take advantage of this relationship. One of the greatest services doctors offer is well-baby care. Well-baby care consists of routine checkups and consultations that will help prepare you for the issues that will arise as your child grows and develops and will also help you prevent as many of the problems that parents face as possible.

Your doctor will go through these early years with your child and you, discussing everything from breast-feeding to teething to walking, solid food to ear infections, temper tantrums to learning how to read, watching with you as your baby grows from an infant into a toddler, starts school, and loses his first teeth, developing an enduring relationship with you and your child over time. At almost every visit, your doctor will counsel you about your child's growth and development, about keeping your child healthy, and about preventing injury (see Chapter 3 and Child Safety and the Home, page 199). In a matter of a few years, your doctor will be asking your child, "How do you like school?" and your child will be chatting with his doctor as with an old friend. Investing in a long-term, positive relationship with your child's doctor will be of great help to both you and your child in the long run.

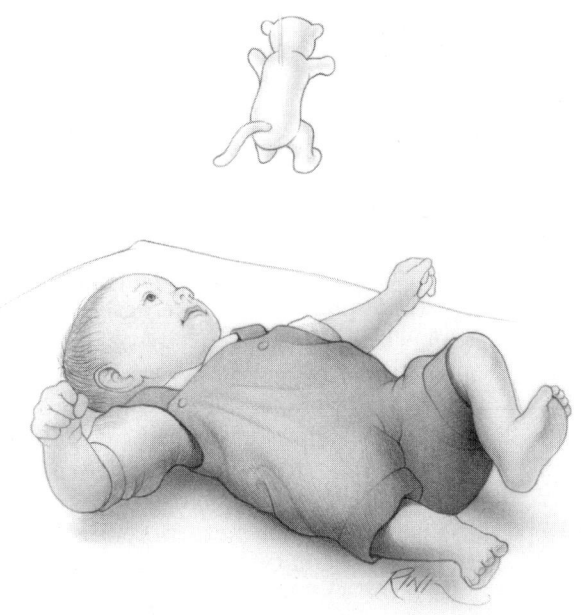

At age 1 month, most babies can focus on their parents' faces and respond to noises by startling or becoming quiet.

Your doctor will want to see your baby on a schedule roughly corresponding to guidelines recommended by the American Academy of Pediatrics, which advocates visits at age 2 to 4 weeks and then, if your baby is healthy and his growth and development are proceeding normally, at age 2, 4, 6, 9, and 12 months. Following is a description of some developmental milestones and what you can expect at these routine checkups (see also page 1583 for standard growth charts).

One month By the time your baby is 1 month old, he will probably be able to focus on your face and briefly lift his head when lying on his stomach. Your baby may also respond to a noise, such as a bell, by crying, startling, or suddenly becoming quiet. He may be able to follow your face moving about 8 in. away from his eyes. He may coo or vocalize in a different way, in addition to crying.

Before your baby's checkup, you will want to make a list of the things you have observed your baby doing and any questions or concerns you might have about your baby's health or development. Your written list will serve as a reminder during the visit of topics to discuss, as it is easy to forget questions when you are trying to manage your baby and consult with the doctor at the same time.

At this month's checkup, your doctor will measure your baby's weight and length and the size of his head. Your doctor will also have the results of the neonatal screening tests. If the doctor does not mention these tests, the results were probably normal, but ask anyway. If the tests were given before your baby was 72 hours old, your doctor will probably repeat them. In some states, testing is always done again. Your doctor will also perform a physical exam and talk to you about what to expect from the next month of life. Your baby may receive a second immunization against hepatitis B at this visit (the first was probably given in the hospital shortly after birth), or it may be deferred until the next visit (see Recommended Childhood Immunization Schedule, page 194, and Immunization, page 851).

Two months By the time your baby is 2 months old, he will be able to smile in response to your smile, coo or vocalize in other ways than crying, recognize your voice, and follow an object in an arc 8 in. in front of the eyes past the midline. Some babies can also lift their head and clear their chest when lying on the stomach, hold their head steady when upright, reach for an object, or hold a rattle.

At this month's checkup, your doctor will measure your baby's length, weight, and head size and perform a physical exam and a developmental assessment to evaluate vision, hearing, and head control. If your baby is in good health, your baby will also receive the appropriate immunizations (see Recommended

Childhood Immunization Schedule, page 194, and Immunization, page 851).

Subjects you will want to address with your doctor include what reactions you should expect to this month's immunization, any feeding or sleeping problems you think your baby may be having, the adjustment of your family to the new baby, what to expect developmentally in the coming months, and, if you are breast-feeding and have not talked about it before, whether or when your doctor recommends supplementing with vitamins, iron, or fluoride.

Four months Unless your doctor is concerned about a particular problem that your baby may have, your next regular well-baby checkup is usually not scheduled until the fourth month. Sometime during the fourth month, your baby will probably be able to prop up on his wrists while lying on his stomach. In addition, during the fourth month, most babies become able to roll over in one direction, grasp a rattle, begin to focus on very small objects and pay attention, or hold the head steady while upright. Some babies turn in the direction of a voice, and some use a vowel or consonant combination, such as "ah-gah." Your baby may also delight everyone in the family by laughing out loud.

Though every doctor will have a personal approach to well-baby care, using more or fewer assessment techniques depending on style, your baby's checkup at 4 months will generally involve much of what the earlier examinations involved, including measuring the baby's length, weight, and head size and a complete physical exam that will include rechecking any problems that may have been of concern earlier. Your doctor will also ask about eating and sleeping patterns and evaluate how your baby is growing and developing, be interested in any reactions to immunizations given at 2 months, and discuss injury prevention. Your baby probably will receive his next immunization doses at this checkup.

When you bring your list of questions to ask your doctor, you may want to include when to introduce your baby to solid foods, what reactions to anticipate to this round of immunizations, and what to do if your baby does experience a reaction to the shots.

Six months Between 6 and 7 months of age, your baby will be able to keep his head level with the body when placed in a sitting

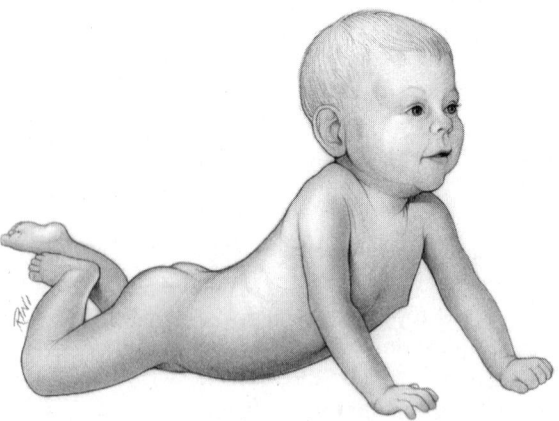

During the fourth month, most babies can hold their heads steady and use their wrists for support while lying on their stomachs.

position and to babble one or more vowel–consonant combinations, such as "baba" and "dada." Your baby will probably also be able to bear some weight on his legs when held in an upright position and to sit without support. He will transfer objects from one hand to another but not yet be firmly right- or left-handed. Some can feed themselves a cracker at this age, and some will express their displeasure if you take away a favorite object or toy. At this age, babies like to look at themselves in the mirror, are fascinated by details, and experiment with cause and effect (such as crumpling newspaper). Though seeing your baby learn to do something new is thrilling, if your baby is not rushing into all these new activities as quickly as you might wish, you need not worry. Every baby develops at a slightly different rate, doing some things sooner and some things later than other babies. However, if you have concerns, these should be discussed with your doctor.

At this checkup, your baby's length, weight, and head circumference will be measured and your baby's growth since birth will be charted. He will be given a physical exam, and his developmental progress will be assessed, including the ability to reach out and grasp objects. Hearing and vision will be checked. If your baby is healthy, another round of immunizations may be given. If your baby was a low-birth-weight baby, a hemoglobin or hematocrit test may be used to check for anemia. This test involves only a prick of the finger for a blood sample.

Questions you might want to ask your doctor this month will include what solid foods to introduce into the diet, whether your baby is ready to drink from a cup, and how you should handle any reactions to this round of immunizations.

Nine months Your baby should have quite a repertoire of physical feats at this point. Your baby not only can sit up and roll over but can crawl and come to a sitting position. Your 9- to 10-month-old may also be able to pull himself up to a standing position from sitting down; stand alone at least momentarily; and walk, holding on to a table, chair, or couch as he goes. Your baby may be able to pick up tiny objects, demand favorite toys or objects that have been taken away, or look for something that has been dropped and work hard to retrieve a toy or favorite object that is just out of reach. He

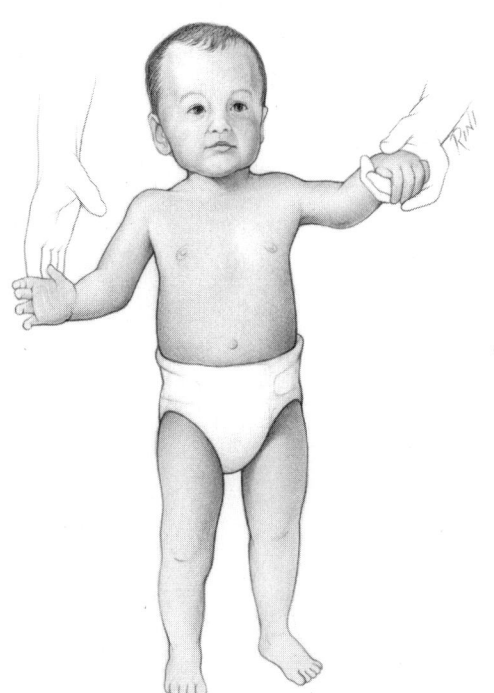

Many 9- or 10 month-old babies can pull themselves to standing positions, stand alone at least momentarily, and walk with assistance.

may be able to say "mama" and "dada" without actually addressing either parent, play peekaboo, and understand the word *no*.

At this checkup, your baby's length, weight, and head size will be measured as usual, and he will receive a physical exam. During the developmental assessment, your doctor may check to see what your baby does, but babies of this age may not respond well to strangers, and your doctor may simply ask you for a report on what your baby has been doing at home. The tuberculin skin test, which is used to indicate whether there has been a previous infection with the tuberculosis organisms, may be administered at this checkup, if you are in a high-risk area or situation. Your baby may also be checked for anemia, a common blood disorder in which hemoglobin is diminished and the red blood cell count is decreased, if he was a low-birth-weight baby.

On your list of questions, you may want to include: Are there any new foods you may introduce into your baby's diet? When should you wean your baby from the breast or the bottle, if you have not already done so? (See Weaning Your Baby, page 206.) Also, if you have any concerns about your baby's progress, particularly regarding hearing and vision, you should share them with your doctor.

RECOMMENDED CHILDHOOD IMMUNIZATION SCHEDULE

AGE	VACCINE
0–2 months	Hepatitis B
1–4 months	Hepatitis B
2 months	DTP (diphtheria-tetanus-pertussis)
	Hib (*Haemophilus influenzae* type B)
	Polio
4 months	DTP
	Hib
	Polio
6 months	DTP
	Hib
6–18 months	Hepatitis B
	Polio
12–15 months	Hib
	MMR (measles-mumps-rubella)
12–18 months	Varicella (chickenpox)
15–18 months	DTP
4–6 years	DTP
	Polio
	MMR
11–12 years	Hepatitis B[a]
	MMR[b]
	Varicella[c]
11–16 years	DT (diphtheria-tetanus booster shot; and then booster shot every 10 to 15 years)

[a] Children who did not have the hepatitis B series in infancy may begin the series at any time but should start or complete the series by the 11–12 year old visit. Unvaccinated older adolescents should be vaccinated whenever possible. The second dose should be administered at least 1 month after the first dose, and the third dose should be administered at least 4 months after the first dose and at least 2 months after the second dose.

[b] Children who have not completed the MMR series should do so by the 11–12 year old visit.

[c] Children who have not received the varicella vaccine or do not have a reliable history of chickenpox should be immunized during the 11–12 year old visit. Susceptible children 13 years of age and older should receive two doses, at least 1 month apart.

The Advisory Committee on Immunization Practices of the Public Health Service, the American Academy of Pediatrics, and the American Academy of Family Physicians have all agreed that all children should be immunized against the following diseases and have agreed upon this schedule, which results in good protection.

Hepatitis B Virus Three vaccine doses are given. The first is usually given shortly after birth before the baby leaves the hospital. The second is given between age 1 and 4 months. The third is given between age 6 and 18 months. Children who are not vaccinated in infancy should receive the series by age 11 or 12 (see table).

Diptheria, Tetanus, and Pertussis (Whooping Cough) These are always given together as one preparation. It usually contains a new acellular type of pertussis vaccine that causes fewer reactions than the old pertussis vaccine did. Five doses are needed in all. Doses are usually given at age 2, 4, and 6 months. A fourth dose is given at age 15 to 18 months. The fourth dose is sometimes given earlier, if 6 months have elapsed since dose number 3. A fifth dose is given at the time the child ▶

One year By the time your baby has his first birthday party, he may be taking a few steps while holding on to furniture. Some babies walk. But most babies will probably spend some of the time crawling at their first birthday party. Your year-old baby will probably be able to drink from a cup, play patty-cake, pick up a tiny object with thumb and forefinger, address mama and/or dada, and perhaps say one other word. Some 1-year-olds, however, may not say their first word until they are 14 or 15 months old. This may be perfectly normal. Some babies may have three or more words at their command, although this does not usually occur until babies are 13 to 16 months old.

After your baby's length, weight, and head size have been measured, your baby will receive another physical exam and developmental assessment. The chart of growth since birth will also be plotted. At this month's checkup, your doctor will note your baby's gross motor skills and, most likely, will inquire about his fine motor and language abilities. The more information

At age 1 year, most babies crawl and some babies are beginning to walk.

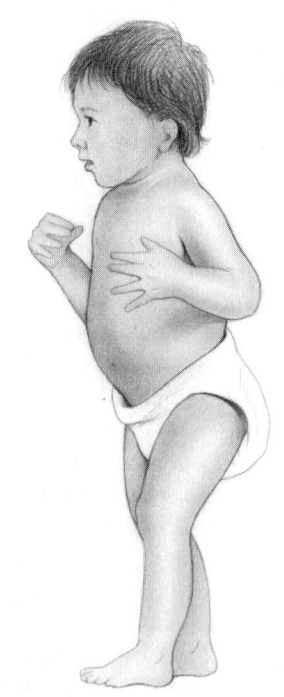

▶ starts school, that is, between age 4 and 6 years. A booster shot should be given to adolescents at age 14 or 16 and then every 10 to 15 years.

Haemophilus Influenzae Type B Four vaccine doses are given. The first three are given at age 2, 4, and 6 months. The fourth is given between age 12 and 15 months. With one currently available vaccine, the dose at 6 months can be omitted.

Polio Four doses are given. Two types of vaccine available, one an oral polio vaccine (OPV) consisting of weakened live virus and the other an inactivated virus given as an injection (IPV). Several different schedules are acceptable. One commonly used schedule requires 2 doses of IPV given at age 2 and 4 months, followed by 2 doses of OPV, one at age 12 to 18 months and one at age 4 to 6 years. Alternatively, a child may receive four doses of IPV by the same schedule of four doses of OPV with the third given between age 6 and 18 months. Children who have weak immune systems or who live in households with persons who are immunosuppressed or immunodeficient should receive IPV only.

Measles, Mumps, and Rubella These are almost always given together in one vaccine preparation that contains live, weakened viruses. Two doses are needed. The first is given at age 12 to 15 months. The second is given at age 4 to 6 years or alternatively at age 11 to 12 years.

Varicella (Chickenpox) One dose is given between age 12 and 18 months. For information on older children who have not been vaccinated see table on page 194.

Other Vaccines Some children, because of special health care problems, need additional vaccines. Most commonly given in special circumstances are vaccines against influenza virus and pneumococcal bacteria. If your child has a chronic illness, ask your doctor whether any additional vaccines are needed. If you plan to take your child to another country, be certain your child's immunizations are up to date and ask whether any other vaccines are recommended or required.

Combination Vaccines Manufacturers are now providing some vaccines in combination preparations so that two of the above vaccines can be given together when they are to be given at the same visit. This minimizes the number of injections. The child's immune system responds to each part just as it would if they were given separately.

Preparing for Immunization Ask your doctor for written information about the vaccines your child will receive. Ask any questions that you have. Although vaccines are not given when a child is seriously ill because the illness might prevent the child's immune system from responding well, colds and other common illnesses are not a reason to delay immunization. Your doctor will want to ask you a few simple questions before administering the vaccines. Take note of any reaction you think your baby has to immunization, and let your doctor know before the next dose is administered. If your baby seems quite ill after an immunization, call your doctor right away.

School Entry Many school systems require that a child be immunized against most or all of the above diseases before entering school. The reason is because high rates of immunization prevent the transmission of these diseases (all but tetanus are communicable) from one person to another. Several months before the first day of kindergarten, check with your doctor to be certain your child is up to date on immunizations.

Side Effects Immunizations sometimes cause fever, and they sometimes cause soreness at the site of injection. More serious side effects, although they do occur, are rare. The risks of serious illness or side effects form the diseases the vaccines prevent far outweigh any possible side effects from the vaccine for almost all children. If you feel your child has had a serious complication from an immunization, you or your doctor should report it to the Vaccine Adverse Event Reporting System. Ask your doctor about it. ■

you can give your doctor about your child, the more smoothly your checkups will proceed. Another set of immunizations will be given at this visit or the next.

Questions you will want to ask your doctor might include: What new foods should I add to my baby's diet? When should I wean him from the bottle or the breast (if you have not done so already)? You should also raise any concerns about behavior, sleeping, eating, hearing, or sight, as you should at every checkup.

Now that your baby is 1 year old, well-baby care checkups will not be as frequent, but this does not mean you should not consult your doctor when you feel there is an issue that concerns you, whether about sleeping, eating, teething, language, behavior, socialization, or any other aspect of your baby's health and development. By now your doctor is a friend and ally in getting your baby off to a good start. Never hesitate to include your doctor when you have questions, and certainly never hesitate to call if you have any concern about your baby's health.

WHEN TO CALL YOUR DOCTOR

All new parents face the dilemma of when to worry and when not to worry. In fact, disagreements between the parents of a newborn often begin over when to call the doctor: One parent's emergency may be the other parent's "let's wait and see." In the case of infants, it is better to be safe than sorry, but before you pick up the phone to call the doctor, be sure you have gathered the information the doctor may ask you about. The doctor is likely to ask you to describe the symptoms, so check your baby's temperature before you call. If your baby has a rash, respi-

WHEN TO CALL THE DOCTOR WITHOUT DELAY: EMERGENCY SYMPTOMS AND SIGNS OF SERIOUS ILLNESS

Seek emergency help if your infant exhibits any of the following:

- Difficulty breathing with
  Drooling
  Grunting
  Gasping
  Rapid breathing
  Troubled breathing

- Blue skin color

- Head injury with
  Loss of consciousness
  Vomiting
  Seizure
  Unequal pupils
  Sore or painful neck

- Burns
  Over a large area of the body
  On the hands, feet, or genitals

- Change in consciousness
  Will not wake up
  Seems disoriented
  Does not seem to recognize the mother

- Eye injury, especially if there is pain or loss of vision

- Rash made up of blood spots on the skin

- Fever greater than 100°F in a baby younger than age 3 months

- Signs of dehydration such as dry mouth, sunken eyes, and infrequent urination

- Unexpected seizures or convulsions

- Complaints of severe pain not responding to reassurance or simple medication

- Possibly broken bone

- If you are worried about your infant, and you think that something bad might be happening

- If you are worried that you might hurt your infant

- Cuts or lacerations that do not stop bleeding after you apply gentle pressure for a few minutes, or look like they need stitches, or are on the hands, face, or genitals

- If you think that your infant has swallowed some kind of poison or drug (you should call your local Poison Control Center first, if possible)

Call your doctor immediately if your infant has any of the following:

- High fever (103°F or higher) in a child who looks or acts sick

- Fever lasting a week or more

- Blood in the stool or urine

- Unexpected, persistent crying that you cannot explain

- Persistent diarrhea, especially if your infant is vomiting or not taking fluids by mouth

- A new limp ■

ratory symptoms, behavior differences, vomiting, or diarrhea, be prepared to describe these symptoms accurately. For more information on symptoms that demand immediate medical attention, see When to Call the Doctor Without Delay, above.

HOW TO HANDLE AN INFANT

Many new parents are afraid to hold their newborn for fear of hurting the baby. It is

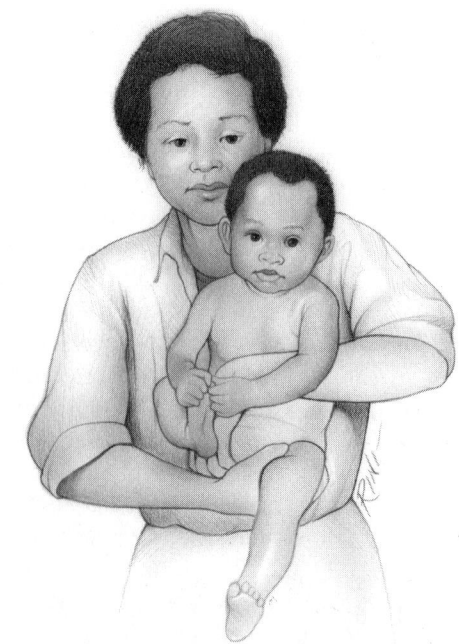

Many babies enjoy facing forward as they are carried. Support the buttocks with one hand while placing the other hand in front of the baby's chest. Transfer the baby slowly and carefully, without sudden movements.

CARING FOR THE UMBILICAL CORD

After the umbilical cord is cut, a remnant of the cord remains. This is referred to as the stump of the umbilical cord. A few days after birth, the stump turns dark and dry. This is normal and part of the process of healing.

Keeping the area dry and exposed to the air will prevent infection and help the healing process. To facilitate healing, you will want to fold your baby's diaper down below the umbilical cord. This will help prevent irritation. Avoid tub baths until the stump falls off. When sponge bathing your baby, you can wash the area with soap and water, but make sure to dry it afterward. Applying alcohol to the base of the stump using a sterile cotton ball, gauze pad, or swab will also help the drying process. If you notice any irritation or redness of the skin of the abdomen around the navel, or if you notice oozing from the stump, call your doctor. The umbilical cord stump generally falls off within 1 or 2 weeks but some take longer. ■

The stump of the umbilical cord turns dark and dry after birth and eventually falls off. During this healing process, fold down the top of the baby's diaper (A) and avoid tub baths until the stump falls off. Gentle washing with soap and water may be done, but the area should be dried carefully afterwards. (B) Apply rubbing alcohol with a cotton ball to aid drying.

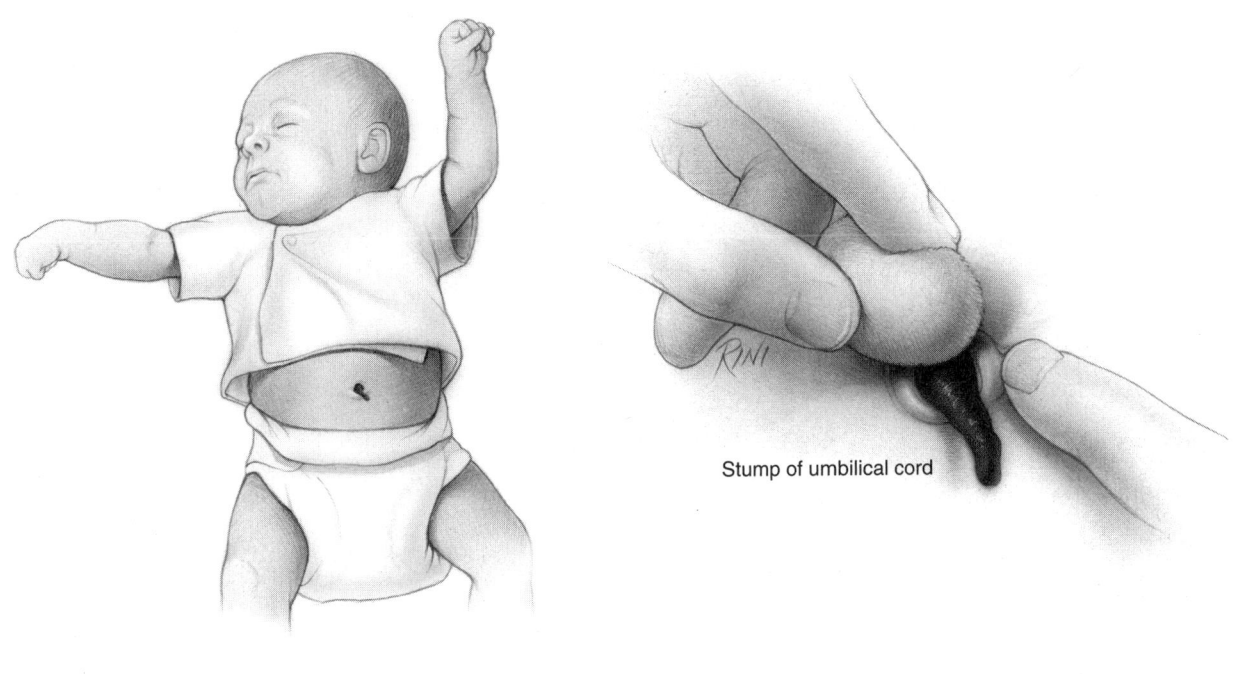

Stump of umbilical cord

comforting to remember that newborn babies are not as fragile as they appear and that they have many instinctual and adaptive behaviors to ensure their own survival. They cry when they are hungry, tired, or wet and if they feel pain. As long as you are careful to always support the head of your newborn, any normal handling of a healthy newborn will not harm the baby. In fact, your baby cannot be held too much. As you are getting to know your baby, your baby is getting to know you and to know the world through you. When you look at your baby, touch your baby, interact with your baby, talk to and hold your baby, you are not only loving your baby, but also aiding your baby's early development. He learns from watching you, hearing you, and being held by you. Holding your baby is an important part of the necessary bonding experience, so you should not neglect this aspect of healthy parenting because you are nervous about holding such a small baby. At this stage of life, holding your baby is what your baby needs most.

Before picking up your baby, make sure he is aware of your presence by making eye contact and talking to him. This will help you avoid startling your baby. When lifting your baby, keep your hands in place under the baby for a few moments before you lift him up. Lift the baby toward

THE FONTANELS

The fontanels are the soft spots on the top of your baby's head. The fontanels are the openings in your baby's skull where the bones of the skull have not yet grown together. Though often referred to as the soft spot, there are two fontanels.

The anterior fontanel is by far the larger of the two openings and is located directly on top of your baby's head. It may be as wide as 2 in. in diameter and may appear diamond or circular in shape. This fontanel is usually completely closed by the time the baby is 13 months old though it may close as early as 7 months. It is flat in appearance, though it sometimes bulges when some babies cry. You may be able to see the fontanel pulse, if your baby's hair is sparse.

The posterior fontanel is usually much smaller than the anterior. It is located toward the back of the head and usually feels triangular. In some babies, it is difficult to locate. The posterior fontanel usually closes completely by the time the baby is 3 months old.

If the anterior fontanel appears sunken, this may be a sign of dehydration. If this occurs even when your baby is lying down, and you doubt whether your baby is feeding well, you should notify your doctor. If the anterior fontanel bulges even when your baby is sitting up and not crying, you should also see your doctor immediately. This may be a sign of increased pressure inside your baby's head.

These fontanels are much sturdier than most nervous new parents think. They are covered by a tough membrane that protects the newborn brain from the occasional touching of older siblings or other children and from daily handling. ■

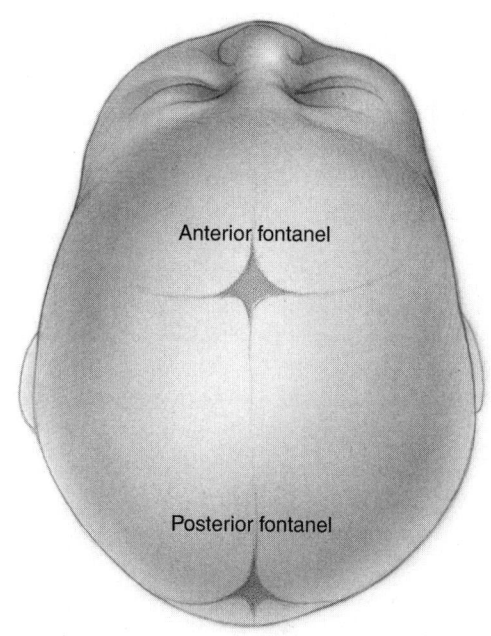

There are two soft spots on the head at birth where bones have not yet grown together. The front (anterior) fontanel is usually larger than the rear (posterior) one. The openings generally close by age 13 months. The anterior fontanel often bulges when a baby cries. A bulge at rest or a sunken appearance of the fontanel can indicate a problem that requires medical attention.

BATHING YOUR BABY

A daily bath is not necessary for a newborn, as long as you clean your baby well when changing the diaper and after feedings of formula or breast milk. A bath two to three times a week is usually adequate, until your baby starts crawling. After the umbilical stump has fallen off, bathing options include a sponge bath, a bath in a baby tub, or in the kitchen sink. When bathing your newborn, never leave your baby alone in the water and never let go of your baby. This is important even if you have your baby in a device that is especially designed for babies.

Before you bathe your baby, make sure you have all the equipment on hand that you need, including baby soap and shampoo, a clean washcloth, sterile cotton balls for swabbing the eyes, a clean towel, a fresh diaper, and a change of clothes. Make sure the room is warm. Be sure your hot water temperature has been turned down to 120°F or less, and use your wrist to test the water in the tub or sink before you begin. Do not remove your baby's diaper until you are ready to begin the bath. If you are bathing your baby in a baby tub, ease him in gently and slowly,

making sure not to startle your baby. If your baby resists the baby tub, return to giving sponge baths.

Wash the face first. Clean the eyes with a sterile cotton ball moistened with water, using a fresh cotton ball for each eye. Wipe the outside of the ears, but do not put anything into the ear. Dry the face. (If you are giving your baby a sponge bath, make sure you dry each area after washing.) Then wash the neck, being certain to get to the bottom of folds, and chest. Wash the arms, making sure to wash the elbow creases. Wash the legs, including the back of the knees.

Wash the diaper area last. Wash a girl's genital area from front to back. If you notice a white, vaginal discharge, do not try to scrub it away. Wash a boy's genitals gently, making sure to wash all the folds of skin. Do not retract the foreskin farther than it will easily go. Dry the diaper area well, apply ointment if needed, diaper and dress your baby.

Shampoo your baby's hair and scalp once or twice a week. On other days, you may want to rinse the scalp with water when you wash the face. ■

your body, cradling the buttocks in one hand and the head in the other. You may use your shoulder to support the baby's head with the baby facing toward you or place the baby against one hip, so the baby is facing sideways with his head against your chest. Babies also love to be carried facing forward, one hand around the baby's chest, the other supporting the buttocks. This allows your baby to look around at his new and exciting world. When putting your baby back down, bend over the bassinets, crib, or carriage to avoid a long transition period from your arms to the mattress. Hold the buttocks with one hand, and support the head, neck, and back with the other until the baby is lying down comfortably. Keep your hands on the baby for a few moments, until he has adjusted to this new position.

CHILD SAFETY AND THE HOME

Having spent 9 months worrying about your pregnancy, you will experience a momentary relief once you have given birth to a healthy baby, only to begin to worry just as much over keeping your baby well. All new parents worry about the safety of their baby, and this concern is justified, as injury is the leading cause of death in children in the United States. There are precautions you can take to help minimize injuries in the home when your baby is an infant.

Always strap your baby into a car safety seat when driving, no matter what the distance, beginning with the ride home from the hospital. Purchase a car seat that is correct for your child's size and that will fit properly into your car. Car seats must be attached securely to your vehicle using the car's seat/shoulder belt and following the seat manufacturer's directions. The back seat of the car is the safest location for the car seat as it is further away from head-on car accidents. Never place a rear-facing car seat in the front passenger seat if your car is equipped with a passenger side air bag. Air bags inflate with enough force to cause serious harm to a child in a rear-facing seat that is placed in the front passenger seat. Even forward-facing car seats, which are used for larger children, are best placed in the rear seat and away from the passenger side air bag. It is against the law to not use a car seat

with your infant and young child. For more information on car seats and car safety, see Chapter 30.

During pregnancy and the first year of your baby's life, you should be an educated consumer when shopping for equipment for the baby, such as a car seat, crib, and also toys (for detailed information on safety requirements in baby furniture and equipment, see Chapter 3). Many parents have been taken by surprise the first time the baby rolls over. So be sure to strap babies into changing tables and carriages even when they are small infants, and do not leave a baby unattended on a surface from which he might fall.

When putting your baby to sleep, lay him on his back. Do not place your baby on his stomach, which may increase the risk of SIDS (see page 190).

Do not smoke in your home or expose your infant to tobacco smoke. There is no way to prevent your infant from inhaling the smoke and the chemicals present in tobacco smoke if you smoke anywhere near your infant or in his surroundings. The child of a smoker is at higher risk of SIDS (see page 190) and more likely to develop ear infections, hearing problems, asthma, upper respiratory infections, and respiratory problems such as bronchitis and pneumonia. Tobacco smoke can make other medical conditions more severe. Later in life, the child of a smoker will be more likely to smoke himself and more likely to develop lung cancer, heart disease, and cataracts. Do everything that you can now to protect your infant from the very preventable consequences of smoking.

Whether or not you smoke, be certain to have a working smoke detector on every floor of your home. Make certain that your hot water temperature does not exceed 120°F; baby skin is easily burned.

Crying babies may be stressful for parents who may already be quite stressed, but it is important to remember that it is never safe to shake a baby. Shaking a baby can cause permanent brain damage or death. If you are feeling overwhelmed and fear you might mishandle your baby, lay the baby down somewhere safe, until you are feeling calmer. If necessary you can let the baby cry in a safe place. But you must never shake your baby.

It is best not to put your baby in a walker. Walkers are responsible for many serious injuries. Before your child starts crawling, you should be planning how to childproof your home for your baby. You will be doing much to secure your baby's health and well-being if you read and apply the detailed safety advice offered in Chapter 3.

NUTRITION

The nutritional needs of your newborn are simple, though time-consuming. While breast milk is the best food there is for most babies, most exclusively breast-fed infants receive supplementary vitamin D and may also receive iron and fluoride supplements as they grow. Your newborn will get all the nutrients he needs if you are breast-feeding and if your baby is feeding well and taking the appropriate supplements. Baby formula approximates breast milk as closely as possible. Formula-fed infants usually do not require supplements. In the first months of life, all the calories, protein, carbohydrates,

Most breast-feeding newborns eat every 2 to 3 hours. Several positions can be used to breastfeed a baby. (A) Mother and baby lying down. (B) Mother upright with baby in a "football hold." (C) Mother upright with baby across the chest.

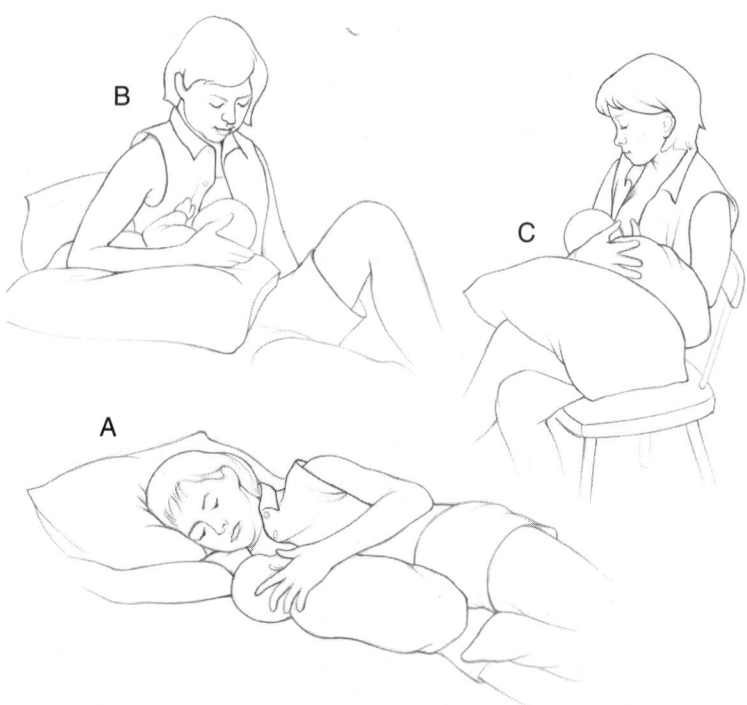

vitamins, and minerals, and liquids your baby needs are provided by breast milk (and supplements) or formula. An infant also needs water, but in most cases your baby will get as much water as is necessary from breast milk or formula. You need not give extra water unless your doctor specifically advises you to do so. If you are breast-feeding, your doctor will advise you to continue taking your prenatal vitamins.

New parents often worry that their babies are not getting enough to eat. Most newborns need to eat every 2 to 4 hours. Most breast-fed infants eat even more often than that in the first few days. As long as your baby is enjoying frequent feedings and gaining weight, your baby is probably getting enough to eat. Newborns usually gain about 2 lb a month during the first 3 months, and have doubled their birth weight by the fifth month of life.

If you are breast-feeding, you may begin to feel as if your baby nurses all day, and at least part of the time, this will be close to the truth. But within the first 3 months of life, your baby will begin to establish a routine to which you will be able to adjust, more or less. This routine usually begins with a feeding in the morning, a period when the baby is up, a nap, another feeding and wakeful period, another nap and another feeding and a final feeding before bed. Almost all newborns wake in the night from hunger and require a bottle or to be nursed. Usually, your baby will need to eat approximately six times a day. If after 6 months, your baby is not sleeping through the night, but instead still crying to be fed in the night, you may want to talk to your pediatrician about ways to wean him from middle-of-the-night feedings, which are no longer necessary, in order that you can get some much needed sleep. When these 3 or 4 AM feedings continue throughout the first year of life, the habit becomes hard to break.

Burping your baby Burping your baby during and after a feeding will help feedings go more efficiently. You can burp the baby when changing breasts or about half-way through a bottle, if your baby is formula fed. If your baby seems to want to stop eating before he usually does, you may also try burping him. Babies need to burp, because along with the breast milk or formula, they are swallowing air, which may make them feel uncomfortable or full before they really are full or may cause them to spit up.

Some babies require only a gentle pat on the back to help them burp, but generally babies require a little more help. You can burp your baby while holding the baby on your shoulder, seated in your lap, or with the baby lying stomach down across your lap. Before burping your baby, place a towel or cloth diaper on your shoulder or lap in case the baby spits up. When burping the baby on your shoulder, hold the buttocks with one hand with the baby's head resting on your shoulder and pat or rub the back gently with the other hand. With your baby seated on your lap, lean the baby forward while you support the chest with one hand and pat the back gently with the other hand. To burp your baby while the baby is lying in your lap, prop the stomach on one knee and the head on the other, holding the baby securely on the buttocks while you gently pat the back.

CRYING: WHAT IS NORMAL AND WHAT IS EXCESSIVE

Crying is your baby's primary tool of communication. Most babies cry when they are hungry and some when they are tired or wet. They may also cry when they are having a bowel movement, and they cry when they are in pain. Babies may also cry just to be held. Sometimes babies cry for no readily identifiable reason, and this can be both frustrating and frightening for new parents.

It may be comforting to know that in most cases when your baby cries for 15 minutes at a time for no apparent reason there is probably nothing in particular that is wrong. In fact, studies show that 80 to 90 percent of babies cry for 15 minutes to an hour on a daily basis for reasons that cannot be readily explained. Some researchers have theorized that life outside the womb is so different from life inside that babies see this as something to cry about as they go through this period of adjustment. In most cases, such crying spells diminish or cease altogether by the time the baby is 3 to 4 months old.

If your baby is prone to episodes of crying, you should first do the obvious: Check whether your baby is hungry, or if the diaper needs to be changed. If you suspect your baby is teething, you may need to offer

PACIFIERS, YES OR NO

There are many ways to comfort your baby. Using a pacifier is one of them, and studies have shown that nearly half of all babies use them. Because babies often need to suck simply for comfort, rather than for nourishment, pacifiers can soothe a crying baby quickly and conveniently. However, once you begin to use a pacifier, it may be hard to stop. And the longer you use a pacifier, the harder getting your baby to do without it will become.

If you do decide to use a pacifier, you will want to choose the right one for your baby and use it safely. The safest pacifiers are constructed of one piece of silicone in an orthodontic shape. They come with a shield with ventilation holes in it, and are easy to clean. Never construct a homemade pacifier from a bottle nipple, because it might pull apart. Never attach your baby's pacifier to a cord or string to be hung around your baby's neck, because it might choke the baby.

If pacifier use continues, it may affect the alignment of your child's teeth. Most dentists agree, however, that the pacifier will do no significant damage as long as it is disposed of before your child's permanent teeth are coming in. ■

more comfort and distraction than your baby usually requires (see Teething, page 202, for more information). If your baby is tired, he may need to cry for a while before falling asleep. Before you pick your baby up, see if this might be the case. You will be doing yourself a favor in the long run by not making your baby dependent on endless, gentle rocking before he falls asleep. When none of the obvious solutions work, try carrying your baby with you in a baby carrier or sling. Sometimes the baby is soothed by being near you and by the rocking motion of your movements—all of which your baby experienced for many months inside the womb.

Excessive and consistent crying may also indicate colic, a condition that may actually refer to a variety of situations in which your baby cries inconsolably on a daily basis for no apparent reason (see Colic and Your Baby, page 202).

If your baby cries frequently for no reason, and you find that nothing seems to help and all you do is worry more, you should

TEETHING

Your baby's first tooth generally arrives at about age 6 months, although the first tooth may appear as early as age 3 months or as late as 12 months. When your baby gets his first teeth is influenced by heredity; so if you or your spouse teethed late, you can expect your baby may do the same. The front teeth on the bottom and top appear first; the molars are the last to arrive, between about 12 and 24 months. There are 20 baby teeth altogether.

The symptoms and duration of teething differ from baby to baby. A lump may appear on the gum and remain for months, or there may be no visible sign until the tooth, itself, appears almost overnight. One baby may be up every night crying in pain, while another baby may not appear to be bothered by teething at all.

Teething stimulates drooling in some babies more than others. If your baby drools a lot, drooling may irritate the skin around the mouth and on the chin, causing chapping or a rash. Wiping away the saliva during the day and placing a towel on the crib sheet to absorb the drool when your baby is sleeping may help prevent irritation.

Doctors debate how much pain teething actually causes. As you get to know your baby during the first months of life, you will become the best judge of how much your baby is suffering. The inflammation of the gum tissue as the tooth is breaking through can cause pain, which usually seems worse with the first teeth. Later on, babies seem to adjust to the sensation and discomfort that was startling at first. Once in a while, teething may cause bleeding inside the gum, called a gum hematoma, but this is rare and not usually a problem.

If your baby is having difficulty with teething, you may offer him something to chew on or rub against or something cool to eat or drink or chew on. If your baby seems to be suffering greatly from teething pain, consult your doctor before offering your baby acetaminophen or other over-the-counter teething pain relievers. Do not rub brandy or anything else on your baby's gums. ■

COLIC AND YOUR BABY

A colicky baby cries inconsolably, sometimes for hours on end. Colic differs from regular crying in that the crying turns to screams, and the baby may be inconsolable for hours. Sometimes, whether or not to label your baby colicky is a tricky question. Many new parents ask about colic, suspecting their baby has it when the baby cries for 10 minutes each day, and other new parents wonder what is wrong with their baby when the baby cries all the time, without suspecting colic. In other words, whether a baby is called colicky sometimes depends on the stamina of the parents.

One in five babies experience crying episodes that are severe enough to be labeled colic. These spells usually begin in the late afternoon and may last well into the evening. A baby suffering from severe colic will clench his fists, pull his knees up to the chest, close his eyes tightly, wrinkle his brow, and wail. Often, the baby will hold his breath briefly. Periods of colic may last for up to 3 hours and in some cases, may go on periodically for 24 hours.

The cause of colic is unknown. Explanations that have been rejected include gastrointestinal disturbance, allergy or sensitivity to something in the mother's diet if they are breast-feeding or in the formula if they are bottle-fed, or parental inexperience. No medication or other treatment approach has been found to relieve colic effectively.

If your baby suffers from colic, you should not blame yourself. Once you and your doctor have ruled out illness or any other physical cause, you must begin by adjusting to your baby's cries, because the more relaxed you are, the better you will be able to help comfort your baby. An agitated parent has little chance of calming a colicky baby. Once you have settled in for the duration, you may want to try the following methods to relieve the problem:

- *Calm your baby.* Sometimes in the excitement of having a new baby in the house, the newborn may become overstimulated.

Try to lower the din and activity at home, and give your baby some hours of peace and quiet where visitors are not always peering and ooing and ahing.

- *Carry your baby.* If you find that your baby's crying time is usually between 5:00 and 7:00 PM, just when you are making dinner, try putting your baby in a sling or baby carrier and go about your business with your baby in tow. Try various carrying positions to see which seems to comfort the baby the most.

- *Check your baby's diet.* First of all, make sure your baby is getting enough to eat. Try an extra bottle or an extra nursing session or two. Your baby may just be hungry. Consult with your doctor before changing formulas.

- *Entertain your baby.* Try to distract your baby with music, pretty objects, interesting, colorful shapes, or gentle bouncing.

- *Give your baby fresh air.* Many babies stop crying the minute they feel the fresh air. Whether it is the air, or the change of scene, or the motion of the stroller is not known, but the quieting effect is often instant.

- *Take a car ride.* Many parents report that a ride in the car instantly quiets the colicky baby. Be sure to use an infant car seat fastened properly in the back seat.

- *Let your baby suck.* Sometimes sucking, itself, comforts a baby. If you are breast-feeding your baby, find a good book or magazine and try letting the baby suck for as long as he wants. If your baby is bottle-fed, try a pacifier (see Pacifiers, Yes or No page 201).

- *When all else fails, give yourself some outside relief.* Sometimes another pair of loving arms may be just what the baby and you need.

Remember, crying itself will not hurt your baby, and colic, too, will pass. It rarely persists beyond about 4 months. ■

call your doctor and share your fears. Your doctor may want to see the baby to be sure there is no medical problem causing your baby's frequent cries. Usually, a checkup will show that your baby is perfectly healthy, and you can begin a new round of tactics to assuage the crying, feeling, if not less tired, at least less worried.

SPITTING UP VERSUS VOMITING

All babies spit up, usually as small wet burps during or immediately after a feeding. This normal process occurs because the muscles at the base of the swallowing tube or esophagus do not tighten well after feedings or when lying down until after the baby is several months old. Spitting up is encountered in both breast-fed and formula-fed babies. The baby is rarely bothered by the spitting up and usually resumes normal feedings easily. The degree of spitting can often be minimized by frequent burping, holding the baby more upright after feedings for a few minutes, and confirming with your doctor that you are not overfeeding the baby. Even when frequent spitting up is a nuisance, the majority of babies have resolved the problem by age 6 to 9 months. If the baby has any coughing or choking during the spit up, or if the baby appears to be in discomfort during or after the feeding, review your concern with your doctor.

In contrast to spitting up, vomiting implies that a larger volume of stomach content comes out. Vomiting may occur during, after, or independent of feeding. While an occasional episode of vomiting may be of

CHOKING

Choking on food and other objects kills more than 200 children each year, most commonly, babies under age 1 year. If your baby is choking, he will begin to cough to clear the airway. If your baby can cough forcefully and can breathe, he will probably be able to clear the airway without assistance. If your baby cannot cough effectively or seems to be struggling for help, call 911 or a local emergency number immediately. If someone is with you, have them call while you try to clear the baby's airway.

To Clear the Airway of a Child Under Age 1 Year

- First, place your baby's face down on your forearm, making sure the head is lower than the torso. If your baby is too big for you to do this comfortably standing up, sit down.

- Then administer four or five strong back blows between the baby's shoulder blades with the palm of your other hand.

- If the baby is still choking and the obstruction has not been dislodged, turn the baby over, making sure, once again, to keep the head lower than the torso, and begin to administer chest thrusts.

  To do this, position your index finger on your baby's sternum (the flat breastbone between your baby's ribs) about 1/2 in. or a finger's width below the nipples. Use two or three fingers to compress this area to a depth of about 1/2 to 1 in. Do this five times.

- If your baby is still conscious, alternate back blows and chest thrusts until the airway is cleared.

- If your baby becomes unconscious, check the airway in the following manner.

  Lay the baby down on a flat, hard surface such as the floor. Tilt the head back, lift the chin up, and administer two breaths, slowly. Make sure your mouth is over the baby's mouth and nose.

  If the chest rises and falls with each breath, the airway is clear.

  Continue rescue breathing until the ambulance arrives or the baby cries and breathes on his own.

  If the chest does not rise, check for a foreign object by opening your baby's mouth and using your thumb to depress the tongue.

  Open the jaw, and look into the throat. If a foreign object is visible, try to dislodge it with one finger. Do not reach for it with two fingers, because you may push it further down the throat.

  After checking for a foreign object, if the baby is still not breathing, repeat the sequence while you wait for the ambulance to arrive.

To help prevent possible choking situations, when you introduce solid foods, avoid foods such as raw carrots or apples. These foods may be parboiled to soften them until your baby is older. Also avoid feeding children under age 4 whole grapes, hotdogs, and hard candy, which are easy to choke on and difficult to dislodge. If your baby likes grapes, cut them in half to avoid choking. Cut hotdogs lengthwise as well as crosswise. When your baby begins to crawl, keep small objects, such as buttons, pins and sewing needles, marbles, button-size batteries, and other siblings' small toys off the floor and off low table tops. Also keep loose balloons or the fragments of a balloon that has popped out of reach of your baby's inquisitive fingers. Plastic bags may also cause asphyxiation very quickly and should be kept out of the baby's reach. Drapery cords are a hazard and should be shortened so that a crawling or climbing baby is not in danger of getting the cord tangled around his neck.

For more information on keeping a baby safe, see Chapter 3. ■

no concern, you should notify your doctor if the vomiting is progressive, contains a greenish-yellow color (bile), or if any blood is noted. If the baby has a swollen or distended abdomen, the vomiting may be of more concern as well. Thus, while spitting up is rarely of concern, vomiting usually requires an evaluation by your doctor and often some additional testing to be sure no bowel obstruction is present. Although many babies will have vomiting with an allergy to the formula or because of a passing mild viral infection, do not assume that you know the cause and waste critical time with multiple feeding changes before calling your doctor.

BOWEL MOVEMENTS

New parents tend to be very concerned about their baby's bowel movements; they wonder if loose, runny stools constitute diarrhea and whether going a day or two without a bowel movement indicates constipation. In most cases, whatever the consistency of your baby's stools and however many times your baby eliminates in a 1- or 2-day period is normal. Newborns, particularly breast-fed babies, often have many bowel movements in 24 hours, and frequent bowel movements are a sign that your child is consuming enough breast milk or formula. The number of bowel movements per day diminishes over the first 2 to 3 months of life. By the third to fourth month of life, many babies have a bowel movement one or two times a day, while others may have a bowel movement up to four times a day or more through the first year of life. It is also common for the stools of a newborn to be loose and runny. This is not the same as diarrhea (see page 213).

DIAPER RASH

Almost all babies develop diaper rash at one time or another during infancy. The incidence of diaper rash usually peaks between 7 and 9 months and can be a problem for as long as your baby wears diapers. There are a number of causes. Diaper rash is related to the chronic moisture present in the diaper area and the presence of urine and stool. Constant cleansing with soap and water, an excessively tight diaper, rubber pants, the taking of oral antibiotics, and problems with diarrhea can make babies prone to diaper rash.

Diaper rash may appear anywhere on the area the diaper covers, from the buttocks to the genitals. The most common form of diaper rash, chafing dermatitis, appears as a rough, red area where friction is most consistent and generally not in the folds of your baby's skin. (See page C-31). The term *diaper rash* is used to describe many different skin irritations in the diaper area including yeast infection, impetigo (bacterial infection), and intertrigo (skin inflammation), which require different treatments.

If your baby has diaper rash, change his diapers more frequently. If the diaper rash persists, zinc oxide or petroleum jelly may be applied to the irritated areas. Many doctors also recommend leaving the diaper off for a while so that the skin can be exposed to air. You might try doing this just after changing a full diaper to lower the chances of accidents. When a diaper rash persists, always call your doctor. In some cases, a very low-dose hydrocortisone cream (0.5 or 1 percent) may be recommended for a short period to eradicate the rash. In other cases, a prescription cream or ointment may be necessary depending on the cause of the rash. Prompt attention to the rash will usually result in healing.

CONSTIPATION

While most babies, especially those that are breast-fed, will have several bowel movements a day, it is equally normal to have only one movement every 2 to 3 days, as long as that bowel movement is large, soft, and empties the lower intestine completely. It is also normal for babies to strain and even turn red when having a normal, soft bowel movement. This is because babies strain and contract all the muscles, forgetting to relax the outer muscle of the rectum to let the movement out.

It is not usually normal for the baby to go beyond 3 days without a bowel movement. When that happens, the first part of the bowel movement becomes very hard, as too much fluid is removed while it sits in the rectum. Sometimes these firm bowel movements actually tear the inside lining of the anal canal, a tear that is called a fissure. Fissures may cause pain and a small amount of bleeding. Fissures heal quickly when stools are softened.

Remember that a bowel movement should empty all the contents of the lower intestine, and if the bowel movement is a small pellet or collection of pellets, much of the bowel movement is still stuck inside. This will eventually cause problems. While some buildup of gas may precede the passage of a normal bowel movement, if your baby's abdomen becomes swollen or distended before or after a bowel movement, call your doctor.

The treatment of firm or infrequent bowel movements usually begins with an effort to soften the composition of the bowel movement without use of a laxative. This may require the use of a small amount of fruit juice or using a barley cereal instead of rice cereal. Do not use honey, because honey given to children younger than 1 year of age can cause botulism, a serious form of food poisoning (see page 467). Many babies become constipated around 1 year of age when increased amounts of cow's milk and starchy foods like pasta are introduced into the diet. If you are concerned about your baby's bowel patterns, check with your doctor.

As Your Baby Grows

Your baby will grow and change more dramatically in the first year of life than at any other time during childhood. During this time, your baby will learn everything from smiling and sitting up to rolling over and holding an object in his hand. Your baby will also begin to eat solid food, hold and sip from a cup, crawl, and even babble his first consonant and vowel sounds or words. By the end of the year, he will also begin to be more independent about eating and sleeping.

INTRODUCING SOLID FOOD

Advice on when to introduce solid foods varies and depends on the individual development of the infant. Years ago, solid foods were introduced as early as the first month of life, but recent research has shown that an infant's digestive system may be too immature to adequately handle solid foods. And very early introduction is not neces-

sary, because breast milk (with vitamin and mineral supplements) or formula meets an infant's nutritional needs. For normal babies, it is usually recommended that strained food be introduced between 4 and 6 months of age when the baby is mature enough to accept the food from a spoon and digest it. You should discuss the introduction of solid food with your doctor during your well-baby care checkups (see Well-Baby Care, page 191).

Doctors often recommend infant rice cereal as the first solid food to introduce into your baby's diet. Rice cereal may be mixed with breast milk, formula, or later on, cow's milk, until it has almost the same consistency as the breast milk or formula your baby is used to, thereby making it easier for your baby to adjust to swallowing the new food. And it is best to let your baby develop a taste for plain foods, rather than relying on sweetening foods to make them more palatable. If your baby is allergic to milk products, consult your doctor regarding alternative choices.

Once your baby is accustomed to eating rice cereal, you can introduce other foods. There are many approaches, but most doctors start with yellow vegetables, like sweet potato, carrots, and yellow squash. Once your baby is consuming one or more of these vegetables, you may try introducing green vegetables, like green beans. It is a good idea to start your baby on vegetables before you introduce him to fruits, so that your baby does not always expect a sweet taste. First fruits to introduce include applesauce, bananas, peaches, and pears. Most doctors recommend introducing meat and poultry only after infants have been weaned from breast milk or formula, which are also high in protein, usually at about 1 year of age.

The texture of all first foods should be smooth, whether you buy baby foods or prepare your own food at home. First foods should be pureed, strained, or mashed. If you need to, you can use water to thin a mashed or pureed food to the consistency of cream. As your baby becomes more familiar with eating solid food, you may offer foods of thicker consistency. When you begin, do not expect him to eat more than about a half a tablespoon of food at first. Eventually, you may expect two to three tablespoons of food to be consumed at a feeding. All first foods may be served at room temperature. Although most adults feel the food will be more palatable if heated, babies are satisfied with room temperature food, and they are less likely to be accidentally burned.

When you do begin to introduce solid foods, only one new food should be fed to your baby at a time, in order to discern whether your baby has any food allergies or intolerance. For example, you may want to try a particular new vegetable one day and another a few days later so you will know which food to blame if your baby seems not to do well with the dietary addition.

Limit the amount of fruit juice you give your baby. Fruit juices can fill a baby up, adding calories with little nutritional value. Too much fruit juice can also lead to diarrhea.

Do not give your baby honey or corn syrup during the first year of life. Both can contain the spores of *Clostridium botulinum*. These spores are harmless to adults but can cause botulism in babies. This illness is sometimes fatal and at the very least can result in paralysis that can lead to pneumonia and dehydration.

WEANING YOUR BABY

Weaning is often not easy and can pose a substantial challenge for parents. The best way to wean your baby is gradually. Most breast-fed babies wean themselves if left to their own devices. It will be easier to wean from the breast when you need or want to if you have helped your baby learn to sip from a cup, eat from a spoon, or suck on a bottle before you begin to reduce breast-feeding sessions.

The first step in the weaning process involves helping your baby become comfortable enough with drinking from a bottle or cup so that you can be confident that he will be able to drink as much from a bottle or cup as from the breast. It takes many breast-fed babies a long time to become willing to try these alternative methods of feeding, so you should introduce these alternatives well before you plan to wean your baby. Using expressed breast milk for practice drinking from a bottle or cup may help your baby adjust more quickly, since this is what he is used to and it will involve fewer new things at one time. You may also use formula or water. If your baby refuses to try anything you offer him, you may want to try skipping one breast-feeding session, so that your baby is hungry enough to give in and try an alternative method of feeding. Often, it helps if someone other than the mother offers the bottle. Mother may even need to be out of the room.

The next step in the weaning process is to reduce the number of breast-feeding sessions. Do not wean your baby too quickly. This can be traumatic for the baby and for you. Gradual weaning will also help protect you from clogged ducts, leaking, breast engorgement, and infection. Try not to begin the process if another major change is occurring in your baby's life. If a decision is made to begin the weaning process near the time of a mother's return to work, or if a new caretaker is being introduced, sufficient time should be allowed between events for your infant to adjust. Weaning is not always necessitated by a return to work, however. It is possible to successfully combine work outside the home with continued breast-feeding, and many workplaces assist a mother in doing so. If an unexpected change occurs just as you begin to wean your baby, curtail your efforts until your baby has adjusted. Weaning goes much more smoothly if your baby is settled and comfortable in a well-established routine. Begin to decrease feedings several weeks before you plan to discontinue them altogether.

The best strategy for weaning is to replace one feeding at a time, then wait approximately a week until you and your baby have adjusted, before replacing the next feeding. If your breasts feel very full, express just enough milk to decrease the tight feeling. Over a few days you will be expressing less and less. If your baby is under 6 months old, replace each feeding with formula, since babies this young are dependent on breast milk for all their calories and nutrients. When your baby is older, a meal or snack may be substituted. Provide other means of closeness and comfort. Which feeding you replace first will depend on which you think it will be easiest for your baby to give up. Usually, the last feedings to go are the early morning and late evening feedings, which give extra comfort as well as nourishment to your baby.

When you wean your baby is an individual decision influenced by your own preferences as well as your baby's. Babies thrive better and usually have fewer colds and other illnesses if they are breast-fed for at least 6 months, though even breast-feeding for as little as a few weeks is beneficial for your baby. Doctors recommend breast-feeding for at least 12 months when possible. It can continue as long as mother and child desire it. In the United States, women breast-feed for a matter of weeks to 2 to 3 years. And as with any other pleasurable habit, the longer you wait, the harder it may be for your baby to give it up. You will probably want to discuss your weaning strategy with your doctor at one of your well-baby visits.

SLEEP PROBLEMS

For the first months of life, your baby will probably not be sleeping through the night. Babies this young get hungry in the night, especially if they are premature. By the time he is 4 or 5 months old, he will no longer need a 2 AM feeding yet may still demand your attention when he wakes in the course of the night. Most babies need to learn how to fall back to sleep on their own before their parents will be able to get a full night's sleep. It is best to start teaching this skill when your baby is 2 months old by putting him in bed awake. The longer you aid your baby in going to sleep or falling back to sleep in the middle of the night with the breast, the bottle, a pacifier, or simply your own presence, the harder it will be to break this pattern.

The first step to take if your baby is not sleeping through the night after age 4 months is to give up the nighttime feeding, if you are still nursing or giving him a night-time bottle. If your baby was premature or a low-birth-weight baby, he may continue to need nighttime feedings longer than other babies, and you should postpone trying to get your baby to fall back to sleep on his own for a few months. Do this gradually, by first shortening the feeding by 1 oz or 1 minute of nursing time per night to give your baby time to adjust. Many doctors recommend letting the baby cry it out if he wakes once or twice in the night, but many parents find this approach difficult. Each parent may feel differently about letting the baby cry in the night. In most cases, letting the baby cry for a couple of nights can lead to peaceful sleep for you both in less than 1 week. If you choose to let your baby cry it out, check on the baby after 5 minutes to make sure he does not have a soggy diaper or some other discomfort. This gives him a chance to settle himself. When checking, do not feed or pick the baby up. Singing may help. When your baby is exhausted, he will eventually fall back to sleep. Some babies may cry for an hour or more, but often it just seems like an hour to the distraught parent. You may check on him every 10 minutes for your own peace of mind. If you are a nursing mother, let the father go reassure the baby to avoid the complication of the baby wanting to eat. No matter how diligent parents may be at letting the baby cry, some babies still do not fall back to sleep. This may be because the baby has learned to be hungry. For these babies, try increasing the time between feedings during the day and be sure to feed late in the evening to avoid nighttime hunger. Still other babies are simply more sensitive to stimuli and more easily awakened.

A different sleep problem frequently begins around 8 to 10 months of age. This is when your baby remembers and calls for you when you are out of sight. Babies this age are also more active and have new fears of strangers. If your baby was sleeping all night and begins waking up, apparently frightened, wait 3 minutes for him to settle himself, then go to him but do not feed or play with him or pick him up. Instead, reassure him briefly, leave a nightlight on, and stay in his room where he can see you, but do not talk to him. This reassures him (and you) without rewarding his night waking. He will stop waking up at night, usually in less than a week, using this strategy. If your baby's sleep problems continue to seem insoluble, consult your doctor.

Illness in Infancy

HIGH FEVER

Fever is an important aspect of the immune system's response to infection. In a newborn, fever can contribute to dehydration and, more importantly, may be a sign of serious bacterial infection requiring notification of your doctor and prompt treatment with antibiotics. You should take your baby's temperature when he seems sick or if he feels warmer than usual to the touch. An infant's

FEBRILE SEIZURES

A very high fever may occasionally cause convulsions in infants. These convulsions are referred to as febrile seizures. Although a febrile seizure in an infant can be extremely frightening for parents, it is important to keep in mind that in most cases the seizure subsides in a matter of moments and that complications due to febrile seizures are rare.

Febrile seizures occur in children between age 6 months and 5 years. About 5 percent of children have at least one febrile seizure, and 50 percent of these children never have another recurrence. When a child has seizures that are not related to fever and recur, this is termed a seizure disorder. A fever need not be excessively high to trigger a febrile seizure, and febrile seizures occur with many different febrile illnesses. Most febrile seizures last for less than 5 minutes, and many occur before the parent is even aware that the child has a fever. For more information on febrile seizures, see Chapter 14.

If your baby has a seizure, try to remain calm, and remember they generally last only a few seconds or minutes and stop on their own. Remove anything from the baby's mouth, such as a pacifier, and hold the baby, unrestrained, in your arms. Work to bring down the baby's fever by removing clothing and sponging the baby's forehead and body with a cool, damp cloth. Do not put your baby in the bathtub or use alcohol to bathe him; either can be dangerous. If your baby begins to vomit, make sure he is facing downward. If your baby is having difficulty breathing, pull the jaw and chin forward gently with your fingers. When the seizure is over, notify your doctor, who will probably want to see the baby immediately to make sure he is okay. If the baby is more than 6 months old, give him acetaminophen when he is awake. If the seizure does not appear to be ending on its own, call 911 or go directly to the emergency room. ■

TAKING YOUR BABY'S TEMPERATURE

The most accurate way to take an infant's temperature is rectally. First, you will want to prepare the thermometer. Wash the thermometer with cool, soapy water. Hot water causes mercury to expand, which may cause the thermometer to burst. Then use a cotton swab with alcohol on it to rub down the thermometer. Check the mercury reading. If it is above 96°F, shake down the thermometer carefully with a firm snap of your wrist. Make sure you have enough room to execute this procedure without breaking the thermometer on a nearby table or other surface. Then lubricate the bulb end of the thermometer with petroleum jelly.

To insert the thermometer, hold your baby on your lap, rear end up with legs dangling, or put your baby on a changing table or bed. With one hand, spread the buttocks. Holding the thermometer in place with thumb and index finger of the other hand, insert the bulb end of the thermometer into the rectum gently and slowly. Insert thermometer approximately 1 in. and no more. Do not force the thermometer into the rectum. Hold the thermometer in place for at least 2 minutes. Never let go of the thermometer while it is in your baby. You may want to use your other hand to hold the buttocks together and keep the thermometer in place. If your baby objects vehemently, withdraw the thermometer immediately. Even if the thermometer has been in place for only 30 seconds, you can get a rough estimate of your baby's temperature to report to your doctor. Very rarely, a thermometer may break while still inserted in your baby's rectum. Although this can be frightening, be assured the mercury in the thermometer is in a nontoxic form, and usually the worst your baby suffers is a slight scratch. You may need a doctor's help in retrieving the broken piece from the rectum.

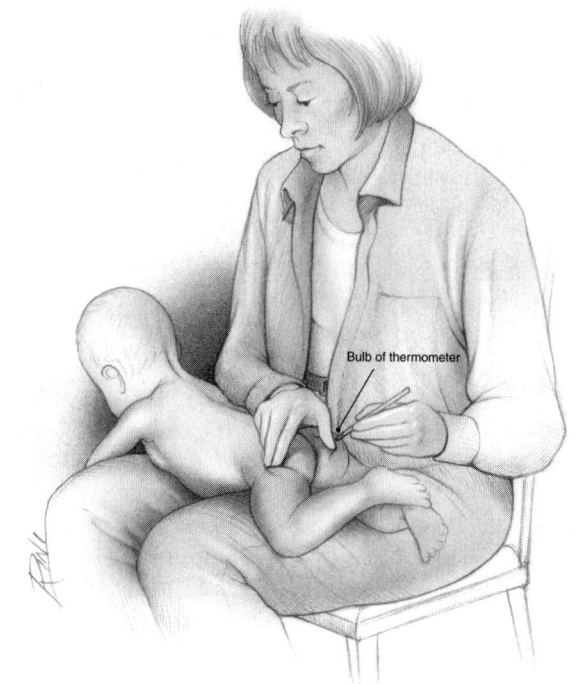

Bulb of thermometer

The rectal temperature is the most accurate for infants. The bulb end of a clean thermometer, lubricated with petroleum jelly, is inserted gently only 1 in. into the anus. Hold the thermometer near the bulb. If the baby is tolerating it well, keep the thermometer in place for 2 minutes, holding it continuously.

A baby's temperature can also be taken in the ear (using the proper equipment) or under the arm. Thermometers with digital readouts are available. You may use one of these. But a basic, inexpensive rectal thermometer is the standard for infants, offering the most accurate reading at the best price. ■

FEVER RELIEF MEDICATIONS AND YOUR BABY

Both aspirin and acetaminophen are effective antipyretics, or fever reducers. Aspirin, however, is linked to a wide range of side effects in infants and children, including Reye's syndrome, and therefore is not recommended for children in most situations. Acetaminophen is the antipyretic found in Tylenol, Tempra, Panadol, Liquiprin, and other brand-name fever reducers on the market for children. While acetaminophen has been associated with liver damage when given in excessive amounts, it is gener-

ally free of side effects when given in the recommended dose. Acetaminophen comes in liquid form for infants and also as suppositories for infants who cannot or will not keep the liquid down. Ibuprofen is also effective at lowering fever and relieving pain, but most doctors reserve it for special situations.

Always check with your doctor before giving acetaminophen to a young infant, and always give the appropriate dose recommended for your baby's age and size. Keep all medications out of reach of children. Any medication can be dangerous in large doses, particularly for babies. ■

---

temperature is best taken rectally; see Taking Your Baby's Temperature, page 208, for information on how to take your infant's temperature safely and accurately. Your baby's temperature varies during the course of the day. It is usually lower in the morning and higher by evening. A rectal temperature over 100.5°F is considered to be a fever, and you should call your doctor even if there are no other symptoms if your baby is less than 3 months old. Your doctor will probably want to examine the baby. If your baby has a fever, do not give him any medicine unless your doctor advises you to do so. Your doctor will usually recommend acetaminophen or ibuprofen.

If your baby has a fever within the first few months of life, your doctor will want to rule out a more serious infection such as bacterial meningitis. Your doctor may want to do some tests on your baby's blood, urine, and spinal fluid. Your baby may need to be hospitalized for treatment with antibiotics by vein and for observation. In most cases, if the samples of blood, urine, and spinal fluid do not grow bacteria, your doctor will determine that your baby has a viral infection, which may not require further treatment.

COLDS

Babies and young children may get colds frequently because their immune systems are immature and they have not yet built up immunity against the many different cold viruses. These viruses are generally transmitted from hand to hand, one reason why washing your hands before touching your baby is important. Colds usually last 6 or 7 days. There is no treatment for the common cold, but you can alleviate the symptoms and make your baby more comfortable while he is recovering.

The most common symptoms of a cold are sneezing, nasal congestion, and a runny nose. The discharge from the nose tends to be watery at first, then thicker and yellowish. If your baby is having nasal discharge, you can use a suction bulb to remove the mucus. If the mucus is hardened, you can use saline nose drops to soften it. You may also want to use a humidifier to moisten the air in your baby's room, which may reduce nasal congestion and make breathing easier. You may also use petroleum jelly under and around the nose to prevent chapped skin, but be careful not to get the ointment in the nostrils. Cough medication, decongestants, and nose drops are not used often in infancy. They can be dangerous, and there is little or no evidence of their efficacy. Do not use any of these preparations unless your doctor recommends their use. Antibiotics cannot cure the common cold and will not be prescribed unless your baby develops a secondary infection that is bacterial.

You should continue to nurse or bottle-feed your baby as usual while he has a cold unless your doctor tells you otherwise. Your baby still needs plenty of liquids while he has a cold.

INFLUENZA

Influenza, also known as the flu, usually occurs during the colder months. Babies and the elderly often are more severely affected. The first sign of flu may be the abrupt onset of a fever that can be as high as 104° F. Your child may have poor appetite, may be irritable, and may be less active. Your baby may also have a dry, hacking cough, sneezing, and nasal stuffiness. Diarrhea or vomiting may also occur but are less common.

If your child appears ill, you should call your doctor immediately. Your doctor will probably recommend acetaminophen for fever relief. If your baby has the flu, you should add extra fluids to the diet. In severe cases, your doctor may recommend antiviral drugs. Complications may include bronchitis, croup (see page 212), otitis media (see below), and pneumonia (see below). If your baby has an underlying medical condition and is more than 6 months old, your child may qualify for yearly immunization with influenza vaccine.

COMMON RESPIRATORY AILMENTS IN INFANTS

For more information on the following conditions see Chapter 18.

Respiratory syncytial virus Respiratory syncytial virus (RSV) infection can occur at any age, but approximately 50 percent of recognized cases occur by age 1 year, and most cases occur before age 2 years. RSV accounts for the majority of hospitalizations of very young children for respiratory disease. RSV infections occur most commonly in late fall to early spring and are rare in summer and early fall. They are transmitted by infected nasal secretions, so meticulous hand washing can help prevent spread. Symptoms of RSV infection may mimic those of the common cold, or they may worsen and result in rapid breathing and wheezing. RSV may lead to bronchiolitis or pneumonia (see below). Especially in premature babies, apnea—a respiratory pause of 20 seconds or longer—may occur. If your baby has the symptoms of a cold and is breathing rapidly, or has a cough, you should call your doctor. Your baby may require hospitalization if the condition is severe.

Bronchiolitis Bronchiolitis is an acute viral infection of the lower respiratory tract. It occurs primarily in babies 2 to 8 months old, and babies with a family history of allergies may be at increased risk. Bronchiolitis is most commonly caused by RSV (see above). A baby with bronchiolitis will have cold symptoms at first and then may develop a cough, wheezing, and rapid, shallow breathing. Your baby may also develop a fever, be irritable, and eat poorly. In severe bronchiolitis, your baby's breathing may be very fast, his face may be pale or even slightly bluish in color, and his lungs may not fully expand when he breathes in. If you suspect your baby has bronchiolitis, call your doctor immediately. If your doctor is unavailable, go to an emergency room. Babies with bronchiolitis sometimes need to be hospitalized and may need extra oxygen. The most serious complications of bronchiolitis are respiratory failure and pneumonia.

Pneumonia Pneumonia is an inflammation of the lung usually caused by an infection. Sometimes it starts out looking like a cold; sometimes it comes on suddenly without preceding symptoms. The presence of fever, cough, and rapid breathing suggests that your baby may have pneumonia. Breathing may be fast and raspy or wheezy, and your baby may look like breathing is difficult. Your baby's cough may sound wet. Sometimes, babies with pneumonia look pale or have a blue tinge to the skin. If your baby develops fever and cough with rapid or difficult breathing, you should call your doctor immediately. If your baby is having persistent difficulty breathing, you should go to an emergency room.

Many different kinds of infectious organisms can cause pneumonia, but most cases of childhood pneumonia are caused by one of a short list of bacteria and viruses. In most cases, the baby can be treated with antibiotics without knowledge of the exact cause. Pneumonia can often be treated at home. Your baby may have trouble eating for a few days, and your doctor may advise you on how to maintain his fluid intake.

OTITIS MEDIA (EAR INFECTION)

Otitis media, inflammation or infection of the middle ear, is one of the most common infectious diseases of infancy. Two of every three children have had at least one case of otitis media before they are 1 year old. Babies are more susceptible to otitis media partly because of the shape and size of their developing eustachian tubes. The function of the eustachian tube is to drain fluids and mucus from the ears down into the back of the throat and to equalize middle ear pressure with the air pressure on the outside. The immature eustachian tubes of an infant are smaller and narrower than when fully developed; they also take a more horizontal path than in older children and adults. The horizontal position of the tubes and their size allow fluid to collect in the middle ear rather than drain into the back of the throat. This fluid is a breeding ground for bacteria that may cause infection.

Symptoms of otitis media may include fever and irritability, sometimes with loss of appetite, and vomiting. Some babies may have no symptoms. Otitis media can be painful, but an infant cannot say that he has pain and may simply cry more than usual or have trouble sleeping. Older babies may rub or tug on their ears. Sometimes, the infection causes a small hole (perforation) in the eardrum, causing fluid to drain from the ear. The baby may feel better when this happens because the pain caused by pressure on the eardrum is relieved; however, your baby will still need an antibiotic and careful follow-up to see that the perforation heals. It is important to have your baby's ears checked whenever you suspect that your baby has an ear infection.

Often, otitis media follows a cold or other viral respiratory infection. Otitis media can be caused either by bacteria or viruses. Allergies may also contribute to inflammation of the middle ear and resulting infections.

In cases of suspected otitis media, your doctor will prescribe an oral antibiotic, because bacterial infection is a common cause. Children's acetaminophen or another fever and pain relief medication may also be recommended. Otitis media can be very painful, so you should not hesitate to give your baby medication for pain.

It is difficult to prevent otitis media. Babies who are breast-fed for at least 3 months have fewer ear infections. Avoid smoking in the home; smoking may contribute to recurrent otitis media. Children with respiratory symptoms from allergies may benefit from the use of an antihistamine. If your child has had many ear infections, your doctor may recommend daily antibiotics at low dosage in an effort to prevent your child from getting additional ear infections.

The use of antibiotics in treating otitis media in children has become an area of some controversy. Because ear infections are so common and antibiotics so commonly prescribed, there has been growing concern that the practice may lead to antibi-

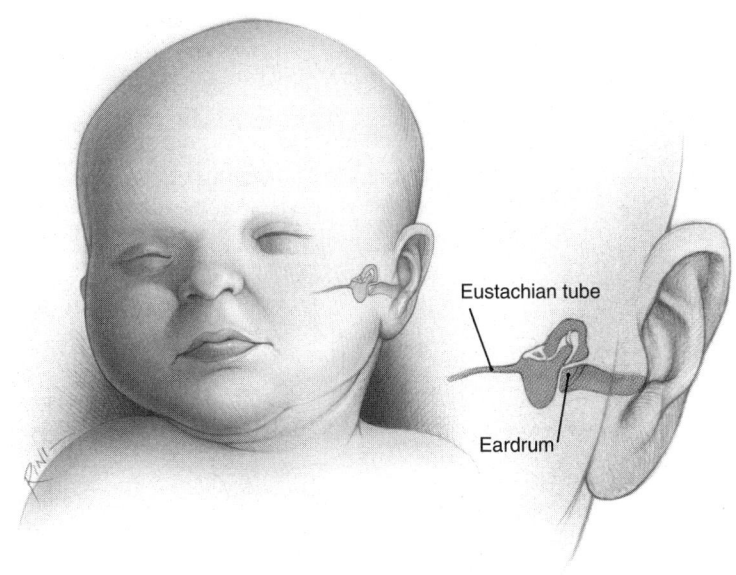

Eustachian tube

Eardrum

Otitis media is a common condition in babies, partly because the baby's straight, narrow eustachian tubes do not drain well. Temporary hearing loss or perforation of the eardrum can occur. Drainage tubes may be needed for recurrent or severe cases.

otic-resistant bacteria. In addition, many ear infections are caused by viruses, and no antibiotic will bring relief, although often several are prescribed in succession. If an antibiotic is prescribed, you should contact your doctor after 3 or 4 days if your child is not getting better. Your doctor may want to change the antibiotic. It is important to give all dosages of antibiotics and for as long as is prescribed. Skipping dosages of antibiotics and not giving them for the right length of time may result in the development of antibiotic-resistant bacteria.

When a baby has chronic and severe otitis media, surgery may be recommended. The surgery involves the insertion of a tiny drainage tube into the eardrum to prevent the buildup of fluid and subsequent infection. The surgery is done under general anesthesia and is generally done if otitis media keeps recurring despite antibiotics and there is documented hearing loss.

Otitis media can lead to a mild-to-moderate hearing loss, which is almost always temporary. While evidence that hearing deficits due to otitis media effect a child's long-term development is scant at best, some experts believe that even a temporary hearing impairment in infancy can adversely affect language and learning skills.

CROUP

Croup, or acute laryngotracheitis, is caused by respiratory viruses and is common in young children, peaking between age 1 and 3 years. Croup is characterized by a hoarse barking cough and wheezy or crowing breath sounds. These occur because swelling narrows the upper part of the airway. Croup is often worse at night. Most children with croup improve without needing medication. To ease your baby's croup, expose him to steam by turning on the hot water in your shower and sitting in the bathroom with your baby with the door closed. Try to keep your baby calm, because crying can make breathing harder. Croup is sometimes so severe it can completely block the airway. Other serious infections (e.g., pneumonia, bacteria tracheitis, and epiglottitis) can mimic croup. If steam does not relieve your baby's breathing difficulties, you should call the doctor right away. In addition, if your baby is drooling, if his lips or face look blue, if he seems to be struggling to breathe or is tiring out, or if you suspect that he has swallowed an object, call 911 immediately. (See Chapter 18 for more information.)

VIRAL MOUTH INFECTIONS

Several common viruses cause fever and sores in the mouth in babies and young children. These illnesses can be quite troublesome, because the mouth sores are exceedingly painful and interfere with the child's willingness to eat and drink. At the same time, fever increases fluid loss, so dehydration is a danger. These infections are usually treated with pain medications and oral fluids, but occasionally hospitalization and intravenous fluids are necessary. Call your doctor if your baby has a fever, is drinking poorly, and has sores in his mouth. Sometimes the sores will not be obvious until the doctor examines your baby's mouth with a tongue blade and light.

Hand-foot-and-mouth disease This is caused by several specific Coxsackie viruses. In the first 2 to 3 days of this febrile illness, small blisters appear inside the cheeks and on the tongue and sometimes on the gums, palate, and lips. Small red sores may then appear on the hands and feet, particularly between the fingers and toes and on the palms and soles. Fever subsides in 2 to 4 days, but the lesions (sores) can last longer (see Chapter 28 for more information).

Herpangina Occurring most commonly in the summer and early fall, herpangina is most often caused by Coxsackie virus infection. Symptoms include high fever, sore throat, difficulty swallowing, and loss of appetite. Some children vomit. Small blisters or ulcers with red halos appear on the tonsils and the back of the throat. The illness usually lasts about a week.

Herpetic gingivostomatitis This is caused by herpes simplex type I virus and is more common in toddlers than infants. Many painful sores appear in the front of the mouth, gums, and lips, and inside of the cheeks. Your child may also have a high fever, be irritable, and, because of the pain, may eat and drink less than usual. Symptoms of herpetic gingivostomatitis usually last no more than 10 days.

ROSEOLA

Roseola infantum occurs most frequently during the first year of life. It is caused by a virus. The most common symptom is a high, seemingly unexplained fever followed by a fleeting rash, often after the fever breaks. (See page C-31.) Faint pinkish spots may occur on the neck, upper arms, and body. Sometimes they may also appear on the face and legs. Rash occurs in 10 to 20 percent of babies with roseola. Other symptoms sometimes include vomiting, diarrhea, and common cold symptoms. Your doctor probably will recommend acetaminophen or ibuprofen for fever relief, because the fever will appear before the diagnosis is clear. Remember to increase fluid intake, as with any fever. Roseola usually lasts from 3 to 7 days (see Chapter 21 for more information).

INFANTILE ECZEMA

Atopic dermatitis, known more commonly as eczema, is a chronic inflammatory disorder of the skin characterized by dry itching skin that may begin in early infancy and almost always by age 5 years. (See page C-31.) Ten to 15 percent of children are eventually affected.

The first signs of infantile eczema generally appear as a rash on the face, arms, legs, and trunk. The diaper area is always spared in infants. Dry, scaly, red patches appear, which are intensely itchy, and frequent scratching may cause oozing and crusting, which may, in turn, lead to infection.

If your baby has infantile eczema, keep his fingernails trimmed, and place his hands in cotton mittens at night to avoid further irritation by scratching. Your baby should wear cotton clothing, and his bedroom should not be overheated, since heat dries out the air and sweating can worsen the rash. Hot baths and vigorous scrubbing with soap frequently make matters worse. Bathe the baby in tepid water instead, and apply a moisturizing ointment right after the bath.

Food sensitivities may play a role in infantile eczema in some infants, so get your doctor's advice about any formula you give your baby and when introducing new foods to your baby.

If you think your baby has infantile eczema, contact your doctor. Because eczema will not heal in most children until later childhood or adolescence (in some people, eczema is a lifelong condition), a carefully thought-out plan is required. Over-the-counter topical corticosteroids often offer relief, but these potent creams and ointments have potential side effects and should not be used except under a doctor's instructions.

The most common complication of infantile eczema is infection with bacteria, which may need to be treated with an antibiotic. Cold sore virus can also be a serious problem that spreads over the entire skin surface. Therefore, infants with eczema should be kept away from siblings or parents with active cold sores until blisters are drying. For more information on atopic dermatitis, see page 1334.

DIARRHEA

While many infants, particularly breast-fed infants, have loose stools, the stools of diarrheal illnesses are usually distinct. They are often liquid in nature, sometimes containing mucus and often occurring with greater frequency and volume. Common childhood causes of diarrhea include infection (bacterial, viral, or parasitic) and dietary problems such as too much fruit juice. Some antibiotics used to treat childhood problems like ear infections precipitate diarrhea. Some parents say they notice diarrhea when their child is teething. Diarrhea is less likely to occur in breast-fed babies because substances present in breast milk appear to offer some protection against infectious diarrhea.

Always wash your hands carefully after handling diapers or going to the bathroom, and pay careful attention to all foods and formula you feed your baby, checking to make sure nothing is spoiled. If your baby is on antibiotics, ask your doctor if it is appropriate to feed your baby yogurt that contains live acidophilus cultures, which may help to prevent diarrhea.

Diarrhea may last for hours or for several days. A baby with diarrhea should have his diapers changed often to prevent diaper rash. If your baby has diarrhea, make sure you increase his fluid intake to avoid dehydration. You can do this by giving your baby extra fluids in addition to regular formula or breast milk. Do not give your baby plain water when he has diarrhea (see Oral Rehydration Therapy, page 245). Dehydration is much more serious than the diarrhea itself. Dehydration can occur in infants after only a few hours of diarrhea. If you notice that your baby has been urinating infrequently, if your baby's diaper is dry for an 8-hour period, or if your baby fails to produce tears when crying, call your doctor. Your doctor will probably want to see the baby and will probably recommend an oral rehydration solution to avoid the complications of dehydration. In some severe cases of dehydration, babies need to be hospitalized to be rehydrated. If your baby has loose, runny stools for 24 hours, if there is blood in the stool, if vomiting accompanies the diarrhea, if your baby stops taking in fluid, or if fever accompanies the diarrhea, call your doctor. Do not try to treat your baby's diarrhea without consulting your doctor. Above all, don't give your baby antidiarrhea medications unless your doctor prescribes this treatment.

BACTERIAL MENINGITIS

Acute bacterial meningitis is characterized by an inflammation of the membranes that encase the brain or the spinal cord and infection of the cerebrospinal fluid (a liquid that surrounds and cushions the brain and

WHEN YOUR BABY IS HOSPITALIZED

The last thing any new parent wants to contemplate is hospitalization, but sometimes hospitalization is necessary for your baby to get the best care.

If your infant is hospitalized for an acute illness, you can help your baby and ease your own anxiety by being with your baby as much as possible. Most hospitals now allow a parent to stay overnight in the hospital with the baby. This is particularly helpful if you are breast-feeding your baby. You will also want to get as much information from the doctor about your baby's condition as possible so that you may become a partner in caring for your baby. Keep track of changes in your baby's condition, so that you can pass any concerns on to doctors and nurses. Your vigilance can ensure that your baby receives the best possible care. When a baby is hospitalized for more than 1 or 2 days, parents may need to take turns staying with the baby and enlist the help of family and friends to avoid becoming too exhausted to care for the baby effectively. ■

spinal cord). The brain can be affected. The symptoms of meningitis include fever, drowsiness, irritability, lack of appetite, vomiting, stiff neck, and sometimes a high-pitched cry. A bulging fontanel, when the fontanel is still open, may also indicate meningitis (see The Fontanels, page 198). While some or all of these symptoms may be present in a variety of lesser infections, you should contact your doctor immediately if your child has these symptoms to ensure the most rapid possible treatment in case your child does have meningitis. Acute bacterial meningitis is a medical emergency.

Although bacterial meningitis is not a common infection, 90 percent of cases occur in children less than 5 years old, and the complications of meningitis can be severe. Babies 6 to 12 months old are at highest risk. If your baby has an apparently mild illness that suddenly takes a turn for the worse, contact your doctor immediately. Immunization against *Haemophilus influenzae B* bacteria has greatly decreased the risk of bacterial meningitis in infancy. (For more information on meningitis, see page 459.)

When Your Baby Has Problems

Although most babies develop normally in the uterus and are born healthy and normally formed, unfortunately, there are exceptions. Any condition present at birth is called congenital regardless of the cause. Many of these are genetic or hereditary conditions—conditions passed on through the genetic material of the mother or the father to the child. Others result from an abnormal development process resulting from any of

COPING WITH CHALLENGES

Giving birth to a baby with a serious disease or disorder can be a devastating experience. After the care and attention you have paid to a healthy pregnancy and the months of waiting to see your child, any imperfection, much less a serious problem, can cause a range of conflicting feelings. Parents may feel angry at the doctors, angry at a stranger with a healthy baby, even angry at the child, and certainly, at times, angry at each other. Feelings of guilt and self-blame are also common, although in most cases there is little, if anything, the parents could have done to change the situation. Such feelings are normal, and the sooner you face them, the sooner you can get on to the work at hand: caring for your baby and taking care of yourself.

If your baby is born with problems, you will need help, and you should not be afraid to ask for it. Coping with a healthy baby is stressful for many parents; coping with a baby with problems can push you to your limit. The best thing you can do for yourself and your family is to ask for help from family and friends and accept it when it is given. When people ask what they can do, do not say "nothing"; give them a concrete task. The more help you have in caring for siblings, if there are any, and the tasks of the day, the more available you will be able to be to your baby.

One of the first things you will have to deal with if you have a baby with problems is what you tell others, from family members to neighbors. People will have a reaction to a baby when there is something visibly wrong. Most people want only to do what is right, but they do not know what that is. By being honest about what is wrong with your child, you may not only help them find the right words to say, you may help yourself get some added support, or at least avoid an uncomfortable moment you don't need.

As the parent of a child with problems, it will be even harder for you than other parents to find and take time for yourself, but more than in any other circumstance, you must. Being with your baby 24 hours a day, every day will not alleviate your baby's problems, and you will be more able to cope with the added burden of caring for a child with problems if you remember to take time for yourself. Spend time with friends, and make sure you and your spouse spend time together alone each week in the first few months of your baby's life, and more and more as time goes on.

Ask your doctor for information on support groups for parents, and try to contact other parents who are facing similar difficulties. For further information on coping with birth disorders, call your local chapter of The March of Dimes, or call the toll-free number, (888) MODIMES (663–4637). ■

a number of stresses like infection, environmental toxins, or maternal nutritional deficiencies. Still others occur during the birth process.

CONGENITAL ABNORMALITIES AND DISORDERS

Cleft palate or lip Sometimes the parts of the upper lip or the palate (roof of the mouth) fail to grow together, and a split, which may be tiny or extensive, remains at birth. About 1 in 1,000 newborns is affected by cleft lip and/or palate. Because sucking is difficult for a baby with cleft lip or palate, feeding can require patience. Your doctors and nurses will advise you about special nipples and positioning for feeding your baby. Ear and sinus infections are more common in babies with a cleft lip or palate, and your baby's hearing should be assessed by a specialist. Surgical closure of cleft lip is usually done when the baby is between 2 and 10 weeks old. Surgical closure of the palate may be done between 6 and 12 months, but sometimes later. The prognosis is excellent. While this is a genetic disorder, the risk for future pregnancy is small. You should consult your doctor for more detailed information.

Abnormalities of the feet *Clubfoot* One of the most common abnormalities of the feet, clubfoot occurs in 1 of 1,000 births. It involves malalignment of the bones of the ankle and foot. The tendons in the area are also tight. Clubfoot may range from mild and easily correctable to severe, and it may affect one or both feet. The technical term is equinovarus. The entire foot is turned inward toward the other leg, and the side of the foot faces down. If it were uncorrected, the child would eventually walk on the side of the foot. The cause of clubfoot remains unknown. Sometimes it is hereditary. Some cases of clubfoot are related to spina bifida, muscle disorders, or neurologic diseases. Treatment for very mild cases may be as simple as stretching of the foot by the parents. In more severe cases, plaster casts that are changed every few days beginning in the newborn period are quite effective. In the remaining cases, surgery, usually performed when the baby is between 6 and 12 months old, may be necessary. Clubfoot is not painful and does not bother the child

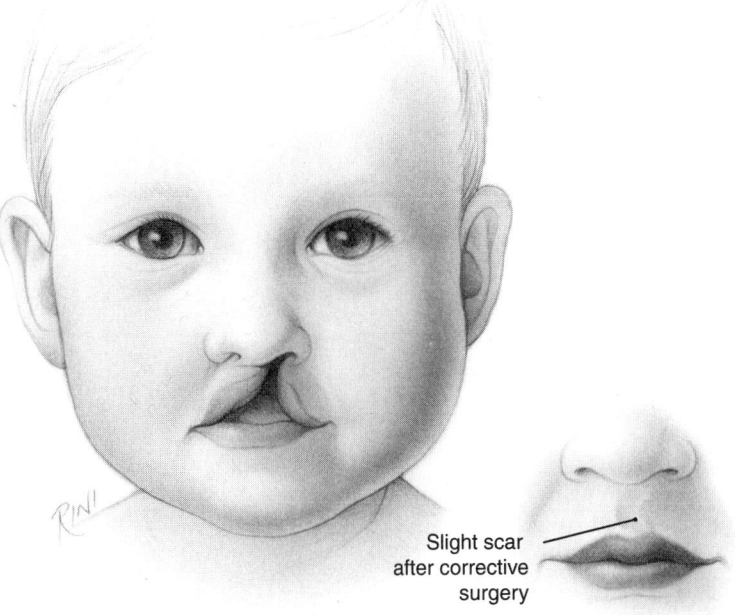

Slight scar after corrective surgery

Cleft lip. (A) In this congenital disorder, parts of the lip or palate may not grow together, leaving a split appearance. This can lead to difficulties with feeding and ear or sinus infections. (B) Surgical closure of a cleft lip can be done between 2 and 10 weeks of age, usually with excellent results.

until it is time to walk. With early, skilled care, the prognosis is good, and the child should be able to walk and run normally. (See page C-33.)

Calcaneovalgus foot The opposite of a clubfoot, the calcaneovalgus foot points up and out. It may be dramatic appearing, with the foot able to touch the leg. It is due to extreme positioning in the womb and resolves on its own after a few days to weeks, because the underlying bones and tendons are normal.

Metatarsus adductus This refers to an inward curvature of the front part of the foot; the back of the foot and ankle are normal. Metatarsus adductus is about three to five times more common than clubfoot. It tends to resolve on its own with growth, either quickly or slowly. For those who are showing no improvement toward the end of the first year, special shoes or casts may be recommended.

In-toeing or out-toeing The turning inward or outward of a newborn's feet and legs are

Webbed (joined) toes usually function normally and represent only a cosmetic problem.

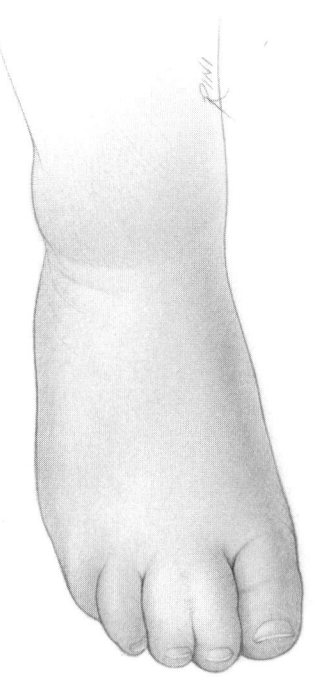

common problems. These positions are part of a developmental process that the legs go through with growth, influenced by heredity and position in the womb. These conditions usually correct themselves, although sometimes this takes several years. They almost never need treatment, a fact recently recognized and in contrast to the older tradition of extensive use of inserts, bars, and braces (to which grandmothers will attest).

Bowed legs and knock-knees These are also normal phases of development that correct themselves, although they can look quite worrisome for a time. Bowed legs do not need medical attention unless they have not started to correct by age 2 years, or unless the child has other medical problems or a family history of bowing. Knock-knees are most common at age 3 years and are virtually never a serious or permanent problem in otherwise normal children. (See page C-32.)

Webbing Webbing, or syndactyly, of the toes is usually only a cosmetic problem. Webbed toes almost always function normally, and surgery is rarely necessary.

Abnormalities of the hands *Polydactyly* This term applies to babies born with an extra finger or thumb. It is most commonly an extra finger at the base of, and smaller than, the fifth finger. It may be attached by skin only or by bone and ligaments to the other fingers. Polydactyly is at least 10 times more common in black children than in other races. If the extra digit is attached by skin only, it can easily be removed by tying it off with a suture. It will come off in a few days. If it is attached by bone, surgery to remove it is recommended when the baby is a few months old.

Webbing Webbing, or syndactyly, of the fingers is more troublesome than webbing of the toes and is usually treated surgically. When fingers are webbed, the individual digits are difficult to use. Surgery is usually recommended at age 6 to 12 months.

Trigger thumb In infants, one or both thumbs may not straighten or may give a soft pop in doing so. This is due to a congenital thickening of the tendon sheath, or covering, which can often be felt. If it does not improve in the first several years, a minor outpatient procedure will take care of this.

Clubhand Clubhand is an extremely rare condition that involves absence of the bone and tissue on the thumb side of the forearm (called radial clubhand). Often, this is associated with other abnormalities. Surgery

In polydactyly, an extra finger is usually present on the side of the hand opposite the thumb. If bone is part of the extra finger, surgery may be needed to remove it.

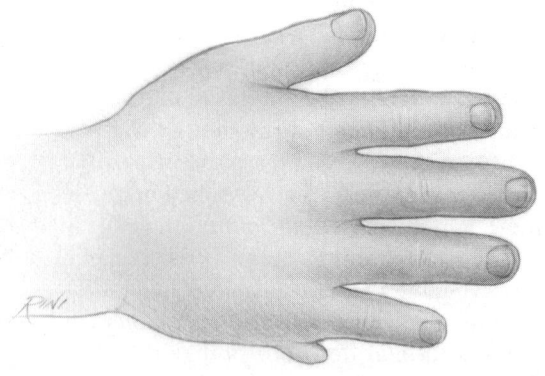

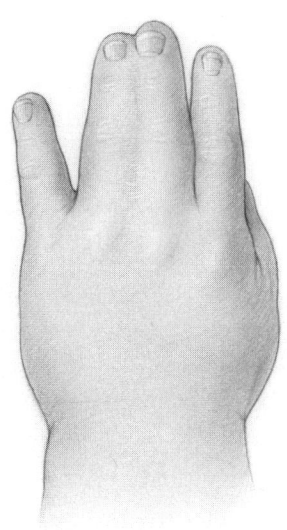

Syndactyly (webbing of fingers). Joined fingers are difficult to use. Surgical treatment can be done between age 6 and 12 months to correct the problem.

may be done in early childhood to reposition the hand. Sometimes several procedures are necessary.

Skeletal disorders The most common serious skeletal disorder of infants is developmental dysplasia of the hip. It is usually caused by abnormal positioning or pressure on the hip joint during development in the uterus. Dislocation occurs before or after birth. It is more common in babies who were in a breech position in the womb just before birth (even if delivered by cesarean section), in girls, or in those who had a relative with the same condition. All babies should be checked for this in the newborn period, although rarely, a dislocation may be impossible to detect. The signs include a hip that does not spread outward (abduct) normally during diaper changing or a thigh that appears foreshortened or has abnormal movement. An ultrasound test may confirm the diagnosis. In many cases, a dislocated hip diagnosed soon after birth may be successfully treated by a brace. In other cases, a cast or surgery may be needed. Early treatment gives the best chance of a good result.

Skeletal dysplasia, or dwarfism, is a more serious skeletal disorder. There are over 100 types of skeletal dysplasia, and most are diagnosable early. By far the most common skeletal dysplasia is achondroplasia. The trunk is short, and the limbs are relatively shorter (see page C-33). Intelligence is normal, and affected children usually achieve independence although they may be delayed in reaching their milestones. Depending on the type of skeletal dysplasia, there may be problems with the spine, hearing, kidneys, or immune system. Parents of a baby with skeletal dysplasia should seek a geneticist to confirm the diagnosis, outline treatment, and estimate the degree of risk that future siblings face.

Down syndrome (trisomy 21) Human cells contain 22 pairs of chromosomes and 2 sex chromosomes, for a total of 46 chromosomes. At conception, the 23 single chromosomes in the egg cell from the mother join with the 23 single chromosomes in the sperm cell from the father to give the fertilized egg 2 copies—or a pair—of each of the 23 different chromosomes. In about 1 in 600 newborns, an error in chromosome division and duplication has occurred such that the infant has inherited not just a pair but three copies of chromosome 21. In the instance of most other chromosomes, presence of a third causes such developmental havoc that the fetus cannot survive, and early miscarriage results. But in trisomy 21, commonly termed Down syndrome, infants usually survive to term, making this abnormality the most common chromosomal malformation-retardation syndrome.

Such errors in duplication or division of chromosomes occur more commonly in old eggs and therefore, the incidence of Down syndrome increases as maternal age increases, from negligible risk in young mothers to 1 in 380 in women who become pregnant at age 35 and increasing to 1 in 30 by age 45. (See page 148 for information on prenatal testing for Down syndrome.)

Infants born with Down syndrome may be normal in size at birth, but they grow more slowly than babies who are not affected and are hypotonic (floppy). They may be difficult to feed. Most babies with Down syndrome show a distinct set of physical features that form a recognizable pattern. These features include a relatively small head that is flat in the back, small ears, extra skin at the neck, upslanting eyes, flat nasal bridge, protruding tongue, wide space between the first and second toe, and short, broad hands with a crease going straight across the palm.

Congenital heart problems—such as valvular malformations, ventricular and atrial septal defects and tetralogy of Fallot—

occur in one third to one half of the children born with Down syndrome (see Congenital Heart Defects, page 224, and Chapter 20) and often require surgical correction. Stomach or intestinal defects such as interruption of the intestine at the level of the duodenum (duodenal atresia) occur much less commonly (in fewer than 10 percent), but when they do occur, they require surgical correction. Such problems as these contribute to the higher than average infant and childhood mortality among children with Down syndrome.

Children with Down syndrome have an increased likelihood of developing pulmonary hypertension, sleep apnea (periodic cessation of breathing during sleep), hypothyroidism (underactive thyroid gland), and gastric acid reflux. They are also more susceptible to respiratory infections, especially pneumonia, and have a higher than average risk of developing leukemia. Vision and hearing problems may also be present. Instability of the cervical spine is common, and x-rays must be taken to detect it, especially before children with Down syndrome play sports. Additional medical problems often develop among people with Down syndrome who survive into adulthood.

Nearly all children with Down syndrome have some degree of mental impairment, often moderate, but sometimes profound. Nevertheless, babies born with Down syndrome are now believed to have greater capabilities than they once were thought to have. Early therapeutic intervention can enhance these capabilities. This new, active approach to treatment has helped to decrease the number of babies with Down syndrome who are severely retarded.

Blindness or visual loss A leading cause of visual loss in infants is retinopathy of prematurity (ROP), previously termed retrolental fibroplasia. ROP occurs in infants born prematurely, by definition, with low birth weights and may be related to the administration of life-sustaining oxygen to the baby after birth.

With thorough ophthalmologic eye examinations provided to premature infants while in the hospital, ROP can be diagnosed earlier and treated promptly by the ophthalmologist. This may prevent further vision loss.

Other causes of decreased vision in infancy include birth trauma directly to the eye, fetal exposure to infection during the

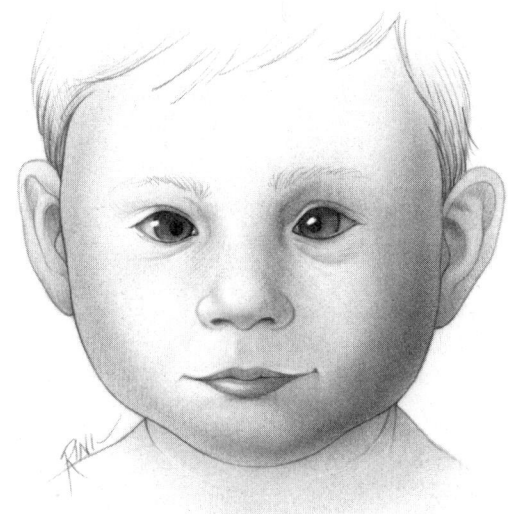

Eyes may cross if one eye wanders inward, toward the nose. This can lead to difficulties with vision, and a doctor should be consulted.

pregnancy or when passing through the birth canal, certain inherited diseases, and damage to the parts of the eyes and brain that process and transfer visual information from the eye through the brain to the vision centers, among others.

Within the first 6 months of life, it may be difficult to recognize that a baby has decreased vision. Sometimes a baby with decreased vision in one eye will object to covering the eye with better vision. The eye with poor vision may also wander in (toward the nose) or out (toward the ear). If a baby has decreased vision in both eyes, the eyes may jiggle and demonstrate rapid, unfocused eye movements. Failure of the baby to reach milestones such as crawling or picking up or reaching for objects suggests poor vision in one or both eyes.

If any symptoms that might indicate poor vision are noted in your baby, do not wait to seek help. Talk with your doctor. Your baby should be evaluated by an opthalmologist, preferably a pediatric opthalmologist, as soon as possible. Rarely, cancer may develop in an eye, causing decreased vision with or without a white pupil or crossed eyes (turning in or out).

If your child has visual difficulties, talk to your doctor about community and social support. (See Chapter 15 for further information.)

Deafness or hearing loss Some babies are at greater risk for hearing impairment than are others and should receive routine audiologic examination. Among those at higher risk are low-birth-weight babies (under 2,500 g or 5 lb, 8 oz); babies who experienced serious complications at birth or shortly thereafter, including asphyxia, intracranial hemorrhage, or seizures; babies who were exposed to drugs or infections known to affect hearing (such as rubella or cytomegalovirus) while in the womb; and infants with a family history of inherited or unexplained deafness. Children who are mentally retarded or blind or who have visible abnormalities of the ears or cerebral palsy are also at greater risk for hearing loss or deafness. If your baby seems not to respond to sounds, you should discuss this with your doctor and ask for testing. The sooner hearing loss or deafness is diagnosed, the better for your child. (See Chapter 16 for more information.)

Ambiguous genitalia During the first 6 weeks of development, the fetus has the potential to develop into either a boy or a girl. Then the sex chromosomes, normally XY for a boy and XX for a girl, begin to orchestrate a delicate process during which the gonads become either testes or ovaries and appropriate ducts form to transport sperm or eggs. A uterus and vagina form in a girl, and the external genitalia become either penis and scrotum (into which the testes descend) or clitoris and labia.

This sexual differentiation depends not only on the right number of chromosomes and correct signals from them but also on the presence and correct amounts of a number of hormones at just the right time, the maternal environment in which the fetus develops, and the ability of fetal tissues to react to chemical signals. Even though the process is complex, it usually works well. However, it can be interrupted in a number of ways, leading to mixed or incomplete development. In these rare situations the baby may be born with genitalia that do not clearly indicate gender. The genitals may look like a small penis and scrotum without testes or, alternatively, an extra large clitoris and labia that could be a scrotum, or there may not be much at all where the genitals should be. The baby is then said to have ambiguous genitalia.

When a baby's sex is not clear at birth, it will take a team of doctors and a series of tests to determine what the baby's genetic gender is, what hormones the baby is making, what internal sexual structures the baby has been born with, and what medical and surgical treatments the baby may need to grow up into an adult with a satisfying gender role and sexual function. Sometimes the abnormalities will also involve the urinary tract. In most cases, this investigation will also provide clues as to what led to the abnormal sexual development.

The parents will want to know as soon as possible whether they should be rearing the child as a girl or a boy. Needless to say, this is an extremely stressful situation for everyone, so it is important for the doctors and the family to work together to make decisions that are well thought out and the best possible ones for the baby's future.

Penile problems Problems of the penis are relatively common in male newborns. While generally not serious, they often require surgical intervention.

Hypospadias Hypospadias is one of the most common congenital anomalies of the penis, occurring in 1 in 300 newborn boys. In hypospadias, the urinary tube (urethra) opens somewhere along the shaft of the penis instead of at the tip. In severe conditions of hypospadias, the opening can be in the scrotum, behind the scrotum, or even near the anus. In addition to the urethra being in the wrong location, the penis can be bent downward, which is a condition known as chordee of the penis. In hypospadias, there is foreskin on the top of the penis

Hypospadias of the penis. In this abnormality of the penis, a boy's urinary tube (urethra) does not open at the penile tip, but more commonly opens along the penile shaft.

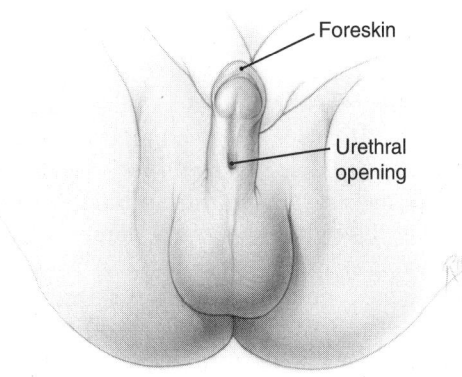

Foreskin

Urethral opening

but no foreskin on the bottom side of the penis.

A newborn with hypospadias should not undergo circumcision, because the foreskin is used in all cases to help repair the hypospadias when the child is older. Surgery is usually performed between age 6 and 18 months. With modern surgical techniques, the repair of hypospadias is very straightforward, and the results are excellent. Occasionally, complications do occur, but these are typically minor. Repair of hypospadias is very important as far as long-term sexual function is concerned so that urination and ejaculation can occur in an appropriate manner.

Phimosis When the foreskin is so tight it cannot be pulled back over the glans of the uncircumcised penis, the condition is called phimosis. Phimosis may be congenital or the result of scarring. Phimosis is not a diagnosis that is typically made in young infants. In the majority of infants, the foreskin is not retractable, and parents must be patient as the foreskin gradually stretches and grows. Most are retractable by the time the child reaches age 5 years. Trying to forcefully retract the foreskin over the glans of the penis when the child is quite young can lead to scarring and the development of secondary phimosis, with the resultant need for later circumcision.

Paraphimosis Paraphimosis occurs when the foreskin is retracted so much that it cannot be drawn back over the end of the penis, and the skin swells. Paraphimosis may cause painful swelling. Treatment involves applying gentle pressure to bring down the swelling and allow the foreskin to be brought over the end of the penis. If this condition persists, circumcision may be necessary. However, this typically occurs in older, uncircumcised children, not in infants.

Undescended testes Like the ovaries in girls, the testes in boys develop within the abdominal cavity near the kidneys. Around the eighth month of pregnancy, the testes make their way from their position in the pelvis through the internal inguinal ring opening in the lower abdominal wall, traverse the inguinal canal and the groin, and enter the scrotal pouch. The purpose of this migration is that the testes lie in an environ-

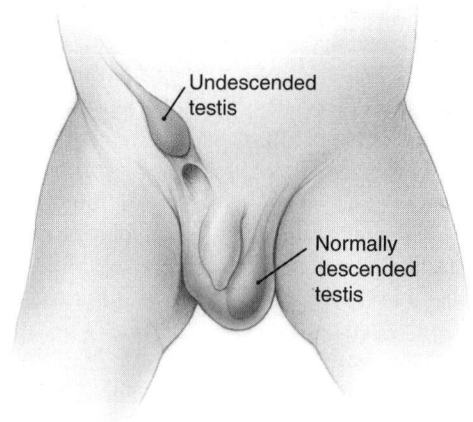

If one or both testes fail to migrate downward from the pelvis through the internal canal and into the scrotum by age 1 year, surgical repair may be needed to prevent decreased fertility and increased risk of testicular cancer later in life.

ment that is slightly cooler than in the body proper, a condition necessary for normal sperm production. In about 1 in 30 full-term newborn boys and 1 in 3 premature babies, the journey of the testes into the groin is arrested, with one or both testes not present in the scrotal sac. In many cases, the testes complete their descent during the first few months of life and can be examined and felt in the scrotum. However, if by age 1 year the testicles are still not in the scrotum, the child will likely need surgical repair to bring the testes down into the scrotum. Hormonal treatment of the undescended testes in North America has only a limited success rate. However, our European colleagues have reported success rates as high as 30 to 40 percent. Surgery to bring the testes into the scrotum is a simple procedure, usually performed on an outpatient basis. It is important to get the testes down before the boy is age 2 years, because some research has shown that changes occur in undescended testes after 2 years and may harm later fertility. Often, with an undescended testis, there is a small hernia present that can easily be repaired at the time the testes are brought down.

Although undescended testes are not painful, if they are not corrected, they carry a significant risk later in life of decreased fertility and testicular cancer. There is an increased risk of testicular cancer in young men whose testes never descend; and while the medical literature does not show that bringing the testes down confers any protection against malignancy, this still should be accomplished. Studies looking at malignancy rates were done in boys who had their testes brought down later in life, typically between ages 7 and 10. Since testes are now being brought down in the first year to 18 months of life, it is likely that in 25 to 30 years the risk of testicular malignancy associated with undescended testes will decrease. Although currently we cannot say that early orchiopexy removes the risk of testicular cancer, it does bring the testis into the scrotum where it can be examined, both by the doctor and by young men when they enter the risk group for testicular tumor, usually between age 25 and 45 (see page 1143).

Extra nipples Sometimes babies are born with one or more extra nipples. These occur along the same line as the normal nipple and may appear as no more than a dark spot. This condition occurs equally in newborn boys and girls. Such nipples are rarely fully developed and rarely present a medical problem. They can be removed for cosmetic purposes if desired.

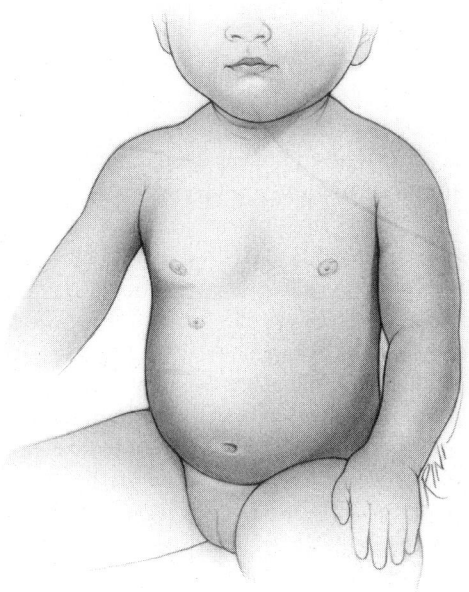

Extra nipples sometimes occur in both boys and girls. They are rarely fully formed but are sometimes removed for cosmetic purposes.

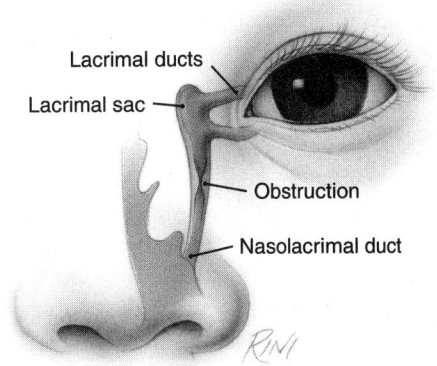

Obstructed nasolacrimal duct. If a duct from the eye to the nose is blocked, tears do not drain effectively, and they may overflow out of the eye and onto the cheek. Swelling, redness, and infections can develop, requiring treatment. The condition often disappears by 1 year of age.

Congenital obstruction of the nasolacrimal duct When a person cries, tears enter the tear ducts, which start at openings in the inner corners of the eyelid margins and travel toward and empty into the nose. If this delicate drainage system becomes partially or totally obstructed, the tears do not effectively drain and instead accumulate on the surface of the eye and overflow onto the cheek. This may affect one or both eyes.

Sometimes, the drainage system is not fully open at birth. The baby's eyes may appear wet, and, in some cases, a mucous discharge may build up in the corners. Sometimes, an infection develops within the blocked tear drainage system, and the area on the nose under the eye may become swollen and red. The doctor may recommend gentle massage of the duct system and may prescribe antibiotic drops to help treat infection. In the majority of infants with congenital blockage of the nasolacrimal duct, the condition resolves on its own by age 1 year; however, in some cases, the ophthalmologist may recommend taking action to open the drainage system sooner.

CONGENITAL CENTRAL NERVOUS SYSTEM DISORDERS

The central nervous system comprises the brain and the spinal cord. It directs all thoughts and actions. The proper construction and functioning of the central nervous system is crucial to normal development and capabilities.

Cerebral palsy Cerebral palsy is the most common childhood disorder of movement and posture. It occurs because of a central nervous system anomaly or because of insult or damage to the immature brain. Cerebral palsy is present in about 1 in 500 babies and ranges greatly in severity. Cerebral palsy may not be apparent at birth and may not be diagnosed until motor delay becomes significant, between age 6 and 18 months. The diagnosis is made on physical examination. Computed tomography (CT) and magnetic resonance imaging (MRI) scans may help to define structural abnormalities and determine the timing of the cerebral palsy.

As yet, it is rarely possible to identify a single, certain cause of cerebral palsy. Sometimes, a careful reconstruction of events during pregnancy or delivery will turn up factors thought to be associated, such as fetal distress during a difficult labor, extreme prematurity or low birth weight, exposure to a toxic substance during pregnancy, lack of oxygen supply to the infant, or some other issue. While birth factors have been noted to be associated with cerebral palsy, these are usually not causal. Babies with unusual nervous systems have unusual prenatal courses, labors, and deliveries.

As they grow, babies with cerebral palsy manifest varying degrees of impairment of central nervous system control over voluntary muscles. Sometimes the results are mild, manifested by nothing more than discoordination in running, for example. Sometimes the results are severe, leading to paralysis or major muscle spasticity. This in turn results in imbalance of opposing muscle groups on the growing skeleton. The imbalanced pull can give rise to bony deformities, joint dislocations (coming out of joint) or contractures (permanently bent position), and often, twisting of the spine.

Cerebral palsy may manifest itself in certain patterns of motor abnormalities. Hemiplegia affects half the body, with the hand usually more involved than the leg. Diplegia, often associated with prematurity, involves both legs but spares hand function. Quadriplegia involves all four extremities. The motor disability of some children extends beyond the limbs and trunk and may affect speech, swallowing, and breathing.

Cerebral palsy is defined by motor disability, but it is associated with other brain-based problems. Visual problems (especially strabismus), hearing loss, learning disabilities, language disorders, spatial problems, and mental retardation are all common, though not invariably present, in children with cerebral palsy.

There is no cure for cerebral palsy. The brain lesion (problem) cannot be repaired. However, much can be done to diminish the motor deficits that arise as a result of the brain lesion. Abnormalities of tone can be addressed by physical therapy, bracing and positioning, medications, nerve blocks, or orthopedic or neurosurgery. Circumvention of many of the motor problems is possible as a result of the ongoing revolution in electronics and computers.

Your role as your child's advocate and caretaker will be a challenging one as treatment continually evolves. Early treatment will concentrate on improving motor function, but in the preschool years, improving communication abilities will become increasingly important. As your child ages, school performance and social acceptance will be of concern. Throughout these years, you will need to ensure that your child receives the services guaranteed by law, as well as any surgical or drug treatments that can prevent deformity and improve motor function. It is crucial in the care of a child with cerebral palsy that the parents and caregivers understand the strengths and weaknesses of that individual child to best help him attain the highest possible level of function through physical and occupational therapy, speech therapy (if needed), and choice of a school environment appropriate to the child's abilities. See page 474 for more information on cerebral palsy.

Hydrocephalus The brain produces a liquid, called cerebrospinal fluid (CSF), which acts as a thin layer of protection, a shock-absorbing cushion in which the brain and spinal cord "float." Occasionally—in about 1 birth in 1,000—reabsorption of CSF is inadequate, resulting in a buildup of excess fluid around the brain. Because the bones of the infant's skull have not yet fused, they can expand as the extra fluid accumulates; the expansion results in the infant's developing an extremely large head, sometimes suffi-

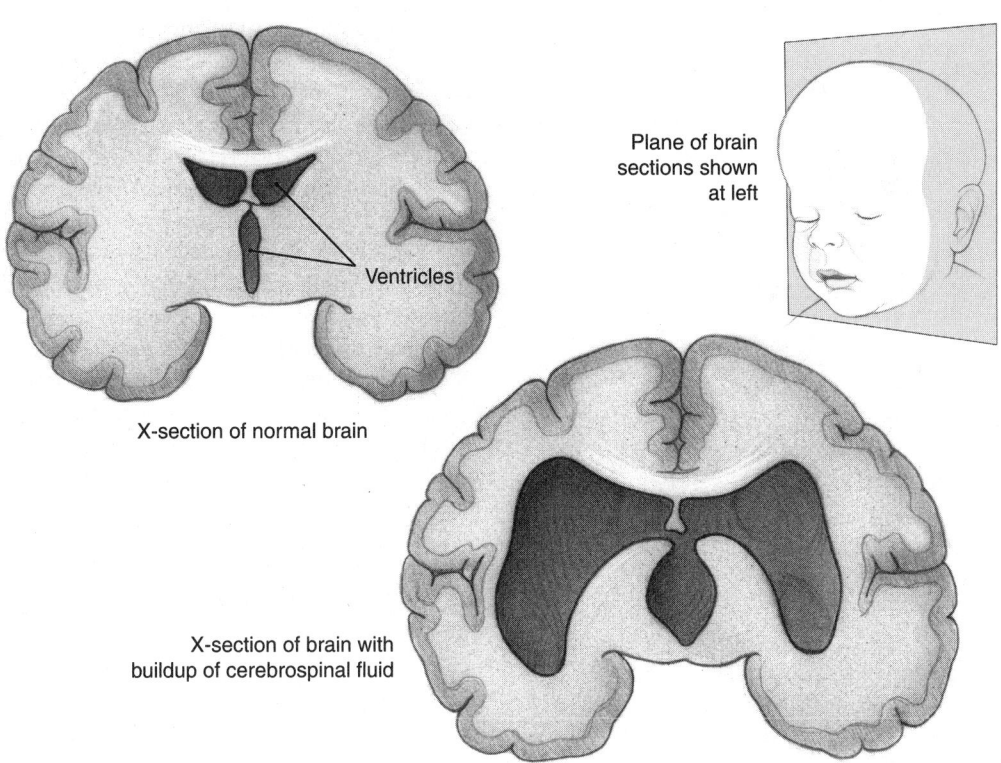

Ventricles

X-section of normal brain

Plane of brain sections shown at left

X-section of brain with buildup of cerebrospinal fluid

Inadequate flow and reabsorption of cerebrospinal fluid may lead to a buildup of fluid inside the brain called hydrocephalus. The baby's soft head can enlarge and make delivery difficult. A tube inserted after birth to shunt the fluid from the ventricles of the brain into the abdomen can improve the outcome significantly.

ciently large to make normal vaginal delivery of the baby impossible. The condition is usually present at birth, but sometimes swelling of the head does not become apparent till after birth.

To decrease the excess fluid, the best and most successful treatment involves surgery to place a permanent drainage tube—called a shunt—in the infant's head. From there, the surgeon burrows a long, thin, flexible catheter beneath the skin, in most cases down to the abdomen, where its tip will enter the abdominal cavity. The excess fluid will then flow through the tube to empty into the abdominal cavity, which can easily absorb it. This method of treatment generally greatly improves outcome for infants born with this disorder, both in terms of survival and quality of life. Without help, over half of infants born with hydrocephalus would die. Treated promptly and appropriately, more than 70 percent will live, and a significant number will have normal intelligence.

Spina bifida The spinal cord of the fetus is formed very early in pregnancy. At birth, it is normally fully enclosed beneath the skin within soft covering tissue layers (meninges) and the bones of the spine. In 1 to 5 births in 1,000, however, the closure is incom-

plete. The resultant opening can be so tiny it is not noticeable except on x-ray—called spina bifida occulta—with a birthmark or tuft of hair as the only visible sign of a problem below. Or the defect can be large enough that part of the spinal cord and its coverings protrude—called myelomeningocele—leading to a variety of problems ranging from lower limb muscle weakness and paralysis to problems with bowel and bladder control (see page C-33). Most commonly, the defect occurs in the lower back, but it can appear anywhere along the course of the spinal cord. The higher up, the more serious and complicated the problem will be. Fortunately, the most severe form of spina bifida is the rarest.

Spina bifida occurs more commonly in girls than boys, tends to run in families, and has been associated with the mother's having had a high fever or low levels of some vitamins, particularly folic acid, during pregnancy. Certain drugs taken during pregnancy can also increase the risk of spina bifida, notably clomiphene (a fertility drug) and valproic acid (taken for control of seizures). If the doctor suspects spina bifida, he can use ultrasound examinations and laboratory tests to confirm the disorder while the baby is still in the womb. A test performed during the third or fourth month

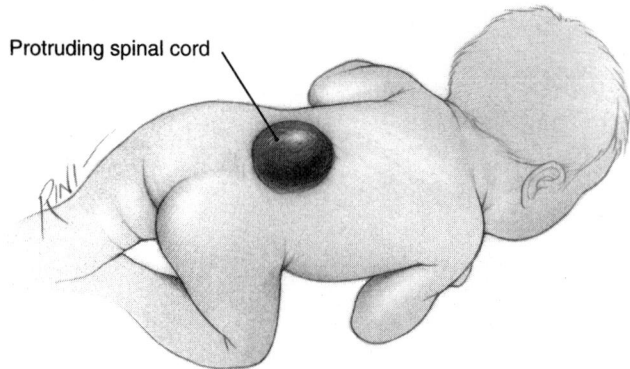

Protruding spinal cord

In spina bifida, the spinal cord can protrude abnormally against or through the skin, leading to weakness or paralysis of the lower extremities and problems with bowel or bladder control. Testing can confirm the existence of this disorder before birth. Treatments include surgery and medical care.

of pregnancy on the mother's blood or on the amniotic fluid that surrounds the baby detects a protein substance, called alpha-fetoprotein, present in high amounts only when CSF leaks from the defect.

Advances in neurosurgery, urologic surgery, and orthopedic and medical care now allow many children with spina bifida to survive with good intelligence and relatively normal longevity. Many factors influence the possibility of one of the most important goals, walking. These include whether there are other skeletal abnormalities, such as hip dislocations, foot deformities, or scoliosis—all of which occur quite commonly and may require surgery to correct; how high along the spinal cord the opening occurred; as well as the degree of motivation and cooperation of the child and family. Early, aggressive orthopedic care—especially physical therapy to strengthen the quadriceps muscles of the thighs and bracing to stabilize the legs—will make walking possible for many children. In higher degrees of paralysis, continued walking may become impossible after the child's body weight exceeds the amount his weakened muscles can support even with bracing. After that time, a wheelchair will allow the child to remain relatively independent and mobile.

Almost all children with spina bifida also suffer some urinary tract and bladder abnormalities that predispose them to infection and incontinence. As a consequence,

they will require regular and ongoing evaluation of the urinary tract. Achieving better bladder control may involve the use of catheters to drain urine regularly or medications to improve bladder muscle tone. For reasons that remain unclear, children with spina bifida have an increased tendency to develop allergy to latex. This may be related to their frequent and early exposure to it in catheters and sterile gloves used in their care. Because such allergies can occasionally develop into a life-threatening reaction (see Anaphylaxis, page 1341), great caution should be exercised in exposing children with spina bifida to latex or latex-containing products.

CONGENITAL HEART DEFECTS

Abnormalities of the heart or blood vessels near the heart are termed congenital when present at birth. Occurring in 1 percent of live births, congenital heart defects are usually of unknown cause, although viral diseases such as German measles contracted by the mother during pregnancy are thought to be contributing factors. Use of drugs and alcohol during pregnancy may also increase risk. Some of the more important congenital heart defects are described below.

Septal defects Occasionally, the muscular partition (septum) that separates the right and left sides of the heart will develop incompletely, leaving a small hole or window in what should be a solid wall. When this occurs between the atria (smaller upper heart chambers), it is called an atrial septal defect; when it occurs between the ventricles (lower pumping chambers), it is called a ventricular septal defect. The hole allows blood to flow abnormally between the atria or ventricles when the heart muscle contracts, sending blood at too high a pressure to the lungs or lessening the effectiveness of the contraction of the chambers and mixing blood that has been to the lungs to pick up oxygen with unoxygenated blood coming back from the lungs. Septal defects usually cause heart murmurs. However, not all murmurs indicate the presence of a septal defect.

If the defect is in the upper chambers or is a small hole in the ventricular chambers,

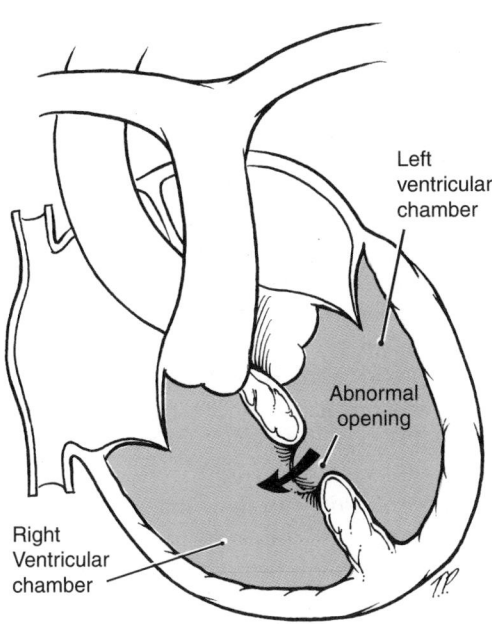

Left ventricular chamber

Abnormal opening

Right Ventricular chamber

Ventricular septal defect. An abnormal communication between a left chamber and a right chamber of the heart causes improper mixing of blood and may change blood pressures. Although some of these holes close without treatment, others can lead to heart failure or lung vessel damage and the need for medication or surgery.

there may be no symptoms, and the abnormality may either close on its own (about 30 to 70 percent of the time) or remain medically insignificant. However, if the defect between the ventricular chambers is large, it may cause difficulties in the first few weeks of life, including symptoms of heart failure such as irritability, poor feeding and growth, and breathing problems and pneumonia.

Treatment of a septal defect will depend on how large it is and how severe are the symptoms it causes. Medications to improve heart function will often be prescribed, followed by surgery to seal the hole with a patch. Ideally, holes in the ventricular septum should be repaired before age 2 years, and those of the atrial septum between age 3 and 6 years.

Tetralogy of Fallot Tetralogy of Fallot refers to a cluster of congenital heart abnormalities that include pulmonary artery obstruction, a shift of the aorta toward the right side of the heart, enlargement of the right heart pumping chamber (the ventricle), and a large hole in the wall between the ventricles (a ventricular septal defect).

The combined effect of these abnormalities results in a decrease in blood flow to the lungs. The right ventricle ordinarily pumps oxygen-poor blood to the lungs to pick up the oxygen for the left ventricle to pump to the brain and body. Poorly oxygenated blood leads to the main symptom of tetralogy of Fallot: cyanotic spells during which the child looks blue and which are relieved in older children by squatting. Depending on severity, tetralogy of Fallot may be discovered only because a baby has an unusual heart murmur, or it may be obvious in the first months of life because the baby has spells of blue skin (cyanosis).

Early treatment is aimed at improving the flow of blood to the lungs to quickly correct the oxygen starvation. The definitive treatment, however, involves surgical correction: open heart surgery to repair the hole in the wall between the ventricles, relieve any obstruction to flow in the pulmonary artery, and reposition the abnormally placed aorta.

Patent ductus arteriosus Before birth, the baby's blood gets its oxygen from the placenta, so the blood does not all need to go to the baby's lungs before being pumped out to the body. While the baby develops in the womb, a connection exists between the pulmonary artery that carries blood to the lungs and the aorta carrying blood to the body. Just after birth, this connection—

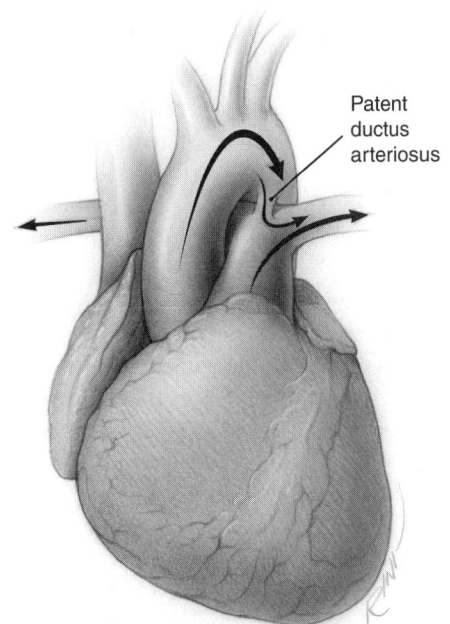

Patent ductus arteriosus

If the connection between the pulmonary arteries and aorta does not close after birth, abnormal blood flow occurs and problems can occur with breathing and growth. The opening often closes without treatment, but medications and surgery can correct the problem if needed.

which is called the ductus arteriosus—usually closes. Occasionally, and especially in infants born prematurely, it remains patent (open), causing abnormal blood flow and a murmur. Sometimes, the flow through the patent ductus to the lungs is so great that it causes breathing problems and interferes with growth. In most instances, especially when associated with prematurity, it will close on its own within a few weeks. If the ductus connection fails to close, indomethacin, an antiprostaglandin drug, may induce it to close. The ductus can also be closed with simple surgery before age 2 years.

The condition occurs more commonly in children born at high altitudes, in female infants, and in babies born to women who contract rubella during the early stages of pregnancy. This is only one of the many problems that rubella can cause. All women of childbearing age who have not had rubella vaccine should receive vaccination against the virus before they become pregnant (see page 143).

Stenosis: pulmonary/aortic Stenosis—abnormal narrowing—of the valve or vessel leading from the heart to the lung (pulmonary stenosis) or from the heart to the body as a whole (aortic stenosis) limits blood flow. Although all such abnormalities are present at birth, mild stenoses may not cause symptoms and may go undetected until a doctor hears a heart murmur on a routine examination. Mild-to-moderate narrowing may not require surgery or even any modification in activity, although the baby may require regular visits to the cardiologist to monitor the situation. Even though mild stenoses may not be of sufficient degree to cause symptoms when the baby is small, as he grows, so does the demand to increase blood flow. And at some future time, the stenosis may limit the ability to meet this demand. (For more information, see also Disorders of the Heart Valves and Lining, page 815). Severe narrowing may cause breathlessness. These more severe degrees of obstruction will require open heart surgery to correct the narrowing as soon as possible.

Coarctation of the aorta Coarctation, or narrowing, of the aorta, if mild, may cause no discernible symptoms and may not be discovered until the teen years or even adulthood or may present with hyperten-

sion (high blood pressure). For more information about this condition, see Chapter 20.

In infants, if the narrowing is extreme, symptoms may be present from birth; the narrowing of the aorta may put such a strain on the heart muscle that it is overloaded. In such cases, surgery (preferably before age 5 years) to open or remove the narrowed segment will be necessary.

Transposition of the great vessels Two main arteries leave the heart. Collectively termed the "great vessels," they are the pulmonary artery, normally carrying oxygen-poor blood from the right side of the heart to the lungs, and the aorta, carrying freshly oxygenated blood from the left side of the heart to the rest of the body as a whole. Rarely, the great vessels develop in a reverse position, a situation that results in sending blood to the body that has not been through the lungs to receive oxygen and eliminate carbon dioxide. The baby's skin will appear blue (cyanotic) from lack of oxygen, and he will require immediate medical attention and urgent surgery to restore the great vessels to their correct positions.

CONGENITAL URINARY AND GASTROINTESTINAL DISORDERS

Hydronephrosis The fetal kidneys begin working to produce urine before birth. As will occur after birth, the urine flows into the kidney's collecting tubes, down the ureters, into the bladder, and out of the urethra. Before birth, it empties into the amniotic fluid. Any obstruction along the way will result in hydronephrosis: urine backing up under pressure, overfilling and stretching the ureters and kidneys. The pressure can permanently damage the kidneys.

An ultrasound test—used to see the baby in the womb—sometimes detects hydronephrosis. Because many pregnant women have routine prenatal ultrasounds, these blockages are often diagnosed before birth. If the ultrasound reveals a problem, serial exams are done to see if the swelling of the kidneys or ureters is increasing. Often, this condition can be watched until delivery, when appropriate diagnostic studies can be completed.

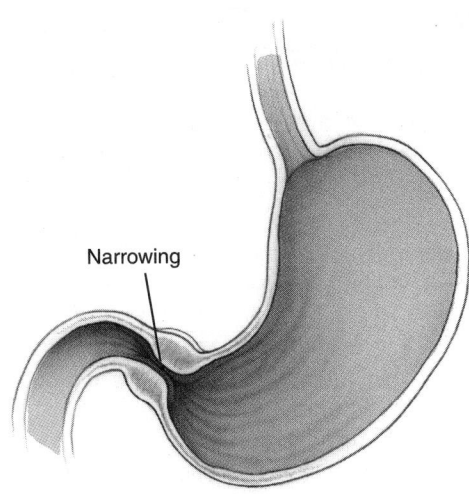

Narrowing

Pyloric stenosis. If the opening at the bottom of the stomach (the pylorus) is narrowed, food does not exit the stomach normally. Vomiting with dehydration can occur, and the baby can fail to gain weight properly. Surgical correction is very effective.

Sometimes, the condition is not discovered until after birth, when the doctor feels enlarged kidneys on abdominal exam or when the baby has problems with urination or urinary infections. Surgery is usually performed to relieve the obstruction (most often caused by a tight constriction where the ureters join the kidney or where the ureters join the bladder) as soon as possible in order to prevent continuing kidney damage.

Pyloric stenosis Narrowing of the pylorus—the bottom portion of the stomach at its outlet to the small intestine—occurs about five times more commonly in baby boys than in baby girls. About 1 in 150 newborn males and 1 in 750 females may develop it. Con-striction of the outlet restricts the normal passage of food from the stomach. The first symptom—forceful vomiting of food shortly after feeding—usually begins during the second or third week of life. After the food comes up, the baby usually seems hungry for more. The baby will usually fail to gain or may even lose weight and may become dehydrated, because most of what goes down comes back up.

The doctor will suspect the diagnosis from the timing and type of vomiting and may even be able to feel a small lump in the abdomen that corresponds to the thickened pylorus muscle. An ultrasound test or gastrointestinal (GI) tract x-ray called an upper GI series can confirm the doctor's suspicion of pyloric stenosis. As soon as the baby receives enough intravenous fluid to correct any dehydration or chemical blood imbalances, the narrowing should be corrected with surgery. Within hours after the opening is widened, the baby usually will begin feeding and within days will be able to take full feedings without vomiting.

Esophageal and intestinal atresia *Atresia* means closure or absence of a normal structure; it can occur in a variety of locations along the GI tract. Atresia of the esophagus—the food tube connecting the mouth to the stomach—occurs in about 1 in 4,500 infants. In this condition, a segment of the esophagus does not fully develop, resulting in a gap between the upper and lower

Esophageal atresia. The esophagus, the food tube that should connect the mouth to the stomach, sometimes fails to grow completely, leading to a sudden "dead end." Esophageal atresia prevents the baby from swallowing normally, and surgery is required to correct the condition.

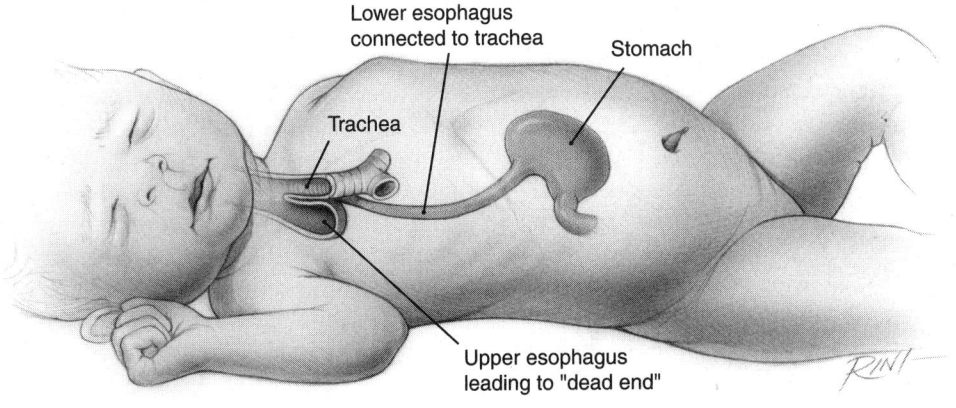

Lower esophagus connected to trachea

Stomach

Trachea

Upper esophagus leading to "dead end"

esophagus. This defect usually occurs along with abnormalities of the trachea (windpipe) or of the heart, urinary tract, and nervous system. Atresia of the esophagus will be apparent right away because the baby is unable to swallow his saliva and feedings and instead coughs and chokes in the first hours after birth. Surgery to reconstruct the esophagus will be performed either right away, when only a short segment is involved, or delayed until the esophagus grows in length. If surgery must be delayed, the surgeon will place a feeding tube directly into the stomach through the abdominal wall.

Atresia of a segment of intestine occurs more commonly than esophageal, in about 1 in 1,500 births. Symptoms include vomiting and a bloated abdomen. If the intestine is totally closed in the segment, the baby won't pass a bowel movement after the first few days of life; however, if the blockage is only partial, it may be more difficult to detect. An x-ray exam following a feeding of special x-ray dye will confirm the suspicion of atresia. Unless the narrowing is quite mild, the baby will require surgery to remove the bad segment. If the problem is identified promptly and corrected, complete recovery is the rule.

Bile duct atresia Very rarely (in about 1 in 75,000 infants), atresia occurs in the bile duct that carries the bile from the liver where it is produced to the gallbladder and the intestine. Buildup of the bile can irritate the liver, causing jaundice (yellowing of the skin) and other symptoms similar to hepatitis (liver inflammation) soon after birth (see Chapter 23). Because the pigments in bile give color to the stool, the bowel movements will be without the normal yellow-brown color. Often, the liver enlarges in size and may distend the abdomen.

Exploratory surgery to pinpoint the site of the underdevelopment will usually be necessary. On occasion, the atresia can be surgically corrected, but more often, there is no single spot of narrowing. The surgeon may endeavor to improve bile drainage by making a special connection—called a hepatoportoenterostomy—best performed within the first 3 months after birth. Up to 75 percent of babies with bile duct atresia continue to develop cirrhosis of the liver, and liver transplantation will be the only recourse to prevent death from liver failure.

Hirschsprung's disease In Hirschsprung's disease, or clonic aganglionosis, the rectum fails to move the stool out of the body through the anus, causing it to back up into the colon (large intestine). This happens because nerve ganglions required for normal movement of the intestine are absent from the last part of the large intestine. As a consequence, the baby cannot pass stool (the earliest sign of the condition), the colon gradually becomes quite dilated, and the baby vomits and feeds poorly. When the doctor examines the baby's rectum with a finger, it may initiate an almost explosive passage of feces. To confirm this suggestive clue, the pediatric surgeon or gastroenterologist will be asked to perform a rectal biopsy—removal of a small bit of the tissue for microscopic examination. If the biopsy confirms the diagnosis, the doctor will recommend surgery.

The surgical correction of Hirschsprung's disease usually occurs in two steps: The first, aimed at relieving the pressure that dilates the colon, creates a colostomy, an artificial opening for the colon through the abdominal wall that redirects the stool into an external plastic pouch; the second, done at about age 1 year, closes this temporary opening and brings the normal colon down to the anus, thus bypassing the abnormal rectum. Sometimes, stable infants of good size may have a one-stage operation before age 1 year that makes a colostomy unnecessary altogether.

Imperforate anus Sometimes, the anus (the opening of the rectum to the outside) fails to develop normally. Usually the abnormality is minor; for example, the opening may be too narrow (about 1 in 500 newborns) or abnormally placed. Less commonly (in about 1 in 5,000 newborns), major abnormalities occur, including total obstruction of the opening—a complete imperforate anus.

With too small an opening or no opening at all, the baby cannot pass stool—a problem that demands prompt correction. If the abnormality is simply narrowing, the pediatric surgeon can use an instrument to dilate the opening. However, if a web or membrane of tissue blocks the opening, solving the problem will mean surgery. Often, a gap occurs between the blind end of the rectum and the outside skin of the buttock. The farther the rectum lies from the outside, the more significant the surgical procedure necessary to correct the problem. Occasionally, the abnormalities are so severe that correction of the problem requires complete surgical reconstruction of the anus. Usually, the doctor will temporarily divert the flow of stool away from the anus to allow the area to properly heal after reconstruction. This usually means temporarily creating an opening through the abdominal wall—a colostomy—so that the stool can pass into a plastic pouch worn on the outside. After 6 to 12 months, a second operation reattaches the colon to the anus and restores normal function. Infants with obstructions low in the anus can usually develop fully normal bowel control, while those with abnormalities higher up may have some persistent difficulty with constipation and soiling.

Diaphragmatic hernia The diaphragm, a powerful fan-like muscle that separates the chest cavity from the abdominal cavity, occasionally develops abnormally with a tear or hole that allows the contents of the abdominal cavity (that is, intestines) to protrude up into the chest cavity. When this happens, the space normally allotted for the heart and lungs is compressed, and the lung on the side of the defect may not fully develop. Most commonly, the infant develops breathing distress shortly after birth. When this potentially life-threatening situation occurs, it requires emergency surgery to bypass the lungs and oxygenate the blood, repair the diaphragm, and relieve the pressure on the heart and lungs.

Other times, however, the defect is not so large, so the growth and function of the lungs are not compromised. As a result, the abnormality may go undetected for some time—perhaps months—when such symp-

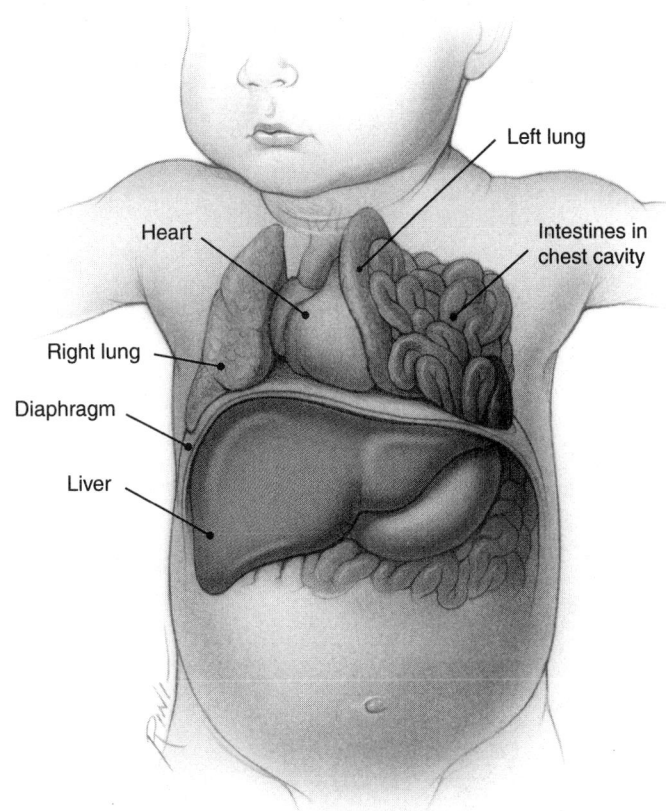

Diaphragmatic hernia. Intestines protrude into the chest if there is a hole in the diaphragm between the two cavities. Vomiting or constipation can occur, the heart and lungs may be compressed, and a lung may develop incompletely. Breathing can be difficult, requiring emergency surgery.

toms as vomiting, constipation, and colicky pain after eating may suggest its presence. The source of the problem may be revealed by chest x-rays that demonstrate the presence of intestine in the chest cavity.

The Preschool to Preteen Years

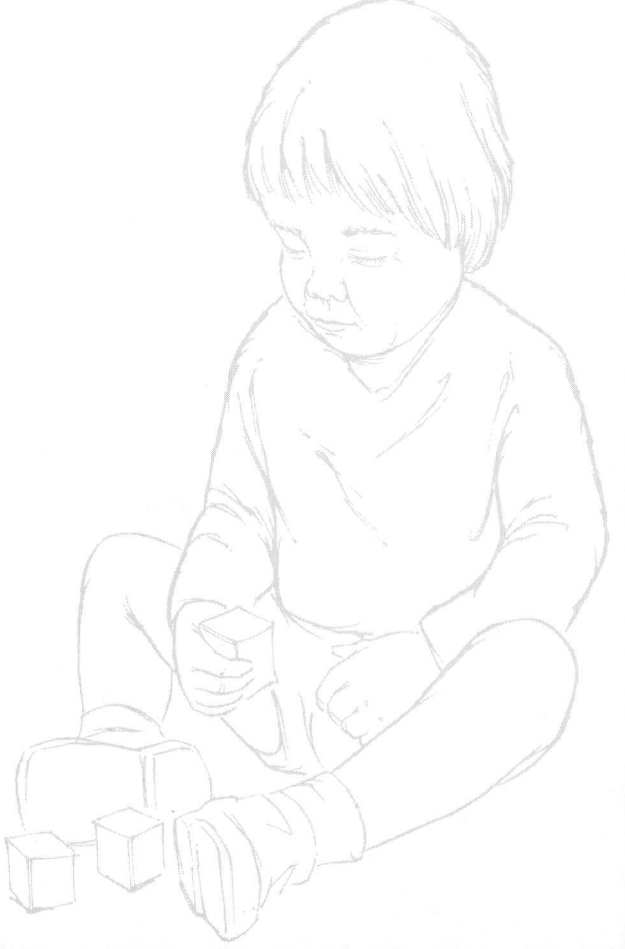

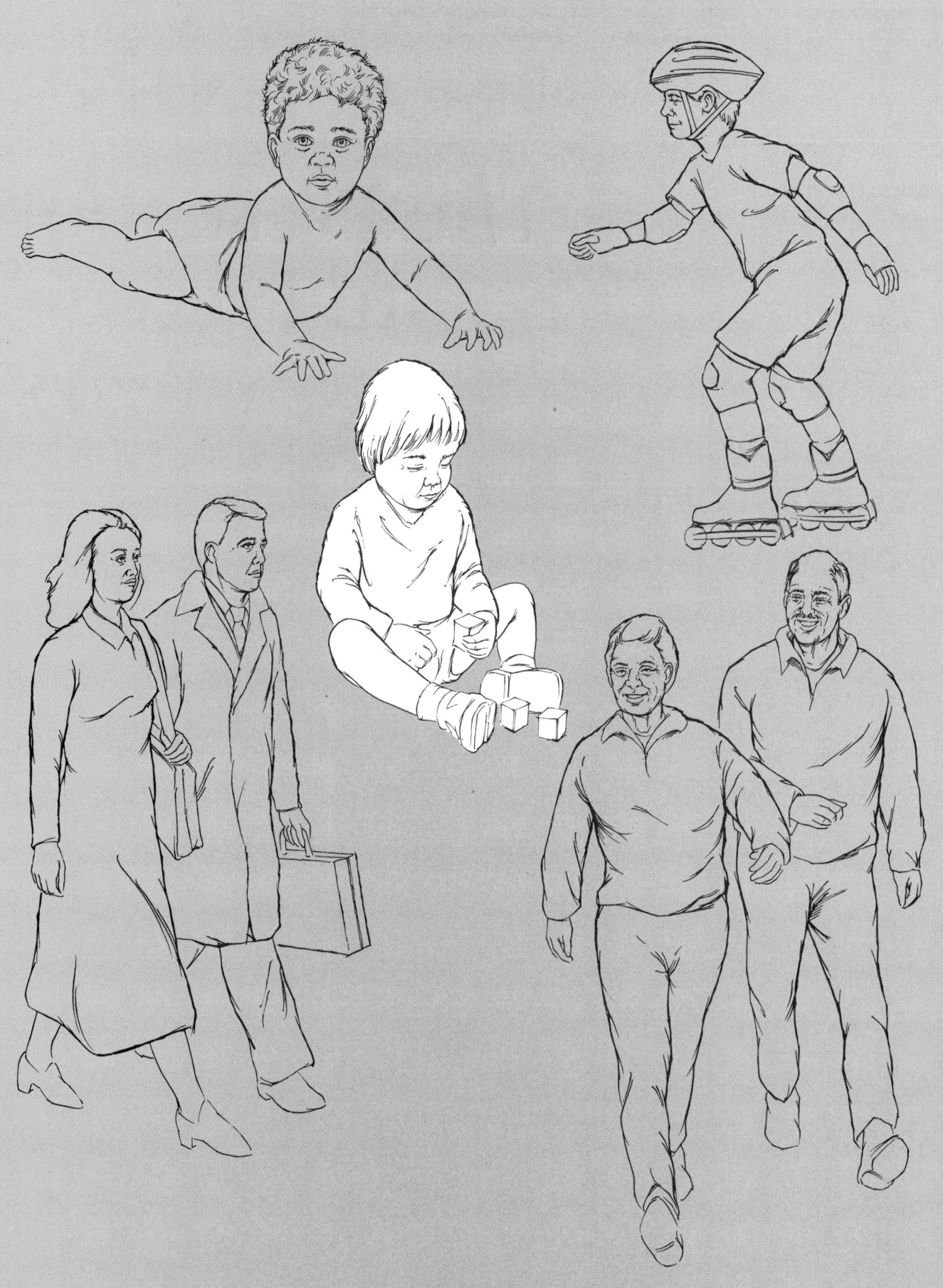

NINE

THE PRESCHOOL TO PRETEEN YEARS

Keeping Your Child Fit

Your doctor will help you maintain your child's good health through regular checkups, visits for occasional illness, information on immunizations, injury prevention, nutrition, exercise, and other needs. But what you, the parent, observe daily will be essential for raising a healthy and fit child. Most likely, you will be the one to spot an impending illness or pick up your child when she falls on the playground. You will be the one deciding when you should take her to the doctor—or even the emergency room—and when you should just give her acetaminophen and put her to bed. This chapter provides information about preventing illness and injury, common childhood illnesses, signs and symptoms of unusual behavior or development, and general advice that will help you ensure your child's health.

Injuries are the leading cause of death of children in the United States. One of the most important things you can do to keep your children well is to follow safety rules at home, in the car, and at play. See Chapter 3 for detailed advice on childproofing your home and preventing injuries in children of all ages. In addition to keeping watch over your children's safety, you will do well by your children to make sure they develop certain habits that will help build the foundation of good health, such as eating properly, getting adequate sleep, and exercising regularly.

IMMUNIZATIONS

The miracle of immunization has produced a kind of cultural amnesia about how very deadly life could be for children in the "good old days." Those who came of age in the years before Dr. Jonas Salk developed the polio vaccine remember the delight of summer's approach being overshadowed by the dread of polio, a crippling, potentially fatal disease that accompanied the onset of warm weather. Through immunization, we have had so much success in taming polio and other illnesses that many have forgotten that not so long ago these diseases disabled and killed large numbers of children and adults.

The proper immunizations are vital to your child's health. The number and type of vaccinations required are complex, but your doctor will advise you when your child is due for a vaccine and will keep an immunization record on your child, beginning at birth. Many vaccines are required by law, and you will be required to provide proof of immunization—usually a standard health form your doctor fills out—whenever your child enrolls in school, daycare, day camp, and such. Be sure to keep your child's immunizations up to date.

In a few situations, the immunization schedule needs to be modified. Most are rare and will be obvious to your doctor, but a few are worth mentioning. If your child has an immune disorder or is on medication that suppresses the immune system or lives with someone who does, you should discuss this with your doctor before having your child immunized. Injectable inactivated polio vaccine rather than oral polio vaccine probably will be chosen in this case. Because of the way some viral vaccines are made—for example, measles vaccine—doctors had been concerned that children with severe egg allergies might react to it. That has not seemed to be much of a problem—if any problem at all with today's measles vaccine—but you should remind your doctor if your child has an egg allergy so it can be taken into consideration. Certainly, if your child has had a severe reaction to a previous dose of vaccine, inform your doctor before your child has another dose.

Some parents have decided to gamble with their children's health and not have them vaccinated out of the misguided notion that vaccines are harmful. Although serious complications from immunization have occurred, they occur very, very rarely, and all vaccines recommended for children are considerably less risky than the diseases they protect against. Most side effects are mild. Fever or soreness can be treated with weight-appropriate doses of a medication, such as acetaminophen, as your doctor directs. Never use aspirin to relieve fever in children unless your doctor specifically prescribes it. Administration of aspirin during certain viral infections has been associated with Reye's syndrome, a rare and potentially deadly form of liver failure (see pages 463 and 854).

Some vaccine reactions, however, can be severe, though these occur only rarely. If you suspect that your child is having one of these reactions, you should contact your doctor immediately.

See Chapter 8, page 194, for specific information on immunization schedule guidelines.

THE IMPORTANCE OF BASIC HYGIENE

Basic hygienic habits can, if adhered to, prevent numerous illnesses. Hand washing is one of the most important things you and your child can do to prevent illness. Quite simply, it helps to prevent the spread of germs that cause disease. Teaching your child to wash her hands after using the bathroom and before meals should be a priority. There is no need to make your child fearful of invisible "bugs," but she should learn to wash her hands before eating and after going to the bathroom as reflexively as she learns to wear her seatbelt in the car.

Children should also learn the importance of regular bathing for hygiene and skin care. Teaching her not to put her fingers in her mouth is also good hygiene. In addition, children should be taught to wash fresh fruits and vegetables before eating them and not to eat food that has fallen on the ground or floor.

CARING FOR CHILDREN'S TEETH

Many adults believe that because baby teeth are going to fall out anyway, there is little need to care for them. Because of this mistaken idea, many young children suffer from significant tooth decay. Decay or premature loss of baby teeth can lead to damage or poor placement of the permanent teeth.

When teeth start to come in, brush them with a soft toothbrush and water, or clean them with a cloth. By age 2½, your child should have all her baby teeth. By age 3, your child should be doing her own brushing, although you will want to continue to help her so that her teeth will be cleaned properly. Using a small amount of toothpaste, start at the gum line and gently massage, then work the toothbrush around the teeth in a gentle, circular motion. Style of brushing is not as crucial as getting all teeth surfaces clean. Many dentists recommend that you begin flossing teeth daily when all the baby teeth are in.

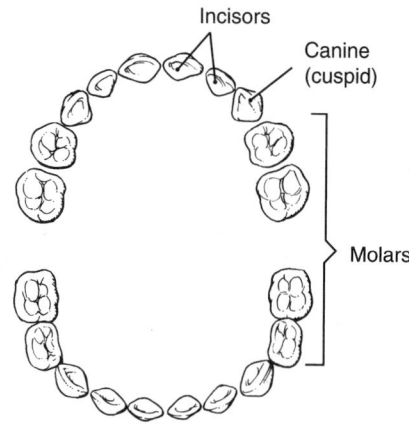

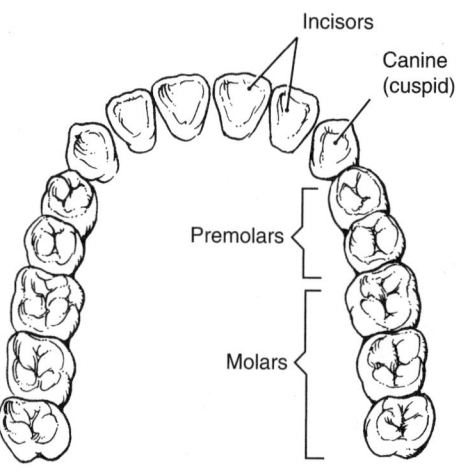

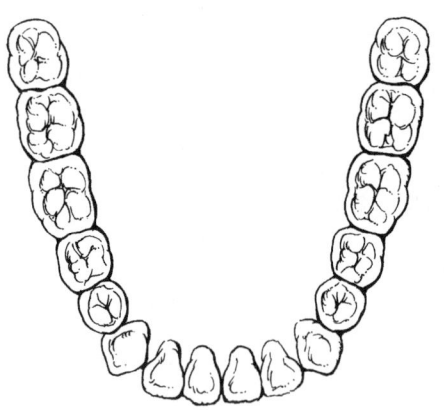

By age 2½ years, babies usually have all of their baby teeth. There are twenty baby (deciduous) teeth and thirty-two adult teeth. The adult has eight additional premolar teeth and four additional molars. Although a baby's teeth are temporary, they still require gentle cleaning.

Thumb sucking is a natural stress-coping mechanism for babies; unfortunately, it can cause dental problems if prolonged into childhood when the adult teeth are beginning to come in. If your child is still sucking her thumb or fingers at age 5 or 6, consult your doctor or your dentist about ways you might divert your child's thumb from her mouth.

The guidelines that follow can help prevent premature tooth decay:

- Never allow your child to fall asleep with a bottle. The sugars in milk, if allowed to pool in your child's mouth, provide perfect growing conditions for bacteria that cause tooth decay; so do the sugars in fruit juices. Acids in fruit juice can dissolve tooth enamel. Premature decay can force your dentist to pull decaying teeth to prevent further decay. Encourage water drinking for thirst quenching.

- Brush regularly, and most important, before bedtime.

- Avoid sugary foods that stick to the teeth. Candy is a big offender.

- Use a fluoride toothpaste. If your water supply is not fluoridated, your child should be taking a fluoride supplement, as prescribed by your doctor.

- Visit the dentist regularly.

When should your child have her first visit to the dentist? If you suspect any problem as her teeth come in, take your child to be examined by a dentist. If she has an accident and teeth are loosened or broken, she should see a dentist promptly.

If all is going well, your child's first regular visit to the dentist should come at about her third birthday. By this time, she should have all of her primary, or baby, teeth, including her molars. The dentist will examine her teeth to ensure that they have come in properly and give her a lesson in dental hygiene. By this time, she should be old enough to understand and cooperate.

Regular trips to the dentist should continue every 6 months to allow your dentist to watch over the growth of your child's mouth and the development of her adult teeth. If your child is not brushing properly or develops cavities or gum disease, your dentist can catch these problems in their nascence and address them quickly. Good dental hygiene, and good dental hygiene habits, will pay off over your child's lifetime.

DIET AND NUTRITION

What your child eats will affect her growth, health, and development. The establishment of good nutrition and eating habits can begin nearly at day one. Statistics show that children who start out obese are much more likely to be obese adults, and obesity has been shown to be a contributing factor in a number of illnesses.

You can work constructively with your child to ensure that she gets a balanced, sensible diet that includes food from each of the following food groups (see The Food Pyramid, page 236):

- Grains (bread, cereal, rice, and pasta)

- Fruit (fresh, dried, or unsweetened canned)

- Vegetables (raw or lightly cooked)

- Meat (meat, poultry, fish, dried beans, eggs, and nuts)

- Dairy (milk, yogurt, and cheese)

For most growing children, three meals a day are not enough; most will likely want and need between-meal snacks. Make sure your child has nutritious choices when it is time to snack. This way you can help her control her own diet. For example, you might offer a choice of an apple, orange, or banana.

Remember that each of the food groups provides some, but not all, of the nutrients a child needs. Foods in one group cannot replace those in another. No one of these major food groups is more important than another; for good health, all are necessary. A child on a balanced diet does not need supplementary vitamins. For more information on healthful eating for the whole family, see Chapter 1.

Some children will eat nearly anything, and some children seem not to like anything you put in front of them. If your child is a finicky eater, you might enlist her help in meal preparation or take her to the grocery store and offer her the chance to pick out fruits and vegetables on her own. Frequently kids trick themselves into eating foods they do not like simply because they have assisted in their preparation. If your child balks at food put before her, do not worry. Studies show that most children will, over time, eat the amount of food that is right for them if they are offered healthful choices.

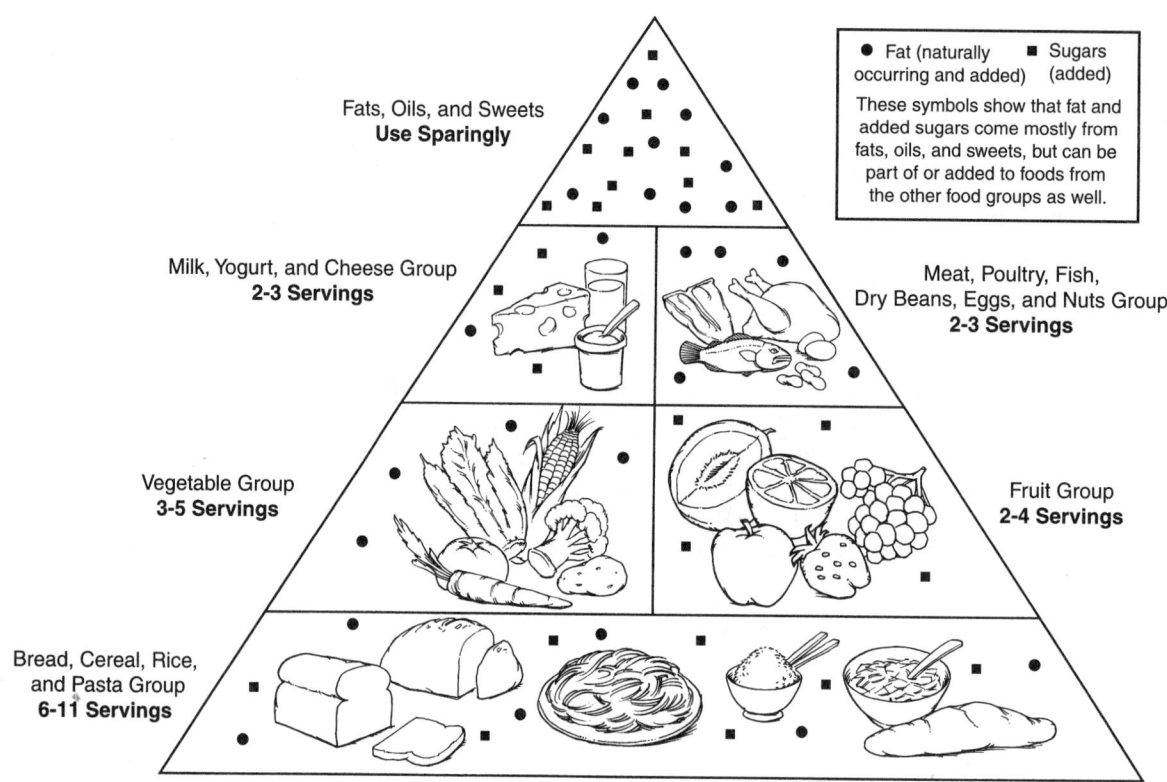

The Food Guide Pyramid. Source: US Department of Agriculture/US Department of Health and Human Services.

Remember that excessive nagging about food or forcing children to clean their plates before leaving the table can lead to problems with eating in the future. And make sure that children do not snack in front of the television. Kids burn about as many calories watching TV as they do sleeping. In fact, preventing obesity is one of many good reasons for limiting the amount of television your child watches.

If your child seems to lack appetite but is growing at a normal rate, there is little reason for concern. However, if your child seems to be eating properly but is failing to grow at the same rate as children of the same age, consult your doctor (see Growth Charts, page 1583).

RECOMMENDED SERVINGS FROM THE FOOD PYRAMID

HOW MANY SERVINGS DOES YOUR CHILD NEED EACH DAY?

FOOD GROUP	NUMBER OF SERVINGS
Bread	9
Vegetable	4
Fruit	3
Milk	2–3
Meat	2, for a total of 6 oz
Total fat (grams)	73

If you choose low-fat, lean foods from the five major food groups and use fats, oils, and sweets sparingly, a child 1 to 3 years old will consume 1,300 calories each day and a 4 to 6 year old will consume 1,800 calories daily assuming average serving size for each age group.

JUVENILE OBESITY

Most babies carry a certain amount of benign, even healthy, chubbiness. Fat, although unhealthy if consumed in excess, is necessary to survival. In children under age 2, restriction of dietary fat generally is not recommended. As your child grows into the toddler years, your doctor can advise you whether you need to begin substituting lower fat foods, for example, 1 percent milk for regular.

Children grow at different rates, but if you are concerned about your child's weight, you should consult your doctor. She will be able to tell you if your child is overweight. Any major effort to overhaul your child's diet should be done under the supervision of your doctor to ensure that your child's nutritional needs are met and that she has the calories needed to grow.

As many as 25 percent of American children are overweight, and statistics show that obese children are more likely to become obese adults. Establishing good eating habits early will pay off throughout your youngster's life. Discuss with your doctor strategies for changing your child's diet in effective but subtle ways. Obese children should not be made to lose weight but instead should be allowed to grow into their weight. This can be accomplished by increasing exercise, limiting TV viewing, and offering the child healthy foods while restricting high-calorie snacks. If your child has a weight problem, be sure to avoid using food as a reward system—candy for cleaning up, ice cream for getting good grades. Be certain that the whole family is on a healthy low-fat diet. And never pressure or humiliate your child into losing weight. Supporting your child's self-image and self-confidence as she struggles to control her weight is the greatest help a parent can provide.

EXERCISE

The average American watches about 6 hours of television a day. If your child plays video games or surfs the Internet, she may be spending even more time sedentary. The importance of physical fitness for children cannot be overestimated, but physical fitness can and should be fun for children—all it has to be is play. Good exercise habits learned early can help your child become an active and healthy adult. Exercise keeps the heart and lungs healthy and helps develop strong, flexible muscles. As your child achieves fitness, her self-confidence will grow along with her body.

Physical Activity Tips for Children

- Set a good example for your children: engage in a regular exercise program; when possible, walk instead of driving.

- When your child is old enough to do so safely, encourage her to walk or ride a bicycle to school or to visit friends. (Don't forget the bike helmet.) Walk or bike with your child.

- Plan physical activities for family time; exercise is more fun with others.

- Limit the time your child spends watching TV to 2 hours or less per day. Encourage going out to a playground, park, gym, or swimming pool instead.

- Encourage your child to participate in sports—instead of merely observing.

- Find out about exercise or sports programs at your child's school and in your community. The important thing is fun. Find out what your child likes—ballet, gymnastics, basketball, tennis—then encourage participation without forcing it.

- Encourage children with disabilities to participate in physical activities as much as possible.

- The goal of sports should not be simply to win. Fun should be at the top of the list, with teamwork and sportsmanship coming in a close second.

DISCIPLINE

Having appropriate boundaries is crucial to healthy child development. Discipline is the way parents define boundaries and expectations for a child, and how you discipline your child will have a direct bearing on how she perceives herself.

Discipline consists not only of punishment for wrong behavior but praise for positive behavior and should seek to teach the child self-discipline. Punishment should never injure a child. Parents can use many more successful alternatives to physical punishment. The most constructive kind of discipline is designed simply to modify behavior while leaving the child's self-esteem intact and to demonstrate to the child that certain kinds of inappropriate actions carry costs. In punishing or disciplining, you should always try to ensure your child's sense of security, belonging, personal competence (it is the behavior that is wrong, not the child), trust (explain the punishment and how it fits the crime), sense of support, and a sense of family self-esteem. It is also helpful to emphasize that failure is okay, even if inappropriate behavior is not.

To avoid situations when punishment is necessary, you can take several helpful steps. Ensure that the goals and expectations that you have for your child are those that she can reasonably be expected to reach and that the adults in the house have agreed on the goals and disciplinary methods. Be sure to acknowledge the child's efforts toward those goals, as well as to reward positive behavior. When your child is old enough to understand, it can be helpful to engage in family meetings to clarify goals and expectations and do as much as you can to diminish misunderstandings. Try to limit punishment to behaviors that truly warrant it. Praise a child who tries to do well, even when the effort falls short.

If you are concerned about your child's behavior, talk with your doctor. You may also want to consult your child's school and other community organizations to see if they have courses on parenting. Seeking help before anger and frustration escalate will benefit the entire family.

How to Treat the Ills You Cannot Prevent

Your child will get sick. All children do. Just as their experiences in the world prepare their minds and bodies for the rigors of life, so do childhood illnesses prepare their immune systems. Being in good physical condition will be of immeasurable value to your child, but everyone has to endure colds, flu, bouts of vomiting, diarrhea, and fever. In the pages that follow, we discuss many of the symptoms your child may experience on those occasions when she gets sick and explain how you can lessen the impact of these conditions and speed your child through them.

Although we will outline general guidelines for when you should call your child's doctor, it is worth saying that when you have concerns, you should call, and you should not worry that you will seem like a hysterical parent. Where children are concerned, it is always better to be safe than sorry. See Symptoms of Common Childhood Illnesses, below, for information on the specific illnesses your child may encounter.

SYMPTOMS OF COMMON EARLY CHILDHOOD ILLNESSES

The following is a list, alphabetically arranged, of common childhood diseases, including symptoms and a brief description of the course of the illness, as well as a cross-reference to the page on which you will find the disorder described in greater detail.

Bronchiolitis An acute viral infection of the lower respiratory tract, bronchiolitis occurs almost exclusively in children under age 2 and primarily in babies 2 to 8 months old. A child with bronchiolitis will have cold symptoms at first and then later may develop a cough; wheezing; rapid, shallow breathing; and fever. In severe bronchiolitis, your child's breathing may be very fast, her face may be pale or even slightly bluish, and the lungs may not fully expand when she breathes in. The most serious complications of bronchiolitis are respiratory failure and pneumonia. If you suspect your child has bronchiolitis, call your doctor immediately (see page 210).

Chickenpox This viral illness caused by the varicella-zoster virus of the herpes family usually begins with a fever (though in many cases it may be negligible or go unnoticed) and runny nose, followed by crops of itchy red bumps that quickly develop into small blisters, then rupture to become crusty sores (see page C-30). These usually appear first along the facial hairline, then on chest, belly, and back, and can spread from head to toe, including the inside of the mouth. Some children will be covered sparsely, others extensively. The child is contagious and should be kept home from school until all the blisters have crusted over completely. Chickenpox can be deadly for people who are immunosuppressed, so they should be told of exposure as soon as possible. (See page 883 for more information on chickenpox.)

Children with chickenpox should not be given aspirin because the combination of chickenpox and aspirin has been associated with Reye's syndrome (see pages 463 and 854).

Conjunctivitis This is an inflammation of the tissues that protect the surface of the eye and inner eyelid. Symptoms of conjunctivitis include crusting or discharge from the eye and redness of the eye. (See page C-45.) Consult your doctor if your child has signs of conjunctivitis. Both bacterial conjunctivitis (pinkeye) and viral conjunctivitis are highly infectious, so your child should be kept home from school until her eyes no longer have a discharge (see Conjunctivitis, page 519).

Croup Croup, or acute laryngotracheitis, is caused by respiratory viruses and is common in young children, peaking between the ages of 1 and 3. It is characterized by a hoarse barking cough and noisy breathing. Croup is often worse at night. Most children with croup improve without medication, but sometimes croup is so severe that the child cannot breath. Some bacterial infections (for example, pneumonia, bacterial tracheitis, and epiglottitis) can mimic croup, so call your doctor if your child has a high fever and noisy breathing. If your child is drooling, her lips or face look blue, or if she seems to be struggling to breathe or is tiring out, or if you suspect your child has swallowed an object, call your doctor or 911 immediately (see Swallowed Objects, page 359).

Ear infection (otitis media) Middle-ear infections often follow respiratory infections in young children; the cause can be viral or bacterial. Symptoms include irritability and severe pain in the ear, a result of fluid buildup in the middle ear caused by a blockage of the eustachian tube. Acetaminophen may ease the pain; when appropriate, your doctor may prescribe antibiotics. An ear infection is not contagious, so if the respiratory infection that may have preceded it has cleared up and if your child is not in pain, she may attend school. (See Otitis Media, page 566).

Fifth disease (erythema infectiosum) This viral illness is caused by the parvovirus B19 and begins with 2 to 3 days of fever, muscle ache, headache, and malaise. The cause becomes apparent 7 to 10 days later when the child breaks out with a characteristic rash. It begins as a fiery-red rash on the cheeks and then extends to the trunk and extremities as a lacy, slightly bumpy rash that may come and go (see page C-30). Joint aches are rare in children but may occur 1 to 6 days after onset of the rash. A child with fifth disease is only contagious before the rash's onset, so a child with the rash can attend school. Any pregnant woman with whom the child was in contact during the contagious stage should be notified because fifth disease can be dangerous to a developing fetus (see page 144).

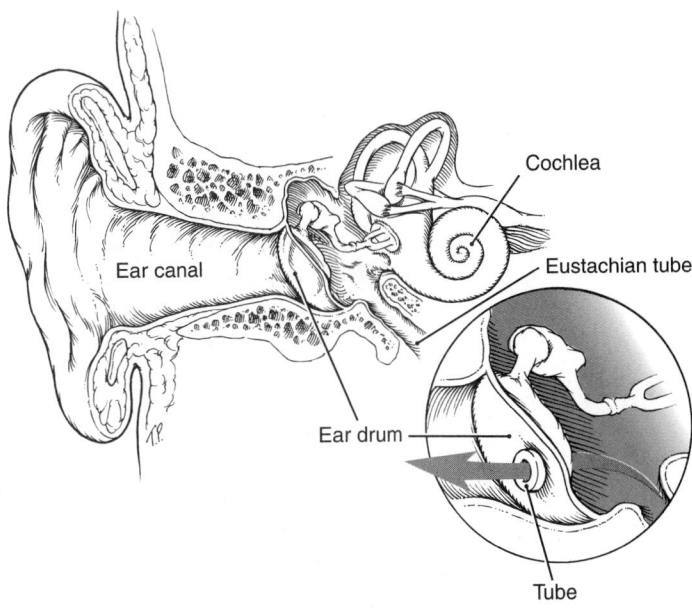

Infections of the middle ear are common in young children, who may become irritable or complain of ear pains or have drainage from the ear. These infections, usually viral or bacterial, often follow respiratory infections. Temporary hearing loss or perforation of the eardrum can occur, and drainage tubes may be needed for recurrent or severe cases. Discuss treatment with your doctor.

Gastroenteritis Commonly called stomach flu and usually viral in origin, gastroenteritis is characterized by vomiting or diarrhea and vomiting. It may also be the result of bacterial toxins or infection, sometimes caused by consuming contaminated food or water. Dehydration can occur from loss of fluids through diarrhea and can be dangerous, especially in young children who are too sick to drink. If your child has sunken eyes, a dry mouth, or decreased urine output, call your doctor. If severe abdominal cramps or pain occur, consult your doctor to rule out other more serious causes. A child with gastroenteritis is often contagious and should be kept home from school until symptoms subside. Good hand washing can decrease spread. (See Oral Rehydration Therapy, page 245, and Viral Gastroenteritis, page 875, for further information.)

Impetigo This is an itchy, sticky, crusty rash caused by staphylococcus or streptococcus bacterial skin infection. The bacteria enter the skin through a break in the skin following an insect bite or small wound. Impetigo occurs most commonly in the warm spring and summer months. It is either bullous (blistery) or nonbullous (no blisters) (see page C-34). Blisters can be large (dime- to quarter-sized) and itchy and can form amber to dark amber crusts. Consult your doctor if your child contracts impetigo; with proper treatment, the infection generally heals within a week. Impetigo is contagious, so a child should not return to school until 24 hours after treatment was begun (see page 1281).

Influenza Caused by the influenza virus, flu (influenza) has the potential to be serious, but most often clears up after about a week of unpleasant symptoms such as fever, headache, sore throat, cough, and muscle aches (see page 730). Because the influenza virus changes rapidly, a new vaccine is prepared each year, but usually vaccination is recommended only for those children in whom the flu might complicate other illnesses. Flu season usually runs from winter to early spring. Children with the flu are contagious and should be kept home for the duration of the illness.

Children with the flu should not be given aspirin because the combination of flu and aspirin has been associated with Reye's syndrome (see pages 463 and 854).

Other viral and bacterial infections can be confused with flu because of the similarity of symptoms.

Pneumonia This is caused by viral or bacterial infection of the lungs. Symptoms include fever; often high, deep cough; and rapid, troubled breathing (see pages 729 and 733). If you suspect pneumonia, call your doctor.

Roseola infantum This primarily strikes children under age 2 but can affect older children as well. This viral illness is most often characterized by several days of high fever followed by a fleeting pink rash on the chest and back (see page C-31) as the fever breaks. (See Roseola Infantum, page 212).

Strep throat An infection of the tonsils and throat caused by group A streptococcus bacteria, strep throat is most likely to occur in mid-winter to early spring. The sore throat of strep infection usually will be accompanied by a fever, and both may have fairly sudden onset. Your child's other symptoms may include headache, stomachache, vomiting, or a general sense of queasiness. She may also have swollen glands in the neck. Some strains of strep also cause a red, sandpapery rash. The illness is then called scarlet fever. Strep causes only a small percentage of sore throats, but if untreated, it can lead to rheumatic fever, which damages the heart. It should be treated promptly, so call your doctor if you suspect strep throat. A child with strep throat is contagious and

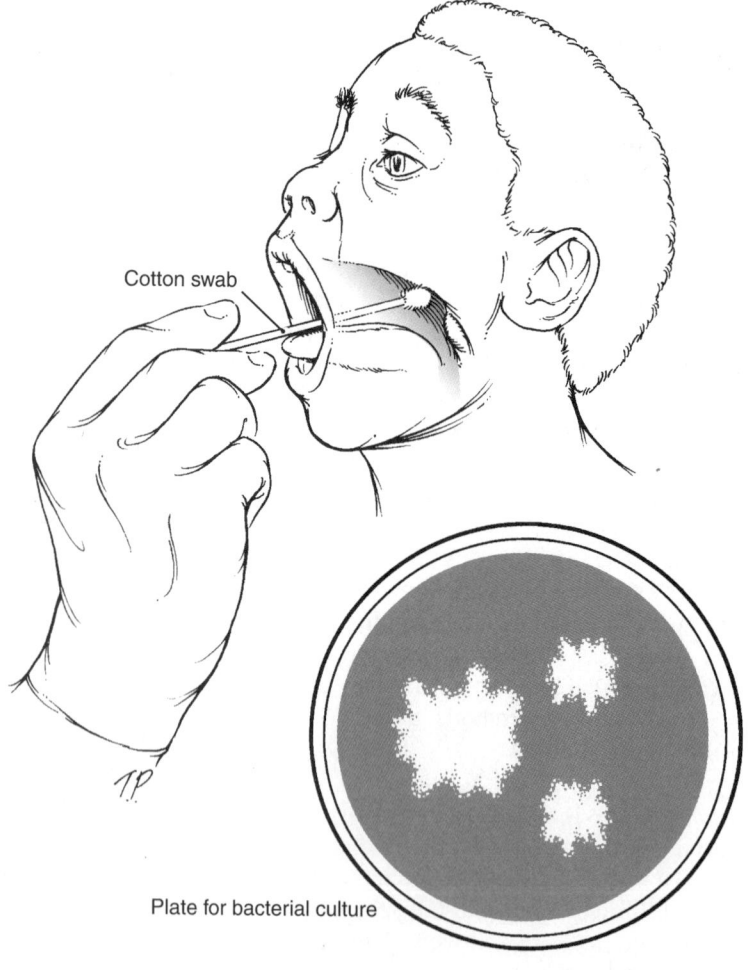

Cotton swab

Plate for bacterial culture

A throat that is infected with group A streptococcus bacteria is generally sore and contagious. Strep throat should be treated to prevent complications such as rheumatic fever and heart damage, so a throat culture may be taken to make the diagnosis. A cotton swab is brushed against the back of the throat and tonsils and then sent to a laboratory where it is brushed across a special plate, on which the bacteria can grow and then be identified.

should be kept home from school until 24 hours after effective antibiotic therapy was begun (see pages 592 and C-40).

Upper respiratory infections Commonly called colds, upper respiratory infections are caused by viruses and are characterized by nasal congestion, coughing, sore throat, sneezing, watery or itchy eyes, and they are often accompanied by a slight fever. They will usually begin to subside in a couple of days, but some symptoms, such as a cough, may linger for several days or as long as 2 weeks. If the symptoms, particularly fever and cough, continue or worsen, contact your doctor. (See page 583.)

Urinary tract infection This is often subtle in young children with few signs other than fever, but symptoms may include frequent, painful urination. The urine may be smelly, cloudy, or bloody. Urinary tract infection can be accompanied by stomachache or pain in the lower abdomen or by backache (see Cystitis, page 1067). Because urinary tract infection can reach as high as the kidneys, you should call your doctor if you suspect it. Kidney infection can be serious.

Other childhood infections Measles, mumps, rubella, and most other diseases that all children are commonly required to be immunized against (excluding chickenpox) are not covered in this section. If you have neglected to immunize your child and you suspect she may have one of these diseases, consult Chapter 21 for more information and contact your doctor immediately.

COLDS, FLU, AND OTHER COMMON INFECTIONS IN CHILDHOOD

By far the most common illnesses your child will experience are occasional viral infections. Because colds, influenza, and a host of other ailments are viral illnesses, not much can be done for them except to relieve their symptoms, such as acetaminophen for fever or aches and pains. Each time you get a cold or flu, it will immunize you against getting that particular virus again. However, because we live with a multitude of different cold and flu viruses, it is normal for a child to become sick frequently.

Colds are mainly annoying and are accompanied only by low-grade fever, if any. Colds in children can lead to ear infections, however, which require the attention of a doctor. Ear infections are common in young children, so be alert for signs of them, including complaints of earache or drainage from the ear. Some earaches are invisible, that is, younger children may show only fever and irritability, or trouble sleeping, without specifically complaining about ear pain (see Chapter 16).

Influenza has the potential to be serious but most often is a week or so of unpleasant symptoms such as high fever, headache, sore throat, cough, and muscle aches. Because the influenza virus changes rapidly, a new vaccine is prepared each year, but usually, vaccination is recommended only for those children in whom the flu might complicate other illnesses. Flu season usually runs from winter to early spring.

Many other viruses exist. Some may cause vomiting and diarrhea; others, fever and a rash. Be sure that you have a clear picture of your child's symptoms when you call the doctor. If there is a rash, for example, be prepared to describe it. The more accurately you describe the symptoms, the more readily the doctor can determine if and how soon she needs to examine your child.

In addition to viruses, your child may occasionally contract a bacterial infection that will require treatment with an antibiotic. Most sore throats are harmless but some are caused by streptococcus bacteria, which will likely be accompanied by a fever and will require the attention of a doctor, who will take a throat culture and will prescribe an antibiotic if strep is found (see Strep Throat, page 240). Fever and cough accompanied by rapid or troubled breathing should prompt immediate medical attention.

Urinary infections are also common in children, particularly girls. If your child needs to urinate frequently and experiences pain when urinating, contact your doctor (see Cystitis, page 1067).

If your child seems to be recovering from an illness and suddenly takes a turn for the worse (seeming lethargic, becoming feverish again, or demonstrating any other symptoms that alarm you), contact your doctor without delay. Simple infections in children sometimes can turn quite serious and should receive immediate attention.

PROPER USE OF ANTIBIOTICS

Antibiotics as a group are one of the most valuable tools we have in fighting illness. Many people, however, have come to take these miracle drugs for granted and are not sufficiently careful about their use. Much of the public is misinformed about what antibiotics can be useful for. Regular antibiotics are only effective in fighting bacterial infections and have no value at all in treating viral disease. If your child has a cold or the flu, for example, antibiotics will do her no good, because colds and flu are caused by viruses. In some cases, as in viral gastrointestinal infections, for example, antibiotics may worsen your child's condition. With viral illness, the virus must run its course, and you should not expect or demand antibiotics that will not improve your child's situation.

When your child has a bacterial infection and an antibiotic medication is prescribed, make sure you follow your doctor's directions to the letter. After a few days on the antibiotic, your child may appear completely well. *Do not discontinue the medication until you have given it as long as your doctor instructed you to.* Your child may appear well yet still harbor bacteria in her body. Stopping the antibiotic before the recommended course has been completed may lead to more serious reinfection. Although it can be difficult to get children to take medicine, you may do your child more harm than good if you don't make sure the prescription is used as directed. If there is any antibiotic remaining once the prescribed course has been completed, throw it away.

If your child suddenly becomes worse after starting an antibiotic, she may be having a bad reaction to the antibiotic, may need a different antibiotic, or may have developed complications of the infection. Contact your doctor immediately.

An antibiotic has a predictable time frame within which it should work for a given infection. When your doctor prescribes it, make sure you know when symptoms should subside, usually after a few days at most. If the symptoms do not subside within that time, contact your doctor. She may want to prescribe a different antibiotic or see your child again. ∎

FEVER

WARNING: *Never give aspirin to a child for relief of fever unless directed to do so by your doctor. Over-the-counter medications may contain aspirin and should not be given to children without consulting your doctor. Aspirin in childhood has been linked to Reye's syndrome (see pages 463 and 854), a potentially fatal illness, the cause of which is unknown.*

If you need to relieve fever, acetaminophen is recommended. Pediatric ibuprofen, which is a nonsteroidal anti-inflammatory drug (NSAID) that contains no aspirin, is also available. Your doctor sometimes may instruct you to give your child ibuprofen for fever or pain.

Although we usually accept 98.6°F as our universal, normal body temperature, temperature varies during the day, reaching its lowest point in the predawn hours and its highest in the afternoon. It also varies modestly between individuals. Small children frequently have a higher normal range of body temperature than adults.

If fever is making your child uncomfortable, you can give her an age- and weight-appropriate dose of acetaminophen or pediatric ibuprofen to help bring it down. Never use rubbing alcohol to cool a feverish child, because the alcohol can be absorbed through the skin; use a tepid bath instead. For complete information on how to bring down a fever, see Understanding a Fever in Chapter 21. Research suggests, however, that reducing fever may actually prolong an illness. For that reason, it can be counterproductive to try to bring down moderate fevers with acetaminophen. It may be best to let nature take its course.

Fever is a common feature of many illnesses. Very young children can spike fevers that will alarm their parents, but fever by itself is not something to be overly concerned about unless it is unusually high and persistent. Fever is most often a signal that the body is fighting an infection; and it is the underlying cause of fever that your doctor will want to determine. For certain illnesses, it is not uncommon for a child to run a fever of 102 to 104°F for a few days. Your biggest concern during this period should be to see that your child does not become dehydrated. Children with fever should get plenty of fluids to compensate for those they may lose. Despite the old adage, "Feed a cold, starve a fever," neither approach is particularly good medicine.

When your child is running a fever, it's a good rule of thumb that she ought to stay home from school to avoid passing along any infection to her classmates.

If you are worried that the fever is too high, or has persisted too long, call your doctor. It will be helpful if you can tell your doctor what your child's temperature is and when any fever-reducing medication was given. (See When to Call the Doctor Without Delay, page 196.)

Touching your child to see if she is warm can be an indicator that her temperature needs to be taken, but it is never a reliable way of measuring fever. Several different kinds of thermometers are now available. At the low-tech and low-cost end of the spectrum is the glass stick thermometer (oral or rectal), which will usually not cost more than a few dollars and is still the gold standard. Glass thermometers can also take readings under the armpit. Used properly (see page 208), they are safe, accurate, and can last for years. In the middle are the newer, battery-operated digital thermometers that are easily read, can be used (with disposable, sanitary plastic covers) to measure temperature orally, rectally, or under the arm; and have built-in mechanisms to signal when a measurement is complete. These usually cost under $10. At the high end of the spectrum are high-tech, digital, tympanic thermometers that measure the temperature at the ear almost instantly and require next to no cooperation from the child. Wax buildup in the ear can cause a low measurement, but generally, these thermometers are quite accurate. Currently, the tympanic thermometers cost between $45 and $75. Some parents may decide that not having to fight with an ill child over the unpleasantness of temperature taking is worth the investment.

COUGHING

Coughing can be caused by any number of different conditions, from pollen allergies to infection to inhalation of irritants like cigarette smoke.

When is coughing a problem, and when should you just ignore it?

The purpose of coughing is to clear the throat or bronchial tubes of anything that might obstruct free breathing. Drinking her milk with supper, your child may inadvertently inhale some, then she will cough. It is the body's way of clearing the air passages. In the case of certain illnesses such as a cold or lung infection (see Viral and Bacterial Infections of the Respiratory System, page 729), the illness itself produces the material—phlegm—that causes the coughing. With other illnesses, such as

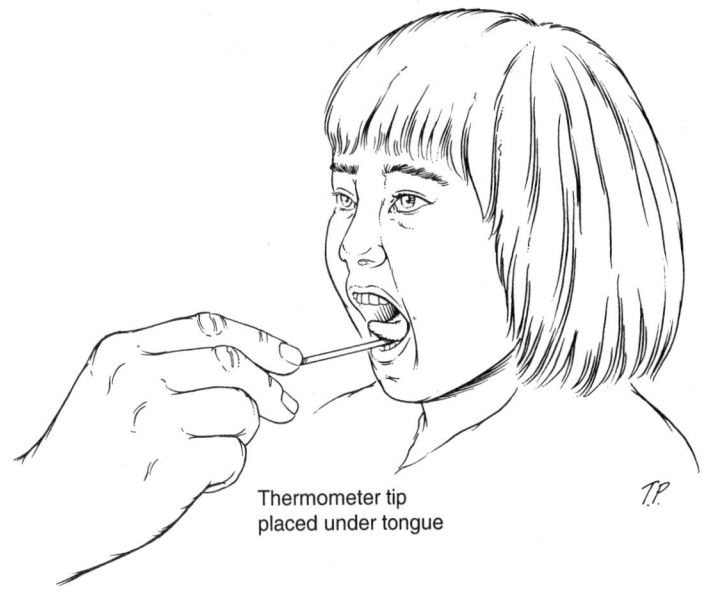

Thermometer tip placed under tongue

There are several ways to take a child's temperature (see text). In the traditional oral method, the tip of a standard glass thermometer is placed under the tongue, where it is left in place for a few minutes with the child's mouth closed before it is read.

croup (see page 212), inflammation can narrow or even obstruct the airways. This kind of cough will make a sharp, barking sound and may cause noisy breathing. When this happens (which will most likely be in winter), what your child needs most is humidity. A humidifier will be helpful during the sleeping hours, but if your child's illness comes on fast, it may frighten both you and the child. The fastest way to humidify dry air is the shower. Do not get in it. Just take your child into the bathroom, close the door, and turn the shower on hot and high. The room will fill with steam in a matter of moments, and breathing should get easier rapidly. If it does not improve quickly, call your doctor. With croup, your child may not need to see the doctor, but if it is accompanied by high fever, if your child is drooling or turns blue, or if your child's breathing does not ease, immediately call the doctor or an ambulance, depending on severity.

Most other coughing will be related to colds or flu or will be caused by postnasal drip (see Viral Rhinitis, page 583) or by the discharge of phlegm. Again, a humidifier in the child's room at night will help, although a cough may still take a couple of weeks to clear. Over-the-counter cough medications are frequently not effective, so do not use one unless your doctor recommends it for your child's cough. If your child is having any trouble breathing, seems ill, or if her cough persists, is accompanied by other worrisome symptoms, or becomes progressively worse, contact your doctor. Cough is sometimes a sign of pneumonia.

HEADACHES

Headaches are a frequent complaint of school-age children. They can be caused by any number of different minor problems, such as sinus problems, stress, colds or flu, or eye problems. Migraine headaches (see Chapter 14) are possible in young children, particularly those whose parents or relatives experience them.

Most headaches in school-aged children are not a cause for worry, but, if they are accompanied by vomiting or are frequent, especially severe, or persistent, you should contact your doctor to rule out eye problems, allergies, sinus infections, migraines, as well as more serious, rare disorders. For a run-of-the-mill headache, an age- and weight-appropriate dose of acetaminophen or pediatric ibuprofen should do the trick.

STOMACHACHES

Many stomachaches will not involve the stomach at all, but the intestines. Some of the stomachaches your child gets will be caused by gas or even hunger. Constipation, food allergy or intolerance, or gastrointestinal infection may also be culprits. Gas pains can sometimes be excruciating.

Some stomachaches may be a warning symptom of a serious disease, such as appendicitis (see page 1015), ulcers, or intestinal disorders. If your child has other symptoms (such as vomiting, blood in the bowel movements, fever) or seems ill, contact your doctor. Most stomachaches, however, will be nothing serious and disappear once the child has eaten or moved her bowels, or even without explanation.

The stomach can be one of the central repositories of anxiety and tension, and some stomachaches may be caused by stress and upheavals in your child's life.

Stomachaches are a frequent complaint of schoolchildren. If your child's routine is changing—is she starting school? are you going through a divorce?—and she suddenly starts experiencing stomachaches, the likelihood is that they are anxiety-induced. Do they occur only on school days? Does she feel fine on weekends or if you keep her at home? Do they happen when she is clearly overwhelmed emotionally?

Just because an illness is psychosomatic does not mean it is not painful or real, but if your child is experiencing stomachaches that are caused by anxiety or stress, it is important to treat the underlying problem and not the symptoms. Stomach medications are not a cure for stress.

Contact your doctor if the stomachaches are ongoing. If you and your doctor decide that they are stress-related (stress can cause diarrhea, too), your doctor can help you to determine ways that you can help relieve your child's stress. Older children (age 7 to 12) may benefit from counseling if the cause of stress is chronic, such as divorce, illness of a sibling, or socialization problems (such as those related to learning disabilities).

It is important to recognize and appreciate the anxiety your youngster is experiencing. Telling young children to toughen up, rather than teaching them coping mechanisms, can worsen their anxiety-induced illness.

DIARRHEA

Common diarrhea, which is characterized by the frequent, often urgent, elimination of loose, watery stools, is relatively easy to treat, but in rare instances diarrhea can be fatal because it robs the body of vital fluids and nutrients and leads to dehydration. Most children will not lose enough fluid to become dehydrated and will not need medication to overcome their diarrhea, only plenty of fluids to replace those lost. Some over-the-counter antidiarrheal agents can harm your child, so *always consult your doctor before giving your child over-the-counter medications.* If your child is having many loose stools, your doctor probably will recommend that you give a young child one of the oral rehydration solutions available in grocery stores and pharmacies.

ORAL REHYDRATION THERAPY

Our bodies and our blood are made up predominantly of fluids. Diarrhea can rapidly rob a child of vital fluids, resulting in dehydration. Lost fluids must be replaced and can be with surprising ease. The best source of fluids are oral rehydration solutions, available under many brand names such as Pedialyte and Infalyte, which include minerals that are lost during bouts of diarrhea or vomiting. Common drinks such as colas, sports drinks, and fruit juices should not be used. They do not contain the best balance of minerals, and many contain too much sugar and can make diarrhea worse. Water alone will not replace lost minerals.

Children with diarrhea need about twice as much fluid as they would normally when well. The most effective method for getting your child to drink oral rehydration solutions is to give her small amounts very frequently. For example, giving your child a teaspoon of an oral rehydration solution every minute will add up to half a pint in less than an hour.

Children never vomit all the fluid that they take in, so continue to give fluids even when your child is still vomiting. Children can usually take a teaspoon or two of oral rehydration solution every few minutes.

Contact your doctor if your child cannot keep down even small amounts of fluid, has a high fever, has blood in her stool, or begins to seem dehydrated. Signs of dehydration include sunken eyes or fontanelle, lack of tears, extreme irritability, cool or pale hands and feet, dry mouth, and decreased urine output. Severe dehydration is life-threatening. ■

Diarrhea can be caused by bacterial or viral organisms. Bacterial diarrhea often causes blood in the stool. If you see blood in your child's stool during diarrhea or at any other time, call your doctor. Blood in the stool always requires medical attention.

In preschoolers, most infectious diarrhea is viral. Diarrhea caused by a viral illness cannot be treated with antibiotics. Letting the condition run its course while you make sure your child gets adequate fluid is the best treatment. If your child does not get adequate fluids to replace those that are lost, dehydration can result. (See Oral Rehydration Therapy, above, for information on how to prevent dehydration.) If your child has persistent diarrhea, be alert for signs of dehydration: decreased urination, no tears, sunken eyes, dry mouth, and lethargy.

Children with diarrhea should continue to eat. A commonly recommended diet for children with diarrhea is the BRAT diet: bananas, rice, apple sauce, and toast. Yogurt with active cultures has been shown to help stop diarrhea and even prevent it in some cases, and it has also been shown to be tolerated more easily by children with intolerance to other milk products.

VOMITING

Generally, vomiting is more unpleasant than dangerous, as long as the child is not in a position to choke on the vomit. Vomiting usually occurs as part of minor illnesses related to the stomach and gastrointestinal tract, but it can also be caused by the gag reflex if your child is coughing. Vomiting is occasionally associated with more serious illnesses, such as meningitis (see page 459) or appendicitis (see page 1015). If your child seems to be quite ill or has severe abdominal pain, or if vomiting occurs with other symptoms, particularly if blood is apparent, or if the vomit is green or brown, contact your doctor immediately.

Even a child who is vomiting can still usually take fluids in a small amount at a time (see Oral Rehydration Therapy, above). If your child continues to be unable to hold down even small amounts of fluids, contact your doctor.

CONSTIPATION

Many children are reluctant to move their bowels away from home. Toilets may not be private enough to give them an adequate sense of security and comfort, or there may be other reasons, fathomable only to your child. Holding back all day long can result in constipation.

Stool is formed in the large intestine. It is part of the large intestine's—or colon's—job to remove moisture from the wet, unformed sludge that comes from the small intestine and turn it into formed stool. But sufficient moisture is necessary in the colon in order for stool to pass comfortably.

If your child becomes self-conscious about moving her bowels and begins to hold back, the holding back can remove too much moisture from the stool and cause it to become painful or at least unpleasant to move her bowels. Once she begins to hold stool back, she can launch into a vicious cycle: The more she holds back, the more painful the unpassed stool can become. The unpassed stool can stretch the walls of the colon and make it more difficult to move her bowels.

How can you tell if your child is constipated? Every child has a different bowel style, partly dictated by genetics, partly by diet, and partly by habit. Some children will move their bowels once every 2 or 3 days and not be constipated. Others may move their bowels every day but still be constipated. In the early years, you should be familiar with your child's bowel habits, the frequency with which she moves her bowels, and the consistency of her stool. You need not be intrusive to learn these facts, or even mention that you are paying much attention.

You should contact your doctor if you notice that your child

- Sometimes goes 3 or more days without moving her bowels and has hard, dense stools
- Seems to be in pain when she moves her bowels
- Has stomachaches that are relieved by bowel movements
- Has bloody stools
- Has leaks of wet, almost diarrhea-like stool between regular bowel movements

More than likely, blood on the stool in a constipated child will prove to be the result of an anal fissure (see page 1024) caused by the rock-hard stool scraping against the wall of the rectum. But it could be an indication of something more serious and should be checked.

What can you do to help your child through constipation? Constipation may have several causes other than stool retention. A likely culprit for constipation is inadequate bulk, or fiber, in the diet. Many of the foods that appeal to children's taste buds, such as cheese and bananas, also plug up their intestines. Try to steer your child toward foods with high fiber content. Prunes, peaches, and apricots are high in fiber (and, like bananas, good sources of potassium), and most children like them because they are sweet. Plenty of beans, broccoli, and leafy vegetables can also help

make softer stools. In addition to being one of the most nutritious fruit juices, prune juice can work effectively as a stool softener. Drinking plenty of water is not only vital to overall good health, it can also help ensure adequate moisture in the bowel.

If these do not help, your doctor may recommend stool softeners or a mild laxative. Do not use medication unless your doctor advises you to do so. If your child has a fear of moving her bowels at school, however, using laxatives and stool softeners may cause accidents that could add to her sense of shame and self-consciousness. If your child has problems with constipation, encourage the development of regular bowel habits. Take advantage of the reflex to move the bowels after meals by making certain there is adequate time after breakfast and the evening meal. Try to be as easygoing as you can about the situation; if it is obvious that you are worried, it will worry your child.

CHRONIC ILLNESS

For most children, illness is a passing storm—frequent but short-lived. For as many as 15 percent of children, however, illness or disabilities persist for a long period of time, even for their lifetime. Some problems are readily apparent; others are diagnosed only after careful investigation or the passage of time. Many need not impair the child's daily activities; others will affect most aspects of life.

If your child has been diagnosed with a chronic disease or disability, you will want to learn all you can about the condition. See Part 4 for detailed information about specific diseases and disorders in all of the body systems; information can be invaluable as you seek effective help for your child. Your doctor will coordinate your child's care, but chronic conditions often require the attention of specialists. Choose a doctor you and your child feel you like and who can spend time with you, because a continuing relationship will serve your child better.

Stress goes hand-in-hand with chronic disease or disability—both for the child and her family. Chronic disease or disability can cause physical stress, psychological stress, social stress, financial stress, the stress of decision making, and a host of other stresses. Seek help before the situation becomes untenable. Community organizations can be an invaluable resource, as can support and advocacy groups. Support groups exist for most chronic diseases; see the entry for the particular disorder. The following organizations can help direct you to an appropriate resource:

- National Information Center for Children and Youth with Disabilities
  PO Box 1492
  Washington, DC 20013
  Phone: (800) 695-0285

- Beach Center on Families and Disability
  c/o Bureau of Child Research
  3111 Haworth Hall
  University of Kansas
  Lawrence, Kansas 66045
  Phone: (913) 864-7600

Developmental Concerns

Developmental difficulties may emerge as your child matures. The presence of a developmental difficulty may explain why a child is unable to do the things or show the behavior expected of her at a certain age. If dealt with promptly and properly, you will be able to help your child reach her maximum potential. You can help your child by spending plenty of time with her, watching her development, and catching unusual behavior or delayed development early, so that it can be evaluated and treated properly. For more information on many of the conditions and disorders discussed here, see the chapters in Part 4: Body Systems and Disorders.

VISION

Severe vision problems may be apparent in your child's infancy (see Blindness or Visual Loss, page 218). However, many defects of sight, including near-sightedness or lazy eye, may not become obvious to parents until later; some will develop as the child grows, while others that have existed will make themselves known over time. Either way, most problems with visual acuity—the sharpness with which your child sees—will not become obvious until your child reaches school age and needs to pay attention to written images. This is why early eye examinations are important—to detect eye

problems and treat them before a child reaches school age. One of the most common and obvious symptoms of a visual difficulty is the need to sit closer to the television than anyone else in the family.

Children whose parents have eye problems or wore glasses in preschool or in the early years of grade school are more likely to have eye problems.

Certain vision problems common to children can and should be caught early and reversed or corrected. Below are some indicators that you should have your child's eyes checked.

- Eyes do not appear to be the same size
- Eyes do not appear straight
- Squints or must be very close to an object to focus on it
- Seems unable to follow moving objects
- Eye looks cloudy
- Pupil of eye looks white instead of red when light flashes in it
- Eyes do not hold steady (jiggle)
- Consistently holds head at an angle
- Complains of headaches
- Complains of blurry or double vision
- Cannot distinguish colors (after age 3 to 4 years)
- Eyes are watering
- Rubs eyes often
- Cannot see distant objects

Any suspected vision problems before age 3 or 4 can and should be evaluated by a pediatric ophthalmologist. Because your child may be able to approach vision testing in a more cooperative and helpful way after age 3 or 4, vision testing may then be conducted during annual checkups with her regular doctor. If your child's vision tests worse than 20/40 before age 5 or 20/30 after age 5, or if there is a difference in acuity between the eyes, she should be referred to a pediatric ophthalmologist.

Important problems affecting vision and the eye are listed below. (See Chapter 15 for more information about these and other vision problems.)

Common vision problems Strabismus, also known as wandering eye, is a condition in which the muscles that control the movement of the eyes do not work in sync. One

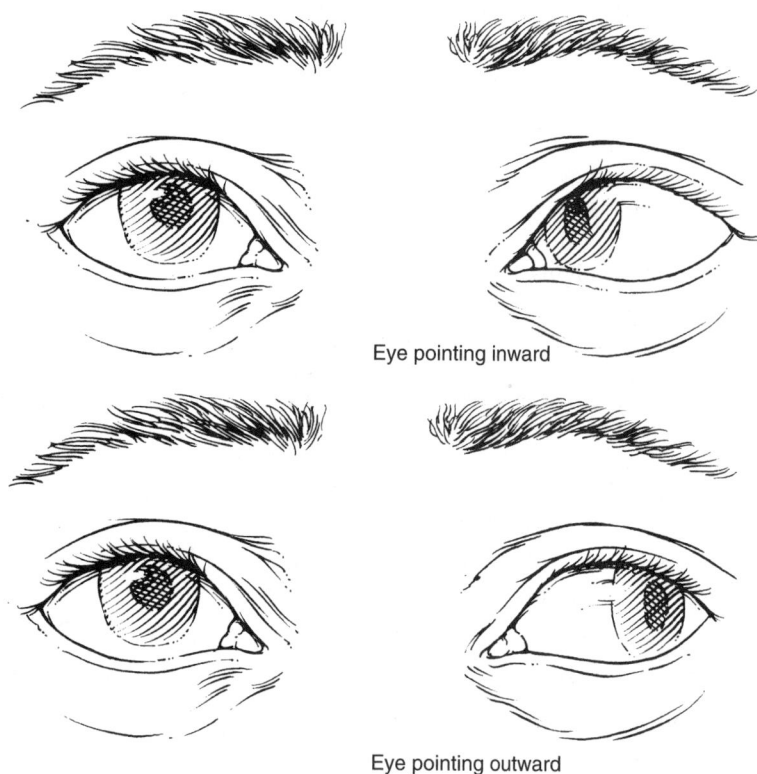

Eye pointing inward

Eye pointing outward

Strabismus is a condition in which the eyes do not converge properly. In esotropia, the eye points inward toward the nose; in exotropia, the eye points outward. If you notice strabismus after the first few months of a baby's life, contact a doctor for prompt evaluation.

eye drifts, and it is impossible for the child to focus on a given point simultaneously with both eyes. Strabismus can be present from birth, can result from an eye injury, or can have a sudden onset. If your child's eyes have seemed perfectly normal, but suddenly one starts to wander, contact your doctor immediately. The earlier strabismus can be detected, the better for your child. While inward-turning and awkward movements of the eyes are common in very young infants, if you notice any signs of strabismus at any time after the first few months of life, you should contact your doctor.

Exercises usually are not adequate treatment for strabismus, and glasses, eyedrops, and surgery may all be necessary to realign the eyes (see Chapter 15).

Amblyopia, or lazy eye, is a common vision problem that, if caught early enough, can often be reversed. It may result from untreated strabismus (another reason for prompt treatment of strabismus), or it may

have other causes. In amblyopia, one eye does not work as well as the other. Over time, the brain compensates, favoring the good eye and ignoring the other. If you notice that your child uses only one eye—always turns her face to one side when looking at something—have her eyes tested. Treatment for lazy eye usually consists of forcing the lazy eye to work by covering the other or deliberately blurring the vision in the good eye. (See Chapter 15 for more detailed information.)

Common eye infections Pinkeye or red eye are common names for *conjunctivitis*, which is an inflammation of the conjunctiva, the tissues that protect the surface of the eyeball and inner eyelid. Conjunctivitis may be the result of a viral or bacterial infection that attacks the eye, or it may be part of a viral infection of the upper respiratory tract that includes the eye. Less frequently, conjunctivitis may signal an allergic reaction (such as to pollen) or a reaction to an irritant (such as cigarette smoke).

Conjunctivitis is common in school-age children, because viral or bacterial conjunctivitis is highly infectious and readily spread from child to child, as is the common cold. A child with conjunctivitis should not be sent to school until the doctor says she is no longer infectious. Other family members should not use linen that the child has used, or the infection may spread throughout the family.

Signs of conjunctivitis may include crusting or discharge from the eye, redness of the eye, swelling of the lids, and itching of the eye. Contact your doctor if your child has signs of conjunctivitis. The doctor may want to prescribe an antibiotic, though conjunctivitis that is part of an upper respiratory infection (a cold) will generally disappear on its own after a few days. If you have medication from someone else's eye infection lying around the house, *never use it on anyone other than for whom it was prescribed* (see Conjunctivitis, page 519, and see page C-45 for an illustration of conjunctivitis.)

Styes are pimple- or boil-like bacterial infections that occur in the glands along the edge of the eyelids. Usually a stye will appear over a period of two or three days as localized reddening of the eyelid with swelling. Like a pimple or boil, the infected area will fill with pus and be sore. The sore-

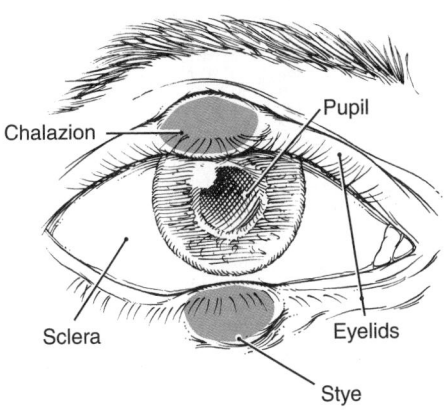

A stye is a lump that occurs when a sebaceous gland at the edge of the eyelid become infected or clogged. It may appear as a red, swollen, sore bump on the eyelid. The eyelid should be cleaned gently and not rubbed. Antibiotic eyedrops are sometimes prescribed. A chalazion is a firm, nontender lump in the eyelid. It may require surgical drainage.

ness will remain until the stye diminishes. The bacteria that causes one stye can cause others, so the eyes should be gently cleansed, and the child should be urged not to rub. Do not apply pressure to the stye or try to pop it. Warm soaks are useful. Talk to your doctor; she may feel antibiotic eyedrops are appropriate, depending upon the severity of the infection.

ORTHOPEDIC CONCERNS

Because we are all formed in the confined space of the womb, it may take some time for our legs to straighten out, when we begin to walk. Most children begin walking in a manner that may seem wobbly and unsteady, often with their legs bowed and their feet pointing outward. As a child grows and gains muscle tone and control, her gait will grow steadier and more natural in appearance. Still, many children retain some leg and foot variation as they move from toddlerhood into the preschool years.

The orthopedic conditions parents notice most readily are bowlegs (one or both legs bent outward at the knee), knock-knees (legs are curved inward, bringing the knees close together), flat feet (flattening of the arch of the foot), and pigeon toes (feet turned inward). These leg and foot variations are generally developmental issues that seldom require any intervention, al-

though severe bowing of the legs that persists as the child matures may require treatment with leg braces. If, however, you notice asymmetry between your child's legs or feet, you should contact your doctor. A new limp that is not attributable to pain due to a simple injury is *urgent* and requires immediate medical attention. This is especially so if there is swelling, pain, or refusal to bear weight or bend a joint; a fracture, bone or joint infection, or tumor may be responsible.

LANGUAGE AND SPEECH

Language development follows predictable patterns. You will probably notice that your child seems to understand some words before being able to say them (see figure on page 250). Each child develops differently, but if your child has not started to speak in simple words, such as "Mama," "Dada," and "bye-bye," by 12 to 14 months, you should contact your doctor. That your child has not spoken by this time does not necessarily indicate a developmental difficulty, but it does suggest the need for evaluation. Even within a single family, children can have surprisingly different rates of speech acquisition.

Speech represents the coming together of a number of different sensory abilities: the ability to hear, the muscular coordination of the mouth, and the cognitive abilities to listen, imitate, and understand language. True late speech or slowed language development is most commonly an indicator of an impairment in the ability of the child to learn. But it can also be an indicator of other, perhaps more subtle things. Usually, if your child has profound hearing loss, you should be aware of it before her first birthday. This could become apparent as early as 3 months. Still, a milder hearing impairment can take longer to detect (see page 578 for more information on early detection of hearing impairment). Some hearing loss is progressive.

If your child seems to lag behind her peers—or if she seems behind where her brothers or sisters were at her age—she may catch up. But it is wise to review the situation with your doctor. It is particularly important to make certain your child is hearing properly, because this is a correctable cause of speech delay.

Each child develops the ability to understand and express language at their own pace, but certain milestones in language development can be tracked by age to determine if learning or hearing disabilities exist in your child. For example, at age 18 months, 90 percent of children will be using two-word sentences. Infants who consistently attain milestones later than the 10th percentile should be evaluated by a doctor. Source: Capute AJ, Palmer AJ, Shapiro BK, et al. Clinical linguistic and auditory milestone scale: Prediction of cognition in infancy. Dev Med Child Neurol 1986;28:762; used with permission.

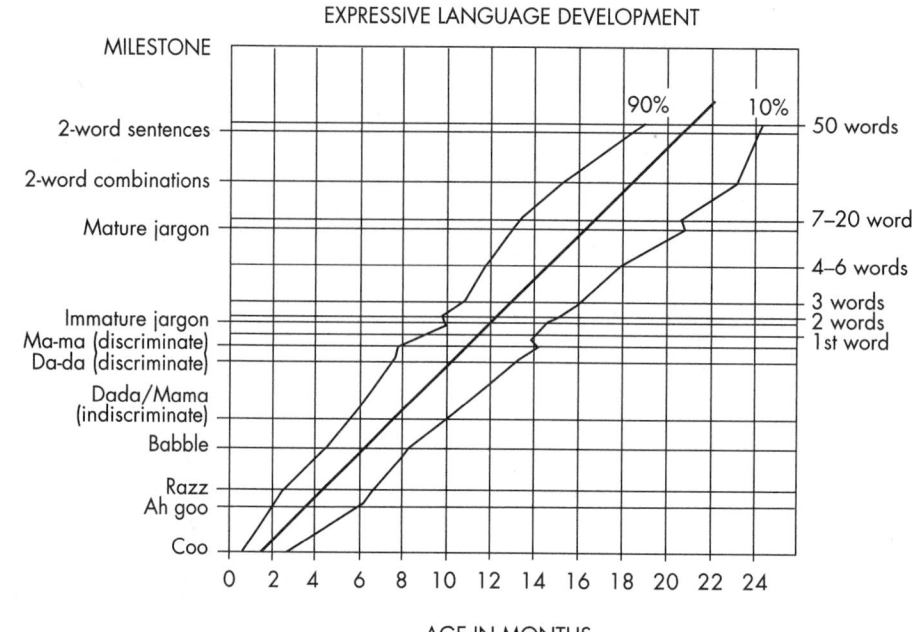

STUTTERING

Many children go through a stuttering phase, usually as their desire to express themselves outstrips their ability to do so. Only about 1 percent of the population, however, becomes genuine stutterers. The problem is most common in boys and tends to run in families.

Hesitations and repetitions in speech that sound like stuttering often surface around 2 to 4 years of age, particularly when your child is excited or feeling stressed, but are usually transitory. In the vast majority of cases, the child will stop stuttering on her own as she matures, and it is best if the parent simply ignores the stuttering so as not to make the child self-conscious. The problem with ignoring it, however, is that early intervention is advisable for those children who are genuine stutterers. The longer the stuttering exists, the harder it is to change. If you are concerned, talk to your doctor, but do not alarm your child or give her reason to become anxious or frustrated, thereby compounding the problem.

Some researchers believe that parents can help their stuttering child best by speaking slowly themselves, particularly at the start and end of sentences. Allow your child time to get out whatever she has to say.

How do you distinguish between the stuttering that is common in toddlers and is eventually outgrown and the stuttering that can become a permanent problem? This is not easily answered, because the causes of stuttering are unknown. If there is a family history of stuttering, the child should be seen by a speech pathologist for evaluation. The following symptoms are characteristic of children whose stuttering is not outgrown:

- The child herself is aware of the stuttering and sees it as a problem.
- The child shows signs of struggle while speaking.
- The child avoids certain words or sounds.
- The child's face contorts or distorts when she has trouble getting her words out.

If these signs are present, consult your doctor and find out about having your child's speech evaluated. Speech therapists can help children who are genuine stutterers overcome stuttering.

ALLERGIES

Allergy, the most common disorder of the immune system, affects as many as one of six children. An allergy occurs when an often otherwise innocuous substance, known as an allergen, is treated by the body as an invading enemy. The body marshals its immune defenses and attacks the allergen, and it is the body's response that results in the inflammation of skin, eyes, or bronchial tubes, or other physical reactions.

Often, allergic reactions to common allergens such as pollen, dust, or molds can appear as cold symptoms: runny nose, nasal congestion, itchy, watery eyes, postnasal drip, and perhaps a cough. Because the condition is an allergic reaction, until the offending allergen is expunged from your child's environment, the so-called cold will not go away. Mucus buildup in your child's sinuses can become a breeding ground for bacteria. A persistent cold that lasts for weeks, or comes and goes, may be an indication that your child should be checked for an allergy.

The most successful treatment for allergy is avoidance. Avoidance of allergens involves first determining what your child is allergic to and then eliminating it from her surroundings or diet, if possible. Determining what your child is allergic to can be tricky and time-consuming, as you eliminate suspect allergens and see if the response disappears. If your child's allergic response is mild, you can try to determine the source of the problem on your own. However, if you think that your child is being made ill by allergies or suffering severe reactions, contact your doctor as soon as possible. You may be referred to a pediatric allergist. An allergist can determine what allergens are responsible and devise a comprehensive treatment plan that may include medication.

The most common foods that some children are allergic to are cow's milk and dairy products, soy protein, eggs (particularly egg whites), citrus fruits and juices, tomatoes, strawberries, wheat products, nuts, shellfish, and fish. The most common symptoms of food allergies are rash around the mouth or bottom; inflammation of the mouth, tongue, or throat; diarrhea; vomiting; general feeling of discomfort; hives; stomachache; and asthma. An allergic reaction to food may occur within a few minutes of ingestion to as much as several hours later.

In addition to dust and pollen, animal dander is another common allergen. Environmental pollutants such as smoke from manufacturing plants and automobile exhaust as well as household sources can be a major cause of allergy-induced asthma, possibly the single most common, severe allergic response in children. (For more information on asthma, see Chapter 18.) Children can also have allergic reactions to medications, insect stings, and certain chemicals.

ACUTE ALLERGIC REACTIONS

Certain allergens, particularly peanuts or peanut butter, nuts, fish, bee stings, eggs, or certain medications, such as penicillin, can cause what is known as an anaphylactic reaction, which potentially can be deadly. These severe, acute allergic reactions happen in adults as well as children and can cause any or all of the following symptoms:

- Hives and swelling

- Vomiting and abdominal cramps

- Sudden difficulty in breathing

- Faintness or dizziness caused by a sudden drop in blood pressure

- Clammy, gray skin

- Loss of consciousness (rarely)

If you know that your child has an allergy that could result in an acute reaction, you should contact your doctor about preventive measures you can take. An allergy such as this is especially dangerous if your child also has asthma. If your child has a history of extreme allergic reactions, your doctor can prescribe a kit with injectable epinephrine to counteract the symptoms until you can get emergency help. Your doctor may ask you to keep an oral antihistamine on hand for less severe reactions.

As with all potentially severe medical conditions, your child's school, teachers, and other caretakers should be alerted to your child's allergies and be warned particularly to strictly avoid foods to which she may have an extreme reaction. You child's school should have a written action plan if your child has a history of severe reactions.

A sensible precaution is to have your child wear a medical identification bracelet that identifies her sensitivity. The Food Allergy Network, (800) 929-4040, can provide excellent support, especially with regard to school. See Chapter 29 for more information on allergies and anaphylactic reactions. ∎

For many allergies, avoidance is not always possible, and long-term medication therapy or immunotherapy (allergy shots) may offer considerable relief. Some children have reactions that are so severe that they need to have emergency medication with them. If you suspect your child has allergies, consult Chapter 29 for complete information on diagnosing and treating the problem.

SLEEP DIFFICULTIES

Some children never seem to have sleep problems, hopping into bed at bedtime and sleeping placidly until sunrise. Others fight going to bed tooth and nail, wake during the night, and can be plagued by nightmares, bedwetting, or night terrors. And both kinds of children can grow up in the same family.

Although sleep difficulties may manifest as a single problem—inability to sleep through the night—they can have many causes, most of them benign, very few of them requiring medical intervention. Usually, a sleep difficulty has one of several particular emotional causes, which can range from fear of wetting the bed while potty training to anxiety or stress caused by family dynamics, and is treatable by establishing a concrete and predictable sleep-time routine for the child.

Although some 5-year-olds can function reasonably well on 8 hours of sleep, the average child really needs about 11 hours, although needs vary from individual to individual. Generally, sleep needs decrease slightly as children get older, with 11- or 12-year-olds needing about 9 hours of sleep. To gauge how much sleep your child needs, observe how long she sleeps on her own when she is not required to wake for school or other reasons. If you watch several nights and then average them, you will have a good idea of how many hours of sleep she requires.

If you have a difficult sleeper, on your own or with the help of your doctor, try to determine the cause of your child's waking. The first thing to do is rule out physical causes, such as the effects of illness or medication (see Night Terrors and Sleep Apnea, page 253). Once you have ruled out a medical cause, you can try to analyze your child's emotional state. It could be as simple as a younger sister wanting recognition and fighting sleep until all older siblings have gone to bed so that she can have her parents' undivided attention. Stress and anxiety may also play roles. A child's worries—about a new sibling, about her parents' arguments—may be perfectly manageable during the day when there are other stimuli, but alone in a darkened room, her worries can come bubbling up and manifest themselves in fears expressed at night. Monsters, for example, can be the embodiment of any number of different fears, from inappropriate TV watching to insecurity rooted in parental tensions.

Here are some steps you can take to help ease young children into a sensible sleep routine:

- Make sure your child has a bedtime routine and sticks to it—a specific bedtime and a particular ritual that helps her wind down toward sleep. Reading to your child at bedtime can be a comforting close to the day. Once a sleep-time routine is established, never waffle and never use staying up late as a reward.

- Make sure your child is not overstimulated at bedtime. Active physical play should cease at least half an hour to 45 minutes before bedtime, and other, quieter activities should follow. Television is usually too stimulating and not a good prebedtime activity. Taking a bath, reading a book, playing soft music, singing to your child, and having quiet conversations are all good activities for winding down.

- If your child prefers, use a night light, or provide a lamp next to her bed that she can turn on and off herself.

- If your child comes to your room in the middle of the night, do not allow her to join you in your bed. Be as reassuring and gentle as you can, but always insist that the child sleep in her own bed. Often, a child will express fear of monsters in her room. You can quiet her fears most effectively by letting your child know gently but firmly that you love her and will protect her and that you will make sure that she is safe in her bed.

- Your child should sleep in her own bed. Different cultures and different economic circumstances can make for different sleep arrangements, but research shows that people who sleep alone sleep more soundly than people who sleep together. It is best for everyone's sleep if your child sleeps alone, in her own bed.

- Use a transitional object. Many children develop strong attachments to objects such as blankets or stuffed animals. Many parents mistakenly believe that their child's dependence on a transitional object is a sign of lack of self-confidence. In fact, the opposite is true. Research shows that children who use transitional objects tend to be more confident in going from one situation to another and will give up their objects when they are ready. Having a transitional object can make bedtime easier for both you and your child.

- Relieve your child's fears about bed-wetting. If your child is potty training, sleep can represent a time when loss of control might occur. Fears that she will wet or soil the bed can keep her from falling deeply asleep. In these instances, be as reassuring as possible: Let her wear disposable underpants or diapers to bed for protection and let her know that everybody at her age loses control once in a while. If she does wet the bed, react in as neutral a fashion as possible. Do not punish her or show disappointment. Her feelings of guilt or anger or inadequacy will only compound her stress. If she can make it the entire night without wetting or soiling, compliment her on her ability. (If your child is over age 5 and wetting the bed, see Enuresis and Encopresis, page 1234, for more information.)

If your school-age child wakes and cries in the middle of night, what should you do?

If your child has a normal sleep routine and is not ill, she may be having nightmares or experiencing night terrors (see below). Nightmares can be quite terrifying and real for children, especially younger ones, so you will need to comfort her and quiet her fears. Reassure her, and, if she wants, leave a light on while she goes back to sleep.

If she is not ill, and the nightmares become continuous, try to sort out what may be bothering her. Has she recently experienced a major upheaval in her life—a family move, a significant change in family circumstances (divorce, death, etc.), loss of a pet? If you cannot help sort out the reasons for her disturbed sleep and it continues, contact your doctor.

❖ NIGHT TERRORS

Symptoms After approximately 2 hours of normal sleep, your child will awaken in a state ranging from mild to extreme agitation; she may seem terrified yet cannot be comforted. The state will usually last only a few minutes, but can be longer. After the period of agitation, your child will usually fall back to sleep and have little or no recollection of the episode.

What is it? The state known as night terrors is different from nightmares and can be quite frightening to parents and family. During night terrors, your child may be thrash-ing about and possibly screaming but will not be consoled or reasoned with. Her eyes may be open, but she is not awake. The fit may last a few moments but can seem like a long time. Because of the child's bizarre behavior and unresponsiveness, many parents mistakenly believe that their children are having seizures or epileptic fits. They are not. Although the cause is not clear, night terrors are more accurately defined as agitation and appear to be a situation in which your child is stuck in a sleep state somewhere between deep sleep and waking and does not recognize you or remember the incident. Night terrors are most common in 5- to 7-year-olds, although they can persist into adolescence and adulthood. They may happen only once, or, very rarely, they could happen nearly every night for a while.

What you can do As frightening as night terrors can be for parents, your child will not remember the episodes, and the phenomenon should go away as she matures. Do not try to wake your child during a night terror. If the child is thrashing violently, holding her could prevent injury, but depending on her age and size, trying to hold her could injure both of you. Try to steer the child out of harm's way. Some children will respond to gentle commands. Eventually, she will settle and resume sleep.

Your child will not remember the night terror in the morning. Do not try to make her remember the situation or sort it out. If you dwell on it, your child may become self-conscious and fearful of sleep.

When to call the doctor Night terrors are likely to be harmless and short-lived. Contact your doctor if the night terrors are frequent, have become disruptive, or if you believe that they began after a traumatic emotional or physical event.

Treatment Night terrors rarely require treatment, though precautions need to be taken to prevent children from injuring themselves. If the problems persists, contact your doctor; she may refer you to a sleep specialist.

❖ SLEEP APNEA

Symptoms *(What your child may experience)* Loud snoring; restless sleep; difficulty breathing—gasps or struggles to breathe—

while asleep; sleeps with mouth open; partially awakens frequently (though may not be completely awake) due to interrupted breathing; thrashes because of breathing difficulties; has morning headaches; daytime sleepiness; bed-wetting (most bed-wetters, however, do not have sleep apnea).

Signs and laboratory findings *(What the doctor looks for)* Enlarged tonsils or adenoids; obesity; craniofacial abnormalities.

What is it? Sleep apnea is the result of a chronic obstruction to breathing. In adults, obesity is a common cause, but in children, the problem often lies with enlarged tonsils and adenoids. It is characterized most notably by snoring and periodic halts in the normal rhythm of breathing, which disturbs the child's sleep. It is not unusual for children to snore when they have colds, so it is important to note the *chronic* nature of snoring in sleep apnea. At times, in the course of a night's sleep, the breathing of a child with sleep apnea becomes so obstructed that it comes to a halt. The child then, in essence, wakes herself, at least partially, to restart breathing. This sleep disturbance is unhealthy for your child in the short term and can over the long term lead to more serious problems, such as stress to the heart, poor growth, or behavioral problems.

It may be your child's loud snoring that draws your attention to her sleep problem. Or you may notice that your child wakens often, sleeps in unusual places or positions, or seems to have difficulty breathing at night. If you bring the problem to your doctor's attention, she can refer you to an appropriate pediatric specialist, depending upon whether the problem is due to obesity, to enlarged tonsils and adenoids, or to some other cause.

What you can do Your child's doctor may ask that you videotape your child asleep or may want to perform tests such as spending the night in a special sleep laboratory to determine if your child is not breathing properly during sleep.

Treatment If the obstruction is caused by abnormally large tonsils and adenoids, the doctor will advise you whether surgery is necessary for your child. Tonsils and adenoids may shrink on their own as the child matures, but if sleep apnea is present, treat-ment is necessary to avoid complications. Surgery usually relieves the problem. The few children who do not respond to surgery or who have additional medical problems are treated with continuous positive airway pressure (CPAP) during sleep. A CPAP machine blows air through a nasal mask to prevent the airway from collapsing.

If the sleep apnea is caused by obesity, your doctor can devise a sensible diet and exercise plan to gradually resolve the problem. However, additional treatment such as CPAP is needed until your child loses sufficient weight.

DEPRESSION

It is natural for children, adolescents, and adults to experience brief periods of sadness ranging from a few hours to days or weeks after difficult life experiences. Depression that results from bereavement or serious life events can last for 2 to 3 months. These symptoms go away with resolution of the crisis or when the child has had time to process the grief or other emotion.

If your child suddenly changes for no reason and begins to withdraw, looks worn or tired, lacks energy or joy, loses her appetite, wants to sleep all the time (or is unable to sleep), or does not seem to care much about herself, these could be signs of depression or other disturbances and should be carefully evaluated by an expert such as a child psychologist or psychiatrist. Your child should be seen by her doctor first, because these can also be signs of a serious medical illness.

Depression can in some children manifest itself in ways that would not necessarily lead a parent to suspect depression. Getting into frequent fights, behaving cruelly toward animals or smaller children—these may not be classic symptoms of depression but do suggest mental health issues. They are cries for help and are cause to talk to your child's doctor. Sometimes just the indication that parents care can be a tremendous boost to a child's mood.

The psychologist or psychiatrist will want to sort out events leading up to the onset of depression to rule out developmental or learning delays and other possible causes (such as inappropriate sexual contact).

CHILD ABUSE

All child abuse has certain aspects in common: It almost always occurs at the hands of a parent, close relative, or other caregiver. It is almost always the result of the adult feeling pushed too far and becoming aggressive and violent to try to stop a child's offending behavior. It often results in the parent feeling guilty and remorseful, with the parent apologizing to the child for what the parent has done. And it almost always is repeated. It can be deadly.

Not all abuse is physical. Emotional abuse is the willful destruction of a child's self-esteem and sense of security by belittling, berating, and ridiculing the child. The long-term results can be destructive and lead to increased rates of depression and substance abuse.

No parent has the patience to be as reasonable as she would like to be at all times. In any given punishment situation, nearly any concerned parent can see how she might have been more effective, less emotional—if only there had not been such confusion; if only everyone was not so tired; if only she had been able to deflect the child's tantrum. No one is going to handle every situation ideally. And different cultures will have differing standards for what is deemed an appropriate response to misbehavior.

Certain parents, however, may suspect that because of their circumstances—their own abuse when they were children, limited financial circumstances, an overwhelming work or school schedule, alcohol or drug abuse—they are not being the most effective parents they can be.

If you feel that you are not in control of your child, if you feel guilty after punishing your child, if you feel that your punishing has become violent, you are not alone. Numerous places can provide you with assistance with parenting and with improving parenting skills. Family counselors are trained in observing family dynamics—how parents relate to children, how children relate to one another—and can offer you sensible, objective advice on how to improve your parenting skills and simultaneously improve the quality of the time you spend with your children.

Many hospitals, as part of their community outreach programs, offer parenting classes. Churches, temples, and community organizations also frequently offer assistance to parents in need of help. Parents Anonymous is an organization specifically created to help parents who have abused their children or fear that they will.

Over 2 million cases of suspected child abuse are reported annually. The true number can only be guessed at, because most cases of child abuse go unreported. Neglect is the most common form of maltreatment, followed by physical abuse, emotional abuse, and sexual abuse. Children who are being abused may have black eyes, bruises, burns, unusual injuries that do not have reasonable explanations, numerous injuries, low self-esteem, aggressive and disruptive behavior, or frightened, passive, or withdrawn behavior.

What should you do if you suspect a child is being abused? You should report the possibility. If you are in doubt—and most people will worry about intruding into the private affairs of others and will want to give the parent the benefit of the doubt—you can call one of the telephone numbers listed below for advice on how you should proceed.

- Child Health USA (800) 4-A-CHILD (422-4453)

- National Clearinghouse on Child Abuse and Neglect Information (800) 394-3366

- National Clearinghouse on Family Support and Children's Mental Health (800) 628-1696

- Parents Anonymous—consult your local telephone directory ■

SEXUAL ABUSE

Sexual abuse is a problem of enormous proportions, although accurate statistics do not exist, because most of it goes unreported. Some statistics indicate that as many as a quarter of all girls experience some kind of inappropriate sexual contact before age 14, and by age 18, that number has increased to one-third. Boys are somewhat less likely to experience sexual abuse, with about one-sixth experiencing some kind of inappropriate sexual contact. But all the numbers are estimations at best.

What do we know about patterns of sexual abuse? It is almost always at the hands of a trusted family member or family friend. Abuse is most often perpetrated by a man, and the victim is usually a girl, although it may be a boy. Abuse does happen at the hands of women, usually to boys. Abuse is most likely to happen at home or close to home. It is likely to continue for an extended period of time before it is uncovered (sometimes it comes to light only in adulthood, after the abuse has long ceased), and its revelation is often met with disbelief or denial or even blaming of the victim.

Those who are sexually abused are at much greater risk for self-destructive behavior, ranging from serious alcohol and other drug abuse to teenage pregnancy and depression. Abused children are at increased risk for becoming promiscuous and engaging in risky, unsafe sexual behavior. They may come to believe that their only value is as a sexual object.

Several signs can point to sexual abuse: injury to the anal or genital area, particularly vaginal bleeding or discharge; sexually transmitted disease; sexual knowledge inappropriate for a child; and sudden and extreme withdrawal by a child who was formerly outgoing. Because children are often coerced into sexual abuse, a child who is suddenly fearful and secretive or asks questions about secrets or legal issues may be sending signals of abuse. Also, fearfulness of a particular adult or an unusual relationship with a particular relative or other adult can be indicative of sexual abuse.

Children should be taught that their bodies are their own. They can be told that no one but a doctor or nurse should touch a part of the body that is normally covered by a bathing suit. ▶

♦ They should also be allowed to refuse kisses and hugs. Children often cannot prevent sexual abuse from happening. However, you can teach children to talk to you when someone touches, or tries to touch, their private parts.

If you suspect your child may be a victim of sexual abuse, do not scare, accuse, or confront her. You should waste no time in contacting your doctor to ask for advice. A careful medical examination is necessary, although in most cases of sexual abuse, the child's physical examination will be completely normal. Your doctor may want a social worker or psychologist to interview your child. A sexually abused child, depending on the duration of the abuse, may need extensive counseling. The child should have no contact with the abuser, and you should seek legal action. If the abuser of a child is a parent or step-parent, separate the child from the abuser, stop unsupervised visits, and seek legal recourse. The entire family may need counseling to process the shame, guilt, anger, and other emotions involved.

Many support groups can give you information, help, and referrals, including

- Child Health USA (800) 4-A-CHILD (422-4453)

- National Clearinghouse on Child Abuse and Neglect Information (800) 394-3366

- National Clearinghouse on Family Support and Children's Mental Health (800) 628-1696 ■

Whatever the cause of the depression, your child may need counseling in order to sort out her feelings and help her regain her self-esteem.

Educational Handicaps

Many developmental difficulties do not become apparent until children are in school, because school makes much more rigorous demands on the child's intellectual, social, and athletic skills.

LEARNING DISABILITIES

Some children make the transition from the easygoing environment of home or daycare or preschool to the more demanding one of grade school with ease. For others, the transition is rocky and difficult. The demands that a more rigorous educational environment place upon these children exceed their ability to meet them. For some, difficulties at this stage may simply be a matter of immaturity, because children develop at different rates. For others, the difficulty may be due to a learning disability or disabilities.

Learning to read and write, add and subtract may seem easy to those of us who already know how to do them, but these skills require a complex interplay between several psychological processes. A learning disability, thus, is defined as a disorder in one or more of the basic psychological processes involved in understanding or using language, spoken or written, which may manifest itself as an imperfect ability to listen, speak, think, write, spell, or do mathematical calculations. There is much we do not know about the causes of learning disabilities or how to prevent them, although we do know that learning problems tend to run in families.

Because learning disabilities can have so many different potential origins, they can be difficult to diagnose and to treat. Although skillful educators can work with children with learning disabilities to circumvent their disability or disabilities, no single treatment can cure the disability.

There are many different types of learning disabilities, but they can be broadly divided into three general categories:

- Academic skills disorders

- Motor skills disorders

- Developmental language and speech disorders

Developmental language and speech disorders Language and speech disorders are subdivided into the following disorders, although each of these disorders may embrace a number of particular conditions.

An *articulation disorder* is a speech disorder in which the child has difficulty producing speech sounds. For example, the child may be unable, at age 6, to form certain sounds and therefore may avoid them or substitute others. This may lead to her being misunderstood.

An *expressive language disorder* is a condition in which the child has difficulty communicating her thoughts to others.

Both articulation and expressive language disorders can lead to behavior problems, as a result of the child's frustration with her inability to communicate in a way that will be understood.

A *receptive language disorder* is a condition in which the child has difficulty understanding what other people say. This may be a sign of more serious brain dysfunction. It usually is accompanied by difficulties with expression and is called receptive-expressive language disorder.

Academic skills disorders A child who is performing at a level significantly below expectation, based on her IQ, in reading, writing, or math, may be diagnosed as having an academic skills disorder. It does not mean that your child is less capable of learning than other normal children. But it does mean that she has trouble learning with standard methods and that her teachers may need to modify conventional teaching strategies so that she can learn and keep up with her peers. Academic skills disorders most often make themselves apparent as the child's school career progresses, and parents may become aware of them only after their child has fallen behind. This can lead to frustration for the student, which may manifest in dislike of school or the development of unhealthy coping mechanisms, such as being class clown or getting into trouble, to compensate for her difficulty in keeping up with her peers. Thus, treatment for an academic skills disorder may require addressing both the academic issues and the resulting self-esteem issues.

Most school systems are now able to cope sensibly with learning disabilities and have programs that can help your child overcome them.

Developmental reading disorder This type of disorder, also known as *dyslexia*, affects 2 to 8 percent of elementary schoolchildren and is more common in boys. A child with a developmental reading disorder may have difficulty distinguishing one letter from another. Her brain may transpose letters—*and* may appear to her as *dna*—or numbers—75 may appear to her as 57. She may have trouble telling a "b" from a "d."

Developmental writing disorder This type of disorder may manifest in an inability to compose complete, grammatical sentences. The child may lack the innate sense of grammar that many researchers believe most of us are born with. Developmental writing disorders may be due to language problems, motor difficulties, or other deficits.

Developmental arithmetic disorder may be indicated by problems with numbers or basic math concepts. These are likely to show up early. Problems involving the calculation of numbers are usually related to reasoning difficulties and occur in older children.

Motor skills disorders Motor skills disorders include problems with gross (big muscle) and fine (small muscle) motor skills. A child with gross motor disabilities, for example, may suffer poor self-esteem as a result of being perceived as clumsy and poor at sports. Fine motor disabilities, for example, can lead to slow, sloppy writing, which can impede progress in school.

What parents can do Our culture and our schools expect children to acquire academic skills at a predetermined rate. But not all children progress at the same pace or in the same ways. In our society, it is difficult for children to feel good about themselves when they fall behind their peers. The parental role is twofold: to have the child's difficulties properly evaluated and addressed, giving her the best possible chance to succeed, and to maintain the child's self-esteem, perhaps with professional help. The first step for parents is to have the child properly evaluated. This can be a complex process involving a variety of tests but generally includes an assessment of the child's abilities using standardized IQ and other tests and comparing these results with the child's educational achievements.

The Individuals with Disabilities Education Act of 1990 guarantees a public education to school-aged children with diagnosed learning disabilities. This act requires public schools to design and implement an individualized educational program tailored to each child's specific needs. The 1991 Individuals with Disabilities Education Act extended services to developmentally delayed children from newborns on. This law makes it possible for young children to receive help even before they begin school. The National Information Center for Children and Youth can provide referrals to appropriate local resources and state agencies. You can contact them at PO Box 1492, Washington, DC 20013, (800) 695-0285. Once a treatment plan that works within your child's abilities is in place, it is up to you as parents to support your child's emotional needs in facing this challenge.

ATTENTION-DEFICIT/ HYPERACTIVITY DISORDER

Attention-deficit/hyperactivity disorder (ADHD), the most common neurobehavioral disorder in children, is a syndrome that affects 3 to 5 percent of all children, perhaps as many as 2 million American children. It has been called a variety of names in the past, including minimal brain dysfunction and hyperkinesis. Two to three times more boys than girls are affected, but part of the difference may be failure to recognize it in girls. On the average, at least one child in every classroom in the United States needs help for the disorder. Most children with ADHD demonstrate the following characteristics: hyperactivity, impulsive behavior, and poor attention; some show inattentiveness alone. Sometimes these children's problems are hard to miss. They cannot sit still. They blurt out answers and interrupt. In games, they cannot wait their turn. Because of their constant motion and explosive energy, hyperactive children often get into trouble with parents, teachers, and peers. Though the hyperactivity may be most noticeable, it is the inability to concentrate that is the most devastating for the child's development. In addition, children with ADHD sometimes have associated conditions that need to be identified and treated, such as learning disorders, depression, anxiety, and other problems.

By adolescence, physical hyperactivity usually subsides into fidgeting and restlessness. About 30 percent of children with ADHD grow out of the disorder; often, the problems with attention and concentration continue into adulthood. At work, some adults with ADHD have trouble organizing tasks or completing their work. They do not seem to listen to or follow directions. Their work may be messy and appear careless. However, many adults who were diagnosed with ADHD during childhood make perfectly satisfactory adjustments to adult life. To ensure the best outcome, it is essential to identify and provide for the special needs (social, academic, and physical) that a child with ADHD may have.

The cause of ADHD remains unknown, but in the last decade, scientists have learned much about the course of the disorder. A variety of medications, behavior-changing therapies, and educational options are available to help people with ADHD focus their attention, build self-esteem, and function in new ways.

Not everyone who is overly active, inattentive, or impulsive has an attention disorder, and there is some concern that the ADHD label is being assigned too readily. ADHD is a diagnosis applied only to children and adults who consistently display certain characteristic behaviors over a period of time and in more than one setting (for example, at school and at home).

If you suspect your child has ADHD, your family doctor may assess her or may refer you to an appropriate specialist. In addition, state and local agencies that serve families and children, as well as some of the volunteer organizations listed in Resources for Families with a Child with Learning Disabilities (see page 259), can help identify an appropriate specialist. Keep in mind that while a variety of specialists can diagnose and treat ADHD, only a doctor can prescribe any medication that may be needed as part of the treatment plan.

Treating ADHD: What are the educational options? Most children with ADHD are able to stay in the regular classroom, and whenever possible, educators prefer not to separate children. But some children with ADHD are too hyperactive or inattentive to function in a regular classroom, even with medication and a behavior management plan. Such children may be placed in a special education class for all or part of the day. In some schools, the special education teacher teams with the classroom teacher to meet each child's unique needs.

Children with ADHD often need some special accommodations to help them learn. Many of the strategies of special education are simply good teaching methods. Telling students in advance what they will learn, providing visual aids, and giving oral as well as written instructions are all ways to help students focus and remember the key parts of the lesson. Small class size and minimizing distractions may also help.

Students with ADHD often need to learn techniques for monitoring and controlling their own attention and behavior.

RESOURCES FOR FAMILIES WITH A CHILD WITH LEARNING DISABILITIES

Support Groups and Organizations

- Attention Deficit Information Network (AD-IN)
  475 Hillside Avenue
  Needham, MA 02194
  Phone: (617) 455-9895
  Provides up-to-date information on current research, regional meetings. Offers aid in finding solutions to practical problems faced by adults and children with an attention disorder.

- ADD Warehouse
  300 NW 70th Avenue
  Plantation, FL 33317
  Phone: (800) 233-9273
  Distributes books, tapes, videos, and assessment on ADHD. Call for catalog.

- Center for Mental Health Services
  Office of Consumer, Family, and Public Information
  5600 Fishers Lane, Room 15-105
  Rockville, MD 20857
  Phone: (301) 443-2792
  This national center, a component of the US Public Health Service, provides a range of information on mental health, treatment, and support services.

- Children and Adults with Attention Deficit Disorders (CH.A.D.D.)
  499 NW 70th Ave., Suite 109
  Plantation, FL 33317
  Phone: (305) 587-3700
  A major advocate and key information source for people dealing with attention disorders. Sponsors support groups and publishes two newsletters concerning attention disorders for parents and professionals.

- Council for Exceptional Children
  11920 Association Drive
  Reston, VA 22091
  Phone: (703) 620-3660
  Provides publications for educators. Can also provide referral to Educational Resource Information Center (ERIC) Clearinghouse for Handicapped and Gifted Children.

- Federation of Families for Children's Mental Health
  1021 Prince Street
  Alexandria, VA 22314
  Phone: (703) 684-7710
  Provides information, support, and referrals through federation chapters throughout the country. This national parent-run organization focuses on the needs of children with broad mental health problems.

- HEATH Resource Center
  American Council on Education
  1 Dupont Circle, Suite 800
  Washington, DC 20036
  Phone: (800) 544-3284
  A national clearinghouse on post-high school education for people with disabilities.

- Learning Disabilities Association of America
  4156 Library Road
  Pittsburgh, PA 15234
  Phone: (412) 341-8077
  Provides information and referral to state chapters, parent resources, and local support groups. Publishes news briefs and a professional journal.

- National Association of Private Schools for Exceptional Children
  1522 K St., NW, Suite 1032
  Washington, DC 20005
  Phone: (202) 408-3338
  Provides referrals to private special education programs.

- National Center for Learning Disabilities
  99 Park Ave., 6th Floor
  New York, NY 10016
  Phone: (212) 687-7211
  Provides referrals and resources. Publishes *Their World* magazine describing true stories on ways children and adults cope with learning disabilities.

- National Information Center for Children and Youth with Disabilities (NICHCY)
  PO Box 1492
  Washington, DC 20013
  Phone: (800) 695-0285
  Publishes free, fact-filled newsletters. Arranges workshops. Advises parents on the laws entitling children with disabilities to special education and other services.

- Sibling Information Network
  A.J. Pappanikou Center
  1776 Ellington Road
  South Windsor, CT 06074
  Phone: (203) 648-1205
  Publishes a newsletter for and about siblings of children with special needs. ■

The process of finding alternatives to interrupting the teacher makes these children more self-sufficient and cooperative, and because they interrupt less, they begin to get more praise than reprimands.

Medical treatments For decades, medication has been used to treat the symptoms of ADHD. The three drugs that seem to be the most effective in both children and adults are methylphenidate (Ritalin), dextroamphetamine (Dexedrine), and pemoline (Cylert). Pemoline can cause liver toxicity. If your child is taking pemoline, she should have liver function tests before and periodically during therapy with this drug. For many children, medication dramatically reduces hyperactivity and improves their ability to focus, work, and learn. Medication may also improve physical coordination, helping children write properly and participate in sports.

Unfortunately, when people see such immediate improvement in hyperactivity, they often think medication is all that is needed. But these medications do not cure the disorder, and they do have side effects. Although medications help people pay better attention and complete their work, they should be combined with other strategies to help people with ADHD feel better about themselves. Many experts believe that the most significant, long-lasting gains appear when medication is combined with behavioral therapy, emotional counseling, and practical support.

DISRUPTIVE BEHAVIOR DISORDERS

Although all children will get in trouble from time to time, certain children seem constantly to be in trouble and even seem to seek out trouble. Often, these children were perceived by their parents as difficult, even from an early age. A certain amount of disruptive behavior is natural in all children, but overly aggressive and antisocial behavior can interfere with a child's education and socialization.

For disruptive behavior to constitute a disorder, it must occur consistently over at least a 6-month period. The behavior may be overly aggressive, antisocial, hostile, negative, or defiant, and it is distinct from the simply disruptive, nondestructive behavior that children with attention disorders may exhibit.

There are two types of conduct disorders, socialized and unsocialized. *Socialized* refers to children making trouble in groups. This may include gang activity but also can include nongang, peer group activity, and it is more common in older and adolescent children. *Unsocialized* refers to the child making trouble on her own, outside of a peer group. This is more common in pread-

olescents. This can indicate difficulties not only within the family (relationships with adults tend to be angry or distant or otherwise hostile) but also problems in socialization, a failure to be accepted by the peer group, or a general feeling of isolation.

If you suspect your child may have a disruptive behavior disorder, contact your doctor, who can refer you to a psychiatrist or psychologist. Both individual and family therapy may be recommended. The earlier the intervention occurs, the better the chances for a successful outcome.

❖ MENTAL RETARDATION

Symptoms *(What your child may experience)* Delayed development in a variety of areas, including language, fine motor skills, emotional maturity; poor overall performance in school.

Signs and laboratory findings *(What the doctor looks for)* An IQ score below 70, based upon reliable, standardized testing.

What is it? Mental retardation is not a disease or illness, just as being gifted is neither disease nor illness. Both are measures of intellectual capacity against a theoretical norm, or average.

Mental retardation affects 3 percent of the population. Eighty percent of those affected are only mildly retarded, which is why many affected children are not recognized until they have entered school, when their incapacity becomes more apparent.

Only a quarter of all slowed mental development is caused either by known inherited defects such as Down syndrome (see Chapter 8) or congenital metabolic disruptions, such as phenylketonuria, which can cause brain damage or limit intellectual capacity if not diagnosed at birth (see Chapter 8). Mental disabilities can also result from environmental, infectious, chemical, and traumatic causes—including poor nutrition, meningitis, exposure to lead or other chemicals, maternal alcohol or other drug abuse during pregnancy, or head injury. The level of disability can range from mild (the child can perform tasks in a mostly average fashion and can grow up to live an independent life but may take longer to learn than others of the same age), to serious (the child maintains a dependence on others to help her live), to profound (the child may not even be able to speak or to perform normal adaptive functions such as feeding, dressing, or toileting, and requires constant care).

The term *mental retardation* has acquired a host of unpleasant associations. No one wants to be thought of, or wants their child to be thought of, as slow. But mental retardation simply signifies a slowing or arresting of certain kinds of intellectual development. Although the label is difficult for any parent to accept, an accurate diagnosis is invaluable in getting your child the help she needs to reach her fullest potential, and it can also help you get the assistance your child is entitled to by law.

If you are concerned that your child's development is not keeping pace with her peers, you should discuss what you have observed with your doctor. She can recommend a complete assessment of your child, including screenings by a variety of medical professionals to evaluate, diagnose, and recommend treatment for your child.

What you can do A great additional handicap faced by children with mental retardation is society's rejection of them. Children with mental handicaps can be the most loving and most loved of children. It is up to parents to value their child and make her feel valued for the unique rewards her life will bring.

Treatment Mental retardation cannot be cured, though special programs can help mentally retarded children achieve their fullest potential. Many parents have difficulty accepting the diagnosis. You can help your child most by working with your doctor and your school to find the best assistance to help her adapt and work around any disability. The goal of any kind of education program—whatever the child's abilities—is to help your child maximize her potential. By law, every child is guaranteed early intervention and appropriate education. If your child is diagnosed as mentally retarded, talk to the specialists you have seen about special education programs in your area, and talk to your local school system to find out how you can use their special education services. Such curricula can be quite valuable in educating mentally handicapped children at a developmentally appropriate pace and in teaching them adaptive skills.

❖ AUTISM

Symptoms *(What your child may experience)* Asocial behavior (not reaching out to parents for comfort when hurt or tired, no interest in playing with peers); the rejection, sometimes violently, of parental or sibling affection; unwillingness to make eye contact; delayed speech; failure to use speech communicatively; unusual responses to sounds, touch, and other sensations; absence of emotional reaction; self-injury, through head-banging or self-biting; engaging in repetitive obsessive or bizarre behavior; lack of fear of realistic dangers.

Signs and laboratory findings *(What the doctor looks for)* Abnormal posture and movements; mental retardation.

What is it? Infantile autism is a permanent mental disorder of unknown cause. Autism generally becomes apparent before age 3; often, problems are apparent in infancy, but some autistic children seem to develop normally at first and then lose the skills they previously acquired. The disorder afflicts boys three to four times more often than girls. Eighty-five percent of autistic children are mentally retarded as well, but some autistic children give signs of occasionally sophisticated intelligence, though autistic children often have no interest in cooperating with an intelligence test.

The autistic child may be unable to develop relationships with others; indeed, she may reject physical signs of affection from her family. She may speak late—or not at all—and when she does speak, she may not use language for the purpose of communicating with others. An autistic child may play with toys in ritualistic ways, lining objects up rather than playing with them imaginatively. She may respond in unusual ways to sounds or touch, yet show no fear in the face of realistic dangers. She may find changes in routine very disturbing. She may walk in unusual ways and express excitement by jumping up and down or flapping her arms. She may injure herself through repetitive head banging or by biting herself.

What you can do There is little a parent can do for autism independently of doctors and therapists. Family therapy may, however, help parents and siblings understand the disorder and cope with its stresses.

Treatment If autism is diagnosed early, your child may be able, depending upon the severity of the disease, to learn many adaptive skills. There is much we do not know about autism, however, and it is difficult to predict how a child will respond to treatment. Treatment seeks to encourage language development and improve social interaction. These are achieved through one-on-one interaction between child and teacher or therapist. Behavior modification methods may be used to discourage particular problems, such as self-injury. Contact your doctor to find a specialist who can develop an individual treatment plan suited to your child's needs.

TEN

The Teen Years

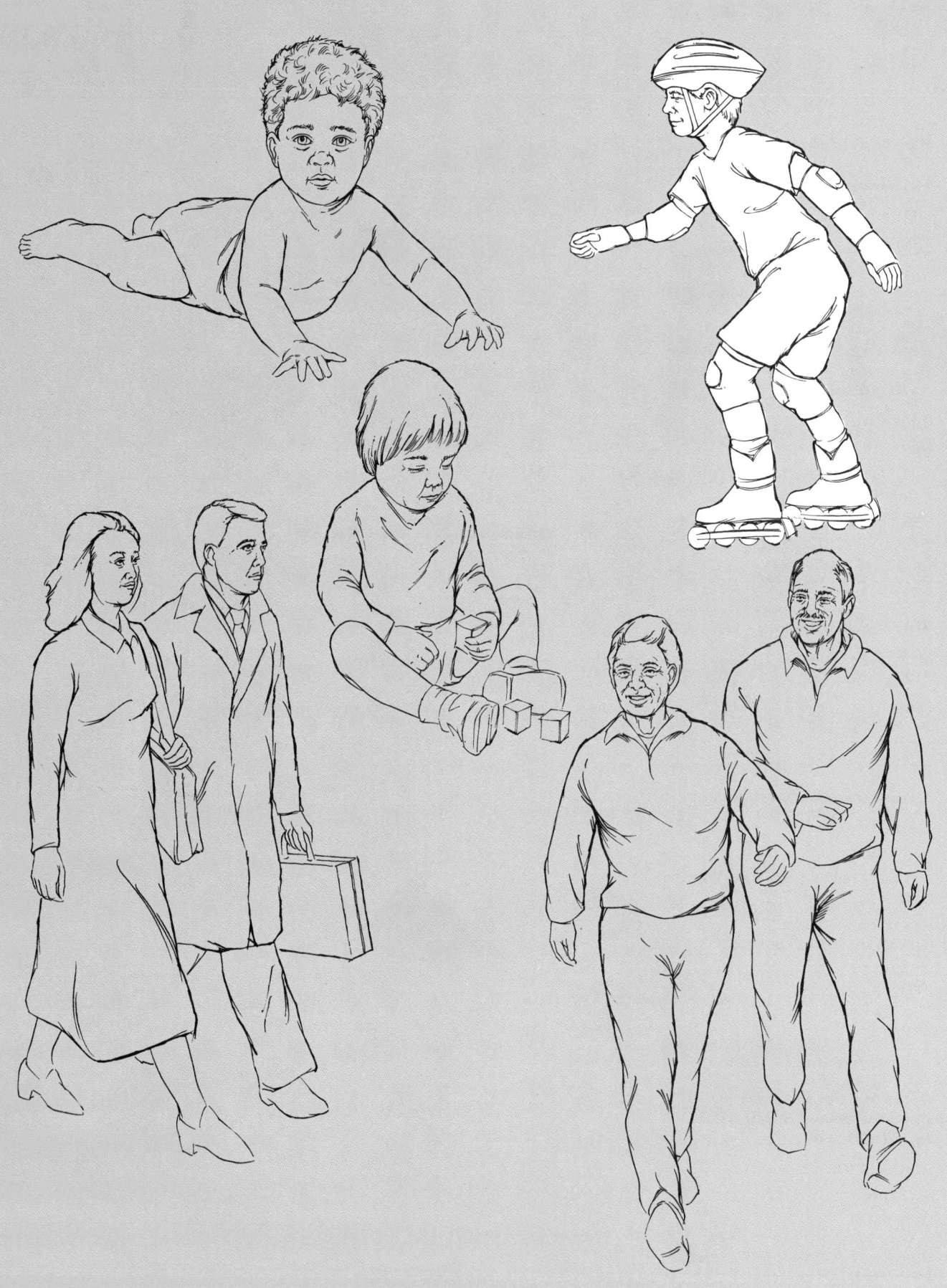

THE TEEN YEARS

What Is Adolescence?

Watching a child turn into an adult can be one of the most astonishing and rewarding experiences a parent can have. And yet, many of us think of adolescence as a time of struggle, a potentially painful time when children seem to reject their parents. In some respects this is so. One of the primary goals of adolescence is the formation of an identity separate and distinct from that of one's family of origin. For an adolescent, the search for self can cause a crisis between conflicting needs. On the one hand, she needs her parents and all that they represent and supply; on the other, she needs to strike out on her own to find herself and build the foundation of self that may eventually become the foundation for her own healthy family.

The adolescent years are transitional years, with many experiences, both for adults and adolescents, occurring for the first time. This chapter aims to give both parent and teen information not only on surviving but on *thriving*. It should be noted that the difficulties and triumphs of a 13-year-old are likely to be significantly different from those of an 18- or 19-year-old. The sections that follow have been broken down not so much by age as by general circumstances that can affect all adolescents and by particular health concerns—both physical and mental—that may be faced by all. If you are a parent worried about your teenager's health and well-being, this chapter will provide essential information. If you are a teenager, with new experiences coming at you at a dizzying rate, this chapter will provide you with answers to questions you may find too embarrassing to ask. You will find important information on how you can stay healthy, as well as advice on dealing with health problems that may occur.

Adolescence—although usually thought of as the teenage years—actually begins with the onset of puberty and does not end until complete adult development is achieved, most often by age 17. In some girls, onset comes as early as age 8 or 9, or as late as age 13 or 14. For boys, the onset of puberty begins roughly 2 years later—at about age 10 or 11, or in some cases, as late as age 14. When puberty begins depends first on genetics—when and how fast parents developed—and then on other factors, such as nutrition, weight, and potential glandular abnormalities. For one person, the entire process of physical maturation can take as little as 12 to 18 months. For others, it can last 3, even 4 years. During adolescence, change occurs more radically and rapidly than at any other time of life, which may be what makes adolescence seem so difficult at times. But these changes can also make adolescent life exciting and rewarding.

The notion of a period called adolescence is actually a fairly recent concept, developed during and after the Industrial Revolution and refined as society has made different demands on young adults. Prior to the 18th century—and indeed to this day in certain cultures—the concept of adolescence, a distinct period between childhood and adulthood, did not exist in the way it does today in our society. There were children, and there were adults. Once children reached a certain age, they were expected to take on adult responsibilities.

As our society has become more complex, the process of adolescence has become much more important. Longer life, the multitude of choices individuals have to make, as well as the variety of difficult concepts that must be mastered, require more sophisticated adults. The process of adolescence is fundamental to acquiring that sophistication, but it can for some young people also make adolescence that much more complex and demanding.

Adolescence, then, is more than the process of physical and sexual maturation. Human adolescence is most importantly emotional and intellectual maturation, including the development of sophisticated, abstract thinking, and the transformation of a child who is dependent upon his parents for nearly all of his needs into a young adult, ready to strike out in the world alone, survive, and prosper.

Physical Maturation

Until puberty, boys' and girls' bodies are shaped essentially the same. Physical maturation is the growth process during which the secondary sexual characteristics of boys and girls appear and reach full development. Primary sexual characteristics are the sex organs themselves. The secondary sexual characteristics—widening hips, breasts, a higher voice, and a higher percentage of body fat in girls; increased physical size and strength, deeper voice, and body and facial hair in boys—begin to make themselves apparent as early as the late preteen years in

265

some children, and as late as the mid- to late-teen years in others, particularly boys. Some children bloom early, and others late.

Most of the physical maturation process is governed by heredity. Most children will resemble their parents not only in how tall they grow and what they look like, but in *how* they grow—when puberty and their growth spurt will begin, whether these will be fast or slow, and so on.

Nearly all children, however, will worry about their development as they go along. Even those who are particularly level-headed, whose growth is proceeding in a perfectly average fashion, will have anxieties about whether they are normal. When children exhibit anxiety about their growth, they may not do so in a direct way; the changes they are undergoing may simply embarrass them. Most adolescents will find it reassuring if parents share with them the anxieties parents experienced during adolescence, though parents should not be surprised if the child acts uninterested. Knowing that parents also worried about weight, about getting their period, about wet dreams, about acne, about being good-looking or athletic enough to be considered attractive may bring a measure of comfort.

If parents are concerned that their children are not developing at the proper rate, they should consult their doctor.

GIRLS

Breast development The beginning of breast development is often the first sign of puberty's onset. Puberty begins about a year before the peak growth spurt, so changes in the breasts may be noticeable some time before a substantial increase in height or weight. The nipple will begin to bud, and the area around it will begin to swell. Quite frequently, the development of one breast may outpace the other, and at full growth, one may be slightly larger than the other. This is normal.

Height and weight gain The growth spurt usually peaks between age 10 and 14, about a year after appearance of pubic hair and breast changes. The body will change as it grows. The hips will widen, breasts will grow, and the body (genetically predisposed to do so) will put away a higher percentage of fat. For a year or two, girls may be taller than boys their own age, but the boys will catch up and then on average surpass the girls in height and weight. Contact your doctor if your daughter's sexual development starts before age 8 or has not begun by age 13.

Hair: pubic, body, and underarm Pubic hair begins to appear about the same time as breast changes. Body hair generally begins to grow in 1 to 2 years after pubic hair, but its amount and distribution on the body vary widely from person to person. Some girls develop almost no body hair, while others can have quite hairy legs, hair surrounding the nipples or extending considerably beyond the bikini line, or a shadow of fine hair above the upper lip. Patterns of hair growth will be mostly governed by heredity.

Consult your doctor if pubic hair has not begun to appear by age 13 or begins before age 8, or if you are concerned that hair growth is not normal.

Perspiration and body odor At about age 12 to 13, the sweat glands mature and adult body odor ensues. Girls may choose to start using deodorant.

Vaginal discharge About a year before the onset of menstruation, the vagina will begin to emit a clear or white odorless fluid. This discharge may be startling initially, but it is completely normal. It will slacken after the onset of menstruation but will never go away entirely. Girls who find the wetness unpleasant may want to wear panty liners. Contact your doctor if the discharge is colored or has a strong odor.

Menstruation The onset of menstruation (menses), or periods, is one of the last markers of puberty in girls, generally occurring about 2 years after breast budding, or between ages 10 and 15. Periods will most often be irregular at first and may take many months or even years to settle into a regular cycle. See What Is Menstruation?, page 267.

BOYS

Height and weight gain The onset of puberty in boys is characterized by enlargement of the testes, followed by growth of

WHAT IS MENSTRUATION?

One of the final signs of puberty in girls is menarche (pronounced like "anarchy"), which is the onset of menses, or menstruation, commonly referred to as a period, because it occurs in monthly periods. For the first few months or years, your period may be irregular, but as the hormone levels stabilize, you are likely to settle into a regular cycle. The average cycle lasts 28 days; each cycle begins with 3 to 7 days of bleeding. Every girl is born with all the eggs she will ever produce, but these eggs only start to reach maturity when menarche begins. At the time of menarche, your two ovaries contain as many as a quarter of a million eggs each. Your ovaries connect to your uterus via the fallopian tubes. It is in your uterus, or womb, where a fertilized egg will one day attach and pregnancy will occur. But before you get to that point, you will have any number of periods, each of which could have resulted in a pregnancy.

During the cycle, your ovaries secrete the sex hormone estrogen, which causes the lining of your uterus (the endometrium) to prepare for a potential pregnancy by thickening and growing. About 7 days into your cycle, an egg is released from one of your ovaries; this is known as ovulation. Both your ovaries alternate randomly. The egg travels down the fallopian tube toward your uterus, a process that can take about a week. During this period, you are fertile and could potentially conceive if sperm were present. As the egg travels toward the uterus, your body continues to produce estrogen and another hormone, progesterone, which together stimulate the lining of your uterus to become even more active, producing nutrients ready to nourish an embryo, should egg and sperm connect. Your menstrual flow results when you do not become pregnant, the egg dissolves, and the uterus sheds its lining. This building and shedding cycle will continue, interrupted only by pregnancy, until menopause.

Before and during your period, you may experience painful cramps. In some cases, this severe cramping, known as dysmenorrhea, may cause you to have an overall feeling of bodily discomfort. Severe dysmenorrhea can prevent you from partaking in your daily activities.

Contrary to what some may believe, dysmenorrhea is a real situation. As you come to understand the various factors that contribute to dysmenorrhea, you will be able to more easily deal with dysmenorrhea as well as find ways to alleviate it.

Physiologically, uterine anatomy may cause one person to experience more severe dysmenorrhea than another person. Each person also has different tolerance levels toward pain. The various hormone levels that your body produces during menstruation may also be a factor.

If you experience dysmenorrhea with your period each month, you will find ways to alleviate the discomfort. Exercise, bedrest,

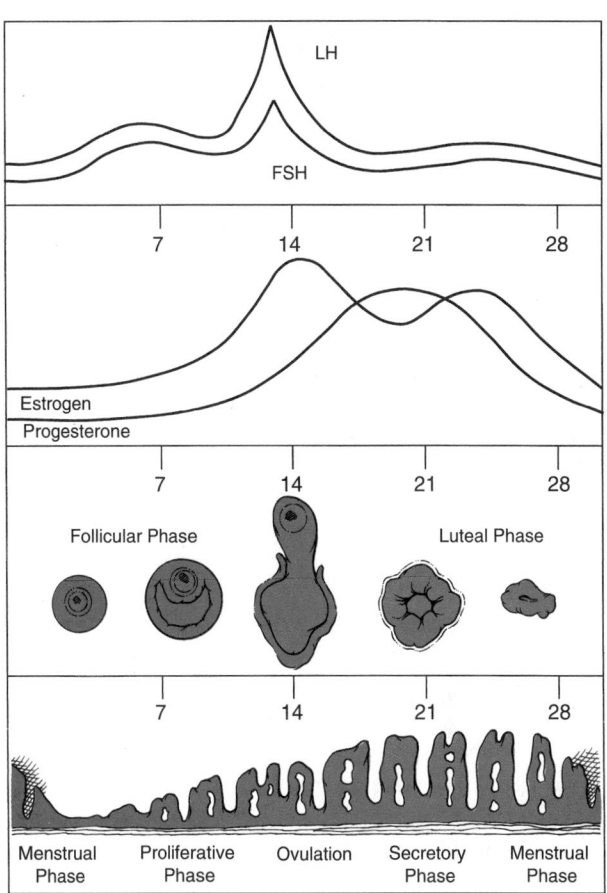

The menstrual cycle consists of three phases and one distinct event. Top to bottom: (1) In the menstrual phase (days 1 to 7), the levels of estrogen and progesterone fall. In response to these hormonal changes, the lining of the uterus sheds and bleeding occurs. (2) During the proliferative phase (days 7 to 14), the levels of estrogen and progesterone rise and support the growth of the lining of the uterus. Follicle-stimulating hormone (FSH) from the pituitary gland in the brain stimulates the development of an unfertilized egg in one of the ovaries (follicular phase). (3) Around day 14 of the cycle, the level of luteinizing hormone (LH) and FSH rise quickly, stimulating the release of the mature egg (ovulation). (4) During the secretory phase (days 14 to 28), the egg secretes estrogen, which further thickens the lining of the endometrium and supports the implantation and development of a fertilized egg. After releasing the egg, the follicle (now called the corpus luteum), secretes progesterone in order to nourish the lining of the uterus. If no egg is fertilized by a sperm, hormone levels fall and the menstrual phase begins again.

and relaxation will help. Various medications are also available to you. ■

pubic hair. The earliest normal age for the onset of puberty in boys is about age 9, the latest, age 14. The growth spurt usually follows onset of puberty by an average of 2 years, or typically at about age 14 (plus or minus 2) years. Boys and parents may notice that boys need new shoes every couple of months because feet grow so fast. Some boys may be fully developed by age 13, while others may not finish growing until

WHAT TO EXPECT DURING YOUR FIRST PELVIC EXAM

Choosing a Doctor for Reproductive Health

As adolescent girls begin to mature and menstruate, their doctors will begin to focus on their reproductive health. Well-health care visits at the pediatrician will include a gynecologic evaluation. Your doctor will also be able to provide you with answers to questions you may have on menstruation, puberty, and if necessary, contraception. Do not be embarrassed if there is a lot you do not know about sexuality and reproduction. Speaking openly with your doctor is the best way to get the information you need to protect your health and well-being.

Alternatively, once their periods have begun, many girls begin seeing a gynecologist. A gynecologist is a doctor whose specialty is the female reproductive system. Specialists certified in adolescent medicine are also capable of providing care for the female reproductive system.

If you are sexually active or considering becoming sexually active, your doctor can advise you on contraceptive methods to prevent pregnancy and on the precautions you need to take to reduce the likelihood of infection with sexually transmitted infections (STIs). The doctor will advise you to have an annual Papanicolaou (Pap) smear (see page 1100). Some experts recommend a semiannual STI screening for sexually active teens. For more information on STIs, see Chapter 21. Teens who are not sexually active and have normal menstrual periods do not necessarily need a pelvic exam until they reach age 18. If you are not sexually active and experiencing no particular problems, a checkup that includes a Pap smear every other year after age 18 will help to protect your reproductive health. However, if you suspect that you have a vaginal or urinary tract infection, you should be seen and treated by a doctor.

What Will the Doctor Do?

Since many pediatricians now incorporate gynecology into their practices, your doctor will begin by reviewing your medical history and expanding on it regarding gynecologic and reproductive issues. If you are seeing a new doctor, she will review your entire medical history with you. You may feel uncomfortable by some of the questions your doctor may ask, but you should be sure to answer as thoroughly and honestly as you can. Your doctor will ask, "Do you have sex with boys, girls, or both?" The doctor will also ask if you have any questions about the specifics of reproductive health. If you are sexually active, your doctor will counsel you on birth control and preventing STIs.

After your history is taken, you may have blood drawn, you may be asked to provide a urine specimen, and you may also be asked to empty your bladder to make your exam more comfortable.

You will then be asked to undress completely and put on a hospital gown. When you are given the gown, ask the nurse whether it should open to the front or the back, a detail most patients find impossible to determine on their own. Standard measurements, such as height, weight, and blood pressure, will be recorded. A nurse may perform many of these preliminary steps.

You will be asked to lie on an examining table. If your doctor is a man, a female nurse will always be present during your examination, and you will never be completely uncovered. The doctor will examine your breasts, feeling for any signs of abnormality, and show you how to perform a breast self-exam. The examining table will have stirrups on the corners for you to place the heels of your feet, as you are directed to lie in a position that allows you to be examined internally.

Your doctor will palpate your abdomen, which means pressing gently around your belly to ensure that everything is in its proper place and that none of your organs are swollen or ▶

---

they are in college. Before or during the beginning of the growth spurt, boys may notice what seems to be some breast development. This is known as gynecomastia and is not abnormal, although its cause is unknown. In general, these changes will be noticeable only to the person they are happening to. Rest assured that swelling or tenderness will go away in a few months, although it is also normal for gynecomastia to last 1 or 2 years.

Contact your doctor if the growth spurt begins before age 11 or has not begun by age 15.

Hair: pubic, underarm, body, and facial
Pubic hair will appear first, usually at age 11 to 12; underarm and body hair will follow at age 13 to 15, and facial hair will usually come last, at about age 13 to 15 or later, depending upon family heredity. Facial hair

usually starts with a mustache, followed by chin hair. Body hair, depending on family genetics, may continue to grow from the belly to the chest for several years, but some men never have a single hair on their chests.

Changes in the testes and scrotum The scrotal sac will darken as pubic hair comes in and the testes enlarge. This will begin on average at about age 11 to 12. If the testicles have not started to enlarge by age 14, or if pubic hair is unaccompanied by enlarging of the testes, or if one testicle is larger than the other, contact your doctor. Size of sexual organs will be governed mainly by family genetics.

Penis growth Generally, at about age 12 to 13, the penis will grow longer, then thicker. Because the rest of you is changing so rapidly, you may not notice the growth—and

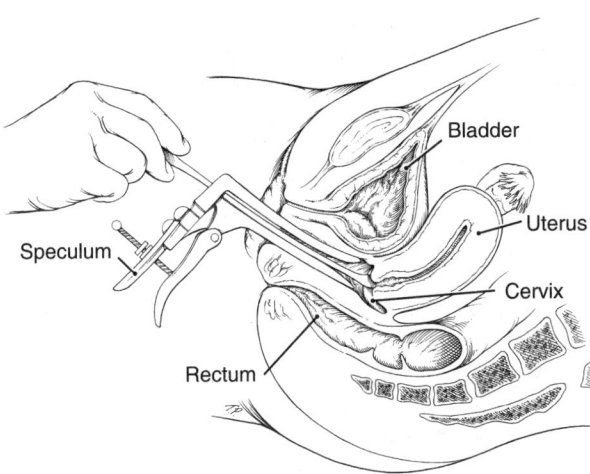

Pap smear. Pap smears are used to check for early signs of cervical cancer. A speculum allows a clear view of the cervix, which is the opening of the uterus. Cells from the surface of the cervix are gently scraped with a wooden spatula or plastic brush. These cells are examined under a microscope to detect changes that may lead to a cancer, so that it can be treated early.

▶ painful. Your doctor will then examine your external genitalia to make sure that all is normal—that, for example, you have no sores, lesions, ulcerations, or inflammation. Then your doctor will perform an internal exam to check the interior components of your reproductive tract. She will be on the lookout for any kind of sores, discharge, or ulceration—anything out of the ordinary. Your doctor will also look at your cervix, which is the opening to your uterus. Your doctor will use an instrument known as a speculum, which is made of either metal or plastic and allows your doctor to gently open your vagina enough to be able to look inside. The vagina is quite elastic, and this should not be painful. If, however, you are quite young or quite small, your doctor may at your first visit only insert a gloved finger to perform a digital exam. She may also simultaneously insert a gloved finger into your rectum to palpate your organs.

With the speculum in place, your doctor will probably insert a cytobrush—a swab that looks a bit like a cotton swab with soft bristles—and rub it against your cervix to obtain cells for a Pap smear. The small amount of cervical tissue removed will be sent to a lab for examination to ensure that there is no abnormal cell growth. Although it is highly unlikely that there would be any abnormal growth at your age, cervical cancer is very treatable, and so Pap smears are an extremely efficient, low-cost method for stopping this disease before it starts. It should be noted that sexually active teens are frequently infected with the human papilloma virus, which causes genital warts, and is a known risk factor for cervical cancer. A Pap smear will be a regular and integral part of your annual checkups.

Like any other sort of checkup, the point of regular pelvic examinations is detecting small problems before they become big problems. ■

---

may in fact consider it slow and inadequate—as it is happening. A fully grown, flaccid—or unerect—penis will range anywhere from an inch or so in length (cold water can make it even smaller) to a few inches, while a fully grown, erect penis will average about 6 inches. Generally, a smaller, flaccid penis will increase in size by a larger percentage when erect than a larger flaccid penis.

Ejaculation Although boys can probably have orgasms as early as in the womb, they will not ejaculate upon orgasm until about age 13 to 14, but it could happen earlier or later. The first ejaculate will likely not have any sperm in it and will be a clear or whitish fluid. If a boy masturbates regularly, this is when he will first note ejaculation. If not, he may first experience ejaculation as a wet dream.

Changes in voice As their voices begin to change, most boys experience a short but difficult period when everyone they speak to on the telephone mistakes them for women. This happens at about age 12 or 13 and will be followed, as the larynx enlarges and the voice deepens, by occasional cracks in the voice. Most boys, unless they are obese, will begin to show their Adam's apple at about age 15 or 16.

Perspiration and body odor At about age 13 to 14, as the sweat glands mature and multiply, and adult body odor ensues, boys may choose to start using deodorant.

Growing Pains: Social and Psychological Development in Adolescents

For some parents, the process of a child's maturing in adolescence can be one of the most difficult phases of parenting. An essential part of adolescence is *individuation*, wherein the child achieves his own identity separate from his parents. One moment, parents may shake their heads in wonder that the toddler who only days ago had trouble saying "spaghetti" is now the poised, intelligent captain of her debate team. The next moment, parents may shake their heads in wonder at how the sensible child of yesterday suddenly, today, can on occasion seem breathtakingly reckless and foolish.

If you are a parent, rest assured that your youngster has not, in all likelihood, really stopped being sensible—or at least not relative to her age. She is, in fact, grappling with a complicated world in which the stability of much of her adulthood is going to depend upon the experiments performed in adolescence. And in some cases, your adolescent is *deliberately* not going to be sensible while you are watching.

INDIVIDUATION

To individuate is to become separate from, to become an individual. The process of individuation is characterized by three essential components: developing a sense of self separate from that of the family; developing independence; and developing intimacy, or the capacity to have close, meaningful relationships outside the family.

Seldom can any human being be truly separate, but during adolescence, many young people want at least the illusion of being separate from their parents, even when they are clearly dependent upon them for food, clothing, and shelter. As dependents, their sense of individuation may come in other ways such as appearing to reject your deeply held values; making clear your presence is an embarrassment; joining groups of which you do not approve. Yet simultaneously, they will do things to be just like you, to show you how much they love you and desire your approval. Arguments can sometimes be the only way a child can express a need for his parents' views and even intervention.

Children begin adolescence closely associated with their family group, accepting its ideas and beliefs unquestioningly. Then, as children become young adults and begin to think in a more abstract and sophisticated way, they start to attach themselves to other groups. Most healthy adolescents will go through a period of perhaps several years during which they assume other ideas and beliefs, some of which may be disturbing to their parents. This stage is fundamental, if temporary. Research has shown, however, that most children eventually adopt behaviors and belief systems similar to those of their parents—this includes good qualities as well as bad.

This modeling of new ideas and beliefs like styles of clothing can sometimes be trying for parents. Keep in mind that there are good, healthy reasons why adolescents will adopt ideas diametrically opposed to yours. This is part of the development of independence, and some children may find it the easiest route to making themselves different from their family of origin.

Finally, as children mature and begin to assume their own ideas and beliefs, assimilating those adopted from the outside with those that come from the family they initially rejected, they become their own person, ready to form deep and lasting attachments in the world outside the family.

REBELLIOUSNESS

The individuation process can sometimes entail degrees of rebellious behavior. How much rebelliousness your adolescent demonstrates will depend in part upon the individual, in part upon values instilled during childhood, and in part upon how parents deal with rebelliousness. A certain amount of rebelliousness is normal and healthy and, most importantly, *transient*. Studies show that most parents get along well with most adolescents most of the time, even during a rebellious phase. How parents react to blue hair or to skirts that leave nothing to the imagination may play a key role in how much rebelliousness parents get. Most experts in adolescent behavior agree that it is better not to back a child into a corner by issuing ultimatums. Rigid dictums reinforce the adolescent's sense that parents are unwilling to listen to his opinions. Best is an approach that allows the young person to save face, leaving his sense of integrity and dignity intact while toeing the parents' line. It is possible to be firm yet give your child the sense that you respect her desires and judgment by allowing compromises that you both can live with. It is important for parents to take the long view and be creative and flexible. A good rule of thumb is to accept or at least ignore things that will not last, but take a harder line on those that can be permanent. You may be embarrassed by a hairstyle, but it will grow out. You may not like a pair of pants, but wearing them is not likely to hurt your child. Cigarette smoking, chronic truancy, alcohol or other drug use, tattoos, a pierced nose or lip—these are dangerous or permanent or both, and can have lasting repercussions. An adolescent does not have the maturity to make decisions alone on such matters.

If parents can find creative solutions while simultaneously showing the child respect, they will help provide good problem-solving tools for future conflicts—some of which may be avoided before they ever reach the living room.

Although children may have some level of conflict with parents over the course of several years, the rebellious phase itself, with pitched battles, peaks during middle adolescence, generally between ages 14 and 17 in both boys and girls. A certain amount of rebellion is a good, healthy thing, because it shows that the adolescent is learning how to reason and how to think for herself; this may mean, however, detailed rational analysis of some of her parents' cherished beliefs.

Some "rebellion," however, is not rebellion at all.

DELINQUENCY

There is no substitute for deep and particular parental involvement in a child's life. Parents' knowing a child's friends and the parents of her friends, and knowing their rules and curfews, can go a long way toward avoiding potential trouble. Monitoring your child's whereabouts at all times can be crucial to the healthy growth of the child. While trust is important, it should not necessarily be blind or automatic. Turning away from potential danger signals should never be thought of as "trusting my child." Younger adolescents simply may not yet have developed the discretion or the sophistication of thought to work out larger, more complex issues. Trust is a complex issue involving not only trust but trustworthiness. The best method for instilling trust and trustworthiness is, of course, by parental example.

Many normal teens will engage in a certain amount of what may be deemed delinquent behavior during adolescence. This can include minor vandalism, graffiti, window breaking, shoplifting, making prank phone calls, or engaging in other nonviolent activity. Usually, these activities take place in groups and are frequently the result of adolescent dares. Usually, the perpetrators of

LEADING CAUSES OF DEATH AND ILLNESS IN ADOLESCENTS

Every one of the leading causes of death in adolescents is avoidable or preventable in some way. Seat belts alone can save the lives of thousands of adolescents each year. See Chapter 3 for detailed advice on safety precautions.

Leading Causes of Death in Adolescents

1. Motor vehicle crashes
2. Suicide (numbers 2 and 3 are approximately equal)
3. Homicide
4. Poisoning (which includes accidental poisonings due to alcohol or other drug overdose)
5. Drowning

Leading Causes of Illness/Injury in Adolescents

1. Trauma (this could be anything from sports-related injuries to gunshot wounds; alcohol or other drug abuse is frequently a factor)
2. Mental health issues (substance abuse, depression, etc.)
3. Sexually transmitted infections
4. Acquired immunodeficiency syndrome (AIDS)
5. Eating disorders

Many of the most common and dangerous sports injuries happen during casual recreation and can be avoided by wearing protective equipment and following safety rules—and by leaving alcohol or other drugs out of the game. Helmets must be worn when engaging in activities such as roller-skating, skateboarding, and cycling. Many states now have laws that require juveniles to wear helmets when bicycling, but they are often not vigorously enforced. Head injuries can be fatal. All young people should be instructed in basic safety for any sport in which they participate. ■

such crimes are otherwise good citizens. When caught, these children are often at a loss to explain why they did what they did. In many instances, such behavior may be seen as a veiled request to have boundaries more firmly drawn.

Certain adolescents seem to have almost a need to break the law. This may be particularly true of children who have lived in households in which rules have been either particularly rigid or particularly lax. As these children begin to question parental authority, they may also question legal authority. If handled sensibly by parents and legal authorities, lessons learned by adolescents in these situations can be positive in the long run. Statistics show, for example, that most of those who experiment with cigarettes or alcohol and other drugs do not go on to become regular users. Some researchers believe that young people who have the mental flexibility to take minor risks to discover why these activities should be wrong or illegal grow up to be healthier, happier adults. Often, however, truly delinquent behavior is not a result of mental flexibility but a result of mental inflexibility.

Breaking the law can be seen as a cry for help or attention, and most children who do so are likely to need and even want appropriate punishment; scrubbing community walls of graffiti; hours of community service to pay for vandalism; getting arrested and even going to trial for shoplifting. Parents should see to it that these children form a clear understanding of what their behavior costs—not only to themselves but to their family and community. If the behavior is a plea to have lax boundaries more firmly drawn and the child's actions have no consequences, the likelihood is more of the same behavior, perhaps escalating in seriousness as time goes on. Similarly, if the behavior is a plea to rethink rigid or overwhelming boundaries and expectations, an overreaction that creates even more rigid boundaries also may lead to repeated and escalated behavior. Counseling may assist both parent and child toward more meaningful and equitable boundaries.

How can you tell what sort of behavior is normal and what is truly delinquent and cause for concern? Certainly, if a child is arrested, it is cause for concern. However, just as it is possible to get pregnant from having sex only once, so it is possible to get arrested for shoplifting only once. If a child does exhibit delinquent behavior, parents need to determine whether the behavior is part of a pattern or is an isolated incident. If it is an isolated incident and the child is truly contrite, then you must decide the best way to approach the situation. If it is part of a pattern—if, for example, it is accompanied by alcohol or other drug use, poor performance in school, repeated truancy, membership in a gang, or running away from home—then you should consult your doctor or the school to seek advice on obtaining appropriate counseling.

Also important to determine is whether the child engaged in such behavior alone or as part of a group. If alone, it may be an indication of a serious underlying problem that calls for intervention. If it is done as part of a group, is the group a gang? Do you know your child's friends? Does your child display gang colors, talk about being a gangster? Although gang violence and the dangers of gangs may in certain localities be somewhat exaggerated by the media, you must discover for yourself the extent of your child's involvement, its underlying reasons, and its potential for endangering your child.

Has your child been involved with guns or alcohol or other drugs? If so, seek counseling for him and for yourself.

A child having problems significant enough to result in delinquent behavior can be reflective of a family having problems, which can range from dysfunctional behavior on the part of parents, such as alcoholism, or lack of parental involvement, such as from working two jobs to make ends meet. Any counseling of a child should therefore involve as much of the family as possible. Such involvement will assist the counselor in treating problem behavior organically, by allowing the counselor to see the family dynamic to find out how overall circumstances can be changed for the better. Such sessions can also serve as a forum for children and parents to share their feelings in a relatively open and objective environment. Refusal of parents to be involved in counseling can signal to the child that counseling—and the child—are not worth the parents' effort and therefore not worthy of the child's effort.

What do you do if your child needs counseling but refuses? Parents and adolescents can try selecting a counselor together, with parents assuring the child that they need counseling as much as she does. You can also try allowing the child to choose the counselor independently, using one, for example, suggested by a teacher or a friend. If nothing you do will get your child to go to counseling, go to counseling on your own. The therapist will be able to offer you strategies for dealing with your adolescent and help you get her into counseling.

THE COMPLICATED DYNAMICS OF PEER PRESSURE

Peer pressure can sometimes be a valuable influence. When your child is being toilet trained, seeing that everyone else is wearing "big girl" or "big boy" underpants can convince your child that it is time to stop wearing diapers. When it comes to adolescents, however, we often associate peer pressure with bad influence.

Peer pressure is intricately tied up with issues of self-esteem and how adolescents perceive themselves. Because young people begin to identify strongly with groups outside their family during adolescence, they begin, consciously as well as unconsciously, to look for strategies for being accepted into those groups. It is from the desire to fit in, to be like others, that most peer pressure arises—not directly from a peer group at all, but from within the adolescent. This is normal, and not very different, in many ways, from adult decisions, which are often influenced by what others are doing or what others will think. For most adults, trying things that "everybody is doing" is of little lasting consequence. In some cases, it can be quite valuable—for example, when "everyone" is having a prostate exam or "everyone" has a retirement plan. Most adults have their value system in place and are less likely to engage in foolish and dangerous behavior to impress others.

Adolescents, particularly those between the ages of 10 and 14, are in the process of developing a concept of who they are, but perhaps more importantly, of who they *appear to be* to others. They are much more influenced by "everyone" and so tend to swing with trends considerably more than adults or older adolescents, precisely because they have not developed a more or less concrete sense of self. Because of their heightened hunger for peer acceptance, adolescents are much more likely to follow the crowd and let others make decisions for them.

Exactly how much an adolescent will feel pressured to be like her desired peer group, or to what lengths she is willing to go to be accepted by that group, will depend partly on temperament but largely on her sense of self-worth. While this may be affected in large part by the values and limits instilled by parents, other factors can play into the acceptance of peer pressure that neither parents nor adolescents can control. The case in point is rate of development. Research has shown that early blooming can heighten boys' sense of self-esteem, while it can have just the opposite effect on girls. Girls who develop earlier have a statistically higher likelihood of risky behavior: drug use, early sexual experimentation, and so on. This may be a result of receiving sexual attention from older boys or men that they simply are not prepared to handle, being taunted by boys their own age, parents' own unprepared-

DISCIPLINE

Much of a teen's sense of self-worth derives first from temperament, second from how valued she feels, and finally from her parents' style of discipline.

Parental discipline can strengthen or undermine a child's sense of self-worth. Excessively strict or rigid parents who have not instilled in their child good decision-making skills should not be surprised if their adolescent decides to risk their displeasure to find favor with her peers. Excessively lax parents who fail to teach their child proper boundaries of behavior should not be surprised if their child learns the hard way that the rest of the world is not so tolerant.

The most effective kind of discipline falls somewhere in the middle. A child knows the rules—and knows that the rules are sensible and enforced—but she also knows that in the gray areas between them parents can be flexible, sympathetic, and creative allies rather than someone who constantly says "no" or someone who always says "whatever." This kind of parent instills strong values by example and demonstrates flexible ways of thinking to find creative solutions. A child decides, for example, that she wants to take advanced placement physics, but halfway through the semester finds herself overwhelmed by the math. Rather than telling the child to study harder, or allowing the child to quit, this style of parent will work with the child to get past her difficulties. By showing that adversity can be overcome, and by demonstrating a willingness to work side-by-side with the child rather than against her, parents reinforce her abilities, and her sense of accomplishment. Children whose parents employ this style demonstrate more facility in dealing with frustration because they understand that they will be listened to and cared for. These children, accustomed to taking limited risks, will feel less pressure from within to conform to a peer group's norms and more freedom to say no. ■

ness to deal with the changes, or a combination of many factors. Early maturing girls tend to hang out with older girls, who of course do older things.

The contrary is true of boys. Early development, with enhanced physical stature and the proliferation of manly attributes, has been shown to increase boys' sense of self-esteem and propel them toward accepting being a man. Boys whose physical manhood comes later, particularly those who are late bloomers, may feel it necessary to try to prove their manhood in different ways, ways that can be risky to their health.

A child's sense of self-worth is nurtured at home. Some of it depends on her own outlook, but much of it depends on how parents act toward her and how her siblings act toward her. If you're a parent and your daughter is an early bloomer, you may do well to work with her to understand and channel the pressure she may feel. If she has never felt popular enough before and enjoys the attention she gets, you may do well to reinforce her sense of dignity, self-worth, and individuality. If you're a parent and your son is a late bloomer, you may do well to reinforce his understanding of what manhood really is—empathy, responsibility—and see to it that he is involved in activities that allow him to pursue a sense of strength and purpose. Parents can monitor the ages of friends and might be concerned if most of a girl's female friends are 1 to 3 years older than her.

If you are an early blooming girl, you should understand that some of the attention you may be receiving, while it may be flattering, may not be particularly healthy. Remember that you are responsible for no one's feelings but your own, and if someone—an older boy, a man—says, "You make me feel …," or "If you loved me you would …" the reality is that they, not you, are responsible for their feelings as well as their actions. If your classmates tease you about your breasts, try to remember that this most often will stem from feelings of fear or inferiority within them, and that by singling you out, they are trying to make themselves feel better.

If you are a late-blooming boy, it may feel as though it will be forever before you start to develop, but remember that the only "children" still out there at age 25 are those who have not matured emotionally, not physically. If you try to prove your manhood by getting in trouble, you will succeed only in getting yourself in trouble.

Most adolescents feel some confusion about their identity. Adolescents who genuinely feel unloved or unwanted by their families regardless of whether it is true or not, are more likely to go to extreme lengths to do what they think will meet a desired peer group's approval.

What can you as a parent do to instill a strong sense of self-worth in your child and help him avoid some of the harmful effects of peer pressure?

- Remember always to criticize the behavior, not the child. When criticizing, avoid ridicule or sarcasm. This produces nothing but anger and resentment. Despite the appearance of rejecting you, your adolescent deeply values your opinion and esteem. Find ways of commenting that are sympathetic. Parents should always try to remember when criticizing children that the reason for their criticism is parental love and concern.

- Keep regular track of your child and her friends, as well as the things they are doing. Make your child feel comfortable bringing friends home. Meet them, and get to know who they are and what they are like.

- Share with your child some of the difficulties you had as an adolescent and the ways you coped with them. Your child may pretend boredom, but you can be sure that, under that veneer, she is always looking for a role model.

- Within reason, and within your own value system, allow your adolescent some freedom to choose what she thinks is right for herself, even if you may occasionally find her choice unappealing.

- Look for ways to encourage her interests, particularly if they are different from your own. This will show your child how much you value her and her opinions.

The complex social and biological dynamics of peer pressure, of individuating and simultaneously yearning for belonging, can be the root of many different social and psychological difficulties. Most of these are transient and will pass like summer storms. Parents should try to keep in mind that as a child's body is maturing, so is her brain, and she is suddenly capable of quite sophisticated thought. This may be troubling to you, particularly if she begins, in the mid-teen years, to dissect and question values and beliefs you had assumed were more or less set in stone. But if this is troubling for parents, it is probably doubly troubling for teens, suddenly to have the sense of seeing through all the failures and foibles of the adults around. It is important for parents to be understanding and patient, to validate the teen's new ideas and opinions while not necessarily agreeing with them. The leap from simplistic, childish thoughts and desires to sophisticated adult thought and desires can be thrilling as well as terrifying. Patience, humor, and sympathy can go a long way toward forging a strong adult–adult friendship between parent and child that will ensue after the adolescent years.

Staying Healthy

NUTRITION

Growing bodies need several things to grow to their maximum potential: adequate exercise, adequate sleep, and substantial amounts of food. Skeletal structure grows first, followed by muscle and fat, and many teenagers may feel and look awkward during their growth spurt.

The average teenage boy needs 2,800 calories daily; the average teenage girl 2,200. Teens who are involved in sports may need an additional 600 to 1,200 calories per day, depending upon the level of exercise. For optimum health, these calories need to come from a balanced diet low in fat (see A Balanced Diet for Teens, this page), rather than from junk food.

For further information on proper nutrition, see Chapter 1.

Remember that each of the food groups provides some, but not all, of the nutrients you need. Foods in one group cannot replace those in another. No one of these major food groups is more important than another; for good health, all are necessary. Most young people tend to get much more protein than they need, while statistically speaking, only about one in four Americans eats the recommended five or more daily servings of vegetables and fruits.

For most individuals, regardless of age, in good health and not suffering from a condition that causes a nutritional deficiency or using a medication that depletes particular nutrients, there should be no need at all for vitamin supplements. Using supplements to replace vegetables and fruit in the diet robs the body of important nutrients it needs and expects. These can be especially important during the growing years.

Some teenage girls, however, may require iron supplements. A recent investigation of iron levels in adolescent girls by Johns Hopkins Children's Center researchers found that as many as 25 percent were iron deficient (but not anemic). Girls given iron supplements tested significantly higher on one test of verbal learning and memory than other girls who were given a placebo. Because of the rapidity of growth and the onset of menstruation, a girl's body has a tremendous need for iron. Those who exer-

A BALANCED DIET FOR TEENS

FOOD GROUP	NUMBER OF SERVINGS NEEDED DAILY FOR TEENAGE GIRLS	NUMBER OF SERVINGS NEEDED DAILY FOR TEENAGE BOYS
Bread, cereal, rice, pasta	9	11
Vegetables	4	5
Fruits	3	4
Milk, yogurt, cheese	3	3
Meat, poultry, fish, dried beans, eggs, nuts	2, for a total of 6 oz	3, for a total of 7 oz
Total fat (grams)	73	93

cise—an important part of anyone's overall fitness—and those who eat a diet low in iron are especially at risk for iron deficiency.

EXERCISE

Exercise is crucial for young people, but because most teenagers are healthy overall, many take their good health for granted and simply will not exercise.

In many cases, adults are in better physical condition than their children because the adults engage in regular exercise programs, while their children do not. Many teens are too busy with academic demands—or the leisure demands of television, computers, and computer games—to find time to exercise. Although sports are an important part of most high school curricula, many young people give up exercise as they enter high school. Often, their reasons have nothing to do with whether or not they enjoy exercise; adolescents may feel self-conscious undressing in locker rooms or may worry that they are not good enough athletes. Unfortunately, too many high schools emphasize team sports played only by the best athletes, rather than a comprehensive fitness program in which all students can keep in shape.

Teens tend to mirror the behavior of their parents (as do most children), and if you do not exercise regularly, chances are your child will not either. If you are concerned that your child is becoming inactive,

ADOLESCENT OBESITY

Adolescents, hungry all the time because of their growth spurt and always looking for independence, can eat a tremendous amount of junk food, and often do so for reasons that have little to do with hunger or caloric needs. Combine this with the sedentary lifestyle that is typical of many adolescents, and as a nation we have a sure-fire plan for obesity. Obesity and overweight tend to run in families. This is not to say that obesity or the propensity toward it is *necessarily* genetic, although research points toward a genetic link. Most children learn by example, and if parents are overweight, snack constantly, and have nothing in the cupboard but junk food, children are likely to become overweight and eat nothing but junk food. While some overweight teens want desperately to lose weight, research shows that most do not.

If your child is overweight, what can you do to help?

The first thing you can do is examine your own physical condition: Are you overweight or obese? What is your physical activity level? Do you lead a sedentary lifestyle—less than 20 minutes per day of strenuous physical activity)?

What kinds of foods do you provide for your children and for yourself? A diet high in fats, animal protein, and highly processed carbohydrates will tend to be weak in vegetables and fruits. Indeed, government statistics show that scarcely a quarter of Americans eat the recommended minimum of five servings of fruits and vegetables per day. A recent survey of children found that up through the teen years, only about 10 percent of children eat according to the government's Food Guide Pyramid, and many get as much as 40 percent of their calories from refined sugars.

If you eat a lot of prepared foods, your diet will likely be high in fat, salt, and lots of other nutrients that can lead to obesity, hypertension—an increasing problem in children—and the attendant problems of obesity, such as diabetes.

If one or both parents are obese, then helping their child attain an appropriate weight must be a family affair. Parents can embark upon an exercise program with children, and all of you can examine together the kinds of foods you eat and why, and more closely model your eating behavior on the food pyramid.

If neither parent is obese, there are many things you can do to help your child lose weight or achieve a weight that is appropriate for your child's size:

- Criticism or jokes about your child's appearance do not help but only further undermine what may already be a fragile sense of self-worth and self-control.

- Try to work *with* your youngster to achieve a balanced, sensible diet.

- If you go to the gym or otherwise exercise regularly, take your child with you.

- Talk to the school to see if there is a fitness program in which your child can participate.

- Talk to a dietitian or your doctor about ways you can be supportive of your child while helping your child slim down.

- If your teen rebels against your suggestions, take your child to the doctor and sit down to talk about dietary goals, the risks of obesity, and a potential exercise plan.

- Emphasize the health benefits of regular exercise.

For further information on appropriate nutrition and weight loss, see Chapter 1.

Counseling may be necessary to get to the root of your child's overeating and to help prevent your child from becoming anorexic or bulimic. It should also address your child's self-perception and self-esteem. ■

take action yourself. Help the child find a fitness activity that interests her—one that she can enjoy with her peers or with her family—and encourage her to keep at it. If you are inactive, become involved in some kind of physical fitness program (even if it is only a daily ½-hour walk). The physical and emotional benefits cannot be overestimated for anyone.

DENTAL HYGIENE

A good dental hygiene program is invaluable for anyone of any age. Teens, who may involuntarily tend to view themselves as immortal, may find themselves neglecting this important aspect of overall health. Brushing and flossing daily and regular dental exams during the teenage years can provide a good foundation for excellent dental health throughout adulthood. Adolescence is a fine time to lay the preventive groundwork against tooth decay and gum disease.

Your dentist may refer your child to an orthodontist if the teeth are out of proper alignment (malocclusion); if there is an underbite where the upper teeth protrude excessively over the lower teeth when the mouth is closed; if there is an overbite, where the lower teeth enclose the upper teeth when the mouth is shut; or if the teeth are crooked, twisted, or crowded in the mouth. The orthodontist will determine if the symptoms are serious enough to warrant the use of an appliance to straighten them out. There are many different kinds of appliances for many different uses, but the most common among teens are braces.

Through slowly exerted pressure on the teeth, braces change the alignment of the teeth and jaw so that in later life dental problems will be minimized. Although most people think of braces as restricted to the adolescent years, many adults wear them to correct a variety of jaw and tooth problems. There are several different kinds, even some that are invisible. You, your child's orthodontist, and your child should discuss which type of brace is best for your child.

If braces are necessary, it may take some time to get used to them and the special care required to keep teeth clean, but the eventual result, straight teeth and a comfortable jaw, will be well worth the energy and anxiety expended. Many teens, because they are concerned with their appearance and their acceptance by others, may worry that their braces will affect their popularity. Most often, this is more a worry than a reality. Wearers of braces may get teased now and again, but such teasing should be taken in stride. Teens should remember that braces are temporary but the results are forever. Talking honestly with parents about feelings toward the appliance can help allay anxiety and fears.

Installation of braces may often be done in stages, and the orthodontist will provide instructions on how to keep teeth clean. Braces will require regularly scheduled visits in order to assess the condition of the mouth and teeth, adjust the fit of braces, and ensure that teeth are clean. In the course of this somewhat lengthy process, most teenagers wearing braces will have matured and will greet the day the braces are removed with a new, more adult, and much-enhanced smile.

Adolescent Sexuality

One of the most dramatic, exciting, and frightening changes that takes place during the adolescent years is sexual maturation. As adolescents grow and their bodies change, boys and girls often feel as though their awareness of sex and sexuality has exploded overnight.

Few things are more difficult for parents and children to talk about, but few things are more important to talk about, than sex. Parents may prefer not to think about their child's sexuality. Adolescents may find it even more difficult to look at parents as sexual creatures. As uncomfortable as teens may be in talking with their parents about sex and sexuality, they really do want to know their parents' feelings and opinions.

Although some people believe that sex education can lead to promiscuity, it has been shown that sex education significantly reduces the likelihood of early, unwanted pregnancy and sexually transmitted infection (STI). Many adolescents feel that sexual curiosity is somehow dirty. It is not; it is perfectly normal. It is part of the process that will eventually have its fulfillment in starting a family. But parents should never rely on the schools to be the sole source of their children's education about sex and sexuality. Sex education should be about considerably more than just how babies are made and how to prevent conception and STIs.

We are all sexual creatures; it is necessary for the survival of the species. But that is not all we are, and despite the power of animal attraction, the healthiest sexual relationships are based *first* on friendship, on intellectual and spiritual connections, and *then* on sex. Sex is serious business, but unfortunately, too many people, perhaps teens in particular, view having sex as business as usual. Television and movies have long used sex as a powerful selling tool, but young people today are exposed to considerably more sexually sophisticated material than their parents were. Many, particularly young adolescents, may not have developed the discrimination to understand the nature of the fantasy life or the commercial longings that television and films create. If an adolescent's only sexual experience is fantasy—watching television, looking at pictures in magazines, or reading romantic stories—he or she may not understand how real-life sex is infinitely more complicated, infinitely more worrisome, and, potentially, more dangerous.

Sexual intercourse requires the participation of two human beings, people equally complex, equally full of doubts and insecurities. And when intercourse is over, there may be many long-lasting repercussions. The decision to have sex is a complicated one, one that should never be entered into lightly. But statistics show that many teens have sex for the first time when they are drunk or otherwise intoxicated. Many young people are surprised that the act is nothing like they thought it would be and

AM I GAY?

Although some gay men and women report knowing for as long as they can remember that they were different, many go through a considerable amount of doubt and even agony before facing what they finally cannot ignore. The high school years can be a particularly confusing time. During the adolescent years, it is common for boys and girls to engage in practice sex play with members of the same sex, sometimes even including kissing and touching. This does not mean that you are a homosexual. As you enter adulthood, it will become clearer to you whether your sexual orientation is heterosexual, homosexual, or bisexual.

Homosexuality is no more a lifestyle choice than being brown-haired. It is a biological condition that has existed for as long as people have, and it affects approximately 1 to 10 percent of the population, with the numbers among men apparently slightly higher. Although it seems clear from the available research that homosexuality has *some* genetic component, researchers remain somewhat at odds over what factors coalesce to make someone gay.

For many gay people, recognition that they are indeed gay comes during college, after having time alone, time to start over with a new group of friends. Because the cultural bias against homosexuality has historically been so great, an admission of homosexuality—either by talking about it or by having sex—can be a source of considerable anxiety and depression.

If you think you might be gay but do not feel you can or want to talk to your family about it, find a sympathetic ear. If you are afraid to confide in friends, call a toll-free crisis hotline. Many high schools and most colleges have gay/lesbian alliances, and they may be able to provide you with empathy, information, and protection. ■

MASTURBATION

It is a word that makes young people giggle, and it is something that most people do not like to admit to, although research shows that most everyone has at one time or another discovered erotic self-stimulation. Your belief systems may strongly influence the way you perceive masturbation and whether or not you engage in it—or are able to engage in it without guilt.

Masturbation is sexual activity in which you stimulate yourself to orgasm. It does not cause any of the ill effects that were claimed in the past—growing hair on your palms, causing acne—and is essentially harmless. It is the safest form of "sex" possible, in that it involves no transmission of bodily fluids from one person to another and carries with it no risk of pregnancy or infection.

Our culture is reluctant to discuss masturbation, but it is not naughty, evil, or sick. On the contrary, most researchers assert that masturbation can be a healthy release of sexual tension for teenagers who are wisely refraining from sexual activity. Masturbation, however, should certainly remain private. ■

are surprised by the unexpected guilt, worry, and disappointment. Sexual intercourse during adolescence may seem grown up, but particularly in the early teen years, the decision to have sex may be more a sign of emotional *im*maturity.

Many younger teens experience a considerable amount of ambivalence and anxiety over sex. It is perfectly normal for young people to wonder whether they are attractive enough, to feel anxiety about being inexperienced, and to feel a certain amount of envy of sexual activity that friends report. Sex requires a great deal of trust between two people, and bragging about something so intimate is likely a signal of immaturity. Like any weighty decision, the decision to have sex should be made after serious thought and consideration. Young people should consider involving parents or other trusted elders in the decision-making process. Parents should, within their own moral and spiritual framework, provide their children with as much information about sexuality, its joys and disappointments, its risks and rewards, as possible. Ignorance serves only those who seek to exploit it.

Speaking strictly from a viewpoint of optimum physical and mental health, one of the best things you can do as an adolescent is *not* to have sex. While a healthy sexual relationship is an important part of adult life, an unhealthy sexual relationship can have consequences that range from mild—guilt—to serious—pregnancy, STIs—to deadly—acquired immunodeficiency syndrome (AIDS). There are at least 40 known STIs, and while risk can be minimized through the use of condoms, there is no such thing as completely safe sex. For more information on STIs and methods of treating or preventing them, see Chapter 25. There is also the risk of pregnancy, and while risk can be minimized by the intelligent use of birth control, every method of birth control (except abstaining) has some failure rate. Condoms, for example, can and do break. For further information on methods of birth control and their reliability, see Chapter 25.

Abstaining from having sexual intercourse does not mean that individuals do not or should not have sexual feelings or that individuals cannot express their sexuality in a healthy, age-appropriate way. Abstinence means putting off a decision to have sexual intercourse until a time when you feel that you have sufficient information, trust, and responsibility to accept the attendant risks. You have to decide for yourself when the time is right.

FOR TEENS: WRONG REASONS TO HAVE SEX

Here are some of the many *wrong* reasons people, young and old alike, have sex:

- Because they are afraid to say no (it is your body and your decision)

- Because they are afraid the other person will not love them unless they do (respect is a fundamental part of love)

- Because they get pressure from their friends

- Because they want to find out what all the fuss is about

- Because "everyone is doing it" (actually, everyone is not doing it—most statistics indicate that fewer than half of all high school students are sexually active)

- Because they believe it will make a man or a woman of them (no, it will not, but it will put them at risk for contracting an STI or getting pregnant)

- Because it feels good (it does, temporarily, but it can feel bad, too; there are other ways to relieve or avert sexual tension)

FOR TEENS: CONSIDER THE IMPLICATIONS OF PREGNANCY

This year more than a million teenage American girls will become pregnant: one in five sexually active teenage girls. These are the highest rates of teen pregnancy in the Western world: twice as high as Canada, England, and France; three times as high as Sweden; and seven times as high as the Netherlands. Research shows that teen pregnancy rates directly correlate with the availability of contraceptives and sex education: Those countries where contraceptives are most available have the lowest rates of teen pregnancy and abortion.

Pregnant teenagers are faced with difficult choices. The decision to carry a baby to term and the decision to keep a baby if carried to term are not easy ones to make and should not be made by a teenager or a teenage couple alone. This decision can influence the rest of your life and should, whenever possible, be made with the help of your parents and with the help of a counselor. Indeed, research shows that most teens involve a parent in the decision-making process.

If you decide to carry a baby to term, you need to decide whether you can parent the baby or make an adoption plan. There are many childless couples desperately wanting to adopt. If you do not want to terminate your pregnancy but also cannot or do not want to raise the child yourself, there are adoption agencies that can help you. Some can even arrange to have health care costs paid during your pregnancy by the adoptive parents. Adoption laws have opened up somewhat in the last several years, and giving up the baby is in many instances not quite as final as it once was. Some birthparents whose babies are adopted may have some sort of ongoing relationship with the child and the adoptive family. Carrying a pregnancy to term and then putting a baby up for adoption may not be an easy decision for most adolescents to make. Counseling and help are available. Many religious groups offer such services, but secular counseling is also available.

For teenage girls who choose to keep their babies, statistics show, unfortunately, that the effect on these young mothers— emotionally, socially, and financially—can be devastating. The effect on the baby as the baby grows can be devastating in other ways. Most pregnant teenage girls will become single mothers, live at home, and be completely dependent upon their parents. The arrival of the baby, statistically speaking, will usually bring the relationship with the baby's father to an end. Most teenage mothers are completely unprepared for the rigors of parenting and the many ways a newborn will limit their freedom and their choices in life. If a couple stays together and keeps the child, statistics demonstrate similar unfortunate consequences for the fathers—considerable social, financial, and emotional difficulties.

RAPE

If anyone—a stranger, a teacher, a relative, a date—forces you to have sex without your consent, it is rape.

Although most rape victims are female and most rapists are male, boys are also raped—by both men and women.

What Should You Do if You Are Raped?

Although your first reaction may be just to keep it a secret and not tell anyone, doing nothing is something you may later come to regret. Doing nothing will not help you and will not help others who might be raped by the same person. The same person may rape you again.

- *Don't bathe.* This may be the first thing you want to do, but don't. The sooner you report the assault and are examined, the better the evidence—and the chances of obtaining a conviction—will be. You may also decide later whether or not you wish to prosecute.

- *Don't blame yourself.* Many people feel a sense of guilt at being raped, especially if they know the rapist, as well as fearfulness. This is natural, but it is not your fault.

- *Tell someone you trust.* Whether you tell your sister or your mother, a teacher, or a rape hotline, report the rape as soon as possible.

- *Retain all evidence.* Don't wash clothing, but keep everything, particularly underwear, that you were wearing as it was. This may be important evidence that will help police catch and put in jail the person who assaulted you.

- *Get examined.* Hospital emergency rooms are equipped to examine people who have been raped, and you should be examined as soon as possible after the assault in order to collect evidence. Some hospitals now have special rape counselors to perform much of the examination and interview. These are usually nurses who have been specially trained to assist rape victims.

- *Consider the "morning after" pill.* If you are concerned that you may get pregnant, do not wait to find out if your next period will come. Within 72 hours of contact, but preferably as soon as possible, you can start this brief regimen, usually of eight pills taken over a 12-hour period. This hormonal treatment is designed to interrupt conception and head off a pregnancy before it happens. See Contraception, page 1161.

- *Get tested.* Speak with your doctor about the STIs you may have been put at risk for. If you are bruised or otherwise injured, see your doctor for treatment.

- *Get assistance.* It's common for victims of rape not to want to be alone for several days after the incident. Someone close to you—a best friend, sister, mother—should try to look after you for the few days following the incident. If the assault leaves you feeling especially depressed or even suicidal, seek counseling as fast as possible. It's important to talk to people. Many people who work in rape crisis centers are women who have been through the trauma of rape themselves and can be of invaluable assistance in getting you started on the road to recovery—as well as help you, if you decide to prosecute, get prepared to attend court and testify. ∎

If you are considering not carrying the baby to term, you should not delay your decision too long, as abortion after the first trimester, or the third month of pregnancy, has more risks and more regulations. First trimester abortions are legal and safe, although each state regulates delivery of abortion services differently. For many teenagers, the decision to abort a pregnancy will not be an easy one, and counseling is available that can assist you in deciding whether this option is appropriate to your situation.

Making a decision to keep, give up, or abort a baby is never easy. Here are some toll-free numbers you can call for help:

- Planned Parenthood, information on contraceptives, maternal health, abortion and other services: (800) 230-7526.

- Information Referrals and Crisis Help Line: (800) 233-4357.

- National Council for Adoption. Pregnant teens can call collect in crisis for counseling and referrals to member adoption agencies in their areas: (202) 328-1200.

- Check telephone directories for these kinds of agencies, which may be able to direct you toward counseling and other services: Family Services Association, Department of Health, counseling services, mental health services.

FOR PARENTS AND TEENS: PREVENTING TEEN PREGNANCY

What can parents do to prevent teen pregnancy? What can young people do to prevent teen pregnancy?

The most important factor for teens is a strong sense of self-worth, knowing they are loved by their families of origin. The second most important factor is thorough and com-

FOR YOUNG MEN: UNDERSTANDING WHEN SEX IS REALLY RAPE

Statistics show that most rapes are committed by men and that most victims are women. Statistics also show that someone the victim knows commits by far the majority of rapes. This may be a relative, but often it is a boyfriend or an acquaintance. It is important not to allow miscommunication or misunderstandings to escalate into a very serious crime.

If she says no, and you have intercourse with her, it's rape. You can go to jail. Your girlfriend may love you, may find you attractive and desirable, but she still may not want to have sexual intercourse with you—even if she has already done so before. Self-control is a fundamental part of growing up. "She got me so excited I couldn't control myself," is no excuse. You and only you are responsible for your actions. If she says no or tells you to stop, it is your responsibility to do so.

Here are some other common misconceptions:

- Since I took her out and paid for the date, she should have sex with me.

- When she says no, she really means yes.

- If she's wet, she wants to have sex.

- She wouldn't go parking with me if she didn't want to have sex.

- If she didn't want to have sex, why did she let me go as far as she did?

- If she gets me erect, then it's her responsibility to do something about it.

- She's slept with other people, so she should sleep with me.

- We've had sex before, and she didn't say no then.

Remember that your feelings of arousal or excitement are your own, and originate within you. If you cannot control them, seek professional help. Counseling can help you control your impulses before they cause pain to others, as well as to you. ■

prehensive education about sexuality, reproduction, emotional attachment, and birth/STI control. Again, ignorance serves only those who seek to exploit it. And statistics show that not only are those who have a good education in sexuality less likely to become pregnant (or get someone pregnant), they are less likely even to become prematurely sexually active.

Common Social and Psychological Difficulties in Adolescence

Rare is the child who slips through adolescence with no difficulty whatsoever. Most adolescents will experience some kind of emotional or academic setback, some kind of unwanted peer pressure, and most will come through, having learned from their experience. Certain difficulties, however, may require intervention.

SCHOOL PHOBIA

Some young people can be so overwhelmed by the many changes they go through in adolescence that they begin to have unreasonable fears of school. These fears can have many root causes (including pubertal timing, or early or late blooming) but are often manifested in the same way.

Most children who develop a school phobia in high school will have shown some tendency toward fear of school in earlier grades. As high school begins, the adolescent's reluctance to attend class can become a full-blown phobia, with outright terror at the prospect of going to school. The most common age for the onset of this condition is about age 14. Full-blown school phobia is relatively rare, because parents and teachers are able to help children work through the underlying problem before medical intervention becomes necessary.

The anxiety that underlies school phobia may be rooted in problems at home or at school. Anxiety over a crisis at home—the death or illness of a parent or sibling, an impending divorce, for example—can make the child afraid to leave the house for long periods in case something momentous or terrible happens while she is not around. Problems at school that may loom large for an adolescent include fear of failure and repeated bullying by other children. Other possibilities include having an ancillary phobia, such as fear of eating in public, panic disorder, or agoraphobia (see Phobia, page 1220).

If your child seems healthy but still misses a lot of school, consult your doctor to rule out any real physical ailment. Consult with school authorities also to assess how your child is faring academically and socially. Talk to your child, and try to get at the root of her anxiety. If you cannot help her work through the fear, counseling may be warranted.

BULLYING

Physical bullying is something that most often takes place between boys. While it often seems clear to adults that bullies are insecure themselves, the experience of being bullied can be terrifying to children and adolescents. The child can feel guilt and shame at being picked on by a bigger classmate and laughed at by friends or peers.

Often, a child is too ashamed of being unable to fend for himself to tell his parents. Or he may believe that parental involvement may make him look more incapable of fending for himself. In some cases, children become so despondent over their humiliation or inability to deal with a situation that they begin having suicidal thoughts. Although most adolescents have thoughts of suicide from time to time, talk of suicide should never be taken lightly (see Warning Signals of Depression and Suicide, page 285).

Sometimes your child may not be able to hide from you that he is being bullied because he comes home bruised and bloodied. Often, however, the signs may be more subtle. He may ask questions that indicate mistreatment—how you might have dealt with bullying when you were his age. He may ask for karate lessons or wish he had a gun. He may become depressed (see Adolescent Depression page 283) or become scared to go to school. Sometimes anxiety over someone threatening him, stealing his lunch money or his homework, or repeatedly challenging him, can create a phobia over going to school.

If you suspect that your child is the victim of bullying, particularly if it seems gang-related, intervention is warranted. If your child has become so depressed and fearful that he has begun to talk of suicide, seek counseling for him immediately. If your family owns guns, they should be under lock and key; if a child becomes depressed or speaks of suicide, any guns that are in the house should be stored somewhere out of the house. If this is not possible, then all guns should be kept under lock and key, with all ammunition kept in a different place under a different lock and key.

Schools have a responsibility to provide a safe learning environment, and it is no more legal for a child to assault another child than it is for an adult to assault another. If you suspect your child is being repeatedly bullied, you should contact school authorities and demand they investigate. If school authorities do not intervene to ensure the child's safety, you should insist upon a meeting with the principal of the school and the bully's parents. This kind of meeting may or may not be useful. Many children become bullies for attention-getting purposes, and their parents may be unaware that there is a problem with their child. Sometimes bullies are the children of bullies.

If the school is unable for whatever reason to provide a safe environment, the next option is to resort to the law. You should contact an attorney or the local Legal Aid Society and ask what steps can be taken to protect your child. If the child has been beaten up, call the police and press charges.

DATE ABUSE

Another kind of bullying that goes almost entirely unreported is that which takes place between adolescent girls and their boyfriends, former boyfriends, or, in some cases, young men they do not even know. In cases of date abuse, abusers are almost always male, and their victims almost always female. Adolescent girls may not have the maturity or the emotional tools to understand exactly what an abusive relationship is or what to do about it.

For parents How would you know if your daughter is in an abusive relationship? Your daughter may not tell you. She may be stuck in victim thinking and believe that she somehow deserves the treatment she is getting; she may be so afraid of her abuser and what he will do that she feels she cannot tell you. If you notice that since she began dating a particular boy she no longer has much contact with her friends, or has unexplained bruises, or has begun to grow depressed, talk to her. If she will tell you nothing, you can try talking to her friends.

Her teachers may have some idea of the dynamics of her peer group, or whether she has suddenly lost interest in school. You can call a local women's shelter or domestic violence center and ask them for information and help. If you suspect some problem but can find no satisfactory answer, consult your doctor or a counselor who specializes in adolescent concerns.

For girls Chances are it did not start out abusively. Chances are it started out just fine: He was charming but maybe a little possessive. But after a while—maybe even just a little while—he began to get moody and jealous. Now he hardly lets you out of his sight, and if he sees you talking to another boy, even if it's just to ask for the homework assignment, he goes ballistic, maybe even threatens the other boy. Maybe at first you felt a little flattered that he cared so much, but now you are starting to feel smothered and a little fearful: What if he starts hitting you? If you think you may be in an abusive relationship, answer the following questions:

- Does he insist on being everything to you and not want you to see your friends?

- Has he hit you, pushed you, or otherwise been physically intimidating?

- Does he follow you and sometimes show up places where you never told him you were going?

- Is he always critical of you—your looks, your abilities, your desirability to other guys?

- Has he ruined things you care about?

- Has he threatened you? Threatened to tell your parents you have had sex?

- Has he forced you to have sex when you didn't want to?

- If you have broken up with him, does he still follow you, or does he follow your friends and threaten them?

If you have answered yes to any of these questions, you should seek help and protection immediately. Your first thought may be to try to take things into your own hands or let your friends take care of him. Do not. Try to talk things over with your parents, or, if you do not feel that you can talk to your parents, immediately contact a women's shelter or a domestic violence center. Counselors will listen compassionately and objectively and tell you where you can go for help.

For boys If you have read the section above and recognize any of the behaviors described in yourself, you should seek counseling. If you are fearful of being abandoned, if you are jealous, and if you cannot trust the girl you say you love, you are much more likely to chase her away than keep her close. Threatening or violent behavior will only make her fearful and resentful of you, perhaps cause her to break up with you, and even have you prosecuted if you hit, stalk, or harass her. Talk to your parents or to your school counselor or a therapist, and try to get to the roots of why you need to be so possessive. This is not love, and she is not responsible for your feelings.

Common Adolescent Mental Health Difficulties

Adolescence is a time of great change, and it is not unusual for problems with self-image and other more serious mental health difficulties to arise. Most of the common mental health difficulties that young people face are mild and transient. Having to deal with them helps young people equip themselves with the emotional tools for dealing with the potentially more trying difficulties they will face in adulthood. Even those difficulties that can be life-threatening, such as depression or eating disorders, although serious, can in many instances be treated and cured. What is most important for parents and adolescents alike is to acknowledge and deal with problems if and when they arise; early intervention can be extremely beneficial.

❖ ADOLESCENT DEPRESSION

Symptoms *(What your child may experience)*

- A lasting sense of despair that either has no root in a life event or arises out of a traumatic event, such as the breakup of a relationship, but does not ease up after 7 to 10 days

- A feeling that everything is hopeless, nothing is enjoyable, and life really is not worth living

- Loss of appetite, loss of weight

- Dramatic changes in normal behavior patterns, such as sleeping, eating, working, or interacting with others

Signs and laboratory findings *(What the doctor looks for)*

- Persistent lethargy and loss of interest in normal pleasure-giving experiences, such as food, friends, pets, sports, and hobbies

- A family history of depression or suicide; previous experience with depression or attempted suicide; alcohol or other drug use; a family pattern of alcohol or other drug use

What is it? Most people experience a certain degree of transient depression. It is perfectly ordinary to get down or blue after some life difficulty: the end of a romance, the death of a friend or family member, the loss of a pet. Such events can be particularly distressing during the younger adolescent years, though it is by no means restricted to that time. A small percentage (perhaps 3 to 5 percent) of the overall population regularly suffers from what is known as major depressive disorder, a condition that often has no root in a life setback or, when it does, grows completely out of proportion to the setback, perhaps even feeds on it. There is a genetic component to depression, though it is impossible to predict who may become truly depressed.

Depressive illness in adolescents can range from mild, persistent blues to profound, lasting despair. Some people with chronic depression are able to function reasonably well but often find doing anything beyond what is expected of them too exhausting to confront. Others may become completely incapacitated and spend their days huddled in bed or hiding in their rooms.

It is now recognized that depression is a brain disorder that has its roots in the physiology of the brain as much as in the emotions—which are, after all, governed by brain chemistry. A major depressive disorder can cause sufferers to descend into an almost completely paralyzing despair that may be difficult for others to comprehend. Well-meaning relatives often try to get sufferers to "just snap out of it," a feat that can be next to impossible.

Another kind of depression is what is known as bipolar disorder, or manic depression. Bipolar disorder is characterized by bouts of mania, or exuberant highs when the affected individual might feel superhuman. These episodes alternate with states of deep depression. This also seems to have a genetic component, but again, it is impossible to predict who might be affected.

What you can do If you suspect that your child is depressed, there are things you can do to try to help her cope, though it should be cautioned that if your child is exhibiting symptoms of depression that include suicidal expressions, you should seek medical assistance immediately. Again, if there is a gun owner in your household, all guns should be moved to another location. If this is not possible, then all guns should be kept under lock and key, with all ammunition stored under separate lock and key. Only a responsible adult should know the location of the key or keys. If your child will talk with you about her feelings, you can try to draw her out. It is likely that she will not be able to explain her feelings, but she may listen. Reassure her that no matter how persistent her sense of isolation or despair feels, *it will not last forever.* Explain that young people are much more likely to suffer from depression than older people and that she will likely learn how to avoid depression as she matures. Try to make sure that she does not isolate herself, but that she continues contact with her close friends. They may not understand her feelings but may be sympathetic; and talking is better than isolation. If she does not feel comfortable talking to you or to her friends, urge her to call a toll-free hotline and talk to someone there (see Toll-Free Help Lines, page 286). She can call anonymously, and chances are the person she will speak to has been through the same thing. If she does not feel like doing any of the things that give her pleasure, encourage her to continue with her interests. Try to get her to exercise, go for a walk, a run, or a swim, and reassure her that exercise is often a good way to sort things out. Urge her to talk to you or to friends if she has dark

WARNING SIGNALS OF DEPRESSION AND SUICIDE

Thousands of young people die each year at their own hands. Suicide is the sixth leading cause of death for 5- to 14-year-olds, and the third leading cause of death for 15- to 24-year-olds. The incidence of adolescent suicide has grown considerably over the last several years.

Many researchers believe that many if not most of those adolescents who commit suicide do not in fact want to die but are depressed and pleading for attention—from parents, from the boyfriend or girlfriend who jilted them, or from anyone at all. Many of the changes of adolescence can seem overwhelming, and high schools and colleges can seem like pressure cookers with their demands to succeed, to be beautiful, popular, and successful. Problems that might seem manageable to adults can sometimes seem completely insurmountable to adolescents.

Depression has been called the "common cold" of mental illness, and most everyone has suffered from it, if only briefly. And most everyone has contemplated what the world would be like if they killed themselves. But most people do not kill themselves or even attempt it.

There are many warning signs of depression, and if you suspect your adolescent may be depressed, consult with your doctor about seeking counseling, not only for your child but also for you, so you can learn how to deal with depression. Pay attention to the danger signals; early intervention can head off a suicide attempt down the road. Consult your doctor if you notice any of these warning signs:

- Dramatic personality change.

- Withdrawal. Someone who was once outgoing turns inward and quiet.

- Alcohol or other drug use.

- Violent behavior. Punching holes in walls, getting into fights, or self-destructive violence.

- Running away from home.

- Significant change in sleeping patterns—sleeping much more, or much less.

- Significant change in weight—either loss or gain.

- Neglect of personal appearance. Most adolescents always want to look their best, even if their idea of looking good is completely at odds with yours.

- Lingering lethargy, a drop-off in school work, loss of interest—cannot concentrate, or everything is boring.

- Loss of interest in recreational activities.

- Lack of interest in praise or rewards.

If a young person is contemplating suicide, she may talk about it, particularly if she is looking for attention. Do not ignore or dismiss the talk, but try to draw the adolescent out. Depressed people may want more than anything to talk about what they are feeling; dismissing their feelings may confirm their sense of worthlessness.

Other adolescents may be so depressed that they may not talk about it directly. Still, there are definite warning signs that you should be alert to. Depressed teens may

- Cry all the time.

- Isolate themselves from all their friends.

- Be unable to explain why they are so blue.

- Express feelings of worthlessness or inherent badness, "I'm just an awful person."

- Give clues in conversation that indicate they will not be around much longer, be a burden any more, or express feelings of being completely overwhelmed, "Nothing makes any difference," or "Life is so useless."

- Give away all their important or favorite possessions, throw out items of significance, and put their affairs in order, such as apologizing or saying good-bye, cleaning their room.

- Suddenly become cheerful or seem relieved after an extended period of depression. This indicates a sense of having made up their mind, and now, with an "answer," the world does not seem so overwhelming. ■

thoughts. Talk to her friends, and enlist their help, explaining your concern and requesting that they report any suicidal talk or behavior to you.

When to call the doctor If your child has been experiencing a persistent state of gloom that has lasted more than 7 to 10 days, and that she cannot explain, contact your doctor. If your child is sleeping excessively, has become isolated from family and friends, or takes little pleasure in the usual things, contact your doctor. See Warning Signals of Depression and Suicide, above, for more information.

Treatment Treatment for mild depression may mean simply seeing a therapist for a few weeks or months to learn mechanisms to cope with life's ups and downs.

Treatment for a major depressive disorder will most often consist of psychotherapy combined with antidepressant drugs. While drugs are very effective, they should

TOLL-FREE HELP LINES

The counselors at the following numbers can help if you need someone to talk to. With any of these, you never have to give your name, tell who you are, or how old you are. The people on the other end are trained to give information to help you, whether it's with depression, drugs, or thoughts of suicide. Call. Sometimes someone who's not from your family or not one of your friends can look at your life in a nonjudgmental way and be a real help. Give them a chance.

Abortion

- (800) 772–9100 National Abortion Federation Hotline
- (800) 230–7526 Planned Parenthood

AIDS

- (800) 342–2437 Centers for Disease Control AIDS Hotline
- (800) 440–8336 Teen AIDS
- (800) 234–8336 Teens Teaching AIDS Prevention (Monday through Friday, 4 to 8 PM Central Standard Time)

Alcohol and Drugs

- (800) 257–7800 Hazelden Foundation (drug and alcohol crisis)

Child Abuse

- (800) 448–4663 Hit Home Hotline for youth crises such as suicide, abuse, pregnancy, depression, counseling, and intervention
- (800) 422–4453 National Child Abuse Hotline

Contraception

- (800) 230–7526 Planned Parenthood

Crisis

- (800) 999–9999 Adolescent Crisis Intervention and Counseling Hotline
- (800) 448–4663 Hit Home Hotline for youth crises such as suicide, abuse, pregnancy, depression, counseling, and intervention
- (800) 448–4663 National Youth Crisis Hotline

Depression

- (888) 782–1000 National Depression Screening Day (October 10)
- (800) 855–2881 National Depression Screening Day (TT—text telephone—for the hearing impaired)

- (800) 826–3632 National Depressive and Manic-Depressive Association

Drugs and Alcohol

- (800) 257–7800 Hazelden Foundation (drug and alcohol crisis)

Gangs

- (800) 999–9999 Gang help line

Gay and Lesbian

- (800) 347–8336 Gay and Lesbian Hotline (this is not a crisis line and is staffed Thursday through Saturday 7 to 11:45 PM Eastern time)

Pregnancy

- (800) 441–2670 Crisis Pregnancy Counseling Center (Dallas, TX)
- (800) 448–4663 Hit Home Hotline for youth crises such as suicide, abuse, pregnancy, depression, counseling, and intervention
- (800) 772–9100 National Abortion Federation Hotline
- (800) 230–7526 Planned Parenthood

Runaway

- (800) 621–4000 National Runaway and Suicide Hotline
- (800) 621-4000 National Runaway Switchboard Hotline (for parents and for runaways)

Sexually Transmitted Infection

- (800) 342–2437 Centers for Disease Control AIDS Hotline
- (800) 234–8337 or (800) 227–8922 Sexually Transmitted Disease Hotline
- (800) 440–8336 Teen AIDS
- (800) 234–8336 Teens Teaching AIDS Prevention (Monday through Friday, 4 to 8 PM Central Standard Time)

Suicide

- (800) 448–4663 Hit Home Hotline for youth crises such as suicide, abuse, pregnancy, depression, counseling, and intervention
- (800) 621–4000 National Runaway and Suicide Hotline ■

never be used alone but should be prescribed and then monitored very closely by a doctor, most often a psychiatrist, who is experienced in treating depression. For adolescents, treatment usually involves some therapy with the whole family.

If your child has tried to kill herself, the doctor is likely to recommend that she be hospitalized and started on drug treatment and therapy and released only when it is clear that she poses no danger to herself.

For many different reasons, treatment with antidepressants takes time to work. These drugs are not like antibiotics; the condition does not clear up in 10 days. Many antidepressants may take several weeks to begin to work properly. Then, because each person is different—and perhaps even each case of depression is different—one drug may not work as desired, and another will have to be tried. This trial and error process can be frustrating, but rest assured that there is usually a combination of medication and therapy that will work for your child.

For the small percentage of people who suffer from bipolar disorder, or manic depression, treatment is usually the drug lithium combined with therapy. Lithium is quite effective in leveling out the highs and lows of bipolar disorder, but it can have side effects. Some people who suffer from bipolar disorder discontinue lithium because they like the high sensation that comes with mania. Your physician will work with your child to keep her on the lowest sensible dose and work to minimize side effects.

Prognosis Good. Recent progress in the development of new drugs that act directly on specific parts of the brain make the treatment of depression much more successful. As knowledge of neurotransmission expands, it is likely that newer and better drugs will become available to make the treatment of depression even more successful. There is no reason for anyone to prolong their suffering from this debilitating disease. Many adolescents and young adults who are treated for depression leave the condition behind them as they enter adulthood, leaving the stresses of adolescence behind. But treatment for many others will be ongoing, and medication may be necessary all their lives. Still, this is a much better prospect than prolonged agony or despair.

❖ ANOREXIA NERVOSA

Symptoms *(What your child may experience)*

- Preoccupation with food, weight, fat, and calories

- Intense and unreasonable fear of being fat

- Continual loss of weight, or failure to gain weight at the appropriate time

- Extreme thinness, while perceiving oneself as fat

- Cessation of menses (the monthly periods stop). If the onset of anorexia nervosa is prior to the beginning of puberty, sexual development will stop and should resume once the child has achieved adequate weight.

- Irritability, depression, and inability to concentrate

- Symptoms of malnutrition. Sufferers can develop iron-deficiency anemia, causing some diminishing of intellectual function—lack of concentration, declining performance in school

What is it? Anorexia nervosa is a potentially fatal eating disorder affecting up to 1 percent of young women in the United States. Those who suffer from anorexia are often quite hungry but willfully suppress it in their pursuit of thinness. Ninety percent of those who suffer from anorexia are female, usually between the ages of 13 and 25, though it can afflict children as young as age 7. Of these, one-third were overweight when they began dieting but kept dieting after they had passed a sensible weight range. Researchers are not in agreement over what causes the disorder, but teenage girls with a shaky self-image who come from a relatively high socioeconomic stratum and participate in activities that require thinness, such as ballet, gymnastics, or modeling, are most vulnerable. New research suggests a link between anorexia and obsessive-compulsive disorder (see Chapter 27).

Our cultural preoccupations with thinness and pressure on adolescents to fit in, to be beautiful, to seek the approval of others, contribute to the problem. It must be kept in mind, however, that 10 percent of people with anorexia are male. Too often, boys are not properly diagnosed as anorectic because of the presumption that only girls suffer from this disorder.

What you can do Adolescents with anorexia rarely acknowledge the problem themselves, so it is up to family and friends to recognize the disorder and get them help. Assess your child's preoccupation with food and with weight. Does your child weigh herself often? Does she describe herself as fat though she is emaciated? Does she wear bulky, long-sleeved, or loose-fitting clothing, even in the summertime, to conceal her thinness? Does she limit the amounts and types of foods she will eat? Seek help to address the emotional and psychological issues that have led to an eating disorder. An eating disorder is a cry for help; it is essential that you respond by seeking professional help for your child.

When to call the doctor Call your doctor if your child exhibits any of the symptoms listed above. She may abuse laxatives or diuretics and the like, which can endanger her life. If she shows signs of this, call your doctor.

Treatment If your youngster has starved herself to the point of emaciation, she will probably have to be hospitalized in order to bring her weight safely back up to normal levels. She will simultaneously receive intensive psychological treatment so that when she is released from the hospital she will be less likely to return to the cycle of weight loss and illness. Treatment involves convincing your child to think differently about her body and her nutritional needs and will also address any coexisting depressive conditions that occur in one-third to one-half of people with anorexia. Treatment of adolescents has the greatest chance of success if the entire family joins counseling.

Prognosis Excellent if identified and treated early in the course of the disease and if the family is supportive. The death rate from anorexia can be as high as 18 percent, mainly due to medical complications and suicide. Most of those who suffer from anorexia are treated successfully and able to develop a healthy, realistic self-image. Some may recover spontaneously. Some may retain peculiar habits or ideas concerning food for many years and may need to continue counseling after they have regained weight and assumed a long-term, normal diet.

❖ BULIMIA NERVOSA

Symptoms (*What your child may experience*)

- Addictive binge eating, resulting from a sense of loss of control, followed by either fasting and unreasonable exercise or self-induced diarrhea or vomiting to purge the body of binged food

- Unreasonable fear of being fat

- Self-image governed almost exclusively by appearance

- Swelling of the parotid glands (the salivary glands, which swell and give mumps its similar, puffy-cheeked appearance)

- Repeated use of diet or water (diuretic) pills, complaints about constipation, and the need for laxatives on a frequent basis

- Usually normal weight

Signs and laboratory findings (*What the doctor looks for*) Because people with bulimia may show few outward symptoms of the illness, the doctor may discover the condition indirectly through blood tests, as improper use of purgatives can lead to dehydration, loss of electrolytes and other significant nutrients; disintegration of teeth from regurgitated stomach acid; and questioning the youngster about her body image or eating habits. Most often, however, it will be the parents of the sufferer or the sufferer herself who tells the doctor of her behavior. The discovery of use of alcohol or other drugs, or sexual promiscuity, may be a clue to the eating disorder.

What is it? There are two types of bulimia nervosa, the purging type and the nonpurging type. A purging bulimic regularly self-induces vomiting and abuses laxatives, enemas, suppositories, or diuretics. The nonpurging type binges and does not regularly use laxatives and the like but uses other behavior to compensate, such as fasting or overexercising. Most males with bulimia are the nonpurging type. Like anorexia nervosa, bulimia is potentially fatal. The use of certain emetics by purging bulimics can cause heart damage. Heart arrhythmia and suicide are major causes of death in people with bulimia.

Bulimia most commonly begins at age 18 to 20 but can develop at an earlier or later age. Unlike those who suffer from anorexia, people with bulimia are aware of but not in control of their eating problem. Many feel trapped in the cycle of bingeing and purging; it may in fact be the only way they keep a normal weight. But the knowledge of the inherent unhealthfulness of the condition, combined with a feeling of helplessness to change it, can lead the sufferer to guilt and, potentially, to depression. People with bulimia have high rates of comorbid depression and often have a drug or alcohol problem.

What you can do If you suspect your child of bingeing and purging behavior—you find, for example, large amounts of purgatives in her bathroom, or notice she seems to have diarrhea frequently, or disappears to the bathroom quickly after eating a meal, or are told by the dentist that your child's tooth enamel has been damaged—you should contact your doctor.

Treatment Most adolescents with bulimia can be treated as outpatients. Antidepressants can be very effective at controlling cravings for food, while therapy provides relief for the underlying problems that led to the disorder.

If bulimic behavior has reached such a severity that the life of your child is in danger, she may have to be hospitalized.

Prognosis Excellent. Most people with bulimia recover with treatment and suffer no long-term ill effects.

For more information on adolescent mental health issues, contact the National Clearinghouse for Mental Health Information at (301) 433-4515.

Common Adolescent Health Concerns

For the most part, adolescents are blessed with wonderful immune systems. They have overcome the diseases of early childhood and no longer are as subject to all the coughs and runny noses that younger children bring home. Yet there are medical conditions that either affect teens most commonly or have their onset during the adolescent years.

ALCOHOL AND OTHER DRUG USE

For the last few years, despite a continuing decline in the use of cocaine and crack cocaine, use of other drugs has been climbing. Although drug use by teens is not as high as it was during the 1970s, the increase, after years of decline, is still alarming to most parents, health care providers, and school administrators.

Although drunk driving arrests and related accidents and fatalities have declined significantly through education programs such as Mothers Against Drunk Driving and Students Against Drunk Driving, alcohol remains the single most popular drug on the planet, as well as one of the most deadly.

Teenagers abuse alcohol more than any other drug, and many report that their abuse has led to such things as unsafe sex, having sex for the first time (usually without protection), drunk driving, and other potentially dangerous behaviors. Those who abuse alcohol are at a statistically higher risk for abuse of other drugs and for smoking tobacco.

Much of the abuse of alcohol and other drugs, particularly marijuana, among young people is linked to the myths that they are "harmless" and "not addictive." While neither drug may be as rapidly addictive as cocaine, heroin or other opioids, or even nicotine, neither is harmless, and both alcohol and marijuana are indeed addictive. However, most of the harm from using alcohol and marijuana comes from teens using them and driving. Marijuana slows reaction time. It also interferes with short-term memory and has a negative effect on learning.

What can parents do to keep teens off alcohol and other drugs?

Many young people will indeed experiment with alcohol or other drugs. It seems to be part of the process of adolescence in this society. Parents should examine their own use of alcohol or other drugs and understand that their children will most likely adapt their attitudes about such things from their parents. There is no substitute for communication and education; every bit of research suggests that the only thing that will keep young people from abusing drugs and alcohol is education. However, research also shows that educating kids about drugs must be coupled with giving them the social skills to resist peer pressure gracefully (that is, without losing face when saying no) in order to be effective. The best place for this learning process to start is at home. Teach your children in frank, age-appropriate terms about the dangers of drugs, about their rightful place in our society, and if at all possible, do so before they reach the experimentation stage. If you suspect your adolescent is using alcohol or other drugs, education is still a good idea, though you may encounter resistance. For more information on the dangers alcohol and other drugs pose, as well as guidance regarding what you can do if you suspect your child is using alcohol or other drugs, see Chapter 5. ■

TOBACCO

Nearly everyone who smokes or uses tobacco products began when they were adolescents. The percentage of those who began after their teen years is so small as to be insignificant. Tobacco companies understand this and target much of their advertising and promotional efforts at young people. Tobacco companies understand that young people are always looking for ways to feel older and to demonstrate their independence and so have learned to exploit this vulnerability. Many states are cracking down on tobacco sales to minors, but as was demonstrated in a recent undercover effort by Virginia authorities, underage teens have little or no problem purchasing tobacco. Many teens have the mistaken belief that use of smokeless tobacco is harmless. This is not true: Use of such products is associated with an increased risk of mouth and esophageal cancers and is as addictive as smoking. It can also lead to permanent damage to teeth and gums.

If you suspect that your adolescent may be smoking cigarettes or using other tobacco products, consult Chapter 4 for detailed information on the dangers of tobacco and what you can do to help your teenager stop. ■

ACNE

Symptoms *(What you may experience)* Whiteheads, blackheads, and pimples, which may be painful. They erupt most often on the face but also on the neck and back and even buttocks. (See page C-26.)

What is it? First, it makes sense to list a few things acne is not. It is not a result of poor hygiene. It is not the result of masturbation or lack of sexual intercourse—it is completely unrelated to sexual activity. Although some researchers recommend against eating certain foods, there is no reliable evidence that acne is caused by diet, although poor diet will not help to heal any infection.

Acne is a skin disease that can be treated. Boys are more likely to get it than girls and more likely to have severe cases, but girls are by no means immune. That acne is most common in adolescents is probably due to the levels of hormones the body releases during this stage of development.

The hormones that stimulate your physical growth also stimulate the growth and activity of sebaceous glands, glands beneath the skin that release a natural oil known as sebum. Increased sebum production supports the proliferation of a bacteria, *Propionibacterium acnes*, as well as sticky skin cells and plugged pores. These sebum plugs become visible as whiteheads or blackheads. If the blocked pores become infected beneath the surface of the skin, a pimple develops.

What you can do Avoid squeezing your pimples, which may lead to the rupture of the follicle beneath the skin, which can lead to a bigger infection (and a bigger pimple or even a cyst). Washing hair and face frequently is helpful.

When to call the doctor Most often, you will not need to call the doctor. Acne can be controlled with over-the-counter preparations. However, if pimples are painful or

Acne. (A) Under normal conditions, the sebaceous glands secrete sebum (oily substance) which passes along the hair shaft and onto the skin to give it protection. (B) During adolescence, changes in the sebum lead to clogging of the pores, which traps the sebum in the hair follicle. Bacteria multiply in the sebum, causing inflammation, redness, and a pustule (a round elevation containing pus) to form on the skin surface.

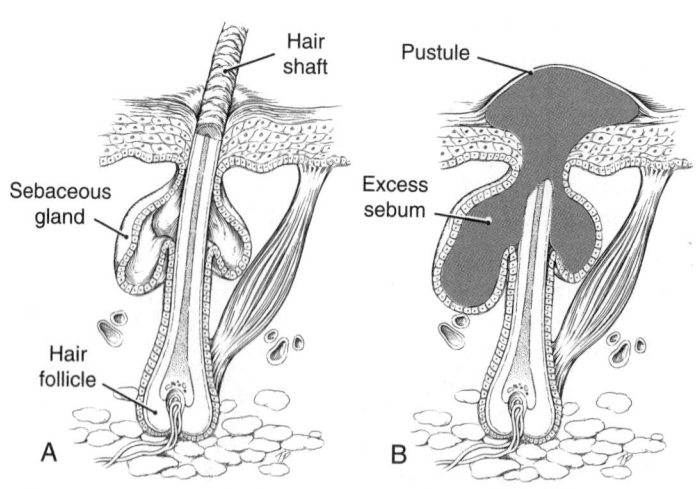

widespread—some can grow as big and painful as boils—or if they are causing scarring or real emotional trauma, you should consult your doctor, who may refer you to dermatologist.

Treatment The first line of treatment for acne is regular washing of the sites where acne appears. This minimizes the presence of oil that can plug pores. Regular hair washing is also important, as it minimizes oil on the scalp and around the hairline. Scrubbing the skin with abrasives or squeezing of pimples is not recommended. Over-the-counter products such as those containing benzoyl peroxide can help to prevent the buildup of sebum.

The next line of treatment is for the doctor to prescribe medication. Preparations using stronger concentrations of benzoyl peroxide can be effective. Tretinoin (Retin A)—topical retinoic acid—is a safe prescription drug that can help in serious cases of acne.

Because acne is a series of small bacterial infections, your doctor can prescribe topical antibiotic creams or lotions containing erythromycin or clindamycin that can be effective in killing bacteria before they can cause infection.

For more serious cases, such as cases of pustular acne, an oral antibiotic, most often tetracycline, can be used over the course of 4 to 6 months, but such preparations should be used judiciously and be closely monitored. Ask your doctor about potential side effects of any medication. Tetra-, mino-, and doxycycline can all cause photosensitivity, which means you will get a sunburn a lot faster than normally and should use a sunscreen. Girls who are taking birth control pills should inform their doctors, because the cyclines can interfere with the effectiveness of oral contraceptives.

Acne can sometimes be reduced in girls by use of hormone treatments (birth control pills) if antibiotics are not successful.

For severe nodulocystic acne (acne involving cysts and hard lumps under the skin surface) the most effective treatment for acne is isotretinoin (Accutane), a vitamin A derivative. Girls who use it must be concerned about sexual activity, because it can cause birth defects in infants conceived while the mother is using the drug. Isotretinoin works by shrinking the sebaceous glands dramatically and thereby reducing the production of sebum, drying up the skin, and reducing inflammation. It can be quite effective, but in the early phase of treatment, it can make acne appear more severe. If you use isotretinoin, you must use sunscreen daily and avoid excessive exposure to the sun. See Chapter 28 for more information on the treatment of acne.

Prognosis Excellent. All but the most severe acne will clear up by late adolescence—late teens or early 20s—as hormonal activity settles down. Some cases may persist into adulthood, but treatment with tretinoin or isotretinoin can help to clear up the most stubborn cases. Scarring can be minimized if treatment is initiated early enough.

❖ INFECTIOUS MONONUCLEOSIS

Symptoms (What you may experience) Mild to high fever; sore throat, usually quite severe; swollen glands; loss of appetite; fatigue and weakness sometimes lasting for weeks; pain or ache in the upper left side of the abdominal area (the location of the spleen, which can become enlarged); generalized aches, chills, flu-like symptoms. Other symptoms that are possible, but not usual, are nausea; vomiting; jaundice (yellow skin/eyes); heart irregularities; rash, especially if taking ampicillin/amoxicillin at the same time; light sensitivity; cough, chest pain, and possibly, difficulty breathing.

Signs and laboratory findings (What the doctor looks for) Swollen glands, enlarged tonsils, enlarged spleen, occasionally jaundice. Your age may lead the doctor to suspect mononucleosis as much as your symptoms. A blood test for antibodies will confirm the diagnosis.

What is it? Mononucleosis, or mono, is called "kissing disease" because it can be transmitted by saliva and most frequently strikes teenagers between the ages of 15 and 17. Caused by the Epstein-Barr virus, infectious mononucleosis has the potential to be dangerous but is mostly not serious, only a nuisance. In some cases, the symptoms will be very mild, and you will not feel or appear very sick. You may, however, feel sluggish and weak for several weeks. Once the fever has abated and the sore throat has cleared, it may take 3 weeks, and in some cases as long as a few months, to get back to feeling like your normal self.

What you can do The best thing you can do is rest, drink plenty of fluids, and keep alert for a worsening of symptoms, which may indicate inflammation of vital organs; this can happen in rare cases and can be dangerous.

When to call the doctor You should call the doctor if you have any sort of flu-like illness with a severe sore throat that doesn't lift within a few days but lingers on or worsens. If you have prolonged flu-like symptoms accompanied by a prolonged or worsening pain in the upper left side of the abdomen—which could indicate inflammation of the spleen—contact your doctor immediately.

Treatment Rest. Like all illnesses caused by viruses, the only cure is the one your body's immune system provides. You should drink plenty of fluids to keep from becoming dehydrated, and even though you may not feel hungry, you should eat. A pain reliever such as acetaminophen or one of the nonsteroidal anti-inflammatory drugs (NSAIDs) will help reduce fever and relieve muscle aches. Most people with mono may have to be out of school for a week or more but can still complete the school year on time with other classmates. Some, however, may be quite affected and may not be able to maintain schoolwork.

Prognosis Excellent. Although it may take a few weeks and you may miss some school, with plenty of rest and proper nutrition and hydration, your body will tackle mono the same way it tackled chickenpox, flu, and other viral illnesses. There is the potential in very rare cases for you to injure vital organs if they become inflamed and you engage in strenuous activities, but this is rare.

❖ SCOLIOSIS

Symptoms *(What you may experience)* The ribs on one side of your body may appear closer together than on the other. A parent or friend may notice that your spine seems curved.

Signs and laboratory findings *(What the doctor looks for)* Usually, x-rays are not required for your doctor to diagnose a curvature of the spine. Most often, the doctor will be able to tell if you have scoliosis using the forward-bending test. Your doctor may x-ray your spine to determine the severity of the curvature. (See page C-42.)

What is it? Scoliosis is a side-to-side curvature of the spine. The normal spine curves inward and outward as it progresses from the skull to the pelvis. It also has a natural side-to-side flexibility. In scoliosis, the spine develops an unnatural curvature from side to side, causing a compression of one side of the body, usually noticeable because the ribs of one side will be closer together and the ribs on the other side will be farther apart. Scoliosis also involves a rotation of the spine, in which the vertebrae twist around the axis of the spine.

Although it is usually associated with adolescent girls, both males and females can get scoliosis. In boys it usually shows up in early childhood. Also associated with poor posture, scoliosis is 99 times out of 100 the *cause* of poor posture rather than caused by it. Its true origins are unknown and are probably genetic.

What you can do Your doctor will determine the severity of your spine's curvature. For truly progressive scoliosis, your doctor will prescribe a brace that will be custom made to extend from the hips to the neck. If you are prescribed a brace, you may have to wear it 23 hours a day. For many young people, having to wear a brace to school can be stressful. Some young people will want to ignore the disease and leave the brace in the back of the closet. Not wearing the brace is a gamble, because surgery may become necessary if the condition is allowed to progress. If you wear the brace, you will probably find that your friends are supportive. If you feel overly self-conscious, you might talk to a counselor or seek support by contacting one of the scoliosis organizations:

- The Scoliosis Association, Inc.
  P.O. Box 811705
  Boca Raton, FL 33481–1705

- National Scoliosis Foundation
  72 Mount Auburn St.
  Watertown, MA 02172
  e-mail: Scoliosis@aol.com

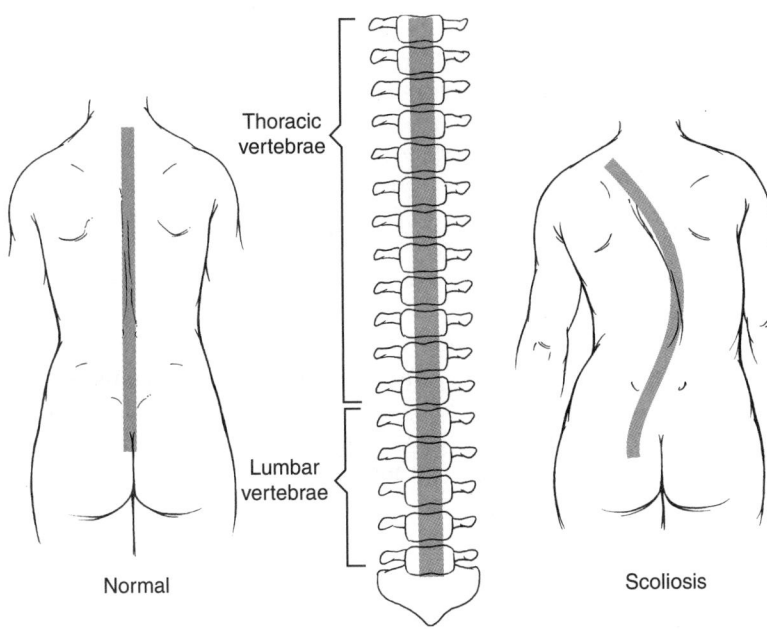

Normal

Thoracic vertebrae

Lumbar vertebrae

Scoliosis

Scoliosis refers to a bend in the spine that is often noticed during adolescence and may worsen during this period of rapid growth. The spine bends to one side or the other and individual bones also rotate around the long axis of the spine. Some cases of scoliosis may need to be treated.

When to call the doctor If you or your family notices any of the above symptoms, contact your doctor. The earlier you begin treatment, the less likely it is that surgery may become necessary.

Treatment Treatment is most often a custom-made brace to hold the spine straight. Surgery may become necessary if the condition is allowed to progress.

Prognosis Mostly very good with treatment. Some cases may be so mild that they need no treatment other than regular follow-up. In some people, the condition can worsen without treatment, and, as time goes on, the compressing of the ribs on one side could also compress the vital organs and cause damage to the heart and lungs.

❖ EPIPHYSITIS

Symptoms *(What you may experience)* Pain in the knee or knees that worsens with strenuous activity and improves after prolonged rest.

Signs and laboratory findings *(What the doctor looks for)* Inflammation of the epiphysis (see below), most commonly around the knees.

What is it? The epiphysis is that portion of the bone that connects the bone shaft to the joint of the longer bones—thigh, upper arm, and shin. While you are growing, the epiphysis can become inflamed if you engage in strenuous physical activity that stresses those particular bones. The most common kind of epiphysitis is Osgood-Schlatter disease (see page 706), which involves the bony prominence just below the knee. The epiphysis near the knee becomes inflamed, and it can be quite painful.

What you can do The best thing you can do is reduce the strenuous physical activity in which you are participating. If you are running cross country or playing football, you should rest and give the inflammation time to subside. You can resume your activity a few days after the pain has subsided, but if it recurs, you should consider changing sports—to swimming, for example, or kayaking—until your growth is complete, at which time the bones should no longer be subject to inflammation. Icing after exercise is also helpful.

When to call the doctor Call the doctor if the pain does not subside after resting for a day or two. There are other potential problems you could be experiencing, and it is sensible to discuss any major or prolonged pain with your doctor, if only to rule out serious injury, such as a hairline fracture.

Treatment Rest is the best treatment, and the pain and inflammation should subside as your strenuous activity subsides. If you are playing on a team, your coach may recommend taking NSAIDs such as ibuprofen or ketoprofen to reduce pain and inflammation and allow you to keep performing. These are worthwhile during a recuperative period, but if you take them consistently or take too many in order to play with an injury, they can have serious consequences.

Prognosis Excellent. With proper rest and the sensible use of over-the-counter pain relievers, epiphysitis should clear up and not return.

❖ MIGRAINE HEADACHES

Symptoms (What you may experience) Intense, throbbing pain, which can last for hours, and is sometimes localized on one side of your head, possibly at the temple, and may spread to your eyes and neck; nausea; occasionally, bizarre visual symptoms, which can include blind spots, hallucinations, patterns, and flashes of light. Some people experience only visual symptoms and nausea, others experience only pain. Because of the strange visual auras and blind spots, the first time you have a migraine, it may be frightening.

Signs and laboratory findings (What the doctor looks for) A family history of migraines.

What is it? While it is unclear exactly what causes migraines, there is a clear genetic connection, and most people who suffer from migraines have a family history of the disorder. Migraines are three times more common in women than in men and can be triggered by any number of factors, from stress to certain foods, such as chocolate, coffee, red wine, foods or beverages containing yeast, and many others. It is believed that migraines occur because of vascular spasms in the brain, though the exact mechanism is unclear. There is no test that will confirm a diagnosis of migraines, so if there is no family history of migraines or if the symptoms are particularly severe or unusual, your doctor may suggest certain tests in order to rule out some more serious condition, such as a brain tumor, aneurysm (see page 435), or other disorder. These tests may include an x-ray of your skull, analysis of your spinal fluid (see Lumbar Puncture, page 429), a computed tomography (CT) scan (see CT Scan, page 427), or your doctor may send you to an ophthalmologist for visual tests.

What you can do Try to determine the particular triggers for your migraines, such as foods, drinks, stress, sleep deprivation, or even exercise, so that you can avoid or minimize them. If you do develop a migraine, try to rest, avoid bright light, and avoid operating an automobile or other heavy machinery.

When to call the doctor Call your doctor if your symptoms do not abate after sleep or after using over-the-counter pain relievers, or if they get worse. You should also call if you are not certain that the symptoms you experience are those of a migraine, particularly if the tendency toward migraine does not run in your family.

Treatment Quite often, the only treatment necessary will be sleep. Some sufferers will respond to over-the-counter pain relievers, although prescription medication is often needed. If you experience more severe symptoms, such as nausea, vomiting, and lingering partial blindness, there are medications your doctor can prescribe that should help quiet your symptoms.

Prognosis Good. For whatever reason, migraines seem to affect children, young adults, and adults, but they lessen in frequency and severity as people get older. This may be due in part to people learning their triggers and avoiding them, or it may involve changes in the brain as it ages, or perhaps a combination of the two. Each person who suffers from migraines will learn the patterns that they follow and probably learn simultaneously how to deal with them.

ELEVEN

Adulthood

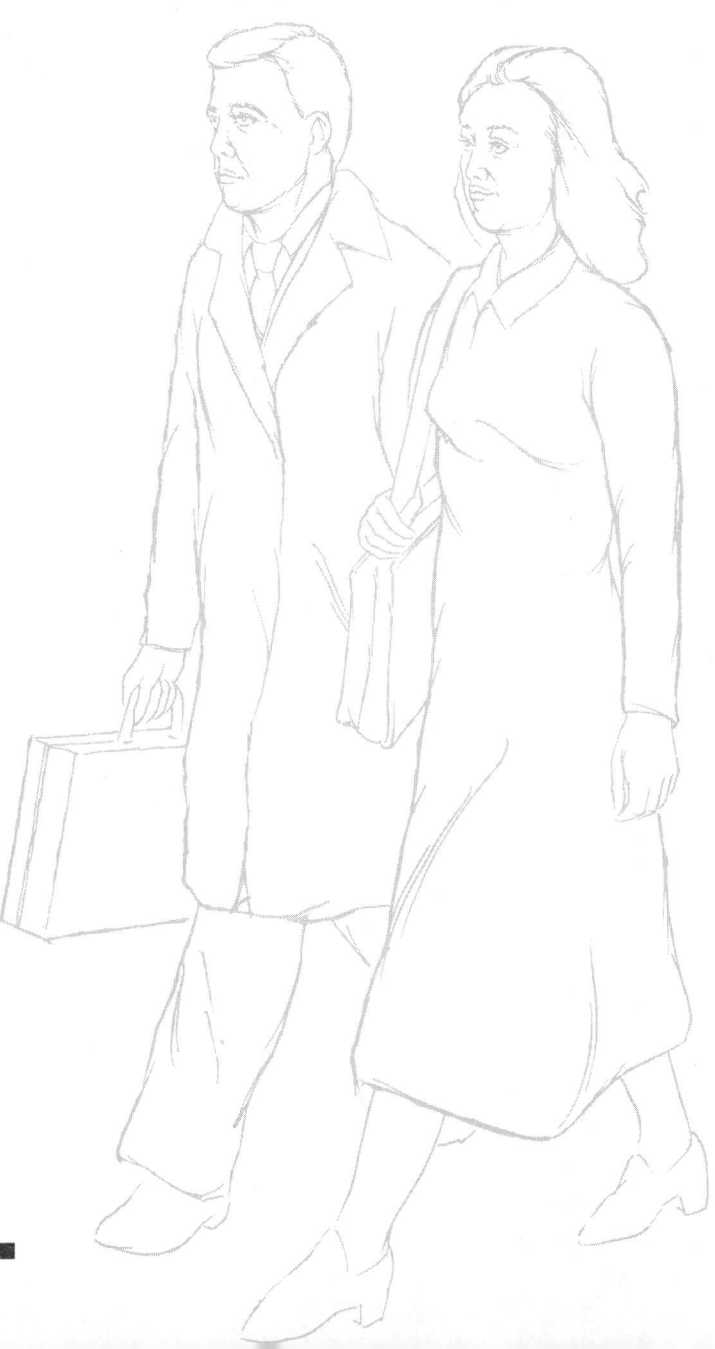

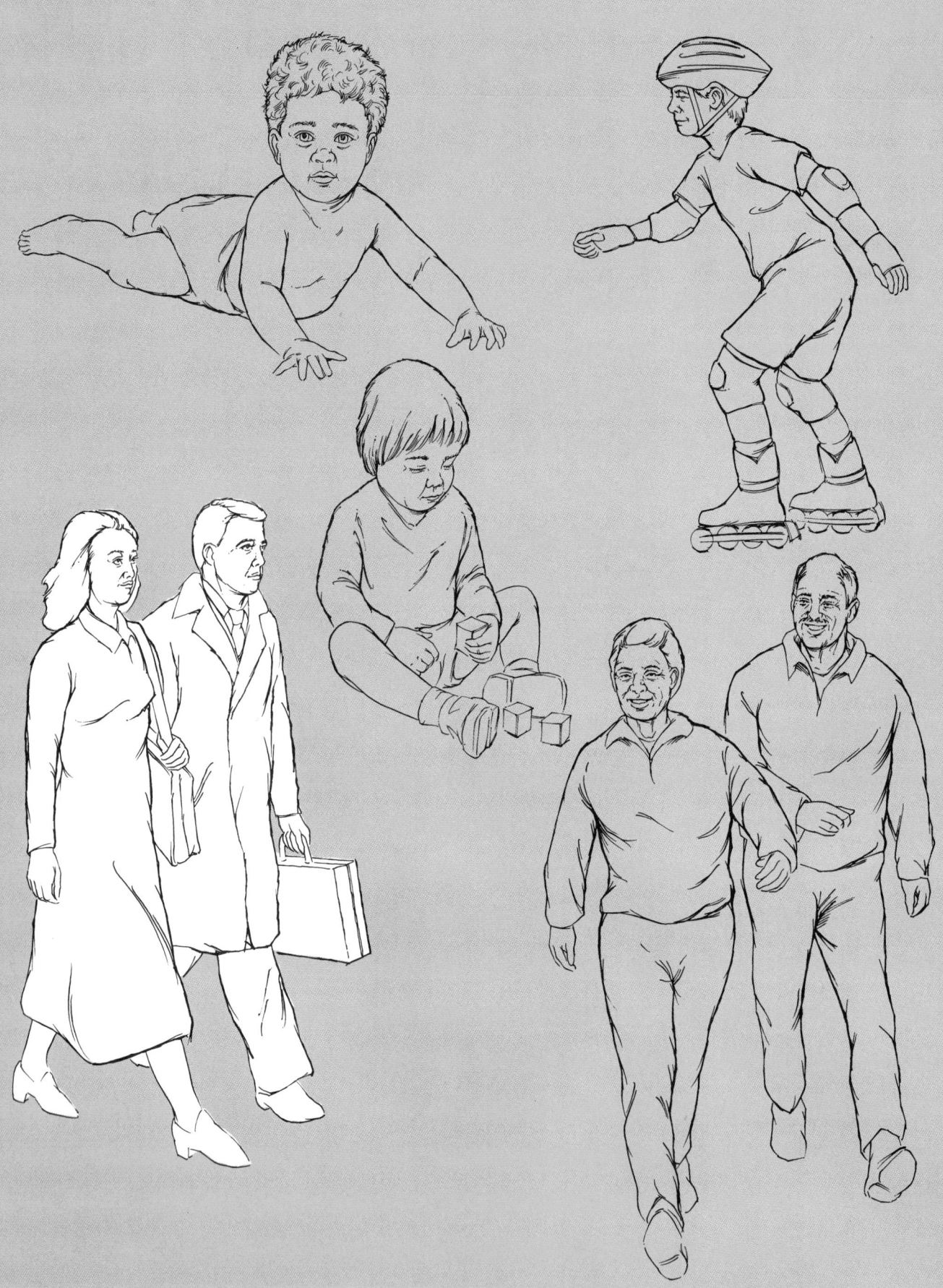

ADULTHOOD

The Busy Years

For many adults, the years that span early to middle adulthood will be some of their best, most fulfilling years. These are the years that establish who we really are—the years when we settle on what we want to become and then become it. These are often the busiest years of our lives, moving from the often intensely social years of our early 20s to the more settled family years of our 30s and 40s, with their steady aggregation of responsibility and rewards.

WHAT IS ADULTHOOD?

Although it is tempting to say that there are three stages of life—childhood, adulthood, and old age—in reality, each of these phases is full of its own stages, each a foundation on which the next is built. Adulthood, usually the longest of the three, is the proving ground of who and what we are, the place where our enduring definitions are forged.

The foundations of our early and adolescent years are built with the help of parents or parent-figures, while the foundations of adulthood are chiefly our own responsibility. In some societies, the choices individuals have as adults are quite restricted; children and adolescents cannot fantasize about being ballerinas or violinists or astronauts, because there are none. In this country, as society has matured from an agrarian to an industrial to a technological culture, the opportunities and possibilities have expanded simultaneously, and the multitude of choices increases the potential for professional and familial enrichment and fulfillment. But at the same time, it also increases the potential for frustration, confusion, failure, and alienation.

For more than a century, research into human development has been weighted heavily on childhood, assuming that who we are is formed and solidified during that time—sometimes as early as age 6. Over the last few decades, researchers have begun to pay much closer attention to adulthood—what it is, how it is attained, what we as human beings seek from it. Indeed, while the world may have its greatest impact on us when we are children, we may have the greatest impact on the world when we are adults. Erik Erikson, a noted theoretician in the study of adulthood, divided the human life cycle into eight ego stages, each of which corresponds to an age range. The stages of adulthood, which, like his other life cycles, Erikson portrayed as dynamic conflicts, consist of three phases: intimacy versus isolation (ages 20 to 40), generativity versus stagnation (ages 40 to 60), and integrity versus despair (age 60 onward).

Since Erikson's work, others have come along to expand and refine our notions of the passages that the adult years constitute. Daniel J. Levinson, in *Seasons of a Man's Life* and *Seasons of a Woman's Life*, considers the impact of the social world on the individual, and the individual's perception of it. Levinson defines the eras of the human life cycle in stages, just as Erikson did. But rather than painting them as conflicts, he depicts a life as stratified: one era of relative emotional stability layered atop an era of change. An individual works toward a particular goal—say, becoming a biologist, a stonemason, or a novelist—and the goal is the end in itself. The attainment of the goal may leave the individual with a sense of satisfaction and fulfillment. But it may also precipitate a reassessment of those aspects of our life that may have been neglected or taken for granted. A period of reevaluation occurs in which the individual negotiates with himself, weighing desires and fantasies against realities, and eventually leading to another goal or set of goals. These varied and continuing goals of adulthood may be the way we each provide order to our adult lives—in a sense, parent ourselves, use our fantasies and dreams and draw on the world around us to shape the lives we want to live. Some of these goals, however—such as the death of parents, the birth of children, loss of employment, and other, unforeseen events of adulthood—are not goals in any traditional sense at all, but simply events that require emotional assimilation. Neither are they necessarily singular: The loss of a parent could coincide with the loss of employment, which could also coincide with the arrival of a child. These crisis moments, which can be more than the unintended consequences of intentional actions, provide an opportunity to explore options, define goals and purposes, and experience the consequences of our actions, both positive and negative. These moments may provide opportunities for some of our most profound spiritual and emotional growth as adults.

EARLY ADULTHOOD: AGES 20 TO 30

Early adulthood is the period when the transition from adolescence to adulthood is mostly completed. We strike out on our own.

The years of the middle 20s constitute what might be called the apprenticeship years, a time of trying on different lives and of apprenticing ourselves to older individuals who serve as role models, who serve as a repository of wisdom and history that we should not ignore. Whether such mentors

THE GOALS AND TASKS OF EARLY ADULTHOOD

In each stage of life, each of us accomplishes several important tasks. There is no single specific way for each of them to be accomplished, although there are probably as many ways that are unhealthy as there are ways that are healthy.

- Recognizing finite opportunities for growth within your family of origin and establishing your own identity

- Starting on the path to a career

- Developing adequate trust and sense of self to begin to establish long-term intimate relationships

- Learning to live independently

- Childbearing and/or parenting (goal of early adulthood for some, middle adulthood for others) ■

WELLNESS GOALS FOR EARLY ADULTHOOD

- Annual health assessments that include screening for alcohol abuse and tobacco use, recommendations for diet and exercise, and advice on birth control and prevention of sexually transmitted infections (STIs)

- Adequate exercise to maintain cardiovascular health and prevent/control obesity

- Balanced diet that does not exceed recommended caloric intake for gender, height, weight, and level of physical activity

- Prevention of STIs

- Regular self-assessment for responsible use of alcohol and other drugs

- Stress prevention such as exercise, meditation, and so on

- Spiritual engagement

- Injury prevention; for example, using seatbelts, firearm safety devices, and proper athletic gear ■

are professors, employers, our own parents, historical figures we admire, or varying combinations, these older individuals help us continue the development of the tools necessary to make important decisions about the many small and large questions that will constitute the foundation of our later adult years.

During these years, the possibilities may seem endless, and as young adults we may fantasize about the myriad of different lives we might lead, visualizing ourselves in different professions, different cities, with different mates. Indeed, this kind of fantasy is one of the hallmarks of our humanity and is by no means restricted to the young adult years. Our ability to reach beyond ourselves is what allows us throughout adult life to consider alternatives, weigh choices, evaluate risks, formulate possibilities, and continually transform ourselves.

The 20s, particularly the early 20s, are often intensely social years. Together with friends, we launch on a voyage of self-discovery—whether that means staying up until dawn talking about the meaning of the universe or dancing the night away. Most in their 20s are at their peak physically and sexually (during the 20s is the healthiest time, physically, to have children, though it may not be the best time emotionally). The old adage has it that youth is wasted on the young, but the tremendous energy expended on socializing can hardly be called wasted. It serves several functions: increasing the exposure of the individual to different ideas and ways of thinking; seeking and perhaps finding a mate (or at least trying out mating behavior); building social and professional networks; establishing the validity of our goals; and refining our ideas through interaction with elders and peers.

During this period, the seeds of problems that can haunt us in later life are often planted. Many begin using alcohol, the single most popular drug in the world, or other drugs. A relatively small percentage may become addicted, although the effects of alcoholism may not become problematic until later in life. Other drug use, particularly illegal drugs such as cocaine, may become problematic almost immediately (see Chapter 5). Also, while skeletal growth has usually been completed by the early 20s, muscular growth often has not, and so caloric requirements are higher than they will be at the end of the 20s. In addition, many people—because they are increasingly busy and take on increasing responsibility but do not work in situations that require intense physical activity—become less active. Eating patterns established in the early 20s can, if not modified, lead to problems with obesity later in life, increasing the risk of hypertension, diabetes, heart disease, and cancer (see Chapter 1). Excessive caloric intake and lack of exercise, when combined with smoking, alcohol consumption, and the aging of the body, can lead to serious health complications.

At the outset of this period, most of us are malleable, full of ideas but open to change. One of the hallmarks of the transition from adolescence to adulthood, Erikson writes, is that we become confident enough in our identity and independence that we can learn to be truly and unselfishly intimate with others, lovers as well as friends. True intimacy is often confused with being able to express our feelings more openly (which we should be able to do) because of the safety of a relationship at the expense of not having to observe many social niceties: being polite, caring, appreciative, thankful, and so on. In truth, real intimacy should actually provide for a heightened expression of these sorts of niceties with those with whom we are intimate. In turn we are rewarded with heightened caring and appreciation from others. So the early 20s can and should be an extremely fertile period for relationships.

As the period nears its end, we may become less flexible as we fall into what may be (good or bad) lifelong patterns of intimacy. Here, however, we have a much surer sense than we did at 20 of who we are, our footing is much more steady, and we have a much clearer eye on where we want to be.

YOUNG ADULTHOOD: AGES 30 TO 40

Levinson writes that we really endure two midlife crises, the first occurring at approximately 30 and the second approximately a decade later. Given that adulthood, like much of life, can be an ongoing process of trying to maintain a sense of mastery of self, the notion of the midlife crisis may be oversimplifying. Still, it is useful to understand that everyone experiences and survives repeated upheavals during the adult years,

THE GOALS AND TASKS OF YOUNG ADULTHOOD

- Developing a long-term, intimate relationship
- Starting a family by finding a mate, perhaps having children
- Refining the career path
- Growing within the career/developing professional responsibility and initiative
- Integrating into a community of your choice
- Assessing and refreshing your relationship with parents and family as an adult ∎

some involving more intense self-examination than others.

For reasons that may be completely arbitrary, we tend to look at new decades (either of our lives or of our century) as thresholds that provoke assessment and reassessment of goals.

By age 30, we have begun to appreciate the privileges and pains of adulthood and recognize that, for better or for worse, adulthood is here to stay. So the years that surround 30 are often a time of assessment and reassessment, questioning of choices and goals, and perhaps reorienting our lives. Real crises (demoralization or the sense of being overwhelmed by adversity)

WELLNESS GOALS FOR YOUNG ADULTHOOD

- Maintenance of intimacy: reinvigoration of intimate relationships (family or couples counseling, parent–child communication)
- Establishment of patterns of healthful behavior: adequate physical activity to maintain relative youth; sensible diet to prevent or curtail obesity
- Establishment or reinvigoration of spiritual life
- Regular assessment of patterns of alcohol use (see Chapter 5)
- Hypertension (high blood pressure) screening
- Stress management through healthy diversion (see Managing Stress, page 307) ∎

can occur when we feel that we are not meeting or mastering the challenges that life presents.

Those who have focused on career goals exclusively during the past decade might, for example, hit 30 (or 28 or 33) and decide that life up to this point has been devoid of meaning and is in serious need of adjusting. A woman in this position may hear her "biologic clock" ticking and suddenly begin to obsess over childbearing. A man may find himself lonely, intimate only with his profession, perhaps not even knowing his wife or children, if he has them. Someone who has married early and expended every waking hour on children and spouse may suddenly wonder where the promise and potential of youth have gone. Another may spend the 20s on binges of alcohol or cocaine, hit 30, and decide that life so far has been wasted. Ideally, such crises provoke us to come to an understanding of how we got to where we are and that life has many different possibilities for meaning. Disappointment in or even being laid off from a particular profession may lead to reevaluation of work goals. The realities of child rearing may lead to spiritual reevaluation. The realization of infertility or the lack of a significant other may provoke other kinds of reevaluation.

Because of the emphasis in this culture on beauty and youth, and the manner in which advertising may play on our fantasy lives and create unrealistic yearnings, some people may confront the increasing inevitability of age during this period—wrinkles, thinning hair, weight gain—with more anguish and even panic than such realities warrant, even before age 40. Others accept these inevitabilities and begin to enjoy the rewards that increasing age, success at work, family life, and community involvement can bring.

It is during these years that we affirm our adult identities and often rededicate ourselves to our need for continual spiritual and emotional growth. As younger people, temperament and environment probably shaped many of the choices we made (career and educational choices, whether or not we married, and so on). The reassessing of life around age 30 can be seen as the natural conflict between the differences in our individual endowments (talents, abilities, and predilections) and our formative experiences. In the resolution of

this conflict, much of the foundation for our later lives is laid. This foundation includes a wide-ranging variety of lifestyle choices including whether we have a solid career to see us to retirement. And it includes the basic building blocks of a healthful middle and senior adult life—a sense of self as shaped by moral, spiritual, and emotional life, as well as sensible nutrition, proper exercise, and regular disease screening and prevention.

MIDDLE ADULTHOOD: AGES 40 TO 60

The second midlife crisis may occur at about age 40. Most people do not begin to feel like adults until their mid-30s, but by the time they have reached 40, they have come to accept the stage of life, even revel in it. But in the years around 40, most adults come to recognize that age has its price as well as its privileges: Staying physically fit requires increasingly more effort. For those who lead a sedentary lifestyle, the age of 40 is when it is recommended to see a doctor before embarking on a strenuous physical fitness program (see Keeping Fit in Midlife, page 301). It is also around 40 when many of us must begin to deal with major life events—the death or illness of parents, perhaps a chronic disease such as diabetes—and many may have to learn to live with the divorces, deaths, and illnesses of close friends and peers (see Depression, page 302).

Although all of us are aware of our mortality, it is around age 40 that many of us begin to really acknowledge it. In our 20s, the possibilities may have seemed endless; now, at 40, the threshold of aging, they may seem much more finite and circumscribed. The second midlife crisis, like the first, is probably not so much a single crisis as it is a more-intense-than-usual assessment of our actual achievements against our youthful dreams, an assessment of the state of our physical and spiritual health that includes preparing for life changes that lie ahead—making sure we have life insurance, retirement plans, and possibly even purchasing cemetery plots.

As well as recognizing our mortality (which some of us may try to evade by indulging in cosmetic surgery or throwing off a long-time spouse for a much younger

KEEPING FIT IN MIDLIFE

Exercise feels good, and exercise helps you feel good about yourself. If you have led a sedentary existence for the last 20 years, starting to exercise may not feel good at first; you may wheeze, and your knees may remind you how old you are. But if you begin with a sensible and moderate exercise program, your body will soon prove to you how young you really are.

Anyone 40 years old or over who has led a sedentary lifestyle, who smokes, or who has diabetes or any other chronic condition should check with his doctor before beginning an exercise program. Many people let their enthusiasm get the better of them and assume more is better, only to injure themselves by not allowing their bodies a chance to acclimate to the increase in exertion. Proper technique—warming up and warming down—is essential. Heart attacks, for example, sometimes happen after exercise.

Your doctor can assist you by helping to gauge the level of exercise you are capable of and can point you toward learning proper technique. You will likely experience some aches in your muscles and possibly joints after first beginning an exercise program. These should go away over a period of time. If they persist, consult your doctor; you may be doing something wrong.

A report from the US Surgeon General concluded that regular, moderate physical activity reduces the risk of developing coronary heart disease, type 2 diabetes mellitus, hypertension, and colon cancer; reduces symptoms of anxiety and depression; contributes to the development and maintenance of healthier bones, muscles, and joints; and helps control weight. Most significantly, the Surgeon General's report concluded that positive health benefits require only a moderate level of activity—sufficient to expend about 150 calories of energy per day, or 1,000 calories per week. To accomplish this, you could walk briskly for 30 minutes each day. Another significant finding was that benefit to health increases in proportion to the amount of activity.

A moderate amount of physical activity can be achieved in many ways and can be incorporated into your lifestyle in a manner appropriate to your personal preferences and life circumstances. Examples of moderate activity include playing volleyball for 45 minutes, raking leaves for 30 minutes, swimming laps for 20 minutes, playing basketball for 15 to 20 minutes, or running 1.5 miles in 15 minutes. These examples illustrate the balance between duration and intensity, with less strenuous activities requiring a longer duration to achieve the same caloric expenditure and health benefit. There is some evidence to indicate that exerting yourself on the weekends and not doing so all week long can lead to health problems—sports injuries—and does not have the benefit of regular exercise. Regular exertion means skipping only 1 or at most 2 days between exercise periods.

See Chapter 2 for more information on exercising safely and effectively. ■

---

lover), many of us also recognize those things that will make up our true immortality, or the lasting legacies of our work, our children, and our charitable works.

How we deal with the emotional and spiritual turmoil that can arise in the middle adult years (what we learn as we come to terms with our accomplishments, or lack of them, and our mortality), as well as how we deal with the ordinary events of midlife, will steer us into the later years and may largely predict how those later years go. If a person is diagnosed with alcoholism, does he ignore the problem or address it head-on and get sober? If someone is chronically depressed, does he seek help and explore all the solutions? If someone is lonely from divorce or from moving with a job, does he seek new relationships in new circumstances or isolate himself (see Building Lasting Relationships, page 310)? If someone notices increasing tension in his most intimate relationships, does he allow the tension to build to the breaking point or address it through couples or family counseling?

These years encompass what Erikson calls generativity versus stagnation. Although generativity and stagnation can start much earlier in life—generativity with child rearing or stagnation with isolation—they grow in importance during the middle years. As Erikson notes, the emphasis is often on the need of the young to learn from their elders, yet little emphasis is put on how much elders need to teach the young—and be needed by them—both spiritually and emotionally. We are a social species, with a valuable and complex web of interconnectivity between the old and young. Studies have shown that social interaction can be an important reliever of stress; studies have also shown that social involvement as well as participation in volunteer organizations such as Big Brothers/Big Sisters can relieve stress, improve healing, and ward off depression. Unfortunately, however, aspects of our culture often work to counter this: Television watching may isolate people by reducing social interaction.

The middle years of adulthood are also a time of many physical changes. Statistics show that most Americans lead sedentary lifestyles. Poor dietary choices and lack of exercise can lead to weight gain and its attendant risks. It can also lead to many conditions we associate with aging. There

DEPRESSION

Depression is a confusing word. People use it for the kinds of unhappiness we all feel. However, we also use the same word when we mean a clinical depression, that is, a disorder that happens to at least 1 in every 25 people during their lifetime. Some higher estimates are that clinical depression will happen to as many as 1 in every 5 people sometime during their lifetime.

Depression referring to unhappiness includes many types of sad feelings, such as boredom, dissatisfaction, and the blues. These feelings occur when difficult things are happening in our lives or when we feel we are making mistakes. We become demoralized and unhappy, and these feelings can be extremely strong. One of the strongest feelings of unhappiness is natural and occurs when we have suffered the loss of a loved one; that is, we experience grief.

When feelings like these are happening to you and are very strong or prolonged, professional help is often extremely useful. Psychotherapy helps you to recover your morale by talking through your problems—by learning effective strategies to handle stress and problems and by learning to think differently about what is happening in your life, your feelings may improve.

Some evidence shows that by helping others you can help yourself. Instead of sitting at home, you can volunteer in your community or get involved with people. Being isolated when you are unhappy usually intensifies your sad feelings. Your energy is better served by being converted to actions that are positive for someone else. This is an excellent way to begin to restore your mood.

Clinical depression is another matter entirely. This type of depression has no origin in events but is a medical condition that can recur throughout life and is different from grief or demoralization. The feeling accompanying this illness may be like one of the feelings described above but more intense. There is a heaviness about the feeling, described by some people as a weight, or black cloud, or fog. The sorrow or sadness is much more severe. It affects everything about the way a person sees himself and his life, extending into the past—so that sometimes it is hard to even recall a good memory—and very much into the future, with feelings of hopelessness and despair. Often, a great deal of anxiety, dread, and even panic accompany this kind of depression. While people with clinical depression search for a reason why they feel so bad and often come up with something in life that they believe must be the cause of such distress, the condition stems primarily from biologic causes. People suffering from clinical depression feel guilt and self-blame and lose confidence. They feel incapable. Energy declines, and there is often a terrible sense of fatigue and bodily discomfort, which makes people believe that they are physically ill. The depression is often more severe in the morning. Sleep and eating patterns are upset, and there may be overeating or loss of appetite, insomnia (difficulty staying asleep at night), and early morning waking. Usual interests are no longer appealing, and there is less or no pleasure in activities that once were enjoyable and entertaining.

There are many levels of clinical depression, from a very mild feeling that allows a person to function in more or less his normal fashion to severe depression, in which the person feels so bad that he believes there is no reason to live. When depression is this severe, suicidal thoughts are very common. It is important to know that depressions are highly treatable. There is always hope, no matter how hopeless it feels.

If you become depressed seek help from your doctor. Remember, depression is a highly treatable condition. Medications are available and may be necessary to correct the chemical imbalances in the brain that cause clinical depression. Moreover, in some forms of depression, vigorous exercise may help reduce the amount of depression you experience, because strenuous exercise releases chemicals that improve mood.

In general, family and friends are confused about clinical depression. They will tell you that you should get active, do something about your problem, and pull yourself up by your bootstraps. It is important to know that this type of depression is a physical disorder caused by chemical imbalances in the brain. You cannot talk or will your way out of a physical problem. It is important to know that it is not your fault. While you should try your best to keep active and to be as positive as you can be, the way you feel is not entirely in your control and is not your fault. You do not deserve to feel the way you do. And you should seek help. (For more information on depression, see Chapter 27.)

is, however, no reason for most people to be sedentary and no reason why anyone should not remain active and fit late into life. (See Chapters 1 and 2 for more information on age- and health-appropriate nutrition and exercise.) Still, some physical changes are inevitable. It is during the years of middle adulthood that women will experience menopause, or the cessation of menses, when periods stop and women become infertile—usually within a few years of age 45 (see page 1104 for more information on menopause).

The knowledge that menopause is approaching or occurring is, depending on circumstances, viewed by some women and some couples as a crisis. Until recently, menopause has been viewed as a taboo subject, leading to misconception and confusion. In terms of health, there is really no reason that menopause should become a crisis. The majority of women experience only mild symptoms, while very few experience severe physical and emotional symptoms. Many are quite happy with the change and continue with their lives, including their sex lives, as before; indeed, some consider having sex without worrying about unwanted pregnancy one of the privileges of age.

COSMETIC SURGERY

Cosmetic surgery, or elective surgery performed to improve appearance and self-image, is a huge industry. Nose jobs, facelifts, tummy tucks, breast enlargement (or reduction), liposuction, and all sorts of body contouring are now nearly as common as dyed hair, although considerably more expensive. And what was once mostly the indulgence of women has now become quite popular among men. In this age- and appearance-conscious society, many people are acutely aware of the social benefits that a young and attractive appearance offers. A survey of American men found that a majority were dissatisfied with some aspect of their looks; a majority also said that if they could improve some part of their appearance, they would be more successful on the job.

Many people object to cosmetic surgery on the grounds that the path to a better self-image is an internal, not an external one. The battle to stay young is one we all lose eventually, and plastic surgery can raise unrealistic expectations. But others view it as the equivalent of good grooming or dressing well: If you can improve your appearance and your self-image, if you can improve your employability, why not do so if you can afford it?

The decision to have cosmetic surgery is one that should not be taken lightly. Unlike dyed hair, it is not something that can easily be undone. Though complications are rare, there is no such thing as risk-free surgery. And quite often, your expectations of the new you will not be met.

Before undertaking plastic surgery, you should discuss your motivations with a counselor and your expectations with your doctor. We all age, and one of the central goals of middle adulthood is the acceptance of that process. ■

Men do not go through a similar onset of infertility and can continue producing viable sperm late into life. However, men do experience increasing numbers of sex-related difficulties during these years, which can also be viewed as crises. Most such difficulties are related to medical conditions that can be treated and in most cases should not be considered an inevitable part of aging. Enlargement of the prostate (see page 1146) and prostate cancer are increasingly being diagnosed due to improved examination methods and new tests (see page 1147). In addition, drugs such as antihypertensives, antidepressants, and antihistamines can affect sexual function (see Impotence, page 1157). Alcoholism can also affect sexual response. Loss of intimacy can also be a significant factor in sexual performance disorders. Diabetes and other chronic diseases can affect sexual response in both men and women. But men do experience hormonal changes as they age, and the aging of the sexual organs, without disease or drugs, may lead to diminished sexual desire.

Everyone ages, but everyone ages differently. Keeping fit and making sensible nutritional choices can go a long way to ensure that although we age, we do not get "old." Our hair may go gray, we may become bald; these are merely the luck of the genetic draw. They do not in and of themselves make us old. There is a lot of truth to the old adage that you are only as old as you feel. Even if your hearing starts to fade or your vision diminishes, there is no reason not to view life as precious and full of possibilities. Regular screening can be invaluable in detecting, preventing, and treating

THE GOALS AND TASKS OF MIDDLE ADULTHOOD

- Reinvigorating your intimate personal relationship, or establishing one

- Helping children into the world and assisting them in becoming responsible and independent adults

- Accepting the reality of the aging process

- Reinventing or revitalizing your relationship with aging parents; accepting their mortality

- Maintaining growth and satisfaction with career

- Coping with life events and stressors—for example, divorce, menopause, retirement, or the deaths of loved ones (see Coping With the Stresses of Adult Life, page 305) ■

WELLNESS GOALS FOR MIDDLE ADULTHOOD

- Maintenance or development of hobbies or other recreational activities to divert stress and maintain social activity

- Maintenance of social activity even in the face of being too busy with personal or professional setbacks (job layoff, death of close relatives)

- Reinvigoration of your love relationship with counseling or self-examination

- Maintenance of personal fitness through appropriate exercise and spiritual pursuits

- Generative behavior and avoidance of stagnation through the pursuit of social and community responsibility ■

RECOMMENDED REGULAR SCREENING AND COUNSELING

SCREENING	COUNSELING
Your doctor should	**Your doctor should**
Assess height and weight.	Counsel you on weight loss if appropriate and emphasize a sensible diet with a caloric intake proportional to your level of physical activity, emphasizing grains, fruits, and vegetables. Advise older people to ensure adequate consumption of bulk fiber to avoid constipation.
Assess fitness.	Advise you on appropriate levels of exercise, risks of obesity.
Assess blood pressure; if you are hypertensive and obese, screen for diabetes.	Offer advice on how to reduce your risk of hypertension-related illness.
Perfom a Papanicolaou (Pap) smear (women).	
Require a mammogram (annually or biannually for women 50 to 69) and annual clinical breast exam	
Perform a fecal occult blood test (for those age 50 and over); sigmoidoscopy every 3 to 5 years for those age 50 and over.	Advise you on dietary ways you can reduce your risk of colon and rectal cancer.
Assess for problem drinking or other drug use.	Advise you on safe levels of alcohol use; advise those with a potential problem on the dangers of addiction and how to get help.
Assess for high-risk sexual behavior and screen you for chlamydia and gonorrhea if you have had more than one sexual partner in the last year; screen you for human immunodeficiency virus (HIV) if you have engaged in high-risk sexual behavior.	Advise you on ways to prevent STIs, unwanted pregnancy, and the benefits of the hepatitis B vaccine.
Assess for tobacco use.	Recommend ways to stop smoking.
Assess your history of immunizations and ensure you have all that are necessary.	
Perform a tuberculin skin test for those at risk.	
Assess rubella (German measles) immunity for women in their childbearing years.	Vaccinate women of childbearing age who are not immune.
Assess your diet.	Advise you on ways to get adequate levels of calcium; for women planning pregnancy, prescribe a multivitamin with folic acid; advise you that your fat intake should be less than 30% of calories.

DENTAL HEALTH

Healthy teeth and gums are an important aspect of overall wellness. With a sensible dental hygiene program, including regular visits to the dentist, you should be able to keep all your teeth for all of your life.

It is important in adulthood not to neglect routine dental hygiene, because periodontal disease can result. *Periodontal* means "around the teeth," but gum diseases, such as gingivitis and periodontitis, can lead to serious problems with your teeth, including tooth loss.

Your gums are known as the *gingiva*; gingivitis is the inflammation of the gums. You can easily tell if your gums are inflamed simply by looking in the mirror: Are they red and swollen? Inflamed gums will not necessarily be painful; indeed, the first indication many people have of gingivitis is bleeding that occurs while they are brushing their teeth.

If you notice such bleeding, consult your dentist. The inflammation of your gums can cause you to brush improperly and can cause buildup of plaque beneath the inflamed portions of your gums. Plaque is the whitish coating on teeth that builds up between brushings; it is the result of oral bacteria feeding on carbohydrates left in your mouth—stuck in or between your teeth or

in your saliva. Plaque can harden into a scaly buildup on the teeth as calculus, or tartar. Both plaque and calculus are slightly acidic and can, with prolonged exposure to the teeth, cause the dissolution of the exterior enamel of the teeth. When plaque and calculus invade beneath the gumline, they can cause considerable tooth decay. Untreated gingivitis can lead to periodontitis, which can, if not treated properly, result in the loss of teeth.

Periodontitis is often painless, but pain in the teeth, particularly when eating hot or cold foods, may also occur. Loose teeth, foul breath, and a bad taste in the mouth are common symptoms.

The best preventive measure you can take against gingivitis and periodontitis is a regular brushing and flossing program—brushing after every meal, and flossing once a day—in order to keep plaque at a minimum. Your dentist should advise you on proper brushing technique; to minimize your intake of sweets, particularly sticky substances; and to brush (or at least rinse your mouth with water) after eating sticky fruits such as raisins or dates, or starchy foods, such as potato chips, which can stick to your teeth.

Your dentist will tell you how often you need to see him, based on your dental history, and will advise you on reducing your risk of periodontal disease. ■

many disorders before they become severe (see Recommended Regular Screening and Counseling, page 304).

Although legally we do not become senior citizens until age 65, we do become in middle adulthood, as Levinson writes, senior members of the adult world—the movers and the shakers of the world at large. Much of whether we are generative or stagnant, to use Erikson's terms, will derive from how we have lived our earlier adult years: decisions we have made about health (emotional, spiritual, and physical) and about giving back to the world that has sustained us, and how we have coped with the various events that have come our way.

THE PERIODIC HEALTH ASSESSMENT

A periodic health assessment is invaluable in maintaining overall wellness. Almost every disease can be helped by early detection, and a periodic health assessment is one of the best means to catch disease early, when it is most treatable, and to identify risk factors that can be modified. Routine urinalysis and blood work can uncover a number of conditions, but your doctor will help you determine, based on your personal history, the specific diseases and disorders that you should be screened for.

Below is a table of screening and counseling services that each of us should have on a regular basis.

Coping With the Stresses of Adult Life

Life today for many of us has become increasingly fast paced and crowded. We juggle the often conflicting demands of our family, work, and social lives with varying degrees of agility, and we find that we have too little time to rest and recuperate from stressors, or the life events that cause stress. Consequently, the words *stressful, stressed out*, and *burned out* have come almost to define much of contemporary adulthood. Despite the prevalence of the term *stress*, however, it is not always clear just what stress means, or how it relates to mental and physical health.

RECOGNIZING STRESS

Different people experience stress in enormously different ways. For some, a fast-paced existence provides the excitement and stimulation they need to be productive and happy. There are even "adrenaline junkies" who find a stressful life so invigorating that they seek out stress in generous doses, doing everything from parachuting to becoming war correspondents in the hottest spots on the globe. For others, the mere thought of confronting stressing events day after day is enough to make them want to hide in a corner with a pillow over their heads. This is all a matter of temperament, and neither kind of temperament can be seen as better or worse than the other.

Most of us, however, are somewhere in between, finding the occasional roller-coaster ride (either real or figurative) invigorating, while finding everyday stressors mostly manageable if not pleasurable.

Stress reactions are rooted in the body's natural fight-or-flight response, without which our ancient ancestors would never have survived. But our stressors today are considerably different from those they experienced. While we still may need to decide whether or not to fight or flee an attacker, we are more likely to have to face a boss we dislike, difficult or unruly children, marital tension, sleep deficits, and other worrisome if not life-threatening events and circumstances.

The body responds, however, in much the same way it has for millennia: In a split-second, in the face of a real or perceived threat, it releases stress hormones, stored energy, and adrenaline, which results in a heightened state of physical and emotional arousal in order to provide the wherewithal either to (in evolutionary terms) stay around and fight or flee. A threat can represent an astonishing variety of different circumstances, from real physical danger, such as being accosted on the street; to unfamiliar situations, such as a blind date or a new job; to troubling or troublesome situations, such as a babysitter quitting, a parent dying, a child leaving for college, or marital difficulties.

Most of us have built up ways over the years of coping with stress and so in some respects may not even recognize its accumulation. Some coping mechanisms are healthy and allow the stress to run itself out. Many, however, are not, and the stress reaction becomes a vicious cycle, with just the threat of a threat provoking a stress reaction. Generally, it is this vicious cycle to which we refer when we commonly talk about "being under stress." Individual stressors come and go, but their effect can easily

linger. Usually, physical reactions to stress are more noticeable than emotional reactions. Symptoms include

- Headaches
- Hyperventilation
- High blood pressure
- Upset stomach
- Digestive distress
- Jitters
- Sleep difficulties
- Nail biting
- Hair twirling
- Jaw clenching
- Teeth grinding
- A sensation of physical illness, nausea
- Fatigue

Psychological symptoms are no less real or troubling, however, and include

- Irritability
- Anxiety
- Pessimistic or resentful feelings
- Feelings of being victimized
- Feelings of being misunderstood or unappreciated
- The desire to withdraw
- Unexpected or unprovoked outbursts of laughing or crying

More severe stress reactions tend to occur when circumstances or events combine to tax your system beyond what you can successfully assimilate. In some instances, you may experience more pronounced symptoms when stress has accumulated over time and you have consistently ignored the signals. For example, you have chosen to tolerate a marriage that has been troubled and angry for a long time, yet when your father dies and you must move your mother to a nursing home, you find yourself unaccountably overwhelmed and emotionally exhausted.

This emotional exhaustion results when pressure from individual stressors has not been dissipated but has accumulated. These situations often do not provide the opportunity for fight or flight in the conventional sense, so your body and mind are aroused to a near-constant state of perceived emergency, but the stress is not released in the sudden vigorous burst of energy the body expects. Consequently, the effects of accumulated stress can be exhibited in many of the symptoms described above.

However unpleasant these symptoms may be—and in some instances you may want to have a thorough examination to rule out any physical condition that could be causing the symptoms—stress, in itself, is not an illness. Yet, when not effectively managed, stress can have serious and long-reaching effects. Accumulated stress can express itself in illness or make an existing illness worse. Indeed, research has shown that accumulated stress can contribute to the development of heart disease and profoundly weaken the immune response. And feelings of helplessness or worthlessness may contribute to careless and even self-destructive choices such as reaching for a cigarette or a drink or other drug, becoming violent, or overindulging in comfort foods, such as fats and sweets—in many respects, exactly those kinds of behaviors that can increase stress rather than decrease it.

MANAGING STRESS

Life is increasingly complex and demanding, and stress is an unavoidable aspect of our existence. Most of our experiences, even the happiest ones, can naturally be accompanied by emotional strain. While in some respects stress can be avoided, in other respects avoiding stress can cause you to miss out on a lot of the pleasures that a full life can afford. If, for example, you are aerophobic, or afraid of flying, you could avoid the stress of dealing with your phobia by never flying. However, by addressing the phobia with the help of a psychiatrist, social worker, psychologist, or other counselor, you could overcome the phobia and open your life to the many pleasures travel can afford. So stress is not something necessarily to be avoided, but something to be recognized and managed.

Many people, perhaps because of the subtle influence of television, in which nearly any problem can be overcome in 23 to 46 minutes, believe that their lives should be smooth, steady, and straight and that disruptions are mere exceptions. If you view stressors as aberrant, you may respond to stress as though it was a sign of failure. Self-

blame only adds to feelings of distress and often contributes to the vicious cycle.

Most of us, however, acknowledge the inevitability of stress. But it is equally important not to view the sources, signs, and symptoms of accumulating stress as things you can do nothing about. Dismissing or ignoring stress-related feelings only defers coping, making it more likely that they will build and spread and have a serious impact on your physical and mental health.

Though we each have our own way of coping with life events, effective stress management generally involves a healthy perspective, a degree of self-awareness, and methods for assimilating and dissipating stress.

When we have confidence in our ability to deal with whatever comes our way, we tend to move through life with fewer stress-related complications. In addition, if we can meet life with humor, flexibility, imagination, and a sense of perspective, we are less likely to develop serious physical or emotional reactions to stress. In most cases, we should try to look at stressful situations as opportunities for personal growth.

The natural question is, of course, how do we turn difficult circumstances around?

The first thing we must accept is that, while there are many things we can change or control, there are also many things we can neither change nor control. Knowing the difference can sometimes be the hard part. Not uncommonly, discomfort arises not only from the reality of a particular stressful event or situation but also from the impression that we are powerless in the face of it. Discovering and exercising the many smaller ways you do have power can ease the burden of helplessness. And giving up attempting to control those situations we cannot control can be a tremendous relief. If, for example, you are experiencing marital difficulties as a result of failing intimacy or failing communication, and these difficulties cause home life to be increasingly stressful, you may not be able to change your spouse, but you most certainly can address the source of the stress. Seeking marital counseling or, if your spouse refuses, seeking individual counseling, can provide you with tools either to communicate more effectively or to channel sensibly the stress you are experiencing (see Communication Strategies for Couples, page 311).

Not everyone responds to the same circumstances with the same degree of comfort (or discomfort). Just knowing what makes you uncomfortable can lessen some of the weight. If you do not already know what makes you feel stressed, and what soothes and rallies you, give it some thought: When you feel yourself having a stress reaction to a particular situation or event, try to analyze what it is that stresses you. Too much stress can make any of us feel as though we are losing control or becoming demoralized. When you have a physical response, it can be comforting to realize that it is stress causing your anxiety or stomach problems.

Also, devise ways of dissipating tension that you cannot avoid. If, for example, your household gets hectic at the end of the day, organize things in a way that anticipates and circumvents the strain. If, for example, your spouse has a habit of getting the kids revved up just as you are trying to get them to go to bed, talk about better ways (for you and the kids) to approach bedtime.

When you do have a distinct stress reaction, resist the temptation to be harsh or critical with yourself. While you may expect to be able to sail smoothly through rough as well as calm waters, and to be in control of yourself regardless of circumstances, such expectations are unrealistic and put you at higher risk for serious and unanticipated stress reactions.

Try not to do things that will increase your tension needlessly. Do you find yourself most tense after a couple of cups of coffee? Cut out the coffee.

For some, feeling stressed out presents the reason to reach for a quick drink or two to help them relax. However, neither alcohol nor other recreational drugs will ease stress in the long run. Indeed, the use of alcohol and other drugs will tend to impair problem-solving capacities, prolonging feelings of stress. In most cases, alcohol and other drugs, particularly central nervous system depressants, intensify feelings of depression, hopelessness, loss of control, and impulsiveness, all of which add to the sense of being out of control, overwhelmed, and demoralized.

Each year, millions of prescriptions are written for tranquilizers such as diazepam (Valium) and chlordiazepoxide (Librium). While these can be valuable in certain circumstances, stress should not be looked at as a disease to be medicated. Medicating stress will likely only numb feelings and, in the long run, do nothing about the circumstances that are causing them. We all experience stress and we all need to learn how to manage it.

Rather than looking for quick fixes and easy solutions outside of yourself, when you begin to feel overloaded or burned out, try breaking the issues confronting you into manageable pieces. Use pen and paper to sort things out. Then work on one piece at a time and consider a variety of solutions.

Coping may entail setting more realistic goals and priorities and being more sensitive to and assertive about your needs. Above all, try slowing down the pace. If you are overcommitted, make fewer commitments. Make time for people, activities, and interests that you value. Join group or people-oriented activities, such as sports, social events, and community service. Find time for introspection, but also make time for friends—particularly those who have experienced the same sorts of things you are experiencing. If part or much of your stress is caused, for example, by a chronic disease such as diabetes, join a support group. If an impending or recent divorce is the cause of difficulties, find a recovery workshop.

For many, exercise, meditation, and relaxation techniques provide considerable relief. Very often, time and a little distance will dissipate enough pressure and immediacy to render even the largest problem manageable.

If you try all these and still feel burdened and out of control, consult a psychiatrist, psychologist, counselor, social worker, or clergyman.

Techniques for managing stress There is no one right way of dealing with stress. Take the time to understand what works for you and what does not. Finding the right balance in your life may be as simple as taking a long walk at the end of each day or as complex as changing jobs and moving out of your urban community. What works for one person or problem will offer no solution for another. As you evaluate your own responses to the stressors in your life, as well as the way you cope, consider the following ways of relaxing and reducing stress:

Exercise People who are physically fit tend to be better able to cope with stress, both physically and emotionally. In many ways, exercise can use the energy and arousal caused by stress reactions and helps dissipate them. Exercise spreads a sense of calm over the body that can last long after the workout is finished. Running and swimming, which require repetitive movement, can produce a mental state similar to that in meditation. Aerobic exercise that increases your heart rate for at least 20 minutes improves cardiovascular health and can decrease feelings of stress. Yoga and nonaerobic stretching exercises are calming and produce a meditation-like state.

Breathing and concentration exercises
Everyone can learn specific skills to lessen the discomfort and duration of stress-related symptoms. Breathing and concentration exercises offer an easy and convenient way of easing tension. You can do such exercises practically any time, any place, without special equipment or clothing.

Set aside 10 to 20 minutes when you won't be interrupted, and find a dark, quiet room. Lie in a comfortable position. Close your eyes and relax your jaw and the muscles around your eyes and mouth. Become aware of your breathing. Inhale and exhale slowly, regularly, and deeply through your nose.

Concentrate on individual parts of your body, checking for tension. Start with your toes and work up through your legs, back, arms, fingers, chest, neck, and scalp. As you focus on each spot, tighten the muscles. Hold for the count of five before moving on to the next area.

After you have moved with your mind through your body, releasing tension at each spot, continue to lie quietly. Resisting the impulse to drift back to your problems and responsibilities, let your mind wander. It may help to repeat a simple word or phrase, such as "one" or "let go," over and over again. Imagine a relaxing color or calm scene. Open your eyes, and lie quietly until you are ready to resume your activities.

Relaxed breathing Learning to breathe in a methodical way can ease tension and soothe discomfort. Many sufferers of chronic pain use breathing exercises to relieve pain and improve quality of life. This can work for stress, too. Sometimes, taking 10 deep, slow breaths can reduce feelings of panic. Usually, relaxed breathing involves using the diaphragm, the spherical muscle that separates the chest and abdomen. When you breathe from the diaphragm, you increase the amount of oxygen and carbon dioxide that are exchanged with each breath.

With relaxed diaphragmatic breathing, you move neither your shoulders up and down nor your chest in and out. Rather than forcefully drawing air in and blowing it out, you allow air to flow smoothly into and out of your lungs as your abdomen rises with each inhalation and falls with each exhalation.

You can teach yourself diaphragmatic breathing. First, notice how you breathe naturally. Lie on your back on a bed, on the floor, or perhaps in a recliner. Make sure your clothes are loose and comfortable. With your feet slightly apart, rest one hand on your stomach and the other on your chest. Draw air in through your nose, and blow it out through your mouth. Notice which hand rises and falls as you inhale and exhale. (If you have trouble breathing through your nose, inhale through your mouth as well.)

Inhale slowly, counting to five. Puff out your stomach slightly. Feel the air flowing in. Imagine air moving throughout your entire body. Pause, holding your breath to the count of five. Slowly exhale to the count of five. As the air flows out, imagine the tension being carried with it. Pause again to the count of five. Repeat the process until your breathing has a slow, even quality. This breathing helps move air throughout your lungs and engages your body in a regular, even rhythm.

Meditation A method of being with yourself, meditation encourages you to live in the moment, rather than living in the future or the past (for example, worrying). Instead of blocking stress, meditation works to put you directly in touch with the moment and your inner resources. As a result, you learn to let go of worry and preoccupation and gain perspective, and perhaps a bit of wisdom.

For many people, meditation begins as a way of relaxing or reducing stress, then with time becomes a way of achieving a deeper level of consciousness. Practically speaking, meditation slows down your breathing and heart rate, reduces oxygen consumption, eases muscle tension, and changes brain-wave patterns. Many people find that, because they meditate regularly, they are able to respond to stressful situations with greater calm and less panic.

There are many ways to meditate. In fact, you can meditate as you stand, walk, dance, jog, do housework, or garden. However, many people prefer to set aside a special time for meditation and to sit or kneel in a quiet environment. By repeating a word or sound over and over again and concentrating on your breathing, you may be able to bring on a sense of serenity.

You can practice meditation alone or with others in a common meditation place. You can learn meditation with the guidance of a book or tape, or you may want to work with a teacher.

Visualization For centuries, people have used consciously created images to soothe and heal. Today, visualization is used for everything from decreasing drug addiction to increasing athletic prowess. Visualizing certain scenes, symbols, or processes seems to relieve tension. In addition, it seems to have a direct effect on the body, acting on the involuntary systems, increasing blood flow to particular areas, and slowing down the heartbeat. Some people find that they can minimize or control pain with visual images.

When you use visualization, you sit or lie in a relaxing position and allow yourself to feel at one with the object, scene, or process you imagine. Allow the image to fill your consciousness until it becomes the only thing in your awareness. If, for example, you feel discomfort or pain, focus on the particular part of the body and imagine relief spreading out.

Most people learn to use visualization on their own, although it sometimes helps to have a guide.

Massage and body work The systematic use of touch has been used for centuries as a way of fostering comfort and calm. When done effectively, massage relaxes the body, increases circulation, releases muscle tension, improves joint flexibility, and improves sensation. Mostly, it enhances a sense of calm.

Massage and manipulative techniques include prolonged and intense touching, pulling, pressing, and rubbing. Sometimes, having a friend knead and stroke your shoulders, feet, hands, neck, and back are all you need to relieve stress and help you feel more relaxed. At other times, you may want to work with a trained massage therapist.

A commonly used method is Swedish massage, which generally applies deep pressure and works the whole body. Other techniques involve applying pressure to energy points within the body or working with muscle trigger points. Some methods emphasize realigning the body to a normal posture. Most practitioners combine aspects of several methods.

Many massage therapists receive their training at nationally accredited schools. Some are certified by professional associations.

Building Lasting Relationships

Adulthood can feel like a juggling act because of the many balls we must keep simultaneously in the air. In early adulthood, we develop careers even as we try to forge meaningful and lasting relationships. In middle and late adulthood, our careers may be even more demanding, yet we have to handle the needs of our families—spouses, children, and often parents and siblings.

COUPLES COUNSELING BEFORE AND DURING MARRIAGE

Marriage is universal. In every human society on the planet, marriage exists as a fundamental institution. In the United States, about half of marriages end in divorce. Most divorced people will marry again, and their subsequent marriages are even more likely to fail than their first. Most marry with every intention to stay with their spouse for life. And yet something happens along the road. Communication breaks down. People grow apart. Having children fundamentally changes a relationship. A couple who were once the best of friends may become mortal enemies.

Alarmed at persistently high divorce rates, some churches have begun to require that those who get married in their congregations complete a course of prenuptial counseling. Most churches, however, do

COMMUNICATION STRATEGIES FOR COUPLES

Us Time Couples should set aside time every day for both partners to communicate. At least 20 minutes per day should be set aside for couples to talk as lovers and partners, not necessarily as parents. More time would be better, but everyone can afford at least 20 minutes. Communication should be allowed to flow naturally, whether it is about work, children, or finances, but it should include hopes and dreams and goals as well. A short walk every evening can provide an excellent opportunity for conversation.

Self Time Each partner should set aside approximately 15 or 20 minutes a day to be alone and quiet. This time can be spent in meditation, prayer, or in simple, relaxed silence, and it should be programmed into every day's schedule. Stress reduction exercises can be employed, such as deep breathing or meditation. You may find that even a small amount of time spent alone will enable you to communicate more clearly with your partner.

Goal Setting Every contractual obligation has some sort of goal—except many marriages. Couples should, together or with the help of a counselor, analyze their goals as a family unit. These can even be written up in a mission statement for the family. Children can be involved, but the backbone of it has to be the parents' invention. Goals can be spiritual (often these are the best, longest lasting goals), which can include family community service, religious involvement, or educational involvement—such as studying something of mutual interest, parents and children together.

Communication Exercises Many couples argue about the same things over and over again; eventually, both partners stop listening. Communication exercises, which a couples therapist can assist you with, help you analyze what you are saying, why, and how it can be expressed more clearly and with more of an understanding of how it will be heard by your partner. Here are some helpful strategies for better communication:

- *Avoid blanket generalizations.* Couples often speak in broad generalizations: "You never take out the garbage." "You're always nagging." With such statements, there is no room left for discussion. Better communication is more specific. "Last week you didn't take out the garbage. I had to do it when I was exhausted, and that left me feeling angry with you."

- *Use "I" statements.* If you can speak in statements that are about yourself and your feelings rather than being accusatory, conversation can flow more smoothly.

- *Mirroring.* This exercise helps couples analyze what each is saying and how the other is hearing what is being said. The speaker makes a statement; the listener then repeats what the speaker said. Many speakers are astounded by what the listener repeats: What the listener understood of the statement is often very different from what the speaker intended.

- *Leaving it and coming back.* Sometimes in the heat of an argument, couples will say things that they not only do not mean but also regret as soon as they are said. While it can be difficult to walk away when something is not resolved, it can also be tremendously helpful to say, "I don't think we're getting anywhere," walk away, and return to the discussion when tempers have cooled. ■

not. And most of those who marry are not counseled. Yet many of those who enter couples therapy when their relationship founders wonder why they did not do so at the outset of their marriage when difficulties in communication could have been resolved more easily and problems might have been averted. Prenuptial counseling, whether it takes place with clergy or with a clinical therapist, has been shown to reduce the rate of divorce significantly.

Prenuptial and marital counseling aim to provide participants with a much better understanding of the backgrounds of each partner and with insight into the patterns that already exist in their lives and into how those patterns might interact as their relationship endures. Couples also learn which issues are most important for them to work on: communication, sexual expression, finances, sense of independence and selfhood, and family relations, all of which will relate to the stages of life.

By looking at themselves objectively, people can gain insight not only into their partner's needs, strengths, and weaknesses, but equally importantly, into their own needs, strengths, and weaknesses. With a strong commitment to the relationship, both partners can use this information as time goes on to avert or reduce their conflicts and crises.

Another of the central goals of prenuptial or marital counseling is to foster communication, perhaps the single most important aspect of any relationship. Men and women think differently, individuals think differently, and people living through the same events can easily see them from astonishingly different perspectives. If the partners recognize the failure of communication and try to facilitate better communication, they can work to remedy problems before they become irreconcilable differences. Marital counseling and what might be called marital refresher courses can help couples significantly reduce their risk of divorce, increase the quality of their lives together, and foster the growth and physical and spiritual health of children.

PREPARING TO PARENT

While parenthood still takes some people by surprise, for most adults today, parenthood is a decision made with deliberation and care. Conscientious parents want to give their children as much of a head start as possible, and therefore they stop smoking, stop using alcohol or other drugs, and try to exercise regularly before becoming pregnant. Most of this effort is centered on the woman; she will after all be bearing and giving birth to the baby. But research suggests that men who are in good physical health improve the odds of their children being in good physical health (for more information, see Chapter 7).

Equally important, couples need to prepare for the many ways becoming parents will change their life together. Both parents live through what is nominally the same experience, but its effects and consequences are profoundly different for each. A new mother may feel isolated and harried. A

new father may feel that his spouse has concentrated all her affection and energy on the baby. The dynamic of the family changes overnight, and both parents can become too tired and upset to work things out. Some couples cease communicating completely, sometimes out of frustration because one person's point of view is so at odds with the other's. It is important to take the time now to find a compromise between differing expectations. Talk about ways you can help one another cope with the changes the baby's arrival has brought about.

Although many of the potential difficulties of childbearing and child rearing can be overcome through sensible communication by the partners, guidance from a trained counselor or from an elder role model from the community (or family) can be invaluable in helping not only to referee but also to provide insight into one another that couples might not derive on their own. Many churches and temples have begun family enrichment programs, designed to bring couples closer together and strengthen family bonds. Often free or offered at nominal cost, these can be a valuable alternative to those who may not be able to afford regular professional therapy.

SLEEP AND YOUR HEALTH

Of all the small steps we can take to ensure good health, getting sufficient sleep may be the easiest one, but the most often overlooked. As adults age, it is agreed that most need fewer hours of sleep, going from approximately 9½ hours during the adolescent years to around 6 in the senior years. Although everyone's sleep needs vary, most adults need approximately 8 hours of sleep a night. Few actually get it. Some people seem to be just fine with fewer hours; others seem to need 9 or 10 to feel truly rested.

Napping rarely makes up for the lack of sleep, even if the total hours slept adds up to 8. Researchers agree that we need to reach the phase of sleep known as rapid eye movement (REM) sleep and stay there for a time. It takes a few hours of sleep to fall deeply enough asleep to reach REM. Waking in the middle of REM and then going back to sleep hours later does not resume that deep sleep. Rarely is a nap of sufficient duration to allow REM sleep.

Research has shown that lack of sleep can result in a weakening of the immune system, poor concentration at work or school, and increased irritability, and it can have potentially dangerous consequences if you operate hazardous machinery, drive distances, or work in circumstances that require a high degree of vigilance for safety.

Consult your doctor if you notice an inexplicable change in your sleeping patterns, or if you suffer from regular insomnia. This may be a signal of a significant medical condition. ■

COPING WITH DIVORCE

Even if a divorce is desired by both partners, it can be one of the most stressful events adults can endure. Indeed, many have likened divorce to the death of a loved one—in this case, the death of more than a relationship, but a way of life, a social structure, and a host of goals and expectations. Even those who are desperate for their freedom go through a grieving process that can last for years.

For many children, a divorce, particularly an acrimonious one, can be a lifelong burden and source of guilt (see Minimizing the Impact of Divorce on Children, page 314). Lingering resentment between ex-spouses can cause even the best-intentioned parents to push their children to take sides. Some studies show that, perhaps as a consequence of this stress, children of divorce have a statistically higher incidence of problem behavior, including delinquency and alcohol and other drug abuse. These studies, however, did not take into account parental psychopathology and substance abuse.

COPING WITH INFERTILITY

Many people who would have been unable to have a child 25 years ago can now have children due to advances in fertility medicine. Unfortunately, undergoing treatment for infertility can be extraordinarily stressful—physically, emotionally, and financially. The quest for a child can consume the life of a couple; some couples are brought together in deeply spiritual ways; others are torn apart.

If you and/or your partner have been diagnosed as infertile, carefully consider all the options available to you in terms of infertility treatment as well as adoption before making a decision. There are self-help groups across the country that can provide essential information and invaluable support.

- American Society for Reproductive Medicine (ASRM)
  Phone: (205) 978–5000

- Childfree Network
  7777 Sunrise Blvd., #1800
  Citrus Heights, CA 95610

- Childless by Choice
  Box 695
  Leavenworth, WA 98826

- Donors Offspring
  Box 33
  Sarcoxie, MO 64862

- Endometriosis Association (USA)
  Phone: (800) 992–3636

- INCIID (International Council on Infertility Information Dissemination)
  Box 91363
  Tucson, AZ 85752–1363
  Phone: (520) 544–9548
  Fax: (520) 509–5251
  e-mail: INCIIDinfo@aol.com
  Web site: www.inciid.org
  President: Linda F. Davey. Support and educational group for the infertile. Annual conference. Newsletter *INCIID Insights.*

- Infertility Focus
  Box 92481
  Rochester, NY 14692
  Paula LaManna, Phone: (716) 385–1628
  Support group. Newsletter *Focal Point.*

- Options National Fertility Registry
  Phone: (800) 786–1786, Monday to Friday 9 to 4 PST
  Egg donor: (800) 886–9373
  A registry/business for donors/patients.

- Organization of Parents Through Surrogacy
  7054 Quito Court
  Camarillo, CA 93012|
  Phone: (805) 482–1566
  Surrogacy referrals and support.

- Resolve National
  1310 Broadway
  Somerville, MA 02144–1731
  Phone: (617) 623–0744
  Fax: (617) 623–0252
  Newsletter, fact sheets, help line, referral services, conferences.

- Resolve of Northern California
  312 Sutter St., Suite 607
  San Francisco, CA 94108
  Phone: (415) 788–6772

- Resolve of Western New York
  5330 Main St., #130
  Williamsville, NY 14221–5380
  Phone: (716) 634–3700
  Newsletter, support groups, help line, seminars.

- Serono Symposia, USA (a division of Serono Labs)
  100 Longwater Circle
  Norwell, MA 02061
  Phone: (800) 283–8088

- Surviving Infertility
  e-mail: jfowler@cris.com (Jim Fowler)
  Web site: www.concentric.net/~jfowler/si/si.shtml
  Infertility support group.

- The American Surrogacy Center (TASC)
  e-mail: joanb@surrogacy.com (Joan Barnes)
  Web site: www.surrogacy.com
  Site for surrogacy; monthly e-mail newsletter, TASCFORCE, available free at the Web site. Also at the Web site, TASC Classifieds: Online advertising for surrogacy, at www.surrogacy.com/classifieds/index.html ■

There are several concrete steps you can take to minimize or ameliorate the inevitable sense of anger, despair, and loneliness you will feel after your divorce. Taking constructive steps to reshape your life may also help your children channel their emotions and rebuild.

- **Accept your responsibility.** As hard a concept as it is for most divorcing people to comprehend, with the exception of those cases of physical or sexual abuse, each of the marital partners is partly responsible for the dissolution of the marriage. Accepting this responsibility is one of the hardest parts of divorce but one of the most fundamental to recovery from the fallout of divorce.

- **Rely on your friends and family.** Indeed, you may discover, going through

MINIMIZING THE IMPACT OF DIVORCE ON CHILDREN

Divorce is an earthquake that shakes children's lives at the core. Though this is a time when you too are under great stress, it is essential to do all you can to address your children's needs. You can provide your children with reassurance and stability in this time of crisis:

- Maintain routines. Children need to have a predictable schedule—predictable meals, predictable homework, bed, and bath times.

- Do not involve your child in discussions about your former spouse. Save conversations about your grief or bitterness until after the children have gone to school or to bed.

- Speak of your former spouse in as positive or neutral a manner as possible. Do not enumerate the other parent's shortcomings or betrayals in front of the children.

- Do not force older children into a parental role.

- Do not force your children to take sides. No matter how wronged you may feel, it will only hurt them.

- Assure your children it is not their fault. Children, particularly younger ones, tend to believe that they are at the center of nearly everything.

- Make sure that your children know you put them first. When and if you begin dating again, make certain that your children know you love them and hold their interests in the highest regard, but also make sure they know that they will not be allowed to dictate your relationships. When you do bring a new person into the children's lives, do so slowly.

- Seek the help of a family counselor if you see signs of distress in your child: frequent illness, failure to maintain friendships, poor performance in school. ■

divorce, who your real friends are. As with any grieving process, many people, particularly those who have not experienced this kind of grief, expect those going through it to just get on with life. But adjusting emotionally can and will take time, and you should let it.

- Use community support resources. Do not allow yourself to become isolated. Many people turn away from their place of worship in shame or guilt at the time when they need it most. Many churches and temples have divorce workshops and self-help recovery programs.

- Establish a support network of people who share your concerns. Getting out and networking may feel like the last thing you want to do, but it is an important step in the recovery process. Find others who have been through what you are going through and talk and listen to them. Divorce workshops, mothers' and fathers' rights organizations, and other self-help programs can offer a community of people.

- Do not resort to alcohol or illegal drug use to assuage your feelings of loss.

- Get involved with volunteer activities. Helping others is often the best way to help yourself.

- When the children are with your former spouse, take time to do things for yourself. Do not define yourself solely as a single parent.

- If you cannot channel your emotions into anything but continued grief, see a counselor (psychiatrist, psychologist, or social worker) who specializes in grief therapy. If you cannot afford counseling, many states sponsor mental health services at little or no cost. Many therapists will waive or reduce fees for those who cannot afford them. If you are so inclined, talk to a member of the clergy, who are often trained as counselors.

Violence and Abuse

Although family violence has been in the news for many years, much family violence goes unreported for many reasons, particularly because victims fear retribution from the perpetrator and believe, despite evidence to the contrary, that the abuse will not happen again and that they are responsible for the abuse. Women are the object of two-thirds of family violence, with husbands or boyfriends typically the abusers. Other abuse affects the elderly, children, and those who are crippled or physically handicapped. A woman is six times more likely to be the victim of violence at the hands of someone she knows than at those of a stranger.

Throughout the country, resources are available to women and children in abusive relationships. Most communities have shelters where women can go to escape abusive relationships. For reasons of guilt, shame, or even upbringing, many people do not even know they are being abused. How can you tell if your relationship is abusive? If your partner/spouse has ever done any of the following, your relationship may be abusive:

- Hit, kicked, choked, slapped, or pushed you

- Bitten or burned you

- Threatened you with a weapon (gun, knife, belt, bat)

- Squeezed you so hard that it left a bruise

- Threatened you with physical violence or death

- Threatened your children with physical violence or death

- Threatened your friends

- Humiliated you in front of friends, family, or significant others

- Punished you by keeping necessities, such as food, medications, money, or transportation from you

- Humiliated or shamed you privately to exert power over you

- Forced you to have sex or perform sexual acts against your will

- Ruined your personal possessions

If this kind of behavior is characteristic of your spouse, you should seek help immediately. There are hotlines you can call in every state, and a national hotline, for referral or protection.

- National Domestic Violence Hotline: (800) 799-SAFE (7233)

- National Resource Center on Domestic Violence: (800) 537-2238 (will provide a listing of domestic violence coalitions nationwide)

- The Department of Justice Information Center: (800) 421-6770 (will provide a copy of The Violence Against Women Act, which was signed into law by President Clinton on September 13, 1994)

RAPE

Anyone can be raped, but women, girls, and boys are most likely to be raped, or forced to have sexual intercourse. Indeed, one study showed that one in four college-age women were subjected to unwanted sexual contact, while one in ten admitted being forced to have sexual intercourse. Most rape, however, goes unreported. Whether it is from shame, a sense of guilt or responsibility for the attack, or threats from the attacker, only a very small percentage of rapes are reported; fewer still are prosecuted.

Although most rape victims are female and most rapists are male, boys are also raped—by both men and women.

What should you do if you are raped?
Although your first reaction may be just to keep it a secret and not tell anyone, doing nothing is something you may later come to regret. It will not help you and will not help others who might be raped by the same person. The same person may rape you again.

- *Don't bathe.* This may be the first thing you want to do, but do not. The sooner you report the assault and are examined, the better the evidence—and the chances of obtaining a conviction—will be. You may also decide later whether or not you wish to prosecute.

- *Don't blame yourself.* Many people feel a sense of guilt at being raped, as well as fearfulness. Rape is *not* your fault.

- *Tell someone you trust.* Tell your sister or your mother, your best friend, or a rape hotline, and report the rape as soon as possible.

- *Retain all evidence.* Do not wash clothing, but keep everything that you were wearing, particularly underwear, as it was. This may be important evidence that will help police catch and put in jail the person who assaulted you.

- *Get examined.* Hospital emergency rooms are equipped to examine people who have been raped, and you should be examined as soon as possible after the assault in order to collect evidence. Some hospitals now have special rape counselors to perform much of the examination and interview. These are usually nurses who have been specially trained to assist rape victims.

- *Consider the "morning-after" pill.* If you are concerned that you may get pregnant, do not wait to find out if your next period will come. Within 72 hours of contact, but preferably as soon as possible, a brief regimen can be started. Usually two Ovral pills (a combination of ethinyl estradiol and levonorgestrel) are taken within 72 hours of the rape and then 12 hours later another two Ovral pills are taken. This hormonal treatment is designed to interrupt conception and head off a pregnancy before it happens (see Contraception, page 1161).

- *Get tested.* Speak with your doctor about the sexually transmitted diseases you may have been put at risk for. If you are bruised or otherwise injured, see your doctor for treatment.

- *Get assistance.* It is common for victims of rape not to want to be alone for several days after the incident. Someone close to you—a best friend, sister, mother—should try to look after you in the days following the incident. If the assault leaves you feeling especially depressed or even suicidal, seek counseling as fast as possible. It is important to talk to people. Many people who work in rape crisis centers are women who have been through the trauma of rape themselves and can be of invaluable assistance in getting you started on the road to recovery—as well as helping you, if you decide to prosecute, get prepared to attend court and testify.

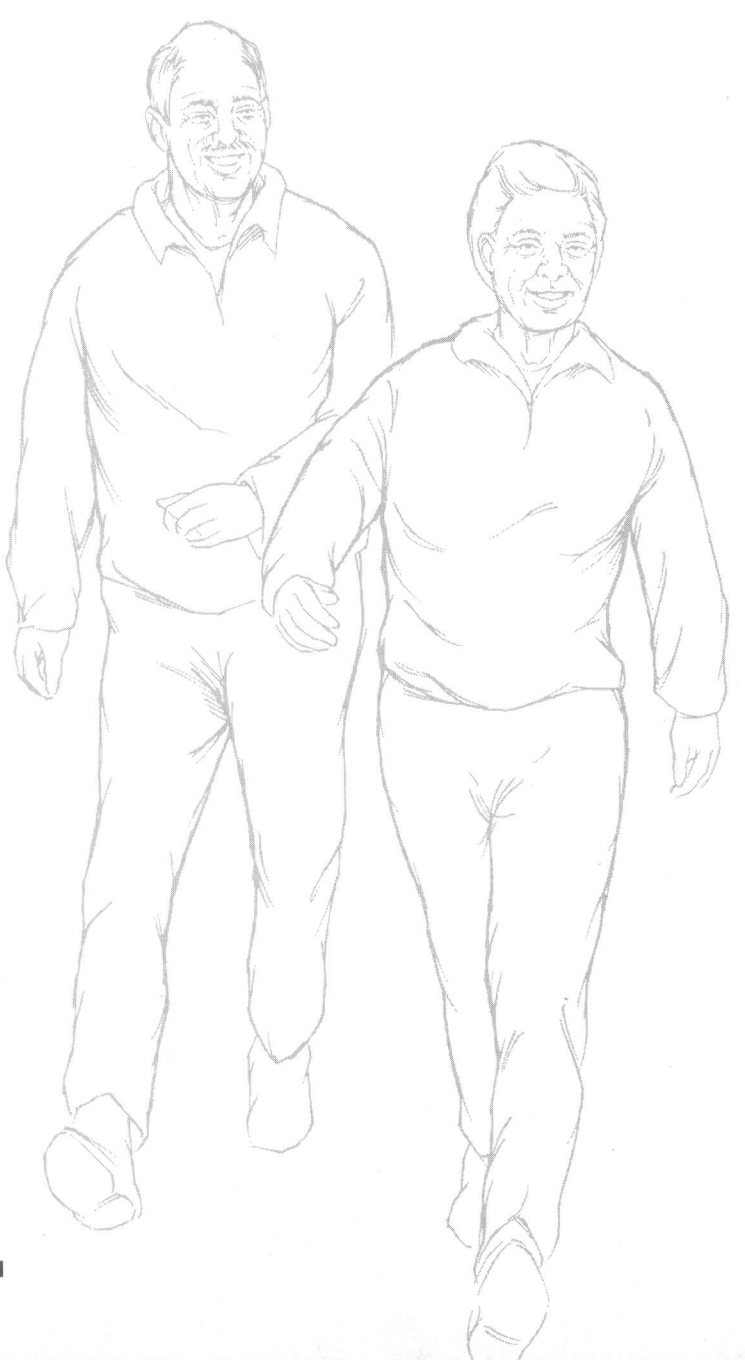

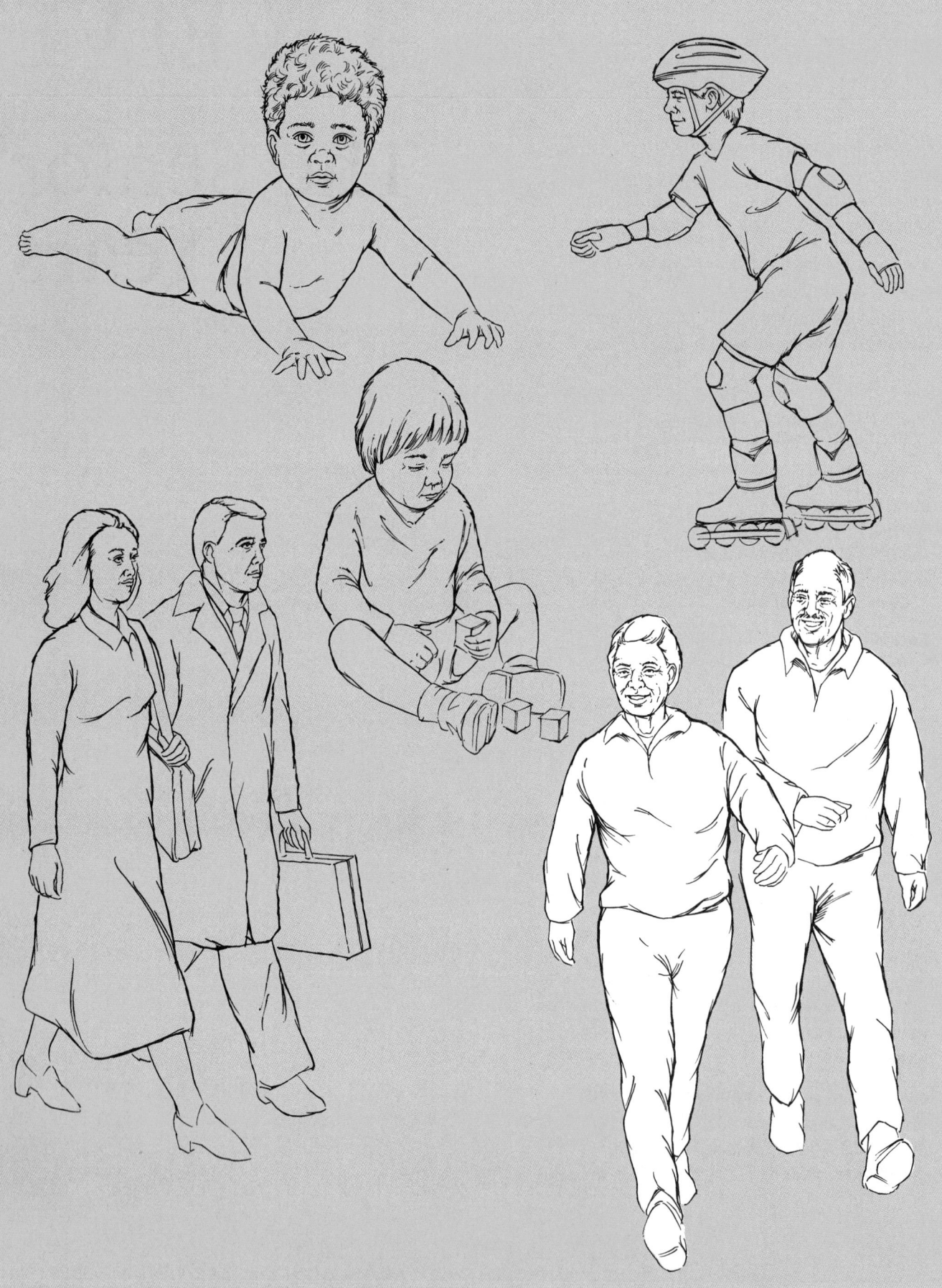

THE SENIOR YEARS

Living Longer, Living Better

The average life expectancy of Americans has soared since the turn of the century from about 47 years in 1900 to about 75 years today. Indeed, for those who live to age 55, life expectancy increases to 85. In many respects, what we think of when we think of "old" people has radically changed over the last several decades. There are triathletes in their 60s, marathon runners in their 80s, and authors on book tours who are more than 100 years old. Still, the fountain of youth has proven elusive, and most researchers believe that there is a fixed upper limit to human life, a point at which the body simply wears out. Depending on genetics, the environmental insults your body has been exposed to, and in many cases just plain luck, the upper limit is believed to range from age 95 to the possible-but-unlikely 110.

Increasing numbers of Americans are living closer and closer to that fixed upper limit, and, more importantly, many are living into ripe old age with a much higher quality of life than was ever possible. Deaths of infants, children, teenagers, and young and middle adults used to be common; now, such premature death is outside the norm in our country. The "graying of America" has been made possible by enormous leaps in the standard of living and quality of health care, which have reduced infant mortality, maternal mortality, and deaths from polio, pertussis, and streptococcal infections. Our health care focus has shifted to chronic and other diseases of the later years: coronary heart disease, atherosclerosis (hardening of the arteries), cancer, and diabetes, to name a few. The good news is that we are living longer, and these chronic diseases are often preventable, treatable, or curable. While a human body may survive only just so long, it would appear to be able to do so in quite healthy fashion almost until the day it quits.

People in their 70s, 80s, and 90s—and even older in some cases—are charting territory that has largely remained unexplored for most of human history, and they are changing our notions of what it means to be "old." When the Social Security Administration was founded during the New Deal years of the 1930s, 65 was set as the age at which Americans could begin to collect retirement benefits. This was at least in part because few Americans lived that long. These days, most Americans stand a very good chance of surviving well into their 80s and even beyond. Indeed, over 13 percent of the population of this country is 65 or over, and as the baby boom generation ages, that number will only grow.

Although illness and infirmity are often thought of as the inevitable results of aging, one does not have to follow the other. Just as many ravaging diseases of childhood can be minimized and prevented by immunization and antibiotics, many of the ravaging diseases of the senior years can be minimized, postponed, or prevented. Should disabilities or chronic disease occur, a variety of treatments and adaptive disciplines can be taught to minimize the effects. Research shows that in many cases those who have good luck and good genes can, through exercise, balanced diet, and good health care, live a high quality of life until their bodies wear out.

Researchers today see what we commonly think of as the senior years as really three distinct periods: young-old, middle-old, and old-old age. None is determined so much by chronologic age as it is by ability.

THE YOUNG-OLD

Young-old age, an arbitrarily determined number of years that spans from approximately age 65 to 74, may often be little more than an extension of adulthood. It is a time when, for many, we are at the peaks of our social and professional lives and not ready for retirement, despite chronologic age. It is a time when many of us, because of grown children and diminished family and professional responsibility, have the opportunity to rediscover things that we may have allowed to slip by the wayside during the busy years—travel and hobbies, recreation and exercise, volunteering and community service. Statistics show that most of us who are 65 and over consider ourselves to be healthy, and the majority of us actually are.

Generally speaking, those age 65 and over are better off financially than those of a similar age in any previous generation; many, with paid-off mortgages, good pensions, and health plans, including Medicare, are better off than their young-adult peers.

During young-old age, and in the absence of disease, we are still essentially capable of almost everything we have always been capable of. If, for example, you walked 15 miles every day at age 50, there is little reason you should not be able to do so at 70. The same is true of most mental tasks. But with age does come some slowing down. In the absence of disease or disability, slowing down should be gradual. In some respects, slowing down may be more a state of mind influenced by our own and society's expectations. In other respects, the slowing down may be the result of a chronic medical condition, such as hypertension (high blood pressure). In many areas, most of us may be capable of much more than we were as younger adults, given the potential for increased financial comfort, our constant growth of knowledge and wisdom, and the seemingly endless capacity of our minds to learn.

THE MIDDLE-OLD

Middle-old age includes the years from 75 to 84. This period can be seen as an extension of young-old age, but with slowing down becoming more apparent. While many in this age group will remain quite healthy during this period, statistics show that many will experience some sort of chronic illness or medical condition. These may range from the serious, such as heart disease or diabetes, to the relatively mild, such as some hearing loss (see page 344) or some diminishing of vision (see page 342).

This period is, like the others, more accurately defined by fitness than it is by age. Someone who is 65 but has had long-standing, untreated hypertension may have a stroke or myocardial infarction (heart attack) and rapidly become old-old, while someone else who is 80 may participate in volunteer activities, walk or run several miles a day, and keep "young" through other means. Still, as we age, our likelihood of having a chronic illness increases. It is therefore important to understand the changes that can occur as we age and to consult a doctor promptly if changes that seem out of the ordinary do occur.

THE OLD-OLD

Even people who become old-old (older than age 85) are often able to function well and fully independently. Nearly all the disabilities and loss of function we commonly associate with age are really related to illness, some of which may be readily prevented. It is possible that some of us may never, into our 90th or even 100th year, experience the loss of function that characterizes old-old age. Indeed, 90-year-old marathoners and other mature athletes are well known. This phenomenon is known as successful aging—health and vitality until the upper limit of one's life span. In fact, to what extent disability will affect each of us is determined by a wide array of factors: Heredity will play a significant part, but so will overall fitness, diet, and lifestyle (see Understanding the Aging Process, page 326). A significant percentage of seniors experiences one or more chronic illnesses. But even having a chronic illness, depending upon its severity, does not mean a senior should give up.

The old-old phase of life begins approximately in the middle 80s—but could, in reality, happen during any time in the senior years—when the individual begins to experience loss of function. For some, it may begin much earlier, for others, later. The onset of frailty and disability common in those in the old-old age group is related largely to the accumulation of diseases and to self-imposed or disease-related deconditioning.

Old-old age is characterized by the gradually increasing loss of certain physiologic functions, which in turn predisposes an individual toward serious complications, such as a case of pneumonia or a fall. Such insults in an old-old individual can greatly increase the possibility of loss of mobility and loss of independence—perhaps the most worrisome possibilities of aging.

Staying Fit in the Senior Years

If there is a fountain of youth, it exists within us. Research has proven that exercise, sensible diet with adequate dietary vitamins and minerals (see Chapter 1), and regular health care can significantly improve your overall health. Working to stay physically and mentally fit can lengthen your vitality and put off or lessen disability and illness. If you are over age 65 and lead an essentially sedentary lifestyle by choice or are over- or underweight, you may have the opportunity to transform your later years and improve your risk factors by starting a program of fitness today. The sections that follow describe aspects of lifestyle that can play a significant role in helping you live longer and better.

STAYING PHYSICALLY ACTIVE

Few 65-year-olds have the raw athletic ability of the best 20-year-old athletes, but the gradual loss of physical edge that can take place as we age is a matter of degree. We do not lose ability as much as we lose the extremes of ability. Jack Nicklaus or Arnold Palmer going tee-to-tee with Tiger Woods would probably lose. Both of them, however, can still leave most 20-year-old golfers in the sand trap. They have not lost the ability. And they have not lost the ability to stay in shape.

There is little reason why anyone in the young-old category should be less active or capable than younger adults (see The Effects of Time on Bodily Systems, page 327). In the absence of chronic disease, nothing in the way the body ages prevents vigorous exercise, and degrees of vigor can be adapted to differing levels of strength.

The difference between the physical activity level of adolescents and that of seniors is due in part to lifestyle. Most of us, as adolescents and young adults, have much more leisure time than we do in adulthood and middle adulthood, as family and professional responsibilities take over. Taking care of ourselves often takes a back seat to taking care of others and taking care of business. The reality is, of course, that we can better take care of others if we take better care of ourselves.

For many older Americans, the loss of the ability to compete or the loss of a certain amount of function may not be of great concern. But the loss of independence—the ability to live on our own, to drive, to get out and do what we want to do—is of paramount concern. This loss can easily result from the progressive deterioration popularly known as "use it or lose it." The corollary to use it or lose it, researchers have discovered, is use it and gain—and this principle applies even late in life.

Physical activity need not be overly strenuous to achieve health benefits. Only 30 minutes a day of brisk walking has been shown to make a considerable difference. This is a goal almost anyone can achieve. Research shows, however, that health benefits increase as the duration, frequency, and strenuousness of exercise increase. At the same time, the risk of injury, particularly to people who are new to exercise, increases as you increase your level of activity, so you should exercise caution as you exercise.

If you have maintained good physical fitness all your life, you have lowered the risk that your senior years will be a time of disability and disease. People who exercise regularly and strenuously have lower levels of low-density lipoprotein (LDL), the "bad" cholesterol, and higher levels of high-density lipoprotein (HDL), the "good" cholesterol, and have a lower risk of atherosclerosis and its attendant complications, such as heart disease. If you can exercise strenuously, within a program supervised and approved by your doctor, you will find that the time you spend is like money in the bank, paying off long-term dividends of good health, increased energy levels, stronger bones, and improved ability to heal and recover from injury or sickness.

For the physically fit, there is little reason why you cannot go on participating in conventional sports activities, such as running, aerobics, tennis, or golf, well into the last stages of life. But what do you do if arthritis, back pain, an injury, or other circumstances prevent you from engaging in these sorts of activities? Must you give up?

The answer is emphatically no. You can do any number of activities that can work around your condition. Indeed, research shows that exercise can help reduce pain. The so-called runner's high is an example of how the body rewards itself by releasing its own natural opiates, endorphins, as we exercise. But you do not need to run to get runner's high. Gardening or walking can offer the same benefits. Physical activity has also been shown to improve the quality of sleep, reduce stress, and alleviate depression.

A recent Stanford University survey of a group of essentially sedentary older adults whose age averaged 70 found that a combination of vigorous physical activity—brisk walking, resistance (weight) training, and low impact aerobics—and more gentle flexibility exercises could increase the ability of the participants to walk farther, lift heavier objects, and improve their overall cardiovascular fitness. The gentler exercise helped them feel more relaxed, comfortable, and flexible.

Increased physical activity has also been shown to boost self-esteem and ward off disease. Other studies have shown that those who regularly exercise vigorously have a lower incidence of breast and other cancers and an improved ability to fight infectious illness by improving overall immune function.

If you cannot tolerate the impact of running or aerobics, one of the most popular options is swimming. Water aerobics also exercises your body aerobically, increasing your cardiovascular fitness, but because it is done in the water, it minimizes impact and helps relieve pain.

If you enjoy walking, but the climate in your area is not suitable for being outdoors many months of the year, local shopping centers often offer seniors special incentives to come walk their malls. It is good for business as well as security to have seniors walking past their stores. Some malls have walking clubs that send out regular newsletters and offer such perks as free periodic blood pressure screening and maps of the mall with mileage measures.

Tai chi chuan, the ancient Chinese art and a gentle stretching exercise, combines meditation with elements of dance and movement in a very low impact routine. It can be an effective way of exercising both mentally and physically. This is something you can do at home, but exercise classes outside the home can have the added benefit of creating new friendships and associations, giving you incentive to get out more and go back to class.

There are also many exercises that are specific to individual difficulties. If you have a chronic condition, talk to your doctor about what kind of exercise is appropriate for you. People with emphysema, diabetes, and other chronic conditions often can still exercise—and improve their condition. Many hospitals have rehabilitation programs you can attend that will supervise and instruct your exercise activity, keep watch on your vital signs, and make sure that you are getting all the exertion you are capable of without overdoing it. Talk to your doctor about goals for fitness that can be tailored to your health, your abilities, and your needs.

There is no excuse. You have everything to gain if you do, and everything to lose if you do not. Research also shows that the sooner you start, the sooner you will feel results, and the better off you will be. See Chapter 2 for more information on the benefits of activity and how to get started safely.

KEEPING MENTALLY FIT

Mental exercise is as important as physical exercise in keeping us healthy and whole as the years go by.

Mental fitness involves two main areas: intellectual capacity, or the ability to learn and keep learning, and emotional capacity, or the ability to keep up with the world and with people.

Over the last couple of decades, many seniors, not content just to sit out the golden years, have gone back to school, earning master's and doctoral degrees. Others have participated in elder hostel programs, taking a week or more during the summer at a university, living on campus, and learning everything from plotting family history to music appreciation to higher math. This sort of mental exercise is not just a pastime, but a good way to keep and hone mental acuity. Indeed, pursuing one's interests, no matter what they are, should be one of the gifts of the golden years.

Maintaining emotional fitness is also crucial. Studies show that people who are socially and emotionally isolated live a shorter life with poorer quality than people who are active in their community, their church, and other social organizations. People who socialize well, who understand the delicate art of asking for help and providing help, are those who tend to survive longest. Many, upon retirement, find themselves missing their jobs not so much for the work they did but for the social structure the job provided. But that sort of structure does not have to fall by the wayside upon retirement. Part-time or consulting jobs in your field can keep you up-to-date. Volunteer jobs with your church, temple, or mosque or with local schools or hospitals can keep you active and involved. And they give you the chance to share your knowledge and experience with children and other adults, to mutual benefit as well as pleasure.

Find out about different possibilities through your local volunteer agencies, through your place of worship, or in the local papers.

AVOIDING UNDERNUTRITION

Although obesity can result when seniors are sedentary and take in excess calories, undernutrition is often a more significant problem. Many factors can lead to this.

As we age, our digestive systems produce lower levels of saliva and gastric juices, which are full of the enzymes that break down food into the nutrients our bodies need. Additionally, the muscles of the digestive tract can lose some of their tone. This can result in less thorough digestion as well as constipation. Seniors have been shown to chew their food less thoroughly than younger people, and if poor dental hygiene and tooth loss are present, which make the thorough chewing of food difficult, you will have more difficulty breaking down your food into the nutrients you need. Even those whose missing teeth are replaced by dentures often lose some of their ability to chew thoroughly. If eating becomes unpleasant or painful because of bad teeth, see your dentist to learn what can be done to improve the situation (see Dental Care for Seniors, page 324).

Changes in the capacity of the vital organs, changes in the production of various enzymes and hormones, and changes in the fat/water ratio that take place in the aging body can all result in the inadequate or even excess metabolization of certain vitamins and minerals (see Vitamin Supplements and Dietary Supplement Drinks, page 325). You may get adequate calories, but you may not get the right vitamins and minerals. If, for example, you are no longer out in the sun at all, you may not get adequate vitamin D, which the skin metabolizes from sunlight.

Risk of vitamin and mineral deficiencies vary from person to person. You may be more susceptible if you take medications, which can deplete particular vitamins and minerals faster or slower, or affect your appetite. When your doctor prescribes medication, inquire how or if it can affect your diet or appetite at the same time you inquire about possible drug interactions.

CONSTIPATION

Constipation is the slowing of bowel motility (the movement of fecal matter through the large intestine) to the point that it is difficult to pass the stool that has accumulated in the colon. Some people find that they have difficulty having a bowel movement at all; others find that when they do move their bowels, they do not have the sense of relief that should normally accompany a satisfactory bowel movement.

Constipation that occurs suddenly and remains chronic or is accompanied by bleeding should always be evaluated by your doctor to rule out the presence of a blockage, polyps, or bowel cancer. This may include the examination by endoscopy of your rectum and the lower portion of your colon (sigmoid colon) to evaluate their condition. See Chapter 23.

Most constipation in seniors is caused by loss of muscle tone in the rectum and colon, which is where stool is formed. Adding to this difficulty is that seniors no longer are able to retain water as well as they once were, and moisture is essential for bowel motility.

Constipation should not be ignored, because the situation can worsen. One of the primary jobs of the colon is to remove moisture from fecal matter, so the longer stool remains in the colon, the drier it becomes, and the harder it becomes to pass. This can lead to the stool becoming impacted. If stool becomes impacted in the colon, the stretching of the colon can cause further loss of muscle tone. Impacted stool can in turn lead to megacolon, or the filling of the colon to such an extent that it becomes distended and enlarged.

What Can You Do?

Diet is one of the most important aspects of good bowel function. Adequate water drinking is essential. Your intake of dietary fiber (wheat bran is a good source, as are prunes, peaches, and apricots) should be between 6 and 15 g per day. Fiber is most useful if taken with sufficient amounts of water. Avoiding foods that slow down digestion can also help: cheeses, certain types of breads, bananas, apple sauce, rice, and fatty foods.

Iron supplements can cause constipation, and your physician should be informed if that becomes a problem. Certain medications, particularly those for parkinsonism and opioid painkillers, can inhibit bowel motility. Have your doctor evaluate all the medications (both prescription and over-the-counter) you use to determine if any of them are a problem.

Your doctor may recommend a bulk-forming fiber laxative such as psyllium husks, available under many brand names, such as Metamucil; stool softeners; or certain other laxatives. One caution about laxatives is noteworthy: Stimulant laxatives, which include castor oil, make your problem worse and should never be used by seniors without talking to their doctor. These laxatives can damage the nerves in the intestines, causing seniors to become permanently dependent upon them. ■

Inquire, too, about all over-the-counter medications you use.

A common cause of undernutrition in seniors is a change in life circumstances that can lead to depression. The loss of a loved one or another profound change—such as an injury or illness—can lead to depression and a sense that food just does not taste

DENTAL CARE FOR SENIORS

For the millennia that preceded modern dental care, loss of teeth and the ensuing inability to eat was a serious danger of aging. Even today, untreated dental problems can lead to poor nutrition and chronic mouth pain, which can affect digestion, mood, and other areas of everyday life. Daily dental hygiene and regular dental care are essential aspects of basic health care for seniors. Too often, regular dental care is neglected because of the expense, but dental problems that are not treated promptly can be far more difficult—and far more expensive—to remedy later.

The main causes of tooth decay are periodontal and gum disease, including gingivitis, or inflammation of the gums, and periodontitis, inflammation and degeneration of the tissue, including bone, that surrounds and underlies the teeth. The main cause of gum disease is poor dental hygiene, all of which can lead to receding gums, cavities in the roots of teeth, and eventual tooth loss. The loss of bone matrix and calcium that results in osteoporosis can also affect teeth. So, calcium supplementation (as used in part to prevent osteoporosis) in both men and women, in addition to a good dental hygiene plan, is crucial. Diminished output of estrogen in women can cause loss of gum tissue, exposing the lower, more delicate parts of the teeth to bacteria, which can cause tooth decay.

Good dental hygiene is actually a pretty simple equation: Brush teeth after meals, floss regularly (at least once a day), and see your dentist as often as he recommends it. Newly available electric and ultrasonic toothbrushes seem to add benefit when used regularly. Remember also that bedtime is the single most important time of the day for tooth brushing. Saliva production decreases while we sleep, and the acids that can disintegrate teeth are at their strongest. Ridding your mouth of plaque before sleep can significantly help your dental health.

Your teeth should be cleaned professionally at least twice a year, at which time your dentist can examine your teeth to see if you have any special dental care needs. See Chapter 16 for more information on periodontal disease and other dental disorders.

Prosthodontics and Dentures

While it is best to practice preventive dental care that will preserve your teeth, permanent teeth are sometimes lost for a variety of reasons, including decay, trauma, and disease. Consult with your dentist as soon as possible about the most effective approach to replacing a lost or decaying tooth. If you delay in replacing a tooth, you may be putting the surrounding teeth at risk.

Partial dentures, or bridges, which are attached to surrounding, healthy teeth, can be used to replace a lost tooth. Other kinds of bridges are removable and consist of false teeth fitted to a metal or plastic footing, and then attached to the surrounding teeth by means of clips. Make sure you understand fully from your doctor how to clean your dentures, as they are more prone to plaque buildup than natural teeth. This plaque buildup can affect the health of your gums and your remaining teeth.

Full dentures are necessary only if, for reasons of disease or tooth decay, all of your permanent teeth must be removed. (If some good teeth remain, a set of overdentures that fit over the remaining teeth can be constructed.) While dentures are commonly removable, a newer technique, known as osseointegration of teeth, has been employed in some cases over the last several years. In this procedure, anchors are placed directly into the bones (the maxilla and mandible) of your mouth, and dentures are screwed into them. This procedure involves a series of steps over a few months but can usually be done on an outpatient basis. This kind of denture gives you teeth that are nearly as effective as the originals, but the procedure is not for everyone. Talk to your dentist to see what procedure is right for you.

For further information on prosthodontics, you can contact

- The American College of Prosthodontists
  211 East Chicago Ave., Suite 1000
  Chicago, IL 60611
  Phone: (312) 573–1260
  acpros@aol.com ■

---

good. If you are suddenly living on your own, you may come to feel that cooking is just not worth it.

If you have never seen a doctor about depression, but have little appetite and no sense that food offers any pleasure, or no sense that life has anything to offer, talk to your doctor about the possibility of depression. Doing nothing about depression—taking the attitude that you should be able to work through your blues by yourself—can often make the situation worse. Excellent treatments are available; see Avoiding Depression, page 339, for more information.

Undernutrition can also be a manifestation of many diseases, which, if treated, can be cured or ameliorated. You should always see your doctor if you lose weight unexpectedly.

If you have become temporarily or permanently disabled and cannot cook for yourself, contact local agencies on aging about meal programs that may be of assistance to you, or contact the National Association of Meal Programs (see below) for information on what is available in your area.

Many people—including those who are neither disabled nor widowed—find that retirement communities in which they can either eat in a community dining room or cook in their own apartments can be great sources of social, cultural, and spiritual companionship. Many communities allow

VITAMIN SUPPLEMENTS AND DIETARY SUPPLEMENT DRINKS

Vitamin Supplements

Many Americans take vitamin supplements without any knowledge of what vitamins they might need and without keeping in mind that vitamin overdoses can be dangerous. We cannot, of course, live without vitamins and minerals, but we should get all we need from our diet. As we age, our needs for and the ability to metabolize certain vitamins change, with some more easily used and others not. Before taking vitamin supplements, you should get the advice of your doctor. The medications you take, the diet you are on, the amount of exercise you get, your level of body fat, your kidney and liver function, the presence of disease—all of these things will affect your levels of absorption and your daily requirements. Not every older person needs to take vitamin supplements.

No over-the-counter vitamin supplement is ideally constituted, though most will not be harmful. Discuss with your doctor the kinds of medications you use, any illnesses you might have, or any other factors that may affect your ability to absorb or eliminate vitamins and minerals. Work with your doctor to make sure you get the vitamins and minerals you need, and do not take those you do not need.

That said, many seniors' diets may need supplements of specific vitamins and minerals.

Calcium Seniors should get at least 1.2 to 1.6 g of calcium carbonate or equivalent per day (1,200 to 1,600 mg). This can be taken in many forms, but the cheapest often comes in antacid tablets such as Tums. Check labels to make sure that the antacid you select uses calcium and not some other chemical. Although some doctors recommend simultaneous supplementation with magnesium and vitamin C, it has not been shown conclusively that these improve metabolization of calcium.

Vitamin D Current minimum daily requirements for seniors are too low. Most older people do not get sufficient sunlight, from which our skin derives vitamin D, or adequate vitamin D from fortified milk. Most seniors should get double the 400 IU recommended for the rest of the population. Research shows that many nursing home patients are seriously deficient in vitamin D.

Iron Seniors should not take iron supplements without a diagnosis from their doctor that they are anemic from iron deficiency and until the reason for the deficiency has been discovered. Seniors should follow the special precautions on iron supplements for children. Iron supplements can be overdosed and cause complications.

Potassium Potassium supplements should only be necessary for heart patients, persons with hypertension, and others who are taking diuretics or other medications that can deplete potassium, such as corticosteroids. Potassium is readily available in meats and fruits and is regulated very carefully by the body.

Vitamin A and Carotenes Carotenes and other antioxidants have been touted as capable of reversing or halting the aging process. Studies have not borne this out. While the consumption of vegetables that are high in carotenes—carrots and leafy green vegetables, for example—has been shown to be of value in preventing certain illnesses, particularly cancers, isolated carotenes have shown no such benefit. In fact, they have been shown to make people sick if taken to excess. Vitamin A and carotenes are not water soluble and can be overdosed, which can result in dermatitis and arthritis. Vitamin A accumulates in the system and can be overdosed. Talk to your doctor about appropriate levels for you.

B Vitamins The B vitamins are water soluble, so overdosing on them is not usually a problem. You also may not need them, so speak with your doctor before starting a multivitamin.

Vitamin C Vitamin C is also water soluble, and so overdosing is not usually a problem, but you should check with your doctor to find out how much you need, if any. ◗

seniors to live with as much or as little assistance as they need.

For the caregivers of the disabled or ill Another source of undernutrition in seniors, particularly in the frail or ill, is neglect. Family members who are sole or primary care providers may become overwhelmed by the responsibility of taking care of the needs of someone frail or ill. If you are the primary caregiver for someone who is ill or disabled, but cannot keep up with the responsibilities, talk this over with the doctor who provides care to the ill or disabled person, and contact local services for the aging to find out what kind of help is available. For seniors who are military veterans or former union members, services may be available from the Veterans Administration or the union. Seniors may also be eligible for services through Social Security or their health insurance provider. Meal-delivery services are available for the homebound elderly, and assistance with elder care is available through state and federal agencies.

- **National Association of Meal Programs**
  1414 Prince St., Suite 202
  Alexandria, VA 22314
  Phone: (703) 548-5558
  To volunteer to help, call toll free
  (888) MEAL HELP (6325 4357)

- **National Association for Area Agencies on Aging**
  Phone: (202) 637-8130

◆ "Fountain of Youth" Supplements

The media have recently been awash with information about various chemicals touted to reverse aging and increase feelings of youth and health. Some of these have been approved by the Food and Drug Administration for certain medical purposes, but most are sold in health food, drug, and grocery stores as "dietary supplements." Certain dietary supplements can be quite powerful chemicals and can potentially be harmful. See Chapter 33 for more information on the potential dangers of "natural" remedies. A few of the most notable dietary supplements are listed below:

Melatonin Melatonin, a hormone that has been used as a treatment for insomnia, has the potential to throw off the balance of other hormones. There is little evidence yet of what its long-term effects may be. It has been known to cause grogginess the day after its use, and its use at this time cannot be recommended.

DHEA DHEA is a precursor to the sex hormones estrogen and testosterone (or a chemical that the body converts into those hormones). Many people hope that by increasing their levels of the precursor, they will increase their level of the hormones, making them more vigorous. No reliable studies to date suggest this is the case, and there is the theoretical possibility that boosting levels of the hormones could lead to hormone-related cancers. Therefore, its use at this time is not recommended.

Human Growth Hormone Human growth hormone is a prescription medication most useful in treating children who fail to grow normally. Abused by body builders and others, it can cause irreversible deformities, diabetes, and heart disease.

Dietary Supplement Drinks

You may have received a rather sweet dietary supplement drink while you were in the hospital, or perhaps seen one of those advertisements on television in which healthy, robust-looking older—and younger—people talk about the wonders of using liquid dietary supplements. Do you need to use them? Or are they just another way of packaging vitamin supplements?

For the most part, they are not a very good idea. They can cause stomach upset and can contain a lot of fat. Unless you are hospitalized or bedridden, or have difficulty eating solid food and need the calories they contain, these are not an appropriate source of vitamin, mineral, or calorie supplementation.

Study after study shows that if there is a fountain of youth, it resides within us, in a lifelong, sensible lifestyle, a balanced, varied diet, regular, vigorous exercise, and constant mental stimulus. But it does not come in tablet, liquid, or capsule form. ■

- National Alliance for Senior Citizens
  1700 18th St. NW
  Washington, DC 20009
  Phone: (202) 986–0117

LOSING WEIGHT TO STAY HEALTHY

Although undernutrition is more likely to be a problem in seniors, particularly older seniors, overweight and obesity can be problems at any time of life.

The two chief culprits in overweight and obesity are overeating and inactivity. Nearly half the adult population of the United States is overweight, and many are obese. Despite the fitness craze, these numbers continue to rise.

The change of lifestyle brought on by retirement can leave some seniors with more time yet less activity than ever. And unfortunately, our society provides far too many opportunities and rationalizations for overeating: senior specials, all-you-can-eat buffets, and constant pressure from commercial television to eat. While the propensity for overweight and obesity may be partly due to genetic inheritance, a significant portion is due to lifestyle choices.

Carrying enough weight, something you should discuss with your doctor, is important, but avoiding obesity, which is defined as being 20 percent over your ideal body weight, can help you in almost every area of your overall health. Obesity may make arthritis worse, strain otherwise healthy joints, strain your heart and lungs, and make it more difficult to go about your everyday tasks. It may make chronic diseases such as diabetes worse and cardiovascular disease more likely.

If you are overweight, speak to your doctor about formulating a safe, effective diet and exercise plan to help you lose the weight and keep it off. For more information, see Chapter 1.

Understanding the Aging Process

We are constructed almost entirely of proteins, from our skeletal structure down to the many hormones that send messages between our cells. Each gene in our cells codes for a protein, or can instruct the body to construct or reconstruct a particular protein out of the materials at hand. So the instructions for building (and rebuilding) our cells and their individual complement of proteins are imprinted in each of our cells. Some proteins are long-lived, others short-lived. In the cells that make up our framework (bones, muscles, cartilage, etc.), the proteins are long-lived and do not turn over frequently. The proteins that make up our vital organs are replaced more frequently. It is believed that our various cells, whether made up of long- or short-lived proteins, can replicate only a finite number of times. So even without disease, the failure of the capacity of the cells to replicate themselves would cause us eventually to age and die. The luck of the genetic draw can play a significant role in how rapidly this happens. But genes are only part of the story: How we use our genetic endowment (fitness, nutrition, mental attitude, and the other factors mentioned above) may in many cases be as or more significant. For more information on genetic heritage, see Chapter 6.

As an example of how genetics interact with environment and lifestyle to affect aging, consider two fair-skinned (heredity) individuals—identical twins. Separate them at birth. Twin number one spends most of his life performing hard physical labor (socioeconomic status) in the sun (environment) and smokes (lifestyle). Twin number two works indoors, exercises three times a week, never smokes, and has avoided excessive exposure to the sun. At age 65, twin number one is likely to appear 5 to 10 years older, with heavy wrinkling, and possibly skin or lung cancer. Twin number two, all other things being equal, may at age 65 appear 5 to 10 years younger. Aging in this case—as in many other cases—has less to do with actual chronologic aging than with a multiplicity of lifestyle choices and the perturbations of disease and injury.

Indeed, we often confuse the effects of disease with the effects of aging. Healthy heart muscle is rarely weakened by increasing age alone, but it is greatly weakened by vascular disease, which can be prevented by making healthy lifestyle choices. Indeed, more Americans die of heart disease than any other single illness—which means more Americans are dying of a disease significantly influenced by lifestyle choices.

The rate of physiologic changes that occur with aging appears in many cases to be quite variable; that is, each person ages in a unique way. Each person's rate of aging is largely genetically driven but is modified by environment and lifestyle-related choices.

THE EFFECTS OF TIME ON BODILY SYSTEMS

No one can turn back the clock, but research shows that we can ameliorate many of the effects commonly associated with aging to prevent or delay the young-old from becoming the frail and disabled. For example, muscle tone is directly related to how much muscles are exercised. In the absence of disease or disability, if we continue to exercise into old age, muscles will not—as is commonly believed—weaken and atrophy with age. Lack of use can cause the muscles of adolescents to weaken and atrophy, and too often does. Indeed, research shows that the muscles of the aged can work as well as those of the young. Even a fitness program established in the later years can be quite beneficial (see Staying Fit in the Senior Years, page 320).

Here is a general overview of what happens to the various areas or systems of the body as the years progress: Aging is not isolated but systemic, that is, it affects the whole body. Loss or disuse in one area is echoed in other areas. Diminished estrogen production after menopause, for example, affects the absorption by the bones of calcium, leading to osteoporosis; it also affects heart health, sometimes leading to impaired circulation and coronary heart disease. These, in turn, affect all other bodily systems.

These "separate" areas are therefore listed that way simply for convenience and clarity's sake. The rates of aging of the bodily systems will vary considerably from person to person. Everyone except identical twins has a different genetic makeup, and everyone has been exposed to different environments. All of us have different lifestyles, and so different parts of different people will age at different rates. Age, after all, is time related, and we cannot change that. One 70-year-old may have the heart of a 40-year-old and the skin of a 90-year-old.

Skin, muscles, and connective tissue As we get older, our skin generally thins, loses some of its blood supply and its collagen (the fiber that gives young skin its tautness), and becomes less resilient and more dry. The skin loses some of its ability to breathe;

it sweats less and reduces production of natural skin oils. Diminished moisture is more or less universal throughout the body. Hair becomes thinner. Wrinkles and blood vessels become more apparent as the layer of fat beneath the skin diminishes. Wrinkling and other skin changes are more pronounced in those who have spent a lot of time in the sun or were smokers. Loss of fat has a number of ramifications. Body fat helps provide a cushion so that we do not bruise as easily and helps us keep warm. It also affects hormone levels and the way alcohol and other drugs are metabolized. For example, research shows that the effect of one glass of wine on a senior is the same as two glasses on a younger adult.

Loss of muscle, if it occurs, is caused by lack of use, a disease affecting muscle, or nutritional deficiency. Research shows that the muscles of the elderly may have a slightly reduced rate of blood flow but remain as efficient in their use of oxygen as those of younger people. The presence of arthritis or another chronic illness, or obesity, can lead to a sedentary lifestyle, which in turn can lead to muscle atrophy.

The cartilage that acts as the cushion and connection between our bones can lose some of its capacity to withstand repetitive impact. Because it has no blood vessels and so depends on blood supply from the surrounding tissues for its nourishment, it can become less resilient with aging.

Bones and teeth   Osteoporosis has become well known as one of the common effects of aging, and indeed, loss of bone density is a problem with lasting consequences for both men and women (see Osteoporosis, page 331). Several different factors account for loss of bone density. First is loss of sex hormone production. Estrogen is markedly reduced in women at menopause. Testosterone levels decline slightly in men as they age, but levels decline more dramatically when testosterone production is compromised by illness or alcoholism. Other causes of bone density loss include lack of exercise, the use of certain medications, and poor nutrition. Osteoporotic bones are weaker and fracture more easily than strong bones. Fractures can lead to severe limitations in physical mobility and can threaten an independent lifestyle.

Bone marrow—which produces the white blood cells that fight infection—diminishes with aging, while marrow fat increases. This does not, however, appear to cause the marrow to be significantly less productive or active. White blood cell counts remain largely unchanged throughout life, and white blood cells retain their ability to fight off bacterial infection.

Although anemia (a deficiency in red blood cells or hemoglobin) is often associated with aging, it is not caused by the loss of capacity of the body to produce red blood cells; rather it is due to other problems, most prominently undernutrition (see Avoiding Undernutrition, page 323), disease, or decreased production of hormones that regulate bone marrow activity.

Dental problems can be a direct cause of poor nutrition. The same circumstances that can lead to osteoporosis and weakening of the bones can also lead to weakening of the teeth.

Circulation   The functioning of the heart does not seem to be significantly diminished by the passing of time itself, and yet cardiovascular disease is the most common cause of death in this country. Many women worry about breast cancer, without realizing that death from heart disease is far more common. Cardiovascular disease on average tends to affect women later in life than men. For reasons not fully understood, the hormone estrogen appears to provide women with protection. After menopause, women are as vulnerable as men to heart disease, due to the narrowing of blood vessels caused by the buildup of plaque deposits that can result in decreased blood flow and increased blood pressure. For men and women alike, diet and exercise can help prevent heart disease (see Chapter 20).

The body's vasculature may lose some of its suppleness, and varicose veins may develop. Some difficulty in circulation to the limbs may occur. Again, however, exercise and diet have been shown to help maintain good circulation.

Lungs   The catchphrase "use it or lose it" is true of muscle mass as well as bone density, and it is also true of lung capacity. Like virtually every other body tissue, lungs can lose some elasticity as we age. They appear to gain volume while losing some of their inner surface area and therefore some of their ability to absorb oxygen from the air we breathe. But research shows that exercise can increase the ability of the lungs to do their job and further demonstrates that seniors who are in good shape already can frequently surpass many young people in lung function. While the ribs and breastbone can fuse, forcing the diaphragm to work harder, loss of lung function does not have to be an inevitable part of aging. The diaphragm does not seem to be adversely affected by normal aging.

Smoking speeds deterioration of the lungs and produces a great amount of heart and lung disease. Stopping smoking now— even late in life—can reduce the risk of many heart- and lung-related illnesses. See Chapter 4 for more information on how to stop smoking.

The gastrointestinal tract Although the gastrointestinal tract remains quite resilient throughout life and does not lose its ability to do its job, there can be some reduction in the capacity of the muscles of the gastrointestinal tract to coordinate their movements. This can lead to constipation (see page 323), a common problem among seniors. The contractions that take place in the upper gastrointestinal tract during swallowing can also weaken and become less well coordinated, which can lead to gastroesophageal reflux, commonly associated with heartburn (see page 969). Over time, the production of gastric juices (hydrochloric acid and pepsin) and saliva tend to decrease. The rate at which different vitamins and minerals are absorbed in the gut can also change over time. Because the ratio of body fat to body water increases as we age, those compounds that are fat soluble, such as vitamin A, may have more rapid absorption and metabolization, while those that are water soluble may not be used as efficiently. Changes can also take place in the way we absorb minerals, particularly calcium and iron.

By compensating with dietary changes and thorough, careful chewing and swallowing, you can enable your digestive tract to work well throughout life.

Another common characteristic of bowels in aging persons is the formation of diverticula in the large intestine. These small, pouch-like formations can result from increased pressure on the walls of the bowel and decreased resilience of the muscles. The disorder can be present in as many as a third of seniors. Often completely

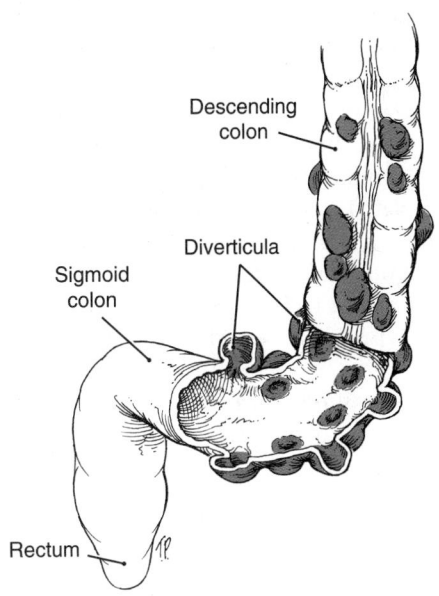

Diverticulosis. Small outpouchings of the inner lining of the intestine (diverticula) can be complicated by obstruction and inflammation (diverticulitis), perforation, or bleeding.

harmless, these diverticula can become inflamed when bits of stool lodge in them and cause infection (see 1016).

Other vital organs Our organs, when we are young, function at a level several times in excess of what is needed in order to do their jobs. As we age, many of our organs gradually lose some of their ability to function to full capacity. Each organ ages at a different rate and differently in each person. The kidneys gradually lose some function but for the most part are able to maintain the delicate balance of water, electrolytes, and other substances in the blood. Loss of organ function may affect the way your body metabolizes certain vitamins. You should check with your doctor to see if you need more or less of particular vitamins (see Vitamin Supplements and Dietary Supplement Drinks, page 325).

The liver becomes somewhat smaller over time and loses some of its blood supply; it is also less capable of renewing damaged tissue. However, the liver should work well throughout life. This is also true of the pancreas, which should work well throughout life, although its position in the body can shift slightly, and it can pick up fat and scar tissue as you age.

Glands of the endocrine system, such as the thyroid, adrenal, pituitary, and hypothalamus—all of which produce necessary hormones—slow down their output by varying degrees. Loss of hormone production can cause a reduction in overall metabolic rate, but noteworthy loss of function in hormone-producing glands is usually associated with serious disorders, such as diabetes, and not the normal aging process. Adult-onset diabetes is usually caused by obesity and lack of exercise, not by aging (see Type 2 Diabetes Mellitus, page 1179).

Genitourinary and reproductive function Men can continue to father children well into old age. Some men, however, experience some kind of transient or chronic impotence, loss of sexual desire, or other impairment of sexual function. This, however, is not a natural consequence of aging but usually is due to illness, such as diabetes mellitus, certain medications, or depression, and can be treated. Because of neural changes, aging is likely to cause some slowing down of sexual response (see Central and Peripheral Nervous Systems, page 331). Despite this, most seniors should be able to continue an active and satisfying sex life throughout life; indeed, it appears that seniors who maintain a healthy sex life are at an advantage for retaining better genitourinary health.

In men, the prostate often becomes enlarged as time passes (see page 1146), and this can cause some urinary and sexual difficulty.

In women, loss of tone in the muscles that govern urinary function can result in incontinence. Incontinence is not an inevitable part of aging, though television commercials for adult diapers may imply otherwise. Incontinence is associated with disorders such as atrophic vaginitis in women or chronic neurologic disease in both men and women. However, lost muscle tone, which is particularly common in women, can almost always be regained with prescribed exercise. About 85 percent of women who are ambulatory and not neurologically impaired can be cured of urinary incontinence or dramatically improved. Both women and men who have incontinence can be helped, so you should discuss the problem with your doctor. If your doctor is not experienced in this problem, many communities have incontinence assessment and treatment programs. For more information, see Urinary Incontinence (Leaky Bladder), page 1071. You can also contact Help for Incontinent People (HIP), (800) BLADDER (252-3337), P.O. Box 544, Union, SC 29379. Another good source is the book *Staying Dry: A Practical Guide to Bladder Control*, written by Bungio, Pearce, and Lucco, Johns Hopkins University Press, 1989.

After menopause, estrogen production diminishes. In the absence of sufficient amounts of the hormone, which you can take supplementally (see Chapter 25), the vulvar region tends to atrophy, with loss of pubic hair and shrinkage of the labia majora.

COMMON MYTHS OF AGING

People become more forgetful as they age Although some loss of short-term memory due to diminishing of neural function can accompany aging, long-term memory generally remains intact. Significant memory loss can be a sign of dementing illness, such as Alzheimer's disease or multi-infarct dementia. If you are worried about your memory or that of someone in your family, contact your physician. In most cases, a little forgetfulness is normal and nothing to worry about (see Benign Forgetfulness, page 458). There are lots of ways to work around short-term memory loss. Posting notes or using a calendar/diary can be helpful reminders.

People become more grouchy and unpleasant as they age Irritability or crotchetiness is not a fundamental part of aging. As we age, we may suffer fools less gladly or grow less inhibited about voicing unpopular opinions, but constant irritability and grumpiness is usually a sign of illness, lack of sleep, chronic pain, or poor diet rather than of aging. Behavioral or personality changes are often a signal of the onset of dementing illness, such as Alzheimer's disease. In the absence of disease, your basic personality persists throughout life.

Urinary incontinence is a natural part of aging Most seniors do not experience incontinence. For those who do, it is usually very effectively treated and need not be a permanent condition.

People naturally become less active as they age In the absence of illness or injury, becoming less active is not an inevitable part of aging. Even in the presence of some types of injury, some exercise is possible and even crucial. Consult your doctor about an exercise program that is appropriate for you.

Age causes loss of muscle and bone mass Americans overall have a calcium-poor diet. That, in tandem with an increasingly sedentary lifestyle and the loss of estrogen in women following menopause, contributes to loss of bone mass. Loss of bone mass can be halted or reversed by hormone replacement therapy, calcium supplementation, and a good exercise program.

Loss of muscle is due not to aging but to lack of use. Continued exercise will lead to continued increases in muscle mass and tone.

Senility is a natural consequence of aging While there is some slowdown in certain mental processes (short-term memory and the ability to learn quickly), most people, in the absence of illness, retain their mental acuity for their entire lives. ■

The labia minora can almost disappear. Certain chemical changes alter the pH of the vagina and lower resistance to some types of infection. The vagina can lose its interior folds and elasticity. An active sex life appears, however, to mitigate these changes.

Even before menopause, the milk-producing glandular tissue in breasts diminishes; menopause causes it to atrophy. Women may notice that their nipples become, over time, smaller and less likely to become erect. Estrogen supplementation may prevent these age-related changes in breast tissue.

Central and peripheral nervous systems The nervous system includes three interacting systems: the central nervous system, or the brain and spinal cord; the peripheral nervous system, which consists of the cranial nerves and spinal nerves; and the autonomic system, which controls the automatic functions of the body, such as breathing and heart rate. With age also comes a slowdown in the rate at which nerves are able to transmit signals to one another. This can affect some types of thought as well as some reflexes and can include a slower response to new information—learning may take more time, but you can do it—and changes in sleep patterns. Forgetfulness may increase slightly, but it is more likely that seniors *notice* forgetfulness more than younger people do. As with muscles and bones, there is a "use it or lose it" mechanism to mental acuity. Just as those who stay physically active tend to stay physically vigorous, those who stay mentally active (taking courses, keeping up with current events) tend to remain mentally vigorous.

For the most part, despite the association of senility with aging, the profound loss of mental acuity is a symptom of a disorder and not a part of the normal aging process (See Common Myths of Aging, page 330 and The Disorders that Cause Dementia, page 339).

As all other bodily systems lose some of their youthful edge, so too can the abilities to see, hear, taste, feel, and react lose some of their acuity. Often, these are not profound changes. They happen only gradually, and perhaps without our noticing; the pupils of our eyes, for example, do not contract as rapidly as we age. And many of the changes that result from disorders—cataracts, hearing loss—can be treated quite effectively (see Visual Impairments, page 342, and Hearing Loss, page 344). Reaction time can diminish as well, and many states now require seniors to undergo driving tests more frequently than younger people. Losing driving privileges can come as a heavy blow to many and represents a considerable loss of freedom—but that loss hardly compares to the potential for loss in automobile accidents. With a positive attitude and some help from family and local agencies, you should still be able to maintain freedom.

Most of the changes listed above are quite gradual in their onset, and many can be quite easily offset by appropriate exercise, sensible diet, and appropriate medical treatment. Others, however, are simply facts of life—but that does not mean that we have to let them turn us into invalids or shut-ins. There are ways to live around and through these changes in order to maintain a high quality of life.

Common Health Concerns of Seniors

While it is true that in the last decades of life serious health problems often occur, too many of us assume that chronic disease and disability are inevitable in the senior years. In many cases, they are not. The benefits of preventive health care—regular exams, early detection of potential problems, and rapid and effective treatment of existing problems as soon as they occur—cannot be overstated.

If a health concern does arise, do not presume that you have to be resigned to it. Seek early diagnosis and treatment, because relief is often available.

OSTEOPOROSIS

Osteoporosis means "holes in the bones" and arises when the diminishment of certain hormones or the use of particular medications alters the body's cycle of replenishing the bone tissue of our skeletons. As time goes on, bones can weaken, leading to the potential for easy fracture. Most debilitating is disintegration of the vertebrae (the disks of bone that make up the spinal column) and hip

ANNUAL HEALTH ASSESSMENT FOR SENIORS: RECOMMENDED REGULAR SCREENING AND COUNSELING

SCREENING	COUNSELING
Your doctor should assess	**Your doctor should**
Height and weight	Counsel you on weight loss if appropriate, and emphasize a sensible diet with a caloric intake proportionate to your level of physical activity, emphasizing grains, fruits, and vegetables
Fitness	Advise you on appropriate levels of exercise, risks of obesity
Your nutritional needs. Are you underweight? Do you need supplemental vitamins or minerals? What kinds of special needs do you have, given existing medical conditions and medications you may take?	Advise you on ways to get adequate levels of calcium, on vitamin supplementation to avoid overdosing, on sensible diet with plenty of soluble fiber to avoid constipation, on ways to increase your saturated fat intake because of loss of body fat
Blood pressure; if you are hypertensive and obese, the doctor should screen for diabetes	Offer advice on how to reduce your risk of hypertension-related illness
Mental acuity	
Vision	
Hearing	Advise on hearing aids and other appropriate devices where necessary
Heart risk	Advise women of potential benefits of hormone replacement therapy, and advise men and woman of lifestyle changes that can reduce their risk of developing heart disease
Osteoporosis	Advise women of potential benefits and risks of hormone replacement therapy
Pap smear (women)	
Mammogram annually or biannually for women over age 50, depending on the doctor's recommendation; annual clinical breast exam	
Fecal occult blood test and/or sigmoidoscopy	Advise you of dietary ways you can reduce your risk of bowel and rectal cancer (more green vegetables, fewer saturated fats, more fiber) and avoid constipation
Genitourinary function; in women, assess for incontinence and relaxation of pelvic muscles with possible drop in position of the uterus; assess high-risk sexual behavior; in men, assess prostate disorders	Advise you on ways to work around aging to continue a healthy sex life; advise you on exercises to help prevent incontinence
Problem drinking or other drug use	Advise you on safe levels of alcohol use; advise seniors with a potential problem on the dangers of addiction and how to get help
Tobacco use	Recommend ways to stop smoking or using tobacco in any form
Tuberculin skin test for those at risk	

Source: Guide to Clinical and Preventive Services, Second Edition. Report of the U.S. Preventive Services Task Force.

fractures, which can significantly reduce mobility and limit independence.

Osteoporosis is estimated to result in nearly a million and a half fractures each year. Some of these fractures are due to falls, but many of them are spontaneous, or occur unprovoked: A bone in the foot breaks while walking down stairs, a vertebra fractures while sitting down in a chair. In fact, it is estimated that a quarter of all women over age 60 develop vertebral deformities and 15 percent develop hip

CONFLICTS IN MEDICATION— AVOIDING A DISASTER

If you see more than one doctor, it is essential that each of your doctors know what medications, both prescription and over-the-counter, you are using so that your medications are coordinated and you will not inadvertently be prescribed one that will harmfully interact with another. Ask your doctor about side effects and possible interactions each time he writes you a new prescription. And be sure to check with your doctor before using any over-the-counter medication. Many people assume that if a drug is sold over the counter it must be safe to use. This simply is not the case, particularly for those with existing conditions or taking other medications.

Dosages and Frequency of Dosages

Whenever a physician writes you a prescription, make certain that you know the proper dosage and exactly how often, and when, you are to take it. Do you need to take it on a full or empty stomach? Should you take it with plenty of water? Can it cause dizziness or fainting?

Drug Counseling and Information

Most pharmacies will provide you with counseling if you request it, either in the form of a discussion with the pharmacist or as literature on the drug. Many pharmacies will provide an information sheet on a prescription the first time they fill it, and most should be able to provide you with one at your request.

If you receive your prescriptions by mail order, you should receive with your order information sheets on each of the medications you receive. Read them carefully. If you have further questions about the drugs you are taking, talk to the pharmacist at your local pharmacy or talk to your doctor.

The Accuracy of Prescriptions

It is an old joke that no one can read doctors' handwriting, but the reality is that prescriptions are written in a medical shorthand that your doctor and pharmacist understand, but that you may not. Still, it is always possible for miscommunication to occur. Always be certain of the name, the dosage, and the frequency of the medication your doctor intends you to take.

If you have been taking 100 mg of a particular medication, and your refill is 200 mg, but your doctor has not discussed a change in dosage with you, check with the doctor before taking the medication. If you see a doctor different from the one you are accustomed to and your prescription changes, talk to the doctor, and find out if the change is intentional or a mistake.

Seniors are the most frequent health care consumers and are often the most vigilant. Always do what you can to assist in your own care. For more detailed information on safe and effective use of medications, see Chapter 33. ■

---

fractures because of loss of bone density. Hip fractures can be especially debilitating, carrying with them considerable pain, loss of mobility, a decrease in social function, and a decrease in expected survival. Vertebral fractures can cause stooping and considerable chronic pain, as well as height loss.

Osteoporosis more commonly affects women, but it can also affect men. Women are more likely to develop it because they have a naturally lower bone density on average throughout life than men, experience a major hormone loss at menopause that causes precipitous losses of skeletal calcium, and have a slightly longer life span. Osteoporosis is particularly common in men with prostate cancer who have undergone antihormonal treatment or who have taken corticosteriods for a long period of time.

What can you do about osteoporosis? Osteoporosis is often not diagnosed until after a fracture has occurred. In these cases, osteoporosis is diagnosed many years after bone loss has begun and when bones have become brittle enough to endure sponta-

IMMUNIZATIONS

Although influenza can sometimes be nothing more than fever, aches, and pains, it can also be deadly, depending on the strain, for young and old, healthy and unhealthy alike. For those age 65 and over, annual flu shots offer protection from the miseries of the flu, both minor and major. Talk to your doctor about scheduling a flu shot at the beginning of flu season. The U.S. government and all preventive task forces recommend immunization for the flu for all those in nursing home facilities, for those who suffer from chronic cardiopulmonary disorders, metabolic diseases such as diabetes, blood disorders, immunosuppressive conditions, or kidney disorders, and for those who are age 65 and older. Those at high risk, who have impaired liver or kidney function, or who experience side effects, may be given other medications to reduce the risk of adverse reaction from the injection.

Pneumococcal vaccine is also recommended for seniors to prevent or reduce the severity of a common form of bacterial pneumonia—that caused by the pneumococcal species. At least a single immunization at approximately age 65 is appropriate. Studies are ongoing to determine the most suitable frequency for booster shots, and currently every 5 years is suggested by most experts.

You should also be certain that your tetanus immunization is up to date. Having a booster every 10 years is recommended. Tetanus can be a fatal disease, and those who are at greatest risk are those who are elderly and have let their immunization lapse and, especially, those who have never received primary immunization.

For more information on immunizations for adults, see Chapter 21. ■

(A) Figures B and C represent cross-sections made through a long bone of the leg. (B) Normal cross-section. (C) Osteoporosis. Cortical and spongy bone are less dense and the central canal is wider, which weakens the structure of the bone and increases the risk of fracture.

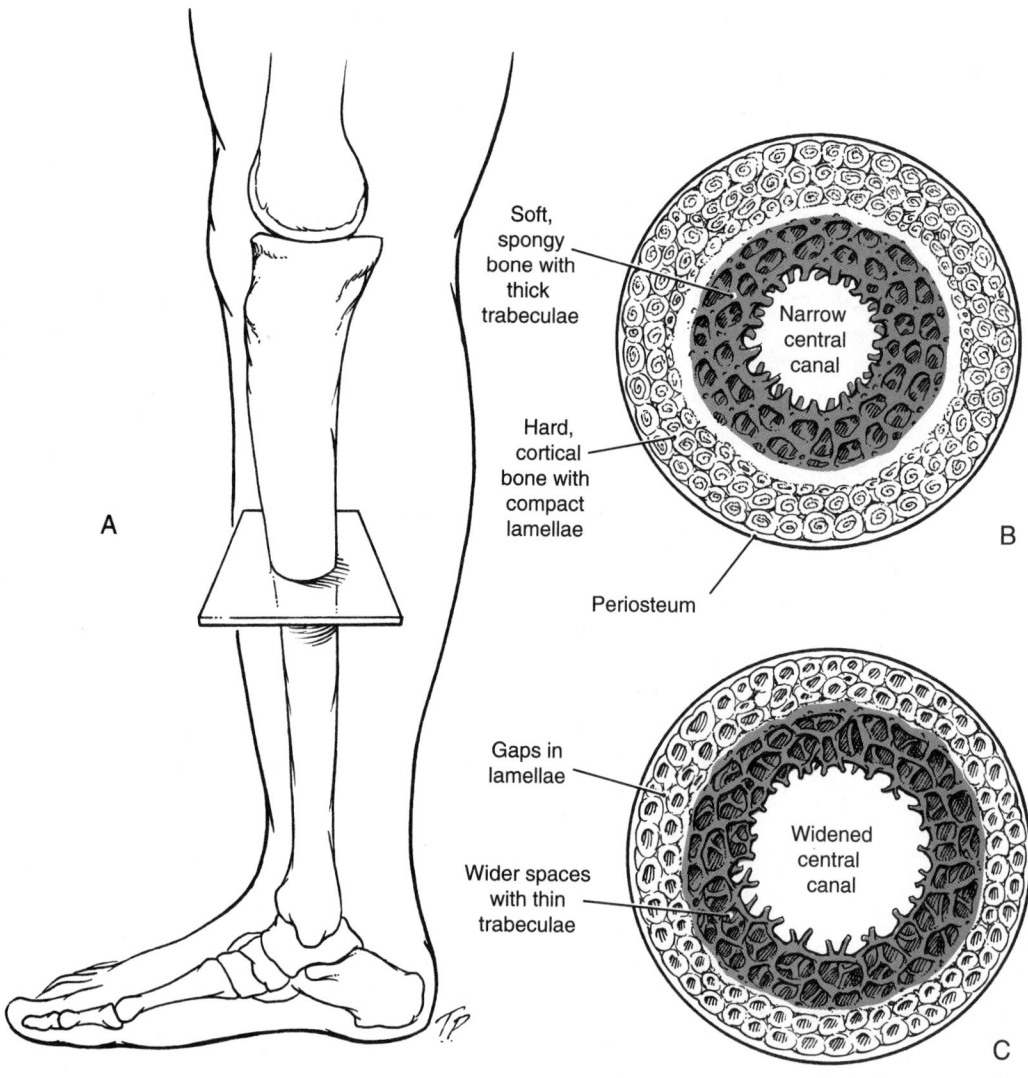

A

Soft, spongy bone with thick trabeculae

Hard, cortical bone with compact lamellae

Narrow central canal

Periosteum

B

Gaps in lamellae

Wider spaces with thin trabeculae

Widened central canal

C

neous fractures. Prevention is paramount. Bone mass can be measured easily and safely using newer scanning techniques such as dual-energy x-ray absorptiometry, which can detect mild degrees of bone loss and can identify candidates for early treatment (prevention) or aggressive therapy. Talk to your doctor about what you can do to help strengthen your bones and keep them strong. Loss of bone density can be halted, and in many cases it can be partially reversed.

In the absence of disease, our bones, like our muscles, tend to be as strong as they are required to be. If you walk or lift weights, your bones will normally be strong enough to support those activities. If you sit and watch television all day, your bones and muscles will be strong enough to support that activity. Astronauts were

found to lose bone density almost immediately upon entering the weightlessness of outer space, and so they now use certain kinds of exercises while in space to slow down or prevent the leaching of minerals from their bones. You also can use exercise to help keep your bones in good shape. Weight-bearing exercise and calcium supplementation can significantly reduce bone mineral loss. Talk to your doctor about what combination of preventive actions is right for you.

In postmenopausal woman, hormone replacement therapy (HRT) with estrogen has been proven effective in preventing loss of bone mineral content, but it has also been statistically linked with uterine cancer. This risk can be eliminated with the addition of progestin to the estrogen. However, controversy remains over whether long-term use of estrogen can increase the risk of breast cancer. Still, the benefits of HRT are clear: Studies have shown that fewer fractures occur in women who begin HRT close to menopause and continue it as they age. If, for example, you begin HRT at menopause and continue with it until you are at age 68 and you do not use corticosteroids or other medications that can deplete bone, at age 68 your bone density will have remained at your premenopausal level. Therapy, even when begun within 10 to 15 years after the onset of menopause, may still offer some protection.

HRT has also shown tremendous health benefits to women in decreasing coronary heart disease. Again, however, there is considerable controversy regarding the potential risks of HRT, particularly an increased risk of certain cancers. Pharmaceutical researchers are attempting to create forms of estrogen that would preserve the bone-building capacity of the hormone without the tissue-building properties that are associated with some of its side effects. Other therapies, such as the bisphosphonates and calcitonin, are also effective at stopping bone loss and preventing fractures. Until then, each woman needs to consider her personal and family history with her doctor to determine whether the benefits of HRT outweigh the risks. (See also Hormone Replacement Therapy, page 1105.)

Dietary calcium intake is important at all ages. There is no easy way to measure the total body calcium content, because the mineral is constantly in flux between the blood and skeleton. The bones are our major store, and if some other system needs it, it comes from that storehouse. The latest research suggests that the Food and Drug Administration's recommended daily allowances—especially of vitamin D and calcium—are too low for seniors (see Vitamin Supplements and Dietary Supplement Drinks, page 325). Calcium supplements may be necessary to achieve these new goals if you cannot tolerate calcium-rich foods.

Using other medication to enhance bone mineral content (such as vitamin D) or medication your doctor can prescribe to prevent mineral loss (calcitonin, bisphosphonates) may also be helpful. Achieving the lowest possible dose or avoiding medication that can cause bone mineral loss (corticosteroids), if possible, is also valuable.

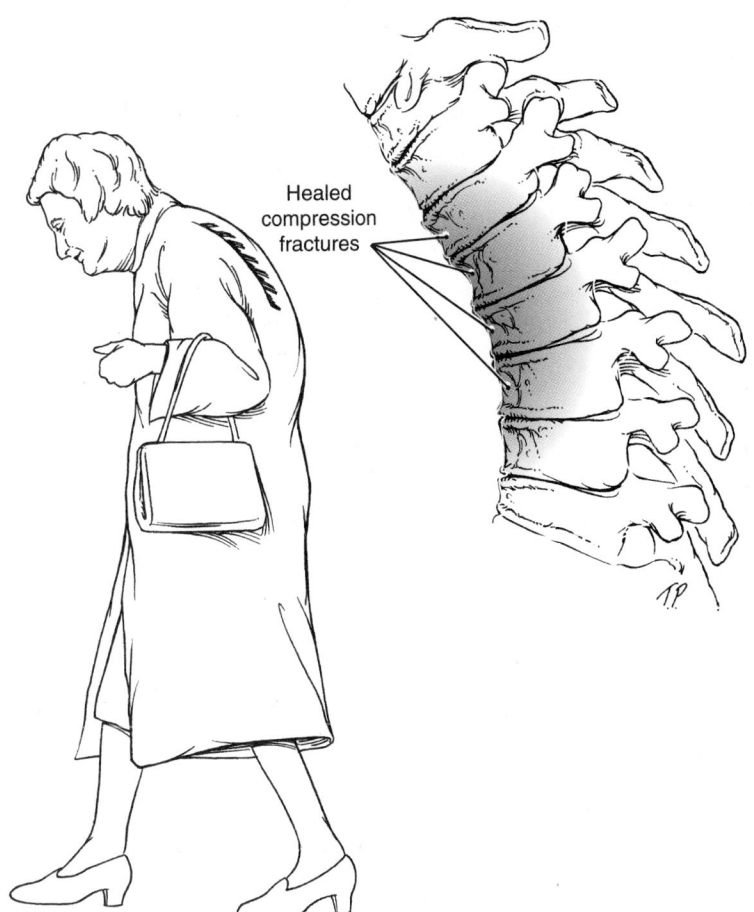

Dowager's hump. Spinal bones weakened by osteoporosis—a common problem in older women—become fractured and compressed in the front giving many older people a hunched-over appearance.

See Osteoporosis, page 654, for more information, or contact

- National Osteoporosis Foundation
  1150 17th St. NW, Suite 500
  Washington, DC 20036
  Phone: (202) 223-2226
  Phone: (800) 223-9994

FALLS

Falls are the leading cause of nonfatal injuries and unintentional injury deaths in older people in the United States. Physiologic changes that can occur as we age—such as postural instability, gait disturbances, diminished vision, and use of certain medications—and environmental circumstances—such as uneven pavement, loose rugs, poor lighting, improper footwear, slippery surfaces, and unexpected objects—all contribute to the increased risk for falls in older people. Those who are more likely to be injured in falls are those who suffer from osteoporosis, fainting, impaired cognitive function (delirium or dementia), and those who use diuretics, vasodilators, or sedatives.

There are ways you can lower your risk of falls and of injury:

- Exercise: Improved strength, muscle tone, and bone density will help keep you from falling and help you avoid injury or speed recovery if you do.

- Make sure that your doctor monitors and fully informs you about the medications you use. If you use any that can make you lightheaded or have vertigo (the feeling that either the environment or your body is revolving), you should be informed of this so that you can take appropriate precautions.

- Talk to your physician about balance training if you experience vertigo or dizziness.

- If you suffer from osteoporosis, make sure it is treated.

- Make sure your home is a haven of safety from falls: if you are frail, avoid stairs. Do not wear slippers that could cause you to slip on bare floors. If you have throw rugs, make sure they are fastened to the floor or have nonskid undersides or nonskid mats beneath them. See Chapter 3 for detailed information on maintaining a safe environment for seniors.

- Make sure you have sensible footwear. If, for example, arthritis in your hands makes it difficult to tie shoelaces properly, look for walking shoes that fasten with Velcro. Avoid shoes that fit too loosely or shoelaces that repeatedly come untied. Talk to your doctor about what is appropriate for your needs.

- Make sure that eye conditions are treated to optimize your vision (see Visual Impairments, page 342). If you have difficulty with peripheral vision, you might try wearing a cap with a bill so that you have a warning system before you bump into cabinets or low overhangs. If you have lost your sight or suffer from partial blindness, make sure your home is arranged in a predictable manner and that any caregiver or housekeeper understands your needs.

- Hip protectors, worn in special undergarments, have been shown to reduce the incidence of hip fractures by 56 percent among seniors. If you believe you may be prone to falls because of medication you may be using, poor eyesight, or other factors, talk to your doctor about the possibility of wearing hip protectors.

For more information on how to prevent falls or how to speed your recovery from a fall, contact

- National Rehabilitation Information Center
  8455 Colesville Rd., Suite 935
  Silver Spring, MD 20910–3319
  Phone: (800) 227–0216

OSTEOARTHRITIS

Osteoarthritis is the most common joint disease in the world. It is caused by the degeneration of the cartilage that cushions the joints and by the secondary bone and tissue reaction to this loss. Cartilage helps to absorb the shock and weight of movement, and it also has the ability to absorb and retain moisture. Though cartilage is resilient, it can break down and begin to affect the underlying bone and joint by causing thickening or distortion of the bone, which can lead to painful movement. Osteoarthritis mainly affects fingers, knees, the spine, and hips. Prevalence of symptomatic osteoarthritis increases sharply after age 65 and is common in both men and women.

While there is as yet no cure for arthritis, there are remedies that may offer relief of symptoms. Ice or warm packs applied to the affected joint may help reduce pain, and over-the-counter pain relievers may help reduce pain and inflammation and make movement more comfortable. Always check with your doctor, however, before starting to use over-the-counter medications. Discuss whether acetaminophen or aspirin or other nonsteroidal anti-inflammatory drugs (NSAIDs), such as ibuprofen or ketoprofen, would be appropriate. Because it causes fewer side effects, acetaminophen is usually suggested over NSAIDs. On rare occasions, injections of corticosteroids directly into the joint or in the tissues surrounding the joint may help reduce inflammation and help you achieve improved function.

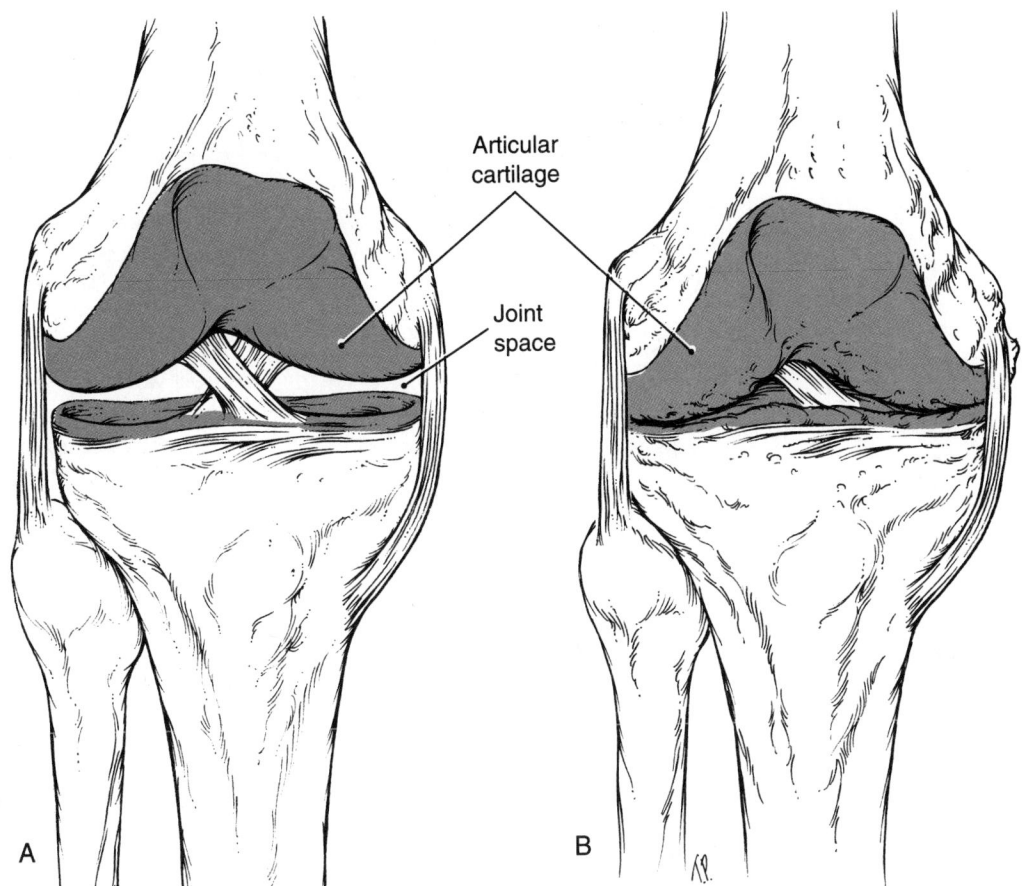

Osteoarthritis of the knee. (A) Normal knee joint. (B) With excessive wearing of joints, the articular cartilage can deteriorate, which narrows the joint space and causes discomfort with activity.

Articular cartilage

Joint space

A

B

See page 651 for more detailed information on osteoarthritis. Or you can contact these organizations:

*   American College of Rheumatology
    60 Executive Park S., Suite 150
    Atlanta, GA 30329
    Phone: (404) 679-5300

*   Arthritis Foundation
    1314 Spring St.
    Atlanta, GA 30309
    Phone: (800) 283-7800

SLEEP DISORDERS

Problem sleep can occur at any time in life, but statistics show that its incidence increases as we age. Nonetheless, poor sleep is not an inevitable development of aging. Healthy seniors do not for the most part have sleep problems.

Although the myth has it that we need less and less sleep the older we get, research shows that our need for rest (7 to 9 hours of sleep per day) does not change throughout adulthood. Many seniors may have more time to nap during the day and may sleep less during the night if they do nap. Research also shows that seniors often spend more time asleep, or trying to sleep, than others do.

Most sleep difficulties are the result of underlying health problems and can be relieved. Occasional difficulty sleeping does not necessarily indicate a sleep disorder.

There are several different primary, nondisease causes of sleep problems in the senior population:

*   Poor sleep habits
*   Daytime napping
*   Stress
*   Lack of exercise
*   Exercise immediately prior to bedtime
*   Use of alcohol or caffeine
*   Unfamiliar or uncomfortable sleeping arrangements

You can make changes to relieve these problems; see Getting a Good Night's Sleep, page 338.

There are also several disorders that are more common among the senior popula-

GETTING A GOOD NIGHT'S SLEEP

If your sleep difficulties are caused by poor sleep habits, you can change them: Is your bed just for sleep, or is it also a place to watch television, read the newspaper, talk on the phone, etc.? Moving the television out of the bedroom and making your bed exclusively for sleep may improve your sleep once you acclimatize yourself to the change. Are your sleeping arrangements comfortable? Try to make your bedroom a haven. Make sure your bed is of a softness or hardness that you find pleasing. Make sure your bedclothes are comfortable, that the room is the right temperature, as dark and quiet as you like it, and that it is free of anything you may be allergic to. If you need to use earplugs or a mask to help, you can find them at your local drugstore.

Napping can turn into a vicious cycle. Some people find themselves quite drowsy in the afternoons and doze off for an hour or more. Many people find that when they do nap, they cannot sleep well at night, yet they need the nap because of last night's sleep deficit. Try eliminating your naps. If you find yourself drowsy in the afternoons, try to exercise then, which will wake you up. On the other hand, a regular nap with an adjusted time for sleep at night can be satisfactory and, indeed, is a healthy pattern used by many.

Coffee or tea or other caffeine-containing beverages or foods can ruin your sleep, particularly if you have them in the evenings. Try decaffeinated beverages, or, for a week or two, eliminate coffee or tea or other caffeine-containing foods and beverages from your diet, and then reevaluate your sleep. Alcohol also makes for poor-quality sleep, and it is best to eliminate alcohol entirely. (Because of the shift in the ratio of body fat to body water, alcohol has about twice the effect on seniors that it has on younger adults.) If you cannot or do not wish to eliminate alcohol entirely, limit consumption to one drink (4 oz of wine or its equivalent) a day.

Do you use sleeping pills? It is best to avoid these. While they may be useful for a few days from time to time, they will, if used for more than a few days, cause a dependence and prevent you from getting to the source of your sleep difficulty and solving it. Also, all sleeping pills have an aftereffect and will lead to fatigue during the following days.

Do you smoke? Stop. Nicotine is a stimulant and causes wakefulness (see Chapter 4). If you smoke, stopping is the single most important thing you can do to improve your health—not just for sleep but in many other ways—no matter how old you are. But not only is nicotine a stimulant, the coughing, throat, and sinus problems that smoking can cause will wake you periodically during the night, thereby ruining your quality of sleep.

Do you exercise? If you do not, talk to your doctor about an exercise program that is suitable for you (see Staying Physically Active, page 321). Mid-day or afternoon exercise can help you feel more tired in the evenings and leave you with more of a sense of satisfaction. Avoid exercising in the late evening hours. The physical arousal that exercise causes can keep you from falling asleep.

If you cannot sleep, do you lie in bed and stare at the ceiling? Get up and read for a while, or try listening to soothing music. Some people find ambient "music," such as forest or ocean sounds, soothing. Others use relaxation techniques, such as deep breathing, to clear their minds and encourage sleep. Discuss your situation with your doctor to see if he recommends seeing a sleep specialist, who can teach you relaxation techniques.

Does your sleep-mate make it difficult for you to sleep? If your partner consistently wakes you with snoring or thrashing, try to change your sleeping arrangements, either by moving to a different room or getting to the root of your partner's sleep difficulty (snoring can be caused by sinus blockage, sleep apnea, obesity, or another treatable medical condition). ■

tion that can adversely affect sleep. If a particular disorder is making it difficult for you to sleep, discuss the problem with your doctor. There is no need simply to accept poor sleep as a "natural" part of aging, because it is not. Rather, you should seek treatment for these problems.

Back pain, arthritic pain, or other forms of chronic pain can all disturb the quality of sleep. Talk to your doctor about seeing a pain specialist who can help you learn techniques for living successfully with chronic pain. There are breathing and other techniques that can be more effective than drugs. See Chapter 14 for more information on dealing with chronic pain. Or your doctor may recommend an appropriate over-the-counter pain reliever to help you get a better night's sleep.

Sleep apnea (periodic cessation of respiration) is often caused by obesity and can be effectively treated. See Chapter 16 for more information.

Heartburn is a common problem in seniors and is usually caused by a loosening of the esophageal muscles, allowing gastric juices to move up. If you experience nocturnal heartburn, eating earlier in the evening may help. Also try elevating the head of your bed while you sleep. If after trying these you still have difficulty, talk to your doctor about possible medications. Examples are antacids, which will neutralize stomach acid; or ranitidine (Zantac) or omeprazole (Prilosec) and other such drugs, which inhibit stomach acid production; and cisapride (Propulsid), which helps diminish nighttime symptoms of heartburn by accelerating the movement of the esophagus and the contractions of the stomach. For more information, see Chapter 23.

Heart disease, even successfully treated, can be a source of sleep difficulty. Talk to your doctor about your medications, and find out why the condition is keeping you up. Some seniors experience rapid heartbeat when they are trying to relax, and this can often be relieved by medication and/or appropriate exercise. Talk to your doctor.

Lung disease, including asthma, can keep you up at night. Talk to your doctor about what you can do to ease your breathing and your stress.

Use of stimulating medication can also cause sleeplessness. Talk to your doctor about your medication, and ask what you can do to control its effects during sleep.

Restless leg syndrome is an involuntary movement of the legs during sleep and is a relatively common cause of sleep disturbance in seniors, although its cause is unknown. It results in fragmented, poor-quality sleep. You may need an aid; your doctor may prescribe for a short period of time a sleeping pill such as a benzodiazepine. This may not halt the movement of your legs but should help you sleep through it, reducing the fragmentation of your sleep and improving its overall quality. See Restless Leg Syndrome, page 492, for more information.

When to call the doctor If you have a sleep difficulty that has lasted more than a couple of weeks and you cannot correct it yourself, talk to your doctor. It could be the result of a new medication you are taking or a symptom of depression or another medical condition. While many disturbances of sleep are transient and can be alleviated by one or more of the remedies described earlier, others can be rooted in serious medical conditions and should be evaluated. Work with your doctor to rule out or treat a serious disorder, such as depression, Alzheimer's disease, or diabetes as a cause of your sleep problems.

THE DISORDERS THAT CAUSE DEMENTIA

As we age, most of us experience some loss of short-term memory and some diminishment of the ability to learn or respond quickly. These changes usually develop imperceptibly, and most of us learn to work around them as they come on. True dementia is a progressive global decline in cognitive function (thinking and memory) that results in significant impairment. Many who suffer from it eventually become incapable of caring for themselves.

There is still much to be learned about causes and potential treatments for disorders that cause dementia, such as Alzheimer's disease. But there is also more hope today than there ever was, as well as real benefits to detecting dementia before individuals are severely impaired. Reversible causes of dementia—such as depression or metabolic disorders—may be identified and treated. Treatments that may temporarily improve memory and other functions can be instituted, but still no drug is available that will change the long-term outcome of dementia. Measures also can be taken to reduce the psychiatric manifestations, such as disruptive behavior or hallucinations, associated with some forms of dementia. Patients and their families can anticipate

AVOIDING DEPRESSION

There is much we do not understand about the illness called depression. Although it is frequently described as being due to a chemical imbalance within the brain, doctors do not know exactly what the imbalance is or how it occurs. What we do know is that persistent depression in an individual is a disease that must be diagnosed and treated to avoid the wide-ranging detrimental effects depression can have on health and well-being.

For seniors, it is essential to understand that depression is not an inevitable part of aging. Loss of loved ones, diminished strength, illness, and changes in lifestyle may be unavoidable in one's senior years, but they need not inevitably lead to full-blown depression. Most seniors will assimilate their losses as they occur and then move forward, renewing their intimate ties and their contact with the world. Others may remain depressed and isolated for months or even years and think it is normal. It is not.

If depression strikes, it should be viewed as a disease that can and should be treated and resolved with the help of medical professionals.

Research indicates that with support from family and friends, most seniors who experience depression unrelated to illness, such as Alzheimer's disease or multi-infarct dementia, can overcome it. Many effective treatments are available, including antidepressant medications that are quite safe and effective. Talk with your doctor if you feel depressed for more than a week or two—if you feel it's just not worth getting out of bed or that food no longer tastes good. There is no reason to live with illness that can be quite effectively treated.

Depression may also occur, especially in the elderly, without much sadness but rather with more nonspecific symptoms of fatigue, loss of energy and motivation, or other widespread physical complaints. You should report such symptoms to your doctor promptly, as this form of depression can also be treated effectively. ■

and prepare for problems that can arise as dementia progresses.

Seniors can also suffer from transient forms of decline of cognitive function. This is known as delirium and can be related to medication, illness, and other causes; see Delirium, below.

There are many different potential causes of dementia, including the following:

- Progressive, degenerative brain disease, such as Alzheimer's disease (see below and page 456).

- Small, multiple strokes that disable portions of the brain (see below and page 429).

- Depression, which may be associated with transient memory impairment but not progressive decline (see page 1223).

- Exposure to poisons (toxins), such as alcohol or drugs (this includes the mixing of too many prescription medications).

- Metabolic imbalances, such as those caused by a vitamin deficiency (B_{12}, for example) or thyroid disease.

- Central nervous system infections, caused by the herpes virus, the human immunodeficiency virus (HIV), or neurosyphilis. Neurosyphilis, though rare, is more common in seniors than is acquired immunodeficiency syndrome (AIDS), because syphilis can be asymptomatic and go undetected for decades. AIDS is not common in seniors, though incidence of AIDS in older people is increasing (see Chapter 21).

- Miscellaneous other causes, such as head injury, subdural hematoma (bleeding between the brain and the membrane that encases the brain), brain tumors, metastatic cancer (spread from other organs), and other illnesses (see Chapter 14).

Delirium Although it may seem like dementia, delirium is a transient form of mental dysfunction characterized by confusion. It is distinguished from true dementia by its rapid onset, fluctuating course, and usually short duration. True dementia typically has a gradual onset over months or years and is often progressive. Delirium usually lasts only hours or days, while dementia lasts much longer.

How can you distinguish between delirium and dementia?

Delirium has a rapid onset and is often characterized by slurring of speech and language that is incoherent, aimless, or disorganized. It may be accompanied by delusions and hallucinations—paranoia is possible—and by disorientation—a lack of understanding of time or place—as well as agitation and extreme irritability. A good example is delirium caused by alcohol intoxication.

Nearly any illness—including fever, infection, hypotension, or low blood pressure, or lack of oxygen in the bloodstream—can throw the chemistry of the brain sufficiently out of balance to cause delirium. Delirium can accompany relatively minor illness as well as quite serious illness; it can occur because of dehydration or be the prelude to a heart attack.

Delirium can also be caused by exposure to a toxic substance, such as the wrong dosage or wrong medication. Indeed, even the right medication in the right dose can cause disturbances in brain chemistry that can lead to delirium. According to the American Geriatrics Society, an unfortunate side effect of some medications taken by nursing home residents as well as seniors in the community is the possibility of delirium. To make matters even more difficult, chronic brain disorders such as Alzheimer's disease predispose patients to delirium from other causes, which is known as superimposed delirium. In fact, delirium is a very common, and often the only, manifestation of a serious underlying illness, such as pneumonia or a myocardial infarction, in a demented patient.

Alzheimer's disease Of all the disorders that cause dementia, probably none is more well known than Alzheimer's disease. Indeed, Alzheimer's disease is responsible for the largest number of cases of dementia in seniors, some 50 to 85 percent. If an individual with Alzheimer's disease lives long enough, then the disease will become full-blown. If not, it may never be discovered. Some estimates are that 50 percent of those over age 85 have a dementing disorder. For Alzheimer's disease, prevalence is about 2 percent at age 65, with a doubling every 5 years, to about 32 percent at age 85.

In its early stages, Alzheimer's disease can easily be overlooked. Patients and doc-

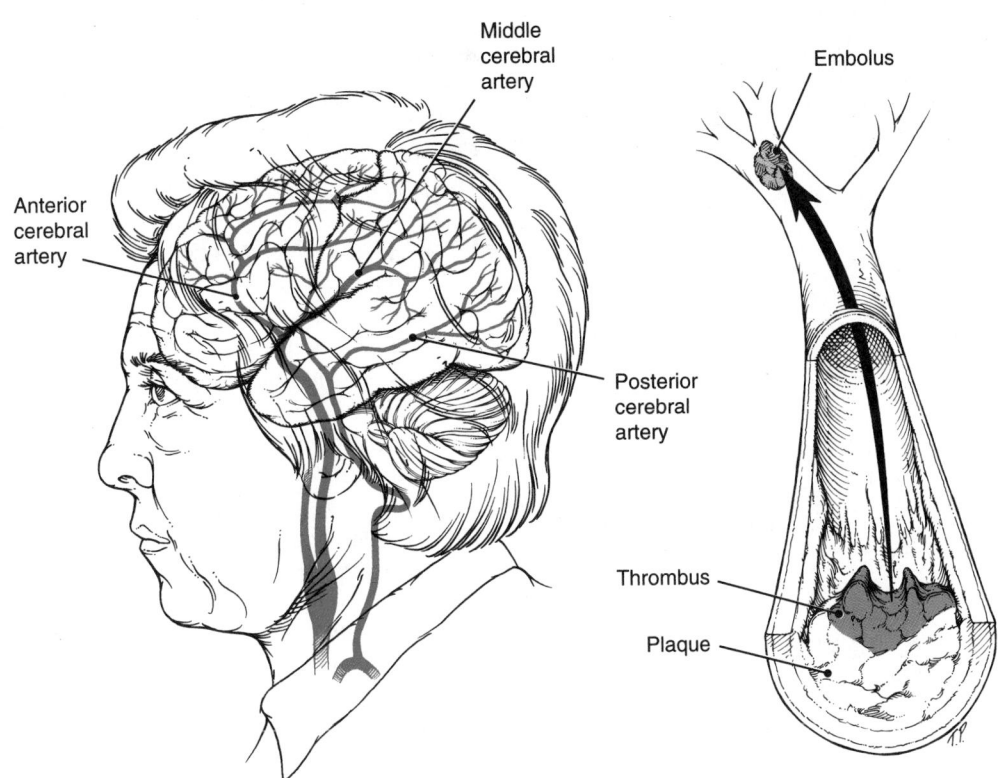

Anterior cerebral artery

Middle cerebral artery

Posterior cerebral artery

Embolus

Thrombus

Plaque

Mechanism of stroke. A stroke represents permanent damage to a section of the brain from an embolism, thrombus, or bleeding. Emboli typically form as blood clots in the heart and travel to the brain where they block a cerebral artery. Plaques (fatty material) form on the walls of blood vessels in the brain and can block the flow of blood when a clot (thrombus) forms on the plaques. The same process in the heart causes a heart attack.

tors alike may mistakenly attribute changes to normal aging. Other patients, fearing the label of Alzheimer's disease, may deliberately minimize symptoms. New treatments, however, offer hope that early detection can delay the onset of the most serious consequences. Recent research indicates that the disease probably has a long latent period of 10, 15, or even 30 years, during which the brain slowly but progressively deteriorates. There is as yet no cure and no way yet to change the eventual outcome, but there are many ways to help individuals who suffer from it. One of the new drugs recently approved that may help with memory problems is donepezil hydrochloride—Aricept. Many other drugs will be approved over the next several years. Even if memory cannot be repaired, associated symptoms can often be effectively treated. For example, the depression and insomnia that often accompany Alzheimer's disease can be alleviated using tricyclic antidepressants, which, unlike the newer antidepressants, can cause drowsiness. Hallucinations and delusions can be quite effectively suppressed using very small dosages of antipsychotic agents such as haloperidol (Haldol) or thioridazine (Mellaril).

Vascular or multi-infarct dementia

Multi-infarct dementia occurs when several small strokes (infarctions) impede or diminish the flow of blood (and therefore oxygen) to areas of the brain (see page 429). This loss of blood supply leads to the destruction of brain tissue and an ensuing loss of cognitive function. Early symptoms include temporary paralysis and speech difficulties. The main causes of strokes are atherosclerosis (arteries clogged by fatty deposits, or plaques), high blood pressure, and heart disease. These conditions can occur on their own or as a secondary result of diseases such as diabetes, or lifestyle choices such as smoking, and obesity.

After Alzheimer's disease, cerebrovascular disease is the most common cause of dementia. Multi-infarct dementia is slightly more common in men than women and most frequently occurs between the ages of 60 and 75. Not all strokes lead to dementia; this depends on whether the areas of the brain that govern cognitive function are affected.

Vascular dementia typically causes a stepwise degenerative decline: Each step is thought to correspond to a stroke, and

INFORMATION SOURCES FOR DEMENTIA-RELATED ILLNESS

- Alzheimer's Disease Education and Referral Center
  P.O. Box 8250
  Silver Spring, MD 20907
  Phone: (800) 438–4380

- Alzheimer's Association
  919 N. Michigan Ave., Suite 1000
  Chicago, IL 60611
  Phone: (800) 272–3900

- National Institute of Neurological Disorders and Stroke
  Building 31, Room 8A06
  9000 Rockville Pike
  Bethesda, MD 20892
  Phone: (301) 496–5751

- National Stroke Association
  300 E. Hampden Ave.,
  Suite 240
  Englewood, CO 80110
  Phone: (303) 762–9922

- Eldercare Locator Service
  Administration on Aging
  Phone: (800) 677–1116 ■

memory is usually affected first. Conversely, the progression of Alzheimer's disease is often more gradual, with varying rates of decline.

Alzheimer's disease cannot be prevented (as far as we know); however, the risk of stroke can be diminished. Discuss with your doctor whether you are at risk for stroke, and make appropriate lifestyle changes: Stop smoking, control hypertension if present, change your diet to include less saturated fat and high-calorie foods and more green vegetables and fruits.

Recent research offers hope for the future. By reversing blood flow in the area of the brain where the stroke occurred, doctors may be able to keep that segment of the brain nourished and dissolve the blockage, preventing or minimizing brain damage and reversing early signs of stroke. This treatment, however, depends on rapid recognition of the problem and immediate treatment. If you suspect someone is having a stroke, consult your doctor or get to the emergency room immediately.

Even if the early signs of stroke go away in a few minutes or hours, talk to your doctor as soon as possible in order to rule out or treat stroke or other serious illness. See Chapter 14 for more information on stroke.

VISUAL IMPAIRMENTS

As we age, many changes occur in the eye. The lens of the eye is made up of long-lived proteins that do not regenerate themselves. They can lose some of their clarity and some of their resilience. As a consequence, nearly all older people require eyeglasses to read. Tear ducts no longer are as productive. There can be some loss in the efficiency of the nerves that transmit visual signals to the brain.

As signals to the brain change or slow down, we can experience a slow but steady diminishing of what are known as static visual acuity (the ability to focus on fixed, or static, objects) and dynamic visual acuity (the ability to focus on moving, or dynamic, objects). Glasses can compensate for most of this loss, but many of us may need more time to sort out visual information, particularly with moving objects.

Like all age-related changes, these changes will vary from person to person depending on genetic heritage, disease, and environmental exposure. Eye protection is just as important to wear in the sunshine as skin protection is, so wear sunglasses with wide spectrum ultraviolet protection—the more of your visual field that is covered, the better.

Visual impairment may be slowly progressive or sudden and acute. It is important to investigate sudden changes in vision promptly to avoid their leading to other problems that can seriously impact your health. Because adaptation to the dark is significantly slower with age and the risk of some visual diseases, such as cataract, increases with age, driving at night may be more difficult and hazardous for seniors. Also, many falls and broken bones are related to visual difficulties; not seeing irregularities in sidewalks or walkways can cause falls. Be sure to have your vision checked regularly. If you suspect your vision is not as good as it was, see your doctor, and ask for a referral to an ophthalmologist.

Most visual problems in seniors are rooted in a few, particular causes: presbyopia, cataracts, macular degeneration, glaucoma, and diabetic retinopathy. See Chapter 15 for detailed information on all these conditions.

Presbyopia Presbyopia is the progressive difficulty in focusing on close objects due to a loss of resilience in the lens of the eye. It affects nearly everyone and begins as early as age 20, though it may not become noticeable until much later, and continues throughout life. It is unavoidable, but is correctable by eyeglasses, usually referred to as reading glasses.

Cataracts A cataract occurs when the lens of the eye becomes clouded. This happens slowly, with vision gradually diminishing. Only when a cataract is fully developed will eyesight be completely obstructed. You may notice that your night vision is diminished or that your vision is impaired in bright sunlight.

Generally, cataracts are treated by removing them surgically. This can usually be done as a simple outpatient procedure. Usually, lens implants, put in at the same time that the cataract is removed, will replace the original lens. Your ophthalmologist will perform the procedure on one eye at a time, sometimes years apart.

If you do not wish to have your cataracts surgically removed, or if because of your health, surgery is dangerous, glasses and contact lenses can be used, as can low vision aids, such as magnifying glasses, although none of the nonsurgical treatments are as effective as removal of the cataracts. If you are developing cataracts related to diabetes, you and your doctor and ophthalmologist will need to work together to monitor your retina to ensure that diabetic retinal changes are recognized early (see Type 1 Diabetes Mellitus, page 1174 and Type 2 Diabetes Mellitus, page 1179). Consistently using eyewear that protects your eyes from ultraviolet rays may also help halt the development or progression of cataracts.

Macular degeneration The macula is the central portion of the retina, and it receives light and sends it to the brain along the optic nerve as neural stimuli. The degeneration of the macula happens for unknown reasons and is characterized by loss of vision in the center of the eye.

There is no treatment to reverse macular degeneration, but many who experience

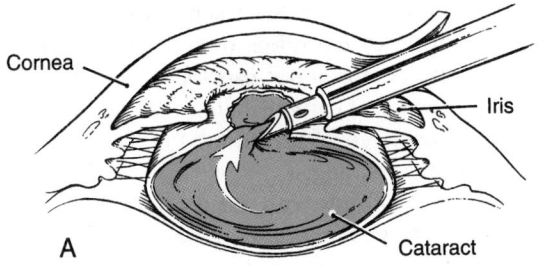

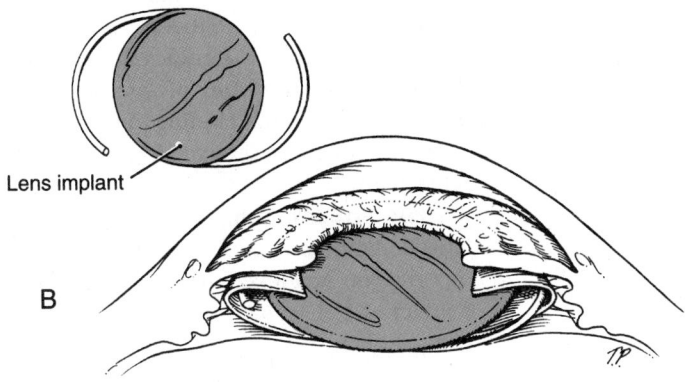

Cataract surgery. (A) Phacoemulsification. A probe, inserted through an incision on the edge of cornea, fragments the cataract with sound waves and suctions out the remains. (B) A plastic replacement lens is implanted and held in place by plastic extensions.

it can learn to work around it. Laser treatment is used to treat some cases, but the vision is usually not restored. Some people with this disorder can be classified as legally blind but still retain quite good peripheral vision (see page 531).

Glaucoma Glaucoma affects less than 5 percent of seniors, but can lead to significant loss of vision from damage to the optic nerve if not treated. It is characterized by increased pressure within the eye, which often goes unnoticed—you will not feel the increase in pressure—until it has affected vision. Visual screening in seniors should include pressure checks of both eyes.

Diabetic retinopathy Like all the complications of diabetes, diabetic retinopathy is caused by chronically high blood sugars. In any given ophthalmologist's office, fully half or even three-quarters of the patients are likely to have diabetes. If you have diabetes, you should work with your primary care doctor to control your blood sugar and blood pressure levels to preserve your vision, and be sure to see an ophthalmologist at least yearly for screening. The examination of the retina done by your primary care doctor is not capable of detecting the changes of early diabetes and should not be considered a substitute for a visit to the ophthalmologist.

Not only can diabetes contribute to cataracts, it can also cause a disease of the retina unique to diabetes, diabetic retinopathy. More often associated with the longevity of the diabetes than with the age of the individual, diabetic retinopathy nonetheless affects a significant number of seniors, who, by virtue of age, are more likely to have long-standing diabetes. See page 537 for more information on diabetic retinopathy.

For further information on vision problems common to seniors, or for information on how you or a loved one can obtain help, contact

- Better Vision Institute
  1800 N. Kent St., Suite 904
  Rosslyn, VA 22209
  Phone: (800) 424-8422

- National Eye Institute
  Information Office
  Building 31, Room 6A32
  Bethesda, MD 20892
  Phone: (301) 496-5248

- Lighthouse National Center for Vision and Aging
  111 E. 59th St.
  New York, NY 10022
  Phone: (212) 821-9200 (Voice)
  Phone: (212) 821-9713 (TT—text telephone)
  Phone: (800) 334-5497 (Voice/TT)

HEARING LOSS

As we age, the inner ear becomes less responsive, and there is a slow reduction in the numbers of nerve fibers within the hearing nerve. As these things happen, the ability to hear at upper and middle tones diminishes, as does the ability to distinguish speech sounds. It is not clear whether the changes that occur are due exclusively to the aging process or to a combination of factors, such as aging and exposure to loud noises. Loud noises can diminish hearing, and there is an accompanying decline in speech discrimination—or the ability to sort speech in noisy listening conditions.

Presbycusis is a pattern of hearing loss that occurs in seniors and is characterized by the slow but progressive loss of ability to hear tones at high and then high and middle frequencies. It occurs simultaneously in both ears and can lead to a diminishing ability to discriminate between the patterns of words.

Hearing disorders have many different causes, including the use of certain medications such as some antibiotics, medicines used in cancer chemotherapy, diuretics, and medications used for malaria. Hearing disorders other than presbycusis are divided into two overall classes: conductive and sensorineural hearing loss. A mixed hearing loss is the combination of these two disorders. For further information on specific hearing disorders, see Chapter 16.

Seniors who fail to recognize and treat their hearing loss are sometimes misperceived as showing early signs of dementia. They appear to be forgetful or appear oblivious to what is being said, when, in fact, they either could not hear what was said or misperceived the verbal message. Because hearing loss often occurs gradually and escapes notice, hearing assessment should be part of your annual health assessment. Fortunately, hearing loss can in many cases be corrected. There is little reason to simply accept hearing loss.

What you can do Many devices are available to assist those with impaired hearing to improve their communication abilities and make their lives easier.

Hearing aids Every year hearing aids get smaller and more sophisticated. Once large devices that amplified all sounds, hearing aids today are quite small and can filter sound through sophisticated electronics. If you have trouble hearing, consult an otolaryngologist or an audiologist about the benefits of hearing aids.

Most hearing specialists recommend that, because of the differing requirements of each person with a hearing impairment, your hearing aid be bought on a 30-day trial basis so that you get the assistance that is right for you and so that you do not purchase a device that is unsuitable.

Devices to assist people with hearing impairments As helpful as hearing aids can be, there are times when other assistance is needed. For example, many hearing aids can produce feedback when used with a telephone receiver, so it is better to use a hearing aid that is fitted with a telephone coil (an inexpensive feature) or a telephone amplifier.

- *Telephone amplifiers* are available in portable, battery-powered models as well as built into your telephone.

- *TDD (telecommunication device for the deaf)/TT (text telephone) machines* are also available for the deaf. These are based on the teletype machines of old and are available in many models and have screens on which you can read incoming conversation. Some print out. Unlike fax machines, they allow two-way communication.

- *Personal television and radio amplifiers* allow you to listen to the television or radio with the volume turned up so that only you can hear.

- *Doorbells, smoke alarms, and telephone-ring devices.* As the ability to hear high frequencies is diminished, it may become difficult to hear doorbells, smoke alarms, or the telephone. Specially designed substitutes replace high-pitched bells with lower frequency sounds that will fall within your hearing range. Others use a visual or tactile alert, such as a flashing light, fan, or a vibrator.

- *Personal amplifications systems* can help you sort out sounds when there is a single speaker or sound source, as during a lecture or watching television.

Some people may feel ashamed of their hearing loss or do not want to think of themselves as deaf, so they just try to manage with their hearing loss. This can lead to frustration, miscommunication, and feelings of isolation. There is no reason not to use the means that are available to help overcome your hearing difficulty. Talk to your doctor about the means of assistance that may be helpful to you. For more information on assistive devices, consult your yellow pages, and see Chapter 16.

Information on hearing loss and assistance is also available from

- Better Hearing Institute
  P.O. Box 180

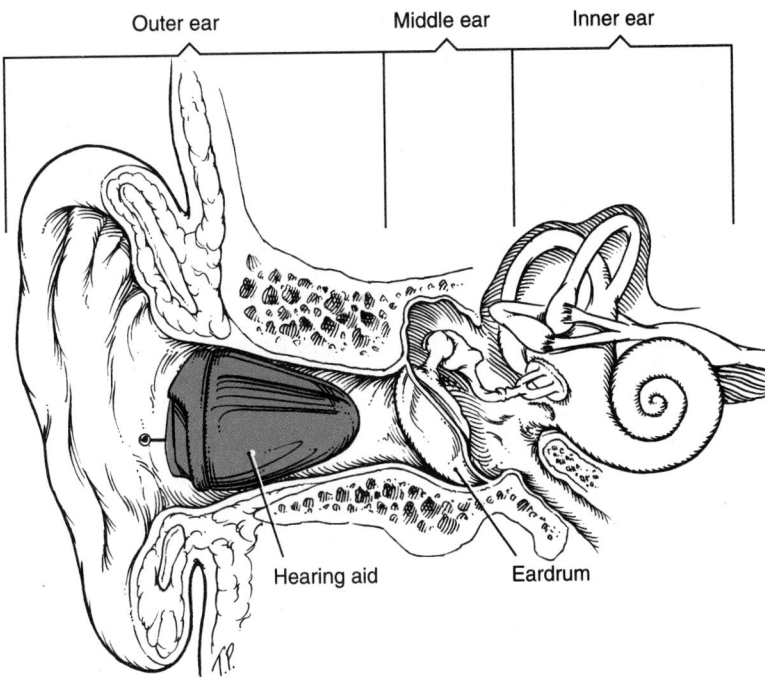

Outer ear   Middle ear   Inner ear

Hearing aid   Eardrum

Three divisions of the ear. Hearing aids, placed in the outer ear canal, amplify sound waves and transmit them to the eardrum (tympanic membrane). The middle ear contains the ear bones (ossicles) and the inner ear converts sensations of the body's movements and vibration from sound into nerve impulses.

Washington, DC 20013
Phone: (800) HEARWELL (432-79355)

- Self-Help for Hard of Hearing, Inc.
  7910 Woodmont Ave., Suite 1200
  Bethesda, MD 20614
  Phone: (301) 657-2248

Caregivers and Caregiving

There may come a time for each of us when we lose a significant enough amount of function that we need care. The situation may be permanent, or for those recovering from surgery or illness, for example, it may simply be temporary. Ideally, each of us will, while still in perfect health with all function intact, set out in writing the kinds of care we want and from whom we would ideally like to have it, as well as set aside funds for that potential rainy day.

Even if we do not have such parameters set down before we need care, there are still many options when we do need care. There are many levels of care, from dropping in and

RESOURCE INFORMATION FOR CAREGIVERS AND CARE RECEIVERS

Caregivers and care receivers should look into resources that exist within the community. To assess the services available in your area, you can start at your local library or health department. Most cities and counties have offices on aging that can provide you with information. Veterans' organizations can be helpful, as can your local hospital or senior center.

Like many other of life's responsibilities, caregiving can have its rewards as well as its challenges, and support groups can be valuable resources of wisdom, help, and information. Contact your local hospital, senior center, library, or office on aging to locate a support group in your area. Places of worship may also be able to offer information.

If you cannot find adequate assistance for your caregiving or care receiving needs, the following organizations may be able to provide more comprehensive information:

- Alzheimer's Association
  919 North Michigan Ave., Suite 100
  Chicago, IL 60611–1676
  Phone: (800) 272–3900

- American Association of Homes and Services for the Aging
  901 E St., NW
  Washington, DC 20004–2937
  Phone: (202) 508–9420

- American Cancer Society
  1599 Clifton Rd., NE
  Atlanta, GA 30329
  Phone: (404) 320–3333

- American Diabetes Association,
  National Center
  P.O. Box 25757
  1660 Duke St.
  Alexandria, VA 22314
  Phone: (703) 549–1500

- American Heart Association
  727 Greenville Ave.
  Dallas, TX 75231–4596
  Phone: (214) 373–6300

- National Association for Home Care
  519 C St., NE
  Washington, DC 20002
  Phone: (202) 547–7424

- National Association of Professional Geriatric Care Managers
  1604 North Country Club Dr.
  Tucson, AZ 85716
  Phone: (602) 881–8008

- National Institute on Adult Daycare, National Council on Aging
  409 Third St., SW, Second Floor
  Washington, DC 20024
  Phone: (202) 479–1200

- National Institute on Aging
  P.O. Box 8057
  Gaithersburg, MD 20898–8057
  Phone: (301) 496–1752

- National Citizens' Coalition for Nursing Home Reform
  1224 M St., NW, Suite 301
  Washington, DC 20005
  Phone: (202) 393–2018

- National Hospice Organization
  1901 North Moore St., Suite 901
  Arlington, VA 22209
  Phone: (800) 658–8898

- National Meals on Wheels Foundation
  2675 44th St., SW, #305
  Grand Rapids, MI 49509
  Phone: (800) 999–6262 ■

checking on the individual to make sure her needs are being met, to assisted living, to nursing home residence. Most seniors do not need aggressive, round-the-clock care, and most people who need care are provided for by family members. According to the American Association for Retired Persons, at least 80 percent of caregivers for seniors are family members. But there are times when family members cannot do everything that needs to be done and times when family simply is not available to help. Outside the family, many options are available, and these are likely to increase as the numbers of Americans over age 65 increase. More caregiving options tend to be available in urban areas than in rural areas, and options will vary according to the area in which you live. For more information on caregiving, see Chapter 34.

TYPES OF CARE AVAILABLE

Depending on where you live, your economic circumstances, and your needs, the following basic types of care may be available. For more information on care both in the home and outside of the home, see Chapter 34.

- *"Gateway" assistance:* provides routine check-in with you—by phone or visit or both—if you are mostly self-sufficient, to ensure that you are getting along well.

- *Chore and personal care:* can assist with household chores, including hygiene and perhaps meal preparation.

- *Meals-On-Wheels/meal delivery:* meal delivery can be arranged as a temporary service until an individual who is mostly self-sufficient is well enough to resume meal preparation.

- *Home maintenance/home sharing:* maintenance services can be arranged if you are no longer able to perform such tasks as yard work, putting up storm windows, and minor home repairs. Such tasks, as well as meal preparation and hygiene assistance, can be arranged in a home-share setup, in which an able individual becomes roommates with you in exchange for services.

- *Senior day care:* an option available to families who want to care for their loved ones but must work during the day. The levels of service in such a setting can be varied, depending on the needs of the senior as well as the needs of the family. For example, caregivers may be able to arrange for overnight or weekend stays (respite care) if they must be out of town and cannot provide the care they normally would. The emphasis in these programs is socialization, hobbies, and health maintenance (including rehabilitative care).

- *Rehabilitative care:* includes programs for helping stroke survivors regain motor and language control, or helping people recuperating from surgery, a fracture, or other temporary disability regain their mobility and independence.

- *Stroke veteran help:* stroke survivors who are recuperating may receive help from individuals who have recovered from strokes themselves.

- *Hospice care:* available in many communities for the terminally ill, not just for cancer but for any fatal disease. Staff in these settings are medically trained but also trained as social workers to provide physical and spiritual care for the dying and their families.

3

PART THREE

First Aid *and* Emergency Care

THIRTEEN

First Aid and Emergency Care

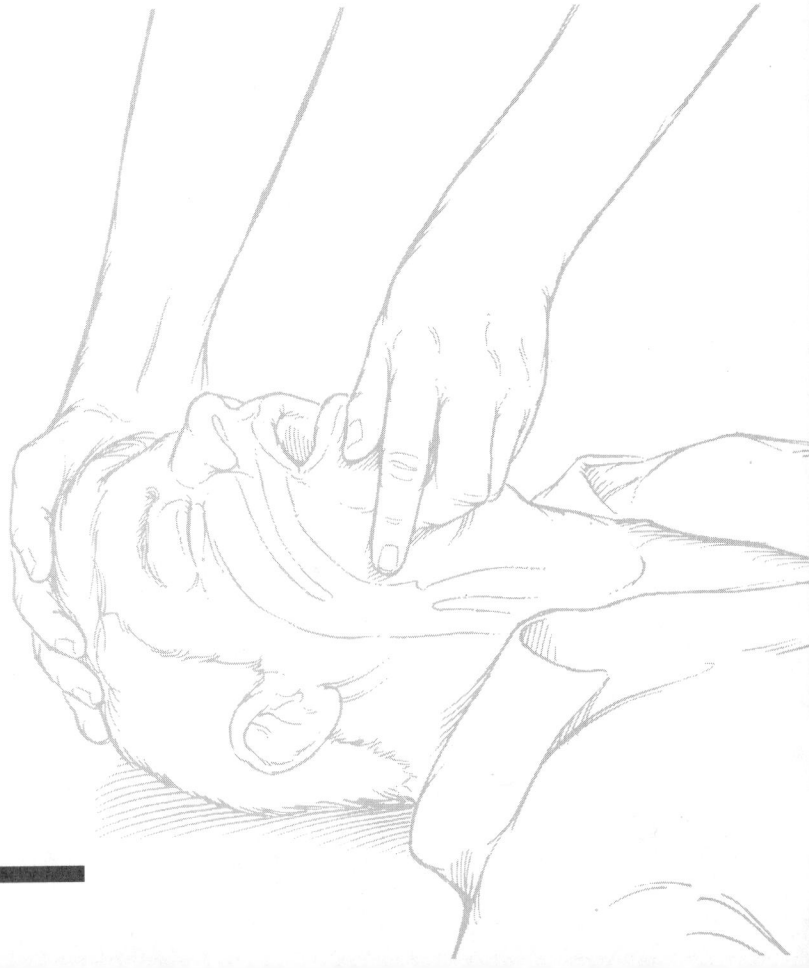

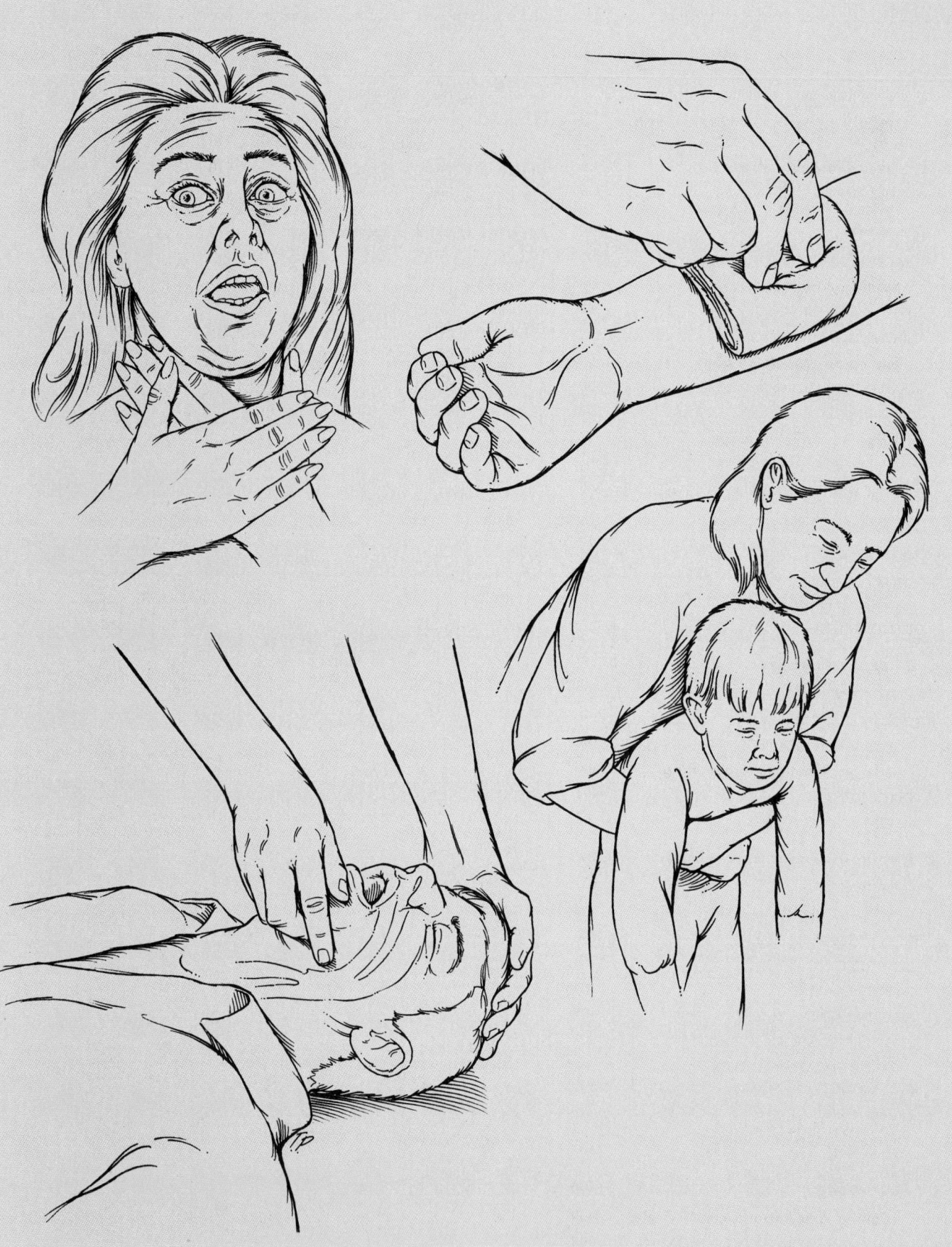

FIRST AID AND EMERGENCY CARE

Be Prepared

First aid is the first link in the chain of survival. First aid can facilitate the care provided by Emergency Medical Services (EMS), emergency doctors, and the hospital. The best time to study first aid is before the need arises. If you have studied first aid in the past, be sure to review the information to periodically refresh and upgrade your skills. A swift response to a sudden injury or illness can mean the difference between life and death, a saved limb and a lost limb, and a quick recovery and long rehabilitation.

It is virtually impossible to prepare in detail for every potential emergency. Setting is a defining factor in an emergency. A deep cut that occurs on the job may be relatively simple to manage if you happen to work near a hospital. The same injury on the top of a mountain or on a boat whose motor has stalled will call for an entirely different plan of action.

However, there are basic guidelines to follow in any situation. While no book can take the place of first aid training and lifesaving courses, this chapter aims to provide you with tools to both assess emergency situations and to address them effectively. Emergencies can be unpredictable and variable; you may need to refer to several different kinds of treatment for a single situation. For this reason, cross-references have been provided to assist you in quickly finding appropriate management strategies for different kinds of injuries (see Where to Find It Fast, above).

FIRST AID BASICS

Get first aid training The time to learn first aid is not during an emergency but before one arises. Since most everyone will be faced with an emergency, everyone should have some first aid training.

Know your first aid ABCs ABC stands for airway, breathing, and circulation, and represents the rule of thumb for all emergencies (see Resuscitation ABCs, page 357). No matter what other injuries a person has, if he is choking, if he has stopped breathing, or if his heart has stopped beating, he will not survive. Always make sure a victim does not have a blocked airway, is breathing, and has a pulse.

WHERE TO FIND IT FAST

Do not panic In emergency situations, panic can turn would-be rescuers into victims and make difficult situations impossible (see Precautions Against Infectious Disease, page 354). Resolve to think clearly, rationally, and coolly. If you feel your emotions getting out of control, stop for a moment and refocus on the situation at hand. Find the internal resources not to panic.

In rendering first aid, there are particular dangers associated with particular situations. In a water emergency, for example, how do you rescue someone without drowning yourself? These kinds of situational precautions are addressed in their specific sections within this chapter. There are, however, general precautions that you can take to avoid contracting bloodborne and other infectious diseases when you are administering first aid (see Precautions Against Infectious Disease, page 354).

Do not try to be heroic Although each of us would probably like to become the person who saved the day, real heroism is often more a case of knowing what not to do than of performing heroic feats. Know your limitations and be able to evaluate situations

353

PRECAUTIONS AGAINST INFECTIOUS DISEASE

Do not let worries about disease stop you from being a Good Samaritan; only a very tiny percentage of people who administer first aid ever become ill from doing so. Still, the following precautions are sensible and relatively easy.

- Avoid getting blood, vomit, or other bodily fluids on you. Generally, unless you have broken skin, you will not contract a blood-borne illness, such as human immunodeficiency virus (HIV), hepatitis B virus (HBV), or hepatitis viruses A or C from direct contact with blood. Still, it is wise to keep several pairs of disposable latex gloves in your first aid kit and to use them when rendering first aid. You can be immunized against HBV; however, there is no vaccine or cure for HIV.

- Improvise another barrier if latex gloves are not available—a plastic bag, for example—as long as it does not prevent you from rendering first aid.

- Keep open wounds covered with proper dressings or bandages whenever possible.

- When possible, use a one-way barrier device when administering artificial respiration.

- There are other infectious diseases, such as tuberculosis (TB), that are virtually impossible to protect against; these you can even get on a bus or walking down the street.

- If you are exposed to blood or other bodily fluids:

  - Wash vigorously as soon as practical with soap and water. Keep alcohol swabs or other moist wipes in your first aid kit and use them to clean your own skin as well as the victim's wounds.

  - Report your exposure to EMS personnel and request relevant information on the health of the victim.

  - See your doctor if you are concerned that you might have been exposed to an infectious disease. ■

FIRST AID SUPPLIES

When purchasing a first aid kit or assembling your own, there are certain basic things you should make sure you have. You can add more, but you should have at least the following, which can be used in a wide array of emergencies:

Home

Bandage Supplies

- Adhesive strips in various sizes

- Butterfly bandages

- Elastic (Ace) bandages

- Adhesive tape

- Rolled gauze for bandaging or for holding other bandages, such as gauze pads, in place

- Gauze pads, 4 × 4 in., sterile, and individually wrapped. Smaller gauze pads are also useful, but the 4 × 4 in. size can be folded for smaller wounds.

- Cotton balls, sterile

- Eye patches, sterile

All your supplies should be sterile. Do not use cotton balls you would buy for makeup removal. If you break open a package, replace it with a new one.

Tools

- Scissors, blunt-tipped for cutting bandages

- Tweezers

- Thermometer. Easy-to-use digital thermometers are now available for less than $10 and are safer in emergency situations than glass thermometers.

General Supplies

- Emergency blanket. A plastic-foil space blanket is good to include even if you have plenty of other blankets in the house.

- Cotton-tipped swabs

- Disposable latex gloves

- Flashlight. Batteries must be periodically checked and replaced.

- Candles and matches. Lighters should not be used because they can be explosive and may lose their fuel over time.

- Paper cups

- Bottled water, in case an emergency occurs during power or water outage

- Roll of duct tape

- Moleskin and mole foam, for burns

Medications

Keep only sealed, unused medications in your first aid kit. Try to purchase medications with similar expiration dates. Twice a year—for example, when the time changes from standard to daylight savings—check the medications in your first aid kit to make sure they have not expired. (You can do this at the same time you check the smoke alarm batteries in your home.) This is also a good time to check the batteries of the flashlight and to replace any supplies that might have been partially used. ▶

▶ • Activated charcoal, in case of poisoning

• Ipecac syrup, in case of poisoning. Only use ipecac syrup when instructed by your local poison control center.

• Antihistamine, such as diphenhydramine (Benadryl)

• Antibiotic cream or ointment

• Antiseptic spray with anesthetic

• Antiseptic wipes, individually packaged, or antiseptic solution to use with cotton balls

• Sterile saline for eye wash

You can keep your first aid kit in any kind of box you find convenient. Put the telephone numbers for your family doctor, your local poison control center, and any other appropriate emergency numbers on the front of the box in easy-to-read print. Make sure that everyone in your household knows where the first aid kit is and that first aid supplies and tools are to be used only in an emergency.

Automobile

Exactly what you keep in your car will depend on whether you live in a climate with severe winters or no winters at all. In any climate a blanket is necessary. It can be used a number of different ways including for warmth in cases of shock, as a pillow, an immobilization device, or as a stretcher. If you live in an area with severe winters, keep a couple of candy bars, extra wool socks, extra blankets, and boots in your car during the winter months in case an emergency occurs during a snow storm.

Bandages see under Home, on page 354

General Supplies

• Blanket

• Cotton-tipped swabs

• Disposable latex gloves

• Face mask or face shield, in case the victim vomits when receiving cardiopulmonary resuscitation (CPR)

• Flashlight

• Candles and matches

• Roll of duct tape

• Moleskin and mole foam, for burns

• Bottled water

• Pencil and pad of paper

Medications

• Antihistamine, such as diphenhydramine (Benadryl)

• Antibiotic cream or ointment

• Antiseptic spray with anesthetic

• Antiseptic wipes, individually packaged, or antiseptic solution to use with cotton balls

• Sterile saline solution for eye wash ∎

clear-headedly. Jumping into the water to save a drowning victim when you do not know how to swim may seem heroic in the heat of the moment, but few things are more foolish.

Evaluate the scene Try to ascertain what happened. Sounds, odors, or unusual sights can help you determine the source of the emergency, how the victims might be injured, and how you can best help. In some cases, it may be simple—a child has put his arm through a window and is bleeding. Other situations may be more difficult to evaluate—an automobile accident has taken place and there is confusion, smoke, and blaring car horns; or an otherwise busy factory is suddenly completely silent.

Determine whether it is safe to act. For example, if victims are overcome by gas or fumes, or injured by electrical equipment, do not risk the same injuries to yourself. Notice how many people are involved and try to judge the relative seriousness of their

injuries. Often, those who are most seriously injured may be unconscious or quiet. Small children may not make any noise at all.

Are there others you can ask for help? If someone else can summon help, send him unless he is better trained at first aid than you are. The sooner EMS is called, the sooner trained help will arrive (see Calling EMS, page 357).

Keep a first aid kit and fire extinguisher in your home and car Being able to implement first aid often requires having the right tools. It is always better to have a first aid kit and no emergency than to have an emergency and no first aid kit. Having the right supplies on hand when a first aid situation arises can often mean the difference between quick, safe treatment and panic, delay, and infection. Every home and automobile should have first aid supplies. The supplies should be kept in a single, central location where they can be easily accessed all at the same time should an emergency arise. Most homes have some

FIRST AID AND THE LAW

Duty to Act

Certain jobs require us to render first aid whether we want to at the moment or not, such as lifeguard, schoolteacher, sports coach, and baby-sitter. This job-related requirement is known as the "duty to act"; if you do not act, you can be found legally liable. There are other relationships that also carry a duty to act, such as parent, driver, and pilot. When a person has assumed responsibility for other people's lives, that person must act if an emergency arises.

Good Samaritan Laws

Most individuals who provide first aid do not get sued and negligence is rarely found even when suits are brought against a person who tried to rescue someone in an emergency. To address this issue most states have enacted what are known as Good Samaritan laws to protect would-be rescuers from becoming the object of lawsuits. Good Samaritan laws are generally based on the following two points.

- Have you obtained permission, when possible, to render first aid?

- Have you acted as a *reasonable* and *prudent* person would under the same conditions?

The question then becomes what is meant by "reasonable and prudent." The following guidelines can help. To find out more about the Good Samaritan laws in your state, contact your local library.

- If the victim is conscious and rational, ask permission to provide help; however, someone who is suicidal, for example, would not be considered rational by a reasonable and prudent person.

- Never move a victim unless his life would be endangered if you did not move him.

- Summon EMS yourself or have someone else summon EMS as soon as possible after arriving at the scene.

- Once you have started first aid, do not stop until someone more qualified—such as a doctor, registered nurse, or EMS technician—arrives and takes over, or unless continuing to give first aid endangers your life.

Although it is important to know your emotional and physical limitations before initiating first aid, do not allow the possibility that you could be sued to prevent you from acting responsibly. If you ask permission and act reasonably, Good Samaritan immunity will generally protect you. ■

first aid supplies scattered about, but medications may be in one place and bandages in another. Take some time to organize your first aid supplies (see page 354).

Use your resources Tapping available resources can often mean the difference between life and death. Using your resources also means improvising. For example, in a fire, a wet towel or piece of cloth wrapped around your nose and mouth can help filter some of the smoke from the air you breathe into your lungs.

BEGIN TO ACT

Before you begin to act in an emergency assess the situation as calmly as you can and formulate a basic plan of action.

Always check the ABCs: Airway—is the victim's airway clear? Breathing—is the victim breathing? Circulation—does the victim have a pulse? The ABCs are indicators of basic functions necessary to sustain life (see Resuscitation ABCs, page 357).

If there is more than one victim, you should treat the most seriously injured person first. This may be difficult to judge;

someone screaming in pain may not be as seriously injured as someone who is unconscious, and vice versa. All you can do is make your best judgment based on the ABCs and begin to act.

If the victim is conscious, tell him your name and ask permission to help. If the victim appears to be unconscious, lean close to him, tap his shoulder, and ask loudly "Do you need help?" If there is no response, check the ABCs. Look for a medical identification bracelet, necklace, or tag on the victim.

If there is only one person involved, treat that person's most serious injury first. Without medical training and equipment, it is often difficult to know which injury is most serious, particularly if the victim is unconscious. Your job is to constantly monitor the ABCs and use your best judgment in deciding which injury needs the most immediate treatment. (see Which Injury Is Most Serious?, page 357).

If you have access to this book, consult Where to Find It Fast on page 353 and turn to the appropriate section for specifics on particular injuries.

Continue rendering first aid until help arrives or the victim recovers.

RESUSCITATION ABCs

ABC—airway, breathing, circulation—is the rule of thumb for all emergencies. If the airway, breathing, or circulation are impaired any other first aid efforts will be useless. Check the ABCs first.

Airway Is the victim's airway clear? Is there any obstruction blocking the victim's breathing? An obstruction may be anything from the victim's tongue to an inhaled foreign body such as food, dentures, or toys.

Breathing Is the victim breathing? Put your ear close to the victim's mouth and nose. Observe the victim's chest by sight or touch to see if it rises and falls. If the victim is not breathing, open the airway and initiate artificial respiration (see Cardiopulmonary Resuscitation, page 361). If the victim is only breathing weakly, make sure the airway is open.

If a victim is not breathing and if you have reason to suspect a neck injury, do not move the victim's head or neck. If at all possible, attempt artificial respiration without moving the victim. If this is not possible, see Moving a Victim of Suspected Spinal Cord Injury, page 369. For victims who do not appear to have a head or neck injury, open the airway following these steps:

1. Roll the victim gently onto his back, making sure that you support his head and neck, as well as any injured areas.

2. Use the chin lift maneuver to open the airway initially (see illustration page 362). Place one hand on the victim's fore-head. Place the fingers of the other hand beneath the victim's chin. Without closing his mouth, simultaneously lift his chin with your fingers and tilt his head back with your hand. Keep the victim's head in this position.

3. Check again for breathing. If the victim is not breathing, initiate artificial respiration (see Cardiopulmonary Resuscitation, page 361).

Circulation Does the victim have a pulse? A pulse means that blood is circulating in the body and to the brain. If the victim is unconscious and not moving, check to see if he has a pulse. To find the pulse, press your index finger gently against the portion of the neck of the victim where the carotid artery travels from the head into the chest. With your index finger and second finger, locate the victim's Adam's apple, then gently draw your fingers toward you into the groove in the side of the neck. If the victim has no pulse, begin CPR immediately (see Cardiopulmonary Resuscitation, page 361).

In an emergency situation, however, it can be very difficult for an inexperienced person to determine whether an unconscious victim has a pulse or not, which may result in the inappropriate interruption or cessation of CPR when a person needs it. Because of this, current thinking holds that if a victim is unconscious, not breathing, and not arousable, CPR should be given. The danger of receiving CPR when a pulse is present is minimal. ■

CALLING EMS

To summon EMS in an emergency, call 911. No matter where you are in the United States, calling 911 will trigger the closest available help.

This national standard emergency number works from cellular phones as well as home, business, and pay phones. Even if you are in an area distant from your cellular phone carrier, dialing "911+send" will bring the help nearest you. The call is always toll free.

When you call 911, try to have as much information as possible for the emergency dispatcher who answers the phone and try to supply it as calmly as you can. Having to repeat yourself will only cause delays.

- Know where you are. Give the address or relative location on a highway—nearest cross street or exit. If you are at a pay telephone with a number listed on it, give the number to the dispatcher.

- Be as descriptive as possible about what happened, how many people are injured, approximate ages of the injured, particularly if there are very young children or senior citizens involved, the nature of the injuries, and how long ago the injuries happened. The dispatcher may ask what seems like a lot of questions when you feel you should be hurrying back to the victims. Answer them. Many times a 911 dispatcher will be able to walk you through first aid steps that you do not know.

- Do not hang up the telephone unless the dispatcher tells you to hang up. If you have left a victim alone, inform the dispatcher and ask what you should do. In most cases, the emergency dispatchers will be able to help you more if you stay on the line. If you are at home or using a cellular phone, the dispatcher may be able to guide you through treating the victim. If you are in a remote area, EMS personnel can use the signal from the cell phone to locate you. *Do not* hang up.

Ask how long it will take for help to arrive. ■

WHICH INJURY IS MOST SERIOUS?

The most serious injury is the most immediately life-threatening. ABC injuries—injuries that involve the airway, breathing, and circulation—pose the greatest threat to survival and should be given priority over other injuries (see above).

If ABC functions are okay, evaluate other injuries as best you can. Is the victim bleeding severely? After injury that affects the airway, breathing, or circulation, bleeding is often the most life-threatening injury.

Has the victim injured his head? If there is no bleeding but the victim has a head injury, there is a risk of accompanying spinal cord injury; immobilizing the victim may be the most important thing you can do. ■

Choking

Choking occurs when breathing is obstructed because the airway has become blocked by a piece of food or other object. The victim may cough or gag in an attempt to dislodge the obstruction. The treatment for choking is essentially the same for most adults and children but is modified for infants, obviously pregnant women, and people who are obese.

There are several ways to recognize that someone is choking. A choking victim:

- Will usually display the universal signal for choking: both hands grasped at the throat, see illustration below

- Usually cannot speak

- May be able to breathe only weakly

- May make snoring, clucking, or high-pitched sounds

- May convulse

- May begin to turn blue in the face or markedly pale

- May faint from lack of oxygen

To remove the blockage, perform the Heimlich maneuver (see below). If you are not succeeding in clearing the airway or are not sure that the foreign body has been

A choking victim often grasps both hands at the throat. The victim may also become unable to speak, develop a blue face, or faint.

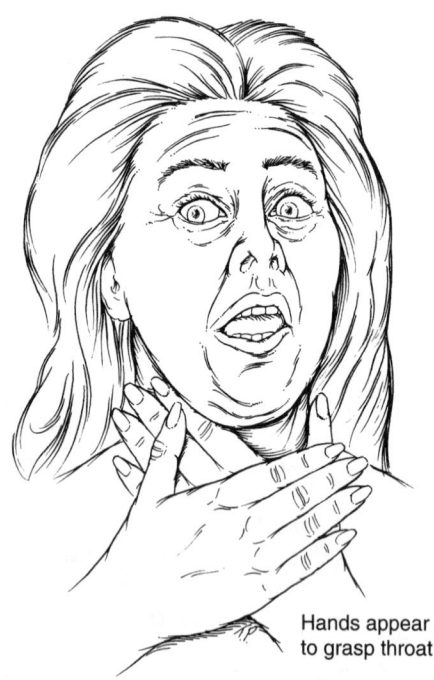

Hands appear
to grasp throat

completely removed, summon EMS. Emergency dispatchers will decide if the victim needs to receive an emergency airway-opening procedure or should be taken to the hospital. It is important to make certain that the victim's airway has been completely cleared and that none of the foreign body has become lodged in the lungs or the bronchial tubes. Aspirating, or breathing in, a foreign object many cause serious complications including a potentially deadly form of pneumonia.

If the choking victim lost consciousness or went without air for more than a few seconds, summon EMS. The victim needs to be evaluated for complications of loss of oxygen, which include potential brain damage. As a matter of course, call EMS if the victim was a child or senior, even if the obstruction was successfully removed.

THE HEIMLICH MANEUVER

The principal treatment for choking in adults and children is the Heimlich maneuver. The Heimlich maneuver is *not* performed on infants. Just below the lungs, right about at the bottom of the ribs, is the diaphragm muscle that expands and contracts the lungs. The Heimlich maneuver helps the diaphragm forcefully push the obstruction out of the airway, allowing the victim to begin breathing. *Never practice the Heimlich maneuver on yourself or another person.*

Heimlich maneuver for a conscious adult or child 1 year old and over First, obtain permission. Then, remain calm and follow the steps below.

1. Approach the victim from behind.
2. "Hug" the victim below the ribs; do not grasp the ribs.
3. Place one hand just above the victim's navel and make a fist with your thumb pointing inwards.
4. Firmly take hold of your fist with your other hand.
5. Using both hands, thrust the fist inward towards you and upwards. Each abdominal thrust should be sharp and distinct. Do not be timid; you are trying to dislodge a stuck object. However, if the victim is a child use more gentle thrusts to avoid injury.

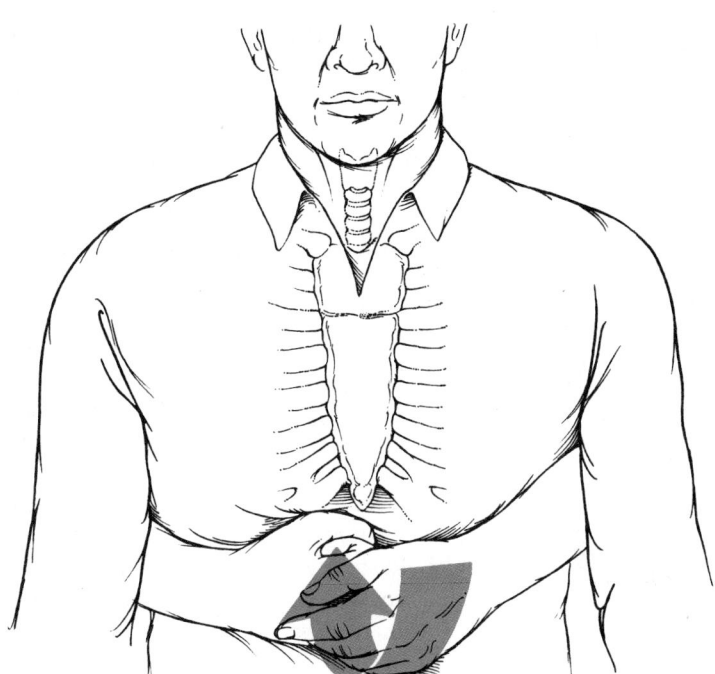

In the Heimlich maneuver, the rescuer's arms are wrapped tightly around the victim's waist from behind, above the navel, with one hand grabbing the other. The fist is then thrust inward and upwards five times in quick succession.

6. Repeat the inward-upward thrust five times in quick succession.

7. If the victim's airway has not cleared and he is still not breathing, evaluate your technique and repeat five quick inward-upward thrusts.

8. Repeat the cycle of five inward-upward thrusts until:
   - The obstruction is coughed out *or*
   - The victim loses consciousness (see below).
   - You are replaced by someone more highly trained than you, such as EMS personnel

Heimlich maneuver for an unconscious adult or child 1 year old and over Call EMS immediately if the victim is unconscious or loses consciousness before coughing up the obstruction. Position the victim on his back, supporting his head and neck, and use the chin lift-head tilt maneuver to open his airway (see Resuscitation ABCs, page 357). After you have tilted his head, perform a careful finger sweep (on adults only) and then attempt to initiate breathing. If airflow cannot be established after attempts to reposition the airway, initiate the Heimlich maneuver.

SWALLOWED OBJECTS

All children go through an oral phase, when their main contact with the world is through their mouths. During this time, usually in the toddler years, it is not uncommon for children to swallow small objects such as buttons, coins, and pieces of toys. Many of these objects will pass through your child without harm. Even though he will probably pass it uneventfully, if you suspect your child has swallowed a coin or other smooth object, it is wise to consult your doctor.

If an object becomes lodged in your child's throat it may cause choking and you may have to perform the Heimlich maneuver (see above). If your child shows signs of an object lodged in his throat but is not choking—symptoms may include difficulty swallowing, vomiting, and abdominal pain—contact your doctor immediately or take the child to the emergency room.

Never reach down the child's throat unless choking occurs; this could force the object deeper and cause it to lodge more firmly.

Sometimes children swallow objects with jagged edges that can damage the gastrointestinal or upper digestive tract, or poisonous objects such as button batteries that are potentially lethal. These kinds of objects may have to be surgically removed. Your child may not be able to communicate to you exactly what he has swallowed. Seek immediate medical attention if you suspect that your child swallowed a battery, because batteries can emit a toxic chemical. Although the battery may pass through your child uneventfully, do not wait for symptoms—which may include vomiting, abdominal pain, tenderness of the abdominal area, and fever—to appear. Contact your doctor as soon as possible or take your child to the emergency room. Do not try to induce vomiting. ■

The Heimlich maneuvers for adults and children are similar (see illustration, page 359), but less force is used on a child.

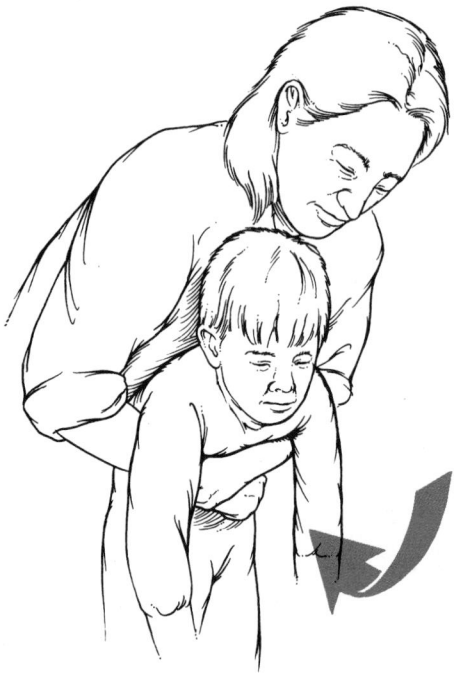

1. Position yourself over the victim, your knees on the ground, straddling his legs.
2. Place the heel of one hand in the center of the victim's abdomen, above the navel but well below the ribs.
3. Place your other hand on top of the hand resting on the abdomen.
4. Push inward and upward against the abdomen. Each abdominal thrust should be sharp and distinct. Do not be timid; you are trying to dislodge a stuck object. However, if the victim is a child use more gentle thrusts to avoid injury.
5. Repeat the thrust five times, keeping your hands in contact with the victim throughout the maneuver.
6. After each cycle of thrusts, perform a finger sweep of the mouth to remove any object that the thrusts may have dislodged. A finger sweep should be done carefully; exercise caution when inspecting the mouth in order to avoid relodging a dislodged object. Never perform a finger sweep on small children.
7. Repeat the cycle of five inward-upward thrusts until:

- The obstruction is coughed out *or*
- You are replaced by someone more highly trained than you, such as EMS personnel

Modified Heimlich maneuver for an obviously pregnant woman or an obese adult When a woman who is obviously pregnant or an obese adult is choking, use chest thrust instead of abdominal thrusts.

1. The victim should either be standing backed up against a wall or other flat surface, or be lying down, in which case your knees should straddle the victim.
2. Place the heel of one hand against the victim's breastbone, the place where the ribs meet in the middle of the chest.
3. Place your other hand on top of the hand resting on the breastbone.
4. Push inward and upward against the chest. Each thrust should be sharp and distinct. Do not be timid; you are trying to dislodge a stuck object.
5. Repeat the thrust five times, keeping your hands in contact with the victim throughout the maneuver.
6. After each cycle of thrusts, perform a finger sweep of the mouth to remove any object that the thrusts may have dislodged. A finger sweep should be done carefully; exercise caution when inspecting the mouth in order to avoid pushing a dislodged object back into the airway.
7. Repeat the cycle of five inward-upward thrusts until:

- The obstruction is coughed out *or*
- The victim loses consciousness (see page 359) *or*
- You are replaced by someone more highly trained than you, such as EMS personnel

How to help a choking infant Contact EMS immediately. Do not use the Heimlich maneuver on a child younger than 1 year old. Follow the steps described below.

1. Turn the infant face down, supporting the chest with your hand; the infant's head should be slightly lower than his body.
2. Using the heel of your hand, slap the infant five times between his shoulder blades. You will actually be hitting rather than pushing against the infant's back. Take care to make your slaps firm but not so hard that you injure the infant.

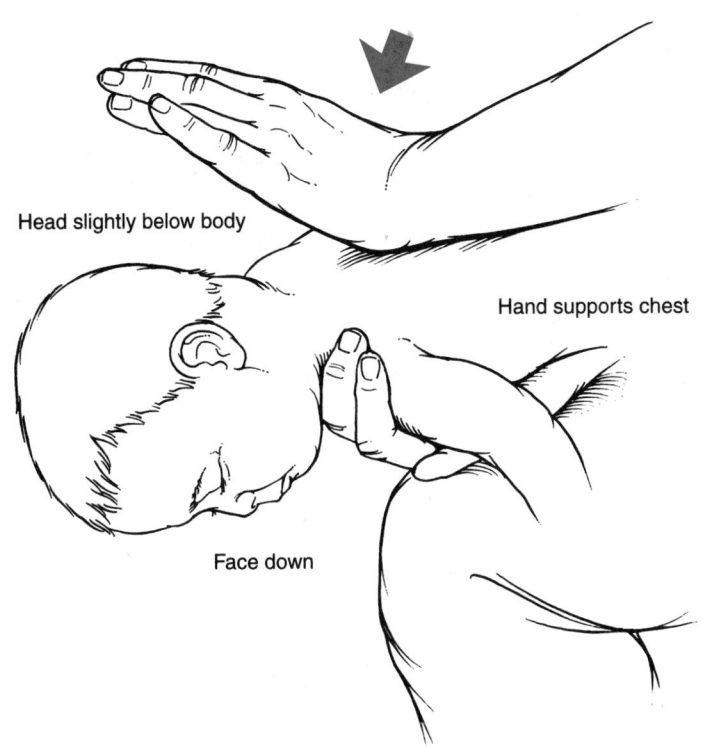

Head slightly below body

Hand supports chest

Face down

To help a choking infant, position the baby with the face down and the head slightly below the body. Support the chest with one hand while hitting the back five times firmly between the shoulder blades.

3. If the back slaps do not clear the airway, turn the baby on his back, keeping his head lower than his body and supporting his back with your hand.
4. With your forefinger and second finger slightly parted, give five thrusts—pushing inward and upward—on the breastbone with your fingertips.
5. Do not perform finger sweeps on a baby because you may inadvertently push a dislodged object back down the throat; instead, perform a visual inspection of mouth and remove the object if you can see it. *Never put your fingers down an infant's throat.*

Self-administered Heimlich maneuver If you choke when you are alone, you can self-administer a variation of the Heimlich maneuver.

1. Remain calm.
2. Place a fist between your navel and ribcage.
3. Grasp your fist firmly with your other hand.
4. Bend over a hard surface such as the back of a chair.

5. Using the surface for pressure, thrust your fist inward and upward.

Cardiopulmonary Resuscitation (CPR)

If a victim is unconscious, not breathing, and not arousable, cardiac arrest (stopping of the heart) may have occurred. Call EMS immediately. In cardiac arrest the heart stops pumping blood; the brain can become damaged very quickly without continuous blood flow. Cardiopulmonary resuscitation (CPR) keeps blood moving through the body until the heart can be restarted. CPR may be followed by more advanced techniques used by EMS technicians. CPR combines chest compression with artificial (mouth-to-mouth) respiration. Even if CPR does not start the heart beating again it can provide a victim with sufficient oxygen to survive until advanced techniques can be applied to restart the heart. CPR does not always result in the survival of the victim, but it increases the chance of survival significantly. No book can be a substitute for a CPR training class, but the technique is relatively simple.

Adult cardiopulmonary resuscitation (CPR). (A) The victim is positioned on his back. The victim's chin is lifted and his head is tilted back to open the airway. (B) Kneeling next to the victim, the rescuer pinches the victim's nose shut and exhales forcibly into the mouth, allowing no air gaps between the rescuer's and the victim's mouths. (C) Place two fingers of your left hand above the breastbone notch. (D) To perform chest compressions, the heel of the rescuer's hand is placed 1 to 1½ in. above the base of the victim's breastbone. The rescuer's other hand provides support as both hands compress the chest by 1½ to 2 in. 15 times rapidly. The rescuer's arms are kept straight.

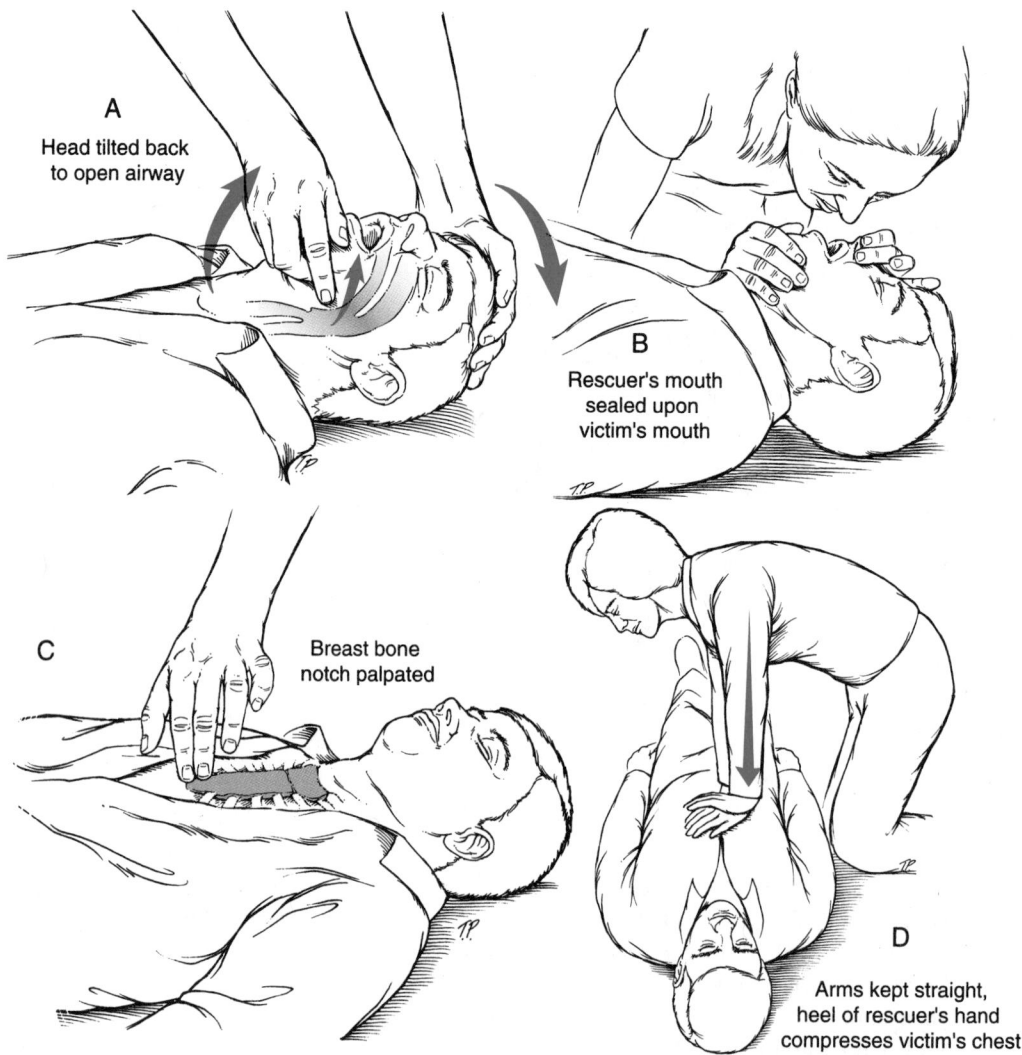

A
Head tilted back to open airway

B
Rescuer's mouth sealed upon victim's mouth

C
Breast bone notch palpated

D
Arms kept straight, heel of rescuer's hand compresses victim's chest

If the victim has a pulse it means that the heart is working and pumping blood through the body and that CPR is not necessary. However, it can be very difficult for a lay person to judge correctly if a pulse is present, especially in an emergency situation. A person giving first aid may mistake his own pulse for the victim's or be unable to locate the victim's pulse correctly. Unless an *obvious* pulse is present, CPR should be given when a victim is unconscious, not breathing, and not arousable.

Adult or child over 8 years old

1. Position the victim on his back with his arms at his side.
2. Use the chin lift maneuver to open the victim's airway. If you have reason to suspect choking, see instructions for performing the Heimlich maneuver when the victim is unconscious (see page 359).
3. Kneel next to the victim's chest.
4. Give two initial breaths into the victim's mouth: Pinch the victim's nose shut, inhale, entirely cover the victim's mouth with your mouth, and then exhale into the victim's mouth.
5. Locate the base of the victim's breastbone, the notch where the ribs meet in the center of the chest.
6. Place two fingers of your left hand above the breastbone notch.
7. Place the heel of your right hand with your fingers extended and bent upwards on the breastbone and just above the fingers of your left hand. This should position your right hand over the victim's heart.
8. Take your left hand and place it over your right hand (you can reverse hands if you are left-handed.) Lean over the victim so that your shoulders are directly above him. Keeping

your arms straight, press downward on the chest with your upper body, compressing the chest by $1\frac{1}{2}$ to 2 in.

9. Allow the chest to rise up again beneath the heel of your hand; do not remove your hands from the victim's chest.

10. Repeat 15 times using the rhythm of a regular heartbeat. Do not rock. Press straight down, keeping your shoulders parallel to the victim.

11. Stop and give two breaths by artificial respiration—your mouth sealed over the victim's mouth, the victim's nose pinched shut.

12. Repeat the cycle of 15 compressions and 2 breaths four to five times a minute for as many as 80 to 100 compressions a minute. CPR can be quite strenuous, but keep it up.

13. Continue giving CPR until you are relieved by a doctor, EMS personnel, or someone trained in CPR; until the victim wakes up or starts to move; or until you cannot continue.

Child between 1 and 8 years old

1. Place the victim flat on his back with his arms at his sides.

2. Use the chin lift maneuver to open up the victim's airway (see Resuscitation ABCs, page 357). If you have reason to suspect choking, see instructions for performing Heimlich maneuver when the victim is unconscious (page 359).

3. Kneel next to the child's chest.

4. Give two initial breaths by artificial respiration: Pinch the victim's nose shut, inhale, entirely cover the victim's mouth with your mouth, and then exhale into the victim's mouth.

5. Place the heel of one hand at the center of the lower portion of the rib cage.

6. Lean over the victim so that your shoulders are directly above him. Keeping your arms straight press downward on the chest with your upper body, compressing the chest by 1 to $1\frac{1}{2}$ in.

7. Allow the chest to rise up again beneath the heel of your hand; do

not remove your hand from the victim's chest.

8. Repeat five times, using the rhythm of a regular heartbeat. Do not rock. Press straight down, keeping your shoulders parallel to the victim.

9. Stop and give one breath by artificial respiration—your mouth sealed over the victim's mouth, the child's nose pinched shut.

10. Repeat the cycle of five compressions and one breath at the rate of about 80 to 100 compressions a minute. CPR can be quite strenuous, but keep it up. Do not worry whether you are fully inflating the lungs each time you give a breath.

11. Continue giving CPR until you are relieved by a doctor, EMS personnel, or someone trained in CPR; until the victim wakes up or starts to move; or until you cannot continue.

Infant younger than 1 year old

1. Place the infant on his back on a firm surface or you can sit in a chair and place him on his back flat against your legs with his head cradled in your left hand.

2. Use the chin lift maneuver to open up the victim's airway (see Resuscitation ABCs, page 357).

3. Give two initial breaths by artificial respiration: Inhale, entirely cover the infant's mouth and nose with your mouth, and exhale into his mouth.

4. Place the index finger of your right or left hand against the breastbone between the baby's nipples; use this finger to position your middle fingers on the breastbone, just below your index finger.

5. Using only the middle fingers of your hand, compress the baby's chest about 1 in.

6. Allow the chest to rise up again beneath your fingers; do not remove your hand from the baby's chest.

7. Repeat five times, using the rhythm of a regular heartbeat. Do not rock; press straight down.

8. Stop and give two breaths by artificial respiration—your mouth sealed over the baby's mouth and nose.

9. Repeat the cycle of five compressions and two breaths at the rate of about 100 compressions a minute. CPR can be quite strenuous, but keep it up.

10. Continue giving CPR until you are relieved by a doctor, EMS personnel, or someone trained in CPR; until the baby wakes up or starts to move; or until you cannot continue.

Sign of a good CPR technique

- Your CPR technique is good if the chest rises and falls each time you give a breath by artificial respiration. If the chest does not rise, make certain the victim's head is tilted properly and the airway is clear.

When you should stop CPR

- A doctor tells you to stop

- The victim wakes up or starts moving. This may require the administration of more advanced heart-starting techniques by EMS personnel; failure of the victim to come to does not mean that you are not doing the right thing.

- You are relieved by EMS personnel or someone trained in CPR

- You cannot continue

CPR precautions

- During resuscitation, a victim may vomit. If this happens, roll the victim onto his left side until it has stopped. If he has revived—has woken up or started to move—leave him in the recovery position illustrated on page 365 until EMS arrives. If he has not revived, wait until the vomiting has stopped then while he is still on his side, wipe off his mouth and, with your hand wrapped in cloth, clear the vomit from the mouth.

- CPR may cause injury, including broken ribs. You can prevent or minimize this by placing your hands in the proper position on the victim's chest—not too low—and by pushing straight down rather than from the side—do not rock. Make sure that your compressions are smooth and even: count them out as you do them—one and two and three, and one and two and three, etc.

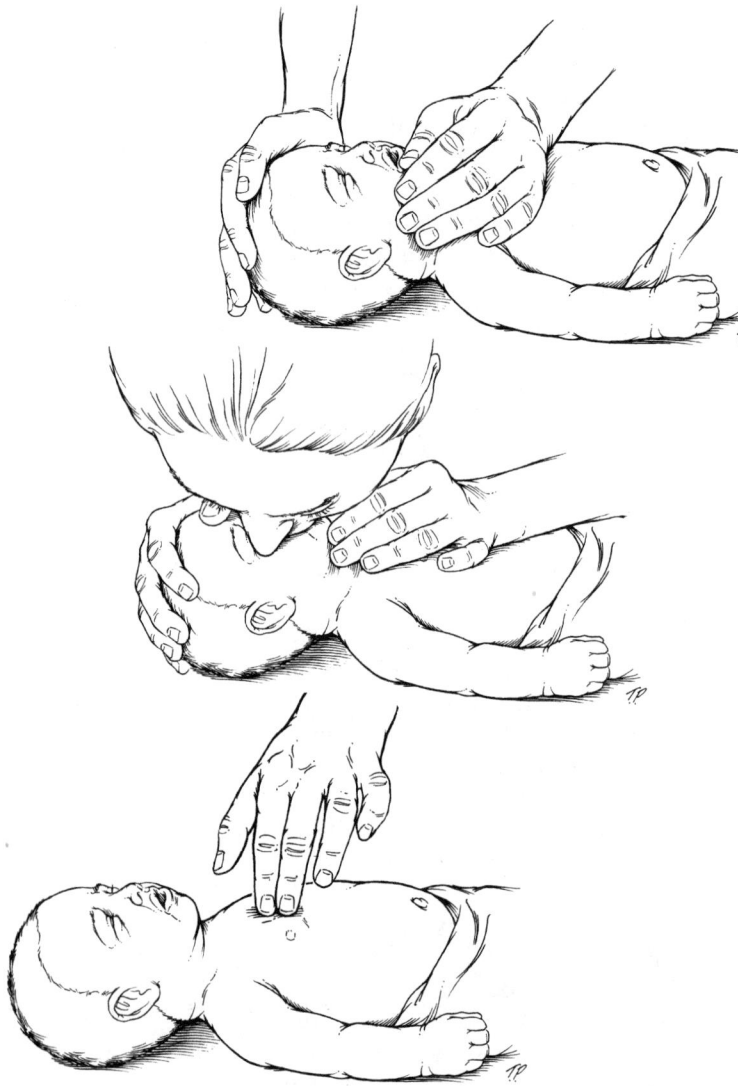

Resuscitating an infant is similar to the procedure for resuscitating an adult, but the infant's chest is compressed only 1 in. using only the middle fingers of the right hand (you can reverse hands if you are left-handed) and the compressions are performed only five times in succession before cycling back to the breathing.

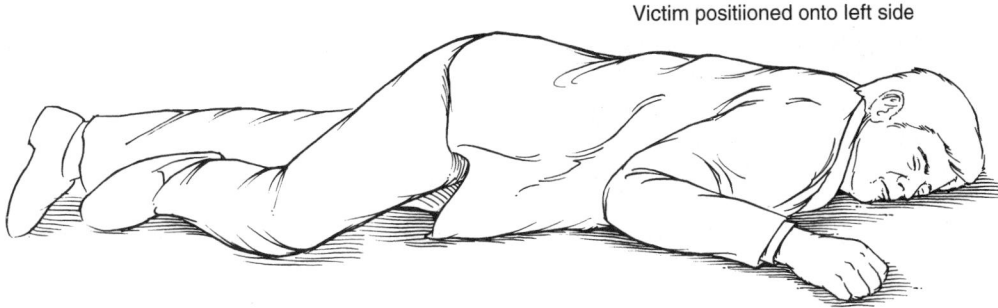

Victim positiioned onto left side

A victim who has vomited during resuscitation should be rolled onto his left side. The rescuer can then clear away the vomited material from the mouth, being careful to avoid direct contact of the vomit with the hands. The rescuer's hands can be wrapped in cloth or another protective barrier for this purpose.

Chest Pain

Chest pain should never be taken lightly. *In the event of chest pain, contact EMS or your doctor at once.* Chest pain may be a sign of a heart attack or other potentially fatal illness related to the heart, circulatory system, and lungs.

EVALUATING CHEST PAIN

Sharp pain of sudden onset If sharp, sudden pain is accompanied by difficulty swallowing, a cough, shortness of breath, bloody sputum, sweating, and/or rapid heartbeat, *contact EMS or your doctor immediately.* The pain may be caused by a pulmonary embolism, or a blood clot in the lung. Death can occur if treatment is delayed (see page 760).

Dull pain If the victim experiences dull pain in the chest accompanied by other signs of heart attack such as breathlessness, dizziness, pale or blue skin, anxiety, and cold or clammy skin, *contact EMS or your doctor immediately.* The faster a heart attack victim gets help, the better his chances for recovery (see Myocardial Infarction, page 811).

Pain in the center of the chest If the victim experiences pain in the center of the chest that extends to the left side of the neck, left shoulder, into the back, and/or down to the belly, and if this pain is accompanied by a feeling of breathlessness, *con-tact EMS or your doctor immediately.* This pain could be caused by pericarditis, an infection of the pericardium, the sac that surrounds the heart (see page 826).

If the victim experiences mild chest pain that is accompanied by a sensation of breathlessness and if the chest pain increases slightly when he inhales, *contact EMS or your doctor immediately.* If the victim is between the age 35 and 40, he could have spontaneous pneumothorax, also known as a collapsed lung (see page 736).

Pain on lying or bending If the victim experiences chest pain only when lying down or bending over and it is accompanied by an acid taste in the mouth and throat or a bloated feeling, he may have heartburn. Try giving an antacid and having him walk around. Heartburn pain should be relieved by the antacid and belching. Heart attack pain may be confused with the pain of heartburn or indigestion. Pain from indigestion can range from the abdomen to the shoulders and neck, and may not be accompanied by a sour taste in the mouth. If the pain continues, worsens, or is accompanied by nausea, dizziness, and intense sweating or if the victim has a known heart condition, *contact EMS or your doctor immediately.*

Sharp pain on the lower left side If the victim is a young, healthy adult and experiences sharp pain on the lower left side of the ribcage that comes and goes, and that increases when he inhales, it may be a precordial catch, a harmless condition of unknown origin that should subside within several minutes to an hour. If the pain does not resolve spontaneously, if it appeared during a cough, or if the victim has recently been involved in some sort of trauma such as a collision, fall, or automobile accident, consult a doctor to rule out broken ribs.

Sharp pain upon movement The victim may have a pulled muscle if he experiences sharp pain that is limited to the chest and associated with movement, especially if he has no history of recent trauma, is age 35 or under, does not have diabetes, and does not have a known family history of cardiovascular disease. A pulled muscle is characterized by moderate to severe chest pain that occurs during exertion. A person will probably know if he has a pulled muscle because the pain will have likely occurred just as he swung a racquet, rake, hammer, or bat. However, if chest pain is accompanied by signs of heart attack such as breathlessness, dizziness, pale or blue skin, anxiety, or cold or clammy skin, *contact EMS or your doctor immediately*.

Pain associated with trauma An automobile accident, sports injury, or a fall may have caused broken or bruised ribs, or a punctured or bruised lung. It is important to be evaluated by EMS personnel or a doctor.

HEART ATTACK

Myocardial infarction (heart attack) occurs when the blood supply to the heart is cut off or significantly diminished, damaging the heart (see page 811).

Someone having a heart attack may experience pain in the region of the chest, neck, jaw, upper abdomen, left shoulder, or left arm.

Is it a heart attack? If you suspect heart attack, it is important to call EMS at once because rapid diagnosis and treatment increase the chances of recovery. A heart attack may sometimes occur with no outward symptoms, although this happens in only 1 in 10 cases. Even then, most people who have had a heart attack report having had some symptoms, which they may have ascribed to heartburn or other causes.

Heart attack is most common among people with heart disease or known risk factors for heart disease, but hidden heart problems may cause heart attack in people who appear otherwise quite and healthy.

Symptoms A heart attack may occur without all of the symptoms listed below. If you think the victim might be having a heart attack, do not delay in getting emergency assistance. Do not wait to see if the pain goes away.

- Chest pain varying from a dull ache to a heavy, crushing pain; sometimes radiating out into the shoulders and left or right arm. Pain may be generalized throughout the chest, and there may be pain in the jaw.

- Breathlessness, lightheadedness, dizziness, giddiness

- Blue or pale skin, particularly around the lips

- Feeling that the heart is not beating properly

- Sense of extreme anxiety—"I think I'm dying"

- Cold sweat or clammy skin

- Overall weakness

What you should do Summon EMS immediately. If the victim is unconscious, check his airway, breathing, and circulation (see Resuscitation ABCs, page 357). If the victim is not breathing and not arousable, initiate CPR (see Cardiopulmonary Resuscitation, page 361). If the victim is conscious position him in a relaxed, half-sitting position, back supported and knees slightly bent; use a pillow or other object to raise the knees slightly. Reassure the victim and encourage him to relax. Let him know that help is on the way. Keep the victim still and do not allow him to move about or eat or drink. Loosen the victim's collar and shirt.

If the victim is conscious ask him if he has been prescribed nitroglycerin for a heart condition; if so, follow his directions or the instructions on the prescription container and place a tablet beneath the victim's tongue. Repeat as prescribed or as directed by the victim. Be aware that nitroglycerin causes the blood vessels to dilate, or open up, which causes a drop in blood pressure and dizziness. Make sure the victim is not standing if you administer nitroglycerin.

Head Pain

Severe head pain of sudden onset should be considered an emergency; call EMS or go to the emergency room immediately. Sudden head pain can indicate a number of conditions ranging in seriousness from tension headache to stroke; the severity of the pain does not necessarily correspond to the severity of the illness. Most head pain does not occur suddenly; a person usually feels a headache coming on. However, head pain due to swelling of the brain that can occur after injury or trauma may build gradually to severe levels and may be a sign of serious injury (see Head Injury, page 390).

EVALUATING HEAD PAIN

Pain associated with a loss of function If the victim experiences head pain accompanied by an inability to walk, talk, or answer questions about who and where he is, *contact EMS immediately.* This pain may be the result of a stroke; the sooner treatment is initiated, the better the chances for recovery (see below). For a complete discussion of stroke see page 429.

Pain accompanied by fever, malaise, nausea, weakness, stiff neck, drowsiness, or disorientation If the victim experiences head pain in conjunction with any of these symptoms, *contact EMS or visit the emergency room immediately.* This combination of symptoms could be a sign of vasculitis, meningitis, or encephalitis. See Chapter 14 for more information on these specific conditions. All of these are serious

illnesses that can result in brain damage; the victim should be evaluated as rapidly as possible. The sooner treatment is initiated, the better the chance for recovery.

Pain in one eye If the victim has pain in an eye that is not associated with an injury and the eye appears normal, *contact EMS or your doctor immediately.* This could be a sign of glaucoma. Failure to get immediate treatment may result in loss of vision in the affected eye.

Intense pain, predominantly on one side of the head, accompanied by nausea and visual disturbances Contact your doctor. These symptoms may be a sign of migraine headache. Migraines can be debilitating and may last for hours or days. The symptoms are also associated with stroke and may indicate a medical emergency if they remain intense.

Intolerable pain that is not responsive to over-the-counter medication If the victim experiences intense head pain that does not begin to get better after taking a pain reliever, *consult your doctor or visit the emergency room.*

Any sudden pain Most headaches do not occur suddenly. Contact your doctor in any case of sudden head pain even if it is not associated with other symptoms.

Loss of Normal Function/Neurologic Emergencies

If someone suddenly loses normal function—tries to speak and cannot, tries to stand and cannot—it is almost always a sign of serious illness. Sudden loss of normal function should be treated as an emergency even if the episode proves to be transient. Do not wait to find out if the episode is transient before summoning EMS; irreparable brain damage may occur.

STROKE

A stroke is a life-threatening medical emergency that requires immediate attention. Stroke is caused by blockage of blood flow to a part of the brain. Without immediate medical intervention, oxygen-starved brain tissue can die.

Symptoms People experiencing stroke often try to minimize their symptoms in the hope that they will pass. However, delaying treatment can be dangerous. If you believe that someone has had or is having a stroke, contact EMS without delay, despite his protests. New treatment offers promise to stroke victims that did not exist in the past, but the treatment is most effective if begun shortly after the stroke occurs.

- Sudden partial paralysis
- Numbness or weakness in a particular area of the body such as the face, arms, or legs, often occurring on only one side
- Sudden onset of complete or partial blindness in one or both eyes; sudden double vision
- Aphasia, or the inability to speak or use language properly
- Sudden loss of coordination or balance, which may resemble intoxication and may include incontinence
- Sudden headache may occur although many strokes do not cause head pain

What you should do Contact EMS immediately. If the victim is unconscious, check his airway, breathing, and circulation (see Resuscitation ABCs, page 357). If the victim is not breathing and not arousable, initiate CPR (see Cardiopulmonary Resuscitation, page 361). If an unconscious victim's airway, breathing, and circulation are fine, lay him out in the recovery position (see page 365) and continue to monitor him until help arrives.

If the victim is conscious lay him on his back, head and shoulders slightly elevated with a pillow or other object. Turn his face toward the side so that he does not choke; if one side is paralyzed, turn his head so the paralyzed side faces up. *Do not give him anything to eat or drink.* Continue to monitor the victim's condition until help arrives.

HYPERTENSIVE CRISIS

Hypertensive crisis results from a sudden, extreme rise in blood pressure and may lead to damage of the heart, brain, eyes, and other organs. Although high blood pressure (hypertension) is quite common, hypertensive crisis is rare. Hypertensive crisis is most common in people with high blood pressure who fail to take their medication as prescribed. Other possible causes of suddenly increased blood pressure include stroke, kidney disease, toxemia of pregnancy, drug interactions, and amphetamine and cocaine use.

Hypertensive crisis is a medical emergency requiring immediate attention. Because of the abnormally high blood pressure that marks hypertensive crisis, blood vessels may rupture and release blood into the tissues of the brain, eyes, and other organs. Blood vessels may also go into spasm. Both these effects can cause stroke, blindness, and other serious problems.

Symptoms

- Severe headache
- Distorted vision
- Confused thinking and nonsensical speech
- Shortness of breath
- Nausea and vomiting
- Chest pain
- Seizure or loss of function of arm or leg

What you should do If you suspect hypertensive crisis, contact EMS immediately. Encourage the victim to lie down and rest until EMS arrives. *Do not give the victim anything to eat or drink.* If the victim displays symptoms of stroke, such as partial paralysis or loss of ability to speak, see page 367. If the victim goes into seizure, see page 369.

SPINAL CORD INJURY

Injury to the spinal cord occurs as a result of trauma, most commonly from a fall, vehicular accident, sports injury, work-related injury, or assault. Because the nerve fibers that make up the spinal cord do not regenerate, many spinal cord injuries result in paralysis. The risk of paralysis is even greater if the victim is moved by someone other than emergency personnel. This is why it is important *to never move anyone suspected of spinal cord injury* unless the victim's life is in immediate danger if he is

MOVING A VICTIM OF SUSPECTED SPINAL CORD INJURY

Do not move anyone you suspect of having suffered a spinal cord, neck, or back injury unless his life is endangered by not being moved. Contact EMS immediately. However, there are times when the victim's life may depend on either a change in position or being taken away from a threatening environment.

If Victim's Airway Is Not Clear Use the log roll technique to place him on his side. *Do not* turn or bend the victim's head or neck unless you turn his whole body simultaneously.

Although it can be done alone, it is safest and easiest to perform the log roll with the help of others. This way one person can support the victim's head and neck and turn it at the same time as others turn his body.

Once you have performed a log roll, do not move the victim again unless his life becomes further endangered.

If Victim Is Unconscious, Not Breathing, and Not Arousable Use the log roll technique to turn the victim onto his back.

Clear the victim's airway (see Resuscitation ABCs, page 357) and perform CPR (see Cardiopulmonary Resuscitation, page 361). If bystanders are available, have someone work to immobilize the victim's body as you give CPR.

If Scene Is Too Dangerous to Remain If the scene of spinal cord injury becomes too dangerous to remain because of fire, toxic fumes, danger of explosion, or other life-threatening hazard, it is reasonable and prudent to move a victim of suspected spinal cord trauma out of harm's way.

If you are the only rescuer, move the victim by means of the clothes-drag technique; drag the victim by the shoulders of his clothing while supporting his head between your arms. Drag the victim either face-up or face-down, depending on the position in which you found him. Crouching low to the ground, grasp the victim's clothing firmly and position your forearms against the sides of the victim's head.

Lift the victim up by his clothes using your hands; with your forearms, lift his head and keep it stable. Drag the victim to safety.

If the victim is not wearing a jacket, sweater, or other substantial garment, log roll the victim onto a substitute cloth such as a blanket.

If you are not alone, enlist the help of others to log roll the victim onto a rescue board. ■

not moved (see Moving a Victim of Suspected Spinal Cord Injury, above). For a complete discussion of spinal cord trauma, see page 483.

Symptoms The following symptoms occurring after trauma are signs of spinal cord injury. Be aware that spinal cord injuries are often accompanied by head injuries (see page 479).

- Sudden head, back, or neck pain
- Sudden difficulty or pain upon moving the arms or legs
- Sudden numbness or prickly, stinging, or burning sensation in the arms or legs
- Incontinence
- Paralysis, or complete inability to move the arms or legs
- Shock

What you should do Contact EMS immediately. Check the victim's airway, breathing, and circulation (see Resuscitation ABCs, page 357).

Do not move victim unless his life is in immediate danger. In some cases, such as spinal cord compression, paralysis may be temporary, with numbness slowly disappearing and movement returning. Even if this happens, do not move the victim or allow the victim to move until EMS arrives.

Do not try to "straighten" the victim's head, neck, or back. If the victim is conscious, keep him completely still. Reassure the victim that help is coming but do not let him move. This means keeping the victim in the car if the injury is the result of an automobile accident, unless remaining in the car would put the victim's life in immediate danger. Use whatever you can find to protect the immobility of the victim: towels, clothing, books—anything that will help ensure that the victim remains in the same position in which you found him until EMS arrives.

Continue monitoring the victim's ABCs—airway, breathing, and circulation—until help arrives.

SEIZURES

Seizures are sudden episodes of involuntary muscular movement usually prompted by abnormal electrical activity in the brain. The most well-known type of seizure is caused by epilepsy. People with epilepsy often wear bracelets or tags to identify their condition and usually carry medication. Seizures can be convulsive or nonconvulsive and range from a grand mal seizure in which convulsions may last as long as 5 minutes, to petit mal seizure, a momentary blackout in which the victim stares blankly for 10 to 30 seconds. Seizures can also be focal (partial), affecting, for example, only the muscles of the leg. For a complete discussion see Seizure Disorders, page 445.

Seizures are often associated with fever, a history of prior seizure, and poisoning. The possibility of poisoning by medication, chemicals, or plants must be considered as a cause of seizure, especially in children (see Poisoning, page 408). *If you suspect poisoning call your local poison control center immediately.* Seizures caused by a fever or a seizure disorder are serious and require medical attention. Seizures are also associated with heat stroke (see page 403); drug overdose (see page 411); venomous bites or stings (see page 397); electric shock (see page 397); diabetic emergencies (see page 371); brain tumor (see page 485), head injury (see page 390), and stroke (see page 367); and heart disease (see Chapter 20).

Symptoms

- Twitching localized to one area of the body

- Blacking out or becoming unaware of surroundings, for a brief period

- Syncope (sudden loss of consciousness)

- Loss of motor control, characterized by intense muscle spasms involving jerking and twitching, or rigid immobility

- Drooling, incontinence, foaming at the mouth

- Uncontrolled noises

- Momentary cessation of breathing

What you should do Call EMS immediately if the victim is not a known epileptic and has a history of high blood pressure or cardiovascular disease; has more than one seizure within a short period; is feverish or becomes injured during the seizure; has a head injury that may have led to the seizure; becomes unconscious and is not arousable after the seizure; is or might be pregnant; has a seizure lasting 2 minutes or more; or has difficulty breathing. Look for a medical ID bracelet or tag.

Once a seizure is underway with uncontrollable muscle spasms, there is nothing you can do to stop it; *do not try to restrain the victim.* Act to make sure that the victim does not injure himself as a result of the convulsions. Remove nearby objects that could cause injury. If possible, cushion the victim's head and loosen tight clothing around the neck.

Do not try to contain the seizure; both you and the victim could be injured. Do not try to perform artificial respiration during the episode even if the victim stops breathing; the seizure should end before brain damage occurs and artificial respiration during the seizure could injure you both. Do not put anything, such as a spoon or your fingers, into the victim's mouth. *Do not give the victim anything to eat or drink.* Do not attempt to move the victim unless he is in danger.

After the seizure has ended put the victim on his side in the recovery position, if he is not injured (see page 365).

Sleep is common after a vigorous seizure and is part of the recovery process. Do not try to wake the victim. Continually monitor airway, breathing, and circulation until the victim wakes up (see Resuscitation ABCs, page 357). Reawakening may take an hour. The victim will likely be disoriented and it may take time for him to regain full use of his faculties.

If the victim is injured, check his airway, breathing, and circulation (see Resuscitation ABCs, page 357). If the ABCs are stable, treat the most serious injuries first (see Which Injury is Most Serious?, page 357). If the victim vomits after the seizure, make sure his airway remains clear.

If the seizure occured during a fever, try to bring the fever down (see page 374) and call EMS.

FAINTING

The medical term for fainting is *syncope.* Although fainting is quite common and probably the least serious sudden loss of function, any loss of consciousness may reflect more serious illness. Fainting is most often due to an abrupt drop in blood pressure that decreases blood to the brain, caused either by postural hypotension (low blood pressure that occurs when standing) or vasovagal hypotension (low blood pressure that occurs when nerves that regulate blood pressure misfire due to emotional overload).

Symptoms

- Sudden paleness or shakiness on standing

- Sudden sensation of weakness, dizziness, or confusion
- Blackout

What you should do Contact EMS immediately if the victim shows signs of stroke, such as inability to speak properly, loss of movement in one side of the face or body, decreased or poor vision, or loss of balance (see page 367); the victim is elderly, has diabetes, cardiovascular disease, or other illness; if the victim does not fully regain function in 1 to 2 minutes; or if the victim complains of a persistent sense of discomfort, shortness of breath, or confusion.

If you see someone who is pale and wavering and appears to be about to faint—after standing, hearing bad news, or seeing the sight of blood—suggest that he lie down immediately. If lying down is not possible, help the victim sit and lower his head between his knees, which will help increase the blood flow to the brain. If someone is already going into a faint, try to cushion his slump or fall.

If someone has already fainted check his airway, breathing, and circulation (see Resuscitation ABCs, page 357); if the victim is not breathing and not arousable initiate CPR (see Cardiopulmonary Resuscitation, page 361).

If ABCs are stable lay the victim back with feet elevated; continually monitor his airway until he regains consciousness. *Do not* splash the victim with water or any other liquid, although you can use a cool damp cloth on the forehead and face.

People who lose consciousness may vomit. If the victim vomits, ensure that his airway is clear and move him onto his side in the recovery position (see page 365).

After a fainting victim regains consciousness encourage him to remain lying down until color and strength return to normal. Check for signs of other illness including injury from falling, chest pain, continued weakness, breathing difficulties, and loss of function that might suggest stroke (see page 367). An episode of fainting, especially in seniors, should be reported to their doctor.

DIABETIC EMERGENCIES

People with diabetes cannot properly regulate their blood sugar levels. Diabetic emergencies may occur with hyperglycemia (abnormally high blood sugar), which can lead to diabetic coma; or with hypoglycemia (abnormally low blood sugar), which can lead to insulin shock. Diabetic coma associated with hyperglycemia and insufficient insulin can indicate either hyperosmolar coma, which is a result of extreme dehydration, or diabetic ketoacidosis (DKA), in which lack of insulin leads to an accumulation of ketone acids in the blood. Hyperglycemia and insulin shock occur with excessive levels of insulin. Both diabetic coma and insulin shock are potentially fatal and should be treated immediately.

Because the symptoms of diabetic emergencies sometimes resemble those of drunkenness, stroke, or even mental illness, they can be difficult to recognize. It can also be difficult to distinguish between the two different types of diabetic emergency, particularly if the victim is unconscious. If the victim is known to be diabetic and has fruity-smelling breath or smells as if he had been drinking, he most likely is suffering from DKA. If the victim is sweating profusely he most likely is having a reaction to too much insulin and may be in danger of insulin shock.

If a victim exhibits symptoms of diabetic emergency and you do not know if he has diabetes, check for a medical alert bracelet or tag; however, be aware that diabetic coma may be the first sign that a person has diabetes.

Symptoms of hyperglycemia and DKA In an unconscious victim, fruity-smelling breath may be the only noticeable symptom of DKA. However, a victim suffering from hyperosmolar coma will not have fruity-smelling breath.

- Extreme thirst (hyperglycemia)
- Frequent urination (hyperglycemia)
- Combative, confused, paranoid, or extremely irritable behavior, increasing in intensity as time goes on (hypoglycemia)
- Vomiting
- Heavy, deep breathing (DKA)
- Fruity-smelling breath (DKA)

What you should do Call EMS immediately. If the victim loses consciousness, check his airway, breathing, and circulation (see Resuscitation ABCs, page 357). Place the victim in the recovery position (see page 365). Look for a medical alert bracelet or tag, which are sometimes engraved with first aid instructions. Do not try to give the victim anything by mouth. Do not try to wake him by splashing him with liquid or by shaking or slapping him.

Symptoms of hypoglycemia and insulin shock Symptoms of hypoglycemia may develop rapidly.

- Extreme hunger
- Pale skin
- Profuse sweating
- Irritable, combative, disoriented, or paranoid behavior
- Seizures (sometimes)

What you should do The victim may have inadvertently taken too much insulin or neglected to eat after taking a dose of insulin, causing his blood sugar to go too low (see the Insulin Reaction—What to Do, page 1177). Many people with diabetes carry food and some form of sugar with them in case they develop low blood sugar.

If the victim is still conscious ask if he has emergency-sugar supplies and help him take them. Be aware that his behavior may be irrational, belligerent, or paranoid—he may think you are trying to poison him—but try to get his cooperation.

If the victim has no emergency supplies, give him orange juice, a nondiet soft drink, or some other sweet substance, such as a candy bar. He should return to a normal state of function about 10 minutes after consuming sugar.

Try not to react to any belligerence on the victim's part and understand that it is a symptom of the illness; reassure him gently without getting angry or panicky.

If the victim is unconscious, summon EMS immediately. Monitor the victim's airway, breathing, and circulation (see Resuscitation ABCs, page 357) until help arrives.

Place the victim in the recovery position (see page 365). Look for a medical alert bracelet or tag, which are sometimes engraved with first aid instructions. Do not try to give the victim anything by mouth. Do not try to wake him by splashing him with liquid or by shaking or slapping him.

Shortness or Loss of Breath

If breathing difficulties occur shortly after an insect bite or sting; after eating fish, peanuts, or other foods to which people are commonly allergic; or are accompanied by redness and puffiness of the face or tongue, nausea, or any other signs of allergic reaction, contact EMS at once, and see Anaphylactic Shock/Severe Allergic Reaction, page 385.

Shortness of breath can accompany conditions from hyperventilation, which can be frightening but is not serious, to truly serious emergencies involving asthma, emphysema, heart failure, acute allergic reaction, or other serious illness or injury such as inhalation burn. These conditions require rapid medical attention and diagnosis.

Nearly every one of these conditions could be fatal to some victim. Unless you are very familiar with dealing with the illness—for example, your child's asthma—seek medical attention immediately by calling EMS, contacting your doctor, or visiting your local emergency room.

SEVERE ASTHMA ATTACKS

Asthma is a common cause of breathing difficulties (see page 745). A chronic condition, asthma afflicts 5 percent of Americans. It is characterized by inflammation of the bronchial tubes, spasm of the muscles surrounding the bronchial tubes, and discharge of mucus into the airway. Asthma attacks can be brought on by many things, including viral infections, cold weather, physical exertion, and exposure to an allergen (substance that causes an allergic reaction). Some attacks are relatively mild, while other attacks can be severe and potentially life-threatening.

Symptoms Wheezy or noisy breathing, tightness in the chest, inability to take a deep breath, and coughing are all symptoms of asthma. A severe asthma attack is signaled by the following:

- Inability to speak without gasping for breath
- Persistence of symptoms despite the use of an inhaler

- Ashen or bluish face, lips, or hands
- Confusion or loss of consciousness

What you should do If you must transport the victim to the emergency room, make sure he is sitting up and not lying down. Do not attempt to monitor the victim's ABCs—airway, breathing, and circulation—while you are driving. Help the victim into a sitting position, either straight up or angled forward slightly with arms supported. If the victim objects to being placed in any position, do not force him into it.

If the victim has an emergency inhaler, help him use the medication. If the medication does not bring relief within 20 minutes, have the victim take a second inhalation and call a doctor's office or emergency room for further instructions. If two inhalations do not provide relief, seek medical care at a doctor's office or hospital emergency room.

If the victim cannot speak or is confused or agitated, contact EMS and reassure the victim that help is on the way. Other than inhalant medication, do not give the victim anything by mouth.

If the victim is unconscious, call EMS and put him in the recovery position (see page 365). Look for a medical alert bracelet or tag which may help clarify the nature of the emergency and are sometimes engraved with first aid instructions.

BREATHING EMERGENCIES IN CHILDREN

Breathing emergencies in children should not be taken lightly. What may be inconsequential for an adult may be life-threatening for a child. If a child in your care is having extreme difficulty breathing, contact EMS at once. A breathing emergency in a child may be the result of an acute illness—often accompanied by fever—such as bronchiolitis, croup, or epiglottitis; it may indicate the emergence of a chronic condition such as asthma; it may indicate a severe allergic reaction (see page 385); or it may indicate choking or blockage of the airway by a swallowed object (see page 359).

Symptoms

- Shortness or loss of breath
- Difficult, very rapid, or labored breathing—sometimes accompanied by tense chest or abdominal muscles
- Frequent cough, either wet and phlegmy, or dry and hacking
- Wheezing, whistling, or croaking sounds
- Ashen, bluish, or pale lips or fingertips
- Unusual chest movements while breathing
- Drooling and reluctance to swallow
- Difficulty feeding by breast or bottle

What you should do If breathing difficulties occur within a few minutes of an insect bite or sting, or after eating a food to which people are commonly allergic, such as peanuts, fish, or eggs, contact EMS immediately (see Anaphylactic Shock/Severe Allergic Reaction, page 385).

If breathing difficulties are severe and accompanied by high fever and bluish lips or fingertips, *contact EMS immediately*.

If you think that a child's breathing difficulties may be the result of choking, call EMS immediately and follow the instructions in this chapter for assisting a choking victim (for a child 1 year old and over, see page 358; for an infant, see page 360).

Help a child with breathing difficulties into an upright sitting position or hold him upright, but do not put him in a position that makes him uncomfortable. If the child is in bed, do not put a pillow beneath his head because it could block his airway; instead, prop up his back, shoulders, and head. Watch his breathing closely until EMS arrives.

HYPERVENTILATION

Hyperventilation is essentially breathing too much and is brought on by anxiety or stress. Someone who is hyperventilating has too much oxygen in his blood, which perpetuates the problem. Hyperventilation can be halted by bringing up the level of carbon dioxide in the blood.

Symptoms

- Rapid breathing
- A sense of not being able to catch one's breath
- A sense of panic, desperation, or anxiety

What you should do Have the victim breathe more slowly; if possible, have the victim hold his breath. Try to calm the victim and encourage him to talk, which may take his mind off his breathing and break the cycle of hyperventilation. Have the victim breathe into a paper bag—*never* a plastic bag—or into his cupped hands

If the victim faints from the effects of hyperventilation, the autonomous nervous system will take over and breathing will return to normal. The victim should regain consciousness shortly (see Fainting, page 370). Monitor airway, breathing, and circulation until the victim revives (see Resuscitation ABCs, page 357).

Fever

Fever is most often a signal that the body is fighting an infection. Most emergency fevers occur in small children, particularly infants; the immunosuppressed; or the elderly. For immunosuppressed adults or for the elderly, particularly the infirm, persistent high fever is probably a signal of a serious infection that the body cannot fight alone. Call the victim's doctor if the fever does not respond to over-the-counter pain relievers. When in doubt, transport the victim to the emergency room.

For children, a high fever does not always mean that the child is seriously ill. It is not uncommon for a child to run a fever of 102° to 104°F for a few days. Very young children may spike fevers that can alarm parents, but fever is not by itself something to be overly concerned about unless it is unusually high and persistent, or is accompanied by a febrile seizure. The biggest concern is that a child not become dehydrated. Call your doctor and see How to Bring a Fever Down Safely, page 853. For more information see Emergency Fever in Children, below.

FEBRILE SEIZURES IN CHILDREN

Most febrile seizures occur as a child's fever is rising; they are relatively common and more frightening than dangerous.

If a seizure is truly caused by fever, it should last no longer than a few minutes. Take your child's temperature once the seizure has lifted, and contact your doctor immediately. Tell your doctor about the seizure and report your child's temperature; ask what kind of medication to give your child and how much, and if he should be seen immediately.

If the seizure lasts longer than a few minutes, if your child turns blue during the seizure or has difficulty breathing, or if you are frightened, call EMS immediately.

WARNING: Never give aspirin to a child for relief of fever unless directed to do so by your doctor. Be aware that some over-the-counter medications contain aspirin and should not be given to children unless directed by a doctor. Aspirin has been linked to Reye's syndrome (see pages 463 and 854), a potentially fatal illness. For relief of fever, children may be given acetaminophen or ibuprofen in an appropriate dosage for their individual weight.

For more information see Febrile Seizures, page 448 and How to Bring a Fever Down Safely, page 853. ∎

EMERGENCY FEVER IN CHILDREN

Fevers accompanied by or characterized by the symptoms below should be evaluated immediately by your doctor or by emergency room personnel. Very young children may not have sufficient immune response to fight some infections, and may require antibiotics or medical supervision. Most often, the fever will not turn out to be a sign of something serious, but never hesitate to call your doctor—immediate action with small children could make the difference between full recovery and serious complications.

Symptoms

- Fever of 100.2°F (measured rectally) in an infant younger than 3 months old
- Fever of 102°F (measured rectally) in an infant 3 to 6 months old
- Any fever at any age accompanied by:
  - Swelling of the soft spot at the top of the infant's head
  - Dotty pink or purple rash
  - Breathing difficulties
  - Pale, blue, or purple skin color
  - Stiff neck
  - Signs of shock (see page 385)
  - Disorientation or difficulty recognizing people

• Dehydration, signaled by sunken eyes, lack of urine, dry mouth, dramatic thirst, weakness or extreme sleepiness, and sinking of the soft spot at the top of the infant's head

What you should do Contact your doctor immediately or bring the child to your local hospital emergency room.

Take steps to relieve the fever. Never give a child aspirin (see warning in Febrile Seizures in Children, page 374). Acetaminophen should be used to bring down fever in children. Pediatric ibuprofen, a nonsteroidal anti-inflammatory drug (NSAID) that contains no aspirin, is also used for children. However, neither acetaminophen nor ibuprofen should be used in infants without a doctor's supervision. Follow your doctor's instructions.

provide a concrete idea of the source of the pain, potential seriousness, and the appropriate level of response.

Abdominal pain related to trauma If abdominal pain is the result of trauma, such as a fall, automobile accident, or other physical injury, call your doctor or EMS immediately. Any abdominal pain related to trauma should be evaluated by a medical professional (see Trauma, page 387).

Intense and persistent abdominal pain Abdominal pain that is persistent, intense, and lasts more than an hour or two should be evaluated by your doctor. It could be an indication of appendicitis or another illness. Generally, you will not have to visit the emergency room or call EMS; however, you should call your doctor immediately.

Abdominal Pain

The abdomen is the area of the body extending from the bottom of the ribcage to the hips. Abdominal pain may indicate an array of conditions from disorders of the digestive tract, including gastroenteritis, ulcer, diverticulitis, appendicitis, colitis, ileitis, hernia, gas, and diarrhea, to problems in any of the abdominal organs, which include the liver, spleen, pancreas, stomach, and intestines. Abdominal pain can also be symptomatic of an allergic reaction (see page 385) or an injury to an abdominal organ (see below). If abdominal pain seems unrelated to trauma, is not accompanied by vomiting or diarrhea and lasts more than 2 hours, or is of sudden onset and lasts more than 2 hours, contact your doctor.

EVALUATING ABDOMINAL PAIN

Abdominal pain can result from either trauma or illness. Because abdominal pain can be symptomatic of so many different illnesses, it must be evaluated in terms of type of pain, relative location, and intensity and duration.

Each of the following sets of symptoms are general and inclusive. The victim may not necessarily experience all the symptoms at once. The descriptions are meant to

VOMITING AND DIARRHEA

In most cases, vomiting and diarrhea are the body's short-term response to infection and will end as the body clears the infection. Persistent diarrhea may, however, cause dehydration; young children and the elderly are particularly vulnerable. If a child or a senior shows signs of dehydration, which include sunken eyes, dry mouth, extreme thirst, irritability, and failure to urinate, consult a doctor immediately.

Give children or seniors small amounts (1 tbl) of water regularly, even during bouts of vomiting. A swallow every 10 or 20 minutes will help keep them from becoming dehydrated. Slightly salty liquids such as clear broth may facilitate absorption of moisture and hydrate better than plain water. Be aware that large amounts of liquid may provoke more vomiting. If severe diarrhea persists longer than 36 hours, consult your doctor. For more information on maintaining fluids during diarrhea in infants, see page 213.

In some cases, vomiting or diarrhea may be a response to medication. If a medication causes nausea and vomiting, check with your doctor to ensure that you are using it properly or ask your doctor to recommend a different medication.

Vomit or diarrhea with blood in it is always a cause for concern. Call your doctor. Vomit that is green, yellow, or red, or is full of dark brown particles with the consistency of coffee grounds is a sign that you should call your doctor immediately.

Diarrhea that is bloody or stool that is bloody or black and tarry-looking may also be a sign of a serious illness and should be evaluated by your doctor as soon as possible. Certain food colorings and medications, such as iron supplements and bismuth-containing compounds like Pepto Bismol, can make stool appear dark, but dark, tarry-looking stool often means bleeding from the stomach or duodendum (upper intestine) and may be a signal of gastritis, peptic ulcer, or other conditions. Bright red blood in the stool indicates bleeding in the lower portion of the gastrointestinal tract and may indicate hemorrhoids, colorectal cancer, ulcerative colitis, or other illness. For more information on these specific conditions, see Chapter 23. ∎

If the abdominal pain is accompanied by high fever and jaundice (yellowing of the skin or whites of the eyes), go to the emergency room. If pain is accompanied by vomiting blood, or a dark, grainy substance with the consistency of coffee grounds, contact your doctor or go to the emergency room.

Abdominal pain that lasts for several hours or even days, particularly following heavy drinking, seems to penetrate all the way through from stomach to back, and increases when the victim lies on his back may be an indication of very serious illness. Contact your doctor or visit the emergency room immediately.

Pain that begins at the navel, progresses to tenderness of the belly and aching at the lower right corner of the abdomen should be evaluated by your doctor.

Abdominal cramping Abdominal cramping may or may not require medical attention. If the cramping is incapacitating and lasts for more than 20 minutes, it may be due to a serious abdominal condition and should be evaluated by your doctor. For more information on disorders of the digestive system that may lead to abdominal cramping, see Chapter 23.

Gastrointestinal conditions that may be unaccompanied by abdominal pain Some illnesses of the gastrointestinal tract may not be accompanied by pain or may be accompanied by transient pain or pain that is easy to ignore. The following symptoms may indicate serious illness that should be evaluated by your doctor, even if you have no pain.

Symptoms

- Change in bowel habits including chronic constipation, loss of regularity, frequent need to move bowels, and loose, unformed stool
- Bloody stool
- Black, tarry-looking stool
- Bright red blood in the toilet water or on toilet paper

Pelvic Pain

The pelvic area is the lowest part of the trunk above the legs and between the hips, and includes the reproductive organs. Pelvic pain is most often related to the genitourinary tract. Some pelvic conditions may be emergencies that require calling EMS. Others, such as kidney stones, can be quite painful but are not necessarily emergencies. Still, you should seek medical attention for any pelvic pain that is more than transitory or is related to injury.

❖ ECTOPIC PREGNANCY

Ectopic pregnancy is also known as tubal pregnancy and happens when a fertilized egg has not descended into the womb but remains in the fallopian tube (see page 150 for more information).

Symptoms

- Abdominal pain and cramps
- Pelvic pain
- Vaginal bleeding (sometimes)
- Urge to urinate or defecate
- Nausea or dizziness

What you should do This is a potentially life-threatening condition and requires immediate attention. *Contact EMS or your doctor immediately.*

❖ OVARIAN CYSTS

As a result of endometriosis, other conditions, and even normally reproductive function cysts can form on the ovaries. In some circumstances, they may cause considerable pain (see page 1124).

Symptoms

- Sudden and severe pain, possibly on one side of the lower abdomen or upper pelvic region (may be mistaken for appendicitis)
- Fever
- Vomiting

What you should do Contact your doctor immediately.

TESTICULAR TORSION

An uncommon but painful and potentially dangerous condition, testicular torsion occurs when one of the testes gets twisted in the scrotal sac. This condition is most common in prepubertal boys but may also occur in men. Because the vas deferens—the vessel that leads from the testicle to the prostate gland and supplies the testicles with blood—can become crimped, loss of blood flow may lead to damage to the testicle (see Testicular Torsion, page 1142).

Symptoms

- Sudden and persistent pain in one of the testes—may occur spontaneously or after physical exertion
- Nausea and vomiting
- Fever (possibly)
- Swelling
- Dizziness or faintness
- Increased pain on lifting the affected testicle

What you should do Because of the potential for damage to the testicle, go to the emergency room or contact your doctor immediately.

❖ KIDNEY STONES

Symptoms

- Sudden onset of intense pain in the flank (side of the torso between the ribs and the hips), likely descending toward the groin
- Painful sense of an urgent need to urinate
- Blood in the urine

What you should do Talk to your doctor. Most cases resolve when the stone is passed out through the bladder and urethra. Passing a kidney stone may be quite painful because stones can be jagged; it is often more painful for men than for women. However, a stone completely blocking the flow of urine may be a medical emergency and you should contact your doctor immediately.

NONSPECIFIC PELVIC OR LOWER ABDOMINAL PAIN

Many conditions, some of which are serious, may cause mild—in some cases very mild—pelvic pain, frequent urination, the sense of

TRAUMA TO THE PELVIC REGION/GENITAL INJURY IN MALES

Most boys are aware from an early age how painful a blow to the groin can be—mild to intense pain accompanied by nausea and even vomiting. But the testicles are resilient and generally pain will subside within a few minutes to an hour. If pain does not subside within an hour, look for:

- Swelling
- Bruising
- Change in shape (swelling of the scrotal sac)

If any of these symptoms is present, contact your doctor. Internal bleeding is always a possibility, so it is wise to have the injury evaluated as soon as possible.

What You Should Do Call your doctor. Keep calm or, if you are helping someone, try to keep the victim calm.

The victim should lie down and not walk around unless absolutely necessary. Use cold compresses on any swelling. You can also gently support injured testicles with a "hammock" of folded towels placed between the legs.

If the trauma was not caused by a blow to the genitals look for the following symptoms:

- Bleeding
- Extreme pain
- Urine leakage
- Urine blockage
- Object imbedded in the urethra

What You Should Do Contact your doctor immediately. Never try to remove an imbedded object; this may cause further injury unless it is done by a medical professional. Treat any external bleeding appropriately (see page 379).

If an injury to the pelvic area occurs in a child and is not accidental, see The Possibility of Sexual Abuse in Children, page 378. ■

needing to urinate frequently, cramps, and dull recurrent pain. These include pelvic inflammatory disease (see page 1116), sexually transmitted infections (see page 861), and cystitis, (see page 1067). Cystitis, or urinary tract infection, may also cause blood in

THE POSSIBILITY OF SEXUAL ABUSE IN CHILDREN

Genital trauma or injury in children may be the result of horseplay, of sexual experimentation by children of similar age, or self-experimentation. But depending on the circumstances—the involvement of older children or adults—and type of injury—genital bleeding or an object imbedded in a body opening—the possibility that the injury could be the result of sexual abuse or assault must be taken seriously. If you suspect sexual abuse or assault there are certain steps you should take.

- Treat external bleeding with direct pressure on the wound using a clean cloth (see page 379).

- Do not try to remove any object that may be imbedded in a body opening.

- Calm the child.

- *Do not* voice opinions about the circumstance; if the child must later be a witness, an adult's comments can color his opinions.

- Do not respond in a confrontational or accusatory manner.

- Try to preserve all potential evidence. Prevent the child from changing clothing, especially underwear; do not allow the child to bathe or wash, unless washing is a part of your cleansing of external wounds.

- Be aware of the possibility of internal bleeding.

- Medical examination is crucial. Take the child to your doctor or to the emergency room immediately. The emergency room may have staff trained to deal with both the physical and emotional aspects of sexual abuse and assault, and may be more thoroughly equipped to preserve evidence and work with the police.

- Be aware of the possibility of sexually transmitted diseases.

- Talk to your doctor, hospital personnel, or other appropriate professionals about counseling for the child. ■

the urine; if cystitis is ignored or neglected, it may lead to kidney damage. All of these conditions should be evaluated and treated as soon as possible. Talk to your doctor. *Any time blood appears in the urine, consult your doctor immediately.*

Pain in the Extremities

If pain in the extremities is related to trauma—a blow, a fall, a sports injury, or other accident—see Fractures and Dislocations, page 387; Strains and Sprains, page 389; and External Bleeding, page 379.

Spontaneous pain in the extremities not related to trauma or injury may indicate a serious medical condition that requires intervention by emergency personnel.

ACUTE PAIN IN THE EXTREMITIES

Sudden pain in the extremities (arms, hands, legs, and feet) that has no external cause such as blow or injury, may indicate that a blood vessel has become blocked either by a blood clot, by an embolus, or by worsening atherosclerosis (see Disorders of the Peripheral Arteries and Veins, page 833).

What you should do Get the victim to the emergency room immediately, even if you are not sure that the problem is an obstruction.

Blockage by plaque is most likely to occur in people suffering from atherosclerosis. More common in diabetics than in the general population, an acute arterial obstruction may lead to very serious complications, including necrosis and gangrene, and the possibility of loss of limb.

Symptoms

- Pain in the leg, possibly near the knee
- Paleness or coolness of the affected limb

ACUTE JOINT PAIN

Spontaneous joint pain may be the result of trauma; arthritis, such as gout; bursitis; or tendonitis. Joint pain caused by arthritis will likely build up over time rather than appear suddenly and will be worse when the joint is moved, especially after resting. Infectious arthritis is a type of arthritis caused by bacteria in the joint. Infectious arthritis is a serious condition and requires emergency medical attention.

What you should do Consult your doctor; any unexplained joint pain needs to be evaluated promptly. Any persistent joint pain following an injury should be evaluated by a doctor. Anti-inflammatory drugs such as aspirin or ibuprofen can provide temporary relief but should only be used if instructed by your doctor.

Bleeding

Blood circulates throughout the body in two loops, one composed of the arteries, which bring blood from the heart to organs and tissue, and the other composed of the veins, which bring blood back to the heart. Coming directly from the heart, blood in the arteries moves at greater pressure; a cut artery will spurt or pulse and is much more serious than a cut vein. A person can bleed to death from a severed artery in a matter of minutes. Veins tend to ooze. Since veins are closer to the skin than arteries, bleeding in most injuries is from veins.

EXTERNAL BLEEDING

Exactly what level of first aid you will need to render for external bleeding problems and whether you will need to contact EMS or use the emergency room depends on the severity of the injury. However, the rule of thumb is to apply direct pressure on the wound to stop the bleeding.

The amount of blood present in a bleeding emergency is *not* a good indicator of whether emergency medical attention is needed. Bleeding from the scalp, for example, where all the blood vessels are close to the surface, may be quite heavy even for a relatively minor cut. A deep puncture or incision wound may not cause profuse external bleeding, yet it may be a serious injury.

There are several different types of soft tissue wounds (wounds to the skin and underlying tissue). Incisions; clean cuts, such as from broken glass, that may go deep; lacerations, jagged or rough cuts; and avulsions, cuts that tear away flesh from the underlying tissue, generally all require the same first aid treatment. Your doctor and EMS personnel may treat each type of wound differently, but the rule of thumb for first aid care providers is direct pressure on the wound to prevent or stop bleeding.

External bleeding emergencies The sight of blood frightens many people, so be aware that even if the victim's wound is relatively minor, he may faint (see page 370). If bleeding is severe, be aware of the possibility of shock (see page 384). If at all possible, have the victim lie down. If you have latex or rubber gloves, use them. If you do not, take precautions by using a few layers of bandages or plastic wrap to minimize your contact with the victim's blood (see Precautions Against Infectious Disease, page

354). If possible, wash your hands before and after treating the victim.

1. Contact EMS immediately.
2. If the victim is conscious, calm him and ask permission to help. If the victim is unconscious, check his airway, breathing, and circulation (see Resuscitation ABCs, page 357).
3. Locate the injury or injuries. Remove any garment that obscures the wound; you may have to cut or tear the clothing. Treat the most severe wound first (see Which Injury Is Most Serious?, page 357).
4. To reduce the danger of infection, try to avoid touching the wound directly with your hands or anything else that is not sterile. If a sterile cloth or gauze is not available, use any cloth; use your hands only as a last resort.
5. Clean the wound.
   - If loose foreign material *surrounds* the wound, remove it by wiping it away from the wound.
   - *Do not* try to clean foreign material out of a serious wound.
   - *Do not* try to remove objects that are imbedded in the wound; leave this to EMS or other medical personnel. Bleeding may worsen when objects are removed.
6. Apply pressure to stop the bleeding (see Controlling Severe Bleeding, page 380)
   - Apply direct pressure to the wound with a sterile dressing or clean cloth.
   - If the bleeding stops with direct pressure but resumes when the pressure is removed, reapply direct pressure.
   - *Do not* use direct pressure to control bleeding if the wound is to the head and there is a possibility of skull fracture, if you suspect a fracture near the wound, or if there are objects imbedded in the wound. Apply indirect pressure (see page 381).
   - *Do not* apply direct pressure or try to stop bleeding from the eyes. Dress and bandage both eyes even if only one is injured; this can help halt eye movement that might further damage the injured eye.
   - If severe bleeding is from the nose see Nosebleeds, page 383.

CONTROLLING SEVERE BLEEDING

In severe bleeding, your object is not necessarily to stop the bleeding entirely, which you may not be able to do. In many cases what you will do is control bleeding so that drastic loss of blood is prevented while you wait for EMS.

Do not use a tourniquet unless all other methods of controlling bleeding fail. A tourniquet can cut off *all* blood flow to the injured area and may do more harm than good.

Direct Pressure

The safest and best method for the control of severe bleeding is applying direct pressure to the wound. If you have latex gloves, use them.

1. Place a sterile gauze dressing, or the cleanest, least fuzzy cloth available, against the source of the bleeding.

2. Apply firm pressure with your hands. This may be painful to the victim.

3. Apply a covering bandage over the gauze or cloth covering the wound. You can do this yourself or have someone else do it while you maintain pressure. Use rolled gauze or the best available material, such as strips of bedsheet, towels, or sack-cloth, making sure that the cloth does not come into contact with the wound but only wraps around the wound to hold the dressing in place.

4. Maintain pressure on the wound until the bandage has been applied.

5. Knot the covering bandage directly over the wound and source of bleeding.

6. Do not remove the bandage. Leave this to EMS personnel or other medical professionals.

7. If the wound bleeds through the dressing, enough pressure may not have been applied. Without removing the bandage,

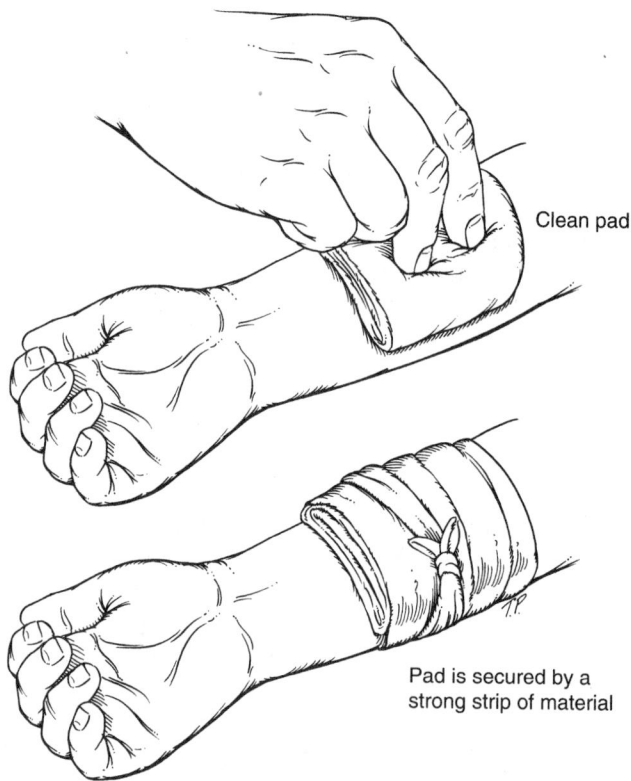

Clean pad

Pad is secured by a strong strip of material

To apply direct pressure to control bleeding, a sterile pad or the cleanest available cloth is applied directly against the wound and held firmly for several minutes. To maintain pressure, a narrow strip of strong material—part of a shirt, sheet, or towel, for example—can be wrapped over the pad and around the limb and then secured.

apply direct pressure again and put a second dressing and bandage over the first. In most cases, this will control the bleeding. ▶

- If severe bleeding is from the mouth see Dental Injury, page 394

- If severe bleeding is the result of a fracture see Fractures and Dislocations, page 387.

7. Elevate the part of the body that is bleeding so that it is above the level of the victim's heart, which can slow the rate of bleeding.

   - *Do not* elevate the body part if it is fractured or if you suspect a fracture.

   - *Do not* elevate the bleeding body part if the victim asks you not to do so.

   - *Do not* elevate the victim's legs if you suspect a spinal injury.

8. Dress and bandage the wound.

- If bandage and gauze are available, completely cover the wound with a sterile bandage and use rolled gauze to secure it in place. If sterile dressings are not available, improvise.

- If there is a large object imbedded in the wound, surround the object with dressings to immobilize it, then bandage around it.

9. Keep the victim as still as possible until EMS arrives or until you arrive at an emergency room. Movement may restart the bleeding.

Nonemergency external bleeding If a wound is minor and not bleeding severely, you can clean it and dress it without the help of emergency personnel. If possible,

▶ 8. If you have nothing to make into a bandage, maintain direct pressure with your hands until EMS arrives.

Indirect Pressure

If direct pressure alone does not control the bleeding, if you suspect fracture, or if there is on object embedded in the wound, you can apply indirect pressure. Indirect pressure is pressure applied to specific arterial pressure points that bring blood to specific areas of the body (see illustration, this page).

1. Use a finger to find the arterial pressure point closest to the wound. If you are using indirect pressure in addition to direct pressure, maintain direct pressure throughout.

2. Apply pressure to the artery with your finger, gently pressing it toward the bone.

3. Maintain pressure only long enough to control bleeding.

Tourniquets

A tourniquet should be used only in cases of life-threatening bleeding, such as may accompany traumatic amputation (see page 390) or other uncontrollable arterial bleeding. Improper use of a tourniquet may lead to further, serious injury including the destruction of tissue.

Never use wire, rope, cable, any other narrow cord, or anything that might cut into the skin to make a tourniquet. A tourniquet should ideally be at least 2 in. wide, which spreads pressure over a wide area of tissue and reduces the risk of tissue damage.

An EMS tool kit will contain a tourniquet, usually a webbed belt with a buckle, but most first aid situations will call for improvisation. You can use your belt, the sleeve of a shirt, a length of towel, or even duct tape. You may have to be resourceful. To make a tourniquet:

1. Wrap the tourniquet tightly just above the wound.

2. If you are using a cloth, try to knot it directly over the pressure point, pressing the artery toward the bone.

3. Do not insert any sort of bar or rod into the device to twist it tight. Pressure from knotting or taping should be sufficient to control the bleeding until EMS arrives.

4. Continue to apply direct pressure and indirect pressure if necessary. ∎

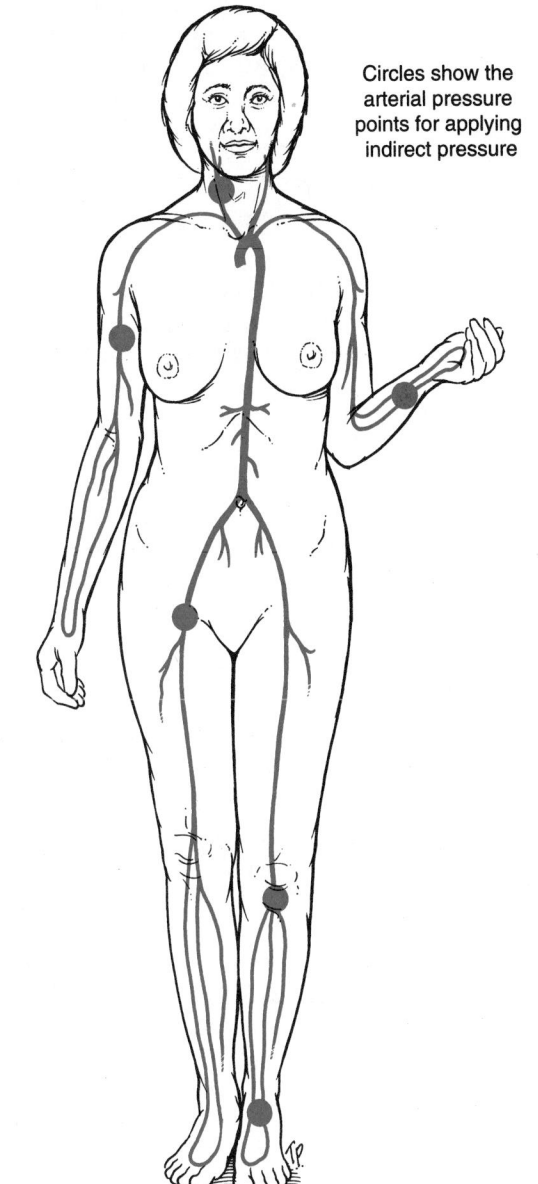

Circles show the arterial pressure points for applying indirect pressure

To slow the blood flow to a wound, arteries supplying blood to a wound can sometimes be compressed at locations other than the wound itself. Find the arterial pressure point closest to the wound and maintain pressure just long enough to control bleeding. Normal pulsations can typically be felt at the pressure points.

wash your hands and wear latex gloves to treat any bleeding wound.

1. Rinse the wound with running water or, if available, a sterile saline solution. If no running water is available, wipe the wound with antiseptic wipes or with sterile gauze or a clean cloth wetted with antiseptic solution. Start in the middle and work outward. If it is not possible to clean the wound thoroughly, bandage it and consult your doctor.

2. When the wound is clean, dry it by dabbing with a clean cloth or, if available, sterile gauze.

3. Apply antiseptic spray or ointment.

4. Use a sterile gauze pad or pads to dress the wound. The dressing is the sterile material placed directly on the wound. Never use cotton balls,

loose cotton, or a similar material directly on an open wound.

5. Bandage the wound; the bandage is the material that holds the dressing in place.

BRUISES

A bruise, or contusion, is an injury caused by a blow that does not break the skin but does break blood vessels beneath the skin. Bruising results in discoloration of the skin in the area of the blow where blood from broken vessels pools.

A severe bruise may be accompanied by considerable, deep pain. Bruises are not usually emergencies. In some cases, however, medical attention is warranted.

What you should do If there is reason to suspect internal bleeding, call EMS (see The Hidden Danger of Internal Bleeding, page 384). Call your doctor if there is loss of function or sensation or if there is reason to suspect a broken bone. When bruises appear spontaneously, without evident injury, they could signal a serious illness. Contact your doctor.

Most bruises do not require treatment and may not be very noticeable once the initial pain has subsided. Treat the injury by applying an ice pack to help reduce swelling and pain, but never put unwrapped ice on bare skin. If the bruise is on the arm or leg elevate the limb above the level of the heart to help reduce swelling and throbbing pain; however, do not elevate the victim's legs or move the victim in any way if you suspect spinal cord injury.

ABRASIONS

When the skin is scraped it has suffered an abrasion. Some abrasions bleed; others leave a welt and are accompanied by a burning sensation, such as a "rug burn." Abrasions are usually more painful than serious. A heavily bleeding abrasion should be treated as any external bleeding wound (see page 379).

What you should do Remove any clothing from the area around the wound. Clean the wound by washing with mild, soapy water. If there are small objects imbedded in the wound such as sand, grit, or twigs, try to flush them away with water. If necessary, carefully remove stubbornly imbedded object with tweezers. Finally, treat the wound with an antibiotic spray or ointment and bandage with sterile gauze to avoid the possibility of infection.

PUNCTURE WOUNDS

Puncture wounds are caused by a penetrating foreign body such as a nail, a thorn, or a bullet. There are two basic types of puncture wounds: perforating and penetrating. Perforating puncture wounds have both an entry and an exit wound; for example, when a bullet goes in through the chest and out through the back. Frequently, the exit wound is the more serious. Penetrating puncture wounds only have an entry wound; the foreign body may remain in the wound.

Puncture wounds include everything from splinters to bullet wounds. Perforating puncture wounds usually bleed externally as well as internally. Penetrating puncture wounds may not bleed externally very profusely; however, this does not mean that the wound is not serious. Depending on its location, a penetrating wound may cause serious internal damage and bleeding.

What you should do Treat puncture wounds for external bleeding (see page 379). If you suspect that the wound may be serious, contact EMS or take the victim to the emergency room.

Penetrating puncture wounds may need to be examined by a doctor and may warrant a tetanus shot. All significant puncture wounds—even if they close rapidly and appear trivial—carry the very real risk of infection, particularly with tetanus (see page 878).

If the foreign body that caused the puncture remains in the wound—the nail that was stepped on, for example—do not try to remove it. Unsuccessful attempts at removal can do more harm than good. Treat for external bleeding and immobilize the foreign body with a sterile dressing (see page 379). Take the victim to the emergency room to have the object removed by medical professionals.

Splinter removal Splinters should always be removed. Except in the case of large or

TETANUS

The bacteria that cause tetanus are most commonly present in soil, but can be found nearly anywhere—on a nail you step on, a can you cut your finger on, or on pavement where you fall. It is not uncommon for these bacteria to enter the skin when it is cut and if the victim is not immunized, tetanus infection may develop. Tetanus can be lethal. Whenever an individual is cut, the possibility of tetanus should be taken seriously.

Shallow incision-type wounds carry the lowest risk of tetanus. Wounds that are left dirty or untreated for long periods of time carry the highest risk. Even if cleaned and treated, puncture wounds still carry a high risk of tetanus because of their very nature—a foreign, potentially bacteria-carrying object that penetrates the body.

Most children in the United States are immunized early against the infection with the diphtheria, pertussis, and tetanus (DPT) vaccine; however, the vaccine's protection is not lifelong and must be renewed every 5 to 10 years.

Who Should Have a Tetanus Vaccine or Booster?

- Anyone with a wound who has never been immunized

- Anyone with a wound who has not had a booster in the last 10 years

- Anyone with a wound that may be considered high risk who has not been immunized or had the booster within the last 5 years should have a tetanus shot.

Check with your doctor if you are unsure or unaware of when you or your child last had a tetanus shot. If necessary a tetanus shot, whether original vaccine or booster, should be given as soon as possible. Immunization works only if it is given within 72 hours of the occurrence of the wound. For further information see Tetanus, page 878. ■

potentially dirty splinters that go deep beneath the skin, splinters are not usually a reason to seek emergency care, although you may want to contact your doctor.

To remove a splinter, first wash your hands. Do not wash the area that contains the splinter; washing may make it more difficult to remove the splinter, particularly if it is wood.

With sterilized tweezers, grasp the protruding end of the splinter and pull it out. Pull at the same angle at which the splinter went in. If the splinter is entirely beneath the skin, use a sterilized, slender sewing needle to open the wound and lift the splinter clear enough of the skin so that you can grasp its end with the tweezers. Do not keep trying if you find you cannot remove the splinter, if the splinter breaks, or if the skin becomes inflamed, is painful, or bleeds; call your doctor or go the emergency room.

Once the splinter is out, wash the area thoroughly and apply an antiseptic spray or ointment. If the wound is more than a pinprick, dress and bandage it. Infection is always possible, particularly with tetanus (see page 878). Make sure the victim is up-to-date on his tetanus immunization. If an infection should develop after a splinter is removed, contact your doctor. If the area becomes inflamed, more painful, or develops pus or if the victim develops a fever, swollen lymph glands, or red streaking on the skin near the wound, an infection may have developed that requires prompt medical attention.

NOSEBLEEDS

Nosebleeds are often more of a nuisance than a life-threatening or emergency condition. They are much more common during cold weather when heated air indoors dries out the nasal passages, and at high altitudes where humidity is consistently at low levels. Use of a saline nasal spray—*not* a medicated nasal spray—during the driest weather helps keep nasal membranes hydrated.

Persistent nosebleeds in an adult may be a sign of high blood pressure and should be evaluated by a doctor.

Nasal bleeding after a blow to the nose may signal a broken nose, particularly if there is swelling or the nose appears disfigured, and requires immediate treatment from a doctor or emergency room (see Fractures and Dislocations, page 387). Bleeding from both nostrils after a blow to the head may signal internal bleeding and the victim should receive emergency medical assistance (see The Hidden Danger of Internal Bleeding, page 384).

What you should do Calm the victim, have him sit down, and encourage him to breathe through his mouth. If there is an object in the nose, see page 384. If the nose is free of foreign objects, gently pinch the nostrils shut. The nostrils should be held shut for 15 minutes. Put a cold compress on the nose and face, which can be done while the nostrils are being held shut.

If bleeding does not stop, after 15 minutes, repeat these steps.

If after a second attempt the nose is still bleeding, contact your doctor. As you treat a nosebleed, try to collect the blood to assess the amount lost.

Removing a foreign object from the nose
Particularly in small children, a nosebleed can be caused by a foreign object lodged in one of the nostrils. The object should be removed immediately and victim should be encouraged not to inhale through the nose but to breathe through the mouth.

Examine the nostrils to determine which one is affected. Pressing the opposite nostril gently closed with a finger, have the victim inhale through his mouth and then blow his nose. To help a very small child or a child who is too upset to inhale through his mouth, gently cover the affected nostril with a finger, taking care not to push the object farther into the nostril. Release the nostril just before he exhales. Once the object is dislodged, treat the nosebleed as described on page 383. If the object does not come out, repeat this procedure. If the object still does not come out, try to induce sneezing. If sneezing does not work, call your doctor.

BLEEDING IN PREGNANCY

Some vaginal bleeding during pregnancy may be more or less routine. During the earliest days of pregnancy, when you may not even know you are pregnant and when your menstrual period would normally be due, you may notice some spotting. In addition, about 20 percent of expectant mothers experience some bleeding during the first trimester that does not indicate miscarriage.

Still, vaginal bleeding at any time during pregnancy is cause for concern and you should always consult your doctor immediately. Bleeding at any time may be a sign of miscarriage; bleeding associated with miscarriage often begins not as bright red blood, but as a brownish discharge. Bleeding in the first trimester may be a sign of tubal, or ectopic, pregnancy. Bleeding after the first trimester is much less common and can signal several potentially dangerous conditions, including miscarriage, premature labor, and abnormal placenta location. For more information see Chapter 7.

BLOODY URINE, STOOL, OR VOMIT

Any time blood appears in the urine, stool, or vomit consult your doctor; the causes range from insignificant to serious. Your doctor will want to rule out severe conditions (see Vomiting and Diarrhea, page 375).

Shock

Shock is an abnormal condition of inadequate blood flow throughout the body, and can be caused by severe injury, loss of blood, electrical shock, sudden illness that shifts fluid from the bloodstream (see Septic Shock, page 386), severe allergic reactions (see Anaphylactic Shock/Severe Allergic Reaction, page 385), poisoning including substance abuse, exposure to extreme temperatures, and even emotional distress. Shock may also result from dehydration. If signs of

---

THE HIDDEN DANGER OF INTERNAL BLEEDING

It is not uncommon for symptoms of internal bleeding to take days or weeks to appear, and every victim of serious trauma should be evaluated by a doctor to rule out internal bleeding. This is especially true of chest, abdominal, head, and pelvic injuries. Nearly any fracture also carries with it the potential for internal bleeding.

Often, internal bleeding will have no symptoms at all. However, there may be bleeding from bodily orifices, for example, vomiting, coughing, or urinating blood; or bleeding from the penis, vagina, or rectum. Following any sort of traumatic injury, even a seemingly insignificant one, suspect internal bleeding if blood appears anywhere it normally does not or should not.

If someone bleeds from the ears or both nostrils after a blow to the head, but not directly to the nose, or after a blow to the back or neck, seek emergency care. Other signs of internal bleeding include tenderness of the abdomen following traumatic injury and tensing or spasm of the abdominal muscles following traumatic injury.

Failure to seek emergency care when there is the possibility of internal bleeding can be life-threatening. ■

SIGNS OF SHOCK

Nearly every physical injury causes some level of shock, although often it is hardly noticeable. What we commonly refer to as shock is severe shock, which can be life-threatening. It is important to recognize the symptoms of shock:

- Dull eyes and dilated pupils

- Confused or dazed expression

- Confusion, anxiety, or loss of mental acuity

- Extremely pale or ashen complexion (often sudden)

- Bluish skin, especially the lips and fingernails

- Clammy skin

- Weakness

- Nausea or vomiting

- Thirst

- Weak but rapid pulse

- Shallow or difficult breathing

- Unconsciousness ■

dehydration—sunken eyes, extreme thirst, dry mouth, lack of urine—accompany symptoms of shock, help the victim drink.

Regardless of the cause, the result is essentially the same: a loss of blood pressure, or volume, that results in the failure of the cardiovascular system to provide enough blood to all tissues. Shock can be life-threatening or it can be transitory depending upon how it is treated, so it is important to treat a victim for shock at the same time as you treat other injuries.

Shock can happen almost instantly upon injury or it can occur hours after the causative event. If untreated, shock may turn a relatively minor injury into a serious one.

TREATING SHOCK/THE SHOCK POSITION

What you should do If you suspect spinal injury, see page 368. If you do not suspect spinal injury call EMS immediately.

Check the victim's airway, breathing, and circulation (see Resuscitation ABCs, page 357). If necessary, begin artificial respiration, CPR (see Cardiopulmonary Resuscitation, page 361), or other treatment for any life-threatening injury, which may have caused shock.

Put the victim in the shock position as shown in the illustration above—flat on his back, arms at his side, and feet elevated above the level of the heart. Do not elevate the victim's head.

The shock position should be used only after you have addressed head, back, neck, and leg injuries. Do not put a victim of suspected spinal cord trauma into the shock position. Do not elevate the legs if a leg injury is a venomous bite—raising

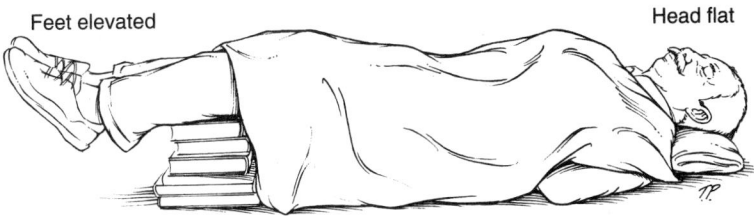

Feet elevated · Head flat

Victims in shock who have not suffered an injury to the spinal cord or a venomous bite to the leg should be placed on the back with the feet elevated above the heart. The head should not be elevated. A blanket may be used to provide additional warmth.

the legs could speed venom through the body.

Loosen any constricting clothing. Keep victim warm; cover him with a blanket. If the victim vomits, turn his head sideways to prevent choking. Care for other injuries as appropriate and continually monitor the victim's airway, breathing, and circulation until EMS arrives.

ANAPHYLACTIC SHOCK/SEVERE ALLERGIC REACTION

Anaphylactic shock occurs when a victim comes into contact with a substance to which he is extremely allergic. It can be life threatening.

Allergies that can lead to anaphylactic shock include those to certain medications such as penicillin, insect bites or stings (see Allergic Reactions to Bee Stings, page 400), fish or shellfish, peanuts, and tree nuts. For more information see Anaphylaxis, page 1341.

(There are many possible allergic reactions to food, most of them mild. It is only

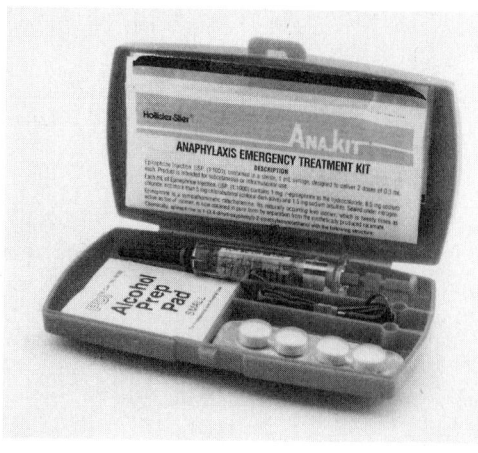

Anaphylactic emergency treatment kits may be prescribed for people who have a definite adverse reaction to certain allergens such as bee venom. Epinephrine injected with a syringe and needle at the time of a reaction can help minimize or prevent severe allergic reactions.

when someone experiences an anaphylactic reaction after exposure to a particular food that an emergency exists.)

Anyone with a known severe allergic sensitivity should wear a medical ID bracelet or tag at all times. A doctor may prescribe injectable epinephrine, also known as adrenaline, for people who have severe allergic sensitivities. Schools should be notified about children with severe allergic reactions and given specific information on what causes the allergic reaction and on how to deal with the reaction if it occurs.

Symptoms An anaphylactic reaction will usually occur within a few seconds or minutes after contact with the allergen. Symptoms may include some or all of the following:

- Swelling of the tongue and face
- Sudden and severe breathing difficulties, especially in people with asthma
- Itching or burning skin or mouth
- Widespread hives
- Weak, rapid pulse
- Dizziness or light-headedness
- Nausea, vomiting, and occasionally diarrhea
- Unconsciousness, which may happen quickly

What you should do Death from anaphylactic shock can occur in as little as 15 minutes. *Contact EMS immediately.*

Anaphylactic shock requires medication, usually epinephrine, in order to counteract the reaction. Some people with severe allergies carry emergency medication with them. If the victim has medication, help him use it. If no medication is available, continually monitor the victim's airway, breathing, and circulation (see Resuscitation ABCs, page 357) while help is on the way. If necessary, perform artificial respiration and CPR (see Cardiopulmonary Resuscitation, page 361). Put the victim in the shock position (see illustration, page 385).

HIVES AND ANGIOEDEMA

Hives are a common external symptom of many different allergic reactions and consist of raised, red, often itchy welts along the skin—much like mosquito bites. Hives can result from almost any allergic reaction. They can occur in areas of the body that do not come in contact with the allergen, as with food allergies. With insect bites, they will often appear in the immediate location of the bite. Depending upon the severity of the allergic reaction, they may spread.

Angioedema is similar to hives, with tissue swelling beneath the skin. This commonly occurs above the neck and frequently involves the lips and eyes, and tongue and throat. Sometimes the hands and feet are involved. Angioedema in the throat can be serious because it can block the airway. If you have known allergic reactions causing hives or angioedema, your doctor may prescribe epinephrine or recommend an over-the-counter antihistamine to counteract the reaction. For chronic or recurrent hives or angioedema it is best to visit an allergist and find out what causes the allergy and avoid future exposure to it. Foods and medications are commonly implicated, but sometimes hives and angioedema are not caused by allergies. There is a rare hereditary form of angioedema that can affect the digestive tract, causing cramping in the gut as well as swelling of the airway. Again, an allergist can help identify, prevent, and treat these reactions.

If angioedema occurs in the mouth or throat, call EMS at once and monitor the victim's airway, breathing, and circulation (see Resuscitation ABCs, page 357) until help arrives. Give the victim epinephrine if available. ■

SEPTIC SHOCK

Septic shock is the result of sepsis, which is an infection that has entered the bloodstream; the symptoms are virtually identical to those of other types of shock (see Signs of Shock, page 385), with the addition of flushing, reddened skin, fever, and chills. The victim may or may not know he has an infection.

Septic shock is a potentially life-threatening condition and must be treated as such. If an infection—such as a kidney infection—is known, and fever is followed by a sudden onset of reddening of skin, chills, and symptoms of shock, such as light-headedness, loss of mental acuity, extreme thirst, rapid but weak pulse, difficult breathing, assume septic shock. If an infection is unknown to the victim, but he displays these symptoms, assume septic shock.

What you should do Place the victim in the shock position and treat for shock (see page 385). Call EMS and monitor the victim's airway, breathing, and circulation (see Resuscitation ABCs, page 357) until help arrives.

Trauma

Traumatic injuries are incurred due to some sort of violence or force—a fall, a collision during athletic competition, an automobile accident—and include broken bones, sprains, dislocated joints, and head, eye, and dental injuries. Some traumatic injuries are serious emergencies that require immediate medical attention; others may be treated at home.

FRACTURES AND DISLOCATIONS

Broken bones range from a fractured skull to a crushed foot to incomplete fractures (stress and greenstick breaks) that may not immediately be recognized as broken bones. Even the slightest break, however, can carry a certain amount of danger because broken bones often have sharp or jagged edges and movement may cause internal bleeding and damage to tendons, muscles, or nerves.

Some fractures, particularly complex fractures, will be quite recognizable as broken bones. Dislocations and sprains, however, often manifest many of the same symptoms as fractures. *When in doubt, treat the injury as a fracture, particularly when discomfort does not resolve within 24 to 48 hours after a traumatic event.*

All breaks have the potential to lead to further complications, including internal bleeding, shock, and further injury if not treated properly. Fractures to the skull, neck, and back carry added risk, chief

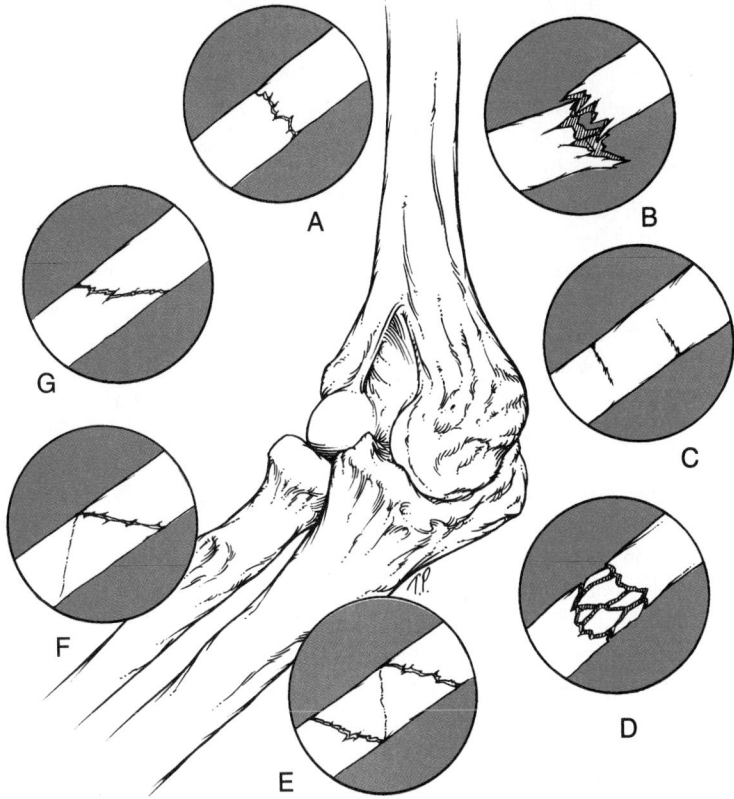

There are many types of fractures depending on shape. (A) Transverse fractures occur at right angles to the long axis of the bone. (B) In compound fractures, the skin is punctured at the site of the fracture and the bone is typically broken completely. (C) Greenstick fractures have incomplete breaks on only one side of the bone, but the fracture actually goes all the way across. (D) Comminuted fractures contain crushed or splintered bone particles. (E) Butterfly fractures are a type of spiral fracture with a central fragment between each spiral. (F) In spinal fractures, the bone has been twisted apart. (G) Oblique fractures do not occur at right angles to the long axis of the bone.

among them damage to the spinal column, which could result in paralysis.

Most fractures can be classified as either simple (a cracked bone, no break in the skin) or compound (a cracked bone, bone puncturing the skin).

Symptoms

- Pain, swelling, and discoloration of the skin in the area of the injury

- Disfigurement of the area—for example, a knee bent at the wrong angle

- Bone protruding through the skin (compound fracture)

SPLINTS AND SLINGS

Splints

The object of a splint is to immobilize a broken bone or suspected broken bone. Use a stiff backing and some kind of lashing to keep the bone in the position in which you found it.

Always treat more serious injuries first, especially bleeding wounds. If the break is compound, treat for bleeding and dress the area of broken skin before splinting.

When applying a splint, make it conform to the shape in which you found the limb, rather than trying to make the limb conform to the splint. Medical professionals will set the bone correctly. Use strong supports—boards, broom handles, baseball bats, rolled newspapers or magazines, folded cardboard, or even an umbrella or cane. If nothing as rigid as any of these is available, use rolled blankets, towels, sheets, or a pillow. You may need to improvise. The splint will ideally extend beyond the area of injury in both directions.

To lash the splint in place, you can use torn cloth, duct tape, or neckties if bandages are not available. Do not allow knots in the bandages to touch the area of injury. Be careful not to lash too tightly or to cut into the skin; circulation should continue normally. Injured areas may swell, so keep a lookout for signs of blocked circulation such as paleness of the limb, numbness, or pain, and loosen the splint if necessary to restore circulation.

Slings

The object of a sling is to support and immobilize a fractured or dislocated shoulder, arm, or wrist. If necessary, a splint can be applied before the sling. A sling will ideally be made from a large, triangular piece of cloth, but they can be improvised from almost any available material. If the injury is to the forearm or the wrist and the injured area is splinted, the sling does not necessarily have to cover the entire area of injury, but can support just the splint.

For shoulder or other injuries, a sling large enough to support the entire arm from elbow to fingertips, is ideal.

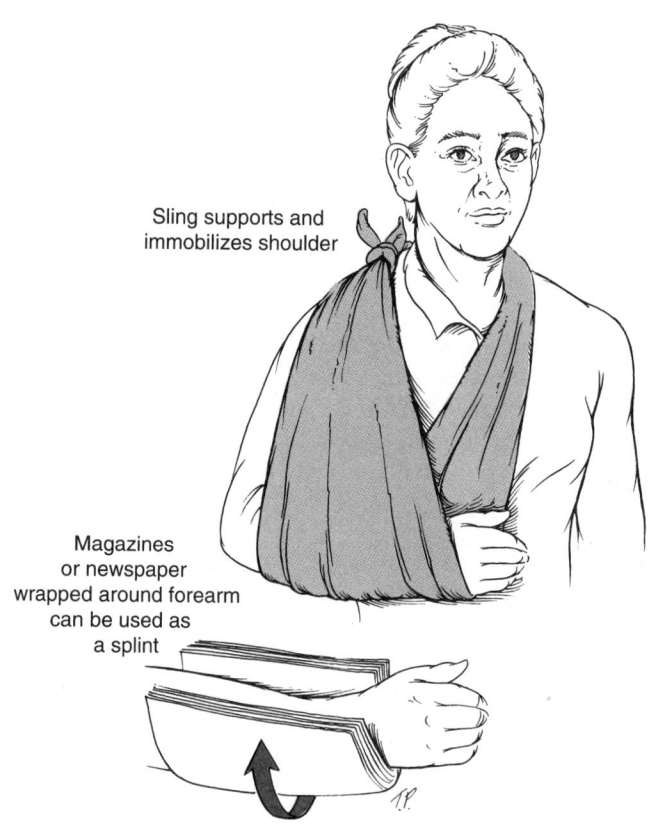

Sling supports and immobilizes shoulder

Magazines or newspaper wrapped around forearm can be used as a splint

A sling can support and immobilize a fractured or dislocated shoulder, arm, or wrist. For a shoulder injury, a large piece of fabric is wrapped around the shoulder and then supports it by covering the entire forearm.

Supporting the injured area, gently drape the material beneath the arm and extend the ends and knot or otherwise attach them around the neck. For more information on splints and slings, see pages 664 and 676. ■

- Loss of movement or persistently painful movement

What you should do Fractures can be either severe or minor. If the break is severe—if there is loss of blood or considerable immediate swelling—contact EMS immediately.

If there is bleeding, cover the wound with sterile dressings and do not move the injured area. If the break is compound and there is bleeding, the danger of shock from loss of blood or drop in blood pressure is very real. Look for signs of shock including cold, clammy skin; weak, rapid pulse; shallow breathing; blue-tinged or pale skin;

thirst; and dazed expression; and treat as necessary (see page 385).

If the suspected break is of the hip, pelvis, or femur (the thigh bone, which runs parallel to a major artery) do not attempt to move the victim or change the victim's position. Moving the victim could result in severe complications, including potentially fatal internal bleeding. If the victim's life is in danger and you must move him, use the clothes-drag technique that is used for moving a victim of spinal cord injury (see page 369).

Never attempt to set a disfigured bone or joint; it could result in further injury to nerves and blood vessels and cause great pain to the victim. Instead, immobilize the area of the break or suspected break. Use pads, blankets, towels, splints, or slings. In some cases, this may be easier to do if the victim is lying down (see Splints and Slings, page 388).

Monitor the victim's airway, breathing, and circulation (see Resuscitation ABCs, page 357) and continue to look for signs of shock until EMS arrives.

If the break is relatively minor, for example, to a toe or finger, and there is no bleeding, immobilize the area. Contact your doctor or bring the victim to the emergency room.

For a fractured nose, jaw, or skull, see Head Injury, page 390.

STRAINS AND SPRAINS

The extension of a joint beyond its normal range of function, or hyperextension, can result in a fracture, but more often it damages the soft tissue that surrounds the joint, resulting in muscle strain or ligament sprain. Strains result from stretching and tearing of muscle fibers. They may swell and can be painful, but they are not usually serious. Sprains result when ligaments or other nonmuscle tissues around joints are torn. Sprains may be quite painful and may swell. Sprains and fractures share similar symptoms and may require the same first aid treatment. Particularly if the joint does not operate properly and appears disfigured, which can happen in a severe sprain, or if the victim is in great pain, treat the injury as a fracture (see page 387).

Suspected muscle strains to the back may cause considerable pain and loss of movement. Victims should consult their doctors to rule out more serious injury to the vertebra bodies or discs.

If severe back pain occurs spontaneously or as a result of trauma, it may be more than muscle strain or stress. Victims should contact their doctors immediately. Back pain that is spontaneous or the result of injury in older women who are at risk for osteoporosis or have been diagnosed with osteoporosis should be evaluated by a doctor as soon as possible.

Symptoms of strain

* Sudden muscle pain, often following the hyperextension of a joint

* Bruising
* Swelling (possible)
* Painful movement

What you should do Remove any constricting clothing—shoes, socks, and rings and other jewelry—from the affected area. If possible elevate the strained area to reduce swelling. Apply an ice pack or cold compress to the affected area, but do not apply ice directly to bare skin.

Rest the affected muscles. Continue with periodic ice packs and rest for 24 hours. If the area feels better, apply heat using a heating pad or hot water bottle as often as possible for the next 3 to 4 days. If the affected area does not feel better within 24 hours, consult your doctor.

A wide elastic bandage can provide support to a minor injury such as a sprain or strain. When wrapping a sprained ankle, keep the elastic bandage slightly stretched but not too tight. Starting behind the toes, the bandage is wrapped smoothly, proceeding to the ankle, where a figure eight pattern is used. Cross the top of the foot, beneath the arch, back across the foot, around the ankle again, and around the lower leg.

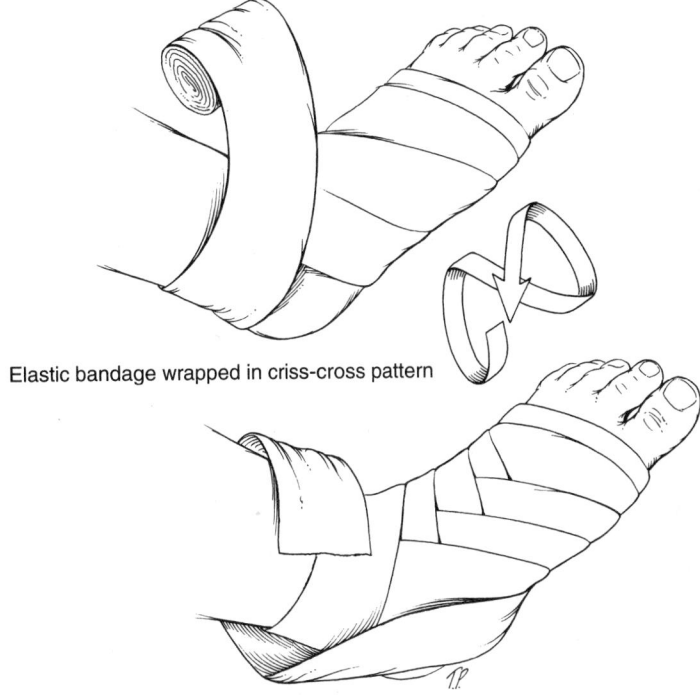

Elastic bandage wrapped in criss-cross pattern

Symptoms of sprain

- Joint pain following hyperextension of the joint
- Bruising
- Swelling
- Pain on movement of the joint
- Joint disfigurement (possible)

What you should do RICE—rest, ice, compression, and elevation—is the accepted treatment for sprains.

Remove any jewelry, especially rings, and constricting clothing from the affected area in case of swelling. Apply cold compresses to the joint as soon as possible after injury. Never apply ice directly to skin; wrap it in an ice pack or cloth, or use a freezable soft compress. An icepack can be bound to the joint with tape or an elastic bandage. Keep the joint as immobile as possible and elevate it with pillows, folded towels, or blankets.

Rest the joint; painful joints should not be used. Nonsteroidal anti-inflammatory drugs (NSAIDs), such as aspirin and ibuprofen, may be used to relieve pain and inflammation. If joint pain does not diminish within 2 to 3 days, does not respond to over-the-counter pain-relievers, is intolerable, or if the joint is misshapen, consult your doctor immediately.

TRAUMATIC AMPUTATION

Traumatic amputation is the partial or complete severing of a body part as the result of an accident. Examples of traumatic amputation are a finger severed by the closing of a car door or a foot or leg severed in an industrial accident.

What you should do Saving the victim's life is more important than locating or saving the body part. Call EMS immediately.

Treat the most serious injuries first, *including* any not related to the traumatic amputation. Check the victim's airway, breathing, and circulation (see Resuscitation ABCs, page 357). Control the bleeding using indirect pressure; use a tourniquet *only if all other attempts to control the bleeding fail* (see Controlling Severe Bleeding, page 380). Watch for signs of shock including cold, clammy skin; weak, rapid pulse; shallow breathing; blue-tinged or pale skin; thirst; and dazed expression; and treat as necessary (see page 385).

Once the victim is stabilized—bleeding has been controlled, the ABCs are stable, and any shock has been treated—then you can try to find and save the severed body part (see Saving an Amputated Body Part, below). Do not attempt to replace a severed or partially severed body part; leave that to medical personnel.

HEAD INJURY

The head is made up of the face, which includes the nose, eyes, ears, mouth, and jaw; the scalp; the skull, the brain; and the spinal fluid in which the brain is immersed; and the blood vessels that provide blood to the head and brain. Head injuries, even those that do not involve a fracture of the skull, can be quite serious. In some cases, a

SAVING AN AMPUTATED BODY PART

After administering first aid to the victim to control bleeding and attending to any life-threatening injuries, try to find and save the severed body part. In many cases it can be reattached by skillful surgeons. Even if the part cannot be completely reattached, it may still be useful to the doctors repairing the wound.

If possible, rinse any dirt or debris from the body part.

If Ice Is Available

- Wrap the body part in a dressing that has been moistened with clean water; a sterile dressing is ideal, but improvise if you must. *Do not place the part directly in ice, wrap it first.*

- Wrap the dressed part in plastic if available; if not, you can improvise by using a clean plastic container.

- Place the *wrapped* part in a bed of ice. Do not use dry ice, which will freeze and damage the part.

If Ice Is Not Available

- Wrap the body part directly in plastic without dressing it first.

- Keep the part away from heat. For example, do not place it in a closed car.

- Label the container with the name of the victim.

Iced body parts may remain viable for as long as 18 hours. Without ice, body parts may remain viable for 4 to 6 hours. ■

head injury without a fracture of the skull may be more dangerous than one with a skull fracture, because of the pressure caused by the swelling brain held within the fixed space of the intact skull.

Head and neck injuries are often related. A blow to the head significant enough to cause head injury may also affect the neck. With all head injuries, always take precautions against the possibility of a spinal cord injury (see page 368).

A child or adult may seem to completely recover from a blow to the head within a few minutes. However, remember that even seemingly mild head injuries carry the possibility of underlying brain injury. The likelihood is that there is no serious damage, but compression of the brain from swelling or bleeding may take time to develop. The victim should be kept quiet and watched for 24 hours for any decline in mental ability or awareness. If the victim wants to sleep let him, but wake him up every 2 to 3 hours to assess his condition. If the victim is hard to arouse or unable to answer specific questions such as what is the address of a friend or the phone number of a family member, call EMS or your doctor immediately. Also call EMS or your doctor if the victim has any of the symptoms listed below.

Symptoms

- Obvious trauma to the head, including disfigurement and bleeding. Bleeding from the scalp may be more profuse than from other areas of the body, even with relatively minor wounds, because of the proximity of the blood vessels to the skin surface.

- Clear or pinkish fluid coming from the ears, nose, or mouth

- Bleeding of the nose or mouth not related to direct trauma to the nose or mouth

- Confused or dazed behavior

- Dilated pupils or pupils of differing sizes

- Severe headache

- Vomiting

- Loss of mental acuity, including slurred speech and confusion. This may occur immediately following trauma or develop over several hours.

- Decline or loss of awareness, which may be either momentary or complete. This may occur immediately following trauma or may develop over several hours.

- Unusual sleepiness or drowsiness

- Anxiety or irritability

- Convulsions

- Swelling of the soft spot in an infant's skull

What you should do Call EMS if you suspect serious head injury. *Do not* move the victim unless his life is endangered; *do not* pick up a child with a head injury. Try to find out the exact nature of the injury either by asking the victim or bystanders.

Check the victim's airway, breathing, and circulation (see Resuscitation ABCs, page 357). If necessary, perform CPR and artificial respiration (see Cardiopulmonary Resuscitation, page 361), or treat for shock (see page 385).

Do not use direct pressure to control bleeding in a victim of head injury unless the bleeding is the product of an identifiably superficial wound to the scalp. If necessary, use indirect pressure to control heavy bleeding (see Controlling Severe Bleeding, page 380). Do not remove lodged foreign bodies.

Victims of head injury may vomit; take precautions to protect the victim's airway. If the victim is a child and vomits after a blow to the head, seek medical attention even if he does not vomit again or appears otherwise normal.

After addressing the victim's airway, breathing, and circulation, and the head injury, treat other injuries or bleeding as necessary (see Where to Find It Fast, page 353).

If the victim is unconscious but his airway, breathing, and circulation are okay, stabilize his head in the position in which you found it by gently placing your hands on either side of the head and keeping the head immobile.

If the victim is *conscious* and his airway, breathing, and circulation are okay, he may still be disoriented, anxious, and even combative. Ensure that the victim stays still and discourage him from trying to stand or move. Try to calm him; tell him your name and that help is on the way. Ask the victim his name and ask him what happened. Be aware that if he cannot tell you what happened, he may have lost consciousness;

inform EMS technicians about this when they arrive.

EYE INJURY

Traumatic injury to the eye may lead to infection, bleeding, laceration, and ultimately, loss of vision. For nontraumatic eye problems, such as infection or vision problems, even sudden ones, see Chapter 15.

Traumatic eye injury includes direct trauma to the eye, such as a scratch, blow, or cut (see below); a foreign body in the eye (see below); penetrating injury to the eye (see page 393); chemical matter in the eye (see page 393); and burns to the eye (see page 394).

❖ DIRECT TRAUMA TO THE EYE

Symptoms

- Pain, stinging, burning, or intense itchiness in the eye or surrounding area
- Signs of trauma including bleeding, cuts, and bruises (see page C-43)
- Presence of a foreign body or the sensation of something in the eye
- Bloodshot appearance, redness, or red spots on the white of the eye
- Tearing or other discharge
- Light sensitivity
- Impaired or lost vision
- Headache
- Uncoordinated pupils, or pupils of differing sizes

What you should do If there is loss of vision, bleeding, or other serious trauma to the eye, contact EMS at once. Never apply pressure to the eye or allow the victim to rub it. Make a homemade eye shield by cutting down a paper cup to a height of approximately 1 in. Use adhesive tape to hold the cut-down cup over the injured eye. Even though the other eye may not be injured, cover it also using an eye patch or dressing; this helps limit eye movement that could further injure the affected eye.

If there is a cut or other injury to the eyelid, the possibility of damage to the eye itself is great: seek emergency medical assis-

tance. As described above, protect the injured eye with an eye shield and also cover the unaffected eye.

If there is internal bleeding of the eye, a pool of blood may become visible behind the cornea, or lens of the eye. If you can see such an area in the iris (the colored part of the eye that surrounds the pupil), seek emergency medical assistance. As described above, protect the injured eye with an eye shield and also cover the unaffected eye. Do not open the eyes once the patches are on, as this may cause further injury.

If the area around the eye is bruised (a black eye), apply an ice pack or cold compress to reduce swelling and pain. Application of raw meat could cause infection. *Do not* apply direct pressure.

If the area around the eye is cut, do not use direct pressure to stop the bleeding. Use sterile dressings to cover the wounds.

Reassure and comfort the victim. Loss of vision, even temporary, can be alarming.

❖ FOREIGN BODY IN THE EYE

If the victim wears contact lenses, do not try to remove them unless the eye is swelling quickly and there is no immediate medical assistance on the way.

Do not attempt to remove any persistent foreign body on the eye or any foreign body that appears to be embedded in the eye; leave this to medical professionals.

Do not use sharp objects, such as tweezers, to try to remove a foreign body from the eye (see page C-44), or dry material, such as cotton balls or swabs.

A corneal abrasion is a scratch to the surface of the eye that gives the sensation of something foreign in the eye. If you find nothing in the eye but the victim still experiences pain and is convinced that there is something there, consult your doctor or visit the emergency room. If you succeed in removing a foreign body, but the victim still experiences pain, swelling, or other symptoms, seek medical attention.

What you should do Strongly discourage the victim from rubbing the eye.

If possible, wash your hands. Examine the eye for the foreign body. If necessary, use a finger to pull down the lower lid of the eye; you can do this by gently tugging on the loose skin beneath the eye. When

IRRIGATING AN INJURED EYE

The safest way to deal with a substance or foreign body in the eye is to irrigate the eye, or flush it thoroughly with a sterile saline solution. Because sterile saline solution may not always be available, you can also use clean tap water. Do not touch the eye or use any other solution than water or sterile saline solution; this could damage the eye further.

If the victim is wearing glasses, remove them, but do not try to remove contact lenses until you have finished the irrigation.

Position the victim's head so that the eye in question is angled downward and the solution will not pool in the area around the eye. With one hand, hold the victim's eyelids open without touch-ing the eye; do this by positioning your thumb and index finger above and below the line of eyelashes.

Pour a gentle, steady stream of irrigating solution into the eye. Pour from the edge of the eye closest to the nose so the solution flows across the eye and out. Continue flushing for 15 or more minutes or until EMS arrives.

If both eyes are affected, put the victim into a very gentle shower and hold both eyes open under a steady stream of *luke-warm* water. If no shower is available, fill a bowl with clean water and have the victim put his head into the bowl and open both eyes.

Remove contact lenses only after the eye has been thoroughly flushed. ■

you locate the object, irrigate the eye thoroughly (see above).

If you still cannot locate the foreign body, examine beneath the upper eyelid either by gently lifting the eyelid at the eyebrow as the victim looks down, or by using the cotton-swab method. To do this, lay a cotton swab just below the eyebrow, across the orbit (bone) of the eye socket. Lift the eyelid, folding it back over the stick of the swab. If you locate the object and there are no other associated eye injuries, irrigate the eye thoroughly to try to expel it (see above). If you are not successful in removing the object by irrigation, and only if medical attention is unavailable, you can try using a clean, dry cotton cloth to "blot" the object out of the eye; do not use cotton balls or swabs.

❖ PENETRATING INJURY TO THE EYE

A penetrating injury to the eye is one in which an object has become embedded in the eye. (See page C-45.) This is potentially quite dangerous and requires immediate medical attention.

As with any other injury with an embedded object, do not try to remove the object; leave this for medical professionals. You could cause further serious injury. Do not attempt to remove contact lenses unless you cannot get immediate medical assistance.

Do not apply pressure to the eye and do not allow the victim to rub it.

What you should do Call EMS immediately. Leave the object embedded in the eye. Dress the eye with an eye shield. Position a cup over the eye and then bandage it in place with adhesive tape. Even though the other eye may not be injured, cover it also with an eye patch or dressing. This helps limit eye movement that could further injure the affected eye.

Try to keep the victim quiet and as calm as possible until medical assistance arrives.

❖ CHEMICAL MATTER IN THE EYE

An eye is naturally wet, and much more sensitive and porous than skin. An eye splashed or otherwise exposed to chemicals requires immediate first aid.

What you should do The eye or eyes should be immediately irrigated in the shower for a prolonged period in order to completely flush out the chemical (see Irrigating an Injured Eye, above). Many materials, such as detergents or solvents, are labeled and the label should have instructions for dealing with eye exposure. If the chemical irritant is known to be harmful to the eye, call EMS at once or your local poison center. However, do not wait to call to begin irrigation. *Immediately* start irrigating the eye; if possible, have someone else call EMS. If the chemical is unknown, it is safest to call EMS, particularly if the victim experiences burning, itching, or any of the other symptoms of eye injury. If the chemical is not labeled as harmful to the eye, which is true of many common kitchen items, it is probably sufficient to irrigate the eye thoroughly. However, if the victim experiences any lingering symptoms after thoroughly flushing the eye, seek medical assistance.

Do not let the victim rub the affected eye. Do not apply pressure to the eye or allow the victim to apply pressure to the eye. Remove contact lenses after irrigation if irrigation does not dislodge them.

If the victim needs emergency medical assistance, dress the affected eye with an eye patch or sterile gauze. Even though the other eye may not be injured, cover it also with an eye patch or dressing. This helps limit eye movement that could further injure the affected eye.

❖ BURNS TO THE EYE

A blast of hot gas, such as from fireworks or a kitchen accident, can severely damage the surface of an exposed eye. Sunlight and sunlamps can burn eyes as readily as they can burn skin. The seriousness of a burn to the eye may not be immediately apparent, particularly those caused by sunlight or sunlamps. If a sunburn is bad enough to cause peeling and blistering and the victim was not wearing ultraviolet eye protection, his eyes should probably be checked by a doctor.

What you should do If the burn was caused by heat from gas or steam, call EMS immediately.

The eye or eyes should be thoroughly irrigated (see page 393). Use cool water to keep swelling to a minimum. Irrigation should be stopped if it causes pain to the eye. After irrigation, a cool compress—not ice—may be helpful in reducing pain and slowing swelling, but never apply direct pressure to the eye. Dress the eye with a shield.

If the burn does not seem serious enough to warrant emergency services, you should still contact your doctor immediately for instructions. Do not wait for the injury to get worse.

FOREIGN OBJECT IN THE EAR

The old adage "Never put anything smaller than your elbow in your ear" is sound advice. In adults, foreign objects in the ear canal usually result from accident, often in conjunction with cleaning the canal; for example, the tip of a cotton-tipped swab breaks loose and lodges in the canal. Occasionally, insects become trapped after flying or crawling into the ear canal. Young children often go through a phase during which they put nearly anything in any body cavity they can reach, which can result in the intentional placement of small beans, rocks, toys, or parts of toys into the ear canal.

What you should do Unless you can see the entire object clearly and can grasp it without inserting an instrument into the ear canal, it is best not to attempt to remove it on your own. Great care must be taken not to push the object deeper, which could possibly damage the delicate ear drum.

Do not irrigate the canal with water or other solutions, particularly if the object is a bean or other vegetable matter; irrigation may cause the object to swell, making its extraction even more difficult.

Insects in the canal can be killed first by putting a few drops of mineral oil into the ear canal. Then you can use a suction bulb—such as those used to suction an infant's nose—to gently extract oil and insect.

If you cannot easily remove the object, contact your doctor immediately. If you can and do remove the object but the victim experiences discomfort in the ear, contact your doctor immediately.

DENTAL INJURY

Dental injuries most often occur from a blow to the mouth and can result in loss or loosening of teeth. Tooth avulsion (accidental removal of a tooth), broken teeth including crown fracture and root fracture, and any loosening or movement of the tooth from its original position are all dental emergencies and require immediate treatment. To avoid these injuries, mouth guards should always be worn while playing sports.

Dental injuries may also be the result of or be accompanied by a broken jaw. If you suspect a fracture of the jaw, it should be treated in the same manner as other fractures (see Fractures and Dislocations, page 387).

❖ TOOTH AVULSION

If the tooth that is lost is a baby tooth, it cannot be reimplanted but it should be saved for evaluation by a dentist. It is possible, however, to reimplant adult teeth if they have been knocked out with the root intact. All teeth that have been knocked out require special care for them to be viable for reimplantation.

The faster the tooth can be reimplanted and then treated by a dentist, the better the chances of success. If the tooth can be reimplanted within 30 minutes, there is a better chance that the tooth can be saved. With proper care, a tooth can sometimes be reimplanted up to several hours after avulsion.

What you should do Seek emergency dental care; call your dentist or go to a hospital emergency room immediately. Save the tooth or teeth as described below; do not touch the root end. To control bleeding, use direct pressure on the wound. Apply an ice pack or cold compress to the wound to reduce pain and swelling.

Pick up the tooth without touching the root end. If water is immediately available, gently rinse off any dirt or debris but do not scrub the root. Holding the tooth by the chewing edge, place it back into the empty tooth socket and hold it in place. If possible, the tooth can be held in place by covering it with gauze or cotton and the victim biting down gently on it. If this is not possible, then the victim or the individual providing first aid can hold it in place by hand.

If putting the tooth back in the socket is not possible, for example, if the jaw is broken and immobilizing the jaw prevents replacing the tooth, rinse the tooth lightly with water to remove dirt or debris and either place it in a sealable container of cool milk or wrap it in milk-soaked sterile gauze. If gauze is not available use cheese cloth or another clean cloth soaked in milk. If milk is not available, place the tooth in a warm saline solution (mild salt water) or in gauze soaked with the victim's saliva. If the victim is an adult, you can also place the tooth in the mouth of the victim between the cheek and gum. *Keeping the avulsed tooth properly moist is essential.*

Burn

You can receive a burn from heat, chemicals, electricity, or the sun (see Sunburn, page 402). Heat burns can be caused by dry heat such as a flame or by wet heat, which results in scalding. First aid varies according to the severity of the burn, location, and the source. Quite often with heat burns, the more severe the burn, the lower the level of pain to the victim.

HEAT BURN

There are three degrees of heat burn:

- First degree: skin surface burned, characterized mainly by faint redness

- Second degree: skin surface burned through and underlying layer burned, characterized by swelling, blistering, deep redness, considerable pain, and swelling

- Third degree: skin burned all the way through, characterized by either whitened or blackened skin and intense pain at or surrounding the burn site

Airway or inhalation burns are heat burns caused by the inhalation of hot gas, smoke, or steam and are also classified by

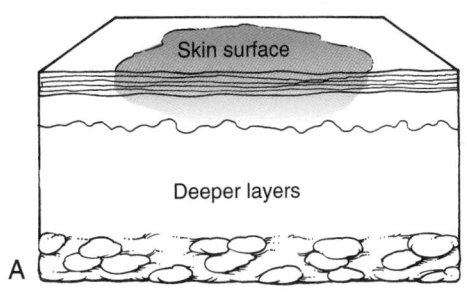

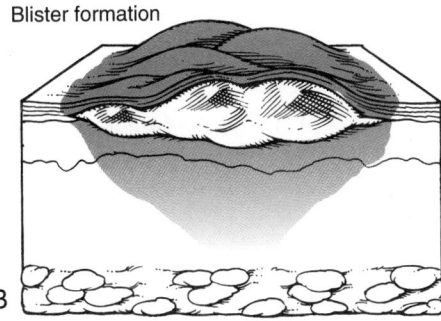

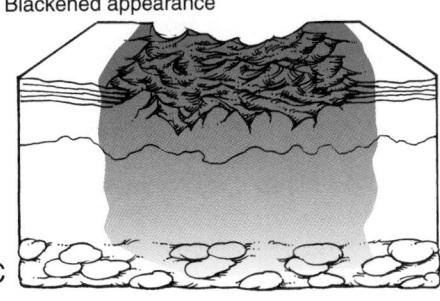

Burns are classified by degree. (A) A first degree burn affects only the skin surface. (B) A second degree burn affects both the skin surface and the layer just under the surface. Blisters and swelling may develop. (C) A third degree burn, which appears white or blackened, affects all skin layers and is extremely painful.

degree. Because swelling of the mouth and throat may cut off the airway, call EMS immediately for all inhalation or airway burns.

All burns need immediate attention, but the extent and severity of burns determine the type of treatment. First degree burns and small second degree burns can usually be treated at home. Second degree burns that are larger than palm size and all third degree burns should be treated by medical personnel.

Symptoms

- Redness of the skin
- Swelling
- Peeling skin
- Pain
- Shock
- Blistering (second degree burn)
- Whitened skin (third degree burn)
- Charred, or blackened, skin (third degree burn)

What you should do Cover the wound to keep out air, relieve pain, treat shock, and prevent infection while emergency assistance is on the way. *Never* use butter, ointment, or any other type of oil or grease on a burn. It must be removed before medical personnel can begin treatment; and its removal can be quite painful.

❖ MAJOR BURN

What you should do Call EMS immediately. Calm the victim and check his airway, breathing, and circulation (see Resuscitation ABCs, page 357). Watch for signs of shock including cold, clammy skin; weak, rapid heartbeat; dizziness; dazed expression; and pale or bluish skin (see page 385).

Remove any garments from around the injured area if they come off very easily. Do not try to remove fabric that may be stuck to the skin; instead, cut around it and leave it attached. Remove any jewelry from the area before swelling sets in unless removing it is difficult and will do more damage. Except for the burned area, keep the victim covered with a blanket; chills can occur following a burn.

Cover the area of the burn as quickly as possible with a cool, moist, loose, and, if pos-

sible, sterile dressing. Use thin material such as gauze or bedsheets. Do not use a blanket or towels unless nothing else is available. If the skin is broken, do not use any kind of sticky or fluffy dressing that may stick to the wound; plastic wrap can be utilized if necessary. Do not allow burned areas to rub against one another. Dress burned toes or fingers separately

❖ MINOR BURN

What you should do Calm the victim. On unbroken skin, run cool water over the burn or immerse the burned area in cool water—not ice water—for about 5 minutes. Use no sprays, salves, or ointments. If the burn is minor but the skin is broken with burst blisters, consult your doctor about how to prevent infection.

Cover the burn with a sterile dressing. Dressings should be loose-fitting and should not put pressure on the burn. Be aware of swelling and loosen dressings if necessary. Try not to break blisters. Use over-the-counter analgesics for pain.

If smaller second degree burns occur in particularly sensitive areas of the body, such as the genitals, face, airway, buttocks, hands, or feet, seek emergency medical care.

CHEMICAL BURN

Chemical burns are those caused by caustic substances. These can be either acidic or alkaline. If the burning agent is alkaline, do not wet because wetting can cause further burning; brush the agent from the surface of the skin before beginning irrigation. If the chemical agent is inhaled, call EMS at once.

Symptoms

- Redness of the skin
- Swelling
- Blistering
- Peeling

What you should do Reassure and calm the victim. Be aware of the possibility of shock (see page 384) and treat if necessary. If the burn is serious or extensive, or leads to shock, call EMS.

Make sure the burned area is clear of the caustic agent. Remove clothing or any article that may contain it. Irrigate the area thoroughly with clean tap water for 20 to 30 minutes. If the victim still experiences a burning sensation in the area after irrigation, continue the irrigation.

Wrap the burned area in a dry sterile dressing or cloth. Use over-the-counter analgesics for pain.

If the burn is to a sensitive area, such as the genitals, hands, feet, or face, or if the agent has burned through the outer layer of skin, contact EMS or take the victim to the emergency room.

ELECTRICAL BURN AND ELECTROCUTION

Because the body is electrically charged and the heart operates on tiny pulses of electricity, even small amounts of electric current supplied over a sufficient period of time can disrupt the heartbeat and cause cardiac and respiratory arrest.

Electrical burns are caused by electric shock. Serious electrical burns may not appear very impressive on the surface layer of skin, despite the presence of considerable tissue damage beneath the surface. Treat an electrical burn to the skin as you would a heat burn (see page 395) and see your doctor to rule out or treat any internal injury.

Electrocution can be a very serious matter. *Never touch anyone you suspect of having been electrocuted if there is any risk of continued contact with the electrical source.*

What you should do Make sure the victim is clear of the source of electric current. Turn off the electricity to the source or roll the victim from the wire or electrical source with a wooden implement such as a broomstick, or one made of another nonconductive material such as plastic or cardboard.

Call EMS immediately.

Check the victim's airway, breathing, and circulation (see Resuscitation ABCs, page 357). If necessary, begin CPR (see Cardiopulmonary Resuscitation, page 361). Continue CPR and monitoring ABCs until help arrives. If necessary, treat for shock (see page 385).

If the victim revives, place him in the recovery position (see page 365) and continue to monitor the ABCs until help arrives.

Bites and Stings

The general category of bites and stings covers a wide range of territory, from human bites—which, emergency room doctors will tell you, are much more common than most of us think and are not limited to those administered by children—to the venomous stings of scorpions and jellyfish. The seriousness of the emergency and the appropriate first aid depend entirely on the source and severity of the bite or sting.

In general, the job of the individual providing first aid is to be on the lookout for signs of severe allergic reaction (see Anaphylactic Shock/Severe Allergic Reaction, page 385), to treat for poisoning from snake or insect venom, to treat bleeding, and to help prevent infection or other disease.

If feasible and safe, capture and kill the offending insect, snake, or marine animal for identification. Transport the insect or animal to the hospital with the victim so that hospital personnel can decide on the proper antivenin to use in treatment. Potentially rabid animals should also be captured or killed, but this should be done by animal control authorities. Be sure to note the geographical location as well as any distinguishing characteristics about the animal. An autopsy of the animal's brain will determine the presence of rabies. If the animal is someone's pet, the animal can be quarantined for 10 days to detect the possibility of rabies.

ANIMAL AND HUMAN BITES

Animal and human bites have similar risks and similar needs for first aid. In both humans and animals, the mouth harbors numerous bacteria and, sometimes, viruses. If a bite breaks the skin there is always a risk of infection. With animal bites, the risk of infection with rabies can be great (see page 398), although human bites also carry the risk of many diseases.

What you should do If the bite does not break the skin, wash the area thoroughly. Because there is the possibility of bruising or contusion, use ice packs or cold compresses on the affected area to help reduce pain and swelling. See your doctor if you are unsure if the bite broke the skin.

RABIES

Rabies is a disease that is fatal if it is allowed to progress. Raccoons, dogs, cats, skunks, bats, squirrels—nearly any animal that lives in the wild or that may come into contact with other animals that live in the wild—may carry the virus that causes rabies. Rabies causes a kind of "madness" in animals, which in turn causes the animal to bite. Foaming at the mouth is often a sign of rabies because the disease makes it difficult for the animal to swallow. The rabies virus is transmitted by the animal's saliva into the wound its bite makes.

The victim of any animal bite should be aware of the possibility of rabies. Local animal control authorities should be alerted; they may be able to help capture the animal and determine whether it is rabid. If the animal is not caught prophylactic (preventive) treatment for rabies will probably be advised. If you have been bitten by an animal whose rabies status is not known or knowable, see your doctor immediately.

Symptoms of rabies infection in humans may appear in a few days, but may also take a long time to develop. The potentially long incubation period can lull bite victims into a false sense of security. By the time the first symptoms of rabies appear, which often include tingling and sensitivity of the skin, the bite may have long since healed and been forgotten. However, for treatment to be effective against rabies, it must be administered before symptoms appear. Once symptoms appear, there is no treatment.

If you are bitten by an animal, wash the wound thoroughly with soap, apply a disinfectant, and treat for bleeding accordingly. *See your doctor immediately.* ■

If the bite breaks the skin wash the wound thoroughly with a disinfectant soap as soon as possible and treat for bleeding. If the wound is severe and bleeding heavily, contact EMS and see Controlling Severe Bleeding, page 380.

Talk to your doctor about the possibility of infection with rabies. If the bite is human, talk to your doctor about the possibility of infection with other illnesses, such as hepatitis or acquired immunodeficiency syndrome (AIDS). Monitor the site for a few days afterwards for signs of infection such as swelling, tenderness, and discharge. Talk to your doctor if infection occurs.

Report all dog or other animal bites to your local animal control authority. Report human bites that occur in school or preschool to the appropriate school authorities.

Animal or human scratches Animal claws often harbor potentially infectious bacteria, as can the fingernails of humans. To treat a scratch, wash the area thoroughly with disinfectant soap. Use a cold compress to help reduce swelling and pain.

In the hours and days that follow the scratch, watch the injury for signs of infection including reddening of the surrounding skin, discharge, inflammation, and fever. If infection occurs contact your doctor.

INSECT AND SPIDER BITES AND STINGS

Insect and spider bites and stings can range from the merely annoying, to the transiently painful, to the potentially deadly, depending upon the type of insect and the victim's sensitivity to allergic reaction.

With the exception of certain scorpion stings and severe allergic reactions from bee stings, most insect stings are minor, if painful, unless they occur to the tongue, mouth, or throat. Although any sting can cause swelling, a sting in the mouth may cause enough swelling to block the airway.

If you do not know what kind of insect stung the victim, try to find out. If the type of insect is unfamiliar to you try to kill it so that, if necessary, medical personnel can identify it for better treatment.

❖ POISONOUS INSECT AND SPIDER BITES

Some insects and spiders carry a venom that is injected by the bite. The venom of some, such as scorpions, black widow spiders, tarantulas, and brown recluse spiders (see illustrations on page 399 and page C-47) can be quite poisonous, even lethal.

Try to identify the insect or spider. If you can capture or kill it without endangering yourself or others, do so. Accurate identification can help medical personnel identify the proper antivenin.

What you should do If the victim experiences an immediate, severe reaction, contact EMS. If you know the kind of insect that bit the victim, tell EMS personnel. Monitor the victim's airway, breathing, and circulation (see Resuscitation ABCs, page 357) until assistance arrives.

If the bite is on a limb, do not elevate the limb above the level of the heart. Do not use a tourniquet, but do use a snug-fitting bandage between the area of the bite and the heart, in order to slow the venom's circulation through the bloodstream. After about 5 minutes, or if the bandage causes the victim to lose sensation in the limb, remove the bandage. Apply an icepack to the area of the bite.

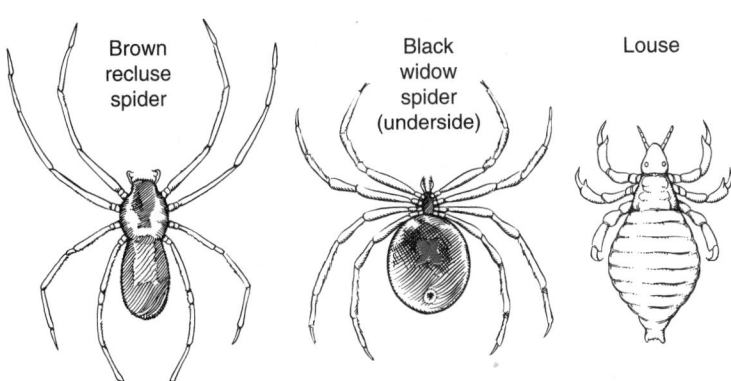

Brown recluse spider

Black widow spider (underside)

Louse

Some insects and spiders have poisonous venom. These include the brown recluse spider and the black widow spider. The louse is a blood-sucking insect that can carry infection.

❖ INSECT STINGS

Only the honey bee will leave its stinger in the victim. The stinger contains bee venom and should be removed as quickly as possible. *Do not* use tweezers to remove the stinger because more venom can be injected into the victim. Use a flat, rigid surface, such as a table knife or a credit card, and brush it across the sting, with the edge against the skin. This should pull out the stinger without injecting more venom.

What you should do If the victim experiences an immediate, severe reaction, contact EMS. Monitor the victim's airway, breathing, and circulation (see Resuscitation ABCs, page 357) until assistance arrives.

For stings in the mouth that do not involve an allergic reaction, give the victim an ice cube to suck or ice water to drink. This will reduce swelling and pain. However, if the airway becomes blocked, call EMS and administer artificial respiration (see Cardiopulmonary Resuscitation, page 361). Monitor the victim's airway, breathing, and circulation (see Resuscitation ABCs, page 357) until assistance arrives.

If the victim has been stung several times by many bees or fire ants, particularly if the victim is a child, contact EMS. Monitor the victim's airway, breathing, and circulation (see Resuscitation ABCs, page 357) until help arrives. Give the victim an antihistamine, preferably in a liquid form such as diphenhydramine elixir.

If the victim does not have multiple stings and experiences only localized pain and swelling, treat him for a minor sting. Wash the area with soap and water to prevent infection. Remove any constricting clothing or jewelry that could aggravate swelling in the area of the sting or stings. An ice pack can be used to reduce pain and swelling. You can also make a baking soda paste and apply it directly to the area of the sting to reduce itching and swelling, or use over-the-counter hydrocortisone lotion or ointment.

Although each of these insects can sting, only the honey bee leaves its stinger in the victim. The stinger contains venom and should be removed. Emergency Medical Services (EMS) should be contacted if many stings occur at the same time from any of these insects.

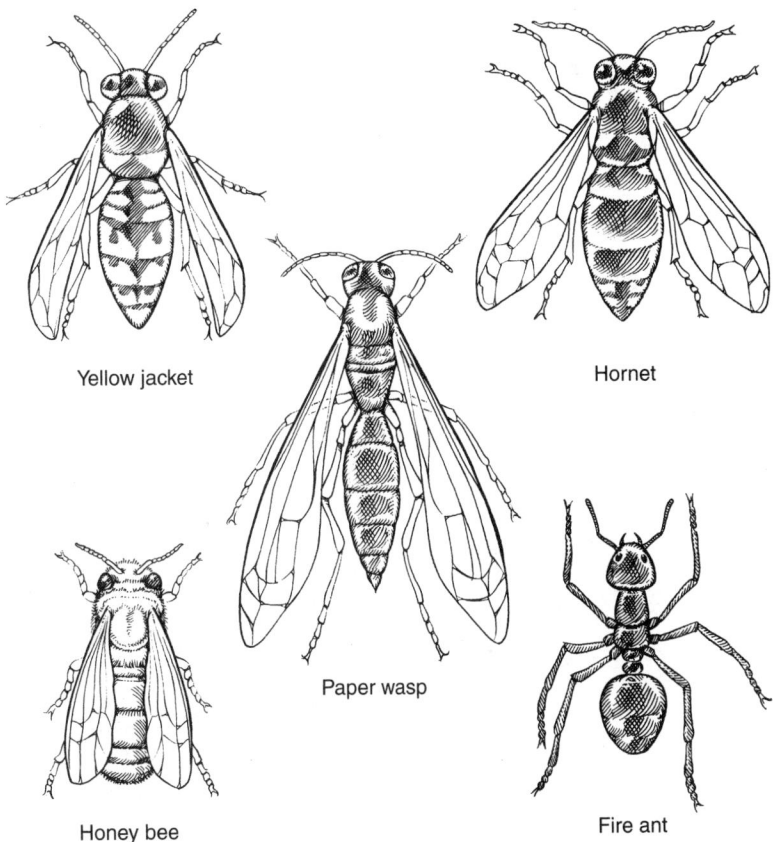

Yellow jacket

Hornet

Paper wasp

Honey bee

Fire ant

ALLERGIC REACTIONS TO BEE STINGS

Severe allergic reactions to bee stings *can* occur in individuals who have been stung before and have not had a severe reaction. Indeed, prior exposure to bee venom can sensitize a person and lead to a severe, anaphylactic reaction. An anaphylactic reaction will usually occur within a few seconds or minutes following a sting.

Symptoms

- Swelling of the tongue and face
- Sudden and severe breathing difficulties, especially in people with asthma
- Itching or burning skin
- Widespread hives
- Weak, rapid pulse
- Dizziness or light-headedness
- Unconsciousness, which may happen quickly

What You Should Do

Death from anaphylactic shock can occur in as little as 15 minutes. *Contact EMS immediately.*

Anaphylactic shock requires medication, usually epinephrine, or adrenaline, in order to counteract the reaction. Some people with severe allergies, including allergy to bee venom, carry emergency medication with them. If the victim has medication, help him use it. Antihistamines may be given to control itching but will not effectively treat anaphylactic shock.

If no epinephrine is available, continually monitor the victim's airway, breathing, and circulation (see Resuscitation ABCs, page 357) while help is on the way. If necessary, perform artificial respiration and CPR (see Cardiopulmonary Resuscitation, page 361). Put the victim in the shock position (see illustration page 385).

See pages 385 and 1341, for more information on severe allergic reactions. ■

❖ BLOOD-SUCKING INSECT BITES

The bites of certain blood-sucking insects can carry serious diseases including encephalitis (see page 458), Rocky Mountain spotted fever (page 888), Lyme disease (page 886), and malaria (page 889). The possibility of tetanus (see page 878) also exists, and for this reason, individuals should always keep up with their tetanus immunization.

Ticks live in grassy and wooded areas. Anyone who spends time in these areas or has pets who spend time in these areas should regularly check for the presence of ticks. Although ticks themselves are not poisonous, they readily transmit infection from one animal to another. Some types of ticks transmit diseases that can affect humans. The deer tick can carry Lyme disease and the wood tick can carry Rocky Mountain spotted fever (see illustration, this page and page C-47).

What you should do If you find a tick on yourself, your child, or a pet, remove it before it embeds its head in the skin. If the tick succeeds in embedding itself in the skin, do not try to pull it off. Cover the tick with oil or petroleum jelly. This impedes its ability to breathe and should cause the tick to remove itself within about half an hour. If the tick has not come out on its own after about 30 minutes, gently remove it with tweezers. Kill it by crushing it on a hard surface. Do not attempt to kill a tick with a lit match, cigarette, or cigarette lighter. Wash the affected area with soap and water and watch the area for any development of a red rash over the next several days. A rash could indicate Lyme disease. Fever, headache, and joint pains can also be symptoms of Lyme disease or of Rocky Mountain spotted fever. If any of

Ticks live in grassy and wooded areas. People who spend time in these areas or who have pets who spend time in these areas should check themselves regularly for ticks, which can carry infections. Deer ticks can carry Lyme disease and wood ticks can carry Rocky Mountain spotted fever, both of which can cause rashes and more severe disease.

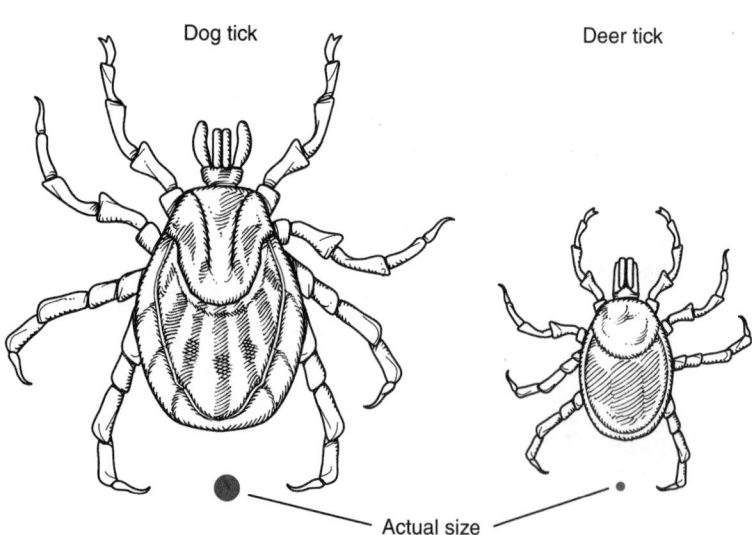

Dog tick

Deer tick

Actual size

these symptoms develop following a tick bite, see your doctor.

Other blood-sucking insects include fleas, mosquitoes, lice, bedbugs, horseflies, and gnats. None is individually poisonous, but all can carry infection. Wash the area of a bite thoroughly with soap and water. If itching and pain are present, use calamine lotion, a baking soda paste, cold compress, or over-the-counter hydrocortisone to reduce itching and inflammation. If signs of infection develop, contact your doctor. For more information on insect stings, see page 1339, and on insect infestations, see page 1304.

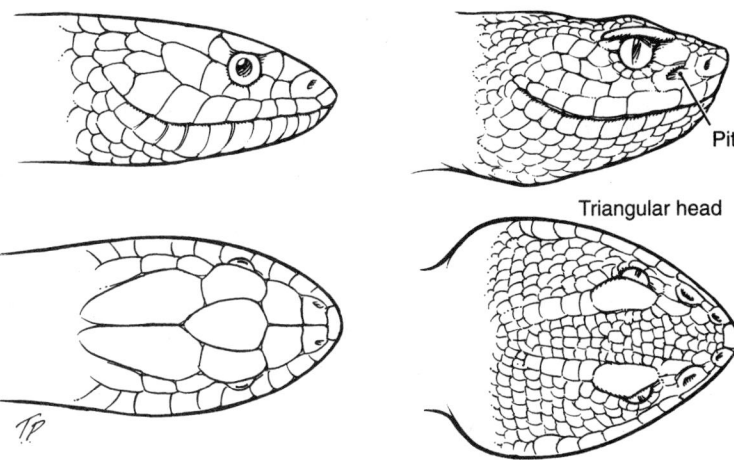

Pit

Triangular head

SNAKE BITES

Of the hundreds of different kinds of snakes that are naturally found in the United States, only four types are poisonous: coral snakes copperheads, rattlesnakes, and water moccasins or cotton mouths. Copperheads, rattlesnakes, and water moccasins are all pit vipers, which are named for the pit in front of the eye on their heads (see illustration, this page). The pit vipers are thick and heavy snakes, with wedge-shaped heads and fangs that inject venom, usually with a single bite. Coral snakes are comparatively small and thin, with small mouths, and usually bite the fingers or toes. Pit vipers, by contrast, can open their mouths quite wide and extend their fangs. Coral snakes have fangs but they are not as visible as are those of pit vipers.

Most snakes, poisonous or nonpoisonous, only bite humans when they are threatened. Snakes use their venom to immobilize and kill the rodents they eat. In humans snake venom causes tissue damage, breathing difficulties, dizziness, nausea, headache, and, perhaps most importantly, shock. The amount of venom that a snake injects when it bites may depend on how recently it has eaten.

Symptoms

- A sharp pain around two small puncture marks although sometimes there is only one mark

- Immediate discoloration, pain, and swelling at the area of the bite (see page C-47.)

- Dizziness and weakness

- Signs of shock including breathing difficulties and weak, rapid pulse

Although various types of snakes can bite, only four snakes found in the United States are poisonous: coral snakes, copperheads, rattlesnakes, and water moccasins. These last three types are pit vipers, characterized by a pit on each side of the head. Compared to coral snakes, pit vipers are thick and heavy and have especially visible fangs. In people, snake venom can cause tissue damage, shock, and a host of symptoms. Do not cut the skin or use suction around a bite without the guidance of a trained professional.

What you should do In the event of a poisonous snake bite notify EMS, but begin treatment first.

Never cut open the skin around a snake bite or use suction to try to remove venom unless directed to do so by an emergency dispatcher. *Never* try to suck venom from a wound with your mouth. Shock is the most frequent cause of death in snakebite victims; look for signs of shock including cold, clammy skin; blue-tinged or pale skin; dazed expression; weak, rapid pulse; shallow breathing; and weakness (see page 385).

Have the victim lie down. If the victim is unconscious, turn his head to the side in case he vomits. Keep the bitten limb immobile and *lower* than the level of heart; do not elevate the limb. Remove all jewelry, watches, and other constricting items, because the area will swell. If medical help is not immediately available, place constricting bandages above the wound, unless the bite is on the finger tip or it is otherwise impossible. If you do not have bandages use duct tape, adhesive tape, or other flat material—never wire. Constricting bandages should be tight enough to restrict circulation but not to cut it off. White or very pale skin below the bandage indicates that circulation has been cut off and that the bandage should be loosened. Monitor the victim's airway, breathing, and circulation (see Resuscitation ABCs, page 357) and treat as necessary. Continue monitoring until help arrives. Do not give the victim anything by mouth.

Try to identify the snake. If you can capture or kill the snake without endangering yourself, do so.

Nonpoisonous snakes also bite. Treat these bites as you would treat any other animal bite (see page 397).

MARINE ANIMAL STINGS

There are many different kinds of marine animals that have venomous bites or stings. Get the victim out of the water as rapidly as possible. In many cases, the chief danger in such stings is drowning resulting from disabling cramps, pain, and even shock in the water.

If possible, identify the stinging animal, or if it does not present serious danger to you, capture and kill it and transport it with the victim to the emergency room.

If the victim has been bitten by a sea snake, it should be treated as you would any poisonous snake bite; see page 401.

❖ JELLYFISH OR PORTUGUESE MAN-OF-WAR STINGS

Perhaps the most common venomous stinging marine animal is the jellyfish, of which there are several types, all with varying degrees of seriousness. Jellyfish tentacles retain their venom even after the animal is dead or even if they have been severed from the animal.

What you should do If the victim has been stung many times or has a severe reaction, contact EMS. Monitor the victim's airway, breathing, and circulation (see Resuscitation ABCs, page 357) and treat for shock (page 385). If you know the kind of animal that stung the victim, report it to the emergency dispatcher, or if you are transporting the victim yourself, call ahead to the emergency room and let them know the type of sting victim you are bringing in.

Rinse stings with seawater, not fresh water. Remove any severed bits of tentacle from the area of the sting. Do not use your hands; use a knife, comb, tweezers, or a seashell, and do not rub. Irrigate the area with white vinegar or make a vinegar compress; a paste made from sugar, salt, or dry sand can also work if vinegar is not available. This should inactivate the stinging within about 30 minutes. If none of these are available, urine, with its salt and ammonia content, is a very effective treatment for marine animal stings and can save a life in an emergency.

Use an over-the-counter hydrocortisone cream or ointment to reduce inflammation and itching; calamine lotion can also be effective in relieving itching. Use an over-the-counter analgesic to relieve pain. Consult your doctor if the sting is severe.

❖ OTHER MARINE ANIMAL STINGS

What you should do If the victim has a severe reaction, contact EMS.

Use tweezers to remove any stingers. For bristleworm stings, place an adhesive tape over the area and pull it off to remove the stinging bristles, then soak the area with rubbing alcohol or a diluted ammonia solution (1 part ammonia to 4 parts water). For stinging fish, sting ray, or sea urchin stings, soak the area in water as hot as the victim can tolerate and seek medical attention. Treat wounds for bleeding and to prevent infection.

Environmental Emergencies

Environmental emergencies are those caused not by trauma but by environmental factors, such as excessive heat or cold, excessive sunlight, high altitudes, or water.

SUNBURN

Prolonged exposure to the ultraviolet rays of the sun without benefit of sunscreen protection can cause painful redness and inflammation of the skin. Because the symptoms of sunburn do not fully appear until a few hours after exposure, people often do not get out of the sun until it is too late. Sunburn can be as bad as or worse than heat burns. Some medications can markedly increase the risk of sunburn by making skin more sensitive to sunlight.

Symptoms

- Tender, inflamed red skin that is hot to the touch

- Blistering

- Pain on touching the skin

- Increased sensitivity to heat. Lukewarm water may feel burning hot.

- Nausea, dizziness, or overall feeling of illness (more severe sunburn)

What you should do Prevention is always the best approach. If anyone is likely to have been severely sunburned, for example, from falling asleep in the sun for several hours, it is wise to contact a doctor immediately before symptoms fully set in. Your doctor may be able to prevent some of the more extreme effects of inflammation and pain with corticosteroids.

If symptoms have fully set in cool the victim in a cool bath or shower; a bath may be easier to endure than a shower. Use aloe vera gel, a numbing antiseptic spray or ointment, or an over-the-counter hydrocortisone ointment or cream several times a day to reduce inflammation and speed healing. If blistering occurs, do not break the blisters. If blisters break, treat them with antiseptic spray or ointment. If the face is severely burned, the eyes should be checked for possible damage. Watch for signs of infection and contact your doctor if infection occurs.

HEAT EXHAUSTION

Heat exhaustion is caused by the loss of fluids and salt through sweating and the failure to drink adequate fluids. The dehydration associated with heat exhaustion can cause shock. Heat exhaustion occurs most often in people who are not accustomed to working or exercising in hot weather, people who are overweight, and people who sweat excessively and do not take the adequate precaution of drinking plenty of water.

Symptoms

- Pale or red, clammy skin

- Intense sweating

- Rapid, shallow breathing

- Rapid, weak pulse

- Weakness, nausea, dizziness, and possibly headache and vomiting

- Confused or irrational behavior (possible)

What you should do Heat exhaustion can cause dehydration, shock, and elevated body temperatures. The object of first aid treatment is to cool and rehydrate the victim. If the victim is vomiting, unconscious, or cannot drink, call EMS immediately.

Move the victim to a cooler place such as into the shade or into air-conditioning. Loosen his clothing. Cool the victim by applying a cool cloth to his face and by fanning him. If you are outdoors and near a source of water, first inform the victim of your intentions and then spray him with a hose or pour cool water over him, avoiding his face. If the victim feels faint, have him lie down and elevate his feet 8 to 12 in. above the level of the heart as you would for shock.

Give the victim electrolyte beverages to sip, such as Gatorade or Pedialyte; if none are available mix a small amount of salt with water. *Do not* give the victim salt tablets.

Treat for shock as necessary (see page 385).

Use extra caution if the victim has high blood pressure, heart disease, or diabetes; seek emergency medical attention.

HEAT STROKE

Heat stroke is an abnormally high body temperature and results in a breakdown of the body's normal ability to cool itself. It is caused by excessive exposure to heat, whether from direct sunlight or from being in an excessively hot place such as occurs when an elderly person is trapped in an apartment without air conditioning at the height of summer. Physical exertion, including exercise and hard work, and high humidity can be contributing factors to heat stroke.

Heat stroke is more common in seniors, people with alcoholism, people who are obese, and people on medications that alter the ability of the body to cool itself.

Symptoms

- Elevated body temperature (over 102°F)

- Hot, dry, and flushed skin
- Initially strong and rapid pulse, which weakens if the condition worsens
- Rapid deep breathing followed by rapid shallow breathing if the condition worsens
- Weakness
- Extreme confusion to loss of arousability
- Convulsions

What you should do Prolonged high body temperature can cause brain damage, so the object of first aid treatment is to bring down body temperature as rapidly as possible.

Move the victim into the shade, a cool room, or an air-conditioned car. Call Emergency Medical Services (EMS). Continuously monitor the victim's airway, breathing, and circulation (see Resuscitation ABCs, page 357) until help arrives. If possible, remove the victim's clothing, wrap him in a cool, wet sheet, and aim a fan at him; evaporation is an extremely efficient method of cooling the body. If you cannot remove the victim's clothing, inform him of your intentions and then immerse him in a bath of cool water, soak him with water from a hose, or immerse him in a stream or lake but use caution to avoid drowning. Continue monitoring the victim's temperature.

FROSTBITE

Frostbite results from exposure to severe cold. Contributing factors include the windchill, wet clothing, alcohol consumption, poor circulation from disease or tight clothing, weariness, some medications, and smoking. The most common sites of frostbite are the nose, toes, fingers, and ears. As long as the sensation of cold is present in the extremities, frostbite has probably not set in.

Symptoms

- Red, painful skin (early stage)
- Whitened, numb skin (middle stage)
- Hard, frozen skin (severe or deep frostbite)
- Blisters and blackened tissue (severe frostbite after thawing with gangrene of dead tissues)

What you should do Call EMS in moderate to severe cases. Do not rewarm or thaw the skin especially if the skin is yellowed, white, or blue-white, and hard to the touch; leave this to medical personnel. Dress frostbitten extremities; to limit movement, pad and splint them. Try not to let frostbitten areas touch one another.

If there will be substantial delay in getting emergency assistance, for example, if the victim is in a remote location and cannot be removed immediately for emergency care, rewarming of severely frostbitten extremities can be done as described below for mild frostbite.

In cases of mild frostbite give first aid and rewarm the area as outlined below, then seek medical assistance. Do not try to thaw out a frostbitten area if there is any danger of it freezing again.

Do not give the victim any warm beverages or any that may contain caffeine and do not allow the victim to smoke; these will constrict the blood vessels. Do not let the victim drink alcohol, which will increase heat loss from the body.

Move the victim to a warm place and remove any potentially constricting clothing such as boots or gloves. Remove any jewelry. Rewarm the area by immersing it in running warm water that is just above body temperature (about 100°F). This can be very painful. Keep the water moving so that it is constantly warm. To rewarm non-immersible areas, use warm compresses (about 100°F); this too can be quite painful. Do not try to thaw out a frostbitten area using direct heat such as a campfire, radiator, heater, or blow dryer. In addition to pain, swelling and color changes may accompany thawing and rewarming. Dry the frostbitten areas gently and then apply dry, sterile dressings. Separate fingers and toes with sterile dressing.

Comfort the victim until help arrives.

HYPOTHERMIA

Hypothermia (loss of body warmth) happens when the body can no longer maintain its core temperature and body temperature drops. Hypothermia most often occurs in infants, seniors, people with poor circulation, people with alcoholism, people in overall poor health, and people with chronic conditions such as diabetes. However, hypothermia can happen to anyone who is exposed to cold for too long, particularly to someone who has been immersed in cold water or has worn wet clothing for any length of time in the cold.

Symptoms

- Shivering
- Loss of coordination, including loss of bladder control
- Usually warm areas of body that are cold to the touch

In extreme cases

- Weakness, dizziness, and confusion, which may include the desire not to be treated
- Muscle rigidity
- Irregular or weak heartbeat
- Sleepiness
- Impaired speech
- Unconsciousness
- Coma
- Cardiac arrest

What you should do Call EMS if symptoms are anything but mild. Check the victim's airway, breathing, and circulation (see Resuscitation ABCs, page 357); as long as the victim is breathing at a rate of more than 6 breaths per minute, treat the hypothermia. Treat the victim gently because hypothermia victims can easily go into cardiac arrest. Initiate CPR if the victim stops breathing or goes into cardiac arrest (see Cardiopulmonary Resuscitation, page 361). If the victim has frostbite and hypothermia, treat hypothermia first. Use only indirect heat to rewarm a victim of hypothermia.

Get the victim into a warm environment and remove wet clothing. Wrap the victim completely in blankets, covering his head and neck as well as his body. Maintain the victim's body heat by moving him near a fire or by placing heat packs, electric heating pads, or hot water bottles in the blankets with him. If necessary use your own body heat to warm up the victim. *Do not* warm the victim too quickly; for example, a frostbitten area should never be placed in a hot bath or directly on or next to a source of heat.

If the victim is conscious, give him warm liquids to drink, but do not give him caffeine-containing beverages and never give alcohol. Keep talking to him to monitor his mental status.

Get the victim to a hospital as soon as possible.

NEAR-DROWNING

Medically speaking, someone either drowns or does not. "Near-drowning" happens when an individual aspirates (breathes in) water but is rescued before drowning. Drowning occurs when either the complete or partial filling of the lungs with water prevents oxygen from being supplied to the brain.

Drowning, or near-drowning, can happen in many ways: a swimmer can suddenly become ill, a non-swimmer can fall into the water, a boater can be knocked unconscious by a capsizing boat, or water can be aspirated into the lungs when snorkeling.

Only a trained life guard should get into the water to try to rescue someone who is drowning. A panicking victim can easily pull you down. It is best to use some sort of implement—a rope, float, ladder, board, or other object—for the victim to grab onto while you remain on dry land or on a boat. If the implement is not of sufficient length to reach the victim, you can wade into shallow water, no deeper than your waist, and extend the implement to the victim. If the victim is a child in shallow water, you must judge the situation to decide whether it is safe for you to venture into the water.

Symptoms

- Bluing of the skin, particularly the face, lips, and ears
- Cold skin
- Respiratory failure

What you should do The focus of first aid for near-drowning is to get oxygen into the victim's lungs and to restart the heart. Never assume that a victim who has stopped breathing and suffered cardiac arrest is dead, particularly if the water is cold. Human beings who appear dead can sometimes be revived, particularly if they have been in very cold water.

Begin first aid immediately, even in the water. Check the victim's airway, breathing, and circulation (see Resuscitation ABCs, page 357) and begin artificial respiration even as the victim is being pulled from the water. Do not try to clear the victim's lungs of water. Simply begin giving breaths; air must reach the lungs.

Once the victim has been pulled from the water call EMS, or if possible, have someone call even before the victim is out of the water.

Position the victim on his back. Check his airway, breathing, and circulation (see Resuscitation ABCs, page 357) again and begin CPR immediately if necessary (see Cardiopulmonary Resuscitation, page 361). When the victim's ABCs are okay, continue with other first aid.

In many swimming accidents, the risk of a spinal cord injury is high, particularly if the victim was found in shallow water or the surf (see Spinal Cord Injury, page 368 and Moving a Victim of Suspected Spinal Cord Injury, page 369). If you suspect spinal cord injury, once the victim is out of the water only move him as necessary to restore breathing and to ensure that his life is not in danger. If there is no danger of a spinal injury, position him in the recovery position (see page 365). Provide first aid for any other injuries or illness as necessary.

When the victim revives, he may cough or vomit and may have difficulty breathing even after his lungs are clear. This is normal. All near-drowning victims should receive medical attention, no matter how they feel afterward. Inhalation of saltwater can cause lung damage and fluid accumulation in the lungs. Reassure the victim until medical assistance arrives.

COMPRESSED-AIR EMERGENCIES

The air tanks that scuba divers use contain compressed air, which can present certain hazards particularly to divers who are not sufficiently trained.

The bends Perhaps the most common compressed-air emergency is "the bends," a painful and potentially deadly mishap. At the extreme pressures that exist underwater, the nitrogen component in the compressed air of the tank becomes liquid in the diver's bloodstream. If the dive is short or not very deep, the small amount of liquid nitrogen in the blood is of little consequence. In longer dives, however, the diver must go through a process of decompression as he surfaces. This means stopping at intervals on the way to the surface so that the nitrogen can gradually be released from the bloodstream. If a diver does not go through decompression, high levels of nitrogen in the bloodstream will cause the bends. The seriousness of the victim's condition depends upon how long and how deep he was underwater.

The only treatment for the bends is decompression, which can be accomplished in two ways. The diver must either go back down underwater with another tank of air and surface again while decompressing, or he must be rushed into a decompression chamber. Before diving, every diver should know where the nearest decompression chamber is or have access to a spare tank of air.

Lung embolism Another common danger associated with compressed air is the potential of an embolism of the lung. Compressed air is delivered at ambient pressure, in other words, at the same pressure as the water surrounding the diver. As the diver surfaces the air he has breathed in expands. If the diver is not constantly exhaling as he surfaces, the expanding air can burst the delicate tissues of the lung.

Symptoms of lung embolism include chest pain and coughing up of blood. The victim needs emergency medical care; call EMS immediately. Make the victim as comfortable as possible and monitor his airway, breathing, and circulation (see Resuscitation ABCs, page 357) until help arrives.

SMOKE INHALATION AND CARBON MONOXIDE POISONING

More people die in fires from smoke inhalation than from burns. When a significant amount of smoke is inhaled, the smoke takes the place of oxygen in the lungs and the victim dies from lack of oxygen. When carbon monoxide is inhaled it has the same effect of depriving the body of oxygen, although by a slightly different mechanism. Carbon monoxide detectors, like smoke detectors, are now readily available for home use and every home should have them. See Safe at Home, page 55.

❖ SMOKE INHALATION

Symptoms

• Breathing difficulties

• Coughing and wheezing

• Irritated eyes

• Respiratory arrest

What you should do Call EMS. Do not endanger yourself; two victims are worse than one.

If possible, get victim clear of the smoky area. Check his airway, breathing, and circulation (see Resuscitation ABCs, page 357) and begin CPR (see Cardiopulmonary Resuscitation, page 361); continue until the victim revives or medical assistance arrives. Loosen any tight clothing and make the victim comfortable.

If the victim is unconscious, position him in the recovery position (see page 365) and monitor his airway, breathing, and circulation until assistance arrives.

❖ CARBON MONOXIDE POISONING

Symptoms

• Flu-like symptoms and headache

• Nausea, dizziness, and vomiting

• Confusion

• Chest pain

What you should do Call EMS.

Do not endanger yourself; two victims are worse than one.

If possible, get the victim clear of the carbon monoxide.

Check his airway, breathing, and circulation (see Resuscitation ABCs, page 357) and if necessary begin CPR (see Cardiopulmonary Resuscitation, page 361); continue until the victim revives or medical assistance arrives. Loosen any tight clothing and make the victim comfortable.

If the victim is unconscious, position him in the recovery position (see page 365) and monitor his airway, breathing, and circulation until assistance arrives.

SEVERE CONTACT DERMATITIS/POISON IVY, OAK, AND SUMAC

Contact dermatitis is an inflammation of the skin that is caused by exposure to an irritant or an allergen (substance that causes an allergic reaction). The leaves, stems, and roots of plants such as poison ivy, oak, and sumac can cause severe contact dermatitis. (See page C-28.) Symptoms include inflammation and blistering in the area that touched the offending agent. Contact dermatitis is often an allergic reaction; some individuals, for example, will not get contact dermatitis from poison ivy.

Inflammation can also be caused internally by inhaling the smoke from burned plants; never attempt to destroy plants by burning them. Plants can retain their toxic potency even after they are dead. If you use an herbicide to kill them, exercise caution in removing the dead plants.

Irritant contact dermatitis can also be caused by chemical agents in products ranging from cosmetics to household cleansers. For more information see Allergic Dermatitis, page 1334, Allergic Skin Conditions, page 1289, and Plant Dermatoses, page 1335.

What you should do If you come in contact with poison ivy, oak, or sumac, you have a few hours in which you can prevent contact dermatitis from developing. Remove and later wash all clothing worn during the contact. Thoroughly wash any area of the body that may be affected.

If you develop contact dermatitis from poison ivy, oak, or sumac, thoroughly wash the affected area. Over-the-counter hydrocortisone cream or ointment or calamine lotion is unlikely to relieve itching or reduce inflammation; talk to your doctor about a prescription-strength hydrocortisone preparation and an antihistamine.

Blistering may develop but, contrary to popular myth, the liquid that weeps from the blisters will not spread the dermatitis. Refrain from scratching the area as much as possible because broken skin can lead to infection. If the skin is broken, use a disinfectant. If signs of infection set in—the presence of pus rather than a clear liquid—consult your doctor.

If you suspect that you may have inhaled fumes from burning poison ivy, oak, or sumac, contact your doctor immediately.

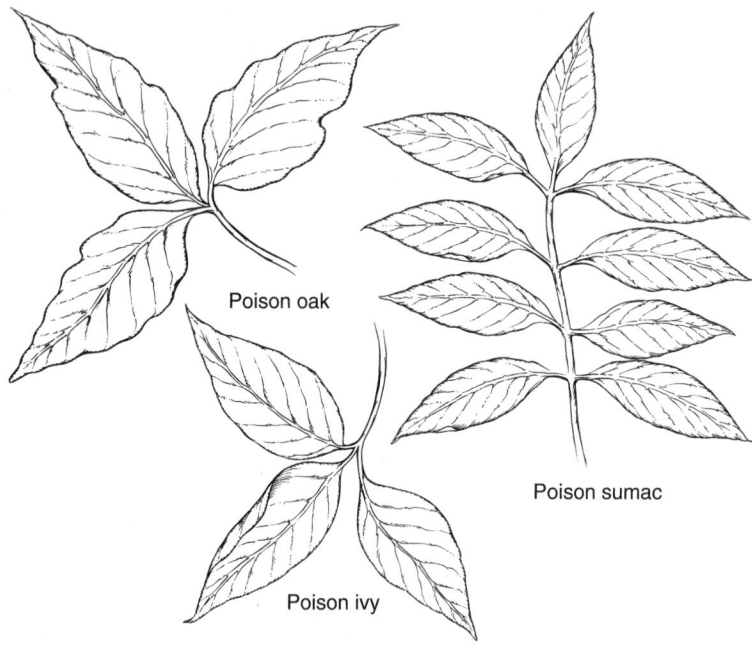

Poison oak

Poison sumac

Poison ivy

Poison oak, poison ivy, and poison sumac plants can cause severe inflammation of the skin (dermatitis).

Poison ivy, oak, or sumac can affect any area of the body, but can be particularly unpleasant in the genital area and the eyes. Treatment is the same, although infection may be more of a problem in moist, warm areas, particularly in the presence of bacteria. Make sure the affected area remains clean and watch for signs of infection. Your doctor may recommend a prescription preparation to reduce itching and inflammation.

Poisoning

Poisoning can occur in a number of ways: from combining medication and alcohol, from drug overdose, from swallowing household chemicals or insecticides, and from ingesting poisonous plants. The seriousness of a poisoning emergency depends on the type of poison, how much was ingested, and whether the victim goes into shock.

Every household, especially households with children, should have the number of the local poison control center near the telephone.

ACCIDENTAL MEDICATION POISONING

There are several ways in which normally beneficial medications can become harmful. Poisoning from medications can result

when they are not used properly, when they are taken with other substances, or when allergic reactions occur. Both over-the-counter and prescription medications can be deadly if they are taken in amounts greater than the recommended dosage. Many prescription medications can be deadly if they are combined with other prescription medications or with alcohol. Some people are allergic to common medications, most notably penicillin. Although these sorts of allergies are not common, if you experience signs of allergic reaction such as hives, angioedema, respiratory distress, or shock after taking a new medication, contact your doctor immediately (see page 1341). In the case of shock contact EMS immediately and see Anaphylactic Shock/Severe Allergic Reaction, page 385.

What you should do For reactions to over-the-counter medications, contact your poison control center immediately. Contact your doctor if you experience any unusual effects from prescription medications. Certain prescription medications can react adversely with common household solvents. If you experience any unusual effects after using paint thinner, for example, contact your doctor. For more information see Chapter 33.

It can never be stressed too strongly that you must follow label instructions and ask your doctor or pharmacist questions about the medications you use.

If someone in your household either takes too much of a medication or takes a medication that they should not have taken at all, give the individual a glass of milk or water to drink, call your poison control center, and follow the instructions that the poison control center gives you.

CHEMICAL POISONING

Almost any household chemical can be poisonous and although all should be kept out of the reach of children, children have remarkable ways of defeating even the most thorough child-proofing. Because many household products are pleasantly scented, they may be inviting to drink. Household poisons, such as rodenticides, insecticides, and other garden chemicals, may also seem appealing to children. Some household poisonings may be quite obvi-

CALLING YOUR POISON CONTROL CENTER

You should have the telephone number of your local poison control center by your phone, particularly if you have children in your household. The number will also be listed in the front section of your local telephone book. Calling 911 or information will not connect you directly with poison control. Emergency or information operators will be able to give you the number of your local poison control center, but they will not have access to detailed information on poisoning and the call could waste valuable time. Only call 911 to summon EMS if the victim is unconscious.

When you call the poison control center, you will be asked a number of questions. Some of them may seem irrelevant or beside the point in the heat of the emergency. You will probably be asked at least the following:

- Name and age of the victim
- Your relationship to the victim
- The address and telephone number of your location
- The substance the victim has swallowed, inhaled, injected, or otherwise taken into his system
- How much of the substance and how long ago
- Any symptoms that may have appeared
- Anything in the way of treatment that you have done so far

Do not hang up. Following the questions, the technician at the poison control center will give you instructions on how to proceed. Follow the directions you are given. *Never induce vomiting unless directed to do so by the poison control center.* ∎

ous—a child with a fistful of aspirin gleefully munching on them—and others may not be so obvious—spilled detergent on the floor and the odor of detergent on the child's breath.

Symptoms Symptoms of more advanced poisoning include:

- Inflammation or burning around the lips
- Difficulty in swallowing
- Pain in the mouth, throat, and belly
- Nausea
- Extreme thirst
- Breathing difficulties
- Any sudden and unexpected medical symptom
- Unconsciousness
- Seizure

What you should do Many household products that contain toxic chemicals have instructions on the label for dealing with a poisoning emergency; look for these instructions while you call your local poison control center. Have the victim drink a glass of milk or water to dilute the poison and slow its absorption. Follow the instructions given by the poison control center.

If the poison is not an acid or alkali, you may be instructed to induce vomiting. Do this by administering a dose of ipecac syrup, an emetic that will provoke vomiting, or by putting your finger to the back of the individual's throat, which will induce the gag reflex and vomiting. If the poison is an acid or an alkali, you may be instructed to give the victim more milk or water and get him to the emergency room or to summon EMS as soon as possible so that his stomach can be pumped.

PLANT POISONING

Symptoms

- Throat or mouth pain
- Breathing difficulties
- Vomiting or other gastrointestinal distress
- Hallucinations
- Convulsions
- Unconsciousness

What you should do Call EMS and then call your local poison control center. If you know the plant that was ingested, have a sample of it with you when you call.

Check the victim's airway, breathing, and circulation (see Resuscitation ABCs, page 357) and, if necessary, begin CPR (see Cardiopulmonary Resuscitation, page 361) until emergency assistance arrives or the victim revives. If the victim's airway, breathing, and circulation are okay, put the victim in the recovery position (see page 365) and continue to monitor them until medical assistance arrives.

COMMONLY INGESTED POISONOUS PLANTS

Many houseplants and plants that may be in your garden or yard can be poisonous. Even some edible plants can have poisonous parts, such as the flora and shoots of potatoes or the leaves of rhubarb. The following is a list of common plants or plant parts that can be poisonous. (See page C-48.)

Berries

- Holly berries
- Mistletoe berries
- Cherry pits
- Daffodil bulbs

Entire Plants

- Poinsettia
- Coleus
- Jimson weed
- Lily of the valley
- Rhododendron
- Mushrooms and toadstools
- Common English ivy

Certain herbal remedies sold as dietary supplements in health food stores can also be dangerous, usually because the ingredient that is supposed to be in the supplement has been confused by the harvester with another, poisonous plant. Many people mistakenly believe that because herbal remedies are called "dietary supplements," they do not pose health hazards. This is not so. Some herbal remedies can be quite toxic when taken in large quantities. If illness occurs after taking an herbal supplement, seek emergency medical attention. Bring the supplement bottle or container with you.

Remedies that use extracts of the ephedra plant can contain large amounts of ephedrine, a powerful stimulant. Ephedra overdose may cause irregular heartbeat and death. If you have used a supplement that contains ephedra extracts and experience palpitations, racing heartbeat, sweating, or similar reactions, seek emergency medical attention.

Although herbal remedies have been useful for humans for tens of thousands of years, unless you are an expert botanist, do not try to mix your own from plants that you have gathered yourself.

Never eat a wild mushroom unless you are absolutely certain what it is. Although most are not poisonous, some that are almost instantly deadly look exactly like nonpoisonous varieties. ■

NICOTINE POISONING

With the recent approval of nicotine gum and patches for over-the-counter sales, there have been several reports of inadvertent nicotine poisoning in children. This can happen if a child finds a piece of nicotine gum and chews it or even if a child falls asleep in the bed of an adult wearing a patch and the patch falls off the adult and adheres to the child.

Symptoms

- Nausea
- Dizziness
- Vomiting
- Unconsciousness (possible)

What you should do Remove the patch or take away the gum and call your local poison control center. Follow their instructions.

Depending upon the strength of the patch or gum and the age of the child, the poisoning may result only in transitory distress.

FOOD POISONING

Food poisoning can be caused by a number of different bacteria or other contaminants and can range from the unpleasantness of gastroenteritis to the potential deadliness of botulism. Generally speaking, the longer the symptoms of food poisoning take to appear, the more serious the poisoning. In addition, the longer symptoms take to appear, the more difficult it can be to ascertain that they indeed are the result of food poisoning. Botulism, for example, can take a day or even longer to produce symptoms; it is usually because more than one person ate the same contaminated food that the symptoms are traced to food poisoning.

Most food poisoning is the result of improperly handled, stored, or cooked food, or food that has been prepared on surfaces that are not clean or by hands that are not clean. As such, most food poisoning can be prevented. Suspect food poisoning if the victim has recently eaten uncooked seafood such as sushi or raw oysters, incompletely cooked eggs, improperly refrigerated or frozen foods, raw honey, home-canned foods, foods that came from a dented can, or any food that "didn't taste right."

The rule of thumb in deciding whether or not to eat a food that has been left unrefrigerated, that is old, or that is in any way questionable, is "When in doubt, throw it out."

❖ GASTROENTERITIS

Gastroenteritis is a general term for what is often called "stomach flu." It is usually transitory and passes in about 24 hours, which is the time it takes the body to clear the infectious agent via vomiting and diarrhea. Gastroenteritis can be caused by *Staphylococcus, Salmonella*, and *Escherichia coli (E. coli)* bacteria.

Symptoms

- Bloating and nausea, 3 to 6 hours after eating
- Stomach cramps
- Vomiting
- Diarrhea
- Dehydration (in extreme cases)

What you should do Usually, gastroenteritis in healthy adults and older children is not an emergency, regardless of how unpleasant it may be.

In seniors or very young children who are more at risk for dehydration, help the victim stay hydrated. Give the victim small servings of broth—as little as 1 tbs every 20 minutes or so if he is having difficulty keeping liquids down. You can also have the victim drink an electrolyte solution such as Pedialyte or Gatorade periodically. Watch for signs of dehydration such as extreme thirst, little or no urination, and sunken eyes, and for signs of shock caused by dehydration (see page 384). If you are unable to keep the victim adequately hydrated, call your doctor. Do not use over-the-counter antidiarrheal medications without consulting your doctor first.

If the victim has an impaired immune system or the symptoms do not clear up within 24 hours, talk to your doctor. Antibiotics may be necessary.

❖ BOTULISM

Botulism is a serious and potentially fatal form of food poisoning. It is often related to improperly canned foods and smoked meats and fish. Symptoms may take as much as a day and a half to develop. Botulism poisoning should be treated as an emergency. The victim will need hospitalization, and health authorities should be notified.

Symptoms

- Headache
- Dizziness
- Breathing difficulties
- Slurred speech
- Blurred vision
- Dry mouth and difficulty swallowing
- Overall weakness
- Urinary retention and constipation
- Unconsciousness
- Paralysis

What you should do Call your local poison control center.

If breathing difficulties are severe, contact EMS. Monitor the victim's airway, breathing, and circulation (see Resuscitation ABCs, page 357). If necessary, begin CPR (see Cardiopulmonary Resuscitation, page 361). If the victim's airway, breathing, and circulation are okay but the victim is unconscious, place him in the recovery position (see page 365) until emergency medical help arrives.

If the victim has not yet begun to experience severe symptoms, take him to the emergency room immediately. If someone has not shown signs of poisoning but ate the same food as others who have, take him to the hospital to rule out infection.

Try to identify the source of the poisoning by questioning the victim or others who may have eaten the same food. Try to get a sample of the contaminated food. Save a sample of the victim's vomit.

Mental Health Emergencies

Certain mental health crises can be as life-threatening or dangerous as any trauma or heart attack, or can lead to trauma, cardiac arrest, or other injury. Some mental health emergencies may be the first overt manifestations of an underlying illness, such as diabetes, severe depression, alcoholism, or other addiction.

ALCOHOL OR OTHER DRUG INTOXICATION

Depending on the level of intoxication, alcohol or other drug intoxication may or may not require emergency care. Regardless of the level of intoxication, however, heavy usage—abuse—of alcohol or other drugs may indicate not only a problem with addiction, but an underlying mental health issue that the individual may be trying to "self-medicate" (see Chapter 5).

Drugs that are commonly abused fall into three general categories: stimulants, depressants, and hallucinogens. Symptoms of intoxication from stimulants and from depressants are essentially opposite. However, abuse of either can lead to death. Hallucinogens are dangerous primarily because they may cause such a level of delusion, confusion, fear, and violence that the user could do considerable harm to himself or others while under their influence.

❖ DEPRESSANTS

Depressants include alcohol, barbiturates, opiates, tranquilizers, and other drugs that suppress the function of the central nervous system. The effects of many of these drugs can be especially heightened by combining it with alcohol. A relatively low dose of a barbiturate, for example, mixed with a relatively low dose of alcohol can result in coma and death.

Symptoms

* Drowsiness
* Slurred speech (some drugs)
* Loss of physical coordination
* Loss of consciousness
* Dilated pupils, even in bright light
* Nausea and vomiting
* Cool, clammy skin
* Shortness of breath

What you should do The most commonly abused drug is alcohol. Acute cases of intoxication by depressants are most often from alcohol; you should be able to tell if the drug is alcohol by the scent of the individual's breath. Alcohol can kill, so do not just put an extremely intoxicated person to bed and leave him there. Alcohol and other depressants can so suppress motor ability that a heavily intoxicated person can smother in a pillow or choke to death on his own vomit.

If the victim is intoxicated to the level of slurred speech, stumbling gait, or unconsciousness, call EMS. If the victim is uncon-

scious, check his airway, breathing, and circulation (see Resuscitation ABCs, page 357). If necessary, begin CPR (see Cardiopulmonary Resuscitation, page 361) and continue until help arrives or the victim revives. If his airway, breathing, and circulation are okay, put the victim in the recovery position (see page 365) and monitor him until help arrives. Be aware of the possibility of shock and treat as necessary (see page 385). If the victim vomits, save some of the vomit for analysis.

If the victim is conscious, try to find out what drug or drugs he took, how much was taken, and how long ago. Call your local poison control center and follow their directions. If the alcohol or other drugs were taken within the last hour, you may be instructed to induce vomiting.

❖ STIMULANTS

Stimulants are drugs that speed up the central nervous system, constrict blood vessels, and cause excitability. Often as the drug wears off, the user experiences a sense of depression. Most stimulants are amphetamines or amphetamine derivatives, but cocaine also has many stimulant effects. There are many dangers of stimulants, not the least of which is overworking of the heart, which may cause palpitations, arrhythmia, and cardiac arrest. Stimulants may also lead to serious mood swings and violent behavior.

Symptoms

* Anxiety
* Agitation
* Sweating
* Constricted pupils, even in dim light
* Aggressive or violent behavior
* Palpitations

What you should do Try to find out from the victim what drug was taken, how much was taken, and when. Phone your local poison control center and follow their instructions. If the drug was taken within the last hour, the poison control center may instruct you to induce vomiting.

If the victim is violent, paranoid, or showing signs of breathing difficulties, call EMS. Try to get the victim to a quiet place and speak to him calmly but never try to subdue a person who is under the influence of stimulants. It could be dangerous to both of you. Reassure the victim that you are trying to help and that help is on the way.

❖ HALLUCINOGENS

Hallucinogens can range from mild to quite powerful. The delusions and hallucinations that these drugs induce can be nightmarish in their intensity.

If a person has a history of alcoholism and has recently stopped drinking, the absence of alcohol in his system can cause delirium tremens, or DTs, which can also cause frightening hallucinations (see Chapter 5).

Symptoms

- Hallucinations
- Bizarre speech and behavior
- Anxiety or paranoia
- Extreme mood swings
- Outbursts of violence

What you should do Try to find out what drug the victim took, how much he took, and when. Call your local poison center and follow their advice. Notify EMS.

Try to talk calmly with the victim in reassuring tones; make eye contact but be gentle and non-threatening. Try to get the victim into quiet surroundings and establish some kind of interaction with him. Get him to concentrate on some particular subject and talk about it. Having the victim perform a simple task, like peeling an orange, is a good way to focus his thoughts. Stay with the victim until emergency help arrives.

Never try to subdue a person who becomes violent. Drugs can have powerful effects on an individual's physical abilities; users of phencyclidine (PCP) have been known to exhibit extraordinary strength, requiring several people to subdue them. Trying to subdue an individual under the influence of a hallucinogen can be dangerous to you both.

SUDDEN VIOLENT PERSONALITY CHANGES

There are many disorders, poisons, and emotional situations that can cause sudden changes in personality, including an adverse reaction to a new medication, drug abuse, stress, stroke, diabetes, and head injury.

If the victim is a known diabetic, is elderly, or suffers from hypertension or other vascular disease, see Diabetic Emergencies, page 371, or Stroke, page 367.

If the victim has a history of drug abuse, he may have taken a "bad" batch of the drug. See if you can find out if this is the case and, if so, find out what the drug was, how much was taken, and how long ago. Call your local poison control center for advice, and call EMS. Often street drugs that claim to be heroin or other drugs are "designer drugs" made in home laboratories, which can be quite dangerous. If the victim still has some of the drug, take it along to the emergency room for analysis.

What you should do If the victim becomes suddenly agitated, starts talking in a bizarre manner, or begins acting peculiarly out of the blue, try to find out why. Get the victim to a quiet place and be gently reassuring. Such behavior could be evidence of poisoning, a psychiatric disorder that needs evaluation, or it could also be the first evidence of an underlying case of diabetes. The victim may or may not be able to tell you what has happened. In any case, be aware of the possibility of paranoid or combative behavior, and call EMS for assistance.

If the victim suddenly becomes violent and threatens you or others with physical harm, notify law enforcement authorities.

SUICIDAL THOUGHTS AND BEHAVIOR

When someone talks about suicide, *it is not just talk*, but a cry for help. Do not ignore it. Sometimes the person simply needs to talk things out, and the best you can do for him is to listen, be gently reassuring, and ask if he really means to kill himself, and why. In talking you may be able to discover if the person has made plans for suicide, such as stockpiled medications or purchased a firearm, or if he is suffering from severe depression. Reassure him that people with severe depression can be helped, no matter how bleak things may seem at the moment. Emphasize that depression is an illness that can be treated effectively.

What you should do If you know that the person is under psychiatric care, ask if he has been taking antidepressants and if he has stopped taking them, for whatever reason. If the person is not under psychiatric care, you can suggest it. Let him know that there are very good medications for treating depression and that it is an illness that no one needs to endure without help. If you have the slightest concern that a person is in danger of committing suicide, seek professional help as soon as possible. Talk to the person's family and try to enlist their help. If the individual is under psychiatric care, convince him to talk to his counselor. However, the situation is often an emergency. You may have to take the person to the emergency room for evaluation. Mental health professionals are available at all emergency rooms to evaluate suicidal patients.

If you believe a person is actively suicidal, has a firearm or other weapon, or has taken an intentional overdose of drugs, call 911 at once. Do not assume that he will come to his senses or that you yourself may not be in danger.

If a person has already attempted suicide—slashed his wrists or begun to lose consciousness from an intentional overdose of drugs—call EMS at once. Administer first aid as appropriate (see Controlling Severe Bleeding, page 380, or Poisoning, page 408).

SEXUAL ASSAULT OR ABUSE

Sexual assault or abuse is an all-too-real fact of life in our society. Nearly anyone can be the victim of assault or abuse, but the most likely victims are children and women.

What you should do if you are sexually assaulted Although your first reaction may be just to keep the assault a secret and not tell anyone, doing nothing is something you may later come to regret. It will not help you and will not help others who might be assaulted by the same person. The same person may attack you again.

If you have been raped *do not bathe* even if it may be first thing that you want to do. The sooner you report the assault and are examined, the more complete the evidence—and the chances of obtaining a conviction—will be. You can decide later whether or not you wish to prosecute.

Do not blame yourself. Many people feel a sense of guilt at being raped, as well as fearfulness. This is natural, but know that it is not your fault.

Tell someone you trust. If it is your sister or your mother, your best friend, or a rape hotline, report the rape as soon as possible.

Retain all evidence. Do not wash clothing. Keep everything that you were wearing, particularly underwear, as it was. It may be important evidence that will help convict and incarcerate the person who assaulted you.

Get examined. Hospital emergency rooms are equipped to examine people who have been raped or otherwise assaulted. You should be examined as soon as possible after the assault in order to collect evidence. Some hospitals now have special rape counselors to conduct much of the examination and interview. Most emergency rooms have nurses who have been specially trained to assist rape victims.

Get emergency contraception (the "morning after" pill). If you are concerned that you may become pregnant, do not wait to find out if your next period will come. Within 72 hours of contact, but preferably as soon as possible, you can start the brief emergency contraceptive regimen, which usually consists of four pills. This hormonal treatment is designed to interrupt conception and head off a pregnancy before it happens (see Postintercourse or Emergency Contraception, page 1164.)

Get tested. Speak with your doctor about the risk of sexually transmitted diseases (STDs). If you are bruised or otherwise injured, see your doctor for treatment.

Get assistance. Most victims of rape do not to want to be alone for several days after the incident. Someone close to you should look after you in the days following the incident. If the assault leaves you feeling especially depressed or even suicidal, seek counseling as soon as possible. It is important to talk to people. Many people who work in rape crisis centers are women who have been through the trauma of rape themselves. They can be of invaluable assistance in getting you started on the road to recovery, as well as help you, if you decide to prosecute, prepare to attend court and testify.

What you should do if you suspect that a child has been sexually assaulted or abused In many instances, our first response to the possibility that a child has been molested is to disbelieve that such a thing could happen. This is particularly true if the molestation was committed by a family member, which in fact is true for most cases of molestation.

You should take anything that a child tells you seriously. You may also discover the molestation indirectly, by blood on the child's underpants, for example.

Do not ask the child leading or suggestive questions. You might inadvertently plant ideas in the child's mind that could become as real to the child as the things that actually occurred, particularly if he is very young.

Do not offer opinions, whether positive or negative, about possible perpetrators.

Allow the child to talk to you and answer his questions honestly. Ask questions only to get enough information to know whether something happened. Do not try to get all the details. Other people with special training will do that.

Call your doctor immediately for advice on where to go for help; there are centers that specialize in helping children who have been assaulted or abused.

If the assault or abuse just occurred, follow the steps described in What You Should Do if You Are Sexually Assaulted, page 414.

Do not try to confront the perpetrator, regardless of how strong that desire may be. Report the assault to the police.

PART FOUR

Body Systems *and* Disorders

FOURTEEN

Brain and Nervous System

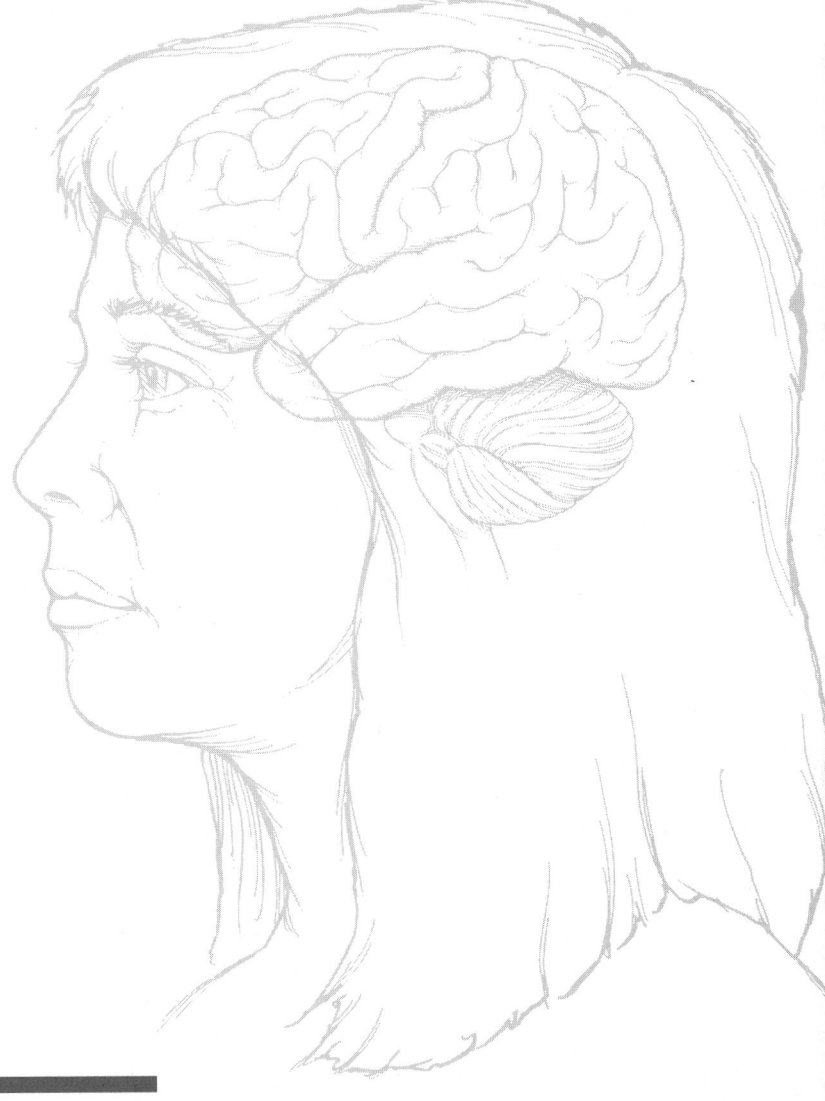

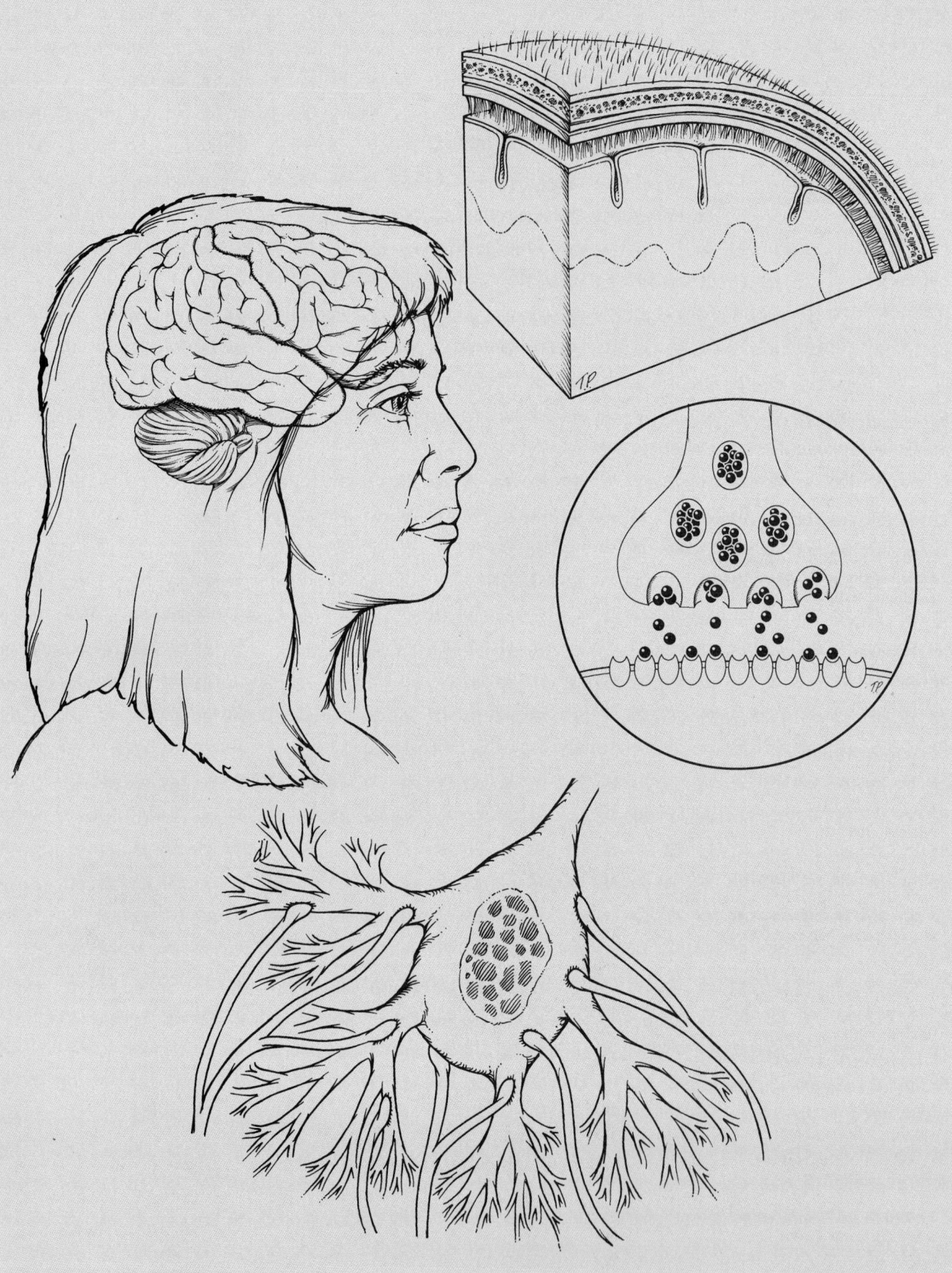

BRAIN AND NERVOUS SYSTEM

How the Brain and Nervous System Work

Information about a beautiful sunset comes through the eyes, the aroma of an exquisite perfume enters the nose, the melody of a song is gathered by our ears, the prickly touch of a thorn is registered via the skin. However, all these sensations are actually centered in the brain. Data from the outside world as well as from the body itself comes to the brain through various nerve pathways, where it is interpreted and acted on.

The basic structural unit of the brain and nervous system is the nerve cell, or neuron. These specialized cells receive and transmit electrochemical impulses. Thread-like fibers extend from the neuron's cell body through major branches called axons to carry impulses away from the cell, and through smaller branches called dendrites to conduct impulses to the cell. The impulses are rapidly transmitted, in an orga-nized pattern, through private channels comprised of dendrites and of axons that are coated with an insulating material called myelin.

Every nerve cell has specialized areas at one end called synapses. Synapses allow cells to communicate with each other. These terminals contain many tiny sacs that hold special chemicals called neurotrans-mitters. Electrical impulses traveling down the axon cause the sacs to release these neurotransmitters. The chemicals bridge the gap between neighboring cells and stimu-late the next cell to produce an electrical charge, carrying the impulse forward. This process repeats again and again (and unbe-lievably swiftly) until a muscle contracts or a sensory impression is noted in the brain.

Sensory neurons transmit signals from special receptors, such as pressure recep-tors in the skin, to the spinal cord or brain. Motor neurons transmit impulses from por-tions of the nervous system to muscles or glands. Other neurons, called interneurons,

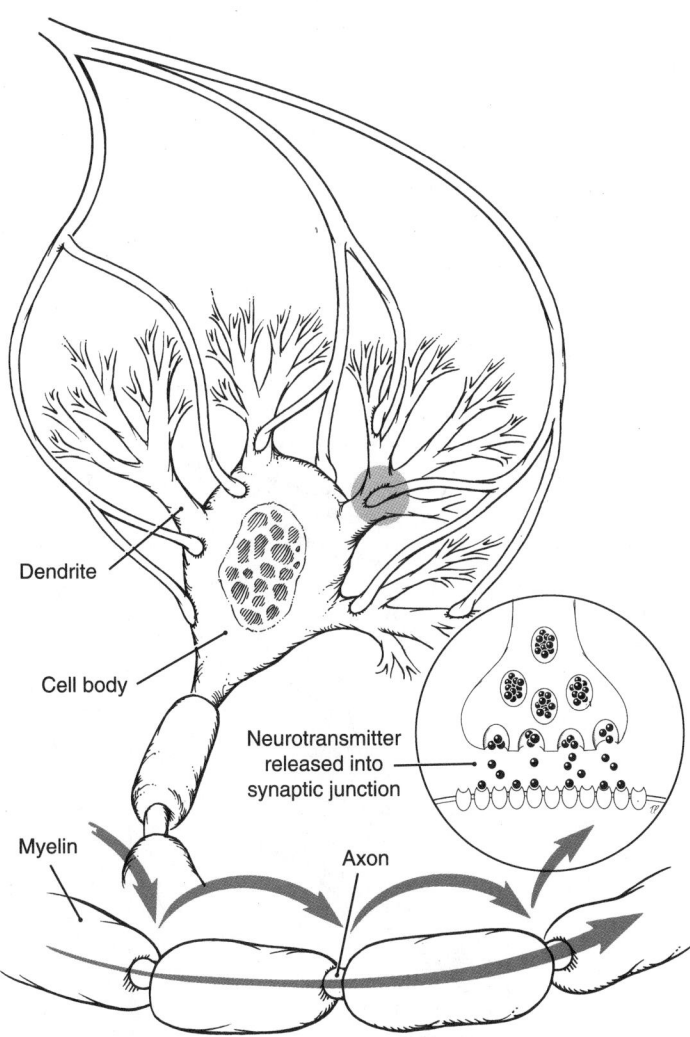

Dendrite

Cell body

Neurotransmitter released into synaptic junction

Myelin

Axon

The nerve cell (neuron) receives and transmits electro-chemical signals. Dendrites make up the receiving end of the neuron, where a signal can be generated depending upon the combined, simulta-neous activities of many other neurons. A signal then pro-ceeds past the cell body and down the long, narrow axon, which is insulated with myelin. At the synapse, where the end of the neuron meets another neuron's dendrites, the electrical signal causes chemical neurotransmitters to be released from tiny sacs. These chemicals are detected at specialized receptor sites on a dendrite of the adjacent neuron. Electrical signals are thus transmitted among large networks of interconnecting neurons.

shuttle the signals through these complex pathways.

These pathways are divided into two main parts: the central nervous system (CNS), made up of the brain and spinal cord, and the peripheral nervous system, which includes nerves that relay messages between the central nervous system and remote parts of the body. The autonomic nervous system is a functional division of the nervous system and has pathways in both the central and peripheral nervous systems. The autonomic nervous system controls involuntary functions such as breathing, digestion, and circulation. The typical human brain weighs about 3 pounds and contains in excess of 10 billion neurons. The brain is more complex than the most sophisticated computer ever built. Protected within the bony confines of the skull, cushioning cerebrospinal fluid (CSF) and three membranes (dura mater, arachnoid membrane, and pia mater), this convoluted mass of white and gray tissue is divided into three main sections: the cerebral hemispheres (together known as the cerebrum), the cerebellum, and the brain stem.

Portions of the cerebrum coordinate such "higher functions" as speech, vision, thought, and memory. If a specific section is damaged—for example, if neurons in the speech center are damaged by a stroke—the ability to speak is impaired. Some functions, such as memory, are not so localized, although structures of the limbic system,

located in the temporal lobe of the brain, have a major role in memory.

The outer surface of the cerebrum is the cerebral cortex, which consists of neuron cell bodies, or gray matter. The inner layers consist of axons, or white matter, plus complexes of nerve cells that control steadiness and motor coordination.

The cerebrum is not a smooth structure; it has elevations and depressions in its many convolutions. Several fissures divide the cerebrum into lobes, which are associated with specific functions. For example, the occipital lobe in the rear of the brain houses the visual area.

The two cerebral hemispheres are connected by a bundle of nerve cells called the corpus callosum. Although connected, the

The brain is divided into three main sections: the cerebrum, the cerebellum, and the brain stem. The cerebrum has four lobes: frontal, parietal, temporal, and occipital. The limbic system plays a major role in memory. Each lobe has specialized functions, such as vision (occipital), sensation (parietal), hearing and speech (temporal), and motor, language, and planning (frontal). A large groove, the central sulcus, separates the frontal lobe from the parietal lobe. Control of coordination and balance occurs in the cerebellum, and the brain stem contains centers involved in eye movements, breathing, digestion, sleep, and cardiovascular function. Major motor and sensory areas are adjacent to each other near the central sulcus. Each major region of the body's skin is represented by a specific region in the sensory cortex. Very sensitive areas of skin, such as fingers and lips, correspond to larger brain regions.

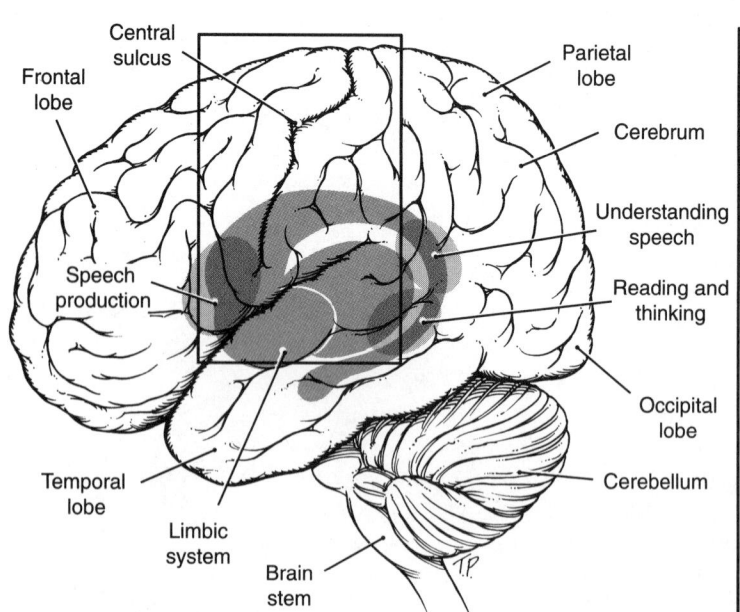

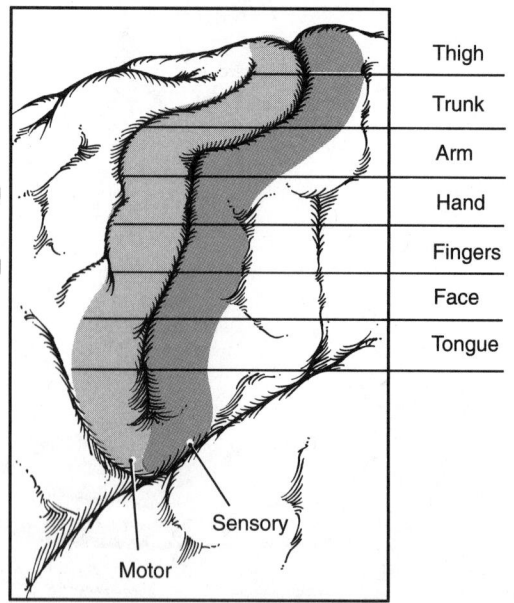

two hemispheres are not equal. The right hemisphere controls the left side of the body; the left hemisphere, the right side of the body. One side almost always dominates. This is how people become left- or right-handed.

Below the corpus callosum lie the thalamus and relay centers, which transmit messages to and from nerve cells in different parts of the cerebrum.

Just beneath the thalamus is the hypothalamus, the body's thermostat, appetite regulator, and blood pressure monitor. Also linked with the pituitary gland, the hypothalamus is involved in stress reactions and nerve impulses related to behavioral and emotional expression.

The cerebellum lies under the cerebrum. It directs certain activities not under conscious control, such as the ability to maintain balance and coordination of movement.

The brain stem sits at the base of the brain and connects it to the spinal cord. Comprised of the medulla, the pons, and the midbrain, it maintains the body's vital functions, such as breathing and heartbeat. Paired cranial nerves exit and enter the brain stem to regulate eye and facial movements and reflexes, as well as chewing, taste, saliva secretion, hearing, and equilibrium.

The roughly elliptical spinal cord is protected by the 33 bony blocks, vertebral bodies that form the spine. These 33 vertebrae are divided into five sections: the cervical, thoracic, and lumbar vertebrae; the sacrum, and the coccyx. Each individual vertebra can move slightly, giving the entire vertebral column significant flexibility. The spinal cord does not run the full length of the spinal column. It ends near the first or second lumbar vertebra in the small of the back. It is about 18 inches long and a half-inch wide. Like the brain, the spinal cord is also cushioned by CSF and membranous dura mater, arachnoid membrane, and pia mater.

Together, the brain and spinal cord make up the central nervous system. The central nervous system communicates with the rest of the body by means of the peripheral nervous system, which originates as 31 pairs of spinal nerves attached to the spinal cord. The spinal nerves pass through openings between the vertebrae. The spinal nerves relay impulses between the spinal

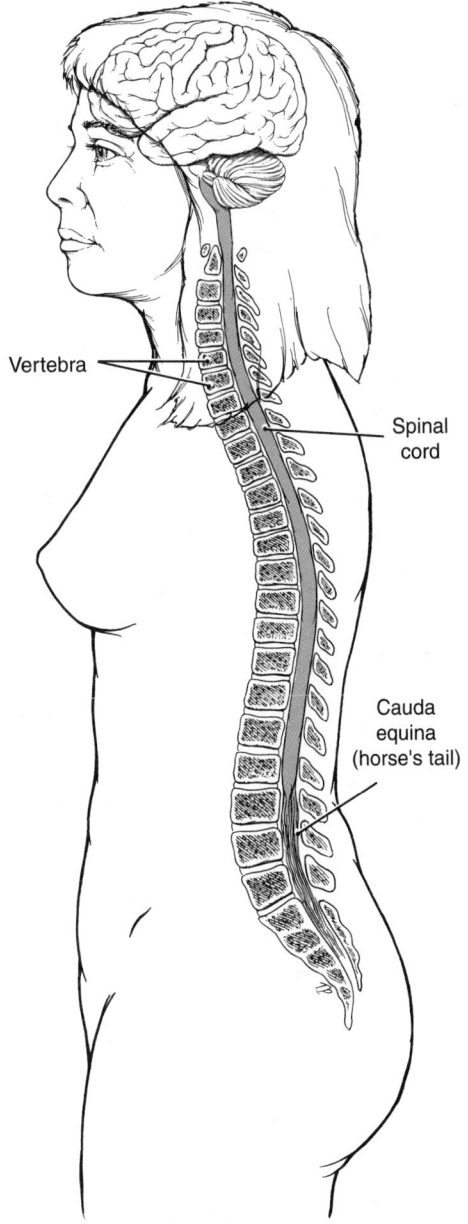

Vertebra

Spinal cord

Cauda equina (horse's tail)

The vertebral column (spine) has 33 bony segments (vertebrae), which give the column both flexibility of movement and protection of the very sensitive, centrally located spinal cord. The spinal roots below the cord are called the cauda equina.

cord and glands, muscles, and sensory organs.

The nervous system is further divided into the somatic (voluntary) nervous system and the autonomic (involuntary) nervous system. The somatic system is responsible for conscious processes such as movement of limbs or sensation of touch. The autonomic system regulates all involuntary body functions. This system is further subdivided into the sympathetic nervous system—which controls blood vessel contraction, increase of heart rate, and regulation of glandular secretions—and the parasympathetic nervous system—which generally has an opposite physiologic effect on the same

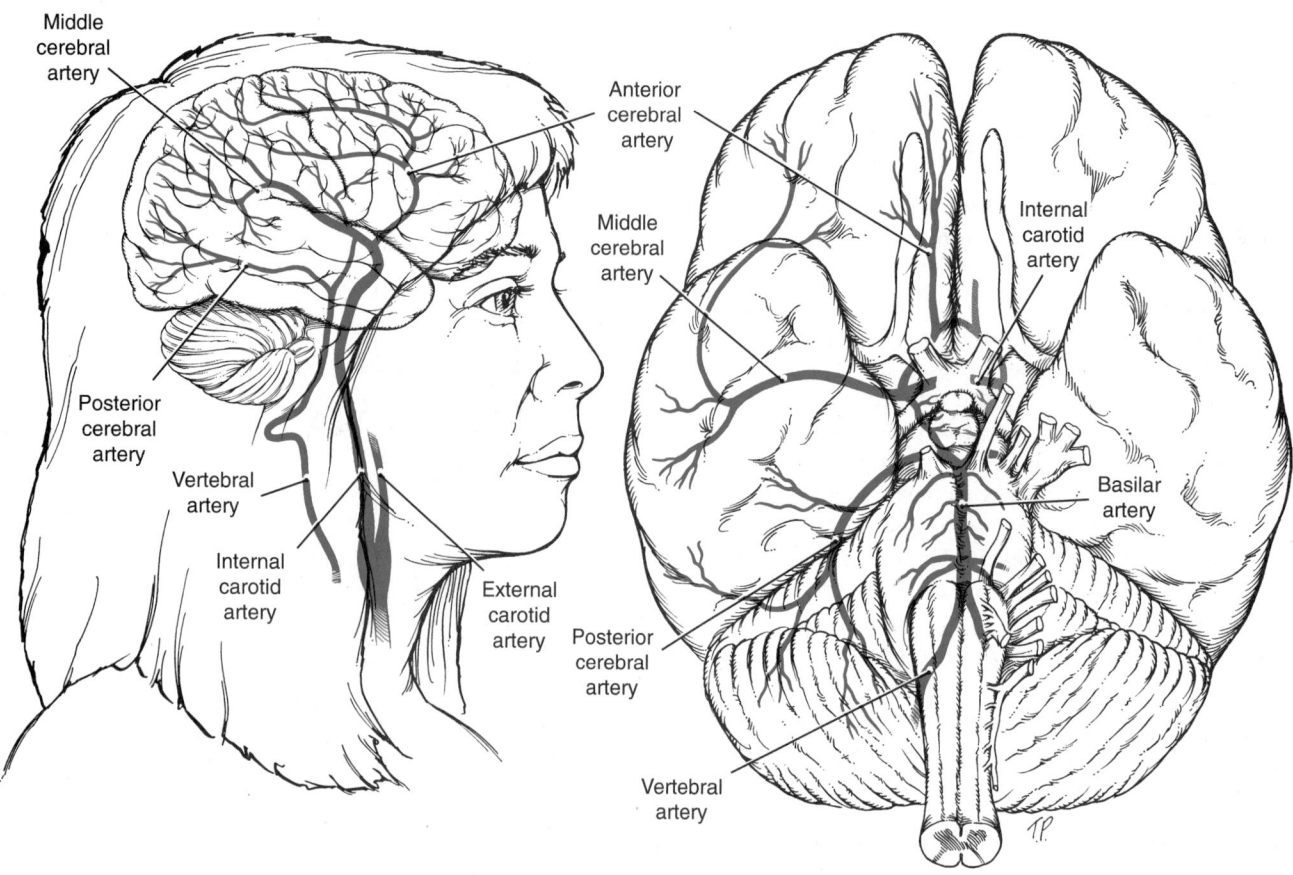

The carotid and vertebral arteries carry blood upward to the brain and eventually branch to serve each region. Branches of arteries on the right and left sides join each other in the circle of Willis, providing multiple possible routes for blood to flow to a given brain region.

structures compared to the sympathetic nervous system. For example, the sympathetic nervous system commands the smooth muscle of blood vessels to contract. It narrows the channel through which blood flows, which raises blood pressure. The parasympathetic nervous system tells those same muscles to relax, widening the vessels and lowering blood pressure.

A steady supply of blood and oxygen is critical to optimum brain function. Blood is carried to the brain by four major arteries, two vertebral and two carotid. These branch off the aorta (the largest artery transporting oxygenated blood from the heart) or from major tributaries of the aorta and run through the neck. They further subdivide to ensure proper blood flow to all parts of the brain.

The brain and nervous system together constitute an overwhelmingly complex, but nonetheless hardy, network. However, they are subject to a variety of disorders, ranging from common and benign (such as tension headache) to progressive and often fatal (such as amyotrophic lateral sclerosis). Disorders of the brain and nervous system can cause extremely varied symptoms, such as head pain, dizziness, loss of balance or coordination, weakness, numbness, shaking, loss of memory, seizures, and difficulty thinking or understanding speech.

Neurologic Examination of The Brain and Nervous System

The growing number of high-tech imaging techniques (see Diagnostic Testing of the Brain and Nervous System, page 426) has created some popular misconceptions about the best way to diagnose problems of the nervous system. Some people may feel cheated if their neurologist (a doctor who specializes in disorders of the nervous system) does not immediately order magnetic resonance imaging (MRI), computed tomography (CT), or other types of sophisticated imaging tests. But the foundation of the diagnosis of neurologic problems is a careful history and physical exam. Thus, most doctors do not begin by ordering high-tech tests but rather by asking the patient to describe all of the symptoms that have led him to seek medical attention, and also to recite a personal medical history. (In the case of children or partially incapacitated persons, the testimony of parents, spouses, or other relatives and friends may be required to supplement the patient's account.) Because many neurologic diseases and disorders have a genetic component, the doctor will also try to learn as much as possible about any family members who have shown similar symptoms.

The doctor will then proceed with a careful examination that is conducted using a few simple tests in the examining room. Systematically, the examiner will assess mental status, sensory function, and motor function. As many as 80 to 90 percent of people with neurologic problems can be diagnosed as a result of the personal history and physical evaluation alone. Despite the amazing complexity of the brain and nervous system, medical science has compiled a rich body of data on various combinations of neurologic symptoms; this enables experienced doctors to pinpoint likely causes after administering the tests described below. Many times, imaging tests will be ordered following the physical exam to give doctor and patient an added measure of confidence in the diagnosis, or to distinguish between one or more closely related disorders that could produce similar sets of symptoms.

Nevertheless, many neurologic diagnoses are, first and foremost, clinical diagnoses that are supported by imaging tests or other laboratory procedures, rather than the other way around. And some neurologic diseases, such as Parkinson's disease, can only be diagnosed on the basis of the clinical exam, because no laboratory test can confirm it.

MENTAL STATUS

While taking your medical history, the doctor already has been gathering data about your mental status. First impressions can come from your behavior and dress. Beyond that, the flow of your conversation—whether quick or halting, rambling or focused—can give the doctor important clues.

The doctor can ask a series of questions designed to test many aspects of your intellectual capacity, including the most fundamental issue of who you are, where you are, and why you are there. The doctor may probe your ability to remember recent events and dates as opposed to events and dates from your distant past. He may ask the names of everyone in your family, their addresses, and what they do, or the name of the president. He may give you a list of three unrelated items (a name, an address, and a color) and ask you to repeat them, both on the spot, and then later in the interview. He may ask you to subtract a series of 7's from 100 or test your ability to do arithmetic in other ways. He may ask you to spell common words backwards.

The particular combination of mental abilities and deficits revealed by these various tests can form a kind of code, pointing the doctor toward the right answer.

CRANIAL NERVES

Next, a series of tests is aimed at testing the functioning of the 12 pairs of cranial nerves, which exert control over sight, hearing, smell, and taste, as well as muscles of the head and neck. These tests can include asking you to identify common aromas with your eyes closed; observing how the eyes respond to light and how smoothly they follow the doctor's finger as it moves from left to right; asking you to look up or to close your eyes so tightly that the doctor cannot open them; asking you to stick out your tongue or clamp your jaws shut; and many other simple tests.

SENSORY TESTS

How you sense certain stimuli—pain, touch, heat, cold, and vibration—is an important indicator of some nervous system disorders. Examples of some sensory tests include: lightly pressing the point of a pin against your skin; placing test tubes filled with hot or cold water against your skin; touching lightly on various parts of your body with a wisp of cotton while your eyes are closed;

touching bony prominences (wrist, elbow, knee) with a tuning fork and asking you to tell your doctor when the fork stops vibrating; moving your toes or fingers up, down, or to the sides and asking you to specify their direction of movement; asking you to identify various textures with your eyes closed; and touching you in two different places simultaneously with sharp objects like calipers and asking if you can sense touch in one or both places.

MOTOR TESTS

In many cases, clinical observation of walking allows the doctor to check posture, balance, and coordination of limb movements. In the same way, tics, tremors, or other motor abnormalities can provide a presumptive diagnosis. Simple tests can provide even more information and help to localize where in the nervous system (brain, spinal cord, or peripheral nerves) the problem lies. Common tests include asking you to: touch your nose with each index finger, alternating hands; tap your index finger and thumb of each hand rapidly together; draw a figure 8 in the air with a foot; walk heel to toe in a straight line; and stand with feet together, arms outstretched, and eyes closed, without falling over. Differences in left- and right-sided functions also can point to central nervous system damage.

To evaluate muscle strength, the doctor will have you grip his hands and squeeze or push against the doctor's palm with a foot. The doctor also will examine your ability to extend and flex your neck, elbows, wrists, fingers, toes, knees, and hips; to contract and relax your abdominal muscles; and to rotate your shoulders.

Muscle tone is examined by analyzing how easy it is for the doctor to move your arms and legs, and the range of motion of your limbs. Assessing the muscles' relative flaccidity or rigidity can point to specific nerve and muscle problems. Checking your reflexes also gives clues about the presence of a nervous system disease. Tapping your ankles, elbows, arms, and knees with a small, rubber-tipped hammer allows the doctors to check your motor nerve functions and connections between the peripheral and central nervous system.

Diagnostic Testing of the Brain and Nervous System

MAGNETIC RESONANCE IMAGING

The magnetic resonance imaging (MRI) scan weds computer technology, high-intensity magnetic fields, and radio waves to provide sharp, clear images of the body's soft tissues. It is used to assess the presence or extent of brain tumors, abscesses, swelling (edema), bleeding, nerve damage, and other disorders that increase tissue fluid content. It also can show spinal diseases including herniated discs or cancer involving the spine.

A closely related test called magnetic resonance angiography (MRA) adds only about 15 minutes to a regular MRI and allows doctors, for example, to evaluate blood vessels in the head and neck in people with stroke or transient ischemic attack (TIA). This is now becoming a standard screening test for arterial blockage.

Some MRI scanners resemble a tube. You lie on a platform that transports you into the center of the device. Others are not enclosed and are better for people who cannot stand tight quarters. These are referred to as "open MRI" units. While open MRI units may be less claustrophobic, the images they produce are less precise than those obtained in "closed" units, and the open units cannot be used in all circumstances. The typical scan takes 30 to 45 minutes to complete. Although the test itself is painless, a dye may be injected into a vein to help doctors better visualize the area under observation. The dye can also enhance detection of tumors and infection. During the scan you may hear knocking noises.

Before entering the scanner, you must remove all metallic objects. Because of the intense magnetic field (many thousands of times more powerful than the earth's magnetic field) magnetic metal objects can become small, unguided missiles in the confines of the scanning chamber. You will also be asked if you have any surgically implanted joints, pins, clips, valves, pumps, or pacemakers that contain metal. If so, you may not be able to undergo the scan.

During an MRI scan, small "slices" of your brain or spinal column are captured on film as the scanner moves down your body. The computer can manipulate this information to provide a three-dimensional image or two-dimensional pictures from different angles or projections.

COMPUTED TOMOGRAPHY

The computed tomography (CT) scan is a system that uses computerized x-rays. In a CT scan, a narrow x-ray beam is projected at the brain. At the same time, a detector is positioned precisely opposite the x-ray source and measures the amount of unabsorbed radiation that passes through the skull and brain. As the projector and the detector revolve around your head, the data are processed by a computer. The pictures that it takes represent thin slices of the brain. These images can be displayed individually on a monitor. In some cases, a special program and equipment can combine the individual slices to create three-dimensional views of the brain, which can be manipulated on a computer screen in three dimensions.

During a CT scan, you lie face up on a table that slides into the center of the machine, which resembles a large doughnut. Your head is held gently by straps that help keep it perfectly still for the duration of the scan, which usually takes about 10 to 15 minutes. A three-dimensional scan can be accomplished, however, in less than a minute. You may hear a lot of noise while you are inside the scanner. This is the x-ray tube rotating inside the machine.

A dye (also known as a contrast medium) may be injected into a vein. This helps enhance the images. If a dye will be used you will be asked to fast for 4 hours before the test. The dye may cause you to feel flushed and warm. It may cause you to experience a metallic taste or nausea and vomiting after it is injected. Newer dyes, called nonionic contrast agents, have milder and much less frequent side effects.

SINGLE-PHOTON EMISSION COMPUTERIZED TOMOGRAPHY

Single-photon emission computerized tomography (SPECT) is a different kind of imaging system. It is used to examine the flow and volume of blood in the brain.

Radioactive tracers can be injected into the bloodsteam. There, they emit tiny particles called photons, which allow their movements throughout the body (in this case, the brain) to be traced by special scanning devices. A computer uses the information to develop a map of the distribution of the radioactive chemical in the brain.

During a SPECT scan the radioactive chemical will be injected into your arm. You will lie face up on a table, and your head will be gently secured by a strap to help keep it absolutely still for the 30 minutes or so of the scan. The table will then be slid partway into what looks like the center of a large doughnut.

SPECT measures the metabolic activity of the brain. It uses radioactive tracers that do not decay quickly, thus making it possible for doctors to image events such as epileptic seizures that may happen hours after the initial injection.

CEREBRAL ANGIOGRAPHY

In cerebral angiography, a dye that shows up on x-rays is injected into the brain's circulatory system. It allows doctors to see how blood flows through the brain's blood vessels. The procedure is useful in detecting such blood vessel problems as aneurysms (weakened areas on blood vessels that resemble blisters on a tire), malformations, and blockages or narrowing. It also is useful in studying blood vessels that may be inflamed due to vasculitis (see page 640).

In this test, which typically lasts from 1 to 2 hours, you will lie on an x-ray table with your arms at your sides. A local anesthetic is injected, usually into the artery in the groin, where a thin, flexible catheter, or tube, will be inserted. This catheter is then snaked through the body's blood vessels to the brain. When it is in place, the dye is injected. This may trigger a brief burning sensation. You may feel warm and flushed, have a brief headache or metallic taste, or even feel nauseated.

You will need to fast for 8 to 10 hours before the test. Be sure to tell the medical personnel if you have ever experienced an allergic reaction to injected dyes, iodine, or iodine-containing substances (such as shellfish).

After the test, you may rest in bed for up to 6 to 12 hours.

CAROTID ULTRASOUND

Harmless, high-frequency sound waves, known as ultrasound, can be used to detect arterial blockages following the same principles used by doctors to form images of a fetus in the uterus. In an ultrasound Doppler test, the examiner applies some gel to the surface of your skin on the neck. Next, the examiner moves a sound-detecting wand (transducer) over the skin surface to monitor the flow of blood in the carotid artery. Measuring the degree of Doppler shift (a change in the pitch of sound waves based on the relative motion of their source) can reveal whether blood is flowing smoothly or turbulently. This study is usually used to screen for disease in the carotid arteries.

ELECTROENCEPHALOGRAPHY

Electroencephalography (EEG), which usually takes about 30 minutes if you are awake, records the brain's electrical activity. It is performed by attaching 16 to 30 small electrodes to your scalp with a special paste as you lie on your back or relax in a reclining chair. The electrodes record the electrical activity and send this information to a machine that traces the brain waves on a paper or a computer screen.

EEG can help determine the presence and type of seizures, as well as evaluate any changes in the brain's electrical activity due to head injury, tumor, stroke, or infection. It is also helpful in the diagnosis of sleep disorders.

Before the recording procedure begins, close your eyes, relax, and remain still. You should not talk while the test is being done. Following the initial recording, you may have more recordings done while brain-stimulating actions are performed. For example, the person administering the test may flash a light in your eyes; or you may be asked to breathe deeply and rapidly for 3 minutes (this may elicit brain wave patterns typical of certain kinds of seizures).

When doctors analyze brain waves, they look for variations in basic waveform patterns, symmetry of brain activity, brief bursts of activity, and responses to stimulation.

The EEG records the brain's activity as waves. Among the basic waveforms are alpha, beta, theta, and delta rhythms. Each of these occur at different frequencies. In seizure disorders, the EEG may identify the specific type of seizure. For example, grand mal (also known as tonic-clonic seizures) are identified by multiple, high-voltage, spiked waves in both hemispheres of the brain. Complex partial seizures are identified by the presence of spiked waves only in the affected region of the brain.

Any condition that causes consciousness to diminish also alters the EEG pattern. For example, someone with a brain infection generally will have diffuse, slow brain waves. If you are going to undergo sleep EEG, you should keep yourself from sleeping as much as possible the night before the test.

ELECTROMYOGRAPHY AND NERVE CONDUCTION STUDY

The electromyography (EMG) and nerve conduction study measures the electrical activity of certain voluntary muscles while they are at rest and while they contract. An EMG takes about an hour to perform. The test is administered to help diagnose carpal tunnel syndrome and other pinched nerves, certain diseases that are characterized by nerve tissue degeneration, such as amyotrophic lateral sclerosis, and neuromuscular diseases, such as myasthenia gravis. It is also useful in identifying muscle disorders, such as muscular dystrophy.

While you are seated or lying down, a doctor inserts a needle electrode into a muscle. He then measures the muscle's electrical discharge, which is recorded electronically. A muscle at rest usually shows little electrical activity. But activity increases significantly while a muscle is working.

A companion to EMG is the nerve conduction study, which measures the speed at which nerves carry electrical messages from the body to the brain. This provides important information in diagnosing peripheral nerve injuries and diseases. In this test, a mild electrical shock is given to stimulate a particular nerve. A recording electrode placed a set distance from the site of the shock detects the response from the stimulated nerve and measures the amount of time it took to arrive. In peripheral nerve diseases and injuries, the time it takes for nerve impulses to travel can be significantly slower than the normal velocity of about 110 miles per hour.

LUMBAR PUNCTURE

Also known as a spinal tap, a lumbar puncture is used when the doctor needs to analyze the cerebrospinal fluid, which is within the spinal cord. The analysis of this fluid may be done to measure the pressure of the fluid, which can help detect obstruction of its circulation, and to help in diagnosing viral or bacterial meningitis, hemorrhage, neurosyphilis, and chronic central nervous system infections.

The test usually takes about 15 to 30 minutes, and is performed under a local anesthetic. Headache is the most common side effect, seen in about 10 to 15 percent of patients. People who get headaches are told to drink fluids and to stay lying down for 24 to 48 hours, which usually resolves the problem.

While you lie on your side with your knees drawn up to your abdomen and your chin on your chest, the doctor administers a local anesthetic and then inserts a needle between the fourth and fifth lumbar vertebrae of your lower spine, allowing the CSF to drip out. You should report any pain or uncomfortable sensation while the fluid is being withdrawn. You should remain still and breathe normally.

Spinal fluid normally is clear. A cloudy appearance can signal infection. Blood in the fluid can indicate hemorrhage, inflammation or a side effect from the test. Fluid pressure that is above normal can imply hemorrhage, tumor, or fluid accumulation caused by injury. Fluid pressure that is below normal can imply an obstruction above the test puncture site. A high white blood cell count can mean meningitis (infection of the coverings of the brain) or another acute infection. It can also mean tumor, abscess, or multiple sclerosis. Protein and sugar levels are also routinely checked. Low glucose levels may indicate bacterial infection and high protein levels may indicate infection, some types of tumors, or some types of neuropathy. Antibody tests may diagnose infections, such as viral infections and Lyme disease. Special protein tests are used to help diagnose multiple sclerosis.

Stroke

A stroke results from any process that impairs blood flow to the brain. The same process that deposits cholesterol and other fatty materials in the wall of coronary arteries can also narrow the channels that bring blood to the brain. This process is called atherosclerosis and is one cause of stroke. Other forms of stroke result from an embolus—a blood clot or material fragment that breaks free from elsewhere in the body and wanders through the bloodstream, eventually lodging in one of the brain's blood vessels. A stroke can also occur when an artery in, or leading to, the brain bursts, due to high blood pressure or a weakened artery wall (aneurysm).

Brain cells deprived of blood begin to die within minutes, resulting in a loss of

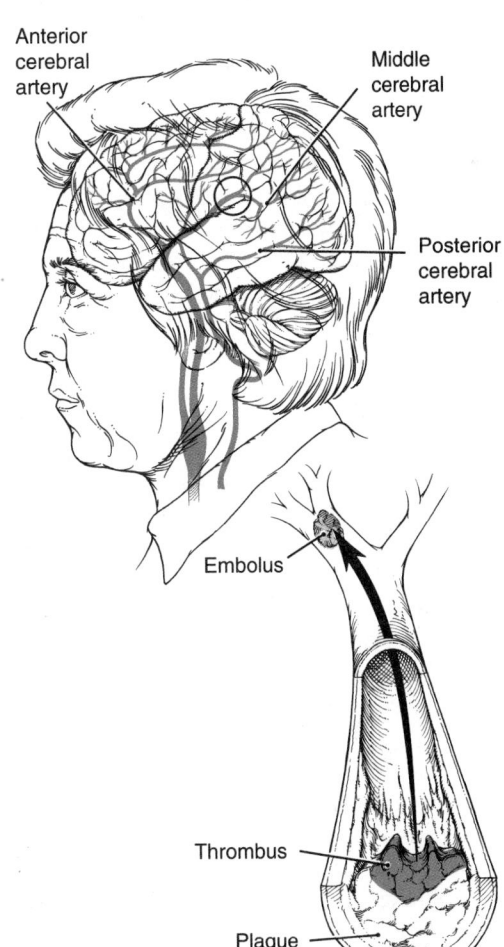

Anterior cerebral artery

Middle cerebral artery

Posterior cerebral artery

Embolus

Thrombus

Plaque

A stroke represents permanent damage to a section of the brain from an embolism, thrombus, or bleeding. Emboli typically form as blood clots in the heart and travel to the brain where they block a cerebral artery. Plaques (fatty material) form on the walls of blood vessels in the brain and can block the flow of blood when a clot (thrombus) forms on the plaques. The same process in the heart causes a heart attack.

HEEDING THE SYMPTOMS OF STROKE

Stroke, also known as "brain attack," is the third leading cause of death in the United States, responsible for about 150,000 deaths every year. On average, someone in the United States suffers a stroke every minute; someone dies of a stroke every 3.4 minutes.

About 500,000 Americans per year experience a new or recurrent stroke. Stroke is the leading cause of serious disability in the United States. About 31 percent of people who survive an initial stroke die within 1 year. About 66 percent die within 12 years.

While the risk of stroke is greater for seniors, being young does not eliminate the risk. About 28 percent of the people who experience a stroke in a given year are under the age of 65.

Thus, it is important to know the warning signals of stroke. They are:

- Sudden weakness or numbness in the face, arm, or leg on one side of the body

- Sudden dimness or loss of vision, especially in one eye

- Loss of speech, or trouble talking or understanding speech

- Sudden, severe headaches with no known cause

- Unexplained dizziness, unsteadiness, or sudden falls, especially along with any of the previous symptoms

If you notice one or more of these signs, do not wait. Call or have someone call your emergency medical service right away.

About 10 percent of strokes are preceded by what doctors call transient ischemic attacks (TIAs), or warning signs. These are short-lived brain attacks— most last fewer than 5 minutes—that occur when a blood clot temporarily clogs an artery and part of the brain does not get the blood it needs. TIA symptoms are similar to those of stroke, but the weakness, numbness, loss of vision, or speech problems are temporary. And, unlike a full-blown stroke, when TIA symptoms disappear people return to normal.

TIA symptoms should not be ignored. If you experience them, you should seek medical attention immediately.

Prompt medical help could prevent a fatal or disabling stroke from occurring. ∎

neurologic control of body parts and body functions. These devastating effects often persist, because brain cells are highly developed, specialized, and evolved cells that do not replace or regenerate themselves. Neurologic impairment may progress over minutes to hours; loss of blood supply to vital areas of the brain can be lethal.

Each year, approximately 500,000 Americans experience a new or recurrent stroke; about 150,000 of these are fatal. Nearly 90,000 women and 60,000 men are struck down annually by these "brain attacks." Stroke is the third leading cause of death in the United States and is the leading cause of serious disability.

Because most strokes are related to high blood pressure and atherosclerosis, it is important to realize that most strokes are also preventable. You can reduce your chances of having a stroke by eating a low-fat diet, engaging in regular physical activity, and not smoking. Keeping your blood pressure within desirable limits through diet, exercise, and medication is probably the most important thing you can do to stave off either type of stroke. For complete information on lifestyle changes to prevent atherosclerosis, see Lifestyle Changes for a Healthy Heart, page 797.

Stroke affects people differently, depending on the type of stroke experienced and the area of the brain affected. If the affected arteries are associated with the brain's vision center, sight can be affected. If the speech center is deprived of blood, the ability to talk or understand speech can be impaired. Muscle strength and motor coordination can be affected, and paralysis on one side of the body is common.

A stroke can also affect the ability to think clearly. Planning and executing once-simple tasks now may require more time and effort. Stroke survivors may not remember how to begin a task, confuse the sequence of steps in performing a job, or even forget how to do something they have done all their lives, such as tying a shoe.

❖ ISCHEMIC STROKE

Symptoms *(What you may experience)*
Sudden weakness or numbness of the face, arm, or leg on one side of the body; sudden dimness or loss of vision, particularly in one eye; loss of speech or trouble talking or understanding speech; unexplained dizziness, unsteadiness, or sudden falls, especially along with any other symptoms.

The loss of feeling in one arm or leg, or the loss of sight in one eye, can result in a loss of awareness of the affected side, a problem referred to as "neglect." Seeing, touching, moving, and thinking can all be affected. Speech can be slowed, slurred, or distorted. Chewing and swallowing food can also become problematic.

In addition, stroke survivors may suffer from depression, both as a result of brain lesions caused by stroke and because they may think of themselves as less than "whole."

Signs and laboratory findings *(What the doctor looks for)* Level of consciousness, orientation, memory, and emotional control; vision loss; muscle weakness; lack of fine muscular dexterity; loss of balance; changes in gait; changes in eye movements. In addition to these signs in the physical exam, imaging tests such as CTs, MRIs, angiograms, and echocardiograms can be decisive in making the diagnosis. Sonograms of the carotid artery can show narrowing secondary to atherosclerotic plaque that causes stroke. Hypercoagulability (an increased tendency of the blood to clot) can be detected using blood tests.

What is it? Ischemic strokes result from inadequate blood flow to the brain or part of the brain. Deprived of oxygen and nutrients, nerve cells in the affected area cannot function, and they die within minutes. When nerve cells cannot function, the part or parts of the body controlled by these cells cannot function. Some effects of stroke are permanent, because dead or damaged neurons in the brain do not regenerate and are not replaced.

There are three principal types of ischemic stroke: cerebral thrombosis, cerebral embolism, and lacunar stroke.

- Cerebral thrombosis is the most common type of ischemic stroke, accounting for an estimated one-third of all strokes. It occurs when a blood clot forms in an artery in the brain or the carotid artery, which carries blood to the brain. Such clots usually form in blood vessels narrowed by atherosclerosis, the process by which cholesterol and other fatty materials are deposited in artery walls. (See Atherosclerotic Disorders, page 806.)

- Cerebral embolism is the second leading type of ischemic stroke, accounting for about another one-third of all strokes. An embolus is a clot or other type of material originating in another

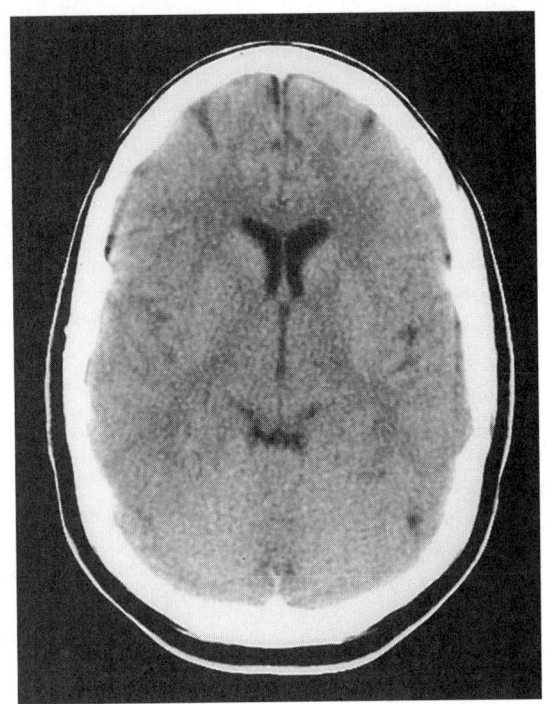

CT scan of a normal brain.

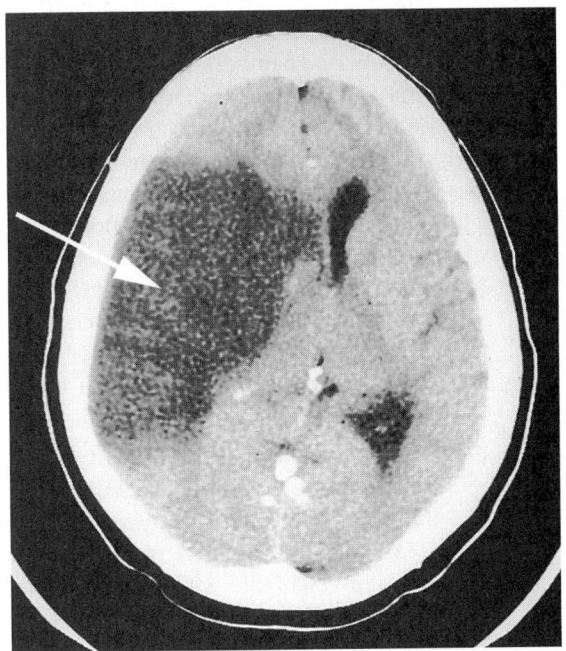

CT scan showing damaged brain tissue (arrow) after an ischemic stroke. Brain cells deprived of blood begin to die within minutes.

part of the body and carried by the bloodstream. When it lodges in an artery, it impedes the blood flow to the brain, causing brain cells to die.

T-PA AND STROKE

Each year about 500,000 Americans experience a stroke. About 400,000 (80 percent) of these strokes are ischemic, meaning that they result from insufficient blood flow to the brain. Usually, the cause of the reduced blood flow is a blood clot that plugs up an artery narrowed by depositions of cholesterol and other fatty materials.

Until recently, little could be done to stop an ischemic stroke in progress. But in June 1996 the US Food and Drug Administration approved the use of the clot-dissolving drug tissue plasminogen activator (t-PA) to treat these "brain attacks."

Although it has been used for several years as an effective treatment for heart attack, its potential as a treatment for stroke was initially unclear because it carries an increased risk of bleeding in the brain. Thus, not every stroke patient should receive t-PA treatment. For the 100,000 patients a year who experience a hemorrhagic, or bleeding, stroke caused by a ruptured blood vessel in the brain, t-PA could only worsen the problem by promoting excess bleeding.

But for some stroke patients, t-PA is the first weapon doctors have at their disposal to attack a stroke while it is occurring.

However, not everyone who experiences an ischemic stroke is a candidate for t-PA treatment.

First of all, the drug is effective only if given promptly. For maximum benefit, the therapy must begin within 3 hours of the onset of stroke symptoms. Therefore, it is critical that people recognize and respond to stroke as an emergency.

Second, t-PA must be administered in a setting where bleeding complications can be managed promptly.

Third, t-PA should be withheld if imaging scans already indicate significant brain damage from the stroke.

T-PA should be administered to patients only after a complete evaluation of the patient that includes a careful examination of a computed tomography (CT) scan.

In addition to educating the public about the signs of stroke and the importance of immediate treatment, substantial efforts by the health care community will be necessary to allow more widespread use of t-PA as a stroke treatment. These include: (1) the organization and training of health care professionals to evaluate and treat stroke patients, and (2) planning for the rapid transport of patients to treatment centers through emergency medical services. ■

The most common cause of these emboli is a heart condition known as atrial fibrillation. In this disorder, the two upper chambers of the heart (the atria) quiver instead of contracting properly. The chambers do not empty completely, and blood is never totally evacuated from them. This stagnation of blood allows clots to form in nooks and crannies of the interior of the atria. (See Abnormal Heart Rhythms, page 828.) Emboli can also result from thickening or infection of the heart valves or from atherosclerosis of the aorta and other arteries.

- Lacunar stroke is the third type of ischemic stroke. Often preceded by a flurry of transient ischemic attacks (TIAs) in the previous 1 to 2 days (see Transient Ischemic Attack, page 434), lacunar stroke was once thought to be uniquely associated with hypertension (high blood pressure). However, it is now known that lacunar strokes can be caused by a variety of factors, including atherosclerosis and blockages from debris (the accumulation of fragments of dead tissue or foreign matter) and other small emboli.

Several factors increase the risk of ischemic stroke. These include: high blood pressure; heart disease; cigarette smoking;

a history of TIAs; abnormal blood clotting factors; a high red blood cell count (this "thickens" the blood and makes blood clots more likely to form); atrial fibrillation; and heart valve disease from rheumatic fever. Ischemic strokes are more likely in seniors, men, African-Americans, persons with diabetes, those who have had a stroke already, or those with a family history of stroke.

Other factors, such as high cholesterol levels, physical inactivity, and obesity, also indirectly increase the risk of a stroke as well as heart disease.

When to call the doctor If you are at high risk for stroke, you and your family members should learn the warning signs. Do not ignore them if they occur. Ignoring mild symptoms in the case of stroke can waste valuable time and have disastrous results. At the first sign of stroke symptoms, call—or have someone call — your local emergency medical service immediately. If you are not sure about the symptoms, call your doctor immediately. Stroke is an emergency situation; every minute spent waiting is time when more brain cells are dying.

It may not be possible to know whether someone is experiencing a stroke or a TIA. Do not wait to contact your local emergency medical service. Even if symptoms

REHABILITATION AFTER STROKE

On average, every minute someone in the United States has a new or recurrent stroke. That translates to approximately 500,000 strokes every year. But approximately 350,000 of those people will survive stroke, and the majority of them will benefit from rehabilitation.

To a large degree, successful rehabilitation depends on the extent of brain damage and the part of the brain affected. But effective rehabilitation also depends on the attitude of the person, the skills of the rehabilitation team, and the cooperation of family and friends. People with little impairment are likely to benefit the most; but even when improvement is slight, rehabilitation can still mean the difference between living at home or living in a long-term care facility.

Rehabilitation does not reverse the effects of a stroke. Instead, its goal is to decrease dependence and build the person's strength, capabilities, and confidence so that daily activities can be continued with a measure of independence.

What is done in rehabilitation depends on what a person needs to move from illness to independence. The person may need to improve self-care skills, such as grooming, bathing, and dressing; mobility skills, such as walking, using a wheelchair, or transferring from a bed or chair to a wheelchair; communications skills in speech and language; cognitive skills, such as memory or problem solving; or the ability to interact favorably with other people.

Rehabilitation will begin when the doctor determines that the stroke survivor is medically stable and able to benefit from it.

Rehabilitation may take place in a hospital, a long-term care facility, at home, or at an outpatient setting.

Under the doctor's direction, rehabilitation specialists form a team to provide a course of treatment specifically suited to the person's needs. Services may include physical therapy, occupational therapy, speech-language therapy, recreational therapy, nutrition education, counseling with a social worker, therapist, or clergy, and educating the family about the effects of stroke and what rehabilitation can achieve.

Family support is important and plays a significant role in stroke rehabilitation. The situation will be easier to handle if the family knows what to expect and how to handle problems that may arise.

The goals of rehabilitation depend on the effects of the stroke; the individual, the family, and the rehabilitation staff work together to set realistic goals. Examples of realistic goals include regaining the ability to walk (perhaps with a walker or cane), regaining the ability to care for oneself (perhaps with special equipment), and being able to drive. Having a job can be a realistic goal for some people, but for others the job they left behind may no longer be suitable. However, another job or volunteer activity may be a realistic goal.

Rehabilitation can benefit the majority of stroke survivors, but it may not be suitable for everyone. Some people are too disabled to benefit. A person who cannot benefit from rehabilitative measures may be better helped by maintenance care at home or in a nursing facility. ■

---

subside after a few minutes, you should still seek medical care immediately.

Treatment If the individual has stopped breathing, cardiopulmonary resuscitation (CPR) may be necessary while you are waiting for emergency medical service (see the inside front cover of this book). If saliva collects in the stroke victim's mouth or vomiting occurs, turn the head to the side. Do not give someone who has suffered a stroke anything to eat or drink.

The most important principle for treatment is to determine the cause of the stroke and institute the therapy that is appropriate for that cause. This may include endarterectomy, anticoagulants, or antiplatelet agents (such as aspirin). Immediate treatment may involve medications to prevent the occurrence of another stroke by reducing clot formation (anticoagulants such as heparin, or antiplatelet medication, such as ticlopidine or aspirin). But anticoagulants increase the possibility of bleeding in the brain and may be dangerous in people with high blood pressure.

To restore blood supply to the brain during an ischemic stroke, doctors can use tissue plasminogen activator (t-PA), a thrombolytic (clot-dissolving) drug. However, t-PA can only be used within 3 hours of the onset of stroke symptoms. It must be used judiciously, because it can increase the risk of bleeding in the brain. (For more information, see T-PA and Stroke, page 432.)

If a patient with a minor stroke or TIA is found to have severe blockage of the carotid, a surgical procedure to remove the fatty material lining the carotid artery walls may be performed. This procedure, called carotid endarterectomy, is used to prevent the further occurrence of stroke. The surgeon isolates a section of diseased artery with clamps and slices it open longitudinally. The material is then removed and the artery is closed. (For more information, see Carotid Endarterectomy, page 434.)

Blockages may recur unless lifestyle changes are made addressing the basic atherosclerotic process. Also, not everyone who has an ischemic stroke is a candidate for surgery. For example, someone whose

CAROTID ENDARTERECTOMY

About 10 to 30 percent of the 500,000 strokes that occur each year in the United States are the result of impeded blood flow through narrowed and clogged arteries that lead to the brain.

The carotid arteries, which supply blood to the brain, can become narrowed due to a process called atherosclerosis. In this process cholesterol and other fatty materials are deposited in the artery walls. But surgeons can remove this material—called plaque—in an operation called carotid endarterectomy.

In the surgery, the affected artery is exposed and clamped at both ends to halt blood flow through it. The blood vessel is then opened longitudinally, and the plaque is withdrawn. Blood flow is carefully restored, and a close watch is kept for any blood clots that might enter the circulation into the brain.

The surgery can be highly beneficial for people who have already experienced a minor stroke, or who have had a transient ischemic attack (a short-lived temporary stroke) and have a narrowing of 70 to 99 percent of the vessel. In this group of people, the surgery reduces the estimated 2-year risk of stroke by more than 60 percent (from greater than one in four to less than one in ten). However, carotid endarterectomy is not without risks and complications.

Although it may be performed soon after stroke symptoms have begun, this is the time of highest risk of death, or a second stroke and attendant disabilities. If the individual has coronary artery disease, the operation may be too risky. High blood pressure must be brought under control before the procedure can be performed. The complication rate at medical centers where surgeons are specially trained to perform the surgery may be as low as 2 or 3 percent, but in hospitals where the surgery is performed less frequently, the risk of complications rises.

A potential complication is the development of an embolus, in which a piece of the plaque breaks off and is carried downstream, where it can lodge in an artery in the brain and cause a stroke.

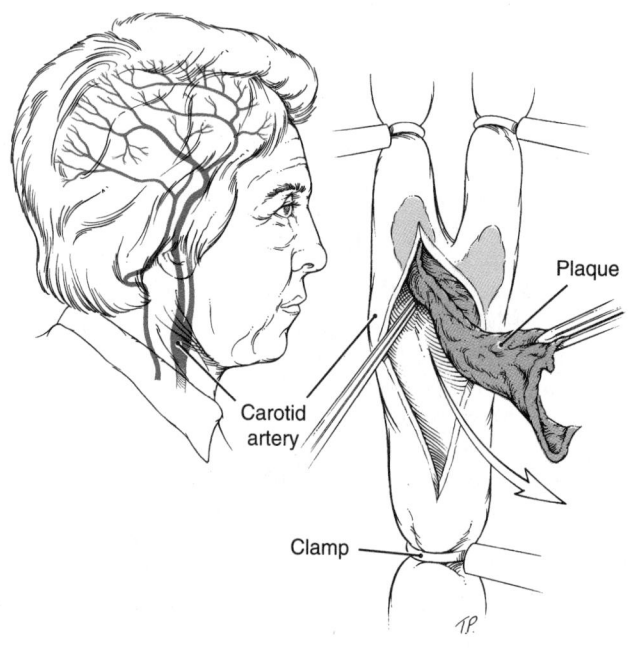

Carotid endarterectomy. In this operation, the narrowed carotid artery in the neck is clamped and cut open, and plaque is removed from the vessel. The vessel is then stitched and unclamped. This operation improves blood flow.

Carotid endarterectomy was first described in the 1950s; its use peaked in the 1980s, when more than 100,000 of the operations were performed each year. Trials were launched in the mid-1980s to identify more closely specific groups of people with carotid artery disease who would clearly benefit from the procedure. Your doctor can help you decide whether carotid endarterectomy may offer benefits in your case. ■

carotid artery is completely blocked generally will not be considered. If high blood pressure is present, it must be corrected before surgery can be considered (for more information, see Managing Hypertension page 799).

Some stroke survivors will need physical, occupational, or speech rehabilitation to relearn lost skills and functions. If the survivor is depressed, counseling or medication to treat the underlying depression can help.

Prognosis Stroke is the leading cause of serious disability in the United States. The outlook for someone who has experienced a stroke depends largely on the extent of

brain damage. Spontaneous recovery in the first 30 days following a stroke probably accounts for most gains in functional ability.

❖ TRANSIENT ISCHEMIC ATTACKS

Symptoms (*What You May Experience*) The symptoms are similar to those of an ischemic stroke—sudden weakness or numbness of the face, arm or leg on one side of the body; sudden dimness or loss of vision, particularly in one eye; loss of speech or trouble talking or understanding speech; unexplained dizziness, unsteadiness, or sudden falls, especially along with any other symptoms.

In a TIA, the symptoms listed on page 434 are transient, lasting from 10 to 15 minutes to less than 24 hours. Patients fully recover after a TIA and may not take these symptoms as seriously as they should; these symptoms are an important early-warning indicator of a more serious stroke ahead if changes are not made.

Signs and laboratory findings *(What the doctor looks for)* TIAs exhibit similar signs to ischemic strokes (see page 431) but typically last only a few minutes, although they can continue for hours. The doctor will pay heightened attention to the patient's medical history. He will also listen for telltale noises (called bruits, the French word for noises) in the carotid arteries. He will examine the heart carefully for irregular beat indicating atrial fibrillation and other signs of disease. Ultrasound of the carotid arteries may be done to look for atherosclerosis. An electrocardiogram (ECG) and an echocardiogram are often helpful to look for sources of emboli.

What is it? TIAs occur when a blood clot temporarily clogs an artery, and part of the brain fails to receive its supply of blood and oxygen. Although symptoms are similar to those of a stroke, TIAs do not result in lasting damage to brain function.

When to call the doctor You should call the doctor or your local emergency medical service immediately upon experiencing any of the symptoms of a TIA.

Treatment The treatment for TIAs is similar to that of ischemic strokes and is aimed at preventing a full-blown stroke from following. The primary means of prevention is to reduce a patient's blood pressure through medications and lifestyle changes. A secondary means of prevention is to introduce antiplatelet therapy using aspirin or other medications. Antiplatelet therapy has been shown to reduce the subsequent risk of stroke by as much as 25 percent. Anticoagulants are also used to prevent stroke.

Prognosis More than one-third of people who have one or more TIAs will later have a full-blown stroke. In fact, someone who has had TIA is 9.5 times more likely to have a stroke than someone of the same age and sex who has not had one. There is no way to tell with any certainty when a stroke will occur; but in approximately half of all cases, it occurs in 1 year.

❖ HEMORRHAGIC STROKE

Symptoms *(What you may experience)* Sudden severe headaches; loss of consciousness; sudden weakness or numbness of the face, arm, or leg on one side of the body; sudden dimness or loss of vision, particularly in one eye; loss of speech or trouble talking or understanding speech; unexplained dizziness, unsteadiness, or sudden falls, especially if they occur with any other symptoms.

Signs and laboratory findings *(What the doctor looks for)* Impaired level of consciousness, confusion, loss of memory and emotional control; vision loss; changes in reflexes and coordination of limbs. Imaging tests will show abnormalities in structure or blood flow. A CT scan of the head will usually show the presence of blood from a hemorrhage in the brain.

What is it? Hemorrhagic or bleeding strokes are caused by ruptured blood vessels in the brain. The two major types of hemorrhagic strokes are subarachnoid hemorrhage and intracerebral hemorrhage.

- A subarachnoid hemorrhage occurs when a blood vessel on the brain surface (below a thin membrane called the arachnoid) ruptures and bleeds into the space between the brain and the brain lining, which contains the cerebral fluid. About 7 to 10 percent of all strokes are of this type. Such hemorrhages are caused by a burst aneurysm. This is a pouch that balloons out from a weak spot on the artery wall. Blood vessels usually are tough and elastic; however, an aneurysm can form on a blood vessel and weaken it in a particular place. Aneurysms often are aggravated by hypertension (high blood pressure), which causes them to stretch and weaken even more, taking them to the bursting point. When a brain artery bursts, the loss of blood supply to some brain cells means that they can no longer function. Accumulated blood in the brain, or between the brain and the skull, may put pressure on the surrounding brain tissue and interfere with brain function.

• An intracerebral hemorrhage occurs when a defective artery in the brain bursts, flooding the surrounding tissue with blood. About 10 percent of all strokes are of this type. Arterial damage due to hypertension or arteriosclerosis usually underlies intracerebral hemorrhage. In young patients, doctors also look for abnormal blood vessels that may be congenital (for example, arteriovenous malformation or AVM). Cocaine or amphetamine abuse may also be a cause of intracranial hemorrhage (as well as ischemic stroke).

What you can do Stroke is often preventable. Damage to the brain can be minimized with prompt medical attention. You can take action to keep a stroke from happening by controlling some risk factors that cause stroke. If you have high blood pressure, for instance, you can control it through medication, diet, exercise, or a combination of these treatments. If you are overweight, see Chapter 2 for information on losing weight. If you smoke, quit; see Chapter 4 for tips on stopping smoking. See Lifestyle Changes for a Healthy Heart in Chapter 20 for more information.

Treatment In hemorrhagic stroke, as in other types of stroke, emergency medical services should be contacted; if necessary, cardiopulmonary resuscitation (CPR) should be initiated.

Tissue plasminogen activator (t-PA) and other drugs that interfere with blood clotting are contraindicated in cases of hemorrhagic stroke. Medications to lower blood pressure should not be administered until after the person has been stabilized.

Supportive care depends on the degree of impairment. An unconscious or comatose person needs nutrients and medications delivered intravenously. A catheter is usually inserted into the bladder to allow urine to drain and to monitor fluid status. Stroke related deficits may impair the ability to swallow. Nutrients can be supplied directly to the stomach through a surgically placed tube for long-term sustenance.

Conscious individuals are confined to bed, advised against any exertion or straining, and given stool softeners. Antiseizure medications, such as phenytoin, may be prescribed. A pain-relieving medication—but not aspirin—may relieve the head discomfort that often follows a hemorrhagic stroke.

In cases of a ruptured aneurysm (subarachnoid hemorrhage), the risk of a further hemorrhage is greatest within a few days of the first bleeding episode. Many individuals (nearly 40 percent) will have another episode within 6 months. To prevent this, surgery is done to clip the aneurysm and prevent rebleeding. This is usually preferred over medical management. X-ray studies called arteriograms will help doctors pinpoint the ruptured artery. This technique requires a catheter to be inserted into major vessels through a puncture site in the groin under local anesthesia (see Cerebral Angiography, page 427).

Prognosis The severity of a cerebral hemorrhage is determined by the amount of bleeding. In half of all cases, people with this type of stroke will die of increased pressure on the brain. There may be partial paralysis, weakness, or numbness, as well as visual or speech deficits. People who survive a hemorrhagic stroke may recover considerable function. This is because much of the damage caused by a hemorrhagic stroke is due to pooled blood, increasing pressure on the brain. As blood is absorbed or removed, pressure gradually diminishes, and the brain may return to its former state.

In general, people with subarachnoid hemorrhagic strokes (burst aneurysms) have about twice the survival rate of people with intracranial hemorrhagic strokes. The most important predictor of the outcome is the level of consciousness of the patient upon admission to the hospital—again emphasizing the need for rapid response if you detect symptoms of a stroke in yourself or someone close to you.

Headache

The brain does not contain sensory nerves, so it cannot feel pain. Pain can be experienced only in the membranes covering the surface of the brain (the meninges), the skin and muscles covering the skull, and the nerves acting as conduits between the brain, head, and face.

Nearly everyone experiences headache. For some it may be a rare occurrence or a minor nuisance. For others, it may be intense, debilitating, and recurring. For some people, headache may be the primary problem; for others, it may be a symptom of a more serious malady.

Most headaches develop slowly, are temporary, are unrelated to any other health problem, and leave no aftereffects. The majority of headaches are tension and migraine headaches. But other factors can induce head pain, including too little or too much sleep, overeating or drinking (especially alcohol), noise, and a stuffy environment.

Headache also can occur as a symptom of another disease, such as sinus infection (see Acute Bacterial Sinusitis, page 585), temporomandibular joint dysfunction, and generalized fever. Headaches also may signal a serious condition, such as an aneurysm or a brain tumor.

- Aneurysm (see Hemorrhagic Stroke, page 435) is a blister-like weakness on the wall of a blood vessel. When such a vascular weakness in the brain ruptures, it causes sudden, unbearable head pain.

- Brain tumor (see page 485) is characterized by pain becoming steadily worse over time (can be weeks to months). It often is accompanied by personality changes, vision changes, speech impediments, seizures, and problems with gait or balance.

Questions a doctor will ask These questions include: When did you first develop these headaches? How often do you have them? In what part of your head is the pain located? How long do your headaches last? Do your parents or grandparents have similar headaches? Do headaches occur at certain times of day or night? Do you have other symptoms that accompany or precede a headache? Do you drink coffee or smoke cigarettes? If you are female, do headaches coincide with your menstrual cycle? What is your sleep pattern?

Although 90 percent of all headaches are typical garden-variety tension headaches, more than 45 million Americans experience chronic, recurring headaches. A chronic headache continues for 6 months or more, disrupting a person's daily routine.

Determining the nature of the pain is important in recognizing the type of headache and selecting appropriate treatment. A throbbing pain is characteristic of migraine; steady, nonthrobbing discomfort

DESCRIBING A HEADACHE TO A DOCTOR

Certain types of headaches have similar traits. Identifying these aspects will allow your doctor to make a proper diagnosis of the kind of headache you have and point the way to appropriate treatment options.

You should be prepared to tell your doctor:

- When you first developed these headaches

- How often you have them

- Where the pain is located

- What the pain is like: Does your head throb? Is the pain a steady consistent pressure? Is it so intense you can not lie quietly and must move around?

- How long the headaches last

- Whether they occur at specific times of the day or night

- Whether the pain has become progressively worse

- Whether the headaches are interfering with your daily routine

- Whether you can associate the onset of your headaches with any activities or foods

- Whether the headache is accompanied by weakness, numbness, dizziness, or other sensation

- Whether you experience any unusual sensory disturbances before the pain starts

- If you are female, whether your headaches occur before, during, or after your menstrual cycle

- Whether any close relatives also have headaches, and if so whether the symptoms are similar

- About your sleep pattern

Knowing if you have recently sustained a head injury or have had a fever or sinus congestion also will help your doctor. ■

indicates probable tension headache; and sudden sharp or burning pain may signal a cluster headache. A sudden "thunderclap" headache may signal a hemorrhagic stroke or burst aneurysm in the brain.

Headaches also can be worsened by stress.

Depending on the type of headache, treatment may involve over-the-counter or prescription painkillers; tranquilizers; or nondrug treatment, such as psychotherapy and biofeedback. Most headaches are treatable; many can even be prevented.

❖ MIGRAINE HEADACHE

Symptoms *(What you may experience)* Throbbing pain on one or both sides of the head; pain severe enough to disrupt normal routine; nausea; vomiting; sensitivity to light and sound; visual, olfactory (related to smell), or other sensory disturbances. People with a "classic" migraine have a premonitory "aura" such as sparkling lights in their vision prior to the onset of the headache. Common migraines can be difficult to distinguish from tension headaches. Indeed, some neurologists believe many so-called tension headaches are mild migraine headaches.

Signs and laboratory findings *(What the doctor looks for)* A normal neurologic exam suggests that the headaches are due to migraine. An abnormal exam, however, will lead the doctor to look for other causes of headache, such as a tumor. A family history of migraine and characteristic symptoms noted above also suggest migraine headaches. If abnormal findings are noted or headaches are worsening over time, the doctor may order a CT scan, vision tests, and a lumbar puncture to rule out other, more serious causes.

What is it? Typically, migraines are severe, recurring headaches that are often accompanied by nausea, vomiting, and sensitivity to light and noise. The word migraine is from Latin *hemicrania*, meaning one-half of the skull.

Doctors used to think a migraine resulted when blood vessels in the head underwent a constriction-dilation, and the widened blood vessels activated pain neurons. Because of this, migraines are referred to as vascular headaches. Some neurologists think it is an inflammatory reaction.

The current theory is that nerve fibers in the brain stem release proteins into the blood circulation of the back of the head. These proteins may induce inflammation of the blood vessels. The inflammation triggers sensory neurons, which send pain signals back to the brain.

The symptoms of a migraine vary from person to person. Some people will have a headache on one side of the head, and others will have it on both sides. Some people will have pain preceded by an aura, and some will not experience an aura. In people who have an aura, the aura may be different.

An aura is a sensory warning that a migraine is on the way. It may be visual. Some people describe a shimmering haze of bright jagged lines that starts as a point of bright light, gradually expands to fill the visual field (except for a narrow tunnel in the center), and then, just as gradually, subsides. Or, it may involve temporary speech impediments, a general sense of confusion, or tingling and numbness in the arms, legs, or face. It may begin 5 minutes or 45 minutes prior to the onset of pain. Auras occur in approximately 20 percent of the 16 to 18 million Americans who suffer from migraines.

Some people may experience what doctors call a migraine prodrome. This is a generalized feeling that a migraine will strike. It may begin 24 hours before the actual migraine process, but it usually occurs 1 or 2 hours before the headache starts. People who experience a prodrome may exhibit mood swings and have food cravings.

The tendency towards migraines often is inherited. If both parents have them, there is a 75 percent chance their children will have them; if one parent has them, there is a 50 percent chance any child will be affected. Women are more likely to have migraines than men. And about 65 percent of women who have migraines have them around the time of menstruation. Pregnancy may hold the headaches at bay.

Certain foods may trigger migraines, including chocolate, red wine, aged cheeses, caffeinated beverages (or withdrawal from caffeine), processed meats, lentils, snow peas, and the flavor-enhancer monosodium glutamate (MSG). Other triggers include changes in barometric pressure and weather, certain chemicals (perfumes, insecticides, and carbon monoxide), missing or delayed meals, altered sleep-wake cycles, stress, depression, altitude changes, bright lights, and excessive noise.

What you can do Once a migraine strikes, you should take a pain reliever, avoid light and noise, apply a cold compress to your head, and try to sleep. Changes in your diet and exercise regimen may reduce migraine frequency.

If migraines are associated with certain foods, note which ones are most likely to produce problems and simply cut them from your diet. Often, dietary triggers are not obvious and require a systematic search.

Regular aerobic exercise increases the brain's production of endorphins. These are chemicals that reduce pain and enhance mood. Exercise also increases levels of serotonin and other chemicals called enkephalins. These also improve pain tolerance. Regular aerobic exercise, three times a week for 20 to 30 minutes, may keep your headaches away.

Exercise also helps people sleep better, thus avoiding the disrupted sleep patterns that can induce migraines.

Biofeedback, a method in which people learn to control body functions such as blood vessel swelling, can significantly reduce the occurrence of headaches; however, success with this method depends on daily practice. Children, who are open to new things and learn quickly, may respond especially well to this technique.

When to call the doctor If headaches are frequent and interfere with your daily routine, consult your doctor.

Treatment Medication treatment of migraine falls into two categories: abortive (treating the headache as soon as symptoms begin) or prophylactic (preventing the headache).

Abortive treatments include:

- Anti-inflammatory prescription (single analgesic), aspirin and nonsteroidal anti-inflammatory drugs (NSAIDs).

- Ergot derivatives (from a plant fungus) are examples of abortive migraine therapy. These can be taken orally, in inhaled form, or as a suppository; one form can be administered by injection. All ergot derivatives may produce such side effects as nausea, vomiting, and muscle cramps.

- Triptans—sumatriptan (Imitrex), zolmitriptan (Zomig), and aratriptan (Amerge)—are one of the newest antimigraine medications and can be taken orally, nasally, or injected. They promote the release of the neurotransmitter serotonin in the brain. Neurotransmitters are chemicals that send messages between nerve cells. Think of these chemicals as "keys" that fit into specific "locks" called receptors on the ends of nerve cells. The specific receptor to which triptan molecules attach is found in high concentrations in several pain-regulating centers in the brain. People with coronary artery disease should not take triptans, because they could constrict already narrowed coronary arteries and cause a heart attack.

- Corticosteroids such as prednisone may help relieve the pain of migraine attacks that are prolonged (lasting 3 to 4 days despite other medications).

Prophylactic treatment includes:

- Beta blockers and calcium channel blockers, originally intended as blood pressure and heart-disease therapies, and tricyclic antidepressant medications such as amitriptyline (Elavil) and nortriptyline (Aventyl, Pamelor).

A medication-free approach to treating migraine will help avoid harmful or irritating side effects. Changes in diet and patterns of physical activity, and learning to manage stress may substantially reduce and even prevent migraine pain (see What you can do, page 438).

❖ CLUSTER HEADACHE

Symptoms *(What you may experience)* Intense one-sided pain; sudden onset; brief duration; pain localized to region around one eye; swollen, watery eye; pain occurring at specific times.

Signs and laboratory findings *(What the doctor looks for)* Characteristic symptoms.

What is it? About 1 million Americans experience cluster headaches, which occur with little or no warning. Cluster headache pain is often described as excruciating, sharp, or burning. The sensation generally is localized to the area behind or around one eye.

People with cluster headaches cannot lie still and are restless and active. This contrasts with migraine sufferers, who often need to go straight to bed in a quiet, dark room. People with cluster headaches also do not experience light sensitivity or gastrointestinal upset common in migraine. One hallmark of cluster headache is its relatively brief duration; it begins abruptly and lasts a short time, usually between 30 and 45 minutes.

The term cluster emphasizes the characteristic grouping of pain attacks with respect to specific time patterns. About 80 to 97 percent of cluster headache sufferers have episodic headaches. This means that they get these headaches at the same time every day for 1 to 3 months. Most get one to four headaches per day during this period. The headaches then disappear for months or years.

The remaining 3 to 20 percent have chronic cluster headaches. Their headaches occur daily for at least 12 months.

Cluster headaches affect about six times more men than women and generally begin around the age of 30. They do not appear to be inherited.

What you can do Altered sleep patterns may trigger these headaches, so people at risk should maintain a regular sleep schedule. Occasionally a food may be associated with the onset of the headache. In such a case, eliminating the food from the diet may prevent the headaches from recurring.

People who experience cluster headaches consistently report greater use of cigarettes and alcohol. The exact nature of this association is unclear. Whether it is a cause-and-effect relationship is uncertain; but the association of cluster headaches with these habits is strong. It is worth the effort to stop smoking and drinking. Your headaches may subside, and your health will certainly improve in other ways.

When to call the doctor If headaches occur frequently or interfere with your daily routine, see your doctor for treatment.

Treatment The short duration of cluster headaches rules out the use of conventional pain-relieving medications. However, breathing oxygen through a face mask for 10 minutes often provides relief. Oxygen needs to be prescribed by a doctor, and oxygen tanks can be obtained from surgical supply stores. An ergot derivative, injected intramuscularly, may provide pain relief.

Other medications that may help reduce the frequency and severity of cluster head-ache include calcium channel blockers, beta blockers, and corticosteroids. But steroids, because of potential adverse reactions, are best reserved for cases in which other treatments have failed or cannot be used. These reactions include personality changes, reduced immunity to infectious disease, gastric ulcers, weight gain, and osteoporosis, a condition in which the bones become brittle and break easily. Triptans are also used.

Lithium, used to treat manic-depressive disorders, also may help people with chronic cluster headache. But be alert to its potential side effects: shaking, weakness, thirst, diarrhea, and nausea. Chronic ingestion of lithium also may affect the thyroid gland and kidneys. Blood tests will be necessary to adjust the amount of lithium taken.

❖ TENSION HEADACHE

Symptoms (*What you may experience*) A dull, nonthrobbing pain on both sides of the head.

Signs and laboratory findings (*What the doctor looks for*) If there are abnormal findings on neurologic and physical exam, a CT or MRI scan may be performed to rule out other, more serious underlying conditions.

What is it? Almost 90 percent of all headaches are classified as tension headaches. Some consider them to be common migraines. Tension headaches occur when muscles of the face, neck, or scalp tighten or contract for extended periods. They can originate from poor posture (such as holding your neck at an awkward angle when reading) or from abnormalities of the neck, teeth, or jaws.

Other triggers include emotional stress, fatigue, and environmental stimuli (such as bright lights and noise).

What you can do Exercising regularly helps increase your body's natural painkillers (chemicals called endorphins and enkephalins). Exercise also helps you sleep and helps you avoid disrupted sleep patterns that can result in tension headaches.

Eat sensibly, according to a regular schedule. People with low blood sugar, or hypoglycemia, often get headaches. Diets rich in refined sugars can produce wide swings in blood sugar level.

When possible, avoid bright or glaring lights.

A massage can relieve not only headache pain, but also tension that can precipitate a headache.

Working for an extended period in a fixed position can trigger a headache. Vary your position often, take breaks as frequently as possible, stretch, and assume correct posture when sitting and standing. Relaxation and deep-breathing exercises also may help relieve tension.

When to call the doctor Consult your doctor to rule out other, more serious, causes, if you find you are taking an excessive amount of pain-relievers; your headache is accompanied by weakness, dizziness or numbness; you become confused or faint; or your headache is associated with ear or eye pain. Otherwise, most tension headaches will resolve on their own and do not need the attention of a doctor.

Treatment Most tension headaches will disappear either by themselves or with the aid of over-the-counter pain-relievers.

Applying hot or cold compresses to your neck or temples may offer relief. You may need to experiment to find which works best for you. Massage can also offer relief.

Tricyclic antidepressants may be prescribed for people with frequent headaches, especially if they are associated with neck pain.

❖ TEMPORAL ARTERITIS

Symptoms *(What you may experience)* Temple pain; dull, throbbing headache on one or both sides of the forehead; vision loss in one eye; jaw pain with prolonged chewing; mild fever; loss of weight and appetite.

Signs and laboratory findings *(What the doctor looks for)* Swollen temporal artery (appears red and is sensitive to touch); blood test revealing a high erythrocyte sedimentation rate (ESR); tissue biopsy of the temporal artery showing characteristic changes under the microscope.

What is it? The temporal arteries run behind your temples in your scalp. They are branches of the carotid arteries, which supply blood to the brain.

When the temporal arteries and the arteries supplying blood to the brain become inflamed, they become thickened, which reduces their ability to transport blood. In severe cases, it can lead to stroke. More often it affects the eyes and can lead to some degree of vision loss—especially in seniors, in whom it often occurs; the typical age for those with this condition is over 70. (For more information on diagnosis and treatment, see Giant Cell (Temporal) Arteritis, page 556.)

Pain

Pain is one of the most common symptoms humans experience, yet it is one of the least understood. Acute pain is the body's smoke alarm, alerting you to a potentially dangerous situation. In fact, people with congenital analgesia, a rare condition that leaves them unable to sense pain, often harm themselves without knowing it. These people commonly die in their mid-30s, usually from injuries they never felt. Because pain plays such a vital role in survival, the brain usually gives it priority over other sensory information.

Acute pain begins when special sense receptors in the skin or internal organs

Some movements are initiated by the spinal cord without input from the brain. These are known as reflexes. A sense of extreme pain in the hand, for example, travels from the skin to the spinal cord, where a long motor neuron triggers the contraction of a muscle in the arm or hand. This contraction typically causes the hand to withdraw from the source of pain.

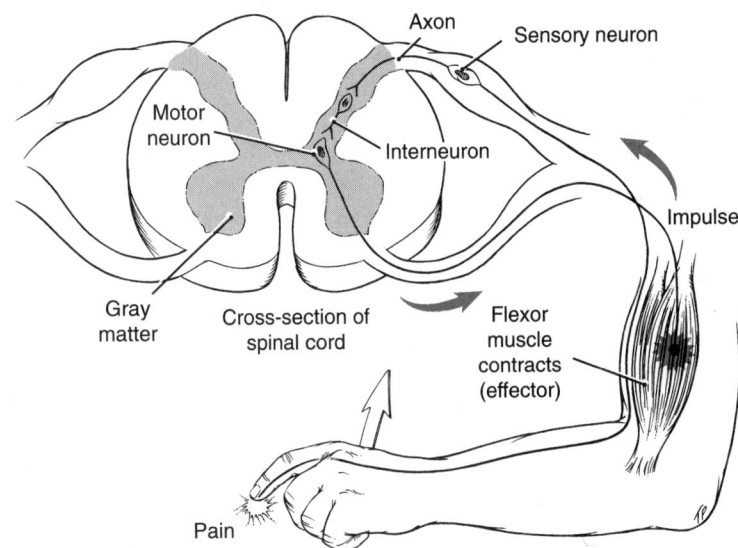

called nociceptors are activated. They receive information about heat, pressure, pricks or cuts, or other injury causing pain. Two types of nerve fibers carry information from the nociceptors to the spinal cord: A-delta fibers, which transmit information quickly; and C-type fibers, which transmit impulses more slowly (and may cause a nagging sense of pain).

At the spinal cord, these pain messages may be modulated by other spinal nerves that enhance or diminish the intensity of the pain stimulus. The impulse travels to different parts of the brain. Some regions determine the location and cause of pain, while other areas integrate the information with additional information to produce a pain sensation, often described as "vicious," "sharp," or "dull."

Chemical couriers, or neurotransmitters, carry the pain messages up and down the nerve tree. Different neurotransmitters activate different receptors on nerve cells. The pain you feel depends on which neurotransmitters and which receptors are involved. For example, when a particular neurotransmitter activates the recently discovered NMDA receptor, nerve cells become so sensitive that even light pressure causes excruciating pain.

Some spinal nerves release neurotransmitters called enkephalins, and some regions of the brain release neurotransmitters called endorphins. These chemicals act as natural painkillers.

❖ ACUTE PAIN

When to call the doctor Tolerance to pain varies among individuals. The degree of pain is associated with the severity of its underlying causes. Underlying causes and symptoms must be evaluated to treat pain. Consult a doctor if you cannot determine why there is pain; it is not temporary; analgesics do not relieve the pain; or you are extremely uncomfortable, or anxious. The doctor will ask what medications you have already taken, they must be considered for an accurate diagnosis and treatment. For example, abdominal pain must be assessed without masking the symptoms with analgesics.

Treatment Analgesics usually relieve pain. Ice on the pain location may reduce discomfort and inflammation. Emotional support for accompanying anxiety is often effective in distracting the individual until the temporary discomfort subsides.

❖ CHRONIC PAIN

Symptoms (*What you may experience*) Persistent pain lasting months or years, with or without an obvious source.

Signs and laboratory findings (*What the doctor looks for*) Medical history reveals previous illness or trauma; underlying causes for the pain such as tumor, infection, a pinched nerve, or arthritis revealed on physical and neurological exams; depression or anxiety shown on psychological exam.

What is it? Chronic pain is persistent discomfort lasting months or years. Persons with chronic pain fall into two groups: those with a specific source of pain, such as

THE SENSE OF TOUCH

The sense of touch pervades our bodies and our lives. It protects us, activating reflexes when we come into contact with something too sharp, too hot, or too cold. Touch helps us manipulate tools and our environment. We could not walk without the sense of touch to tell us when one foot hits the ground and one pushes off.

Nerve endings just beneath your skin's surface transmit messages to your spinal cord and brain about texture, temperature, and pressure. As the brain interprets these messages it fires back signals telling your muscles to tighten or relax. The process is in a constant feedback loop; information is constantly being sent through a complete circuit, allowing you to constantly adjust, say, your grip on a pen. Touch receptors in the tongue, fingertips, and lips are more sensitive than those in other parts of the body. Each fingertip has more than 3,000 touch receptors, while the skin of your entire trunk contains about that many. Hairy skin has special receptors that deal with the movement of the hairs. That is why we say things like, "I felt my hair stand on end."

Nociceptors, which are nerve receptors in the skin that sense temperature and pain, are sensation subspecialists. Two kinds sense temperature (one senses only cold, the other senses only heat) and two kinds sense different types of pain (rapid, pricking pain or slow, burning pain). Each group of temperature nociceptors can sense changes in hot or cold as little as a hundredth of a degree.

Some of the fibers carrying touch information pass through the spinal cord and, without stopping, proceed to the brain stem. Other nerve fibers carry information to the gray matter of the spinal cord, where it is analyzed and filtered before being sent up to the brain. Messages regarding pain are analyzed in the spinal cord as well, allowing for the assimilation of touch and pain messages.

Whether the touch sensations come by the direct or indirect route, they eventually wind up deep in the thalamus, where various different types of information are assimilated, enabling the cerebral cortex to put together an accurate picture of what our touch receptors have sensed. ■

THE PROPER USE OF ANALGESICS

Analgesics are medications that relieve pain. Non-narcotic analgesics are used for mild to moderate pain. They act at the site of pain, do not cause dependency, and do not alter the individual's perception as narcotics might. The old standby in pain control is aspirin. A part of our medicine chests for about 100 years, this medication (also known by its tongue-twisting technical name, acetylsalicylic acid or ASA) works in part by suppressing the production of prostaglandins, hormone-like substances involved in inflammatory reactions.

But aspirin is not for everyone. For example, you should not take aspirin if you have ulcers, because it can worsen symptoms, or if you have asthma, because it may trigger an attack. Aspirin also could worsen kidney or liver disease. And, a history of taking high doses of aspirin on a regular basis could place you at risk for tinnitus, also known as "ringing in the ears."

Children should never be given aspirin if they have evidence of a viral infection, because of the possibility of Reye's syndrome—a rare, potentially fatal disorder that may cause seizures and brain damage.

Pregnant women should not use aspirin during their last trimester because of the increased risk of bleeding during childbirth.

Acetaminophen is an analgesic aspirin substitute that is thought to act directly on nerve endings to suppress pain. It is usually taken in the same adult dose as aspirin.

Acetaminophen is gentler on the stomach than aspirin and carries no risk of Reye's syndrome in children. However, if taken in excess, it can cause lethal liver damage in heavy drinkers.

Ibuprofen and naproxen sodium are extremely powerful pain relievers. Like aspirin, they also inhibit prostaglandin production. The Food and Drug Administration (FDA) approved ibuprofen as an over-the-counter pain remedy in 1984 and naproxen sodium in 1994. Although ibuprofen and naproxen sodium both are comparatively gentler on the stomach than aspirin, they should be avoided by people with ulcers or those who are allergic to aspirin. They also can impair liver function and interfere with blood clotting.

The most important reminder about over-the-counter analgesics is that they are intended as medications to be taken on a short-term basis. If you find you are taking these drugs for more than 10 days to relieve pain or more than 3 days to reduce fever, you should see your doctor. Children should not take such medication for more than 5 days.

You also should seek medical attention if your symptoms worsen or other symptoms develop.

Narcotic analgesics act on the central nervous system and alter the individual's perception. If your doctor prescribes a stronger pain medication for you, make sure that what the pharmacist gives you is what your doctor prescribed. If you are unsure of the actual name of the drug, ask you doctor to spell it for you.

Two classes of narcotics are opiates and opioids. Opiates come from naturally occurring substances, while opioids are synthetic but with similar pharmacologic properties. The prototypical opiate is morphine. In addition to relieving pain, opiates also reduce fear and anxiety. Other examples of opiates and opioids are codeine, meperidine (Demerol), and methadone. Codeine derivatives often are combined with acetaminophen or aspirin.

Narcotics are also known for their sedating effects. But their most troubling problems are tolerance and dependence. A person who takes such medications over an extended period requires higher and higher doses to obtain the same effect. However, physical dependence is rare when these drugs are used briefly and properly.

Under the Controlled Substances Act of 1970, such drugs are classified into five schedules (non-narcotics are marked with an*):

- Schedule I – have a high abuse potential and no proven medical use. Examples are heroin and lysergic acid diethylamide (LSD).*

- Schedule II – have a high potential for severe dependence but are medically useful. Examples are morphine, short-acting barbiturates,* amphetamines,* and cocaine.*

- Schedule III – have less potential for severe dependence and are medically useful. Examples are longer-acting barbiturates*, certain nonamphetamine stimulants,* and combination drugs that contain small amounts of opioids.

- Schedule IV – have a low potential for dependence and are medically useful. Examples are valium* and phenobarbital.*

- Schedule V – have limited potential for dependence and are medically useful. Examples are analgesic mixtures with small amounts of opioids and other non-narcotic ingredients, such as acetaminophen (Tylenol) with codeine.

You should also learn from your doctor how much of the drug you should take and how many times each day you should take it; any side effects you may expect; what length of time you should expect to take it; and any special information (for example, if you should take it before eating, after eating, or before bedtime).

One of the most important rules involved in taking medication is to never take someone else's prescription medication. This can lead to serious adverse reactions, medication interactions, or other forms of drug poisoning. (For more information, see Chapter 33.) ■

nervous system injury or a systemic disease like arthritis, and those without an obvious source. Some people who experience chronic pain but do not have an obvious source of their discomfort may have forgotten an injury that has healed. For reasons not well understood, nerves sometimes "remember" acute pain, transmitting the sensation even though the cause no longer exists.

In some cases, pain can spread through the body to sites far removed from the site of injury. In a condition known as reflex sympathetic dystrophy, pain usually spreads over one limb but can involve much of the body. Scientists think pain signals arriving at the spinal cord send a recruiting call out to neighboring nerve cells. These cells then respond as though they are receiving pain signals.

About 34 million people in the United States experience chronic pain. About one-third of these people suffer from back pain, and another one-third have arthritis. Various forms of cancer also cause persistent pain. Many people have developed dependencies on strong pain-killing medications and have fallen into a cycle of pain, depression, and inactivity.

When to call the doctor If you experience persistent pain for several weeks or months, seek help from your doctor. If relief is not achieved, consult a specialist at a pain clinic.

Treatment The medical management of chronic pain depends largely on the underlying problem. The first step is to identify the underlying cause of the pain and determine if it is remediable. If possible, treatment is given for the underlying cause. If not possible, non-narcotic analgesics usually relieve the pain. Antidepressant medications also alter the transmission of pain impulses to the brain. Some recurrent pain associated with facial tics responds to medications commonly used to treat seizure disorders.

Narcotics also can be used to dull or relieve chronic pain. Many doctors, however, are reluctant to prescribe these medications because of possible addiction. However, narcotic medications taken by mouth or absorbed through the skin may not be as addictive as medications injected directly into the bloodstream.

Well-motivated people may benefit from relaxation or biofeedback techniques to help manage pain more effectively. (See Chapter 11 for more information on relaxation and biofeedback techniques.)

In extreme cases, surgically interrupting the nerve pathways carrying pain messages to the spinal cord may be considered. A trigeminal ganglion section may alleviate facial pain in tic douloureux; a dorsal rhizotomy, or section of the dorsal roots, relieves limb pain, but often only for a few months,

when the roots grow back. Transcutaneous electrical nerve stimulation (TENS) may provide relief of pain. In TENS, an electronic device delivers an electric current up the spinal cord or to specific neural sites. This stimulation may fatigue the neural pathway transporting the pain messages and diminish its effectiveness, or disrupt neural traffic patterns and prevent the messages from getting through. It may also distract the sufferer from the pain and trigger other biofeedback or behavior modifications.

People who experience chronic pain but have no remediable underlying cause may be treated initially with aspirin or a nonsteroidal anti-inflammatory drug (NSAID). Certain antidepressants may help.

A number of special clinics or pain centers are successfully treating people who suffer chronic pain.

Because chronic pain intrudes on every aspect of a person's life, physical and occupational therapy may help, as could psychological or psychiatric intervention.

❖ TRIGEMINAL NEURALGIA—TIC DOULOUREUX

Symptoms (*What you may experience*) Lightning-like jabs of burning or searing pain on one side of the face, usually triggered by touch, cold wind, or trying to eat.

Signs and laboratory findings (*What the doctor looks for*) Patient history of pain; patient will point to affected area but never touch it; MRI scan to rule out tumors or signs of inflammation around the nerve.

What is it? Trigeminal neuralgia is a painful disorder of the fifth cranial (trigeminal) nerve. In some cases it is related to multiple sclerosis or a herpes zoster infection. Some cases are felt to be due to irritation of the nerve by a crooked blood vessel. Usually, however, the cause is unknown.

Trigeminal neuralgia produces pain attacks shooting through one side of the face along the length of the nerve. The pain is so sharp that it will frequently cause a facial spasm. The name tic douloureux is from the French word for painful. It can be triggered by merely touching an affected area or even by a gentle breeze. The pain lasts from seconds to minutes and can also be triggered by eating, drinking hot or cold beverages, smiling, or talking. The frequency of attacks varies from many times a day to several times a month or year.

Trigeminal neuralgia occurs mostly in people older than 40, in women more often than men, and on the right side of the face more often than the left.

In some cases the pain is accompanied by muscular spasms and a facial tic. Sometimes it is associated with an underlying disease such as multiple sclerosis, tumor, infection, or an aneurysm.

Treatment Carbamazepine, gabapentin (Neurontin), or phenytoin (Dilantin), usually prescribed to control seizures, may relieve or prevent pain; however, these drugs need to be monitored because of potential side effects. Baclofen (Lioresal) and narcotics may also be helpful.

If medication therapy fails or painful attacks increase in frequency, neurosurgical intervention can provide permanent relief. Nerve roots can be destroyed by applying heat via electricity or radio wave energy. Surgically severing the nerve also may be an option. However, destruction of the nerve can leave the face permanently numb.

Prognosis This is not a life-threatening condition. However, the agonizing pain can be distressing and disabling.

If someone with trigeminal neuralgia undergoes a procedure to destroy the nerve, he should avoid hot foods and drinks, which could burn the mouth; and he also should see a dentist regularly to detect any problems that might arise in the numbed area.

Seizure Disorders

Brain cells normally produce electrical patterns. Seizures are physical effects of unusual electrical energy bursts in the brain. The type of seizure produced by these electrical disturbances depends on where in the brain they occur and how much of the brain they affect. Chronic seizure disorders are generically referred to as epilepsy.

Seizures may be so brief and mild they are not noticeable to someone else; or they may be prolonged and involve generalized muscular convulsions and loss of consciousness.

A single seizure episode may have a host of causes. But when seizures recur, the condition is described as epilepsy. About 2.5 million Americans have some form of seizure disorder; 30 percent of these people are younger than 18. About 125,000 new cases are diagnosed each year.

In about 70 percent of cases there is no known cause. Of the remaining 30 percent, the most common causes are head trauma, brain tumor, stroke, poisoning (for example, lead poisoning or alcoholism), infection, and injury to the brain during fetal development due to maternal infection or illness during pregnancy. With exceptions, seizure disorders are not themselves inherited, although there may be a familial predisposition to seizures. However, seizures may be associated with certain genetic diseases, such as tuberous sclerosis.

About 85 percent of cases can be fully or partially controlled. The major form of treatment involves anticonvulsant medication therapy. More than one medication may be necessary, but single-medication therapy is common and is the first goal of management. When medication fails, surgery may offer hope if the affected brain area is small and its removal or destruction does not jeopardize personality or function. For children with hard-to-control seizures, the high-fat ketogenic diet has also been used at Johns Hopkins and other epilepsy centers.

TONIC-CLONIC SEIZURES—GRAND MAL

Symptoms *(What you may experience)* Loss of consciousness; whole-body spasms and muscular convulsions; tongue biting; incontinence; apnea (inability to breathe). After the seizure there may be fatigue, daze, and confusion. Headache or muscle soreness and weakness may be present.

Signs and laboratory findings *(What the doctor looks for)* A detailed description of seizure activity: how often the seizures take place, under what circumstances they occur, and how they appear. For example, does the person exhibit loss of consciousness and generalized twitching and jerking, or does the person "go blank"? Patient history of trauma and/or recent fevers; abnormal findings on neurologic examination may indicate the need for an MRI to look at brain structure and an EEG to assess brain electrical activity; other tests including serum glucose (sugar) and calcium, and sometimes lumbar puncture to look for infection in the cerebrospinal fluid.

What is it? A tonic-clonic seizure is a generalized convulsion resulting from a global electrical abnormality within the brain. In some cases a partial, or focal, seizure, which usually affects one area of the brain, becomes generalized and leads to a tonic-clonic seizure. A tonic-clonic seizure often begins with a cry, caused by air suddenly forced from the lungs as the individual loses consciousness. Tonic refers to the initial 15- to 20-second period characterized by muscle rigidity. The clonic phase then begins with an average 1- to 2-minute period of rhythmic, jerking, muscular contractions. During this time, the individual may bite his tongue repeatedly or lose control of bladder and bowels. The tonic-clonic phase is usually followed by a short period of deep sleep, from which the individual awakens with no memory of the seizure.

Tonic-clonic seizures usually occur at seemingly random moments, but may be triggered by external stimuli such as certain sounds, patterns of light, stress, missed meals, and altered sleep cycles. Menstruation also may be involved in the onset of such a seizure.

Although they can be well controlled, grand mal seizures can be extremely dangerous if they occur while you are driving. Check with your state's division of motor vehicles to find out about any license restrictions.

Because most seizures have no known or identifiable cause, they may not be prevented, only controlled. However, some seizures may result from an underlying infection or other reversible disorder—in which case treating the underlying cause can make the seizures disappear.

What you can do Taking prescribed medication regularly, getting adequate rest, and avoiding excess alcohol can help keep a seizure disorder under control. Also, wearing a medical bracelet advising of the condition, whom to contact, and medications to be used in treatment is important.

Family members should know how to administer aid to someone in the throes of a grand mal seizure. Do not restrain the individual, and loosen any tight clothing. Place something flat and soft under the person's head. If the mouth is open place a soft object between the teeth to protect the tongue. Turn the head to allow breathing and permit saliva to drain. When the seizure passes, assure the person he is all right, orient him to time and place, and inform him of what has occurred.

When to call the doctor If this is the first seizure experience; if the seizure is prolonged; or if another seizure begins soon after the first, consult your doctor.

Treatment Anticonvulsant medication therapy can control seizures in many people. Traditional medications include carbamazepine, phenytoin, valproate, or phenobarbital. Some people may do well on one medication, while others may need to take more than one. Anticonvulsant medication therapy needs regular medical supervision. The medication may have undesirable side effects, so patients must be monitored for such symptoms as lethargy, dizziness, drowsiness, slurred speech, irritability, nausea, vomiting, loss or lack of muscular coordination, or involuntary eye movements. A woman of childbearing age should discuss the possibility of pregnancy with her doctor, who may recommend a change in medication. Some anticonvulsants have a higher risk of birth defects than others and may also impair the effect of birth control pills.

Sometimes medication may not be enough to control seizures. In such cases, the area of the brain responsible for the seizures can be located and removed surgically. Seizures caused by brain tumors or hemorrhages may cease after surgical treatment.

Prognosis Short, infrequent seizures have little, if any, effect on brain function. However, cognition may be affected by prolonged, severe, frequent seizures or seizures associated with oxygen deprivation or head injury.

About half of all cases of grand mal seizures can be controlled completely by medication therapy. In another 35 percent, medications will significantly reduce seizure frequency. Medications allow most people with grand mal seizures to lead normal lives. Children can engage in organized sports activities with minimal restrictions emphasizing safety and supervision. Adults with active seizures work in many professions but should avoid careers where they may place themselves or others in danger.

Seizure disorder is a chronic condition that often accompanies a person throughout life. In some cases, the need for medication may be reduced or even eliminated over time.

ABSENCE SEIZURES— PETIT MAL

Symptoms *(What you may experience)* Brief 10- to 30-second loss of consciousness with eye or muscle fluttering.

Signs and laboratory findings *(What the doctor looks for)* Blanking out episodes reported by family; neurologic examination is often unremarkable between episodes; abnormal brain wave activity as demonstrated by EEG; abnormal brain images shown on CT scan or MRI.

What is it? Absence seizures are short periods of "blanking out." The seizures generally begin and end abruptly and last only a few seconds, but they may occur dozens or even hundreds of times daily. Such seizures often happen so quickly that the person having them, as well as people nearby, may not notice anything unusual.

Absence seizures are most common in children over age 2 years, and rarely begin after the age of 20. Parents and teachers may think a child having these seizures is daydreaming or just being inattentive. During the brief lapse of consciousness, the person stares straight ahead. Sometimes the stare is accompanied by rhythmic twitching of muscles around the eye. When the attack is over, the person picks up right where he left off.

Some children, though, have atypical petit mal seizures, marked by more intense muscle involvement similar to grand mal seizures and a longer recovery time. Unlike typical seizures, for which a cause is rarely found, atypical absence seizure may be associated with some other neurologic condition, such as congenital defect in brain anatomy or a metabolic problem that, for example, results from liver illness.

What you can do Make sure your child takes prescribed medication, gets adequate rest, and wears a medical bracelet with treatment instructions. An adult with this condition should also avoid excess alcohol.

When to call the doctor If your child seems to "lose touch" several times a day, or if his ability to learn appears to be decreasing, consult a doctor.

Treatment Petit mal seizures may be treated with valproate (Depakene), ethosuximide (Zarontin), or clonazepam (Klonopin). Because any medication may have undesirable side effects, it is important to carefully observe the child to watch for symptoms such as lethargy, dizziness, drowsiness, slurred speech, irritability, nausea, vomiting, loss or lack of muscular coordination, or involuntary eye movements.

Prognosis Medication therapy will control or greatly reduce petit mal attacks in about 75 percent of people. About 30 percent of children with petit mal seizures will outgrow the condition and cease having seizures in adulthood. Children with these seizures should be encouraged to participate in normal, everyday activities as much as possible. Consult with your doctor to see what restrictions should be observed.

❖ PARTIAL SEIZURES

There are two main types of partial seizures. Temporal lobe (or complex partial) seizures are produced in the temporal lobe region of the brain (this is on each side of the head between the temple and a point just behind the ear); and Jacksonian (or simple partial) seizures, named for John Hughlings Jackson, who first described them.

Symptoms *(What you may experience)* An "aura," or sensory warning that precedes the seizure; stiffening or jerking in a portion of a limb; a glassy stare; picking at one's clothes; aimless wandering; lip-smacking or chewing motions; unintelligible speech.

Signs and laboratory findings *(What the doctor looks for)* Reports from family and observers about described behavior. Neurologic examination is often unremarkable between episodes. Brainwave analysis by EEG; brain images via MRI or CT.

What is it? People with temporal lobe seizures often have a sensory warning called an aura that precedes their attacks by seconds or minutes. They may hallucinate, have a sense of fear for no apparent reason, smell something unpleasant, or have a distorted perception of what is happening around them. The seizures generally last about 2 minutes, and the person will briefly lose touch with reality and make automatic movements, such as hand fidgeting chewing, repetitive swallowing, and aimless wandering. They will not remember what happened during the seizure. Mental confusion may persist for a few minutes after the seizure. The seizure may be mistaken for psychosis, or drug or alcohol intoxication.

Someone with a Jacksonian seizure remains conscious and aware but loses control of some body motion. It generally begins with a tingling sensation and jerking or trembling motion of an arm or leg. Sometimes the movements start in a finger and slowly march upward until the hand and whole arm are shaking.

A lesion or tumor in the temporal lobe of the brain may cause these seizures. Destroying or removing these potential causes may prevent future seizures. But in many cases, the cause of the seizures is unknown.

What you can do Wear a medical bracelet advising of the condition, whom to contact, and medications to be used in treatment. Compliance with medication is very important; stopping medication abruptly can cause seizures.

Treatment If the source of the seizures is identified—a tumor, scar tissue, or lesion in the brain—it may be destroyed or removed surgically, resulting in significant reduction of seizures in most cases. Long-term medication therapy can control attacks in 35 percent of people and reduce the frequency of seizures in 50 percent; however, complex partial seizures are less responsive to medical treatment than other types of seizures. The medication frequently produces side effects and must be closely managed and supervised.

Prognosis About 85 percent of people with complex or partial seizures can expect some relief from management with medication. However, epilepsy is a chronic and often life-long condition.

❖ FEBRILE SEIZURES

Symptoms *(What your child may experience)* Febrile seizures are associated with onset of fever-producing illness; symptoms may include muscle rigidity, sometimes followed by generalized convulsions lasting less than 15 minutes and brief loss of consciousness. Seizure is usually followed by a long period of sleep. The seizures often occur when the temperature is rising rapidly but may also take place as the temperature is going down.

Signs and laboratory findings *(What the doctor looks for)* The history and neurologic exam may indicate a lumbar puncture to rule out brain infection; simple febrile seizures may not require further examination. Complex febrile seizures may require EEG and CT.

What is it? Fever-induced seizures are the most common type of seizure encountered in infants and young children. Three out of every 100 children experience febrile seizures, primarily between the ages of 3 months and 5 years. Although the initial seizure, and even subsequent seizures, can be extremely frightening to parents of a young child, febrile seizures are rarely harmful. "Simple" febrile seizures are brief (often lasting less than a minute) and solitary. "Complicated" febrile seizures last longer than 15 minutes and recur two or more times over 24 hours. A child who experiences simple febrile seizures has a slightly increased chance of subsequent seizures not associated with fever. Those who experience complicated febrile seizures have an even greater risk. A family history of seizure is apparent in about 25 percent of cases.

About 2 to 4 percent of children who develop these seizures will go on to experience seizures without accompanying fever.

What you can do When a seizure occurs, place the child on a flat surface and turn the head to one side so saliva flows out. Do not put anything in the child's mouth. Remove nearby objects that could harm the child.

Reduce and control the fever with acetaminophen or ibuprofen and tepid sponge baths. For more information, see page 208.

Children prone to febrile seizures should always be properly supervised in situations where a sudden seizure poses great risk, such as in the bath.

When to call the doctor If your child has a convulsion, seek medical help right away whether or not a fever is present.

Treatment Learning to react properly and calmly to a child in the throes of a seizure, and using acetaminophen or ibuprofen to control fever may be the only intervention necessary.

Anticonvulsant medications can reduce the chances of seizure occurrence and can be given at the start of a fever to children with severe or frequent febrile seizures. Approach prophylactic use of antiseizure medication with caution, however, because these medication can affect the child's learning ability.

Prognosis Febrile seizures are usually a common but benign occurrence during childhood. A child who has experienced at least two episodes of febrile seizure may be placed on anticonvulsant therapy. If the child remains seizure-free for a few years, he may be gradually weaned off the medication. Most children outgrow febrile seizures.

Movement Disorders

Our movements are under control of the central nervous system (CNS). Nervous impulses flow from the brain and spinal cord to receptors on voluntary muscles. These innervate the muscles and make them contract, forming movement.

But sometimes this control breaks down. The impulses travel and muscles contract, but the end result is muscle movement that appears random, uncoordinated, and without conscious control.

This can be distressing, because a number of these disorders have no cure. But as scientific research progresses and our understanding of illness proceeds, there is hope of increasingly more effective treatments.

❖ TOURETTE'S SYNDROME

Symptoms *(What you may experience)* Facial tics; other muscular tics involving the head and shoulders; vocal tics (grunts, barks, hisses); coprolalia (uttering "dirty" words and phrases); echolalia (repeating what someone else said); palilalia (repeating words and phrases); obsessive-compulsive behavior.

Signs and laboratory findings *(What the doctor looks for)* Existence of muscle/vocal tics for at least 1 year; tics that occur many times each day; tics that began prior to age 18; careful neurologic exam; blood tests to rule out Wilson's disease (due to excess copper); and psychiatric exam to rule out schizophrenia.

What is it? Tourette's syndrome (also known as Gilles de la Tourette syndrome) is a motor behavioral disorder caused by a probable genetic disturbance affecting the central nervous system. It is one of a number of tic disorders characterized by twitchy muscular movements and involuntary utterances. It occurs more often in boys (generally beginning around the age of 7 or 8). Tics often occur in "bouts," with many tics over a brief period. Concentration may enable a person to inhibit the tics; for example, a surgeon who has Tourette's syndrome may exhibit no tics at all while performing an operation. Later, however, the tics may erupt violently.

Motor tics are rapid, involuntary, and sometimes, quite complex movements. Facial tics signal the onset of Tourette's syndrome in about 80 percent of individuals with the disorder. Vocal tics—grunts, barks, and hisses, for example—show up initially in the remaining 20 percent. Other muscle tics often include the face, head, and shoulders—sniffing, blinking, frowning, and shrugging. When Tourette's syndrome occurs in girls, behavioral problems such as obsessive-compulsive behavior are more common than facial or vocal tics. The severity of symptoms may wax and wane over weeks and months. In many cases, tics diminish with age. In others, they become more severe in adulthood.

In some cases, tics may involve such behavior as hair-pulling. Diagnosis of tics may be delayed, because they may be interpreted as a sign of psychiatric illness or some other movement disorder. This subjects patients to unnecessary treatments before Tourette's syndrome is recognized.

What you can do Avoid fatigue and stress, which can bring on or intensify symptoms. Emotional support from friends and family can lessen feelings of societal isolation. Psychotherapy may help resolve anxiety and conflicts created by the disease.

Treatment Therapy consists of medication to reduce the frequency and severity of tics. The medication of choice is generally haloperidol (Haldol), but fluphenazine (Permitil or Prolixin) or pimozide (Orap) may be better tolerated in some cases. Other medications that may be helpful include clonidine (Catapres) and fluoxetine (Prozac).

Prognosis Many people with Tourette's syndrome adjust well, although they may have emotional pain. Social adaptation depends greatly on family acceptance and support, and on the individual's personal strength of character.

❖ TRANSIENT FACIAL TICS AND SIMPLE MOTOR TICS

Symptoms and Signs *(What you may experience)* Involuntary muscular movements that typically involve the areas around the mouth or one eye; head twitching; shrugging of the shoulders.

What is it? These are involuntary, repetitive movements, usually involving the muscles of the upper body and head. They generally become apparent during childhood. Indeed, 25 percent of all children experience transient tics. They often disappear as the person gets older. They may be induced by head injury, or by certain drugs, such as nervous system stimulants.

In addition to simple motor tics that include eye blinking, neck jerking, shoulder shrugging, and facial grimacing, children also may have complex motor tics. Examples of these include self-hitting or self-biting, jumping and hopping, and twirling when walking.

Tics may also be vocal. Simple vocal tics include coughing, hissing, and barking. Complex motor tics may involve repeating words out of context, echoing what someone said, or using socially unacceptable words.

All tic disorders are more common in boys than girls. Some children outgrow tics. Chronic, multiple tics, such as those in Tourette's syndrome, are distinguished from other tics that are a temporary, developmental glitch that do not require treatment.

Treatment Mild tics require no treatment unless other difficulties develop. In more severe cases, emotional support is important for children who feel "different." Counseling may be helpful.

Prognosis In most cases, prognosis is excellent.

❖ BENIGN ESSENTIAL TREMOR

Symptoms *(What you may experience)* Uncontrollable shaking of one or both hands and/or the head; sometimes, quavering speech.

Signs and laboratory findings *(What the doctor looks for)* Uncontrollable shaking that worsens when maintaining a posture; family history of tremor; medical history that includes medications that cause tremor (stimulants, lithium, valproate).

What is it? Tremor, or uncontrollable shaking, is common in some neurologic diseases, such as Parkinson's and stroke. However, many people have benign essential tremor. This occurs when shaking is the only symptom of the disorder. Unlike Parkinson's shaking, which eases during movement, essential tremor usually intensifies when maintaining a posture (for example when holding a cup).

Essential tremor is most prominent when the hands are in use. It may involve other parts of the body, but the hands and head are most often affected. Shaking often begins in the dominant hand (the one used for writing, for example) and may spread to both hands, which affects the ability to eat, as well. Some people also develop quavering speech.

Stress or caffeine may exacerbate the tremor.

Benign essential tremor affects about 3 to 4 million people in the United States. Men and women are affected equally. It most commonly begins in midlife, but many cases begin in early adolescence; some begin in infancy, early adulthood, or when the person is a senior. In more than half of cases, the disease is inherited. Children of an affected person will have a 50 percent chance of developing it.

The cause of the disease is unknown in cases that are not hereditary.

Treatment The beta blocker medication propranolol may be helpful. The antiseizure drug primidone also may be helpful. Many people discover that small amounts of alcohol may temporarily relieve tremor, but heavy drinking should be avoided.

Prognosis Essential tremor is slowly progressive, and shaking often worsens over time. The condition itself is benign, but in some cases the tremor interferes with many daily activities, such as writing, speaking, and eating, and can be socially debilitating.

❖ PARKINSON'S DISEASE

Symptoms (What you may experience) Tremor; stiff muscles or cramping; falling, unstable gait; change in handwriting; drooling; reduced ability to chew, eat, and swallow; depression; fatigue or general malaise.

Signs and laboratory findings (What the doctor looks for) Rigidity, tremor, absence of spasticity; "cogwheel rigidity" (when the arm is pulled straight it seems to jerk as if controlled by a ratchet in a cogwheel); reduced blinking; a mask-like, expressionless face; a shuffling walk and walking with the body bent forward.

What is it? First described by James Parkinson in 1817, the disease that now bears his name is a chronic, progressive "shaking palsy" that usually begins when a person is between 50 and 65 years old. As symptoms become more pronounced over time, people may have trouble walking, talking, or completing other simple tasks that involve smooth movements. Symptoms may involve only one side of the body or both sides. Tension or fatigue can intensify muscle tremors.

People with severe symptoms may have a fixed facial expression, unblinking eyes, and a slightly open mouth with saliva dribbling at the corners. Other symptoms include stooped posture and rigid trunk and limbs. Some people "freeze" while moving.

Parkinson's disease is not contagious, nor is it usually inherited.

Early symptoms may be ignored. Initial symptoms may be a stiff sensation in an arm or leg, dragging one foot slightly when walking, or mild shaking in the fingers of one hand.

Parkinson's disease is caused by the gradual deterioration of nerves in a region of the brain called the substantia nigra. This region controls movement, especially the somewhat automatic movements such as arm swinging while walking. When nerve cells in this area die or become impaired, production of a brain chemical called dopamine, which aids in transmitting signals, decreases resulting in impaired movement.

Although Parkinson's disease is due to degeneration limited to the substantia nigra, other degenerative diseases can produce "secondary Parkinsonism" with similar symptoms. A detailed examination is required to tell the difference; in early stages it may be impossible to tell.

In later stages of the disease, there may be some intellectual deterioration and memory loss.

Depression often accompanies the disease. People in late stages of Parkinson's may have visual and auditory hallucinations, which may be triggered by medications to control other symptoms.

Parkinson's disease strikes about one in every 100 people over the age of 60. About 50,000 to 60,000 new cases are diagnosed in the United States each year.

What you can do Currently, Parkinson's disease cannot be prevented, although research is making progress in identifying preventative agents. There are things you can do, however, to ease movement in and around the house. Practical changes include bath rail supports, an elevated toilet seat, banisters along walls, and chairs with high arms to facilitate rising. Regular exercise also can give a physical and psychological boost.

Because a slowly progressing disability can give rise to depression, psychological counseling may be of value. Support groups offer encouragement and emotional support.

When to call the doctor Many people develop a mild tremor after age 50 or 55 and do not have Parkinson's. There are many other possible causes of tremor. However, you should consult your doctor if the tremor worsens or if you have unexplained walking difficulty or falling, or if you develop other symptoms.

Treatment The primary aim of treatment is to relieve symptoms and keep the individual functional for as long as possible. Medication, physical therapy, and, in some cases, surgery can help. The disease's early symptoms may require no treatment at all.

The antiviral medication amantadine (Symmetrel) may help reduce symptoms of

Parkinson's disease, but its effectiveness wears off after several months in about one-half to one-third of individuals taking it.

Dopamine cannot be absorbed directly into the brain from the bloodstream, so a compound called levodopa (Dopar, Larodopa) is given to help the brain boost its own production of dopamine. Levodopa is often given in tandem with another medication called carbidopa (Lodosyn, Sinemet, Sinemet CR) which keeps levodopa from being destroyed before it reaches the brain. Although beneficial for thousands of people, levodopa has some side effects. The most common ones are nausea, vomiting, low blood pressure, involuntary movements, and restlessness. But combining the medication with carbidopa enables a lower dose of levodopa to be given and thus reduces some of the side effects.

Bromocriptine (Parlodel) and pergolide (Permax) are medications that stimulate the action of dopamine. Anticholinergic drugs such as trihexyphenidyl, which counter the relative excess of acetylcholine, also may be prescribed.

Young, otherwise healthy persons with one-sided muscle tremor or rigidity may benefit from a surgical procedure in which a portion of the thalamus is destroyed to prevent involuntary movement.

Electrodes similar in function to a heart pacemaker can be placed in the brain to achieve some degree of control over the involuntary muscle movements.

Some researchers have claimed some success in transplanting fetal brain tissue into the brains of people with Parkinson's disease. However, questions about the efficacy of the surgery and, to some extent, ethical concerns raised by this type of tissue transplant have kept it from being widely practiced. Genetically engineered cells producing dopamine may make tissue implantation more acceptable.

Prognosis Because Parkinson's disease does not affect nerves connected with vital organs such as the heart, it is not directly life-threatening, but is eventually disabling. It can be present in a mild form for 20 or 30 years. Independence should be encouraged as much as possible in people with the disease. Usually after 10 to 15 years, people with Parkinson's will need assistance with routines of daily living.

❖ HUNTINGTON'S DISEASE OR CHOREA

Symptoms *(What you may experience)* In progressive chorea, the individual's movements become more and more rapid, seemingly violent, and purposeless. Dementia; personality changes.

Signs and laboratory findings *(What the doctor looks for)* Chorea (a pattern of irregular, uncontrolled movements) and muscular deterioration or compromised intellectual function as shown by physical exam. Genetic defect as shown by DNA analysis; family history of the disease; CT and MRI to show brain atrophy in specific areas characteristic of Huntington's disease.

What is it? Huntington's disease is a hereditary disease marked by degeneration of the basal ganglia in the cerebral cortex. It was described by an American doctor, George Huntington, and called Huntington's chorea, from the Greek word for dance, because of the jerky, almost dance-like motions of the individuals stricken with it. Individuals develop progressive mental deterioration, ending in dementia, along with loss of the ability to control major muscle movements.

If either parent has the disease, there is a 50 percent chance a child will inherit it. Symptoms usually do not become apparent until the age of about 35; however, there have been instances in which symptoms have developed in children or in persons as old as 60. Because of this it is possible to transmit the gene to children before you know you have the disease.

Huntington's disease is relatively uncommon, with an incidence of about 10 to 20 per 100,000 people.

Onset of the disease is slow and subtle. Initially abnormal motions occur on one side of the body and are more likely to involve the face and arms. Facial movements resemble mild grimacing, and speech is fidgety and indistinct. Symptoms may be more severe with emotional upset.

When to call the doctor If you have a family history of Huntington's disease, you may want to consider genetic testing before having children.

Treatment Because there is no cure, treatment involves lessening the severity of symptoms. Tranquilizers and other medications such as benzodiazepines and neuroleptics can help control muscular movements.

Prognosis After the onset of symptoms, people with Huntington's disease will need assistance performing daily functions for an average of 10 to 15 years, after which death usually occurs. This is often from suicide—or, once the person is bedridden, from congestive heart failure or pneumonia.

Demyelinating Disorders

Electrical impulses race along nerves at high speeds. In fact, these transmissions travel at such high velocities that we can jerk a finger away from a hot stove before we even feel the burning pain. Sometimes, however, something interrupts the flow of nerve transmissions. This can have an adverse effect on muscle strength and movement as well as the ability to perceive sensory information.

Nerves consist of a central body, short extensions of the cell body called dendrites, and an elongated extension called the axon. The axon is especially important in transmitting nerve impulses from the cell body to other neurons.

A membranous covering, called the myelin sheath, insulates the axon. In healthy nerves, this keeps the impulse from short-circuiting. But if this covering or even the nerves themselves deteriorate, the electrical impulses cannot continue to their destinations. Muscles cannot contract to their full ability and movements become weak and uncoordinated.

❖ MULTIPLE SCLEROSIS

Symptoms *(What you may experience)* Partial loss of vision; blurred vision; pain in one eye; numbness and tingling sensations in the arms and legs; muscle weakness and spasms; problems with urinary incontinence or urgency; mood swings; problems with speech or swallowing; fatigue with little exertion.

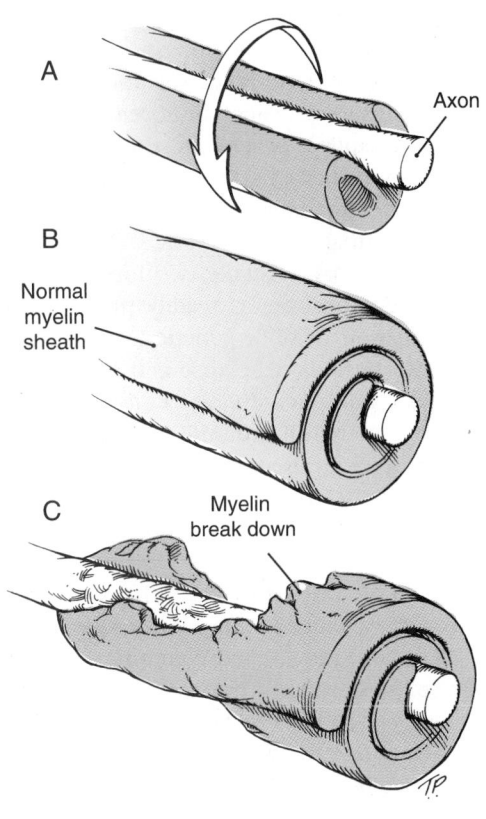

A
Axon

B
Normal myelin sheath

C
Myelin break down

(A) In a normal neuron, myelin insulates the axon and helps to ensure proper conduction of electrical signals down the axon. (B) In some neurologic diseases, such as multiple sclerosis, myelin breaks down, causing abnormal signal conduction. This can lead to problems with strength, sensation, and coordination.

Signs and laboratory findings *(What the doctor looks for)* Physical examination and observation of the patient shows altered reflexes; history of multiple occurrences of symptoms located at multiple sites within the central nervous system; characteristic lesions of the brain and upper portion of the spinal cord revealed by MRI; immunoglobulin G in spinal fluid as revealed by lumbar puncture; electrical tests called evoked potentials show slowing of nerve conduction from past demyelination (sometimes).

What is it? Multiple sclerosis (MS), which affects about 200,000 people in the United States, is a chronic disease of the central nervous system. In multiple sclerosis, the myelin sheath that covers and insulates the axons of nerve cells breaks down. This causes numerous electrical short circuits and interrupts the free flow of nerve impulses. Because this happens at multiple sites within the brain and nervous system, the symptoms vary from person to person and are extremely diverse.

The disease usually begins to appear between the ages of 20 and 40 and may be so mild as to go almost unnoticed. In most people, months or years may separate the initial episode from the appearance of new symptoms or recurrence of the original signs. Thus, diagnosing the disease is difficult and requires periodic testing and close observation, perhaps for years. Frequency of episodes may reach a peak 3 to 4 years after the initial attack.

The disease can take two forms. Some people demonstrate a steadily progressing deterioration of body function, while others have periods of relapse and remission. Relapses and incomplete remissions can lead to increasing disability. Stress and increased body temperature may worsen symptoms. Relapses also are more common 2 to 3 months following the end of pregnancy.

Multiple sclerosis affects three women for every two men and five whites for every black. It also may be more common in persons of western European descent who live in temperate climates. There appears to be an association between multiple sclerosis and specific biochemical markers called human leukocyte antigens, which provides support for a theory of inherited susceptibility. However, the risk of developing the disease is only mildly increased if a relative is affected. The current theory is that multiple sclerosis results from an immune-related injury to the myelin sheath.

What you can do Actions can be taken to make the person more comfortable. These include massages and relaxing baths and active, resistive, and stretching exercises to maintain muscle tone and joint mobility, improve coordination, and give a psychological boost.

People with multiple sclerosis should avoid stress and exposure to infections. They should also avoid heat (hot tubs or unairconditioned rooms in summer months). Constipation is often a problem in people with advanced multiple sclerosis because they are sedentary and may loose control of bowel function. Eating a nutritious diet rich in roughage can help prevent constipation.

Treatment The aim of treatment is to relieve and decrease the severity of symptoms, allowing the individual to resume his lifestyle. The severity of attacks may be lessened by ACTH (adrenocorticotrophic hormone), prednisone, or dexamethasone. Sometimes high doses of intravenous steroids

are used for severe attacks. Baclofen, dantrolene (Dantrium), or a new medication, tizanidine (Zanaflex) may decrease spasticity, and bethanechol (Urecholine, Duvoid, Myotonachol) or oxybutynin (Ditropan) may relieve urinary problems.

Beta interferon has helped some people who experience relapsing symptoms. Although generally well tolerated, it is associated with several side effects, including pain and inflammation at the site of injection, flu-like symptoms, and changes in liver function.

There have recently been major advances. Whereas symptomatic treatment had been the only relief available, there is increasing evidence that alteration of immune response will slow progression of multiple sclerosis.

Prognosis The course of MS is highly variable. However, as many as 70 percent of people with MS lead active, productive lives with prolonged remissions. Most affected people remain able to walk, and life expectancy after the first episode may be 40 years. Less frequently, the disease progresses rapidly, disabling the person or causing death within months of onset.

Spinocerebellar Degeneration Disorders

Spinocerebellar degeneration disorder is a family of mainly hereditary disorders characterized by ataxia—that is, poor muscle coordination, especially when attempting a voluntary movement. Three major groups of ataxia are spinal ataxias, cerebellar ataxias, and multiple system atrophy (wasting away). Each results from degeneration of a specific area of the brain. Symptoms can appear at varying ages.

❖ CEREBELLAR DEGENERATION

Symptoms (*What you may experience*) Loss of balance and coordination; weakness in arms and legs; slurred speech; staring. Dementia may appear in some cases.

Signs and laboratory findings (*What the doctor looks for*) Tremor; staring or loss of peripheral vision; change in color or pigment of retina; slurred speech; unstable gait; muscle weakness or loss of control.

What is it? Cerebellar degeneration is a broad category of ataxias that occur during teen years or through middle adult life. It worsens progressively, and there is no known treatment. It is usually inherited.

Treatment There is no specific treatment for this disorder. Doctors may try different medications to treat the symptoms. Physical therapy may be helpful.

Prognosis Cerebellar degeneration is slowly progressive. Death usually occurs about 20 years after onset.

❖ FRIEDREICH'S ATAXIA

Symptoms *(What you may experience)* Unsteadiness while standing; shaking in hands or feet; speech problems; difficulty walking; occasional curvature of the spine.

Signs and laboratory findings *(What the doctor looks for)* Loss of reflex and sensory responses; slowing of conduction shown by electromyogram; examination of the tissues with nerve and muscle biopsies; heart block revealed by electrocardiogram; diabetes and B_{12} deficiency as ruled out by blood and urine tests.

What is it? Friedreich's ataxia (FA), named for the German doctor who first identified it in the 1860s, is a spinal ataxia disorder that generally emerges during childhood or early adult life, usually between the ages of 5 and 15. It is a slowly progressive illness resulting in the inability to coordinate voluntary muscle movements. It is caused by degeneration of nerve tissue in the spinal cord and of nerves extending to the arms and legs. In addition to loss of voluntary muscle movement, there may also be loss of sensations of touch and pressure in the limbs. Friedreich's ataxia weakens the heart muscle (see Cardiomyopathies, page 824), preventing the heart from pumping effectively. Friedreich's ataxia may be accompanied by cardiomyopathy and, rarely, heart failure and diabetes.

Friedreich's ataxia is caused by a genetic defect on the long arm of chromosome 9. It does not affect intelligence. It is caused by a recessive trait; the disease appears only when a defective gene is transmitted from both parents. A child who receives the defective gene from one parent and a normal gene from the other will become a "carrier" and never develop the disease. When both parents are carriers, the child's chance of inheriting the defective gene from both is 25 percent.

When to call the doctor If there is a history of the disease in both families, seek genetic counseling. Genetic testing for the FA gene in utero is available.

Treatment There is no known cure, but many of accompanying symptoms can be treated. Orthopedic appliances or surgery can correct spinal deformities and help improve ability to walk. Assistive devices and occupational therapy will help maintain physical activity. Attendant heart problems and diabetes can be treated with medication.

Prognosis The disease is invariably fatal; most patients succumb to respiratory failure in their middle 30's.

Dementia

Dementia is a general term for a number of diseases characterized by nerve cell deterioration. This degeneration can come about from some as-yet-unknown cause, as in Alzheimer's disease, or from an encounter with an infectious agent, as in Creutzfeldt-Jakob disease, or by poor blood flow to the brain.

Dementia is defined as a loss in at least two areas of complex behavior, such as language, memory, visual and spatial abilities, and judgment, that significantly interferes with a person's daily activities.

It is usually a slow process, taking months or years. Symptoms of various diseases differ widely in individuals, depending on what area or areas of the brain are involved.

Dementia affects more than 4 million Americans. Alzheimer's disease accounts for about half of all diagnoses of dementia. Other causes are Creutzfeldt-Jakob disease; vascular causes, such as stroke or heart disease; metabolic diseases, such as thyroid or liver diseases; infectious diseases, such as acquired immunodeficiency syndrome (AIDS); head trauma; toxins such as alcohol; and brain tumors.

Although dementia affects multiple areas of mental performance, initial symptoms may occur in only one area. For example, you may notice that remembering things like today's date is becoming more difficult. Although all dementia-disordered people forget, being forgetful is not necessarily a sign of dementia. A slight decrease in short-term memory often occurs with aging (see Common Myths of Aging, page 330), and occasional forgetfulness should not be confused with the severe decline in memory that characterizes dementia. Dementia is failure to retain mental capabilities once enjoyed, such as abstract thinking, judgment, or cognitive orientation. Many people with advanced dementia are not aware of or will not admit to a problem.

In many instances, dementia cannot be prevented. For example, only some of the factors involved in Alzheimer's disease are now known. But, because some dementia can be related to preventable diseases, keeping those illnesses at bay can keep dementia from developing. For example, exercising regularly, not smoking, and keeping an eye on blood cholesterol level can reduce the risk for stroke (see Stroke, page 429); abstaining from alcohol or drinking only moderately may help decrease the risk of liver disease which can cause dementia.

Therapy generally involves managing various symptoms. Tranquilizers can lessen agitation, anxiety, and aggression. Keeping a familiar routine, encouraging social and physical activity, and maintaining a safe environment can enable the person to maintain comfort and dignity. A person with dementia should wear a medical identification bracelet in the event of wandering or disorientation. In cases where the underlying cause of dementia is untreatable, it may eventually be necessary to place the person in a health facility providing care on a 24-hour basis.

People have a good chance of recovering mental functioning if a treatable cause of their dementia is discovered, such as metabolic disorder, brain tumor, or cerebrovascular disease. But most people with dementia will experience gradually deteriorating mental function.

❖ ALZHEIMER'S DISEASE

Symptoms *(What you may experience)* Forgetfulness; memory loss; difficulty learning and remembering new information; inability to concentrate; personality changes; language difficulties; disorientation; susceptibility to infection and accidents. Symptoms are progressive.

Signs and laboratory findings *(What the doctor looks for)* Alzheimer's disease is diagnosed through a clinical assessment, patient history, and a neurologic exam. Definitive diagnosis is possible only upon autopsy. However, doctors rule out other possible causes using tests, which include: detailed medical history; CT or MRI to rule out any structural abnormality, such as a tumor; blood chemistry rules out liver or kidney disease or other metabolic disorders that cause cognitive impairment; EEG to examine patterns of brain wave activity (sometimes). Doctors should also rule out the possibility that medications are causing the "dementia" in seniors.

What is it? First described in the early 1900s by the German neurologist Alois Alzheimer, the disease that now bears his name is a progressive, degenerative brain disease that results in impaired memory, thinking, and behavior. Alzheimer's disease affects about 4 million people in the United States. Primarily a disease of seniors, the prevalence of Alzheimer's disease increases with age. About 3 percent of men and women between the ages of 65 to 74 have it, and nearly 20 percent of those 85 and older may be affected by it.

Alzheimer's disease is the most common cause of dementia in older people, accounting for about half of all cases. Dementia is the medical term for a condition that disrupts the normal working processes of the brain (see Dementia, page 455). Alzheimer's disease affects parts of the brain that control thought, memory, and language. But it is important to note this disease is not a normal consequence of aging.

The cause of Alzheimer's disease remains a mystery. However, researchers are exploring several factors to determine whether they play a role in the development of this disease.

A hallmark of the disease is the visualization of specific microscopic features in the brain. These are plaques, which are abnormal deposits of proteins, and neurofibrillary tangles, which are abnormally twisted fibers inside nerve cells. Although plaques and tangles are seen in the brains of normal people, they are found in significantly greater concentrations in the brains of people with Alzheimer's disease. These plaques can only be uncovered in autopsy, however, so Alzheimer's is usually diagnosed by eliminating other possible causes of dementia.

The illness proceeds through three distinct stages. In the first stage, diagnosis is difficult because symptoms are subtle and the individual may still have the ability to cover mistakes. (There is some evidence that Alzheimer's may be so slowly progressive that it begins decades before diagnosis.) In the second—or moderate—stage, impairment becomes more obvious. Finally in the third—or severe—stage, the person is unable to care for himself and may become bedridden. The rate at which symptoms progress varies among individuals. Depending on the stage of the illness at diagnosis, the lifespan of a person with Alzheimer's can be as short as 4 years or as long as 20.

What you can do Alzheimer's is not an acute condition; in the early stages, care can be provided at home under a doctor's supervision. When possible, maintain familiar daily routines and encourage physical and social activity. It is important that the environment be safe, and bathing or showering be supervised to avoid accidents. It is advisable that a person with Alzheimer's wear a medical identification bracelet, in case he wanders off on his own.

Alzheimer's disease does not affect just one person; the whole family has to adjust to the situation. Open communication between family members can be invaluable in providing emotional support to all concerned. Support groups and community services can be invaluable sources of advice and assistance.

Treatment There is no available therapy to stop or reverse the mental deterioration of Alzheimer's disease. A calm and well-structured environment can allow the person with Alzheimer's to live in comfort and dignity. In later stages, 'round-the-clock care or institutionalization may become necessary.

APOLIPOPROTEIN E AS A RISK FACTOR FOR ALZHEIMER'S DISEASE

To fully explain the role of apolipoprotein E (apo E) as a risk factor for Alzheimer's disease, we need to talk a little bit about cholesterol.

Cholesterol is a waxy, fatty material that is involved in the disease process called atherosclerosis. In this process, cholesterol and other fatty materials are deposited in the artery walls, narrowing them and laying the groundwork for a heart attack or stroke.

Cholesterol and other fats cannot dissolve in blood and must be transported by special carriers called lipoproteins. Two of the better known are high-density lipoprotein (HDL), known as the "good" cholesterol because it is thought to be protective against heart attacks, and low-density lipoprotein (LDL), known as the "bad" cholesterol because it is the one that deposits cholesterol in artery walls.

Another kind of lipoprotein is very-low-density lipoprotein (VLDL), which is the largest kind of lipoprotein. One of the protein constituents of VLDL is apolipoprotein E.

Apo E plays an important role in helping the body metabolize these blood fats. The gene that directs production of apo E is called a polymorphic gene—that is, it can call for the production of three apo E proteins that are just slightly different from each other. These proteins are designated as apo E2, apo E3, and apo E4. Because of the way we inherit genes—one from each parent—our apo E genes can be E2/E2, E2/E3, E2/E4, E3/E3, E4/E4, and so on.

The brains of people with Alzheimer's disease are characterized by the abnormal deposition of another protein called beta-amyloid. These accumulate as senile plaques. Scientists have shown that beta-amyloid is brought into the brain by apo E. However, the speed with which someone develops Alzheimer's disease depends upon which of the apo E gene variants he inherits.

The apo E4 variant is the one that appears to be most involved in the development of Alzheimer's disease. It is more adept than the other variants at pulling bits of amyloid from the bloodstream and depositing them in brain cells. However, this is what doctors call a *susceptibility* characteristic. For example, having a high blood cholesterol level increases the risk of having a heart attack, but it does not mean that you certainly will get one. Inheriting an apo E4 variant from each parent increases the likelihood of developing Alzheimer's disease; it does not mean that you will definitely develop the condition. ■

Some doctors believe that a medication called tacrine (Cognex) can temporarily help memory problems. Donepezil hydrochloride (Aricept)—a newer version of tacrine with fewer side effects—may slow deterioration of memory and reasoning. Mild sedatives or antidepressants may be necessary if the person's behavior is disruptive within the household. Proper nutrition and health maintenance are important, as most people succumb to infection.

BENIGN FORGETFULNESS

There are three categories of memory—short-term, long-term/recent, and long-term/remote.

Short-term memory involves learning and remembering new information for a few seconds or minutes—for example, remembering the license number of a car long enough to write it down.

Long-term/recent memory is remembering what you had for dinner last night or who was in that meeting with you a few days ago.

Long-term/remote memory has to do with events from your distant past, such as your childhood.

The type of memory that most often is affected by aging is long-term/recent memory. Most complaints of memory loss are the result of normal memory loss due to aging.

But other factors can contribute to loss of memory. In some people, memory loss might be due to such things as drug side effects, a thyroid gland that is not operating normally, or a number of conditions that can be detected and treated. Depression and anxiety, for example, can impair memory.

Little actually is known about the physiology of memory storage in the brain. It is unclear whether memories are stored at specific sites or if memory involves widespread brain regions working in harmony. Some researchers have suggested that different storage mechanisms exist for long-term and short-term memory.

If the extent of your memory loss is that you occasionally forget if you locked the front door at night or where you put your glasses, do not worry. But you should see your doctor if you or someone close to you senses that your memory is getting progressively worse. If your doctor perceives a problem with your memory he will refer you to a neurologist, psychiatrist, or clinical psychologist for additional testing.

As you age, there are some things you can do to improve or enhance your memory. Make sure you hear and see well; hearing or vision aids can help you focus on what is being shown or said to you. Have your doctor review with you all of the medications you are taking; some may dull your mind or memory.

You also can use memory aids, such as a pocket recorder or lists. Sometimes, just writing something down can engrave it in your memory.

Do not be afraid of a slight memory lapse. The less you worry about it, the less likely you are to experience it. You may forget the name of a casual acquaintance, but relax. Chances are, that person has forgotten your name, too. ■

Prognosis Long-term outlook is poor. People with Alzheimer's can, with proper treatment, survive for as long as 15 to 20 years; however, mental and physical deterioration is inevitable.

Infections of the Brain and Nervous System

Because the brain and spinal cord have no contact with the external environment, the likelihood of their becoming infected is less than that seen with other organ systems, such as the respiratory system. But sometimes infectious agents do gain access to the nervous system via the bloodstream, the air spaces in the sinuses or ears, or through fractures. Viruses, bacteria, protozoans, fungi, and almost any infectious agent can invade the central nervous system (CNS) if given the opportunity.

Most CNS infections have certain symptoms in common: headache, fever, confusion, sensory disturbances, neck and back stiffness, and abnormalities of cerebrospinal fluid (CSF). Infections of the brain and nervous system constitute a medical emergency. Early diagnosis may not only be lifesaving, but could also prevent long-term damage to the brain, spinal cord, or nerves.

❖ ENCEPHALITIS

Symptoms *(What you may experience)* Sudden fever; headache; vomiting; stiff neck and back; drowsiness; seizures; coma; paralysis; inability to coordinate muscle movements; convulsions.

Signs and laboratory findings *(What the doctor looks for)* Confusion, altered consciousness, and fever will be apparent in a clinical exam. Inflammatory cells in CSF as revealed by lumbar puncture; abnormal EEG; areas of swelling and fluid accumulation in the brain as denoted by CT and MRI. Some viruses can be detected by DNA tests of cerebrospinal fluid.

What is it? Encephalitis is a viral infection of the brain and has many causes. One group of viruses (arboviruses) grow in both insects and man. They are usually transmitted by mosquito bites and are therefore highly seasonal and geographically localized. Enteroviruses are the most common cause of encephalitis in the United States; they are relatives of poliovirus and spread from one person to another by the fecal-oral route. Like other enteric infections, they are most common in summer. Herpes simplex encephalitis occurs year 'round; it is the only treatable form of encephalitis. Before the days of universal vaccination, cases of encephalitis used to occur after common childhood infections such as measles and mumps. Such cases are now rare in the United States, but they still occur in developing countries.

What you can do Outbreaks are more likely to occur in parts of the world outside of the United States. Travelers should check if any outbreaks are occurring at their destination. There is a good vaccine for Japanese B encephalitis. Mosquitoes are known to carry the viruses that transmit the disease, so removing pools of standing water from property can keep mosquitoes from breeding more insects to distribute the virus. Use mosquito repellent when exposure is a risk.

When to call the doctor Contact the doctor if someone in your family has confusion, inability to arouse, stupor, fever, mental disturbances, coma, or severe headaches. Signs of infection that warrant immediate attention in older children and adults include mental disturbances, severe headache, and sensitivity to light (photophobia). In infants, important symptoms are a bulging in the fontanelle (the soft spot of the skull) and a stiff neck.

Treatment The antiviral medication acyclovir (Zovirax) is effective against herpes simplex encephalitis. Treatment of other forms of the disease includes anticonvulsant medication, sedatives to induce sleep and rest, analgesics to relieve headache, and antipyretics to reduce fever. Sometimes steroids are given intravenously to reduce brain inflammation and accumulation of fluid.

Prognosis Encephalitis in babies and seniors can be fatal. People in other age groups are likely to recover, although the illness may be serious and prolonged. Recovery may be slow, and special therapy may be required to regain certain skills. Certain viruses are associated with a very bad prognosis. Eastern equine encephalitis is rare (less than 10 cases per year in the United States). However, the mortality rate is 50 to 60 percent; and most survivors are neurologic cripples.

❖ MENINGITIS

Symptoms *(What you may experience)* Fever, chills, malaise; headache; vomiting; stiff neck; inability to tolerate bright light; deep red or purplish skin rash.

Signs and laboratory findings *(What the doctor looks for)* Resistance to bending in the neck; lumbar puncture to analyze (CSF) for white blood cells and glucose and culturing to identify bacteria type; signs of bacterial infiltrate revealed by chest x-rays; and CT of head to assess presence or absence of abscess or fluid accumulation.

What is it? Meningitis is an inflammation of the meninges, the membranes that surround the brain and spinal cord. Most meningitis is acute; the patient becomes sick abruptly and the whole course of the illness may run from 48 hours to 1 or 2 weeks. The most dangerous form of acute meningitis occurs when bacteria traveling through the bloodstream (septicemia or blood poisoning) gain access to the meninges. Most acute bacterial meningitis is due to bacteria in the blood that passes from the bloodstream into the space between the meninges. Over 90 percent of cases of this type of meningitis are due to one of these organisms: *pneumococcus,* *meningococcus,* or *Haemophilus influenzae.* Other bacteria that are in the bloodstream, such as staphylococci or gram-negative rods, do cause meningitis occasionally. Newborn infants may develop septicemia and meningitis from Group B streptococci or gram-negative rods aquired from their mother's genital tract during delivery.

Another kind of acute bacterial meningitis occurs when there is a hole between the meninges and the outside world that allows bacteria to transit. Surgical operations or penetrating skull injury may allow bacteria to enter the brain directly. Infection of the nasal sinuses or the middle ear may also erode through the bone into the brain. Similar cases may follow nasal surgery or basal skull fracture.

Acute meningitis may also be caused by viruses—most usually by enteroviruses (which are cousins of polioviruses). In general, viral meningitis is clinically mild, and spontaneous recovery without complications is the norm. Often it is difficult and expensive to find out which virus is present, and because there is no treatment available, the effort is not made. Such cases are called "aseptic" meningitis to distinguish them the bacterial cases.

Chronic meningitis occurs when slow-growing organisms such as tubercle bacilli (which causes tuberculosis) or fungi gain access to the meninges. This disease develops over weeks, sometimes months, and occasionally years. The symptoms are fever, headache, vomiting, cranial nerve palsies, and mental clouding, just as for bacterial cases. However, all symptoms develop gradually.

What you can do Vaccines are available for *Haemophilus influenzae* and pneumococci. The number of cases of *H. influenzae* meningitis in this country has fallen from 10,000 cases per year to less than 1,000 since the *Haemophilus* vaccine came into general use. Pneumococcal vaccine is not in general use, but it is recommended for particular groups, such as children with sickle cell anemia.

Seek medical care at the first sign of what may be a bacterial infection. If you are given antibiotics, make sure you comply with your doctor's instructions and take all the medication. People with skull fractures or penetrating head wounds may be given antibiotics in an attempt to keep meningitis from developing.

When to call the doctor This is a medical emergency. Contact your doctor if you suspect that a child or senior has contracted the disease. Be alert to the symptoms of fever with neck or spine pain and stiffness.

Treatment Bacterial meningitis is usually fatal if not treated; if an untreated patient does manage to survive, he is generally severely disabled. The most important factor in changing that dismal outlook is to treat the patient with powerful intravenous antibiotics as rapidly as possible. It is important to know the bacterial species; blood cultures and a lumbar puncture are done as rapidly as possible to provide specimens for culture. Then the patient is given some kind of antibiotic, preferably within an hour of presenting to the hospital. The antibiotic choice is subsequently modified in the light of blood culture results and the patient's progress. In addition to antibiotics, the patient may need treatment for shock, seizures, or severe headache. Most patients with meningitis are unable to eat or drink, and need parenteral fluid therapy (fluids entering the body someplace other than the mouth, usually through a vein or a tube in the stomach).

Prognosis With good treatment, few people die of meningitis. However, patients whose treatment is delayed still die, or may recover with permanent disabilities. Even children who have apparently completely recovered may prove, on detailed examination, to have mild deafness, cognitive defects, and emotionality leading to behavior problems in school.

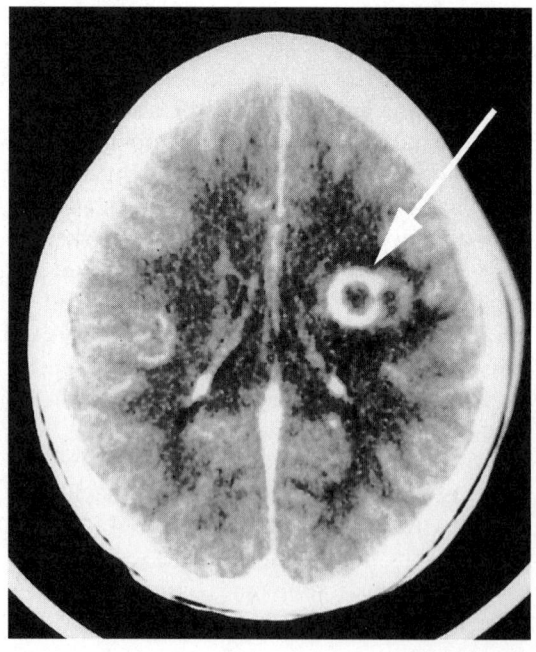

Brain abscess (arrow) as shown on a CT scan. Bacteria from infection in another part of the body can travel to the brain through the bloodstream. The pus that develops as a result of the infection collects in the brain forming an abscess.

❖ **BRAIN ABSCESS**

Symptoms *(What you may experience)* Persistent headache; nausea; vomiting; focal or generalized seizures; visual disturbances. Symptoms depend on where in the brain the abscess lies: infection in the temporal lobe may affect the ability to understand speech, or cause central face weakness or partial paralysis on one side of the body; infection in the cerebellum may cause dizziness, tremor, inability to coordinate voluntary muscle movements; infection in the frontal lobe may cause inability to articulate words, partial paralysis on one side of the body, drowsiness, inattention, or cognitive impairment.

Signs and laboratory findings *(What the doctor looks for)* The major sign for the doctor is rapidly developing dysfunction of part of the brain. The neurologic signs will be specific for the brain functions in the region of the abscess and will vary with the site. Other signs include heart murmur, history of infection, especially of the middle ear, nasal sinuses, heart, or lungs. Tests include CT scan and CT-guided biopsy of brain tissue.

What is it? A brain abscess is a free or encapsulated collection of pus developing from bacterial infection, usually involving the ear, sinus, or teeth. Bacteria from an infection in another part of the body—gum, heart, or lung—may travel to the brain via the bloodstream. Pus forms as a result of this infection. As pus collects in the brain, it puts pressure on surrounding tissue.

Although a brain abscess can occur at any age, they usually are seen in people between the ages of 10 and 35 and rarely in seniors. A small percentage of children with congenital heart disease develop them. People with AIDS can develop a brain abcess from organisms that do not affect people whose immune system is normal.

What you can do If you have been prescribed antibiotics to treat an infection, take all the medication as directed. Antibiotics may be given to someone with a penetrating head wound or a heart murmur to prevent infection. If you have a heart murmur or implanted hardware, take antibiotics before undergoing dental work.

When to call the doctor A brain abscess is a medical emergency; seek immediate help.

Treatment Intravenous antibiotics will be started immediately to fight the infection; surgical drainage of the abscess is frequently necessary. The surgeon opens the skull and removes the collection of pus. Anticonvulsant medications may help prevent seizures. Other medications may be used to combat fluid accumulation in the brain and increased pressure in the brain.

Prognosis If untreated, brain abscess usually is fatal. Even with treatment, about 30 percent of people with a brain abscess will develop focal seizures (seizures that affect a portion of the body).

❖ CREUTZFELDT-JAKOB DISEASE

Symptoms *(What you may experience)* Personality changes; hallucinations; muscle twitching and muscle stiffness; gait changes; poor coordination; trouble speaking; drowsiness; dementia; memory loss; anxiety.

Signs and laboratory findings *(What the doctor looks for)* Muscle twitching and stiffness as revealed by a complete clinical exam; gait changes; poor coordination and impaired cognitive ability. Changes in brain wave activity as assessed by EEG; CT scan to examine brain structure and rule out other causes of the symptoms, such as a tumor; bacterial infection of the brain and nervous system as ruled out by lumbar puncture; brain biopsy may be done to confirm diagnosis; postmortem examination of the brain to show the spongelike appearance of tissue characteristic of the disease.

What is it? Creutzfeldt-Jakob disease is an example of a group of diseases called spongiform encephalopathies. A hallmark of these diseases—which also include scrapie, bovine spongiform encephalopathy (BSE, also known as "mad cow disease"), and kuru—is that the brain develops numerous tiny holes. These are too small for the naked eye to see, and the entire appearance is that of a microscopic sponge.

Creutzfeldt-Jakob disease occurs worldwide but is exceedingly rare. There is approximately one new case for every 2 million people per year. It most commonly appears in people over age 55, and rarely in people over age 80.

It is thought to be transmitted by a virus-like organism (a transmissible protein) called a prion. In recent years, it has been demonstrated that the disease can be transmitted by grafting of corneas and brain tissue from infected donors. Now potential donors are screened for the possibility of Creutzfeldt-Jakob disease. The disease was also linked to treatment with contaminated natural human growth hormone. This is no longer a danger, because now genetically engineered human growth hormone is used.

Some cases appear to be genetic; there also have been a few documented cases in which people contracted the disease via improperly or nonsterilized surgical instruments. It is now standard practice to destroy or use a more extensive sterilization process for all instruments used during an operation on a person with Creutzfeldt-Jakob disease. In Great Britain, 16 unusual cases of Creutzfeldt-Jakob disease have been diagnosed since 1994 in people much younger than the average patient. It was suspected, though not proven, that the cases were related to cattle that had been infected by eating the processed carcasses of sheep. However, the government there has since banned the feeding of sheep meat in any form to cattle. Thus the rate of bovine spongiform encephalopathy in British cows is decreasing and should pose no threat to the country's human population. According to the US Department of Agriculture, BSE has not been diagnosed in the United States.

Treatment There is no cure for the disease. Medications can control aggressive behaviors. The shakiness or jerky muscle movements can be treated with sedatives.

Prognosis Creutzfeldt-Jakob disease follows a rapid course, with most people succumbing to pneumonia within 6 months of the appearance of symptoms. In about 10 percent of cases the disease runs a more prolonged course of 2 to 5 years.

Neurologic Disorders Related to Infection

❖ POSTPOLIO SYNDROME

Symptoms *(What you may experience)* Weakness; fatigue; pain in muscles and joints; breathing difficulties; swallowing problems; sleep disturbances.

Signs and laboratory findings *(What the doctor looks for)* Evidence of past polio infections; neurologic exams to exclude all other possibilities; electrophysiologic studies of muscles and nerves, spinal fluid analysis, and muscle and nerve biopsy to exclude other conditions.

What is it? Postpolio syndrome is a condition that can strike polio survivors decades after recovery from an initial bout with the poliomyelitis virus. It is characterized by a further weakening of muscles previously injured by a polio infection. Some people experience only minor symptoms, while others experience a more severe course. About 25 percent of the estimated 300,000 polio survivors in the United States may be affected.

The cause of postpolio syndrome is not known, but it is not caused by reactivation of the virus. During the initial attack, nerve cells in the spinal cord controlling voluntary muscles are damaged or destroyed. Fortunately, some of these cells survive and send out new nerve connections to the orphaned muscle cells. This enables the individual to regain some muscle use. Researchers theorize that after many years these overburdened nerve cells may begin to fail, resulting in new muscle weakness.

Symptoms are most likely to appear 25 to 35 years after the initial polio attack. The risk of postpolio syndrome is significantly higher in people who sustained permanent paralysis from their initial bout. Women also appear more likely than men to experience symptoms of postpolio syndrome.

When to call the doctor If you had polio and gradually experience any of the symptoms of postpolio syndrome, consult your doctor.

Treatment Individualized exercise programs can help improve muscle strength and function. Medications may help reduce fatigue and increase strength, but they are experimental. Over-the-counter medications, such as aspirin and other nonsteroidal anti-inflammatory drugs (NSAIDs) may reduce pain and inflammation. Changing leg braces, decreasing activity levels, or treating other conditions that may be present, such as arthritis, may help.

Prognosis Postpolio syndrome is seldom disabling. In one study, only about 20 percent of affected people reported a need to use aids for mobility and breathing.

❖ NEUROLOGIC COMPLICATIONS OF AIDS

Symptoms *(What you may experience)* Fatigue; difficulty speaking; vision problems; fever; headache; stiff neck; cognitive impairment; paralysis; convulsions; loss of consciousness.

Signs and laboratory findings *(What the doctor looks for)* Abnormalities in the brain as visualized by MRI; evidence of infection as detected by lumbar puncture.

What is it? At some point about 40 percent of people with acquired immune deficiency syndrome (AIDS) will experience some form of neurologic complication. Because of the ability of the underlying virus to compromise the immune system, persons with AIDS can develop certain unusual infections and malignancies of the brain. These include: toxoplasmosis (a parasitic infection), progressive multifocal leukoencephalopathy (an infection with a "slow" virus), cryptococcal meningitis (a fungal infection), and primary brain lymphoma (a malignancy). Brain abscesses also may develop as a result of a bacterial infection.

In addition, the human immunodeficiency virus type 1 (HIV-1), the virus responsible for AIDS, can directly invade the brain. This can lead to meningitis or encephalitis.

HIV-1 also causes a slowly progressive dementia in about 30 percent of infected children and adults that is characterized by apathy, withdrawal, and progressive memory loss. About 20 percent of AIDS patients develop a spinal cord syndrome with progressive, spastic leg weakness and loss of sensation. The virus also can cause peripheral nerve and muscle disorders.

Treatment If you have AIDS and you get a secondary bacterial infection, it may be treatable with antibiotics; however, effectiveness may be related to the degree to which your immune system is depressed. Research on new therapies continues.

Drugs that suppress HIV and improve the immune system often indirectly help in the treatment or prevention of central nervous system problems in AIDS.

There are strategies caretakers can implement to minimize the effects of AIDS-related dementia. These include: keeping the environment as structured and routine as possible; keep many clocks and calendars around the house; not rearranging furniture; leaving some lights on at night; not allowing clutter to pile up; giving instructions slowly and one step at a time; simplifying tasks by breaking them into small parts; allowing lots of time for small tasks.

See Chapters 21 and 22 for more information on AIDS.

Prognosis The long-term outlook for people with AIDS has improved with newer, combination drug therapies. New medications and therapies are being investigated that may increase survival and may even offer hope of neurologic improvement.

❖ REYE'S SYNDROME

Symptoms *(What you may experience)* Sudden continuous vomiting; lethargy; agitation; confusion; irritability; delirium; loss of consciousness; rising blood pressure, respiratory rate, and pulse; hyperactive reflexes.

Signs and laboratory findings *(What the doctor looks for)* Recent viral infection and use of aspirin to reduce fever; serum ammonia level, clotting factors, and liver function verified by blood tests; the presence of fatty droplets as checked by liver biopsy; lumbar cerebrospinal fluid (CSF) pressure and presence of white blood cells checked by lumbar puncture.

What is it Reye's syndrome is an extremely rare, acute childhood illness characterized by brain swelling and fatty deposit in the liver. It most commonly affects children between the ages of 5 and 11.

Its exact cause is unknown, but it almost always follows a viral infection, such as influenza or chickenpox. Use of aspirin during a viral infection appears to greatly increase the risk of Reye's syndrome. After a sudden upsurge of Reye's syndrome in the 1970s, the American Academy of Pediatrics issued a warning against the use of aspirin in children. As a result, Reye's syndrome has once again become a rare disease.

What you can do To prevent Reye's syndrome, do not give aspirin to children or adolescents unless specifically instructed to do so by a doctor. If medication is needed, use acetaminophen or ibuprofen.

When to call the doctor Reye's syndrome is a medical emergency. If your child has had a viral infection within the past week and exhibits the symptoms of Reye's syndrome, consult your doctor immediately.

Treatment Intensive care hospitalization may be required so that the child can be monitored and stabilized. Glucose and electrolyte solutions will be given intravenously to normalize the child's blood chemistry. In more severe cases, additional aggressive therapy may be necessary to relieve pressure inside the skull.

Prognosis About 80 percent of children who contract the disease survive. If death occurs, it usually results from respiratory arrest or from accumulation of fluid and pressure in the brain. Children who survive coma may have some degree of brain damage.

Neuromuscular Disorders

Neuromuscular disorders are characterized by a failure in the key communications link between nerve endings and muscle cells. Nerve endings order muscle cells to contract by releasing a chemical neurotransmitter known as acetylcholine. This neurotransmitter bridges the gap between nerve ending and muscle receptors, translating impulse to action. This vital signaling process can be short-circuited by various causes, ranging from an autoimmune response in which the body's own antibodies attack the receptors, to infection by botulism. Some of the key symptoms of neuromuscular disorders are weakness and muscle wasting, loss of motor control, and severe muscle fatigue that accompanies exertion.

Other incapacitating neuromuscular disorders are caused by breakdowns in the nerve cells that initiate muscle movement. In poliomyelitis (now, fortunately, extremely rare in North America) a virus attacks the motor neurons in the brain stem and spinal cord. In amyotrophic lateral sclerosis—indelibly associated with the name of baseball great Lou Gehrig—unknown causes lead to widespread, progressive degeneration of the cells in the spinal cord that control muscles.

❖ MYASTHENIA GRAVIS

Symptoms *(What you may experience)* Fatigue; drooping eyelids; double vision; difficulty talking, chewing, and swallowing; weakness in limbs; respiratory difficulties that get worse late in the day or when fatigue develops.

Signs and laboratory findings *(What the doctor looks for)* Examination of muscle reflexes and muscle strength as well as eye movement and eyelid strength; decrease in muscle contraction, strength, and stamina as shown by electromyography; demonstration of improved muscle strength 30 to 60 seconds after injection of edrophonium or neostigmine; the specific antibodies that cause the disorder present in the blood as revealed by blood tests.

What is it? This uncommon neuromuscular disease primarily strikes young adults between the ages of 20 and 40. It affects about one in every 25,000 people, rarely children. It is about three times more common in young women, but in adults older than 40 the incidence is similar in men and women.

Myasthenia gravis is due to an antibody that blocks the pathways connecting motor neurons and muscles. The space between the nerve ending and the muscle fiber is called the neuromuscular junction. When the nerve impulse arrives at the nerve ending, it stimulates the release of the neurotransmitter acetylcholine. This chemical travels across the gap to the muscle fiber, where it attaches to specific receptor sites. When enough of these receptor sites are activated the muscle contracts. But in myasthenia gravis, an abnormal immune system response generates antibodies that attack these receptors and reduce their number by as much as 80 percent. The thymus gland, which helps form a person's developing immune system, appears to be somehow involved.

Cranial nerves that stimulate the muscles of the face, eyes, tongue, neck, and throat are almost universally affected; they are the first and most severely weakened. Later, other muscles can be involved as well. Maximum extent of muscle involvement is generally seen within the first 5 to 7 years after the appearance of symptoms. Crisis periods of weakness so intense that the person needs help breathing can be triggered by other illnesses, such as infection.

Typically, an individual with untreated myasthenia gravis feels strong on awakening from a night's sleep or a nap. Weakness develops progressively over the course of the day.

Women with myasthenia gravis are not advised against becoming pregnant, however, they should be closely supervised by a doctor. About 12 percent of babies born to mothers with the disease develop signs of neonatal myasthenia, but these signs disappear during the first few months of life.

This disease led to the name of the mechanical arms that scientists and technicians use to manipulate dangerous compounds behind shields of glass and other materials. The science fiction writer Robert Heinlein, in his short story *Waldo*, created a protagonist afflicted with myasthenia gravis. He invented these devices to help him pick up and move objects. Hence, these arms are now called waldoes.

Another form of neuromuscular signaling breakdown, Eaton-Lambert syndrome, can produce symptoms very much like those of myasthenia gravis. However, Eaton-Lambert syndrome is caused by failure of the body to release the messenger acetylcholine, and is associated with lung cancer and other diseases.

What you can do When possible, avoid exposure to infection, excessive heat and cold, overexertion, and emotional stress, all of which intensify muscle weakness. Plan your daily routine around energy peaks, and allow opportunities for rest.

When to call the doctor When the disease involves the respiratory system, it can be life-threatening, so call the doctor at the first sign of respiratory infection. If you have difficulty breathing or swallowing, seek immediate treatment.

Treatment Anticholinesterase medications allow acetylcholine to remain at the neuromuscular junction a little longer than usual so more receptor sites can be activated. Corticosteroids and other immune-system suppressive medications can help.

About 10 to 15 percent of patients have tumors of the thymus gland, so surgical removal of the thymus in such cases may be necessary.

A blood-cleansing process called plasmapheresis, in which abnormal antibodies in the blood plasma are removed and replaced, offers temporary improvement in muscle strength and is used if a patient is in a crisis.

Prognosis Although the disease cannot be cured, treatments cause significant improve-

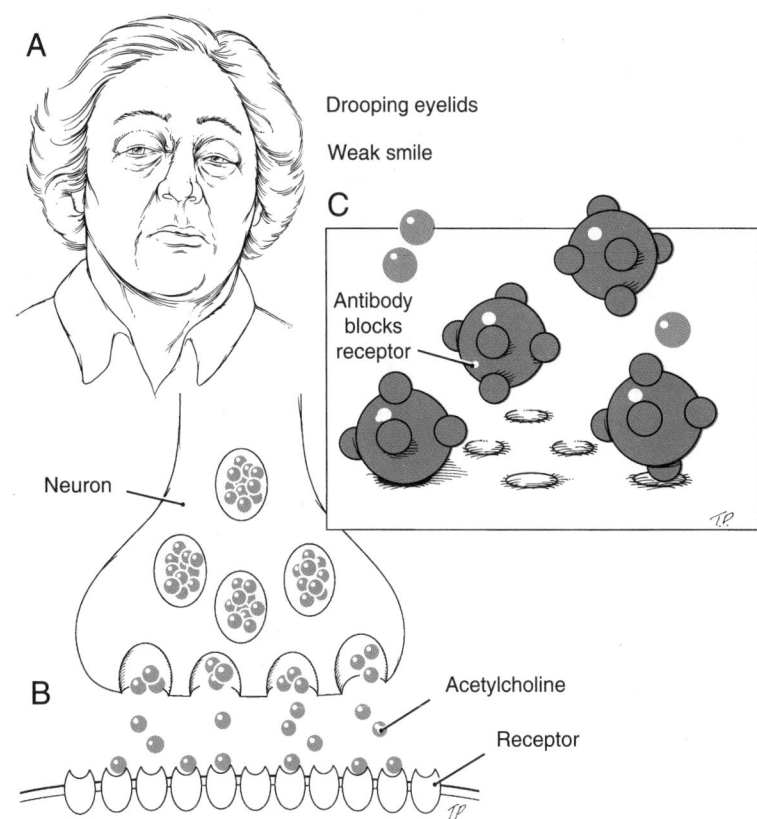

Myasthenia gravis. Signs of this neuromuscular disease may include difficulty smiling, speaking, chewing, or keeping the eyes wide open. The disease affects the junction between a nerve and a muscle. (A) Acetylcholine is released by a neuron and, after being sensed by a muscle's receptors, initiates a muscle contraction. (B) In myasthenia gravis, antibodies block many of the muscle's acetylcholine receptors, decreasing the number of receptors available to sense the acetylcholine released from the neuron.

ments, and most people can expect to lead normal or nearly normal lives. In some cases, the disease may go into remission and muscle weakness disappears. But remission is not a cure; people in remission should take the same precautions as they would if they still had symptoms.

❖ AMYOTROPHIC LATERAL SCLEROSIS

Symptoms (*What you may experience*) Gradual muscle weakness and progressive decrease in strength and coordination (typically starts in the hands and arms or, sometimes, in the tongue and pharynx); paralysis and muscle cramping; hoarseness; difficulty swallowing; gagging or choking; trouble breathing; muscle atrophy.

Signs and laboratory findings *(What the doctor looks for)* Amyotrophic lateral sclerosis (ALS) is diagnosed by a set of characteristic physical findings. These are upper and lower motor neuron signs that include muscle weakness, atrophy, involuntary or spastic movements, or cramping. Testing may rule out other diseases whose symptoms mimic the ALS pattern. These tests include: electromyography and nerve conduction velocity tests to determine motor neuron abnormalities and analyze distribution patterns of nerve cell abnormalities; a panel of blood tests for toxins and biochemical abnormalities that may cause similar symptoms; measuring levels of cerebrospinal fluid protein through a lumbar puncture.

What is it? ALS, also known as Lou Gehrig's disease after the famed New York Yankee who died of ALS, is a progressive degeneration of nerve cells that control voluntary motor functions. When the nerves that govern the use and control of muscles shrink and disappear, muscle mass diminishes due to lack of nerve stimulation. This leads to loss of muscle strength. More muscle groups become involved over time. There is no effect on intelligence or the ability to think and reason. Its cause is unknown, but an inherited genetic defect seems to be involved in 5 to 10 percent of affected individuals.

More than 30,000 people in the United States have ALS, and about 5,000 new cases are diagnosed each year. It affects men and women equally and usually appears between the ages of 40 and 70.

What you can do Individuals with ALS depend upon the emotional and physical support of family and friends.

When possible, care should be taken to avoid physical stress or infection that might exacerbate the condition.

A rehabilitation program can prolong independence. Programs should not include weight lifting or resistance training. Stationary bicycle riding, water exercises, and walking on an even surface may be suitable. Devices such as button hooks and zipper pulls may help upper-limb function.

Support items such as wheelchairs and walkers also help maintain independence. Bathrooms and other sites in the home where falls may occur should be modified. Because swallowing may be affected, individuals with ALS have to learn how to suction fluids to avoid choking or drowning. Soft, solid foods and upright positioning during meals helps digestion.

Treatment The disease cannot be cured, but symptoms can be treated. Immediate relief of pain may be possible. Long-term treatment options must be carefully considered and discussed. The medication Riluzole (Rilutek), recently approved by the Food and Drug Administration, may slow the course of the disease in certain people.

Anti-inflammatory medications or wet heat may relieve joint pain due to extra stress caused by muscle weakness.

Supportive measures must be administered in the face of respiratory dysfunction. All infections must be treated promptly. Supplemental oxygen can be given, if necessary.

If swallowing problems are present, special diets minimize the possibility of inhaling food particles into the lungs. A feeding tube inserted into the stomach through the abdomen bypasses the swallowing problem and provides a more direct route for liquid nourishment. If the person has excess salivation, medications that decrease saliva production can be given, or suction devices can be used.

Sometimes, a person with ALS may exhibit inappropriate crying and laughing. This is not a psychological problem; it is associated with upper motor neuron dysfunction and may be treated with medication.

In diseases like ALS for which there is no cure, fraudulent therapies may be promoted by quacks. Individuals can do more to help themselves and others by participating in scientific, controlled clinical trials. Contact the Muscular Dystrophy Association for information about current clinical trials.

Prognosis There is no cure for ALS. Death often occurs within 2 to 10 years of the onset of symptoms. About 20 percent of people with ALS live longer than 5 years, and some survive for much longer.

❖ BOTULISM

Symptoms *(What you may experience)* Within hours, symptoms may develop that include double or blurred vision; lack of saliva; difficulty swallowing; paralysis of arms and chest muscles; paralysis of legs; abdominal pain and vomiting; difficulty breathing.

Signs and laboratory findings *(What the doctor looks for)* Paralysis of throat and eye muscles as revealed by clinical exam; paralysis of legs and arms; identification of specific toxin in patient's serum, stool, gastric contents or suspected food; imaging and laboratory tests to rule out other possible causes, such as myasthenia gravis or Guillain-Barré syndrome; EMG tests can be helpful in diagnosis.

What is it? Botulism is a life-threatening paralytic illness caused by a toxin produced by the anaerobic bacillus *Clostridium botulinum*. It usually results from eating contaminated foods that have been improperly cooked. *C. botulinum* thrives in the absence of air, so improperly prepared canned foods are a major cause of the illness. Because the offending organism also lives in soil, an open wound that comes into contact with infected dirt can become infected.

Approximately 250 cases of botulism are reported each year in the United States.

Infants can become infected by eating raw honey, though this will not affect adults. In infant botulism, the toxin is formed in the gastrointestinal tract after the ingestion of honey that contains botulinal spores (in food-borne botulism, the toxin is formed in the food).

The poison produced by the bacteria inhibits the transmission of nerve impulses to muscles and the salivary glands, which can cause respiratory failure.

What you can do Botulism is rare in commercially prepared food, but has occurred. Do not use foods from cans with bulging lids or sides. Home canning and preserving of food must be done carefully at the correct temperature, pressure, and time settings. As an extra precaution, boil home-preserved food for 10 minutes before serving. Do not feed infants raw honey. Be sure wounds are covered when you are walking barefoot.

When to call the doctor Symptoms can appear between 6 hours and 8 days after eating contaminated food. If symptoms show up within 24 hours, the illness is potentially fatal, so seek medical help immediately.

Treatment Intravenous or intramuscular administration of antitoxin is the mainstay of treatment. Intravenous fluids will be given as appropriate to prevent dehydration. Treatment is supportive until toxin is slowly removed by the body.

Prognosis Seventy-five to 90 percent of people who contract botulism survive and make a complete recovery. Death most often occurs from respiratory failure during the first week.

❖ POLIOMYELITIS

Symptoms *(What you may experience)* Most infections are subclinical, having no symptoms, or abortive (not completely developed), which causes slight fever, malaise, headache, sore throat, and vomiting. Major polio involves the central nervous system and takes two forms: nonparalytic, with moderate fever, headache, vomiting, lethargy, irritability, and pain in the neck, back, arms, legs, and abdomen; and paralytic, with the same symptoms as nonparalytic plus asymmetrical muscle weakness, loss of reflexes, urine retention, constipation, a tingling or burning sensation on the skin, and paralysis.

Signs and laboratory findings *(What the doctor looks for)* Arm or leg paralysis but no numbness; analysis of CSF for protein level through lumbar puncture.

What is it? Poliomyelitis is an infectious disease caused by poliovirus. As recently as 1950, between 50,000 and 60,000 cases of poliomyelitis were diagnosed in the United States every year. Because of the widespread use of polio vaccines, there are now fewer than 10 cases per year; most of the cases that do occur are due to the vaccine. Wild poliovirus has not been found in the United States since 1979 and has not been found in the Western Hemisphere since

MYOPATHIES

Myopathies are muscle diseases that are traceable to deficits in the "motor unit." Unlike other neuromuscular disorders the primary disease in myopathies is in the muscles themselves rather than in the nerves or the neurotransmitters. All myopathies result in muscle weakness—often in the pelvic region, face, neck, and trunk. Other frequently encountered symptoms are: exercise-induced fatigue; muscle atrophy or shrinkage (which may not, however, be as great as the degree of weakness would lead one to expect); tenderness to touch; and myotonia, or the inability of a muscle to relax properly after it has contracted.

The causes of myopathies are many and varied; they have a wide range of treatments and outcomes, depending on their causes. Some of the leading types of myopathy are: congenital, endocrine, nutritional or toxic, and inflammatory.

Congenital Myopathy can result from defects in the way muscles store and use glycogen (a carbohydrate that can be changed to glucose, a primary form of energy). An even larger number of myopathies represent congenital diseases of the mitochondria. Mitochondria are small organelles that are located in the body's cells outside the nucleus. Their job is to produce energy. Mitochondria have their own genes which are passed down exclusively by the mother.

Endocrine Myopathy can result from endocrine diseases that cause overproduction or underproduction of hormone by the thyroid gland or overproduction of hormones by the parathyroid or pituitary glands.

Nutritional Or Toxic Myopathy can be caused by alcoholism, leading to shortages of potassium in the blood and muscles. It can also be caused by a number of prescribed (or nonprescribed) medications, including the corticosteroids—which, ironically, can be indicated to treat inflammatory myopathies (see below). In that case, the use of steroids needs to be closely monitored to make sure they do not lead to secondary myopathies.

Inflammatory Polymyositis and dermatomyositis are both considered to be autoimmune diseases, characterized by inflammatory changes in the muscle (polymyositis) and skin and muscle (dermatomyositis). Some cases of dermatomyositis are believed to be associated with lung or breast cancer, while polymyositis may be an expression of systemic lupus erythematosus, sclerosis, or other connective tissue disorders.

The clinical evaluation of myopathic muscle diseases may not be able to differentiate them from many other neuromuscular disorders. But blood tests will frequently show elevated levels of the enzyme creatine kinase or, significantly, no elevated levels of the enzyme lactate following exercise. Needle electromyography tests can usually distinguish between myopathies, which are based primarily in the muscle, and neuropathies, which are based in the peripheral nerves. Finally, muscle biopsy results, showing characteristic abnormalities in the muscle fibers, are definitive in the diagnosis of myopathies. ■

1991. The World Health Organization has set the goal of eliminating poliovirus worldwide by the year 2000.

What you can do When a child is born, arrange for immunization against polio with a pediatrician. If you or another member of your family has not been immunized, consult your doctor. Check with your doctor or a specialist in travel medicine if you plan to visit a country where the disease is more common.

Treatment Treatment is for the problems polio may cause, rather than for the polio itself.

Prognosis Long-term outlook depends on the part of the body affected. If the central nervous system (CNS) is spared, prognosis is excellent. But even with CNS involvement, 90 to 95 percent of affected people survive, although various disabilities may result.

Neuropathies

Damage to peripheral nerves (the nerves that are not in the brain and spinal cord) is called peripheral neuropathy. Peripheral neuropathy can affect the sensory nerves in arms, hands, fingers, legs, feet, and toes that convey information to the brain; the autonomic nerves that control function of the heart, sexual organs, stomach, and digestive system; and motor nerves, through which the brain sends commands to control muscle movements. Damage to these can affect your ability to feel sensations or move a certain body part. Causes of peripheral neuropathy include: alcoholism; diabetes; inherited conditions; B_{12} and thiamine vitamin deficiencies; and exposure to certain chemicals, such as arsenic, mercury, lead, and insecticides. Destruction of nerves also can result from invasion by microorganisms.

Anything that places undue pressure on a nerve also can cause damage, resulting in burning, numbness, or abnormal sensitivity. Causes of such peripheral neuropathies are abnormal bone growths, tumors, and rheumatoid arthritis.

Symptoms of peripheral neuropathy generally build up gradually over many months. It often begins with a tingling sensation along the periphery of all four limbs that travels inward to the trunk. Numbness may follow the same path; or, the skin may become very sensitive, and sharp pain, known as neuralgia, may develop. There also may be a sense of gradual muscular weakening throughout the body. Peripheral neuropathies also pose the risk that if a numbed part of the body becomes injured, the injury may not be properly perceived by the body until other damage, such as infection, has occurred.

❖ BELL'S PALSY

Symptoms *(What you may experience)* Facial weakness on one side; drooping eyelid or inability to close one eye; numbness or heavy feeling in the face; alteration of taste; tearing; producing an amount of saliva that may be more or less than normal. Pain behind the ear.

Signs and laboratory findings *(What the doctor looks for)* History of abrupt onset of pain behind the ear; facial paralysis observed on clinical exam; testing is done if the palsy does not resolve with time or if other neurodeficits are found.

What is it? Facial paralysis, probably due to a viral infection of the nerve. The facial nerve is compressed within the temporal bone. Bell's palsy usually appears abruptly, over a 24- to 48-hour period, and affects one side of the face. Bell's palsy may result from a primary infection with herpes simplex type I virus and can also be a manifestation of Lyme disease. Many times the cause is unknown.

When to call the doctor Facial weakness can signal many neurologic diseases. If there is abrupt onset of facial paralysis, a consultation with your doctor can rule out other diseases. If the eye remains open, some protection for it will be necessary. If pain is present, analgesics may help.

Treatment Because the cornea is exposed, an eye patch should be worn to prevent injury. Methycellulose eye drops should be used to lubricate the eye. Steroids can enhance recovery if started within 48 hours of onset of paralysis. In persistent cases, surgery to decompress the facial nerve may be recommended.

Prognosis A full recovery usually occurs within a few months after partial paralysis. After complete paralysis, there is 90 percent chance of full recovery if nerves are undamaged. If nerves are damaged, full recovery falls to a 20 percent chance. Some residual involuntary movement or contraction of facial muscles may remain or develop when fatigue or stress occurs.

❖ ALCOHOLIC NEUROPATHY

Symptoms *(What you may experience)* Tingling of hands and feet slowly spreading along arms and legs; numbness; pain; cramps and muscle tenderness more pronounced in the legs.

Signs and laboratory findings *(What the doctor looks for)* Physical findings of alcohol consumption, alteration in temperature sensation. Red blood cell appearance as inspected by blood tests; history of exposure to toxic chemicals; liver function analyzed through blood tests; a specific pattern of nerve injury (axonal degeneration) as shown in electromyography and nerve conduction velocity tests.

What is it? This is a form of peripheral neuropathy. It is common in alcoholics because they often do not consume a sufficiently nutritious diet.

What you can do Recognizing early signs of alcoholism can put you on the path to recovery. Your doctor can help you locate an alcoholic recovery program that may be right for you.

Treatment Vitamin replacement, tricyclic antidepressants, and anticonvulsants for pain if necessary. Alcoholic neuropathies are treated by addressing the cause. (See Chapter 5 for more information on stopping alcohol abuse.)

Prognosis Early diagnosis is important, because peripheral nerves, unlike nerves of the central nervous system, can show gradual improvement with proper care. However, if drinking begins again, the neuropathy may return.

❖ DIABETIC NEUROPATHY

Symptoms *(What you may experience)* Numbness, prickling or tingling sensations in the toes and feet; pain in the foot; difficulty or pain on walking; double vision. These symptoms may be symmetric or localized to one region. There may be problems with urination, digestion, or erection, or frequent urinary tract infections.

Signs and laboratory findings *(What the doctor looks for)* Presence of diabetes; patient description of symptoms; analysis of muscle strength; degree of sensation loss, or numbness; nerve conduction velocity; presence of footdrop (dragging the foot when walking); diminished activity of autonomic function as shown by testing heart rate and blood pressure responses, gastrointestinal (GI) tract, and genitourinary function.

What is it In diabetes, the body either fails to produce insulin, or produces varying amounts of the hormone but cannot use it effectively to break down sugar. Problems associated with diabetes can affect the entire body.

Diabetes-related disorders of the nervous system can include impotence, loss of sensation, episodes of pain, and worsening of vascular problems. Its early signs include tingling in toes and fingers and muscular weakness. Because numbness is a key symptom, a person with diabetes may injure his feet and not know it until it has become serious. Just how diabetes damages peripheral nerves is not known, but it is very likely tied to insulin deficiency and high blood glucose levels. (See Chapter 26 for more information on diabetes.)

What you can do Many diabetic neuropathies can be prevented by proper management of the disease through tight control of blood sugar levels. Persons with noninsulin-dependent (type 2) diabetes, in particular, can often control the disease by losing weight and engaging in regular physical activity. (See Chapter 26 for more information.)

When to call the doctor If you have diabetes, see your doctor when you first feel the tingling sensation that signals the beginning of neuropathy.

Treatment If diabetes has caused peripheral neuropathies, specific symptoms can be relieved. Pain-killing medications can alleviate the discomfort; mechanical assistive devices can help the individual regain muscle control and mobility. Regularly inspect the skin of the feet and lower legs. Any break in the skin should be treated promptly and aggressively. Men who are impotent can consult a doctor about a number of options available to help them maintain erections, enabling sexual intercourse. These include implantation of a penile prosthesis, injections, and the oral drug silfenadil (Viagra).

❖ GUILLAIN-BARRÉ SYNDROME

Symptoms *(What you may experience)* Weakness rapidly evolving over days; tingling sensation in toes, feet and legs; sensory loss; difficulty breathing; paralysis of the legs, arms, respiratory muscles, and face.

Signs and laboratory findings *(What the doctor looks for)* History of illness with fever preceding clinical symptoms; ascending paralysis, loss of muscle tone, or loss of muscle reflexes revealed by physical exam; CSF protein level as revealed by lumbar puncture; slowed conduction and "blocked" nerve impulses as shown on electromyography and nerve conduction velocity test.

What is it? Guillain-Barré syndrome is a disorder in which the body's immune system attacks the peripheral nerves, (which are outside the brain and spinal cord). Initial symptoms are typically tingling sensations or weakness in the legs. In many instances, these spread to the arms, upper body, and face within 24 to 72 hours. Symptoms can increase in intensity until the muscles cannot be used at all and the person is almost completely paralyzed.

Guillain-Barré syndrome is rare, affecting an estimated one in every 100,000 persons. It can strike anyone at any age but is most common between the ages of 30 and 50. It usually occurs a few days or weeks following a febrile (fever) illness, usually a viral infection that affected the respiratory or GI system, but it can follow bacterial infections as well. Surgery or pregnancy can sometimes trigger it.

The course of the disease runs through three phases: The initial phase starts with the appearance of the first clinical symptoms; the plateau phase begins 1 to 3 weeks later and lasts several days to 2 weeks; the recovery phase can extend from 4 to 6 months or may take as long as 2 years. If the initial phase is severe, it can lead to paralysis of the respiratory and swallowing muscles, an emergency situation requiring immediate and intensive care.

The exact cause of the disease remains a mystery. However, doctors and scientists believe the immune system destroys the myelin sheath surrounding the axons of nerve cells, or the axon itself. When this happens, the nerve cells cannot transmit signals efficiently, and muscles that they control lose their ability to respond to commands. The brain also receives fewer sensory signals, resulting in an inability to feel textures, heat/cold, pain, and other sensations.

When to call the doctor If, after a febrile illness, you perceive a tingling sensation in the toes, feet, or legs followed by muscular weakness—especially if it evolves over days—consult your doctor as soon as possible. If you live alone, failure to see a doctor promptly can lead to progression of the disorder and paralysis, which can leave you unable to seek help.

Treatment High-dose immunoglobulin therapy—in which doctors administer intravenous, high doses of the proteins that the immune system uses to attack invading organisms—can, for reasons not well understood, lessen the immune attack on the nervous system. More serious cases are treated by plasmapheresis, in which the blood is removed and "cleansed" of its own plasma and antibodies that may be contributing to the attack.

Much of the treatment is supportive and consists of keeping the body functioning, especially the respiratory system, while the nervous system recovers. Once the initial crisis phase is over, rehabilitative therapy begins, first with passive exercise, and as soon as possible, with active exercise to promote recovery of muscle strength.

Psychological counseling can help relieve the emotional difficulties affected people may face with sudden paralysis and dependence on others.

Prognosis Recovery from this disease occurs in the vast majority of cases, taking as little as a few weeks or as long as a few years. About 30 percent of affected people still feel residual weakness after 3 years. About 3 to 5 percent may suffer a relapse of muscle weakness and tingling many years after the initial attack. People who die of

Guillain-Barré do so because of respiratory collapse, infection, or blood clots in the legs and lungs.

❖ CHARCOT-MARIE-TOOTH DISEASE/ HEREDITARY NEUROPATHY

Symptoms *(What you may experience)* Muscle weakness in hands, forearms, lower legs, and feet; clumsiness, frequent falls, and tripping over one's own feet.

Signs and laboratory findings *(What the doctor looks for)* Muscle atrophy producing a characteristic stork-like shape of the legs; mild curvature of the spine (scoliosis); foot deformities, such as a high arch and flexed toes; difficulty in maintaining balance while standing; other signs of muscular weakness. Feet or hands may be cold with blotching of the skin. Reflexes, such as the knee jerk, may be lost. Electrical activity of muscle cells as measured by electromyogram; slowed nerve conductions as shown by nerve conduction velocity test.

What is it? Named for three doctors who identified it in 1886, Charcot-Marie-Tooth disease is one of a group of diseases known as hereditary motor-sensory neuropathies. It is a genetic disorder marked by slowly progressive muscle weakness in the lower limbs and a mild loss of sensation in the fingers and toes. It usually becomes apparent in adolescence, but it may first appear in people at any age through the fifth decade. The weakness results from the disease of nerves or myelin sheath that stimulate muscle and not from a degenerative process of the muscle itself.

Charcot-Marie-Tooth disease is genetic and can be detected in utero. If one parent carries the defective gene, there is a 50 percent chance the child will inherit the disease.

Early symptoms are foot deformities, such as a high arch and flexed toes, and difficulty in walking because of these structural changes.

There are several types of hereditary neuropathies; the two most common are hypertrophic and neuronal. Hypertrophic is the predominant form and has an earlier onset (in childhood). In both, the muscles of the feet are initially affected, and sensory alterations are apparent. Later small muscles of the hands become involved.

Treatment There is no known cure, nor can the disease be prevented. Foot deformities can be treated with carefully fitted shoes and proper foot care. A regular program of moderate exercise can build up muscles and increase joint mobility. Surgery may be helpful for very highly arched feet. Surgery usually is not needed to correct the spinal curvature, but it may be considered in severe cases. Adaptive hand devices can be used to help an affected individual handle table utensils and writing implements. It is especially important to take good care of numb feet, inspecting them regularly for small ulcers. Shoes should be inspected for proper fit.

Prognosis Affected individuals can expect a normal lifespan; most remain able to walk.

Birth and Developmental Disorders and Muscular Dystrophies

The brain and spinal cord develop in the fetus within the first 2 months after conception. Along the back of the embryo is a strip of cells that gradually curls inward to form what is called the neural tube. The brain forms at the front of the tube; the rear of the tube becomes the spinal cord.

It is possible for abnormalities of the brain and spinal cord to form while the fetus develops. Such congenital disorders tend to be genetic. Blood tests can be conducted early in pregnancy to find out whether certain disorders exist (see Chapter 6, Family History, Genetics and Your Health). Sometimes a problem can be detected by using ultrasound to generate an image of the fetus inside the uterus.

For some defects, little can be done. The fetus develops from its DNA blueprint. If the genetic code is distorted, the infant may have a serious problem that can hamper intelligence, physical form, and possibly, life. On the other hand, many developmental problems can be easily corrected or may even be inconsequential.

Some defects can be prevented if the mother eats well, exercises moderately, and generally takes good care of herself during pregnancy. (See Chapter 7 for more information.)

❖ SPINA BIFIDA

Symptoms (*What you may experience*) A depression or dimple, tuft of hair, soft fatty deposits on the skin over the spinal defect; or a sac-like structure (cyst) that protrudes over the spine. (See page C-33.)

Signs and laboratory findings (*What the doctor looks for*) Weakness in the feet, change in reflexes, spinal defects. Visualization of the defect on the infant's back; spinal cord involvement as shown by MRI; x-ray if verification of a spinal bone defect is needed; fluid accumulation in the brain as shown by skull x-rays and CT; kidney function as revealed by urinary tests.

What is it? Spina bifida is a spinal cord defect characterized by incomplete closure of one or more vertebrae. In its most benign form, spina bifida occulta, there is no protrusion of the spinal cord or its covering (the meninges) through the vertebral opening. But in its more severe forms, there is protrusion. In spina bifida with meningocele, the sac contains meninges and cerebrospinal fluid (CSF), and the cyst can be as small as a nut or as large as a grapefruit. In spina bifida with myelomeningocele, the sac contains meninges, CSF, and a portion of the spinal cord. Myelomeningocele is the most severe form of spina bifida; there may be no cyst at all, only the exposed section of spinal cord and nerves.

Developmentally, these defects arise as a result of the neural tube's failure to seal. Though genetics may play a role, 95 percent of babies with spina bifida are born to parents with no family history of the disorder. Viruses, radiation, and other environmental factors may contribute, as may vitamin deficiency, especially folate, a form of folic acid (a vitamin of the B complex).

Every year in the United States, about 1,500 babies—one in every 2,000 live births—are born with spina bifida. It occurs more frequently among Hispanics and whites of European descent and is less common among Ashkenazi Jews, most Asians, and blacks. (See Chapter 8 for more information on spina bifida.)

Prevention The development of spina bifida can be greatly influenced by the mother's diet during pregnancy. In 1992 the US Public Health Service issued recommendations that all women of childbearing age (15 to 44 years) who are capable of becoming pregnant should consume 400 mcg (0.4 mg) of folic acid every day to reduce the risk of having a baby with spina bifida. It may be difficult to consume this much folic acid through diet alone—even though flour, corn meal, rice, and pasta should be fortified with this compound. Your doctor can recommend an appropriate prenatal multivitamin that will ensure that you receive the necessary amount of folic acid.

Women who have already had babies with spina bifida can talk with their doctors about taking higher doses of folic acid before attempting to conceive again.

When to call the doctor Spina bifida can be detected prenatally. The alpha-fetoprotein screening test can detect a higher-than-average risk that a fetus will have spina bifida, but most mothers with high levels in their blood will have normal babies. Additional tests include a detailed ultrasound examination of the fetal spine, and amniocentesis, in which a small amount of amniotic fluid is withdrawn so levels of alpha-fetoprotein can be directly measured.

Treatment Spina bifida usually requires no treatment. Meningocele can be treated surgically, and there usually is no paralysis. But babies born with myelomeningocele usually undergo surgery within 24 to 48 hours after birth. Such prompt surgery can help prevent additional damage to the open spine from infection or physical injury. Such children, though, will have limb paralysis and bladder and bowel problems.

Physical therapists will teach the parents how to exercise their baby's legs and feet to prepare for walking with leg braces and crutches. Some children may need wheelchairs. The degree of paralysis will depend on which spinal nerves were involved. The higher the openings on the spine, the more severe the paralysis.

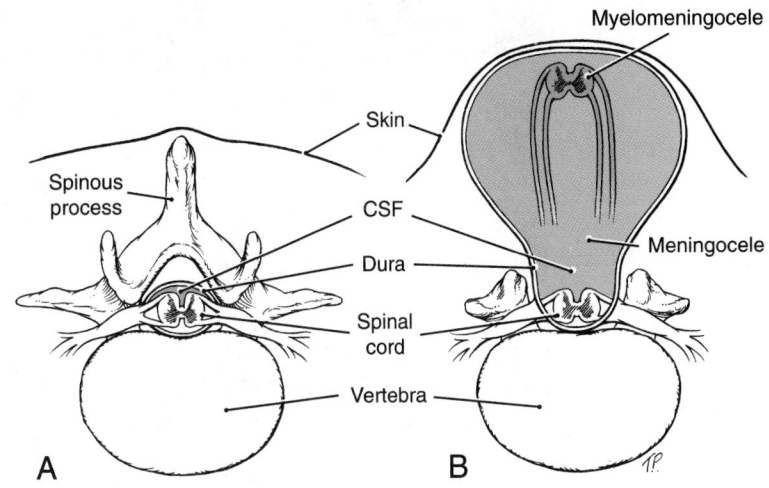

(A) Normal vertebra. (B) In spina bifida, one or more vertebrae are not completely closed, and thus can have the appearance of two branches (bifid). In severe cases, a sac (meningocele) containing cerebrospinal fluid (CFS) and meninges protrudes from the skin of the back. A portion of the spinal cord is sometimes included in the sac (myelomeningocele).

Prognosis With treatment children with spina bifida usually can lead active lives. Most affected women can bear children, although such pregnancies are considered high risk.

❖ HYDROCEPHALUS

Symptoms *(What you may experience)* Global deficits in neurologic function. In newborns, enlarged head; slowed development; lethargy. In adults, headache; vomiting; mental or psychological dysfunction.

Signs and laboratory findings *(What the doctor looks for)* In newborns, enlarged head; distended scalp veins; thin, fragile, shiny scalp skin; underdeveloped neck muscles. In adults, head injury as detected by physical exam; previous disease; gait disorder. In newborns and adults, differentiation of hydrocephalus from brain lesions as revealed by CT and MRI.

What is it? Hydrocephalus is also known as fluid or water on the brain. It occurs when cerebrospinal fluid, which cushions and protects the brain and spinal cord, is unable to drain properly. The fluid collects in and around the brain, causing the head to enlarge.

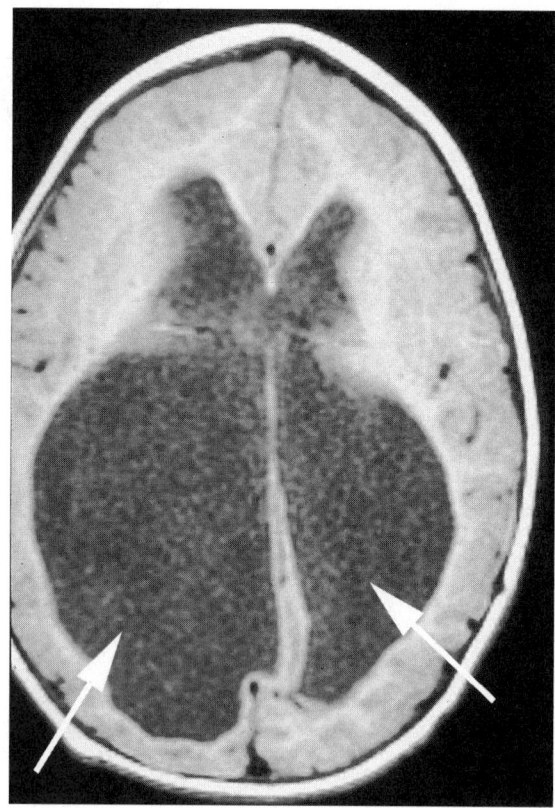

Hydrocephalus. Arrows indicate a buildup of fluid in the ventricles inside the brain as shown on MRI.

What you can do Adults participating in contact sports need head protection to prevent head trauma. Careful treatment and monitoring of illness such as meningitis, or encephalitis.

When to call the doctor You should have your child examined if you notice developmental delay and lethargy. In adults, medical consultation is advised when headaches, vomiting, and lethargy appear, or after experiencing head trauma, meningitis, or encephalitis (see pages 459 and 458).

Treatment Surgical implantation of a shunt that transports excess fluid into the abdomen is the primary treatment. Less commonly a shunt that transports the fluid into the right atrium of the heart is used. (See page 222 for more information.)

Prognosis With proper treatment, about 70 percent of infants with hydrocephalus survive, and nearly 50 percent will have normal intelligence. But even after surgery, mental retardation, impaired motor function, and loss of vision can persist.

❖ CEREBRAL PALSY

Symptoms *(What you may experience)* In infants: floppy muscles (in older children, stiffening of the limbs); legs crossed like scissors, feet pointing down; arms tucked into the side with arms and wrists bent; clumsy movements; difficulty sucking and swallowing; developmental delays, especially walking and talking.

In children: distorted speech; motor control problems of arms, hands, feet, and legs; frustration in children of high or normal intelligence.

Signs and laboratory findings *(What the doctor looks for)* Abnormal motor tone; spasticity. In ataxic cerebral palsy, which accounts for about 10 percent of cases, tremor in arms or legs with voluntary movement; crossed legs in infant picked up from behind; legs are hard to separate; persistent use of one hand; low birth weight; history of seizures. In other types of cerebral palsy, involuntary movements.

What is it? Cerebral palsy is a group of nonprogressive disorders that result from damage to the cerebrum before birth, during birth, or soon after birth. Spastic cerebral palsy, which affects about 70 percent of people with cerebral palsy, is characterized by various degrees of partial paralysis (palsy) of the arm and leg on one side of the body, partial paralysis of all four limbs, or partial paralysis of both legs but no paralysis of the arms. Dyskinetic cerebral palsy, which affects about 20 percent of people with cerebral palsy, involves abnormal involuntary movements of the limbs. Ataxic cerebral palsy, which accounts for about 10 percent of all cases, is characterized by disturbed balance, lack of coordination, reflexes that are less active than normal, muscle weakness, and muscle tremor. Children with cerebral palsy may have a combination of symptoms.

In infants, possible causes include: infection during pregnancy (especially with rubella, or German measles); radiation during pregnancy; maternal diabetes; malnutrition during pregnancy; forceps delivery; multiple birth (especially the last infant in a multiple birth). Older children may develop it as a result of a head injury, severe seizure, brain tumor, blood vessel abnormality in the brain, or brain infection.

Cerebral palsy occurs in an estimated 7,000 live births each year. It is seen most often in premature infants and in those who are small for their gestational age. Lack of oxygen before birth or during birth is the greatest contributor to cerebral palsy. Children with cerebral palsy also may have such associated symptoms as seizures, speech disorders, mental retardation, dental abnormalities, and hearing and vision defects such as crossed eyes.

The condition is not inherited, and having one affected child does not increase the chances of having another.

What you can do Regular prenatal care can help prevent many cases of cerebral palsy. Eat a well-balanced diet and follow your doctor's instructions.

When to call the doctor Although damage causing cerebral palsy occurs before, during, or after birth, cerebral palsy is rarely diagnosed before 6 months of age, and often later. Talk with your doctor if you are concerned with your baby's development. Tests can be performed to exclude other possible disorders.

Treatment Cerebral palsy cannot be cured, but many steps can be taken to help affected children achieve their full potential. Treatment may include: braces, splints, or other adaptive devices to assist in walking and more controlled arm movements; use of wheelchairs for children and young adults unable to walk; adapted eating utensils; range-of-motion exercises and orthopedic surgery to minimize stiffening of limbs, fingers, and toes; hearing aids to improve hearing; surgery for crossed eyes; muscle relaxants to ease limb stiffness; and medications to treat seizures.

Emotional support is vital. Encourage the child to ask for things he wants. Teach him to place food far back in his mouth so he can swallow more easily. Encourage the child to chew food thoroughly and drink through a straw (this helps develop mouth muscles to control drooling). Allow the child to choose his own clothes and dress independently, if possible.

Parents may feel unreasonably guilty about their child's condition. Psychological counseling can help. Programs of special education and support groups can foster heightened independence and productivity.

Caring for an affected child is a team effort, uniting the efforts of parents, doctors, physical therapists, speech therapists, and teachers. (For more information, see Cerebral Palsy, page 222.)

Prognosis Cerebral palsy is chronic but not life-threatening. Long-term prospects for children with cerebral palsy depend on the type and degree of handicap severity. With guidance and help, people with cerebral palsy can lead long, rich lives.

MENTAL RETARDATION

Mental retardation is a feature of many disorders. It is a general term for low intelligence (IQ of 70 or under) and adaptive functioning. Many things can cause mental retardation. Infections, injury during birth, ingesting toxic substances during pregnancy, physical trauma during pregnancy, metabolic or hormonal disorders, and nutritional deficiencies are just some possibilities. Sometimes retardation is determined genetically. The cause of retardation is unknown in about 80 percent of cases, but a woman can reduce the risk of carrying a child who will be retarded by eating a healthy and balanced diet, refraining from using alcohol and drugs, taking steps to avoid infections, and receiving proper prenatal care.

Most instances of mental retardation may not become apparent until a child is several years old or even in school. About 90 percent of retarded people are considered mildly retarded; they can learn basic elementary reading and number skills and may be able to function independently as adults. Those considered moderately retarded can learn to perform certain tasks and may be able to live semi-independently in supervised housing. Those who are severely retarded can learn simple conversational skills but only minimal self-care skills (such as eating, dressing, and toilet training) and need to have their activities supervised. People who are profoundly retarded cannot interact in society and may have only minimal skills in caring for themselves. Such individuals may have to live in an institution.

❖ DOWN SYNDROME

Symptoms *(What you may experience)* Deficit in intellectual capacity and developmental skills (see Well-Baby Care, page 191).

Signs and laboratory findings *(What the doctor looks for)* Cognitive impairment and delayed motor and language development revealed by assessment of neurologic function; an IQ score of 70 or below. Physical characteristics of Down syndrome: slanted eyes; a small, short head flattened at back and front; flat bridge of the nose; a thick tongue; short hands, feet, and limbs; crease across the top of the palm; poor muscle tone in arms and legs.

What is it? Down syndrome is a genetic disorder characterized by varying degrees of mental retardation. People with Down syndrome have a limited potential to learn and develop skills needed to care for themselves. As with many disorders, there are degrees of mental retardation and varied characteristics and levels of development. People with Down syndrome have 47 chromosomes in their body cells instead of the usual 46. This extra chromosome, a condition known as trisomy 21, causes all of the unusual characteristics of Down syndrome.

People with Down syndrome often suffer from associated problems, including hearing and vision impairment, and cardiac and GI problems—sometimes life-threatening and requiring extensive surgeries. (For more information on Down syndrome, see page 217.)

What you can do The chances of having a child with Down syndrome increase as a woman ages. At age 20, the risk is one in 2,000 live births; by the age of 40, the risk is one in 100. For this reason, it is recommended that women who become pregnant after age 35 should consider genetic testing. Amniocentesis and chorionic villus sampling are genetic tests that can be performed during pregnancy and can tell you if the child you are carrying has Down syndrome. Amniocentesis can be performed within the 16th to 18th week of pregnancy; chorionic villus sampling can be performed earlier, at about the 8th or 9th week.

Treatment Down syndrome cannot be cured, but children can be encouraged to reach their full potential. Retarded children and adults are entitled to a variety of special services that can help them develop special skills and achieve some independence. Some children can attend special classes in public or private schools; others can attend special schools. (For more information, see Mental Retardation, page 260.)

Having a mentally disabled child often introduces stress into the family environment. Seek the support of community services, support groups, and counseling, if necessary.

Prognosis Prognosis depends upon the degree of disability. Many Down syndrome men and women have enough intellectual ability to function with a reasonable degree of success and achieve varying degrees of independence as adults.

❖ FRAGILE X SYNDROME

Symptoms *(What you may experience)* Deficits in intellectual capacity, motor function, and speech and language development.

Signs and laboratory findings *(What the doctor looks for)* In boys, elongated face; large, protuberant ears; prominent chin and forehead; and large testes, especially after puberty. Females have only a slightly abnormal appearance, sometimes including protruding ears and other subtle features.

What is it? Fragile X syndrome is a form of mental retardation caused by a mutant X chromosome at a fragile site. It follows Down syndrome as the second leading cause of mental retardation, and it occurs more often in males than females.

What you can do There is no preventative action for this genetic disorder, which is carried by the mothers.

Treatment Treatment depends on the degree of mental retardation accompanying fragile X. Education and training opportunities are available and professional special education teachers are often able to teach mentally retarded people reading, numbers, and self-help skills.

Prognosis As with Down syndrome, men and women are often able to function successfully and live moderately independent lives.

OTHER GENETIC DISORDERS

Other genetic disorders include the muscular dystrophies, Tay-Sachs disease, phenylketonuria, adrenoleuko dystrophy, andrenomyeloneuropathy, and these are discussed below.

❖ MUSCULAR DYSTROPHY

Symptoms *(What you may experience)* Weak muscles in hips, leg, and shoulders of a child (in Duchenne's and Becker's dystrophies, almost always a male child); difficulty walking or standing.

Signs and laboratory findings *(What the doctor looks for)* Muscle weakness, muscle bulk; excessive levels of the enzyme creatine kinase as revealed by blood test; muscle biopsy shows characteristic pattern of muscular dystrophy and reduction or absence of the protein dystrophin, characteristic of people with Duchenne's and Becker's muscular dystrophy; electromyography shows "myopathic" pattern indicating the weakness is due to the muscles, not the nerves; large calf muscles, other muscles poorly developed.

What is it? The muscular dystrophies (MDs) are a group of inherited diseases characterized by progressive symmetric wasting of skeletal muscles.

The most common muscular dystrophies of childhood are Duchenne's and Becker's muscular dystrophies. They are X-linked recessive disorders (see Prevention, below) that affect boys almost exclusively. Duchenne's muscular dystrophy strikes about 13 to 33 boys per 100,000; Becker's muscular dystrophy occurs in 1 to 3 boys per 100,000.

Duchenne's muscular dystrophy begins gradually, initially affecting the leg muscles of boys between the ages of 3 and 5 years. It then spreads to the pelvic muscles. Children develop a waddling walk and have difficulty walking up steps or stairs. They usually also have an exaggeration of the forward curve of the lower back. As they get a little older, they develop a tendency to stand and walk on the forward part of the foot with the heels off the ground. Later they depend on wheelchairs for mobility.

The large calf muscles seen in these children are due to pseudohypertrophy (deposits of fat and other materials).

Some children with Duchenne's muscular dystrophy have other medical problems. These include impaired cognition and problems of the joints, spine, heart, and lungs.

Becker's muscular dystrophy is less disabling than Duchenne's. An arbitrary means of distinguishing between the two is whether the child can still walk at age 16 years. Symptoms generally begin to show up around the age of 5 years. There is no adverse effect on intellect in people with Becker's muscular dystrophy. Joint, lung, and spinal problems are milder.

Both conditions are due to defects in the same gene, which is involved in the production of the protein dystrophin. Dystrophin is absent from muscles in Duchenne's and reduced in Becker's.

Facioscapulohumeral dystrophy is a slowly progressive and relatively benign form of muscular dystrophy that usually is apparent by the age of 10 years but may develop a few years later. It causes weakening of the muscles of the face, shoulders, and upper arms. Eventually it spreads to all voluntary muscles. Early symptoms include the inability to pucker the mouth or whistle, abnormal facial movements, and absence of facial movements when crying or laughing.

The limb-girdle dystrophies are also slow to appear and progress. They cause only slight disability. They usually appear when the child is between 6 and 10 years of age, but they sometimes do not appear until early adulthood. The upper-arm and pelvic muscles are first affected. People with this form of muscular dystrophy have spinal problems, a waddling gait, poor balance, and cannot raise their arms.

Myotonic dystrophy is the most common form of inherited muscular dystrophy in adults. It is characterized by myotonia (delayed relaxation of muscle after contraction). It is called multisystemic because it affects the organs and tissues of many body systems in addition to causing muscle weakness and wasting. Fifty percent of people with this disorder will show visible signs by about age 20, but some do not develop clear-cut symptoms until after 50.

Many dystrophies are X-linked recessive disorders or genetic disorders that mothers can transmit to their sons, though the mothers themselves are unaffected by the disease. (Females have two X chromosomes, so the only way for a female to get the disease is from a mother who is a carrier and a father who has the disease, an extremely rare occurrence. Men who have the disease cannot transmit it to their sons, because they donate a Y chromosome to sons.) Female relatives of affected males may carry the gene for Duchenne's muscular dystrophy and Becker's muscular dystrophy. The son of a carrier has a 50 percent probability of being affected, and the daughter of a carrier has a 50 percent chance of being a carrier. Because the gene is linked to the X chromosome, the son of an affected male will be unaffected. Family members who are carriers should discuss the risk of transmitting the disease to their sons with a genetic counselor.

About one-third of Duchenne's cases are caused by new gene mutations not carried by the mother.

When to call the doctor If a young boy exhibits trouble walking or standing; if there is a family history of muscular dystrophy and you plan to have children.

Treatment No accepted therapy exists that can halt the progression of any form of muscular dystrophy. But there are treatments for some of the problems people with the disease may experience. Physical therapy and surgery can help with joint problems. Curvature of the spine also may be treated surgically by inserting a steel rod through the spine to straighten it. When muscles of the chest that assist in breathing become very weak, mechanical assistance in the form of a face mask to deliver oxygen may be helpful.

Prognosis Most people affected by Duchenne's muscular dystrophy are almost totally dependent on wheelchairs by their early teens; few survive beyond their 20s. People with Becker's muscular dystrophy usually can still walk by their 20s and some into their 40s; many survive well into their 40s.

❖ TAY-SACHS DISEASE

Symptoms *(What you may perceive in your baby)* By age 6 to 12 months, infant is apathetic and responds only to loud noise; weak neck, arm, trunk, and leg muscles; difficulty turning over; unable to grasp objects; loss of vision; eventual paralysis.

Signs and laboratory findings *(What the doctor looks for)* Evidence of poor responsiveness and low muscle tone on neurologic exam. Atrophy (wasting away) of the optic nerve and a distinctive cherry-red spot on the retina shown by ophthalmic examination; deficiency of an enzyme called hexosaminidase A as revealed by blood test.

What is it? Tay-Sachs is a rare genetic disease that affects people of Eastern European Jewish descent about 100 times more often than the general population. Children with the disease are deficient in producing the particular enzyme necessary for certain metabolic processes in the tissues of the central nervous system.

What you can do If you are a couple of Eastern European Jewish descent and plan to have a child, speak with your doctor about genetic testing. If both parents are carriers of the defective gene, there is a 25 percent chance that children will be born with the genetic defect causing the disease.

Treatment There is no cure; treatment is supportive.

Prognosis The disease is characterized by progressive mental and motor deterioration. Usually it is fatal by the age of 5 years.

❖ PHENYLKETONURIA

Symptoms *(What you may perceive in your baby)* Seizures at about 6 to 12 months of age; small head; dry skin; musty odor; hyperactivity; irritability; purposeless, repetitive voluntary muscle movements.

Signs and laboratory findings *(What the doctor looks for)* Blood screening of newborns is nearly universal in hospital births. Abnormal blood and urine levels of phenylalanine; abnormal brain wave pattern shown by EEG.

What is it? Phenylketonuria (PKU) is a hereditary disease characterized by increased amounts of certain amino acids in the blood and urine. Children born with the disease cannot convert phenylalanine (an amino acid essential for growth in infants) into the amino acid tyrosine. Thus, levels of phenylalanine accumulate and lead to mental deterioration.

The disease occurs in one out of every 14,000 births in the United States. Its incidence is lowest among Jews of Eastern European descent and African-Americans.

By the time phenylalanine levels are significant—usually within a few days after birth—damage to the brain has begun. Most states require screening for PKU at birth, so therapy can begin before brain deterioration occurs.

What you can do Make sure your baby is tested for PKU. Seek genetic counseling if you are a woman of reproductive age and have the disease. You may be able to minimize heart and central nervous system damage in your children by adhering strictly to a low-phenylalanine diet—including avoiding milk, which is high in phenylalanine.

When to call the doctor If your child, by the age of 4 months, is poorly aroused or in a stupor and exhibits signs of arrested mental development, personality changes, dry skin, and a musty odor.

Treatment A diet that restricts consumption of phenylalanine. Your doctor can help you or recommend a dietitian who can steer you through the maze of desirable and undesirable foods in a diet that needs to be maintained throughout life. Milk is high in phenylalanine and should be avoided.

Prognosis Early detection and treatment can minimize brain damage and allow the child to develop normally.

❖ ADRENOLEUKO-DYSTROPHY AND ADRENOMYELO-NEUROPATHY

Symptoms *(What you may experience)* In boys 3 to 16 years old: altered school performance; perceptual problems; attention deficit disorder; memory loss; personality changes; leg stiffness; loss of control of the lower limbs; in some cases, seizures.

Signs and laboratory findings *(What the doctor looks for)* Changes in the neurologic exam of tone and coordination of legs. Characteristic changes on CT or MRI (white matter lesions); abnormal levels of long-chain fatty acids in blood and skin cells; abnormal adrenal gland function.

What is it? Adrenoleukodystrophy (ALD) is a progressive genetic disorder that affects the adrenal gland and the white matter of the nervous system. In ALD the accumulation of long-chain fatty acids causes damage to the tissues (but the mechanism is not well understood). ALD is linked to the X chromosome, so it affects only boys and is transmitted by the mother. It afflicts about one in every 20,000 males.

In its classic childhood form, ALD strikes boys between the ages of 3 and 16 years. Neonatal ALD is an autosomal recessive form (not X-linked), which occurs in early infancy and includes seizures, severe muscle weakness, and an enlarged, impaired liver. Neonatal ALD progresses rapidly, with death usually by 1 year of age.

Adrenomyeloneuropathy (AMN), which affects the spinal cord or bone marrow, is an adult form of ALD in men between the ages of 21 and 35. AMN progresses more slowly than the childhood form, but it also results in nervous system deterioration.

Sometimes a woman who is a carrier of the gene develops mild symptoms of the disease.

What you can do Genetic counseling is recommended for female relatives of a known case of ALD who plan to have children.

Treatment Treatment options are still experimental. They include a diet restricted in very-long-chain fatty acids and bone marrow transplantation. These treatments have shown promise in delaying disease onset in presymptomatic individuals, but they have been ineffective in halting the progress of the disease.

Prognosis There is no cure for ALD. Death usually occurs within 10 years of diagnosis.

Traumatic Injuries to the Brain and Spinal Cord

The components of the central nervous system are susceptible to traumatic injury, despite the bony encasement provided by the skull and spinal column. A blow to the head can jolt and bruise the soft tissues of the central nervous system, even though the skull is not fractured. This is known as a closed head injury. For example, a motor vehicle accident can cause the brain to crash against the skull. Attendant bruising and swelling can cause additional brain damage. Injuries in which the skull itself sustains fracture are even more likely to cause brain damage.

Loss of consciousness following a head injury requires immediate medical attention. The damage produced by brain injuries varies widely and appears to be directly related to the mechanism and site of the injury. Symptoms may be headache, confusion, and loss of memory or consciousness. Other symptoms may include speech difficulties, bleeding from the ears or nose, paralysis, and coma. Late complications, such as the development of a blood clot between layers of tissue that surround the brain, can develop weeks or months after a head injury. Seizure disorders also may result.

Damage to the spinal cord almost always produces obvious neurologic deficiencies. The most common causes include motor vehicle accidents and diving accidents.

❖ CONCUSSION

Symptoms *(What you may experience)* Short-term loss of consciousness; vomiting; memory loss; behavioral changes; dizziness; nausea; headache.

Signs and laboratory findings *(What the doctor looks for)* Level of consciousness as evaluated by neurologic examination, mental status, reflexes, and orientation to time, place, and identity; possible skull fracture and bleeding in or around the brain as identified by CT.

What is it? Concussion is the most common head injury, resulting from a blow to the head. The blow causes the brain to strike the skull, but not hard enough for the organ to sustain a bruise. It can result from a punch, a car accident, a fall, or being shaken severely (more commonly seen in child abuse). Post-concussion syndrome is a constellation of symptoms characterized by headache, dizziness, vertigo, anxiety, and fatigue and it may persist for several weeks after an injury.

What you can do To prevent concussion, wear your seat belt if you are driving or riding in a motor vehicle; wear a helmet if you are driving or riding on a motorcycle or a bicycle.

When to call the doctor A concussion usually resolves on its own; however, any head injury causing loss of consciousness merits investigation by a doctor. The possibility of more serious injury should be eliminated. Sluggishness and sleepiness after a head injury require immediate medical attention.

Treatment An over-the-counter painkiller, such as acetaminophen, can help alleviate head pain. Avoid aspirin because of the risk of bleeding. The condition generally will resolve itself with 24 to 48 hours.

Prognosis The outlook for a person who has experienced an isolated concussion is excellent. Repeated concussions, however, could be damaging over time.

❖ TRAUMATIC BRAIN INJURY

Symptoms *(What you may experience)* Loss of consciousness; drowsiness; confusion; disorientation; there may be paralysis on one side of the body; there may be temporary speech difficulties.

WARNING SIGNS OF SERIOUS HEAD INJURY

Car and motorcycle accidents are two of the leading causes of head injury in the United States. Observing speed limits and wearing a seat belt or a motorcycle helmet could prevent many serious head injuries.

The skull does not need to fracture for the brain to be injured. Although the skull offers protection against an outside assault, it can turn into a foe if the brain batters into it with the considerable force that often develops in an auto accident. The windshield can put a halt to the forward motion of your head, but your brain is still moving at high speed when it crashes into its bony shelter.

Similarly, an adult who shakes a child violently can cause a serious injury to the child's brain.

Symptoms of a brain injury vary and are directly related to the severity of the damage. Concussion is the mildest form of head injury, it may be accompanied by headache, dizziness, and inability to recall events immediately before or after the injury.

Signs of a more serious head injury include difficulty speaking, bleeding from the nose or ears, muscle weakness, paralysis on one side of the body, convulsive seizures, and coma.

If you or someone you are with suffers a loss of consciousness as a result of a head injury, you should seek medical attention immediately. (For information on emergency first aid for someone with a head injury, see page 390.) ∎

Signs and laboratory findings *(What the doctor looks for)* Changes in neurologic examination, particularily impaired mental status and orientation to time, place, or identity; differing responses of the pupils to light; damaged areas of the brain as shown by CT scan.

What is it? Traumatic brain injury implies injury beyond a concussion and involves bruising and shearing of brain tissue, which disrupts normal function of the involved pathways.

Such an injury can occur directly beneath a blow when the brain rebounds against the skull. The force of the blow can cause the brain to impact the inner table of the opposite side of the head. Injury can occur when the head is hurled forward and stopped abruptly (as in striking a windshield). In this case, the brain continues moving even though the head has stopped, slaps against the skull, and rebounds. If the brain strikes against bony ridges on the inside of the skull, it can cause bleeding and pooling of blood between the brain and skull. Direct injury results when an object, such as a bullet, penetrates the skull and injures the brain.

What you can do You can dramatically cut your risk of this type of brain injury by wearing a seat belt in a car and a helmet if you are engaging in a high-velocity activity (rollerblading, skateboarding, riding a motorcycle or bicycle). It is important to wear protective gear, such as a hard hat, in any situation where your head may sustain a damaging blow.

When to call the doctor If you have had a head injury and have not lost consciousness but begin to feel lethargic or have trouble seeing or talking, consult your doctor immediately. If you have had a head injury, lost consciousness, but were not taken to an emergency room, you should contact your doctor.

Treatment Surgery is performed to drain blood clots when a CT scan indicates sizeable accumulations.

Prognosis Chances for recovery depend on the severity of brain injury but improve with prompt treatment. Recovery may take weeks to months. Possible outcomes include memory loss, intellectual impairment, muscular weakness in an arm or leg, or slurred speech, but patterns of recovery vary. Physical therapy may be necessary for weakness, stiffness, and poor coordination. The injury may be fatal in cases of damage to the vital centers that regulate breathing and blood flow.

❖ SUBDURAL HEMATOMA

Symptoms *(What you may experience)* Convulsions; loss of consciousness with weakness or paralysis after a head injury; numbness on one side of the body; headache; nausea.

Signs and laboratory findings *(What the doctor looks for)* Weakness; decrease in level of consciousness; changes in the fundus (the back of the interior of the eye) noted on retinal inspection; areas of pooled blood identified by CT scan; abnormal blood clotting tests; use of anticoagulants.

What is it? In a subdural hemorrhage or hematoma, blood slowly accumulates in the space between the dura sheath and the underlying subarachnoid membrane, the two

Subdural hematoma (arrow). CT scan shows how accumulation of blood puts pressure on the brain after a head injury.

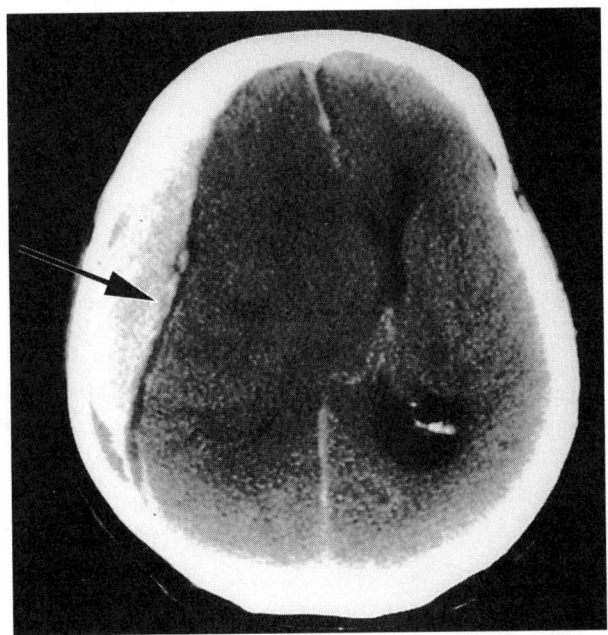

outermost layers of the meninges (the membranes covering the brain). The blood vessels that rupture are usually veins on the underside of the dura mater. A head injury—either from something as traumatic as an automobile accident or, in seniors, as apparently benign as bumping your head—can cause these veins to tear and form a blood clot, squeezing against the brain. The pressure placed on the brain by this mass, known as a hematoma, can cause the brain to shift and produces a spectrum of mental disturbances and neural defects.

Subdural hemorrhage or hematoma is seen most often in seniors who have sustained a fall and struck their head. Symptoms may emerge weeks to many months after the original trauma. The person may not remember the head injury, especially if alcohol was involved.

The degree of severity is associated with the amount of time elapsed between the initial development of symptoms and loss of consciousness. If the interval is less than 48 hours, the injury is considered acute. If it is between 48 hours and 2 weeks, it is subacute. If the interval is longer than 2 weeks, it is considered chronic.

Acute subdural hematoma often is fatal, despite prompt medical attention and surgical intervention. Subacute and chronic forms are not as dangerous but require medical attention when symptoms develop. Brain damage can result if untreated.

Aspirin and other types of anticoagulants increase the risk of bleeding in or around the brain.

What you can do If you are a senior, you can guard against falls by installing a series of rails in your home, especially in the tub or shower. Keep passageways well lit and free of obstacles. (See Chapter 3 for more information.) Be sure to wear a seat belt if you drive or ride in a motor vehicle, and a helmet if you ride a motorcycle or bicycle. Children who participate in sports or other physical activities, should wear head protection when there is risk of head injury.

When to call the doctor Any head injury that causes loss of consciousness should be investigated by a doctor.

Treatment Diuretic medications control brain swelling caused by sudden accumulations of fluid. Surgery may be necessary to locate and control bleeding, as well as to remove any accumulation of blood or clotted blood. If neurologic symptoms dictate, anticonvulsant drugs may be prescribed after surgery to control or prevent seizures that otherwise might develop. Such medications might have to be taken long-term because seizures may develop even 2 years following the injury.

Prognosis When the problem is promptly identified and treated, chances for a full recovery are excellent.

❖ EPIDURAL HEMORRHAGE AND HEMATOMA

Symptoms (What you may experience) Immediate loss of consciousness followed by a lucid interval for minutes or hours, giving way to rapid decrease in level of consciousness; progressively severe headache; nausea; vomiting.

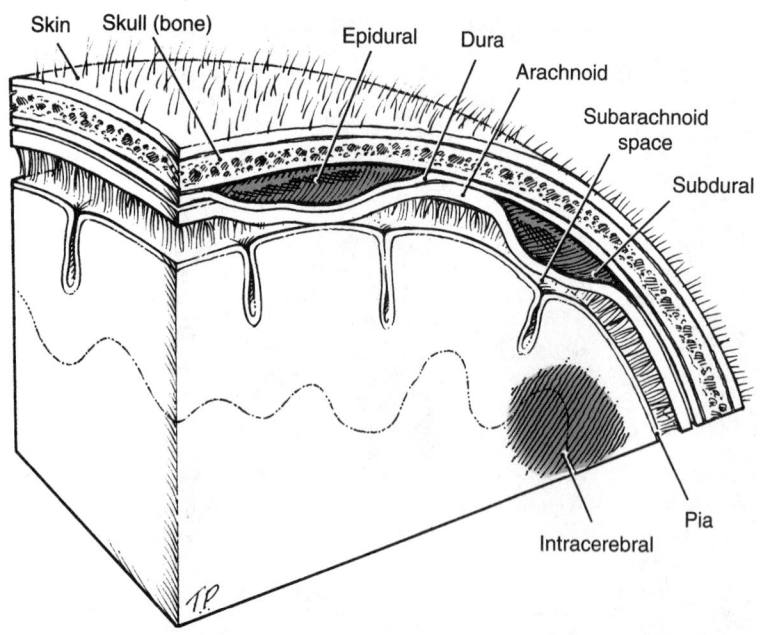

Types of brain hematoma. A collection of blood (hematoma) in or around the brain can be classified depending on its location. An intracerebral hematoma occurs within the tissue of the brain. A subdural hematoma occurs just under the dura, which is the outermost layer of the meninges covering the brain. An epidural hematoma occurs between the dura and the bone of the skull.

Signs and laboratory findings *(What the doctor looks for)* Specific neurologic deficits to pinpoint localization of the deficit; areas of pooled blood identified by CT scan.

What is it? Epidural hemorrhage and hematoma occur after severe head trauma usually involving a skull fracture, when blood vessels rupture on the upper side of the dura mater, the outermost meningeal layer that covers the brain. Blood flows over the surface of the brain between the dura mater and the skull. Because these are large blood vessels, blood accumulates rapidly and symptoms develop just as quickly.

The swift pooling of blood on the surface of the brain creates an emergency situation, because the fluid places increased pressure on the brain. If not relieved, it can cause permanent brain damage or even death.

What you can do To prevent head injury, wear your seat belt while traveling in a motor vehicle; wear a helmet if on a motorcycle or bicycle.

When to call the doctor Any head injury that causes loss of consciousness merits investigation by a doctor.

Treatment A craniotomy will be performed, wherein an opening is cut in the skull through which the damaged blood vessels are repaired, the pooled blood removed, and pressure on the brain relieved.

Prognosis If detected early and treated promptly, chances for recovery are good. Convalescence make take 6 months or longer, during which symptoms such as headache and difficulty in concentration may persist.

❖ SPINAL CORD TRAUMA

Symptoms *(What you may experience)* Symptoms are dependent on the location of spinal cord damage; there may be numbness and weakness; paralysis from the shoulders down; paralysis from the waist down; pain from injury to nearby nerves; loss of bladder or bowel control. Symptoms almost always appear immediately after the injury.

Signs and laboratory findings *(What the doctor looks for)* Deficits on neurologic examination; evaluation of ability to move or feel pressure; level of damage as assessed by MRI or CT scan; x-rays of the cervical spine are taken with the head and neck immobilized to check for neck fracture or displacement.

What is it? The spinal cord is a flexible conduit encased within the vertebral bones of the spinal column. Discs of cartilage separate these bones from each other. This permits you to bend and twist your back.

Unfortunately, your spinal cord is not invulnerable. Many things can pressure, damage, or even completely sever the spinal cord. These include: traffic accidents (44 percent of all spinal cord injuries), acts of violence (24 percent), falls (22 percent), sports injuries (8 percent), as well as other causes (2 percent). About 7,800 people sustain spinal cord injuries in the United States each year.

About 80 percent of people with spinal cord injuries are male. People between the ages of 16 and 30 have the highest rate of spinal cord injury.

The degree of injury depends on the site of the damage to the spinal cord. Generally, the lower on the cord the point of damage, the less severe the disability. The results may not be life-threatening, but spinal cord injury can result in total or partial disability that often is permanent. Weak and numb extremities are especially susceptible to other kinds of injuries. If nerves controlling bladder function are paralyzed, the individual may have recurrent bladder infections.

What you can do If you are driving or riding in a car, wear a seat belt. Never dive into shallow water. Hold railings when using stairs; use mats or rails that prevent slipping in the bath or shower. Be careful on slippery surfaces. Adults and older teens should not dive on children's water slide mats.

Because alcohol is involved in many spinal cord accidents, drink responsibly.

When to call the doctor Call for emergency help immediately. Do not move an injured person who may have a spinal injury. This is a job for emergency medical personnel. (See page 368 for information on emergency first aid precautions for spinal injury.)

Treatment Spinal injury is a life-threatening emergency requiring intensive medical

REHABILITATION AFTER PARALYZING TRAUMA

You, a friend, or a loved one may have recently become one of the 7,800 Americans who sustain spinal cord injuries each year. Thus, you may be one of the estimated 250,000 to 400,000 people currently living in the United States with some degree of paralysis.

Chances are you were in a motor vehicle accident, on the receiving end of an act of violence, or fell (these cause 90 percent of all spinal cord injuries). Only about 8 percent of spinal cord injuries result from sports activities (and two-thirds of those are from diving).

Slightly more than half of all spinal cord injuries result in quadriplegia, which is spinal and motor dysfunction in all four limbs. About 67 percent of people over the age of 45 who experience spinal cord injury are quadriplegics.

Overall, about 85 percent of people who survive the first 24 hours after a spinal cord injury are still alive 10 years later.

The aim of a spinal cord rehabilitation program is to teach people how to regain their independence. At most rehabilitation treatment centers, therapy is coordinated by a team that includes neurosurgeons, urologists, internists, physical therapists, and vocational rehabilitation specialists.

Psychological counseling may be an integral part of the rehabilitation program, because people with paralysis may experience intense sadness, frustration, and anger. Intense depression and anger can impede rehabilitation, but translating that anger into vigorous rehabilitative activity can often help relieve feelings of anger, depression, and helplessness. Motivation is a major factor in successful rehabilitation.

Physical therapy after a paralyzing injury often includes progressive resistive exercises done with weights, pulleys, and special exercise machines; a tilt table, which can be repositioned at various angles to help the cardiovascular system readjust after the person has been in bed for an extended time; mat classes, where, on mats, people relearn and practice skills needed for independent living (such as changing position in bed, getting dressed, and moving from one place to another); wheelchair classes, in which people learn how to negotiate obstacles while in a wheelchair; and, when appropriate, driver evaluation and training that will allow you to drive your own properly adapted motor vehicle.

Some questions you may wish to ask when evaluating a rehabilitation program are: Do people in the program have similar levels and kinds of spinal cord injuries? How many people are admitted to the program each year? Is the program accredited by the Commission on the Accreditation of Rehabilitation Facilities or the Joint Commission on Accreditation of Healthcare Organizations? Are there treatment specialists in the program who speak the same primary language as the person seeking treatment? Will the treatment team develop short-term and long-term goals? Is the doctor in charge a specialist in rehabilitation medicine (a physiatrist)? Is a doctor on duty around the clock all week? Are nursing and respiratory care available on a 24-hour basis? Will occupational and physical therapy be administered at least 3 hours each day?

You may also want to ask other questions about psychological and social counseling, facility policies regarding family members, and discharge planning. ■

care. The course of treatment will depend upon the nature and extent of the injury. Several recent advances in acute care of spinal cord injury, including massive steroid doses, are improving therapeutic outlook.

A neck injury can paralyze breathing. Immediate emergency care is necessary to prevent additional damage and even death. A severed spinal cord cannot be repaired, and nerves do not regenerate. If the spinal cord is damaged, but not severed, recovery will depend upon the extent of the damage.

Hospitalization after a spinal injury is usually prolonged, lasting from several days to several months. Keeping the spine stable and allowing time to heal is the primary therapy. Traction may be necessary to allow the back to heal. If necessary, antibiotics will be given for urinary tract infections and steroids to reduce pressure on the spinal cord. Surgery may be advised to stabilize injured vertebrae or drain accumulated fluid or bony fragments that can compress the spinal cord. As injuries heal, the extent of permanent disability and the possibilities for rehabilitation are assessed. Depending upon the extent of spinal injury, assistance may be needed for breathing, eating, moving on the bed to prevent bedsores, and for bladder and bowel relief. Once the body has healed, rehabilitation will begin. (See Rehabilitation after Paralyzing Trauma, above, for more information.)

Prognosis Spinal cord injury requires major adjustment and accommodation for daily routines. However, people who are paralyzed from the neck down can lead rewarding lives.

Tumors of the Brain and Spinal Cord

Any tumor of the brain or spinal cord—whether benign or malignant—can be dangerous, because of the potential for

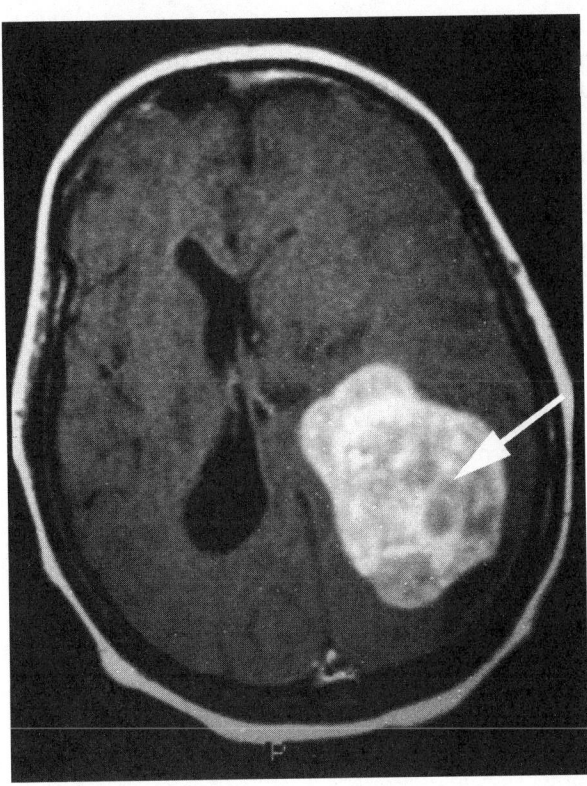

Brain tumor (arrow) as shown on MRI scan. This tumor originated elsewhere in the body and spread (metastasized) to the brain through the bloodstream.

compression of the brain or spinal cord. The damage done by tumors of the brain and spinal cord is due to their size. The vertebrae and bones of the skull cannot expand to accommodate even a small mass. As a result, the tumor presses on and displaces normal brain and spinal cord tissue. This may damage or destroy delicate tissue. Typically, neural deficits progress slowly.

These tumors most often arise from support cells of the central nervous system or as the result of metastasis (spreading of malignant cells from other sites in the body, such as the breast, lung, and skin).

❖ BRAIN TUMORS

Symptoms *(What you may experience)* Frequent headaches, which are most painful while lying down; nausea; vomiting; blurred or double vision; weakness or numbness on one side; hearing loss, unsteadiness; loss of smell; memory disturbances; personality changes; seizures.

Signs and laboratory findings *(What the doctor looks for)* Deficits on neurologic examination; signs of increased intracranial pressure, particularly as reflected on visual examination; CT and MRI are particularly helpful when contrast agents are used to visualize the tumor; identification of the tumor by brain biopsy.

What is it? A tumor is an abnormal growth of tissue. About 70 percent of primary brain tumors are benign (noncancerous), do not spread, and have distinct boundaries. The other 30 percent are malignant (cancerous), which is always life-threatening. They may, but usually do not, spread to other locations in the brain or spinal cord.

Brain tumors are either primary or metastatic. Primary tumors develop in the brain and, with one notable exception, do not travel to other parts of the body (the exception is medulloblastoma, which can spread to the lymph nodes, bone marrow, lungs, or elsewhere). Primary tumors are classified into two groups: gliomas, which are composed of glial cells that invade neighboring tissue; and nonglial tumors, which compress neighboring tissue rather than invade it.

Metastatic tumors originate elsewhere in the body but spread to the brain via the bloodstream. They are the most common form of brain tumor, outnumbering primary brain tumors by about 100,000 new cases each year.

Primary malignant brain tumors are the second most common cause of cancer death in children and adults up to age 34; they are the third most common form of cancer death in men 35 to 54 years of age.

The most common childhood primary central nervous system tumors are astrocytoma, medulloblastoma, and ependymoma. The most common adult tumors are metastatic brain tumors from the lung, breast, melanoma, and other cancers; glioblastoma multiforme; malignant astrocytoma; and meningioma.

About half of all brain tumors and about one-fifth of all primary spinal cord tumors are gliomas, growing from support cells called glial cells. An example of gliomas is:

- Astrocytoma—the most common type of primary brain tumor. They develop from star-shaped cells called astrocytes. They also may occur in the brain stem and spinal cord.

Examples of brain tumors that are not gliomas are:

- Chordoma—more common in people in their 20s and 30s. They are often slow-growing.

- Medulloblastoma—represent more than 25 percent of all childhood brain tumors. They occur more often in children than adults and often arise in the cerebellum in the lower part of the brain.

- Meningioma—benign; originate from the membranes covering the brain and spinal cord in favored sites along the under surface and front face of the brain. They account for 15 percent of all brain tumors and about 25 percent of all primary spinal cord tumors. They affect people of all ages but are most common in people in their 40s.

- Schwannoma—benign. They arise from cells covering the cranial nerve fibers, particularly the hearing and balance nerve and vagus nerve. They may grow on one or both sides of the brain.

Treatment Surgical removal is often the best means of treating a brain tumor, even if it involves a crucial part of the brain. Surgery can be guided by MRI studies that map out crucial functional areas to lessen postoperative disabilities. Sometimes it may be possible only to remove a portion of the tumor. In either case, surgery generally is followed by radiation or chemotherapy to kill remaining tumor cells. (See Chapter 30 for more information on the treatment of cancer.) Steroid drugs may help reduce brain tissue swelling. Anticonvulsant drugs can control seizures, and analgesics can relieve headache pain. Surgery is not necessary for small, asymptomatic meningiomas, a common finding on MRI.

Children with brain tumors are likely to receive the best possible treatment and care at pediatric cancer centers. Brain surgery in adults is likely to be most successful when performed at major teaching hospitals that perform these operations frequently.

Prognosis Long-term outlook depends on a number of factors—what type of tumor is involved, where in the brain is it located, what stage it is in (that is, how long and fast it has been growing). Both benign and malignant tumors can cause neurologic impairment by compression and invasion, respectively. Benign tumors are often curable; however, if they are located in an inaccessible spot, complete removal may be difficult, making recurrence possible. Some tumors grow so fast that treatment is not possible. However, in many cases, a tumor found at an early stage can be removed completely. Tumor removal by surgery is increasingly guided by preoperative imaging studies and monitoring during surgery to limit neural injury from cutting or stretching areas of the brain and cranial and peripheral nerves.

❖ SPINAL CORD TUMORS

Symptoms (*What you may experience*) Persistent back pain; numbness or cold sensations; muscle weakness in one or more limbs; urinary or bowel problems.

Signs and laboratory findings (*What the doctor looks for*) Sensory numbness; spasticity (stiffness) of muscle tone; weakness; loss of coordination; abnormal reflexes shown on neurologic exam; visualization of tumor on CT or MRI scan.

What is it Spinal cord tumors are similar to brain tumors in that they are tissue masses that develop in the central nervous system. As they grow, they place more and more pressure on the delicate network of nerves that makes up the spinal cord. Spinal cord tumors occur far less frequently than brain tumors, and are benign in 60 percent of all cases.

When to call the doctor If you have persistent back pain for no apparent reason, along with a numbing sensation or muscle weakness in one or more limbs, consult your doctor as soon as possible. Prompt treatment can minimize the possibility of permanent disability.

Treatment Surgery to remove bone and tumors will decompress the spine and spinal cord contained in it. Spine may need stabilizing. Treatment depends on tumor size, location, and stage of growth. Some tumors may be removed surgically, but others may be inaccessible; in these cases, radiation therapy may be needed. Corticosteroids may be administered to reduce swelling. If pain is a symptom, analgesics may be prescribed. As with most forms of cancer, early detection and treatment offer the best chance for cure. Because there may be some residual damage following treatment, a program of physical therapy may improve mobility and strengthen muscles that may have weakened from nonuse. (See Chapter 30 for more information on the treatment of cancer.)

Prognosis Long-term outlook depends on the type of tumor, its exact location, and how long it has existed. Removing the tumor could result in neurologic impairment if the spinal cord is damaged. Benign tumors are often curable, but complete removal may be difficult, making recurrence possible. This emphasizes the need for long-term follow-up imaging studies.

EVALUATING SLEEP

You may find that you are excessively sleepy during the day or that you just can not seem to get to sleep at night. You have tried counting sheep, drinking warm milk before bedtime, and taking over-the-counter sleep aids. Nothing seems to work.

Your next bet may be to ask your doctor to refer you to a sleep disorders center, where specialists in this field of medicine can evaluate your specific problem.

After hearing your specific complaints and your sleep partner's description of your sleep patterns and behavior, the sleep specialists will administer a night-long test called polysomnography.

The test usually is carried out during the night so that normal sleep patterns can be reproduced. Technicians will place electrodes on your scalp, the outer edge of your eyelids, and the skin on your chin. These electrodes will record your brainwave activity and eye movements during sleep. Other measurements taken while you sleep are your respiratory rate, blood pressure, how well your blood is saturated with oxygen, and heart rhythm.

In addition, a video recording will be made of you so that there is a record of your movements during sleep.

You should not take any sleeping medication or drink alcohol or a caffeinated beverage before the test.

The test will allow doctors to evaluate your rapid eye movement (REM) sleep and your nonrapid eye movement (NREM) sleep. REM sleep is associated with dreaming and generalized muscle paralysis (except for the eye muscles and diaphragm). NREM sleep has four distinct stages identifiable by specific brainwave patterns. REM sleep and NREM sleep alternate with each other about every 90 minutes. A person with normal sleep has about four to five cycles of REM and NREM sleep during a night.

Costs vary depending on the measurements made, how often the tests are to be repeated, and fees for the sleep laboratory.

Polysomnography is useful in diagnosing sleep apnea (a condition in which breathing can stop many times each night during sleep, leading to multiple waking episodes); other breathing difficulties during sleep; and insomnia. The video recordings are helpful in assessing movement problems such as restless legs syndrome and sleepwalking.

In some cases you may also undergo another sleep assessment called a multiple sleep latency test. This follows an overnight sleep study with a series of similar analyses during daytime naps to assess the degree of daytime sleepiness. This test is useful in diagnosing narcolepsy. ■

Sleep Disorders

About one-eighth to one-quarter of the population of the United States has some form of sleep difficulty. Poor sleep adversely affects daytime mood and performance. Persistent insomnia has been associated with a higher risk of clinical anxiety or depression. (For more information on the healthy benefits of proper sleep, see Sleep and Your Health, page 312.)

Sleep consists of a rapid-eye-movement (REM) phase and a nonrapid eye movement (NREM) phase. We dream during REM sleep.

The brain is active and requires more blood and oxygen. NREM sleep is the quiet and restful stage of sleep. The stages of sleep occur in a repetitive cycle of NREM followed by REM, with each phase lasting about 90 minutes. Thus, the sleep cycle is repeated 4 to 6 times during a 7- to 8-hour sleep period.

When our sleep patterns are interrupted, we can feel "fuzzy," tired, apathetic, and unenthusiastic. We may think less clearly and our social interactions may not proceed smoothly. People deprived of sleep for a long period can become psychologically disturbed.

Disorders of initiating and maintaining sleep are the most common, but disorders of excessive sleepiness, disorders of the sleep-wake cycle, and disorders during sleep also occur.

❖ INSOMNIA

***Symptoms** (What you may experience)* Difficulty falling asleep; frequent awakening with difficulty returning to sleep; awakening earlier than desired. Daytime somnolence and depression can occur as a result of insomnia.

***Signs and laboratory findings** (What the doctor looks for)* Illnesses that could affect sleep as identified by medical history; a sleep diary filled out by the person or bed partner.

What is it? Men and women of all age groups suffer from insomnia, although women and seniors seem to be more susceptible. Because people need a varying amount of sleep, insomnia is not defined by the failure to sleep a specific number of hours. It is, however, regarded as not getting "enough" sleep. Some people with insomnia may actually sleep more than they perceive; but for unknown reasons, possibly related to the quality and nature of their sleep cycle, their sleep is inadequate, producing daytime fatigue and lethargy.

The causes of transient insomnia are varied, but can often be readily identified and remedied. Causes include stress, environmental noise, extreme temperatures, changes in the surrounding environment, and medications.

Chronic insomnia persists for longer than 3 weeks. It is more complex and often results from a combination of factors that can include depression; arthritis; kidney disease; heart failure; asthma; and other sleep disorders, such as sleep apnea (brief interruptions of breathing during sleep; see page 490). Behavioral factors also may be involved. These include caffeine use; alcohol or other substance abuse; shift work or other sleep/wake disruption; chronic stress. Smoking cigarettes before attempting sleep and excessive daytime napping can contribute to chronic insomnia.

What you can do Temporary insomnia can be addressed by isolating and dealing with the cause. For example, cutting out coffee after dinner may work wonders. Stress counseling may enhance quality of sleep.

Other practices will help you sleep better. Go to bed at the same time each night; rise at the same time each day; exercise regularly; keep your bedroom temperature at a comfortable level; make sure your bedroom is dark and quiet enough. Avoid using over-the-counter sleeping pills; eventually, they can worsen the problem. (For more information, see Tips for a Better Night's Sleep, this page.)

When to call the doctor If you cannot identify the cause of your inability to sleep and/or daytime sleepiness is interfering with daily activities, consult your doctor.

TIPS FOR A BETTER NIGHT'S SLEEP

Do you relax with a cup of coffee or an alcoholic nightcap before bed? Do you watch TV in bed before going to sleep? Do you go to bed at a different time every night? If so, you may be contributing to your insomnia.

Here are some things you can do that may help you get a more restful night:

- Go to bed at the same time every night.

- Get up at the same time every day.

- Get regular exercise every day.

- Keep the temperature in your bedroom at a comfortable setting.

- Make sure your bedroom is dark enough and quiet enough for sleep.

- Use your bed only for sleep and sex.

- Take medications only as directed.

- When you go to bed, relax your muscles, beginning with your feet and working your way up to your head.

There are also some things you should avoid doing to get a better night's sleep. These are as follows:

- Avoid exercising just before you go to bed.

- Avoid stimulating activity just before bed (such as a competitive game).

- Avoid caffeine.

- Do not watch television in bed.

- Do not use alcohol as a sleep aid.

- Do not take another person's sleeping pills.

- Do not lie in bed awake for more than 30 minutes. If you cannot sleep, get out of bed and read, or drink some warm milk, or do something else you find relaxing. After a while, return to bed to sleep. ■

SLEEPING PILLS

Medication to help you sleep, whether over-the-counter or prescription, is not appropriate for nightly use. Sleeping pills can be helpful for occasional use when you are having difficulty sleeping, but they are not safe for use night after night. If you are unable to fall asleep nightly without taking a pill, you should consult your doctor in search of possible causes and more effective and safe solutions.

Over-the-counter sleeping pills are not always effective, and they may cause seniors to be confused. If your doctor prescribes sleeping pills for you, use them only as directed. If taken for more than 2 weeks, they may actually worsen insomnia. Do not drink alcohol if you take sleeping pills.

If you are older and taking sleeping pills, you may be more likely to fall if you get up during the night. If you have to get up at night, do so slowly. Sit on the edge of the bed for a minute and walk carefully to where you have to go. Either turn on the lights or use a flashlight.

Barbiturates, such as Seconal, and benzodiazepines, such as Valium, are sedative-hypnotic medications that can be used as tranquilizers and as sleep aids. They are prescribed to reduce anxiety, make a person less fretful, and promote sleep.

But some people can become psychologically and physically dependent on these medications. People begin to depend on the medications for their stress-reduction effects and to enjoy the "good" feelings the medications bring with them. They find that they cannot sleep without them. Then, as the body becomes tolerant of them, larger doses are needed to produce similar effects. Discontinuation of the medication at this stage results in withdrawal.

Withdrawal from these medications can be severe and life-threatening. Symptoms include rapid pulse, weakness, convulsions, hallucinations, anxiety, restlessness, and temporary psychoses. Withdrawal should only be attempted in a controlled setting under the care and supervision of a doctor.

One substance that has received attention as a potential sleep aid is melatonin. Melatonin is a naturally occurring hormone produced by the pineal gland, which is located at the base of the brain. Scientists are investigating whether it plays a role in promoting sleep and regulating daily rhythms, but this has not been proven.

Health food stores sell synthetic melatonin as a nutritional supplement; because of this, it is not subject to regulation by the Food and Drug Administration (FDA). However, the FDA's Office of Consumer Affairs states it is "not aware of any substantial published scientific evidence which documents that any melatonin products are generally recognized as safe and effective for sleeplessness and other conditions." Most doctors recommend that you exercise caution in using melatonin, since its safety has not been established. And keep in mind that most melatonin pills come in larger doses than may be necessary to aid sleep. Like other sleeping aids, melatonin's efficacy seems to diminish with continued use. If you are using melatonin, be sure to check with your doctor or pharmacist. Mixing melatonin with certain drugs can cause potentially dangerous reactions.

Certain foods contain melatonin, so you might want to think about including such foods in your evening meal. These include oats, sweet corn, rice, barley, ginger, tomatoes, and bananas. ■

Your doctor can offer treatment for insomnia, but will also want to rule out more serious disorders as the cause.

Treatment Your doctor will first determine if there is obstructive sleep apnea present. Asthma, heart disease, kidney disease, arthritis, or depression can cause insomnia; proper treatment of the underlying cause may offer relief. Sometimes medications prescribed for other conditions can cause insomnia. Review with your doctor all medications you are currently taking to determine if substitutions may bring relief. If discomfort from pain or illness is keeping you up at night, speak to your doctor about pain relief that can improve your sleep.

Daytime naps can contribute to nighttime insomnia. But daytime naps may be a way to make up for lost sleep for those who have chronic conditions, such as arthritis, that cause pain when they maintain one position for too long. If painful joints wake you up, do not lie in bed waiting for sleep to return. Get up, stretch, read, drink warm milk, and then return to bed to complete your sleep.

When dealing with chronic insomnia not caused by some other physical disorder, the first step is to diagnose and treat any underlying psychological problem or behavior that can interfere with sleep. Behavioral techniques, such as relaxation therapy, sleep restriction therapy, or reconditioning, may offer more promise than drug therapy.

In relaxation therapy, specific techniques are taught to reduce or eliminate tension and induce restful sleep.

Some people who experience insomnia spend too much time in bed unsuccessfully trying to sleep. A sleep-restriction program begins by limiting time spent in bed. Gradually, the allotted time increases until a "normal" night's sleep is achieved.

OVERCOMING JET LAG

If you have ever traveled through different time zones, chances are you have experienced jet lag. It is characterized by feelings of fatigue, disorientation and fuzziness, becoming irrational or unreasonable, and having broken sleep after arriving at your destination.

Just about everyone who travels on a long flight suffers jet lag to some degree. People who stick to a rigid daily routine and who are bothered by changes to that routine often suffer worst. People whose normal lives involve highly varied routines can often adjust better and adapt to a disruption of normal sleeping and eating patterns. People who sleep easily also can better cope with crossing multiple time zones.

If you have jet lag, perhaps the best thing you can do is try to step back into your normal routine as soon as possible. For instance, if you have just arrived at your hotel at 10 AM local time after an overnight 8-hour flight, try staying up until evening. If you go to sleep as soon as you arrive, you may be unable to sleep that night.

There are techniques to reduce jet lag. First, get a good night's sleep just prior to departure and make sure your personal and business affairs are in order. Get plenty of exercise in the days just before you leave.

Some studies have indicated that taking melatonin can combat jet lag; indeed, this is one of the few uses for which melatonin is recommended. Melatonin is a naturally occurring hormone produced in the pineal gland, which sits at the base of the brain. Peak levels of melatonin correlate with darkness, indicating that it plays a role in scheduling daily biologic rhythms (for more information, see Sleeping Pills, page 489).

Things you can do onboard an aircraft that can help you relax:

- Blindfolds, ear plugs, and pillows can help you get some quality onboard sleep.

- Walk up and down the aisle, stand, and do small stretching and twisting exercises in your seat.

- If you have an extended stop-over on a long flight, take a shower if facilities are available. ■

In reconditioning, a person learns to associate a bed only with sleeping and sex, and is advised to go to bed only when sleepy. If he is unable to fall asleep, he should get up and not return to bed until he is sleepy.

In some cases, a doctor may prescribe medication to help you sleep. Medication should be taken only as directed. Sometimes, the dose is gradually lowered until the medication is discontinued. Insomnia can recur if medications are stopped abruptly. (See Sleeping Pills, page 489, for more information.)

Prognosis Transient insomnia usually resolves itself. Chronic insomnia takes a little more work, but it often can be treated successfully.

❖ SLEEP APNEA

Symptoms *(What you may experience)* Daytime sleepiness; loud snoring; cessation of breathing during sleep; headache upon awakening.

Signs and laboratory findings *(What the doctor looks for)* Periods of decreased air flow (apneas) and drop in blood oxygen shown on polysomnography (electronic recording of body functions during sleep).

What is it? Sleep apnea is characterized by brief interruptions of breathing during sleep. Central sleep apnea is the less common of two types. It occurs when the brain fails to send appropriate signals to the respiratory muscles that initiate breathing. Obstructive sleep apnea occurs when air cannot flow in or out of the person's nose or mouth although efforts to breathe continue.

In a given night, breathing "pauses" may number as many as 30 per hour. These are almost always accompanied by snoring. Some people may experience choking sensations. Frequent sleep interruptions lead to early morning headaches and excessive daytime sleepiness. There is some question whether sleep apnea unduly stresses the heart. Because obesity contributes to both heart disease and sleep apnea, it is unclear whether high rates of heart disease in adults with sleep apnea are due to obesity or to sleep apnea.

Sleep apnea is common to all age groups and both sexes, but it seems to attack men with a somewhat higher frequency. As many as 18 million Americans suffer from sleep apnea, which sometimes runs in families. (For information on sleep apnea in children, see page 253.)

People most likely to have obstructive sleep apnea are overweight and snore loudly; they also have high blood pressure or some physical abnormality of the nose, throat, or other part of the upper airway.

Obstructive sleep apnea occurs when the throat muscles and tongue relax during sleep and partially block the opening of the airway. Obesity can play a role by narrowing the airway with an excess amount of tissue.

Alcohol and sleeping pills increase the frequency and duration of breathing pauses in people with sleep apnea.

What you can do If you are overweight, see Chapter 2 for information on losing weight. Avoid alcohol and sleeping pills.

When to call the doctor People are generally unaware of their own sleep apnea. If you observe the symptoms of sleep apnea in someone, alert him to the problem so he can consult his doctor.

Treatment Specific therapy is individualized, based on medical history, physical examination, and results of sleep studies. Medications usually are ineffective. Behavioral changes, such as losing weight and abstaining from alcohol and drugs, may solve the problem. In some people, breathing pauses only occur when they sleep on their backs. In such cases, devices that force them to sleep on their sides are helpful.

If behavioral changes are not successful, continuous positive airway pressure (CPAP) is the most common effective treatment. The person wears a mask over his nose during sleep. An air-blower forces air through the mask into the nasal passages. The air pressure keeps the throat from collapsing during sleep.

Surgery to increase the size of the airway may help some people. Other common procedures are removing the adenoids and tonsils, nasal polyps, and other tissue in the airway, and correcting structural deformities. In some cases, the person may undergo a procedure called uvulopalatopharyngoplasty to remove excess tissue at the back of the throat. However, this procedure is successful only 30 to 50 percent of the time, and success is difficult to predict.

People with severe, life-threatening sleep apnea can benefit from a tracheostomy. This involves placing a small tube into a small hole cut into the windpipe. During the day, the hole is closed and breathing and speaking are normal. At night the hole is opened, allowing air directly into the breathing passages, bypassing whatever obstructions exist in the upper airways.

People who are morbidly obese may benefit from surgery to treat the obesity.

Prognosis Once the problem is correctly identified, treatment options provide a good long-term outlook.

❖ NARCOLEPSY

Symptoms *(What you may experience)* Excessive and overwhelming daytime sleepiness; falling asleep at inappropriate times and places; cataplexy (loss of muscle function); sleep paralysis (temporary inability to talk or move when falling asleep or waking up); hypnagogic hallucinations (vivid, dream-like experiences that occur while dozing or falling asleep).

Signs and laboratory findings *(What the doctor looks for)* Abnormal results of polysomnography (electronic recordings of body functions during sleep) and multiple sleep latency test (which shows time needed to reach different stages of sleep).

What is it? Narcolepsy is a chronic sleep disorder characterized by excessive and overwhelming daytime sleepiness that leads to a person's falling asleep at inappropriate times and places. Daytime sleep attacks may occur without warning and may be irresistible. Attacks can occur repeatedly during the day.

Only about 20 to 25 percent of narcoleptics experience cataplexy, sleep paralysis, and hypnagogic hallucinations.

Narcolepsy can occur in men and women at any age, although its symptoms are usually first noticed in teenagers and young adults. About 10 percent of people with the disorder have a close relative who also has it. Narcolepsy may affect as many as 200,000 Americans, but fewer than 50,000 have been diagnosed. It often is mistaken for depression, a seizure disorder, or side effects of medication.

Although the cause of narcolepsy is unknown, it appears to be related to a neurologic problem affecting the sleep-wake cycle. During normal sleep, brain waves follow a conventional pattern. In the initial stage of sleep called non–rapid eye movement (NREM) brain waves becomes slower and less regular. After about 90 minutes, the person enters rapid eye movement (REM) sleep, where the brain waves become more active. In narcolepsy, the order and length of NREM and REM sleep are disturbed. REM (and dreaming) occur at the onset of sleep instead of after NREM sleep.

What you can do Schedule short naps throughout the day so that you feel rested.

Be sure to leave yourself plenty of time for sleep at night.

When to call the doctor If the disorder becomes severe enough to cause serious disruptions in your social, personal, and professional life, or if you have a close relative who has been diagnosed with the disorder, consult your doctor.

Treatment Treatment of narcolepsy consists of medication and behavioral changes. Excessive daytime sleepiness can be treated with a family of drugs called central nervous system stimulants. Antidepressants can be used to treat cataplexy and other REM-sleep disturbances.

Taking 15-minute naps a few times each day also can help control daytime sleepiness.

Avoid eating a heavy meal just before an important activity. Drinking caffeinated beverages also may help you stay awake during the day.

❖ SLEEPWALKING

Symptoms (*What you may experience*) Rising from bed in a state of altered consciousness, and walking around or performing other activities. Can last for 5 to 30 minutes; usually, there is no recollection of the episode when awakened.

Signs and laboratory findings (*What the doctor looks for*) A patient history is usually adequate, especially in children. More difficult cases require a polysomnography (electronic recording of body functions during sleep).

What is it? Sleepwalking, which most commonly affects children between ages 6 and 12 years, usually is a response to an emotional concern. It is more common in boys than girls, and it is estimated to occur in 1 to 6 percent of all children. Sleepwalking is not just walking, but is a term used to employ a host of activities a person can perform during a state of altered consciousness. They may include moving furniture, eating, and dressing. A sleepwalker has a blank expression and opened eyes and is usually difficult to awaken. He may awaken spontaneously, however, and is usually disoriented upon awakening—or he may return to bed and fall asleep again. If he falls asleep again away from his bed, he will be surprised to find himself there upon awakening.

Sleep terror, also known as night terror, is a related sleep disorder also seen in children: Sleep terror can occur with sleepwalking. The child sits up suddenly, expressing intense fear, and may scream or cry out. The child's eyes are open, and he is difficult to arouse or comfort. The disturbance subsides as he awakens. Sleep terrors, which occur during NREM sleep, are not the same as nightmares, which occur during REM sleep.

Sleepwalking and sleep terrors sometimes run in families.

What you can do The main risk to sleepwalkers is injury to themselves. So, if a family member is known to sleepwalk, make the house as safe as possible. Remove phone or electrical cords so the sleepwalker doesn't trip. Don't rearrange furniture. If there are stairways, you may want to install a gate at the top of each stairway.

Treatment Most children outgrow sleepwalking. Other than the chance of self-injury, the condition is harmless, and there is no need to call the doctor. If stress is contributing to the problem, however, counseling may be beneficial. Short-acting tranquilizers also may help.

Prognosis Most children outgrow sleepwalking by their late teens or early 20s.

❖ RESTLESS LEG SYNDROME

Symptoms (*What you may experience*) Unpleasant creeping or crawling sensations in the legs while lying down—often relieved by walking, stretching, knee bends, massage; involuntary leg movements while sleeping.

Signs and laboratory findings (*What the doctor looks for*) Diagnosis depends on descriptions of symptoms.

What is it? Restless leg syndrome is a disorder in which a person experiences unpleasant sensations in the legs. These sensations may be felt anywhere from thigh to ankle, but most commonly are perceived in the calf. One or both legs may be affected. Some people experience these symptoms in the arms as well. People describe an irresistible urge to move their limbs when they feel these sensations. Symptoms tend to worsen when relaxing or inactive. They also seem to follow a daily cycle, being more troublesome during evening and nighttime hours than during the day. Because the discomfort is most common at night, it disrupts sleep.

Restless leg syndrome can start any time, but it is more common and usually more pronounced in middle-age and older adults. Children and adolescents may be thought of as hyperactive because they cannot sit still. Symptom severity varies from day to day and year to year.

Although its cause is unknown, certain factors are associated with its appearance. These include: family history; pregnancy (symptoms usually disappear after delivery); low blood levels of iron (anemia); chronic diseases such as kidney failure, diabetes, rheumatoid arthritis, and peripheral neuropathy; and caffeine intake.

Because people with restless leg syndrome and a related disorder, called periodic limb movements in sleep, have trouble falling asleep and staying asleep, they may experience excessive daytime sleepiness.

What you can do Decreasing intake of caffeine may reduce symptoms. Supplemental iron (with doctor's approval) may improve anemia.

When to call the doctor If restless leg syndrome is affecting your job, social life, or recreational activities, consult your doctor.

Treatment In mild cases, a hot bath, massage, exercise, and heating pad or ice pack help alleviate symptoms. More severe cases require medication that includes benzodiazepines, dopaminergic agents, and opioids.

❖ BRUXISM

Symptoms *(What you may experience)* Frequent muscle contractions on the side of the face; tooth grinding noises during sleep; damaged teeth, gums, and bone; headaches.

Signs and laboratory findings *(What the doctor looks for)* Mouth x-rays and dental examination showing damaged teeth and bone.

What is it? Bruxism is the term for teeth grinding. It most often occurs during sleep but can happen during waking hours. Sometimes the noise made while sleeping is loud enough to awaken others. Continual tooth grinding can cause the gums and supporting bones in the mouth to erode.

Bruxism can be associated with a spastic motor disorder. It may be caused by stress and anxiety or by unconscious attempts to correct a faulty bite, which is the dental term for the contact between the upper and lower jaws when the mouth is closed. Alcohol can intensify it.

The condition affects between 30 and 40 million people of all ages and races in the United States.

What you can do Avoid alcohol.

When to call the doctor If you or your partner or child grind their teeth at night, seek help. Ignoring the condition can lead to permanent damage of your teeth and jaw bones.

Treatment If bruxism is a symptom of stress, seek counseling to help you deal with your anxiety. If it is due to a faulty bite, your dentist may be able to correct the problem. If you continue to grind your teeth, your dentist may construct a night-guard prosthesis to prevent tooth grinding while sleeping. The prosthesis consists of plastic splints that fit over the tops of the teeth to eliminate incorrect biting pressure.

Prognosis With proper treatment, prognosis is excellent.

FIFTEEN

Eyes

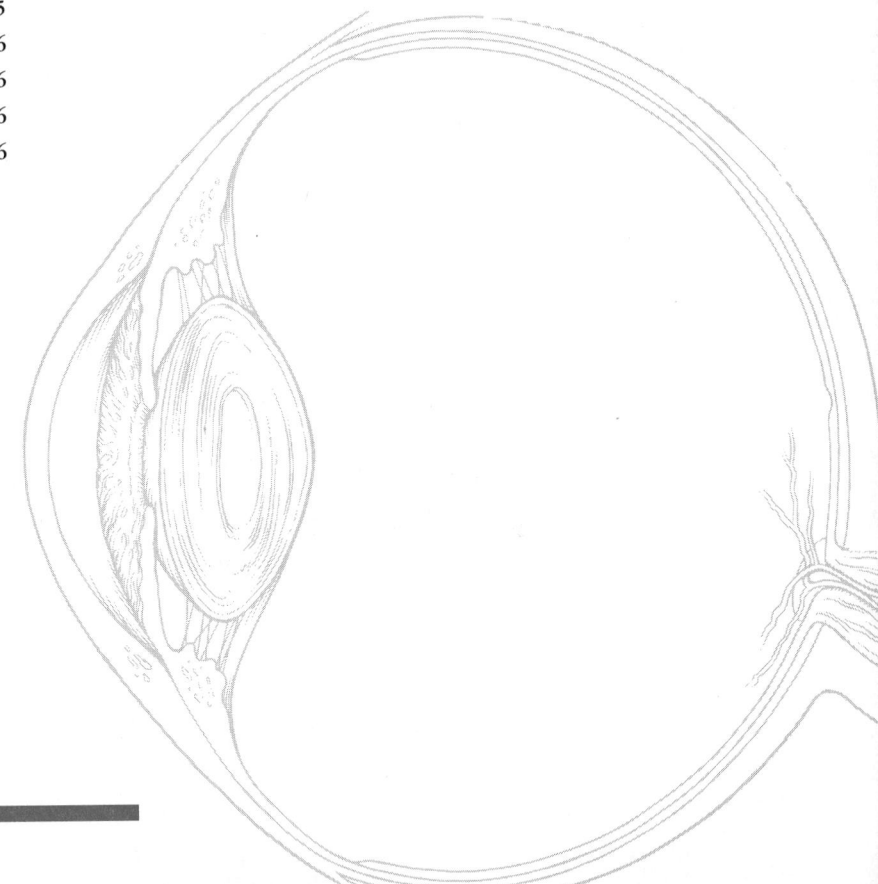

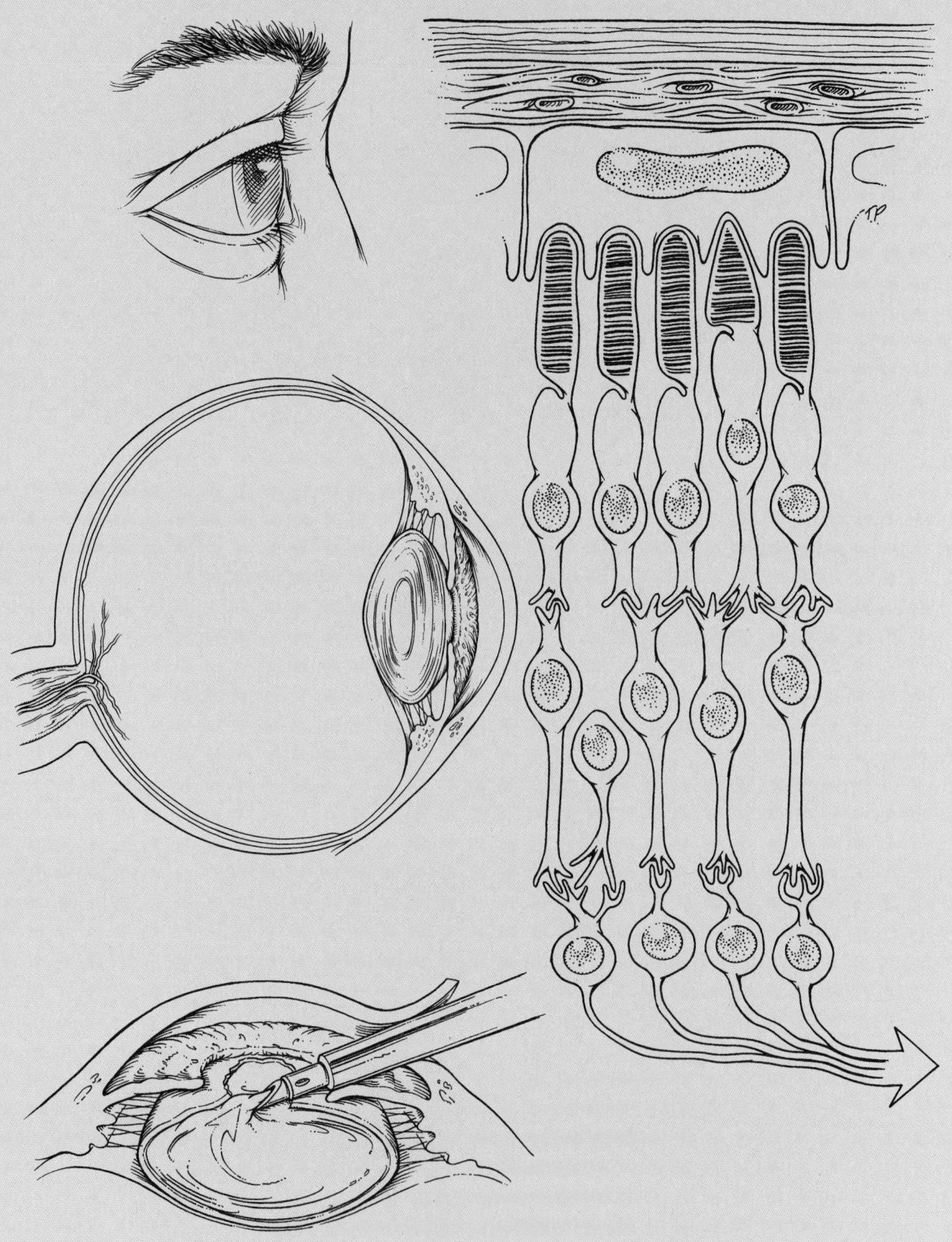

EYES

Anatomy of the Eye

Our eyes connect us to the physical world. They provide perception of light and dark and shade, color and movement and depth, from the small type on the page of a book to the vast panoramas of nature. They process millions of stimuli every day, both simple and complex, providing the input for our brains to paint an ongoing picture of our environment.

Vision is a complex process that involves gathering, directing, focusing, and translating light into images. The eye is an intricate structure composed of delicate tissues and blood vessels, some solid, some liquid, some viscous gel. Each of the parts of the eye is susceptible to disease or injury. Our eyes require attention all our lives and increasing attention as we get older, like many parts of our body.

The eye lies within a cavity called the orbit, which in the average adult is about 33 mm high (1.37 in.), 45 mm wide (1.77 in.), and 40 to 45 mm deep.

The bony orbit—the circle of seven facial bones where the cheekbone, the bridge of the nose, and the eyebrow surround the eye—is one of the main protectors of the eye. The others are the eyelids, both upper and lower. The eyelids contain the thinnest skin on the body and are controlled by muscles that open and shut involuntarily to protect the eyes from foreign particles, bright light, and trauma. The lashes along the upper and lower lids also help protect the eye.

The eyelids not only protect when they close reflexively but also serve the additional function of spreading the tear film. A properly functioning tear film nourishes the eye and is important for its health. There are three layers to the tear film: an oily top layer, a watery middle layer, and an inner mucous layer. Tears perform several purposes; they provide a smooth surface where the eye meets the air, carry debris off the eye, and supply oxygen to the outermost layer of the cornea, the front window of the eye through which light enters and begins to be focused. Tears also prevent eye surfaces from drying out and carry antibodies that help fight infection. Tears are primarily secreted by glands in your eyelids and orbit—the lacrimal glands—and they drain from your eyes into your nose through tiny openings in the eyelids.

Eye movement is controlled by six muscles around each eye in three pairs that are attached to different areas of the sphere of each eye. These muscles control side-to-side and up-and-down motion of the eye. The muscles of the two eyes act together so that the eyes move together, although in some conditions this coordination is impaired.

To understand how we see, it helps to know about the eye's components.

EYELIDS

The upper and lower eyelids provide dynamic coverage of the eye for physical protection and lubrication. The "windshield wiper" action of the eyelids cleans and nourishes the eye surface. The eyelids consist of delicate skin overlying fibrous tissue and the muscles of lid retraction and closure.

CONJUNCTIVA

This mucous membrane covers the inner surface of the upper and lower eyelids and the sclera. It stops at the limbus, where the white of the eye (the sclera) ends and the colored part (iris) covered by the cornea begins. The conjunctiva is nourished by a dense network of tiny blood vessels.

CORNEA

This curved surface in the center of the front of the eye is made up of layers of clear tissue. It contains no blood vessels, and part of the cornea, the anterior (front) stroma, is packed with tiny nerve endings, making the cornea very sensitive to pain when abraded. Light enters the eye through the cornea, which bends or refracts the rays of light through the pupil, where it is focused on the back of the eye. The cornea is responsible for approximately 65 percent of the focusing that the eye does. The center of the cornea is thinner than the edges.

IRIS

The iris is the colored part of the eye, the round, pigmented structure containing blood vessels and connective tissue that adjusts the size of the pupil. The iris works quickly and precisely in reaction to light and other stimuli (for example, drugs) to regulate the amount of light that reaches the retina in the back of the eye.

PUPIL

The pupil is the dark spot in the middle of the iris. It is actually an opening in the iris that changes size to accommodate the amount of light that enters the eye. The pupil contracts in bright light to limit the light that is entering the eye and protect the retina from too much light, and dilates (expands) in dim light or in response to certain drugs to allow more light to enter. In normal indoor light, the average pupil is about 3 mm in diameter.

SCLERA

The sclera is the tough white outer membrane that covers most of the surface of the eyeball, with the exception of the portion covered by the cornea. In contrast to the transparent cornea, the sclera is white and opaque. The sclera is covered by the overlying conjunctiva.

CHAMBERS

The anterior chamber is located between the cornea and the iris and pupil. It contains the aqueous humor, a clear watery fluid that is manufactured in the posterior (back) chamber. The posterior chamber is located between the lens and the iris. Behind that is the vitreous cavity, the largest section of the eye, which is filled with the vitreous humor, a clear, gelatinous substance.

LENS

The crystalline lens is comprised of two curved sections that meet in an ellipse. It is located directly behind the pupil. After the cornea, the lens bends and further focuses light. The lens does not contain nerves or blood vessels and is nourished by the aqueous and vitreous humors. It is contained within a capsule and is attached by a network of elastic fibers, called zonular fibers, to the wall of the eye.

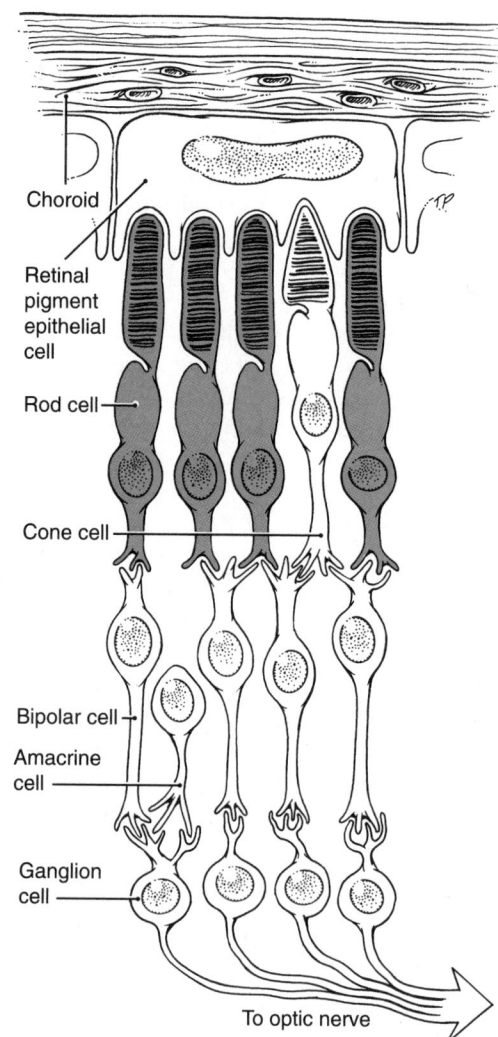

Choroid

Retinal pigment epithelial cell

Rod cell

Cone cell

Bipolar cell

Amacrine cell

Ganglion cell

To optic nerve

The retina is a layer at the back of the eye, similar to the film in a camera, which changes light into electrical signals that eventually reach the brain. The numerous rods provide peripheral vision and vision in dim light. Cones perceive light and color in the center of the retina. Other cells in the retina relay signals to the optic nerve.

The lens focuses light rays on the retina by changing the shape of its curvature, depending on the distance of the object being viewed. It thickens to focus on a nearby object and thins when perceiving something in the distance. The process by which the eye changes refractive power—refraction involves the way that light is bent by the cornea or lens—by altering the shape of the lens is called accommodation. As we grow older the lens accumulates more crystallines and becomes less flexible and less capable of focusing on nearby objects. This is why most people over age 40 have trouble reading small print or performing tasks that require seeing small things close-up without the assistance of reading glasses.

RETINA

You might compare the retina of the eye to the film of a camera, the place where the image is processed. The retina is a thin layer of transparent tissue at the back of the vitreous cavity and lines the inside of the back part of the eye. This tissue contains millions of light-sensing nerve cells, the rods and cones. Rod cells, which outnumber cone cells 20 to 1, perceive light; cone cells perceive light and color. The rods and cones change light images into electrical impulses, which are then sent to the brain via the optic nerve. The macula of the retina is a central area that contains the fovea where sharp central vision occurs.

FOVEA

The fovea is a depression in the center of the macula that is packed with cone cells and provides our sharpest vision. No blood vessels normally exist in the fovea. Cones, which are concentrated in the fovea, provide sharp central vision and perception of color and details. Rods are spread from the edge of the fovea through the rest of the retina and give us peripheral vision, perception of motion, and the ability to see in dim light.

RETINAL PIGMENT EPITHELIUM

The retinal pigment epithelium (RPE) lies under the retina and prevents blood vessels and blood products from the choroid from entering the retinal tissue and vitreous cavity.

CHOROID

The choroid is the layer of tissue rich with blood vessels that lies under the RPE. It also nourishes the retina. The choroid dissipates heat from the eye.

OPTIC NERVE

The optic nerve connects the eye to the brain. It transmits the impulses created by the retina to the visual cortex of the brain, which translates the impulses into an image.

How the Eye Works

With these basic structural relationships in mind, we can understand how the eye works and how we see. These are the basic steps in the process:

- Light rays reflect off an object and enter the eye through the cornea.
- The cornea bends or refracts the rays to pass through the pupil.
- The light rays then pass through the lens, which changes shape to further refract them. The convex lens inverts the image, turning it upside down.
- From the lens, the light rays pass through the vitreous humor to the fovea in the retina.
- The photosensitive cells of the retina transform the light into impulses that are sent through the optic nerve to the brain.
- The brain, in processing the impulses, turns the image right-side-up and translates it into a recognizable image.

Preventive Eye Care

Eye exams are recommended for people of all ages, beginning in childhood and continuing throughout life. Many serious and potentially blinding eye diseases hardly affect vision at all until their damage is done, and regular eye exams are the best preventive measure you can take for your eye health.

Most eye exams are painless with only a minimal amount of discomfort. However, the eye exam may seem like a mysterious process. The examiner looks at your eyes with different instruments, asks you to read or identify objects on various charts, and asks you to make a series of choices about whether you see one object better than another.

RECOMMENDED SCHEDULE FOR EYE EXAMS

The American Academy of Ophthalmology (AAO) recommends vision and eye health screening beginning in infancy and continuing through life for a normal child.

- Newborn baby: eye examination by a pediatrician or family doctor to determine general eye health

- 3 years old: screening for visual acuity (sharpness) by a pediatrician, family doctor, or ophthalmologist

- Age 5: preschool vision and ocular motility (eye movement) evaluation

- Ages 6 to 39: One initial comprehensive eye exam, then subsequent exams in the case of ocular symptoms, visual changes, or injury. People with risk factors should have more frequent exams

- Age 40: baseline comprehensive eye exam by an ophthalmologist

- Ages 41 to 65: Eye exam by an ophthalmologist every 2 to 4 years

- Over age 65: Eye exam by an ophthalmologist every 1 to 2 years

Risk factors indicating the need for more frequent eye exams.

- Low-birth-weight infants

- Infants whose mothers had rubella or a history of substance abuse, sexually transmitted diseases, or other medical problems during pregnancy

- Severe nearsightedness (see page 504), farsightedness (see page 505), or astigmatism (see page 505)

- Diabetes (see pages 1174 and 1179)

- Family history of diabetes, hypertension (high blood pressure), or glaucoma (see page 526)

- Blacks and Native Americans are considered at increased risk for glaucoma, because of a high incidence of this disease in these populations ■

EYE CARE SPECIALISTS

Ophthalmologist This is a doctor of medicine (MD) who specializes in diseases and conditions of the eye. In addition to 4 years of medical school after completion of an undergraduate degree, the ophthalmologist also has 3 to 4 years of specialty training in an ophthalmology residency program. An ophthalmologist treats eye injury and disease, performs surgery on the eye, and may prescribe glasses or contact lenses to correct vision. An ophthalmologist also manages disorders of the eye caused by many diseases such as diabetes or the acquired immunodeficiency syndrome (AIDS).

WHEN TO SEE AN OPHTHALMOLOGIST

Regular eye exams are important for everyone. In addition, if you experience any of the following, consult an ophthalmologist or ask your doctor for a referral.

- A change in vision in one or both eyes; may include a decrease in visual acuity, blind spots, double vision, flashes (see Floaters and Flashes, page 534), or new floaters

- Pain or persistent irritation (for example, itching, discharge, or a sensation of a foreign body) in one or both eyes

- Persistent problems with excessive tearing, or not enough tearing

- Recurrent conjunctivitis (see page 519)

- Any growth on the eyelid

- You are currently taking oral steroids. Cataract (see page 524) and glaucoma can develop as a result ■

Optometrist The optometrist, a doctor of optometry (OD), may be the first person you see when seeking help for vision problems. Optometrists specialize in correcting vision with glasses or other nonsurgical means (see Common Vision Problems, page 503). They prescribe glasses, contact lenses, low vision therapy, or other optical aids. An optometrist is not trained to perform invasive procedures such as laser therapy or surgery. Optometrists must complete a 4-year program in a certified school of optometry and be licensed by the state in which they are practicing. In some states, optometrists are licensed to prescribe certain medications for evaluating and treating eye conditions. If an optometry exam indicates signs of eye disease or other underlying health problems, your optometrist will refer you to an ophthalmologist for further evaluation.

Optician This is a technician who grinds and fits lenses, filling the prescriptions for glasses or contact lenses written by the optometrist or ophthalmologist. The optician will not examine your eyes or prescribe the correction needed, but will fit glasses and contact lenses to your face and eyes.

Ocularist An ocularist specializes in making artificial eyes and prosthetic devices for people who have lost their eyes because of disease, injury, or congenital (present at birth) defect.

THE EYE EXAM

The eye exam varies somewhat from person to person and from practice to practice. Some tests may not be given until a person is a certain age, for example, or unless certain indications are present. If you are seeing an ophthalmologist, parts of the exam may be conducted by a technician or nurse in the office.

Like any general medical exam, the eye exam begins with a personal health history. The examiner will ask about the reason you are having the exam and if there are any specific complaints. The examiner will also want to know if you have a history of previous and current eye problems. The history should also include your general health background; family history of diseases such as diabetes, hypertension, or glaucoma; any medications you are taking; and any allergies of which you are aware. The examiner may also want to know how you use your eyes at work and in your leisure activities to determine any special issues that must be considered.

After the history, the eye exam consists of eight parts, which may proceed in the following order.

Visual acuity Visual acuity (the sharpness of your vision)—also called refractive status—is measured by having you read lines of progressively smaller letters on a chart, known as the Snellen chart, in most instances. To test distance visual acuity, you will be asked to read the smallest line of letters you can discern on a chart 20 feet away. To test near visual acuity, you will read small print on a card close to your eyes. If you wear glasses or contact lenses, you will be examined with your already prescribed correction. Your eyes will be tested individually, with a paddle held over the eye not being tested. If you need correction, you will read the chart through a phoropter, an instrument with a combination of lenses of different strengths, and the examiner will be able to determine what strength lens gives you the clearest vision.

For small children who cannot yet read the letters on an eye chart, simple pictures on object-recognition cards are used. However, the child must be old enough for some sort of verbal communication before acuity tests can generally be meaningful. Babies can be checked for vision by evaluating their response to bright light or by determining if they can fix on and follow an object.

Normal vision has been determined as the ability to read letters 3/8-inch high at a distance of 20 feet. This is called 20/20 vision, and deviations from normal vision are measured against the 20/20 norm. For example, if you can see from 20 feet what a person with normal vision can see from 40 feet, you have 20/40 vision. A person with 20/200 vision in the better eye is considered legally blind.

Abnormal results of visual acuity testing may indicate nearsightedness, farsightedness, astigmatism, or presbyopia (age-related inability to focus on close objects). See Common Vision Problems for information on these conditions.

The part of the eye exam in which the examiner flips different lenses in front of your eyes and asks which is better, number one or number two, is to subjectively check your need for glasses by determining what the numerical value of the refractive error is. While there are no right or wrong answers, it is important to be as accurate as possible; if you can discern no difference between number one and number two, you should say so. This exam tells the doctor which lens the person has better vision with and consequently what prescription for glasses is needed.

The strength of the lenses needed to correct your vision problem is measured in units called diopters. The degree of nearsightedness is measured in negative numbers; the degree of farsightedness is measured in positive numbers.

The retinoscope is a handheld instrument that may be used in this portion of the

COLOR BLINDNESS

Color blindness—the inability to perceive or differentiate color, or some colors—is usually an inherited disorder. It is a vision problem that does not often present serious difficulties in life but can be restrictive. The name is misleading—few people with color blindness see the world entirely in black and white; only achromatopsia, the most severe form of color blindness, causes a complete inability to see colors. It is very rare and usually associated with serious refraction problems and other eye diseases. More commonly, people with color blindness do not see colors as brightly as do others or have difficulty discerning certain shades.

Most inherited color blindness is related to genes that are carried on the X chromosome and passed from mother to son. Color blindness is much more common in males than in females; 8 percent of men are color blind compared to 0.5 percent of women. Acquired color blindness can come from retinal disease, cataract, optic nerve disorders, or simply the process of aging, which dims colors for many people.

The cones enable us to see colors. Healthy cones distinguish among red, blue, and green and the multitude of combinations that comprise the spectrum. With red/green color blindness, the most common inherited variation, there is difficulty seeing red or green. Blue/yellow color blindness (trouble seeing blue and yellow) is almost always acquired. Few people will confuse bright red with bright green or bright blue with bright yellow. Rather, someone with a red/green defect may find that pastel shades of pink, yellow, and green look similar. With a blue/yellow defect, dark blue and green may look alike.

Color blindness cannot be prevented or treated and presents very little handicap to most people. In some cases, specific coping techniques are recommended, for example, a color filter placed over an eyeglass or contact lens to highlight color contrasts. Many cases of color blindness go undetected, although there are a number of color vision tests to diagnose and measure a person's color blindness. Color blindness is often tested for in routine vision screening. (See page C-46.) ∎

eye exam to objectively check the need for glasses and determine the refractive error. Through the peephole in the scope, the examiner will observe the reflex in your eye from a streak of light while you fix your eyes on a distant point in the room (often the Snellen chart).

The visual acuity portion of your eye exam may also test for color vision.

External exam As part of the external exam, the examiner will inspect and perhaps touch the various parts of the eye that are externally accessible: the rims of the orbit, eyelids and lashes, and tear ducts. The examiner will check for lid swelling, proptosis (protruding eyeballs), masses, and other problems.

Ocular motility This part of the exam concerns the movement of the eye, how the eye muscles are working, and if they are working as a team. It determines the presence of crossed eyes, also called strabismus, a condition in which the eyes are misaligned and only one eye focuses on the object being viewed. The examiner makes these determinations by closely observing the movement of the eyes as each is alternately covered and uncovered in a series of cover tests. Corneal light reflex tests are also used to assess eye movement, particularly in young or uncooperative patients.

Pupils The examiner will look at your pupils in both a lighted and semidarkened room to see if there are any irregularities in the normally round symmetric shape of the pupil. If there are, they will be investigated more thoroughly with the slit-lamp. Pupillary response will be further evaluated by flashing a bright light obliquely at the eye several times and observing the way the pupils dilate and constrict. Impaired response may be a sign of a neurological problem. Another test is the swinging flashlight test, in which the light source is swung back and forth from one eye to another. This determines how well the pupils work together and may help uncover optic nerve disease.

Visual fields In a visual field test, you will track a target (either handheld or through an automated electronic instrument) to determine the limits of your central and peripheral vision. Normal ranges vary, depending on the brightness, color, size, and speed of movement of the test object. For some visual field tests, you will be seated in front of a screen with your head positioned on a chin rest and press a buzzer or button when you see the target. Visual field disorders may indicate glaucoma, retinitis pigmentosa (see page 535), a brain tumor, or other serious eye or systemic diseases.

Slit-lamp exam The slit-lamp is a special microscope used for viewing parts of the eye. It provides a magnified, three-dimensional view of the structure of the eye and surrounding tissue. Light can be directed at the eye at various angles and intensities to view different parts. Usually the slit-lamp is set up so that you pull your chair up to it and put your chin in a chin rest. Through the slit-lamp, the examiner can see signs of infection or inflammation of the eye and detect early signs of cataracts or problems with the cornea. With special lenses, the slit-lamp can also be used to examine the retina. The slit-lamp can be used for diagnosing problems with contact lenses as well.

Tonometry The tonometer is an instrument used to measure the fluid pressure within the globe of the eye. This is an important test in the diagnosis of glaucoma, a disease characterized by increased pressure in the eye. There are several types of tonometers. The most widely used tonometer is attached to the slit-lamp and directs a puff of air against the cornea. The air is automatically turned off when light is reflected from the cornea; the amount of time it takes is a measure of the intraocular pressure. This test has some limits; while it does not cause pain, some people are uncomfortable with it, and it is also ineffective if there are any scars on the cornea. Other tonometry methods involve placing a drop of anesthetic on the surface of the eye and bringing the tonometer into brief, direct contact with the cornea.

Fundus exam The fundus (back of the eye) is viewed through an ophthalmoscope, a device consisting of a light that is usually strapped to the examiner's forehead and a magnifier that is handheld. The examiner can see through the pupil to the retina, retinal blood vessels, and the optic nerve head, where the nerve is attached to the eye. The ophthalmoscope is the only device that allows direct observation of a network of blood vessels in the body without surgery. Through the ophthalmoscope, the examiner can see early signs of certain systemic conditions that affect the retina such as diabetes, atherosclerosis (hardening of the arteries), and hypertension.

When your eye is to be viewed through the ophthalmoscope, you will usually be given dilating drops that open the pupil to give the examiner a better view. Find out in advance if you will be given dilating drops because your vision will be blurry after the exam and you may need someone to drive you home. Wearing sunglasses is a good idea after a daytime exam because dilation may cause an increased sensitivity to light that lasts for hours. The administration of dilating drops will lengthen the duration of your exam since

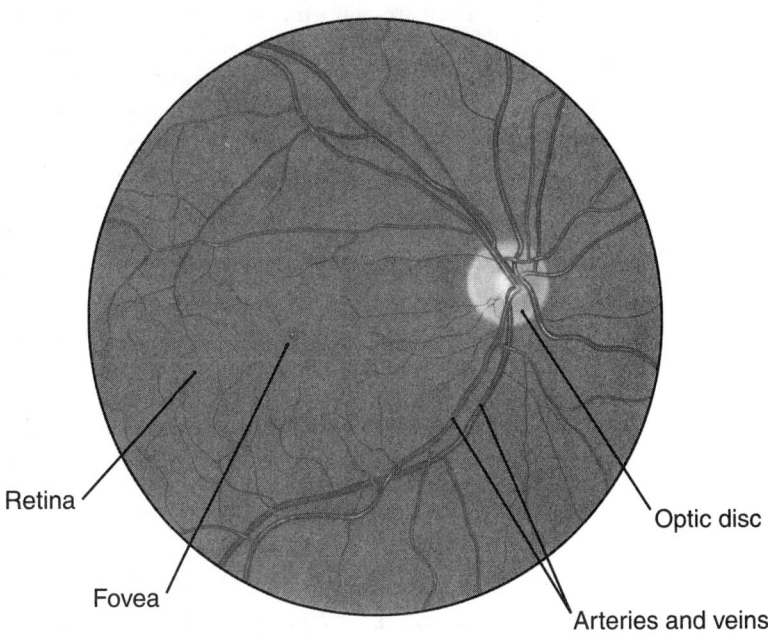

Retina

Fovea

Optic disc

Arteries and veins

The back of the eye appears this way when viewed through an ophthalmoscope, after using dilating drops to open the pupil. Signs of many diseases can be found in the blood vessels (arteries and veins), optic disk, and retina, which occupies most of the field. The optic disk has no sensory receptors, so is known as the blind spot. The macula contains fewer blood vessels, and vision is sharpest in its center (the fovea), which contains no blood vessels at all.

you will have to wait 20 to 45 minutes for your eyes to dilate.

The above tests are what you can expect in a thorough eye exam. If you are being examined for a specific problem, other tests may also be done.

Common Vision Problems

The most common eye problems occur due to errors of refraction including those caused by an eye that is too short or too long. In these cases, the light rays that hit the cornea or lens are not focused directly on the retina, where the photosensitive rods and cones can turn them into electrical impulses and send them to the brain. Instead, they are focused either in front of or behind the retina, or diffused. These refractive errors are not diseases of the eye;

they are abnormalities that are usually correctable at any time in adults. In children less than 8 years old, uncorrected refractive errors can lead to serious and permanent vision problems such as lazy eye—also called amblyopia—if not promptly diagnosed and treated.

Emmetropia is the term used to refer to normal or ideal vision—an eye that requires no refractive correction. Abnormal vision is called ametropia. Ametropia encompasses the four most common vision problems—nearsightedness, farsightedness, astigmatism, and presbyopia. More than 150 million Americans have a need for vision correction.

❖ NEARSIGHTEDNESS

Symptoms *(What you may experience)* Persistently blurred distance vision almost always accompanied by near vision that is clear. A nearsighted child whose vision is not corrected often sits close to the chalkboard or television screen in order to see, holds books very close to the eyes, is unaware of objects in the distance, or squints frequently. Parents often become aware of a child's nearsightedness when the child is unable to read words on signs or billboards.

Signs and laboratory findings *(What the doctor looks for)* Failure to see at a distance in the eye exam. Nearsightedness is easily diagnosed by visual acuity tests and by checking for the need for glasses. See Preventive Eye Care, page 499, for information on the eye exam.

What is it? Nearsightedness, also called myopia, is the ability to see near but not in the distance without glasses or contact lenses. The nearsighted eye focuses in front of the retina. The cause of this abnormality is unknown but there appears to be a genetic component because the condition runs in families. It is the most common vision problem, affecting more than 25 percent of the population in the United States (about 66 million Americans). Much higher rates exist in other parts of the world (in Asia, for example, the rate of nearsightedness is much higher than it is in North America).

Nearsightedness usually begins in childhood or early adolescence. Most children

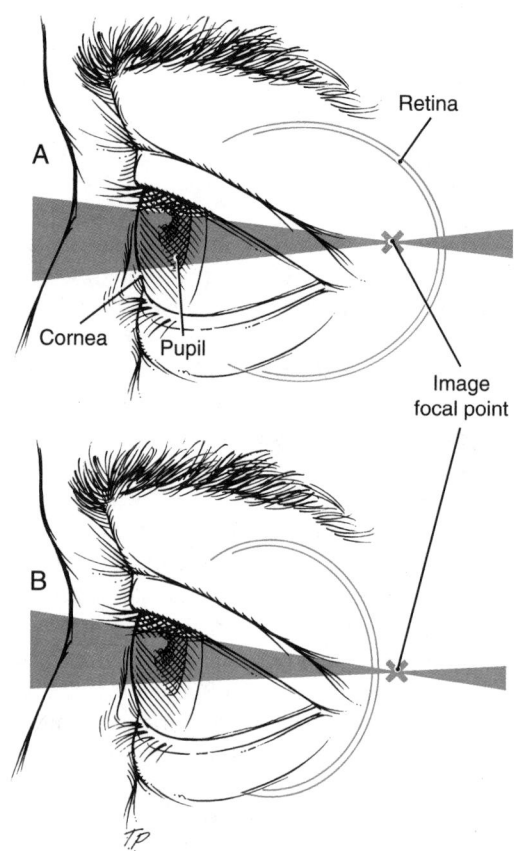

(A) In farsightedness, a short eye with a flatter, underpowered cornea or lens causes the image to focus behind the retina, blurring close objects. (B) In nearsightedness, the eye is longer than average and the curvature of the cornea greater. Thus the image focuses in front of the retina, blurring distant objects.

get progressively more nearsighted until their late teens or early twenties, when the condition stabilizes. The younger a child is when nearsightedness begins, the greater the progression is likely to be.

Acquired nearsightedness is much less common. Many diseases of the eye can cause it. These include keratoconus (see page 522), congenital glaucoma, diabetes, cataract, anterior lens dislocation (see Dislocated Lens, page 526), posterior staphyloma, scleral buckle placement (see Detached Retina, page 533), retinopathy of prematurity (page 538), and spasm of accommodation.

Anatomically, nearsightedness can be classified in two types. With axial myopia, the globe of the eye is not spherical, but elongated, causing the focus point to be in front of the retina. In the case of refractive myopia, the refractive power of the cornea or lens is too strong, causing the same effect.

When to call the doctor Because nearsightedness usually develops in childhood, it is up to parents, teachers, and health care providers to be alert to the symptoms. A child who experiences any difficulties seeing distant objects should have a prompt eye exam to prevent the development of a lazy eye and to exclude other potential causes of blurred vision.

Treatment Properly prescribed glasses or contact lenses can correct nearsightedness; surgical procedures may be an option for some people (see Options for Correcting Vision, page 506).

Prognosis Nearsightedness may be corrected with glasses or contact lenses. Most nearsighted people can expect to have their vision fully corrected.

❖ FARSIGHTEDNESS

Symptoms *(What you may experience)* Blurred near vision usually accompanied by clear distance vision. Common: headache; fatigue; eye strain; blurred vision after prolonged reading or close work.

Signs and laboratory findings *(What the doctor looks for)* Blurred near vision that slowly progresses until distance vision is also blurred; visual acuity test results. The signs may vary depending on a person's age.

What is it? Farsightedness (also called hyperopia or longsightedness) is the inability to focus on near objects. Close objects are blurred because the image is focused behind the retina. It is thought to be an inherited condition and tends to run in families. With axial hyperopia, the farsighted eye is shorter than the normal eye. With refractive hyperopia, the refractive power of the cornea or lens is insufficient for the image to be focused on the retina.

Farsightedness is usually congenital. Mild cases may not need correction and may go undiagnosed until adulthood. Children and young adults have an elastic lens that will accommodate for the short eye or deficiency in corneal refraction, and it may not even be noticeable. However, the lens of a person between the ages of 20 and 30 starts a process of slow and gradual hardening that will continue through adulthood, and this lessens its ability to accommodate.

Farsightedness is sometimes diagnosed when this process begins.

Certain diseases and disorders of the eye can lead to acquired farsightedness. These include some forms of retinopathy, tumors (tissue masses) in the eye, and lens dislocation.

When to call the doctor Visual screening in school may detect farsightedness. If a child experiences eye strain, headache, or has difficulty reading or doing other close work, an eye exam should be promptly scheduled.

Treatment Properly prescribed glasses or contact lenses can correct farsightedness. Surgical procedures are being used increasingly to treat farsightedness and may be an option for some people although they are more commonly used for nearsightedness (see Options for Correcting Vision, page 506).

Prognosis Farsightedness is usually easily corrected with glasses or contact lenses. Most farsighted people can have their vision corrected.

❖ ASTIGMATISM

Symptoms *(What you may experience)* Blurred vision, both near and distant; eye strain, headaches; frequent squinting may occur as a result of eye strain and headache.

Signs and laboratory findings *(What the doctor looks for)* Blurred portions on vision testing as detected in an eye exam. See Preventive Eye Care, page 499, for information on the eye exam.

What is it? Astigmatism results from variations or irregularities in the curvature of the cornea or lens. In the astigmatic eye, the cornea is oval or football shaped as compared to the normal cornea, which is round. In the astigmatic eye, the variations in the curvature of the cornea prevent all the light rays of a source from focusing at a single point, thus causing blurred vision. Astigmatism is a common problem; in many people it is mild and does not need correction. It is thought to be hereditary and runs in families. Astigmatism may also occur with other refractive disorders; approximately half of all nearsighted people, for example, also have astigmatism.

Astigmatism can also be acquired due to certain diseases and disorders. These include keratoconus, chalazion (see Stye and Chalazion, page 514), drooping eyelid (see page 516), and lenticonus, among others.

When to call the doctor Schedule an eye exam if your vision is blurred or if your child complains of blurred vision, eye strain, or headache.

Treatment Astigmatism can be corrected with glasses, certain contact lenses, or surgery (see Options for Correcting Vision, page 506).

Prognosis Astigmatism may increase slowly as a person ages but usually remains stable throughout life. The prognosis for excellent vision is good for people with astigmatism with glasses or contact lenses alone, unless it is caused by certain eye diseases and disorders such as keratoconus.

❖ PRESBYOPIA

Symptoms *(What you may experience)* Blurred near vision and increased difficulty in focusing on close objects; in people over age 40, eye strain and fatigue when doing close work. Distance vision is usually unaffected.

Signs and laboratory findings *(What the doctor looks for)* Decreased close-range acuity as detected in a visual acuity test.

What is it? Presbyopia—derived from the Greek words for "old eye"—is the diminished ability of the lens to focus, primarily on close objects such as the words on the page of a book. Through the years, the lens loses elasticity. This stiffened, aging lens becomes less capable of thickening, which is necessary to bring close objects into focus. Presbyopia is a normal part of the aging process and affects nearly everyone.

What you can do There is no way to prevent presbyopia. By age 50, nearly everyone has some degree of it. Good lighting when reading or doing other close work is one way to counter the effects of early presbyopia.

Treatment Properly prescribed glasses or contact lenses can correct presbyopia (see Options for Correcting Vision, page 506).

Prognosis Presbyopia will worsen through the years until about age 65 when the lens has lost most of its elasticity. A number of different options for correction—depending on presence of other refractory problems such as nearsightedness—make presbyopia mostly correctable.

Options for Correcting Vision

There are three main ways that refractive errors of vision can be corrected: glasses, contact lenses, or surgery.

GLASSES

Glasses have been used since antiquity and are still the most common method of correcting vision. While the science of optics is complex, the basic principle governing how glasses work is simple. The curvature of the lenses in the glasses compensates for the refractive error of your eye.

- If you are nearsighted, you will need a concave lens, which will adjust the focal point of your eye so that it is on the retina rather than in front of the retina.

- If you are farsighted, a convex lens will refract the light so that the focal point is on the retina rather than behind it.

- A cylindrical lens corrects astigmatism by sharpening the blurred image caused by the uneven cornea. For some people with astigmatism, cylindrical lenses cause problems of distortion, but adjustments in prescription and the way the glasses are fitted to the face can usually overcome these problems. If not, contact lenses usually are effective.

Simple magnifying glasses—the reading glasses you might buy off the rack in a pharmacy—are helpful for many people with presbyopia. However, when presbyopia is combined with nearsightedness or farsightedness, correction becomes more complicated. For some nearsighted people, the disorders cancel each other out, and they can read comfortably without correction. (Distance vision, however, still must be corrected.) Bifocals and trifocals are other options to make the corrections necessary for middle-aged and elderly eyes.

Bifocals correct for distance and near vision. The top and outer rim of the lens corrects for distance vision, while a smaller lens set into the inside bottom quadrant of the frame—the section you usually look through for reading or other close work—corrects for near vision. However, bifocals can be custom designed for a user's specific needs—for example, a reversed design for an airline pilot who may need to read through the upper part of the lenses when looking up at an instrument panel.

Some people, particularly as they grow older, need a third level of correction for intermediate, arm's length work (2 to 4 ft) that allows them to work comfortably at a computer terminal or read the prices on the supermarket shelf. If you find yourself straining your neck as you peer through the bottom part of your bifocals to read something that will not focus with your distance correction, you may need trifocals. Trifocals allow a person to focus on objects that are beyond reading distance but are closer than about 3 ft.

Traditionally, the lenses in bifocal and trifocal glasses have been separated by a line. This necessitates a jump, a quick change in focus, when you move from one section to another. Some people adjust to this very well but others find the jump disorienting. Progressive lenses offer an alternative and are becoming increasingly popular. In progressive lenses, also called multifocals, there is no visible line between the sections. A narrow—and invisible—band of gradual change separates the sections. Some people find that this seamless change translates into better vision while others prefer progressive lenses for cosmetic reasons, believing that the line in the lenses of traditional bifocals and trifocals is an unattractive sign of aging.

For some conditions, such as crossed eyes, prisms are incorporated into the lens. Prisms play a role in helping align the eyes. Clip-on or stick-on prisms can be tried before having the prescription ground into the lens.

Lenses in glasses are made of glass or plastic. Although glass is stronger, government regulations require that all lenses pass a test for impact resistance; they must be able to withstand the impact of a 5/8-inch steel ball dropped from a height of 50 in. Plastic lenses are more likely to scratch but they are 30 to 40 percent lighter in weight than are those of glass.

Coatings for lenses are available for several purposes. Coatings can reduce reflective glare, block ultraviolet light, and make the lenses scratch resistant. These are all useful features to protect your eyes and your eyewear. Sunglasses are recommended for anyone spending extended periods of time in bright sunlight. Dark sunglasses absorb as much as 80 percent of ultraviolet rays, which are known to cause tissue damage and may contribute to eye disease. Try to choose sunglasses that provide protection from ultraviolet A (UVA) and ultraviolet B (UVB) light. The higher the UVA or UVB rating on the glasses, the more protection they offer.

The fit of glasses is important for the best correction for your refractive problem. Lenses sitting too far or too close to your face can make glasses ineffective. When you get glasses, be sure to get them from a qualified optician who has experience in fitting glasses and offers a wide selection of frames.

Protective eyewear is manufactured for many purposes. A plastic called polycarbonate is used in lenses when special protection is needed for the eye—for example, by athletes, people in certain workplaces, or people who have already injured one eye. Polycarbonate is extremely tough and impact resistant; however, it is more expensive than is the material used to make conventional lenses. Safety glasses made of polycarbonate provide side shields to protect the eye and have other safety features.

Glasses work well for most people and are easy to maintain and relatively inexpensive. The disadvantages of glasses are that they may restrict peripheral vision and may interfere with some physical activities. Some people also do not like the way glasses change their appearance; others are bothered by the weight and presence of glasses on the face, and they are easy to lose or damage.

CONTACT LENSES

Contact lenses have developed as an increasingly popular and versatile alternative to glasses. Contact lenses—often just called contacts—came into widespread usage in the 1960s and today are used by more than 25 million Americans. They are suitable for correcting nearsightedness, farsightedness, and astigmatism. They are also used to correct blurred vision in eyes with keratoconus, and may be better than glasses at enhancing vision for people without artificial lenses implanted as part of cataract surgery. Contacts are also used therapeutically as part of recovery from some types of eye surgery.

A contact lens is a thin, delicate disc, smaller than a dime. Held directly on the cornea by the tear film, contacts provide a larger field of vision than glasses, without the peripheral distortion caused by some strong prescriptions for glasses. Technical advances have made contacts increasingly more comfortable to wear and a viable vision correction option for more and more people.

Wearing contacts, however, is not quite as effortless as simply slipping a pair of glasses on your face. According to the Contact Lens Manufacturers Association, as many as 20 percent of people who attempt to wear contacts stop wearing them. Using contacts requires a commitment to proper care of the lenses (see Proper Care of Contact Lenses, page 510), some manual dexterity in handling very small objects, and the willingness to tolerate some discomfort during a short adjustment period. Contacts are usually less feasible in small children but may be necessary in some cases.

With the increasing use of contacts, there are many reports of problems that result from their usage, and in some cases, these can be severe. In fact, infection is more commonly caused by contacts than it is by corrective eye surgery. It is important to be aware of early signs of problems from contacts and respond to them promptly by discontinuing usage and consulting an ophthalmologist. Sleeping with contacts on is not recommended.

There are three major types of contact lenses: hard lenses, soft lenses, and rigid gas permeable (RGP) lenses. Soft lenses may be disposable. When contacts were first developed, one of the biggest problems to overcome was keeping the cornea oxygenated. The different types of lenses address this in different ways.

- *Hard contact lenses* are made from a substance called polymethylmethacrylate. These were the first type of contact lenses used, but currently account for only about 2 percent of the American market. Hard lenses are rigid and thus more resistant to scratches and rips than are soft lenses. However, because of their rigidity, these lenses can feel uncomfortable on the eye, can be difficult to keep sufficiently wet, and may slip out of place. They also may have a tendency to pop out. With hard contacts, oxygen reaches the cornea only during blinking when the lens moves slightly.

- *Soft contact lenses*, also called hydrophilic lenses, are more comfortable to wear. About 85 percent of the contact lenses worn by people in the United States are soft lenses. They are made of hydroxyethylmethacrylate, a soft plastic that absorbs water. Because of their flexibility, soft contacts conform to the shape of the cornea. They are a bit larger than hard lenses. The water in soft lenses gives oxygen a medium to travel through to get to the cornea. The disadvantage of soft contacts is that bacteria will grow more easily on their surfaces than on hard lenses, and soft lenses must be regularly disinfected (see Proper Care of Contact Lenses, page 510). Soft lenses are also very fragile and wear out relatively quickly. In most cases, they must be replaced at least every 2 years. Some soft contacts are considered disposable and designed to be replaced after days or weeks of usage. Disposable contacts are thinner and more fragile than are other lenses but are very useful for users who have problems with allergies or chemical deposits on their lenses.

- *RGP lenses* are rigid like hard lenses but have pores in the rigid surface that allow oxygen to pass through. Because of their firm structure, these lenses often provide the sharp focus needed for people with astigmatism. RGP lenses are more durable than are soft lenses and are less likely to lead to infection or dry eye. They are also sometimes useful in treating people with extreme nearsightedness, with keratoconus, or following eye surgery.

The disadvantage of these contacts is that they may require a longer period of adaptation, but after a period of time most users report that RGP lenses are as comfortable as are soft lenses.

- *Toric lenses* are a kind of soft contact lens designed to correct for astigmatism. They have two different curvatures (like a donut) and the toric (curved) surface on the back of the lens helps correct the astigmatism. Toric lenses are weighted or are designed to stabilize the lens in place on the cornea so that it does not rotate with each blink, providing a sharper and more constant correction.

- *Extended-wear contact lenses* are soft lenses that are designed to be worn for days at a time, even while sleeping. However, most doctors now warn against round-the-clock contact lens wear. Studies by researchers from the Johns Hopkins Wilmer Eye Institute and other institutions found that people who wear contacts while sleeping are at least eight times more likely to develop damage to their corneas than are people who take their lenses out when they sleep.

Contacts also have cosmetic uses. Tinted lenses will change your eye color. Lenses with opaque tints completely cover the natural color of the iris and can give you the aqua, violet, or amber eyes you were not born with. Tinted lenses are clear in the center, though, and do not tint the world that you see.

Tinted lenses can also serve a more medical cosmetic purpose to mask iris or cornea malformations or an irregular pupil. Another use of tint is to color lenses so they are easier to see when handling. This light tint is not visible when the lenses are on the eye. Many contacts are also treated with shield that protects the eye by absorbing ultraviolet rays.

As you grow older and presbyopia develops, vision correction becomes more complicated. There are several options available for contact lens wearers. The simplest is to wear reading glasses over your contacts when you need to read or do close work.

Bifocal contacts are also available. While bifocal contacts have posed problems in the past, they have become increasingly refined and effective. There are two systems available. With simultaneous vision bifocals, the lens corrects for both near and distant vision at the same time. With these lenses, you look through both the reading and distance parts at all times, and your brain learns to suppress the blurred image and focus on the clear one. Translating bifocal lenses work in a similar way as bifocal glasses, with a divided prescription for each lens. These lenses generally have a thick lower edge, which keeps the reading correction in the lower part of the lens when you look down to read.

Another system that many middle-aged contact lens wearers with nearsightedness find effective is called monovision. With monovision, as the name suggests, one of your eyes—the dominant eye—will be fitted with the lens you need to see at a distance. The other will be fitted with the lens you need for close vision. For most people, the brain will automatically make the choice of which eye to use, and they will not be aware of the adjustments they are making. However, using just one eye at a time does pose problems with depth perception for some people. Often people will use a modified monovision system, using distance lenses in both eyes for tasks such as driving, which require maximum distance visual acuity.

Wearing contacts is not risk free. There are a number of medical problems that can occur as a complication of wearing contacts. The most important thing to remember is that if you wear contacts and experience any problems or symptoms, you should immediately stop wearing your lenses and get a medical evaluation of the problem. All contact lens wearers should have a backup pair of glasses for this purpose.

- *Giant papillary conjunctivitis (GPC)* appears as swelling on the inner surface of the upper eyelid and is often a result of a reaction to lens protein deposits, the lens itself, or the solution. The eye is itchy with a sticky discharge and reduced vision and makes lens wearing extremely uncomfortable.

- *Corneal abrasion* can occur when a tiny particle gets between the contact lens and the cornea or during improper technique when inserting or removing a contact lens. You will feel something foreign in your eye. It is

PROPER CARE OF CONTACT LENSES

In caring properly for your contacts, you are essentially caring for your eye. If you think of a contact lens as a foreign body that you regularly put in your eye, you can appreciate the need for meticulous hygiene and conscientious care when handling your contacts. An infection from a contact lens can cause serious vision impairment or blindness.

Always wash, rinse, and dry your hands before touching your lenses. If you wear makeup, insert your contacts before applying makeup, and remove them before taking it off. Water-based cosmetics do less harm to contacts than do oil-based. Try not to get lotions or sprays in your eyes. If you are experiencing any kind of irritation or problems with your eyes, stop wearing your lenses and see your doctor.

Use only the solutions your doctor has recommended. Use fresh, sterile solutions, and do not touch bottle tips to any surface. Never use tap water or saliva. Take your lenses out every night, clean and disinfect them, and let them soak overnight in a clean case with fresh solution. Avoid sleeping with your lenses on.

There are a number of solutions on the market, serving a variety of functions for different types of lenses. Talk to your doctor about what type and brand will work best for you. The basic types of solutions available include the following:

- Daily cleaners remove dirt and debris that accumulate on the lens. When you remove a contact, put it on your palm, put a couple drops of daily cleaning solution on the lens, and rub very gently with your finger on both sides.

- Rinsing and storing solutions further remove debris and provide a clean environment in which to store the lens.

- Disinfectants kill bacteria on the lens.

- Multipurpose solutions may combine the cleaning, rinsing, and disinfectant purposes.

- Rewetting solutions are like artificial tears to put in the eyes while wearing contacts to keep them lubricated.

- Enzyme solutions remove the protein film that deposits on your contacts. Some people tend to build up more protein than do others, but enzyme cleaning is usually recommended once a week. Enzyme cleaners are in the form of dissolvable tablets. ■

more common with RGP lenses than with soft lenses.

- *Corneal neovascularization*, the growth of abnormal blood vessels into the cornea (which normally does not have blood vessels), occurs when the cornea is deprived of oxygen. Usually a new type of lens or discontinuation of contact lens wear is suggested when this develops.

- *Corneal swelling* occurs because of insufficient oxygen to the cornea and may be associated with extended wear lenses. There are often no symptoms,

although some users experience blurred vision, halos, and pain when they remove their lenses. Avoiding overnight wear is the best prevention.

- *Infectious keratitis*, also called corneal ulcer, is potentially the most dangerous complication of wearing contacts. It may be caused by bacteria, fungi, or parasitic agents, and is often traced to improper cleaning and disinfection of contacts or to extended wear. Acute eye pain, the sensation of a foreign body in the eye, discharge, or red eye should be a signal to immediately discontinue lens wear and consult your doctor. Permanent scarring and decreased vision may result despite immediate treatment.

REFRACTIVE SURGERY

As anyone who wears glasses or contact lenses knows, the necessity for vision correction can be bothersome, inconvenient, or uncomfortable. This is particularly true if you require a strong refractive prescription and heavy lenses. Many wish for 20/20 vision without glasses or contacts. The idea of a cure for refractive errors of vision was little more than a dream until about 20 years ago, when a surgical technique called radial keratotomy came into use for correcting nearsightedness.

Advances in techniques of microsurgery have not only made radial keratotomy surgery safer and more effective, but have also opened the doors for a number of new procedures and improvements in refractive surgery. We are now entering a new era of refractive surgery, with increasingly refined and varied techniques and options available to improve visual acuity.

Bear in mind, however, that refractive surgery is not for everyone, and successful outcomes cannot be guaranteed. You should consult your doctor if you are considering this option and carefully go over the benefits and risks. One essential precaution is to never have both eyes operated on at the same time. Only an ophthalmologist can perform this surgery; seek someone with experience and a good track record. See Chapter 32 for information on selecting a surgeon.

Each procedure poses its own set of possible side effects or complications, but there are a number of side effects common to the different types of refractive surgery. In the immediate postoperative period, these include the following:

- Pain
- Sensitivity to light
- Blurred vision
- Overcorrection or undercorrection
- Glare or haze
- Starburst effect
- Induced astigmatism

These problems usually diminish and disappear during the healing period. More serious complications are rare and include the following:

- Infection
- Inadequate healing
- Persistent, irregular astigmatism
- Unstable vision
- Progressive overcorrection

The most common forms of refractive surgery are radial keratotomy and photorefractive keratectomy (PRK), which is done with a laser. Other techniques are still in research phases, but show much promise for people with severe or complicated vision problems.

Radial Keratotomy After more than a million procedures worldwide and a decade of follow-up, it is clear that radial keratotomy can allow many people with mild to moderate nearsightedness to lead their lives without glasses or contacts. At least 85 percent of people who have radial keratotomy can pass a standard eye exam for a driver's license (requiring at least 20/40 vision) without glasses or contacts. While people with mild nearsightedness usually have the best results, the final visual outcome for any person cannot be predicted.

Radial keratotomy surgery is performed on an outpatient basis, and the procedure itself takes less than a half hour to complete. Some people may be given medication to help them relax before the surgery. Anesthesia in the form of eyedrops will numb the eye. Then the doctor will make a series of incisions (usually four to eight, depending on the severity of the nearsightedness) starting near the center of the cornea and radiating outward like the spokes of a wheel. The incisions are the depth of about 80 to 90 percent of the thickness of the cornea. The center of the cornea through which light passes, known as the central optic zone, is not cut.

The effect of these incisions is to relax the edges of the cornea, which will then bulge slightly because of the normal pressure of the eye. This microscopic bulge allows the central cornea to flatten, reducing the refractive power of the cornea so that light rays are focused closer to or directly on the retina.

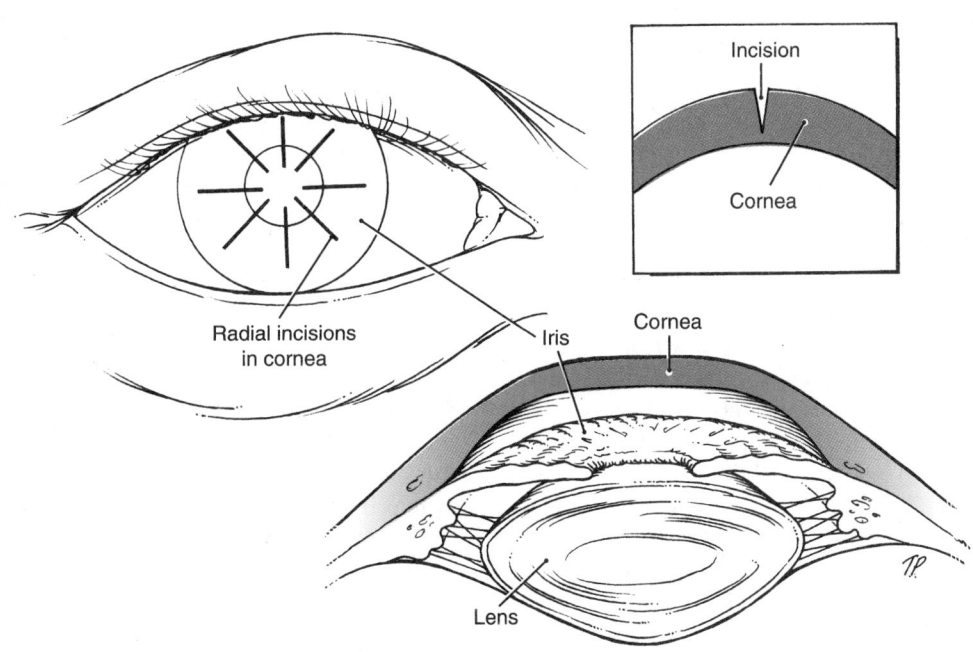

Radial keratotomy surgery can improve nearsightedness and some types of astigmatism. Several deep incisions in the cornea are created, radiating outward. As the edges of the cornea relax, the center becomes flattened.

Astigmatic keratotomy Astigmatic keratotomy is a procedure used to reduce or correct astigmatism. It is similar to radial keratotomy, but the incisions are made in a curved rather than radial pattern in the periphery of the cornea. The irregular cornea of the person with astigmatism is smoothed with these incisions, which are placed concentrically in the quadrant with the steepest corneal curvature, allowing that section of the cornea to relax and flatten.

Automated lamellar keratoplasty (ALK)
This is a more complex procedure that is used to reduce high levels of nearsightedness and some farsightedness. It is a two-stage operation, but like radial keratotomy, it is done as an outpatient procedure, uses local anesthesia, and generally takes less than an hour.

The doctor makes an incision across the front of the cornea with a microkeratome, a tiny precision instrument that functions in much the same way as does a carpenter's plane. This creates a smooth, thin flap of tissue that looks something like a contact lens. It is folded back. To correct nearsightedness, a small amount of tissue is then removed from the underlying cornea, flattening the curvature of the central optical zone and reducing nearsightedness. The original flap of tissue is then put back in place; the replaced tissue reattaches in a matter of minutes, and there is no need for stitches.

To correct farsightedness, the cornea is sliced at a deeper level. The internal pressure of the eye causes it to bulge forward against the remaining thin surface of the cornea, providing the steeper refractive angle that is needed in farsighted eyes. The surface flap is laid back into place with no need to remove any corneal tissue. Again, no stitches are used.

Photorefractive keratectomy (PRK)
This is a relatively new form of refractive surgery, approved for use in the United States in 1995. It uses laser pulses to vaporize small amounts of tissue in the cornea in order to reshape it. The special type of laser used for this is called an excimer laser. No incision is necessary. Usually the tissue that is removed amounts to a layer that is less than one-third the thickness of a human hair. The laser is capable of precision sculpt-

ing, removing a few cells at a time without causing any damage to the surrounding tissue.

Although it is a recently developed form of refractive surgery, PRK has been extensively tested and more than a half-million people worldwide have benefited from it. It is an outpatient surgery and takes less than an hour, with the actual laser exposure lasting less than a minute. Anesthetic drops are used on the eye and the procedure is painless. Recovery is slower than that from radial keratotomy, but since PRK is performed on the front surface of the cornea, it poses very little risk of damaging the structure of the cornea. Visual acuity will improve in the months after the surgery, reaching its peak in 6 to 12 months. About 95 percent of PRK patients ultimately achieve 20/40 vision or better.

PRK works best for mild to moderate nearsightedness but has demonstrated success in treating more serious cases of nearsightedness than has radial keratotomy. PRK has also proved to be safe and effective in correcting mild farsightedness. Another variation, photoastigmatic refractive keratectomy, promises success in treating astigmatism.

Laser-assisted in-situ keratomileusis (LASIK) LASIK is an investigative technique that combines two forms of refractive surgery—ALK and PRK. A corneal flap is created with the microkeratome. When the flap is folded back to expose the underlying corneal tissue, the excimer laser is used to remove precise amounts of tissue from the center of the cornea. LASIK is a promising procedure that may be useful to correct severe nearsightedness and astigmatism. Since the two component parts of it have been approved, doctors can perform LASIK surgery at their medical discretion, but more extensive testing and study is necessary before its role and safety are fully determined.

Eyelids and Eyelashes

Our eyelids are remarkable structures. They contain the thinnest skin in the body with no fat layer underneath, and they are subject to constant movement with each blink. They are packed with tiny blood vessels that promote health and help prevent infection. The lashes originate from the front edge of the lid in two or three irregular rows, about 100 in the upper lid and 50 in the lower. At the inner edge of each eyelid by the nose are the lacrimal ducts, which drain the tears from the eyes into the nose.

Most medical problems in the eyelids and lashes involve infections, but muscle and nerve damage and tumors can also affect the eyelids.

❖ BLEPHARITIS

Symptoms *(What you may experience)* Swollen, red, and irritated eyelids with itching, tearing, and burning; sensation of a foreign body in the eye; crusting around the eyes upon awakening; dandruff-like flakes. (See page C-45.)

Signs and laboratory findings *(What the doctor looks for)* Crusty, red, thickened eyelid margins with pronounced blood vessels and thickened oil glands; mild mucous discharge. In more serious cases, small ulcers may develop along the edge of the lid (ulcerative blepharitis).

What is it? Blepharitis is an inflammation of the edges of the eyelids. It is a common problem for both children and adults and can be chronic. It can involve the lids, the lashes, the meibomian glands (which secrete the oil layer of the tear film and help lubricate the eye), and the conjunctiva. There are two main types of blepharitis: seborrheic, which is caused by excessive secretion from the glands in the eyelid, and staphylococcal, which is caused by a smoldering bacterial infection. Many cases are a combination of the two types because excess oil secretion creates an environment favorable for bacterial growth. Less commonly, blepharitis may be caused by lice.

What you can do Frequent hand washing and general good hygiene can help prevent some cases of blepharitis. If you use eye makeup, a hypoallergenic formula may help prevent blepharitis. If you have blepharitis, soak your eyelids with a warm washcloth to dissolve the crusty discharge. Keep the eyelid edges and surrounding skin clean by washing regularly with warm water and a mild soap (a 20 to 1 mixture of baby shampoo and water is recommended), rubbing the solution over your eyelid margins, where the eyelashes come out, with a cotton swab.

Some over-the-counter (OTC) remedies are available; consult your doctor about them.

When to call the doctor Call your doctor if you experience the symptoms of blepharitis or if symptoms do not clear quickly with OTC medications.

Treatment In many cases, blepharitis can be controlled with good eyelid hygiene and regular cleaning. Warm compresses for 15 minutes four times a day are recommended. The heat causes blood vessels to dilate, improving blood circulation, cleaning out infected glands, and promoting healing. For more serious cases, a topical antibiotic ointment is applied to the eyelid. Cortisone drops may relieve the itching and irritation. Stubborn and recurrent cases may be treated with oral antibiotics.

Prognosis Blepharitis is usually not serious but it can be a recurring condition that is difficult to completely eliminate. With conscientious treatment, however, it can almost always be controlled. However, if left untreated, staphylococcal blepharitis can lead to infection of the cornea.

❖ OCULAR ROSACEA

Symptoms *(What you may experience)* Irritation; redness; burning; sensation of a foreign body in one or both eyes.

Signs and laboratory findings *(What the doctor looks for)* Erythema (inflammatory redness) on the cheeks, forehead, and nose; pimply bumps on the facial skin, which are sometimes pus filled; dilated blood vessels just under the skin. Blood vessels may also grow in the cornea, and blepharitis, chalazion (see Stye and Chalazion, page 514), and conjunctivitis (see page 519) are also often present.

What is it? Rosacea is a chronic skin inflammation with unknown cause. It usually occurs around the center of the face, involving the nose, cheeks, and eyelids. If untreated, this dermatological problem can involve the eyeballs, causing corneal scarring and vision problems. See Chapter 28 for more information on rosacea.

When to call the doctor Rosacea is likely to be diagnosed by a dermatologist or general doctor; if there is any eye involvement, an ophthalmologist should be consulted.

Treatment Rosacea is usually responsive to oral antibiotics, particularly tetracycline. Metronidazole cream, an antibacterial, helps reduce the face rash, and topical corticosteroids can reduce inflammation of the eye. Warm compresses may reduce the blepharitis symptoms. Treatment should be multidisciplinary to address all the systems involved.

Prognosis Ocular rosacea has the potential to cause blindness, but treatment is usually effective. Follow your doctor's advice for regular medical follow-up, since this can be a recurrent condition. If there is corneal involvement, the follow-up should be more frequent.

❖ STYE AND CHALAZION

Symptoms *(What you may experience)* Lump or swelling in the eyelid that may or may not have pain associated with it (a chalazion is generally painless while a stye is more tender and sensitive); light sensitivity; excessive tearing. (See page C-46.)

Signs and laboratory findings *(What the doctor looks for)* A lump on the eyelid that is apparent in an eye exam; blockage of the ducts of the meibomian glands as revealed by microscopic examination; eyelid swelling; redness and tenderness.

What is it? Stye, also called hordeolum, and chalazion are two common conditions that can cause lumps on your eyelids. Hordeolum can be external or internal. A stye is an external hordeolum. It occurs when the eyelid glands and their ducts become infected or clogged. Styes are most often seen on the edge of the upper lid but may also occur on the lower lid. An internal hordeolum is the same thing but involves an internally located gland, and the swelling is further back in the eyelid. Because of its location, it is usually more painful than a stye.

A chalazion is lump that can be as large as a pea. It is caused by the blockage of one or more of the meibomian glands in the eyelid. The accumulated secretions harden and form the bump. Usually it is painless, but it may become infected. If the chalazion becomes large enough, it can press on the cornea, distorting the globe and resulting in blurred vision.

Carcinoma of sebaceous (oil) glands (see Carcinoma of the Eyelid, page 518) may masquerade as an eyelid disorder with symptoms similar to recurring chalazion or blepharitis, such as swollen, red, or irritated eyelids; lump in the eyelid; or crusting around the eyes.

What you can do Conscientious eye hygiene may help prevent styes and chalazia. Wash the eyelid daily with water and diluted baby shampoo, applied with a cotton swab.

Compresses are an important tool for treatment. At the first indication of eyelid irritation, apply warm compresses. Generally, compresses should be applied for about 15 minutes four times a day. A stye will usually burst on its own, and the pus will drain out. Carefully wash your eye when this happens. Do not attempt to squeeze out the infection yourself.

When to call the doctor Consult your doctor if a stye or chalazion causes discomfort or visual impairment, shows no sign of improvement, or worsens. Any swelling that is not localized to one site and involves more of the lid should be evaluated by a doctor; the same is true if fever accompanies these symptoms.

Treatment With warm compresses, a stye or chalazion usually disappears on its own within a few weeks. Antibiotic ointment or drops may also be prescribed and less commonly an oral antibiotic. If a chalazion does not disappear after about a month of treat-

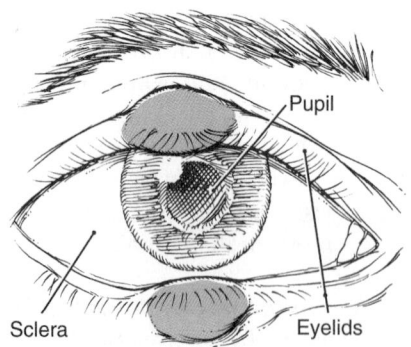

A stye is a lump that forms when glands and ducts at the edge of the eyelid become infected or clogged. In a chalazion, secretions harden abnormally and the meibomian glands of the eyelid become blocked.

Pupil

Sclera

Eyelids

ment, it can be removed through a minor surgical procedure. Sometimes steroids are injected into the chalazion to dissolve it. Styes also can be drained surgically but this is rarely necessary.

Prognosis Most styes and chalazia resolve spontaneously and have no consequences. In the case of a persistent or recurring chalazion, a biopsy (tissue sample analysis) to rule out a tumor is recommended.

❖ DACRYOCYSTITIS/TEAR DUCT AND SAC INFECTION

Symptoms *(What you may experience)* Acute dacryocystitis: pain; redness; swelling over the innermost part of the lower eyelid (near the nose); tearing; discharge; fever. Chronic dacryocystitis: slight swelling of the lacrimal (tear) sac.

Signs and laboratory findings *(What the doctor looks for)* Discharge of mucus or pus when applying pressure on the lacrimal sac near the punctum (present in both eyelids, it is the tiny opening of the tear duct in the eyelid near the nose); an obstruction in the tear duct between the eye and the nose; in chronic cases, a cyst (fluid-filled cavity) in the tear sac.

What is it? Dacryocystitis is an inflammation of the tear sac. It usually occurs when there is an obstruction in the nasolacrimal duct, the tiny tube that the tears pass through from the eye to the nose. This may be due to an abnormality in the duct, an infection, nasal polyps, or trauma, particularly fracture of the nose or facial bones. It is often seen in children.

What you can do As with many problems involving the eyelid and related structures, warm compresses can help relieve the pain and resolve the infection. Gentle massage over the tear duct may also help loosen the duct and clear the infection.

When to call the doctor Call the doctor at any sign of a tear duct blockage or infection.

Treatment Most cases of dacryocystitis are successfully treated with oral antibiotics. For severe cases, intravenous (IV) antibiotics may be used. Sometimes the doctor will irrigate the duct to help clear and dilate it. For stubborn or severe cases, surgery may be necessary to clear the obstructed tear duct. Usually the acute infection will be treated with antibiotics before surgery is attempted.

Prognosis Most of the time dacryocystitis will heal completely with medication. The surgery for this condition has a high success rate.

❖ DRY EYE SYNDROME

Symptoms *(What you may experience)* Burning; itchy, gritty-feeling eyes; excess tearing (sometimes). Symptoms may be aggravated by smoke, wind, heat, low humidity, or eye strain.

Signs and laboratory findings *(What the doctor looks for)* Dry spots on the cornea, revealed by putting a stain in the eye (a painless process); the affected layer of tears—aqueous, lipid, or mucous—as revealed by tear analysis.

What is it? Dry eye syndrome is one of the most common eye problems. It is a condition that increases with age and is more common in women than in men. There are many causes of dry eye syndrome. In women it is often associated with hormonal activity and is seen at menopause and other times of hormonal alteration such as during pregnancy or lactation, after menstruation, or when taking birth control pills. Other medications may also contribute to dry eye, including antidepressants, antihistamines, decongestants, antianxiety agents, and blood pressure medications. Dry eye may also be an allergic reaction to medications for other conditions that are being used in the eye.

Deficiencies in the tear film are also associated with a number of systemic diseases including Sjögren's syndrome, rheumatoid arthritis and other autoimmune disorders, Bell's palsy and myasthenia gravis, and thyroid dysfunction. People with Sjögren's syndrome will have dry mouth due to degeneration of the salivary glands too.

The symptom of excessive tearing may seem strange in a syndrome called dry eye. But what seems to be excessive tearing is usually just one layer, the aqueous layer, pro-

HOW TO APPLY ARTIFICIAL TEARS

Artificial tears, which are available without prescription, are often the only medication needed to treat dry eye syndrome. Drops should be applied frequently—as often as every 1 to 2 hours if needed. How frequently depends on the severity of your condition, and you should consult your doctor about this.

Put the drops in by gently pulling down the lower lid, creating a pocket that you can squeeze one drop into. Do not let the tip of the dropper touch your eye or your fingers. Close your eyes slowly after you put the drop in, open and blink once to mix the artificial tears with your natural tears, then close your eyes and keep them closed for about 30 seconds.

There are two types of artificial tears, preserved and nonpreserved. For some people, the preservatives in these products may worsen symptoms; however, products that are not preserved have a limited shelf life or may be in single-use containers. Consult your doctor about which type of artificial tear will work best for you. Usually if the drops are to be used more than every 3 hours, preservative-free drops will be recommended.

Continue using eyedrops for 1 or 2 weeks, depending on the severity of the problem. As the symptoms go away, taper off the drops to every 4 hours, then every 6 hours, to a level that feels comfortable to you. Long-term use is likely. ■

duced as a reflex reaction to the destabilized tear film. These watery irritant tears simply run off and are not capable of performing the lubricating function of healthy tears.

What you can do If you use contacts, stop wearing them if you experience any symptoms of dry eye syndrome. In fact, dry eye syndrome is one of the main reasons people stop wearing contacts.

It helps to be aware of some of the contributing causes to dry eye syndrome, including medications you are taking and exposure to environmental conditions such as low humidity, dry heat, smoke, or chemical vapors. It has also been found that long hours of close work or work at a computer screen may lead to decreased blinking, exacerbating the symptoms of dry eye syndrome.

People with severe dry eye syndrome can wear swimming or ski goggles or moisture chamber glasses for outdoor activities.

When to call the doctor Call your doctor if you have dry eye symptoms that persist for more than several days. Even though the primary treatment is an OTC medication, you should not begin treatment without consulting a doctor.

Treatment Treatment consists of either replacing or conserving tears. For mild to moderate dry eye syndrome, the treatment is the application of artificial tears, which are available over the counter (see How to Apply Artificial Tears, this page). Lubricating ointments are also available for more severe cases; these usually blur vision and are intended to be used at bedtime.

In severe cases, when replacement of tears with eyedrops does not relieve symptoms, the tears are conserved by plugging the openings through which they drain. These four holes in the four eyelids—the puncta—can be blocked with dissolvable collagen plugs or longer-term silicone plugs. For the most serious cases, the puncta can be permanently closed with electric cauterization.

If you have an underlying systemic disease that is causing or contributing to dry eye syndrome, make sure you are receiving appropriate treatment for it.

Prognosis There is no known cure for the dry eye syndrome, although treatment can successfully alleviate most symptoms for most people.

❖ DROOPING EYELID

Symptoms (*What you may experience*) Drooping eyelid—either one or both eyelids may be affected.

Signs and laboratory findings (*What the doctor looks for*) Related visual disturbances such as lazy eye or crossed eyes; head positioning; chin level; the way the eyebrows move when the person is looking up, down, or straight ahead; the severity of the condition as assessed by eyelid measurements.

COSMETIC SURGERY ON THE EYELIDS

As we grow older, the skin in our eyelids may begin to droop and sag, leading to wrinkles and heavy looking bags under the eyes. In some cases, upper eyelids may droop over the eyes enough to impair vision. These changes in the eye may be inherited or due to a number of environmental causes including sun exposure, nutritional factors, fatigue, prior eye surgery, and allergies.

A surgical procedure called blepharoplasty—sometimes called an eye lift or eyelid tuck—removes excess skin and fat deposits around the eyes. While most people have this procedure done for cosmetic reasons, there are also medical purposes, such as when vision is impaired or the drooping lids cause muscle strain.

Blepharoplasty is usually done in a doctor's office or outpatient center under local anesthesia and will generally take from 1 to 2 hours, depending on how extensive the procedure is. Often, the patient will also be given a sedative for relaxation, sometimes intravenously.

A tiny incision that follows the natural folds of the eye (to avoid obvious scarring) is made in the eyelid crease. Excess skin and fat is then removed, and the incision is stitched closed. For younger patients with more elastic skin, the incision can be made inside the eyelid, and there will be no stitches needed and no scarring. This is called transconjunctival blepharoplasty.

Antibiotics are usually recommended after eyelid surgery to prevent infection, and cool compresses will help reduce swelling and bruising. Stitches will be removed within a week of surgery, although it may take several weeks for complete healing to occur. You will be advised to avoid vigorous exercise during the healing period.

Some doctors are now using lasers for blepharoplasty. In general, laser surgery has a shorter recovery period and less risk of complications than does incisional surgery.

As is the case with any surgical procedure, there are risks and complications associated with blepharoplasty, but if they occur, they are usually mild. Most people experience bruising, because of the many small blood vessels that are disturbed during the surgery. This usually disappears after a few days. Disturbance of an eye muscle can lead to double vision. In most cases, this will resolve within hours; if it persists longer, there may have been some damage to the muscles that control the eye, and that should be evaluated. If too much skin is removed, it can lead to an inability to completely close the eye or to turning out of the eyelid (ectropion), which interferes with effective tearing and lubrication of the eye. In some cases, further surgery is needed to correct these conditions. The most disastrous complication of eye surgery is blindness—this can occur in the case of severe hemorrhage, but is extremely rare in blepharoplasty.

Always have eye surgery performed by a qualified, experienced doctor. For blepharoplasty, you may want to consider using a doctor who has training in both ophthalmology and plastic surgery. See Chapter 32 for information on selecting a surgeon. ■

What is it? Drooping eyelid, also called blepharoptosis and more commonly known as ptosis (pronounced *to sis*) is either a congenital or acquired disorder in which one or both of the upper eyelids droops so that it covers part or all of the pupil, impairing vision and ocular functioning. It is usually caused by a problem with the levator muscle, the muscle that raises the eyelid. Congenital ptosis is due to faulty development of the levator muscle; it usually affects only one upper lid. Acquired ptosis, which is more common, may result from stretching of the tendon between the levator and the eyelid. It may occur after eye surgery or trauma or may be a result of aging.

Both congenital and age-related acquired ptosis may run in families, suggesting a genetic tendency to the disorder. Acquired ptosis can also arise in children or adults as a result of other diseases including chronic eye inflammation, myasthenia gravis, muscular dystrophy, diabetes, or brain tumor.

When to call the doctor When congenital ptosis interferes with a child's vision, treatment should begin at a very early age to prevent lasting damage to the vision such as lazy eye. If congenital ptosis does not cause vision problems, surgery can be delayed until the child is 3 to 5 years old, but the child should be closely monitored. If acquired ptosis occurs in a child, it merits prompt investigation by a doctor to determine if it is a sign of potentially serious underlying disease. Adults with acquired ptosis should see a doctor if the droop occurs suddenly or if the drooping eyelid interferes at all with vision.

Treatment For some people, eyelid crutches attached to glasses work to hold up the drooping eyelid. However, the primary treatment for drooping eyelid is surgery. For congenital ptosis, the levator muscle is tightened. In acquired ptosis, the tendon is tightened. Surgery for drooping eyelid usually done under local anesthesia as an outpatient procedure.

Prognosis The drooping eyelid itself is a correctable disorder and surgery is generally successful.

❖ ENTROPION AND ECTROPION/INVERTED AND EVERTED LIDS

Symptoms *(What you may experience)* Entropion: eye irritation; sensation of a foreign body in the eye; tearing; red-looking eye; in some cases, there may be no symptoms. Ectropion: tearing; eye or eyelid irritation; in some cases, there may be no symptoms.

Signs and laboratory findings *(What the doctor looks for)* Inward turning of the edge of the eyelid (usually lower) for entropion, often with lashes rubbing against the cornea, causing corneal inflammation; outward turning of the edge of the eyelid (usually lower) for ectropion, observed during the eyelid exam with forcible blinking. There may be signs of a secondary corneal or conjunctival infection.

What is it? Entropion is an inward turning of the eyelid. Ectropion is a sagging and turning out. Both of these conditions are found much more commonly in the lower than in the upper eyelids. Usually both conditions are a result of aging and the loss of tone in the muscles that keep the lower eyelids in place. Sometimes (but rarely) they are congenital. They can also result from chronic eye infection that creates scar tissue in the lid, trauma, burns, tumors, paralysis, or previous eyelid surgery.

The primary concern with entropion is that the turned-in lashes will irritate and scratch the cornea and cause permanent scarring of the cornea. With ectropion, the turned-out lids may pull the punctum out of place so that tears do not drain properly.

What you can do Get prompt medical attention for any eye infection. Apply warm compresses several times a day to reduce inflammation and relieve discomfort.

When to call the doctor Call the doctor at any sign of eye infection or if symptoms occur.

Treatment Artificial tears may be a preliminary treatment for entropion, to keep the cornea lubricated (see How to Apply Artificial Tears, page 516). Symptoms of both conditions may be also treated with antibiotic ointment. Taping the eyelids in place may provide temporary relief. The primary way of correcting entropion and ectropion is with surgery, which is usually done under local anesthesia on an outpatient basis. In general, the surgery shortens or tightens the muscle or tendon of the eyelid, but there are a number of surgical variations.

Prognosis Entropion and ectropion are usually curable with surgery. Recurrences are not uncommon and emphasize the importance of individualized treatment.

❖ CARCINOMA OF THE EYELID

Symptoms *(What you may experience)* Basal cell or squamous cell carcinoma: mildly irritating eyelid lump; there may be no symptoms at all. Carcinoma of the sebaceous glands: swollen, red, or irritated eyelids; lump in the eyelid; and crusting around the eyes. Carcinoma of the sebaceous glands may masquerade as an eyelid disorder with symptoms similar to recurring chalazion or blepharitis. Melanoma: irregular mole or mole that changes or grows—may not be pigmented.

Signs and laboratory findings *(What the doctor looks for)* Inflammation, ulceration, or distortion of the eyelid. A basal cell carcinoma may appear as a firm, raised, pearly-colored bump, usually on the lower eyelid. Inflammation on the edge of the lid may occur. Eyelashes may fall out. If cancer is suspected, the doctor will confirm the diagnosis with a biopsy.

What is it? Malignant tumors can develop on the eyelid just as they can on the skin of any other part of the body. The most common type of eyelid malignancy is basal cell carcinoma, which accounts for at least 90 percent of malignant eyelid tumors. Basal cell and squamous cell cancers are usually localized and do not metastasize (spread) to other parts of the body, although they may grow very deep and spread locally. Cancer of the sebaceous glands and melanoma are much less common, but they do present the danger of metastasizing if they are not treated.

What you can do Skin cancers are related to sun exposure, and staying out of the sun or shielding your eyes with sunglasses can be an effective preventive measure. People with fair hair and light skin are more likely to develop skin cancer than are darker skinned people. To prevent cancer spread, be alert to symptoms and seek early treatment. See Chapter 30 for more information on prevention and treatment of skin cancer.

When to call the doctor Consult your doctor if any of the symptoms are noted. Cancer of the eyelid may cause mild symptoms or none at all, confirming the need for routine eye exams.

Treatment Treatment for eyelid cancer is surgical removal of the tumor. It is important that the entire tumor be removed. Often after removal of an eyelid malignancy, reconstructive surgery is needed. The eyelid can be repaired and reconstructed by an ophthalmic plastic surgeon.

Prognosis Basal cell and squamous cell cancers usually grow very slowly and usually do not metastasize, and the prognosis for a complete cure is good. Cancer of the sebaceous glands or melanoma are much more aggressive and can metastasize to other parts of the body if not treated in a timely manner. Cure is also possible for these cancers.

Conjunctiva

The conjunctiva is the thin, transparent tissue that lines the inner surface of both eyelids, and the sclera of the eyeball until it meets the cornea. There is only one disease that is commonly discussed that affects the conjunctiva, but it can have a number of different causes and is one of the most common eye diseases.

❖ CONJUNCTIVITIS (PINKEYE)

Symptoms *(What you may experience)* Sticky discharge from the eye that causes the lids to stick together, particularly upon awakening; excessive tearing; red- or pink-looking eye; sensitivity to light; gritty feeling in the eye; pain; itching (particularly with allergic conjunctivitis); blurred vision. Often symptoms will start in one eye and soon spread to the other. (See page C-45.)

Signs and laboratory findings *(What the doctor looks for)* Cause of infection as determined by laboratory culture of eye discharge.

What is it? Conjunctivitis is an inflammation of the conjunctiva. It is a common disease, particularly in children. It can be contagious and is known to spread quickly in school or daycare settings. Conjunctivitis is commonly referred to as pinkeye because of the pink, bloodshot appearance of the eye.

There are a number of agents that cause conjunctivitis, including viruses, bacteria, chemical exposure, and allergic reaction. Newborns sometimes have a form of conjunctivitis that is caused by an incompletely open tear duct. Infants can also get noninfectious conjunctivitis from a reaction to silver nitrate, the medication that used to be routinely placed in the eyes of newborns to prevent infection.

Viral conjunctivitis is frequently caused by adenovirus, which is easily spread through person-to-person contact. Adenovirus is often associated with an upper respiratory infection, and it can be spread by coughing, sneezing, or direct contact with infected surfaces, such as pillows or towels used by a person with the virus. Herpes simplex viruses (the viruses that cause cold sores on the lips), chickenpox, and shingles can also cause conjunctivitis, as can the viruses that cause influenza, or measles. Gonorrhea, a sexually transmitted disease, can also cause conjunctivitis. Chronic conjunctivitis is often associated with the bacteria *Chlamydia*, that causes another sexually transmitted disease. See Chapter 21 for information on infectious diseases.

Allergic conjunctivitis is caused by common allergens, such as pollen, and other environmental factors, such as smoke.

Giant papillary conjunctivitis (GPC) is another form of conjunctivitis; it is associated with contact lens use, specifically soft contact lenses (see page 507). Inflamed red bumps are usually visible on the underside of the upper eyelid, especially while contacts are being worn, and the contact tends to ride up on the eye with blinking. GPC is thought to be an allergic reaction to solutions used with contact lenses, chemicals absorbed by the lens, or protein deposits on the lens, and is becoming less common as newer, more hypoallergenic, solutions come on the market.

What you can do Since conjunctivitis can be caused by bacteria, including *Hemophilus* B, vaccination against this bacterium during infancy, as recommended, can prevent the condition. Allergic conjunctivitis can be prevented by avoiding known allergens. (See Chapter 29 for information on avoiding allergens.) Proper care of contact lenses, including regular enzymatic cleaning of lenses, can prevent GPC.

The spread of infectious conjunctivitis can be prevented by keeping your hands away from your eyes, thoroughly washing your hands after you touch your eyes, and not sharing washcloths, eye cosmetics, or eyedrops. Dispose of used tissues. Children with conjunctivitis should be kept home from school or daycare and should not go into swimming pools. Adults may be required to stay home from work.

Warm compresses can dissolve the crusty discharge associated with conjunctivitis; cool compresses can relieve the scratchy, burning feeling of allergic conjunctivitis. Resist the temptation to rub your eyes; this will only make the symptoms worse. At the first symptom of conjunctivitis, contact lens wearers should stop wearing their lenses. Soft contact lens users who have chronic GPC should consider switching to rigid gas permeable (RGP) lenses, or discontinue contact lens wear, either temporarily or permanently.

When to call the doctor While conjunctivitis is common, it should not be ignored or taken lightly. Consult the doctor if symptoms do not go away in 1 or 2 days. Call the doctor right away if there is redness, swelling, or blurred vision. Sometimes symptoms of more serious diseases resemble those of conjunctivitis, and it is important to have an eye exam to rule out other problems.

Treatment Bacterial conjunctivitis is treated with antibiotic drops or ointment, which generally clear the symptoms within a few days. For more stubborn cases, an oral antibiotic may be prescribed. Oral antibiotics are needed for all cases of conjunctivitis caused by gonorrhea or chlamydia and all sex partners also need treatment.

Viral conjunctivitis does not respond to antibiotics, and generally you have to wait for the infection to run its course—usually 1 to 2 weeks. Artificial tears can help relieve the symptoms. Conjunctivitis caused by herpes simplex virus may be treated with antiviral eyedrops or ointment; steroid drops should not be used because they can spread the infection and potentially damage the cornea.

Allergic conjunctivitis is treated with antihistamine or nonsteroidal anti-inflammatory drops and removal of the allergen, if possible.

Prognosis Conjunctivitis is usually not a serious disease and responds well to medication or clears up on its own. However, some forms may spread to the cornea and impair vision if not treated appropriately.

Cornea

The cornea consists of five layers of clear tissue. On the outside is the skin-like layer, the epithelium. Below the epithelium is an elastic, fiber-like layer called Bowman's layer. The thickest layer, the stroma, comes next. It is made of collagen. The next thin elastic layer is Descemet's membrane. The endothelium, a layer only one cell thick, is the innermost layer; it maintains the cornea's transparency and water balance. The cells of this layer cannot regenerate if damaged, so injury can lead to permanent vision loss.

The cornea is the front clear window of the eye, bending the light as it enters the eye. The cornea is responsible for about 65 percent of the eye's focusing ability, so a diseased or damaged cornea will almost always impair vision. The cornea can be the site of a number of infections, ulcers, or injuries, but the latest technology offers treatment or repair for most conditions and corneal transplantation as an alternative for the most severely damaged corneas. The prefix *kerato* is Greek for cornea and will be part of the name of most disorders involving the cornea.

❖ KERATITIS

Symptoms *(What you may experience)* Red eye; sensation of a foreign body in the eye; blurred vision; pain; sensitivity to light; watery eye.

Signs and laboratory findings *(What the doctor looks for)* Vesicles (fluid-containing blisters) on the eyelid; ulcers on the cornea that may develop dendrites (distinctively shaped branches), visible upon microscopic examination. The doctor will test the visual acuity and pupil response, look at the eye through a slit-lamp, and take measurements of the cornea. Laboratory cultures are sometimes taken to confirm the diagnosis.

What is it? Keratitis is an inflammation of the cornea. It can be caused by bacterial or fungal infection or overwear of contact lenses, but the most common cause of keratitis is the herpes simplex virus type 1, the virus that causes cold sores. Other viral causes of keratitis include the varicella zoster virus (also a herpes virus), which is associated with chickenpox and shingles, and the adenoviruses, which cause upper respiratory infections.

What you can do Some types of keratitis may be linked to vitamin A insufficiency, so eat a well-balanced diet or ask your doctor about vitamin supplements.

Contact lens wear, particularly extended wear, is associated with a large percentage of cases of bacterial keratitis. It is recommended that you never wear contacts while you are sleeping.

When to call the doctor The seriousness of a keratitis is quite variable, but you should call the doctor promptly if symptoms develop or in the case of pain or vision impairment.

Treatment Antibacterial or antifungal drops can effectively treat keratitis caused by bacteria or fungi. Sometimes oral antibiotics are also used.

Prognosis Infectious keratitis may be curable when diagnosed and treated early, although some cases are resistant to treatment and may require long-term care by the doctor.

❖ CORNEAL ULCER

Symptoms (*What you may experience*) Red eye; mild to severe pain in the eye; sensitivity to light; decreased vision; discharge from the eye.

Signs and laboratory findings (*What the doctor looks for*) Opaque, white spot on

the cornea; evidence of other infection in the eye; culture to identify cause of infection. (See page C-44.)

What is it? A corneal ulcer is an open sore on the cornea. It is an infectious keratitis, most commonly bacterial keratitis. If a stain is put in the eye, the ulcer can be clearly seen.

What you can do Prompt attention to early signs of eye infection can prevent progression to corneal ulcer. Good hygiene when handling contact lenses is essential. Do not wear contacts overnight, and stop wearing them at the first signs of inflammation or discomfort.

When to call the doctor A corneal ulcer is a medical emergency and requires immediate treatment by an ophthalmologist.

Treatment Corneal ulcers are treated as an infectious keratitis, with antibiotic, antifungal, or antiviral drops or ointments. They are treated aggressively and sometimes require hospitalization. The doctor will evaluate daily the response to treatment, examining and measuring the ulcer to make sure it is getting smaller. If it does not respond to treatment or is getting so big that the cornea is in danger of perforating, corneal transplantation will be considered.

Prognosis Complete recovery from a corneal ulcer is likely if it is treated promptly and appropriately. But if left untreated, diagnosed late, or is an aggressive infection, it can cause serious vision impairment.

❖ HERPES SIMPLEX VIRUS KERATITIS

Symptoms (*What you may experience*) Red eye; sensation of a foreign body in the eye; blurred vision; pain; sensitivity to light; watery eye. In most cases, herpes simplex virus (HSV) keratitis affects only one eye.

Signs and laboratory findings (*What the doctor looks for*) Vesicles on the eyelid; ulcers on the cornea that may develop dendrites, visible upon microscopic examination. The doctor will test the visual acuity and pupil response, look at the eye through a slit-lamp, and take measurements of the cornea. Laboratory cultures are sometimes taken to confirm the diagnosis and determine the cause.

What is it? Keratitis is an inflammation of the cornea. The most common cause of keratitis is the herpes simplex virus type 1, the virus that causes cold sores. HSV keratitis is also called ocular herpes. People who are infected with the herpes simplex virus and get cold sores on their mouths know that the infection tends to recur but can remain dormant for months or years. However, not all herpes infections affect the eye. When the eye is involved, HSV usually affects the epithelial (outermost) layer of the cornea initially, but it can progress into the inner stroma, the largest part of the cornea located behind the epithelium. When the stroma becomes involved, the risk of vision impairment increases. Other viral causes of keratitis include the varicella zoster virus, (also a herpes virus) which is associated with chickenpox and shingles, and the adenoviruses, which cause upper respiratory infections.

What you can do If you have a cold sore, do not put your fingers to your eyes. If there is any suspicion that you have HSV, avoid OTC steroid eyedrops, which cause HSV keratitis to worsen.

When to call the doctor The seriousness of keratitis is quite variable, but you should call the doctor promptly if symptoms develop or in the case of pain or vision impairment.

Treatment Antiviral drops effectively clear the symptoms of HSV, but this is not a cure because the virus remains in your system and can flare up again. Sometimes in more serious cases the doctor will apply anesthetic drops and debride (gently scrape off) the diseased tissue of the cornea. Often after debridement, you will wear an eye patch for a couple of days. The doctor may put on a therapeutic soft contact lens after debridement to help relieve symptoms until the infection subsides.

Prognosis HSV keratitis is controllable but incurable. A person who has had HSV keratitis has a 50 percent chance that the infection will recur. Factors that can trigger a recurrence include fever, stress, sunlight, and trauma, but often there is no known cause for a recurrence. This emphasizes the importance of being attentive to early symptoms and warning signs, so that treatment can begin promptly. An untreated corneal infection can permanently damage the eye. When keratitis progresses to the stroma, it can cause permanent corneal scarring and decreased vision.

❖ KERATOCONUS

Symptoms (*What you may experience*) Slowly progressive visual blurring and distortion, usually beginning in adolescence or the early 20s; pain; light sensitivity; profuse tearing; sudden clouding of vision that clears over weeks or months. In advanced cases, vision may deteriorate rapidly.

Signs and laboratory findings (*What the doctor looks for*) Irregular astigmatism in the visual acuity exam; thinning of the cornea with bulging of the central portion into a cone shape; scarring on the cornea (sometimes); corneal swelling in the case of acute hydrops (the sudden infusion of fluid into the stretched portion of the cornea).

What is it? Keratoconus is a disease in which the normally round cornea thins and develops a cone-like bulge. This can have a significant impact on vision, causing blurriness and distortion. Its effects range from mild to severe. It is a progressive condition, usually beginning in the teens or 20s, but often stabilizing after a few years. It usually occurs in both eyes.

The cause of keratoconus is unknown, but it runs in families and may have genetic origins; about 7 percent of people with keratoconus have a family history of the disease. Some research has indicated that frequent and firm eye rubbing may contribute to the development of keratoconus. Keratoconus is also associated with other diseases including Down's syndrome, atopy, Marfan's syndrome, and mitral valve prolapse; and certain eye diseases, including retinitis pigmentosa and retinopathy of prematurity (ROP), among others.

What you can do Do not rub your eyes, since aggressive and frequent eye rubbing can damage the epithelium of the cornea.

When to call the doctor See an eye doctor for a visual acuity exam whenever there are changes in your vision.

CORNEAL TRANSPLANT

Corneal transplantation—also called penetrating kerato-plasty—is the most successful form of organ transplantation. More than 40,000 vision-restoring cornea transplants are performed each year in the United States with a success rate of 90 percent or higher.

Corneas are transplanted to replace diseased or damaged corneas that result from keratoconus, trauma, congenital malformations of the cornea (also called dystrophies), or other diseases of the cornea. Replacement corneas come from human donors. Because the cornea does not have blood vessels, there is much lower risk of rejection, compared to other organ transplants. Corneas are preserved and stored in eye banks around the country; increasingly refined storage solutions developed over the past 25 years make it possible for corneas to be kept safely for as long as 2 weeks. Corneas are screened for transmissible diseases, such as AIDS, before they are transplanted.

A corneal transplant can be done under local or general anesthesia. The diseased cornea is removed with a cookie-cutter-type instrument called a trephine, and the transplant—called a button—is laid in place and secured with microscopic stitches.

Your eye will have a protective shield over it after surgery, and your postoperative care has as much to do with the success of the transplant as the surgery itself. You should see your doctor frequently and use topical antibiotics and steroids as prescribed. While this procedure has a very high success rate, there are also many possible complications. These include glaucoma, infection, problems with stitches, graft rejection, and serious astigmatism.

A corneal transplant takes months to completely heal, and it is important to continue using the prescribed drops and see your doctor frequently during the recovery period. Vision will remain blurred for several weeks or sometimes months. Rejection, while not common, has been known to occur as long as 20 years after the transplant. Usually symptoms of rejection can be successfully treated with medication. ■

Treatment The first stages of keratoconus can usually be corrected with glasses (see Options for Correcting Vision, page 506). For most cases, RGP contact lenses are effective for correcting the blurred vision of keratoconus, helping to neutralize the astigmatism of the cornea. An alternative for people for whom rigid lenses are not comfortable is a piggyback arrangement with a soft lens next to the cornea and an RGP lens on top of that. Good lens fit is essential for people with keratoconus, since a poor fit could aggravate the condition.

In about 10 percent of people, the cornea becomes too steep, or scarred, and contacts can no longer be tolerated or cannot provide the necessary correction. In these cases a corneal transplant is performed (see Corneal Transplant, above). In another operation called epikeratophakia, a layer of epithelial cells is surgically grafted to the cornea to flatten it.

Prognosis Often keratoconus stabilizes on its own in a few years without causing serious vision problems. Glasses or RGP lenses offer a permanent solution for most people, although some accommodations may be necessary—for example, frequent adjustment of contact lens prescriptions and planned rest periods during the day when contacts can be removed. Corneal transplantation has success rates of about 90 percent, although 60 percent of people who receive corneal transplants need to wear contacts or glasses after surgery to correct nearsighted-ness or astigmatism. Epikeratophakia has similar success rates to transplantation and can be followed with corneal transplantation if it is unsuccessful.

❖ RECURRENT CORNEAL EROSION

Symptoms (*What you may experience*) Acute pain, often beginning upon awakening; sensitivity to light; tearing, especially upon awakening or while sleeping.

Signs and laboratory findings (*What the doctor looks for*) Rough or swollen cornea, but this may resolve quickly and not be apparent at the time of examination. The pain and discomfort experienced may seem out of proportion to what is seen in the exam. Examination with the slit-lamp often shows that the corneal epithelium is only loosely attached to Bowman's membrane, which connects it to the rest of the cornea.

What is it? Recurrent corneal erosion is a common disease of the cornea, distinguished by acute pain that comes and goes quickly. The pain probably results from the poor attachment of the epithelium and exposure of underlying corneal nerves. When the eye can be examined during an acute episode, part of the epithelium may be heaped up.

In many instances, the condition is related to a prior abrasion to the cornea, as from a fingernail scratch or paper cut, but many people who experience this recurrent pain do not remember ever having had the initial corneal injury. It may also be associated with a disorder of the cornea called map-dot-fingerprint dystrophy, in which the adhesion between the epithelium and Bowman's membrane is not normal. This is a very common condition. Many people experience no symptoms at all.

When to call the doctor Call the doctor if you experience acute pain in your eye, even if it goes away quickly.

Treatment For the mildest cases, artificial tears will relieve the symptoms. An antibiotic or salt-based ointment with or without a pressure patch on the eye may be used for less mild cases. For some people, a therapeutic contact lens reduces the pain and permits healing. For people with painful and frequently recurring corneal erosions, a salt-based drop or ointment applied nightly can prevent recurrences. A new surgical laser procedure called phototherapeutic keratectomy (PTK) may also provide relief.

Prognosis For many people, this condition resolves on its own or responds quickly to simple treatments. For more difficult cases, new laser technology offers hope for a permanent solution.

Lens

The crystalline lens is the clear, soft structure behind the pupil. Its two convex surfaces provide the second phase of focusing for light (after the cornea) before it reaches the retina. With age, the lens stiffens and leads to presbyopia. Another common problem is clouding of the lens, which needs to be transparent for clear vision. The resulting cataracts are a major cause of blindness but can be surgically removed and an artificial lens inserted.

❖ CATARACT

Symptoms *(What you may experience)* Slowly progressive blurring or dimming of vision, over months or years; sensitivity to bright light or glare (for example, oncoming headlights at night); worsening nearsighted-ness, requiring prescription change; distorted vision; double vision.

Signs and laboratory findings *(What the doctor looks for)* Opaque areas within the lens. The shape of the opaque areas depends on the type of cataract. In examination, it will be difficult for the doctor to see the retina with the ophthalmoscope when looking through some cataracts. (See page C-43.)

What is it? Cataract, the progressive clouding of the eye's normally clear lens, is one of the most common disorders related to aging. Besides aging, cataracts can also result from injury, some chronic eye diseases, and systemic diseases such as diabetes. In some cases (1 in 2,000 live births), babies are born with cataracts due to metabolic disorders or exposure to rubella (German measles) or other harmful agents during gestation. However, aging is by far the most common cause—by the time you reach age 65, you have a 50 percent chance of developing a cataract, and when you are age 75, you have a 70 percent chance.

Cataracts progress at varying speeds and may cause very little vision impairment. Sometimes they remain small and do not disturb vision at all. But in other cases, the vision loss is significant. More than a million cataract operations are performed each year in the United States. Cataract surgery is the most frequently done surgery on people over age 60 in the United States.

There are three types of cataracts, described by the location in the lens. The lens has three main parts: an outer membrane, the capsule; an inner layer, the cortex; and the center of the lens, the nucleus. A nuclear cataract is found in the center of the lens. A cortical cataract appears as wedge-shaped spokes in the cortex, extending from the perimeter of the lens toward the center. A subcapsular cataract is a small opaque area under the capsule, usually at the back of the lens. This is the type of cataract that is often found in people with other contributing conditions, such as diabetes, retinitis pigmentosa, or prior oral or topical corticosteroid use.

What you can do There is not much that can be done to prevent a cataract, although some researchers think that wearing sunglasses that filter out ultraviolet light from sunlight may reduce cataract formation.

When to call the doctor Call the doctor when cataract symptoms begin interfering with your vision.

Treatment In early stages of cataract development, a change in your prescription for glasses may improve vision, but that improvement will be temporary if the cataract progresses. For some people with presbyopia, as a cataract begins to develop, the mild to moderate nearsightedness it causes will lessen the need for reading glasses. However, this phenomenon—called second sight—is temporary. Another measure that provides temporary relief for some people is dilation of the pupils, which allows light to pass around parts of the cataract.

The treatment for cataracts is surgical removal. The lens is then replaced with a permanent intraocular lens (IOL) implant.

Cataracts are often referred to as ripe when vision is totally clouded. The decision about when to have surgery is a personal and lifestyle judgment, not a technical medical finding. Each person must decide when a cataract is interfering with the activities of daily living and when it should be removed. If both eyes have cataracts, the eye that is more severely impaired will be operated on first. Surgery on the second eye will be scheduled after the procedure on the first eye appears to be successful.

Surgery is usually done as an outpatient procedure under local anesthesia. It usually takes about an hour. A small incision is made in the eye, and the impaired lens is broken into tiny pieces and aspirated (suctioned out). The back membrane of the lens (posterior capsule) is left in place and helps support the plastic-like IOL implant that is then inserted.

In earlier versions of cataract surgery, the nucleus of the lens was removed in one piece through a big incision, and the remaining softer parts of the lens aspirated. This technique is being replaced by a procedure called phacoemulsification, in which sound waves are used to break up the hard nucleus and the rest of the lens. Phacoemulsification allows for a smaller incision. The surgery is referred to as no-stitch or one-stitch, depending on whether a stitch is needed to make the incision watertight after surgery. Stitches usually do not have to be removed and are eventually absorbed by the body.

Cataract surgery once left people without a lens, and they had to depend on thick

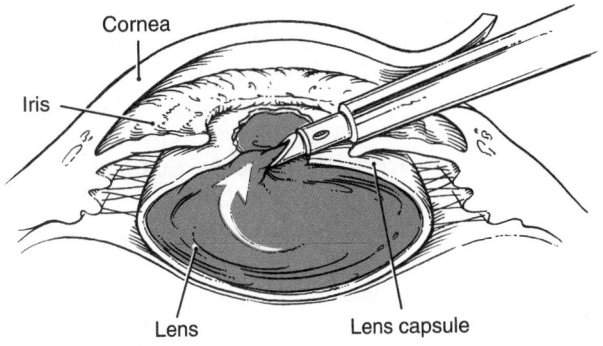

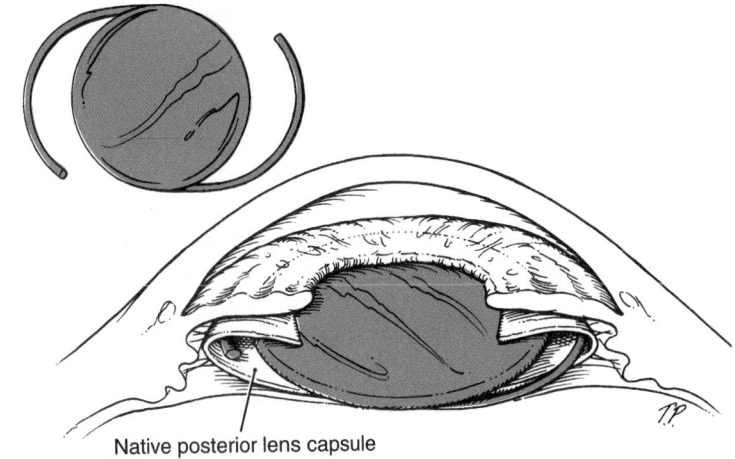

Native posterior lens capsule

The phacoemulsification procedure involves using sound waves to break up most of the lens, which is then suctioned out of the eye. An artificial lens can be implanted in its place.

glasses to help make up for the absent lens. With modern materials and surgical techniques, an intraocular lens is now installed in 98 percent of people who have cataract surgery in the United States. These IOLs are made of plastics which the body tolerates very well, and the newest materials being used are flexible enough for the IOL to be bent and inserted through the same tiny incision through which the cataract is removed. IOLs have different refractive powers, and you will receive an IOL with a refractive power that is based on the length of your eye and the curvature of your cornea. It cannot be felt or seen when it is properly in place.

In some cases, the posterior capsule turns cloudy in the months or years after cataract surgery. When this happens, a laser procedure can clear the membrane. However, a laser is not used to actually remove cataracts.

Prognosis Cataract surgery has an excellent success rate, with more than 90 percent of people achieving 20/40 vision with or without glasses after surgery. People who have cataract surgery report significant improvement in many areas of their lives. Usually the eye is stabilized within 6 to 12 weeks after surgery, and the optimum correction through glasses or contact lenses can be prescribed.

Complications of cataract surgery are rare but include infection, bleeding, glaucoma, inflammation in the eye, corneal problems, and retinal detachment.

❖ DISLOCATED LENS

Symptoms (What you may experience) Decreased vision; blurred or double vision.

Signs and laboratory findings (What the doctor looks for) Displaced or off-center lens apparent in eye exam; iris may quiver because of lack of support from lens.

What is it? A dislocated lens is a lens, either your own lens or an IOL, that is out of place. The condition can be congenital; people with certain genetic disorders such as Marfan's syndrome are born with or are likely to develop displaced lenses. Acquired lens dislocation is most commonly caused by trauma but is also associated with other diseases such as syphilis. Usually the reason for the dislocation, whether congenital or acquired, is weakness or dysfunction of the fibers that hold the lens in place.

Lens dislocation is also the term used to describe fragments of the lens that get into the vitreous cavity during cataract surgery. An implanted IOL may also become displaced, either due to insufficient support or trauma.

When to call the doctor Call the doctor if there is any change in your vision. Usually people with genetic conditions associated with a dislocated lens are under continuing medical care.

Treatment Treatment depends on the position of the dislocated lens and whether it affects vision. In some cases, when vision is not impaired, the doctor can monitor the situation, taking no action unless it worsens. If the lens is in the anterior chamber, it may be possible for the doctor to physically manipulate it into place, using a local anesthetic on the eye. If causing problems, the lens or IOL should be surgically removed. Either can be replaced with an IOL implant.

Prognosis A dislocated lens can be successfully treated surgically.

Optic Nerve

Cells in the retina are connected to the brain via nerve fibers that collect at the back of each eye to form the cable called the optic nerve. The optic nerve is a vital conduit in the process of turning light into images. Disease or injury to this collection of nerve fibers—connected to the globe of the eye at the optic disc—can pose a serious threat to vision. Glaucoma, one of the world's leading preventable cause of blindness, ultimately affects this part of the eye.

❖ GLAUCOMA

Symptoms (What you may experience) Primary open-angle glaucoma. Blind spots with progressively decreasing peripheral vision to ultimately result in loss of central vision if not successfully treated; symptoms usually appear in the late stages. Acute angle-closure glaucoma: eye pain; blurred vision; colored halos around lights; headache; nausea and vomiting.

Signs and laboratory findings (What the doctor looks for) Elevated intraocular pressure (IOP) as indicated by an exam with a tonometer; irregularities in drainage angle for fluids within the eye, as observed through a gonioscope (a special mirrored lens); deterioration of optic nerve fibers, as seen through the ophthalmoscope; the extent to which peripheral vision is impaired as determined by visual field tests. Normal average IOP ranges are from 10 to 21 mm of mercury (mm Hg), and any measure above 22 is considered suspicious. The doctor will also ask questions about family medical history, since there are hereditary tendencies for some types of glaucoma.

What is it? Glaucoma is not a single disease but a group of eye diseases characterized by damage to the optic nerve, usually because of increased pressure in the eye. It is the

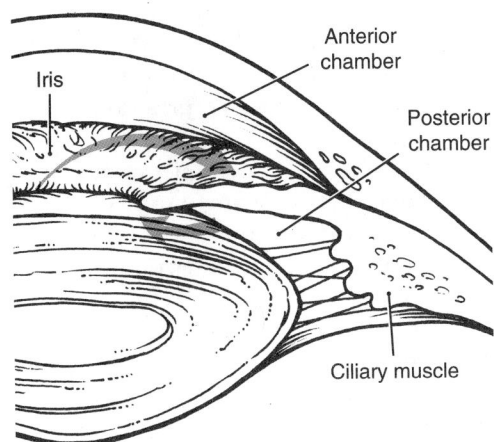

Fluid (aqueous humor) in the eye flows through the pupil from the posterior chamber to the anterior chamber, and then into the bloodstream via the trabecular meshwork at the angle between the cornea and iris.

leading cause of blindness in the United States, and more than a million people in this country have some vision loss due to glaucoma. In its most common form, it is a progressive, chronic disease. Approximately 2.3 million Americans have glaucoma, most of them over age 60, but there are also forms that affect children and young adults.

Glaucoma has been called the sneak thief of sight because in many cases there are no apparent symptoms before vision loss actually begins. However, subsequent loss can be prevented with prompt and continuing treatment. Because of availability of eye care in this country, only 4 percent of Americans with glaucoma become blind. But glaucoma is a lifelong disease; once a person has it, the need for monitoring and treatment will be lifelong, as for diabetes and hypertension.

The two main types of glaucoma are classified by the mechanisms that cause the pressure buildup and optic nerve damage.

- *Open-angle glaucoma.* This is the most common form. The aqueous humor is the fluid in the eye that flows through the pupil into the anterior chamber of the eye, passing through a filtration system between the iris and cornea called the trabecular meshwork, and then draining through tiny drainage canals and ultimately into the bloodstream. In open-angle glaucoma, the trabecular meshwork does not function normally, backing up the fluid, building up the

IOP, and eventually damaging the optic nerve, resulting in loss of visual field. This type of glaucoma has a tendency to affect nearsighted people; blacks are four to five times more likely to get it than whites.

- *Angle-closure glaucoma.* In this form of the disease, the trabecular meshwork is blocked by the iris. This can be a chronic, slowly developing blockage or an acute and sudden blockage. Angle-closure glaucoma is more common in Asians, and Eskimos have the highest rate in the world. It is more common in farsighted people. Acute angle-closure glaucoma—a rare form of the disease—can develop very quickly; it should be considered a medical emergency because vision-impairing optic nerve damage can occur within hours of the blockage. Some cases of acute angle-closure glaucoma are associated with the use of certain medications, including antidepressants, cold medications, antihistamines, and some antinausea medications, in predisposed people.

Childhood glaucomas are rare, but they do occur, and can start in infancy, childhood, or adolescence. Glaucoma in young people is thought to be genetically based, and there may be hereditary aspects to age-related glaucoma as well. If a close relative has glaucoma, you are four times more likely to have it than is someone with no affected family members.

There are other types and subtypes of glaucoma. Some people have normal IOP (below 22 mm Hg) but still develop optic nerve damage; this has been called normal-tension glaucoma. Conversely, some people have elevated IOP—called ocular hypertension—but no optic nerve involvement or vision impairment. It is important for these people to be closely monitored. Visual field tests are used to determine if peripheral vision has been affected.

Pigment dispersion syndrome is a genetic disorder that leads to glaucoma in about 5 to 10 percent of young adults who carry the gene. In these people, who are usually nearsighted, the iris is floppy and pigment is released into the aqueous, clogging the trabecular meshwork. In pseudoexfoliation glaucoma, both pigment and grayish-white material in the eye clog the trabecular meshwork. Congenital glaucoma may be the result of developmental abnormalities that block the drain in the eye. Glaucoma sometimes develops following eye surgery, in conjunction with other diseases of the eye such as uveitis (see page 544), or after taking certain oral or topical medications such as steroids.

What you can do The most effective way to detect the earliest signs of glaucoma is to have regular eye exams which include measurement of IOP with a tonometer. Also be aware of any risk factors you may have. If you think you are at risk, you should have regular and frequent eye exams, beginning at a young age. Risk factors include a family history, race, diabetes, previous eye injury, and age (over age 50).

When to call the doctor Acute glaucoma is a medical emergency; if you experience symptoms, contact your doctor immediately or go to the emergency room. Chronic glaucoma may have no symptoms; should any change in your vision or acute pain in your eye occur, however, contact your doctor.

Treatment Since the vision loss attributed to glaucoma cannot be reversed, the aim of treatment is to prevent further damage. There is some disagreement about when to begin treatment, with some doctors taking a wait-and-see attitude, while others take a more aggressive approach. There are three levels of treatment for open-angle glaucoma.

Medication This is usually in the form of eyedrops. Two types of eyedrops used to treat glaucoma are beta blockers and miotics. Most beta blockers decrease the rate at which fluid flows into the eye. They have fewer side effects in the eye than do miotics, but may have systemic effects including worsening pulmonary disease, difficulty breathing, slowing of heart rate, decreased blood pressure, and impotence. Miotics cause the pupil to contract, helping open the drain and increasing the rate of fluid flowing out of the eye. Possible side effects include pain around that eye for the first few days of use, blurred vision, or nearsightedness. Some miotic drops also produce a burning sensation.

Latanoprost solution (Xalatan) is a new medication (a prostaglandin analog) that increases the rate at which fluid flows out of the eye. Epinephrine is another medication in drop form that lowers IOP by increasing the rate of the flow of fluid out of the eye. Apraclonidine (Iopidine) is another eyedrop that lowers eye pressure, among others.

Systemic side effects of eyedrops can be minimized by pressing on the corner of your eye near the nose and keeping the eyelids closed for a minute after putting in the drop.

For people who do not get relief from eyedrops, another class of medication, carbonic anhydrase inhibitors, may be prescribed in pill form. These reduce the fluid flow into the eye. They may have side effects, including frequent urination, tingling in fingers and toes, rash, depression, fatigue, or rarely, a sometimes fatal anemia. Carbonic anhydrase inhibitors also are available in eyedrop form.

Laser treatment Laser surgery is used for people who do not get the desired lowering of IOP using medication or who find the side effects of medication intolerable. Laser procedures are done on an outpatient basis with local anesthesia (eyedrops) and are usually painless.

Laser trabeculoplasty is the procedure usually used to treat types of open-angle glaucoma, including pigment dispersion and pseudoexfoliation glaucoma. The heat of the laser on the trabecular meshwork causes some areas to shrink, with adjacent areas then opening to permit better drainage of aqueous humor. Effects vary from person to person and many people continue or resume using eyedrops. As more and more evidence builds about the safety of laser trabeculoplasty, many doctors are recommending its use earlier in the treatment of glaucoma.

Laser iridotomy is used to treat angle-closure glaucoma. The laser makes a small hole in the iris to let aqueous flow through. A variation, laser peripheral iridoplasty, lifts the iris off the drain it is clogging.

For advanced or aggressive cases of glaucoma, a procedure called cyclophotocoagulation uses a laser beam or a freezing treatment to destroy parts of the ciliary body, the part of the eye that produces aqueous humor.

Surgery Conventional incisional surgery may be the best option for people whose IOP is not sufficiently lowered by medication or laser procedures. This is usually done on an outpatient basis with local anesthesia, although the procedure generally takes longer than does laser treatment and may have more risks. In filtering surgery, the doctor removes a tiny piece of the sclera with an overlying trap door (also made out of sclera) creating a new drain for the aqueous. Sometimes a small tube or valve is placed through an incision in the sclera to regulate the outflow of aqueous fluid.

Prognosis The vision that is lost to glaucoma cannot be restored, but the prognosis is good for retaining vision once the diagnosis is made and treatment begun. This emphasizes the importance of regular and preventative eye exams.

❖ OPTIC NEURITIS

Symptoms (What you may experience) Acute visual loss or blurring, over days or, more rarely, hours; pain in the orbit; loss of color vision; reduced perception of light intensity. Usually vision will steadily worsen for a week before stabilizing, and generally symptoms are just in one eye, but may be in both.

Signs and laboratory findings (What the doctor looks for) Decreased visual acuity; uneven reaction of pupils to light (called relative afferent pupillary defect and tested with a swinging light). Upon examination, the optic nerve may or may not appear swollen.

What is it? Optic neuritis is an inflammation of the optic nerve. It is often an early sign of multiple sclerosis, a more generalized nerve disease (see Multiple Sclerosis, page 453). It is sometimes called retrobulbar neuritis—*retro* for behind and *bulbar* for the bulb of the eye. Most of the 25,000 Americans who are diagnosed with optic neuritis each year are women between the ages of 18 and 45, and studies show that more than half will go on to develop multiple sclerosis within 15 years. In some people with multiple sclerosis, even though there have been no symptoms of optic neuritis, there is evidence of damage to the optic nerve. The cause is unknown but may be due to inflammation of the myelin sheath of the optic nerve. Optic neuritis may also be seen in people with Lyme disease (see page 886).

See General Diseases that Affect the Eye, page 553, for more information on the connection between eye disorders and other diseases such as multiple sclerosis.

When to call the doctor Call the doctor at any sign of decreased vision.

Treatment Treatment for optic neuritis is somewhat controversial, since the inflammation subsides and the condition heals spontaneously almost all the time. Traditionally, oral corticosteroids have been used. Recent studies have found, however, that taking corticosteroids orally may worsen the disease, or be associated with recurrences. Intravenous (IV) steroids, however, have been shown to speed the restoration of vision and also may play a role in preventing or delaying the onset of multiple sclerosis.

Prognosis About 95 percent of people return to at least 20/40 vision within a year after an attack of optic neuritis with or without corticosteroids. The visual benefit from the treatment of acute optic neuritis with IV corticosteroids is short term, limited to an accelerated recovery rate. Treatment must be individualized. However, 50 to 60 percent of people who have optic neuritis go on to develop MS.

❖ OPTIC NEUROPATHY

Symptoms (What you may experience) Painless loss of vision in one or both eyes that may be progressive or swift, depending on the type of neuropathy. Arteritic optic neuropathy may be preceded by headache, fever, weight loss, or general malaise.

Signs and laboratory findings (What the doctor looks for) Extent of vision loss as determined by visual acuity and visual field tests; slow pupil constriction, indicating damage to the optic nerve; photographs of the nerves; amount of swelling of the optic disc as determined by examination with the ophthalmoscope.

What is it? Optic neuropathy is a group of disorders, the most common of which is ischemic optic neuropathy. Ischemic optic neuropathy is sometimes compared to a stroke of the eye because the blood supply to the optic nerve is cut off, causing neuropathy (degeneration) of the nerve. In the most serious forms, it can progress to optic atrophy, in which all or part of the optic nerve wastes away.

Optic neuropathy usually affects the anterior optic nerve, thus the abbreviation AION for anterior ischemic optic neuropathy. The disorder is further differentiated by what causes the ischemia (decrease in blood supply). In some cases, it is arteritic, caused by a disease called temporal or giant cell arteritis (see page 556), which inflames large and medium-sized arteries throughout the body, including those that provide the blood supply for the optic nerve. This generally occurs in people over age 55 and affects women twice as often as it does men. People with nonarteritic AION are usually younger and generally experience less severe vision loss. About 50 percent of people with nonarteritic AION have hypertension. Nonarteritic AION may be caused by arteriosclerosis. See General Diseases that Affect the Eye, page 553, for more information on the connection between eye disorders and other diseases such as temporal arteritis.

When to call the doctor Call the doctor at any sign of vision loss.

Treatment Oral steroids are given for arteritic AION. In severe cases, they may be given intravenously for 1 or 2 days. The steroids work to reduce swelling in the affected arteries.

There is no known effective treatment for nonarteritic AION. In the past, a surgical procedure called optic nerve decompression was used to treat people with nonarteritic AION, but studies found that it was no more effective in restoring vision than was careful monitoring, and this surgery is not currently recommended.

Prognosis Optic neuropathy rarely resolves spontaneously; most cases remain stable while some cases progress. Without treatment, arteritic AION may progress to affect the second eye within 6 weeks of symptoms in the first eye.

❖ PAPILLEDEMA (OPTIC NERVE SWELLING)

Symptoms *(What you may experience)* Brief episodes (lasting just seconds) of vision loss, often in both eyes; headache; double vision; nausea; vomiting; a decrease in visual acuity (less commonly).

Signs and laboratory findings *(What the doctor looks for)* Swelling of the disks where the optic nerve connects to the globe of the eye, blurring of the edges of the disks, and dilation of the small blood vessels; in later stages, retinal hemorrhage, fatty accumulations near the optic disk, and atrophy of the nerve.

What is it? Papilledema is swelling of the optic nerve due to increased pressure within the skull. Increased intracranial pressure may be a sign of such serious conditions as a brain tumor, cerebral hemorrhage, brain trauma, meningitis, severe hypertension, subdural hematoma (blood clot in the brain), or encephalitis.

When to call the doctor Call the doctor or go to the emergency room at the first sign of any of these symptoms.

Treatment Treatment is for the underlying condition causing the elevated intracranial pressure.

Prognosis The conditions causing papilledema are very serious, sometimes life threatening. If the intracranial pressure is not reduced, the optic nerve will eventually atrophy and permanent vision loss will occur.

Retina

The retina is the thin delicate structure of tissue that lines the back inner surface of the eye and is similar to the film of a camera. It is packed with millions of rods and cones, the light- and color-sensitive nerve cells that translate light into impulses that move through the optic nerve to the brain.

Looking with an ophthalmoscope through the dilated pupil, the retina is wholly visible to the doctor. It is divided into two sections: the macula in the center, which is responsible for central vision; and the peripheral zones, which give us peripheral and night vision. Also important to the healthy functioning of the retina is the retinal pigment epithelium (RPE), an outer pigmented layer of tissue, and the choroid, the

LOW VISION AIDS

Vision that is not correctable to better than 20/70 in the affected eye is considered low vision. Low vision may result from disease, injury, or aging; macular degeneration is the most common cause. Even when there are no refractive, medical, laser, or surgical alterations to improve low vision, there are a variety of devices that can help people live independent and productive lives. Different aids are used for different purposes.

Optical low vision devices use lenses to provide magnification. Magnifying spectacles are stronger than regular prescription glasses, but you will need to hold reading material very close when you use them. With hand magnifiers, you can hold reading material at a normal distance. Stand magnifiers rest on reading material and may have a built-in light source. Telescopes are used for distance vision, and they too can be mounted in frames or hand-held. Closed-circuit TV projects an enlarged image on a television screen; this is the most expensive of the low vision aids, but it can be the most useful, especially for someone with severe low vision.

Nonoptical low vision devices include large-print books and newspapers, talking books (books on tape), watch faces with high contrast, large-numbered telephone dials and calculators, large-size playing cards, and machines that talk. Computers provide a number of options for people with low vision—large font screen types, for example, or text-to-voice functions.

Lighting is another important consideration for people with low vision. When reading, place the light source close to the reading material. Use a visor or hat with a brim to block the glare of overhead light. Sometimes special absorptive lenses help control glare.

Living with low vision is a matter of optimizing the vision you have by using a device and learning to adjust and make necessary lifestyle changes. Some people find it helpful to share their experiences, and many support groups exist for this purpose. For example, there are support groups for people and their families with the major diseases causing visual loss (macular degeneration and glaucoma).

Following is a list of organizations that provide support and information for people with visual impairments:

- American Foundation for the Blind
  11 Penn Plaza, Suite 300
  New York, NY 10001
  Phone: (800) 232-5463

- Foundation Fighting Blindness
  Executive Plaza I, Suite 800
  11350 McCormick Rd.
  Hunt Valley, MD 21031-1014
  Phone: (888) 394-3937

- The Glaucoma Foundation
  33 Maiden Ln.
  New York, NY 10038
  Phone: (800) GLAUCOMA (800-452-8266)

- The Lighthouse National Center for Vision and Aging
  111 East 59th St.
  New York, NY 10022
  Phone: (800) 334-5497

- Macular Degeneration Foundation
  P.O. Box 9752
  San Jose, CA 95157
  Phone: (888) MDF-EYES (888-633-3937)

- National Association for the Visually Handicapped
  22 West 21st St.
  New York, NY 10010
  (212) Phone: (212) 889-3141

- National Library Service for the Blind and Physically Handicapped
  Library of Congress
  Washington, DC 20542
  Phone: (800) 424-8567 ■

layer rich in blood vessels that envelops and nourishes the retina and RPE.

❖ AGE-RELATED MACULAR DEGENERATION

Symptoms *(What you may experience)* Dry (non-neovascular): gradual loss of central vision. Wet (neovascular): distortion of straight lines or edges; rapid loss of vision; blind spot in the center of the field of vision.

Signs and laboratory findings *(What the doctor looks for)* Amsler grid results; drusen deposits (abnormal deposits of cellular material and debris that collect where the RPE meets the choroid) within the macula; in the case of wet age-related macular degeneration (AMD), blood vessel growth and leakage. The doctor may use a fluorescein angiogram to visualize these vessels more precisely; in this test, a nontoxic dye injected into the arm makes its way to the eye and highlights these blood vessels in special pictures taken with a camera.

What is it? AMD is a progressive disease in which the macula degenerates, becoming dotted with drusen underneath the photoreceptor cells that may cause localized detachment of the RPE. This may slowly impair central vision. It usually occurs in both eyes, although one may be affected more than the other.

AMD is one of the most common reasons for vision loss in people over age 60. Nearly 20 percent of people over age 75 have some vision impairment because of macular degeneration. It affects more than 13 million Americans. It is seen most commonly in people with light-colored eyes, and less frequently in blacks.

About 90 percent of AMD is dry, the milder type, also called non-neovascular or atrophic. It is characterized by the buildup of drusen, which eventually causes the photoreceptor cells to atrophy. Drusen may build up for many years before causing damage, and some people have drusen deposits without ever experiencing symptoms.

Wet, also called neovascular, AMD is associated with choroidal neovascularization (CNV). In wet AMD, new and fragile blood vessels begin to grow from the choroid, leaking blood and fluid and causing damage to the retina and deterioration of the photoreceptor cells. Scar tissue often also develops in the macula. Wet AMD is likely to progress more quickly than is dry AMD and to lead to greater vision loss.

There are also some forms of macular degeneration that are not age related. Juvenile macular degeneration is inherited from a parent who carries a gene for the disease; several genes have been identified that are responsible for different types of juvenile macular degeneration. Heredity is also thought to be a factor in AMD.

What you can do While medical science has not yet come up with a way to prevent macular degeneration, this has been an area of intense research, particularly as more and more baby boomers approach the age when AMD is likely to occur. There are a number of areas under study that suggest some possibilities about how AMD might be prevented, or its progression slowed or halted.

- *Cigarette smoking.* Studies have found that smokers have more than twice the risk as do nonsmokers of developing AMD. Smoking poses many health risks and blindness may be one of them. See Chapter 4 for information on how to stop smoking.

- *Nutrition.* Some studies have found lower rates of AMD in people who eat diets rich in antioxidant vitamins, but further research is necessary to determine if there is an actual cause and effect, and what role vitamin supplements may play. Zinc and selenium are also hypothesized to have a role. In the years ahead, studies such as the National Eye Institute's long-range Age-Related Eye Diseases Study will provide more definitive answers about these relations, and perhaps clues to the causes of AMD. A diet rich in foods that supply antioxidants—vegetables and fruits, particularly dark green leafy vegetables and orange vegetables like carrots and sweet potatoes—is a healthy diet for many other reasons. Talk to your doctor about the advisability of vitamin or mineral supplements to prevent AMD.

- *Sunlight.* Studies have not shown a definite relationship between exposure to sunlight and development of AMD.

The most important thing you can do to prevent disabling vision damage from AMD is to get regular eye exams, particularly after drusen deposits or AMD have been diagnosed. Your doctor may give you an Amsler grid to use at home daily, so that you can be quickly aware of any change in

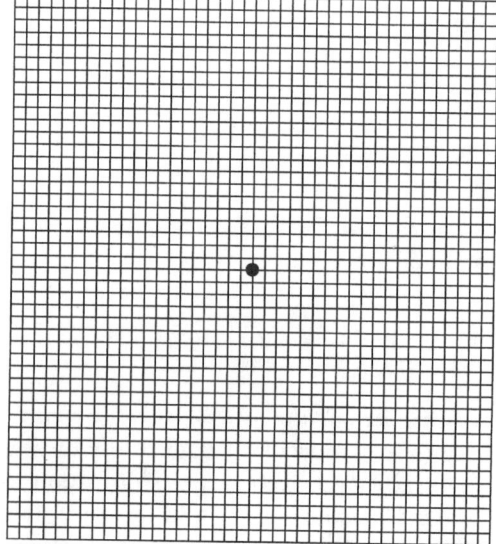

The Amsler grid aids in the detection of central visual field defects, such as those seen with age-related macular degeneration. A defect exists if the central spot is invisible when looking directly at it, or if any of the grid lines appear absent, curved, or distorted.

your vision. The Amsler grid looks like graph paper. You must determine if any of the lines look wavy or are absent, and if a central spot in the middle is visible when looking straight at it.

When to call the doctor Call the doctor at any sign of blurred central vision, or straight lines that appear wavy.

Treatment There is no treatment to prevent or reverse the process of dry AMD. Low vision aids are prescribed for people in whom vision loss is severe (see Low Vision Aids, page 531).

In people with wet AMD, a process called laser photocoagulation can prevent further deterioration of the macula and possibly preserve some vision in the long run, if it is done early enough in the course of the disease. Laser rays destroy the blood vessels growing in the choroid below the retina and seal leaky areas; the rays also destroy the overlying retinal tissue creating a blind spot in the area of treatment. However, if the blood vessels have already grown under the macula, the laser procedure may be effective at limiting the size of the blind spot, but will not restore any vision. It also leaves a blind spot, but most people learn to adjust to this, and it is usually preferable to the vision loss that the progressing disease would ultimately cause.

Prognosis People with macular degeneration may experience mild to severe central vision loss, but it does not affect peripheral vision. Peripheral vision is useful, and someone with macular degeneration can learn to maximize it, sometimes with the help of low vision aids.

Scientists at Johns Hopkins and other medical institutions are involved in research on macular degeneration that offers promise for future treatment. One process, macular translocation surgery, moves the macula of the retina to a new location away from the area affected by CNV to permit laser treatment of the CNV without destroying the fovea. Another possible treatment option, photodynamic therapy, involves the IV administration of a medication which accumulates in the abnormal blood vessels in the eye. When it is activated by a light from a nonthermal laser, the blood vessels which cause wet AMD can be closed. These procedures are in experimental phases but represent hope for the future for people with AMD.

❖ DETACHED RETINA

Symptoms *(What you may experience)* Sensation like a shade being drawn over the eye; bright flashes of light, especially in the periphery; translucent specks called floaters (see Floaters and Flashes, page 534); peripheral or central visual loss. There is no pain, and tears or small detachments of the retina may have no symptoms at all.

Signs and laboratory findings *(What the doctor looks for)* Evidence of elevation of the retina; separation of the retina from the RPE and choroid; buildup of vitreous liquid between the retina and RPE, as seen with the ophthalmoscope. Often the detached retina has a corrugated appearance to the eye doctor.

What is it? A detached retina is a separation of the retina from the wall of the eye. There are several types, classified according to how the detachment occurs. It may be caused by trauma, nearsightedness, disease, or aging, but frequently develops sponta-

A separation of the retina from the wall of the eye is often spontaneous and is a life-threatening emergency requiring immediate treatment.

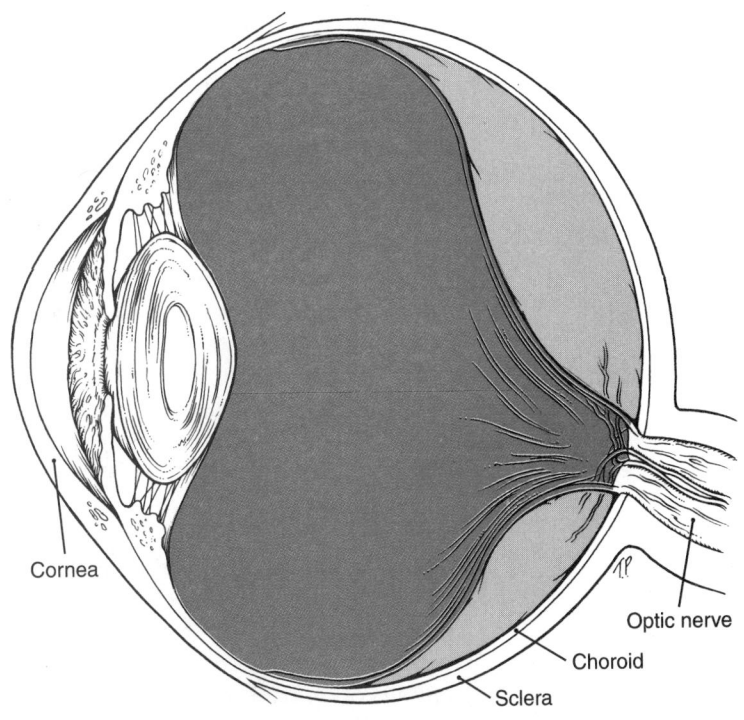

Cornea

Optic nerve

Choroid

Sclera

FLOATERS AND FLASHES

Many people notice small specks or strands that move in their field of vision, especially when looking at a plain background. These are called floaters. They look like they are in front of your eye. Actually they are clumps of gelatinous cells floating in the vitreous, the clear gel that fills the inside of the eye behind the pupil.

Floaters are a result of the vitreous liquefying, shrinking and pulling away from the retina on the back wall of the eye. This happens with age and is called a posterior vitreous detachment. Floaters can be disturbing, especially if they appear suddenly, but they may or may not be indicative of serious problems. If floaters are annoying or get in the way of reading or other activities, it is sometimes helpful to move your eyes, looking up and then down, to displace the floaters. However, a posterior vitreous detachment can lead to tearing of the retina and retinal detachment, so if you have floaters you should see your doctor quickly, particularly if new floaters suddenly appear.

Flashes occur when the vitreous tugs at the retina as the vitreous shrinks. The brain interprets this as a flash of light. If you see sudden flashes, you should see your doctor to make sure that the retina is not torn. ■

neously. Retinal detachment is a serious, vision-threatening medical emergency that requires immediate treatment.

The most common type of retinal detachment is a rhegmatogenous detachment (from *rhegma*, the Greek word for break). It occurs when there is a break or tear in the retina, allowing vitreous fluid to leak between the retina and the RPE. The buildup of fluid lifts the retina up off the back wall of the eye. Untreated retinal detachment can lead to the development of proliferative vitreoretinopathy, when cells grow on the inner and outer surfaces of the retina, causing it to contract, fold, and scar.

People with severe nearsightedness, a family history of retinal detachment, or a previous retinal detachment have greater risk of having a detached retina. Some people also have a thinning of the retinal tissue called lattice degeneration which may put them at increased risk for retinal detachment.

What you can do Prompt attention to symptoms of retinal breaks (flashes of light or floaters) may prevent this from progressing to a retinal detachment.

When to call the doctor Call the doctor if you experience any of the symptoms of retinal tear or detachment. Retinal detachment is a medical emergency that requires immediate attention.

Treatment Tears in the retina that are discovered before detachment has occurred can be sealed with laser treatment or cryotherapy, a procedure using a freezing probe. These methods may also be used for small peripheral detachments, but most detachments need more extensive eye surgery.

There are two surgeries used for retinal detachment. Scleral buckling surgery may be performed under general or local anesthesia in the operating room. The tear is treated, excess fluid may be drained, and then the sclera is indented toward the retina with a hard silicone band called a buckle. The buckle, which may be wrapped around the entire circumference of the eye or just a portion, is stitched in place and left in the eye permanently. It cannot be seen. In some cases, a gas bubble is injected into the vitreous cavity; when properly positioned it pushes the retinal tear against the scleral buckle to help keep the tear closed. In other cases, additional surgery, called a vitrectomy, may also be needed to remove the vitreous gel and reattach the retina. Pneumatic retinopexy is the injection of the gas bubble after cryotherapy but without the use of a scleral buckle. This can be done under local anesthesia in the office. The person is instructed to position the head in a way that allows the gas bubble to press the detached retina against the back of the eye. Not all configurations of a detached retina can be treated with the pneumatic method.

Antibiotic drops are usually prescribed after surgery, and people are advised to limit their physical activities for several weeks to avoid disturbing the retina.

Prognosis Modern surgical techniques have considerably improved the prognosis for retinal detachment. About 90 percent can be repaired; however, this does not always guarantee good vision. Sometimes multiple surgeries are needed. The return of good vision depends on whether the part of the retina containing the macula was detached, and for how long. If the macula was not detached, outcomes are generally very good. However, if left untreated, loss of vision can occur. Despite successful reattachment, proliferative vitreoretinopathy or scarring can develop and detach the retina again.

❖ RETINITIS PIGMENTOSA

Symptoms *(What you may experience)* Difficulty seeing in the dark or in dimly lit places; loss of peripheral vision; less commonly, decreased central vision and loss of ability to discern colors.

Signs and laboratory findings *(What the doctor looks for)* Clumps of pigment spread throughout the peripheral retina; atrophy of the RPE; progressive loss of peripheral vision in a visual field test. People at risk for retinitis pigmentosa may be given a test called an electroretinogram (ERG). In an ERG, the eye response to a light stimulus is recorded; an ERG in someone with retinitis pigmentosa will show decreased signals from the rods and cones, particularly the rods.

What is it? Retinitis pigmentosa is a group of progressive, inherited diseases characterized by degeneration of the rods and cones, the photosensitive cells in the retina that perceive light and color. It is the major cause of blindness in people under age 60. Retinitis pigmentosa affects about 100,000 people in the United States and 1.5 million worldwide.

There are a number of variations of retinitis pigmentosa, but usually the rods, which are responsible for peripheral and night vision, begin to deteriorate. The process can be very slow. Often the first signs of the disease begin in childhood, but may not be recognized for years. As the disease progresses, the person is left with tunnel vision, just able to see what is straight ahead.

Most people with retinitis pigmentosa will be legally blind by age 40. This means visual acuity less than 20/200 even with correction in the better eye, and a field of vision (regardless of acuity) that is restricted to a 20° diameter in the better eye. However, most people with retinitis pigmentosa still have enough vision to walk, even though they are legally blind and are unable to read or drive a car.

What you can do There is no way to prevent retinitis pigmentosa, but for some forms of the disease, the gene that causes it has been identified. For some people with retinitis pigmentosa, or with family histories of the disease, genetic counseling can provide useful information to make decisions about whether to have children.

When to call the doctor Call the doctor if you have trouble seeing in the dark or begin to lose your peripheral vision. If you have a family history of retinitis pigmentosa, you should have regular eye exams to test for the disease.

Treatment There is currently no treatment for retinitis pigmentosa, and no way to prevent its progression. Low vision aids (see Low Vision Aids, page 531) are helpful for many people. Some research has suggested that large daily doses of vitamin A may slow the onset and progression of the disease, but these findings are controversial and there may be long-term side effects of large doses, particularly to the liver. Talk to your doctor about the advisability of taking vitamin A if you have retinitis pigmentosa.

Prognosis Most people with retinitis pigmentosa lose most of their vision, so the prognosis is not very positive. However, work is being done to explore ways to restore vision in eyes with retinitis pigmentosa. In one promising procedure, tiny chips of silicone with light-sensitive electrodes may be temporarily attached to the retina to substitute for the damaged photoreceptors. This is still in the early experimental stages.

❖ RETINAL ARTERY/VEIN OCCLUSION

Symptoms *(What you may experience)* Sudden and acute blurring of vision, painless and usually just in one eye.

Signs and laboratory findings *(What the doctor looks for)* Artery occlusion: whitening of the retina. Vein occlusion: hemorrhage in the retina; dilation and twisting of the retinal blood vessels apparent upon examination of the eyes. Fluorescein angiography (enhanced visualization of the retinal vessels after injecting a dye in the arm) will be used to determine the status of retinal blood circulation in the eye.

What is it? Retinal artery or vein occlusion is a blockage of the blood supply either coming (artery) or leaving (vein) the retina. Blockage may occur because of a blood clot or lipid (fat) deposit, and it may be in the central or branch blood vessels. The location and type of blockage will have a great deal to do with the damage to the eye.

The cells of the retina will decay and die without the nourishment they get from the blood the arteries bring to them. When veins that carry blood away become blocked, it also results in decreased vision but to varying degrees. Swelling of the macula also occurs when retinal veins become blocked, and sometimes a painful glaucoma can develop.

Retinal blood vessel occlusion may be associated with other eye diseases such as glaucoma or systemic diseases including hypertension, diabetes, and atherosclerosis. Some types of medication (oral contraceptives) have also been associated with occlusion.

What you can do Good control of diseases such as diabetes, atherosclerosis, and hypertension may have a role in preventing retinal vessel occlusions.

When to call the doctor Call the doctor or go to the emergency room if sudden and acute blurring or loss of vision occurs.

Treatment Treatment depends on the location of the occlusion. A central retinal arterial occlusion is a medical emergency that requires immediate treatment within 90 minutes of the onset of symptoms to withdraw fluid from the eye. This is done to unclog the artery and prevent permanent vision damage. Massage of the eye is the first step and then withdrawal of fluid from the eye through a needle, after a local anesthetic has been administered. Medication will also be given to decrease the pressure in the eye. Sometimes patients will inhale a combination of oxygen and carbon dioxide; this may dilate the retinal artery to allow the obstruction to move.

Laser photocoagulation can be used for central vein occlusion to remove abnormal blood vessels that can grow in these eyes and in some cases, the laser can help to reduce macular swelling. Retinal specialists at the Wilmer Eye Institute at Johns Hopkins are studying the effectiveness of laser surgery to bypass the blocked retinal vein and improve the circulation.

Treatment of underlying conditions such as hypertension and diabetes is very important.

Prognosis Outcomes vary for retinal vessel occlusions, depending on where in the eye they occur and how quickly they are treated. With quick treatment, vision loss may be lessened, but these disorders usually result in vision loss. A number of experimental treatments are under investigation, including bypass of blocked vessels with lasers and use of synthetic proteins to dissolve the occlusions.

❖ ENDOPHTHALMITIS

Symptoms *(What you may experience)* Decreased vision; redness; light sensitivity. Sometimes: pain; swelling in the conjunctiva, eyelid, and cornea.

Signs and laboratory findings *(What the doctor looks for)* Inflammation in the eye; white blood cells in the vitreous; reduced visual acuity; a history of recent eye surgery, trauma, or infections elsewhere in the body. The fundus may not be visible in an exam because of inflammation of the vitreous. (See page C-44.)

What is it? Endophthalmitis is inflammation inside the eyeball and is usually caused by an infectious agent such as a bacteria or fungus. It is a serious condition that can result in loss of sight and even loss of the eye.

Endophthalmitis usually develops after eye surgery or penetrating trauma. In some cases, bacteria are introduced into the eye with the implantation of intraocular lenses (IOLs) resulting in endophthalmitis. Cases develop at variable rates, depending on the infectious agent, and are of varying degrees of severity.

What you can do Postoperative endophthalmitis has been less common in recent years, as doctors have learned more about how infectious agents get into the eye and how this can be prevented. Researchers continue to study and refine the use of antibiotics during and immediately following surgery to prevent infection.

When to call the doctor Call the doctor if any symptoms of endophthalmitis appear.

This is a serious infection and prompt medical attention is necessary to prevent permanent damage to the eye.

Treatment Antibiotics are given, usually in the form of injections into the eye and as eyedrops. Corticosteroids may also be applied topically, unless a fungus is the cause of the infection. Hospitalization may be required. A recent study of eyes that developed endophthalmitis after recent eye surgery by the National Eye Institute found that removing a small sample of vitreous gel from the eye for culture is just as good as removing all of the vitreous gel from the eye in most cases. The study also found that topical and intraocular antibiotics are sufficient to treat these eyes, and that IV antibiotics are not necessary or beneficial; however, treatment must be individualized.

Prognosis This is a serious disease that can cause permanent vision loss. However, with prompt and appropriate treatment, it may be successfully treated, with some visual improvement.

❖ DIABETIC RETINOPATHY

Symptoms (*What you may experience*) Blurred vision; slowly progressive vision loss, usually in both eyes, but it may affect one eye more than it does the other. It may cause no symptoms in the early stages.

Signs and laboratory findings (*What the doctor looks for*) Nonproliferative: microaneurysms (tiny outpouchings of blood vessels); lipid deposits called hard exudates, which look like white or yellowish deposits in the retina; dot hemorrhages. These are detected with examination and fundus photographs. Swelling of the macula may also be present in any of the stages. Intraretinal microvascular abnormalities may also be present. Proliferative: new abnormal blood vessels and fibrous (scar) tissue growing into the vitreous; vessels may be unstable and bleed. The fibrous tissue may pull on the retina and detach it.

What is it? Diabetic retinopathy is damage to the normal blood vessels of the retina caused by high blood glucose (sugar) levels. The effects of high blood glucose are cumulative, and the longer a person has had diabetes and the higher the blood glucose levels, the more likely is that person to develop diabetic retinopathy. In people who have had diabetes for 10 years or longer, nearly half have some degree of diabetic retinopathy. In some cases, people are unaware that they have type 2 diabetes (also called noninsulin-dependent or adult-onset diabetes) until a diagnosis of retinopathy leads to diagnosis of the diabetes.

Diabetic retinopathy is classified in progressive stages—nonproliferative and proliferative—but the first stage does not inevitably lead to the next, particularly if optimum blood glucose control is practiced. In the nonproliferative stage, blood vessels may leak a clear fluid which causes macular edema (swelling). Macular edema is responsible for blurred vision, which may come and go as the fluid fluctuates. In many cases, nonproliferative diabetic retinopathy presents no symptoms.

As the condition progresses, new abnormal blood vessels proliferate in the retina, bleed into the vitreous, and result in cloudy vision. The vessels are accompanied by the growth of fibrous (scar) tissue. This fibrosis can cause the retina to contract, pulling it from the back wall of the eye and causing a retinal detachment. The new blood vessels can also grow on the iris and into the trabecular meshwork, increasing pressure in the eye and causing a painful glaucoma.

What you can do Like most of the complications of diabetes, diabetic retinopathy is at least partially preventable by practicing good blood glucose control with the guidance of your doctor. This means frequent daily monitoring of blood glucose levels, making the necessary changes in diet, insulin dose or other medication, and exercise to keep the levels in the target range.

Everyone with type 1 diabetes (also called insulin-dependent or juvenile-onset diabetes) and type 2 diabetes should have regular ophthalmologic exams. Retinopathy usually does not develop in childhood or adolescence, but every child with diabetes should have a baseline eye exam within a year of being diagnosed with diabetes, and annual exams thereafter. The American Academy of Ophthalmology (AAO) recommends yearly dilated exams for everyone with diabetes. Fluorescein angiography is a very effective way to guide the treatment of specific problems in the eye due to diabetes, such as macular edema and new blood vessels.

When to call the doctor Call the doctor at any sign of blurred or failing vision. People with diabetes should be attentive to any changes in vision, and each eye should be checked separately.

Treatment Laser photocoagulation has become the standard treatment for proliferative diabetic retinopathy and diabetic macular edema. Laser treatment, administered in time, has been shown to reduce the risk of severe vision loss from proliferative diabetic retinopathy by as much as 90 percent.

In this procedure, the laser is used to decrease the production of a substance that makes blood vessels grow. The leaking blood vessels then close off and the retina is lasered down to the back of the eye. More than one laser procedure is usually needed.

In some cases of proliferative diabetic retinopathy when the fibrous tissue causes a retinal detachment, a vitrectomy may be recommended. In this operation, the vitreous fluid—which may be cloudy due to bleeding—is extracted and replaced either with a saline solution or a gas bubble that will hold the retina in place. The fibrous tissue is peeled off and the retina reattached with a laser. Eventually the body's natural fluid will fill the vitreous cavity.

Prognosis In many cases, good blood glucose control can prevent diabetic retinopathy. If detected early enough, laser treatment can prevent serious vision loss. However, in some cases diabetic retinopathy does progress to severe vision loss or blindness. Diabetes is one of the leading causes of new cases of blindness in adults under age 65 in this country.

❖ RETINOPATHY OF PREMATURITY

Symptoms *(What you may experience)* The subtle retinal changes of retinopathy of prematurity (ROP) in an infant apparent only through an exam by an experienced ophthalmologist with an ophthalmoscope. Premature and low-birth-weight infants should be screened if they are born at less than 36 weeks gestational age or weigh less than 4 lbs 6 oz (2000 g) at birth.

Signs and laboratory findings *(What the doctor looks for)* Visible border or ridge between peripheral and central retina; abnormal growth of blood vessels in the retina that proliferate and leak; retinal detachment.

What is it? ROP leads to an abnormal growth of blood vessels in the retina that is seen in some premature or low-birth-weight babies. It probably occurs because of inadequate development of the vascular system in the eye and may be triggered or worsened by external conditions such as too much or too little oxygen at birth or pulmonary distress. Risk factors for ROP include the following:

- Prematurity, especially babies born at 36 weeks or less gestation
- Birthweight less than 4 lbs, 6 oz (2000 g); the lower the weight, the greater the risk
- Supplemental oxygen after birth

ROP is classified according to the stage of severity. In early stages, only subtle changes in the retina are apparent, but in progressively severe cases, there will be growth and leaking of the abnormal blood vessels into the vitreous. Abnormal growth leads to scarring, and contraction of fibrous tissue pulls the retina loose from the wall of the eye. Stage 5, the most severe, is retinal detachment. Treatment is based on the severity. The timing of treatment is critical.

What you can do Comprehensive and regular prenatal care to prevent prematurity or complications of childbirth is the first line of defense against ROP. See Chapter 7 for information on prenatal care and preventing prematurity.

There is some controversy over the causes of ROP, and some people think that giving oxygen to premature babies or the lighting in neonatal intensive care nurseries may contribute to ROP. While the administration of oxygen does seem to play a role, the role of lighting has not been confirmed.

Treatment In the early stages, no treatment is recommended but the baby should be closely monitored. These infants should be examined by a doctor every 1 to 2 weeks until they are 14 weeks of age, and then every 1 to 2 months.

In more advanced stages, cryotherapy, a freezing technique, has shown to be effective in stopping the abnormal growth of blood vessels. Laser treatment is also used. In the case of a detached retina, a surgical technique called scleral buckle or vitrectomy techniques may be used.

Some studies have shown that vitamin E may reduce the severity of ROP, but this is still under investigation.

Prognosis In as many as 85 percent of affected babies, ROP gets better on its own without treatment, and the abnormal vessels disappear or regress spontaneously. However, more advanced cases may lead to a number of different eye problems, including blindness. Other eye problems that pose a risk later in life for children with ROP include subsequent retinal detachment, cataract, glaucoma, crossed eyes, lazy eye, and nearsightedness.

❖ CENTRAL SEROUS RETINOPATHY

Symptoms *(What you may experience)* Blurred or dim vision, sometimes with sudden onset; a blind spot; distortion of shapes; reduced visual acuity.

Signs and laboratory findings *(What the doctor looks for)* Leak of serous (watery) fluid between the retina and the retinal pigment epithelium (RPE) leading to areas of retinal detachment. A fluorescein angiogram may be obtained to find the source of the leak.

What is it? Central serous retinopathy (also called chorioretinopathy) is a disorder in which fluid gathers under the retina, resulting in visual distortion. It is primarily seen in young adults between the ages of 20 and 45, and men are 10 times more likely to get it than are women. It results from improper functioning of the RPE, but the cause is unknown. Many cases have been associated with a high level of stress, and it has been suggested that high blood levels of epinephrine and cortisol hormones may play a role.

When to call the doctor Call the doctor at any blurring of vision, especially if it happens suddenly.

Treatment Most cases of central serous retinopathy heal spontaneously, and often no treatment is recommended. However, laser photocoagulation is sometimes used to speed healing. If you have this condition, your doctor will probably follow you closely for about 4 to 6 months. If it does not clear up on its own in this period, if the affected eye is your only eye, or if this is the second episode, your doctor may suggest the laser procedure.

Prognosis The average time for spontaneous recovery from central serous retinopathy is 3 to 4 months, and most people recover their former visual acuity within 6 months. Some people have residual symptoms such as distortion, decreased sensitivity to contrast, or difficulty seeing at night, and as many as half may experience future recurrences of the condition.

❖ RETINOBLASTOMA

Symptoms *(What you may experience)* Whitish light reflection in pupil (also called leukocoria or cat's eye); crossed eyes or other abnormal eye movements; red or swollen eye (occasionally). Less commonly: difference in pupil size or iris color; bulging eye.

Signs and laboratory findings *(What the doctor looks for)* White lesion in the retina, which may be accompanied by white particles in the vitreous; retinal detachment; white tumor visible on fundus examination.

What is it? Retinoblastoma is a malignancy that occurs in the eye, almost always in young children. More than 80 percent of cases are diagnosed in children less than 5 years old. In 70 percent of cases, the tumor is in one eye. Some cases of this cancer (including all cases when it occurs in both eyes) may be genetically linked.

Retinoblastoma may be intraocular, which is confined to the inside of the eye; extraocular, which has spread to tissues around the eye or other parts of the body; or recurrent, when the cancer has come back after treatment, either in the eye or elsewhere in the body.

What you can do There is no known way to prevent retinoblastoma, but if there is a family history of the disease, genetic counseling can help predict the risk. Siblings of children with retinoblastoma should be examined periodically for signs of the disease.

When to call the doctor Call the doctor at any symptoms. Babies should be screened for retinoblastoma routinely at birth and at all well baby exams. If there is a family history, more frequent eye exams should be performed.

Treatment Treatment for retinoblastoma depends on how advanced it is when diagnosed. The goals of treatment are to cure the disease, prevent the cancer from spreading, and to preserve as much vision as possible.

For smaller tumors, cryotherapy can kill the cancer cells by freezing them. Laser photocoagulation is also used for small tumors. In the case of larger tumors filling more than half of the eye, or if tumor cells are seen in the vitreous, the entire eye is removed in a procedure called an enucleation. When an enucleation is performed, the child is fitted with a prosthetic implant in place of the eye.

In the past 40 years, as other anti-cancer techniques have been developed, enucleation has been used less to treat retinoblastoma. Radiation and systemic chemotherapy (administration of a combination of powerful anticancer medications) are also used to treat retinoblastoma. See Chapter 30 for a more detailed discussion of these anticancer therapies.

Prognosis With earlier diagnosis and improved treatment, the recovery and survival rate of children with retinoblastoma continues to improve. More than 90 percent of children survive this disease, and when it occurs in one eye, the vision in the other eye is usually unaffected.

However, if not diagnosed and treated early enough, retinoblastoma can spread to the brain or other parts of the body. Also, survivors of retinoblastoma have an increased incidence of other malignancies later in life.

❖ CHOROIDAL MELANOMA

Symptoms *(What you may experience)* Decreased vision; visual field defect; floaters; flashes; pain. Often there are no symptoms.

Signs and laboratory findings *(What the doctor looks for)* Gray-green, brown, or yellow mass in the choroid (under the retina/RPE complex); large amount of fluid under the retina causing retinal detachment; ill-defined area of orange pigment; thickened-looking choroid without a mass. Since the mass is completely visible through the pupil with an ophthalmoscope, a biopsy is usually not necessary; however, sometimes the diagnosis may be facilitated with fluorescein angiography or ultrasound.

What is it? Choroidal melanoma is a cancer of the eye. In adults, it is the most common tumor seen in the eye. It originates in the pigmented cells of the choroid, the tissue rich in blood vessels that nourishes the retina. It may begin from a choroidal nevus, which resembles a small freckle and is often benign but may become cancerous. Choroidal melanoma is a primary cancer of the eye, meaning it originates in the eye. It may spread to other parts of the body, either by growing out into the optic nerve, or by cells breaking loose and traveling through the bloodstream. It is classified by size and by different cell types, spindles (named for their shape) and epithelioid (named for the epithelial cells they resemble).

What you can do If an eye exam shows that you have a choroidal nevus, schedule frequent eye exams (every 6 months) for monitoring purposes. Since choroidal melanomas can be asymptomatic, regular eye exams with a dilated fundus examination are important for early detection.

When to call the doctor Call the doctor at any sign of vision loss or pain in the eye.

Treatment While laser photocoagulation, cryotherapy, or surgical excision are sometimes used for smaller tumors, the two most commonly used treatments for choroidal melanoma are radiation or enucleation. Enucleation has been the standard treatment, but refinements in radiation procedures in the past 20 years have expanded the role of radiation. Also, some studies suggest that removing the eye may cause cancer cells to spread in some cases, but none of the studies have been conclusive.

The goal of radiation is to destroy the tumor and save the eye, and at least some vision. In a radiation procedure called brachytherapy, a piece of radioactive material, called a plaque, is sewn under the conjunctiva, the tissue lining the white of the eyeball. The plaque is shielded with gold to prevent the radiation from harming the structures around the eye, and it stays in place for about 3 days.

It is unclear which treatment provides the best long-term outcome for choroidal melanoma, and the National Eye Institute is conducting a study, the Collaborative Ocular Melanoma Study, to determine the relative benefits of enucleation, radiation, or a combination of the two therapies.

Prognosis The size of the tumor and the type of cells it contains influence the prognosis. The prognosis is better for spindle cell tumors than it is for epithelioid cell tumors. Many people with small to medium-sized tumors have complete recovery and retention of vision after treatment; treatment is also effective for many larger tumors. However, the prognosis is poor for melanomas that have spread within the eye, metastasized to other parts of the body, or recurred. In these people, there is a little more than 50 percent survival rate after 15 years.

❖ CYTOMEGALOVIRUS RETINITIS

Symptoms *(What you may experience)* Blurred or decreased vision; loss of peripheral or central vision; floaters; pain behind the eye.

Signs and laboratory findings *(What the doctor looks for)* Large yellow-white lesions on the retina, with exudates and hemorrhaging that spread along the paths of blood vessels. (See page C-44.)

What is it? Cytomegalovirus (CMV) is a very common type of herpes virus, present in more than half the adult population of the United States. It is transmitted in body fluids, including saliva, blood, urine, semen, and breast milk. Most people have been infected by the virus by age 3. In a healthy person, CMV has no effect: The immune system inactivates the virus, leaving it in a dormant state within the body. But if the immune system is severely weakened by a disease, such as acquired immunodeficiency syndrome (AIDS), or suppressed by medications, such as those used in organ transplantation or chemotherapy, CMV can be reactivated, causing serious disease of the eyes, gastrointestinal tract, lungs, and other organs.

CMV retinitis is one of the earliest signs of CMV disease. It is commonly found in people infected with the human immunodeficiency virus (HIV) and usually appears late in the disease, when HIV has almost totally destroyed the immune system. The infection can result in limited vision and even total blindness if damage to the retina is extensive. CMV retinitis is the most common cause of blindness in people with AIDS.

What you can do Good hygiene, including handwashing, can reduce the risk of transmission of CMV. However, because people with normal immune systems can retain the latent virus throughout their lives without ill effects, there is no need for intensive infection-control measures for healthy people. In immunocompromised people, regular eye exams every 4 to 6 months can help catch CMV retinitis in its early stages.

When to call the doctor People with weakened immune systems should call their doctors immediately if any unusual problems with vision occur. Untreated CMV retinitis can progress rapidly, and the infection can spread to other parts of the eye. Prompt treatment is essential to prevent loss of vision.

Treatment In March 1998, three antiviral medications—cidofovir, foscarnet, and ganciclovir—were approved by the Food and Drug Administration (FDA) for treatment of CMV retinitis in people with AIDS or those with compromised immune systems. These medications can cause serious side effects, including impaired kidney function, seizures, and lowered white blood cell count. Careful monitoring by a doctor is necessary.

Prognosis Treatment of CMV retinitis can slow or even stop spread of the infection, but in most cases lost vision cannot be restored. People with CMV retinitis need lifelong maintenance therapy to prevent progression of the disease and loss of vision. Even with maintenance therapy, however, the disease progresses in many people.

Eye Muscles

Six muscles control the movement and positioning of each eye. Three taut, elastic pairs of muscles hold the eye in place, opposing each other and providing tension that allows the eye muscles to move faster than do any other muscles of the body.

When you are looking straight ahead and your head is straight, this is considered the primary position of the eye. The eye muscles can move the globe of the eye about 50° in each direction (up, down, right, and left), but generally when you move your eyes 15 to 20°, you will also begin to move your head. In the healthy eye, the eye muscles of the two eyes work together, but disorders of the muscles can lead to vision problems.

❖ CROSSED EYES

Symptoms (*What you may experience*) Misaligned eyes and uncoordinated eye movements, either constant or intermittent; squinting; tilting head to look at things; frequent eye movements; headache; rubbing of eyes; tearing; double vision.

Signs and laboratory findings (*What the doctor looks for*) Deviations in eye movement; inability to keep one eye fixed on an object; poor visual acuity in one or both eyes. The doctor will use a number of different tests including cover tests to determine how the eyes move.

What is it? Crossed eyes, also called strabismus, occur when there is a misalignment or lack of coordination between the two eyes. Generally with this condition, the two eyes point in different directions. The misalignment is a result of the failure of the eye muscles to work together properly. It is usually diagnosed in childhood, but can also occur later in life. An estimated 4 percent of American children have some degree of crossed eyes; it affects boys and girls equally.

Most children with crossed eyes are otherwise normal, but there is a high incidence of this disorder in children with cerebral palsy (see page 474) and hydrocephalus (see page 473). Crossed eyes often worsen when eye muscles are tired—for example, late in the day, in bright sunshine, or during the course of an illness. Crossed eyes sometimes cause double vision in children (see Double Vision, this page), but commonly does in adults. If untreated, crossed eyes are likely to worsen with age.

Crossed eyes are classified by the way the eye deviates. The most common form is esotropia or convergent strabismus, which occurs when the eye turns in toward the nose. More than half of children with crossed eyes have the esotropic form. Accommodative esotropia is a variation in

---

DOUBLE VISION

Diplopia is the medical term for double vision, and it can be caused by a number of different problems in the eye. Treatment depends on the cause and severity of the condition.

When our eyes are working properly, we experience stereovision—the images seen by the two eyes fuse together as they are interpreted by the brain so that only one image results. This gives us depth perception, which can be lost to double vision. With double vision, the second image is sometimes distinct or sometimes shadowed or blurred.

There are two types of double vision—monocular and binocular. In the case of monocular diplopia, if you cover one eye, you will still see two images. This is less common than is binocular diplopia, where a double image is seen through two eyes, but only one image is seen if either eye is covered. Monocular diplopia is usually associated with a problem within the eye itself such as an irregularity in the cornea or lens, or severe astigmatism. Binocular diplopia is more likely to have a neurologic basis, and a tumor or aneurysm should be ruled out. Sometimes binocular diplopia is associated with crossed eyes.

Double vision is treated by diagnosing and treating the underlying disorder. Conditions that can cause it include trauma, brain tumor, cranial nerve palsy, diabetes, myasthenia gravis, thyroid disorder, or multiple sclerosis (MS), among others. In some cases, double vision can be alleviated by putting a patch over one eye. For some people, glasses containing prisms correct the double vision and bring together the two images. Surgery to strengthen an eye muscle is recommended in some cases. ■

farsighted children whose eyes cross because of the effort to focus. Exotropia or divergent strabismus, sometimes called wall-eye, occurs when the eye drifts outward. Sometimes eyes will drift up or down.

Crossed eyes can be caused by muscle weakness in the eye (leading to uneven muscle development), injury, other eye diseases, a brain tumor, or a tumor in the eye.

False or pseudo-strabismus is a condition in infants that looks like crossed eyes but is not; the appearance of crossed eyes is caused by an extra fold of skin that some children have near the inner eye, a broad flat nose, or eyes that are unusually close together. Pseudo-strabismus will disappear as the child's face grows. Your doctor should decide if a crossed eye is true strabismus or pseudostrabismus.

What you can do Parents should pay attention to early symptoms—early diagnosis is important to prevent lazy eye. Proper diagnosis is also important—without treatment a child will not outgrow crossed eyes.

When to call the doctor Call the doctor at the first sign of misalignment of a child's eyes. This can be difficult for a parent to detect because an infant's eyes may wander before coordination of the muscles develops, but it can be diagnosed by a doctor even in young babies. Babies should have eye exams by 6 months old, or sooner if a problem is suspected.

Treatment Treatments range from glasses to surgery. Glasses can be used to correct mild crossed eyes, by improving focusing and redirecting the line of vision. Sometimes an eye patch over the strong eye helps the weak eye focus. Exercises may also be prescribed to strengthen the weak eye. In some cases, drops are put in one eye, clouding vision and forcing the weaker eye to take over.

Surgery either strengthens or weakens an eye muscle in order to balance a pair of muscles. Usually it is done under general anesthesia. The incision is through the conjunctiva, and the exact place depends on which muscle is being treated. In some procedures, adjustable stitches are used to allow further adjustments after surgery. Sometimes, more than one operation is needed.

In a relatively new medical technique, a medication called botulinum (Botox) is

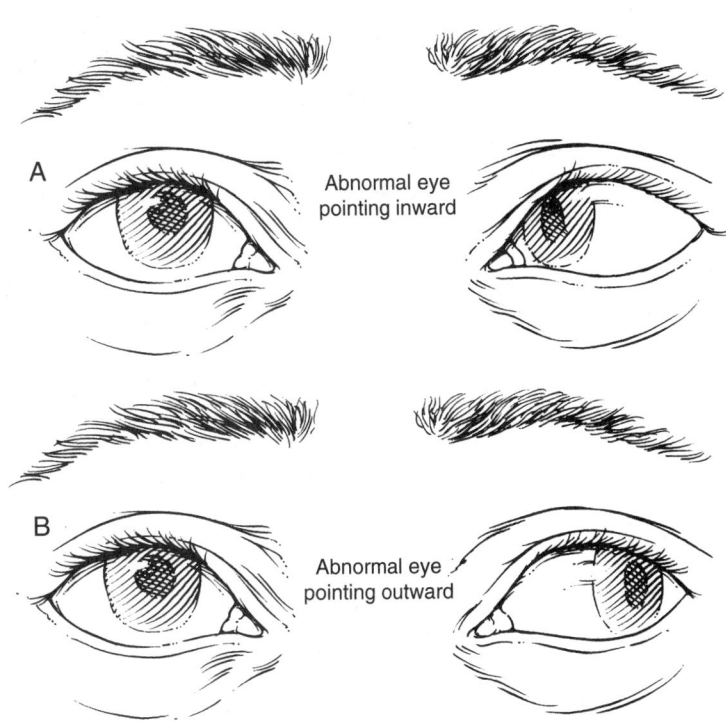

Strabismus is a disorder of eye muscles that leads the eyes to "cross," or point in different directions. (A) In esotropia, one eye turns inward toward the nose. (B) In exotropia, one eye points outward, away from the nose.

injected into an eye muscle. This temporarily weakens and relaxes the muscle and allows the opposing muscle to tighten. The effect of the medication wears off in several weeks, but the correction may be permanent.

Prognosis With timely and appropriate treatment, the prognosis is excellent. Most of the time crossed eyes can be corrected, both for visual and cosmetic effects.

❖ LAZY EYE

Symptoms (*What you may experience*) Closing one eye; tilting head to see; inability to gauge depth.

Signs and laboratory findings (*What the doctor looks for*) Reduced visual acuity (in one eye or both) that is not correctable with glasses or contact lenses in the late stages.

What is it? Lazy eye, also called amblyopia, is a condition in which vision becomes significantly impaired in an otherwise healthy eye because of lack of use of that eye. It affects about 2 percent of the population and usually develops in children less than 8 years old, as vision is still developing.

The most frequent cause of lazy eye is misalignment of the eyes or crossed eyes; about half of children with crossed eyes develop lazy eye. Another frequent cause is uneven visual acuity in the two eyes. If one eye is severely nearsighted or farsighted, the brain will favor the visual input of the stronger eye over the weaker, and the visual pathways of the brain will not develop normally. Lazy eye can also be caused by cataracts, drooping eyelid, or any other eye condition that impairs vision in one or both eyes.

There are three progressive stages of lazy eye: suspension, when the brain turns the weaker eye on and off; suppression, when the weaker eye is turned off indefinitely but still has usable vision and will be used if the other eye is covered; and amblyopia, when the misuse has continued for so long that the vision impairment cannot be corrected.

What you can do It is important to treat crossed eyes, childhood cataracts, refractive errors, drooping eyelid, and other underlying causes of lazy eye promptly and aggressively.

When to call the doctor Be attentive to the early signs of lazy eye and seek treatment. Prompt treatment may prevent vision loss.

Treatment There are three major treatment options: correcting the underlying problem, correcting refractive errors (see Options for Correcting Vision, page 506), and occlusion to force the use of the lazy eye by limiting use of the better eye. Occlusion is usually done by having the child wear a patch over the nonlazy eye. Sometimes (particularly in the case of small children who may object to a patch), drops or ointment are used to blur vision in the stronger eye, so that the lazy eye will take over. Occlusion may be full or part time, depending on the seriousness of the lazy eye. It is important to guard against overtreatment, so that lazy eye does not develop in the previously stronger eye.

Prognosis If lazy eye is detected and treated early enough, treatment is usually successful. Sometimes after successful treat-ment, the condition will recur, and another course of treatment will be necessary. If the cause of lazy eye is not treated, some degree of permanent vision loss in one or both eyes is likely.

Eyeball Inflammation

Within the globe of the eye, there are a number of areas that are subject to inflammation. One is the uvea, which lies between the sclera and the retina. The uvea is composed of the iris, the colored part of the eye that controls the intensity of light reaching the retina by dilating or constricting the pupil; the ciliary body, a muscular tissue that contracts the zones of the lens and also plays a role in the manufacturing of fluid in the eye; and the choroid, the tissue rich in blood vessels that lines the eye and nourishes the retina. Another is the sclera, the tough, white outer membrane that makes up the white of the eye.

UVEITIS

Symptoms *(What you may experience)* Anterior: pain; red eye; sensitivity to light; slight decrease in vision; tearing. Posterior: blurred vision; floaters. Less frequently: redness, pain, and sensitivity to light. Uveitis can occur suddenly, with a painless blurring of vision.

Signs and laboratory findings *(What the doctor looks for)* Anterior: contraction of the pupil; inflammatory cells visible on slit-lamp exam; deposits called keratic precipitates on the back of the cornea. Posterior: inflammatory cells; fuzzy white lesions in the retina; inflammation of the choroid.

What is it? Uveitis is an inflammation of the uvea, the iris, ciliary body, or choroid. It may be associated with other infections or diseases in the body and has many different causes.

The uvea is divided into different areas, and the inflammation is classified according to where it is. Anterior uveitis involves the iris; when the inflammation is confined to the iris, it is called iritis or iridocyclitis. Posterior uveitis involves the choroid and is sometimes called choroiditis. If the uvea is inflamed in the middle of the eye, it may be called pars planitis.

Sometimes the specific cause of uveitis can be determined, but often it is unknown. Approximately 40 percent of cases are associated with a systemic disease. This is why it is important for someone diagnosed with uveitis to have a complete physical exam to try to find the underlying cause if it is not already known.

The diseases that are associated with uveitis include tuberculosis, herpes simplex and herpes zoster, Lyme disease, rheumatoid arthritis, sarcoidosis, syphilis, inflammatory bowel disease, and toxoplasmosis. This is only a partial list—more than 100 different diseases have been linked to uveitis.

When to call the doctor Call the doctor if any symptoms of uveitis appear. This is a serious disease that can scar the eye if treatment is delayed and cause cataracts and glaucoma.

Treatment Treatment of uveitis includes the use of topical or systemic medication, depending on the severity of the condition. Treatment must be multidisciplinary to treat the associated disease.

Steroid drops or ointment on the eye are the primary medications used to treat uveitis. Anti-inflammatory drops may also be used, and cycloplegics, drops that paralyze the ciliary muscle. If the inflammation does not respond to topical steroids, steroids may be injected around the eye or taken orally.

Warm compresses may provide relief from symptoms, and wearing sunglasses will help with sensitivity to light.

In some cases of uveitis, oral immunosuppressive medications are used. These medications often have serious systemic side effects, however, and if they are used, the person receiving them should be closely monitored by an internist as well as the ophthalmologist.

Surgery may be used to treat some of the complications of uveitis, such as cataracts, glaucoma, or detached retina.

Prognosis The prognosis for recovery from uveitis is good if the inflammation is diagnosed and treated promptly, and the underlying systemic disease is also treated. However, uveitis can become chronic and recur, and can lead to scarring in the eye. With treatment, anterior uveitis usually gets better in days to weeks, but relapses are common. Posterior uveitis is likely to be more stubborn, and the inflammation may last months and require aggressive treatment.

VASOCONSTRICTORS

Doctors advise caution in using eye drops containing vasoconstrictors. These eyedrops (available under a host of brand names, such as Visine and Murine) are among the most popular over-the-counter (OTC) medications on the market—more than 15 million bottles are sold each year in the United States. They are used to self-treat redness in the eye.

A vasoconstrictor is a medication that causes blood vessels to narrow. This can provide temporary relief for mild redness in the eyes. However, many people continue to use the drops for long periods—years, even—and this can lead to problems. Prolonged use of vasoconstrictor eye drops can cause dryness in the eye, increased swelling, rebound redness, and conjunctivitis.

Most of the time these symptoms disappear once a person stops using the drops, but recovery may take weeks, particularly for long-term users. If you feel you need to continue using vasoconstrictor eye drops for more than a couple of days, you should consult your doctor about your symptoms. ∎

❖ EPISCLERITIS

Symptoms *(What you may experience)* Sudden redness; mild pain in one or both eyes; pink or purple color to the eyeball; sensitivity to light; tearing.

Signs and laboratory findings *(What the doctor looks for)* Inflamed blood vessels in the episclera, a tissue between the conjunctiva and sclera.

What is it? Episcleritis is an inflammation of the episclera. It is most often seen in adults between the ages of 20 and 50, and usually lasts for 1 to 3 days before clearing up on its own. The cause is usually not known, but it is sometimes associated with connective tissue diseases, such as rheumatoid arthritis and systemic lupus erythematosus. See Chapter 17 for information on connective tissue diseases.

When to call the doctor Call the doctor if symptoms persist for more than a couple of days, if the pain is bothersome, or if vision is affected.

Treatment Generally, episcleritis is self-limiting and will clear up without treatment. Artificial tears may relieve the symptoms of mild episcleritis. In more serious cases, steroid drops or ointment may be prescribed. Oral nonsteroidal anti-inflammatory drugs (for example, ibuprofen) may also provide relief.

Prognosis Episcleritis is generally a mild condition that responds well to treatment and usually clears up spontaneously. Sometimes there are recurrences.

❖ SCLERITIS

Symptoms *(What you may experience)* Severe piercing pain which may radiate to the forehead, brow, or jaw; red-looking eye; tearing; sensitivity to light; gradual decrease in vision; bulging of the eye (less frequently). Pain may be mild at first and increase gradually. Pain may worsen at night and disturb sleep. In more than half of cases, symptoms are in both eyes.

Signs and laboratory findings *(What the doctor looks for)* Inflammation of the sclera. The sclera may appear swollen and purplish; nodules (small bumps) may be apparent.

What is it? Scleritis is an inflammation of the sclera, the tough outer membrane that we call the white of the eye. It is usually a much more serious condition than episcleritis and can lead to damage to the eyeball itself. It is most common in adults between the ages of 30 and 60 and is seen more often in women than it is in men. While the cause of scleritis is unknown, it is often associated with rheumatoid arthritis, Crohn's disease (see page 1007), and other autoimmune disorders.

Scleritis is classified according to its location (anterior or posterior) and the appearance and severity of the inflammation. The most dangerous form is necrotizing, which means cell death is evident.

Treatment For mild cases of scleritis, oral nonsteroidal anti-inflammatory drugs are given. For more severe cases, oral steroids are prescribed. Topical steroids are usually not effective, but they may reduce inflammation and pain. If the examination shows thinning of the sclera due to scleritis, be sure to use protective glasses or an eye shield to prevent additional damage from trauma. Sometimes immunosuppressant medications are used. Treatment of the underlying disorder is an important part of the treatment plan.

Prognosis Scleritis usually responds to treatment, but it may recur. Ocular complications are not uncommon and may include keratitis, cataracts, uveitis, and glaucoma. If untreated, scleritis can lead to perforation of the eyeball. About 40 percent of people with necrotizing scleritis have some loss of vision.

❖ ORBITAL CELLULITIS

Symptoms *(What you may experience)* Swollen, shiny, taut eyelids; red eye; pain; bulging of the eye; blurred or double vision; fever; headache; general malaise.

Signs and laboratory findings *(What the doctor looks for)* Swelling, redness, warmth, and tenderness to the eye; restricted or painful eye movement; infection in the blood as determined by blood cultures; evaluation of the extent of infection using computed tomography (CT) scan.

What is it? Orbital cellulitis is a bacterial or fungal infection in the orbit behind the eye. It is very serious and potentially life threatening, if it goes untreated. Most frequently, orbital cellulitis is a complication of a progressing sinus infection. Orbital cellulitis is not common, but may be seen in children who are infected with *Haemophilus influenzae* B (HiB) or in adults with sinusitis. It is also seen sometimes after trauma to the eye. Besides HiB, orbital cellulitis is caused by staphylococcus, streptococcus, or other bacteria and rarely some fungi.

What you can do Immunization with HiB vaccination according to recommended schedules is an effective measure to prevent HiB-related orbital cellulitis. Prompt evaluation and treatment of sinus infections is another important preventive step. See

Chapter 8 for information on vaccination schedules.

When to call the doctor If symptoms of orbital cellulitis are present, call the doctor immediately or go to the emergency room.

Treatment Orbital cellulitis can progress rapidly and should be treated promptly and aggressively. It is usually caused by a bacterial infection, often an infection that spreads from the sinuses. Hospitalization is usually necessary, and treatment will usually include intravenous (IV) antibiotics. If an abscess (accumulation of pus) has developed, it may be drained surgically. Because of sinus involvement, usually your doctor will consult with an otolaryngologist. Once the condition is clearly improving, oral antibiotics can be used. The CT scan is an important tool for evaluating the status of the orbit and sinuses; if improvement is not timely, further CT scans will be taken to evaluate the problem.

Prognosis If orbital cellulitis is diagnosed and treated in a timely manner, full recovery can be expected. If it is allowed to progress untreated, however, it can cause optic nerve damage and vision loss, or brain infection and death, in the most severe cases.

Eye Injury

The delicate tissues of the eye can be injured by many agents in many ways. There are more than 2.5 million eye injuries each year in the United States, leaving 40,000 people with significant visual defects (defined as the inability to read newspaper print).

Trauma to the eye poses a threat to vision and eye health and should never be taken lightly or neglected. Retinal detachment is often a consequence of trauma to the eye, and significant eye injury merits evaluation by a doctor (see Detached Retina, page 533). See Eye Injury, page 392, for information on emergency first aid treatment for eye injuries, including burns.

❖ BLOWOUT FRACTURE OF THE ORBIT

Symptoms (*What you may experience*) Following a blunt blow to the eye: pain, especially when trying to move the eye up

PROTECTIVE EYEWEAR

One of the most important things you can do to protect your eyes is also one of the easiest. Wearing glasses or goggles or special shields is the most effective way to protect your eyes from injury. Whenever you are engaged in an activity that poses a threat to your eyes—whether it is your occupation, a hobby, or participation in a sport—you should use protective eyewear.

Protective eyewear ranges from simple glasses or sunglasses to specially manufactured gear designed for specific purposes. Nearly all prescription glasses can be made of polycarbonate, which is an extremely tough plastic much more resistant to impact than is standard lens material. Goggles seal against the face and provide better protection from flying objects.

For many sports, an integrated helmet and face mask offer the best protection for your eyes and from head injury. Special care should be taken for contact and stick sports like football, hockey, and lacrosse. Safety glasses with polycarbonate lenses and side shields are recommended in many industrial settings. Sometimes polycarbonate safety goggles are worn over a person's regular eyewear. Polycarbonate lenses are also recommended for a person with only one eye, since failure to protect the good eye from injury can lead to blindness. ■

and down; tenderness; binocular double vision (resolves when one eye is covered); swelling of the eyelid, especially after blowing nose.

Signs and laboratory findings (*What the doctor looks for*) Restricted eye movement; presence of air in tissues of the orbit; numbness or diminished feeling in cheek or lip on the side where the injury occurred; recession of the eyeball into the orbit.

What is it? A blowout fracture is a unique type of fracture to the orbit, the structure of facial bones that protects the eye (see also page 624). It is caused by a blunt blow to the eye; for example, being hit directly in the eye by a round object such as a baseball. The pressure to the eye can force the soft tissues downward. The thin floor of the orbit offers the path of least resistance and fractures downward. Fractures may also occur in other walls of the orbit.

The blowout fracture may trap the lower muscles of the eye or the tissues around the muscle, causing double vision, particularly when trying to look upward. Approximately one-fourth of blowout fractures are associated with some damage to the eyeball.

What you can do   Wear protective glasses or goggles when playing sports or involved in activities or occupations where the orbit could be injured (see Protective Eyewear, page 547.)

When to call the doctor   Consult your doctor following any forceful blunt blow to the eye, particularly if you experience any of the symptoms of blowout fracture.

Treatment   In three-quarters of cases, blowout fractures will heal themselves, but they need to be carefully followed medically. Upon diagnosis, a complete ophthalmologic workup should be done to detect any damage to the eye. Nasal decongestants are usually recommended for your comfort, and oral antibiotics will be prescribed to prevent infection. You may be instructed to keep ice packs on the orbit for 1 to 2 days and to avoid blowing your nose.

In some cases, surgical repair is necessary. This is usually required when an eye muscle (the muscle controlling the movement of the eye) or its associated tissues are trapped in the bone, if the eyeball has the potential to recede, or if there is extensive involvement of the floor of the orbit. Usually surgery is performed 1 to 2 weeks after the injury or sooner if the eye muscle is trapped. The doctor will remove bone fragments, elevate the eye, and reinforce the orbit with a plastic implant or bone graft.

Prognosis   The prognosis is excellent for recovery from a blowout fracture of the orbit, but the person should be monitored throughout the recovery period for associated eye problems such as orbital cellulitis (see page 546) or bleeding, among others.

❖ OPEN GLOBE

Symptoms (*What you may experience*)
Following blunt or penetrating trauma: pain and decreased vision.

Signs and laboratory findings (*What the doctor looks for*)   Significant swelling and hemorrhage under the conjunctiva; abnormally deep anterior chamber; blood in the anterior chamber, sometimes clotted; limited eye movement; blood in the vitreous; low eye pressure. In the case of an open globe due to a penetrating injury, a laceration in the sclera or cornea will be evident. In some cases, some of the internal contents of the eye will be outside the wall of the eye. (See page C-43.)

What is it?   The globe of the eye can rupture or break open from blunt trauma, such as the impact of a baseball, or from a penetrating injury such as being pierced by a dart. Blunt trauma can cause serious damage to any of the delicate tissues of the eye if it is forceful enough. Some of the thinner spots of the sclera are where the rupture is likely to occur. Ruptures can vary in severity, and this is usually a very serious and sight-threatening injury.

What you can do   Wear protective glasses or goggles when playing sports or involved in activities or occupations where the eye could be injured.

When to call the doctor   Seek emergency care for any penetrating injury or blunt trauma to the eye. If an object becomes stuck in your eye, you should not touch it, apply pressure, or try to remove it, but seek emergency medical help. See pages 392 and 393, for information on emergency first aid following blunt trauma or penetrating injury.

Treatment   As soon as an open globe is diagnosed, the eye should be protected with a shield, and no pressure put on it. The person will be hospitalized with no food or drink, and given IV antibiotics and a tetanus shot (if inoculation is not up to date). A CT scan may be taken, and surgery will be scheduled promptly. The nature of the surgery will depend on the location and extent of the rupture. In rare cases, the eye will have to be removed at this time (see Eye Prosthesis, page 549). In other cases, vision will be destroyed but the integrity of the globe can be sufficiently maintained. If the eye becomes blind, its removal is sometimes recommended to prevent any sympathetic inflammation in the other eye.

Prognosis   Prognosis depends on the location and severity of the injury. An open

EYE PROSTHESIS

In generations past, losing an eye to injury or disease was an all too common occurrence. Modern medicine and surgery have done much to reduce this risk. But sometimes enucleation is the only solution to an ophthalmologic crisis.

Once the eye is removed, an artificial eye—called a prosthesis—is put in for both cosmetic and physical reasons. The use of artificial eyes can be documented as far back as the Renaissance, when glassblowers made an art of the manufacture of glass eyes. After World War II, plastic replaced glass as the material of choice for artificial eyes.

Today, the art and science of eye prostheses are so advanced that you can tell the difference between an artificial and natural eye only upon very close examination. Artificial eyes are manufactured and fitted by technical specialists called ocularists, who will work with your doctor to achieve an optimum fit.

The installation of an eye prosthesis is a surgical procedure that is done in several stages; it may take as long as a year before the final device is in place. It begins with the enucleation procedure, when an implant is placed in the orbit followed by a conformer to maintain the shape of the eyelids. A temporary prosthesis will be fitted 2 to 6 weeks after surgery, when swelling has subsided, and then a permanent one, usually within a few months.

The newest generation of eye prostheses are used with a material called hydroxyapatite, which comes from coral. The hydroxyapatite implant is inserted in the orbit following enucleation, and the muscles that move the eye are stitched to it. Blood vessels will grow around and into the implant. A conformer is also put into place. After about 6 months, a prosthesis will be attached over the implant by means of a peg that fits into a hole drilled into the implant. The conformer is removed. This arrangement allows the eye muscles to actually move the artificial eye, and the two eyes can move together. ∎

---

globe can lead to loss of vision and loss of the eye as well.

❖ BLACK EYE

Symptoms *(What you may experience)* Following trauma: purplish bruising around the eyelids and sides of the eye after trauma, gradually fading to greenish-yellow; swelling of the eyelid; soreness around the eyelids.

What is it? A black eye, also called a periorbital hematoma, results from blunt trauma to the eye. It is caused by bleeding underneath the skin. Black eyes are very common injuries and are usually external; however, the eye may also have been injured.

What you can do Wear protective glasses or goggles when playing sports or involved in activities or occupations where the eye could be injured.

When to call the doctor Call the doctor if the black eye is accompanied by blurred or double vision, pain, floaters, light sensitivity, or other irregularities in vision, or if the bruising does not start to fade in a couple of days. See the doctor if there is any indication that the injury is more extensive than bruising of the eyelids.

Treatment Apply cold packs to the bruised area frequently (15 minutes of every hour) to reduce swelling and numb the pain. Apply gently to avoid further bruising.

Prognosis Black eyes rarely cause serious or lasting medical problems and heal spontaneously within about 2 weeks from the time of injury.

❖ HYPHEMA

Symptoms *(What you may experience)* Usually following trauma: bloodshot eyes; pain; blurred vision.

Signs and laboratory findings *(What the doctor looks for)* Blood in the anterior chamber of the eye, between the cornea and the iris.

What is it? Hyphema is an accumulation of blood in the anterior chamber of the eye, between the cornea and iris. It may be caused by blunt trauma or an injury that penetrates any of the tissues of the eye. Hyphema is often related to a sports injury, but it also sometimes occurs spontaneously, without a history of trauma.

Hyphemas vary in size and shape and are classified by grades (1 to 4) according to severity. Hyphema is the most common reason children are hospitalized following eye trauma. It is a serious condition that requires restriction of physical activity to prevent rebleeding. Recurring hemorrhage increases the risk of complications such as glaucoma and corneal blood staining, which can permanently cloud vision and require a corneal transplant.

Hyphema occurs when the vessels of the iris or the ciliary body are injured, but the causes are not always apparent, even under microscopic examination. In many cases, the accumulated blood elevates intraocular pressure and can lead to glaucoma. Concern about pressure is greatest in people with sickle cell disease or trait, and black individuals with hyphema should be screened for sickle cell disease or trait. See Chapter 22 for information on sickle cell disease or trait.

What you can do Wear protective glasses or goggles when playing sports or involved in activities or occupations where the eye could be injured.

When to call the doctor Call the doctor at any sign of blood in the front of the eye after a traumatic injury. See Eye Injury, page 392, for first aid information relating to traumatic injury to the eye.

Treatment The first goal of treatment of hyphema is to prevent further hemorrhage. This often means hospitalization or enforced bed rest for a week. The head of the bed should be elevated 30°. The injured eye should be shielded but not patched because there should be no pressure on it.

There is some controversy among doctors about the medications to treat hyphema. Atropine drops, which dilate the pupil and relax the eye, are often prescribed. Sometimes steroid drops or oral steroids are also used, or an oral or topical medication (aminocaproic acid) may be used to prevent rebleeding. Mild analgesics (painkillers) may be used (for example, acetaminophen), but no products containing aspirin should be used because aspirin thins the blood. If intraocular pressure is elevated, it will be treated with a topical beta blocker or other medication. See Glaucoma, page 526, for more information on lowering intraocular pressure.

In the case of rebleeding or elevated intraocular pressure that will not go down, surgery may be necessary to drain the blood.

Prognosis The outcome of hyphema depends on the extent of the injury to the eye, but most uncomplicated cases heal successfully within a week or so. With mild grade 1 hyphemas, 80 percent of people recover their pre-injury visual acuity if there are no other associated eye injuries, but that number drops to 30 percent for larger grade 4 hyphemas. Complications are most likely when there has been rebleeding, and the most common complications are elevated eye pressure and impaired vision due to staining of the cornea.

❖ CORNEAL ABRASION

Symptoms *(What you may experience)* Sudden sharp pain; sensation of a foreign body in the eye; tearing; sensitivity to light; discomfort when blinking.

Signs and laboratory findings *What the doctor looks for)* An abrasion evident when fluorescein dye is applied to the eye; redness of the conjunctiva; swelling of the eyelid.

What is it? A corneal abrasion is the most common corneal injury, and one of the most common injuries to the eye. It can be caused by a number of events—contact with a finger or fingernail, the edge of a piece of paper, something that hits the eye, or by improper fit or excessive wear of contacts. Corneal abrasions are among the most common sports-related eye injuries.

An abrasion is the loss of the epithelium of the cornea, like a scratch on the front surface of the eye. The outermost tissue of the cornea is the epithelium; loss of this exposes the corneal nerves. That is why a corneal abrasion can be very painful, even though the trauma seems minor. It is possible for corneal injury to occur without your being aware of when it happened or what caused it.

The thin layer of the epithelium plays an important role in preventing bacteria from entering the cornea. A scratch in the epithelium exposes the inner layers of the cornea to bacteria, and this can lead to infectious keratitis, a more serious problem. Another type of wound to the cornea called welder's burn results from exposure to ultraviolet light, which can come from the welder's torch but also from the sun or, more commonly, a sun lamp. Welder's burn usually does not become symptomatic until approximately 12 hours after exposure, so the cause and effect may not be immediately apparent.

What you can do Certain common sense steps can help prevent a corneal abrasion; for example, keep a baby's fingernails trimmed short and smooth; avoid putting anything sharp (even something as seemingly harmless as a piece of paper) near your eyes; use care with contacts; and use protective eyewear when working with any materials that may fly into the eye or when exposing the eye to a sun lamp or any other source of ultraviolet light rays.

If you experience a corneal abrasion, close the eye and avoid rubbing. Remove contacts immediately. Sometimes blinking several times will remove small, irritating particles in the eye, and sometimes pulling the upper eyelid over the lower eyelid can dislodge a foreign body. However, do not take any further steps to remove anything from your eye—that could lead to a more extensive abrasion.

When to call the doctor See the doctor for symptoms of corneal abrasion.

Treatment Corneal abrasions are treated with cycloplegic drops that dilate and relax the eye, and antibiotic drops or ointment. Often a snug-fitting pressure patch is put on the eye for a day to keep the eye from moving and prevent further abrasion to the cornea. *Do not attempt to place this patch yourself.* If not properly bolstered, the patch may worsen the condition by directly contacting the surface of the eye. However, a pressure patch is not recommended for contact lens wearers with abrasions; patching in these people increases the risk of infection. If you wear contacts you should not resume wearing contacts until you are symptom free for 3 or 4 days and you have had your lenses checked for scratches, protein buildup, or other problems.

See Keratitis, page 520, and Herpes Simplex Virus Keratitis, page 521, for information about treating infectious kertatitis.

Prognosis Corneal abrasion is one of the simplest eye emergencies to treat, and outcomes are almost always successful. Many corneal abrasions heal on their own within 48 hours. However, corneal abrasions can turn into infections with the risk of perforation (see Recurrent Corneal Erosion, page 523).

❖ FOREIGN BODY

Symptoms *(What you may experience)* Sensation of a foreign body in the eye; tearing; blurred vision; light sensitivity; irritation in the eye.

Signs and laboratory findings *(What the doctor looks for)* Presence of a foreign body; eyelid swelling; irritation in the eye; red-looking eye. (See page C-44.)

What is it? Foreign bodies can injure the eye from any number of sources: soot, dirt, or chemical particles in the air; cosmetics; debris from yard work or building projects; even your own eyelash. If not removed, they can cause irritation, inflammation, abrasion, and possibly infection.

The presence of foreign objects will cause increased flow of tears, and this often washes away the offending substance. However, sometimes more intervention is necessary to remove it.

What you can do As with other eye injuries, using protective eyewear can prevent foreign bodies on and in the eye.

When you feel a foreign body become lodged on the eye, flush the eye with clean water, for 15 minutes if possible. It may help to hold the eyelids apart. Sometimes you can dislodge a foreign body by drawing the upper lid down over the lower lid. If the object is visible, you (or someone helping you) can very carefully try to remove it by lightly touching a moistened cotton swab or corner of a clean cloth to it. Do not persist if it does not come out easily, because you could cause it to become more deeply embedded. Never rub the eye. See page 392 for more information on emergency first aid for foreign bodies in the eye.

When to call the doctor Call the doctor if you cannot remove the foreign body, or if pain or irritation persist.

Treatment The doctor locates the foreign object usually by examining the eye through the slit-lamp microscope. The object is then removed either through irrigation or with a sterile needle, forceps, or blunt spatula. Antibiotic ointment will be applied to prevent infection, and cycloplegic drops to relax the ciliary muscle. A patch may be placed to keep the eyelids closed and prevent further injury, usually for about a day.

In rare cases if the foreign body enters the inside of the eyeball, more extensive surgery is needed to remove the foreign body.

Prognosis With the microscopes and advanced imaging equipment that are available today to examine the eye, it is relatively simple for foreign objects on or in the eye to be found and removed. The location of the foreign object will determine the visual outcome.

❖ CHEMICAL INJURY

Symptoms *(What you may experience)* Burning sensation in the eye after being splashed with a chemical; tearing; pain.

Signs and laboratory findings *(What the doctor looks for)* Swelling in the cornea

EMERGENCY EYE WASHING

A simple rule of thumb for eye care and eye safety: When in doubt, wash it out. And keep on washing.

A steady stream of clean water over the eye will remove many foreign particles on the surface of the eye and help wash away chemicals to which you have been exposed. For chemical exposure, flood the eyes and eyelids and continue rinsing for at least 15 minutes.

Emergency eyewash equipment is required in industrial and laboratory workplaces in the United States. The American National Standards Institute regulates this equipment and requires that a controlled flow of clean water be available for both eyes, at a velocity that will not injure the eye. Water should be between 60 and 90°F.

Continuing eye irrigation is one of the principles of treatment for some kinds of ocular trauma. Special ocular irrigation devices are used, with tubing running into a cup that holds the eyelid open, so that neither the patient nor the doctor has to be concerned with the keeping the eye open for irrigation.

See page 393 for more information on how to wash an eye in an emergency. ■

and conjunctiva; opaque area in the cornea that may block the view of the anterior chamber, iris, or lens. After copious irrigation, the doctor will measure the pH of the eye to assess the nature of the chemical substance.

What is it? Chemical injuries to the eye occur frequently, and their effects vary in severity from mild irritation to loss of vision and sometimes loss of the eye. Damage can be caused by chemicals in solid, liquid, powder, or mist form. Chemical injuries that happen in the home are most likely to be caused by detergents, disinfectants, solvents, cosmetics, drain cleaners, oven cleaners, ammonia, bleach, or other household supplies. In agriculture settings, fertilizers or pesticides can cause eye damage; in industry, caustic chemicals and solvents are the usual culprits.

Most chemical exposures to the eye will cause only superficial damage and no structural or visual impairment. Strong alkalis and acids will cause the worst damage, and alkalis are generally more of a threat to the eye than are acids. Acid damage may be somewhat self-limiting, but alkaline agents can quickly work their way into the eye and continue to cause further damage.

What you can do To prevent chemical damage to the eye, wear protective goggles whenever working with chemicals.

The most important thing to remember when a chemical exposure occurs is the need for immediate and continuous irrigation. Flush the eye with clean water, a strong steady stream that should continue, if possible, until medical evaluation can take place (see Emergency Eye Washing, this page). See page 393 for more information on emergency first aid for chemical matter in the eye.

When to call the doctor Chemical injury to the eye is serious and potentially threatening to vision. Seek immediate emergency medical care in the case of any chemical exposure to the eye.

Treatment The doctor or emergency medical technician will continue irrigation of the eye, with a saline or Ringer's solution if available. Usually an anesthetic drop will be applied to the eye and the irrigation done through tubing or a special apparatus for this function. The eyelids may be immobilized with a retractor or similar instrument. After a period of irrigation, the pH of the exposed eye will be tested. Irrigation will continue until the pH is normal or near normal. In some cases, particularly severe alkali burns, irrigation may continue for as long as 24 hours.

After irrigation, the doctor will examine the eye, remove any foreign particles, and check intraocular pressure. Cycloplegic drops will be applied to relax the ciliary muscle, and topical antibiotic ointment to prevent infection. Sometimes damaged corneal tissue will be debrided. Sometimes a needle will remove poisoned fluid from inside the eye. Usually a pressure patch is applied. Antiglaucoma medications will be given if the intraocular pressure is elevated. See Glaucoma, page 526, for more information on lowering intraocular pressure.

Serious cases of chemical injury may require hospitalization in order to closely monitor intraocular pressure and healing of the cornea.

Prognosis The prognosis for recovery from chemical injury varies, depending on the nature and extent of the exposure. Most people experience full recovery. However, complications can result, including glaucoma, corneal damage, and dry eye syndrome. In the most severe cases, chemical exposure can lead to vision loss or loss of the eye itself.

LACERATION OF THE EYELID

Symptoms (*What you may experience*) Cut to the eyelid; pain; swelling; bleeding.

Signs and laboratory findings (*What the doctor looks for*) Laceration evident in the eye exam. The doctor will also look for related eye damage.

What is it? Laceration of the eyelid is a tear or jagged wound to the upper or lower eyelid. It can result from traffic accidents, dog bites, or a variety of other accidents. Severity can range from mild to serious, depending on how extensive the wound is and whether structures within the eyelid, such as the tear glands or ducts or muscles, are damaged.

When to call the doctor Seek emergency treatment for any injury involving laceration of the eyelid. See page 392 for information on emergency first aid for eyelid laceration.

Treatment The first step in treating the eyelid is to determine whether there is any damage to the eyeball itself. If there is, treatment of the eyeball will take precedence over the eyelid injury. If the injury is the result of an animal bite, the need for rabies vaccine should be investigated. A tetanus shot will be given to people who have not had one within 5 years. The wound will be cleaned and irrigated, and a topical antibiotic applied.

Surgical repair is necessary for eyelid lacerations; it should be done by a qualified ophthalmic plastic surgeon. Often surgery is delayed for 24 to 48 hours to allow swelling to diminish. Complicated eyelid surgery will be done in the operating room, but simpler procedures (for example, when there is no gland, duct, or muscle involvement and no significant loss of tissue) can be done in the doctor's office or emergency room. The eyelid is stitched together; the number of stitches needed depends on the extent of the injury. The goal of surgery is a smooth outer edge of the eyelid, for both cosmetic and functional reasons.

After surgery, the doctor may prescribe cold compresses or ice packs to decrease swelling. Antibiotic ointment will be applied, and often oral antibiotics are also prescribed. The stitches are removed in 4 to 6 days, except for those on the margin of the lid, which may be removed in 10 to 14 days.

Prognosis When appropriately treated, eyelid lacerations usually heal in 1 to 2 weeks. Unattended lacerations can result in scarring of the eyelid.

General Diseases that Affect the Eye

Various systemic diseases exhibit manifestations in the eye. Treatment of these disorders requires collaboration between the doctor who is treating the systemic condition and an ophthalmologist.

❖ GRAVES' DISEASE

Ocular symptoms *(What you may experience)* Early symptoms: feeling of irritation in the eyes; double vision; excessive tearing or dry eye; proptosis; sensitivity to light. Late symptoms: swelling of the eye; inability to move the eye; corneal ulceration; loss of vision in severe cases (rarely).

Ocular signs and laboratory findings *(What the doctor looks for)* Swelling behind the eye; retraction of the eyelid; enlarged extraocular muscles.

What is it? Graves' disease (see page 1185) is a thyroid disorder characterized by hyperthyroidism (hyperactivity of the thyroid gland). An excess of the hormone thyroxine is produced, resulting in a range of hyperthyroid symptoms including jitteriness, weight loss, rapid heartbeat, heat intolerance, muscle weakness, and changes in the menstrual cycle. It is a fairly uncommon disease, striking about a million Americans each year, and women are more than five times more likely than are men to get it.

About half of people with Graves' disease develop eye symptoms, known as Graves' eye disease or Graves' ophthalmopa-thy. The eye symptoms are not a result of the hyperthyroidism but of a related autoimmune process. The thyroid and eye diseases run independent courses, and both must be treated.

Usually the eye symptoms are mild and easily treated. Eye problems arise when tissues, muscles, and fat in the orbit behind the eye increase in volume. This swelling causes the proptosis or pop-eyed look associated with Graves' disease. In serious cases, the swelling may cause paralysis of the muscles that move the eyeball or may compress the optic nerve. As the eyelids and conjunctiva swell, they may retract, which can lead to corneal exposure and infection.

Treatment In mild cases, cool compresses, sunglasses, and artificial tears provide relief for the symptoms of Graves' eye disease. People with Graves' eye disease are often advised to sleep with their heads elevated to alleviate eyelid swelling. If double vision is a continuing problem, glasses containing prisms may be prescribed (see Double Vision, page 542).

Oral corticosteroids may help with early stages of eye muscle problems, but are not effective later in the course of the dis-

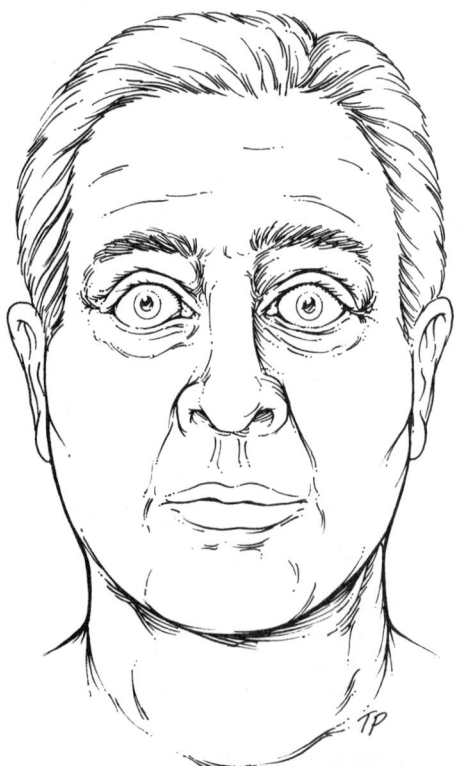

In Graves' disease, an autoimmune process causes the tissues behind the eye to increase in volume, which makes the eye appear to pop out of the sockets (orbits). This can lead to problems with vision and eye movement.

ease. Oral or IV steroids may be used to treat compression of the optic nerve, which is the most serious complication of Graves' eye disease.

In more stubborn cases, radiation treatment to the orbit eases orbital swelling, and in the most serious cases when more conservative approaches fail, orbital decompression surgery is done. In this procedure, a bone between the orbit and sinuses is removed to allow more space for the orbital tissues. Other operations that may be done for serious Graves' eye disease are extraocular muscle surgery to realign the eyes, and eyelid surgery to reposition the eyelid.

Prognosis Most of the symptoms of Graves' disease, including eye symptoms, can be successfully treated.

❖ MULTIPLE SCLEROSIS

Ocular symptoms *(What you may experience)* Blurring or dimming of vision; blindness in one eye; pain in the orbit; loss of color vision; reduced perception of light intensity; nystagmus (uncontrolled horizontal or vertical eye movements).

Ocular signs and laboratory findings *(What the doctor looks for)* Decreased visual acuity; uneven reaction of pupils to light; swollen optic nerve; uncontrolled horizontal or vertical eye movements.

What is it? Multiple sclerosis (MS—see page 453) is a chronic neurological disease with a variable course—some people are very disabled from it, while others enjoy long spontaneous remissions. It is characterized by destruction of myelin, the fatty white substance that coats nerve fibers. The ophthalmologic manifestation of MS is usually optic neuritis (see Optic Neuritis, page 529). Optic neuritis is sometimes an early sign of MS and probably results from destruction of the myelin sheath of the optic nerve.

Prognosis Optic neuritis is usually a self-limiting condition. MS has a variable course and is difficult to predict, but approximately one-third of people with MS live a normal life span without significant disability. Crossed eyes as a result of MS is usually self-limiting.

❖ DIABETES MELLITUS

Ocular symptoms *(What you may experience)* Blurred vision; slowly progressive vision loss, usually in both eyes. In the early stages, there may be no symptoms.

What is it? Diabetes mellitus is a disease in which the pancreas either fails to produce insulin (type 1, also called insulin-dependent diabetes) or the body cannot adequately utilize the insulin that is produced (type 2, also called non-insulin-dependent diabetes). Insulin is necessary for the metabolism of glucose, and high blood glucose levels can have a cumulative effect that impacts many body systems, including the eyes. A person with diabetes is 25 times more likely than is a person without diabetes to experience vision loss, and the longer the duration of the disease, the greater the chance of visual impairment. See Chapter 26 for more information on diabetes.

The eye disease most commonly associated with diabetes is diabetic retinopathy (see Diabetic Retinopathy, page 537). People with diabetes are also at increased risk for cataract (see Cataract, page 524), and the retinopathy can also lead to a painful glaucoma (see Glaucoma, page 526).

What you can do The eye complications of diabetes can be prevented, at least in part, with good blood glucose control. This means monitoring of blood glucose levels several times a day, making the necessary changes in diet, insulin dose or other medication, and exercising to keep the glucose levels in the target range. Treatment of hypertension, if present, can also prevent progression of diabetic retinopathy.

Everyone with diabetes (type 1 and type 2) should have regular ophthalmologic exams. Retinopathy usually does not develop in childhood or adolescence, but every child with diabetes should have a baseline eye exam within 1 year of being diagnosed with diabetes and annual exams thereafter. The American Academy of Ophthalmology (AAO) recommends at least yearly dilated exams for everyone with diabetes.

❖ HYPERTENSION

Ocular symptoms *(What you may experience)* Headache; visual disturbances.

Ocular signs and laboratory findings (What the doctor looks for) Constricting of the arteries in the retina; small retinal hemorrhages; exudates that have leaked from the blood vessels. Through the ophthalmoscope, the blood vessels of the eye are easily observed and they can be highlighted by fluorescein angiography.

What is it? Hypertensive retinopathy, the damage done to the retina in someone who has hypertension, is a risk of untreated or poorly controlled hypertension (see page 799). People with hypertension rarely experience visual symptoms, but in severe cases, such as a hypertensive crisis, the retinal blood vessels can become so constricted that vision loss results. The longer the duration of hypertension, the more damage there will be to the blood vessels in the eye. Retinal vessel occlusion (see Retinal Artery/Vein Occlusion, page 535) is another possible consequence. The amount of retinal damage is graded, ranging from barely detectable arterial narrowing at Grade I to hemorrhage, exudates, and swelling of the optic disk and possible visual loss at Grade IV.

What you can do Hypertensive retinopathy can be prevented by the early detection and control of hypertension.

Treatment Treatment is the same as that for hypertension.

Prognosis If hypertensive retinopathy has progressed to Grade IV, some visual loss is likely. This grade of retinopathy is also associated with advanced heart and kidney complications from hypertension.

❖ MIGRAINE

Ocular symptoms (What you may experience) Visual field disturbances, such as wavy, shimmering lights, the aura that is characteristic of migraine headaches.

What is it? Migraines (see page 438) are persistent headaches, usually accompanied by nausea, that may be preceded by visual symptoms. The aura perceived by the person with a migraine will usually last less than 45 minutes and is not usually associated with pain, but the subsequent headache is likely to last several hours and can be very painful. Some people report the visual symptoms of migraine without headache, and they should be evaluated for underlying ophthalmologic or neurologic disorders. An ophthalmoplegic migraine involves partial paralysis of the eyes and can cause double vision. The eye symptoms of migraines do not require treatment.

❖ GIANT CELL (TEMPORAL) ARTERITIS

Ocular symptoms (What you may experience) Double vision; sudden and transient vision loss, either partial or total.

Ocular signs and laboratory findings (What the doctor looks for) Definitive diagnosis is through biopsy and examination of one or both the temporal arteries.

What is it? Giant cell arteritis (see page 639) is an inflammatory disease of the large and medium-sized arteries. The disease almost always strikes people over age 55, and women are twice as likely as are men to get it. It influences the eye when the inflammation affects the posterior ciliary arteries, feeding blood to part of the eye. If untreated, it can cause blindness, and it should be treated as an ophthalmologic emergency.

Treatment Giant cell arteritis is very responsive to treatment with prednisone, a corticosteroid. Prednisone is usually given orally, but sometimes it is administered intravenously. Immediate treatment is very important, particularly if there is already vision loss, since it may prevent vision loss in the other eye.

FRONTAL LOBE TUMORS

Tumors on the frontal lobe of the brain may show symptoms in the eye, including impaired vision and papilledema. See Chapter 14 for more information about brain tumors.

SEXUALLY TRANSMITTED INFECTIONS

Some sexually transmitted infections have ophthalmologic symptoms and consequences in the eye that can lead to blindness. These include syphilis, gonorrhea, chlamydia, and the acquired immunodeficiency syndrome (AIDS). See Chapter 21 for information on these diseases.

Syphilis can cause uveitis, optic neuritis, conjunctivitis, retinitis, dacryocystitis, scleritis, and other eye diseases. Babies born to mothers with syphilis may have inflammation of the cornea or uvea, and there may be atrophy of the optic nerve. Babies born to women with chlamydia often have chlamydial conjunctivitis. Someone with gonorrhea can spread the infection to the eyes from secretions on the fingers, and this can result in gonococcal conjunctivitis and even perforation of the cornea.

One of the opportunistic infections associated with AIDS is cytomegalovirus (CMV), which can lead to CMV-related retinitis or optic neuropathy. Untreated CMV retinitis can lead to blindness, and even with treatment, blindness cannot always be prevented. People with AIDS, who have compromised immune systems, are also subject to a number of other viral, bacterial, and fungal infections that can affect the eye (see CMV retinitis, page 541).

Sixteen

Ear, Nose, and Throat

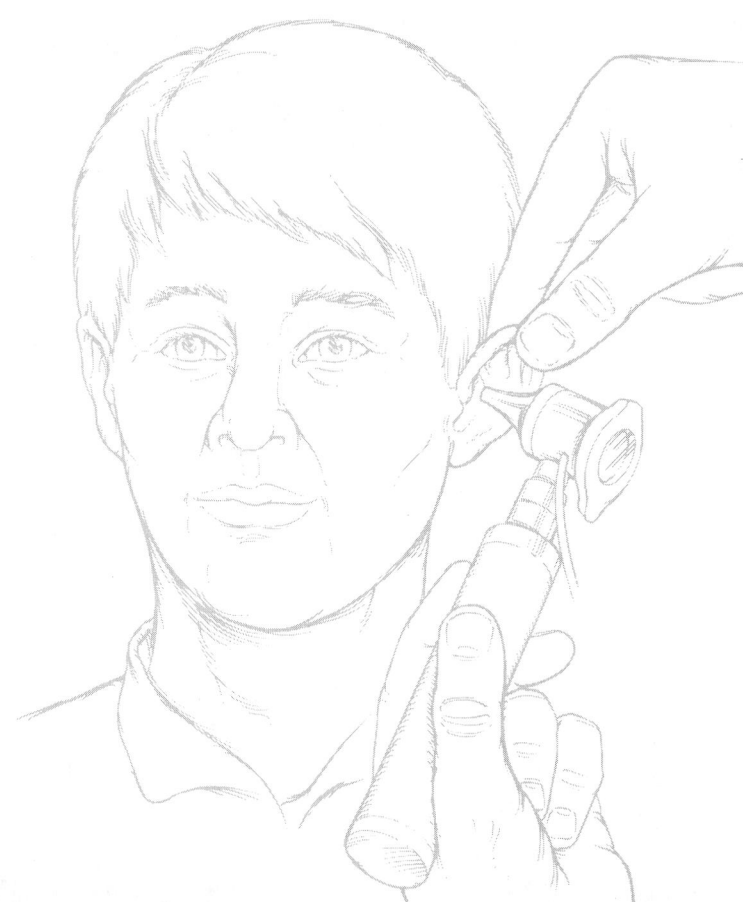

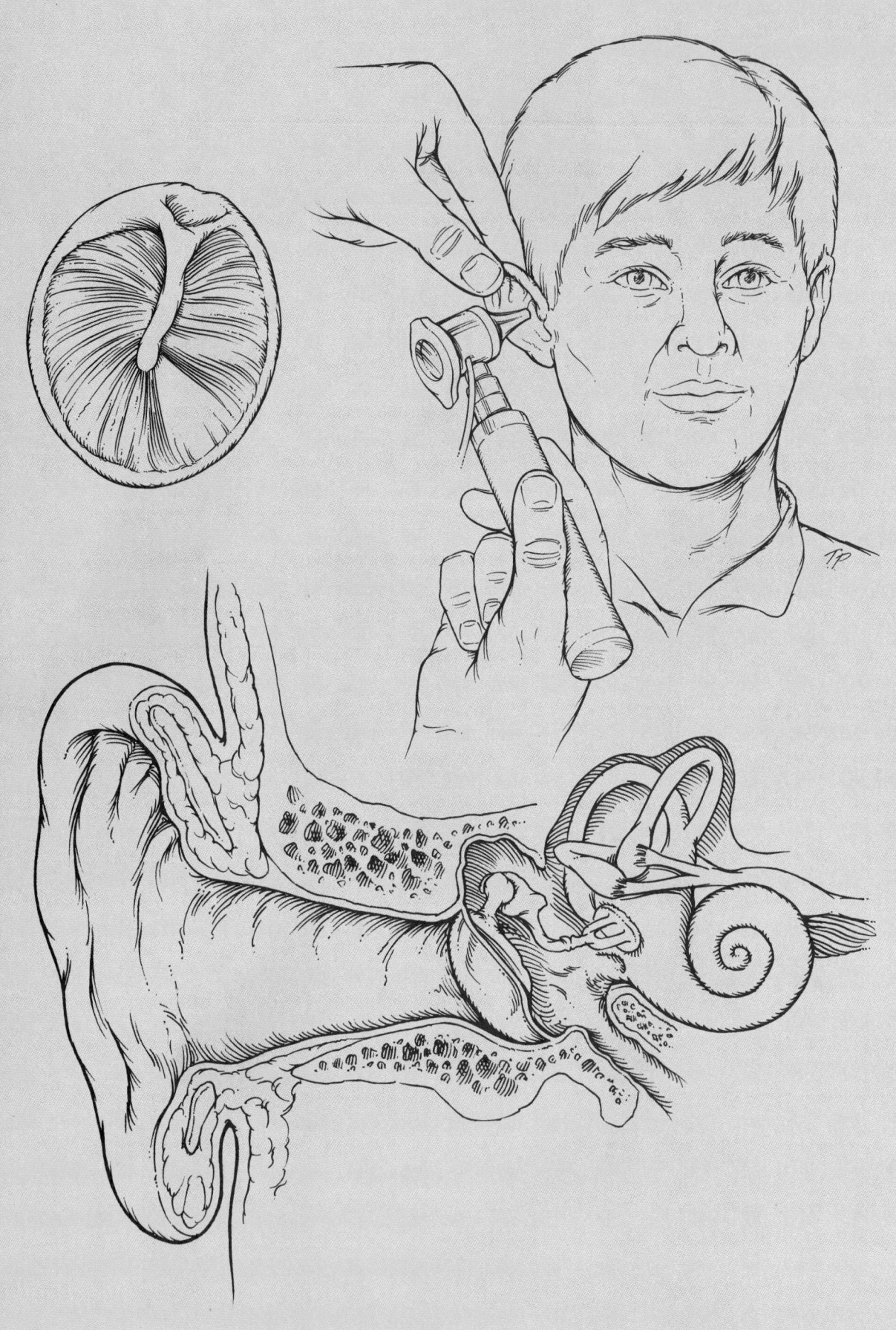

EAR, NOSE, AND THROAT

D isorders of the ear, nose, throat, and other parts of the head and neck are usually treated by an otolaryngologist (ear, nose, and throat or ENT doctor). The ear, nose, and throat are closely interrelated in structure and function. For example, the ear chamber communicates with the throat through the eustachian tube. The nose and sinuses drain into the throat and from there into two passages: the airway (larynx, bronchial passages, and lungs) and the digestive tract (esophagus). Infections and tumors in one area may spread to others because of these connections. Although each structure will be addressed separately, you should be mindful of the relationship between them.

THE EAR

T he ear is responsible for the sense of balance as well as for hearing. It is a complex organ consisting of three separate parts: the external ear, middle ear, and inner ear. The outer visible portion of the ear gathers sound, the middle ear amplifies sound vibration, and the inner ear translates sound vibration and head movement into nerve impulses that the brain interprets as sound and position, respectively.

Sound waves, produced by the vibrations of molecules, are gathered by the outer ear and funneled toward the eardrum. The size and energy of the waves determine loudness; the number of vibrations per second determines pitch. When sound waves strike the drum, they cause vibrations that are picked up and intensified by the bones involved in hearing. The waves are transmitted to the oval window, the entrance to the inner ear. The hearing portion of the inner ear, called the cochlea, is a hollow, bony canal filled with fluid and lined with specialized cells that have tiny hair-like tufts. Movement creates fluid waves in the hearing portion of the inner ear that stimulate these cells, triggering activity in nerve fibers; these fibers in turn transmit nerve signals through the hearing nerve to the brain, which interprets them and allows us to perceive sound. Interruption of any step in this chain of events can impair or destroy the ability to hear.

The External Ear

The outer crescent-shaped portion of the ear, called the auricle or pinna, gathers sound waves like a radar scanner and funnels them to the eardrum, also called the tympanic membrane. The outer portion of the canal is lined with skin and a protective waxy substance called cerumen that is designed to trap particles and debris that enter the canal. Nearer to the eardrum, the lining skin is thin and vulnerable to trauma.

❖ OTITIS EXTERNA (SWIMMER'S EAR)

Symptoms *(What you may experience)* Itching of the ear canal; pain when tugging on the external ear or when moving the jaw; muffled hearing; drainage from the canal (often greenish or yellow).

Signs and laboratory findings *(What the doctor looks for)* Swollen, red external canal; debris and draining fluid. A culture of drainage is occasionally necessary.

What is it? Otitis externa occurs most commonly in the summer months when heat, moisture, and in many cases frequent swimming may promote infection of the lining of the ear canal, making it more vulnerable to infection. Often the first indication of a problem will be itching of the ear canal—in fact, vigorous scratching may contribute to the infection by abrading the canal skin. Commonly, the infection is caused by bacteria—usually either *Pseudomonas* (which characteristically causes a greenish discharge) or *Staphylococcus* (which usually produces a yellow crusty discharge). Fungal infection usually does not produce a weepy discharge but rather a fluffy white or black

561

material that remains within the canal and may only be visible through a lighted otoscope (instrument used to examine the ear).

Occasionally, the problem is caused not by infection but by eczema. This type of ear infection occurs in people prone to dry skin and other conditions such as seborrheic dermatitis and eczema of other sites. See Chapter 28 for more information about this kind of canal disorder.

What you can do Keep the ear canal dry (see Care and Prevention of Swimmer's Ear, below).

When to call the doctor If fever or severe pain accompanies the disorder—particularly in people who have diabetes or have an immune system impairment such as those with acquired immunodeficiency syndrome (AIDS) or who have had organ transplants—or if the canal fills with reddish,

CARE AND PREVENTION OF SWIMMER'S EAR

In most areas of the country, summer means water sports. For some people, particularly children and teens who may spend many hours in the swimming pool, lake, or river, summer brings with it bouts of otitis externa or swimmer's ear. To avoid swimmer's ear, never swim in polluted waters. Drying the ear canal after swimming also can help prevent swimmer's ear. Follow these steps to reduce your risk, especially if you are prone to ear canal infections.

- Upon coming out of the water, spend a few moments with each ear resting on a dry towel to allow the bulk of the water to drain from the canal. Tug gently on the ear in an upward and backward direction to drain the canal.

- Instill a few drops of an over-the-counter acetic acid drying agent such as VoSoL or Swim-EAR or make your own after-swim solution from equal parts of white vinegar (which is acetic acid) and rubbing alcohol. Note that acetic acid eardrops are not antibiotic drops; antibiotic drops should not be used on a routine basis but only when prescribed by a doctor for a specific infectious ear disorder. The skin of the ear canal is quite thin and absorbs the medication well. The neomycin contained in many antibiotic eardrops can cause an allergic reaction, swelling the canal shut and making the canal and surrounding tissues and skin red and inflamed.

- An alternative to drops of any kind is to gently air dry the canal with an electric handheld hair dryer on the lowest setting. Do not use the high setting or hot air since excessive heat can dry and irritate the thin skin of the canal.

- Hair spray and hair dyes can also irritate the ear canal so be sure to protect your ears when using these products. ■

swollen tissue that bleeds easily, seek medical help. These findings can signal the development of an urgently serious form of this disorder, termed malignant otitis externa, that often requires hospitalization and antibiotics administered intravenously.

Treatment The most important step at the start of therapy for otitis externa is to thoroughly clean the ear canal. After cleaning, medicated eardrops or creams may be applied. In some cases, severe swelling of the canal prevents adequate delivery of medication to the deeper reaches of the ear canal. In these cases a soft, compressed sponge "wick" can be placed gently into the canal, leaving only the end visible. The wick will absorb the drops and transport them into the recesses of the canal. After 2 or 3 days, usually the swelling will have resolved sufficiently to remove the wick.

The appropriate choice of medication depends on the cause of the infection. Bacterial infections are best treated three or four times daily for 5 to 7 days with drops of an antimicrobial-steroid solution such as polymyxin B neomycin hydrocortisone (Cortisporin Otic Suspension) or acetic acid (VoSoL or VoSoL HC). *Note:* neomycin, contained in some eardrops, causes severe allergic reactions of the ear canal skin in susceptible people, resulting in severe sudden redness and swelling of the canal and sometimes accompanied by the formation of blisters. The reaction may extend out of the canal to the outer ear and even to the facial skin. Long-term use of the drops can also increase the risk of fungal infection.

Fungal infections respond to a single light dusting of sulfanilamide powder on the surface of the canal or to antifungal drops (clotrimazole) twice a day for 2 weeks. However, the most important treatment for fungal infections of the ear canal involves cleaning of the canal and avoidance of unnecessary antibiotic treatment. Eczema, a common precursor condition to fungal otitis, is best treated by daily application of topical steroid cream such as triamcinolone or hydrocortisone to the skin of the canal for 2 weeks.

Prognosis Uncomplicated cases of swimmer's ear should resolve in 5 to 7 days with appropriate treatment. Muffled hearing should return to normal as swelling subsides.

❖ INFECTION OF THE EAR CANAL AND EARLOBE

Symptoms and signs Localized swelling, redness, and tenderness in the ear canal or earlobe.

What is it? The small glands that produce oil to lubricate the skin of the ear canal or earlobe can sometimes become obstructed and a small cyst can form. Bacteria can enter the occluded canal and begin to multiply. Their invasion alerts the immune system, which sends immune defense cells to the area. Pus forms within the cyst, which increases in volume, causing swelling and pain.

Some cases of infection result from piercing the ear for cosmetic reasons. Such infections can arise in the earlobe but there is an even greater risk of infection if the cartilage (tissue) found in the external ear is pierced. Cartilage has less of a blood supply than the earlobe and is more vulnerable to infection at the site of piercing, especially after swimming.

What you can do Keep the boil clean with mild antibacterial soap and water. Apply warm packs to the boil to consolidate it and bring it to a head. The boil may rupture and drain on its own. Removing a pierced earring from an infected area may worsen the condition. Consult a doctor first.

Do not pierce your ears, especially the outer ear, if you have a skin condition of the external ear. Never have your ear pierced by an inexperienced practitioner.

When to call the doctor If conservative measures fail to resolve the boil, if fever develops, or if pain is significant, consult your doctor.

Treatment The definitive treatment is surgically opening and draining the boil. In some cases, early in the course of its development, antibiotic medication may resolve a boil; once it has softened, antibiotics may fail to penetrate to the liquid center to effectively kill the bacteria.

Prognosis Excellent, following drainage. Pain relief is almost immediate upon releasing the pressure. Healing usually takes about 1 week.

❖ FOREIGN OBJECTS IN THE EAR CANAL

Symptoms *(What you may experience)* Fullness; muffled hearing; pain (sometimes); or noise in the ear canal (occasionally).

Signs *(What the doctor looks for)* Object visible in canal on examination with an otoscope.

What is it? In adults, foreign objects in the canal are usually the result of an accidental insertion, often in conjunction with cleaning the canal—for example, the tip of a cotton-tipped swab breaks loose and lodges in the canal. In children, the insertion may result from intentional placement of small beans, rocks, toys, or parts of toys into the canal. Occasionally, insects become trapped after flying or crawling into the canal.

Obstruction of the canal by a foreign object causes a muffling of hearing and often a sense of fullness or discomfort. Insects in the canal can cause irritation or a tickling sensation with movement and may produce an audible buzzing sound.

What you can do See Safe Removal of Objects from the Ear, below.

SAFE REMOVAL OF OBJECTS FROM THE EAR

- Unless you can see the object clearly and grasp it without inserting an instrument into the canal, it is best not to attempt removal of the object on your own.

- Great care must be taken not to push the object deeper, which could possibly damage the delicate eardrum beyond it.

- Do not irrigate the canal with water or other solutions, particularly if the object is a bean or other vegetable matter; irrigation may cause the object to swell, making its extraction even more difficult.

- Insects in the canal can be killed by instilling mineral oil into the canal. Use a suction bulb (such as would be used to suction an infant's nose) to gently extract the insect. ■

When to call the doctor As soon as possible after discovery. Contact the doctor immediately if there is pain, bleeding, discharge of fluid or pus, or dizziness.

Treatment The doctor can usually remove the object with forceps or a wax-removal instrument. Safe removal of objects tightly or deeply imbedded in the canal sometimes requires a local anesthetic; in children, general anesthesia may be necessary.

Prognosis Hearing should return promptly upon removal.

❖ LACERATION AND CONTUSION OF THE EXTERNAL EAR

Symptoms and signs Bruising, bleeding, or swelling of the external ear.

What is it? Trauma to the ear commonly occurs from a direct blow to the ear; the external ear can also be the subject of tearing or biting.

Because the external ear consists of contours of cartilage covered with skin and little

else, lacerations need not be deep to be serious. Injury to the ear—both direct blows and cuts—often leads to the development of a hematoma (an accumulation of blood or fluid beneath the skin) which can hamper healing of the wound and increase the risk of infection. Damaged cartilage can become thickened during healing, resulting in a traumatic deformity called cauliflower ear.

What you can do For bruises and swelling, apply a cold pack to the ear.

When to call the doctor Significant swelling or a laceration of the ear should always be evaluated by a doctor.

Treatment Careful anatomic repair of all lacerations by an experienced doctor is a must. Measures should be taken to drain away fluid that accumulates under the wound so that it can heal.

Formation of a large clot, even in the absence of a cut, usually requires surgical drainage to remove the accumulated blood.

Deformation of the cartilage may require plastic surgery to reshape or replace the cartilage and restore a normal appearance.

Prognosis Excellent if promptly and appropriately treated.

❖ WAX BLOCKAGE OF THE CANAL

Symptoms (*What you may experience*) Intermittent fullness and muffled hearing that are worse after swimming or showering.

Signs (*What the doctor looks for*) Wax obstructing the canal visible on examination with an otoscope.

What is it? Glands in the skin of the outer portion of the ear canal produce a protective wax that lubricates the skin of the canal and traps foreign particles. Some people produce a wax that is stiff and dry while others produce a softer, moister variety. Accumulated wax can sometimes reach a volume sufficient to occlude the canal but more often blockage, also called occlusion, occurs when the wax is pressed into the canal with cleaning attempts or when heat and humidity cause the coating to collapse, filling the canal.

HOW TO SAFELY CLEAN THE EAR CANAL

Warning: If there is any possibility that the eardrum has been perforated, do not flush with water or any other liquid. Doing so could cause infection or damage to the bones involved in hearing. Also, do not attempt to remove wax from an ear that can hear normally if the hearing of the other ear is impaired.

Soft wax can easily be removed by flushing the ear canal with a bulb syringe and warm water. You may assemble your own kit for this purpose (composed of a bulb syringe, hydrogen peroxide, and perhaps a bottle of Debrox, an over-the-counter wax-dissolving solution) or there are several earwax removal kits sold over the counter that contain bulb syringes and usually some drops to dissolve the wax. Note: Solutions that dissolve wax should be used with caution since some can trigger an allergic reaction in the ear canal.

- Use water that is approximately body temperature—neither too warm nor cool. Significant variation from normal body temperature can stimulate dizziness if the water strikes the eardrum.

- Direct the stream of water upward and backward against the canal wall. You may gently pull the ear slightly up and back to help direct the stream of water.

- Stiffer, drier wax should be softened first with a few drops of hydrogen peroxide (or over-the-counter earwax softening agents such as Debrox) used twice daily for 1 week before flushing the canal. ■

Once blockage occurs, sound waves cannot pass to the eardrum and hearing becomes suddenly muffled. The muffling may come and go, worsening after swimming or showering.

What you can do See How to Safely Clean the Ear Canal, page 564.

When to call the doctor Consult a doctor if the home removal methods outlined in How to Safely Clean the Ear Canal fail to relieve the blockage, if there is drainage of blood or pus, if there is fever or pain associated with the blockage, or if there is concern that the eardrum has been punctured.

Treatment Occasionally—in cases that cannot be relieved by self-treatment or when there is hearing loss or suspected or known perforation of the eardrum—the doctor will have to remove the plug of wax with a special instrument under direct magnified vision.

Prognosis Excellent.

❖ PROTRUDING EARS

Symptoms and signs Large ears or ears that stick out.

What is it? Each year about 10,000 Americans undergo the procedure known as otoplasty, the pinning back of large or protruding ears. Children are especially vulnerable to unkind teasing regarding protruding ears and sometimes become introverted or develop self-image problems as a result.

Several types of external-ear aesthetic defects can occur, ranging from lax cartilage that allows the ear to flop down, to defects in the shape of the outer portion of the ear or ear canal. In some cases the bowl of the ear lacks the normal folds and may be quite deep and round; as a result it will push out from the head instead of laying more flatly back.

What you can do Taping or strapping the ears to the side of the head at night will have no effect whatsoever. Changing hairstyle, however, may successfully disguise the problem.

When to call the doctor An ear can be considered protruding only in the context of the overall shape of the head. Generally, ears that stick out more than four-fifths of an inch (about 2 cm) from the back of the head are considered to be protruding; in such a case, you may wish to speak to a doctor. Often, waiting until a child reaches age 5 or 6, at which time the ear approaches full size, will improve the final result.

Treatment During surgery, the surgeon reshapes the cartilage structure of the external ear to maintain the ear's shape and anchor the ear to the scalp, pulling the bowl portion of the ear flush with the head.

Prognosis Excellent.

❖ CANCER OF THE EXTERNAL EAR

Symptoms *(What you may experience)* Nonhealing sore or scaly patch on the skin of the ear; in later stages, a firm swelling in front of or behind the ear.

Signs and laboratory findings *(What the doctor looks for)* Abnormal cells revealed by microscopic examination of a skin biopsy specimen.

What is it? Like skin cancers elsewhere (see Chapter 28), those involving the outer portion of the ear most commonly are of the basal cell or squamous cell variety. Basal cell tumors tend to remain localized for a longer period of time; the squamous cell type tends to be aggressive, invading the surrounding tissues and spreading to lymph nodes in front of and behind the ear, the nearby parotid gland in the cheek, the mastoid bone (behind the ear), or the external ear canal.

When to call the doctor Consult a doctor regarding any sore or scaly spot on the ear that fails to heal promptly (within 1 month).

Treatment Complete surgical removal of the cancerous tissue is the treatment of choice and should be done early to prevent spreading. The structure of the outer ear makes this surgery technically and cosmetically challenging and it is best performed by a specialist. If the cancer is extensive, radiation therapy may be used in combination with surgery. See Chapter 30 for more information on the diagnosis and treatment of cancer and Chapter 28 for more information on skin cancer.

Prognosis Good if diagnosed promptly and treated appropriately. Spreading of the cancer to lymph nodes or adjacent areas worsens this prognosis.

The Eardrum, Middle Ear, and Mastoid

The eardrum is a cone-shaped, thin membrane located at the end of the external canal. The middle-ear chamber, an air space that lies behind the eardrum, contains the ossicles, three tiny bones involved in hearing: the hammer, also called the malleus; the stirrup, also called the stapes; and the anvil, also called the incus. The hammer is con-

nected to the eardrum; the stirrup-shaped bone is connected to the inner ear; and the anvil connects the hammer to the stirrup. They form a bony chain that conducts sound waves from the eardrum to the hearing portion of the inner ear, amplifying the sound by a factor of almost 30. The lining of the middle-ear chamber is similar to the tissue lining the nose and produces a mucus-like fluid; normally, the fluid drains from the middle ear down the eustachian tube into the back of the throat. Blockage of the eustachian tube can cause fluid to build up and become infected. This tube also provides a means to equalize the pressure in the middle-ear chamber with that of the external environment. For example, ear-popping, which often happens when flying in an airplane, is due to pressure changes mediated by the eustachian tube. The chamber also communicates with the mastoids, a bony cavity behind the ear perforated throughout with air chambers.

To examine the eardrum, the doctor uses an otoscope.

How sound is heard. (A) Sound waves that enter the external ear are amplified by the eardrum (tympanic membrane). Three small bones (incus, malleus, and stapes) transmit the sound vibrations to fluid in three tubes (cochlear duct, scala tympani, and scala vestibuli). Fluid motion is converted to nerve impulses that travel along the cochlear nerve to the brain. (B) Hair cells in the cochlea convert the motion of fluid in the inner ear into impulses.

❖ ACUTE OTITIS MEDIA (MIDDLE-EAR INFECTION)

Symptoms (*What you may experience*) Sense of fullness in the ear; decreased hearing; pain (severe pain indicates infection).

Signs and laboratory findings (*What the doctor looks for*) Bulging of eardrum or fluid visible behind the eardrum on examination with an otoscope; sometimes, drainage of pus or fluid from the canal, hearing loss, or tenderness of the mastoid bone.

What is it? The mucous membrane lining the middle-ear space, like that of the nasal chamber, produces fluid. Normally, the fluid drains from the middle ear down the eustachian tube into the back of the nasopharynx, the area where the nose and throat meet. Viral infections of the upper respiratory tract (for example, a cold) can result in increased production of mucus from the middle-ear lining and swelling of the eustachian tube, a combination that allows fluid to build up in the middle-ear chamber. (Because this uninfected straw-colored fluid is termed serous fluid, this condition is termed serous otitis media.) Fluid in the chamber dampens vibration of the eardrum and movement of the middle-ear

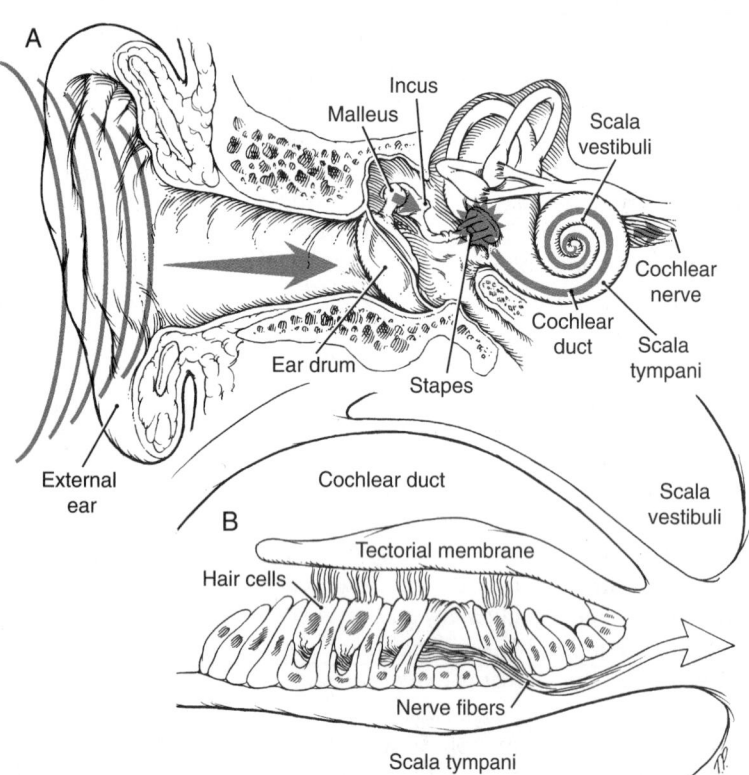

A

Incus
Malleus
Scala vestibuli

Cochlear nerve

Cochlear duct

Scala tympani

Ear drum
Stapes

External ear

B

Cochlear duct

Scala vestibuli

Tectorial membrane

Hair cells

Nerve fibers

Scala tympani

bones, leading to a temporary decrease in or loss of hearing.

Further accumulation of fluid will cause the eardrum to bulge and create a sense of fullness or pressure in the ear, sometimes accompanied by mild pain. Because of direct communication to the throat via the eustachian tube, bacteria can contaminate the middle-ear fluid and create a pus-producing—also called suppurative—infection in the middle-ear space called suppurative otitis media. The pressure from the rapid expansion of pus stretches and stresses the nerve-rich eardrum, resulting in extreme ear pain. Continued stress can rupture the eardrum, an event signaled by drainage of pus or blood from the ear canal.

Middle-ear infection is most common in young children: By age three, 80 percent of children have had at least one episode of otitis media and almost 50 percent of children have had three or more episodes. Because the angle of the eustachian tube is almost horizontal in infants and young children, it fails to drain fluid adequately. As the head grows, the angle increases and the tube drains fluid into the throat more effectively. The immature immune systems of young children may also contribute to the problem, making them more prone to the upper respiratory infections that can lead to middle-ear infection.

Complications of otitis media are rare but potentially serious. Infection can spread to the mastoid air cells, to other bones and sinuses nearby, and to the brain causing meningitis (infection of the coverings of the brain) or brain abscess. Tenderness of the bone of the skull behind the ear may signal the development of mastoiditis and should be reported to the doctor immediately. Paralysis of the facial nerve can occur, signaled by difficulty completely closing the eye and weakness of the muscles around the mouth and eye.

What you can do A number of devices are now commercially available to screen for middle-ear infection. Keep in mind that these devices are difficult to use. A child's small ear canals are angled in such a way that the eardrum is difficult to see. Note that ear infection is best detected by looking for fever, fussiness, ear tugging, and loss of sleep and appetite, especially after a cold or sore throat. Use of over-the-counter (OTC) decongestant nasal sprays or drops such as Afrin or

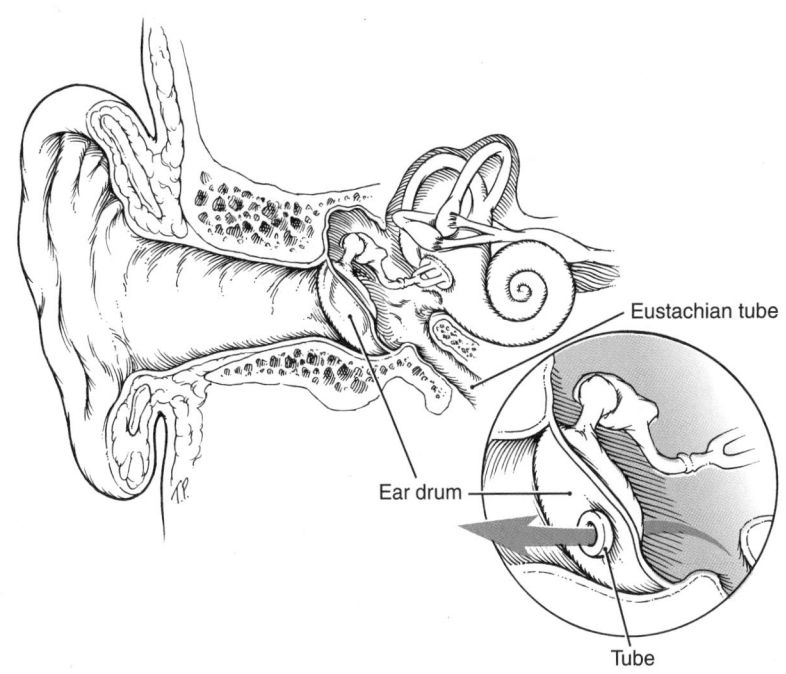

Eustachian tube

Ear drum

Tube

Recurrent middle-ear infections in children (otitis media) can be helped by placing a tube in the eardrum (tympanic membrane) that allows drainage of infected fluid, thus decreasing the frequency and severity of reinfections and improving hearing.

Neo-Synephrine up to four times daily can help to open the swollen eustachian tube but their use should be limited to no longer than 3 days (see Nasal Spray Abuse and How to Kick the Habit, page 1338). Application of warm packs and use of analgesic (pain-relieving) anti-inflammatory medications such as ibuprofen or acetaminophen (Tylenol) can help to relieve pain.

If drainage occurs, gently cleanse the fluid from the skin of the ear and face with a soft cloth moistened with mild antibacterial soap and warm water, taking care not to allow water into the ear. To protect the skin from irritation, you can apply an OTC antibacterial ointment to the outer portion of the ear and skin of the nearby cheek (do not put ointment or other drops into the ear canal until instructed to do so by a doctor); place a cotton ball loosely in the canal to absorb the drainage. Contact your doctor.

When to call the doctor See your doctor if the pain worsens or fails to resolve; if muffling of hearing persists; if sudden blurring of vision, dizziness, or loss of balance develops; or if drainage of pus, fluid, or blood occurs. In children, muffled hearing may be indicated by delayed development of speech, particularly the ability to produce crisp-sounding consonants.

Treatment Appropriate use of antibiotics is important in the treatment of this condition. Initial medical treatment of serous otitis media often consists of antibiotic therapy for 10 days, usually with erythromycin ethylsuccinate (EES), sulfisoxazole (Gantrisin), the combination medication trimethoprim sulfamethoxazole (Bactrim or Septra), or amoxicillin alone or with addition of clavulanate (Augmentin). It may be necessary to increase dosage once the infection has become established.

Occasionally, the accumulation of pus behind the eardrum may cause symptoms—pain and vertigo—(the sensation of spinning in the absence of head or body movement)—sufficiently severe to warrant a controlled rupture of the eardrum. This procedure, called a myringotomy, creates a slit in the eardrum to allow removal or drainage of pus and to prevent extension of the infection to adjacent areas. The incision usually heals within 1 to 4 weeks.

Your doctor will follow the condition to its resolution to be certain that the fluid drains or reabsorbs and that hearing returns to normal. If the fluid or loss of hearing persists longer than 3 months, surgical treatment (myringotomy) may be necessary, often followed by the placement of a pressure-equalization (PE) tube (drainage tube) into the eardrum to prevent recurrence. In adults, this procedure can be performed in the doctor's office using a local anesthetic (see also Ear Tubes For Children, page 569).

Prognosis Prompt resolution of pain occurs in almost all cases once treatment is begun. Fever (if present) should resolve in 48 hours after antibiotic treatment has begun. Restoration of hearing results from drainage or reabsorption of middle-ear fluid, healing, and the return of the eardrum to its normal shape and position. This process may take 1 to 4 weeks. A hearing test is often advised to assess the slight possibility of long-term (permanent) effects on hearing.

❖ CHRONIC OTITIS MEDIA, CHOLESTEATOMA, AND MASTOIDITIS

Symptoms (What you may experience) Intermittent or persistent drainage of cloudy fluid or foul-smelling pus from the ear; loss or reduction of hearing for longer than 6 weeks.

Signs and laboratory findings (What the doctor looks for) Perforation of the eardrum or a skin cyst—also called a cholesteatoma—within the eardrum or middle ear (visible on examination with an otoscope); conductive hearing loss; drainage of cloudy fluid or foul-smelling pus from the ear; or destruction of mastoid air cells as shown by x-rays (sometimes).

What is it? Otitis media is said to be chronic when, despite treatment, drainage of fluid or pus and hearing loss persist longer than 6 weeks. Chronic otitis media can take two forms: inactive and active.

In the inactive form, symptoms include persistent drainage of cloudy fluid from a perforation usually in the center of the eardrum and muffling of hearing.

In the active form, a skin cyst in the middle-ear space erodes and destroys the bone in the mastoid air cells and promotes the spread of infection to adjacent structures. The growing cyst may damage the inner ear, producing disturbances in hearing or balance. Damage to the facial nerve may result in weakness of the muscles that control smiling, frowning, pursing the lips, and tightly closing the eyelids on the affected side.

When to call the doctor Persistence of drainage from the ear or hearing loss should always be evaluated by a doctor. Development of dizziness, loss of balance, or facial muscle weakness should also prompt immediate medical attention.

Treatment In the inactive form of the disorder, extending the course of treatment with antibiotic medication may be sufficient to resolve the problem. If fluid accumulation does not improve, surgical treatment may be necessary. The surgery is usually a simple myringotomy and placement of PE tubes.

The active form always requires surgical treatment. The type of surgery depends on the extent to which the infection has spread or on the amount of destruction done by the growing cyst. These procedures can usually be performed as outpatient surgery followed by 2 to 3 days of moderate discomfort that can usually be adequately treated with prescription-strength pain medication. After surgery, most doctors will recommend that for 4 to 6 weeks you avoid heavy lifting, strenuous exercise, or any other activity that might increase the pressure in the middle ear. The specific surgery is dictated by the extent of the infection. Options include the following:

- Myringoplasty is a procedure designed to close the hole in the eardrum by using a graft that serves as a foundation for the eardrum to form a permanent membrane. It can be performed under local or general anesthesia depending upon age and other factors.

- Tympanoplasty is a procedure designed to repair the hole in the eardrum and to repair any disruption of the bones involved in hearing. This procedure may require general anesthesia but might also be possible using a local anesthetic. If performed under local anesthesia, the hearing result can be assessed at the time of surgery to determine if refinements are needed.

- Simple mastoidectomy involves removal of the mastoid air cells and the scraping away of the cyst, usually through an incision behind the ear, leaving the bony wall of the ear canal intact. This operation requires general anesthesia.

- Modified radical mastoidectomy involves removing the cyst, fully exposing the mastoid air cells, and creating a common cavity between the mastoid and the external ear canal to drain and eradicate infection due to the cyst. It also requires general anesthesia.

Prognosis Excellent for infection control, although additional surgery is occasionally needed to address new pockets of infection or provide refinements in hearing once infection has been cleared. Useful hearing is often achievable.

❖ PERFORATION (RUPTURE) OF THE EARDRUM

Symptoms (*What you may experience*) Hearing loss, tinnitus (ringing in the ears), pain, and bleeding.

Signs and laboratory findings (*What the doctor looks for*) Perforation of the ear-

EAR TUBES FOR CHILDREN

For young children who are prone to frequent, painful bouts of otitis media and who have undergone extended courses of antibiotic therapy, the surgical insertion of ventilation tubes into the eardrum may be recommended as a solution to the problem.

The tubes themselves are similar to tiny plastic bobbins, a hollow central tube flared on each end. Placement of the tubes requires making a slit in the eardrum into which the tube is seated. In adults, this procedure can usually be done in the office under local anesthesia; in children, it is usually performed in the operating room under general anesthesia.

While the surgery can break the cycle of recurrent and persistent otitis media, it should not be performed unless you are aware of the few risks related to the surgery. For children, there is a small risk associated with any surgery performed under general anesthesia. In addition, while the tubes allow accumulated fluid to freely drain into the ear canal, they also provide a route for water to enter the middle-ear space from outside. Therefore, for the entire time the tubes remain in place, precautions such as the use of ear plugs must be taken to keep contaminated water out of the ears when bathing or swimming.

In most cases, the tubes do not have to be removed. Usually within a period of 6 to 18 months the eardrum will extrude them and the slits will seal closed. If the tubes have not fallen out within 18 months, they will need to be removed, usually in the doctor's office. If the tubes are allowed to remain in place too long, the slits may not seal shut. ■

drum seen on examination with an otoscope; loss of mobility of the eardrum, which may be documented by tympanogram.

What is it? Rupture of the eardrum may be caused by any pressure against the membrane. The pressure could come from direct puncture by an object such as a cotton-tipped applicator, stick, hairpin, or other foreign object; a forceful stream of water; or a blast of air pressure against the eardrum, such as might occur from a hard blow against the ear. Symptoms—including hearing loss, ringing in the ears, pain, and bleeding—may begin immediately following the perforation.

(Alternately, an infection within the middle ear leading to an accumulation of fluid and pus may cause rupture of the eardrum. See Acute Otitis Media, page 566.)

What you can do If you suspect that you may have damaged the eardrum, place only a dry cotton ball in the opening of the canal. Under no circumstances should you instill any kind of liquid, drop, or oil. OTC analgesics such as ibuprofen or aceta-

An infection of the inner ear or trauma to the ear are among several causes of a perforated (ruptured) eardrum (tympanic membrane). Pain and decreased hearing are common symptoms.

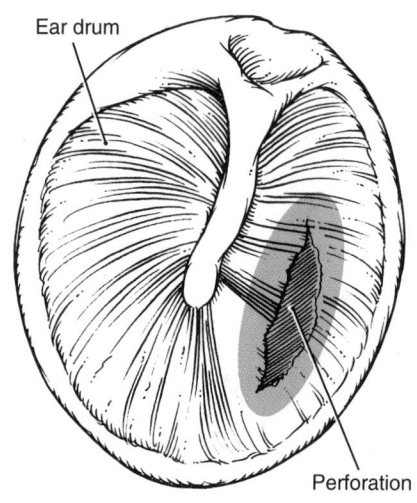

Ear drum

Perforation

minophen (Tylenol) can help relieve the pain until you see the doctor.

When to call the doctor If you sustain physical trauma to the ear, followed by symptoms associated with perforation—particularly bleeding or pain—contact your doctor right away. Persistent ringing in the ears or vertigo are signs of inner ear damage and require referral to an otolaryngologist.

Treatment If the perforation is small, it may heal on its own in several weeks. Larger holes may require myringoplasty.

Antibiotics such as amoxicillin or erythromycin are necessary if there is a risk of contamination and infection.

Afterward, prevent water from entering the ear by inserting a petroleum-jelly-covered cotton plug when bathing or showering. Do not swim until your doctor says it is permissible.

Prognosis Hearing loss usually resolves completely after either spontaneous healing or myringoplasty and within a few months the appearance of the eardrum should return to normal.

❖ BAROTRAUMA (EAR PRESSURE WITH FLYING OR DIVING)

Symptoms *(What you may experience)* Sudden fullness, pain, and decreased hearing in one or both ears.

Signs and laboratory findings *(What the doctor looks for)* Retracted eardrum,

blood behind the eardrum, or perforation of the eardrum on examination with an otoscope.

What is it? Proper function of the ear requires that the air pressure within the middle ear is equal to that of the surrounding atmosphere. Sudden changes in pressure can either put outward traction on the eardrum or cause it to collapse. In either event, the result can be pain and diminished or muffled hearing. Any pressure change can damage the eardrum; most commonly it occurs with descents when flying or scuba diving. Allergic or infectious upper respiratory tract conditions can block the venting function of the eustachian tube, making barotrauma during these activities more likely. Damage can range from painful traction to bleeding and rupture of the eardrum.

What you can do If possible, do not fly or engage in scuba diving when you suffer from allergic or infectious upper respiratory conditions. If you must fly, try to resolve these conditions beforehand by chewing gum, swallowing, yawning, or using a nasal decongestant (spray is preferable to oral form) an hour before takeoff. Use the decongestant again before landing when on an overseas flight.

When to call the doctor Sudden hearing loss, pain, or drainage of blood from the ear associated with pressure changes should prompt a visit to the doctor.

Treatment In many cases, decongestant nasal sprays or tablets may relieve symptoms. Occasionally, myringotomy may be necessary if there is bleeding behind the eardrum. If a perforation occurs, a small myringotomy will usually heal uneventfully; larger ones may require a graft. (See Perforation (Rupture) of the Eardrum, page 569.)

❖ OTOSCLEROSIS

Symptoms *(What you may experience)* Progressive hearing loss, often accelerating during pregnancy.

Signs and laboratory findings *(What the doctor looks for)* Examination is usually normal.

What is it? In otosclerosis, abnormal growth of sponge-like bone occurs in the vicinity of the inner ear. This bony tissue gradually fixes the stirrup (one of the bones involved in hearing), limiting and finally preventing its motion. Since the motion of the bone is essential for efficient transmission of vibrations to the inner ear, the result is progressive hearing loss (the rate is slow) at which hearing is lost. The disorder, which usually affects both ears, occurs more commonly in adults in their 20s and 30s and is the most common cause of hearing loss in young adults regardless of whether or not there is a history of the disorder in the family. Women are affected more often than men and the condition may accelerate during pregnancy. The hearing loss associated with otosclerosis is usually a conductive hearing loss, so called because it is related to the sound-conducting mechanisms of the ear. Conductive hearing loss is often reversible with surgery. The disorder may extend to affect inner-ear function, producing a combined conductive and sensorineural (nerve) hearing loss.

When to call the doctor Progressive hearing loss should always be evaluated by a doctor.

Treatment The best treatment is surgery, either with a procedure called a stapedotomy, which bypasses the stirrup by making a small opening in the inner ear, or with a stapedectomy, which involves removal of the stirrup and replacement with an artificial bone. The surgery usually can be performed under local anesthesia and is typically done in the operating room of a hospital. Hearing is usually regained quickly.

In a very small percentage of cases (1 to 2 percent in most reported series), people who undergo stapedectomy experience complete hearing loss. Therefore, if otosclerosis is affecting both ears, you should consider the procedure of hearing restoration in two stages. After the operation on one ear, have your hearing evaluated before embarking on the procedure for the second ear.

Hearing aids can also be used to minimize hearing loss caused by otosclerosis, particularly when a combined conductive and sensorineural hearing loss is present (see Hearing Aids, page 574). For the nerve component of such hearing loss, fluoride therapy may be prescribed.

Prognosis Excellent for restoration of hearing after either surgery.

The Inner Ear

Encased in the protective bones of the skull, the inner ear houses sensory organs that serve two very different purposes: hearing and balance. The hearing portion of the inner ear is called the cochlea and the balance portion the vestibule. Diseases and disorders of these two parts of the inner ear are discussed separately in the following sections.

The Cochlea or Hearing Inner Ear

The inner ear, also called the cochlea, is shaped like the shell of a snail. It is lined with thousands of specialized hair cells that are connected to thousands of nerve fibers. The pressure waves that have been intensified by the bones of the middle ear are carried into a chamber filled with fluid called the endolymph, making the hair cells that line the inner ear vibrate. These vibrations produce nerve impulses that are carried to the hearing centers of the brain. Sensorineural hearing loss due to disorders of the sensory mechanism of the inner ear is covered in this section.

❖ AGE-RELATED HEARING LOSS

Symptoms *(What you may experience)* Progressive hearing loss. The ability to hear, first, high-frequency sounds and then conversational speech is affected.

Signs and laboratory findings *(What the doctor looks for)* Sensorineural hearing loss as determined by audiometric and tuning fork testing.

What is it? A certain degree of hearing loss, beginning first in the high-pitched range, is nearly universal among the elderly. It is likely that it results from a combination of genetic vulnerability, the effects of diseases such as hypertension (high blood pressure), and nonoccupational noise exposure. It represents the most common cause of deafness in the United States. One in four

AUDIOMETRY—MEASURING HEARING LOSS

Precise determination of the level of hearing loss requires an audiometric evaluation by an accredited audiologist (hearing specialist). Usually, a doctor will recommend an audiologist who either works in the clinic or to whom the doctor customarily directs patients. You can locate an accredited audiologist by telephoning the referral source of the American Speech-Language-Hearing Association at (800) 638–8255.

The audiogram is a simple, painless test that takes about 20 or 30 minutes. In a soundproof room, the audiologist presents a series of pure tones to each ear independently through earphones. The person being tested then notes each time a sound is heard. The audiologist can determine whether the loss affects one ear or both and whether it is a consequence of problems with the nerve (a sensorineural loss) or the conductive mechanisms (a conductive loss).

The intensity of sound is measured in decibels (dB). The louder the sound, the higher the number of dB. The lowest audible intensity for normal ears to hear ranges from 0 to 20 dB. Conversational speech is typically about 45 to 55 dB. Since ears when functioning normally can usually hear a sound at 10 to 20 dB, someone who cannot hear sounds until the intensity reaches 50 dB has a 30 to 40 dB loss. The American Speech-Language-Hearing Association has devised categories to grade degrees of hearing loss.

- Mild loss (at 26 to 40 dB) indicates difficulty with long distance speech (such as occurs in group meetings, social gatherings, or the theater).

- Moderate loss (at 41 to 55 dB) indicates difficulty with short distance speech and normal conversation.

- Moderately severe loss (at 56 to 70 dB) indicates difficulty with conversation even at close range.

- Severe loss (at 71 to 90 dB) indicates no understanding of the conversational voice but an ability to hear speech amplified by raising the voice or with assisted-listening devices or hearing aids.

- Profound loss (at greater than 91 dB) indicates inability to hear and understand the spoken voice despite maximal amplification. ■

people age 65 to 75 and nearly half of those over age 75 experience some hearing difficulty. The majority of these people do not complain of deafness; rather, their family members are often the first to note the deficit. Both the life circumstances and the level of disability the loss of hearing creates will dictate appropriate measures of evaluation and therapy. For example, a self-sufficient elderly person living alone may experience a greater degree of disruption from the loss—not hearing the doorbell, the telephone, the timer on the oven, or an intruder—than a person living in the protective environment of a retirement or rehabilitation facility. Ignoring a hearing loss is

unwise. Continued participation in the mainstream of life relies on effective social interaction.

The cause of age-related hearing loss is not clearly understood but may result from a genetic predisposition superimposed on a lifetime of exposure to the moderate noise levels found in most cities and towns.

When to call the doctor When loss of hearing begins to interfere with quality of life, particularly with the quality of your social interactions, contact your doctor for referral to an audiologist (hearing specialist) for audiometric testing.

Treatment The usual treatment is a prescription for a hearing aid (see Auditory Rehabilitation Measures, page 573).

Prognosis The disorder is usually progressive but correctable to a degree with a properly fitted hearing aid.

❖ TRAUMATIC (OCCUPATIONAL AND NOISE) HEARING LOSS

Symptoms *(What you may experience)* First, loss of perception of high-frequency sounds (may include normally spoken voice tones, particularly the consonant sounds); later, loss of perception of low-frequency sounds.

Signs and laboratory findings *(What the doctor looks for)* Hearing loss verified by audiometric testing; nerve loss verified by tuning fork testing.

What is it? Chronic, usually occupational, noise trauma accounts for nearly 20 percent of all cases of impaired hearing. Chronic exposure to loud, intense noise—whether in an industrial or employment setting from power tools, firearms, or heavy equipment or from recreational exposure to gunfire or loud music—can damage the sensitive and delicate structure of hearing: the inner ear's hair cells and the nerve fibers they contact. The first loss occurs in the high-frequency register (high-pitched sounds) but with continued exposure and aging the loss will progress to involve lower-register sounds as well. At first, perception of conversational speech may only be a problem in settings in which there is a significant amount of back-

AUDITORY REHABILITATION MEASURES

Several technological advances have made communication easier for people with impaired hearing.

- Assisted-listening devices—composed of portable microphones, amplifiers, and earphones—magnify sound, enabling the hearing-impaired listener to perceive it. These devices can be useful in interview settings in which the hearing-impaired person must respond to questions—for example, in the doctor's office or hospital or at a job interview. Such instruments are available at many electronics stores or directly from the manufacturers. Similar devices are available to augment the amplifier of the telephone.

- Hearing aids are battery-powered devices that filter and amplify sound. Modern hearing aids condition the amplified sound to improve clarity of the signal. These devices can assist a person with sensorineural loss or irreversible conductive loss. The design of hearing aids has improved dramatically; some models are small enough to be hidden completely in the ear canal or behind the ear.

Hearing aids can increase the intensity of sound by 70 decibels (dB). Using one successfully will require some practice. It should be custom-fitted to ensure comfort and performance. The majority of hearing-impaired people will benefit from hearing aids but only trial and adjustment will determine how useful a hearing aid is in a particular person. Unfortunately, only a minority of those people who would benefit own a hearing aid. Sometimes the problem is financial although most dealers will allow a trial rental period of 30 days to assess the benefit of a hearing aid. Some people perceive that wearing a hearing aid will be cumbersome or embarrassing. Nothing could be further from the truth with a properly fitted and well-functioning hearing aid. Speak to your doctor to see if a hearing aid would benefit you (see Hearing Aids, page 574).

Cochlear implants consist of two parts: a device known as the receiver/stimulator that is implanted surgically in the part of the skull that houses the inner ear and an external processor worn by the individual. The implanted receiver/stimulator acts as the control tower and directs the signal from the antenna and processing unit worn externally. Although not everyone with hearing loss is a good candidate for a cochlear implant, those who are likely to benefit include people such as the profoundly deaf who are unable to derive significant benefit even from the use of powerful hearing aids, those who have lost their hearing after developing some language skills or have been profoundly deaf for a short period, and those who possess sufficient motivation and family or social support to complete the postoperative rehabilitation. Rehabilitation consists of learning to adjust to the new signals and associating the new sound patterns with perceptions that were recognized previously as meaningful sounds. For this reason, the rehabilitation process will prove easier for people whose hearing impairment occurred after the learning of some language skills. Results can be dramatic including phone use and music appreciation. The vast majority of implant users find great benefit in improved access to spoken language. ■

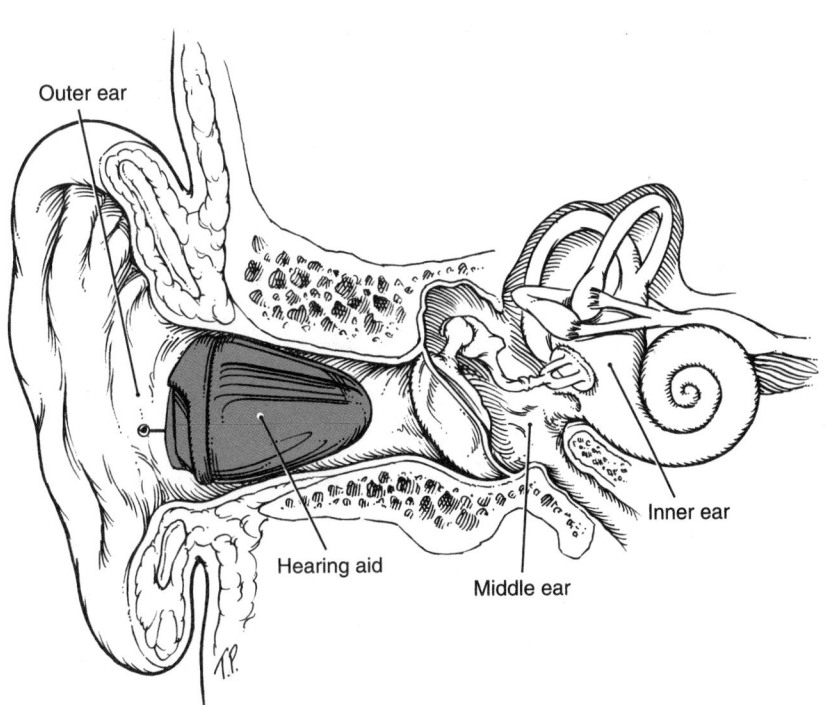

Three divisions of the ear. Hearing aids, placed in the outer ear canal, amplify sound waves and transmit them to the eardrum (tympanic membrane). The middle ear contains the ear bones (ossicles) and the inner ear converts movements of the body and vibrations from sound into nerve impulses.

Outer ear

Hearing aid

Middle ear

Inner ear

HEARING AIDS

In the United States, one out of every nine people will develop permanent hearing loss; the problem is most common in the senior years. Because only 5 to 10 percent of adult hearing problems can be treated medically or surgically, for most individuals with hearing loss relief can be found in the use of a well-fitted hearing aid. Hearing aids cannot restore normal hearing but they can reduce the effects of hearing loss by making soft sounds louder and listening to speech easier.

Hearing aids will offer the most benefit if fitted properly. Your ears should first be examined by a doctor; in fact, federal law requires that an ear examination be performed by a doctor no more than 6 months before the purchase of a hearing aid (unless you are age 18 or over and sign a waiver). Your doctor will refer you to an audiologist for a hearing evaluation. If your hearing loss cannot be medically or surgically treated, the audiologist will advise you on the type and model of hearing aid that is best for you.

Hearing aids today are small and technologically sophisticated. They consist of a microphone to pick up sound, an amplifier to make the sound louder, a receiver to deliver the sound to the ear, and batteries. Hearing aids often have earmolds to hold the hearing aid in place and improve sound quality. Modern hearing aids come in three basic styles:

- Canal aids, the smallest type of hearing aid available, fit partially or completely in the ear canal.

- All-in-the-ear aids are larger than canal aids but fit within the external ear.

- Behind-the-ear aids sit behind the ear and are connected to an earmold by clear plastic tubing.

Over 75 percent of hearing aids sold today are canal or all-in-the-ear models; eyeglass and body aids used in the past are rarely dispensed. In most cases of hearing loss in both ears, two hearing aids are recommended; the audiologist will discuss with you whether one or two hearing aids will serve you best. The technical characteristics of a particular hearing aid—the amount of amplification at each frequency and the specialized signal processing—as well as convenient features such as volume control will be taken into consideration in determining which type of hearing aid will offer you the most benefit. A mold will be made of your ear canal so that the earpiece will fit comfortably and work efficiently.

Cost of hearing aids can range from hundreds to thousands of dollars but reliability of the product and the replacement cost of the particular type of battery should be taken into consideration in making cost comparisons. If you are concerned that you cannot afford a hearing aid, your doctor may be able to refer you to community-based service organizations that can offer help. Some health care plans will cover the cost of the hearing evaluation and hearing aid; check with your plan representative.

Because a hearing aid requires individual fitting and adjustment as well as a period in which to grow accustomed to its use, you should only purchase a hearing aid that offers a 30-day trial period as recommended by the Food and Drug Administration (FDA). Allow yourself some time to get used to the new technology but consult your audiologist if you have any concerns. Ask whether a seminar in hearing, orientation, and listening strategies is available. The audiologist has several testing techniques that evaluate whether the hearing aid is working properly and whether it is offering the expected hearing improvement. If the hearing aid is not comfortable or does not improve your hearing even after adjustment, you should return it. Your audiologist may be able to recommend an alternative model that may work better for you.

Give yourself a few weeks to adjust to your hearing aid. You may be disconcerted initially to find that it will make your own voice louder and the speech of others seem somehow different. You will also need to learn how to tune out the background noise that will be amplified along with the sounds to which you are trying to listen. If you use your hearing aid daily, you will soon grow accustomed to it and will enjoy hearing sounds that you may not have heard for some time.

After you have been fitted with a hearing aid, you should have your hearing re-evaluated regularly by your doctor, usually on an annual basis. ■

COMMUNICATING EFFECTIVELY WITH A HEARING-IMPAIRED PERSON

To avoid the frustration of miscommunication, follow these suggestions when speaking with a hearing-impaired person:

- Face the person you are addressing. Be sure you have the person's attention before speaking.

- Speak slowly, pausing frequently.

- If the person is wearing a hearing aid, do not raise your voice. If not, speak a bit louder than normal but do not shout.

- Use gestures and facial expressions to reinforce what you are saying. Make sure lighting is adequate to assist in lip reading.

- Decrease background noise, if possible, or move to a quieter environment to speak. If there is background noise, stand closer to the person when you speak.

- If the listener does not seem to understand you, rephrase your question or statement using different words.

- Be patient and ask your listener to suggest ways that you can communicate more effectively. ■

ground noise—for example, in a noisy, crowded restaurant or party—but with continued exposure, the hearing loss will become apparent in everyday conversational interactions whenever the topic of conversation is unfamiliar and direct face-to-face contact is not possible.

While chronic damage from noise cannot be reversed, progression of the hearing loss can be prevented by protecting the ears from further high-noise exposure (see Protecting Your Hearing, this page).

Sudden, single loud noises (gunfire or explosions) may cause a reversible loss called temporary threshold shift that will correct given time and protection from further noise trauma. Continued exposure to both steady and intermittent noise will produce a permanent threshold shift.

What you can do Always protect your ears from noise, whether occupational or recreational, by use of earplugs or sound-dampening muffs. Muffs are more effective than earplugs. Beware of excessively amplified music. The sound frequencies typical of rock music cause a slower loss that may not be evident for 10 to 15 years after repeated exposure. If you have already sustained some degree of loss, it is of paramount importance that you avoid further exposure to loud noise. Note that a preexisting hearing loss does *not* protect your ears from noise damage (see Protecting Your Hearing, this page).

When to call the doctor If you have difficulty perceiving certain sounds—especially if you have been exposed chronically to high noise levels—contact your doctor.

Treatment There is no treatment to reverse sensorineural hearing loss; however, a hearing aid may help.

Prognosis There is no reversal of this problem once it occurs but management strategies (use of amplification, auditory training, and communication skills) can be of immense benefit.

❖ INFLAMMATORY CAUSES OF HEARING LOSS

Symptoms *(What you may experience)* Increasing trouble with hearing in one or both ears, usually developing slowly but

PROTECTING YOUR HEARING

After age, noise trauma is the most common cause of hearing loss from nerve damage. Any noise that exceeds 85 decibels (dB), especially with ongoing exposure, can damage the hearing center. Typical industrial noise is usually in the mid-90 dB range; rock concerts are even louder.

Protecting your hearing—which is exceedingly important if you already suffer from some degree of hearing loss—can be done by using simple earplugs, custom earplugs, or earmuffs. All types of hearing protectors reduce high-pitched noise better than noise of lower pitch and, except for specially equipped muffs, they block all noise—both harmful loud noise as well as more moderate surrounding noise and speech—which can itself be a safety hazard.

- Simple plugs, typically fashioned from waxed wool or foam polyurethane, reduce sound by 7 to 10 dB. They work well for most people but it can take a few days to get used to wearing them. They may also be difficult to fit into a small ear canal.

- Custom-fitted plugs can reduce noise levels by about 10 to 15 dB, which is often enough to reduce noise levels below the critical damaging threshold of 85 dB.

- Properly insulated earmuffs offer excellent damping of noise, reducing levels by 15 to 25 dB. Protective earmuffs, usually fashioned from a solid cup filled with sound-absorbing material, protect better but in many instances are less comfortable to wear. In industrial settings, in particular, when hard hats may also be required, the muffs may not fit properly. ■

sometimes occurring rapidly; dizziness; possibly facial paralysis. Some patients experience flu-like symptoms (fever, malaise, loss of appetite, fatigue). Rash, joint pain, and other symptoms may develop depending on the nature of the underlying illness.

Signs and laboratory findings *(What the doctor looks for)* Blood and urine tests can reveal signs of bacterial or viral infection. Specialized blood tests can reveal immune system proteins that indicate whether an autoimmune response is taking place. Audiometric tests can detect the extent of hearing loss.

TINNITUS (RINGING IN THE EARS)—A SYMPTOM OF HEARING DISTURBANCE

The Latin root of the word tinnitus means "to tinkle or ring like a bell." Related to the ears, it refers to the perception of sound—a buzzing or ringing—in the absence of a source for the sound. This phenomenon is referred to as subjective tinnitus—the sound is heard by the person affected with subjective tinnitus but is inaudible to a bystander. Almost everyone has experienced a brief episode of ringing in the ears at one time or another, and these transient episodes are usually of no significance. It is currently estimated that 50 million American adults have ringing in the ear to some degree. Of that number, 12 million have it severely enough to seek medical help. This persistent, more severe ringing can often be traced to one of a variety of specific problems related to the eardrum, the nerve of hearing, or the bones of the hearing portion of the inner ear.

Does this ringing indicate the onset of deafness? No, but quite often it represents an early symptom of hearing impairment, thought to be caused by removal of the normal masking effect of low-level noise around us. When the ear no longer perceives this low-level background noise from outside the body, the normally inaudible noises from inside the body created by the flow of blood, movement of muscles, and vibrations of the eardrum may be heard as a buzz, ring, or hum. Often this kind of ringing is pulsatile, ebbing and flowing with the rhythm of blood flow.

Sometimes, the ringing is not merely subjective—it is a buzz or ring that another person standing close by can appreciate. This form, called objective tinnitus, often arises as a consequence of abnormalities of the arteries near the ear including the development of aneurysms of the internal carotid artery or benign tumors of the blood vessels in the region. Other causes of objective tinnitus include instability of the temporomandibular joint (TMJ)—which connects the lower jaw to the skull just in front of the ear—or spasm of the muscles of the roof of the mouth.

Ringing in the ears can be frustrating for the sufferer because even when the cause can be found there may not be a treatment available that stops the ringing. Sometimes sedation at bedtime (when the relative silence makes the ringing more obvious) will help. Some people find that the sound of an FM radio helps them sleep by creating competing noise. Patients with severe ringing may be good candidates for a masking apparatus—one that generates white noise at a low level to compete with the ringing even during the day. Behavioral training using biofeedback can be of help to some. If symptoms of depression such as sleeplessness, lack of appetite, or loss of motivation are present, discuss the situation with your doctor. Treating the underlying depression can often aid coping ability. The distressing nature of the problem has given rise in most large cities to newsletters, support groups, and clinics devoted to the disorder.

If you suffer from persistent ringing, see a doctor for evaluation and for more information about the resources available to help you cope with this problem. ■

What is it? Infections caused by bacteria or viruses trigger the body's immune response, in which immune cells destroy the infectious agent. In the process, certain substances such as histamine are released from cells. These substances produce inflammation, which involves pain, swelling, redness, and irritation of affected tissues. Unless the inflammation is treated, there is a risk that it can lead to long-term damage of tissues and structures in the ear, especially the blood vessels. The result is sensorineural hearing loss.

In some cases, autoimmune diseases can lead to loss of hearing. An autoimmune disease such as rheumatoid arthritis is one in which a person's own immune system attacks the cells and tissues of the body as if they were foreign invaders. Many such diseases cause inflammation. Inflammation that affects the ear can cause loss of hearing; the longer the condition persists, the greater the threat to hearing. Among the autoimmune diseases associated with hearing loss are Cogan's syndrome, Meniere's disease, systemic lupus erythematosus, and Wegener's granulomatosis.

When to call the doctor Contact your doctor if you notice loss of hearing, especially if the problem arises following a bout with an infectious disease.

Treatment Steroid drugs can relieve symptoms of inflammation. If a bacterial infection is found to be the cause, treatment also calls for the use of antibiotics. Depending on the type of underlying autoimmune disease involved, anti-inflammatory medications, steroids, or other methods may be used in treatment. Hospitalization may be required and in many cases use of steroids must continue indefinitely.

Prognosis Between 40 and 70 percent of people recover functional hearing without treatment. A return to complete hearing following a severe infectious disease is rare. The outcome depends on various factors such as age, extent of deafness, and the presence of other problems involving the blood vessels.

❖ OTOTOXICITY—TOXIC CAUSES OF HEARING LOSS

Symptoms (*What you may experience*) Ringing in the ears or loss of normal perception of sounds during or following courses of certain medication.

Signs and laboratory findings (*What the doctor looks for*) History of current or recent medication intake and sensorineural hearing loss indicated by audiometry and tuning fork tests.

What is it? Several classes of medication may produce sensorineural hearing loss in both ears because they are toxic to the hearing nerve. Temporary hearing loss is associated with use of aspirin and other non-steroidal anti-inflammatory drugs, quinine (used for leg cramps and to prevent or treat malaria), and diuretics. Permanent loss sometimes occurs with aminoglycoside antibiotics (gentamicin, tobramycin, streptomycin, neomycin, vancomycin, and chloramphenicol), and certain cancer drugs (antineoplastics, especially cisplatin). For most of these drugs, toxic damage to the hearing nerve—also called ototoxicity—is related to the amount of medication taken, with higher dosages causing more risk for hearing loss, but even normal dosages of certain medication can cause problems. For example, a mild degree of impairment to hearing occurs in as many as 10 percent of people taking normal therapeutic dosages of antibiotics of the aminoglycoside group. This loss may occur quite suddenly after only a few doses and may be permanent. Ototoxicity especially affects people with renal insufficiency (poor kidney function), those who have preexisting hearing loss, and those whose treatment requires concurrent administration of several ototoxic substances. The risk can be limited by identifying people who are likely to be affected. If possible, alternate medication should be chosen; if no substitution is possible, the levels of these drugs in the blood during therapy should be monitored and assessments of the ability to hear should be performed with audiometry.

The hearing loss from anticancer drugs or aminoglycoside antibiotics may be permanent but the prognosis varies according to the drug. For example, quinine, quinidine (a heart rhythm drug), and high dosages of salicylates such as aspirin commonly cause temporary hearing loss and ringing in the ears. These symptoms usually resolve after stopping the drug; however, following accidental overdose of these substances (especially in children) cases of permanent loss have been reported. Intravenous administration of extremely high dosages of diuretic medication such as ethacrynic acid or furosemide (Lasix) that might be used to treat severe hypertension or congestive heart failure in the hospital have been associated with sudden hearing loss that may be permanent.

What you can do If you are taking OTC medication such as aspirin or quinine and you develop ringing in the ears, stop using the medication. If you already have some degree of mild hearing loss, be sure to inform your doctor.

When to call the doctor If your perception of sounds or your balance changes while on medication, notify your doctor immediately.

Treatment Beyond stopping medication and allowing the symptoms to subside if they will, there is no treatment to reverse toxic damage to hearing. Hearing rehabilitation is often useful.

Prognosis Excellent in cases of aspirin or quinine toxicity, variable when other drugs are the cause. In some cases, the loss may be permanent.

❖ ACOUSTIC NEUROMA (ACOUSTIC TUMORS AND VESTIBULAR SCHWANNOMA)

Symptoms *(What you may experience)* Hearing loss usually in one ear only, with reduced understanding of speech such as with telephone use; mild vertigo; loss of balance; occasionally, facial numbness, twitching of the eyelids or eyebrow, or an unbalanced smile.

Signs and laboratory findings *(What the doctor looks for)* Significant sensorineural hearing loss with impaired speech comprehension as demonstrated by audiometric testing; difficulty walking with a tendency to fall to one side; hyperactivity or weakness of the facial muscles as revealed by neurologic testing; tumor on the nerve as shown by computed tomography (CT) or magnetic resonance imaging (MRI).

What is it? This uncommon, benign tumor arises from the hearing and balance nerve (cranial nerve VIII), usually originating in those fibers mainly involved in maintaining balance and physical orientation. People who develop such a tumor will complain of loss of hearing in one ear, mild vertigo with change of position (see What is True Vertigo?, page 580), and loss of balance. The cranial nerves, those that send signals for sensation and motion of the head and neck, arise within the brain rather than the spinal cord. Several of these (numbers V, VI, VII, and VIII) travel in close proximity within the skull. For this reason, a growth on one of them (in this case, number VIII) can put pressure on its neighbors, causing loss of function. Deafness and vertigo are symptoms related to cranial nerve VIII; numbness and weakness of the face relate to pressure on neighboring nerves. Occasionally the pressure of a large acoustic neuroma on the cranial nerves and portions of the brain can cause weakness and paralysis, which may be mistaken as symptoms of stroke.

When to call the doctor   Loss of hearing on one side should always prompt a visit to your doctor.

Treatment   Although these slow-growing tumors are benign, their growth threatens the auditory, balance, facial, and other cranial nerves. Surgery to remove the tumor is the treatment of choice. The procedure will require hospitalization, as it must be performed in the operating room under general anesthesia. Best results are usually obtained at a major medical center, as it can be difficult to remove the tumor while preserving hearing as well as the facial nerves. Recovery following surgery will usually include a 5- to 7-day stay in the hospital. See Chapter 32 for more information on selecting a surgeon.

Recently radiation therapy has been used as an alternate method. It is not curative; instead, it induces scarring of the tumor. The goal is to prevent further tumor growth. Hearing loss and facial paralysis occur following radiation therapy at rates that exceed those of surgery performed by experienced teams.

Prognosis   Surgery stops further loss of nerve function. Resolution of facial weakness and numbness may occur. In people with good hearing before surgery, it may be possible to preserve hearing, but often the hearing loss is permanent.

❖ CONGENITAL HEARING LOSS

Symptoms   *(What you may experience)*
It can be difficult for parents to recognize hearing loss or deafness in their baby. Early identification is important for appropriate intervention that can reduce the impact of the condition in later life. By 3 months old, a baby with normal hearing startles or jumps when there is a sudden, loud sound; stirs, wakes, or cries when someone talks or makes a noise; and recognizes parents' voices and quiets when they speak. By 6 months old the baby with normal hearing looks toward interesting sounds, appears to listen, and awakens easily to sounds. By 1 year of age, the child turns toward soft sounds, understands "no" and "bye-bye," and begins to imitate speech sounds or says simple words. If these developmental milestones do not occur, the child should be tested.

Signs and laboratory findings   *(What the doctor looks for)*   Even mild degrees of hearing loss may be identified by otoacoustic emission testing and the auditory brainstem response. Children who have reached the developmental age of 6 months or over can be assessed by traditional methods (monitored behavioral responses to sound) that permit identification of most levels of hearing loss. At the first sign of hearing loss, children, even newborns, should receive a formal audiologic evaluation by an audiologist.

What is it?   Every year in the United States, over 4,000 babies are born with severe but treatable hearing disorders. Over 90 percent of them are born to hearing parents. Because only about 3 percent of newborn infants are screened for hearing disorders, many hearing-impaired babies unfortunately go undiagnosed until 2 or 3 years of age. By that time, the risk of fully overcoming the impairment is diminished.

Stimulation of the hearing nerve by sound is crucial. If the condition is not recognized early and if steps are not taken to amplify sound or otherwise stimulate the nerve, permanent deprivation effects on the brain can result. Hearing aids can be fit as early as a few months of age to provide early sound exposure. Because detecting and processing sound is an integral part of language development, children who cannot hear have an extremely difficult time learning how to read, write, and speak.

What you can do   If you suspect hearing loss, insist on screening and early intervention with hearing aids or surgery as indicated for your newborn. Learn as much as possible about options for developing your child's communication abilities. Deafness is not inevitable for most children born with severe hearing impairments. Your actions will make a difference.

When to call the doctor If you suspect that your newborn or infant cannot hear normally, contact a doctor right away.

Treatment Auditory stimulation is critical during early development of the auditory system in particular; such stimulation also affects many other aspects of cognitive development as well. For many infants born with hearing impairment, sufficient auditory stimulation can be provided through the use of hearing aids or through surgical intervention (see Auditory Rehabilitation Measures, page 573).

Prognosis Early intervention and early exposure to sound significantly increase the likelihood that children with severe hearing impairments can learn how to read, write, speak, and succeed in mainstream society. Strong evidence suggests that failure to provide early stimulation may do irrevocable damage to the hearing pathways within the central nervous system.

The Vestibular Inner Ear (the Balance Center)

The balance center, also called the vestibular labyrinth because of its curving, twisting, cloverleaf structure, lies encased deep within protective bones on either side of the skull. This portion of the inner ear helps to maintain our equilibrium and balance with respect to movement and to orient us as to our location and position in the world around us. It gives us our sense of the horizon, even when it is not visible, and is critical to maintaining eye position to produce a stable visual field.

The balancing mechanism within each ear consists of the utricle, the saccule, and the semicircular canals, all of which continually monitor the position and movement of the head, which allows the body to adjust itself and remain balanced. The utricle and saccule are jelly-filled organs lined with sensitive cells that have hair-like caps. These caps act as motion detectors. They contain tiny "rocks" called otoliths that

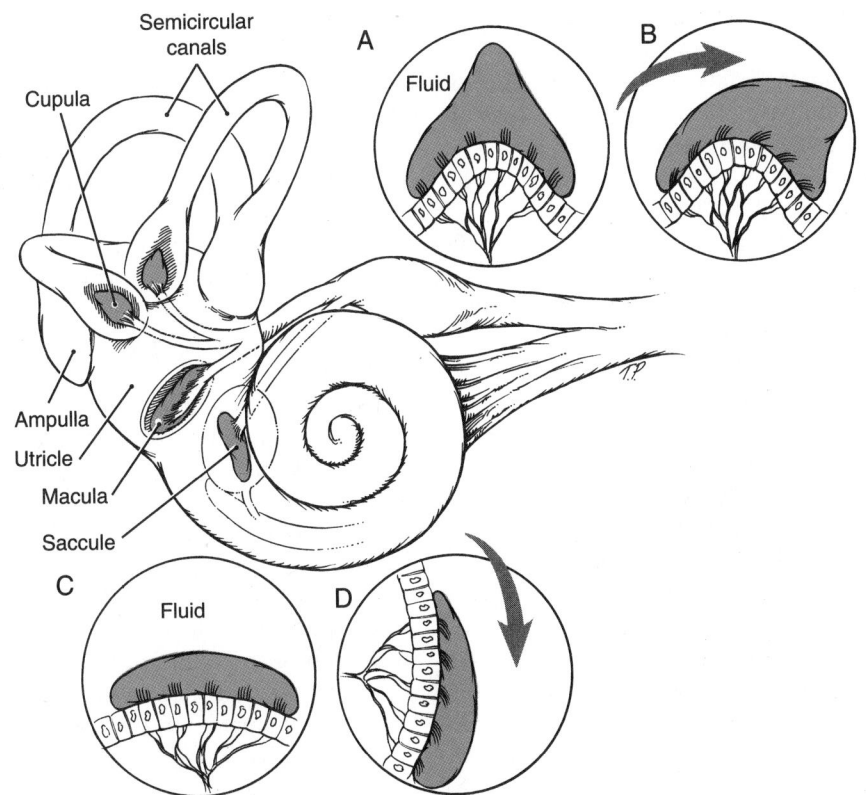

(A & B) Fluid in the semicircular canals flows in response to rotation of the head and body, moving the cupula. Hair cells inside the cupula convert that motion into nerve impulses that are sent to the brain. (C & D) Acceleration of the body in one direction, such as from the force of gravity, causes movement in the fluid of the utricle and saccule. Fluid motion displaces hair cells in the macula and converts the acceleration into nerve impulses.

WHAT IS TRUE VERTIGO?

Many conditions cause a sensation of lightheadedness or dizziness. Common causes include disturbances of electrolytes in the blood such as low potassium or sodium; sudden drops in blood pressure when rising quickly from sitting to standing; insufficient blood flow to the brain from atherosclerotic blockage of the arteries; and side effects of medication. But the lightheaded feeling common to these conditions is not true vertigo. Vertigo occurs when you experience a sense of rotation—that is, spinning—in the absence of head or body movement. The spinning may seem to come from within, as if you are spinning while the world stands still. The sensation may be that the world is spinning around you. The sensation can be so powerful that it is accompanied by motion sickness, with nausea and vomiting. You may feel so disorientated that walking becomes difficult or impossible—as if you were trying to walk on the deck of a ship being tossed on the sea.

The symptoms may last a few moments or several hours to days. In some cases, the vertigo may occur only if stimulated by movement of the head while in others it may occur without movement. Sleepiness may follow for several hours after the attack of vertigo has subsided and a sense of being somewhat off-balance may persist for days.

Vertigo is most often a symptom of inner-ear dysfunction but is also associated with disorders of the central nervous system ranging from infection to tumors. For this reason, evaluation of true vertigo by a doctor who can determine its cause is important. ■

accentuate movement in the fluid. Movement of the head causes the otoliths to shift, bending the hair-like sensors and stimulating the nerve endings. The three fluid-filled semicircular canals are oriented in three planes at right angles to each other: up and down, front and back, and side to side. At the base of each canal is a mass of jelly encasing tiny hair-like nerve endings. Movement of the head in any direction will cause the fluid to move, stimulating the nerve endings. (If, for example, you are spinning around and stop suddenly, the fluid continues to move in the canals, causing momentary dizziness.)

The brain integrates the movement of the fluid and otoliths in the vestibular system of the inner ear and translates those nerve signals into a perception of the body's position in relation to the world around it, resulting in a sense of balance or equilibrium.

The design of the balancing mechanism is elegant in its simplicity, functioning flawlessly in most of us most of the time. When problems arise within the balance center—usually from infection, inflammation, or trauma—we feel out of balance and disoriented. This sense of spinning around in the world or the world spinning around us we call vertigo (see What is True Vertigo, this page).

❖ ACUTE LABYRINTHITIS

Symptoms (*What you may experience*) Sudden onset of continuous, severe vertigo; decreased ability to hear; nausea and vomiting; difficulty maintaining a fixed gaze or scanning eye movements.

Signs and laboratory findings (*What the doctor looks for*) Nystagmus (characteristic sign on examination of jerking eye movements with head movement or occasionally spontaneously, usually in association with a spell of vertigo).

What is it? Acute labyrinthitis, a term meaning sudden infection or inflammation of the labyrinth, begins abruptly with severe vertigo that may last several days to 1 week. The vertigo may be sufficiently severe to cause nausea and vomiting and to make walking or standing (or even lifting your head from a pillow) difficult. The sudden onset of these symptoms can be frightening, though the condition is not dangerous. Hearing loss and ringing (often of just one ear) may accompany the disturbance of balance but this is less likely.

Some people suffer a severe attack of vertigo that lasts several days to weeks but is not associated with hearing loss or ringing in the ears. Although research has yet to discover a certain cause since the disorder frequently follows an upper respiratory infection such as a cold, it is often referred to as viral or infectious labyrinthitis. The disorder may represent viral vestibular neuritis (infection of the vestibular nerve by a virus.)

What you can do Bed rest with limited head motion will help to minimize the sense of spinning. OTC medication for motion sickness such as Dramamine or Bonine may help to reduce symptoms.

When to call the doctor If sudden vertigo following an upper respiratory illness fails to resolve within a day or two or if symptoms become severe, contact a doctor. Although in most instances the cause will be benign, a thorough evaluation is necessary to eliminate more serious potential causes such as a brain tumor or aneurysm (abnormal enlargement of a blood vessel).

Treatment Even severe vertigo usually resolves without further treatment in a few days. However, if severe nausea and vomiting accompany the vertigo, medication to quiet these symptoms such as prochlorperazine (Compazine), hydroxyzine (Vistaril), or promethazine hydrochloride (Phenergan) may help. Symptoms may linger for weeks although gradual improvement is the rule. Some doctors may recommend prescription tranquilizers such as benzodiazepines (Valium, Klonopin). Meclizine (Antivert) can also help somewhat to reduce vertigo.

Prognosis Excellent for resolution of vertigo. If there is associated sudden hearing loss in the affected ear, further follow-up and evaluation are needed to rule out other causes (related to the inner ear or brain) of the vertigo.

❖ MENIERE'S DISEASE (ENDOLYMPHATIC HYDROPS)

Symptoms *(What you may experience)* Episodes of vertigo lasting minutes to hours that may be accompanied by nausea and vomiting; variable hearing loss; ringing in the ears; ear pressure or fullness.

Signs and laboratory findings *(What the doctor looks for)* Abnormal caloric test (stimulation with warm and cold water) of the inner ear.

What is it? Meniere's disease, also called Meniere's syndrome or endolymphatic hydrops, is a disorder of the inner ear that causes episodic bouts of severe vertigo and fluctuant hearing levels. It typically begins between the ages of 20 and 50, affecting men and women equally. The problem appears to arise from an abnormality of the tissue lining the canals of the inner ear. This lining produces and filters the endolymph—the fluid that fills the balancing and hearing mechanisms of the inner ear. See The Vestibular Inner Ear (the Balance Center), page 579, for more information about these structures. When an excessive amount of fluid distends the labyrinth, the pattern of stimulation of the hair-like nerve fibers within the canals may become distorted. The brain cannot properly interpret these conflicting signals—it would be as if one canal were telling the brain that the person were reclining and another were telling the brain that the person stood erect. Unable to determine the correct signal, the brain attempts to incorporate all of them, with the result being a sensation of spinning. The symptoms wax and wane as the pressure in the fluid rises and falls.

Along with the episodic vertigo, people suffering from Meniere's disease often have other symptoms including impaired hearing of low-frequency tones that may worsen with time, ringing in the ears (in this case, a ringing that takes on a low-tone blowing quality), and a sense of fullness in the ear. The disorder usually affects only one ear but in one-third of cases it may affect both ears; the second ear affected is typically less seriously impaired. Although the above cluster of symptoms is characteristic of typical Meniere's disease, atypical forms of the disorder have also been identified and may respond to the therapy used to treat Meniere's disease.

What causes the problem to develop is unclear in most cases, but two causes are known: head trauma and syphilis. Sometimes a variant of migraine accompanies episodic bouts of vertigo; it resembles Meniere's disease but lacks hearing impairment and ringing in the ears. The cause of this variant, called recurrent vestibulopathy, is also unknown but it is likely that it is mediated by blood vessel spasms.

This disorder may cause an increased visual dependency—that is, people with Meniere's disease may become more dependent on information received visually to help them keep their balance.

What you can do Because of increased visual dependency, it is a good idea not to walk through dark rooms; keep lights or night-lights on at all times; do not drive a car at night or during stormy weather when visibility is poor.

A salt-restricted diet may help to reduce the frequency of attacks. The usual recommendation is to keep intake below 2 g a day.

Avoid caffeine, smoking, and alcohol since these substances may aggravate symptoms. Avoid the additive monosodium glutamate (MSG), often present in Chinese food, as it may trigger symptoms. Stress may aggravate the vertigo and ringing in the ears associated with Meniere's disease and undermines the ability to cope with these symptoms. Stress reduction techniques may be helpful.

When to call the doctor The onset of symptoms suggestive of Meniere's disease should prompt a visit to your doctor. Evaluation to determine the cause of vertigo should always be done.

Treatment Medication such as meclizine (Antivert) or diazepam (Valium) used to control vertigo may provide temporary relief.

The use of diuretic medication such as hydrochlorothiazide may help to reduce fluid buildup in the inner ear. If diuretic therapy prevents recurrence of the vertigo, it can be discontinued after 1 year. In those people for whom dietary salt restriction and diuretics fail to adequately control symptoms, inner ear surgery to control the vertigo may be necessary. A procedure called endolymphatic sac drainage usually preserves hearing; attacks of vertigo are controlled in one-half to two-thirds of cases.

Other surgical options include cutting the balance nerve (a vestibular neurectomy) as it leaves the inner ear and courses to the brain. This procedure may permanently cure the vertigo and often preserves hearing.

In cases in which the hearing is already poor in the affected ear, the surgeon may recommend a labyrinthectomy, in which the balance canals are removed completely. This procedure results in the highest rates of control of vertigo but will render the affected ear permanently deaf. Surgical treatment is more difficult in those people with Meniere's disease affecting both ears. Depending on test results, your doctor may recommend the surgery for the ear that is most affected, which may prevent recurrence of the most severe attacks of vertigo. More recently, techniques involving the judicious application of ototoxic medication to the ear have been refined, providing a valuable form of treatment of vertigo for patients who are not candidates for surgery.

Prognosis In general, although the disease cannot be cured, vertigo can be controlled in most cases with diet and medication. Although reserved for the most severe cases, surgery provides a viable treatment option.

❖ POSITIONAL VERTIGO

Symptoms and signs Transient vertigo following changes in head position.

What is it? In some people, head movement, particularly quick changes of position, can prompt vertigo lasting from 10 to 60 seconds. The symptoms may occur in clusters, persisting for a few days and then disappearing. The cause of this disorder is unclear but may arise from otoliths free-floating within the semicircular canals of the balance center.

What you can do Avoiding the head positions that typically trigger vertigo can minimize symptoms.

When to call the doctor Persistence of positional vertigo lasting longer than a few days should prompt a visit to the doctor. Consistent development of vertigo when tipping the head back to look up should also be investigated since this symptom suggests insufficient blood flow through the arteries (in the back of the head and neck) to the brain.

Treatment A form of physical therapy called single-session habituation that aims at repositioning the free-floating otoliths has proved to be of great help. A new surgical technique under investigation is designed to interrupt the semicircular canal positioned toward the back of the head. The purpose of this surgery is to minimize the inner-ear response caused by tilting the head at an angle—a motion that often prompts a sense of spinning.

Prognosis The disorder may recur despite treatment but recurrence may well be responsive to repeated treatment involving physical therapy.

THE NOSE AND PARANASAL SINUSES

The nose serves as the natural opening to the respiratory tree. It consists of two nostrils that open into chambers divided by a central wall called the septum. The two

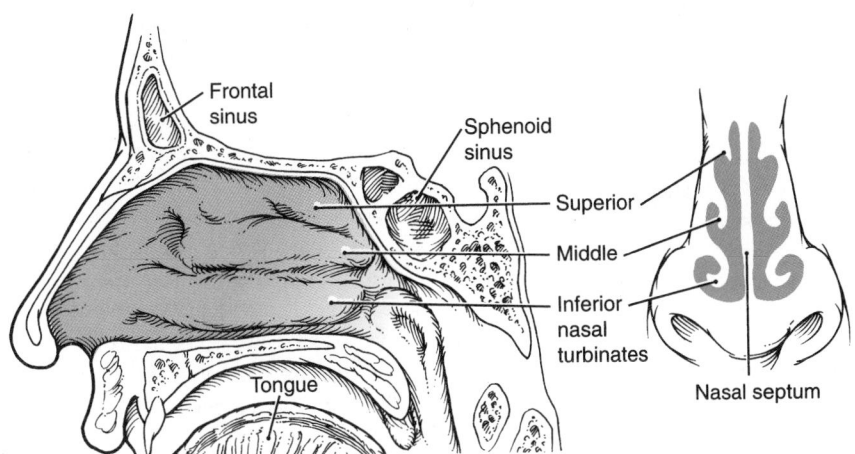

Normal nasal anatomy.

chambers merge into one where the nasal passageway meets the back of the oral cavity and throat. Within each chamber, thin shelves of bone called nasal turbinates jut from the sides of the chamber, providing filtering and humidification to the nasal passageway.

Mucus-producing tissue lines and moistens the passageways, and protective hairs guard the entrance at the nostril; both structures clean and filter the incoming air. The lining of the nose also contains a rich supply of blood vessels to warm the air as it enters.

The nasal passageways connect to the nearby paranasal sinuses, a series of air-filled chambers in the bones of the skull on either side of the nose and in the forehead. By this route, problems affecting one area can spread to the other.

Sinuses in the skull bones are airspaces that are lined with tissue. Drainage into the nose can become blocked, which leads to infection of the sinuses (sinusitis).

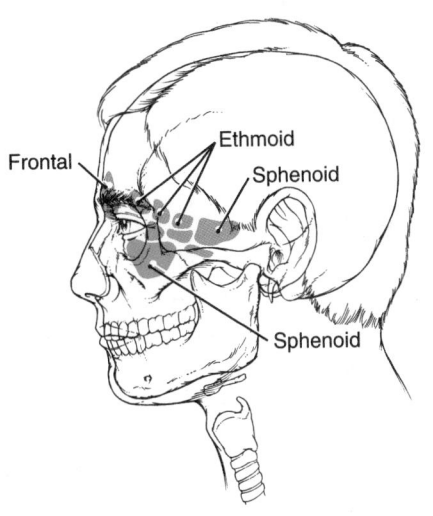

The upper portion of the nose also houses the fine and very sensitive fibers of the olfactory nerve, which is responsible for detecting odors. See The Sense of Smell, page 584, for more information about how this sensory system operates—or fails to operate.

❖ VIRAL RHINITIS (THE COMMON COLD)

Symptoms *(What you may experience)* Watery nasal discharge, sneezing, stuffiness, sore throat, fatigue, muscle aches, and headache; low-grade fever (occasionally).

Signs and laboratory findings *(What the doctor looks for)* Inflamed nasal lining; swollen turbinates; clear mucus; red throat.

What is it? What we call the common cold is actually a constellation of symptoms of upper respiratory infection caused by one of hundreds of different viruses. Because of the large number of viruses that can cause viral rhinitis, it is impossible for the body to develop solid immunity against a cold. The immune system may be prepared to defend against a certain virus to which it has been exposed, but if another comes along, even though it causes the same symptoms, immune defenses will fail to recognize it. For that reason, a person can have multiple colds, one after another. The wide range of infectious agents that can cause the common cold has thwarted development of a preventive vaccine.

THE SENSE OF SMELL

Like hearing, the ability to smell depends on adequate functioning of a system of structures, in this case a gathering device (the nose) and a detection system (the olfactory nerve). Impairment to either part of the system will diminish the ability to smell.

Swelling of the nasal lining (whether from trauma, infection, or allergic disorders), polyps, tumors, or other causes of obstruction can prevent odor-bearing air from being gathered in sufficient quantity for detection. Blocked access for scented air to reach the detection area is the most common cause for loss of the ability to smell, also called anosmia, or diminishment of the sense of smell, also called hyposmia.

At the sensory end of the system, the first cranial (olfactory) nerve controls the ability to smell. From its origin in the brain, it branches into finer and finer segments that ultimately terminate in nerve endings that penetrate into an area very near the back recesses of the nasal cavity.

Odoriferous molecules must travel through the nasal chamber to reach this area, which is bounded by a thin plate of bone punched through with many small holes. There the molecules must dissolve in the mucus that coats the exposed olfactory nerve endings in order for the odor to be perceived.

Transient loss of smell accompanies many self-limiting conditions such as viral upper respiratory infections but the causes can vary widely. Persistent loss of the ability to smell can occur with brain tumors, following head trauma, as a consequence of nutritional deficiencies, or with disorders of the endocrine system.

Because the sense of smell augments the sense of taste, permanent loss of the ability to smell or diminishment of the sense of smell may reduce your enjoyment of food. Seasoning foods with pungent spices such as pepper can help by stimulating the endings of other nerves in the area (cranial nerve V, for example) to augment taste. Important safety issues may arise when a person loses the ability to smell—for example, smoke or natural gas may go unnoticed. Equipping the home with smoke detectors and electrical appliances is recommended to ensure safety.

Sense of smell. Odor molecules must first dissolve in a mucus layer in the nose. The shape of the odor molecule determines which receptors are stimulated. The molecules fit into specific receptors on the cilia, which are the swollen ends of receptor cells. The receptor cells convert the odor molecule into a nerve impulse, which travels via the olfactory bulb and nerve to the brain.

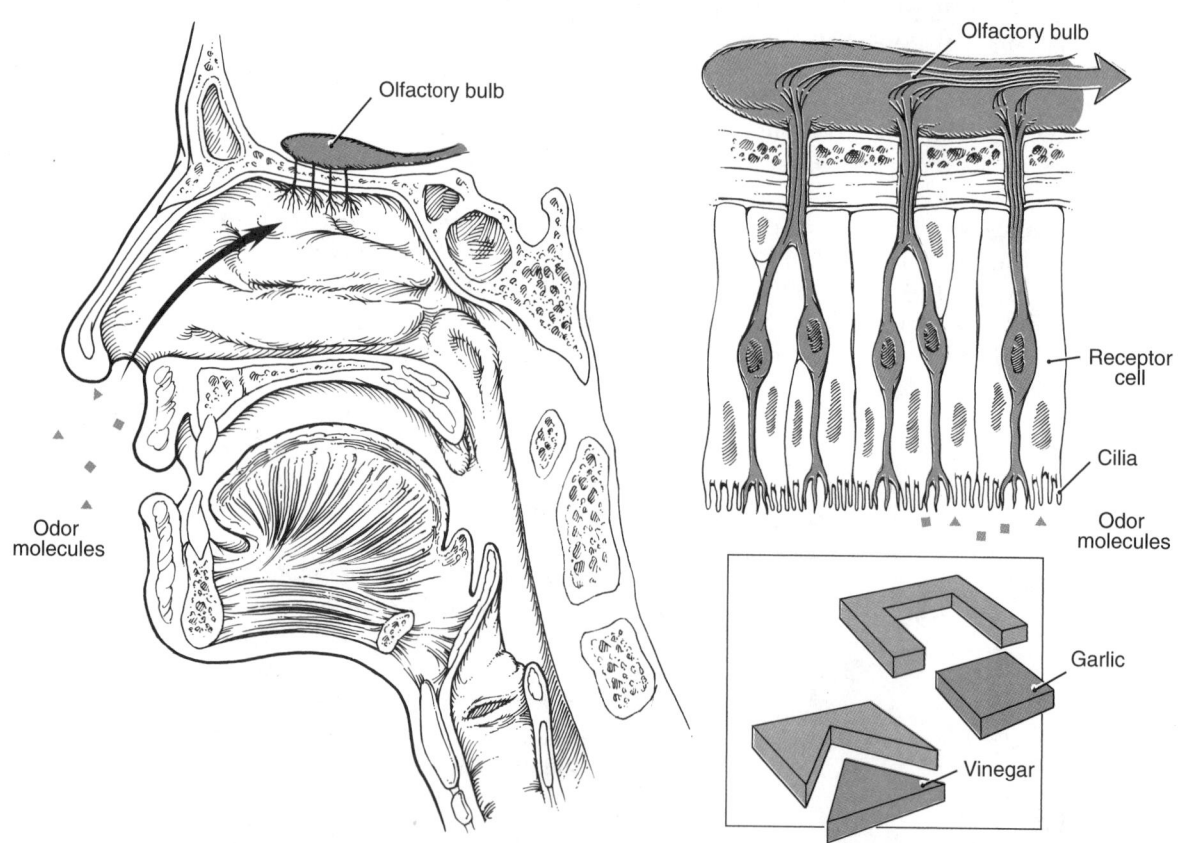

Despite popular belief, colds do not arise because you become chilled or wet. The viruses that cause colds pass from person to person, usually through hand contact with nasal secretions or because viruses come into contact with respiratory membranes. From the onset of symptoms, the cold syndrome usually builds over a few days to a peak and persists, slowly resolving, over the next 7 to 10 days.

Occasionally, bacterial infection of the upper respiratory system may follow a cold (see Acute Bacterial Sinusitis, page 585).

What you can do Prevention of colds is the best defense against them (see Preventing a Cold, this page).

Only your immune system can eradicate a virus but OTC cold remedies, decongestant medication, and acetaminophen can temporarily reduce the misery of the symptoms. Recent studies suggest that the mineral nutrient zinc, taken as a lozenge dissolved in the mouth three or four times a day for a few days, may help reduce the length of the cold; however, the benefits of taking zinc lozenges remain inconclusive and should be discussed with your doctor.

When to call the doctor Call your doctor if your fever fails to resolve in 48 to 72 hours or if it exceeds 102°F. Also call if you experience focused facial or forehead pain; if the character of the mucus changes, becoming thick and discolored or bloody; if you develop severe pain in the sinuses or ears; or if you develop a severe cough productive of discolored or bloody phlegm.

Treatment Except for symptomatic treatment, there is no effective medical therapy.

Prognosis Full recovery is the rule.

❖ ACUTE BACTERIAL SINUSITIS

Symptoms *(What you may experience)* Thick nasal discharge, usually colored or tinged with blood; pressure and pain over the cheek or forehead; headache. Sometimes: nonspecific aching of nearby teeth; fever.

Signs and laboratory findings *(What the doctor looks for)* Causative bacteria demonstrated by a culture of discharge fluid accumulation and swollen tissues in the sinuses shown by x-rays or CT scans. An MRI scan may be necessary to rule out the possibility of sinus malignancy in some cases.

What is it? When viral infections or allergies swell the sinus-lining tissues, causing blockage of the drainage openings, mucus becomes trapped inside. The stagnant secretions provide a fertile medium for bacterial growth, and pus forms within the sinus. Pressure within the cavity increases as the infection builds. Pain may be felt over the affected sinus—over the cheeks in the large

PREVENTING A COLD

There are hundreds of cold viruses, each of which can cause stuffy or runny nose, watery eyes, and scratchy throat as well as other symptoms. Cold viruses are spread by direct contact with infected respiratory secretions—either person-to-person contact or contact with contaminated surfaces such as tissues or doorknobs on which the viruses may lie. People with colds frequently wipe their noses and cover their mouths when they cough; in this way, hands can spread the virus to anything touched.

Careful handwashing is the best prevention against catching a cold. During the winter cold season, wash hands in soap and water several times daily, particularly after handling potentially contaminated surfaces or coming in contact with infected people. Avoid touching the nasal chambers with the hands. Cleaning the nose should always be done with a tissue, followed by washing the hands and discarding the tissue appropriately. ■

maxillary sinuses or across the forehead in the frontal sinus.

Deep within the skull lie the ethmoid and sphenoid sinuses, which can sometimes become infected in conjunction with infection of the other larger sinuses. Sinusitis in these areas may cause a headache difficult to localize but often perceived as being in the middle of the head or sometimes on the top or crown of the head. Eyelid swelling may be a danger sign that infection has spread to the eye socket.

The bacteria that infect the sinuses, in general, are the same ones that commonly cause middle-ear infections—typical respiratory invaders such as *Streptococcus pneumoniae*, *Haemophilus influenzae*, and less commonly *Staphylococcus aureus* and *Moraxella catarrhalis*. Occasionally, other less typical bacterial strains infect the areas and these may resist common antibiotic treatments. These stubborn infections may require culture to identify the offending bacterium and sensitivity testing to determine the best antibacterial medication to kill it.

Complications may arise from sinus infections. For example, osteomyelitis occurs when the infection extends to involve the bones of the sinus cavity, or a mucus-filled cyst may form. These expanding cysts may erode the bone by pressure. More seriously, bacteria from the infected sinus can enter the bloodstream and cause meningitis or thrombosis (a clot) in the venous sinuses in the brain.

What you can do See Preventing a Cold, page 585, and Chapter 29 for tips on reducing the occurrence of colds and allergies which can lead to sinusitis. If you experience a cold or allergy, try taking Robitussin or a similar mucus-thinning agent along with drinking plenty of fluids to keep the mucus from becoming thick and sticky. Also keep the nasal mucosa (lining) adequately moisturized (especially during the winter months) with humidification and OTC saltwater nasal sprays. A dry, cracking nasal lining is susceptible to bacterial invasion. Saltwater nasal sprays and a bedroom humidifier can help to keep these tissues moist and can aid the removal of thick mucus with nose blowing.

When to call the doctor Some people develop some form of sinusitis every time they get a cold. This can lead to a tendency to ignore sinusitis the way one ignores colds. However, if symptoms of sinus infection persist beyond 2 weeks or if high fever or other symptoms arise, a doctor should be consulted.

Warning: If you develop high fever, severe headache, inability to move your eyes in all directions, severe swelling of the eyelids, double vision, or loss of vision in conjunction with a sinus infection, seek immediate medical help.

Treatment Oral decongestants such as pseudoephedrine or nasal decongestant sprays may help relieve congestion. An appropriate antibiotic will usually be sufficient to eradicate the common bacterial causes. The regimens should be continued for longer periods than those required for most infections due to the fluid accumulation that typically accompanies sinusitis.

Prognosis Excellent if promptly diagnosed and adequately and appropriately treated with antibiotic medication.

❖ CHRONIC SINUSITIS

Symptoms (*What you may experience*) Nasal congestion with nasal discharge and postnasal drip; localized masses of swollen tissue known as a nasal polyps (see page 587), reduced sense of smell; inflammation leading to sense of fullness or heaviness in the forehead and cheek area; headache; drainage of thick, irritating phlegm into the throat that leads to cough, bad breath, mild throat pain, and sense of fullness in the throat. Coughing and the need to clear the throat is most severe upon arising from sleep.

Signs and laboratory findings (*What the doctor looks for*) Redness or irritation in the throat, drainage of phlegm, and nasal polyps.

What is it? Sinusitis is an inflammation of the sinuses resulting in impaired airflow into the sinuses and inadequate drainage of mucus produced by the sinus lining. The inflammation results from an infection by viruses, bacteria, or fungi or arises due to allergy. Chronic sinusitis persists for a long time or occurs in repeated episodes.

What you can do The goal is to improve sinus drainage and relieve the underlying cause of inflammation. Steam inhalation soothes nasal passages and promotes drainage. Avoiding exposure to substances or environments that trigger allergic responses can also help. If you smoke, quit.

When to call the doctor Consult a doctor if symptoms persist longer than 2 weeks or if a persistent high fever develops.

Treatment Therapy depends on identification of the infected sinus or sinuses by x-ray. Treatment addresses the cause of infection or the underlying condition such as allergy or exposure to chemicals or smoking.

In some cases, if antibiotic therapy is ineffective, surgery may be needed to remove the infection or to provide portals for sinus drainage and exposure to air. One technique is known as endoscopic sinus surgery. Surgery is usually performed under local anesthesia on an outpatient basis although sometimes the procedure involves an overnight hospital stay (see Endoscopic Windows Surgery for Sinusitis, page 587).

Prognosis When the source of the underlying infection is properly identified, treatment is usually very effective. Some people who undergo surgery may need additional minor endoscopic procedures. In rare cases, more extensive surgery may be required.

❖ NASAL POLYPS

Symptoms *(What you may experience)* Difficulty breathing through the nose; persistent stuffiness and facial discomfort; nasal drainage; recurrent sinus infections.

Signs and laboratory findings *(What the doctor looks for)* Translucent, grape-like masses (yellow to gray) visible on examination of the nasal chambers; an associated history of asthma and aspirin allergy (sometimes).

What is it? How and why nasal polyps develop is still unknown but they may be a consequence of chronic inflammation of the nasal lining. Polyps occur commonly in people with chronic vasomotor and allergic rhinitis and frequently occur in children with cystic fibrosis. They obstruct the nasal airway producing symptoms of stuffiness and chronic nasal drainage. Because of the frequent association of nasal polyps, asthma, and aspirin allergy, people with nasal polyps should avoid aspirin products, which can stimulate a sudden and sometimes severe shortness of breath from spasm of the bronchial tree.

What you can do Avoid aspirin-containing products.

When to call the doctor Chronic nasal obstruction symptoms should prompt an evaluation by a doctor to determine the cause.

Treatment Small polyps may respond to topical nasal steroid sprays. Larger, better established polyps generally do not respond well to medication, whether it is topical steroid sprays or courses of systemic steroids taken by mouth or injection.

Surgery is the treatment of choice. It is usually performed in an outpatient operating room under local anesthesia unless computed tomography (CT) scans have shown that the polyps extend deeply to involve the sphenoid sinus. In these cases, a more aggressive surgery to remove the polyps from these deeper areas must be performed although the surgery is usually still done in an outpatient setting. In most

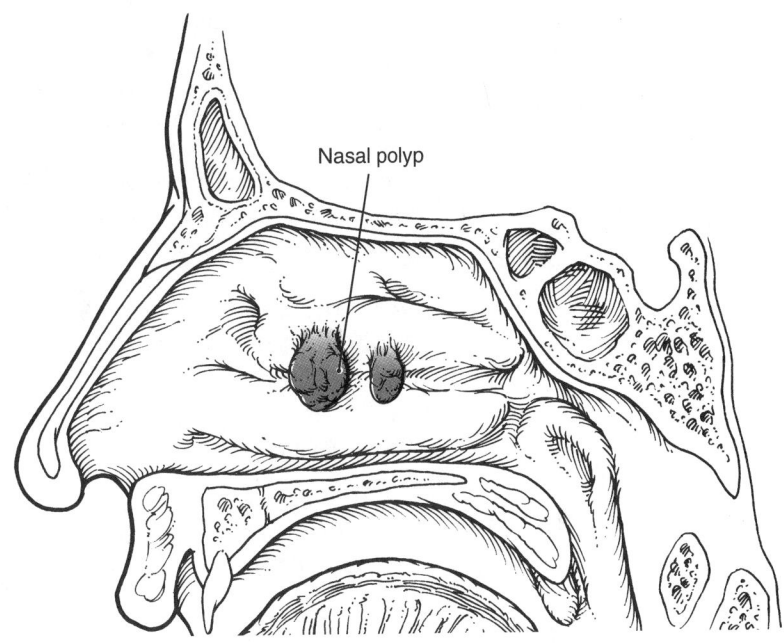

Teardrop-shaped pouches of nasal tissue filled with mucus (nasal polyps) can cause breathing problems and recurrent sinus infections (sinusitis). In these cases, they can be removed by a simple surgical procedure.

ENDOSCOPIC WINDOWS SURGERY FOR SINUSITIS

Surgery is not required in the majority of people with sinus problems, but for those whose chronic sinus problems do not respond to medical therapy, endoscopic sinus surgery may be recommended. Endoscopic surgery uses lighted scopes and tiny cutting instruments, offering less invasive surgical approaches by providing relief without the need for incisions and removal of surrounding normal tissue. In addition to removing disease from the sinuses, the endoscope often allows the surgeon to open a permanent window to facilitate sinus drainage and sinus aeration.

Endoscopic surgery allows direct examination of the lesser sinus areas—particularly the ethmoid area—where chronic infection can smolder, evading antibiotic treatment and re-igniting recurrent infection into the maxillary or frontal areas. Endoscopic sinus surgery can be performed on an outpatient basis without a hospital stay and usually without the necessity and discomfort of nasal packing.

Recovery occurs at home with return to most normal activities being possible right away although you should not blow your nose for approximately 5 days following surgery. Although endoscopic surgery reduces the risk of bleeding, nasal secretions may be tinged with blood for 1 or 2 weeks as the sinuses heal. ■

cases, polyps can be removed by a new, less extensive surgery performed with an endoscope (see Endoscopic Windows Surgery for Sinusitis, page 587). All polyp tissue should be sent to the pathologist for examination under a microscope; rarely, what appears on the surface to be a simple, benign polyp proves to be cancerous.

Prognosis Although surgery may be curative, the disease may recur and subsequent procedures may prove necessary.

❖ DEVIATED SEPTUM

Symptoms *(What you may experience)* Obstruction to nasal breathing (usually one-sided); head pain in the deep forehead (rarely).

Signs and laboratory findings *(What the doctor looks for)* Observable bending of the nasal septum on examination.

What is it? Obstruction of the nasal airway sometimes occurs because of structural changes in the bone or cartilage. These changes usually result from trauma that may occasionally occur during childbirth but more often from an accident—a fall on or blow to the nose—during childhood or later in life. Mild bending of the septum occurs so frequently as to be considered normal. Greater degrees of deviation may cause complete or partial obstruction of one nasal chamber and impede airflow and the normal passage of mucus.

Mild cases may cause no noticeable airflow disturbance but more severe deviation (or when swelling from colds or allergies complicates mild cases) can cause considerable difficulty including mouth breathing, restless sleep, irritability, and persistent sinus infection.

What you can do When a cold or acute allergic swelling complicates a mild deviation, judicious use of topical decongestant sprays may make breathing easier. These types of medication can be overused; their use for longer than 3 consecutive days can lead to an almost addictive abuse (see Nasal Spray Abuse and How to Kick the Habit, page 1338).

When to call the doctor If you have persistent difficulty breathing from one nostril, particularly if difficulty breathing at night causes sleep disturbances, contact your doctor.

Treatment Mild deviation may cause no difficulty except when complicated by swelling. The more severe the deviation, the more likely that surgery will be the best option for relieving the obstruction. See Rhinoplasty—the Nose Job, page 589, for more information about the option for corrective procedures. In addition to deviation, other indications for nasal septal reconstruction surgery include chronic nosebleeds and chronic sinus infections brought on by sinus blockage resulting from the deformity.

Prognosis Improvement of the nasal airway occurs in 80 to 90 percent of cases treated by surgery. There is a 5 to 15 percent chance that a second surgery may be necessary to achieve optimal function and the desired cosmetic result.

❖ NASAL TRAUMA
(BROKEN NOSE)

Symptoms *(What you may experience)* Pain, swelling, bruising, obstruction to nasal airflow, and sometimes bleeding following nasal trauma.

Signs and laboratory findings *(What the doctor looks for)* A deformity or fracture revealed by nasal examination and occasionally x-ray studies.

What is it? A blow to the nose can damage any of the nasal tissues: breaking the nasal septum or support cartilages on either side of the nose, dislocating the nasal cartilage from the bones of the skull, or causing a hematoma (blood clot) on the septum or inside the nose. Of all the facial bones, the nose is the most commonly broken. In fact, nasal injuries occur so commonly that they often go undiagnosed and untreated. Evaluation is important if the trauma is severe and deformity is present. Failure to realign a deformity or address a septal blood clot can result in long-term breathing difficulty and cosmetic deformity and can predispose the person to more frequent sinus infections (see Deviated Septum, above). Brain fluid leakage can occur with severe trauma.

Swelling from the trauma (both externally and internally) can hamper initial assessment of the degree of deformity. Since soft tissue swelling will subside, the degree of bone and cartilage architectural disruption will determine whether the injury will leave a lasting cosmetic deformity or obstruction to nasal breathing.

In certain sports, boxing in particular, blows to the nose exact a heavy toll on the nasal profile. (The term "pug nose" comes from "pugilist," the technical name for a boxer.) Repeated battering and multiple fractures of the delicate nasal bones and cartilage can in time result in collapse of the support bone high on the nose. This damage causes a typical deformity—called a saddle deformity—in which the middle of the nose sags like a saddle in the middle of a horse's back. This deformity requires more extensive plastic and reconstructive surgery to repair than does a simple nasal fracture.

What you can do As soon as possible after the injury, apply cold packs. If the nose is bleeding, compress the nostrils between your fingers padded with a clean cloth for 5 minutes without releasing. (Breathe through your mouth during this time.) Cleanse any abrasion to the skin with mild antibacterial soap and water.

When to call the doctor Seek medical help if there is significant deformity, persistent bleeding, laceration of the skin or inside the nose, or if there was any period of unconsciousness following the injury. The fracture should be set soon after the injury, so do not delay seeking treatment.

Treatment In most instances, a technique involving manipulation and realignment of the support structures is often done in the emergency room or an outpatient clinic; sometimes the procedure may need to take place in the operating room where the tissues can be adequately decongested, anesthetized, and realigned. In agitated patients or in children or if the injuries are extensive, setting the fracture will probably be done under general anesthesia.

Prognosis Excellent if evaluated thoroughly and treated appropriately as soon as possible. Delay of treatment will make future relocation of the fractured tissues more difficult and may increase the risk of cosmetic or breathing abnormalities in the future.

RHINOPLASTY—THE NOSE JOB

Rhinoplasty is the name of the operation that corrects deformities of the external nose. A hump on the nose, a nose that is too long or wide, a nose that is deformed through injury or because of birth defects, or a nose that is obstructed and causes breathing and sinus problems and headaches are some of the external and internal conditions of the nose that can be corrected by plastic surgery. If rhinoplasty is being performed for cosmetic reasons, it is important to have realistic expectations of what the surgery can accomplish. The surgery can only transform the appearance of the nose; too often, people expect that the surgery will transform their lives.

In this procedure, the surgeon places incisions just inside the rim of the nostrils where they will not be visible. Occasionally, a very short incision across the skin between the nostrils may also be necessary. The soft tissues of the nose are then carefully lifted up, exposing the underlying cartilage and bone. The surgeon can then remove the offending structures and reshape the remaining bone and cartilage.

Rhinoplasty can be performed in conjunction with reconstruction of a deviated nasal septum to relieve obstruction inside the nose. In this procedure, called a septorhinoplasty, the surgeon removes the obstruction and reconstructs the interior of the nose through incisions inside the nose.

The procedures usually last 2 to 3 hours depending on the amount of work to be done. It can be performed under general anesthesia in the doctor's office or as outpatient surgery in the hospital. Following the surgery, a small splint is usually placed on the outside of the nose for several days and light packing may be necessary inside. Significant pain is rare but there is some mild discomfort easily controlled with medication.

Some swelling or bruising of the nose and eyelids can be expected; sometimes, the eyes will be bloodshot. The swelling usually subsides in a few days and the bruises generally clear in a couple of weeks. Significant improvement may be noted right away but it will take several weeks to months before the final result can be seen. ■

❖ EPISTAXIS (NOSEBLEED)

Symptoms (*What you may experience*) Passage of bright blood from the nose.

Signs and laboratory findings (*What the doctor looks for*) Dryness and chafing of the nasal mucous membranes (often); changes in blood pressure (sometimes); abnormalities in blood clotting (occasionally).

What is it? Nosebleeds can occur spontaneously or from trauma, with the flow of blood ranging in severity from minor to life-threatening. Drying of the nasal lining in the winter often contributes to minor spontaneous nosebleeds. Most episodes of epistaxis—the medical term for a nosebleed—occur because the person inserts a finger into the nostril and disrupts the rich network of blood vessels located in the nasal

POSTNASAL DRIP AND STUFFY NOSE

The lining of the respiratory passages, from the nose to the sinuses and bronchial tree, produces a protective mucus designed to coat and moisturize the lining and to trap inhaled particles of dust. In fact, the lining produces about 1 cup of mucus every day under normal conditions. When conditions depart from the norm—heavy pollen, allergic swelling, or pollution in the air causes irritation—the amount of mucus produced will increase. This extra amount of mucus generated in response to irritants in the air will create postnasal drip, which is nothing more than mucus flowing in greater-than-normal volume down the back of the throat.

Any condition that swells the interior of the nose can cause stuffiness—allergies and infection are common ones. Many people suffer intermittent or sometimes chronic episodes of sneezing, nasal stuffiness, and watery drainage that are unrelated to either of these causes. This form of nasal obstruction is known as vasomotor rhinitis, a condition that arises due to dilation of the blood vessels that supply the nasal interior. When these vessels dilate, they swell the lining of the nose, taking up more space within an already limited area. The mechanism of this dilation is through the autonomic nervous system (see Chapter 14 for more information). The vasomotor reaction can be precipitated by many factors including environmental irritants such as smoke, dust, smog, or lack of humidity; temperature changes, as in the drippy nose of cold weather; emotions such as anxiety, rage, guilt, or sexual arousal; hormonal changes in the body such as occur in pregnancy, diabetes, hypothyroidism, or menstrual cycling; food stuffs such as spices and peppers, which can cause a drippy nose and sneezing; beer or wine, which can cause stuffiness; and certain medications, particularly blood pressure medications such as reserpine or propranolol, both of which can cause nasal stuffiness.

Treatment of the disorder depends on its severity. No treatment may be appropriate in mild cases. Removal of known identifiable triggers, if possible, should be routine. Although sometimes antihistamine/decongestant (anti-allergy) medications help, in many cases they do not. Nasal steroid sprays such as beclomethasone may help dramatically—they are most effective against allergic nasal symptoms—and these may be worth trying if the symptoms are severe. Cromolyn sprays and allergen desensitizing injections—immunotherapy—offer no relief in this condition.

Complications of chronic vasomotor rhinitis include the development of polyps and asthma. People with chronic vasomotor rhinitis are more likely to develop these associated conditions than are people with allergic rhinitis. ∎

septum between the nostrils, near the front of the nose. Usually, simple home remedies can control nosebleeds arising in the anterior (forward) part of the nose without medical intervention, because the blood vessels in this area are much more accessible to treatment.

Occasionally, the bleeding arises from blood vessels in the back of the nose—a posterior nosebleed. The location of these blood vessels makes them especially difficult to view or to compress to stop the bleeding. Because some of the blood escaping from these posterior vessels drains down the throat instead of forward and out of the nose, the volume of blood lost is usually underestimated. Especially in the elderly (in whom this type of nosebleed is more common), the lack of significant quantities of visible blood may delay seeking medical help. Posterior nosebleeds are potentially life-threatening unless recognized and treated promptly.

What you can do In the winter months or in dry climates moisturizing the nasal membranes by the use of home humidifiers, a moisturizing ointment, or nasal saltwater sprays can maintain the moisture of the nasal membranes and minimize spontaneous bleeding.

Avoid vigorous nose blowing if you have recently had a nosebleed or are prone to them. Keep fingers out of the nose. In addition to causing nosebleeds, this habit is a common method for spreading bacteria and viruses.

If the bleeding appears to be from the front of the nose, apply pressure by pinching the nostrils between the fingers padded with a clean cloth or tissue. Sit as you apply the pressure; lying down will only increase the bleeding. Breathe through your mouth as you hold the pressure firmly for 5 minutes before releasing to check the effectiveness of the remedy. If bleeding persists, try a second application of 5 minutes pressure. Collect the blood in a bowl to more accurately gauge the amount lost.

When to call the doctor If pressure fails to stem the flow, seek medical attention. If you take blood-thinning medication or have blood-clotting abnormalities or significant hypertension, seek medical help right away. If the bleeding seems to be coming from the back of the nose, with significant quantities draining down the throat, seek medical attention right away.

Treatment Topical preparations to constrict the blood vessels—usually medicinal cocaine, epinephrine, or oxymetazoline—applied with a cotton-tipped applicator may stop the flow of persistent anterior nosebleeds. Afterward, the doctor may apply one of several topical substances to speed up clotting.

If topical remedies fail, the next measure is cautery—the use of heat, generated either chemically (using silver nitrate or

Monsel's solution) or electrically, to coagulate the blood and seal the point of bleeding. Because this method can be painful, it requires the use of a topical anesthetic beforehand.

When other measures fail, packing the nasal cavity with a sponge-like pack or lubricated gauze ribbon will control almost any anterior nosebleed.

Packing is almost always necessary for posterior nosebleeds. A rolled mass of lamb's wool or folded gauze or a balloon pack is pulled snugly against the back of the nasal chamber where it meets the throat. The posterior pack should only be put in place by a doctor or emergency specialist with appropriate experience. It must be secured with sturdy tapes through the nose and anchored to the front, lest it become loose and block the airway in sleep. For this and other reasons, application and use of posterior packs must be monitored in the hospital.

If packing fails, a dye-enhanced x-ray study with delivery of clotting materials or surgery may be necessary to halt the bleeding.

Prognosis Excellent for most anterior nosebleeds; good for posterior nosebleeds identified promptly and treated appropriately. A life-threatening loss of blood can occur in vigorous posterior nosebleeds if treatment is delayed.

❖ RHINOPHYMA

Symptoms and signs Enlarged, bulbous, red nose.

What is it? For many years, this disorder was thought to occur from heavy drinking. More careful research has shown that rhinophyma has no association whatsoever with alcohol consumption. It occurs more commonly in men and is an inflammatory condition of the skin of the nose, in which the skin thickens excessively, causing it to take on a distorted, bulbous shape. The reason for the change is unclear but the disorder poses no threat to breathing or general health. It is primarily a cosmetic problem.

When to call the doctor If the condition arises and progresses (which it usually does) and is troublesome to you, contact your doctor. It is not a health-threatening or serious condition.

Treatment In the early stages, the skin thickening may be controlled by treating the infection and reducing inflammation in the oil-producing glands of the skin with topical and oral antibiotics.

Surgery is the only effective remedy for advanced rhinophyma. Following removal of the excess tissue—which sometimes can be done using a local anesthetic but usually requires general anesthesia in the operating room—the nose heals in its normal, previous shape.

Prognosis Excellent.

❖ CANCERS OF THE NOSE AND PARANASAL SINUSES

Symptoms *(What you may experience)* Nasal airway obstruction; nosebleed; sometimes, numbness of portions of the face, bulging of one eye, pain in the forehead, eye, or facial bones.

Signs and laboratory findings *(What the doctor looks for)* A growth as revealed by nasal examination, x-ray studies, or CT scans; a biopsy of any visible growth may contain cancerous cells.

What is it? Most cancers of this area arise locally—from the superficial cells lining the cavities (squamous cell carcinoma) or from the glandular, mucus-producing tissues (adenocarcinoma). Occasionally a cancer found in the sinus or nose can represent a metastasis, or spreading, of cancer that originated elsewhere such as the breast, gastrointestinal tract, or reproductive or urinary tracts.

Hidden from view, cancers of the nose and sinuses may grow to fairly large size before causing symptoms. Growth of the tumor puts pressure on surrounding structures, causing symptoms that will vary depending on location. Long periods of undetected growth of these cancers can allow substantial growth before detection. For that reason, anyone who develops nasal obstruction, facial pain or numbness, and nosebleeds, should be fully evaluated for the possibility of cancer in these areas.

What you can do Do not attribute chronic nasal or sinus symptoms to colds or allergies without an evaluation.

When to call the doctor Sudden development of nasal stuffiness—unexplained by infection or allergy—should prompt a visit to the doctor, especially if the stuffiness is associated with nosebleeds or with numbness or pain in the face or eye.

Treatment Treatment is surgical, with removal of the cancer and a wide margin of surrounding tissue. Surgery coupled with radiation offers the only chance for improving an otherwise dismal survival picture.

High-voltage radiation may be useful in containing cancers considered inoperable.

The possibility of local recurrence of the cancer demands continued surveillance and may require repeat surgery. See Chapter 30 for more information on the diagnosis and treatment of cancer.

Prognosis Five-year survival rates for treatment of cancer of these areas varies but in general is less than 50 percent. Early detection is essential and may improve prognosis.

THE THROAT

In the back of the oral cavity where the nasal chamber joins it lies the throat. Medically termed the pharynx, the throat functions as the common pathway for the respiratory and gastrointestinal systems. To pass from mouth to esophagus and stomach, food and drink must traverse the throat as must air on its way from the nose or mouth to the lungs. The throat, then, is the main portal into the body. Nature has endowed the throat with a protective ring of immune defense tissues, which serve to apprehend and deactivate infectious invaders. The immune tissues congregate to form the two sets of tonsils—the palatine tonsils at the back of the throat (familiar to everyone) and the lingual tonsils seated at the base of the tongue—the pair of adenoids located far in the back of the nasal passageway at its junction with the throat, and bits of tonsil-like tissue scattered across the back wall of throat.

The throat ends at the level of the epiglottis, the flap-like cover that closes with swallowing to prevent food and liquid from entering the respiratory passages but opens to admit air. Here, the single cavity divides again into two passageways: the respiratory tree (becoming the larynx, then trachea, bronchi, and lungs) and the gastrointestinal tract (becoming the esophagus, then stomach and intestines).

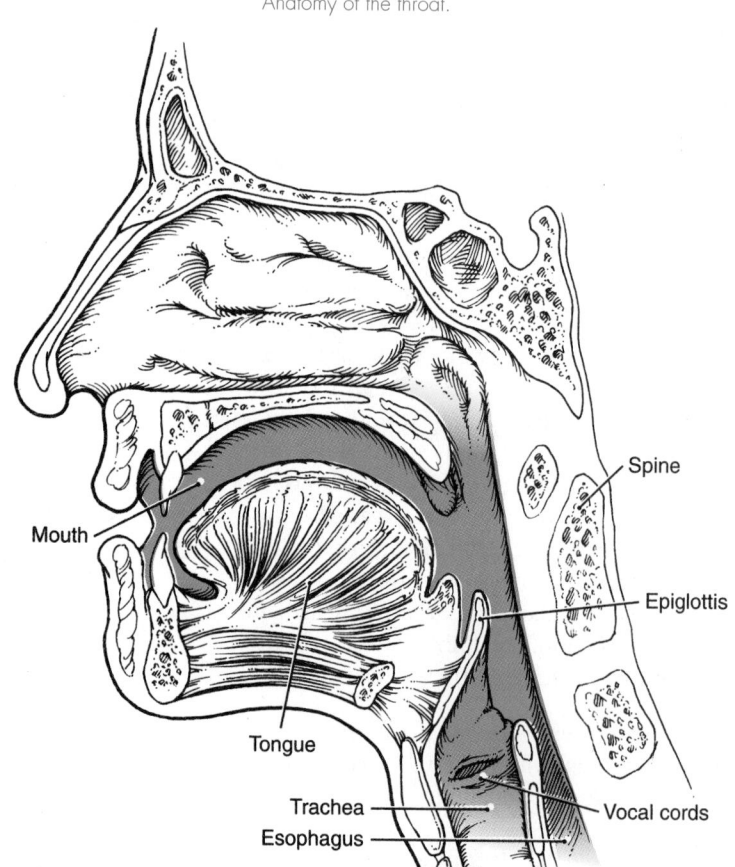

Anatomy of the throat.

Mouth

Spine

Epiglottis

Tongue

Trachea

Esophagus

Vocal cords

❖ PHARYNGITIS (SORE THROAT, STREP THROAT, AND TONSILLITIS)

Symptoms *(What you may experience)* Sore throat, difficulty or pain with swallowing, and swollen lymph nodes in the neck; often body aches, fever, headache, ear discomfort; diminished sense of well-being; rash (occasionally). (See page C-40.)

Signs and laboratory findings *(What the doctor looks for)* Red throat, swollen tonsils, pus or white patches on the tonsils (sometimes); or a causative agent identified by a screening test.

What is it? The tonsils and adenoids serve an immune protective function and are fashioned of tissue similar to lymph nodes. Positioned strategically at the entrance to the breathing and swallowing passages, they sample bacteria and viruses that enter the nose and mouth. These samplings result in a low-level infection of the tonsils designed to help the immune system form antibodies to defend against future infections. Sometimes the response is not localized to the tonsils but spreads to involve other organs, particularly the kidneys and the heart.

When such infections occur frequently, when the swelling of the tonsils or adenoids blocks the breathing passageways, or when swollen adenoids block the eustachian tubes resulting in frequent fluid accumulation or infection of the middle-ear space (which can impair hearing and consequently language development in children), the doctor may recommend removal of the tissue—a tonsillectomy and/or adenoidectomy also called a T & A (see Tonsillectomy, page 594). Once the child is about 3 years old, when the immune system has matured, removal of the tonsils poses no risk to immune function. (The tonsils and adenoids shrink throughout childhood; by puberty, the adenoids have almost disappeared.)

Infection by bacteria most often causes pharyngitis or tonsillitis, the most common bacterial cause being beta-hemolytic group A streptococcus. This infection—known commonly as strep throat—can be detected by either culturing the bacteria from samples of pus collected from the throat or by the rapid strep tests, now almost universally available in doctors' offices and emergency rooms (see The Importance of the Strep Test, above).

Viruses can also infect the throat but in general do not cause the formation of white patches and pus on the tonsils. There are exceptions, however. The most important viral throat infection is mononucleosis, caused by the Epstein-Barr virus (see Chapter 21). This infectious agent can be differentiated from bacterial causes by a simple rapid screen of a small blood sample. This test, called the monospot test or heterophile antibody test, can detect mononucleosis in

THE IMPORTANCE OF THE STREP TEST

Prior to the advent of effective antibiotics to eradicate them, infections with group A streptococcus could be deadly. Scarlet fever, which describes a strep infection with a florid red rash and a high fever, shot fear through the hearts of parents concerned about a sick child. Before effective treatments, strep infection was understood to be potentially deadly—predisposing to rheumatic fever and kidney disease. Antibiotics have changed that outlook but unless they are taken right away and continued for a sufficient length of time, the disease may not fully respond—and it is still potentially deadly. Untreated or under-treated strep infections still lead to rheumatic fever and acute inflammation of the kidney.

Even an experienced doctor has difficulty making a definitive identification of what organism is responsible for a fiery red throat or a pair of swollen tonsils covered in pus. Is it bacterial or viral? Are antibiotics necessary? Features that increase the likelihood that a sore throat is due to strep infection are the coexistence of fever, headache, and swollen lymph nodes in the neck. These criteria, however, are not foolproof.

The development of in-office rapid strep tests now allows doctors to make immediate and correct diagnoses and to begin treatment promptly. It is no longer necessary in many cases to wait 24 to 48 hours for bacteria to grow—or not grow—on an incubated culture plate before prescribing antibiotics. Keep in mind, however, that the rapid strep test can fail to detect a small percentage of strep infections. If a rapid strep test is negative but strep infection is likely, the culture test may be positive for strep 24 to 48 hours later. Prompt, correct treatment continued for at least 10 days will prevent the complications of strep infection. That makes the test worthwhile. ■

the doctor's office. However, 15 percent of cases of Epstein-Barr virus infection have a negative monospot test.

What you can do Gargle with warm salt water (1 to 2 tsp of table salt dissolved in 8 oz of warm water) to help relieve the discomfort.

The use of OTC anesthetic sprays or lozenges such as Cepastat or Nice can offer symptomatic relief.

When to call the doctor Failure of symptomatic treatment to resolve the problem within 1 or 2 days, the presence of fever for more than 24 hours, or the appearance of a rash should prompt a visit to the doctor.

Treatment Bacterial pharyngitis or tonsillitis requires a minimum of 10 days of antibiotic treatment to be certain that the bacteria have been completely eradicated. Even though fever and signs of illness may disappear in 2 or 3 days, do not fail to complete the course of medication.

TONSILLECTOMY

Removal of the tonsils and/or adenoids may be recommended for some children and occasionally for adults because of frequent infection, severe infection such as abscess formation, or breathing obstruction. Although not occurring as commonly as before the advent of antibiotics to treat tonsillitis, removal of the tonsils or adenoids still occurs almost 400,000 times per year in the United States alone.

The procedure is quite simple in children and slightly more difficult in adults. The doctor performs the surgery using a general anesthetic in the operating room. Prior to surgery (generally after midnight the night before), the patient should have nothing to eat or drink; this restriction applies to gum, mouthwashes, throat lozenges, toothpaste, and water. (If you take daily medication, notify your doctor in advance for specific instructions about whether to take your regular medication on the day of surgery.) Following the procedure, in most cases after 4 to 6 hours of recovery and observation, the patient can go home. Some doctors prefer to keep patients overnight to ascertain that all risk of postoperative bleeding has passed.

Following the surgery, several symptoms may occur including difficulty swallowing, vomiting, fever, throat pain, and ear pain. These unpleasant symptoms do not occur commonly and usually last only a few days. Occasionally bleeding may occur postoperatively; if it does, notify your doctor immediately.

Removal of the tonsils or adenoids does not guarantee that throat infections will no longer occur, though they usually occur much less frequently. ∎

For viral causes including mononucleosis no effective medical treatment—other than symptomatic—yet exists. Eradication of the virus is the job of the immune system; doing that job may take 7 to 10 days or longer.

For frequent episodes of infection, the doctor may recommend tonsillectomy or tonsillectomy and adenoidectomy.

Prognosis Excellent in most cases. Untreated or undertreated bacterial pharyngitis caused by strep (most often the consequence of stopping the medication) increases the risk of complications such as rheumatic fever or poststreptococcal nephritis (kidney disease).

❖ PERITONSILLAR ABSCESS

Symptoms *(What you may experience)* Severe throat pain, swelling of one tonsil, swollen lymph nodes in the neck; sometimes, fever, headache, ear discomfort.

Signs and laboratory findings *(What the doctor looks for)* Dramatic swelling and exquisite tenderness of one tonsil.

What is it? Sometimes bacterial infection extends deeper into the tissues around the tonsils, forming an expanding abscess cavity. Within the cavity, the bacteria continue to grow and multiply resulting in an increasing volume of pus contained within the cavity walls. The expanding volume of pus distends the surrounding structures and can be seen as an asymmetric bulging of the area around the affected tonsil.

A peritonsillar abscess requires immediate attention by a doctor since the abscess can extend further within the soft tissues of the head and neck, resulting in potentially serious complications.

When to call the doctor If you develop a sore throat and upon self-examination note asymmetric swelling inside the throat, seek medical help right away.

Treatment Drainage of the abscess is the only effective treatment. Antibiotics will not reach sufficient levels within the abscess cavity to eradicate the infection. The doctor can sometimes perform the lancing procedure—which is much like lancing a boil to drain pus—in the office but occasionally will recommend hospitalization and drainage in the operating room.

Following the drainage, a course of antibiotics to eradicate the bacteria usually will be recommended.

Prognosis Excellent if promptly diagnosed and appropriately treated.

❖ EPIGLOTTITIS

Symptoms *(What you may experience)* Sore throat; fever; difficult or painful swallowing; hoarseness. In infants and young children: whistling or crowing sounds with breathing; shortness of breath and progressive difficulty with breathing; refusal of food or water; sometimes drooling of saliva (refusal to swallow saliva).

Signs and laboratory findings

(What the doctor looks for) Diagnosis is based on x-ray studies. There is a danger that physical examination may trigger sudden and potentially fatal closing of the throat. During the exam a person with epiglottitis often assumes a posture of leaning forward and stretching the neck out to make breathing easier. Once the doctor has made sure that the airway will stay open, a physical exam may be done under anesthesia. The swollen, red epiglottis will be visible.

What is it?

A special form of rapidly progressive inflammation of the throat. The epiglottis is the flap-like cartilage at the base of the tongue that acts as a valve to protect the larynx (voice box) and trachea (windpipe). Normally, it remains in an open (forward) position to permit the passage of air into the larynx and trachea. During swallowing it closes the laryngeal inlet to prevent the passage of food and liquid into the airway, directing it instead to the esophagus.

The epiglottis may become infected, usually by the common bacterial invaders of the throat and respiratory tree (most prominently *Haemophilus influenzae*). Infection inflames and swells the epiglottis, limiting its motion. In young children (usually between 2 and 7 years old, in whom these structures are smaller) and occasionally in older children as well as teens and adults, the swelling can become pronounced enough to block the airway entirely, creating a life-threatening situation. When this occurs, immediate emergency treatment at the hospital is necessary to insert an endotracheal tube (to bypass the obstructing epiglottis) or tracheotomy tube to secure an open passageway for air. It is unusual for swelling of the epiglottis to cause pronounced respiratory distress in an adult but the seriousness of this disorder requires that the diagnosis be considered in all age groups.

Although the disease can occur in anyone, it most commonly afflicts children between ages 2 and 5, occurring more often in females than in males and in whites more often than in other races.

What you can do

See Pharyngitis (Sore Throat, Strep Throat, and Tonsillitis), page 592.

When to call the doctor

A sore throat accompanied by even the slightest degree of restricted breathing should prompt a visit to the doctor. In children, progressive hoarseness or refusal to swallow food, drink, or saliva should prompt you to seek immediate medical evaluation. The doctor may order x-ray studies of the neck to determine how swollen the epiglottis has become.

Treatment

Antibiotics to eradicate the infection are the mainstay of treatment. Severe difficulty in breathing requires immediate measures to preserve or restore the airway. Sometimes this can mean an emergency tracheostomy (opening of the trachea) in order to insert a tube through the neck directly into the windpipe. Hospitalization for at least a few days usually follows this procedure. The tube is removed when the infection is under control and the swelling of the epiglottis subsides. The opening will usually heal completely and seal the airway within days.

Prognosis

Prompt and appropriate treatment should result in complete recovery within 2 weeks. If an endotracheal tube has been placed for breathing, hoarseness may persist for a few weeks.

❖ QUINCKE'S ANGINA

Symptoms

(What you may experience) Painful, raw throat; difficulty swallowing; muffled speech.

Signs and laboratory findings

(What the doctor looks for) Dramatic swelling of the uvula (see below); a red throat (usually).

What is it?

Occasionally in cases of viral pharyngitis there is sudden and tremendous swelling of the uvula (the pendulum of tissue that hangs down in the center of the back of the throat). In some cases the normally unobtrusive uvula may swell sufficiently to cause gagging, muffling of speech, and a sense of needing to lean forward to keep the breathing passage open. The condition is usually accompanied by an extremely sore, raw throat.

What you can do

Lean forward to reduce the tendency to gag. Sip cold water to help reduce the swelling.

When to call the doctor See the doctor as soon as possible.

Treatment Administration of medication such as injections of epinephrine (adrenaline) to reduce swelling may be beneficial.

Anesthetic/analgesic (pain-relieving) mouth sprays may help.

Prognosis Excellent. As is the case with most viral illnesses of the throat and respiratory tree, the immune system will respond and contain the infection in about 7 to 10 days. The dramatic swelling usually only persists for a day or two.

❖ CHRONIC SORE THROAT

Symptoms *(What you may experience)* Frequently recurrent or persistent scratchiness or burning pain in the throat; persistent discomfort in swallowing (this symptom is nonspecific and may occur in several other conditions).

Signs and laboratory findings *(What the doctor looks for)* Often no specific signs; sometimes general redness of the oropharynx (back of the throat).

What is it? Persistent sore throat can occur for a variety of reasons. For example, breathing through the mouth because of nasal stuffiness and repeated throat-clearing due to chronic postnasal drip from allergies can leave the throat irritated and raw (see Chapter 29 for more information about allergies). More commonly, however, the persistent burning or scratchy throat results from reflux, the backing up of stomach acid into the esophagus and throat. Although the stomach lining is suitably equipped to handle the acid in the gastric juices, the esophagus and throat are not. People who suffer gastroesophageal reflux may experience burning or irritation of the throat from caustic stomach acid that flows into these vulnerable areas upon lying down or bending over.

The chronic sore throat of reflux is not associated with symptoms of inflammation such as fever, fatigue, or malaise that accompany infectious sore throats.

What you can do If the sore throat is due to reflux, see Gastroesophageal Reflux Disease, page 969, for detailed information on ways to relieve gastroesophageal reflux. Weight loss and avoidance of eating for 3 to 4 hours prior to bedtime are important.

When to call the doctor If the symptoms persist for longer than a few weeks despite OTC remedies, contact your doctor; rarely, other more serious conditions such as cancer could be the cause.

Treatment If OTC remedies fail, the doctor may recommend either higher (prescription-strength) doses of these or similar medications or Prilosec, a medication developed specifically to combat gastroesophageal reflux (see Gastroesophageal Reflux Disease, page 969).

Prognosis Excellent once the underlying cause has been appropriately treated.

❖ CANCER OF THE THROAT (PHARYNX AND LARYNX)

Symptoms *(What you may experience)* Painful or difficult swallowing; hoarseness; swelling of the neck or lymph nodes; pain radiating to the upper neck, jaw, or ear; sense of something sticking in the throat.

Signs and laboratory findings *(What the doctor looks for)* Abnormal growth visible by examination with a laryngoscope.

What is it? Cancers of the throat may be roughly divided into those that involve the throat (swallowing chamber of the throat) and those that involve the larynx (speaking chamber of the throat). The two chambers share a common wall and drain into a common network of lymph nodes. Cancers of the larynx and the pharynx share many of the same risk factors and often cause similar symptoms. Throat cancer is most often a cancer of the larynx that begins in one area and that spreads to involve the pharynx. Because of these many shared features, cancers of the larynx and the pharynx will be discussed together here.

These cancers usually develop after age 60 and are about 10 times more common in men than they are in women. Lifestyle plays an important role in their occurrence: Those who smoke and those who drink alcohol excessively develop cancer of the throat far more often that those who do not.

SWOLLEN LYMPH NODES IN THE NECK

Lymph nodes (glands) are small, round or bean-shaped structures designed to filter lymph, trap foreign invaders carried therein, and to produce certain types of infection-fighting white blood cells (see Chapter 22 for more information about lymph nodes and the immune system). Swollen lymph nodes can indicate the presence of infection, or in some cases cancer, in a region.

When viruses, bacteria, or fungi infect the body, their presence may cause activity in the lymph nodes guarding that area. Lymph nodes that perform this protective function for the ears, nose, sinuses, throat, and skin of the scalp and face lie in chains down either side of the front of the neck, down either side of the back of the neck, and in front of and behind each ear.

Infection usually causes dramatic swelling and tenderness of multiple lymph nodes in a group. For example, mononucleosis and strep throat will usually cause tenderness and swelling in the clusters of lymph nodes on either side of the neck. Lymph node swelling from infectious causes usually appears suddenly along with the illness; the tenderness usually abates as other symptoms diminish but the swelling may linger for several weeks following recovery. In some cases, the small remnant of a formerly swollen node may persist indefinitely. This is particularly true in children, who may have frequent enough infections of the nose, throat, and ears to keep the lymph nodes in this region actively inflamed most of the time.

Swollen lymph nodes can also occur with spread of a cancer in that area and for this reason should never be ignored. A cancerous lymph node usually appears as a single, firm, painlessly swollen gland that gradually increases in size and may become fixed by adhering to the surrounding tissues. Its appearance will bear no relationship to a recent infection; it will not wax and wane.

Discovery of a swollen lymph node should always prompt a visit to the doctor. In the majority of cases the swelling will prove to be of infectious origin but only a thorough evaluation can determine the cause. ■

The onset of these cancers is often marked by chronic, unexplained hoarseness or persistent difficulty or pain with swallowing. The hoarseness develops if the cancer either involves the vocal cords themselves or damages the nerve that supplies the vocal cords, impairing cord movement. Occasionally a chronic, irritating, dry cough may occur from irritation of the nerve that supplies sensation to the larynx.

When to call the doctor If you develop hoarseness or difficulty or pain with swallowing that lasts for more than 2 weeks, contact your doctor.

Treatment Caught early, cancers of the throat can often be cured by radiation therapy or limited surgery (removal of only a part of a vocal cord, for example). Cancers that have metastasized or spread to other areas of the throat may require extensive surgery that completely removes the larynx (called a laryngectomy) and/or large sections of the pharynx. Removal of the larynx will require a period of retraining to learn how to speak. Methods include using voice aids or a device that shunts a stream of air into the upper esophagus and throat to produce "esophageal speech." Because the pharynx conveys food, drink, and saliva to the esophagus and stomach, removal of the pharynx necessitates surgical reconstruction of the connection, usually by placement of a tubed segment of tissue with either its original ("native") blood supply or a newly connected set of blood vessels. See Chapter 30 for more information on the diagnosis and treatment of cancer.

Prognosis Caught early and treated appropriately, cancer of the throat is frequently curable; once it has spread to adjacent or distant areas, the chance of cure is reduced. Smoking cessation is critical to remaining disease-free after treatment.

Larynx and Vocal Cords

The larynx lies in the neck at the point where the throat separates into the airway and the esophagus; it is in line with the trachea below and opens to the pharynx above. Although its most well known function concerns the production of sound by the vocal cords, the larynx also serves the important role of protecting the lower airways. The epiglottis closes during swallowing to prevent aspiration, the entrance of food and fluid into the lungs. The muscles of the larynx also assist in clearing the lungs by generating the forces needed to cough. To generate sufficient pressure to clear fluid or mucus from the airway, the larynx must close tightly in order to temporarily trap and then release an air column.

The larynx contains several structures made of cartilage, suspended in sling-like fashion by slender strap muscles and ten-

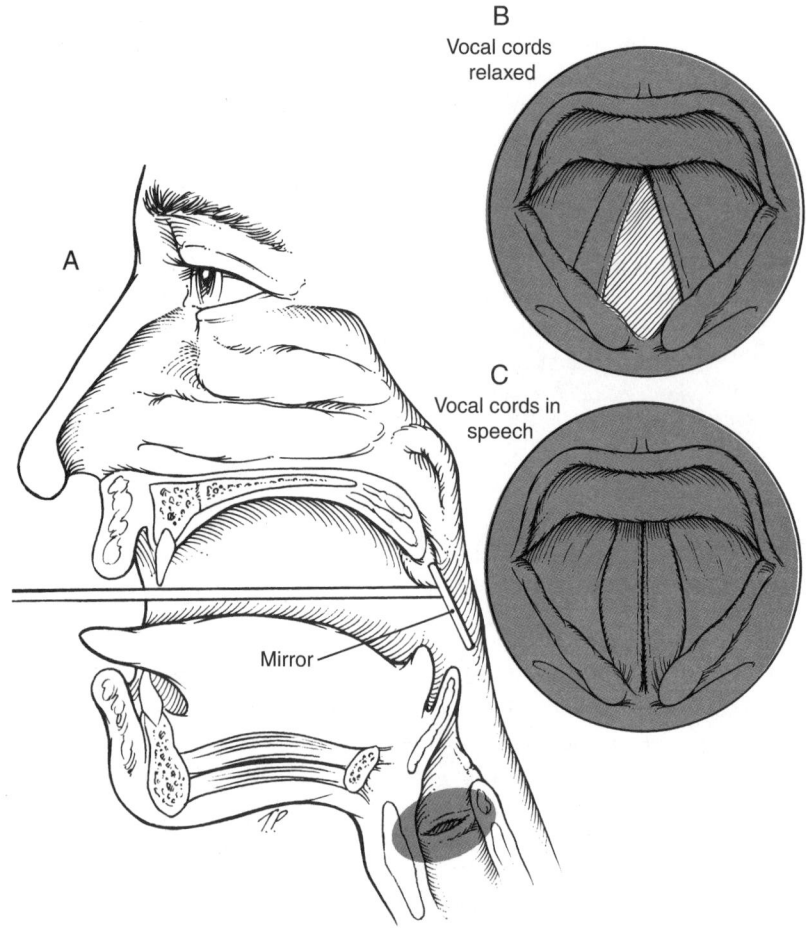

B
Vocal cords
relaxed

C
Vocal cords in
speech

A

Mirror

(A) The vocal cords can be viewed by your doctor with a mirror and light source, a procedure known as indirect laryngoscopy. (B & C) The vocal cords convert air coming from the lungs into sound by vibrating. Muscles control the vibration of the vocal cords by changing their length and tension, determining the quality of the sound produced (phonation).

dons. The internal chamber of the larynx forms the inlet to the airway and is lined with membranes. The largest of the cartilage structures is the thyroid cartilage that protrudes to form the Adam's apple.

The vocal cords are a pair of strong bands of elastic tissue covered with a thin mucous membrane, that span the windpipe from front to back. A small protected airspace lies above them to ensure their free vibration as air from the lungs passes across them; it is by this means that voiced sounds are produced. The quality, pitch, and intensity (or loudness) produced depends on the speed of their vibration and the resonance within the upper air chambers: the throat, oral cavity, and the air spaces within the skull. The human capacity to speak, however, hinges on a complex and coordinated

interplay between the vocal cords, the laryngeal muscles, the highly flexible tongue, and the changing shape of the oral cavity generated by movement of the jaws, teeth, and lips.

❖ ACUTE LARYNGITIS

Symptoms *(What you may experience)* Hoarseness; raw throat; the sensation of needing to clear the throat; associated upper respiratory infection (often).

Signs and laboratory findings *(What the doctor looks for)* Often no specific signs; sometimes general redness of the throat and vocal cords as demonstrated by inspection with a laryngoscope or mirror.

What is it? Laryngitis implies inflammation or infection of the vocal cords. When the cords swell, they do not vibrate normally, so the quality of sound they produce changes. With minimal swelling, the hoarseness may be mild, but as the swelling increases the voice may temporarily be reduced to little more than a harsh whisper.

Laryngitis often occurs in association with viral infections such as a cold or influenza, with the hoarseness often appearing as the sore throat begins to resolve. These simple viral cases usually clear up in a few days. Sometimes, however, the infecting agent is bacterial, with laryngitis preceding, accompanying, or following a lower respiratory tree infection such as bronchitis or pneumonia.

What you can do Warm saltwater gargles can offer symptomatic relief during the phase of throat soreness. Moisturizing the air with a humidifier may also help. You can run a hot shower for several minutes and inhale the moisturized air. Allow your vocal cords to rest by talking as little as possible. Whispering is not helpful as it requires just as much vocal cord activity.

When to call the doctor If hoarseness is associated with persistent fever, difficulty breathing, or a cough productive of colored phlegm or blood, contact your doctor.

Treatment Viral laryngitis rarely requires medical treatment. To determine the presence of bacterial infection the doctor usually will take a throat swab for culture and identification in the laboratory. Following identification of the bacterium, treatment usually consists of antibiotics to eradicate the infection.

Prognosis Acute laryngitis is usually a brief, self-limiting infection that resolves completely within a few days to 1 week.

❖ CHRONIC LARYNGITIS

Symptoms *(What you may experience)* Persistent hoarseness without other symptoms of illness.

Signs and laboratory findings *(What the doctor looks for)* Thickening or inflammation of the vocal cords on inspection with a laryngoscope or mirror.

What is it? Chronic vocal cord irritation can occur for a variety of reasons such as heavy drinking or smoking, chronic postnasal drip, or reflux of stomach acid into the back of the throat during sleep. Exposure in the workplace to irritating chemicals, dust, or other airborne pollutants can also contribute to persistent hoarseness. Chronic irritation from these and other sources leads to vocal cord thickening, which limits vibration of the cords, leading to alteration of voice quality.

Chronic trauma from voice overuse or allergies can also contribute to persistent hoarseness (see Voice Abuse and Hoarseness, page 600).

What you can do Stop smoking and reduce or eliminate alcohol intake since these substances can promote chronic laryngitis. Reduce or eliminate workplace exposure to dust, chemicals, and airborne pollutants by wearing a protective respirator (a surgical mask will provide no protection). Gastroesophageal reflux disease may contribute to the problem.

When to call the doctor Persistent hoarseness always merits investigation by a doctor to be certain of its cause. Although usually the cause is relatively benign and correctable, it could be more serious. For example, damage to the nerve that causes the vocal cords to move can alter voice quality. That damage could represent invasion of the nerve by a cancer and it is for this reason that persistent hoarseness should never

ACUTE VOCAL CORD SWELLING (ANAPHYLAXIS)

In some people, response to an allergy-provoking substance can be sudden, severe, and life-threatening. Allergens commonly causing such an exaggerated response include bee stings, peanuts, nuts or seeds, shrimp or other shellfish, or medication such as penicillin, aspirin, or certain antihypertensive medications

The reaction usually begins with swelling of the lips, eyes, and a sensation of the throat closing. Hives usually appear as irregularly shaped, raised, itchy patches on the skin. Breathing becomes difficult and respiration takes on a strident crowing sound as swelling narrows the windpipe and closes the vocal cords. This syndrome—called anaphylaxis—is life-threatening and can prove fatal in a matter of minutes in the absence of medical intervention. *Immediate medical treatment is necessary.*

People who have experienced this response to any allergen should always keep an emergency epinephrine injection kit—commonly called a bee sting kit—with them at all times (see page 1341 for more information). Having a ready dose of epinephrine at hand can literally mean the difference between life and death. ■

be ignored (see Cancer of the Larynx, **page 601**).

Treatment Treatment of the underlying cause—reflux, postnasal drip, or allergy—will usually resolve the hoarseness. See specific disorders and their treatments for more information.

Prognosis Very good in most cases. Chronic hoarseness related to recurrent laryngeal nerve trauma or cancer usually does not fully resolve.

❖ VOCAL CORD NODULES, POLYPS, AND ULCERS

Symptoms *(What you may experience)* Breathy, hoarse voice; in the case of ulcers, mild pain with swallowing or speaking.

Signs and laboratory findings *(What the doctor looks for)* An irregularity of the vocal cord surface such as nodular swelling,

VOICE ABUSE AND HOARSENESS

Most disorders of the voice result in a change in the quality of its sound—usually a harshness, huskiness, or hoarseness. Misuse of the voice is often responsible. A normal voice depends on the proper control of air flow of an amount sufficient to establish the right degree of vibration of the vocal cords without overly constricting the muscles. Sometimes in order to develop a louder or more powerful voice—the typical example is a child predisposed to shouting such as a cheerleader or avid sports fan—the person contracts the laryngeal muscles to increase the pressure of the air as it enters the larynx, much like crimping a water hose to create a more forceful jet steam. Creating pressure by this method can lead to the development of vocal cord irritation, nodules, or polyps, all of which can further alter voice quality.

In many cases, learning to use the abdominal muscles rather than squeezing the larynx to produce a louder or more powerful voice will solve the problem. A qualified speech pathologist can assist in voice retraining, which begins with identification of the areas of misuse and involves designing appropriate rehabilitation to correct them. Behavioral modification is important in controlling childhood behaviors that are likely to be associated with voice abuse. ∎

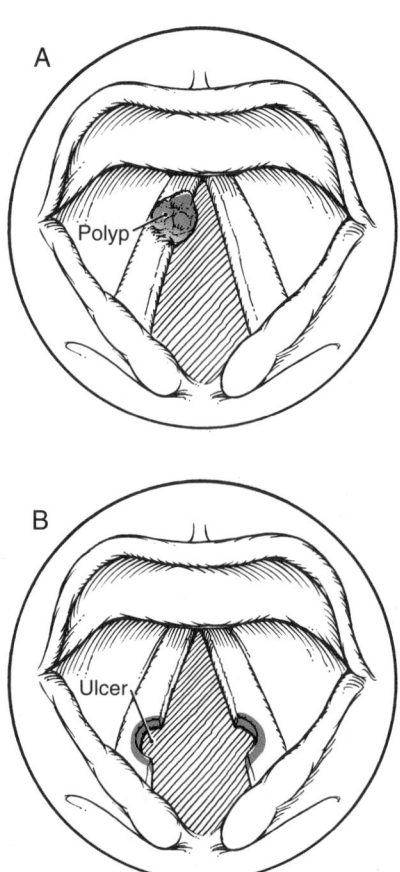

(A) Vocal cord polyps are growths typically caused by overuse of your voice through prolonged singing or yelling. Polyps are often removed to distinguish them from a cancerous growth. Voice training can help prevent their recurrence. (B) Vocal cord ulcers are areas of superficial damage caused by overuse of your voice or regurgitation of gastric juices, including acid, into the esophagus. Ulcers on the vocal cords can cause discomfort when swallowing and hoarseness.

a polypoid mass, or an ulcerated pit or crater as revealed by examination with a laryngoscope or mirror.

What is it? The vocal cords are vulnerable to damage from chronic abuse, whether from chronic irritation by cigarette smoke or from overuse or misuse of the voice. Nodules develop at sites of chronic irritation much in the same way that calluses develop on hands or feet exposed to constant friction or pressure. Occupations such as professional singer, auctioneer, member of the clergy, salesperson, telemarketer, or teacher predispose to the development of nodules because of a heavy reliance on the voice. Inappropriate use of the voice can also lead to damage of the vocal cords. Voice abuse occurs in children who scream often, in cheerleaders, and in sports fans who shout excessively.

Ulcerations can form on the vocal cords with voice abuse and with overexposure to acid from the stomach. This condition develops in people who suffer from gastric acid reflux (chronic heartburn) and in people who purge by vomiting such as those with bulimia. Damage to the vocal cords can also occur accidentally during intubation (putting a breathing tube into the larynx) in preparation for anesthetic delivery for surgery.

What you can do Rest your voice for 4 to 6 weeks. Do not scream or sing and keep even quiet talking to a minimum. Whispering is not advised and may even be harmful. Avoid irritants such as cigarette smoke or chemical or particulate aerosols.

When to call the doctor If hoarseness persists, see your doctor to evaluate the problem. If it is associated with significant discomfort in swallowing or speaking, see your doctor right away.

Treatment In most cases, nodules, polyps, or ulcers respond to voice rest and retraining by a speech pathologist. If gastric acid reflux seems to be a contributing cause, administration of a gastric acid blocker such as Tagamet, Axid, Zantac, or Pepcid may resolve the problem (see page 969).

In stubborn cases, laser surgery to remove the growth is necessary.

Prognosis Very good once the underlying cause is identified and properly treated.

❖ VOCAL CORD PARALYSIS

Symptoms *(What you may experience)* Breathy or hoarse voice without apparent cause.

Signs and laboratory findings *(What the doctor looks for)* Immobility of the vocal cord on laryngoscopic examination.

What is it? The vocal cords are designed to move, to tense and relax in response to the coordinated pull of the muscles of the larynx that are attached to them. When something interrupts the neural activation of the vocal cord, the affected vocal cord will be paralyzed, which alters the quality of sound produced. Most cases of paralysis of the vocal cords result from damage to the recurrent laryngeal nerve (the nerve responsible for vocal cord movement); this condition most commonly occurs following surgery to the thyroid because of the nerve's proximity to the gland and the arteries that feed it. Another frequent cause is viral infection leading to temporary paralysis. In rare instances, paralysis of the left vocal cord can result from invasion of the nerve by spreading cancers of the thyroid gland, chest, or lung; and aneurysm should always be suspected as a possibility in cases of isolated left vocal cord paralysis.

Immobility of the cords can also be a consequence of arthritis in the small cricoarytenoid cartilages to which muscles that operate the cords are attached.

Voice quality may be surprisingly good. However, paralysis of both cords will usually cause audible respirations, with a strident crowing sound produced as breath moves in and out through the narrowed space.

When to call the doctor The sudden or gradual development of a hoarse, breathy quality to the voice should prompt a visit to the doctor for evaluation of the cause. *Warning: If the onset of difficult or noisy breathing is sudden, seek medical help immediately.*

REHABILITATION OF A PARALYZED VOCAL CORD

Paralysis of the vocal cord alters voice quality and breathing patterns and may hamper swallowing and cause choking. Because the paralyzed cord is usually frozen in a position at the side of the larynx, procedures designed to move it toward the center of the opening are integral to improving the quality of the voice.

In most instances, the affected vocal cord is injected with a stable substance that will make it bulge toward the center of the laryngeal opening. In the past, the preferred substance was Teflon although it has an unfavorable tendency to migrate into surrounding tissues and cause an exaggerated immune system response called a foreign body reaction. Recent work by Johns Hopkins surgeons Charles Cummings and Paul Flint suggests that better alternatives to Teflon may exist. Implants with hydroxyapatite (a bone-like material) incite a less dramatic immune response, appear to resist migration to surrounding tissues, and may stimulate stabilizing bone growth. Advances such as these in implant technology and materials offer greater hope and better rehabilitation outcome for people who suffer vocal cord paralysis. ■

Treatment In paralysis of a single vocal cord, voice quality can sometimes be improved by injection of substances into the cord to medialize it (bring it closer to the other vocal cord). Surgical procedures to alter the shape of the immobile vocal cord (laryngoplasty) may also improve voice quality.

Sudden closure of the cords that compromises breathing requires emergency tracheotomy (opening a passage for air directly through the neck into the windpipe). See Rehabilitation of a Paralyzed Vocal Cord, above.

Prognosis Good for a certain degree of improvement.

❖ CANCER OF THE LARYNX

Symptoms *(What you may experience)* Persistent hoarseness, pain when swallowing or speaking, ear pain (referred pain), coughing up of blood; weight loss (later).

SPEAKING AGAIN AFTER LARYNGECTOMY

Removal of the larynx means the loss of the natural speaking mechanism but does not mean the end of being able to speak. A combination of surgical and rehabilitative techniques can restore speech in almost every case.

Most surgical methods involve creating a passageway to direct air first brought into the lungs through a tracheostomy stoma, back up from the lungs and into an artificial larynx that may be a hand-held device pressed against the neck, inserted into the mouth, or a device that is fitted into the stoma called a tracheoaesophageal prosthesis or a voice prosthesis. This artificial larynx sends vibrated air into the pharynx that can then be molded by mouth shape and tongue to produce more natural speech.

Many people are able to learn another method, termed esophageal speech, in which air is taken into the mouth and compressed into the esophagus. The compressed air is then released, somewhat as in a burp, sending vibrating air into the pharynx where the lips, tongue, and oral cavity mold it into spoken sounds.

People who have had recent laryngectomies often find it motivating and helpful to visit with others who have learned to speak with an artificial larynx or mastered esophageal speech. ∎

Signs and laboratory findings *(What the doctor looks for)* Enlarged (usually painless) lymph nodes in the neck; cancerous cells confirmed by laryngoscopy and biopsy.

What is it? Cancer of the larynx arises most often between ages 50 and 70, predominantly in heavy smokers. Alcohol consumption appears to enhance the risk of laryngeal cancer from smoking but by itself may be a less potent laryngeal carcinogen. The most common type of laryngeal cancer is squamous cell carcinoma arising from the superficial layer of the lining.

The earliest symptom is usually persistent hoarseness that lasts more than 2 to 3 weeks and develops in the absence of infection or other apparent explanation. Subsequently other symptoms will usually appear including sometimes significant pain when speaking or swallowing and coughing up of bloody phlegm. Weight loss and the painless enlargement of lymph nodes in the neck are later, more ominous signs that the cancer may have spread to distant sites.

What you can do If you smoke, stop. See Chapter 4 for information on how to quit smoking.

When to call the doctor Hoarseness that persists longer than 2 weeks should always be evaluated by a doctor.

Treatment Early squamous cell cancers respond well to radiation or limited surgical procedures. In more advanced stages of the disease or if radiation fails, treatment requires partial or total laryngectomy (removal of all or part of the larynx). See Chapter 30 for more information on cancer diagnosis and treatment.

Following surgery, rehabilitation can restore useful speech to most people.

Prognosis Detected early and treated promptly, cure rates exceed 85 to 90 percent. As is so often the case, delay of diagnosis worsens the prognosis; advanced lesions are associated with low cure rates.

The Tongue, Lips, and Oral Cavity

The lips and oral cavity form the gateway to the gastrointestinal tract; digestion begins here and the sense of taste resides here. Our ability to speak depends in great measure on highly flexible and maneuverable tongue and lips. Trauma or disease affecting these structures can therefore have an impact on two critical human activities: eating and speaking. The oral cavity is a relatively common site for manifestations of systemic disease.

The lips, a pair of fleshy folds that surround the mouth, have hairless, more deeply pigmented skin on the outside, a layer of highly mobile muscles in the middle, and the slick mucous membrane lining of the mouth on the inside. The sharply demarcated junction of the richer, pigmented skin of the lip with the surrounding facial skin is called the vermilion border.

The oral cavity is roofed by the palate—the hard (bony) palate in the front and the soft palate in the back. The entire cavity is

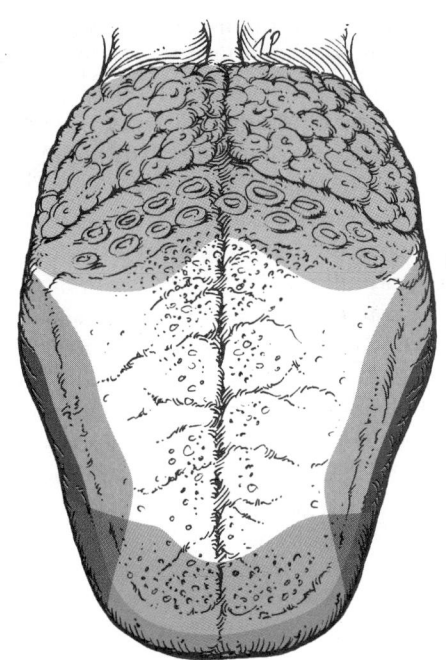

The tongue is covered with projections called papillae that contain special taste receptors called "taste buds." Taste buds are specialized: those in the front of the tongue sense sweet and salty foods, sour foods are sensed on the sides, and bitter foods are sensed toward the back of the tongue.

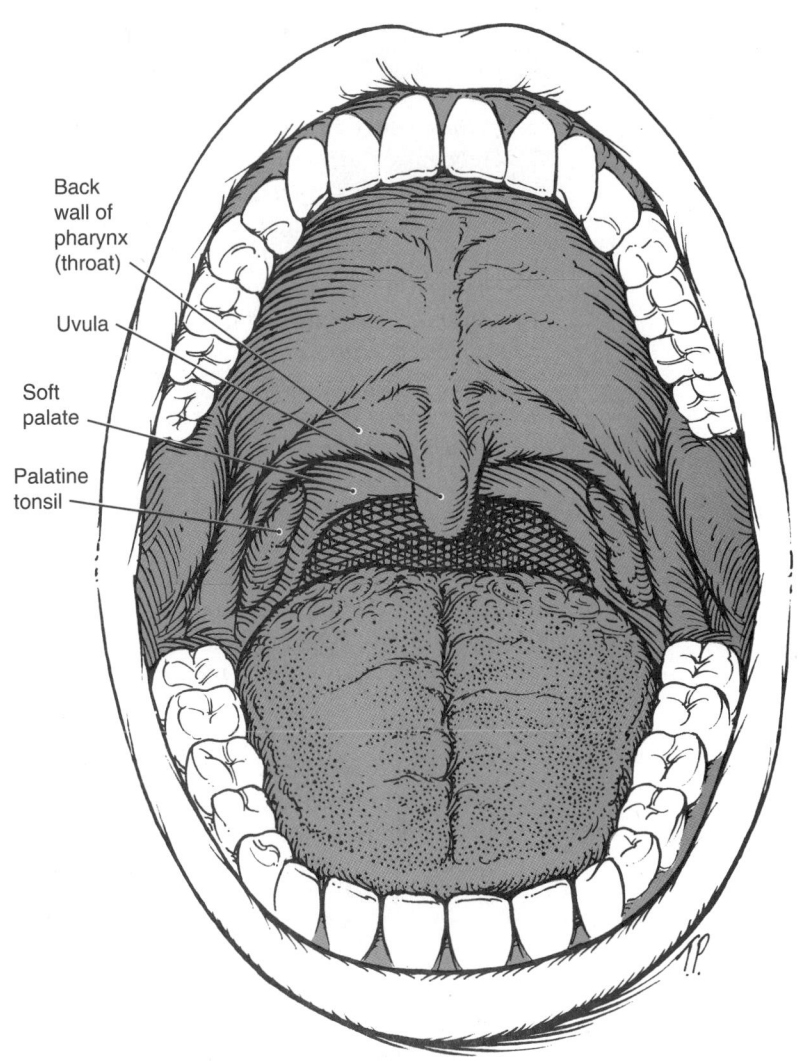

Back wall of pharynx (throat)

Uvula

Soft palate

Palatine tonsil

Normal anatomy of the oral cavity.

lined by a slick mucous membrane. The cheeks form the side walls of the oral cavity and within them lie the large parotid (salivary) glands.

The entire oral cavity is richly supplied with blood vessels—so richly supplied, in fact, that some types of medication can be absorbed through the mouth lining directly into the bloodstream.

❖ ORAL HERPES SIMPLEX (COLD SORES)

Symptoms (*What you may experience*) Tingling and tightness of the lip or drawing (a gathering sensation within the lip); later, painful clusters of small water blisters on the lip; occasionally associated with fatigue and malaise. (See page C-40.)

Signs and laboratory findings (*What the doctor looks for*) Clusters of blisters on a red base on or near the lips; laboratory testing may identify the causative virus.

What is it? Herpes simplex virus is a member of the herpes virus family, the same fam-

ily of viruses that causes chicken pox and shingles. These viruses have an affinity for peripheral nerve roots and ascend via the nerve to its origin, where they rest dormant, until reactivated. In the case of herpes simplex infection of the lips, the nerve supplying this area originates in a ganglion in the brain. Under certain stimuli—such as ultraviolet light, fever, or impairment of the immune system—the dormant virus is reactivated. It travels down the nerve covering and erupts in a subsequent infection commonly described as cold sores or fever blisters.

The reactivation is often heralded by a sensation of tingling or drawing in the area previously infected. Sufferers learn to recognize this prodromal sensation as a cold sore or fever blister coming on. Viruses—potentially infectious—begin to shed from the area at this time and continue to do so until the blisters that subsequently form have crusted over and begun to heal.

What you can do The moment that you recognize the prodromal sensation, begin to treat the virus as instructed by your doctor. Since ultraviolet light can stimulate a recurrence, protect your lips with strong (30 to 45 spf) ultraviolet sunblock for lips when outdoors for extended periods.

Each eruption sheds potentially infectious herpes viruses. For this reason, wash your hands thoroughly after applying medicated cream or touching the sores in order to prevent the spread of the virus to the nose or eyes or to other people.

When to call the doctor If you develop an outbreak for the first time, see the doctor immediately. Quick, aggressive treatment may sometimes prevent recurrences.

Treatment Acyclovir (Zovirax) tablets and ointment have been shown to abort or reduce viral shedding and speed healing of herpes simplex outbreaks. Initial outbreaks should be treated for 10 days. Recurrences should be treated for 4 to 5 days.

Prognosis The disorder usually recurs periodically but outbreaks can be controlled with medication in many instances. In immunocompromised people, such as those with acquired immunodeficiency syndrome (AIDS), infection can spread to the central nervous system (brain), a condition that carries a less optimistic prognosis. See Chapter 21 for more information on infectious diseases.

❖ APHTHOUS STOMATITIS (CANKER SORES OR MOUTH ULCERS)

Symptoms (*What you may experience*) Recurrent painful ulcers inside the mouth.

Signs and laboratory findings (*What the doctor looks for*) Cream-colored to yellowish ulcer craters on the lining of the lips or cheeks.

What is it? These painful, small (usually 1 to 2 mm) and round ulcers can develop on the mucosal lining of the cheeks and lips, on the tongue, or on the base of the gums. They occur quite commonly in healthy people and, apart from the discomfort they cause, they pose no risk to health. They are sometimes single, sometimes multiple, and usually recurrent. Multiple discrete ulcers are scattered across the lining of the mouth, not clustered in groups. (Clustering more typically occurs with herpes-related ulcers; the large groups coalesce to form a single large ulcer.) Aphthous ulcers appear as yellowish ulcer craters rimmed with a red halo. It is not known what causes canker sores. They sometimes occur after an injury or irritation to the mouth; stress, dietary deficiencies, and hormonal fluctuation may also be factors. The painful stage lasts 3 to 10 days but up to 3 weeks may pass before the ulcer disappears completely.

What you can do Topical analgesic medications such as Anbesol may help to relieve the discomfort.

When to call the doctor Persistent or large ulcers can occur as a part of other, more significant, disorders. Among these are inflammatory bowel disease, herpes virus infection, drug allergies, arthritic disorders, inflammatory skin disorders, and cancer. If the ulcers persist longer than 3 weeks or are larger than $1/2$ in., see your doctor, particularly if you are or have been a smoker.

Treatment Treatment is mainly symptomatic. Topical application of steroid cream or ointment may help. To adhere inside the mouth, medicated cream or ointment should be mixed in a special dental base called Orabase.

If there is doubt about the identification of the ulcers, the doctor may recommend a biopsy. A pathologist can examine the specimen under the microscope and identify the exact type of ulcer.

Prognosis The disorder is self-limiting and the ulcers usually heal without scarring or long-term problems; the disorder tends to recur.

❖ CHEILOSIS

Symptoms (*What you may experience*) Painful redness, cracking, and sometimes weeping from the corners of the mouth.

Signs and laboratory findings (*What the doctor looks for*) Specific nutritional deficiencies as demonstrated on blood testing;

bacterial or yeast infection as revealed by microscopic examination or culture of fluid from the area.

What is it? Painful cracking of the corners of the mouth—sometimes on one side only but usually involving both—that occurs when there is a loss of facial support. Such loss commonly occurs in the elderly, in whom laxity of tissues coupled with ill-fitting dentures or the absence of teeth or other forms of dental support may keep the angles of the mouth moist from saliva. The disorder also occurs in people who habitually lick the corners of the mouth.

Moisture where skin presses against skin provides a fertile environment for the growth of *Candida* (skin yeast) which will increase the redness, irritation, and cracking.

Especially vulnerable are people with underlying health disorders such as anemia, neutropenia (low levels of certain types of white blood cells), diabetes mellitus, and AIDS. Taking excessive amounts of supplemental vitamin A can also cause cracking at the corners of the mouth.

What you can do If you wear dentures, check to see that they fit properly. Toothless people should obtain properly fitting dentures. Keep the corners of the mouth protected from saliva with topical application of a small amount of mild, soothing ointment; those made for diaper changes in babies are usually mild and protective.

When to call the doctor If the condition persists despite topical remedies and dental fitting, contact the doctor.

Treatment *Candida* infection associated with cheilosis requires topical or systemic antifungal medication. Recurrent or persistent cases call for a search for underlying conditions that compromise the local immune system and allow the fungus to grow.

Prognosis Once the underlying cause—whether due to facial architecture or a systemic disease—is determined and appropriately treated, this condition usually can be remedied.

❖ *CANDIDA* (THRUSH)

Symptoms *(What you may experience)* Whitish, elevated patches on the tongue and lining of the mouth; irritation or pain in the mouth. (See page C-40.)

Signs and laboratory findings *(What the doctor looks for)* White patches atop the fragile, bleeding oral cavity lining.

What is it? The yeast fungus, *Candida albicans*, lives in as many as two-thirds of healthy mouths as a normal inhabitant. Most people are exposed to this organism at an early age and carry the yeast in the gastrointestinal tract from that point forward. Usually the organism causes no problems but in the presence of certain predisposing conditions it can overgrow and cause disease. (It is the same organism that causes vaginal yeast infections.) The yeast overgrowth in the mouth—termed thrush—appears as painful, irregularly shaped, whitish patches on the tongue or lining of the mouth that can be wiped away easily with a tongue depressor or piece of gauze. Below the patch, the tongue or lining of the mouth will be red, irritated, and will bleed easily. The doctor can examine the yeast by collecting a specimen of the patch and placing it under a microscope.

The environment of the oral cavity plays a role in the development of thrush; dry mouth, smoking, and wearing dentures can make the mouth vulnerable to *Candida* overgrowth. Also, the use of broad-spectrum antibiotics wipes out the bacterial competitors in the gastrointestinal tract, allowing unrestricted growth of yeast and the development of thrush. When normal immune function is impaired—as it is in people receiving cancer chemotherapy or radiation or in people with AIDS or who have had organ transplants—there is a predisposition to the development of thrush. Systemic diseases, especially diabetes mellitus, make the overgrowth more likely as does the long-term use of corticosteroid medication associated with severe inflammatory arthritis or autoimmune diseases.

What you can do Rinsing the mouth with a solution of one part water and one part hydrogen peroxide may provide some symptomatic relief. Swish the mixture in the mouth for 1 minute—it will foam—then spit it out. Do not swallow the rinse.

If you smoke, stop. See Chapter 4 for information on how to stop smoking.

COATED OR DISCOLORED TONGUE

Sometimes the tongue becomes coated or discolored and this change can be alarming. Usually the causes are simple and, for the most part, benign. Here are the major causes.

- *Black or brown tongue.* Overgrowth of the normal "friendly" bacteria that inhabit the mouth can sometimes accumulate in the cracks and buds of the surface of the tongue giving it a brown-streaked appearance. Tobacco smoking can worsen this phenomenon. Use of bismuth-containing medications such as Pepto-Bismol can cause the tongue to appear black. The condition is most easily remedied by simply brushing the tongue twice daily with a toothbrush or scraping it with a tongue scraper available in some pharmacies, followed by rinsing the mouth with an antiseptic mouthwash.

- *Strawberry tongue.* The tongue appears red (although it sometimes appears coated with a whitish film) with enlarged red papillae scattered across its surface that resemble the seeds on a strawberry. Although the condition is not a symptom of illness, it is often seen in streptococcal pharyngitis. If an illness, a sore throat, and fever are present, see your doctor for testing to pinpoint strep infection and to receive treatment with antibiotics if it is present.

- *Hairy tongue.* Rarely, the papillae of the tongue grow excessively, making the surface appear to be covered with fur. It may occur in conjunction with antibiotic therapy, dry mouth, dehydration with fever, excessive use of certain mouthwashes, or lack of attention to oral hygiene. It is not serious and responds to brushing the tongue twice daily with a soft toothbrush.

- *Geographic tongue.* Irregularly shaped patches of smooth tissue (absent the papillae) will intermingle with the surface of the tongue to create an appearance similar to a map. The appearance may change from day to day or may persist; in some cases, the tongue may burn (see Glossitis and Glossodynia [Painful Tongue], this page). The cause is poorly understood and no effective treatment has emerged. Avoiding irritants such as tobacco, alcohol, or spicy food may give symptomatic relief. Allergies may be responsible in some cases (see Chapter 29 for more information on allergies). ■

When to call the doctor If the condition persists despite conservative home treatment or if you think that you may be predisposed to thrush, contact your doctor as soon as possible.

Treatment Antifungal medication such as fluconazole, ketoconazole, clotrimazole, or nystatin can contain the yeast. These medications can be administered as tablets, mouth rinses, or dissolving lozenges (called troches). For denture wearers, application of nystatin powder to the dentures three or four times daily for several weeks may help to heal the tender tissues beneath the plates.

Addressing predisposing factors will make treating thrush easier.

Prognosis Excellent for individual outbreaks; the disorder tends to recur in people with underlying systemic disorders.

❖ GLOSSITIS AND GLOSSODYNIA (PAINFUL TONGUE)

Symptoms and signs Painful, red, smooth-surfaced tongue; difficulty chewing, swallowing, or speaking due to tongue pain.

What is it? In the disorder called glossitis, the tongue becomes red and inflamed, losing its papillae (the rough-looking "buds") and taking on a smooth appearance. This condition sometimes occurs in response to nutritional deficiencies (especially of niacin, riboflavin, and vitamin E) but also may occur with dehydration or as a reaction to medication, irritants, or pollutants. Although glossitis usually causes no pain, a related disorder termed glossodynia does. Glossodynia, a condition marked by burning pain in the tongue, is often associated with glossitis. It can occur in conjunction with diabetes, dry mouth, or thrush and is also associated with tobacco smoke and the use of certain medications such as diuretics (fluid pills).

What you can do If you smoke, stop. See Chapter 4 for information on how to stop smoking.

When to call the doctor Although glossodynia is a painful condition, it is not a serious threat to health. If the condition causes

HALITOSIS (BAD BREATH)

The mouth is normally self-cleaning courtesy of the production of adequate amounts of saliva. As a result, breath should normally be unremarkable. Breath may sometimes take on an unpleasant odor, which may relate to nothing more than having eaten pungent foods (such as onions or garlic whose volatile oils enter the bloodstream and are exhaled through the lungs), smoked tobacco, or consumed alcoholic beverages. However, halitosis could signal an underlying medical disorder.

- *Foul-smelling breath.* Poor dental hygiene can cause foul-smelling breath that results from the decomposition of trapped food particles or pockets of infection around teeth (periodontitis). Growth of bacteria on the posterior portion of the tongue is a major cause of bad breath. Bad breath can result from infection in the nasal sinuses or even deeper in the respiratory tract (the bronchi or lung). Fetid- or putrid-smelling breath sometimes occurs when there is poor stomach movement, and belching brings forth the odors of fermenting stomach contents. Lack of sufficient saliva to cleanse the mouth (dry mouth) can also cause bad breath.

- *Fishy odor.* A fishy odor may accompany severe liver disorders such as liver failure; it is also the result of an inherited genetic disorder.

- *Fruity breath.* A scent similar to nail polish remover may occur in diabetes mellitus and can be an important sign of developing ketoacidosis, a potentially serious problem for an adult or child with type I diabetes mellitus.

- *Urine-like odor.* A urine-like odor sometimes occurs in kidney failure.

In most cases, halitosis can be eliminated with daily oral hygiene: brushing after each meal, flossing between teeth regularly, brushing the tongue, and keeping the teeth in a good state of repair. Drinking plenty of water to keep the mouth moist (especially important for people with dry mouth) can also help. Recent studies have pointed to the role the tongue may play in the development of bad breath in some healthy individuals. The tongue becomes coated with bacteria that ferment proteins producing odorous gases. The solution is to scrape the tongue as far back as you can go using a tongue scraper (which can be found in some pharmacies) or a bent metal spoon.

In those cases resulting from an underlying medical disorder, treatment of the disorder will help to resolve the bad breath. ∎

significant pain or persists longer than a few weeks, contact your doctor.

Treatment Treatment of the underlying disorder will help to resolve the problem. Symptomatic relief can sometimes be obtained with anesthetic mouth rinses such as lidocaine (Xylocaine Viscous 2%).

Prognosis Good once the underlying cause is identified and appropriately treated.

❖ TRAUMA TO THE LIPS AND TONGUE

Symptoms and signs Bruising, swelling, or a cut on the lips or tongue.

What is it? Trauma to the lips, oral cavity, and tongue occurs commonly. The lips are especially vulnerable to trauma by virtue of their soft, fleshy consistency and exposed location. A blow to the face (from a fist during a fight or from a hard surface during a fall) can crush the lip between the hard surface from without and the teeth from within. The person's own tooth can lacerate the inside of the lip and cause a through-and-through puncture laceration that penetrates the covering skin. Many tongue lacerations occur as a result of people biting their own tongues due to blows or falls.

Lacerations to the inside of the mouth can bleed profusely because of the extensive network of blood vessels supplying the oral cavity, but this rich blood supply also results in quick healing—often within just a few days.

Lacerations that cross the vermilion border of the lip require meticulous closure to ensure that the architecture of this distinctive boundary is preserved. Even a small irregularity in the border will be permanently noticeable.

What you can do Cleanse the traumatized skin surfaces with mild soapy water and a soft clean cloth. Rinse the inside of the mouth with cool water or half-strength hydrogen peroxide (one part hydrogen peroxide and one part water); do not be alarmed that the bacteria normally in the mouth cause the peroxide to foam. Do not swallow the peroxide rinse.

Apply a cold compress to a swollen or bruised lip. Apply pressure with a clean cloth for at least 5 minutes to stop bleeding. Holding crushed ice in the mouth (or wrapping ice in a small square of clean gauze held inside the cheek) may help to minimize swelling, bleeding, and discomfort.

When to call the doctor Seek medical care if bleeding cannot be controlled with pressure and a cold compress, if the trauma punctures the lip through and through, if a laceration crosses the vermilion border, or if infection (symptoms include redness, tenderness, and drainage of pus) develops following the injury.

If a tooth is loose, contact a dentist (see If a Tooth is Knocked Out or Broken, page 617).

Treatment Puncture lacerations that extend to the outside skin may only require closure of the skin outside but often at least a single stitch may be necessary inside the mouth.

Small puncture lacerations to the tongue usually heal without incident if kept clean with antiseptic or half-strength hydrogen peroxide mouth rinses. Although larger lacerations may require sutures, because the tongue is so mobile in talking and chewing they may not remain securely in place for long.

Damage involving the vermilion border requires closure by an experienced surgeon to obtain the best cosmetic result.

Prognosis Excellent. The rich blood supply encourages rapid healing, often with minimal scarring, following trauma to the oral cavity, lips, or tongue.

❖ TRENCH MOUTH

Symptoms and signs Painful swelling, bleeding, and shaggy coating on gums; foul breath; fever; swollen lymph nodes in the neck.

What is it? Trench mouth—also called Vincent's angina or necrotizing ulcerative gingivitis—is an inflammatory and infectious disease of the gums, usually caused by the combination of two bacterial species. It occurs in people debilitated by stress or underlying disease. It is most common in teens and young adults under stress and is not contagious.

The infection swells the gums and they bleed easily and profusely when brushed or touched. Loss of adequate oxygenation to the gum tissue may cause necrosis (tissue death) and sloughing or shedding of dead tissue as a grayish membrane-like coating. Fever and putrid breath may accompany the disorder along with swelling of the regional lymph nodes in the neck.

What you can do A warm mouth rinse made with equal parts of warm water and hydrogen peroxide may help.

When to call the doctor As soon as such a condition develops, contact your dentist for evaluation.

Treatment Antibiotics—usually penicillin in those who can take it—may help to eradicate the bacteria. But it is also important to rest, eat a balanced diet, and avoid mouth irritants such as spicy foods and smoking. Sometimes dental curettage (scraping away the dead tissue) may be necessary.

Prognosis Excellent with appropriate treatment and time to allow healing.

❖ ORAL LICHEN PLANUS

Symptoms (*What you may experience*) Sore, dry mouth; metallic taste; painful ulcerated areas (rarely). (See page C-40.)

Signs and laboratory findings (*What the doctor looks for*) Pale bumps and a lacy white network on the cheeks and tongue; shiny, slightly raised red patches on the cheeks and tongue.

What is it? This disorder, which can occur in any adult, affects women of middle age more than it does any other group. It develops for uncertain reasons; in some cases it appears to be triggered by emotional stress while other times it seems to occur as a reaction to medication or in association with cigarette smoking. Lichen planus can also involve the skin (see Chapter 28 for information on skin disorders) and although about half of the time the two forms occur together, they may also occur separately.

When to call the doctor The appearance of this condition should prompt a visit to your doctor or dentist, especially if you are a smoker or you have begun a new medication prior to its onset.

Treatment If the condition appears to be related to the use of a new medication, treatment consists of stopping the offending drug. Smokers should make an effort to quit. Occasionally the doctor may prescribe pain medication for discomfort sometimes associated with oral lichen planus. Usually, no treatment is required.

Prognosis Good.

❖ ORAL CAVITY CANCERS

Symptoms *(What you may experience)* A lump or discolored patch or ulcer in the mouth or on the tongue. The patch or ulcer is acutely sore on exposure to acidic liquids such as citrus juice.

Signs and laboratory findings *(What the doctor looks for)* Swollen lymph nodes in the neck (sometimes); cancerous cells confirmed by a biopsy.

What is it? Cancers of the oral cavity typically occur on the floor of the mouth or the sides of the tongue, although they can occur on the cheeks, gums, or roof of the mouth. Cancers of the lip (see page 610) and throat (see page 596) are also oral cancers. Most of the cancers that occur in this area arise from the squamous cells—the most superficial layer of the lining.

In the United States, oral cancers occur almost twice as commonly in men than in women and account for about 2 percent of all cancer deaths. Over 90 percent of these cancers are traced to two major lifestyle risk factors, tobacco and alcohol, which probably account for the gender disparity. The risk of oral cancer is almost 30 times higher among smokers. Because smokeless tobacco products such as chewing tobacco cause more direct, locally toxic effects on the lining of the mouth, the risk associated with using these products is even higher. Alcohol, while not as potent a risk factor as tobacco, contributes to the occurrence of oral cancer and potentiates the harmful effect of smoking.

Since this cancer may not be readily apparent without specific inspection of the floor of the mouth and the sides and bottom of the tongue, it may go undetected and spread to adjacent or distant sites before discovery.

What you can do If you smoke or use smokeless tobacco, you should stop now (see The Dangers of Smokeless Tobacco, page 610).

If you are or have been a tobacco user, perform regular self-examinations—both

LEUKOPLAKIA (WHITE PATCHES IN THE MOUTH)

Derived from the Greek words *leukos* (white) and *plax* (plate), leukoplakia describes any white patch in the oral cavity that simple rubbing will not remove. Most often the patches are small but can reach several centimeters (an inch or more) in size. Usually they form in response to chronic irritation—such as from poorly fitting dentures or smokeless tobacco—much like a callous forms on the feet or hands. Although most leukoplakia are benign, in as many as 6 percent of cases they may represent a precancerous or early cancerous lesion and should never be ignored.

In most cases the patches cause no discomfort and are usually discovered by a dentist, doctor, or oral hygienist during a routine examination or occasionally by the person with the leukoplakia when something else has drawn attention to the lining of the mouth. Depending on the size and appearance of the lesion, the doctor or dentist may suggest watching the area closely for a period of time or may recommend biopsy to rule out cancerous cells.

Because the risk for oral cancer increases with the use of smokeless tobacco, cigarette smoking, and excessive alcohol intake, people in these groups should regularly inspect the entire oral cavity and report any white patches or unusual areas to their doctors or dentists. See Oral Cavity Cancers, this page, and The Dangers of Smokeless Tobacco, page 610, for more information. ■

visually and by feeling with your fingers—of the entire oral cavity. See Leukoplakia (White Patches in the Mouth), above, for more information on precancerous lesions.

When to call the doctor If you discover a thickened or discolored area in your mouth or on your tongue, contact your doctor as soon as possible.

Treatment The doctor will usually recommend biopsy of the area, under local anesthesia, to confirm the diagnosis.

Early surgical removal of the cancer offers the best rate of cure, particularly for tumors found early. Early detection will limit the extent of surgical resection. Once the tumor is large or has spread to adjacent

THE DANGERS OF SMOKELESS TOBACCO

Smokeless tobacco has been viewed—especially by young men—as a safe alternative to cigarette smoking or as a way to emulate their favorite sports stars or country western entertainers. However, nothing could be further from the truth. Here are the facts:

- A can of smokeless tobacco (snuff) delivers as much nicotine as do three packs of cigarettes.

- Smokeless tobacco users become dependent on continued use because nicotine, an addictive drug, gives them a "buzz."

- When the supply runs out or the users try to quit, they may become moody, experience headaches, and have trouble sleeping and concentrating.

- Some users become so addicted that they keep a pinch of snuff in place all day long and during the night when they sleep.

- Many users find that when they want to quit, they cannot. Smokeless tobacco is harder to give up than are cigarettes.

- Sore, receding gums and tobacco stains on the teeth result from using smokeless tobacco.

- Receding gums leave the delicate root exposed and more vulnerable to decay.

- Long-term users have a 50 percent greater risk of developing oral cancer than nonusers because the tobacco contains cancer-causing agents such as nitrosamines.

- Cancer of the tongue and oral cavity can spread to the neck, where treatment will involve disfiguring surgery to remove portions of the face, jaw, and neck.

- Advanced cancers caused by smokeless tobacco may fail to respond to surgery. ■

or distant areas, radiation therapy may be recommended in addition to surgery.

Depending on the extent of removal, a period of rehabilitation to restore the ability to speak and chew may be necessary. Plastic and reconstructive surgery to restore a more normal appearance may also be required. See Chapter 30 for more information on the diagnosis and treatment of cancer.

Prognosis With early detection (before spread) and appropriate treatment, 79 percent of people are still alive at 5 years. Once distant spread has occurred, the prognosis falls to 19 percent; this shows the importance of finding and treating such cancers early.

❖ CANCER OF THE LIP

Symptoms (*What you may experience*) Nonhealing sore or scaling patch on the lip; a persistent pale bump with a depressed center resembling a crater.

Signs and laboratory findings (*What the doctor looks for*) Cancerous cells confirmed by a biopsy.

What is it? Cancers on the lip usually arise from one of two types of skin cells: those from the most superficial layer, the squamous cell cancers, and those from the deeper layer, the basal cell cancers.

The most important risk factor for cancers involving the lip is chronic exposure to solar radiation—especially in fair-skinned people who burn easily. Lip cancer most commonly affects the lower lip which, by virtue of its position, receives the most sun; this association holds especially true for the squamous cell type. And as with other cancers of the mouth, tobacco use—in this case, particularly cigar smoking—increases the risk for developing lip cancer.

What you can do If you spend significant time outdoors, either at work or play, protect your lips with frequent application of a strong (spf 20 or higher) sunblock for lips.

If you use tobacco, stop. See Chapter 4 for more information on how to stop smoking.

When to call the doctor Any sore or unusual bump on the lips that persists longer than a few weeks should prompt a visit to the doctor.

Treatment Removal of cancer, if detected early, can be accomplished by conventional surgery, cutting away the tumor and a wedge-shaped margin around it and then bringing the two sides of the gap back together to heal. If the cancer has become large, its removal by this method can distort the shape of the lip. In these cases, to effect a more pleasant cosmetic result, the doctor may recommend a special surgery called Mohs' microsurgery. This procedure employs magnification and concurrent microscopic evaluation that allow the surgeon to remove very thin layers of the tumor in succession until all microscopic evidence of cancer is gone. Mohs' microsurgery offers the advantage of less disruption of the lip architecture.

Very small basal cell cancers, which tend to be less aggressive, can sometimes be removed by cautery (burning away) if they do not cross the vermilion border that demarcates the more darkly pigmented portion of the lip from the skin of the face.

Prognosis Very good if detected early and treated appropriately.

THE SALIVARY GLANDS

The glands that produce saliva primarily reside in the cheeks and in the floor of the mouth. The largest and best known pair of these glands—the parotid glands—are embedded high on the cheeks, near the ear. Their ducts open into the mouth on the cheek near the upper rear molar teeth. Other, smaller glands lie in the tissues of the floor of the mouth, opening in numerous bumps on either side of the tongue on the floor of the mouth.

These glands produce saliva. Saliva plays an important role in the digestion of food, moistening it to make swallowing easier and containing enzymes that begin the initial work of breaking down the food during chewing. Saliva also functions to cleanse the mouth, tongue, and teeth.

❖ VIRAL INFECTIONS (MUMPS)

Symptoms *(What you may experience)* Chipmunk-like swelling of one or both cheeks; often accompanied by runny nose, watery eyes, fever, malaise, and possibly hearing loss.

Signs and laboratory findings *(What the doctor looks for)* Redness and swelling of Stensen's duct (the opening of the parotid gland inside the mouth); tenderness of the gland to touch or to the administration of substances that stimulate the flow of saliva.

What is it? Infection of the parotid gland by the mumps virus once occurred commonly in children. The advent of effective vaccines to prevent it has reduced significantly the incidence of this disease. In susceptible children or adults, viral infection of the gland causes dramatic swelling, creating a facial appearance reminiscent of a chipmunk with fully stuffed cheek pouches. The gland sits in the cheek on either side, extending to the area just in front of the ear (where the swelling may be most dramatic). The swelling and discomfort usually last 7 to 10 days.

Transmission of the virus to other susceptible people occurs through direct contact with infected saliva and respiratory

Three sets of salivary glands (parotid, sublingual, and submandibular) secrete saliva into the mouth through ducts.

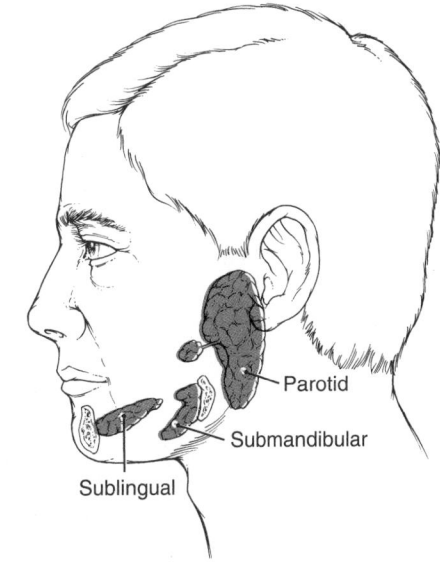

secretions during the first 3 to 5 days of the illness. A case of mumps infection confers immunity against future infection with the virus. Vaccination against the virus is quite effective.

The swelling of the parotid gland can compress nerves in the area and in rare instances can spread to cause permanent hearing impairment. Fortunately, in most cases hearing is affected on only one side. The virus can progress beyond the salivary glands to infect other organs such as the ovaries or breasts in females or the testicles in males. Mumps orchitis (testicular infection) occurs in as many as 20 to 30 percent of males infected with the mumps virus, resulting not only in considerable discomfort but in an increased risk for testicular cancer. In as many as 10 percent of cases, the mumps virus can spread to the coverings of the brain, causing meningitis.

What you can do Susceptible individuals should ensure immunity to the disease by taking the mumps vaccine. MMR (a combination of measles, mumps, and rubella vaccines) is now a part of the standard recommended series of pediatric injections. Ideally the first MMR should be given at age 15 months and the second at the start of school (between the ages of 4 and 6) but it is safe to take at any time—except during pregnancy.

Once infected with the mumps virus, rest and take ibuprofen or acetaminophen to relieve fever and body aches. Avoid sour foods or beverages; the sour taste causes excessive production of saliva and can cause pain when the infected gland and its ducts constrict to expel the saliva.

When to call the doctor The appearance of swelling in the parotid glands should prompt a visit to the doctor to determine the cause. The development of testicular pain or severe headache with mumps infection also merits evaluation by the doctor right away.

Treatment Only symptoms can be treated as there is no effective medication to eradicate the virus.

Prognosis In the absence of complications, recovery from mumps is complete and uneventful.

❖ BACTERIAL INFECTION OF THE SALIVARY GLAND (SIALADENITIS)

Symptoms *(What you may experience)* A tender, red lump in the cheek or under the chin; drainage of pus from the duct of a salivary gland; fever; malaise.

Signs and laboratory findings *(What the doctor looks for)* Pus expelled from the duct opening of a salivary gland on the application of pressure.

What is it? The salivary glands contain a complex and interconnecting meshwork of ducts continually flushed with saliva. Sialadenitis, or bacterial infection of a salivary gland, usually occurs when the flow of saliva is obstructed or reduced for some reason. In people debilitated by illness, people recovering from surgery, or in certain elderly people, dehydration can reduce salivary production, allowing infection to develop. Development of an obstructive stone or kink in the duct can also diminish normal flow and predispose to infection (see Salivary Duct Stones, page 613).

Bacterial invasion alerts the immune system, which moves huge numbers of white blood cells to the area to contain the infection; the result is pus—the debris of the struggle between the bacteria and the immune defenses. As the pus develops, its increasing volume expands the gland, causing pain and tense swelling; the increased pressure forces some of the pus out through the duct of the gland and into the mouth—the hallmark diagnostic sign of this disorder. Some bacteria may escape the confines of the gland and pass into and infect the blood, causing high fever, chills, and system-wide illness.

What you can do Drink plenty of fluid to maintain adequate hydration; this is especially important following surgery or during illness or in an elderly person.

Warm packs and massage of the gland can help relieve some of the discomfort.

When to call the doctor The development of tender, red swelling of a salivary gland, particularly in those people at higher risk for developing infection, should prompt a call to the doctor right away.

Treatment Adequate hydration, by intravenous administration of fluid if necessary, is the first step. Eradication with antibiotics of the responsible bacteria (*Haemophilus influenzae*, *Staphylococcus aureus*, or *Streptococcus pneumoniae*) should begin immediately. Typical antibiotic choices include cephalosporins or penicillin.

Once fluid balance has been restored, the use of substances such as sour candies that stimulate saliva production may be recommended if they do not cause discomfort to the person.

If aggressive medical therapy does not resolve the fever and bring the infection under control within 24 to 48 hours, surgery to open and drain the gland may be required.

Prognosis Very good with prompt diagnosis and appropriate and aggressive medical or surgical therapy.

❖ SALIVARY DUCT STONES

Symptoms (*What you may experience*) Sudden swelling in the cheek or under the chin; pain when eating sour foods; sudden drainage of pus or saliva into the mouth (occasionally).

Signs and laboratory findings (*What the doctor looks for*) Tense swelling of one salivary gland on examination with fingers; occasionally, isolated firmness (the stone) on examination with fingers.

What is it? The salivary glands constantly produce a flow of saliva that flushes through their interconnecting meshwork of ducts and empties into the mouth. When the volume of saliva or the rate of its flow decreases, solids in the saliva may coalesce or crystallize to form solid bits of gravel (sometimes even sizable stones) that can obstruct entirely the flow through the duct. Once obstruction is complete, swelling of the duct behind the stone can occur suddenly. Salivation that occurs during a meal can balloon the duct to the size of a walnut or larger in a matter of minutes. If the stone does not obstruct the duct totally, the back up of saliva will slowly drain away and the swelling will subside; with the next meal or sour-tasting food, it may return.

Persistent entrapment of saliva in the duct behind the stone can lead to bacterial infection in the gland. See Bacterial Infection of the Salivary Gland (Sialadenitis), page 612.

What you can do Apply cool compresses to the area and gently massage the swollen area to help drain the accumulated saliva. Drink plenty of fluids to ensure that normal levels of saliva are maintained. Avoid sour foods if they promote sudden swelling and discomfort.

When to call the doctor Sudden swelling of one of the salivary glands should prompt a visit to the doctor for evaluation.

Treatment Usually the doctor can gently manipulate the stone within the duct, working it toward and through the opening. Occasionally, with large stones, surgery is used to open the affected duct and extract the stone.

Prognosis Excellent once the stone is removed.

❖ CANCERS AND BENIGN LUMPS

Symptoms (*What you may experience*) Slowly enlarging lump in the cheek, under the chin, or on the tongue or roof of the mouth; occasionally there is pain in the lump.

Signs and laboratory findings (*What the doctor looks for*) Palpable lump in a salivary gland; a fine needle biopsy is used to test for cancerous cells in the gland and magnetic resonance imaging (MRI) may be used to reveal a tumor in a salivary gland.

What is it? Tumors in the salivary glands occur rarely, representing only about 3 percent of all tumors. About 80 percent arise in the largest salivary gland, the parotid gland, with the remainder divided among the smaller glands under the chin and scattered throughout the mouth on the roof and tongue. Of those arising in the parotid, about 80 percent are benign; of those in the glands under the chin, about half are benign; of those under the tongue, about 20 percent are benign.

Malignant tumors occur much more rarely, usually arising between the ages of 50 and 60. Pain can occur in both benign and malignant tumors; when the tumor is found

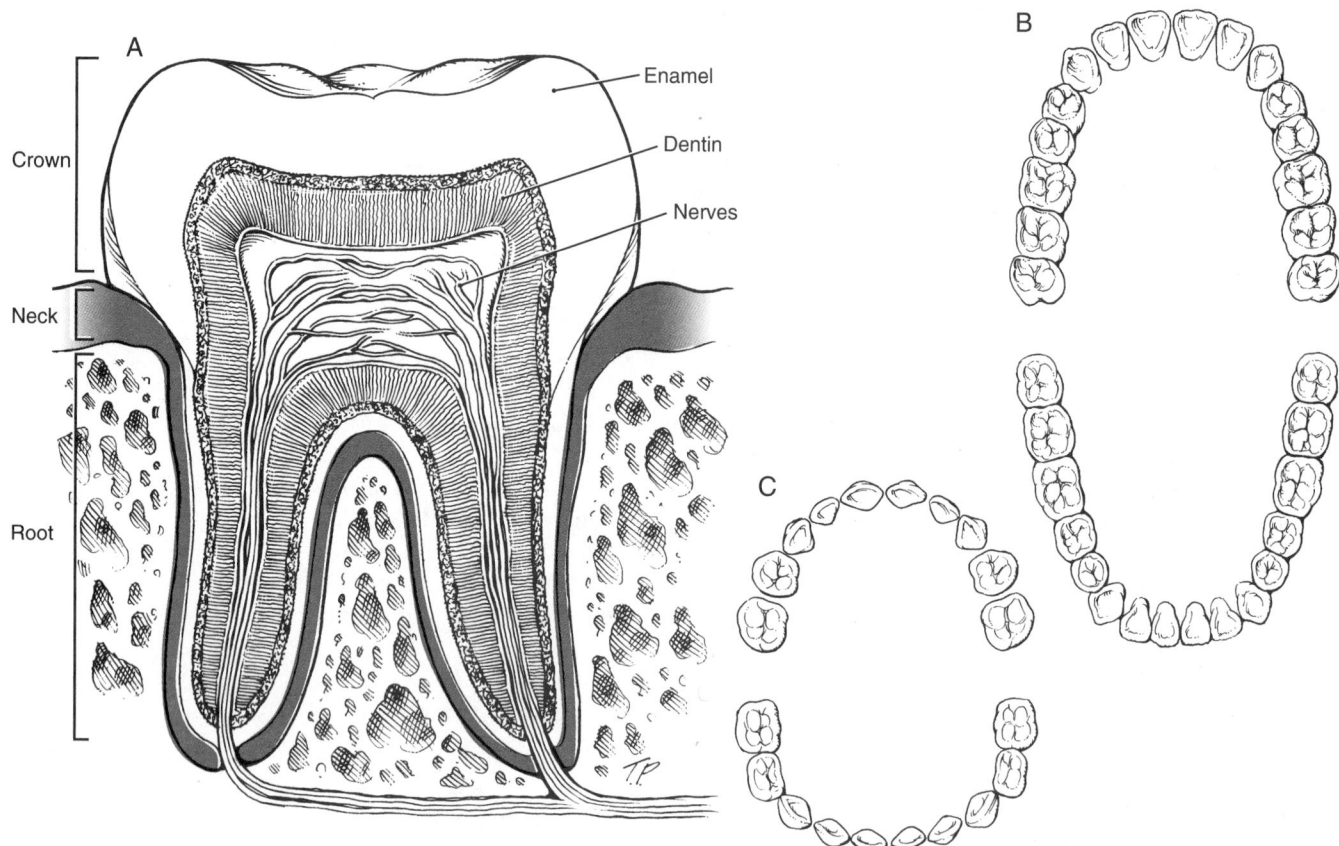

(A) Normal tooth anatomy; (B) permanent adult teeth;
(C) primary (baby) teeth.

to be malignant, the presence of pain may worsen the prognosis.

The only known risk factor is radiation exposure.

TOOTH AND GUM ANATOMY

The outside of each tooth crown is made of a hard, compact layer called enamel. The enamel has no sensation and cannot repair itself if it is damaged. The enamel covers the main body of the tooth called the dentine. Within the dentine lies a central chamber filled with soft, sensitive pulp, rich in blood vessels and nerve fibers. Below gum level, the dentine is covered by a special layer of tissue called cementum. The tooth is anchored in the bone of the jaw by a strong root that is held firmly in place by the periodontal ligament.

The gums consist of tough, fibrous supportive tissue that covers the bone of the jaw and a slick mucous membrane that forms the outer covering. ■

When to call the doctor The appearance of a slowly enlarging mass in a salivary gland should prompt a visit to the doctor.

Treatment For small lesions, surgical excision is often curative. An experienced otolaryngologist or head and neck surgeon will offer the best chance for complete excision with nerve sparing. Combined therapy with surgery and radiation offers the best hope for survival in the case of large, cancerous salivary gland tumors. See Chapter 30 for more information on the diagnosis and treatment of cancer. Simple surgical removal is sufficient for benign tumors although they may recur.

Prognosis Excellent for benign tumors. In cancers not associated with pain, the overall 5-year survival rate is 66 percent; the survival rate falls to 33 percent if the cancer causes pain. The reasons for this association are unclear.

Teeth and Gums

We are provided with two complete sets of teeth. None are usually visible at birth, but an initial set of 20 deciduous or primary

CARING FOR YOUR TEETH

To keep your teeth sound and healthy for a lifetime, practice good dental care methods yourself and teach your children good dental care habits at an early age. For dental health, follow these simple rules.

- Brush teeth daily. Proper tooth care depends on removing the sticky plaque that develops each day on the teeth. Brush the teeth and gums with a fluoride toothpaste, ideally after each meal and before bed but at least in the morning and at night. Plaque removal before bed is especially important since the flow of saliva is less while sleeping so the natural cleansing effect is diminished. If you are unable to brush after meals or snacks, at least rinse your mouth with water.

- Floss between teeth daily. Flossing removes the plaque between teeth and below the gum line.

- Reduce your intake of sugars and starches. These substances promote tooth decay by providing food for the bacteria that normally inhabit the mouth. The bacteria digest the sugars and produce acids that damage tooth enamel.

- See your dentist or dental hygienist twice yearly for a professional checkup and cleaning.

- Children (as well as other groups who are at risk of a high incidence of cavities such as the disabled) may benefit from tooth sealing procedures, in which a plastic-like protective coating is applied to the chewing surfaces of the teeth. The coating acts as a shield to block buildup of plaque in the crevices and pits in the teeth. Dental sealants normally remain effective for about 10 years. Periodic touch-ups can extend their useful life.

- Make sure that children are receiving adequate fluoride supplements either through drinking water or by a dietary supplement (usually in the form of a liquid or chewable tablet).

teeth erupts in childhood. A second permanent set of 32 teeth begins to erupt when a child is 6 years old and is usually complete by age 18.

Each tooth has three parts: the crown, the part that sticks up above the gum line; the root, firmly embedded entirely within the bone of the jaw; and the narrow neck between the two.

The permanent set of teeth consists of 8 incisors in front, for biting or cutting food; 4 canines, slightly larger and stronger than the incisors for stabilizing larger chunks of food; and 8 premolars and 12 molars, for crushing or grinding food.

The gums protect the bone that supports the teeth. The gums also provide a protective seal to prevent bacteria from penetrating to the root.

Disorders affecting the teeth and gums include infection, erosion (cavities), discoloration, trauma, and developmental problems.

❖ DENTAL CARIES (CAVITIES)

Symptoms (*What you may experience*) Sensitivity to hot, cold, or sweet foods.

Signs and laboratory findings (*What the doctor looks for*) Discolored or eroded areas on the crown or root; cavity formation within the tooth as shown by x-rays.

DENTISTS AND DENTAL SPECIALISTS

The practice of dentistry has become specialized. Some practitioners focus solely on certain aspects of tooth care. The primary divisions in dentistry include:

- *General dentist.* Much like a general practitioner in medicine, the general dentist will render basic care for virtually all adult (and often childhood) dental problems. The general dentist will usually have a general understanding of all the specialties and often have special expertise in one or more of them. The general dentist will refer to specialists when necessary.

- *Pediatric dentist.* More and more, delivery of dental care to children has become the province of dentists who limit their practice only to children, usually from birth through adolescence. The pediatric dentist is also a general dentist but has a special focus on children's disorders.

- *Periodontist.* This specialist diagnoses and treats disease of the tissues around the tooth—the gums, supportive ligaments, and underlying bone.

- *Endodontist.* This specialist diagnoses and treats disease within the tooth cavity, in the area of the pulp and nerve. This dental surgeon performs root canal surgery.

- *Oral and maxillofacial surgeon.* This specialist is usually a medical doctor with a specialization in tooth extraction and treatment of injuries and disease of the jaw, face, and mouth. Severe dental trauma, extraction of wisdom teeth, and plastic surgery of the oral cavity fall within this specialty.

- *Prosthodontists.* These specialists create artificial replacements such as crowns, bridgework, or dentures for missing or defective teeth.

- *Orthodontist.* The orthodontist specializes in the diagnosis and treatment of abnormalities in tooth position and jawbone growth in children and adults. ■

What is it? Dental caries—or cavities as they are more commonly known—develop from acid erosion of tooth enamel. A host of bacteria normally live in the human mouth; some of them convert into acids the sugar and carbohydrates (starches) in the foods we eat. The bacteria and acids, along with saliva and food particles, form a sticky film—called plaque—that coats the surfaces of the teeth. You can feel this slightly textured coating with your tongue within a few hours of brushing. The plaque forms especially readily in cracks, pits, or fissures in the back teeth, between teeth, around dental fillings or bridgework, and near the gum line.

The acid in the plaque damages the outer enamel coating on the tooth crown, forming microscopic pits or erosions that enlarge over time. Penetration of the protective enamel exposes the softer, vulnerable dentin (main body of the tooth) beneath to acid and bacteria. Beneath the dentin lies the soft tooth pulp and the sensitive nerve fibers within it. Inflammation from entering bacteria causes swelling and pain.

What you can do   Daily brushing and flossing and regular visits to the dentist for professional cleaning twice a year are essential (see Caring for Your Teeth, page 615).

When to call the doctor   The early stages of decay are usually painless; only regular professional examination and x-rays can detect early trouble. Tooth pain is not normal. If you develop sensitivity to chewing or to hot, cold, or sweet foods or beverages, contact your dentist.

Treatment   The standard treatment for most cavities is to fill the tooth. After the dentist removes the decayed material in the cavity (usually following use of anesthesia to obliterate the pain), the cavity is filled. Fillings can be a composite resin for front and back teeth or a silver-mercury amalgam material alloyed with copper and other metals in order to improve durability. Gold inlay may be used if greater strength is needed but this is a more expensive restoration. Increasingly, especially in front teeth, composite resins or bonded porcelains are preferred for strengthening the tooth structure and reducing the amount of natural tooth removed compared with silver alloys.

The amount of filling material required to repair a large cavity with extensive erosion may be more than the remaining tooth can support. In these cases, the dentist will remove the decay, fill the cavity, and replace the crown with an artificial one.

Sometimes the crown of the tooth remains relatively intact, with greater damage existing in the interior of the tooth. In these cases, the dentist may recommend referral to a dental specialist for a root canal. In this procedure, the endodontist removes the pulp including the nerve and replaces it with an inert material. The natural crown may have reduced support and may need to be replaced with an artificial permanent crown.

❖ TOOTH ABSCESS

Symptoms *(What you may experience)* Persistent, throbbing tooth pain; sometimes, sensitivity to hot food, tenderness to tooth pressure (as with chewing); later, fever, tenderness of lymph nodes under the jaw or in the neck, sudden rush of foul-smelling and foul-tasting fluid into the mouth.

Signs and laboratory findings *(What the doctor looks for)* Localized tenderness and swelling of the gum near the tooth line; visible decay of a tooth; swelling of lymph nodes under the jaw or in the neck; evidence of bone erosion around the root of the tooth as shown by x-rays.

What is it? When bacterial infection within a cavity elicits a response by the body's immune system, white blood cells rush to the area to attempt to eradicate the bacteria; pus forms within the tooth pulp as a result of this confrontation between the immune system and bacteria—a condition called a tooth abscess. The infection can spread to the root and surrounding bone and may loosen the tooth in its socket. The body tries to contain the infection and keep it localized but the inflammation of the dental pulp in a confined area and bacteria in the supporting bone cause intense pain. As the infection escalates, it can burrow through to the gum, forming a visible boil that may rupture and spill foul-tasting, foul-smelling pus into the mouth. Once the boil ruptures, the intensity of the pain often immediately decreases. Infection can spread to other areas of the head and neck from teeth that do not drain. These can become serious, life-threatening infections.

When to call the doctor Intense throbbing pain in the tooth should always prompt a visit to the dentist. Even though the pain may diminish with spontaneous drainage of pus, a visit to the dentist for definitive treatment of the abscess is crucial.

Treatment Antibiotics to eradicate the infection will usually be the first step in treatment. Although tooth extraction was once the only therapy—and still may be used on occasion—dentists today can save many abscessed teeth with root canal therapy.

Saving an abscessed tooth begins with draining the infected pulp chamber in order to relieve the pressure and remove the bulk of the infection. Once the cavity is cleared, the dentist uses piles to enlarge the canal and may then fill it or treat it in stages. Later the dentist places a permanent filling. Dental x-rays 12 months later are necessary to confirm that healthy bone and tissue are filling the abscess. If the bone is not healed after the treatment, referral to a dental specialist may be required to address infection or inflammation at the tooth root.

Prognosis Excellent if detected promptly and treated appropriately.

❖ IMPACTED WISDOM TEETH

Symptoms *(What you may experience)* Swelling of the gum; unpleasant taste in the mouth; halitosis; pain or irritation on opening the mouth; pain on biting.

Signs and laboratory findings *(What the doctor looks for)* Tenderness and swelling of the gum over an unerupted tooth; tooth visible below the gum line on an x-ray.

What is it? The last molar teeth, called third molars or wisdom teeth, usually begin to erupt during the late teen years or early 20s, often causing considerable pain in the process. The teeth frequently are mispositioned (malposed) in the jaw and as a consequence they fail to emerge properly, coming in rotated, tilted, or out of line. If the wisdom tooth pushes in at an angle, it can press on the neighboring tooth, causing

IF A TOOTH IS KNOCKED OUT OR BROKEN

The knocking out of a sound tooth—whether primary or permanent—should prompt an immediate visit to the dentist or hospital for emergency treatment. Quick action can lead to successful reimplantation of a sound tooth lost to injury. Follow these steps:

1. Gently pick up the tooth by its crown—avoid handling the root.

2. Rinse very gently by dipping it by the crown in tap water—do not hold it under a running stream of water and do not attempt to rub or brush away any dirt, as these maneuvers may harm the root.

3. If possible, try to carefully replace the tooth in its socket and bite down with gentle pressure on a piece of clean gauze, a moistened cotton ball, or several layers of a moistened paper towel or a folded, moistened coffee filter.

4. Telephone your dentist immediately. If your dentist is not available, go straight to the nearest hospital emergency room.

5. If you are not able to return the tooth to its socket, you must keep it moist. Protect it on the way to the dentist or emergency room by placing it gently in a jar of one of the following liquids: milk; warm, mild salt water ($1/2$ tsp salt in 1 cup warm water); or saliva from the mouth the tooth came from.

Unfortunately, broken teeth cannot be reimplanted; nonetheless, a dentist should evaluate the injury right away. Repair of a broken tooth usually entails replacement with an artificial restoration. Small chips may only require filing in order to restore the shape. ■

pain or damaging the tooth. Food particles can become trapped in the soft gum tissue surrounding the erupting tooth and then the area becomes vulnerable for infection and tooth decay. A bad taste in the mouth, particularly when chewing on the affected side, betrays the presence of infection or decay surrounding an unerupted tooth. Dental x-rays will confirm its location and position.

As in infancy when the tooth attempts to erupt, the overlying gum may swell and cause pain. Pain can be referred (transmitted) to other teeth in the area or to the ear.

What you can do Careful dental hygiene—brushing, flossing, or the use of water-jet devices—that removes trapped food particles from the soft gum tissue after meals can reduce the risk of infection.

Application of topical OTC anesthetic gels, warm-water mouth rinses, and massaging the gums (one method involves chewing sugarless chewing gum) can provide symptomatic relief of gum pain.

When to call the doctor The eruption process for wisdom teeth may wax and wane. Pain may occur for several days and then subside for months only to recur at a later time. Because an impacted tooth can damage neighboring healthy teeth or distort the bite, even if the pain subsides temporarily it is prudent to consult the dentist for x-ray determination of the extent of the problem and make a treatment plan. If the pain becomes severe or persists longer than a few days, see your dentist right away.

Treatment Infection surrounding the tooth will usually require antibiotics. The typical treatment for impacted teeth is extraction because the location of the teeth in the back of the mouth makes it difficult to clean them properly and so they are vulnerable to decay and periodontal disease.

Often the extraction can be carried out in the dentist's office with a local anesthetic. If several of the wisdom teeth are impacted (difficult to remove), the dentist may recommend referral to an oral surgeon who will remove them using an intravenous sedative and a local anesthetic or in the hospital operating room under general anesthesia.

Prognosis Excellent.

❖ TOOTH DISCOLORATION

Symptoms and signs Discoloration of the tooth enamel or dentin.

What is it? As the tooth enamel develops, whether of baby teeth or permanent teeth, the color of the enamel covering can be affected by many factors. Teeth can darken over time due to stains from foods and drink. Illness can discolor dentin; heredity or environmental factors can discolor both dentin and enamel and in rare cases injury can discolor either dentin or enamel. Excessive use of fluoride—in drinking water containing greater than two parts per million or in fluoride mouth rinses—can cause mottled bleaching of the enamel. Although many cities add fluoride to drinking water, such excessive amounts usually do not result from municipal water treatment but occur naturally in the water in some areas. Maternal use of certain antibiotics, notably those of the tetracycline family, during pregnancy can cause brown or gray discoloration of the baby's tooth enamel. Children who take this medication during the period of permanent tooth development may have similar discoloration of the permanent teeth.

What you can do Prevent discoloration by avoiding excessive fluoride use. You may want to check the fluoride level with water quality agencies in your community. If you are pregnant do not take antibiotics of the tetracycline family. Do not give such antibiotics to children less than 8 years old.

When to call the doctor Discoloration of enamel may be a cosmetic problem but it can also be a structural one. Contact a dentist to obtain a proper diagnosis and to learn what treatment options are available.

Treatment Professional tooth-whitening products can improve enamel color in many instances. Severe discoloration may require enamel-bonding procedures for good cos-

TOOTH-WHITENING PROCEDURES

Methods for whitening teeth range from inexpensive (and less effective) to very costly. At the lower end of the spectrum are simple OTC whitening toothpastes that may remove simple stains due to coffee or tea oils.

Deeper stains of the enamel may respond to professional tray bleaching compounds. For success with this procedure, the teeth should be healthy and not sensitive. It is not advisable for people with crowns in their front teeth and may require replacement of fillings. For those people deemed good candidates, the dentist will mold a vinyl tray to fit the upper and lower teeth. The tray holds a bleaching gel solution next to the teeth for several hours. At home, the process is gradual and depending on the degree of staining may take a few days to several weeks of regular application.

In-office bleaching offers the most immediate and best cosmetic result but is more expensive. With in-office bleaching procedures, it is possible for some stained teeth to become whiter teeth in as little as an hour and a half.

Your dentist can advise you on which procedure would best benefit you. ■

DENTURES AND PROSTHETICS

Loss of teeth and reliance on dentures was a normal part of growing older for generations past. Modern dental care and the discovery that fluoride could substantially reduce tooth decay have freed subsequent generations from the inevitability of toothlessness. In the future, far fewer people will require removal of their natural teeth and replacement with artificial ones.

Partial Dentures

Occasionally one or more teeth may be lost to decay or trauma. If you lose a tooth but do not replace it promptly, the surrounding teeth may begin to shift, altering your bite and leading to potential problems that will be more difficult to remedy. To fill in the space left by the lost tooth, your dentist can fashion a bridge (partial denture). A fixed partial denture consists of an artificial tooth retained by the natural teeth on either side of the missing tooth or teeth space. The healthy teeth on either side of the missing tooth are reduced in size by the dentist so that the bridge can be cemented onto them. Alternatively, your dentist may recommend a removable partial denture (which may be less expensive) that consists of an artificial tooth on a metal or plastic base that clips to the surrounding teeth.

Bridges are prone to plaque buildup. A fixed partial denture should be brushed carefully. Removable bridges should be removed before you brush and floss your natural teeth. They need to be brushed regularly and removed at bedtime.

Complete Dentures

Although decay has become a less common cause for extensive tooth replacement, full dentures may be necessary in certain cases. Replacement of all upper or lower teeth can be done, as in times past, with removable dentures or with dental implants.

Removable complete dentures are made of acrylic resin and metal and are removable replacements for all the teeth. There are two methods for fitting dentures: conventional and immediate. In the conventional method, the teeth are extracted and the gums and jaw allowed to heal for several weeks before the dentures are fitted. In the immediate method, the dentures are prepared in advance and inserted as soon as the teeth are removed. The disadvantage of the conventional method is that the person has no teeth for several weeks; the disadvantage of the immediate method is that the dentures may not fit as well and may need considerable adjustment or to be completely redone after the gums and jaw heal. Your dentist can help you decide which method is more appropriate in your case.

When a few healthy teeth remain, an overdenture can be fitted over them. Each of the covered teeth may first need to have the nerve removed in a root canal procedure but the covered teeth will help keep the denture in place, which is particularly helpful for the lower denture. Be sure to floss and brush the remaining teeth regularly.

Learning to wear a new denture will take time, particularly in the case of a lower denture, which may feel strange to the tongue at first. Speaking may feel different for the first few hours; practice aloud in private until you adjust. Eat only soft foods for the first few days. As you begin eating solid food, cut it up into small bites, chewing slowly and carefully. It is normal to have some soreness during the adjustment period until the gum tissues accommodate to the denture. If discomfort persists beyond a couple of weeks, however, consult your dentist. A well-fitting denture should not be uncomfortable.

Even when you have adjusted to your dentures, you may need to exercise caution in eating certain foods. Corn may need to be cut off the cob; apples should be eaten sliced. Follow your dentist's directions. You may find that dentures slightly diminish your sense of taste because they cover the sensitive tissue on the roof of your mouth. In addition, the chewing pressure you can exert is not as strong and effective as that of your natural teeth. Take the time to eat slowly and carefully with your dentures; proper chewing of food aids in digestion.

Caring for Your Dentures

Dentures are delicate but will last longer if cared for properly. While you may be told to wear your dentures continuously during the first few weeks, subsequently you should always remove them at night. Research has shown that removing dentures for a minimum of 8 hours during the day or night allows gum tissues to rest and the mouth to be cleansed by the tongue and saliva. Your mouth and gums should be cleaned each day with a brush or cloth.

Remove and brush your dentures daily with a brush designed for cleaning dentures. Check with your dentist about which cleanser is appropriate for your dentures. Never use harsh cleansers, bleach, or abrasive toothpastes; never sterilize them in boiling water or clean them in a dishwasher or the dentures will warp.

When you are not using your dentures, they should be soaking in water to prevent drying which may affect the fit. An appropriate cleaning agent can be added to the water. Some removable partial dentures cannot soak in cleanser overnight; check with your dentist.

You should have an annual examination by a dentist to evaluate the dentures and the oral cavity and to have an oral cancer screening exam. Because your gum tissues change constantly but your dentures do not, your dentures will need to be relined periodically for a proper fit. Dentures generally need to be relined or remade every 3 to 5 years.

Dental Implants

Placement of dental implants—a procedure called osseointegration—involves surgically imbedding titanium fixtures or root forms into the bone of the jaw. The dental surgeon can then attach individual teeth or full dentures to the fixture with screws. This secure attachment provides chewing power roughly equal to natural teeth and there is less risk of deterioration of the jaw bone.

Osseointegration is a complicated procedure that can take several months. Depending upon the degree of complexity, the surgery may be performed under general anesthesia and require hospitalization or it may be performed in the dentist's office. Holes are drilled in the upper and lower jaw bones and hollow titanium cylinders are inserted. Several months later (during which time your old dentures may be worn), metal posts are screwed into the cylinders. A few weeks after that, artificial teeth are fashioned and screwed into the posts. The procedure is expensive but the long-term results can be very satisfactory. ■

ORTHODONTICS (BRACES)

Chewing—and by extension, digestion—suffer when teeth do not fit together properly. Malalignment of teeth affects more than appearance; it can contribute to the development of periodontal disease or could damage the temporomandibular joint (TMJ) of the jaw.

Disorders of alignment fall generally into two broad categories: underbite and overbite. In an underbite, the lower jaw is larger than the upper one, causing the upper front teeth to bite behind the lower ones. Conversely, an overbite occurs when the upper front teeth protrude too far over the lower ones, failing to make an effective bite. Malalignment also can result from rotation, overlapping, or incorrect spacing of the teeth.

A dentist will usually refer cases of malalignment to the orthodontist, the dental specialist who deals with this facet of care. The orthodontist will examine the teeth and will usually make plaster impressions of the current bite and take special x-rays of the head, jaw, and teeth to determine the extent of the problem and what treatment will be necessary to produce an even bite and the best cosmetic result.

Correction of alignment involves using appliances such as braces, also called orthodontics. Significant discrepancy in jaw size may require surgery to better align the bite in conjunction with placement of dental appliances. (Corrective jaw surgery is necessary more commonly in adults than it is in children.) Severe overcrowding of teeth may require selective removal of certain teeth (usually premolars) to make more room for the remaining teeth.

Fixed braces, usually made of metal, either encircle the teeth with sleeve-like bands or are attached with adhesive to the outside surface of the tooth. The orthodontist may be able to use clear plastic or tooth-colored ceramic materials from which to fashion less conspicuous braces.

Strategically placed interconnecting wires and rubber bands put varying amounts of tension on individual teeth to gradually shift them into new positions; the bone of the jaw responds by reabsorbing bone in front of the tooth movement and laying it down behind. When more tension is needed to guide the movement, the orthodontist may fashion external appliances, called headgear, to be worn at night or during specific periods during the day.

The shifting of teeth and remodeling of the jawbone causes discomfort for a few days each time the braces are tightened or the tension is altered. OTC pain relievers such as ibuprofen or acetaminophen and warm packs can usually assuage the discomfort. ∎

metic result (see Tooth-Whitening Procedures, page 618).

Prognosis Excellent with cosmetic treatments.

❖ GINGIVITIS

Symptoms (What you may experience) Red, swollen gums; bleeding gums.

Signs and laboratory findings (What the doctor looks for) Plaque deposits at the tooth base; later, early separation of the gum from the tooth.

What is it? Normal, healthy gums should be firm and adherent to the underlying bone; their color will vary with ethnic origin, usually appearing pale pink except in races with darker pigmentation, in which normal gums may be brown, gray, or mottled. When gingivitis occurs, the gums become inflamed, red, and swollen and bleed easily. The disorder may go unrecognized because it causes little pain in the early stages.

Adolescents and adults develop mild gingivitis quite commonly. If left unchecked, it may become severe and progress to periodontal disease, a more serious gum disorder that can progress to tooth loss. People with poorly controlled diabetes mellitus and pregnant women are especially at risk for its development.

Plaque can inflame and irritate the gum. If not removed regularly, plaque can harden and form mineral deposits called tartar or *calculus* (a Latin word meaning stone), which irritate the gums even more by providing a place for bacteria to grow. Poorly fitting bridgework, rough or broken fillings, or misaligned teeth may provide crevices that easily trap food particles and are difficult to clean; these areas provide fertile ground for the accumulation of plaque and tartar and promote the development of gingivitis.

What you can do Brush and floss teeth regularly, not only in the morning but more importantly before bed. Brushing and flossing remove plaque and nightly brushing reduces the buildup during sleep. Have your teeth professionally cleaned regularly (every 6 months to 1 year) to prevent plaque from becoming tartar and to remove any tartar that may have already formed.

When to call the doctor If your gums bleed easily when you brush them or they become tender, contact your dentist.

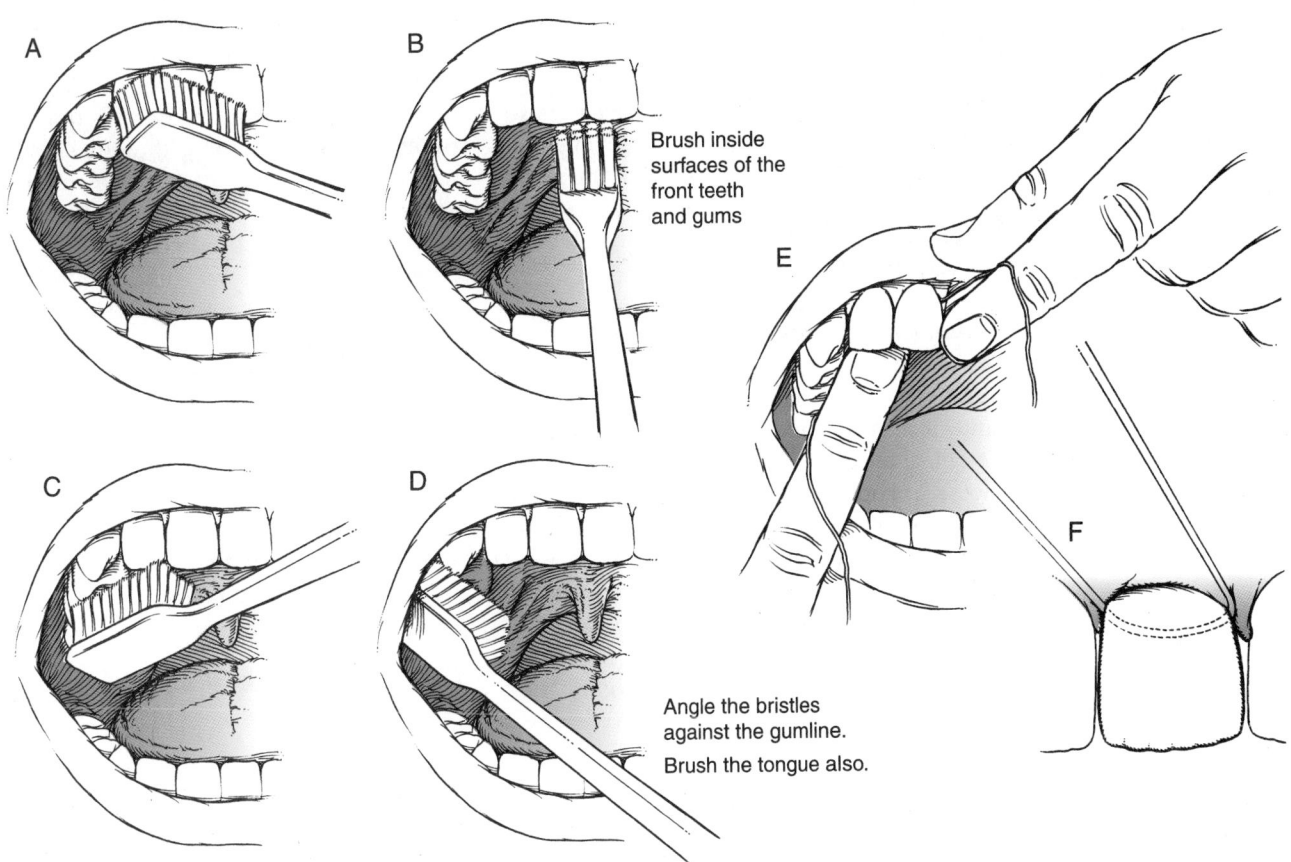

A

B

Brush inside
surfaces of the
front teeth
and gums

E

C

D

F

Angle the bristles
against the gumline.
Brush the tongue also.

(A–E) Proper brushing technique. (F) Proper flossing technique includes passing the floss below the level of the gum line.

Treatment Gingivitis is reversible by daily effective removal of bacteria from the teeth. The dentist usually will first recommend removing all plaque and tartar. The dentist also can provide information on effective oral hygiene methods.

Controlling underlying medical conditions such as diabetes mellitus can make gingivitis easier to treat. Repair of fillings and restorations to improve their fit can remove a chronic source of irritation.

Prognosis Excellent once a program of good dental hygiene has been instituted.

❖ PERIODONTITIS

Symptom (*What you may experience*) Swollen, receding gums; bad breath; an unpleasant taste in the mouth.

Signs and laboratory findings (*What the doctor looks for*) Periodontal pocketing evident on examination; loss of supporting bone shown on x-rays; loose teeth; gum recession causing the neck of the tooth to be visible.

What is it? The name *periodontitis* comes from *peri* (around), *odont* (tooth), and *itis* (inflammation). The inflammation results from a combination of bacterial activity and immune system response. If not treated, chronic inflammation of the gums will usually progress to involve not only the gums but the underlying bone and supportive ligaments around the tooth (see Gingivitis, page 620, for more information on inflammation of the gums). As plaque accumulates at the base of the tooth, it creates a space between the tooth and the gum. Long-standing infection will finally erode the bone surrounding the tooth, weakening its attachment and loosening the tooth. At its most severe, periodontitis can cause the tooth to be lost.

Periodontitis usually is relatively painless. The onset of significant pain may signal development of an abscess.

What you can do Daily brushing and flossing (morning and night) and regular visits for professional cleaning can help prevent periodontitis.

When to call the doctor If you have persistent bleeding of the gums, swelling, or drainage of pus, call your dentist. The dentist should perform a periodontal disease screening examination during initial and subsequent dental visits.

Treatment The first treatment usually will be nonsurgical: a meticulous cleaning and removal of the tartar deposits from the root and neck of the teeth. Following this professional cleaning, a strict regimen of daily flossing and brushing is recommended. Within several weeks, the gums should return to a normal, healthy appearance in color and firmness. If pocketing persists, surgical treatment may be recommended.

In severe cases of periodontitis, the gums are lifted surgically from around the teeth to expose the deeper root structures

for extensive cleaning. Following the procedure the gum tissue is put back in place and tacked into position with sutures.

Excess gum tissue may sometimes be trimmed away; reshaping the gums makes the roots of the teeth easier to keep clean. Occasionally operating more deeply is necessary to correct deformity in bone shape or to scrape away underlying bone damaged by chronic infection. Bone regeneration techniques allow the surgeon to fill bony defects and cause the bone to regrow.

Prognosis Good if recognized promptly and treated aggressively. Once bone loss occurs the prognosis is less favorable depending on the severity of loss. Lifelong periodontal maintenance may be required once the disease is controlled.

The Jaw and Facial Bones

The front portion of the skull consists of the facial bones, irregularly shaped flattened bones that interlock to form the contours of the brow ridges, eye sockets, cheeks, nose, and jaw. The facial bones vary in thickness and strength, from the robust zygoma (cheekbone) to the paper thin bone that forms the floor of the orbit (eye socket).

The lower jaw—called the mandible—attaches to the skull only by means of a hinge joint called the temporomandibular joint (TMJ). The upper and lower jaws serve as the bony anchors for the teeth and the powerful masseter (chewing) muscles. See TMJ Dysfunction Syndrome, below, for more information on the upper and lower jaws.

Disorders related to the jaw and facial bones primarily result from trauma—for example, fractures, dislocations, or overuse injuries. Nerves that supply sensation to the face and the teeth and oral cavity course through channels in the bones and are also vulnerable to injury if the bone is broken or crushed.

❖ TMJ DYSFUNCTION SYNDROME

Symptoms *(What you may experience)* Aching discomfort in front of the ear; popping or clicking sounds of the jaw with motion; loss of free mobility of the TMJ; pain on movement of the jaw.

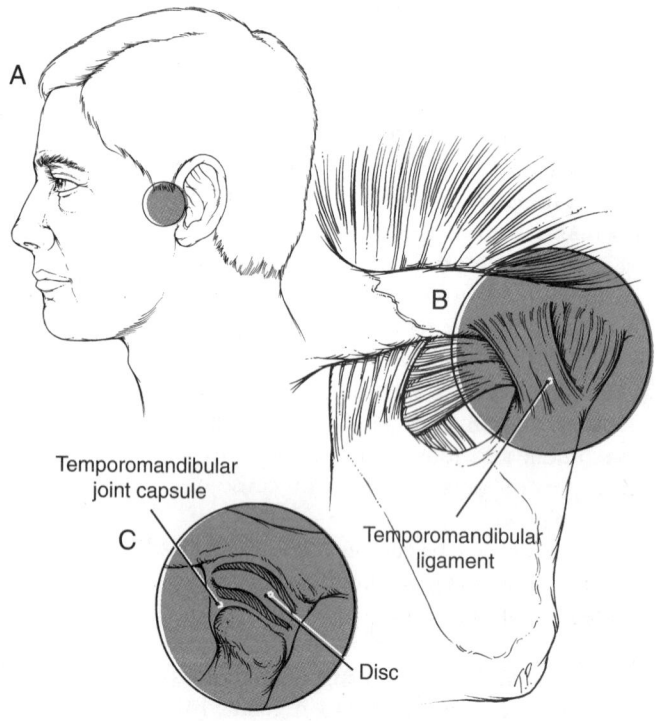

(A–C) The temporomandibular joint, or TMJ, is covered by a capsule and supported by the temporomandibular ligament, connecting the temporal bone of the skull to the mandible (jaw). Inside the bones and within the capsule is a disc — (C) — that allows for smooth motion between the bones in the joint. TMJ disorders are commonly caused by muscle tension and displacement of the disk.

A

B

Temporomandibular joint capsule

C

Temporomandibular ligament

Disc

Signs and laboratory findings *(What the doctor looks for)* Tenderness in response to direct pressure on the TMJ; grinding or clicking when opening and closing the TMJ; x-ray evidence of joint damage (occasionally).

What is it? The joint of the jaw operates like a hinge, permitting the mouth to open and close but limiting side-to-side movement. The lower jaw has a round hingeball at its ends that fits within sockets in the upper jaw to attach it to the skull proper; this hinge forms the TMJ.

To reduce friction between the bones, the gliding surfaces of the ball and socket of the TMJ (as is the case with all joints) are covered with slick cartilage and a thin film of joint fluid. A protective disk within the joint prevents the bones from rubbing against each other.

Ideally, the right and left hinges open or close in synchrony, limiting wear and tear of the joint that occurs with chewing or talking. Sometimes habitual tooth-grinding or jaw-clenching damages the TMJs. Damage also can occur on the gliding surface, causing the joint to make cracking sounds as the jaw opens and closes. Chronic damage can lead to the development of the disorder commonly called TMJ dysfunction syndrome, which is associated with inflammation and pain in the hinge. Spasm of the powerful chewing muscles that attach to the bone around the joint can cause facial and head pain and may limit the degree to which the mouth can open.

What you can do During episodes of discomfort, application of warm packs to the painful joint can give symptomatic relief. Anti-inflammatory medication such as aspirin or ibuprofen can help reduce pain.

Stick to easier-to-chew, soft foods for a few days to reduce the demand on the joint. If you have TMJ dysfunction syndrome, avoid overuse of chewing gum or chewing on ice or hard candies. Avoid wide-open yawning and do not lean the jaw on your hand when you rest your head.

When to call the doctor Inability to open or close the jaw, significant popping of the joint with chewing or talking, the development of tenderness of the joint, or spasm of the muscles around the joint should prompt

a visit to the doctor. If the hinge slips out of joint and the jaw will not close, it is dislocated. Go directly to the doctor or hospital emergency facility.

Treatment In the short term, prescription strength anti-inflammatory medication and, sometimes, muscle relaxants may be necessary to combat pain and muscle spasm. Physical therapy is also needed in many cases. Given time, most cases of TMJ dysfunction syndrome resolve.

Short-term treatment to relieve TMJ dysfunction syndrome may involve the use of a bite-guard appliance inserted between the teeth. This device may help to prevent joint damage in people who grind their teeth while sleeping or who clench their jaws during the day. Low-dose antidepressant medication is sometimes used to reduce nighttime grinding.

If the problem continues despite these remedies, referral to an oral surgeon for surgical repair or removal of the disk within the joint may be necessary. Most surgeons will not operate due to high failure rates unless the person has already had surgery.

Prognosis TMJ problems tend to be chronic and recurrent, although treatment can help alleviate discomfort and slow progression of wear on the joint.

❖ DISLOCATION OF THE TMJ

Symptoms and signs Locking of the jaw; inability to close the jaw.

What is it? Occasionally, the TMJ can slip out of joint and lock. Locking sometimes occurs unexpectedly with yawning, which opens the joint widely, allowing the ball of the lower jaw to slip out of place. When this happens, the joint is locked in the open position and cannot be closed. As with any dislocated joint, dislocation of the jaw causes considerable discomfort until it is put back into place.

When to call the doctor Dislocation of the jaw should prompt an immediate visit to the doctor or hospital emergency room to have the hinge put back in place.

Treatment As with all dislocated joints, relaxation of surrounding muscles that usually develop spasm with the unaccustomed stretch is helpful in returning the ball of the hinge to its original position. Relocation of the joint involves pulling the body of the lower jaw downward and tipping the chin upward to free the ball of the joint from its entrapment. For a moment, the jaw floats free, held only by the muscular and ligamentous tissues, until the doctor can guide the ball back into the socket.

Following relocation, minimize jaw movement and stress by eating a soft or liquid diet for several days. Avoid foods that are hard to chew such as tough meats, carrots, hard candies, or ice cubes. Avoid wide yawning or opening the mouth too widely.

Prognosis Excellent.

Fractures of the Facial Bones

Fractures of the facial bones commonly occur from a blow to the face such as that from a fist or blunt instrument or as a result of a fall or vehicular accident. Symptoms and treatment will depend on which bone has been broken.

❖ FRACTURE OF THE LOWER JAW (BROKEN JAW)

Symptoms *(What you may experience)* Swelling, tenderness, bruising of the jaw following injury; a sudden abnormality in bite following a jaw injury.

Signs and laboratory findings *(What the doctor looks for)* Movement of the teeth at the fracture line; point tenderness along the jaw bone; the fracture is confirmed by CT or panoramic x-ray.

What is it? This injury commonly occurs during a boxing match or fist fight in which a moving object strikes the lower jaw or as a result of direct trauma to the jaw as in an unsupported fall with fainting. The body of the lower jaw is usually the point that gives and cracks although fractures also occur just below the ball of the TMJ as well. The most telling symptom betraying a fracture of the lower jaw is malocclusion of the teeth: Even a crack in the jaw bone will alter

the bite so that the teeth do not feel like they fit together properly.

What you can do Apply a cold pack and use a soft bandage such as roll gauze to immobilize the jaw.

When to call the doctor Development of a bite abnormality following a blow to the jaw should prompt an immediate visit to the dentist or oral and maxillofacial surgeon for a certain kind of x-ray (panoramic x-ray of the jaws) that offers the best picture of the lower jaw.

Treatment In most cases treatment is surgical and involves realignment of the fracture with wiring of the fragments to allow them to heal properly. Usually the surgeon will immobilize the jaw for 1 or 2 months by wiring it closed. With the jaws immobilized, nutrition will need to come in liquid or semiliquid form, such as soups, juices, shakes, and possibly junior baby foods, such as strained meats and vegetables that require no chewing and can be taken through a straw. Sometimes the jaw can be repaired with internal metal plates and screws; the diet is often more liberal if this technique is employed.

Prognosis Excellent with prompt diagnosis and appropriate medical and surgical treatment.

❖ FRACTURE OF THE ORBIT (EYE SOCKET)

Symptoms *(What you may experience)* Pain, swelling, bruising around the eye following direct trauma; an inability to look up following a blow to the eye (often).

Signs and laboratory findings *(What the doctor looks for)* Fracture confirmed by x-rays or CT (see also page 547).

What is it? The orbit, commonly called the eye socket, is fashioned of paper-thin bone that cradles the eyeball. A direct blow to the eyeball such as that delivered by a fist, baseball, softball, or football compresses the soft eye tissues and transmits a shock wave of energy that literally blows out the thin walls of the eye socket, giving rise to the common name of this injury: a blow-out fracture.

As the soft tissues around the eyeball swell, they become entrapped in the blown-out floor of the socket, preventing the free movement of the eyeball in the upward direction. When entrapment occurs, although vision is usually unaffected, the eye on the injured side cannot move to look up.

What you can do Apply a cold pack—not ice—to the area. Protect the delicate eyelids with a soft cloth between the cold pack and the skin.

When to call the doctor A direct blow to the eye merits evaluation by a doctor. If upward eye motion is not equal to the other eye, seek immediate medical attention. Any change in vision associated with a direct blow to the eyeball deserves immediate medical evaluation.

Treatment Surgical repair of the fracture to free any entrapped tissue should be done right away. Delay can make repair more difficult and result in combined functional and cosmetic defects such as a misalignment of the eyes.

FACIAL PARALYSIS

Paralysis of the facial muscles results from inflammation or damage to the facial nerve (cranial nerve VII). It manifests itself as an inability to smile on the affected side (the corner of the mouth will not rise), in loss of the normal contours of the facial folds, and in loss of the ability to tightly close the eye on the affected side. Dysfunction of the facial nerve can occur in association with a middle-ear infection (see Acute Otitis Media, page 566); because of inflammation or viral infection of the nerve; because of pressure on the nerve as it passes through the bone of the skull; due to pressure from an acoustic neuroma, a benign tumor of the adjacent cranial nerve VIII (the hearing nerve); or as a component of other systemic diseases such as sarcoidosis, Lyme disease, or human immunodeficiency virus (HIV) infection. See Chapter 14 and Chapter 21 for more information on conditions associated with facial paralysis.

Treatment of facial paralysis depends on its cause. Any facial paralysis should be assessed by a doctor immediately. ■

SEVENTEEN

Musculoskeletal System

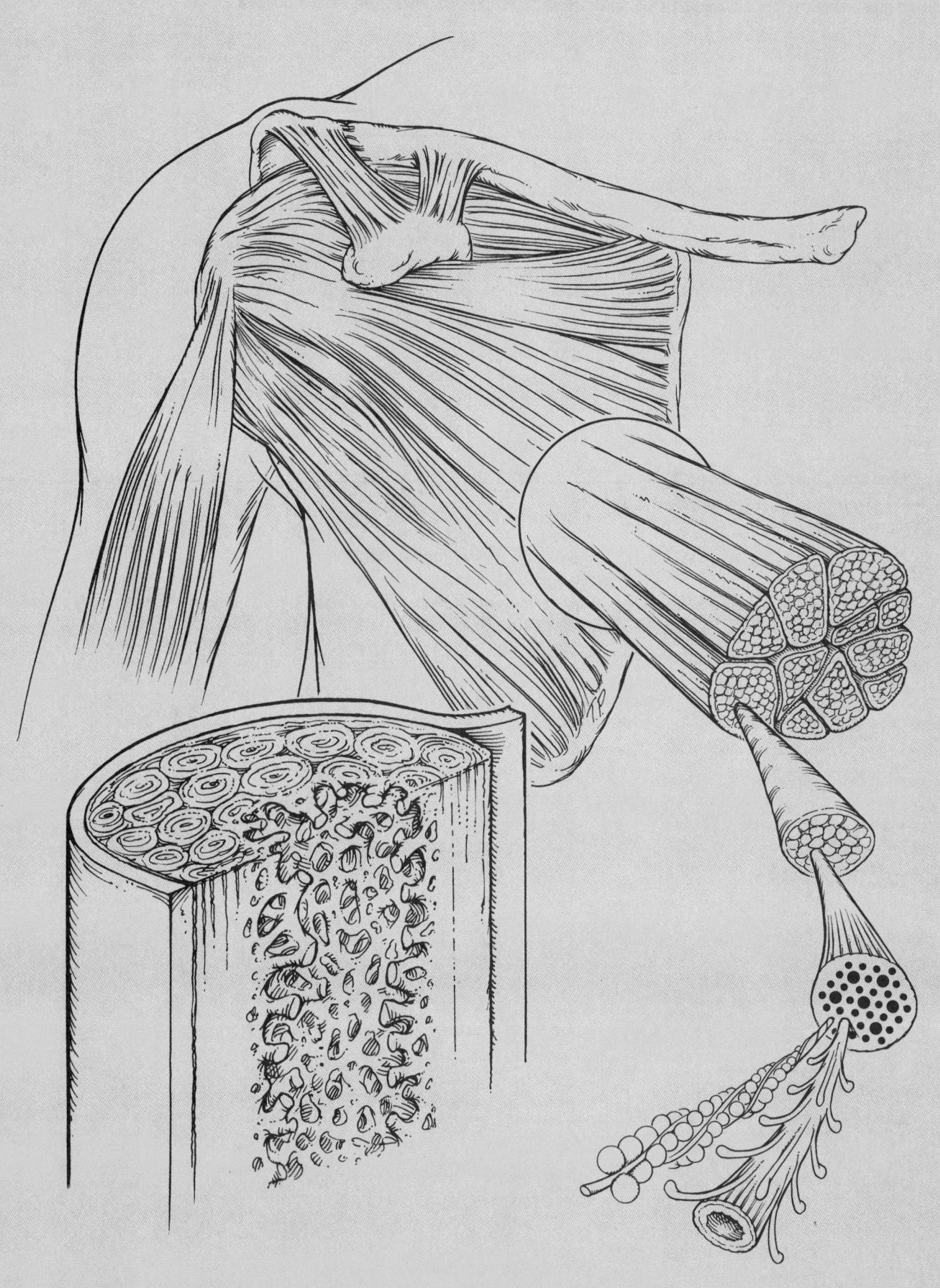

MUSCULOSKELETAL SYSTEM

How the Musculoskeletal System Works

A framework of interconnected bones supports the soft tissues of the body and gives them their basic shape. The system is uniquely designed to impart both load-bearing strength and a high degree of flexibility and mobility. The components of the musculoskeletal system include bones, cartilage, joints, tendons, ligaments, bursae (protective fluid-filled pouches near large joints), and muscles. The bones impart strength and structure; slick, resilient cartilage covers the ends of the bones, where one bone meets its neighbor; lubricating joint fluid enables the surfaces to move smoothly and with minimal friction; and flexible, tough ligaments attach one bone to another.

Muscle and tendon groups attach to the bones and their soft tissues across the joints—much like an elaborate system of opposing pulleys—enabling the body to perform tasks as varied as lifting a heavy load, leaping into the air, running a marathon, climbing a tree, threading a needle, writing with a pen, or playing the piano.

The signals necessary to coordinate the intricate movements of the musculoskeletal system—the ability to think about what movement we desire and then do it—come from the nervous system. Our conscious thought may be something as seemingly simple as picking up a glass of water with our left hand, but that simple thought must be translated by the brain and nervous system into a complex and integrated motion from the shoulder to the fingertips, all without conscious direction. Each muscle, from the larger arm and shoulder muscles to the tiny lumbrical muscles between the bones of the hand, must receive nerve signals that originate in the brain and travel along the super highway of the nervous system. Interruption of these signals at any point along the way will leave the muscle useless and immobile—unable to perform a task as simple as picking up the glass of water. Lack of regular nerve stimulation will cause any muscle to shrink (a process called atrophy); this phenomenon occurs following trauma, such as spinal cord injury or a stroke.

THE BONES

The adult skeleton is composed of more than 200 bones, connected to one another at joints. A newborn has far more bones than does an adult—about 350. As the child develops, many of the bones fuse together, reducing the overall number. Although it is readily apparent during infancy and childhood that bones change in size and shape, once we have attained full adult stature we may think of the bones as solid, fixed structures; in reality, they continually change. The bones of an adult are made of living bone remodeling cells (called osteoblasts and osteoclasts) and mineral compounds (mainly calcium and phosphate) attached to a fibrous (protein) framework.

The outer portion of the bones—called the cortex—forms as a resilient, strong tube of densely packed tissue, capable of bearing enormous stress. The inner layers develop as a honeycomb of more porous bony tissue interwoven with hollow spaces. These spaces serve to lighten the weight of the bone.

Providing the body's structure and protecting organs from injury are not the only functions of bones. The hollow spaces in porous bony tissue provide nourishment channels and storage for blood, blood cells, and bone cells. Deep within the cavity of some bones lies the bone marrow, a core of fatty tissue that houses the body's reservoir of blood stem cells—the cells that divide to produce a continuing supply of red and white blood cells throughout life. Bone also serves as the storehouse for calcium, which is essential for healthy body functioning. See page 947 for more information on bone marrow.

THE SOFT TISSUES

The nonbony tissues of the musculoskeletal system include muscles, tendons, bursae, ligaments, and joint cartilage. Each of these tissues serves a specific function.

- *Muscle*. These tissues contain specialized cells (called actin and myosin filaments) with the unique ability to shorten and lengthen. The filaments group together into larger and larger bundles that, under the control of the nervous system, shorten or lengthen in a coordinated fashion, causing the muscle to contract or relax. The muscles of

EVALUATION OF THE MUSCULOSKELETAL SYSTEM

Methods used in routine evaluation of the musculoskeletal system include blood tests, x-ray studies, chemical analysis of joint fluid, and arthroscopic examination of joints. The tests necessary to appropriately evaluate a specific condition will depend on the nature of the problem.

Blood Tests

Laboratory testing of blood will usually be necessary for diagnosis of inflammatory rheumatic and joint disorders such as rheumatoid arthritis (see page 646), gout (see page 652), scleroderma (see page 643), systemic lupus erythematosus, known as lupus or SLE (see page 642), polymyalgia rheumatica (see page 639), and reactive arthritic disorders (see page 648) and in bone thinning conditions such as osteoporosis (see page 654) and hyperparathyroidism (see page 1193). Common blood tests include the following:

- Erythrocyte sedimentation rate (ESR) or sed rate gives a measurement of inflammation or infection but it will not localize the cause of inflammation. It is commonly used in diagnosing and tracking progression of inflammatory rheumatic conditions. An elevation of the ESR implies an active ongoing disease process, while a falling measurement indicates improvement or resolution of the problem.

- Arthritis profiles are groups of blood tests used to differentiate various arthritic conditions. The profile will usually include some or all of the following tests designed to measure antibodies against certain body proteins: rheumatoid arthritis (RA) factor titer, antinuclear antibody (ANA) test, antinative DNA test, anticardiolipin antibodies, lupus anticoagulant, and others. Elevation of one or more of these substances helps distinguish one rheumatic tissue condition from another with similar symptoms.

- Elevated uric acid levels in the blood occur in gout; when crystals of uric acid deposit inside the joints, they cause a painful inflammatory arthritis.

- Complete blood count gives the number and type of white blood cells and concentration of red blood cells. Certain musculoskeletal conditions may be associated with anemia (low numbers of red blood cells) or with changes in white-blood-cell number or type.

Imaging Studies

These include standard plain film x-rays as well as computed tomography (CT), magnetic resonance imaging (MRI), and bone scans (radioactive isotope scanning).

- Plain films are the standard type of x-ray pictures used to detect breaks and dislocations of bones and to follow their healing. The standard plain film relies on the fact that the x-ray beam will penetrate some body tissues more easily than others. Bone is very dense and will permit few x-rays to pass through it, appearing as a white unexposed area on the x-ray film. Softer tissues—blood, muscle, ligament, or tendon—are mainly made of water and will allow more x-rays to pass, casting a gray shadow on the x-ray film. Unfortunately, almost all these tissues appear alike to the plain x-ray beam. Air within the body allows the x-rays to pass virtually unobstructed and appears black on the x-ray film. Once the only method of looking at the bones, the use of plain film x-ray to assess tumors (tissue masses), infections, and hidden fractures has been eclipsed by newer methods such as CT, MRI, and bone scans. However, plain films are usually needed before other types of scans are performed.

- CT scan relies on a computer to more precisely differentiate the various densities of soft tissues, giving much greater detail than a plain film x-ray. CT scans can be better used to detect small occult (difficult to detect) fractures previously invisible to standard x-ray, infection within the bone, tiny bone erosions, loose bodies within the joint, cervical spine fractures, and complex fractures of the hip socket, knee, ankle, heel, and wrist. Some cancers of the bone are well identified on CT scans.

- MRI studies, like CT, rely on computer assistance to assemble a three-dimensional picture of the tissue under inspection. This study offers excellent details of the soft tissue and bone. MRI has eclipsed CT as a tool to study herniated disks, compression of or bleeding into the spinal cord, tumors of the bone and soft tissues, and avascular necrosis of bone (bone death from lack of blood supply). The MRI shows the soft tissue along with the bone.

- Radionuclide bone scan involves the intravenous (IV) administration of a radioactive substance (usually technetium-99m) that travels through the blood and accumulates in areas of abnormal bone. Once there, a highly sensitive scanning technique illuminates the accumulations, highlighting hidden fractures, areas of inflammation or infection, or bone cancers. Bone scanning permits the doctor to accurately locate bone abnormalities for biopsy (tissue sample analysis), removal, or irradiation.

Chemical and Microscopic Analysis of Joint Fluid

In many arthritic conditions, the doctor may remove joint fluid (with a needle and syringe) to send for chemical analysis, culture of bacteria, or microscopic evaluation. Such an evaluation includes the density of the fluid, its color, and the presence of crystals of uric acid, blood, infecting bacteria, or infection-fighting white blood cells.

Arthroscopy

The arthroscope is a slender, lighted tube about the width of a pencil, fitted with a miniature camera. Working something like a periscope, it enables the doctor to look directly into a joint to assess the damage through small incisions. With an operating arthroscope, the orthopedic (relating to the prevention and treatment of skeletal abnormalities) surgeon can pass tiny instruments into the joint, to perform such procedures as shaving the meniscus of the knee (the menisci are a pair of crescent-shaped cushioning cartilage pads), removing loose or torn cartilage, and even repairing or reconstructing ligaments within the joint. For years this instrument has proven especially useful in evaluating and repairing knees, hips, ankles, wrists, and shoulders, as well as smaller joints. ■

the skeletal system are called voluntary muscles, meaning that they perform upon our conscious command, as opposed to the involuntary muscles of the wall of the gastrointestinal tract or the heart, which operate without regard to conscious direction. Voluntary muscles are spread throughout the body, and compose up to 25 percent of our weight.

The muscles of the skeletal system in general operate as opposing pairs. For example, the biceps muscle on the front of the upper arm contracts to bend the arm at the elbow, while contraction of the triceps muscle on the back of the arm straightens the elbow. When one contracts, its opponent must relax in order to perform a smooth motion. Such paired interaction occurs across most joints throughout the system.

- *Tendons.* Tough, flexible fibrous tissue bundles that anchor muscles to bone, tendons vary in size from the delicate strings of tissue in the minute muscles of the hands to the heavy tendons, thick as ropes, that anchor the thigh or calf muscles. A slick, filmy covering allows the tendon to glide freely, with minimal friction, in its space.

- *Bursa.* Where a tendon crosses a joint or bony prominence, the surrounding tissues form a fluid-filled pouch, called a bursa, to cushion and protect the tendon from wear. The lining of the bursa can respond to trauma by producing yet more fluid to expand the pouch, forming an internal cushion to protect an injured or inflamed joint or tendon. Bursae also exist between bones and the skin.

- *Joint capsule.* The fibrous tissue that surrounds a joint is lined with a special membrane that produces a viscous, slippery fluid called synovial fluid. The synovial fluid lubricates the joint and promotes nearly frictionless movement.

- *Ligaments.* These tough fibrous tissues serve to connect neighboring bones to one another for increased stability or to limit the motion of a joint. They may be inside a joint, attached to the capsule of the joint, or outside the joint altogether. They are the tethers that hold the bones together and help control how

much motion occurs between the bones.

- *Cartilage.* Joint cartilage covers the ends of bones where they face one another in a joint. Cartilage has the unique ability to deform under the pressure of weight bearing to minimize the stress on the bone beneath it, then to regain its original shape when the load is removed. Young, healthy cartilage provides an almost frictionless surface, allowing smooth motion of the joint.

Disorders of the Soft Tissues

❖ RHEUMATISM OF THE SOFT TISSUE (BURSITIS, TENDINITIS, TENOSYNOVITIS, AND CHONDRITIS)

Symptoms *(What you may experience)* Pain in the tissues around a joint, often following excessive, unusual, or unaccustomed use.

Signs and laboratory findings *(What the doctor looks for)* Painful motion, tenderness to palpation (pressing on), or swelling of specific muscle groups, tendons, ligaments, bursae, or cartilage.

What is it? Whether it is a painful shoulder from throwing a softball or painting the ceiling, a painful elbow from casting a fishing rod or hitting a tennis ball, or a painful hip from too much work in the yard, the cause is essentially the same: rheumatism (inflammation or injury) of the soft tissues surrounding the joint. (See Rheumatoid Arthritis and Juvenile Rheumatoid Arthritis, page 646, for information on arthritis, which is rheumatism of the joint itself.) While other causes of pain in the tissues near a joint must always be eliminated by specific testing (which can include evaluation of joint motion and muscle strength, blood tests to rule out the possibility of inflammatory arthritic conditions such as gout, and possibly x-ray studies to ascertain that there is no bone cancer, small fracture, or dislocation of the joint), such pain that follows excessive or unaccustomed demands is usually the result of self-limiting soft tissue injury or inflammation. The name given to the disorder depends on which of the soft tissues around the joint has become inflamed, and will derive from the name of the structure, followed by *-itis* (a suffix meaning inflammation or infection of). Common ones include the following:

- *Bursitis*. The bursae can swell and become inflamed and painful with unusual or repetitive use of the joint. Commonly involved areas of bursitis include the shoulder, hip, knee, and elbow.

- *Tendinitis*. Inflammation of the tendon that attaches muscle to bone can occur in any joint, but commonly occurs in the shoulder, elbow, knee, and wrist.

- *Tenosynovitis*. When the inflammation involving a tendon also includes the synovium (joint lining), the disorder is referred to as a tenosynovitis. Areas of small, numerous joints, such as hands or feet, are often affected by this variant of soft tissue rheumatism.

- *Chondritis*. Inflammation of the cartilage surface or its covering is termed chondritis. Typical sites for cartilage inflammation include the junction of the ribs and the breast bone.

What you can do Apply ice packs to the affected area daily until the pain is gone. Rest the affected joint by supporting it. Support a painful shoulder with an arm sling; rest knees or hips by limiting weight bearing activity; rest wrists and elbows by limiting motion with a soft splint or supportive elastic bandage. Following the period of rest, begin to gently move the joint through its full range of motion. Do not force the joint beyond the point of pain. Frozen joints can result if you do not move soon enough.

Rest and taking acetaminophen for 24 to 48 hours may help. If your symptoms persist you should take an over-the-counter (OTC) nonsteroidal anti-inflammatory drug (NSAID) to help to relieve the discomfort.

When to call the doctor You should contact your doctor if you experience an increase in pain, swelling, or loss of function despite ice and rest.

Treatment When OTC medications and range-of-motion exercises have failed to resolve the problem, the doctor may recom-

mend a prescription strength anti-inflammatory agent or may elect to infiltrate the joint, bursa, or tendon with an injection of a potent and long-acting anti-inflammatory corticosteroid medication (synthetic form of the body's natural stress hormone, cortisol). A course of more intensive professional physical therapy may also be necessary.

Prognosis Excellent with appropriate medical management, although the condition may recur with repeated overuse.

❖ FIBROMYALGIA SYNDROME

Symptoms (*What you may experience*) Symmetrical pain in specific trigger spots. Sometimes: migraine; difficulty sleeping; irritable bowel syndrome (alternating bouts of constipation or diarrhea); fatigue.

Signs and laboratory findings (*What the doctor looks for*) Tenderness to pressure over specific trigger points; physical and laboratory examination results.

What is it? This common disorder of the musculoskeletal system typically afflicts women, who may complain of total body pain or hurting all over. Applying pressure over certain symmetrical trigger points (the same spot on the right and left sides of the affected structure) elicits substantial pain. These paired trigger points commonly include the neck, shoulder girdle, either side of the breast bone, the lower back at the sacroiliac joints (located an either side of the pelvis), the outsides of the elbows and hips, and either side of the knees. Laboratory evaluation is usually normal; the disorder is neither destructive nor deforming, but may wax and wane chronically and be quite disabling and frustrating. Fibromyalgia syndrome may be associated with sleep disturbances, migraine, and irritable bowel syndrome.

A disorder that can mimic fibromyalgia is polymyalgia rheumatica. It differs from fibromyalgia in age distribution (typically affecting the elderly) and in causing certain laboratory abnormalities, including anemia and an elevation of ESR (see Polymyalgia Rheumatica and Giant Cell Arteritis, page 639).

What you can do Recognize triggers: stress, lack of exercise, poor sleep, and other health problems. Remain physically active. One component of the syndrome is that it worsens during periods of deconditioning. Low impact aerobic exercise or swimming can be quite helpful. Restful sleep is also critical.

When to call the doctor A thorough medical evaluation is necessary in all instances of chronic musculoskeletal pain to eliminate other more serious causes, such as hypothyroidism (see page 1188), lupus, or inflammatory arthritis. Once the diagnosis of fibromyalgia has been definitively made by your doctor, you should call if the quality of the pain changes, its intensity increases, or it fails to respond to your prescribed treatment regimen.

Treatment Low doses of tricyclic antidepressant medications at bedtime may be helpful in treating the sleep disturbances and in reducing pain. Often a team approach is used, including behavioral therapy to aid in stress management, physical therapy for planned exercise, and prescription medications for pain and sleep.

Prognosis The condition waxes and wanes in its severity. It may persist for many years, but is neither destructive nor fatal. It may disappear spontaneously in some cases.

❖ SOFT TISSUE TRAUMA (PULLED MUSCLES, CONTUSIONS, LIGAMENT TEARS, AND MUSCLE OR TENDON RUPTURES)

Symptoms *(What you may experience)* Acute pain in a discrete area (hand, foot, back, neck, leg, hip, shoulder, etc.) immediately following an injury; an audible pop at the moment of injury (sometimes); swelling and bruising within 24 hours (usually).

Signs and laboratory findings *(What the doctor looks for)* Specific tenderness over the injury; loss of normal motion (in muscle or tendon ruptures).

What is it? When physical activity stretches a muscle, tendon, or ligament beyond its limits, these soft tissues will fail, tearing or, in some cases, snapping in two. The type of injury sustained depends in large measure on the kind of stress applied.

Ligaments function to connect bones to one another as well as to define the limits of joint motion in both amount and direction. Ligament tears commonly occur when a sudden force is applied to a joint beyond its defined limits or in a direction in which it is not designed to move. For example, stability of the knees hinges on ligament support from both sides—the medial (inner) and lateral (outer) collateral ligaments—and from within—the anterior and posterior cruciate ligaments. The knee is designed to move like a hinge, opening and closing front to back, but not to twist or rock side to side. An injury that traps the foot and lower leg, but allows the thigh and hip to continue to twist (such as commonly happens in a fall on snow skis or in the tackling of a running back in football), applies an unnatural twisting or side-to-side force on the knee and often ruptures the cruciate or collateral ligaments.

Tendon ruptures often occur with a sudden, strong stretch of the muscle. These tend to occur more commonly with age, as the tendons become less elastic and flexible. Rupture of a tendon is usually accompanied by the sound or sensation of a pop. Some common ruptures include those of

IMMEDIATE CARE OF SOFT TISSUE INJURIES

Any contusion (direct blow), crush, or twisting injury to the soft tissues can tear blood vessels, allowing bleeding into the tissues and the formation of a bruise. To properly render immediate care following any such injury, use the rest-ice-compress-elevate (RICE) regimen.

Rest Avoid any activities that may cause pain or swelling. Rest is essential to promote tissue healing.

Ice the Injury Place crushed ice in a zip-closure bag. Protect the skin with a soft cotton washcloth (or a few turns of an elastic bandage) and lay the bag atop it. Ice the area for 15 to 20 minutes, repeating the procedure as often as is necessary until the swelling goes down.

Compress the Swelling Use an elastic bandage applied evenly but not too tightly to hands, feet, arms, or legs to prevent swelling of the injury. After making a few turns of the elastic bandage over the injured part, apply the zip-closure ice bag, then secure it with the remaining length of the elastic bandage to keep it from sliding off.

Elevate the Injured Part To help relieve swelling, lie down on a sofa, recliner, bed, or even the floor. Elevate the affected part using pillows, the sofa back, or a nearby chair so the injured area is higher than the joint above it. (The foot should be higher than the knee which should be higher than the hip; the hand should be higher than the elbow which should be higher than the shoulder, etc.) ■

SPRAIN AND STRAIN— WHICH IS WHICH?

Although these two terms may seem interchangeable, they actually represent two distinct injuries. A sprain implies the tearing of a ligament—those tough fibrous structures that attach one bone to another; a strain involves a tearing injury to a muscle or tendon. Both of these injuries are termed soft tissue injuries and the immediate treatment for them is essentially the same (RICE, rest, apply ice, compress the swelling, and elevate the injured part). The long-term outlook, too, is similar, with both strains and sprains requiring a few weeks to 1 or 2 months to heal depending on severity. ■

the biceps tendon in the upper arm (see Biceps Tendinitis and Biceps Tendon Rupture, page 679); the gastrocnemius, soleus, or plantaris tendons in the calf (see Calf Muscle Tears, page 710), and the Achilles tendon—the large tendon at the back of the heel (see Achilles Tendinitis, page 717, and Achilles Tendon Rupture, page 717).

Pulling a muscle means suddenly stretching a portion of it beyond its limits. Those limits increase with muscle conditioning exercise and when the muscle has been prewarmed by gentle motion to increase blood flow to it. Sudden lengthening creates minute tears within the body of the muscle, not of sufficient magnitude to rupture the muscle as a whole but enough to cause discomfort each time that muscle bundle is asked to perform. The movement necessary to elicit pain in a pulled muscle may be very specific; when at rest, the muscle will not hurt.

Contusion of muscles occurs from a direct blow to the soft tissues—for example, being hit with a baseball or falling and landing on a hard surface. The blow crushes the soft tissues, ruptures blood vessels within, and allows blood to seep into the tissues, forming a bruise, also called a hematoma. The blood forms a hard knot in the tissues that, depending on its depth from the surface, may bruise immediately or may not become visibly discolored for hours or even days later. Large bruises may remain as firm areas in the muscle for many months. The blood, once free in the tissues, can migrate under the influence of gravity along the tissue bundles, an event that can be alarming to the layman but is expected. For example, what began as a swollen knot on the shin after a few days becomes a green and then yellowish discoloration around the back of the ankle or on the top of the foot. Likewise, the blood collection of a large bruise on the forehead (so common to toddlers) after 1 or 2 days, drifts downward to become two black eyes. While such a change in an injury might merit a discussion with your doctor, in the absence of other symptoms it should not unduly alarm you when it occurs.

Occasionally, the contused area of muscle may calcify during healing (a condition termed myositis ossificans). This causes the area to become very firm and hard. If it continues to enlarge, you should see your doctor.

What you can do Follow the RICE rule for the first 48 hours following any acute soft tissue injury (see Immediate Care of Soft Tissue Injuries, page 633). See Chapter 13 for more information on treating injuries.

For discomfort, take acetaminophen. Avoid aspirin or other NSAIDs in acute soft tissue injury, because their blood thinning effect can worsen the bruising by increasing the tendency for blood to seep into the tissues.

Ice should be applied daily until the pain and swelling are gone. Gentle, controlled motion of an injured joint or muscle at this time is advisable; early mobility improves outcome.

When to call the doctor Following an injury, consult a doctor if you cannot move a joint through its full, normal range of motion (compared to its partner on the opposite side), if you feel or hear a pop at the moment of injury, if a joint swells and discolors immediately, if significant discomfort accompanies the injury, or if discomfort lasts longer than 48 hours.

Treatment Appropriate treatment depends on the injury sustained. Complete rupture of muscles or tendons usually requires surgery to repair the injury. Some ligament injuries that cannot or need not be surgically repaired will be temporarily immobilized (in splints or casts) to protect the area and allow it to heal. In most instances, the period of "immobilization" includes a course of physical therapy to work the tissues through a controlled and safe range of motion or the use of electrical stimulation or ultrasound to provide ongoing stimulation to the injured muscle and thereby minimize the consequences of limited activity; muscles quickly shrink and become weak with lack of use.

Prognosis Prognosis depends on the severity of the injury. Most injuries to the soft tissues heal within a matter of weeks, although some take longer. Ligament and tendon injuries—with or without surgery—may require several months of rehabilitation with exercise and physical therapy. Deep muscle contusions that form large bruises may persist as firm areas (to the touch) for many months. In some cases, they may calcify (harden due to the deposit of calcium salts) and persist indefinitely.

❖ REFLEX SYMPATHETIC DYSTROPHY

Symptoms *(What you may experience)* Moderate to intense nagging, tearing, or stinging pain, (usually); burning (occasionally); loss of motion; swelling; tenderness; excess sweating of any body area weeks or months following trauma (sometimes); later, shiny coolness of the skin of the area.

Signs and laboratory findings *(What the doctor looks for)* Thinning (loss of mineralization) of the bones as detected by x-ray studies.

What is it? Reflex sympathetic dystrophy is the term applied to a syndrome that may develop in the weeks or months following an injury, usually in the regions of the shoulder, chest, pelvis, or leg and, in some cases, following heart attack or stroke. Usually striking an older population, but affecting men and women equally, its onset is heralded by the appearance of symptoms in the hand or foot (or occasionally in the kneecap or hip) that include burning pain, loss of motion, tenderness of the joints, swelling resulting in a shiny appearance of the skin of the painful area, and excessive sweating, particularly of the limbs toward the hands and feet. It usually involves just one side of the body. The part may be cool or warmer to the touch and may exhibit loss or increased hair growth. After a period of weeks or months, the skin of the region

becomes shiny and cool. When it involves the hands, the tendons of the fourth and fifth fingers may draw into a flexed position (see Dupuytren's Contracture, page 668).

When to call the doctor The unusual appearance of these symptoms in the weeks or months following a heart attack or stroke or an injury to the arm, shoulder, chest, pelvis, or hips should prompt a visit to the doctor as soon as possible. Unless treated promptly, the syndrome can lead to irreversible damage to and possibly permanent loss of function of the affected part.

Treatment Your doctor should recommend ice and NSAIDs at full dose, and possibly an exercise program. If conservative remedies cannot resolve the syndrome, the doctor may prescribe a course of calcitonin or corticosteroid medications to control the process. Continued movement of the affected parts or areas is also recommended.

Prognosis The syndrome, although it develops somewhat suddenly, usually pursues a course of gradual progression that left untreated may culminate in permanent loss of function. With prompt and appropriate treatment, it usually resolves within weeks or months.

❖ TENDON SHEATH GANGLIA

Symptoms *(What you may experience)* Rapidly developing, usually painless but sometimes tender lump (often at the base of the finger or thumb).

Signs and laboratory findings *(What the doctor looks for)* Diagnosis can be confirmed by the withdrawal of thick, clear, jelly-like fluid, but this is seldom necessary.

What is it? These benign swellings can occur at any age, but most often develop between the ages of 20 and 50, with women affected twice as often as are men.

Tendon sheath ganglia may occur in response to minor (often unrecognized) injury of tendons, particularly those that flex the fingers. These small round lumps most commonly form in the crease at the base of the finger where it joins the palm,

WHEN AND HOW TO APPLY ICE

The application of ice or cold to an injury or an area after surgery has been shown to decrease pain and to help prevent swelling. Sports medicine specialists now recommend that ice be used not just for 24 to 48 hours after an injury or after surgery but for as many days as necessary to reduce pain and swelling and that ice be used instead of heat for relief of pain and swelling due to many causes.

There are basically two ways to apply ice to an area, and these are known as ice massage and ice bags/packs. During ice massage, the injured area is rubbed with ice directly, using either ice cubes or paper cups filled with water and frozen. Ice packs can be made with cubed or crushed ice in a plastic bag, or a bag of frozen peas can be used. Other forms of ice packs include gel packs or other devices available in the store.

Injuries on which Ice Should Be Used

- Bruises

- Sprains (such as ankle, knee, or jammed finger)

- Any injury that begins to swell

- Arthritic joints that hurt or are swollen

- The spine, joints, or arms or legs after surgery

- Stiff joints during physical therapy

How to Apply Ice

- It is recommended that ice not be applied directly to skin but with a washcloth placed in between. If you choose not to cover the skin, the ice should not be left on as long, since it can freeze the skin and result in frostbite.

- Ice packs should be left on for 15 to 20 minutes at a time.

- Ice should be applied to an area as often as every 2 hours. The more severe the pain and swelling, the more often ice should be applied.

- Ice may be used for many days in a row or until the pain and swelling subside. Ice may be used longer than just the 48 hours following injury or surgery.

- Ice massage is performed by rubbing the injured area with an ice cube or cup of ice for 10 to 15 minutes or until the skin is slightly numb. An ice cup is made by putting paper cups of water in the freezer until the water freezes. When ready to use, the paper cup is peeled away enough to expose the ice, and the cup is held while icing the involved area. This type of icing is typically used for very small areas of inflammation, such as tennis elbow or a localized inflammation of the knee or ankle. Ice massage may be performed as often as every 2 hours and may be used until the pain and swelling go away.

Injuries on which Ice Should Not Be Used

- Areas of the skin where sensation is not normal, such as in paraplegia, diabetes, or neuropathy. This type of skin does not have protective sensation and the skin can be easily frozen.

- Skin without normal blood supply due to injury, vascular disease, or surgery. Ice may decrease blood flow and further damage the area.

- Injuries to people with contraindications to the use of ice (very rare).

If there is any question about whether ice should be used or not, contact your doctor.

Signs that Ice Has Been Applied Too Long

- Pinkness of skin does not return after ice has been removed for a few minutes.

- Tingling or numbness beyond the area being iced (indicates that nerves are being frozen).

- Increasing pain despite ice and pain medication could be serious. Contact your doctor if you have any doubts.

Continuous Ice Devices, Cold Sprays, and Balms

Some doctors may recommend continuous ice devices, which usually do not get as cold as a regular ice pack and can be left on the area for longer periods of time. Cold sprays or balms that promote cold are generally not as good as ice bags or ice massage to produce cold. Usually the cold produced is of short duration and they can be expensive and cannot be used every few hours as ice can. ■

Source: McFarland EG, Cosgarea AJ: Patient Guide to Ice Techniques. Johns Hopkins Sports Medicine, Baltimore, Maryland.

---

but could occur in other tendons as well. Tendon sheath ganglia on the finger or thumb are the same as ganglia that occur on tendons elsewhere on the body, such as on the wrist. Should such a lump occur at the wrist, see Ganglion Cyst, page 673. Tendon sheath ganglia can become painful, especially if handled frequently; it is better to leave them alone as much as is possible.

What you can do Minimize handling the ganglia to prevent its becoming irritated and somewhat painful. Should periods of increased size and discomfort occur, limit excessive use of the affected joint.

Ice massage (see When and How to Apply Ice, above) and OTC anti-inflammatory medication (such as ibuprofen) may help relieve discomfort.

When to call the doctor The initial appearance of such a swelling should prompt evaluation by a doctor for identification. Your doctor may want to perform tests to make sure the swelling is not being caused by a tumor of the tendon or another problem.

Once diagnosed as a ganglion, it can safely be ignored, unless increased pain or limitation of motion occur.

Treatment No treatment is necessary in the absence of pain, grip weakness, or unsightly appearance; this swelling does not pose a threat to health.

Withdrawal of the jelly-like contents of the ganglia (under local anesthesia in the doctor's office) is curative in about half the cases.

Surgery to remove the ganglion results in 95 percent success.

Prognosis The prognosis is excellent, although the ganglia occasionally recur even following removal.

❖ MUSCLE CANCERS

Symptoms *(What you may experience)* Slowly enlarging, usually painless lump deep within a muscle.

Signs and laboratory findings *(What the doctor looks for)* Identification of the tumor using x-rays; diagnosis as confirmed by a microscopic examination of surgical biopsy specimen.

What is it? While cancerous growths rarely originate within the muscle tissue, they represent the most common tumor of this type in children and adolescents (in whom soft tissue cancers are quite rare); they can develop in all age groups. These cancers, also called rhabdomyosarcomas, rarely cause pain or tenderness of the muscle and are usually noticed as enlarging masses, deep within the muscle tissue.

When to call the doctor Any steadily enlarging lump in a muscle—particularly in children—should prompt evaluation by a doctor.

Treatment Treatment consists of surgical removal of the tumor, or as much of it as is possible. If metastasis (spread) of the cancer is suspected, surgery will be accompanied by radiation or chemotherapy (administration of a combination of powerful anticancer medications), which can also help prevent recurrences. See Chapter 30 for more information on the treatment of cancer.

Prognosis Early detection improves prognosis, which depends upon the location and stage of the cancer at the time of diagnosis. Tumors of the head and neck and genitourinary tract have a better prognosis than do tumors that originate in some other parts of the body. Five-year survival rates are as high as 82 percent in cancer cases diagnosed at an early stage, and as low as 27 percent in cases in which tumors have metastasized at the time of diagnosis.

Immunologic Rheumatic Disorders

The musculoskeletal system can be roughly divided into the bones, the soft tissues (muscles, tendons, ligaments, bursae, and cartilage), and the tissues that connect them. This varied group of connecting tissues includes the supportive fibrous material that surrounds the blood vessels, the synovial tissues that line the joints, and the fascia (the fibrous material that covers muscle bundles). These tissues and the soft tissues share a common risk in that they are subject to the development of generalized inflammatory disorders that were once lumped together under the rubric of rheumatism. Although the rheumatic disorders discussed in this section are themselves distinct entities, broad overlap exists among them. They share a common underlying cause: an exaggerated response on the part of the immune system in which it mistakenly attacks its own normal body tissues. These kinds of disorders are referred to as autoimmune disease. See page 946 for more information on autoimmunity and the immune system.

❖ POLYMYOSITIS/ DERMATOMYOSITIS

Symptoms *(What you may experience)* Muscle weakness, especially of the hips and shoulders; patchy reddish rash on face, around eyes, on knuckles, knees, ankles, and elbows; occasionally, fever, weight loss, and muscle and joint tenderness; sometimes Raynaud's syndrome (symptoms include an extreme sensitivity of the fingers to cold).

Signs and laboratory findings *(What the doctor looks for)* Elevated levels of muscle enzymes (a confirmation of muscle fiber breakdown) as well as elevated levels of certain autoantibodies, particularly the Anti-Jo-1, as shown by blood tests; confirmation of damage as shown by microscopic examination of muscle tissue biopsy; abnormal electrical patterns on an electromyogram (EMG)—a test that makes a tracing of electrical activity in muscles, much like the electrocardiogram (ECG) does for the heart—that occur in 90 percent of people with polymyositis or dermatomyositis. Abnormal electrical patterns on an EMG are not specific for this condition.

What is it? Polymyositis is an inflammatory rheumatic autoimmune disease that strikes the muscles; if it is accompanied by an inflammatory process that strikes the skin as well, it is called dermatomyositis. Although the exact nature of the disease is unknown, current research suggests that it may occur because certain types of the body's own white blood cells infiltrate and attack the tissues. These two conditions are quite rare, but as with most rheumatic diseases, the occurrence in women outnumbers that in men (by about two to one). These disorders can occur at any age but tend to strike adults between the ages of 30 and 70 and children between the ages of 5 years old and 15 years old.

In most cases the onset is gradual, with symptoms developing over a period of 3 to 6 months; occasionally, however, the development is sudden. In either case, the symptoms may disappear and reappear without identifiable cause.

Myositis means inflammation of the muscles. One of the first symptoms of the disorders may be muscle weakness, manifest in the hips and thighs as a difficulty in climbing stairs or getting into or out of a bathtub. With shoulder muscle involvement, raising the arms to reach high shelves or brushing or combing hair may prove daunting. The leg muscles are involved more commonly than are the arms. The muscles usually appear normal until very late in the evolution of the disorder when they may shrink in size. The pattern of muscle involvement and the normal appearance helps to differentiate this disorder from neurologic disorders such as amyotrophic lateral sclerosis (Lou Gehrig's disease) or myasthenia gravis that may also cause weakness of muscles.

Muscle weakness seen in polymyositis may affect other groups besides those in the legs or arms, bringing with it a variety of symptoms. For example, involvement of the chest muscles or diaphragm may make it hard to take a deep breath. When the muscles of the neck are involved, swallowing, speaking for long intervals, or even lifting the weight of the head off a pillow may prove difficult.

In addition to the muscle inflammation, some people also develop an inflammation of the dermis (deep layers of skin) that results in a patchy red rash, typically seen on the face, around the eyes, and over the bends of joints, such as the elbows, knees, ankles, and knuckles. When this occurs a diagnosis of dermatomyositis is made.

Although the muscles and joints may not be particularly tender in some people with this disorder, in others they are. A few people may also develop Raynaud's phenomenon (see Raynaud's Syndrome/Phenomenon, page 1227) a condition in which cool temperatures cause an exaggerated spasm of the blood vessels supplying the fingers. Upon exposure to cold, the fingers become quite pale, then almost blue. Upon rewarming, they blush and sometimes throb.

In about 10 percent of people, a vasculitis (inflammation of the blood vessels) may accompany the disease; typical symptoms associated with the vasculitis are small areas of tissue damage (dark spots) around the fingernails, ulcerated sores on the pads of the fingers, or tender red bumps under the skin.

Polymyositis, or more likely, dermatomyositis, can develop in conjunction with an underlying malignancy in about 5 to 10 percent of people who have these disorders, especially so after age 50—the most common forms of cancer associated with these disorders being lung, breast, ovary, prostate, and colon. The development of vasculitis makes the possibility of malignancy as a cause more likely, increasing the need for your doctor to search for a possible undiagnosed cancer.

What you can do Adhering to a schedule of regular physical therapy can keep muscles stronger and more mobile; therapy can include heat and massage, whirlpool baths, and gentle range-of-motion exercise during times of disease activity. Remember that inactivity can worsen muscle weakness, too.

Avoid deep muscle massage or heavy physical workouts during these periods, since the inflamed muscle fibers are fragile and more easily damaged by such activities.

Take frequent rest breaks during times of disease activity; the amount of rest needed is proportional to the severity of symptoms.

When to call the doctor Persistent muscle weakness—particularly of the arm and leg muscle groups closest to the trunk (thighs and hips, shoulders and upper arms)—should prompt a visit to the doctor. Because there is muscle weakness, but little pain, early symptoms are too often ignored, which can be unfortunate, since polymyositis and dermatomyositis respond well to early treatment.

Treatment The mainstays of therapy are the corticosteroid medications, most commonly prednisone. In the early stages of the disease, the dose may be quite high, tapering after several weeks as the symptoms improve and follow-up blood tests show lower levels of muscle enzymes. At some point, the corticosteroid may be dropped completely.

The doctor may turn to stronger immunosuppressive medications, such as methotrexate, azathioprine, cyclosporine, or cyclophosphamide, to slow down the immune system's attack. Both corticosteroids and other immunosuppresive medications are potent, and can have serious side effects, among them weight gain, easy bruising, bone thinning, hypertension (high blood pressure), cataract formation, diabetes mellitus, stomach ulcers, depression, and increased risk of infection. IV gamma globulin has been reported to be helpful in treating dermatomyositis.

Do not discontinue or reduce your steroid medication without your doctor's guidance. Because of the high doses needed to arrest the disease progress, the body temporarily stops making its own natural steroids.

Prognosis These conditions are chronic, waxing and waning over many years, but can be suppressed and controlled with proper medical management. Those people who develop the condition in association with a malignancy may not respond as favorably. In general, older age and involvement of the heart muscle worsens the prognosis.

❖ POLYMYALGIA RHEUMATICA AND GIANT CELL ARTERITIS

Symptoms *(What you may experience)* Persistent stiffness and pain in the muscles of the neck, shoulders, and pelvis; headache; cramping of the jaw muscles; vision changes; frequently, fatigue, fever, and malaise.

Signs and laboratory findings *(What the doctor looks for)* Tenderness and diminished pulse felt over the temporal artery; elevated erythrocyte sedimentation rate (ESR) (see Evaluation of the Musculoskeletal System, page 630); anemia as detected by blood testing (possibly); confirmation of diagnosis via surgical biopsy of temporal artery.

What is it? Giant cell arteritis, so named because of the presence of giant cells seen on microscopic examination of biopsy specimens, is an autoimmune inflammatory disorder of medium to large blood vessels and the most common form of vasculitis in the Northern Hemisphere. It most often develops in whites of northern European or Scandinavian descent and less frequently among Hispanic, Asian, and black populations. Polymyalgia rheumatica, a closely related inflammatory disorder of certain muscle groups, occurs in the same general population groups, typically striking people over age 50, but the average age of onset is around age 70. Although the disorders usually develop abruptly, occasionally they may come on gradually.

The two disorders commonly (but not invariably) occur together. Polymyalgia is more likely to occur alone; it occurs two to three times more commonly than does giant cell arteritis. They also share many common general symptoms: fatigue, malaise, weight loss, depression, anemia, and elevation of the ESR, which is a nonspecific measure of inflammation in the body.

In 90 percent of people, the inflammatory damage of giant cell arteritis occurs in the medium-sized branches of the aorta, the main artery carrying blood from the heart to the rest of the body. Although giant cell arteritis could develop in any medium-sized or large artery and thereby produce some very unusual symptoms, those most commonly involved are the temporal, vertebral, and ophthalmic (eye) arteries supplying blood to the head and eyes. This pattern gives rise to the common symptoms of headache, tenderness in the temporal area, cramping of the jaw muscles on chewing, and visual disturbances. The tenderness over the temporal area may be of significant enough degree to make combing hair or wearing glasses uncomfortable in some instances. Cramping of the jaw, while chewing (especially meat) or during prolonged talking, occurs because the inflammation of the arteries reduces blood flow to the jaw muscles. Inflammation of the ophthalmic arteries can lead to blindness if undetected and untreated. See page 556 for more information on giant cell arteritis.

In polymyalgia, the inflammation of muscles primarily involves those of the shoulders and pelvis. The disorder causes painful stiffness of these muscles, rather than weakness. The discomfort of the shoulder muscles may make it difficult to lift the head and shoulders to get out of bed, shampoo hair, or put on a heavy jacket or coat. Pain in the pelvic muscles may be evident when trying to arise from a chair, climb stairs, or get out of the bathtub.

The systemic symptoms—fever, malaise, unexplained weight loss, fatigue, and depression—may occur temporarily and disappear, despite continued progression of the inflammatory disorder of the muscles or arteries.

What you can do Remaining physically active can improve the pain and stiffness associated with polymyalgia, which seems to worsen with inactivity. A daily routine of walking, swimming, or gentle range of motion exercise of affected muscles may help.

When to call the doctor Polymyalgia rheumatica and giant cell arteritis are very serious diseases and require immediate medical attention. Development of any vision change should prompt an immediate visit to the doctor, as it may indicate inflammation of the arteries to the eye.

Development of fever, malaise, or loss of appetite or weight should prompt a doctor's evaluation to rule out other possible causes for these nonspecific symptoms, including occult infection or cancer.

Treatment In giant cell arteritis, high dose

therapy with prednisone should begin as soon as a diagnosis is suspected—before the results of biopsy have returned—because of the risk of blindness and other vascular events. Once on treatment, most people feel better within just a few days. Doses must be slowly tapered over a long period of 6 months to 2 years.

In polymyalgia rheumatica alone (without symptoms of giant cell arteritis) lower dose prednisone is usually sufficient. Response is quick, within 1 to 3 days; in fact, failure to respond quickly to treatment should prompt investigation for other causes for the symptoms. Tapering the prednisone could prompt a return of symptoms; if this occurs your doctor will increase the medication to the lowest dose that controls symptoms or consider steroid spacing anti-inflammatory medications.

Prognosis Although the disorder is chronic, prompt and proper medical management is essential because it can prevent blindness and ongoing care can keep symptoms abated.

❖ VASCULITIS (POLYARTERITIS NODOSA, WEGENER'S GRANULOMATOSIS, TAKAYASU'S ARTERITIS, AND KAWASAKI DISEASE)

Symptoms *(What you may experience)* General symptoms: fever; weakness; fatigue; weight loss. Symptoms vary depending on the organ system involved.

Signs and laboratory findings *(What the doctor looks for)* Usually an elevation of the ESR; confirmation of diagnosis via microscopic examination of surgical biopsy of an artery segment.

What is it? In a vasculitis, inflammation destroys blood vessels. This process occurs in a variety of uncommon disorders including polyarteritis nodosa, Takayasu's arteritis, giant cell arteritis, polymyalgia rheumatica, Wegener's granulomatosis, Kawasaki disease, and Henoch-Schönlein purpura. See page 1085 for more information on Henoch-Schönlein purpura.

The development of signs or symptoms that suggest a vasculitis should prompt a visit to the doctor, since in most cases the effectiveness of treatment diminishes if delayed.

Polyarteritis nodosa The term polyarteritis means inflammation of many blood vessels. The cause of the inflammation in polyarteritis nodosa is not clearly understood, but evidence suggests it may follow infection with hepatitis B. Unlike many of the inflammatory rheumatic disorders, this condition is twice as likely to develop in men—usually after age 45—than in women.

The common symptoms include muscle aches (much like the flu), fever, and weakness. Although muscle inflammation may be the most common symptom, the disorder can affect virtually any organ in the body: the lungs, skin, intestines, and nerves. If the kidneys become affected, hypertension can result.

Because of the vague nature of the early symptoms, diagnosis may prove difficult, and biopsy of affected tissues (skin, muscle, nerve, or kidney) may be necessary to confirm the condition. Angiograms (x-ray dye studies of the arteries) may also be helpful in making the diagnosis.

Treatment with corticosteroids will quiet the inflammation, although other immunosupressive medications are often needed to control this life-threatening disease. Serious side effects can arise from long-term use, such as increased risk for infection, easy bruising, bone weakness, and a heightened risk for fracture.

Takayasu's arteritis Thickening of the artery walls that occurs in this disease diminishes the pulse in the wrists, giving rise to its other name: pulseless disease. It affects more women than men, and primarily strikes young adults in their 20s and 30s.

Fever, muscle and joint pain, and fatigue may occur as early symptoms. As inflammation of the blood vessels progresses, the narrowing of the artery will ultimately block the flow of blood.

The absence of palpable (feelable) pulses at the wrists suggests the condition; angiography will confirm the diagnosis.

Early treatment with corticosteroid medications can stop the inflammation and prevent the narrowing of the arteries. Other immunosuppressive drugs may be necessary. Once narrowing has occurred, medications will not prove as beneficial, and

surgery may be necessary to restore blood flow by bypassing the blocked arteries.

Wegener's granulomatosis This form of vasculitis primarily involves blood vessels in the sinuses, lungs, and kidneys. Almost always, the condition begins with persistent symptoms of the upper and lower respiratory tracts, including chronic sinusitis, nasal crusting, congestion, ulceration in the nasal passages, nosebleeds, repeated ear infections, chronic cough, production of bloody phlegm, a sense of breathlessness, and pleurisy (chest pain with breathing). Not uncommonly, arthritis and fever may also accompany the onset of the disease. Diagnosis hinges on specific blood abnormalities (elevated ESR and positive antineurophil cytoplasmic antibody test and characteristic abnormalities on chest x-ray or computed tomography (CT) scan. Occasionally, only lung biopsy can confirm the diagnosis. Treatment with cyclophosphamide (a powerful cancer-killing drug) has altered the prognosis of this once quickly fatal disease to a manageable chronic condition characterized by flares and long periods of remission. The disease strikes men and women with equal vigor, and although it can arise at any time in life, usually develops after age 40.

Kawasaki disease This inflammatory disorder of blood vessels occurs in young children less than 5 years old; boys are more likely to develop it than are girls. Although the cause is not known with certainty, evidence points to a viral infection.

The disorder begins with a few days of high spiking fever followed by swelling of the eyelids, palms of the hands, and soles of the feet. Redness of the lips and tongue along with a rash on the back and buttocks develop during this period. Many children experience muscle and joint aches. Lymph glands may become swollen. In a minority of children, the inflammation may involve the coronary arteries that supply blood to the heart.

Diagnosis can prove difficult since a wide range of childhood viral illnesses can cause similar symptoms; however, the development of the specific signs listed above suggests this condition.

Treatment with aspirin is usually sufficient to reduce the inflammation and fever. Two-dimensional echocardiography should be done to rule out coronary artery involvement which, if present, is treated with IV gammaglobulin. Although in most instances the child will recover without any major problem within a few weeks, late cases of coronary artery disease have been reported, so careful follow-up is essential. *Always seek your doctor's advice before administering aspirin to a child because of the risk of Reye's syndrome (see pages 463 and 854).*

❖ SYSTEMIC LUPUS ERYTHEMATOSUS

Symptoms *(What you may experience)* Swelling and tenderness of the joints of the hands, feet, knees, hips, elbows, and shoulders; red malar rash (across bridge of the nose) or a generalized, spotty red rash; fever; spotty hair loss; swollen lymph glands; pleuritis (chest pain associated with taking a deep breath).

Signs and laboratory findings *(What the doctor looks for)* Malar rash (see page C-27); discoid (disk-shaped) rash; photosensitivity (unusual sensitivity to the sun); mouth ulcers; arthritis; serositis; kidney disease as detected by the presence of red blood cell casts or proteinuria; neurologic disorders (seizures or psychosis); hemolytic anemia, anemia, or low white blood count; immunologic disturbances as detected by antibodies to DNA or false positive syphilis test results; positive antinuclear antibody (ANA) test. Diagnosis is made by identifying at least 4 of these 11 common findings.

What is it? Systemic lupus erythematosus (SLE, lupus) is an autoimmune rheumatic disorder of unknown cause that typically strikes young women. Women are, in fact, nine times more likely to develop lupus than are men, though when the disease does strike men it is likely to be severe. The disease also has a genetic basis; there is a 10 percent chance that any person with lupus will have another family member who also has lupus: a 100-fold greater risk than that found in the general population.

The disease typically follows a waxing and waning course, with cycles of flares and remissions occurring repeatedly over many years after its onset. For the first 50 years following its discovery in the 1890s, it was considered impossible to treat and invariably fatal within 5 years. That bleak prognosis changed with the discovery of cortisone as an effective therapy to halt the progression of the disease. Today it is rarely fatal.

Lupus involves multiple body systems (hence the term systemic), but its effects on the joints and skin are most apparent. Its skin manifestations are what give lupus its name. The classic red rash of lupus, called a malar or butterfly rash, erupts across the bridge of the nose and cheeks. The word lupus, meaning wolf, derives from this characteristic rash that was thought to resemble a wolf's markings; erythematosus is derived from the Latin word for redness. Other common sites of involvement include the lining over the heart and lungs, the nervous system, the blood clotting system, the kidney, the intestinal tract, and the heart. Because of the wide variety and potential mildness of symptoms, lupus can be difficult to diagnose. The initial episode of lupus usually causes more symptoms than do subsequent flares, but fever, malaise, fatigue, weight loss, and swollen lymph glands typically accompany flares regardless of which organ system the disease involves. In the first decade of the disorder, a flare may occur every 1 or 2 years, with the frequency decreasing as time goes by. Although many organ systems may be involved initially, the disorder usually settles into a pattern of one or two chief problem areas with time.

The damage of lupus occurs when the immune system responds by producing antibodies that attack the body's own tissues. The development of these autoantibodies harms the body in several ways. Sometimes, for example, when lupus causes anemia, the antibodies attach to body proteins (in this case, red blood cells) and destroy them. The attachment of autoantibody to body protein can also form large immune molecules that circulate in the blood and then deposit in the blood vessels of the skin, joints, and other organs, causing vasculitis. Circulation may also be impaired when the inflammation causes the blood to clot more easily.

Abnormalities of the immune system also make people with lupus somewhat more vulnerable to certain infections (a problem made even worse by the corticosteroid and immunosuppressive medications used to alleviate their symptoms). See page 945 for information on precautions to take to minimize the risk of infection.

The most potentially life-threatening and least evident damage occurs in the kidneys with the development of lupus glomerulonephritis. For more information on glomerulonephritis, see page 1084.

Certain medications can trigger a condition called drug-induced lupus. This variant of lupus usually occurs in a slightly older group of people and affects men and women almost equally. A large group of medications has been implicated in possibly causing lupus, but those medications definitely associated with this disorder include chlorpromazine (a tranquilizer), hydralazine (a blood pressure medication), isoniazid (used to treat tuberculosis), methyldopa (used to treat Parkinson's disease), and procainamide and quinidine (used to stabilize abnormal heart rhythms).

What you can do Avoid significant sun exposure—wear sunscreen and broad-brimmed hats when outdoors. Be compliant with medications, rest, exercise, and good diet.

When to call the doctor Report to your doctor any symptoms that suggest active lupus. Development of shortness of breath or significant tissue swelling of the feet and ankles could indicate kidney involvement and should be evaluated. Coughing up blood should also prompt a visit to the doctor as soon as possible.

Recurrence of fever, malaise, fatigue, unexplained weight loss, and lymph gland swelling usually signals a flare and should be reported to your doctor.

Treatment Because the disease is so variable in both its symptoms and their severity, treatment must be matched to the severity at that time.

Minor joint complaints usually respond to nonsteroidal anti-inflammatory drugs, or NSAIDs. More severe symptoms involving joints and skin may merit hydroxychloroquine (a medication used to treat malaria but that works well in lupus). Major flares may require tapering courses of corticosteroid medications or immunosuppressive medications (commonly, cyclophosphamide or azathioprine).

Prognosis Today the disease is quite manageable, with 97 percent of people surviving at 5 years and 90 percent at 10 years.

Serious kidney disease, especially early in the course of the disease, worsens the prognosis. The disease also appears to progress more rapidly and fatally in those people who develop bleeding in the lung.

❖ SCLERODERMA

Symptoms *(What you may experience)* Cold sensitivity in the fingers and toes with color changes or skin ulcers; hardening or thickening and shiny appearance of the skin, especially of the hands, arms, and face; skin tightness (difficulty bending fingers); pain, stiffness, warmth, or swelling in joints; small reddish spots on fingers, palms, face, lips, or tongue; gastrointestinal symptoms, such as difficulty swallowing, heartburn, constipation, diarrhea, nausea, vomiting, or bloating; occasionally, shortness of breath or a persistent cough.

Signs and laboratory findings *(What the doctor looks for)* Intense Raynaud's phenomenon with sores or ulcerations on the fingers; changes in the thickness and texture of the skin of the hands, arms, and face; loss of hair over the thickened areas; telangiectasias (bursts or tufts of tiny blood vessels visible through the skin); calcinosis (hard white calcium deposits under the skin); associated Raynaud's phenomenon.

What is it? Scleroderma means hard skin. Although it can appear in children or the elderly, this rare disorder usually begins between ages 30 and 50, affecting women more commonly than men. In scleroderma, the body begins to lay down excessive amounts of collagen (the main protein component of fibrous tissues) in certain areas, most visibly in the fingers and hands, toes and feet, and the face. The reason for this deposition is not clearly understood, but researchers believe that injury to small blood vessels (causing Raynaud's phenomenon) and an abnormal response of the body's immune system—called an autoimmune reaction—play a role. New evidence suggests that abnormal function of small blood vessels causes low oxygen to the tissues. This low oxygen state triggers tissue injury that provokes an autoimmune response.

Scleroderma occurs in two basic types: localized and generalized. The localized variant mainly involves the skin, and to a lesser degree the muscles and bones, but does not affect the internal organs. The generalized variety involves many body parts: the skin, blood vessels, esophagus (pipe connecting the throat and stomach), stomach, bowel, heart, lungs, kidneys, muscles, and joints. In some rare instances, scleroderma may involve only the internal organs, leaving the skin unaffected.

Within the generalized variety, further subdivision includes two types of disease: limited and diffuse. The acronym CREST stands for the typical spectrum of symptoms that occur with this variant of limited disease disorder: calcinosis; Raynaud's phenomenon; esophageal dysfunction (difficulty swallowing); sclerodactyly (hardening and stiffness of the skin of the fingers); and telangiectasia. This form of scleroderma appears slowly, with the first symptoms appearing 10 to 20 years before any serious internal organ involvement. It usually involves the skin of the fingers and face and leaves a mild expression of disuse in the internal organs.

In diffuse generalized scleroderma, the collagen deposition may go on throughout the body, usually involving the skin of the arms, thighs, chest, and abdomen as well as the face and hands. This form may progress more rapidly in some people and may involve many body systems, among them the lungs, kidneys, heart, bowels, blood vessels, and joints. Symptoms related to involvement of these organs include difficulty swallowing, shortness of breath, persistent cough, hypertension, muscle weakness, and arthritis.

Involvement of the kidney often occurs in the first year of the disease and can be a particularly hard to detect problem. This is a greater risk for those people who develop hypertension related to scleroderma. Important symptoms that could signal kidney involvement include persistent severe headache, shortness of breath, visual disturbances, chest pain, and mental confusion.

Because of its widespread and variable nature, scleroderma may be difficult to diagnose. Although specific blood tests and physical findings can be quite definitive, it may take several visits to the doctor (or often to several different types of specialists—rheumatologist and dermatologist) before a diagnosis is confirmed. Special tests can identify esophageal involvement, and now tests are available to detect lung problems much earlier in their development.

What you can do Take the following measures:

- Keep warm; avoid exposure to the cold.

- Remain active; regular exercise improves mobility, keeping the skin and joints more flexible, improving blood flow to these tissues, and helping to prevent contractures (fixation of the joints): Good exercises include swimming (in warm water), cycling, and walking. Try to perform range-of-motion exercises for particular joints—opening and closing the affected joints, moving the shoulder or hip through its full motion in all directions—twice daily. For example, stretch your fingers flat on a table top to keep them from becoming stiff in a flexed position. Gently flatten them with your other hand.

- Muscle and joint pain and swelling may benefit from acetaminophen or over-the-counter (OTC) anti-inflammatory medications such as ibuprofen.

- Protect your joints from excessive trauma; avoid lifting and carrying heavy loads. Rest and protect painful joints in soft removable splints or slings.

- Protect your skin from extreme cold. Dress warmly (in several layers of insulating material) and wear warm gloves in cold weather to protect skin and maintain good blood flow. Cover exposed facial skin with a warm scarf.

- Keep skin moist by using nondrying bath soaps and oils—avoid strong detergents that may dry the skin. Use a mist humidifier during cold weather or in dry climates to assist in keeping skin moist.

- *Do not* attempt to excise or remove the calcium deposits that form; on occasion, they may be injured or may rupture spontaneously and drain a chalky white liquid. They are harmless and opening them (even by spontaneous rupture) could lead to infection.

- If you suffer from gastrointestinal disturbances, it may help to eat smaller portions of food more often—for example, six small meals a day as opposed to three larger ones. Chew the food well to reduce the risk of choking as you swallow larger bites. Eat your largest meals early in the day, avoiding heavy meals before bedtime. Prop the head of your bedframe up on 6 in. blocks to elevate you slightly during sleep to prevent acid reflux into the esophagus.

- Dry eyes may benefit from the use of such OTC products as artificial tear solutions (lubricating eyedrops to replenish the moisture normally provided by natural tears. See Dry Eye Syndrome, page 515, for more information on treating dry eyes.

- Vaginal dryness may respond to OTC vaginal lubricants.

When to call the doctor Worsening of any of the problems associated with this disorder—or the appearance of new ones—merits a consultation with your doctor as soon as possible.

Treatment Medications that control the disease or permanently soften the skin do not exist but many treatments are available that can improve quality of life and prolong survival. Treatment of the disease varies depending on the symptoms. When OTC remedies for inflammatory pain have proven insufficient, prescription-strength medications may offer relief of inflammation and pain. On occasion, the judicious use of steroid medications may be necessary to quiet the arthritis or muscle inflamation. The development of hypertension usually demands medication to contain it, since, left untreated, hypertension can damage the kidneys. Medications that improve blood flow may be helpful in combating Raynaud's phenomenon. New medications can control gastrointestinal malfunction and reflux disease. Pulmonary complications can be treated by immunosuppressive medications.

Prognosis Scleroderma is a chronic disease, meaning it can last for months, years, or a lifetime. Although there is no cure for it, it can be treated; and with prompt and appropriate medical management, many people with the disease can lead full, productive lives. It is recommended that people with scleroderma consult regularly with a rheumatologist and that they visit a special scleroderma center.

❖ SJOGREN'S SYNDROME

Symptoms (*What you may experience*) Dry eyes, dry mouth, dry skin, dryness in the vagina, and musculoskeletal pain.

Signs and laboratory findings (*What the doctor looks for*) Increased numbers of decayed teeth; decreased tear formation as detected by Schirmer's test; confirmation of diagnosis by microscopic analysis of biopsy specimens from the small salivary glands within the lips; low white-blood-cell count, mild anemia, elevated ESR, the presence of certain antibodies (anti-Ro) suggestive of the disease, or hyperglobulinemia (presence of excess immune system components called gamma-globulin) as detected by blood testing.

What is it? Sjogren's syndrome—also called sicca syndrome—typically occurs after age 50, although it can begin at any time in life. It affects women more frequently than it does men. Its cardinal symptom—eye dryness, a condition called xerophthalmia—reflects failure of the lacrimal (tear) glands to produce sufficient fluid. The same failure can be seen in the salivary glands as in dry mouth, and in fact the biopsy proof of the condition usually comes from specimens of tissue taken from the lip lining where the minor salivary glands lie. The condition is believed to have an autoimmune basis—the body's defenses mistakenly attack its own tissues—and microscopic analysis of specimens of tissue taken from these areas show an invasion of white blood cells around the glands that produce saliva (or tears). A less invasive test can document insufficient production of tears. In this procedure, called the Schirmer test, absorbent paper strips are placed between the lower eyelid and the anesthetized eyeball, allowing measurement of the amount of tears produced (absorbed through the strip).

Lack of tear production will leave the eyes feeling gritty, dry, and irritated, and can make the nerve-rich cornea (the clear portion over the iris and pupil) vulnerable to damage. Lack of salivary production impairs the natural cleansing of the mouth and teeth, and as a consequence, the incidence of dental cavities rises as food particles more easily adhere to the teeth. Moistening a bite of food for thorough chewing can also become difficult. Dryness of the skin and airways of the respiratory tract, arthritis, and fatigue are common. Swelling of the parotid gland can mimic mumps.

Sjogren's syndrome may occur alone or in association with other autoimmune disorders, including systemic lupus erythematosus, rheumatoid arthritis, polymyositis (see Polymyositis/Dermatomyositis, page 637), scleroderma, Hashimoto's thyroiditis (see page 1189), autoimmune hepatitis (see Chronic Active Hepatitis, page 1042), and primary biliary cirrhosis (see page 1058).

What you can do To relieve gritty dryness of the eyes, use any of the OTC artificial tear eyedrop solutions as frequently as needed to prevent symptoms and keep the cornea moist.

Dry mouth is more difficult to relieve, but it helps to increase fluid intake, chew sugarless gum, or use sour sugarless mints or lozenges. Avoid candies, drinks, or desserts containing sugar, since the lack of natural saliva creates an environment much more favorable for the development of dental cavities. Regular dental checkups for cleaning and fluoride treatment will also help to minimize their formation. Recent studies have shown that pilocarpine can improve saliva production.

When to call the doctor Sjogren's syndrome is a system disorder (affecting many systems of the body) so it is appropriate to call your doctor if new symptoms occur. Recurrent or pronounced enlargement or firm swelling of the salivary glands (either the parotid glands in the cheek or those under the chin) merits a visit to the doctor to investigate the possibility of lymphoma (a cancer of the lymph glands) or a salivary gland tumor.

Development of significant eye pain may indicate a corneal erosion from overdrying and should prompt a visit to your doctor or an ophthalmologist.

Treatment Since this condition is associated with several other autoimmune disorders, treating the chief problem will usually be the focus of medical therapy.

Occasionally, the doctor may recommend a course of phaguenil or a corticosteroid medication to relieve significant enlargement of the parotid glands or the symptoms of dry mouth. Pilocarpine may help dry mouth.

Prognosis The disorder, while causing discomfort, is usually not life threatening. Persistence or slow progression of the drying of the eyes, mouth, and vaginal tissues can

occur. A minority of people who develop Sjogren's syndrome—particularly those who suffer recurrent bouts of salivary gland enlargement—may develop vasculitis or lymphoma.

Generalized Disorders of the Joints

❖ RHEUMATOID ARTHRITIS AND JUVENILE RHEUMATOID ARTHRITIS

Symptoms *(What you may experience)* Persistent pain, swelling, warmth, and limited motion of the shoulders, elbows, wrists, ankles, or the joints of the hands and feet or neck; unusual tendency to become fatigued (often); fever (usually of low grade, but can be high in children); lack of energy; rheumatoid nodules (tender soft lumps) near the joints (occasionally).

Signs and laboratory findings *(What the doctor looks for)* Characteristic pattern of joint involvement; elevated ESR; high levels of particular antibodies (anti-IgG or rheumatoid factor) or other markers of inflammation such as C-reactive protein or alpha$_2$-globulins (often); mild anemia; later, development of bony changes visible on x-ray.

What is it? Rheumatoid arthritis (RA) is a relatively common autoimmune inflammatory disorder affecting about 1 percent of the adult population. The majority of people who develop RA are young to middle-aged adults, but it can arise at any age, affecting infants and young children—where it is called juvenile rheumatoid arthritis (JRA)—as well as the elderly. Twice as many women as men develop it in adulthood, but the gender disparity disappears among the elderly.

What triggers the development of RA has not been clearly identified, but the tendency to develop it appears to have a genetic basis—in other words, susceptibility to the disease may be inherited.

The disease may begin with systemic symptoms, such as low-grade fever, unusually pronounced fatigability, and lack of energy, which may precede the joint involvement. A systemic presentation with high fever and rash is commonly seen in the juvenile form. The hallmark of the disease, however, is the development of persistent arthritis, usually persisting at least 6 to 12 weeks—in a symmetrical or paired fashion: both knees, both wrists, both ankles, both elbows, both shoulders. Such symmetry is not common in any other arthritic disorder.

The inflammation and pain of RA can be extreme, with significant swelling, warmth, and visible redness of the tissues over the joint. With periods of immobility (such as overnight) the fluid within the arthritic joints becomes semisolid—a phenomenon known as gelling. The gelling causes morning stiffness of joints lasting more than an hour. This significant loss of motion and stiffness often troubles people more than does the pain.

Exuberant growth of the synovium causes a mushy feel to the swollen joints; the synovial overgrowth erodes the cartilage surface of the bone and can also compress nerves or blood vessels nearby. In the wrist, the compression can lead to carpal tunnel syndrome and in the knee to the development of large cysts (fluid-filled cavities), called Baker's cysts (see Baker's Cyst of the Knee, page 701), that can cause lower leg edema (swelling). Swelling and inflammation of tendons—particularly those at the wrist—is quite common. Dislocation, rupture, or contraction of tendons causes joint deformities characteristic of this disease.

While RA primarily affects the joints, it can also involve other organ systems, including the coverings of the heart and lungs and the lymph glands, spleen, blood vessels, and eyes. Enlargement of the spleen occurs in about 5 to 10 percent of people with RA, a combination dubbed Felty's syndrome.

Because of the variable nature of RA, early diagnosis can be difficult; it may take many months before the condition can be identified with certainty.

What you can do Maintain mobility of affected joints by daily nontraumatic exercise, such as swimming or water walking or gentle range-of-motion exercises to carefully move the joint through its full range.

Balance exercise with rest of the affected joints. Protecting and resting joints is especially important during flares of disease activity.

Apply warm or cold packs to inflamed joints; they may give symptomatic relief.

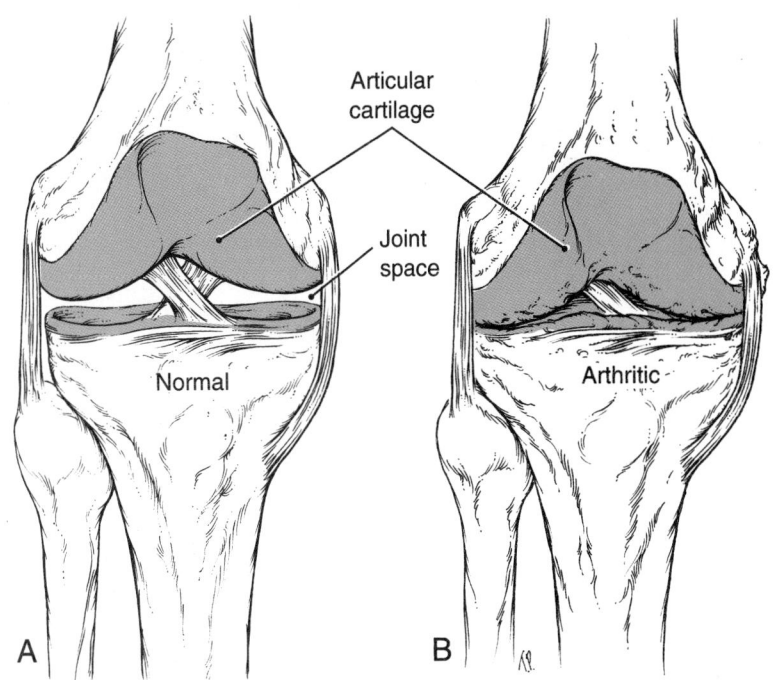

(A) Normal knee joint. (B) Arthritis can be related to inflammation or degeneration of tissues, which can lead to pain, stiffness, and swelling as well as deformities of bone, cartilage, or the space between bones.

When to call the doctor Persistent joint pain, lasting more than a few days, accompanied by joint swelling, warmth, or redness should prompt an evaluation by a doctor. Once diagnosed, notify your doctor of the appearance of new or worsening symptoms.

Treatment Controlling the inflammatory process—usually with potent anti-inflammatory medications (ranging from high-dose aspirin to the prescription medications called nonsteroidal anti-inflammatory drugs or NSAIDs), corticosteroid medications (usually prednisone), or immune-system-suppressing medications (such as methotrexate)—is the cornerstone of treatment for RA. All these medications have the potential for serious side effects, such as gastritis (stomach inflammation) or the development of ulcer disease, easy bruising, increased risk for infections, or bone weakness and an increased tendency for fracture. Their aggressive use early in the course of the disease can arrest it, sometimes for long periods, and help to preserve joint structure and function.

TOTAL WRIST REPLACEMENT SURGERY

The development of artificial replacement joints has revolutionized the field of orthopedic surgery and improved the quality of life for countless millions of people who would otherwise have been physically disabled by their condition.

Although the total wrist can be used to replace a joint damaged by major trauma, its chief use has been in people with arthritis. One of the most onerous disabilities that faces people who suffer from the joint destruction of rheumatoid arthritis is the hand deformities that result from joint damage to the bones of the wrist. In this condition, instability of the wrist joint allows the tendons and muscles of the forearm, wrist, and hand to pull the hands and fingers to the sides (toward the little finger), resulting in a deformity—called ulnar deviation—that renders the hands almost useless in time. In people with rheumatoid arthritis, the installation of an artificial total wrist prior to the development of the ulnar deviation can preserve the normal configuration of hand and wrist and prevent the loss of hand function. ■

Preserving function and mobility of joints is of paramount importance. To achieve that goal, the doctor may also prescribe courses of physical therapy and sometimes splinting of affected joints to prevent the malalignment that can occur from shortening, dislocation, or rupture of tendons.

If the disease process destroys the joint cartilage of knees, hips, ankles, or wrists, the doctor may recommend total joint replacement surgery (see Total Wrist Replacement Surgery, above, Total Knee Replacement Surgery, page 702, and Total Hip Replacement Surgery, see page 694).

Prognosis RA is a chronic disease. Early diagnosis and vigorous treatment—both medical and surgical—can prevent disability. On average, people with RA have a life expectancy about 10 years shorter than do those without it, but the course and severity of the disease are quite variable. High levels of rheumatoid factor in the blood, the development of rheumatoid nodules, and bone erosions visible on x-ray worsen the prognosis.

❖ REACTIVE ARTHRITIC DISORDERS (ANKYLOSING SPONDYLITIS, REITER'S SYNDROME, PSORIATIC ARTHRITIS, AND ENTERIC ARTHRITIS)

Symptoms *(What you may experience)* Back stiffness and pain; swollen, tender, warm large joints (especially in the hips, knees, or ankles); heel pain; swelling of the Achilles tendon; sausage-like swelling of an entire finger or toe. Ankylosing spondylitis: eye redness and pain. Reiter's syndrome: painful, frequent urination. Psoriatic arthritis: scaly rash and thick silvery patches over the elbows, knees, or knuckles. Enteric arthritis: abdominal cramping with bouts of diarrhea and blood in the stool.

Signs and laboratory findings *(What the doctor looks for)* Arthritis of the bones of the spine and often the sacroiliac joints as detected by x-rays; presence of specific histocompatibility antigens, such as human leukocyte antigen (HLA) B27, as detected by blood tests.

What is it? Development of inflammatory arthritis in the bones of the spine occurs in four related disorders: ankylosing spondylitis, Reiter's syndrome, psoriatic arthritis, and enteric arthritis. They are called reactive arthritic diseases because they seem to develop in response to—or as a reaction to—infectious triggers in susceptible people. Susceptibility appears to be inherited; among people who develop these conditions, there is a tendency to carry HLA-B27. This is especially true for ankylosing spondylitis, in which 90 percent carry this inherited marker.

These disorders also share many clinical, x-ray, and blood test findings. Among them are arthritic involvement of the spine and large joints and inflammation of the entheses, the area where tendons, ligaments, and connective tissue bands attach to the bone. A discussion of the characteristics of each of these disorders follows.

Ankylosing spondylitis This disorder occurs three times more commonly in men than in women. The term ankylosing means bony fusion and the most serious consequence of this spinal arthritis is a progressive fusion of the vertebrae (bones of the spine) with stiffening and bowing of the back. Arthritic pain of the sacroiliac joints, the hips, and shoulders is typical. The problem is more one of limitation of motion than of severe pain, but joints were made to move; when they do not, they may become fixed in position and create significant disability. This problem occurs quite commonly in the back joints.

Inflammation of the plantar fascia (a connective tissue band that forms the sole of the foot and attaches to the heel) results in heel pain. The Achilles tendon also commonly becomes inflamed.

Outside the skeleton, the disease may involve the eye, causing pain by inflaming the iris and the muscle that controls the thickness of the lens of the eye (see Uveitis, page 544). These complicating symptoms can occur at any time in the course of the disease. Other organ systems may not become involved for many years, but include the heart (causing incompetence of the aortic valve or sometimes heart rhythm disturbances), the lung (causing a fibrosis of the top portions of the lung and restriction of breathing), and the nervous system (mainly the spinal cord from compression of nerve roots by the fusing spine).

The treatment hinges on maintaining posture and mobility of the hips and shoulders. What happens during the first 10 years of the disease predicts its course. The prognosis is generally good for most people.

Reiter's syndrome This form of reactive arthritis occurs primarily in young men—it is, in fact, the most common form of chronic arthritis in this group. It clearly occurs in reaction to infections of the gastrointestinal tract (commonly caused by *Salmonella, Shigella, Campylobacter,* or *Yersinia*) or by sexually transmitted organisms (especially *Chlamydia trachomatis*).

In the classic onset, symptoms of Reiter's syndrome begin within 2 to 6 weeks following a triggering infection. In the early phase, some people may be extremely ill, with high fever, shaking chills, and rapid heartbeat. Other times, the first symptom may be nothing more than a mild discomfort or increased frequency of urination and perhaps a slight discharge of pus or mucus from the urine tube. Redness and scratchy discomfort of the eyes may also occur early on; uveitis, with significant eye

pain, redness, and sensitivity to light, may occur as well. Arthritis typically occurs last—sometimes several weeks later—usually involving joints of the legs and feet. It may persist for several months and resolve. Heel pain occurs quite commonly from inflammation of the plantar fascia or Achilles tendon. While many people with Reiter's syndrome develop low back pain from inflammation of the sacroiliac joints, only about one-fourth will show visible changes on x-ray. Often, the disorder involves the entheses, causing sausage digits in which the entire finger or toe swells.

Occasionally, people develop a rash on the palms, soles, or trunk. It begins as red blotches or clear blisters on a red base. Later the areas become thickened and scaly or form pustules (small pus-filled blisters).

Treatment consists of stopping the inflammation, usually first with a NSAID and, in some cases, with other anti-inflammatory drugs such as corticosteroids (prednisone) or a low dose methotrexate (Rheumatrex). Some doctors advocate the use of antibiotics. Although infection triggers the disorder, antibiotics to kill the bacteria may not stop the inflammation once it has begun.

In most cases, the illness subsides after several weeks or months. But its course is unpredictable; it may recur after many disease-free years. A small minority of people suffer persistent and unremitting arthritis requiring ongoing treatment.

Psoriatic arthritis This disorder, familiar as a problem of the skin, may also cause arthritis in the spine and other joints. Approximately 2 percent of the world's population suffers from the skin disorder psoriasis, but approximately 5 percent of these people will have arthritis associated with it. Usually beginning in early adulthood, this form of reactive arthritis affects men and women about equally.

Although there is an inherited component for this condition, it is much less commonly associated with antigen HLA-B27 than are the other reactive arthritic disorders. Psoriatic arthritis rarely involves organs other than the skin and skeleton.

It tends to strike one joint of a pair, but often not the other; inflammation of the entheses causes swelling of an entire finger or toe. Spinal arthritis occurs in about one in five cases and usually involves mainly the sacroiliac joints and the very low part of the lumbosacral spine.

Treatment is aimed at arresting the inflammation with potent NSAIDs or, when necessary, disease modifying agents such as methotrexate.

This form of reactive arthritis tends to be more slowly progressive and more easily controlled than are others.

Enteric arthritis   In conjunction with two inflammatory disorders of the bowel— ulcerative colitis (see page 1010) and Crohn's disease (see page 1007)—about 20 percent of people develop an arthritis. It usually occurs transiently, may migrate (affecting first one joint and then another), and is rarely destructive. Arthritis of the spine can occur, particularly of the sacroiliac joint.

Because of the associated bowel disease, treatment with aspirin or other NSAIDs should be approached with caution in this group of people. Injection of corticosteroids into specific affected joints may be helpful in reducing the inflammation locally.

Arthritic pain may wax and wane in conjunction with activity of the intestinal disease. In most cases, the arthritic symptoms may last a few weeks to a few months and then resolve without permanent joint damage. Arthritic episodes tend to be more severe and more frequent in the first few years of the bowel disease and abate somewhat with time.

What you can do   Physical therapy to keep the spine and joints mobile is of paramount importance. In preventing deformity of the spine (especially in ankylosing spondylitis) the following guidelines may prove helpful:

- Use a firm mattress

- Avoid sleeping on a pillow, which promotes forward bending of the neck

- Be conscious of posture; continually stand straight

❖ INFECTIOUS ARTHRITIS

Symptoms *(What you may experience)* Stiffness and pain in the joint; fever. Most frequently affected joints are the knee, hip, shoulder, wrist, ankle, elbow, finger, or toe.

Signs and laboratory findings *(What the doctor looks for)* Inflammation, generally of only one joint; infection as confirmed by laboratory tests on fluid extracted from the joint.

What is it? Infectious arthritis is most often caused by bacteria traveling from another source of infection through the blood-stream to the joint. It can also be caused by bacteria entering the body through an open wound. It is rarely found in healthy people who do not have a penetrating injury, previous joint surgery, prosthetic joints or an immunocompromised state. There are several types of infectious arthritis.

Gonococcal arthritis is caused by the same organism that causes gonorrhea. It is one of the most serious complications of gonorrhea as it can cause permanent damage in the joint if not treated immediately with antibiotics. Unlike nongonococcal arthritis, it affects otherwise healthy people. About a third of people with gonorrhea develop gonacoccal arthritis, and it more often affects women than it does men. It is rarely found in people over age 45.

Staphylococcal and streptococcal bacteria account for about 80 percent of non-gonococcal infectious arthritis. People whose resistance is compromised by other conditions such as rheumatoid arthritis, diabetes, alcoholism, or long-term steroid use are more susceptible to having a staph infection spread to the joint through the blood.

Lyme disease is named for the town in Connecticut where it was first discovered. It is contracted through the bite of a particular tick which leaves a ring-shaped rash around the site of the bite. Fever, muscular aching, and fatigue may accompany the arthritis.

Some viral infections may cause arthritis, such as hepatitis B, rubella (German measles), and mumps. Antibiotic treatment is not effective in viral cases and anti-inflammatory medication is usually sufficient.

When to call the doctor   Infectious arthritis can lead to permanent joint damage if left untreated. The joint can become stiff and useless due to damaged cartilage. You should be concerned about infectious arthritis if you suffer from pain in a single joint accompanied by fever; contact your doctor. If you have gonorrhea and experience joint pain, you should contact your doctor immediately as permanent joint damage can occur within days of the first sign of pain in the joint.

Treatment Antibiotics specific for the type of bacteria should be prescribed. The doctor may use a needle to drain the infected joint or surgically open the joint to remove fluid and damaged tissue. After the infection is eliminated, the joint should be exercised to prevent permanent stiffness.

Prognosis Good with immediate treatment.

❖ OSTEOARTHRITIS

Symptoms *(What you may experience)* Pain and stiffness of specific joints; knobby deformity, especially of finger joints. (See page C-42.)

Signs and laboratory findings *(What the doctor looks for)* Enlargement of the joint with little inflammation such as Heberden's nodes (knobby deformities on finger joints), which are typical of osteoarthritis (OA); x-ray studies showing characteristic bone changes. Blood tests are generally unremarkable.

What is it? The most common form of arthritis, OA has been recognized for thousands of years and is in part the consequence of years of wear and tear of joint surfaces over time. It produces symptoms most common in women and in the elderly. Although it can strike multiple joints, it may trouble only one or two. The neck and back are often involved, as are the knees, hips, and hands. Previous significant trauma to a joint may predispose to the development of arthritis in it with age. In addition, the weight-bearing joints of obese people of both genders tend to develop OA more commonly.

In OA, a wearing away of the slick cartilage surface that coats the bone ends develops in conjunction with the new growth of bone spurs, also called osteophytes, that may contribute to limitation of joint mobility. The narrowed joint spaces (from loss of cushioning cartilage) and the bony spurs are evident on x-ray. Although the bone spurs may deform the external appearance of the bones of the hands and make the joints stiff and painful, this form of arthritis rarely causes significant crippling or the destruction of joints that can occur with RA; and even severe osteoarthritis will not shorten your life span.

Although it is well documented that wear and tear plays an important role in its development, there are a number of complex biological changes of the cartilage that cause it to fail over time. Some of these may be inherited.

What you can do Allow extra time in the morning to warm and mobilize the stiff joints. In most cases of OA, morning stiffness lasts only a few minutes to perhaps a half hour. Try to develop a regular regimen of exercise (nonimpact) to keep the joints mobile. Walking, swimming, biking, and light weight training are good activities for larger joints; playing piano, typing, washing dishes, and kneading bread dough are varied activities to keep the small joints of the hands mobile.

COPING WITH THE CHRONIC PAIN OF ARTHRITIS

Once arthritis has developed in a joint (or in many joints) the condition usually persists, waxing and waning in severity to some degree, but present at some level most of the time. For that reason, it is important for any person suffering with an arthritic illness to learn to deal with the day to day stiffness and discomfort. Here are some helpful guidelines:

- Allow extra time in the morning to mobilize and warm the joints. Develop a routine of heating the joints (in the bath or shower) followed by gentle range-of-motion, stretching, and strengthening exercises.

- Recognize that arthritic pain waxes and wanes, often worsening in cold weather or during periods of barometric upheaval as storm fronts move through an area.

- Recognize that during periods of stress and emotional upheaval (depression, grief, or personal loss) the pain of arthritis may be worse. Treatment directed toward relief of the emotional disturbance will help to alleviate the arthritic discomfort.

- Since as many as 8 hours a day are spent sleeping, make an effort to find a supportive but cushioned and comfortable bed. Use extra pillows to cushion and support painful joints during sleep. ■

Shedding excess weight can help to take stress off arthritic joints.

Use acetaminophen for pain relief. If that does not work, then use OTC anti-inflammatory medications (aspirin, ibuprofen, etc.) to help reduce pain and inflammation.

Use hot pads, hot water soaks, or hot wax dipping tubs (for hands and feet) to relieve pain.

When to call the doctor The appearance of pain in a previously pain-free joint, worsening pain, or pain that limits daily activities in spite of the conservative remedies outlined above should prompt a visit to the doctor.

Treatment People with severe inflammation or pain may benefit from physical and occupational therapy that can help them learn how to protect their joints, perform daily activities, and learn more about the therapeutic use of exercise, heat, and massage.

Occasionally, inflammation may become severe enough to warrant administration of a single injection of corticosteroid medication into an arthritic joint. Recently, compounds of joint fluid have been made into an injectible form for temporary relief of knee pain. Severe destruction and loss of mobility that affect walking or spontaneous pain at night may indicate a need to demand joint replacement (the wrist, knee, and hip joints are the most commonly replaced). Recent studies suggest that arthoscopic surgery can be helpful to reduce pain—especially in the knees.

Prognosis OA is a chronic disorder that waxes and wanes. There is no cure, but the symptoms can be controlled with medication, physical therapy, exercise, and at times surgery.

❖ GOUT

Symptoms *(What you may experience)* Intermittent attacks of intense pain in the first great toe joint or other large joints (ankles, knees, or instep of the foot); tender, swollen red nodules (called tophi) under the skin near joints. (See page C-42.)

Signs and laboratory findings *(What the doctor looks for)* Elevated level of uric acid in the blood; uric acid crystals seen in microscopic examination of joint fluid; arthritic changes in joints (later) as detected by x-rays; kidney stones.

What is it? Gout has been known since antiquity. It is an inflammatory disease of joints caused by the deposition of needle-like crystals of uric acid in the joints. It usually begins after age 30 in men and age 45 in women, occurring in men more commonly than in women until menopause, when the disparity narrows.

In over half the people, the initial episode of gout occurs in the first joint of the great toe, where it joins the foot—a condition called podagra. Ultimately, up to 90 percent of people with gout will develop inflammation in this joint. Why this particular joint is so prone to gout is unclear, but it may be because the joint is more vulnerable to trauma and is cooler. Cool temperatures and trauma—even of a minor nature, such as stubbing the toe—can precipitate an attack of gout in susceptible people. Susceptibility may be inherited.

A person may suffer a series of small attacks of gout as the disorder develops, leading up to a major attack; the pain of a severe attack can be excruciating, with the inflamed joint so tender that the weight of bed coverings on it is too much to bear. Untreated, the attack can last from days to weeks and lead to damage of the joint.

A disease characterized by calcium (not uric acid) crystals in the joints resembles gout so closely that it is called pseudogout. Pseudogout is equally common in men and in women, but only half as common as is gout. It also usually strikes in different joints such as the knee or the wrist. Pseudogout begins later than does gout, generally occurring after age 65.

Uric acid—found normally in the blood—can become elevated in the blood in two ways. In about 15 percent of cases, it is the result of overproduction of urate (the salt of uric acid). In the vast majority of cases (85 percent) the elevation comes about as a result of underexcretion—that is, the kidneys fail to get rid of uric acid as effectively as they should. Most often, this inefficiency in excretion is inherited, but sometimes it is acquired, such as when the kidneys have been damaged and fail to work properly for other reasons. One of those reasons is lead toxicity, which both impairs the kidneys' ability to excrete uric acid as well as making it more likely to form crystals in the joint fluid; the gout it causes is termed saturnine gout. Many years ago, it occurred in people who drank alcohol heavily—especially sherry, which was stored in lead-lined casks. Nowadays, saturnine gout still occurs, but usually in people who drink illegally manufactured whiskey, distilled in lead-lined stills. Environmental exposure to lead in other forms, such as the lead-based paint in old houses, could be another route for the development of gout. Overproduction of urate may occur after eating too many foods containing purines, which the body metabolizes into uric acid. These foods include shellfish, sardines, and organ meats such as liver, kidney, and pancreas (sweetbreads).

Uric acid crystals can also deposit under the skin, especially near joints on the feet and hands, forming nodules—called gouty tophi. The nodules—filled with chalky white material—often become inflamed, red, warm, and painful, and may be mistaken for boils. A sample of the material, examined under the microscope, will clearly show the presence of needle-like crystals of uric acid. The tophi can erode the bone near the joints; on x-ray studies the erosion creates a characteristic picture, called a rat bite erosion because it looks like a rat has nibbled the bone away. Tophi usually only develop in untreated or inadequately treated gout.

Deposition of uric acid crystals in the kidney can also cause kidney stones (see page 1088).

What you can do Avoid eating large quantities of foods high in purines, including shellfish, sardines, and organ meats. Avoid consumption of alcohol, which increases uric acid production and inhibits uric acid excretion.

When to call the doctor At the first twinges of pain in the great toe, it would be wise to see your doctor and have uric acid levels checked, particularly if gout runs in the family. Controlling the problem before a severe attack occurs will save you from tremendous discomfort.

People with gout often have hypertension and elevated lipids (blood fats). If you have experienced gout, your doctor may want to investigate whether you have hypertension or abnormal fats in your blood.

Treatment In an acute attack, the first priority is to stop the severe inflammation and pain. The usual remedy is an NSAID, most often indomethacin, which substantially relieves the pain in the first 48 hours. Usually by 5 days, the pain is eliminated. In people who cannot take NSAIDs (usually because of peptic ulcer disease or a specific medication intolerance or allergy) the attack can be stopped with corticosteroids (by pill or local injection into the joint). Another alternative is the medication colchicine, which is effective if it is begun promptly, but not as good once the inflammation is fully established. Although once the standard of treatment, it is no longer widely used because of toxic side effects, including nausea and diarrhea.

After the acute attack has subsided, therapy focuses on reducing the excess uric acid in those people with very high levels or who have had multiple attacks. One method is to encourage the kidney to excrete more uric acid (by administering uricosuric agents, such as probenecid or sulfinpyrazone along with plenty of water) or by reducing production of uric acid. The medication most commonly employed to achieve this goal is allopurinol. The choice of which therapy to use depends on the cause of the elevation of uric acid. Long-term therapy should be reserved for people who have had multiple attacks and a uric acid kidney stone.

Prognosis The disease tends to occur in intermittent episodes over many years, but in most instances can be controlled with proper medical and dietary management. Left unmanaged, gout can cause significant disability and pain.

❖ ASEPTIC NECROSIS

Symptoms *(What you may experience)* Gradually worsening discomfort in a joint, most commonly the hip, apparently unrelated to recent trauma; development of a limp (related to hip pain); persistent discomfort in a joint long after trauma.

Signs and laboratory findings *(What the doctor looks for)* Medical history indicates alcohol abuse, prolonged use of steriods, or trauma. Motion of the affected joint may be painful; x-rays or scans—nuclear bone scan, magnetic resonance imaging (MRI) or computed tomography (CT)—confirm the diagnosis.

What is it? The term aseptic means clean or free of bacteria. While it is not uncommon for a bacterial infection in bone to destroy it (a process called necrosis), occasionally a similar appearing disorder arises unrelated to infection.

This disorder, termed aseptic necrosis, implies the death of an area of bone, caused not by infection, but most commonly by some process that impairs the blood supply that nourishes the bone. The initiating insult that prompts the damage could be trauma—a strategically located fracture, for example, that shears an important feeder artery within the bone (not an uncommon cause of this process in bones of the wrist). In the hip, another cause is long-term use of corticosteroid medications, for example, when used to treat chronic allergic inflammatory conditions.

By whatever means, when an area of bone fails to receive sufficient nourishment, as with any living thing, it will weaken and finally die. The dead (necrotic) bone no longer has the strength and resilience of healthy bone and will collapse and deform. When this occurs in the head of the femur (thigh bone), chronic hip pain and a limp most often result. In the wrist, the syndrome may cause persistently painful motion and sometimes loss of grip strength secondary to the pain.

The condition may strike young adults, and is the most common cause for hip replacement in that group.

When to call the doctor Persistent pain in a joint, limited motion, or the appearance of a limp should prompt an evaluation by a doctor.

Treatment Studies suggest that severe bone collapse can be prevented by drilling a hole into the involved bone to decompress it. In most instances, the best remedy is surgical. Opening the joint and removing the dead and damaged bone may be necessary and, in some cases (especially the hip), joint replacement may prove the best option.

Prognosis Untreated, the condition will persist indefinitely and may worsen. Surgical treatment offers the best chance for a return to normal or near-normal function.

Generalized Problems of the Bones

❖ OSTEOPOROSIS

Symptoms *(What you may experience)* Loss of height and severe bone pain. Often there are no symptoms until bone fracture occurs.

Signs and laboratory findings *(What the doctor looks for)* Loss of height; dowager's hump (curving of the spine); bone thinning as detected by x-rays; bone mass deficiency as detected by specialized x-ray or bone density studies; elevation of breakdown products of bone collagen as detected by blood or urine tests; elevated level of calcium in the blood or urine (occasionally); elevated levels of parathyroid hormone (rarely).

What is it? Postmenopausal osteoporosis, also called type 1 osteoporosis, afflicts an estimated 25 million Americans, primarily women. Although some men develop the disorder, it is usually a consequence of reproductive hormone deficiency. The female reproductive hormones play an important role in maintaining the density and integrity of the bony skeleton in women. The disorder typically appears in the first decade or two following menopause, when reproductive hormone output wanes. Among whites, it strikes one in four women. Senile osteoporosis, also called type 2 osteoporosis, affects both men and women over age 70, though women are twice as likely to have the disorder.

Throughout early adult life, both the mineral portion and the framework of bone is in constant balanced flux—with old tissue being broken down and reabsorbed and new bone being laid down at approximately the same rate. With advancing age, however, the rate of renewal begins to lag behind the rate of removal, leaving the bones thinner and more fragile.

In osteoporosis, the thinning of bone creates vulnerability to fracture even from relatively minor trauma. The most common areas of fracture include the vertebrae of the spine (compression or collapse), the hip, and the wrist. By age 65, one-third of women have sustained the most common fracture—collapse of a vertebra—but the cost in both suffering and dollars is highest for hip fracture, from which as many as 2 in 10 women do not survive.

Both heredity and environment play roles in determining risk for osteoporosis. There is a genetic component to the peak density that bones develop, with white and Asian women having the lowest general bone density and therefore greater risk of thinning as compared to blacks. But lifestyle plays an important role as well: Being sedentary promotes loss, as does smoking, excessive intake of caffeine, and heavy alcohol intake. Physical activity and weight bearing exercise seem to protect against bone loss to some degree (and will also enhance renewal once loss has begun).

What you can do Alter your lifestyle to reduce risk.

- Calcium plays an important role in skeletal metabolism, and may preserve bone mass. To avoid a calcium deficiency, make certain that your intake of calcium in the diet is at least 1,000 mg; if you are not taking estrogen, 1,500 mg daily is recommended. Supplements may be used if these goals cannot be met through your diet. The recommended daily allowance (RDA) of vitamin D (400 IU) taken along with the calcium supplement will enhance its absorption.

- Develop a regular regimen for careful weight bearing exercise to strengthen your bones. Good types of exercise include nonimpact or low-impact aerobics, dancing (ballroom, square-dance, or country-western dancing), housecleaning, hiking, cross-country skiing, walking, stair climbing, and tennis. Try to exercise for a total of 20 to 30 minutes three or four times a week. See page 42 for more information on exercise to prevent bone loss.

- If you smoke, stop. See Chapter 4 for information on how to stop smoking.

- Reduce your intake of caffeine and limit alcohol to no more than two drinks per day. (A "drink" of alcohol equals an oz of liquor, 12 oz of beer, or 5 oz of wine.)

- Particularly in older people, it is important to reduce the risk of falling by making the house a safer place: Be sure handrails on stairs are secure; remove

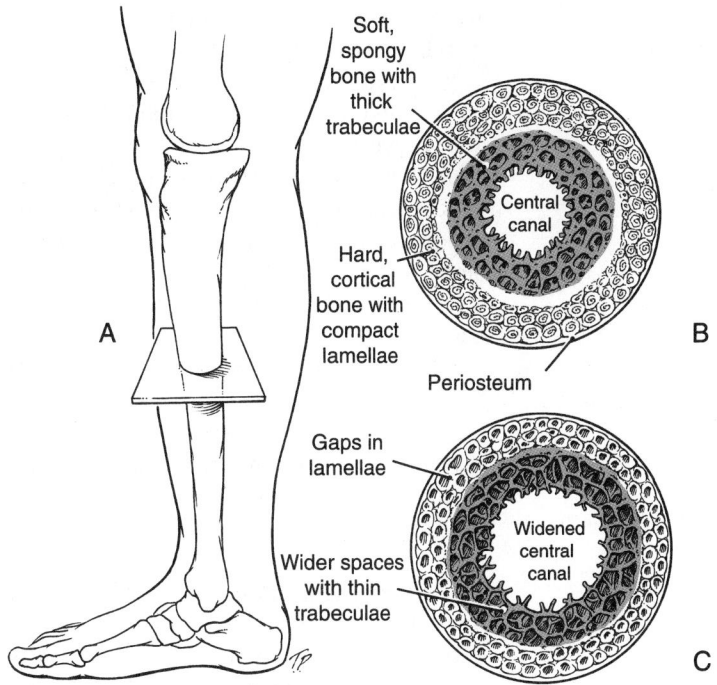

Normal (B) and osteoporotic bone (C) as it would appear if sliced through its long axis is shown. Although osteoporotic bone may appear normal, the inside has less bone and more space. Loss of density increases the risk of fracture.

loose throw rugs from the house; keep all rooms well lit; light hallways, bedrooms, and bathrooms with nightlights; install handrails beside the tub/shower and toilet; place nonskid rubber suction mats in the bathtub/shower and on slick bathroom floors. See page 58 for more information on safety at home for older people.

When to call the doctor Development of significant back pain could signal the development of a compression fracture of the spine and should prompt a visit to the doctor.

Because of the heightened risk of fracture, see a doctor for any continued pain, discoloration, or swelling following even minor trauma.

Treatment Prevention of bone fracture is the focus of treatment for osteoporosis. To minimize the likelihood of fracture, present efforts focus on preservation of bone mass in people with normal bone density (prevention) or improvement of bone mass in people with low bone density (treatment). Estrogen is a very effective option for women with postmenopausal osteoporosis; it helps to halt the bone loss and exerts a very modest bone-building effect. Studies have shown that a combination of estrogen and progestin is as effective as estrogen alone, and can lower the risk of endometrial cancer. Estrogen's beneficial effects last only as long as the hormone is taken, however. Since stopping estrogen will restart bone loss, long-term treatment (10 to 15 years) is usually recommended.

Estrogen is usually not recommended for women who have had breast cancer; tamoxifen (Nolvadex) or raloxifene (Evista) may be prescribed instead. See Hormone Replacement Therapy, page 1105, for more information on the pros and cons of estrogen therapy.

Other medications can also inhibit bone loss. Salmon calcitonin, a hormone that regulates calcium levels in the blood, is available in nasal spray and injection forms, and may be beneficial in women with established osteoporosis.

Alendronate (Fosamax), one of a new class of medications called biphosphonates, may be used to prevent bone loss or to increase bone mass. Alendronate has also been shown to significantly increase bone mass and reduce the risk of fractures.

If fractures should occur, treatment may take substantially longer and may require casts, braces, physical therapy and even surgery, since bone building is necessary for effective bone healing. Osteoporotic fractures generally heal well.

Prognosis Left untreated, the disorder causes serious disability. With proper medical and self-care, it can be managed quite effectively.

❖ OSTEOMALACIA

Symptoms *(What you may experience)* Generalized muscle weakness; bone pain.

Signs and laboratory findings *(What the doctor looks for)* Decrease in bone density as detected by x-rays; pseudofractures (radiologic evidence of new bone formation over what looks like incomplete fractures) on the long bones, ribs, pubic bone, and shoulder blades, also called the scapulae; confirmation of diagnosis via bone biopsy; low level of calcium in the blood or urine; decreased vitamin D levels.

What is it? Osteomalacia is much less common than is osteoporosis and rare in people who maintain a good diet. It is the adult counterpart to the childhood disease rickets and occurs when there is a dietary deficiency of vitamin D, calcium, or phosphate, or in some instances from inherited or acquired abnormalities in vitamin D or phosphate metabolism. Most cases of deficiency arise either as a consequence of the body's inability to absorb fat (required for proper vitamin D absorption) or because of excess acid in the body from poorly functioning kidneys (resulting in loss of calcium in the urine). People who avoid dairy products, multivitamins, and sunlight are at risk as well.

In children, inadequate mineralization of bones results in skeletal deformities (usually bowing of the lower legs). In adults, because bone growth and development have already occurred, the inadequacy rarely causes deformity of bone shape, but does weaken the bones, leading to pain.

In the past, deficiency of vitamin D and calcium occurred from dietary shortage, but the fortification of dairy products with vitamin D has virtually eliminated this cause. However, children and adults who cannot tolerate dairy products may require supplementation to prevent deficiency.

The body can manufacture vitamin D from substances in the skin, activated by exposure to sun; this pathway provides most of the body's daily needs for vitamin D.

What you can do Eat a diet adequate to provide the RDA for calcium (1,000 mg to 1,500 mg daily) and vitamin D (400 IU daily). Foods rich in these nutrients include low-fat dairy products (such as milk, yogurt, and cottage cheese) and sardines. If you cannot eat these foods and do not have sufficient sunlight exposure (about 15 minutes of direct sunlight per week on the face, hands, and arms) you may need a vitamin D supplement or a daily multivitamin tablet that contains 400 IU of vitamin D.

When to call the doctor Development of new bone pain or significant new muscle weakness should be reported to your doctor.

Because of bone weakness and the consequent heightened risk for fracture, see your doctor if you experience persistent pain following even minor falls or other trauma.

Treatment If osteomalacia arises as a consequence of poor fat absorption or kidney problems, initial therapy should focus on their correction. Thereafter, therapy is aimed at correcting the mineral deficiency with supplemental vitamin D and calcium.

Prognosis In most cases, the symptoms resolve upon correcting the vitamin or mineral deficiency. Even in children, ultimately the bone changes will usually disappear.

❖ OSTEOMYELITIS

Symptoms *(What you may experience)* Fever and chills; pain or tenderness of a bone. Symptoms are likely to be more dramatic in children than in adults.

Signs and laboratory findings *(What the doctor looks for)* Culture of a blood sample during fever that grows infecting bacteria (often); confirmation of diagnosis via aspiration (removal of tissue with a needle and syringe) of pus. X-rays may not show changes until late in the condition.

What is it? Infection in bone—osteomyelitis—can occur directly by introduction of bacteria through puncture of the skin and into the bone, such as might happen with a gunshot wound, an open bone fracture, a surgical procedure, or IV drug administration (either for medical therapy or, more likely, by illicit use where concern for sterile conditions may be minimal). Infection in the bone can also occur due to spreading through the blood of infection that originates in other parts of the body.

In most cases not due to trauma, the infection comes from a single strain of bacteria, most often staphylococci or group A hemolytic streptococci. In IV drug abusers, because of the lack of hygiene that may attend needle use, the common causative bacteria are *Staphylococcus aureus* (a pathologic skin bacterium) and *Escherichia coli* (a normal inhabitant of the large intestine, found in feces).

Infection within a bone can cause significant pain, as the body's attempt to defend itself against the invasion results in the formation of pus. The expanding volume of pus within the bone presses against the nerve-rich covering, stretching it and causing discomfort. When the bacteria seed into the bloodstream, they cause spiking fevers and chills.

Spread of the infection through the blood to other bones is possible, as are chronic, slowly progresssive infections, or recurrences.

When to call the doctor Persistent bone pain or the appearance of recurrent spiking fever and chills always merit a doctor's investigation for cause.

Treatment The doctor may obtain a specimen of the pus (by needle aspiration under local anesthesia) to identify the bacterial strain and which antibiotic will most effectively destroy it. Initially, the choice of antibiotic is aimed at the most probable organism, then changed if necessary based on the susceptibility tests which may take 48 hours to complete. A common regimen is ciprofloxacin taken twice daily for up to 2 months. This medication, taken by mouth, may be as effective as IV administration of many antibiotics.

Drainage of the pus speeds healing. Medication for pain, and rest and elevation of the affected body part also are beneficial to speedy recovery and comfort.

Recurrent or chronic infections may demand surgical saucerization, scraping away the infected bone down to a healthy base under general anesthesia.

Prognosis In many cases, if the infection is treated aggressively, it can be eradicated quickly—usually within 4 days. Complete resolution is much more likely in these cases. When the immune system is not functioning properly—such as in people under treatment for cancer, those receiving immunosuppressive medications, or people with acquired immunodeficiency syndrome (AIDS)—the possibility of a chronic, smoldering infection is higher.

Failure to receive antibiotic treatment, treatment for too short a period of time, or treatment with the wrong antibiotics leads to destruction of bone. Once bone death occurs, it is impossible to eliminate the infection and chronic osteomyelitis develops. This condition can be marked by continuous symptoms or intermittent symptoms over many years. Chronic osteomyelitis is best treated with surgery to remove the dead bone and intensive antibiotic treatment. Sometimes reconstructive surgery is possible. If the infection cannot be eliminated, amputation, although rare, may be necessary.

❖ OSTEOGENESIS IMPERFECTA

Symptoms *(What you may experience)* Bones break from minimal trauma; bluish cast to the whites of the eyes.

Signs and laboratory findings *(What the doctor looks for)* Blue cast to the sclera (the eye's outer membrane); evidence of fractures in the womb as detected by x-rays or during birth process.

What is it? This rare inherited syndrome causes a defect in bone development that makes bones very fragile and easily broken. The syndrome may be readily apparent at birth—osteogenesis imperfecta type 2—with fractures of bones occurring while in the womb. This most severe form occurs in 1 in 50,000 births and most babies born with it do not survive infancy. In the case of the milder form, osteogenesis imperfecta type 1, which occurs in 1 in 20,000 births, its appearance may be delayed with fractures occurring after birth.

Although fragility of bones is the hallmark, several other symptoms may accompany the syndrome, among them a blue color to the whites of the eyes, conductive hearing loss, scoliosis (twisting of the spine) or kyphosis (bending of the spine), and abnormality of the teeth.

What you can do Take care to prevent even minor injuries; even minimal trauma can result in fracture.

When to call the doctor Following even minor trauma, if pain, significant swelling, or discoloration persists more than a few days, call the doctor.

Treatment To date there is no effective treatment to strengthen the bones or improve their formation in this condition.

The condition is genetic. Most cases of the very severe type 2 neonatal osteogenesis imperfecta represent new mutations. There is a low risk of recurrence in the family. The milder type 1 is inherited as an autosomal dominant; it may be transmitted through several generations.

Prognosis In its most severe forms, babies with osteogenesis imperfecta are unlikely to survive infancy. For children with milder forms, the condition persists and must be managed for life. Fractures usually become less of a problem after puberty.

❖ PAGET'S DISEASE OF BONE

Symptoms *(What you may experience)* Pain and joint stiffness in hip and lower back (sometimes); headache; tinnitus (ringing in the ears). Usually there are no symptoms.

Signs and laboratory findings *(What the doctor looks for)* Characteristic appearance on x-ray studies (often discovered coincidentally, when radiographic evaluation is performed for an unrelated condition); elevated blood level of alkaline phosphatase (usually); confirmation of diagnosis via bone biopsy.

What is it? Paget's disease—also called osteitis deformans—is a bone weakening disorder involving abnormal growth and remodeling of bone tissue. It usually arises in older people, and is quite common in the elderly. One in 1,500 adults over age 45 may have the disorder, rising to 1 in 20 over age 75. The cause of the disorder is unknown, though a viral infection of certain bone cells is a possible cause. It can affect any part of the skeleton, but most commonly involves the leg (femur or tibia), skull, spine, and pelvis. Under normal conditions, bone continually undergoes a process of being broken down (reabsorbed) and replaced by new healthy bone. Early in the course of this disorder, areas of increased bone reabsorption develop, followed by an exaggerated phase of rebuilding of dense, irregular, and haphazardly constructed new bone. Even though it is dense, this new bone is weak, lacking the strength of normal bone, and therefore prone to fracture. As Paget's disease progresses, it can lead to hearing loss because of its effects on the bones and nerves in the skull; it can also cause other neurologic and cardiac complications in the elderly. Rarely, malignant cancers of bone arise in the areas of Paget's disease, but this possibility must always be excluded by the doctor.

What you can do Acetaminophen or OTC nonsteroidal anti-inflammatory drugs (NSAIDs), such as ibuprofen, can be taken to relieve pain should it occur.

Treatment Mild Paget's disease can be treated as described above. In more severe cases, such as those with severe bone pain, hearing loss, or congestive heart failure, other treatments will be necessary. Treatment with calcitonin (a hormone that regulates calcium levels in the blood) may restore normal bone growth. Biphosphonates, such as alendronate, pamidronate, or tiludronate may help slow bone resorption.

In some cases, the abnormal bone can be surgically removed or modified and if needed, healthy bone can be grafted into the defect to strengthen it. In some cases, Paget's disease can cause the hip or knee to wear out prematurely; these damaged joints can often be replaced surgically.

If you experience increasing pain or swelling in an area affected by Paget's disease, you should contact your doctor.

Prognosis There is no cure for this disorder, but with proper management it need not significantly impair quality or length of life.

❖ FIBROUS DYSPLASIA

Symptoms *(What you may experience)* Pain in the lower leg bones or other bones (sometimes); difficulty walking; bowed legs. Often there are no symptoms.

Signs and laboratory findings *(What the doctor looks for)* Characteristic appearance on x-ray studies; confirmation of diagnosis via bone biopsy.

What is it? Fibrous dysplasia, a rare disorder involving abnormal bone formation, typically appears in childhood. Although its cause is not clearly understood, in some cases it is associated with precocious sexual development in girls.

Under normal conditions, bone continually undergoes a process of being broken down (reabsorbed) and replaced by new healthy bone. In this case, bone is reabsorbed at an accelerated pace and is replaced by fibrous tissue instead of healthy bone. These cystic areas of fibrous replacement weaken the bone and can cause bone pain. It usually affects only one bone—commonly a lower leg bone, which may cause difficulty walking.

When to call the doctor Although many children complain of growing pains in the lower legs, persistent bone pain (longer than a few weeks) or a fracture in a lower leg, especially in children, merits evaluation by the doctor.

Treatment In some cases, the fibrous areas can be surgically removed and if needed, healthy bone can be grafted into the defect to strengthen it.

Prognosis There is no cure for this disorder, but with proper management it need not significantly impair quality or length of life.

❖ ACHONDROPLASIA (DWARFISM)

Symptoms *(What you may experience)* Disproportionately short arms and legs at birth; enlargement of the skull; small middle face; flat nasal bridge. (See page C-33.)

Signs and laboratory findings *(What the doctor looks for)* Accentuated bowing of the middle and lower back on x-ray at birth; diminished muscle tone; ligament laxity; narrowing of the lumbar spinal canal as detected by x-ray; trident hands (enlarged space between the middle and ring fingers); bowed legs.

What is it? This condition, representing the most common form of disproportionate dwarfism, occurs because of a single genetic defect. It is a dominant trait, meaning that passage of a single copy of the defective gene from one parent to a child will result in dwarfism. On the other hand, because we receive two copies of every gene (one from each parent), a parent who suffers from dwarfism has a 50 percent chance of passing the normal gene to his child, and if the normal gene is passed on to the child he would be of normal stature. In most instances, however, the disorder arises not by passage of a defective gene but by spontaneous mutation of the defective gene occurring in the germ cells of one parent who is normal, and passed to the affected child. That affected child can then transmit the gene to half of his offspring. The condition is usually apparent at birth.

The disorder results in growth disturbance of the cartilage cells, primarily affecting the capacity for lengthening of the long bones (arm and leg bones). Characteristically, the head develops slightly larger than normal, with a particularly prominent forehead and chin. The middle of the face may be somewhat underdeveloped. This is because the cartilage that forms the base of the skull does not develop properly.

The most common spinal problem is lumbar stenosis (narrowing of the spinal canal in the lower back). This narrowing can compress nerves and nerve roots in the region giving rise to such symptoms as aching pain and tiredness of the legs with prolonged standing or walking, lower back or leg pain; numbness or pins-and-needles sensations, and, at advanced stages, bowel or bladder incontinence.

The disproportionate shortness of the limbs may create difficulty in performing personal care activities, such as dressing and personal hygiene, since the fingertips may barely reach the level of the hips. Assistance in learning to cope creatively with this challenge should be a priority for caregivers.

What you can do   Squatting, because it flattens the curve of the lower back, may help the nerve symptoms in the back and legs. Similarly, bicycle riding is well tolerated even by an achondroplastic with severe restrictions in walking.

Weight loss (if overweight) can help take added stress off the lower back and legs.

Treatment   Therapy should be aimed at minimizing the impact of dwarfism socially, psychologically, and physically on the child.

Lumbar stenosis and spinal deformities, because of their attendant neurologic complications, may require surgery to widen the spinal canal or stabilize the spine.

Tibial osteotomy (surgery to correct bone alignment in the legs) may improve cosmetic appearance, relieve leg pain, and improve gait.

Leg lengthening procedures, more frequently performed in Europe than in America, can sometimes increase leg length up to 30 cm (about 10 to 12 in.) if begun early, but require prolonged treatment. Before embarking on such a therapy, many factors must come into play—social, psychological, and economic.

Prognosis   The disorder is present from birth and cannot be cured. Its effects can be minimized by thoughtful medical, surgical, and social management.

❖ PRIMARY BONE CANCER: OSTEOSARCOMA

Symptoms   *(What you may experience)* Persistent sharp and progressively increasing localized pain in a bone; bone pain that wakes you from your sleep; a slowly enlarging, firm lump on a bone (often); fracture of a bone with minimal trauma; pain that increases over time despite treatment.

Signs and laboratory findings   *(What the doctor looks for)* Characteristic x-ray appearance of bone reabsorption and disorganized new bone formation.

What is it?   Although most cancers of bone are metastatic from cancers elsewhere in the body, primary bone cancers do occur. Malignant tumors of bone (much less common—only 2 to 4 percent of all tumors) can arise from the bone producing cells (osteosarcomas), the cartilage-producing cells (chondrosarcomas), or from cells within the marrow cavity (see Multiple Myeloma, page 951).

Cancers that originate from the bone producing cells usually develop in the long bones of the arm or leg, but can occur in any bone and sometimes even in the soft tissues. The most commonly involved areas include the femur, the tibia (lower leg), and the humerus (upper arm and shoulder). These cancers may arise from within the bone, on the surface of the bone, or from the soft tissues next to the bone or those near the bone.

Those arising within the bone almost always behave aggressively, rapidly destroying normal bone and surrounding soft tissues; they may metastasize to the lung, so prompt aggressive treatment is of paramount importance.

Those developing from the surface of the bone tend to occur in young adults, and although they may not be as aggressive in their course, still grow into the soft tissues and into the interior of the bone. The first symptom may be a slowly enlarging firm lump affixed to the bone or chronic pain that gradually worsens. Almost half of all cases of osteosarcoma in children involve the region of the knee.

Those in the adjacent soft tissues (the most common site is the thigh) may grow slowly for years with a little swelling, but little pain. They tend to carry a better prognosis than do those in the bone, but early treatment is beneficial.

Tumors arising farther from the bone in the soft tissues tend to occur in young adults near the shoulder and pelvis and are less aggressive than are those in the bone itself.

When to call the doctor The development of significant localized bone pain that is not associated with trauma or persists longer than a few weeks should be evaluated by a doctor.

Treatment Surgical removal of the tumor followed by either radiation therapy or chemotherapy is the usual course of therapy. In most instances, the tumors that arise within or on the bone itself demand aggressive surgical removal of the entire affected bone and the joints at either end to offer the best hope of containing the malignancy. Surgery is followed by high-dose chemotherapy.

For children with osteosarcoma, treatment at a cancer center may offer the greatest possibility of survival, as well as the most refined prosthetic techniques for replacement with an artificial limb.

Soft-tissue tumors can usually be removed surgically; the doctor may also recommend a course of chemotherapy in some cases.

See Chapter 30 for more information on the treatment of cancer.

Prognosis With early aggressive surgical removal of the tumor followed by high-dose chemotherapy, about 60 to 65 percent of children with these cancers survive the disease. For those whose cancer has spread, aggressive treatment may result in a 25 to 50 percent chance of survival.

❖ PRIMARY BONE CANCER: CHONDROSARCOMA

Symptoms *(What you may experience)* Slow-growing firm lump. Often there is little or no discomfort.

Signs and laboratory findings *(What the doctor looks for)* Identification of the mass by x-ray or CT scan.

What is it? Although most cancers of bone are metastatic from cancers elsewhere in the body, primary bone cancers do occur. Malignant tumors of bone can arise from the bone-producing cells (osteosarcomas), the cartilage-producing cells (chondrosarcomas), or from cells within the marrow cavity (see Multiple Myeloma, page 951).

Cancers arising from the cartilage producing cells of the bone occur in adults and in the elderly; they may occasionally develop in areas of known cartilage or bone abnormality (such as cartilage or bone cysts) or where cartilage appears normal. The most common sites for chondrosarcoma development include the pelvis, shoulder blade, upper arm (humerus), femur, and tibia. Their course can be quite

MYOSITIS OSSIFICANS

This condition develops in adolescents and young adults following a deep muscle bruise, such as may occur with a direct blow to the muscle. Common sites include the quadriceps and adductor muscles on the front and inner portion of the thighs, the deltoid muscle on the side of the shoulder, and the brachialis muscle in the forearm.

Hemorrhage deep within the muscle incites inflammation, tenderness, and swelling. Then, for reasons not clearly understood, formation of bone, cartilage, or fibrous tissue begins within the damaged area. In time, the inflammation subsides but leaves a permanent hard mass—often containing bone—within the muscle.

Though this condition is entirely benign during its development phase, this new growth in the muscle can be mistaken for a malignancy on x-ray or microscopic examination of a biopsy specimen. Always be sure to notify your doctor if you experience increasing pain or swelling at the site of a contusion to a muscle. ∎

LIMB AMPUTATION AND ARTIFICIAL LIMBS

Amputation of a limb can occur because of injury or disease. While loss of a limb may not be life threatening, the emotional consequences and lifestyle changes it engenders can be more difficult to deal with. Immediate and ongoing care by psychiatrists, rehabilitation specialist doctors (physiatrists), and physical therapists can facilitate both physical and emotional recovery.

In general, loss of a limb occurs either by accidental trauma or for other causes. The reasons for the intentional removal of a limb by surgery are several, including cancer and infection, but chief among them is diabetes mellitus and its complications. When a crushing or tearing injury results in the traumatic amputation of a limb, immediate medical attention can be lifesaving. See page 390 for information on what to do in the case of a crushing or tearing injury.

Advancements in microsurgical techniques now permit many severed parts, ranging from fingers to entire limbs, to be surgically reattached. The success of such a reattachment and the extent of recovery of normal function and sensation depend on the degree of trauma to the severed part as well as how it is treated en route to the hospital. When possible, find the amputated part, rinse any dirt or debris from it, and wrap it in a clean cloth moistened with clean water. The cloth-covered limb should be wrapped in plastic, if available, and placed in a bed of ice for transportation to the hospital. Not all severed parts can be saved; severe mangling of the limb may so damage vital arteries, veins, and nerves that successful reattachment is not possible.

A limb lost because of amputation can be replaced with a prosthesis. Advancements in prosthetic technology have led to better fitting and more useful replacement limbs, which although they cannot match the intricacies of motion, strength, and flexibility of natural limbs, can allow a person to live a normal life following amputation.

Successful use of an artificial limb hinges on achieving and maintaining good physical conditioning of the remaining muscles in the limb. After the initial period of tissue healing, physical therapy must be the primary focus of treatment.

At first, a temporary prosthesis worn for progressively longer periods each day will condition the tissues to the unaccustomed feel of the new limb. The construction of a custom-fitted permanent replacement limb will follow, with its exact design tailored to fit individual needs. Some people may have more than one prosthesis for varying circumstances, such as to accommodate different types of physical activity or to be more aesthetically pleasing. ■

variable; sometimes they behave aggressively and destructively, quick to spread throughout the body and cause death. In other cases, they slowly enlarge, do little damage to surrounding structures, and spread after many years to distant sites or may not metastasize at all.

Although most chondrosarcomas eventually cause some discomfort, they may grow quite large without causing pain. Those that arise from the pelvic bones, for example, may grow into the abdominal cavity, gain tremendous size, be present for years, and often be found incidentally on x-ray studies or scans performed for other reasons.

When to call the doctor The presence of a firm lump in the tissues, even if not tender, should prompt evaluation by a doctor.

Treatment Surgical removal of the growth and a wide margin of healthy tissue around it offer the best possibility of cure. Neither radiation or chemotherapy has proven effective in treating this cancer.

Prognosis Early diagnosis and prompt, aggressive surgical attention improve prognosis.

❖ CANCERS METASTATIC TO THE BONE

Symptoms (*What you may experience*) Persistent (although sometimes vague) bone pain; fracture of bone with minimal trauma.

Signs and laboratory findings (*What the doctor looks for*) Characteristic areas of the tumor as detected by standard and specialized x-ray studies; confirmation of diagnosis via microscopic examination of bone biopsy specimen.

What is it? This condition occurs when cells from a cancer elsewhere in the body spread through the blood to take root in the bone. Nearly all malignant tumors can metastasize to the bone, but the most common ones (making up 80 percent of all bone metastases) include carcinomas of the lung, breast, and prostate. The other 20 percent arise primarily from the kidney, gastrointestinal tract, female reproductive organs, and thyroid gland.

When cancers spread to bone, although they can occasionally incite excessive, new, and dense bone production in an area, they usually cause destruction of normal bone, leaving the areas demineralized and weaker. These areas of cancerous replacement of bone show up as dark spots on standard x-rays, but not until the cancer has destroyed a substantial portion of the bone. Newer radiologic techniques, such as a bone scan, computed tomography (CT), or magnetic resonance imaging (MRI) can detect the spread earlier and can provide the clearest details of the metastasis.

The weakened areas are vulnerable to easy fracture with even minor trauma—a phenomenon termed a pathologic fracture. When a bone breaks from minimal stress, the possibility of its being a consequence of the spread of a malignant tumor to the bone must always be thoroughly investigated, especially in middle-aged and elderly people; in some cases, the bone metastasis may be the first indication of the underlying cancer. Surgical biopsy for microscopic examination of the fractured area is warranted.

Although any bone can be involved, common areas include the vertebrae, the humerus (upper arm or shoulder), and the femur.

When to call the doctor Do not ignore persistent bone pain especially if you have a history of cancer; see your doctor for evaluation.

Treatment The first thing is to see a doctor to get an exact diagnosis of what is causing your pain. The basic treatment is aimed at the underlying primary cancer, but additional treatment of metastases may focus on preserving function and relieving pain. Use of internal fixation (surgical application of reinforcing screws, plates, or wires) to stabilize a site of potential fracture risk may be recommended. Additionally, radiation therapy, chemotherapy, or hormonal therapy (depending on the type of primary cancer involved) may also prove beneficial. See Chapter 30 for more information on the treatment of cancer.

Prognosis The prognosis for any cancer that has spread to the bone is not always an optimistic one, however, the specific prognosis depends on the primary cancer involved.

Fractures, Sprains, and Other Common Injuries and Disorders of the Musculoskeletal System

This section contains primarily orthopedic information concerning the major common injuries that befall specific areas of the body. The section, organized by body area—that is, hand, wrist, or arm—describes how these common injuries typically occur, any special instructions on their care, as well as quick methods of emergency immobilization of such injuries.

See Chapter 13 for more information on emergency care for common injuries of the musculoskeletal system.

The Hands

❖ BALL CATCHER'S FRACTURE

Symptoms *(What you may experience)* Tenderness, swelling, bruising, and loss of normal motion over a finger joint, usually the last joint nearest the nail.

Signs and laboratory findings *(What the doctor looks for)* The end of the finger drooping with an inability to straighten the finger; bone chip fragment along joint line as detected by x-ray.

What is it? This injury occurs when the fingertip sustains a sharp direct blow, often during an attempt to catch a baseball or other ball, hence the name. The force of the blow can stretch the ligaments of the finger joint where they attach or the blow can pull the tendon off the bone, sometimes with a piece of bone attached.

Pain will be immediate and usually more pronounced over top of the knuckle or the crease of the joint than the sides. Bruising may also occur right away.

The seriousness of the injury correlates with the size fragment of bone cleaved away and how much the fingertip droops.

What you can do Apply ice right away. Splint with tape to the adjacent finger.

When to call the doctor As soon as possible, see the doctor. Only an x-ray can determine the extent of this injury.

Treatment If the fragment is small (involves less than 10 to 20 percent of the joint surface) or if the tendon is torn, it can be treated by simple splinting for 5 to 6 weeks. Larger fragments may require surgical fixation to wire the fragment in place.

SKELETAL TRAUMA—FRACTURES AND DISLOCATIONS

The broken bone is one of the most common ailments of the skeletal system. The body is quite efficient at repairing injury to the bones. When a break occurs, the body mobilizes specialized bone cells called osteoclasts whose job is to enter the area and reabsorb the damaged bone cells and debris from the injury. During the first or second week following a break, this clean-up process proceeds; during this time, x-rays of the fracture may look worse. In fact, some small fractures not visible at the time of injury will become more easily seen a week or 10 days later. At the same time, a second type of specialized bone cells called osteoblasts enter the area and begin to quickly lay down new bone in a somewhat haphazard way, making an internal bony splint around the break. This process, called callus formation, continues for the next few weeks. Finally, over the next several months or more, the body will remodel and refine the repair, resculpting the bone into its normal shape, leaving only x-ray evidence of the old injury.

People sometimes become confused about their injuries because of vague terminology. Although not all breaks are the same, there is no difference between the terms break and fracture. A fractured bone is a broken bone. The terms are interchangeable. The following paragraphs will briefly examine the different types.

- *Closed fractures.* These are cracks or clean breaks through the bone that do not penetrate the skin.

- *Open or compound fractures.* This type of fracture occurs when the broken bone pierces the skin, exposing the bone to the outside environment. These fractures are highly more likely to become infected.

- *Compression fractures.* These occur when the outer hard shell of bone collapses into the spongier cavity within. These fractures commonly occur in the vertebrae of the spine and in the skull.

- *Dislocation.* Dislocation implies that a joint has shifted from its proper alignment and the bones that make up the joint no longer touch each other. In most instances, the dislocating force stretches or tears the ligaments around the joint, causing bleeding into the joint, bruising externally, loss of normal motion, and significant pain, which will continue until it is put back into its proper place.

Subluxation. These occur when the bones of the joints shift but do not totally dislocate. Although the bones usually go back to their original position, subluxation can cause symptoms similar to a dislocation.

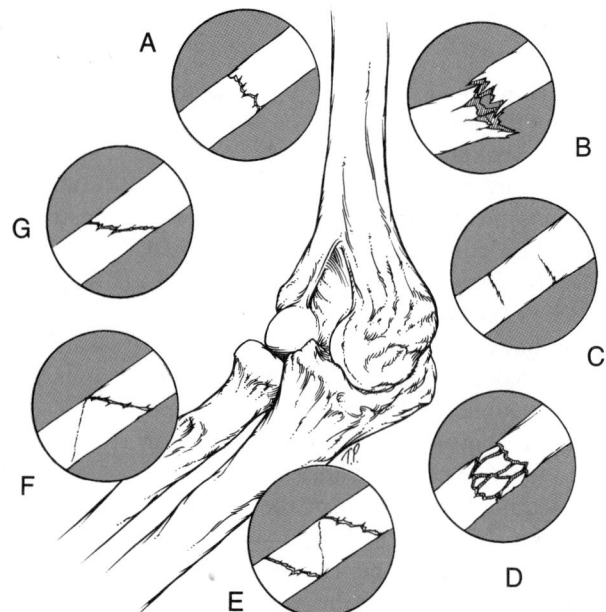

There are many types of fractures depending upon shape. (A) Transverse fractures occur at right angles to the long axis of the bone. (B) In compound fractures, the skin is punctured at the site of the fracture, and the bone is typically broken completely. (C) Greenstick fractures have incomplete breaks on only one side of the bone, but the fracture actually goes all the way across. (D) Comminuted fractures contain crushed or splintered bone particles. (E) Butterfly fractures are a type of spiral fracture with a central fragment between each spiral. (F) In spiral fractures, the bone has been twisted apart. (G) Oblique fractures do not occur at right angles to the long axis of the bone.

Children can break their bones just like adults. Because their bones are a little more flexible and can bend more before the fracture is completed, their fractures sometimes look different on x-rays. However, do not be deceived—the bone is broken and must be treated.

- *Buckle or torus fracture.* The bone has a sharp bend or buckle when the outer cortex of the bone is deformed. This can involve one or both sides of the bone.

- *Greenstick fracture.* In this pattern of fracture only one side of the bone appears broken and the other side appears bent. Sometimes the bend is so great the doctor must manipulate the break to straighten the bone. This is done with anesthesia so that the setting of the bone is not painful. Most greenstick fractures heal well with casting. ■

MAKING AN EMERGENCY SPLINT

Whether the injury is a twisted knee or ankle or a potentially broken arm or leg, the first order of business is to keep the injured part as immobile as possible on the way to the hospital or clinic to prevent further injury. Use what is available at the site of the injury.

- Use a magazine to support an injured wrist, a child's arm, or a toddler's leg. Slip it gently under the part, with minimal movement of the injury, wrap it lengthwise around the injury (attempt to span the joints at either end of a bone), and secure it with string or tape. Do not wrap it too tightly or the blood supply may be cut off.

- Use a length of thick corrugated cardboard for wrists, arms, or legs. For legs, place a length on either side and tape around the splints.

- A length of heavy corrugated cardboard, folded at a right angle, can splint a twisted ankle. Place it behind the ankle and secure with tape or an elastic bandage.

See page 388 for further information on splints. ■

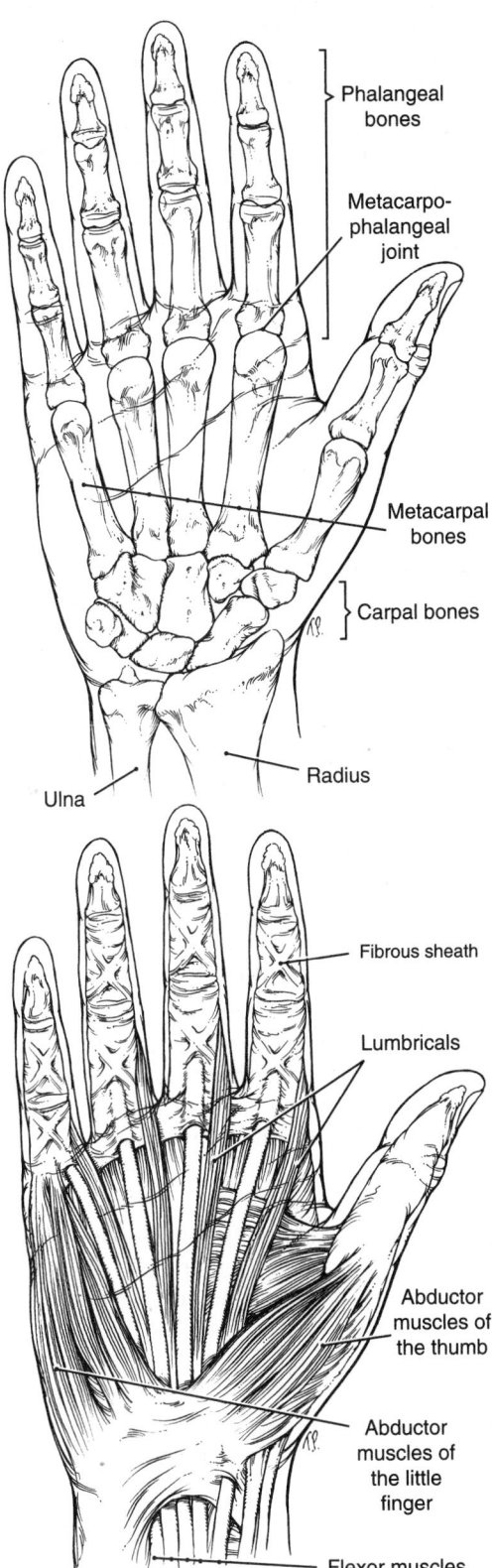

Phalangeal bones

Metacarpo-phalangeal joint

Metacarpal bones

Carpal bones

Radius

Ulna

Fibrous sheath

Lumbricals

Abductor muscles of the thumb

Abductor muscles of the little finger

Flexor muscles

The human hand can perform thousands of activities and contains numerous structures. Carpal bones are in the wrist, metacarpals are in the hands, and phalanges are in the fingers (digits). The thumb has two phalanges and the other digits each have three. Knuckles are known as metacarpophalangeal joints. An intricate system of muscles and tendons allows very fine movements.

Prognosis Prognosis is excellent with prompt and appropriate orthopedic attention.

❖ TRIGGER FINGER

Symptoms *(What you may experience)* Finger joint becomes stuck or pops when opening and closing.

Signs and laboratory findings *(What the doctor looks for)* Tenderness of the joint where the finger meets the hand (usually on the palm side only) and pain with stretching the tendon. Usually a tender lump on the hand near the crease can be felt. The condition does not show on standard x-rays.

What is it? Chronic overuse (repetitive gripping, grasping, or pressure on the palm) rather than acute injury usually causes this inflammatory condition involving the tendons that bend the finger (including the thumb). The tendons run in tunnels of tissue called a pulley. As the inflammation swells the tendons and the tendon sheath (their covering layers), they can no longer glide smoothly through the pulleys that anchor them close to the bone. When the swollen area attempts to glide through the pulley, it catches and sometimes locks the finger in a flexed or bent position, usually at the joint nearest the palm.

What you can do Avoid activities which seem to make it worse, including the use of vibrating hand tools. It is important not to let the affected finger get stuck and stay there. Apply ice (two to three times a day, for several weeks if necessary) to the palm in the area where the hand and finger meet. Buddy tape the painful finger to its neighbor (see Immobilizing an Injured Hand or Finger, page 666). Acetaminophen or OTC anti-inflammatory medications, such as ibuprofen, may help reduce the discomfort of the inflammation.

When to call the doctor If the condition persists or worsens despite home care remedies, or if the finger locks and will not open, consult the doctor.

Treatment The doctor may recommend injection of a mixture of local anesthetic (for numbing) and corticosteroid medications into the tendon. Failure to reap signifi-

IMMOBILIZING AN INJURED HAND OR FINGER

To immobilize an injured finger, the easiest method is to fashion a buddy tape splint, using the neighboring finger as the splint. To make a buddy splint follow these guidelines:

- Pad between the injured finger and its largest nonthumb neighboring finger with cotton balls, a small roll of soft cloth, or a folded tissue or paper towel to absorb moisture.

- Tear two pieces of tape (½ to 1 in. width works best) about 4 to 5 in. long.

- Wrap the tape snugly but not tightly around both fingers, binding the injured finger to its neighbor. Wrap one piece of tape between the middle knuckle and the finger tip and the second between the middle knuckle and the knuckle of the hand, leaving the middle knuckle uncovered by tape. This allows some protection and very slight movement.

- To prevent any movement, secure a piece of stiff corrugated cardboard or a wooden stick to the underside of the fingers and tape in place, wrapping tape around fingers and cardboard.

To make an emergency splint for the hand, follow these guidelines:

- Crumple a soft cloth (a wash cloth, gauze, scarf, or paper towel) and place it in the hollow of the palm to softly pad the hand. Allow the hand and fingers to gently assume their naturally curved shape.

- Gently wrap roll gauze, an elastic bandage, strips of cloth, or adhesive tape around hand, thumb, and fingers. Do not tightly bind the hand or fingers; allow a bit of slack to accommodate any swelling that might occur. ■

cant improvement may necessitate a second injection.

In some cases, surgical release to free the tendon from the overlying tunnel or band may prove necessary. This surgery can usually be performed as an outpatient procedure, followed by physical therapy to stretch and strengthen the tendon and restore its mobility.

Prognosis Prognosis is excellent. In two-thirds of cases, a single injection of steroid medication provides effective long-lasting relief. About 25 percent of cases require repeat injection within a year. Only about 10 percent need surgery; recovery in 3 to 4 weeks is the rule following the surgical procedure.

❖ BENNETT'S FRACTURE OF THE BASE OF THE THUMB

Symptoms (*What you may experience*) Pain, swelling, and bruising in the hand where the thumb joins the wrist; limitation of grip or motion of the thumb following trauma.

Signs and laboratory findings (*What the doctor looks for*) Confirmation of fracture via x-ray.

What is it? Because mobility of the thumb in all directions is of extreme importance to effective hand function and grip, all injuries involving the thumb demand evaluation. Fractures to the base of the thumb's metacarpal (the area where the bone of the thumb extends into the hand to meet the wrist) demand an extra measure of care. The attachment of small muscle groups within the hand to the first (thumb) metacarpal tend to pull broken pieces of the bone apart and prevent stable realignment. If the bone fragments are not held securely together, healing is not possible; without strong union of the bone fragments, long-term pain and weakness of grip may result.

What you can do Apply ice (intermittently) and elevate the injured hand for 24 to 48 hours. It may be helpful to splint the thumb and the wrist.

When to call the doctor If significant pain and loss of mobility occur and last more than a few hours, consult a doctor.

Treatment Because of the risk that casting alone will not maintain the fracture fragments in proper alignment, the treatment most often employed in this injury is surgery to realign the fracture and place internal fixation devices (wires, pins, or screws) to hold the position securely.

Prognosis Prognosis is good if identified promptly and treated aggressively; long-term pain, weakness of grip, and loss of full function may occur if the condition is improperly treated.

❖ GAMEKEEPER'S THUMB OR SKI POLE INJURY

Symptoms *(What you may experience)* Severe localized tenderness on the medial side of the first joint of the thumb (where it joins the hand) following trauma; pain, weakness, or instability when making a pinch between the thumb and forefinger.

Signs and laboratory findings *(What the doctor looks for)* Instability of first metacarpal-phalangeal joint ligaments. Usually, the injury is not visible on x-ray.

What is it? Two ligaments on either side of the first thumb joint maintain its stability and fix the joint to allow the thumb to oppose the fingers (which enables the hand to pinch or to grasp), a function that sets the human hand apart from those of other mammals. The high degree of mobility this arrangement affords makes the thumb extremely useful, but also vulnerable to injury.

When the force of an injury pulls the thumb in a direction away from the hand, it stretches or tears the ligament stabilizing the inner side of the joint. This type of injury occurs often in the sport of snow skiing, when during a fall, the thumb becomes caught on the ski pole and twisted away from the body of the hand. Damage to the medial ligament prevents the strong, stable opposition of the thumb necessary to make a pinch, grasp and pick up small objects, and write or draw.

The injury derives its older name—Gamekeeper's thumb—from feudal times in Britain when a chronic form of the injury was common among the keepers of the royal game preserves. A part of the keeper's job was to thin the populations of small game animals (rabbits, pheasant, etc.), which was accomplished by holding the game with the hand and snapping its neck with a sharp shake. The maneuver placed stress on the thumb ligaments, which over time stretched them sufficiently to render the thumb unstable.

What you can do Temporarily splint the thumb to the hand: Place a roll of cotton or soft cloth between the thumb and hand to absorb moisture and wrap the hand and thumb with an elastic bandage or adhesive tape. Elevate and apply ice—a zipper lock bag filled with ice can be placed on the injured thumb and incorporated into the last wrap of the bandage or tape—to reduce swelling and bruising.

When to call the doctor An injury that weakens pinch should be seen by a doctor as soon as possible for examination and x-rays to rule out associated fracture and to definitively treat the injury.

Treatment A gamekeeper's injury is a ligament injury, not a fracture, but healing the important thumb ligament requires immobilization in a specially constructed cast (called a thumb spica splint) for 6 to 8 weeks. During immobilization, physical therapy to restore thumb function is critical. Newer treatment methods allow for physical therapy sooner, which improves long-term outcome.

If the ligament has been completely torn away from the bone, surgery to reattach the ligament will be necessary.

Prognosis Prognosis is excellent if promptly diagnosed and appropriately treated.

❖ BOXER'S FRACTURE

Symptoms *(What you may experience)* Pain, swelling, bruising, and a sunken appearance of the back of the hand over a knuckle near the outer edge of the hand; limited motion of the ring or small fingers.

Signs and laboratory findings *(What the doctor looks for)* Deformity of the head of the fourth or fifth metacarpal bone near the finger; fracture of the metacarpal just below the head as detected by x-ray.

What is it? As its name implies, this injury occurs commonly in boxers, but can also occur from other common traumas, such as punching a wall or falling on the knuckles of a fisted hand. When a loose fist strikes a hard object, the force of the blow against the end of the more mobile fourth or fifth bone of the hand breaks the bone and bends its end downward toward the palm. The break leaves a depression on the back of the hand over the knuckle, but it may not be clearly apparent until the swelling subsides. The angled head of the bone does not properly align and the misplacement makes normal motion of the fourth or fifth finger painful and difficult.

What you can do Apply ice immediately. If possible, cleanse any skin abrasions or cuts with clean, mild soapy water and pat dry. If there are deep cuts over the knuckle you should seek treatment immediately because the joint may get infected. Temporarily splint the injured hand by crumpling a clean washcloth or other soft cloth, placing it in the palm, and securing it with an elastic bandage or tape wrapped around the fingers and hand (leaving the thumb out).

When to call the doctor Significant pain over the fourth or fifth knuckle following punch injury should prompt a visit to the emergency room or doctor's office for x-rays.

Treatment Realigning the head of the bone and immobilizing the break for 4 to 6 weeks is usually sufficient. A small degree of angle in these more mobile bones does not significantly impair their normal function. A greater degree, however, is unacceptable. Rarely, surgical fixation of the bone head with wires or pins proves necessary.

Prognosis Prognosis is excellent if promptly diagnosed and properly treated.

❖ DUPUYTREN'S CONTRACTURE

Signs and symptoms Inability to straighten the ring and small finger, although other fingers may be involved; painless knots or lumps in the palm or the sole of the foot.

What is it? Dupuytren's contracture is a gradually progressive condition of fibrous thickening of the palmar fascia (the connective tissue of the palm) predominantly in the region of the tendons that flex the fourth and fifth fingers. As the thickening progresses, it creates a pull on the tendons, gradually drawing the fingers they serve into a bent position in the palm of the hand. Thickened areas along the palmar fascia account for the knots that develop in the palm.

Although the condition is usually painless and no threat to life or health, it can create disability by limiting normal hand function—for example, holding a hammer or other hand tool can become difficult.

What you can do The goal of self-care is to improve flexibility of the tendons; daily stretching exercises will help. Warm the hand (in warm water or if available in a paraffin wax dip device) and gently stretch the fingers into a straighter position using the other hand; massage the tendons in the palm with a good quality lanolin massage cream. Because the condition is progressive, the sooner stretching exercise is instituted, the longer surgery to release the tendons may be delayed.

When to call the doctor If the knotty areas in the palm or the tendons themselves become painful or inflamed, consult your doctor. When the contraction of the fingers is severe, exercise and massage alone will not usually be sufficient to restore mobility. See your doctor for an evaluation for the need for surgery.

Treatment Painful inflammation of the tendon coverings can sometimes occur and is best treated by injection of the area with a corticosteroid medication, such as Kenalog.

Surgical release—cleaning away the fibrous overgrowth from around the tendons—should be considered when the bending interferes with normal hand function. Physical therapy before and after surgery to improve and restore mobility is imperative.

Prognosis Surgery can be very successful for this condition, but in some cases it may continue to progress.

❖ SUBUNGUAL HEMATOMA (BLOOD UNDER THE NAIL)

Symptoms *(What you may experience)* Black discoloration under the nail; throbbing pain of the nail following trauma.

Signs and laboratory findings *(What the doctor looks for)* Associated fracture of bone as detected by x-ray.

What is it? The nails sit on a bed of tissue rich in blood vessels and nerves. A direct blow to the nail—such as hitting the finger with a hammer or slamming it in a car

CARE OF CASTED AND SPLINTED PARTS

Proper care of a cast or splint will speed healing of a casted or splinted injury. Here are some important guidelines:

- Keep the cast or splint dry. Use a double layer of plastic (trash bags or bread wrappers secured with a large rubber band or shoelace work well) or a commercial waterproof shield when bathing or showering. Moisture weakens plaster. Even if your cast or splint is made of waterproof material, remember that damp padding beneath the cast or splint can cause skin irritation.

- Allow the cast to dry completely before placing a weight stress on it. Do not walk on a walking cast until it has cured completely—about an hour for a fiberglass cast/splint and about 48 to 72 hours for a plaster cast/splint.

- Keep dirt, sand, or powder (including anti-itching or deodorant powders) away from the inside of the cast/splint. Once inside, they can chafe and irritate the skin.

- Do not pull the padding away from your cast/splint. Padding is placed there to prevent pressure over bony areas or to allow room for swelling.

- Do not insert objects, such as coat hangers or sticks into the cast/splint to scratch an itch. You could damage the skin and an infection could occur where it cannot be seen. Report itching to your doctor if it persists.

- Do not trim away or break off rough edges without first consulting your doctor. Never attempt to remove your cast yourself.

- Pay careful attention to the skin around the cast/splint. If it becomes red, raw, or painful, call your doctor.

- Inspect finger or toe tips or nails for signs that the cast may be too tight. With slight pressure applied with the thumbnail, the finger- or toenail or digit tip should blanch white and when the pressure is released should immediately return to its normal color. If it does not, it could indicate insufficient blood flow from too tight a cast/splint. Other signs that a cast is too tight include burning-type pain and increasing pain despite elevation and pain medication. Call your doctor right away.

- Regularly inspect your cast/splint. If it becomes cracked or develops soft spots, contact the doctor. A weak cast/splint cannot properly protect your injury.

- If your hand or foot swells you should elevate it. If swelling continues and pain increases despite elevating the limb, you should contact your doctor. ■

door—can often tear small blood vessels in the bed, allowing blood to leak under the nail. Separation of the nail from its bed and the buildup of blood under pressure beneath the nail cause intense throbbing pain (see Subungual Hematoma, page 1323, for more information).

Sometimes, the blow breaks the terminal phalanx (small finger bone) beneath the nail. X-rays can determine whether this has occurred. Puncturing the nail to relieve the accumulated blood potentially leaves a route open for bacteria to penetrate to the broken bone although this is rare.

What you can do Elevate the finger and apply ice immediately to reduce the leakage of blood beneath the nail.

When to call the doctor As soon as is possible, see the doctor for x-rays and evaluation as well as for definitive treatment of the hematoma.

Treatment Puncturing the nail will relieve the intense pressure and pain almost immediately. This procedure is best accomplished by use of a cautery needle (electric wand with a hot tip). The procedure is quick (a matter of seconds) and painless. An alternative method—not as quick—involves use of a special tiny drill to bore a hole in the nail. By either method, the collected blood drains out right away. Waiting too long to seek treatment could allow sufficient time for the blood to clot firmly, in which case the collection of blood cannot be relieved by simple puncture.

If x-rays have shown the presence of a fracture of the tip of the finger, the doctor may prescribe a course of antibiotics to prevent infection.

Prognosis Prognosis is excellent when treated promptly and appropriately. In some cases, the nail can be saved. In others, the nail will be lost, but will regrow over several months. In some cases the nail that grows back may be slightly deformed.

The Wrist

❖ COLLE'S FRACTURE

Symptoms (What you may experience)
Pain, swelling (often), bruising (often), and deformity of the forearm at the bend of the wrist; pain with attempted movement of the wrist.

Colle's fracture. Falling on an outstretched hand can cause the large bone (radius) in the forearm to break near the wrist.

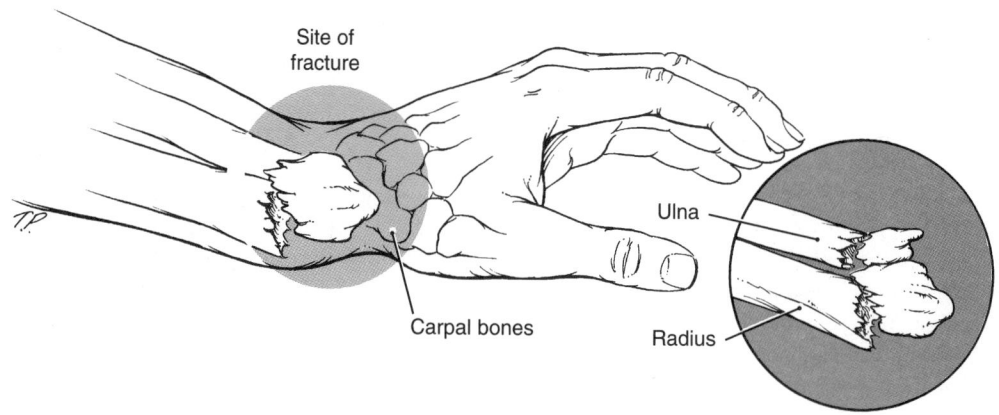

Site of fracture

Ulna

Carpal bones

Radius

Signs and laboratory findings *(What the doctor looks for)* Point tenderness to pressure over the radius and ulna (forearm bones) at the wrist; typical fracture of the end of the radius and often the tip of the ulna as detected by x-ray.

What is it? Landing on an outstretched hand during a fall forward is the most common means of sustaining this injury, also sometimes called a fracture of the distal radius. The force of the weight of the falling body jams the end of the radius into the hard surface and, in some cases, the bone breaks. The severity of the injury is dictated by where the fracture line occurs. In the simplest form, the break extends only into the joint between the radius and its forearm partner, the ulna. If it extends into the joint where the radius meets the bones of the wrist, it is a more severe injury. If the tip of the ulna (also called the ulnar styloid) is

sheered off as well, that worsens the degree of injury.

As with any fractured bone—but especially so in the wrist where many veins, arteries, nerves, and tendons gather in a small space—damage to these important structures from the break or from the swelling that follows can be a major threat. Compromising the blood supply in the hand can have catastrophic consequences. Care must be taken to ensure that there is always good circulation—both blood flow into and return of blood from the hand following injury.

What you can do Apply ice. Move the wrist as little as possible. Make an emergency splint to stabilize the wrist (see Splinting the Injured Wrist and Forearm, page 670).

Check the pulse at the wrist—found easily on the thumb side of the underside. To check circulation in the fingers, gently press each nail on the injured hand with a thumb or fingernail; the nail should be pink and with pressure should blanch white. Upon release of the pressure the nail should immediately return to pink. You should have normal sensation as well when you touch your fingers.

When to call the doctor Call the doctor as soon as possible; only an x-ray can determine the extent of a Colle's fracture. If the elbow is painful, x-rays of that joint may be needed as well.

Treatment Usually, in simple fractures that are not displaced, properly splinting or casting the injury is all that is needed, immobilizing the break for 4 to 6 weeks. Elevation and ice during the first 24 to 48 hours is the

SPLINTING THE INJURED WRIST AND FOREARM

Splinting a wrist in an emergency situation may mean using whatever material is at hand. In accidents that happen at home or the office, one good method is to use a thick magazine or a large section of newspaper. Bend the magazine or newspaper lengthwise to form a cradle for the wrist, forearm, and hand. Lift the wrist, hand, and forearm as a unit just enough to slide the magazine or newspaper (or other splint material, such as stiff cardboard or a piece of wood) under it. Be sure the length of the splint will be sufficient to support the entire length of the forearm from elbow down to the fingers. Secure the splint in place snugly but not too tightly with tape, an elastic bandage, heavy string, or strips of cloth tied at intervals around it.

Support the splinted arm with the other hand or with an arm sling (see How to Make and Use a Sling, page 676). See page 383 for more information on splints. ■

rule. Then about 3 to 5 days into the period of immobility, active exercise of the fingers and the shoulder should begin as a part of therapy.

Complicated fractures—or those involving the bones at the elbow—may require surgical fixation to properly hold the realigned bones in place internally. Wires used to affix the bone fragments remain in place for several weeks and then are removed in the office by the doctor who applied them. Sometimes the surgeon may need to use plates with screws or a device called an external fixator (pins or wires placed through the skin from the outside) to stabilize the fracture.

Prognosis Prognosis is excellent in young people with simple fractures; the fractures heal without consequence in just a few weeks. Prognosis is good even in complicated fractures if properly diagnosed and appropriately treated by the doctor.

❖ SCAPHOID FRACTURE

Symptoms *(What you may experience)* Persistent pain in the wrist or persistently painful grip following a fall; limitation of normal wrist motion.

Signs and laboratory findings *(What the doctor looks for)* Tenderness in the anatomic snuff box of the wrist (the hollow at the base of the thumb as it joins the wrist); evidence of fracture of the scaphoid (also called navicular) bone as detected by x-ray.

What is it? Falling backward on an outstretched hand is the classic means of sustaining a fracture of the scaphoid bone of the wrist; common circumstances include slipping on ice or a wet floor. However, any sharp blow against the palm of a bent hand could also cause this injury to the wrist.

The small, irregularly shaped bones of the wrist are loosely arranged in two rows—one nearest the body of the hand and the other nearest the bones of the forearm. The scaphoid bone lies closest to the forearm on the side of the thumb. To prevent a backward fall, the natural inclination is to catch the weight on an outstretched hand. This maneuver traps the scaphoid between the radius and the first row of wrist bones, often cracking the scaphoid.

Unlike other bones in the wrist, the scaphoid is especially vulnerable to poor healing because of its blood supply. Failure to discover the crack and obtain proper medical treatment could also allow too much movement along the fracture and prevent the bone from strongly knitting back together, termed nonunion of the fracture.

What you can do Initially, apply ice and elevate the wrist. Limit motion by splinting the wrist in a functional position (see Splinting the Injured Wrist and Forearm, page 670).

When to call the doctor What may seem like a persistent, bad wrist sprain could be a much more serious injury if the scaphoid is injured. Initial x-rays (taken at the time of injury) may not show a crack. Persistent pain indicates a need for repeat x-ray, by which time the crack may have widened and be more visible. A bone scan is the second test after x-ray.

Treatment Immobilization of the fracture in a special cast that includes the thumb (called a thumb spica cast) is mandatory. The wrist should be cocked slightly backward and the hand turned slightly toward the thumb. Immobilization for 10 to 12 weeks is the rule, but complete x-ray healing of the scaphoid may require up to 4 to 6 months.

Nonunion of the fracture or avascular necrosis require surgical repair, either a bone graft (placement of shavings of live, healthy bone into the unhealed area to stimulate new bone formation) or excision of smaller unhealed parts of the bone.

Prognosis If diagnosed promptly and treated appropriately, greater than 90 percent of scaphoid fractures heal. Long-term discomfort, painful grip, stiffness, and loss of wrist mobility can result if left untreated.

❖ CARPAL TUNNEL SYNDROME

Symptoms *(What you may experience)* Numb sensation in the first three fingers; shooting pain up and down the arm following use of the hands or wrist; loss of ability to oppose the thumb (to make the pad of the thumb meet the pad of another finger).

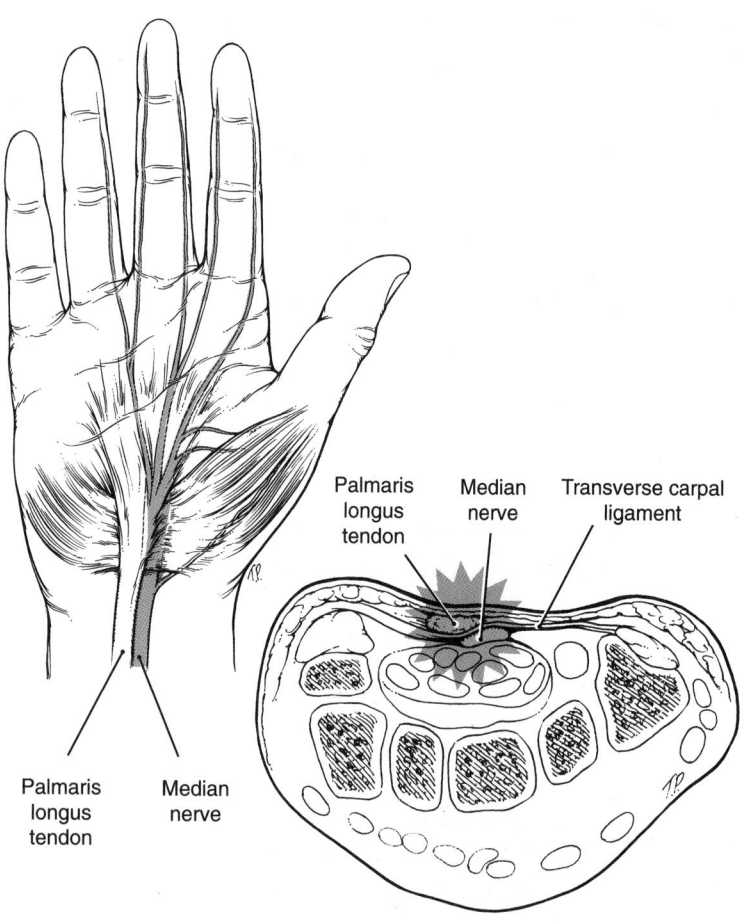

Palmaris longus tendon

Median nerve

Transverse carpal ligament

Palmaris longus tendon

Median nerve

Compression or entrapment of the median nerve in the arm or under the carpal ligament in the wrist can cause numbness and pain. The risk of getting carpal tunnel syndrome increases with repetitive motions of the hands and wrists.

Signs and laboratory findings *(What the doctor looks for)* Compression of the nerve with with thumb; positive nerve conduction velocity test (in about three-fourths of cases); tinel sign (sharp shooting pain into the fingers from tapping over the underside of the wrist); temporary relief of pain with regional anesthetic block (in about 90 percent of cases).

What is it? Carpal tunnel syndrome occurs as a result of compression or entrapment of the median nerve—the one primarily responsible for supplying feeling to the palm side of the thumb and first two fingers. This nerve, along with other vital nerves, blood vessels, and tendons, passes from the arm into the hand beneath the carpal ligament. The carpal ligament's tough, band-like struc-

ture spans the wrist from side to side, forming the roof of what is termed the carpal tunnel. Although entrapment or compression occurs most commonly in this location, it can also occur higher in the arm, nearer the elbow, usually following trauma to that area.

Chronic, repetitive use of the hands and wrists is a common cause of overuse trauma that may increase the risk of development of carpal tunnel nerve compression. For example, overuse may occur with such activities as typing, playing the piano or other fingered instrument, working on an assembly line, or operating motorized lawn/ garden or construction tools, but may also occur in a wide variety of other activities. Carpal tunnel syndrome can occur secondary to inflammatory arthritis involving the wrist or other conditions that affect the carpal tunnel. Carpel tunnel syndrome is common among pregnant women, people with hypothyroidism, and those who have had a wrist fracture.

Compression of the nerve usually first leads to a sensation of numbness in the thumb and first two fingers with inactivity, as though they have fallen asleep. With some activities, pain can occur, radiating in lightning bolts down the hand to the fingers or sometimes upward toward the elbow. Grip strength may suffer, at first because of the pain that motion may cause, but later from true weakness and atrophy (wasting) of the muscles. Pain may also occur with the development of inflammation in the tendons and joint linings (a tenosynovitis) of the hands and wrist.

What you can do Try to eliminate chronic repetitive stress to the hands and wrists. For example, use wrist supports when typing at a keyboard; use wrist splints at night or during periods of heavy physical activity. Protect the hands and wrists against vibration stress when operating lawn/garden or construction tools with antivibrational padded gloves.

When to call the doctor If symptoms persist or weakness develops, see the doctor as soon as possible for testing and evaluation.

Treatment Injection of corticosteroid medication into the carpal tunnel followed by resting the wrist in a splint day and night for 30 days may help. The doctor may recommend repeating the injection in 4 to 6 weeks if symptoms have not improved by at least 50 percent. Nonsteroidal anti-inflammatory drugs (NSAIDs) may also help in some cases.

Persistence of symptoms or the development of weakness of the fingers, thumb, or wrist may necessitate surgery to free the nerve from its compression.

Prognosis Medical therapy (injections, splinting, and exercise) controls the symptoms long term in only about 25 percent of the cases of carpal tunnel syndrome, but is highly effective in the short term (a few months). Surgical release cures about 90 percent of the cases; in the remaining 10 percent, some permanent damage or inflammation to the nerve from long-standing compression or further compression from newly formed scar tissue may cause symptoms to persist.

❖ GANGLION CYST

Symptoms (*What you may experience*) Rapidly developing, usually painless but occasionally tender lump, most often at the wrist; painful or weak grip (sometimes).

Signs and laboratory findings (*What the doctor looks for*) No specific x-ray or laboratory studies are helpful except to exclude other problems.

What is it? A ganglion cyst develops as a soft or rubbery swelling over the wrist (or occasionally the top of the foot or a finger) usually in response to minor (often unrecognized) injury that damages the joint capsule. The injury inspires excessive production of joint fluid that collects in a sac-like structure adjacent to the joint. The cyst increases in size rapidly—sometimes seemingly overnight—and may wax and wane with the level of activity. (These characteristics differentiate it from cancers, which usually grow much more slowly and do not wax and wane.) Its size may vary but in most instances is about 1 cm (about the size of a dime).

These benign swellings can occur at any age, but most often develop between ages 20 and 50, with women affected twice as often as are men.

What you can do Apply ice daily for 2 to 3 weeks. Minimize handling the cyst to pre-

vent its becoming irritated and somewhat painful. During periods of increased size and discomfort (should they occur), limit excessive use of the affected wrist or hand.

Acetaminophen or over-the-counter (OTC) anti-inflammatory medication (such as ibuprofen) may help relieve discomfort.

When to call the doctor In most cases, a ganglion can safely be ignored, but to be certain that the lump is indeed a ganglion cyst and that no other problem is causing the lump, consult your doctor.

Treatment No treatment is necessary in the absence of pain, grip weakness, or unsightly appearance; ganglion cyst do not pose a threat to health. Ice and NSAIDs can help decrease swelling.

Aspiration (removing fluid with a syringe) of the cyst (under local anesthesia in the doctor's office) is curative in about half the cases. Because of its close proximity to the radial artery, aspiration of cysts on the underside of the wrist should be done with more caution.

Surgery to remove the cyst contents as well as the joint lining is usually successful.

Prognosis Prognosis is excellent, although the cysts sometimes recur even following excision.

❖ DE QUERVAIN'S TENDINITIS

Symptoms (*What you may experience*) Painful grip with loss of grip strength; pain and swelling of the wrist on the thumb side.

Signs and laboratory findings (*What the doctor looks for*) Swelling over the radial styloid (end of the forearm bone nearest the base of the thumb); positive Finklestein maneuver (stretching the tendon by moving the wrist in a direction away from the thumb causes extreme pain); resisted upward motion of the extended thumb causes pain. X-ray studies are of use in this condition to rule out other causes of the pain.

What is it? Excessive or unaccustomed use of the thumb to grip or grasp causes irritation and inflammation of the thumb's tendons that extend it (pull it toward the back of the hand) and abduct it (move it perpendicular to the palm). With the pain of inflammation, gripping or grasping can prove difficult. The inflammatory process usually

The humerus is the long bone in the arm, and it is supported by four muscles, including the biceps brachii and the triceps brachii muscles. The biceps flexes the elbow and the triceps extends it. Many shoulder muscles, including the deltoid, also surround the top end of the bone, which rests in the shoulder's socket. The socket allows rotation of the bone in multiple directions. Dislocation of the shoulder can occur under severe physical stress.

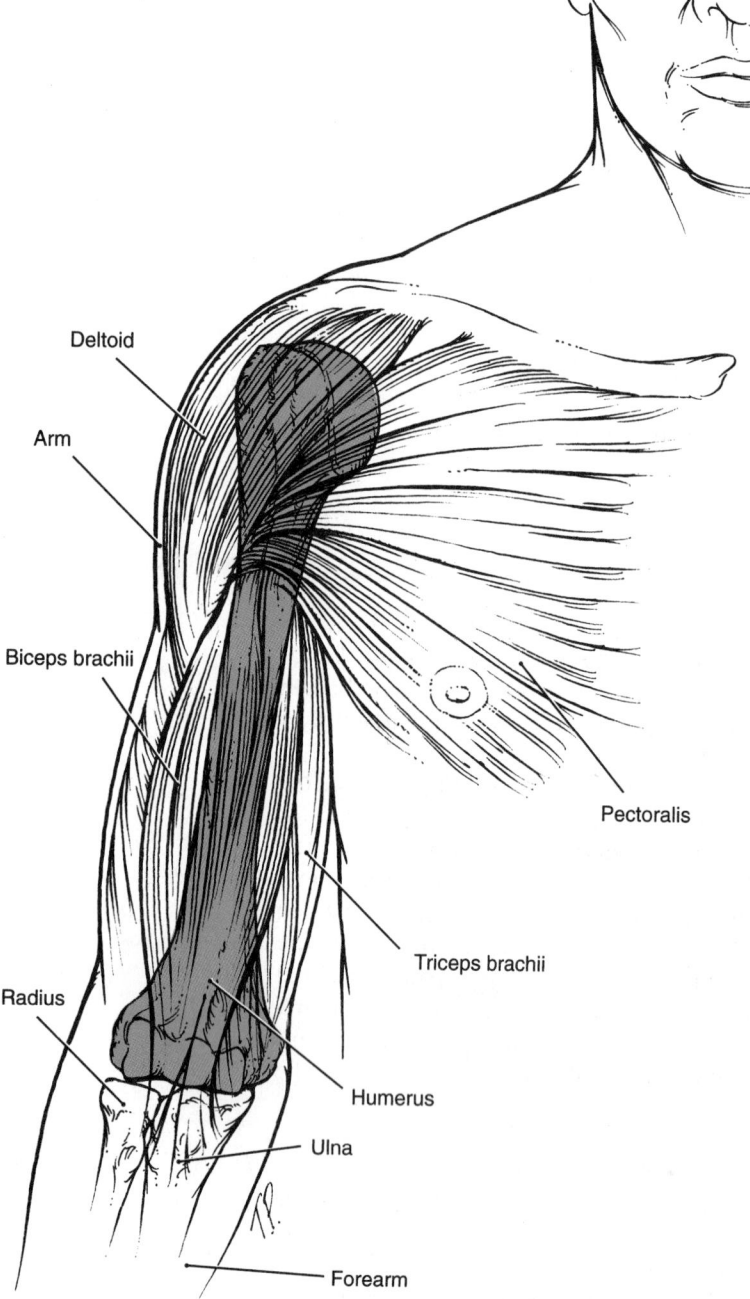

Deltoid

Arm

Biceps brachii

Radius

Triceps brachii

Humerus

Ulna

Pectoralis

Forearm

causes swelling of the tissues of the wrist near the base of the thumb. Left untreated, it may even incite the laying down of fibrous tissue around the tendon coverings, binding the tendon and limiting motion of the thumb.

What you can do Rest the thumb—avoid gripping or grasping. Apply ice to the wrist and base of the thumb. Acetaminophen or OTC anti-inflammatory medications, such as ibuprofen, may help reduce the pain. Splint the thumb to its neighbor—the index finger—with a strip of adhesive tape that encircles the end of the thumb and the base of the index finger (see Immobilizing an Injured Hand or Finger, page 666).

When to call the doctor If the simple remedies outlined above fail to resolve the pain within 4 weeks, consult your doctor.

Treatment The doctor may recommend full doses of an anti-inflammatory medication or an injection of corticosteroid medication and anesthetic into the sheath covering the tendon as it crosses the radial styloid. The injection can be repeated at 4 to 6 weeks if it has failed to relieve the discomfort by half. If a second injection proves necessary, it should be followed by more elaborate splinting or casting to completely immobilize the thumb (a thumb spica splint or cast) for 4 to 6 weeks. Following immobilization, exercise to stretch the thumb across the palm helps to restore normal function. Surgical release of a scarred tendon should be considered if medical treatments fail.

Prognosis Medical measures (full doses of an NSAID, injection, immobilization, and exercise) resolve the pain significantly in 90 percent of cases. About one-third may require a second injection after a year. Only about 10 percent of cases fail to respond to medical therapies and require surgery to release the tendon.

The Arm

❖ RADIUS OR ULNA SHAFT FRACTURE (FRACTURED FOREARM)

Symptoms *(What you may experience)*
Pain, swelling, and often deformity of the

lower arm following trauma; numbness or loss of normal motion (sometimes).

Signs and laboratory findings *(What the doctor looks for)* Confirmation and delineation of the break via x-rays.

What is it? Two long bones—the radius and ulna—form the skeleton of the forearm. A fall or direct blow to the forearm can snap one or both of these bones along their shafts. In some instances, the jagged broken ends pierce the skin and tissues of the arm (an open or compound fracture), an occurrence that heightens the risk for bone infection and worsens the prognosis for uncomplicated healing.

Depending on the location of the break, vital nerve or blood vessels in the area could sustain damage. For this reason—as with any fracture—careful examination to check the integrity of circulation and sensation in the arm and hand beyond the break is mandatory.

What you can do Carefully—with as little movement as possible—splint the injured arm (see Splinting the Injured Wrist and Forearm, page 670). Apply ice and elevate on a pillow, folded towels, or blanket to cushion jarring en route to the emergency room or doctor's office. Do not eat or drink anything—in some cases, anesthesia and surgical fixation might be necessary and would be delayed by a stomach full of fluid or food.

When to call the doctor Call the doctor immediately.

Treatment In children, after x-rays have determined the nature of the break, the doctor (usually an orthopedist) will manipulate the bone back into good alignment and set the fracture in a cast extending from the knuckles to midway up the arm beyond the elbow (a long arm cast). In most adults, surgery is necessary to properly align the bone before casting. It is usually necessary to immobilize the entire length of the broken bone, which implies immobilizing the joint above the break and the joint below the break to ensure stability along the fracture site. In this case, that means immobilizing both the elbow and the wrist. The length of immobilization varies, but in most cases will last 10 to 12 weeks—until the

bone has begun to visibly repair itself. Repeat x-rays will show the formation of bony callus (like the body's internal splint) around the fracture site in about 4 to 6 weeks—sooner in growing children and longer in the elderly or in women with osteoporosis.

Some fractures may require surgical fixation (with placement of wires, screws, or plates) to properly and securely align the bone ends. Open fractures will need an operation for surgical debridement (cutting away damaged tissue) to remove or cleanse mangled or potentially dirty tissue. IV antibiotics—given in the hospital after surgery and occasionally longer for open fractures—will reduce the risk of infection into the bone.

Prognosis Prognosis is excellent in most cases.

❖ NURSEMAID'S ELBOW

Symptoms and signs This condition occurs in toddlers. Arm held bent at the elbow and pulled close to the chest; tearful resistance of attempts to straighten the arm.

What is it? The end of the radius nearest the elbow narrows to form a round disk that is flattened on one side—called the head of the radius—that is free to rotate in an encircling ligament that binds it to its partner bone, the ulna. In young children, the ligament is somewhat lax, and the bone still fairly pliable. A sharp pull on the hand or lower arm—such as a nursemaid, parent, or older sibling might employ to pull the child along the street or up the stairs—can pop the head of the radius free from the ligament that binds it. Pain is immediate, and the child quickly bends the arm and pulls it in toward the chest in a protected posture. The pain diminishes in this position and crying may stop, but the child will not use that arm normally. Attempts to straighten the arm will incite tearful resistance.

What you can do Sling the arm or simply allow the child to keep it in a comfortable position. Apply ice if the child will allow it.

When to call the doctor Proceed to the emergency room or doctor's office right away.

HOW TO MAKE AND USE A SLING

To support an injured arm or shoulder, you can fashion an emergency sling from a scarf, square or length of cloth, piece of rope, or an elastic bandage. Do the following:

- Fold a large scarf or square of cloth into a triangle. Tie two ends of the triangle around the neck snugly enough to support the arm bent at a comfortable angle with the hand slightly higher than the elbow.

- Tie the ends of a long length of cloth or rope, place the tied end around the neck and the loop under the arm just below the wrist. Be sure the full length of the forearm is supported by a splint (see Splinting the Injured Wrist and Forearm, page 670).

- An elastic bandage can also be used to immobilize the shoulder. Tuck the bent arm closely to your chest and firmly (but not too tightly) wrap the elastic bandage around both arm and body, going from the uninjured shoulder, across the chest, around the affected arm, around the body and across the back returning to the uninjured shoulder. Make as many loops as the length of bandage allows and secure with clips or a safety pin. This form of splinting should only be used as a stop gap during transport to a medical facility.

See page 388 for more information on slings. ■

A sling can support and immobilize a fractured or dislocated shoulder, arm, or wrist. For a shoulder injury, a large piece of fabric is wrapped around the shoulder and then supports it by covering the entire forearm.

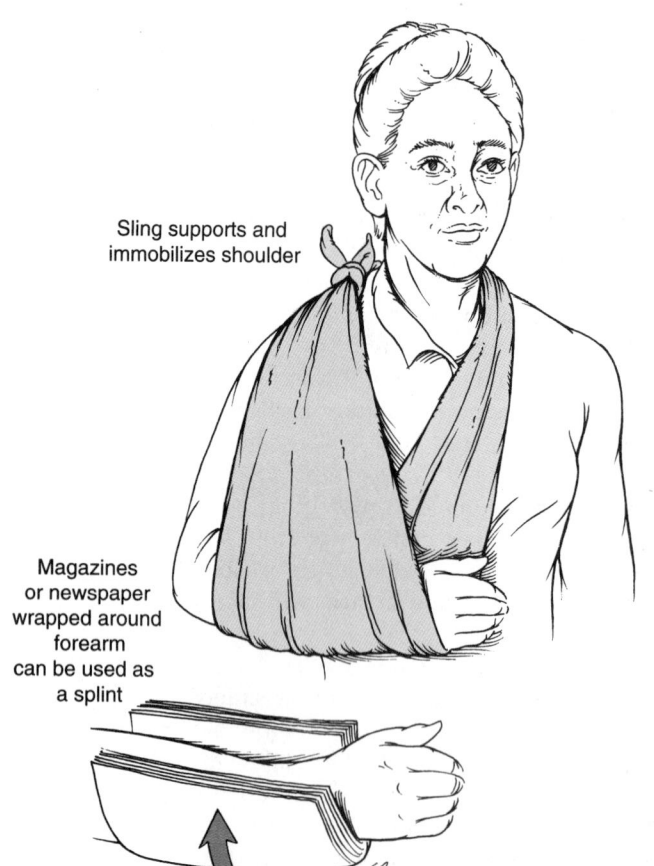

Sling supports and immobilizes shoulder

Magazines or newspaper wrapped around forearm can be used as a splint

Treatment Relocating the misplaced head is a simple and quick procedure that involves pulling on the hand to pull the radial head out a bit further and then quickly twisting it back into place. Properly performed it is relatively painless and as soon as the head pops back into place, the pain (and crying) stop and normal function returns to the arm.

Prognosis Prognosis is excellent. Recurrence is unusual unless the arm is pulled on again.

❖ FRACTURE OF THE RADIAL HEAD

Symptoms *(What you may experience)* Pain and swelling of the outside aspect of the elbow following trauma; worsening pain on turning the hand palm up.

Signs and laboratory findings *(What the doctor looks for)* Loss of range of motion, especially rotation; swelling, especially on the outer side; tenderness upon pushing on the side of the elbow over the radial head; confirmation of fracture by x-rays.

What is it? The radius of the forearm narrows at the elbow to form the radial head encircled by a tough ligament that binds it to the ulna. The radial head is usually broken by falling on an outstretched arm. Occasionally, a direct blow to the side of the elbow can break the head of the radius.

What you can do Sling the arm for comfort, keeping it as still as possible (see How to Make and Use a Sling, this page). Apply ice and elevate on a pillow or on folded towels or blankets. Check pulses at the wrist and evaluate for any loss of feeling.

When to call the doctor Proceed to the emergency room or doctor's office right away for evaluation.

Treatment In some cases, immobilization in a sling for several weeks is all that is needed. A splint is recommended (one extending from the knuckles of the hand to midway up the arm beyond the elbow) to permit healing to take place for only a week or so. Displaced or severe fracture may demand surgical fixation with placement of wires to hold the radial head in place securely.

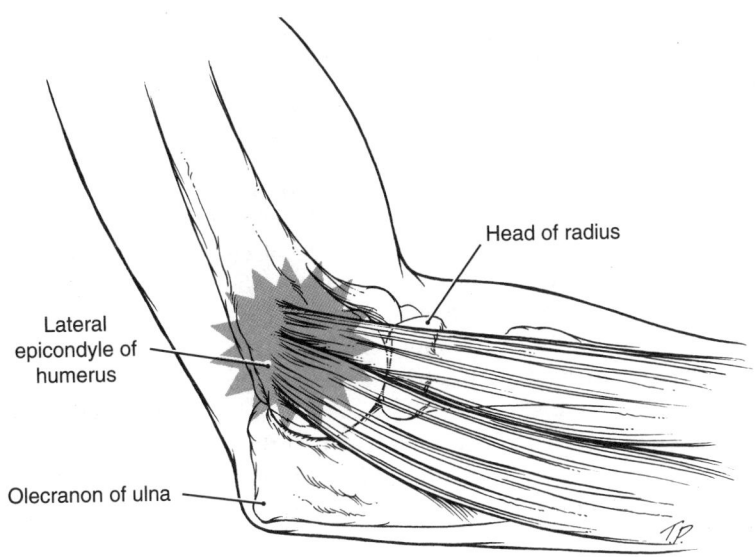

Head of radius

Lateral epicondyle of humerus

Olecranon of ulna

Extensive performance of certain activities such as gripping or twisting can cause microscopic tears of muscle tendons where they are attached to bones in the elbow. Inflammation and pain can then develop.

Prognosis Prognosis is excellent if promptly identified and treated. Left untreated, although the bone may knit together, it may do so improperly aligned, leaving the radial head unable to rotate properly and painlessly in its groove. The result is limitation in turning the hand palm up. The biggest problem is loss of motion, so it is important to begin motion within 7 to 10 days of the injury.

❖ EPICONDYLITIS (TENNIS ELBOW)

Symptoms *(What you may experience)* Aching pain on the outside aspect of the elbow without preceding trauma; sharp pain in the outside of the elbow with gripping or twisting motions of the hand and forearm.

Signs and laboratory findings *(What the doctor looks for)* Tenderness over the lateral epicondyle; worsening pain with attempts to resist wrist extension (bending wrist back) and radial deviation (turning it toward the thumb side). X-rays usually are normal and help to exclude other causes.

What is it? The muscles of the forearm used to grip, make a fist, and twist the hand palm side down attach to the elbow in the region of the lateral epicondyle. Unaccustomed use or overuse of these muscles—in such activities as gripping a tennis racquet, driving nails, or using a screwdriver—can cause microscopic tears of the muscular attachments to the bone (the tendons) and bring on an acute inflammation of the epi-

condyle. Because of its common association with playing tennis, this condition has become known as tennis elbow, even though it can develop following a wide variety of other activities.

What you can do Limit lifting, gripping, twisting, hammering, or other repetitive motions of the wrist or hand. Apply ice to the epicondyle for 20 to 30 minutes several times a day and after exercise. Use of OTC anti-inflammatory agents, such as ibuprofen, may help relieve discomfort. A splint to limit motion of the wrist may help by resting the muscles.

When to call the doctor If the conservative remedies outlined above fail to resolve the condition in 2 to 3 weeks, consult a doctor.

Treatment Most people with tennis elbow respond to rest and full doses of NSAIDs. If these measures fail to resolve the problem, an injection of corticosteroid medication into the region of the epicondyle may be necessary to resolve the inflammation and pain.

Persistence of pain or significant impairment of grip strength may require orthopedic referral for surgery to repair the tendinitis.

Prognosis Prognosis is very good with adequate treatment. Recurrence of symptoms occurs in at least one quarter of cases as a consequence of poor healing, often brought about by inadequate treatment. In those cases requiring it, surgery eliminates pain and restores normal strength about 90 to 95 percent of the time.

❖ OLECRANON BURSITIS (WATER ON THE ELBOW)

Symptoms *(What you may experience)* Often sudden (sometimes gradual) development of redness, warmth, and golf-ball–sized swelling just below the point of the elbow without known trauma; development of a painless fluid-filled sack just below the point of the elbow.

Signs and laboratory findings *(What the doctor looks for)* X-rays are not helpful except to rule out other conditions.

What is it? The underside of the point of the elbow—called the olecranon process of the ulna—is cushioned by a bursa. Repetitive trauma to this area—most commonly sustained by pressure from constantly resting the elbows on a hard surface—causes the bursa to swell and become inflamed, resulting in bursitis. (See Rheumatism of the Soft Tissue [Bursitis, Tendinitis, Tenosynovitis, and Chondritis] for more information on bursitis.) The speed with which the swelling occurs can be impressive; sometimes within just a few hours a lump the size of a golf ball can arise. In 90 percent of cases, repetitive trauma is at the root of the problem, in 5 percent gout causes the swelling, and in another 5 percent the bursa has become infected by bacteria, most commonly *Staphylococcus aureus*.

In some cases that look infected or that do not respond to treatment, aspiration of the fluid in the sac may be necessary. The fluid is sent to the laboratory for analysis to determine the presence of bacteria, uric acid crystals, or blood. The in-office procedure, usually performed under local anesthetic with an injection to numb the skin, is relatively painless.

What you can do Apply ice to relieve pain and inflammation. An elbow pad may help prevent further irritation by rubbing. Acetaminophen or ibuprofen can help.

When to call the doctor As soon as possible, consult your doctor for complete evaluation, especially if you have signs of infection (increasing pain, warmth, redness, fevers, chills). Because of the small risk that infection could be the cause, it is not safe to delay.

Treatment In simple bursitis caused by repetitive or chronic trauma, ice, padding, NSAIDs, or immobilization may be required. In some instances, the doctor may recommend an injection of corticosteroid medication into the bursa. Injection is a last resort, as it may cause infection.

Those cases caused by infection require treatment with antibiotics sufficient to kill the most likely bacterial cause, *Staphylococcus aureus*, until culture results are final (about 48 hours). Surgery is rarely needed unless these treatments fail.

Cases caused by gout require immediate and ongoing treatment for this condition (see Gout, page 652).

Prognosis Prognosis is excellent if promptly and appropriately treated.

❖ HUMERUS FRACTURE

Symptoms *(What you may experience)* Pain and limitation of motion of the arm just at the shoulder following trauma (usually a fall or direct blow); discoloration and swelling (sometimes).

Signs and laboratory findings *(What the doctor looks for)* Confirmation of the fracture via x-rays.

What is it? The bone of the upper arm—called the humerus—flares at its end to form a ball shape that fits into a hollow socket at the shoulder. Soft tissues, such as tendons, muscles, and ligaments, attach the ball and socket leaving the arm fairly free to rotate and move in many directions.

Fractures to the humerus from a fall or a direct blow to the side of the shoulder, such as might happen in a broadside automobile accident, commonly occur in the area of bone just beneath the ball, called the head of the humerus. These fractures occur more commonly in the elderly or in people with osteoporosis.

The fracture, depending on its exact location, can jeopardize vital nerves and blood vessels that course along the under surface of the humerus on the way to the lower part of the arm.

What you can do Move the arm as little as possible. Support it with an arm sling or wrap it, bent at the elbow, close to the body with an elastic bandage, gauze bandage, or long strips of cloth (see How to Make and Use a Sling, page 676). Apply ice. Check pulses at the wrist and note any area of numbness.

When to call the doctor Proceed immediately to the emergency room or doctor's office for x-rays and evaluation.

Treatment In some instances, uncomplicated humeral fractures heal with simple immobilization in a shoulder immobilizer, collar and cuff sling, or sling-and-swathe bandage—all soft, padded devices that support the bent arm and prevent its moving too far away from the body.

In fractures of the humeral shaft the weight of the arm itself is usually all that is needed to keep the fracture properly aligned. Rarely, maintaining proper position of the fracture requires more weight to pull downward. In these instances, the doctor places a cast on the forearm and suspends it on a collar around the neck—called a hanging cast. In some cases, the doctor must operate on the ends of the broken bone to place them closer together with pins or a plate with screws to allow the fracture to heal. In some cases the humeral head must be replaced by an artificial joint.

Finger, wrist, and elbow range of motion exercises should begin within a few days after the fracture. Gentle shoulder exercises should begin at about 2 to 4 weeks following the fracture to prevent the development of a frozen shoulder—starting with 5 minutes of pendulum swinging several times a day and progressing to strengthening exercises for the shoulder muscles (see Frozen Shoulder, page 681).

Prognosis Prognosis good if promptly diagnosed and treated, with aggressive pursuit of physical therapy. Complete healing may take as long as 12 weeks.

❖ BICEPS TENDINITIS AND BICEPS TENDON RUPTURE

Symptoms *(What you may experience)* Pain in the front of the shoulder, aggravated by lifting or overhead pushing or pulling. Rupture: loud pop near the front of the

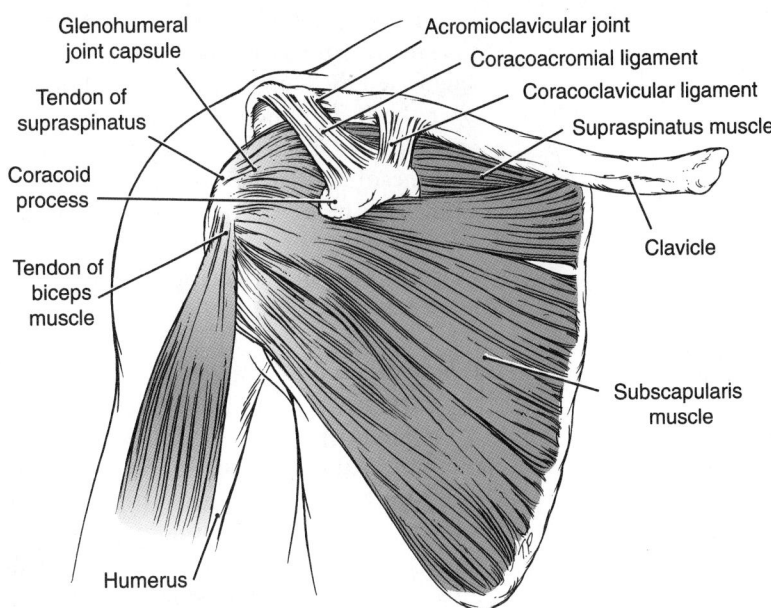

The ball-shaped top end of the arm's humerus (the bone that extends from the shoulder to the elbow) lies inside the shoulder's socket and is surrounded by numerous muscles connected to bones via strong tendons.

shoulder during lifting or straining the arm; suddenly enlarged biceps muscle hump; bruise over biceps near elbow. Tendinitis of the biceps is considered a manifestation of rotator cuff tendinitis. See Painful Shoulder (Tendinitis, Bursitis, Rotator Cuff Injuries, and Impingement Syndromes), page 681, for information on rotator cuff tendinitis.

Signs and laboratory findings *(What the doctor looks for)* Calcification near path of biceps tendon (sometimes). X-rays usually are not helpful for tendon rupture but can be helpful to evaluate tendonitis.

What is it? The biceps muscle, located on the front of the upper arm, functions to bend the arm and to support a carried load. The muscle has two parts (called a long head and a short head), each of which attaches to the bone via a tough tendon. The long head attaches high on the front of the shoulder. In some people, this tendon becomes irritated and inflamed from overuse or repetitive lifting and can develop microscopic tears and chronic pain (biceps tendinitis). Sudden heavy lifting can place enough strain on the inflamed tendon to rupture it—and in fact, the biceps tendon is the tendon in the body that is most commonly ruptured spontaneously.

Inflammation may lead to chronic soreness in the front of the shoulder, particularly aggravated by lifting or pushing and pulling over the head. When rupture occurs, it is accompanied by a loud pop that can be both heard and felt and the sudden diminishment of pain. Since the muscle has two heads, even though one has failed, the arm can still bend, and usually with only slightly less strength.

What you can do   Apply ice to the front of the shoulder to limit bruising and swelling. Avoid lifting or overhead pushing or pulling motions, although range-of-motion exercises are helpful to prevent stiffness (see Stretching the Painful Shoulder, page 682). During the inflammatory phase, OTC anti-inflammatory medications (such as ibuprofen) may help reduce inflammation.

When to call the doctor   If the conservative remedies outlined above fail to resolve the discomfort, or if rupture of the tendon has occurred, consult your doctor.

Treatment   In tendinitis, rest and full doses of an NSAID or local injection of corticosteroid medication into the groove on the bone where the biceps tendon runs may help. If symptoms fail to diminish, the doctor may recommend a repeat injection.

When rupture does occur, repair of the tendon surgically is not mandatory, but may be advisable in certain instances, depending on the physical demands of the person.

Prognosis   Tendinitis is painful but not a threat to life or health. Proper management controls discomfort, and oddly, rupture often cures the symptoms. Little to no disability results from rupture, and consequently the prognosis is favorable.

The Shoulder Girdle

❖ FRACTURED CLAVICLE (COLLAR BONE)

Symptoms (*What you may experience*)   Pain, swelling, and bruising of the collar bone following trauma.

Signs and laboratory findings (*What the doctor looks for*)   Confirmation of the fracture via x-rays.

What is it?   The most commonly broken bone in the body, the collar bone, also called the clavicle, bridges the front of the chest, from the shoulder to the breast bone. A fall on an outstretched arm transmits the force of the weight of the falling body up the arm, through the collar bone, to the central bone of the chest. The weak link in the chain is often the collar bone, which snaps in two or buckles under the stress, with the break usually in the middle.

In the vast majority of cases, healing occurs without incident, but it is important to remember that many large blood vessels and nerves pass just below the collar bone on their way to the arm, and the topmost part of the lung sits just behind. Although very rare, jagged ends of bone could potentially tear or puncture these vital structures, leading to such symptoms as shortness of breath, coughing up of bloody secretions, discoloration, loss of pulses, or loss of normal sensation in the hand or arm on that side.

What you can do   Apply ice and immobilize the shoulder (see Stretching the Painful Shoulder, page 682).

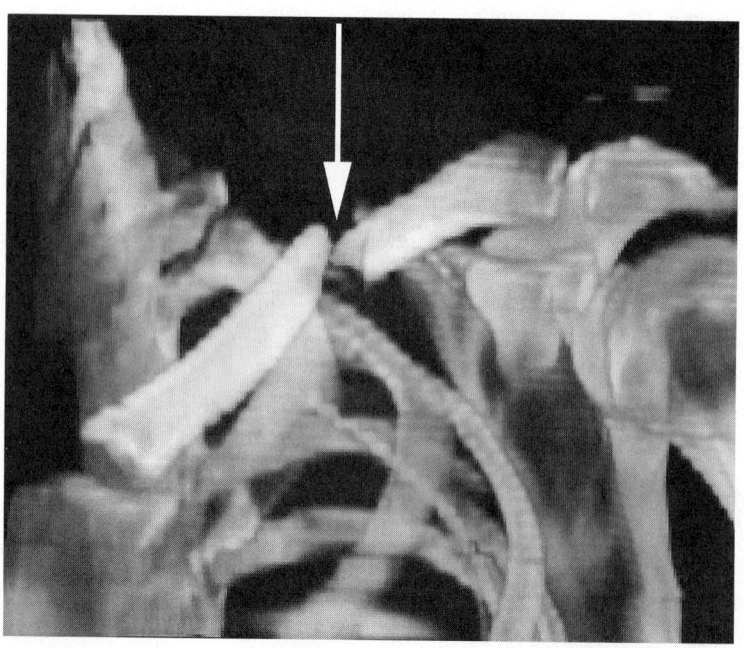

A clavicle (collar bone) fracture is shown on this CT scan (arrow). The clavicle is the most commonly broken bone in the body and nearly always heals without incident with the aid of a splint.

When to call the doctor Because of the risk to important structures, consult a doctor for evaluation and x-rays as soon as possible. Development of shortness of breath, coughing up of bloody secretions, or loss of pulses or normal sensation in the hand or arm require immediate medical attention.

Treatment In most cases, adequate healing occurs with only simple immobilization, using a simple sling. Rarely—except when damage to underlying structures complicates the picture—is surgical pinning or plating necessary to realign the bone ends. Range of motion of the fingers, wrist, and elbow can begin right away; shoulder range of motion should begin in a week.

Prognosis Prognosis is excellent in virtually all cases. A small percentage (less than 5 percent) do not heal and may require surgery.

❖ PAINFUL SHOULDER (TENDINITIS, BURSITIS, ROTATOR CUFF INJURIES, AND IMPINGEMENT SYNDROMES)

Symptoms *(What you may experience)* Pain, sometimes sharp and severe, during specific shoulder motions, most commonly reaching above shoulder level; weakness and limitation of motion of the shoulder in certain motions.

Signs and laboratory findings *(What the doctor looks for)* Standard x-rays are necessary first to exclude other causes. Rotator cuff tears detected by magnetic resonance imaging (MRI) or special x-ray studies.

What is it? The shoulder joint is a highly mobile ball-and-socket joint formed by the head of the humerus (the ball) and a hollowed depression in the shoulder blade that forms the socket. Soft tissues stabilize and attach the two bones, the primary ones being a group of strong muscles—called the rotator cuff—that encircle the joint and function to rotate the ball in its socket, allowing the arm to twist palm up to palm down, almost 360°. The muscles of the upper arm—the biceps and deltoid muscles—also attach nearby. Between the bony prominences and the tendons of these muscles lie protective bursae to cushion the

friction attendant with so great a range of motion.

Pain in the shoulder joint can originate from inflammation of the tendons themselves (tendinitis), from inflammation and swelling of the bursa (bursitis), from limitation of motion as a consequence of swelling or bony spurs (an impingement), or from tears of the rotator cuff muscles (rotator cuff tear).

The location of the inflammation or tear dictates which directions of shoulder motion cause the most pain. Quite often, motions such as reaching behind the body (either above the head or below the back) or raising the arm to the side cause the most discomfort. These motions in particular rotate the head of the humerus into a constricted position and pinch (or impinge on) the inflamed tissues.

While bursitis, tendinitis, and impingement syndromes usually develop as a consequence of overuse or unaccustomed stress, tears of the rotator cuff occur by either wearing out over time or from specific trauma. Overhead activities, such as spiking a volley ball, executing an overhead smash in tennis, or throwing a ball, are often the cause of tendinitis, but tears of the tendons can occur following long-standing rotator

FROZEN SHOULDER

The term frozen shoulder implies a stiffened shoulder joint, restricted in motion. When painful conditions cause people to limit use of the shoulder joint to protect against the discomfort, the result can be progressive stiffness of the joint. The shoulder's normal flexibility and mobility are lost. The condition can follow such injuries as rotator cuff tendinitis, shoulder bursitis, stroke, or fractures of the humeral head. Sometimes it occurs with no injury and this is called idiopathic frozen shoulder.

Preventing a frozen shoulder demands rapid mobilization of the injured joint as soon as the doctor gives permission—usually just 48 hours following most injuries.

The process of rehabilitation of a frozen shoulder is a long one—sometimes taking 6 to 9 months. Exercise and physical therapy sometimes fail to resolve the problem; in these cases surgery may be indicated. A manipulation under anesthesia tears the scar but the same regimen of physical therapy is necessary after the surgery. Sometimes arthroscopy is needed in conjunction with the manipulation.

See Stretching the Painful Shoulder, page 682, for more information about how to mobilize the shoulder.

The best treatment is prevention. Frozen shoulder is best treated with ice to decrease the pain, NSAIDs to decrease the inflammation, pain pills to help decrease the pain when stretching the joint, and occasionally steroids (prednisone) by mouth. Physical therapy is helpful and a home program of stretching should be done daily. ■

STRETCHING THE PAINFUL SHOULDER

A few simple steps can keep a painful shoulder mobile. First, warm the shoulder joint with moist hot packs or in the bathtub or shower. If motion is still too painful, or in the early stages following an acute injury, try applying ice to numb the pain. Then, perform the following exercises:

- *Pendulum stretches.* Standing or sitting on a chair, bend slightly at the waist toward the injured side. Hold your arm out straight and make slow swings or circles, reaching out no more than a few inches from the body. Try to perform the exercise for 5 minutes twice daily to stretch the shoulder joint open.

- *Wall-walking exercise.* Stand facing the wall. Place the fingertips of the hand on the painful side onto the wall and begin to creep them upward, raising the arm toward the front. Push yourself slightly to extend the walk a little higher each time. Try to perform 15 walks a day. Turn with your painful shoulder next to the wall and repeat the 15 walks raising the arm to the side. As before, push to extend the length of the walk a bit higher each time.

- *Toning exercises for the shoulder muscles.* Using an elastic exercise band or bungee cord, perform the following exercises in sets of 15 to 20: With elbows bent and held close to the body, grasp one end of the band or cord in each hand. Keeping the elbows tucked to your sides, stretch it 5 to 7 in. with an outward motion, as though opening a pair of swinging doors, hold the position for a count of five, then slowly return to starting position. Repeat for a total of 15 counts. Next, fasten the ends of the band or cord to make a circle. Place both arms inside the circle and position the band or cord a few inches below the elbows. Now stretch the band or cord by pulling the elbows out from the body about 5 in., hold the position for a count of five, and slowly return to the starting position. Repeat the exercise for a total of 15 counts. When done with the exercise, ice the shoulder. ■

cuff tendinitis. If due to trauma, the tear causes pain that begins immediately, but often intensifies over time.

What you can do In acute injury, apply ice immediately. Supporting the shoulder with an arm sling should only be done for a brief interval, as it may encourage immobility. Limit overhead reaching. See Stretching the Painful Shoulder, above, for details on keeping the shoulder mobile safely. Do not keep the shoulder immobile; frozen shoulder can result.

When to call the doctor If discomfort or limitation of motion persist longer than 1 or 2 weeks despite the remedies outlined above, a visit to the doctor is in order.

Treatment Reducing inflammation and swelling and preventing the development of a frozen shoulder are the main goals of treatment. These can be accomplished by applying ice to your shoulder for 20 minutes 2 to 3 times a day until the pain is gone, by taking NSAIDs, and by gentle range-of-motion exercises. An injection of anesthetic and corticosteroid medication into the bursa, joint, or tissues around the tendon may be necessary if the above treatments are not effective. Physical therapy may be recommended by your doctor to strengthen the shoulder muscle and keep it mobile.

If the muscles of the rotator cuff are still weak even with freedom from pain, you should see your doctor for further testing; MRI scans or arthrograms may be needed to determine the location and extent of the tear. Surgery to repair the tear may be necessary if treatment fails or the tendon tear is acute.

Prognosis Prognosis is good with proper adherence to therapy.

❖ SHOULDER DISLOCATION

Symptoms *(What you may experience)* Sudden, painful, limited motion of the shoulder joint following injury; a sensation of the shoulder giving way following specific motions of the arm (often throwing or reaching behind the body).

Signs and laboratory findings *(What the doctor looks for)* Confirmation of dislocation via x-rays.

What is it? While the shoulder has great range of motion, it can lose its stability and the head of the humerus can sometimes pop out of its proper position in the socket of the joint. Movement out of the joint can occur partially (called subluxation) or completely (called dislocation) and can occur toward the front of the body (an anterior subluxation or dislocation), toward the back of the body (a posterior one), or out of the bottom of the joint (an inferior one). The most common directions are toward the front of the joint.

Although some people are born with somewhat loose shoulder ligaments that allow the shoulder to sublux or dislocate without trauma, most initial instances of subluxation or dislocation in normal shoulders follow significant trauma. After the joint has dislocated or subluxed the first time, however, repeated episodes can occur more easily.

What you can do Keep the arm in as comfortable a position as possible, using a sling or elastic bandage (see How to Make and Use a Sling, page 676). Apply ice or cold packs to reduce swelling and pain, take ibuprofen or other over-the-counter (OTC) anti-inflammatory medication to reduce discomfort.

When to call the doctor The shoulder must be relocated as quickly as possible—see your doctor or proceed to the emergency room right away.

Treatment Relocation of the joint may involve the use of medications to relax the spasm of the muscles around the shoulder. Once the joint has been put back into place, a course of supervised physical therapy restores normal shoulder motion and increases the strength of the muscles; these muscles protect the joint and help to prevent repeat dislocation or subluxation.

If the shoulder remains loose and unstable following a course of physical therapy, surgery may be needed. Often the doctor inspects the joint (under anesthesia prior to the operation) using the arthroscope to assess the extent of damage to the interior of the joint and its cartilage. The type of surgery that is done depends upon what structures are damaged. Severely unstable shoulder joints require open surgery to repair, reattach, or tighten supportive tissues around the joint. In some instances, stability can be restored from within the joint, using just the arthroscope.

Physical therapy to mobilize the hand, wrist, and elbow may begin the day after surgery. Supervised physical therapy of the shoulder usually begins within 1 to 4 weeks following surgery.

Prognosis Most people can write and use the arm to eat within 3 to 7 days following surgery and drive within several weeks.

Full range of motion usually returns within 6 to 8 weeks following rehabilitation with physical therapy or surgery. Strength usually returns within 3 months. Return to physical shoulder activity with work or sports may take 4 to 6 months, and full strength recovery may take 9 to 12 months. With surgery the risk of recurrence is low (3 to 5 percent).

❖ ACROMIOCLAVICULAR JOINT SEPARATION (SEPARATED SHOULDER)

Symptoms (*What you may experience*) Pain and sensation of grinding on the top of the shoulder (usually with reaching up and across the body); persistent shoulder pain and swelling following landing on the shoulder in a fall; sharp pain that disrupts sleep when lying on the affected shoulder.

Signs and laboratory findings (*What the doctor looks for*) Results of standard x-ray.

What is it? The acromion—the bony lump on the top of the shoulder—is a part of the shoulder blade. It joins the collar bone, to which it is connected by a tough ligament called the acromioclavicular ligament. The acromioclavicular ligament and another ligament that binds the collar bone from below to another bony knob of the shoulder blade (called the coracoid process) stabilize the shoulder.

These ligaments are susceptible to injury and overuse and can be strained, partially torn, or completely ruptured. These injuries are termed shoulder separations and are graded respectively as first-, second-, or third-degree separations.

Pain occurs when the injured ligament is compressed by raising the arm to the side and moving it above shoulder level or by stretching it, such as in reaching across the chest to scratch the opposite shoulder blade.

What you can do Apply ice to reduce swelling and pain as often as four to five times a day. Take a nonsteroidal anti-inflammatory drug (NSAID) do not reach overhead or across the chest. Immobilize the shoulder (see How to Make and Use a Sling, page 676). Gentle exercise to keep the shoulder joint mobile (see Stretching the Painful Shoulder, page 682) should be done carefully to prevent frozen shoulder.

When to call the doctor Severe pain, limitation of motion, and swelling should prompt a visit to the emergency room or doctor right away. Lesser injuries that fail to respond within 2 weeks to conservative measures suggested above merit evaluation.

Treatment In first- or second-degree injuries that are painful after recovering from the injury, local injection of anesthetic and corticosteroid medication may help, although it is not curative. Immobilization of the shoulder for 3 to 4 weeks is the rule.

Surgery is usually not necessary in cases of complete tear (third-degree injury), but surgery may be needed in physically active people or in cases where there is lesser degrees of disruption but which are painful with limitation of motion despite treatment.

Prognosis Outcome of this injury is usually good, with most people able to return to work and sports with few limitations.

The Neck, Back, and Spine

❖ CERVICAL SPASM (CRICK IN THE NECK)

Symptoms *(What you may experience)* Aching, tightness, sharp or stabbing pain, and muscle spasm in neck; limitation of motion, usually in turning the head to one side; spasm in neck muscles following trauma (usually a fall or motor vehicle accident); headache along with neck tightness (sometimes). Many people just wake up with it.

Signs and laboratory findings *(What the doctor looks for)* Tenderness, lumps in the muscle, and pain on motion; loss of normal curve of the spine secondary to muscle spasm as detected by x-rays. X-rays will also diagnose arthritis or fracture following trauma.

What is it? Irritation and spasm of the cervical (neck) muscles can occur for a variety of reasons, among them: muscle tension from physical or emotion stress, abnormal position during sleep, whiplash injury from a fall or motor vehicle accident, abnormal alignment of the cervical spine, or arthritis of the cervical spine. Doctors often refer to arthritis of the spine as degenerative disk disease or spondylosis.

Whatever its cause, when it occurs the neck loses its normal flexibility, and motions in specific directions can be quite painful. The muscles of the neck are strong, as they must be to support the

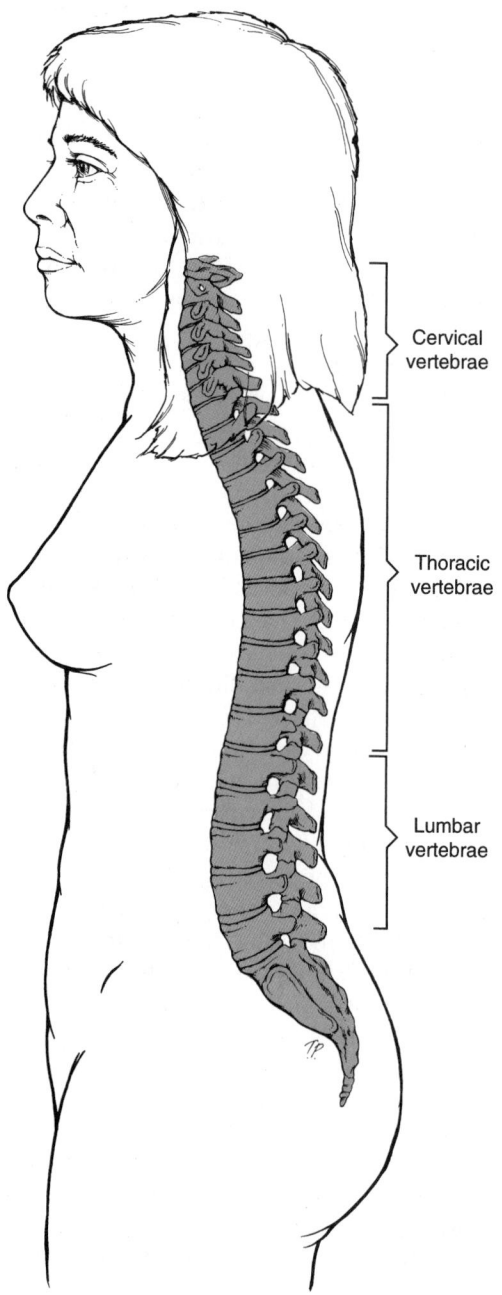

Cervical vertebrae

Thoracic vertebrae

Lumbar vertebrae

The spine has a natural curvature from front to back. Many problems can arise in the neck, back, or spine such as muscle tension, whiplash injury, abnormal spinal alignment, and arthritis. Neck pain following trauma should always be evaluated immediately.

weight of the head, and their contraction in spasm cannot only cause pain, but can pull strongly enough to straighten the normal gentle curve of the spine or even pull the head to the side (a condition called torticollis or wry neck).

What you can do In severe injury, proceed directly to the hospital emergency room to rule out a fracture or severe ligament damage. Weakness, tingling, or numbness are serious signs and you should seek immediate treatment. In lesser injuries or those spasms not caused by trauma, take stress off the neck muscles by supporting the weight of the head using a soft cervical collar (available at most full service pharmacies) or using a bath towel, folded lengthwise three or four times, wrapped softly around the neck and secured with a safety pin. Cervical collars should be used for only a short period of time. In these acute strains, apply ice packs to the neck and upper back muscles. OTC anti-inflammatory medications may help.

Ongoing neck care should include the following:

- Sleeping on your back, with the head, neck, and shoulders aligned, supporting the curve of the neck with a cervical pillow and the lower back with a pillow under the bend of the knees.

- Avoidance of carrying heavy bags or purses by shoulder straps. Do not lift heavy items.

- Gentle daily exercise to stretch the neck, such as shoulder rolls, shoulder shrugs, pinching the shoulder blades together, and cervical stretches—tipping the head forward, backward, side to side, and rotating the face to one shoulder and then the other.

When to call the doctor Neck pain following trauma—particularly if accompanied by numbness, tingling, or weakness in the hands or arms—should always be evaluated immediately by a doctor. Severe pain which lasts more than a day, or any weakness or numbness which develops, should be evaluated by a doctor.

Treatment Treatment focuses on reducing pain and muscle spasm, strengthening injured muscles, and restoring normal neck curvature and flexibility. Full doses of an NSAID with rest is recommended.

Physical therapy with ultrasound, deep massage, and cervical traction may help.

Local injection with anesthetic and sometimes corticosteroid medication into trigger points can often reduce irritation and spasm when pain persists.

Long-standing neck discomfort may respond to home therapy with a transcutaneous electrical nerve stimulator (TENS) unit. This device helps to reduce spasm and pain through use of a low-level electrical current transmitted through adhesive patches placed near the trigger area.

Prognosis Symptoms respond to therapy, but unfortunately often recur. If symptoms are not gone in one month or if they remain severe, see your doctor.

❖ SCOLIOSIS (CURVATURE OF THE SPINE)

Symptoms *(What you may experience)* Vague back muscle pain or stiffness (sometimes). Usually there are no symptoms.

Signs and laboratory findings *(What the doctor looks for)* Uneven bulge of the shoulder blades; visible or palpable curve or twist of the spinal alignment; x-rays confirm the condition. (See page C-42.)

What is it? The normal spine has several gentle curves if viewed from the side. In the neck it sags slightly forward, gently sweeps backward between the shoulder blades, sags toward the front again at the level of the hips, and curves backward again to terminate in the tail bone. Viewed from the back, however, it should be straight, without a curve or twist to the right or left, but this perfect alignment is not always present.

In some people—more commonly in adolescent girls than in boys—for reasons that are not entirely clear, a curve or twist develops as the spine grows. A bend to one side will occur in the back and in an effort to maintain upright posture, a compensating bend in the other direction will occur elsewhere in the spine. The twisting effect can usually be noted only by careful inspection or screening. In a scoliosis screening examination—often performed by schools—the examiner watches the levels of the shoulders and shoulder blades as the child bends slowly forward. A greater dip of one shoulder could indicate scoliosis and the need for x-ray studies.

Developing scoliosis may go undetected until adolescence, when the child enters the period of rapid growth at puberty; at this time, the degree of spinal bending can increase so dramatically that

A curvature of the spine to the right or left, called scoliosis, can be detected through careful inspection or routine screenings in the childhood and teenage years. A back brace or surgery can sometimes help correct the problem.

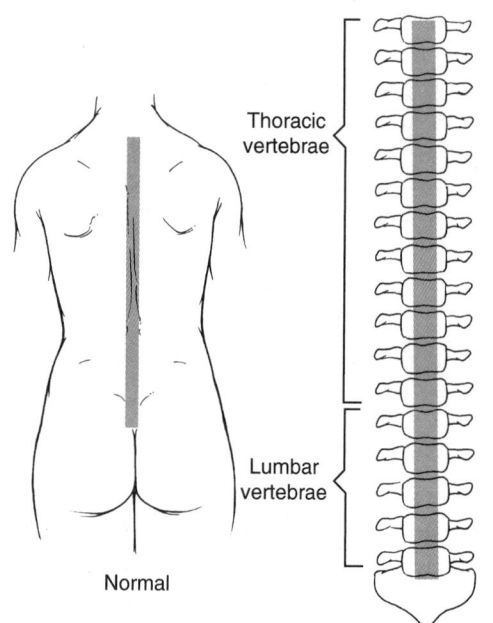

Thoracic vertebrae

Lumbar vertebrae

Normal

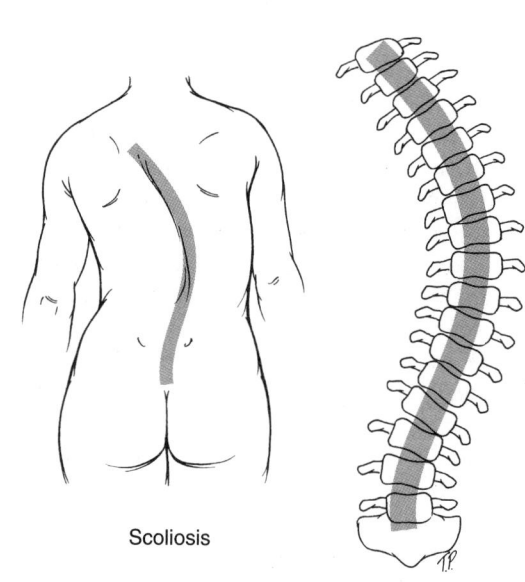

Scoliosis

PROPER POSTURE

The muscles of the back, neck, and shoulders are designed to keep the spine properly aligned and straight. The natural curves of the spine permit erect posture with the least muscle work. Even though it may sometimes seem more difficult to maintain a straight posture, slouching (either while seated or standing) increases the work the muscles must do and, consequently, aggravates back problems. People who make an effort to stand and sit with a straight back and square shoulders suffer fewer back aches.

To envision what proper posture should be, imagine the body in profile with a solid rod connecting the center of the top of the head, the shoulders, the hips, and the middle of the feet (just in front of the ankle) all in a straight line. In this posture, the shoulders do not hunch or droop and the lower back does not sway forward.

Particularly in people who suffer back problems, sitting can be uncomfortable, since sitting places even more stress on the back than does standing. Proper posture while sitting is made more difficult in overstuffed, low chairs. Opt for straight backed chairs or those fitted with a lumbar (lower back) pillow or support, especially if sitting for prolonged periods. Sit up straight with the buttocks and thighs well supported. ■

measurable changes can occur in as little as a month.

While the cause of scoliosis is not clearly understood, at least in some cases, there may be genetic factors at work.

What you can do A family history of scoliosis is an important risk factor. Early screening of children by either a pediatrician or the school is important. Do exercises to improve posture and strengthen the muscles that support the spine. (See Caring for the Back and Keeping it Mobile, page 687.)

Treatment Initially, the doctor may recommend a specially molded spinal brace, padded and fitted to apply pressure to correct the curve. If conservative measures fail, surgical correction—with the temporary placement of fixation rods to straighten the spine—may prove necessary in severe cases.

Prognosis Caught early and treated appropriately, the condition may not progress or cause disability.

❖ PARASPINOUS MUSCLE SPASM (LOWER BACK STRAIN)

Symptoms (What you may experience) Aching pain and stiffness in the muscles of the lower back; limitation in bending; lower back discomfort with sitting for prolonged periods.

CARING FOR THE BACK AND KEEPING IT MOBILE

People with chronic back problems should avoid certain activities that can place excess stress on the bones and soft tissues of the back, including the following:

- Bending or stooping deeply or for prolonged periods.

- Touching the toes.

- Use of rowing machines.

- Heavy weight workouts. (Note: Proper use of light weights at high numbers of repetitions can actually be beneficial.)

- Sleeping on a soft or sagging mattress.

- Sleeping positioned on the stomach.

Always lift any object with great care following these rules:

- Avoid lifting heavy or unbalanced loads.

- Keep the load close to the body, lifting with the legs, knees, and hips and not the back.

- Do not twist the back during lifting; keep the load squarely in front of the body.

Keep the back muscles toned and well stretched with the following exercises:

- *Knee-to-chest stretch.* Lying on the back, slowly bend one knee and bring it as near to the chest as possible, holding it with the hands for a few seconds. Repeat with the left knee to finish the set. Aim for 10 repetitions. Stop immediately if severe pain occurs and consult your doctor. See Chapter 2 for more information on back exercises.

- *Side bends.* Lying on the back with shoulders square, knees slightly bent, and arms at the side, walk the fingers along the floor beside the body toward the knees; this motion should bend the back slightly to one side. Hold the bent position for a few seconds and return to the straight position. Repeat with the other side to finish the set. Aim for 10 repetitions. Stop immediately if severe pain occurs and consult your doctor.

After 4 to 6 weeks of daily stretching, begin these exercises to strengthen and tone the muscles of the back:

- *Modified crunches.* Lie on the back keeping the knees bent, feet flat on the floor, and small of the back pressed into the floor. Hold arms crossed loosely over the chest, a hand at each shoulder. Raise the head, neck, and shoulders only 3 or 4 in. off the floor, hold the position for a few seconds and gently lower them back to the rest position. Repeat. Aim for a set of 15 to 20 daily.

- *Weighted side bends.* Stand, holding a 5 to 15 lb weight in one hand. (A gallon container of milk or water weighs about 8 lbs and will do nicely.) Gently tip the shoulder of the weighted side to tilt the spine just a few inches and smoothly return to a straight posture—do not jerk, but rather rock smoothly down and back up. Keep the weight close to the body at first—the farther away from the body the weight is held, the greater the amount of muscle work required. Repeat the tilt 15 to 20 times on one side, then move to the other side for a set of 15 to 20 repetitions. Perform the exercise daily. ■

Signs and laboratory findings *(What the doctor looks for)* Scoliosis, tender muscles, lumps in muscles, tightness, and loss of bendability. X-rays are usually normal and done to exclude other causes.

What is it? Powerful overlapping sets of muscles lie on either side of the spine, functioning to keep it upright and permit the spine to bend forward, backward, tilt side to side, and twist. The activities of daily living—sitting, stooping, lifting, and bending—all place stress on the lower part of the back in the region where the spine meets the pelvic bones.

Most commonly, irritation from overuse or unaccustomed use of improperly toned or stretched muscles causes spasm in these muscle groups. Other underlying causes include an old, unrecognized compression injury to a vertebra (see Compression Fracture, page 688), malalignment or slipping of the bones of the spine (see Mechanical Back Problems, page 689), or arthritis. Acute injury—from a fall or motor vehicle accident—can also cause spasm in these muscles.

When strong muscles contract in spasm, they cannot only cause stiffness and pain with attempted movement, but can alter the alignment and normal curve of the spine, further worsening the problem.

What you can do Avoid lifting or doing exercises to a degree you are not accustomed to. Ask your doctor about proper lifting techniques. Avoid sudden or extreme twisting, tilting, or bending motions. In acute injuries, apply ice or cold packs to reduce swelling.

Avoid sleeping on the stomach. Allow the back muscles to relax fully during the night by sleeping on the back with the hips and knees slightly bent and supported by a pillow or foam roll.

Keep the back mobile with gentle stretching exercises (see Caring for the Back and Keeping it Mobile, page 687).

When to call the doctor Severe or persistent discomfort or the presence of such symptoms as tingling, numbness, or weakness in the legs or feet should prompt an immediate medical evaluation to rule out a disk problem, nerve compression, or tumor.

Pain higher in the back (near where the rib cage ends) can sometimes be caused by kidney infection, stones, a fracture due to osteoporosis, or other disorders. See the doctor right away.

Treatment Therapy focuses on relieving the spasm and irritation which may temporarily require stronger medication to relax muscle spasm or relieve pain. In acute injury, 3 or 4 days of bedrest are in order. The use of potent pain relievers (especially narcotics) should be limited to 7 to 10 days.

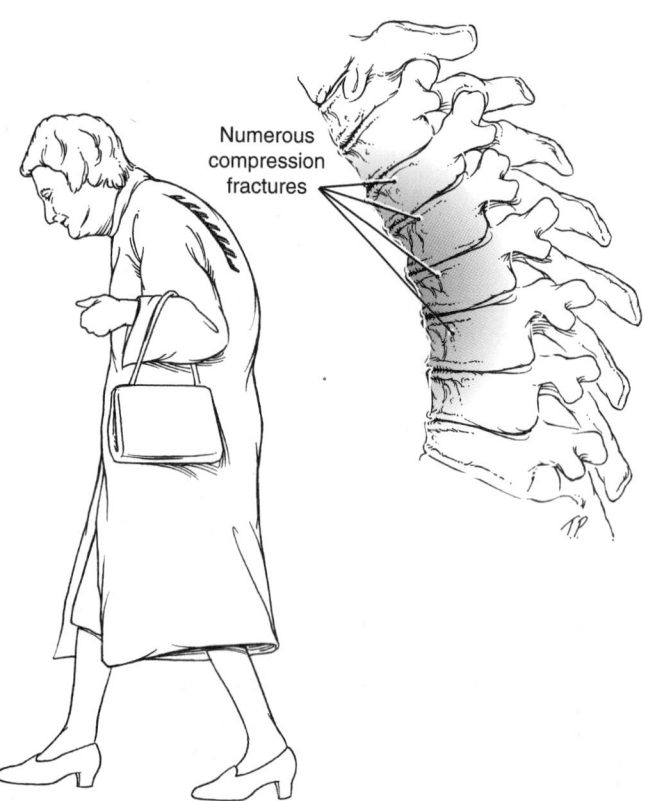

Compression fracture. The spinal bones (vertebrae) can be broken from an injury or osteoporosis. This type of fracture can cause distortion of the spinal column, pain, spasm, and compression of a nerve root.

Numerous compression fractures

Full doses of NSAIDs help relieve pain and inflammation.

The cornerstone of treatment should be physical therapy and exercise—initially, ice packs followed by ultrasound treatments and stretching. After a few weeks of gentle stretching, the focus of exercise shifts to those that strengthen the muscles, and then to those that improve their tone and flexibility (such as low-impact aerobics, walking, or swimming).

Local injection of anesthetic with or without corticosteroid medication into trigger points in the region may prove helpful for some people.

Chronic back pain and stiffness may respond to low level electrical stimulation with a TENS unit. Intractable chronic back pain may also necessitate referral to a pain management clinic. See Alternative Management of Chronic Back Pain, page 692, for information on other approaches to back pain.

Prognosis Prognosis depends on the cause and to a large degree on the person's willingness to stretch and exercise the back. In general, the prognosis for acute injuries is better than that for chronic back pain. Most go away in weeks to a few months. Surgery is only indicated for cases of structural abnormality (see Mechanical Back Problems, page 689).

❖ COMPRESSION FRACTURES

Symptoms (*What you may experience*) Acute, severe onset of pain which persists (often without significant trauma).

Signs and laboratory findings (*What the doctor looks for*) Localized tenderness over the collapsed vertebrae; confirmation of the fracture via x-rays.

What is it? The vertebrae—the squarely shaped bones of the spine—are made of a dense outer cylinder of bone surrounding a core of softer spongy bone. Occasionally, a sudden stress placed on the bones (in a sit-down fall, often) is sufficient to cause one or more of the vertebrae to collapse on one side, turning the stable square configuration into a wedge.

The wedging of the vertebra distorts the normal curves of the spinal column, and this can cause abnormal muscle traction, and with that, worsening back pain and spasm. This phenomenon occur in older women with osteoporosis, leading to a dowager's hump.

In addition, collapse of a vertebra can compress the nerve root. Spinal nerve roots exit the spinal column between the vertebrae, with sufficient but not abundant room. Compression can cause loss of nerve function, manifested as numbness, tingling, or weakness.

What you can do Bedrest for the first 3 to 5 days is in order. Once the acute pain has subsided, use crutches to help support weight when walking. As the pain begins to lessen, begin exercises to hyperextend the back (bend it backward) and strengthen the muscles.

When to call the doctor Significant pain or the development of numbness, tingling, weakness, or changes in bowel or bladder function should prompt a visit to the doctor right away.

Treatment Pain may be severe enough to require strong prescriptive pain medication, such as narcotics. A supportive brace may be needed for a few months to prevent excessive flexion (forward bending) of the spine. Surgery is indicated if the wedging of the vertebra exceeds an angle of 35°, if the fracture has rendered the spine unstable and likely to shift, or if nerve root compression has occurred. Newer bone injection techniques may prevent surgery and relieve pain.

Prognosis Healing may take 4 to 6 months. In people who suffer from osteoporosis (bone thinning) the course to healing may be prolonged and difficult.

❖ MECHANICAL BACK PROBLEMS (RUPTURED OR BULGING DISK, SPONDYLOSIS, AND SPONDYLOLISTHESIS)

Symptoms *(What you may experience)* Tenderness and limitation of mobility; tingling, numbness, or weakness or sharp shooting pains in the buttock, leg, or back.

Signs and laboratory findings *(What the doctor looks for)* Loss of normal nerve

DANGER SIGNS OF LOWER BACK PAIN

The back bears the brunt of living: sitting, stooping, standing erect, walking or running, lifting, and carrying. Consequently, lower back pain is one of the most common complaints brought to a doctor's attention. In the vast majority of cases, the cause is simply misuse or overuse of the back and poses no real threat to health or mobility. Here are some important warning signs of back pain that could mean danger:

- Pain that shoots down the buttock or leg.
- Numbness or tingling in the leg, foot, or toes.
- Weakness of the muscles of the leg, foot, or ankle.
- Inability to raise the foot or great toe (foot drop).
- Loss of control over bowel or bladder function.
- Numbness or tingling in the perineum (genitalia and anal regions). ■

function, such as weakness, loss of sensation, or loss of reflexes as demonstrated by neurologic examination; confirmation of the cause via x-ray, MRI scan, or computed tomography (CT) scan.

What is it? The structure of the back is resilient, flexible, and complex, with interlocking irregularly shaped bones, carefully interconnected and stabilized with tough ligaments, and separated by cushioning disks. Protected within a bony canal inside the spine lies the spinal cord, the nerve center responsible for directing all function from the neck down, its nerve roots projecting out between the vertebrae. Because of its intricate construction and the vital structures it houses, mechanical problems involving the back can be not only painful but potentially dangerous as well.

Conditions include those that cause laxity or instability of the spine such as spondylolisthesis, compromise its flexibility such as ankylosing spondylitis, scoliosis, or spondylosis that causes stiffening of the spine, or encroach on the spinal canal and cord within it such as arthritis, lumbar stenosis, or a bulging or ruptured disk.

- *Spondylolisthesis.* In this disorder, the stabilizing ligaments of the spinal column and the smaller bones in the back of the spinal column fail in their job of holding the vertebrae securely in position. This permits one vertebra to slip forward or backward relative to its neighbor above or below it. A bony abnormality (fracture of the small bones of the spine) must be present for this to occur. The predisposing causes for such fractures to occur could be traumatic (back injury) or congenital (present at birth). While slippage of a mild degree (less than 50 percent) may pose no risk to the spinal cord or nerves within the column, greater movement could potentially cause crimping or crushing of the cord and with it loss of nerve function. Therefore, spondylolisthesis of significant degree may require surgical stabilization.

- *Spondylosis.* This disorder—also called degenerative joint disease, degenerative disk disease, or arthritis of the spine— refers to the condition in which the spine loses its flexibility when age, overuse, or injury causes the disks between the vertebrae to wear thin. The result is painful stiffness of the back. Thinning of the disks, designed to cushion the junction between vertebrae, results in narrowing of the spaces and less room for the spinal nerve roots to pass between them. X-rays confirm the diagnosis; treatment involves a combination of pain relief with anti-inflammatory medications (aspirin or ibuprofen) and physical therapy.

- *Lumbar stenosis.* This condition occurs when the lower end of the spinal canal becomes narrowed from trauma, arthritis, or in some cases as a congenital condition. Narrowing squeezes the spinal cord or the collection of nerve roots (called the cauda equina, meaning horse's tail) that trails away from the lower end of the spinal cord. Compression of the cord or the tail causes cramping pain in the legs and feet, not unlike the symptoms caused by blockage of the blood supply from atherosclerosis (see page 836); for that reason, tests on the blood vessels to assess their status are in order. Treatment of severe narrowing involves removal of some of the bone of the spinal column (a procedure called a laminectomy) to make more room for the cord.

- *Ruptured disk.* This relatively common condition occurs when one (or occasionally more) of the spacing disks between the vertebrae fail. The job of

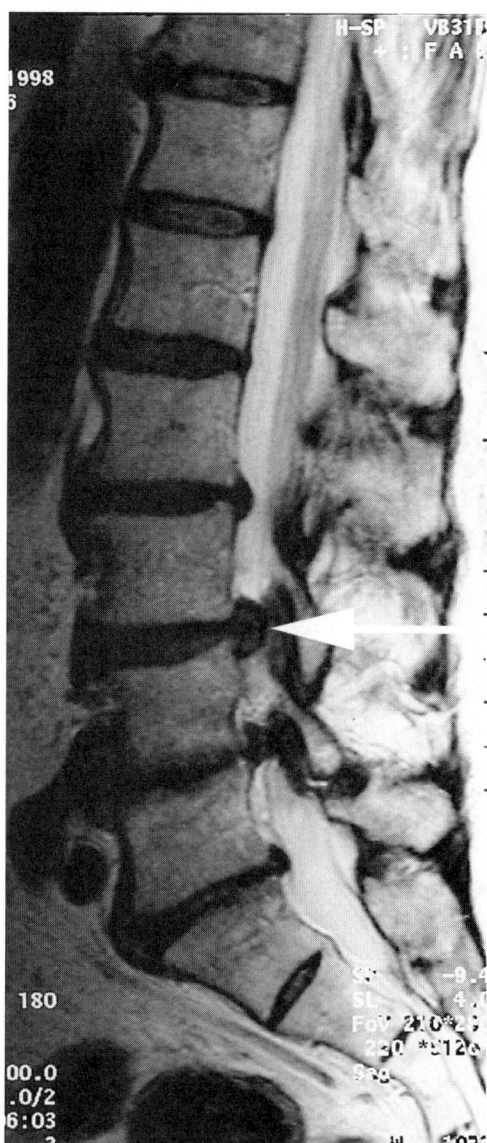

Ruptured disk (arrow). Disks between the vertebrae cushion the junction of the bones of the spine and compress slightly to allow for flexibility. Age or strain can cause the outer shell of the disk to weaken allowing the gel inside to bulge or rupture. This MRI scan shows a ruptured disk between the lumbar vertebrae (arrow) with smaller disk bulges at other levels.

the disk is to cushion the junction of the bones of the spine in weight bearing and to compress and deform slightly to permit flexibility in bending and leaning side to side. The disks themselves are made of a tough fibrous outer shell surrounding a cushioning gel core. Age or excessive strain can cause a rent or weakness in the fibrous shell that

DEBATING DISK SURGERY

The benefits of surgery for lower back pain are not at all clear cut. Even when x-rays or scans seem to confirm the presence of a bulging disk, the disk may not be the cause of the particular condition for which the person is seeking relief. Surgery may not relieve the pain, and it is not without significant risk. These factors must be weighed carefully and discussed at length with the doctor before accepting or rejecting the notion of surgery.

In general, a responsible doctor (even one whose practice primarily involves surgery) will not recommend an operation on the back unless all other less invasive options have proven ineffective in resolving the condition. Nonetheless, there are some clear indications where surgery must be performed. For example, surgery might be the best option for acute rupture of a disk with clear and definable loss of nerve function (sensation or strength) that correlates with the location of a bulge seen on an MRI scan. In most cases, when there is documented loss of nerve function from disk pressure that cannot be relieved by conservative means, surgery may be the only means to prevent permanent nerve damage. ■

---

allows the gel within to bulge or extrude (rupture or herniate). Herniation of the core into the spinal canal compresses the spinal cord or tail, causing pain in the areas of the body controlled by those nerve roots. Typical symptoms include sharp shooting pain into the buttock or down the leg, worsened with a cough or sneeze or by bending at the hips with the knees kept straight.

Treatment of disk problems may be as simple as bedrest and pain relieving medications until the inflammation subsides; however, when the symptoms involve compression of nerve roots, surgery to remove the pressure on the nerve (laminectomy or full or partial disk removal) may be recommended to prevent long-term nerve damage. The potential benefits and risks of surgery should be discussed with your doctor. Most herniated disks recover without surgery.

Alternatives to standard surgery such as percutaneous discectomy, laser discectomy, and endoscopic discectomy are being developed. They allow disk removal with a large needle or tube inserted through the skin. Some doctors use these techniques now but they are new enough that comparisons with proven surgical techniques is not yet possible.

Prognosis Mechanical back problems vary in their prognosis, but some degree of stiffness, loss of flexibility, and mild discomfort should be expected intermitently for the long term even after surgical interventions. The long-term symptoms vary widely in degree depending upon the cause of the problem.

❖ SACROILIITIS

Symptoms *(What you may experience)* Stiffness very low in the back in bending or leaning side to side; aching or occasionally sharp pain localized high on the buttock or hip.

Signs and laboratory findings *(What the doctor looks for)* X-rays may confirm sclerosis (bony scarring) of the sacroiliac joint.

What is it? Inflammation of the sacroiliac joint can occur as a component of a number of conditions, among them inflammatory bowel diseases such as ulcerative colitis (see page 1010) and rheumatic disorders involving the spine. See Reactive Arthritic Disorders (Ankylosing Spondylitis, Reiter's Syndrome, Psoriatic Arthritis, and Enteric Arthritis), page 648, for information on rheumatic disorders involving the spine.

The two sacroiliac joints form the junction of the pelvic bones low in the back, joining the ilia (a pair of bones forming the wings on either side of the pelvis) with the sacrum (a roughly heart-shaped bone at the end of the spinal column, which is in reality the fusion of the bottom five vertebrae of the spine).

The sacral nerve roots run in close to the sacroiliac joints, a proximity that explains why irritation or inflammation of the joint can cause shooting, nerve-root-like pain into the buttock at times.

Chronic inflammation can sometimes cause sclerosis of the joint on one or both sides, leading to aching and stiffness in the lower back.

ALTERNATIVE MANAGEMENT OF CHRONIC BACK PAIN

Chronic back pain can be disabling, physically and emotionally. Because chronic back pain can result from literally dozens of potential causes, ranging from structural and mechanical problems to disorders of the kidneys, abdominal or pelvic organs, or cancers, it merits a thorough evaluation by a doctor. In many instances, the underlying cause cannot be simply identified, and in other instances it can be identified but not cured; the pain continues despite orthodox medical treatments. In these cases, many people seek other treatments that offer the possibility of relief.

Physical Therapy The physical therapist serves a key role in the care of both injured backs and those cases of chronic back pain that are primarily mechanical or structural in nature—spinal arthritis, degenerative disk problems, and compression fractures of the vertebrae. The modalities the physical therapist may employ include massage, hot or cold packs or baths, ultrasound, iontophoresis (a procedure in which ultrasound waves are used to drive anti-inflammatory medication directly to the site of the injury), electrical stimulation, and joint range-of-motion exercise. The primary goals of physical therapy are to overcome muscle spasm, improve muscle tone and strength, and preserve maximum mobility and flexibility of the back.

Chiropractic The practice of chiropractic involves the restoration of health through manipulation of the spine. According to recommendations by the Agency for Health Care Policy and Research, such manipulation can be helpful for some people in the first month of lower back symptoms. If your symptoms do not improve after 4 weeks of spinal manipulation, you should be re-evaluated by your doctor. The laws governing what sorts of therapies a chiropractic doctor may perform vary from one state to another; check with the local medical governing board for more information.

Acupuncture The art of acupuncture—the placement of fine needles through the skin to achieve freedom from pain (as well as many other applications)—originated in China, where it is currently an accepted method of treatment and local anesthesia in orthodox medical circles.

In the United States, acupuncture is also used by trained practitioners (from chiropractic doctors to medical doctors) as a tool of pain relief, but be warned that this may not always be the case. People without adequate training may call themselves acupuncturists, making it important to check the credentials of the practitioner prior to receiving treatment. In this country, the effectiveness of acupuncture is regarded as controversial at best.

Biofeedback The body has an enormous capacity for self-regulation of seemingly unconscious functions, ranging from heart rate or blood pressure to the perception of pain. Learning how to control the traffic of these incoming and outgoing nerve signals forms the basis for the technique of biofeedback. Many pain clinics (both private facilities and those affiliated with hospitals) now have practitioners (often psychiatrists or psychologists) experienced in teaching this method of pain control; becoming proficient in performing the technique may take many weeks of practice. Be aware that biofeedback does not cure the cause of the pain, rather it teaches the person experiencing it how to alter their perception of it. ■

What you can do See Caring for the Back and Keeping it Mobile, page 687.

When to call the doctor Persistent, sudden, or significant pain in this area—particularly associated with tingling, numbness, or weakness of the lower extremity—should prompt a visit to the doctor for evaluation. Chronic pain in this area which is worsening or unrelieved by self-care should be evaluated by a doctor.

Treatment If the condition is associated with an underlying disorder, therapy focuses on treating that disorder. Anti-inflammatory medications may offer some help, as may brief courses of corticosteroid medication or trigger point injections.

Prognosis This condition is frequently chronic, although symptoms may come and go and at times may even disappear completely.

The Hips and Pelvis

❖ HIP FRACTURE OR DISLOCATION

Symptoms *(What you may experience)* Severe pain and limitation of motion of the hip following trauma (usually a fall); inability to bear weight following a fall.

Signs and laboratory findings *(What the doctor looks for)* Confirmation and identification of the specific nature of the fracture via x-rays.

What is it? Fractures of the hip (actually the ball end of the femur) can be divided into the following three categories:

- *Femoral neck fractures.* The neck of the femur is the slender curved area that joins the vertical shaft with the ball end. Breaks in this area typically occur in falls

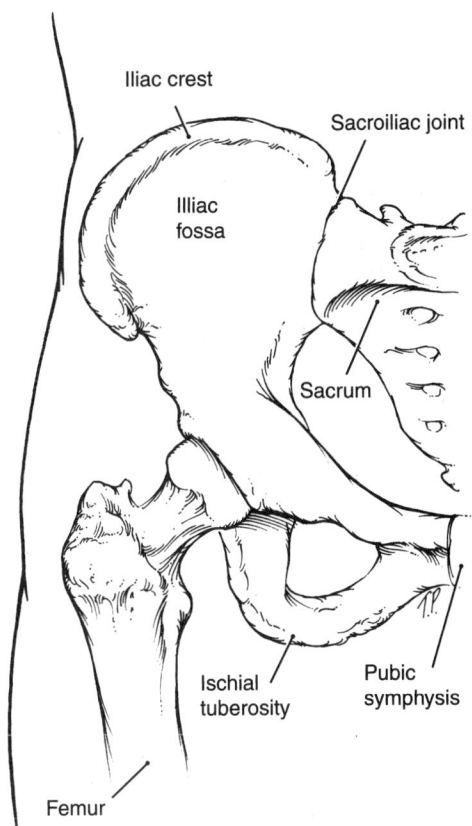

The centrally located sacrum joins the left and right iliac bones at the two sacroiliac joints. Sacral nerve roots run across the joints. Inflammation or injury can cause pain or sclerosis (scarring).

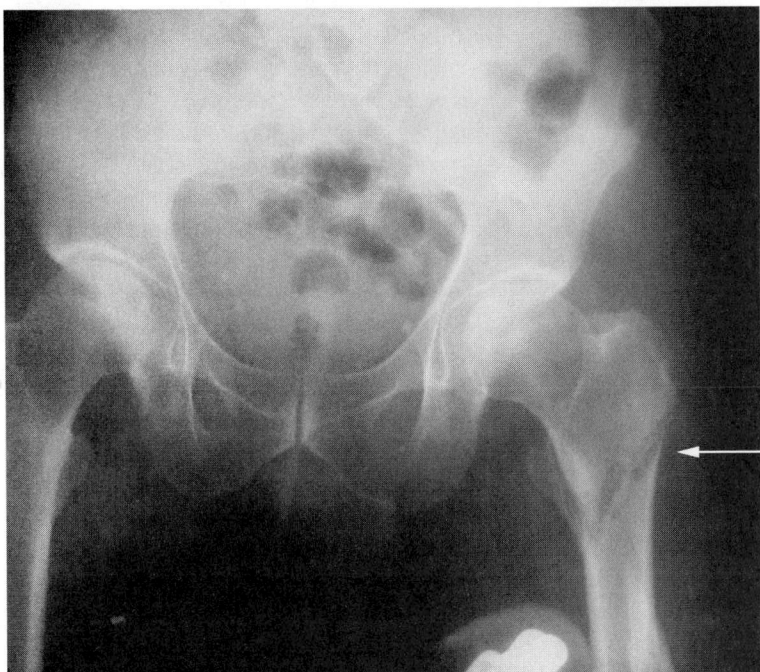

Hip fracture. This x-ray shows a subtrochanteric fracture (arrow).

in people over age 50; they may also occur in younger people involved in high energy trauma (such as motor vehicle accidents, falls from heights, or crushing injuries) and in response to chronic stress in athletes. The danger in these fractures is that their location heightens the risk of injury to the blood vessels in the area. Compromise of the blood supply increases the likelihood of poor healing and osteonecrosis (death of bone) in the ball or head of the femur.

- *Intertrochanteric fractures.* The femur has two prominent humps on its surface near the hip. These humps, called the greater and lesser trochanters, represent sites where powerful muscles arise or attach to the bone. When the femur breaks between these two humps, it is said to be an intertrochanteric (between the trochanters) fracture. Such injuries usually result

from a fall, and often in elderly people with thin bones weakened by osteoporosis. Swelling and bruising may be apparent on the outside of the hip, over the prominent bony hump found there. Movement of the limb causes pain and should not be attempted. The leg usually seems shorter than its mate and will often be held in a position that rotates the foot outward, away from the midline of the body.

- *Subtrochanteric fractures.* Fractures below the trochanters usually occur in young people involved in high energy trauma, but as with other hip fractures, in the elderly they may occur from simple falls. Immediate pain and swelling generally occur and movement of the hip in any direction causes extreme pain. As with fractures between the trochanters, the pull of muscles in the region will shorten the injured leg somewhat and rotate the leg and foot outward, away from the body.

When to call the doctor Do not attempt to move a person who may have sustained a hip fracture, if at all possible. Keep them warm and still and seek emergency help.

Treatment Treatment varies according to the type of fracture.

TOTAL HIP REPLACEMENT SURGERY

When the hip joint is destroyed or severely damaged— whether from arthritis, infection, inflammation, or trauma—successful treatment may demand its replacement with an artificial joint. When this procedure is necessary, the doctor will surgically remove the damaged ball of the hip and firmly cement an artificial metal or ceramic ball into the bone end. The new ball, which usually is made of metal, will fit into a new artificial socket. The socket consists of hard plastic inside a metal cup, which is either pressed into or cemented into the bone socket. Total hip and knee joint replacement is considered the major advance in the treatment of osteoarthritis (OA) in the last 30 years.

Most people stay 3 to 7 days in the hospital after surgery. Physical therapy is begun while you are still in the hospital to restore normal mobility and strength to the hip and thigh. Compliance with physical therapy recommendations during the weeks and months following the surgery can make the difference between a poor result and a successful recovery of function. Despite the pain following surgery and the demands of physical therapy, the operation has a very high satisfaction rate, with studies showing that 90 to 95 percent of people undergoing the operation were satisfied with the pain relief and improved mobility. Most people say they would have the surgery again, if necessary.

The major complication of total hip replacement is the loosening of the prosthetic joint after 10 to 15 years causing pain and perhaps requiring another surgery. Another technique called noncement fixation was developed in response to this problem. The cementless implant has a porous surface into which bone can grow holding the new joint in place.

People who have undergone hip replacement need to keep in mind certain long-term precautions. Since there is no blood supply at the new joint, the body is unable to fight infection should it occur at the artificial hip. As a result, if you have an infection any-

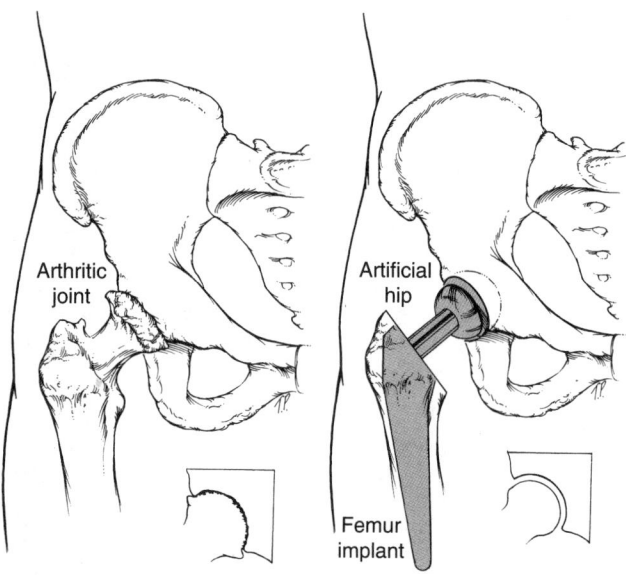

Bones in the hip can be replaced with artificial parts to treat some cases of arthritis or cartilage damage. A metal ball is cemented into the femur, and a socket of bone and plastic is inserted into the native socket. Improvement in pain nearly always results. Risks of hip replacement include infections and loosening of the joint.

where in your body, including your teeth or mouth, you should be on antibiotics immediately. In the past it was recommended that you be on antibiotics before and after dental procedures. This is controversial but you should always tell your dentist if you have a hip replacement. Antibiotics are usually recommended for people with total joints who are undergoing surgery of any type, but you should ask your doctor. ■

- *Femoral neck fracture.* The treatment depends upon the severity of the fracture. If the bones are aligned and the ball is still on the neck, the fracture can be treated with pins. These are usually fixed with several long screws, although a plate with screws is sometimes necessary. If the fracture is severe, especially in older people where healing may be poor, the hip may be replaced with an artificial joint replacement.

- *Intertrochanteric fractures.* The leg must immediately (even before x-rays) be placed in weighted traction to prevent further damage to the soft tissues. Treatment choices are dictated by the prefracture status of the person; in most cases, surgery with placement of internal fixation devices (plates and screws) followed by early mobilization is the preferred method. In those with senile

dementia who are completely bedridden, surgery may not be a viable option; continued traction may suffice. The goal of treatment is to attempt to return the person to the previous level of activity as soon as possible. Surgery with internal fixation or in some cases a prosthetic hip replacement allows for a rapid return to mobility and in large measure prevents many of the attendant complications.

- *Subtrochanteric fractures.* In adults the standard treatment involves surgery to align the bone ends and the placement of internal fixation devices, such as a long rod down the inside of the bone or a long plate with screws on the surface of the bone to hold the fracture in place. In children 10 to 12 years old, the fracture may be treated with traction and immobilization in a long-leg hip cast.

Prognosis The prognosis depends on the site of the fracture, the development of secondary complications, and the age of the person. If the surgery is successful, many people can walk and be active with few restrictions.

❖ TROCHANTERIC BURSITIS

Symptoms *(What you may experience)* Aching pain or tenderness in the upper outer hip with walking or prolonged standing or when rolling onto the hip in sleep; hip discomfort when climbing stairs.

Signs and laboratory findings *(What the doctor looks for)* Tenderness directly on the greater trochanter, increased pain with resisted hip motion in certain directions. X-rays may be normal or rarely may show calcium deposits; x-rays or scans may also be done to exclude other causes of hip pain.

What is it? The hip, like many large joints, is protected by a bursa. In some instances, the bursa becomes inflamed. The inflamed bursa aches with prolonged walking or standing, with the pain felt on the outer upper area of the thigh and hip. Not uncommonly, a sharp pain, sufficient to disrupt sleep, occurs when rolling over onto the affected hip in bed.

What you can do Avoid direct pressure over the affected hip; limit weight bearing while the discomfort persists; limit bending of the hip (stair climbing, rising from a chair, or squatting); apply ice packs to the affected area; take NSAIDs for pain relief.

Perform daily stretching exercises of the buttock muscles as follows:

- *Hip stretch*. Stand with your side an arm's length from the wall, with your feet together and firmly planted on the floor. Put your arm straight out so that your palm is flat on the wall. Gently push the side of your hip toward the wall. Hold gently in this position for a few seconds, then relax. Repeat five times.

- *Knee to chest pulls*. Lying on the floor, bend the knee of the affected side and pull it as closely as possible to the chest—stopping when more than a gentle pulling sensation is felt. Hold the gently pulling position a few seconds, then relax. Repeat five times.

- *Leg cross over stretch*. Sitting on the floor or in a chair, cross the affected leg over the other knee. Using the hands, pull the affected leg to cross it a bit more until a gentle pulling sensation is felt in the buttock. A sharp pain indicates too much pull. Hold the gently pulling position a few seconds, then relax. Repeat five times. See Chapter 2, page 38, for more information on stretching exercises.

When to call the doctor Sharp pain, a sensation of grinding in the joint, or impaired joint mobility should signal a visit to the doctor.

Treatment First try applying ice packs to the affected area and NSAIDs. If anti-inflammatory medications taken by mouth and physical therapy fail to resolve the pain, injection of a corticosteroid medication into the bursa may be necessary. Continued pain should warrant a doctor's examination.

Prognosis Prognosis is excellent with appropriate care; surgery is almost never needed.

❖ ILIAC CREST CONTUSION (HIP POINTER)

Symptoms *(What you may experience)* Localized point tenderness of the bony crest of the pelvis following trauma (usually a fall or other direct blow); often bruising over the area.

Signs and laboratory findings *(What the doctor looks for)* Tenderness over the area hit; bone chip fracture (possibly). X-rays are usually normal.

What is it? In several places in the body— most notably the shins—the bony skeleton comes very close to the surface of the body with very little soft tissue padding over it. This is the case with the wings of the iliac bones of the pelvic girdle. These areas are commonly referred to as the hip bones, although the true hip joint lies much lower, where the leg joins the body. Despite the anatomic incorrectness, the name hip pointer persists to describe this injury.

The lean padding over this area of the skeleton makes it vulnerable to injury, usually a hard fall landing directly on the bone or a direct blow to the area. The soft tissue or even the bone may be bruised.

In general, pain is worst when applying pressure over the injury, although motion can also cause some pain.

What you can do As soon as possible, apply ice to the area to reduce swelling and bleeding into the tissues. You should ice the area daily until pain and swelling are gone.

When to call the doctor Pain with hip motion or a sensation of grinding should prompt a visit to the doctor right away. Although usually the injury is limited to the tender spot of the impact, in pointers resulting from severe falls or crushing injuries to the pelvis, other pelvic injury is possible and should be ruled out by a doctor. Depending on the severity of the fall or blow, be alert for any signs of urinary tract injury, such as painful urination or blood in the urine.

Treatment Usually only medication to relieve pain and time to allow the injury to heal are all the treatment necessary.

Prognosis The discomfort of hip pointers can remain for many weeks, sometimes even months, but ultimately resolves.

❖ FRACTURED COCCYX (BROKEN TAILBONE)

Symptoms *(What you may experience)* Pain over the tailbone (tip end of the spine) following trauma; pain worsened by walking, sitting, lowering the body to sit, rising from sitting, or straining with urination or bowel movements.

Signs and laboratory findings *(What the doctor looks for)* Tenderness over the coccyx. X-rays may confirm fracture or appear normal.

What is it? Below the sacrum, the spine's last few bony segments dwindle and curl slightly to form a short chain of irregularly shaped bones collectively termed the coccyx (tailbone). The coccyx no longer has a function—since humans do not have tails—but it can be injured, typically in a hard sit-down fall. Such accidents occur commonly in slips on ice or when going down a flight of stairs.

Pain is immediate and sometimes severe, but the injury itself is rarely serious—qualifying more as a painful nuisance than a risk to health. Because a number of muscles within the pelvic cavity anchor on or near this bone, several movements can be quite uncomfortable, among them sitting, lowering the body into a sitting position, rising from a seated position, walking, climbing stairs, and any activity that requires a bearing down action, such as coughing, sneezing, or straining to urinate or defecate. The discomfort with passage of wastes occasioned by the injury can lead to urinary retention, constipation, and rectal impaction (on occasion).

What you can do Apply an ice pack immediately and continue to do so intermittently until the pain is gone. Take over-the-counter (OTC) pain relieving medication, such as ibuprofen or acetaminophen. Use of an OTC stool softener, such as Surfak or Colace, may reduce the discomfort of bowel movements. (Note: Use a softener, not a laxative; the latter will stimulate an increased urge to defecate, which could prove painful.)

Use of an inflatable or foam donut-shaped seat cushion may help, particularly in jobs necessitating prolonged sitting.

When to call the doctor Call the doctor right away if you experience severe discomfort with an inability to sleep; tingling, numbness, or weakness in the legs; the presence of blood in urine or stool; or difficulty passing urine or stool.

Treatment Except in rare instances, these injuries require only symptomatic treatment and time to heal completely. In a few cases, a syndrome of chronic tailbone discomfort—termed coccydynia—develops, which may respond to local injection of corticosteroid and anesthetic medications directly into the painful area.

Prognosis These injuries generally heal uneventfully. Freedom from all discomfort could take several months to achieve.

❖ PEDIATRIC HIP DISORDERS

Symptoms *(What you may experience)*
Slipped capital femoral epiphysis: knee pain, especially on the inside where the knees touch (often the only warning sign); intermittent pain in the groin; awkward outward twist of the leg and foot; limited range of motion of the hip. Perthes disease: painless limp in a preschooler. Congenital hip dysplasia and dislocation: delayed walking; limited hip motion; assymetrical motion in the hips when putting on diapers.

Signs and laboratory findings *(What the doctor looks for)* Confirmation and identification of the abnormality via x-rays.

What is it? As the hip joint develops from infancy to early adolescence a number of abnormalities can arise. The three most common of these abnormalities are slipped capital femoral epiphysis, Perthes' disease, and congenital hip dysplasia and dislocation.

- *Slipped capital femoral epiphysis*. This developmental disorder primarily arises in obese boys at or near puberty. Sometimes, for reasons that are not clearly understood but may involve excess weight or hormonal stimulation, the thighbone's insertion into the hip slips out of position. In as many as 25 percent of cases, both hips slip. In some cases, the slip occurs gradually, but in others abruptly. If a substantial degree of displacement occurs suddenly, the risk of problems increases. Symptoms may range from mild complaints of intermittent groin or knee pain to the development of an awkward rotation of the leg and foot outward.

- *Perthes' disease*. Also called Legg-Calvé-Perthes disease, this hip disorder usually strikes young children 3 to 6 years old. Most commonly, the child is a male, usually somewhat smaller than his peers. This condition arises as a developmental inflammation of the growth plate and the junction of the cartilage and bone that may be the result of abnormal pressure, compression, tension, or traction on the ball of the femur. In most cases, the first sign of a problem is the development of a painless still-legged limp. The condition is readily identified with standard x-rays that will show the characteristic changes in the bone. Examination will usually uncover a moderate degree of spasm of the hip muscles and a limitation in the ability to roll the hip and leg toward the middle of the body.

- *Hip dysplasia and dislocation*. In this disorder, the fit of the ball of the hip joint into its socket is abnormal from birth. The poor fit can more easily allow the ball to dislocate (slip out of the socket), an event that may occur in the womb prior to birth or occur during birth or shortly thereafter. The infant may hold the affected limb in an unusual or awkward position and may resist its being moved through a normal arc; however, the abnormality can sometimes go undetected until the child reaches the stage of walking. With an unstable hip or one already out of place, walking is problematic. The child may not even attempt to walk, and this should serve as a strong signal that something is amiss. Most pediatricians check for this routinely in infants.

When to call the doctor Difficulty in or refusal of bearing weight normally on one leg in a child of any age should prompt evaluation by a doctor.

Treatment Treatment for pediatric hip disorders varies.

- *Slipped capital femoral epiphysis*. The usual treatment is surgery to the hip to place a fixation screw to hold the ball of the thigh bone to the neck portion of the thigh bone. The goal is to prevent further slippage.

- *Perthes' disease*. The use of crutches or braces to reduce the weight bearing load is helpful and routine. Physical therapy to improve mobility of the hip is of paramount importance. Surgery may be necessary depending on the degree of deformity and the age of the person.

- *Hip dysplasia and dislocation*. Relocation of the ball into the socket is the first priority. Surgery to better seat the bone securely in place may also be necessary. Depending on the degree of dysplasia, surgical correction may prove necessary to prevent future dislocations. In very young babies a harness can be worn, which is successful in most cases.

Prognosis Prognosis is good if identified early and treated promptly and appropriately.

The Buttock and Thigh

❖ SCIATICA

Symptoms *(What you may experience)* Sharp, shooting pain down the thigh and leg

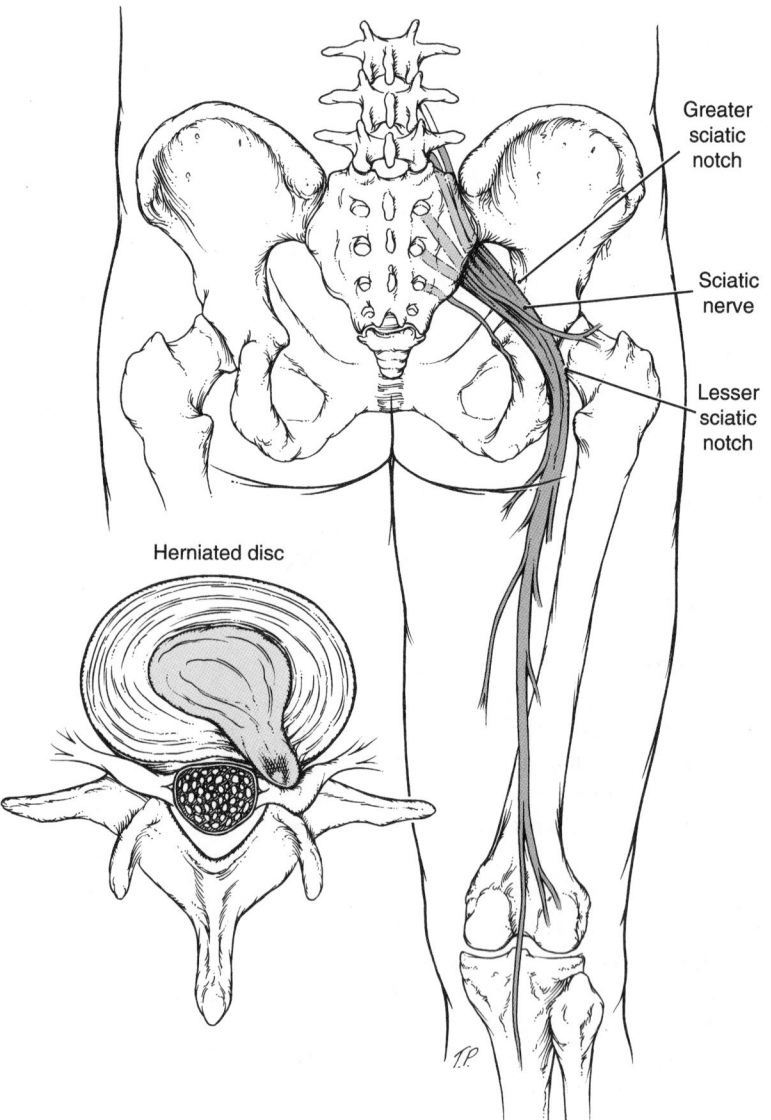

The sciatic nerve that runs down the buttock and thigh can become pinched in the sciatic notches, which causes a condition called sciatica. Numbness, weakness, tingling, and pain can occur along that region.

Greater sciatic notch

Sciatic nerve

Lesser sciatic notch

Herniated disc

especially noted when walking or with a cough or sneeze; weakness, numbness, or tingling in the foot or leg. Back pain may accompany these symptoms.

Signs and laboratory findings *(What the doctor looks for)* Specific pain with straight-leg-raise maneuver and often neurologic deficits, such as sensory loss, motor weakness, or diminished deep tendon reflexes. X-rays or CT scans are usually normal but done to exclude other causes.

What is it? The many nerve roots that exit the spine in the lower back join to form several large nerves, one of which is called the sciatic nerve. Pressure on the nerve due to herniated disks, lumbar disorders, or other problems causes both pain and loss of nerve function, demonstrated by such symptoms as numbness, tingling, and weakness of the muscle groups of the buttock and leg on that side.

The pain—called sciatica—worsens with any maneuver that causes a sudden increase in pressure within the abdomen, such as a cough or sneeze, as well as with those motions that stretch the nerve, such as flexing the hip with the leg straight. In some cases, the piriformis muscle (a muscle deep in the buttock) traps the sciatic nerve. Pressure over the nerve can also occur from outside the body—one common cause being a large wallet carried in the back pocket. From whatever cause, sciatic pain is usually sharp and shoots into the buttock and often down the leg along the path of the sciatic nerve supply. Continued pressure may cause tingling, numbness, or even weakness of the lower extremity, demonstrated as a foot drag or clumsiness of the lower leg. In the most extreme cases, loss of nerve function affects bowel or bladder control.

What you can do Get bed rest for 3 to 5 days. Limit walking and standing to a half hour per day; crutches may help reduce the pressure of weight bearing. (They will also facilitate getting from bed to bath during the period of bed rest.) Taking NSAIDs and applying a heating pad to the affected area also helps.

Use hand weights to keep the upper body muscles toned during the period of bed rest. Once pain subsides (about 1 week) begin gentle stretching exercises (see Caring for the Back and Keeping it Mobile, page 687).

Swimming—once the acute pain and symptoms have subsided—helps to tone the muscles without placing undue stress on the lower back.

When to call the doctor Call the doctor if you experience persistent or severe pain or loss of strength or sensation of the leg or foot. The loss of bowel or bladder control is an emergency and you should go to the emergency room or see your doctor immediately.

Treatment Bed rest and NSAIDs; pain medication; oral steroids; and occasionally muscle relaxants may be prescribed.

Physical therapy plays a critical role in prevention of recurrent episodes. Piriformis syndrome, in particular, can be relieved by supervised physical therapy. Surgery is utilized when the pain will not decrease with treatment or if the episodes of pain are very frequent. If there is nerve damage with weakness the doctor should monitor your nerve function. Loss of bowel or bladder control is considered a surgical emergency.

Prognosis Ninety-five percent or more of people with pain and numbness but only minimal weakness will respond favorably to conservative medical therapy and will not require surgery. Most people requiring surgery respond well and recover fully with time.

❖ HAMSTRING AND QUADRICEP MUSCLE STRAIN OR TEAR

Symptoms and signs Sudden pain in the thigh following abrupt and excessive stretching of the muscle; an audible pop with the injury (sometimes); continuing pain with specific use of the injured muscle.

What is it? Strain or tear of any muscle can occur when the muscle is stressed or stretched beyond its limits. The quadriceps at the front of the thigh and the hamstrings at the back are muscles that control the extension and contraction of the knee. Pain is usually immediate at the moment of strain or tear of these muscles, and if the tendon of the muscle ruptures, there may also be a

THIGH MUSCLE STRENGTHENING EXERCISES

These exercises should be performed as follows:

- *Straight leg raises.* Lying on the back or sitting in a chair, keep one leg bent at the knee and one leg straight. Raise the straight leg slowly 3 to 4 in., hold for a few seconds, and slowly return to the starting position. Repeat 15 to 20 times.

- *Leg extensions.* Lying on the stomach or raised up on the hands and knees, extend one leg straight and raise it about 3 to 4 in. from the floor. Hold it for a few seconds and then lower to the starting position. Repeat 15 to 20 times. ∎

pop, either felt or heard. Damage levels range from grades 1 to 3, grade 1 being a mild stretch and grade 3 a complete tear—these include swelling, black and blue discoloration, and difficulty walking.

Attempts to make the muscle contract—such as might occur during activities like walking and rising from a seated position—can cause discomfort.

What you can do Apply ice or cold packs immediately following the injury to reduce the risk of bleeding into the injured muscle; limit use of the injured muscle.

Rehabilitation of the strength and tone of the muscle is important as soon as the muscle is no longer acutely tender. Within the limitations of discomfort, perform thigh muscle strengthening exercises (see above).

Once you have recovered from the muscle strain or tear, be sure to warm up and stretch those muscles before beginning any strenuous physical activity.

When to call the doctor Significant swelling, significant pain, or inability to use the muscle normally despite pain should prompt a visit to the doctor.

Treatment Application of ice; NSAIDs; stretching exercises; and occasionally physical therapy may be advised. Crutches may be needed in severe cases.

Prognosis Healing varies according to the degree of damage. Severe muscle tears (grade 3) can take months to recover while grade-1 strains will usually take only a few weeks; grade-2 injuries fall somewhere in between.

❖ DEEP THIGH BRUISE

Symptoms and signs Tender, firm swelling and discoloration (bruising) of the thigh following a direct blow (often).

What is it? The muscles of the thigh are large and rich in blood supply. A direct blow to the front of the thigh—commonly seen when running into the corner of a table or counter or being hit by a ball or other thrown object—can rupture blood vessels in the thigh muscles and result in not only a visible surface bruise but often significant accumulation of blood deep in the muscle. Unlike surface bruising which usually resolves over 2 or 3 weeks, a large, deep collection of blood may take many months to reabsorb. Rarely, this collection of fluid may become infected or inflamed, demonstrated by overlying redness and heat. Sometimes, the bruise contracts or even calcifies to form a firm mass in the muscle that persists for years.

What you can do Apply ice packs and pressure to the area immediately following the trauma to reduce bleeding. Ice the injury for 15 to 20 minutes several times a day for the next week or so. Wrap the thigh—firmly but not constrictively—with an elastic bandage to apply pressure during this period. Try to bend and straighten the knee as pain subsides.

When to call the doctor Severe swelling or pain or difficulty bearing weight should prompt a visit to the doctor as soon as possible.

Treatment Usually no special treatment is necessary. Occasionally, if the bruise becomes infected or inflamed and you have a fever, call your doctor.

Prognosis Deep bruises to the thigh may take many months to completely resolve and will usually be tender for quite some time. In most cases, the bruise ultimately resolves without incident or long-term problems.

❖ FEMORAL SHAFT FRACTURE (BROKEN THIGH BONE)

Symptoms (What you may experience) Severe pain, swelling, and bruising of the thigh; inability to bear weight without severe pain.

Signs and laboratory findings (What the doctor looks for) Confirmation of the fracture and delineation of its extent via x-rays; estimation of blood loss as measured by blood tests.

What is it? Severe, high energy trauma is usually necessary to break the body of the femur. But when a femoral fracture occurs, it can be fraught with complications, including significant and sometimes even life-threatening loss of blood into the area of the fracture. Blood clots can form in the veins of the thigh which can travel to the lungs and brain where they interrupt blood flow. Chest pain after this injury should be evaluated immediately. (See Pulmonary Embolism, page 760, and Stroke, page 429, for more information about embolism.) Even in a young and healthy person, femoral fracture represents a potentially life-threatening injury that demands expert orthopedic care.

What you can do Immobilize the leg and if possible apply ice and compression. Proceed to the nearest emergency room for treatment.

Treatment In most instances, a femoral shaft fracture will require surgery to place an internal fixation device (a rod) in the marrow cavity to hold the cylindrical bone properly in place. The use of the femoral rod speeds healing and permits earlier mobilization and a quicker and more painless recovery than does immobilizing in a full-leg-and-hip plaster cast. The rod remains in place until the fracture heals. It can be removed at a later date but often is left in the bone.

Following surgery, recovery requires a period on crutches (non-weight bearing) with gradual progression to full weight-bearing activities, a process that takes several months to complete depending on the type of fracture. During this time, adherence to the prescribed physical therapy regimen will improve mobility and strength and speed your return to normal or near-normal activities.

Prognosis Prognosis is very good, except in some older people with weakened, thin bones (see Osteoporosis, page 654).

The Knee, Calf, and Shin

❖ ARTHRITIS OF THE KNEE

Symptoms (*What you may experience*) Aching, pain, stiffness, and swelling of the knee, especially after use; popping or crackling with bending; loss of full knee motion to bend or straighten (sometimes); sometimes water on the knee (swelling).

Signs and laboratory findings (*What the doctor looks for*) Tenderness along the joint line of the knee (inside more frequently worse than outside); fluid or swelling of the knee; confirmation of diagnosis via x-rays.

What is it? Osteoarthritis (OA) of the knees causes a progressive wearing away of the cushioning cartilage that normally covers the bone ends and provides smooth and nearly frictionless motion. There may also be the development of bone spurs that reflect that the joint cartilage is wearing out.

The knees, because of their role both in weight bearing and locomotion, are especially susceptible to the development of arthritis. A number of risk factors can predispose to the disorder, including family history, previous injury (particularly damage of the cartilage inside the knee), obesity, or abnormalities of knee alignment (such as *genu valgum*, commonly called knock knee, or *genu varum*, called bow leg). It is not clear exactly why there is an association of OA and obesity, but obesity may cause excessive wear and tear with weight bearing and possibly abnormal alignment.

Arthritis can affect the knee joint on its inner aspect, the outside of the knee, or the area where the knee meets the knee cap. The disorder tends to worsen with time and to erupt in periodic flares of discomfort and swelling after periods of relative quiet.

What you can do Exercise regularly in such activities as swimming, cross-country skiing or ski machines, but limit deep knee bending, kneeling, or squatting; avoid weight-bearing sports that pound the joints such as biking and aerobic dancing. After exercise, apply ice to limit swelling. Use heat before exercise to warm the joint, followed by gentle range-of-motion exercises. Keep the muscles that support the knee (the hamstrings and quadriceps) strong and toned (see Thigh Muscle Strengthening Exercises, page 699).

Use OTC pain-relieving medications, such as ibuprofen, acetaminophen, or aspirin to relieve discomfort.

When to call the doctor Significant pain, a change in the quality of the pain, significant joint swelling, development of redness or heat around the joint, grinding of the joint with motion, inability to walk or participate

---

BAKER'S CYST OF THE KNEE

A Baker's cyst is an abnormal pouch of joint fluid behind the bend of the knee. Compression of the pouch with bending may exaggerate awareness of the mass, a feeling somewhat like bending the knee around a hard boiled egg. Because the cyst takes up space, it may make the knee joint feel tight or swollen. This cyst is benign and may wax and wane in size. Ice and NSAIDs can help when the cyst swells. If it continues to grow you should see your doctor.

The most common cause for development of a Baker's cyst is OA or rheumatoid arthritis (RA) of the knee, and although x-rays may confirm these associated diagnoses, the cyst itself usually cannot be seen on standard x-rays. Ultrasound or magnetic resonance imaging (MRI) examination will confirm the fluid-filled nature of the mass. Although uncommonly needed, the ultrasound can be used to guide the doctor in aspirating the fluid to deflate the cyst. Injection of the cyst or the knee with corticosteroid medication following removal of fluid may be helpful, although these cysts tend to recur. These cysts very rarely are excised with surgery.

Physical therapy to strengthen and tone the muscles that support the knee—the hamstring and quadriceps—may help prevent recurrence (see Thigh Muscle Strengthening Exercises, page 699). ∎

TOTAL KNEE REPLACEMENT SURGERY

When arthritis of the knee becomes painful enough to decrease joint mobility and to effect or disrupt normal activities, the doctor may recommend knee replacement surgery.

Unlike many knee operations that can be performed with the arthroscope as single day surgery, replacement of any large joint requires major surgery, usually under either a general anesthetic or special anesthetic techniques that put only the legs to sleep (spinal or epidural). A 3- to 5-day hospital stay to begin rehabilitation generally follows.

During surgery, the doctor opens the skin of the knee with an incision and removes the entire joint surfaces, including the knobby end of the femur and a portion of the upper flat end of the tibia (lower leg bone), to prepare a suitable base on which to attach the new joint surfaces.

The femur is replaced with a metal component while the top of the tibia is replaced with a plastic or metal piece. The surfaces of these components are designed to glide across each other with almost no friction; this way the joint moves easily and with as little wear as possible. The artificial materials are cemented in place with a special bonding material that acts like a mortar to hold the components to the bone.

Following surgery, there is some discomfort, but medications sufficient to handle the pain are available if needed. Suction drains remain in place for 1 or 2 days to evacuate accumulated blood and fluid from the surgical site. Physical therapy begins to mobilize the joint and restore muscle tone and strength usually the day after surgery.

The process of physical rehabilitation is of paramount importance to success; it will continue both in the hospital and during the weeks and months that follow. The goals of physical therapy are to increase the strength and motion of the knee and to train the person to walk with supports. The more effort put into the therapy, the greater the chance for a complete recovery and a return to full or near-full activity.

Most total knee replacement patients do very well in decreasing pain and restoring motion and function. A majority of knee replacements will last 15 to 20 years, but young (under age 45), highly active people may shake the knee replacement loose over time. It is important that you ask your doctor about what activities you should not do in order to optimize the lifespan of your joint. ■

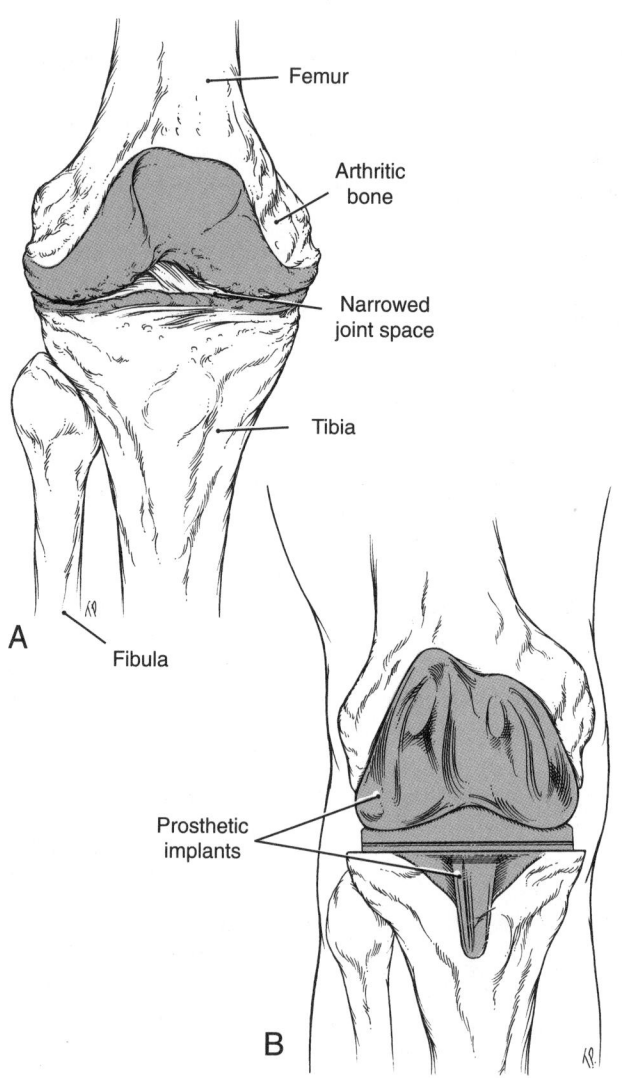

(A) Degenerative osteoarthritis is characterized by major changes in the bony structures. (B) Severe disabling arthritis may benefit from an artificial knee replacement. An artificial knee replacement requires major surgery. During surgery, parts of the tibia and femur bones and the knee joint surfaces are removed. Artificial pieces that fit together and allow smooth motion are inserted and cemented into the femur and tibia and can often last 15 to 20 years.

in your usual sports should prompt a visit to the doctor.

Treatment Most cases get relief with ice, NSAIDs, and activity modification. If not effective then local injection of the joint with anesthetic or corticosteroid medication can offer dramatic relief in some cases. The doctor may recommend tapping the knee to remove large collections of fluid when the water on the knee causes pain and limitation of motion.

In active people in whom knee arthritis causes significant pain, loss of mobility, or diminishes quality of life, the doctor may recommend arthroscopy or, in more severe cases, arthroplasty (total replacement with an artificial joint). (See Total Knee Replacement Surgery, above.)

Prognosis The disorder tends to wax and wane in severity, but can progress depending upon a variety of factors. With care, surgery may not be necessary. Total knee replacement is very effective at providing pain relief.

❖ TORN MENISCUS

Symptoms *(What you may experience)* Initially, pain and swelling following twisting injury of the knee. Later, snapping, popping, locking, or pain or swelling of the knee joint.

Signs and laboratory findings *(What the doctor looks for)* Popping felt with bending and straightening of the knee by the doctor; the tear as demonstrated by MRI (sometimes).

What is it? The knee joint is formed where the lower dual-knobbed end of the femur meets the flat dual-plateaus of the tibia. The menisci are a pair of crescent-shaped, cushioning cartilage pads that cradle each knob of the femur. Twisting forces on the knee (which can occur with falls in active sports such as snow skiing or basketball or contact sports such as football or soccer) tear the meniscal cartilages, causing immediate swelling and pain of the knee. Later, with movement, the torn piece of cartilage can become trapped under the knob of the femur as the knee bends and straightens. Trapping of the torn cartilage can cause the knee to lock, pop, and become painfully stiff and swollen.

Grinding of the offending piece, left unattended, can cause irreparable damage to the smooth joint cartilage that covers the end of the bone, leading to the development of wear-and-tear arthritis of the knee.

What you can do Immediately after the injury, apply ice and elevate the leg. Limit weight bearing by using crutches to rest the knee.

When to call the doctor Immediate swelling following injury should merit a visit to the doctor. Persistent or recurrent locking or popping should also be evaluated.

Treatment Using the arthroscope, the doctor can view the interior of the joint and identify the damage and use tiny instruments that can pass through the flexible arthroscope tubing to remove or repair broken pieces. Recovery from arthroscopic surgery is rapid in most cases, with ice packs, rest, and elevation following the operation. Depending on the extent of repair, most people can go home the day of surgery and, using crutches for the next 3 to 7 days, can begin bearing weight right away. Return to sedentary work (in sitting jobs) and driving (automatic transmissions) may be as soon as a week. Total recovery often takes longer and varies from 4 to 8 weeks.

Prognosis Prognosis depends entirely upon what was found and what was done at the time of surgery. People with significant arthritis of the knee may not be able to return to such activities as running or jogging. People with removal or repair of simple acute meniscus tears can usually return to previous athletic endeavors. With a part of the cartilage removed, future arthritis is still a possibility with continued heavy knee stress.

❖ KNEE LIGAMENT INJURY

Symptoms *(What you may experience)* Popping sound and sometimes sudden pain in the knee following injury; tenderness and swelling of the knee.

Signs and laboratory findings *(What the doctor looks for)* The doctor can usually tell what ligaments are torn by examining the knee. In some cases an MRI is needed to detect the damage.

What is it? Several tough ligaments support and stabilize the knee. On the two sides lie the collateral ligaments; the lateral collateral on the outer aspect is a dense collection of tough ligament fibers that forms a cable-like structure about the size of a fat pencil. It is not easily torn, except with severe trauma. The medial collateral ligament spreads out like a thin fan across the inner aspect of the knee; it is more easily injured than is its lateral mate, with any stress that forces the knee into a knocked knee position.

Deep inside the knee, a pair of tough ligaments called the anterior and posterior cruciate ligaments (commonly referred to as the ACL and PCL) crisscross from back to front and front to back to stabilize the

These strong ligaments support and stabilize the knee. The lateral (fibular) collateral ligament is like a cable, and the medial (tibial) collateral ligament is spread like a fan across the knee. The anterior and posterior cruciate ligaments criss-cross to stabilize the knee further; these can be damaged by twisting or pivoting motions.

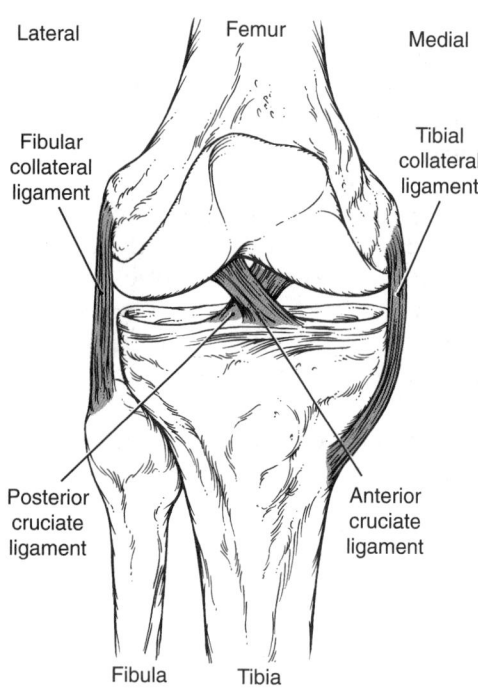

Lateral Femur Medial

Fibular collateral ligament

Tibial collateral ligament

Posterior cruciate ligament

Anterior cruciate ligament

Fibula Tibia

What you can do Apply ice and elevate the leg to limit or reduce swelling; limit or avoid weight bearing, using crutches to prevent the injured knee from further stress. For discomfort, take NSAIDs or acetaminophen; if you choose to take aspirin, do not take more than six a day because of its blood-thinning characteristic.

When to call the doctor Significant pain, immediate swelling, or the sensation of joint instability—a feeling as though the knee would give way with weight bearing—should prompt a visit to the doctor.

Treatment Injuries to the medial collateral ligament, while painful, usually do not need to be repaired with surgery; time and the natural healing forces of the body are the best remedy. Significant tears of the lateral ligament, however, usually require repair with surgery. Arthroscopy can identify the extent of damage to the ligaments within the knee and through this instrument, replacement of the anterior cruciate ligament (using a tendon graft) is possible. Recovery from arthroscopic surgery is much quicker than is surgery that requires a total opening of the knee. Pain control can usually be managed by application of ice and taking medication for pain. Usually, IV antibiotics are given at first to ensure that the joint does not become infected after surgery.

knee against stresses in those planes. They can be injured by cutting, twisting, or pivoting maneuvers, commonly performed in such sports as football, basketball, soccer, and skiing.

The intensity of pain experienced in a knee ligament tear can vary widely, but can sometimes be severe. Swelling is usually immediate (within the first few hours).

ARTHROSCOPIC KNEE LIGAMENT RECONSTRUCTION SURGERY

Once the anterior cruciate ligament tears, attempts to repair it are usually not successful. Consequently, better outcomes usually result if the ligament is surgically replaced (or reconstructed) with another tendon from around the knee. The procedure once required fully opening the knee joint during surgery, a major surgical procedure fraught with many months of disability and rehabilitation; however, it can now be performed through the arthroscope.

Through a small incision on the front of the knee, the doctor harvests a section of the patellar (knee cap) tendon to be used as the replacement. Occasionally a donor tendon from another person (called a cadaver tendon or allograft because it is taken and banked after a donor's death) is used instead. Although these donated tissues are carefully screened for infectious diseases—such as hepatitis or acquired immunodeficiency syndrome (AIDS)—a low potential risk (estimated at 1 in 500,000) exists for infection from a donor tendon graft; consequently, many doc-

tors recommend grafting with a person's own tendon when possible.

From whatever source, once the graft is available, the doctor drills a tunnel through the ends of the femur and tibia and then threads the graft through the tunnel and secures it in position with screws, staples, or stitches. These fixation devices are left permanently in place within the knee.

This surgery can be done on an outpatient basis, or patients often stay one night. Following an initial session with the physical therapist the patient can be discharged. Most people are on crutches for 5 to 10 days, progressing to full weight bearing as swelling, mobility, and strength allow. Ongoing compliance with physical therapy recommendations and the prescribed exercise regimen can make the difference between a poor result and a successful return to full or nearly full knee function. During this period of rehabilitation, a hinged knee brace protects the knee from twisting and re-injury.

Depending on the nature of a person's surgery and future activity level, recovery to full activity may take 4 to 9 months. ■

Regular physical therapy during the weeks following surgery is necessary to restore normal function. Usually people wear a sturdy hinged brace on the injured knee for several months following surgery to permit controlled bending and straightening but prevent side-to-side motion or twisting.

Prognosis Return to full activity following knee ligament injuries usually requires 4 to 12 months, depending on the person and the nature of future activities.

❖ PATELLAR (KNEE CAP) PAIN SYNDROME

Symptoms (What you may experience) Aching of the knee cap after activity; pain with squatting or kneeling; grinding sensation with bending the knee; swelling of the knees (occasionally).

Signs and laboratory findings (What the doctor looks for) Abnormal tracking of the knee cap in its groove; abnormalities as detected by x-rays.

What is it? Knee cap pain can occur for a variety of reasons, some traumatic and others that occur over a longer interval of time. Sudden trauma to the patella (knee cap), sufficient to dislocate it or to break it, may occur with a kneeling landing from a fall. In these instances of sudden injury, severe pain and usually considerable swelling and discoloration of the knee cap usually occur immediately.

More gradual onset of knee cap pain occurs with inflammation of the patellar tendon from abnormal or unaccustomed use over an extended period of time. Another cause of ongoing knee cap pain arises from abnormalities of the knee cap itself. Chronic knee cap disorders usually cause pain (and sometimes swelling) in the hours following use, such as after jogging, hiking, or biking. Activities that cause stress on the knee cap, such as stair climbing, squatting, or kneeling, can also cause discomfort.

What you can do For acute injuries, apply ice, elevate the leg, and restrict weight bearing with crutches for at least 48 hours. For chronic knee cap disorders, apply ice to reduce swelling when needed and after sports activities. Avoid knee bends, squat-

ting, and, as much as possible, stair climbing. Daily straight-leg-raising exercises to tone and strengthen the quadriceps muscles of the thigh that support the knee are helpful (see Thigh Muscle Strengthening Exercises, page 699). Use of OTC anti-inflammatory medications, such as ibuprofen, may help.

When to call the doctor Following a fall that injuries the knee cap, see your doctor or seek emergency treatment if the pain is severe, if it persists at a significant level longer than 48 hours, if you cannot bear weight without pain, or if the knee cap appears displaced from its normal position.

Chronic knee cap disorders merit investigation by a doctor if the character or intensity of the discomfort changes appreciably or if the disorder interferes with normal activities.

Treatment Fractures of the knee cap require immobilization in a splint, brace, or cast and often need repair (sometimes with surgical placement of wires to hold the fragments together properly). Dislocated knee caps must be put back into their proper position; in some cases, surgery to realign the track of the knee cap in its groove may be necessary to prevent repeat dislocation. These procedures (called a lateral retinacular release and a tibial tubercle transposition) revise the architecture of the front of the knee, allowing the knee cap to fit more securely into the valley or groove between the knobs of the femur.

Chronic knee cap disorders respond best to physical therapy exercise to tone and strengthen the thigh muscles that support the knee.

Arthroscopic evaluation may be necessary in some cases to evaluate the cartilage in the knee and to rule out other causes of the pain.

In all cases, the cornerstone of recovery is treatment with ice, NSAIDs, and a physical therapy regimen designed to tone and strengthen the quadriceps muscles of the thigh; the best are daily straight leg raises in sets of 20.

Prognosis Acute injuries of the knee cap may require as long as 12 weeks to completely heal and, even then, discomfort may come and go. Chronic knee cap disorders tend to occur in flares of swelling and discomfort (particularly with overuse) followed by relatively symptom-free periods. Most people with the latter can return to sports with treatment.

❖ PRE-PATELLAR BURSITIS (HOUSEMAID'S KNEES)

Symptoms *(What you may experience)* Painful redness, warmth, and swelling over the knee cap.

Signs and laboratory findings *(What the doctor looks for)* Swollen bursa as detected by x-rays (x-rays are not necessary for the diagnosis); clear or translucent yellow fluid from the bursa as removed by aspiration.

What is it? The knee cap is protected by several bursae. The sac that lies between the knee cap and the overlying skin is called the prepatellar (meaning before the patella) bursa. It bears the brunt of chronic, unaccustomed, or overuse trauma involving kneeling and commonly becomes thickened, inflamed, and swollen from such activities as scrubbing or waxing floors—hence the name housemaid's knees—although many other activities can contribute to its development. The condition can also arise from infection of the bursa (usually by bacteria of the *Staphylococcus* family) or as a consequence of gout (see page 652).

What you can do Avoid direct pressure on the knee cap; limit squatting and kneeling. A padded knee sleeve may be helpful as well as the application of ice packs to decrease the pain and swelling. Take OTC anti-inflammatory medications, such as ibuprofen, for discomfort.

When to call the doctor If the condition fails to respond to the conservative measures outlined above, consult your doctor; if the pain or swelling becomes worse or fever develops signalling infection, consult the doctor right away.

Treatment If symptoms persist or indicate infection, the doctor will aspirate to relieve the pressure as well as to permit lab examination of the fluid. Lab tests on the specimen will determine whether the cause is infectious, gouty, or simply inflammatory. Use full doses of nonsteroidal anti-inflammatory drugs (NSAIDs) and rest.

Infectious bursitis requires the administration of antibiotic medication sufficient to eradicate *Staphylococcus* while the culture grows in the lab (a process that usually takes 48 hours to complete).

Prognosis The condition may wax and wane and be of a chronic nature but, with proper management, it resolves completely in many cases.

❖ OVERUSE SYNDROMES OF THE KNEE (JUMPER'S KNEE AND OSGOOD-SCHLATTER'S DISEASE)

Symptoms *(What you may experience)* Pain, tenderness, and swelling (sometimes) of the tendon running from the kneecap to the leg—worse with activity, especially jumping or running.

Signs and laboratory findings *(What the doctor looks for)* Site of most tenderness as pinpointed by examination. X-rays may be helpful, especially in Osgood-Schlatter's disease.

What is it? Overuse of the knee—as in competitive running or jumping—can cause inflammation and pain. In young people, still actively growing, repetitive running or jumping motions can stress the weakened growth area where the patellar tendon attaches to the tibia just below the knee cap; this stress may be sufficient to irritate the growth plate where the tendon attaches to the tibia. As a result, Osgood-Schlatter's disease is seen only in children with open growth plates. The overlying area may become visibly inflamed, with redness and warmth; the pain may be minimal at rest but usually worsens with running or jumping.

Jumper's knee results from stress on the attachments of the tendon of the knee from repetitive jumping in such sports as basketball, volleyball, or high-impact aerobics. The microscopic tears of these attachments cause tendinitis to develop and with it, chronic knee pain. The disorder often affects only one knee—when both knees are involved, the cause may be more than simple jumper's knee and merits investigation by a doctor.

What you can do Limit activities that provoke the pain, such as jumping or repetitive bending. Apply ice packs throughout the day and after sports activities. Over-the-counter (OTC) anti-inflammatory medications—such as ibuprofen—may help. Wearing a neoprene knee brace, padded above the kneecap, may reduce discomfort during activities that cannot be curtailed. Exercise to strengthen and tone the thigh muscles may help improve the efficiency of knee mobility (see Thigh Muscle Strengthening Exercises, page 699).

When to call the doctor Persistent discomfort or bilateral discomfort (involving both knees), large swelling, or severe pain should prompt a visit to the doctor.

Treatment Apply ice packs and take NSAIDs daily for 4 to 6 weeks. Physical therapy is recommended if the pain continues. In Osgood-Schlatter's disease, the doctor may recommend surgical removal of bone fragments that fail to fuse to the main body of the bone after the growth plate is closed.

Prognosis In most cases, the prognosis is very good with therapy. Most adolescents with Osgood-Schlatter's disease will resolve their symptoms when they reach bone maturity and growth has been completed. Tendinitis in adults usually waxes and wanes with treatment. Rarely, surgery can be done on the tendon to decrease the pain.

❖ KNEE EFFUSION (WATER ON THE KNEE)

Symptoms *(What you may experience)* Swelling, tightness, and limitation to full motion of the knee.

Signs and laboratory findings *(What the doctor looks for)* Fluid within the knee as detected by physical examination; associated causes, such as degenerative arthritis, as determined by x-rays; a fluid specimen removed by aspiration for lab analysis.

What is it? Water on the knee, also called a knee effusion, occurs when an abnormally large amount of joint fluid accumulates within the joint. The most common causes of such an accumulation include osteoarthritis (OA), inflammatory arthritic disorders such as rheumatoid arthritis (RA), torn meniscal cartilage, and, rarely, infection. Sudden swelling in the joint can also occur with bleeding into the joint with injury (called a hemarthrosis). The appearance of blood in the joint fluid following injury can mean a tear of a meniscus or one of the ligaments within the knee and demands referral to an orthopedic specialist for further treatment.

Whatever its source, as the fluid accumulates within the joint, its bulk creates a tightness or fullness that limits smooth motion, making it difficult to fully flex or bend the knee.

What you can do Apply ice, elevate the leg, and take acetaminophen or ibuprofen to reduce swelling. Limit squatting or kneeling. Perform daily straight-leg-raising exercises to strengthen the muscle groups of the thigh that support the knee (see Thigh Muscle Strengthening Exercises, page 699). Crutches may be needed.

When to call the doctor Significant or worsening pain, discomfort with weight bearing, or the appearance of warmth, redness, or fever should prompt a visit to the doctor right away. Swelling of the joint following trauma should be evaluated right away.

Treatment If ice and NSAIDs fail, it is necessary to identify and treat the underlying causes of water on the knee. Removal of the fluid for microscopic and culture analysis is necessary to determine the presence of blood, infection-fighting white blood cells, bacteria, or crystals. Aspiration relieves the tightness and discomfort, although the fluid may reaccumulate and require repeat aspiration in a few days to weeks. It is recommended that you apply ice packs frequently after aspiration. In noninfectious cases of water on the knee, use of full doses of an NSAID is usually effective. If not then aspiration may be accompanied by an injection of corticosteroid medication into the joint to reduce inflammation; this treatment can be repeated in 4 to 6 weeks if symptoms are severe enough.

In persistent cases, examination of the joint with an MRI scan or by arthroscopy may prove necessary. With the arthroscope, the doctor can identify and remove loose pieces of cartilage or repair tears of the meniscus that might be causing the condition to recur or persist.

Prognosis The prognosis depends on the underlying cause. Those cases of water on the knee caused by mild to moderate inflammatory arthritis (OA or RA) respond most favorably to aspiration and injection, often with many months of relief of symptoms. Failure to respond may indicate a non-inflammatory cause, one more likely to require arthroscopic surgery.

❖ SHIN SPLINTS

Symptoms and signs Pain in the shin following repetitive trauma from running or walking; tenderness to pressure on the inside of the tibia. X-rays confirm diagnosis.

What is it? The exact cause of shin splints is unknown. The repetitive motion occasioned by unaccustomed running or walking can cause excessive stress on the attachment of the posterior tibial muscle (the muscle on the front of the shin) to the tibia. This condition, commonly referred to as shin splints, can result in pain with continuing activity.

What you can do Stretching and exercises to strengthen the muscle of the front of the shin (such as flexing your ankle upward) will help to prevent this condition. Decreasing weight-bearing activity and running on softer surfaces should help. Wear comfortable shoes with a good arch and heel support. It has been suggested, though not proven, that frequently changing shoe inserts may also help. Apply ice and take acetaminophen or ibuprofen for pain.

When to call the doctor Significant or persistent pain or the presence of swelling (lasting longer than a few weeks) should prompt a visit to the doctor.

Treatment In cases that result from malalignment of the foot and lower leg, an orthotic splint (arch-supporting shoe insert) may help. The doctor may also prescribe a special heel wedge insert for the shoe to alter the pattern of weight bearing. For continued pain, a bone scan may be needed to rule out a stress fracture.

Prognosis The pain may come and go; surgery is rarely needed.

❖ CONTUSION OF THE SHIN

Symptoms (What you may experience) Pain, swelling, and discoloration of the shin following a direct blow.

Signs and laboratory findings (What the doctor looks for) X-rays may be done to rule out the possibility of a fracture.

What is it? Because little soft tissue padding covers the shin, a direct blow—such as might occur from being struck with a baseball or car door or being kicked—can be very painful. Rupture of small blood vessels in the soft tissues and bone covering can result in a discolored bruise. Because this blood is outside the blood vessels and therefore free to move about in the tissue, it may migrate with gravity over the days following the injury, resulting in bruises lower in the shin, around the ankles, and in the foot. The appearance of bruising in these areas can cause alarm, but the condition is not dangerous. The bruises—wherever they appear—will disappear in the course of healing over 1 or 2 weeks.

What you can do Immediately apply ice and compress the injured area with an elastic bandage to limit swelling. Take acetaminophen or ibuprofen for pain; avoid aspirin as it may thin the blood and increase the tendency to bruise.

When to call the doctor Significant pain, limitation of normal motion, or difficulty bearing weight without pain should prompt a visit to the doctor for evaluation of possible associated fracture. Pain which worsens despite rest and medication should be evaluated.

Treatment Generally only ice and compression of the injured area are needed for the injury to heal on its own, once other complications (such as fracture) are ruled out.

Prognosis Prognosis is excellent, although the contused area may be tender to the touch or to pressure for several weeks. A firm lump on the bone can sometimes persist for months, and may even calcify and remain permanently.

❖ LEG OR CALF CRAMPS

Symptoms *(What you may experience)* Grabbing pain in the calf at rest, at night, or with activity.

Signs and laboratory findings *(What the doctor looks for)* Mineral imbalances, especially low potassium, calcium, or magnesium (sometimes): blockage as detected by Doppler ultrasound or x-ray dye studies of the arteries supplying the legs (in some cases).

What is it? The muscles of the calf are strong enough to cause substantial discomfort when they contract sharply. A wide variety of factors can cause the calf muscles to spasm or cramp, but among the most common are low levels of critical minerals (such as potassium, magnesium, or calcium) or fluid depletion that may accompany intense athletic competition; excessive use of the muscles in cold weather; and obstruction to blood flow in the arteries supplying the calf muscles.

Blockage to blood flow can occur from within or without. Buildup of atherosclerotic plaque within the interior of the blood vessel can narrow the artery and restrict blood flow through the artery (a condition termed claudication). This condition typically develops gradually in older people. The calf cramping of claudication occurs during an activity, such as walking or jogging, and unlike a simple cramp which may persist after ceasing the activity, the pain of claudication usually subsides immediately with rest. A rough measure of the degree of blockage can be determined by how far a person can walk or jog prior to the onset of cramping symptoms.

Rarely, interference of blood flow from outside the artery can occur in the bend of the knee where muscular or fibrous bands of tissue can compress it (a condition called popliteal entrapment syndrome). The pain begins during calf muscle activity and like the claudication caused by arterial blockage, subsides with rest. Unlike atherosclerotic buildup, popliteal entrapment is congenital and usually identified in young adults.

Nocturnal leg cramps occur in the middle of the night, usually disrupting sleep. The cause, while not clearly understood, may stem from sluggish blood flow that may occur with the legs elevated.

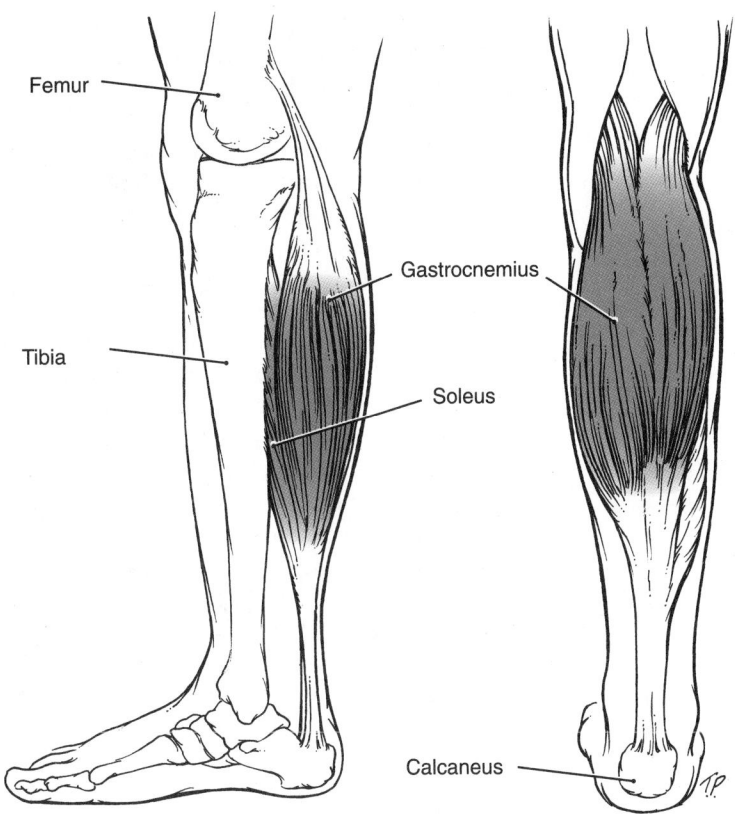

Several muscles support the structures in the leg (calf). The gastrocnemius is the large muscle in the back of the calf, originating in the femur and inserting into the calcaneus. The soleus muscle connects the tibia and fibula to the calcaneus via the achilles tendon, and also assists with ankle flexion.

What you can do Drink plenty of water to prevent dehydration. When exercising during hot weather, rehydrate with fluids that replace both water and mineral electrolytes to restore balance of potassium, sodium, and other minerals lost in sweat. In cold weather, always warm up and stretch muscles prior to heavy use.

Nocturnal leg cramps may respond to OTC medications containing quinine; consult your pharmacist for recommendations. Should a nocturnal leg cramp occur, flexing your toes upward (toward your head) while stretching the leg may help resolve the cramp.

When to call the doctor Pain that suggests atherosclerotic obstruction—that comes on at a generally predictable interval during exercise and is relieved immediately with cessation of the activity—should prompt an evaluation by a doctor. Occasional nocturnal leg cramping is no cause for alarm; frequently recurring cramping of any muscle, however, merits investigation.

Treatment Mineral or electrolyte imbalances are corrected by replenishing the deficient substance, either in pill or capsule form or, in severe cases, by IV infusion.

Correction of popliteal artery entrapment requires surgery to relieve the compression on the artery. The treatment for claudication arising from atherosclerotic blockage in the arteries is to clean out the buildup of plaque inside the artery (a procedure called endarterectomy) or to bypass the obstruction with natural or artificial artery grafts. Medications to improve circulation may bring some relief of symptoms and increase the capacity for exercise before the onset of discomfort.

Prognosis The prognosis depends on the specific cause. Mineral or electrolyte imbalances usually resolve quickly and completely upon correction of the deficiency. Nocturnal cramping responds less predictably and may come and go for many years. Atherosclerotic claudication tends to progress if untreated; however, appropriate treatment can substantially improve quality of life.

❖ CALF MUSCLE TEARS

Symptoms (*What you may experience*) Sudden pain, swelling, discoloration (sometimes), and tenderness in the calf, usually during activity; an audible pop at the moment of injury (sometimes).

Signs and laboratory findings (*What the doctor looks for*) Special x-ray dye studies or Doppler ultrasound studies to exclude the possibility of a blood clot may be necessary.

What is it? With sudden unaccustomed or excessive stretching stress, especially in middle-aged male athletes, the calf muscles (or their connecting tendons) can suddenly rupture. The tear often occurs during such calf-intensive activities as jogging or playing tennis, but can also occur in any instance where the foot is sharply flexed upward, suddenly stretching the calf. A typical cause is stepping unaware into a hole or off a curb. Often, an audible pop accompanies

the rupture, followed by pain and swelling. Because sudden pain and swelling of the calf are also typical symptoms of a blood clot in the deep veins of the lower leg, this possibility must be often excluded by special testing (see Deep Vein Thrombosis, page 834).

What you can do Apply ice, elevate the leg, and apply slight compression. Rest the calf and limit any activity that flexes the foot upward, stretching the calf muscles; try to keep the foot at 90° (a right angle) to preserve a normal angle for walking. OTC anti-inflammatory remedies—such as ibuprofen—can offer some relief. Crutches may be necessary.

When to call the doctor If the symptoms did not occur in association with injury during physical activity, see the doctor right away. If the symptoms worsen or fail to resolve in 48 hours with the conservative treatments outlined above, consult the doctor.

Treatment Usually no repair is necessary, and time will heal the injury. Severe tears can take months to recover. A gradual return to activity should be dictated by the level of discomfort—when an activity no longer causes pain, it is permitted.

Prognosis Prognosis is excellent for complete recovery and in most cases an eventual return to sports.

❖ KNEE AND LOWER LEG FRACTURES

Symptoms (*What you may experience*) Significant pain and often swelling following trauma to the lower leg; deformity of shape and bruising (often); penetration of the bone through the skin (occasionally).

Signs and laboratory findings (*What the doctor looks for*) Nature and exact location of the fracture as determined by x-rays.

What is it? The bones of the lower leg—the tibia and fibula—are the most commonly broken bones in the United States (estimated at 185,000 per year). The causes are various ranging from severe motor vehicular trauma to a fall to a direct blow to the bone. Fractures can be closed (meaning the skin over the break is intact) or open (a laceration of the skin over the break has occurred, leaving the broken bone open to the environment and increasing the likelihood of infection). The fracture may also be comminuted (broken into multiple fragments).

Fractures that occur in the end of the tibia where it flares to meet the femur at the knee joint can be especially troublesome. Restoring normal function to the joint demands near-perfect surgical realignment of the fractured fragments.

The risks of a broken tibia or fibula are several, with damage to nearby nerves or blood vessels being the most immediately significant. In closed fractures, bleeding and swelling within the soft tissues can also cause pressure on these structures and must be vigorously treated.

What you can do Do not attempt to bear weight. Immobilize the leg, using whatever materials are at hand, such as a board or several lengths of heavy corrugated cardboard long enough to span from above the knee to below the foot. Lift the leg as a unit, moving the fractured area as little as possible to slide the splint under it. Affix the splint securely with an elastic bandage, packing tape, duct tape, scarves, or belts. Apply ice to limit swelling on the way to the hospital emergency room. If there is a skin break, cover it with a clean cloth bandage.

When to call the doctor See your doctor immediately or go to the emergency room. In open fractures, call emergency service for assistance, if possible.

Treatment Assessment of any damage to nerves or blood supply is imperative, followed by x-rays to determine the extent of injury. In some cases, only splinting or casting the injured leg is needed. More complicated cases (especially those involving the portion of the tibia near the knee or ankle) may require surgery with placement of internal fixation rods, plates and screws, or wires to hold the fractured bone in proper position for healing. Open fractures require debridement and antibiotics to prevent infection. Pressure buildup within the calf may require surgical release by splitting the calf muscle to relieve the pressure before nerve or blood supply damage occurs.

Prognosis In most cases the outcome is very good if treated immediately and adequately. Delay of treatment, especially in open fractures, can result in serious infection that could threaten life or limb. Fractures closer to the ankle are more likely to result in deformity and a longer period of recovery than are those closer to the knee. Tibia fractures can take up to 3 to 6 months to heal.

The Ankle

❖ ANKLE SPRAINS

Symptoms (*What you may experience*) Pain, swelling, and bruising over the ankle following injury; ankle pain with weight bearing or motion following injury.

Signs and laboratory findings (*What the doctor looks for*) Excessive laxity of ligaments; x-rays are often done to exclude the possibility of fracture; MRI rules out other injuries if ankle does not improve with treatment.

What is it? Of all ligaments in the body, the most commonly injured are those in the ankle. On either side of the ankle, groups of tough ligaments span the space between the bones of the lower leg and the bones of the foot and the heel. The ligaments on the outer aspect of the ankle are weaker and more vulnerable to injury with a twist of the ankle than the broader and tougher group on the inner side.

Ankle sprains are classified based on severity as grade I, II, or III, representing mild, moderate, or severe damage to ligaments. Damage to the medial (inner side) ligaments is almost always a more serious injury than the lateral (outer) ligaments.

In a groove just behind the bone that forms the outer side of the ankle, runs the peroneal tendon (tendon of one of the small muscles of the calf). It is anchored to the bone by a ligament sleeve that permits the tendon to glide smoothly, but holds it securely in place. Sometimes twisting injuries to the outer side of the ankle also tear the ligament sheath away from the bone, leaving the tendon vulnerable to dislocation.

What you can do Apply ice several times a day until the swelling is down (may take

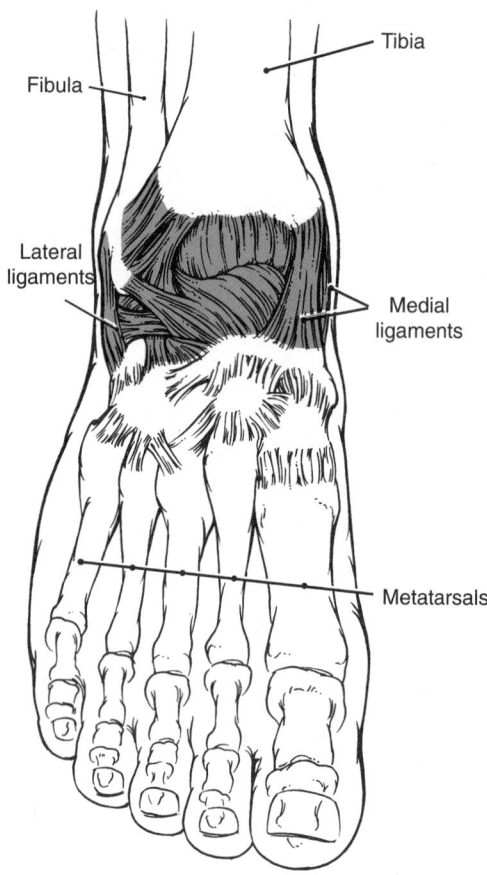

The ankle and foot bear significant weight, and the most commonly injured ligaments are those in the ankle, especially ligaments on the lateral side. Metatarsal bones are the longest bones in the foot.

several weeks), compress with an elastic bandage, and elevate the injured ankle (see Wrapping the Injured Ankle, page 713). Take OTC ibuprofen or acetaminophen for pain. Do not bear weight on the injured ankle if it causes pain—use crutches (see How to Properly Use Crutches or a Walker, below).

When to call the doctor Dramatic swelling, limitation of motion, significant pain, or inability to bear weight on the injured ankle without pain should prompt a visit to the doctor for evaluation.

Treatment Range-of-motion exercises and weight bearing as tolerated will aid in recovery. Physical therapy may be recommended for cases that do not respond to ice and exercises.

During the first or second month of rehabilitation, the doctor may recommend taping the ankle or using a brace for additional support to the injured ankle. People who wish to pursue athletic endeavors may need to continue taping or wearing a supportive brace during such activities for up to 6 months following injury or indefinitely depending on the injury.

Surgical repair or reconstruction is usually reserved for cases that demonstrate chronic ankle instability with activity.

Prognosis Grade I injuries should heal suf-

HOW TO PROPERLY USE CRUTCHES OR A WALKER

Although the way to use crutches may seem obvious, all too often people use them incorrectly and injure themselves in the attempt. If you have problems with crutches or a walker then you should discuss them with your doctor or physical therapist. However, a few simple guidelines may help.

Size Crutches should be properly fitted for size, with the crook high enough to touch the arm pit and the hand rests at a level where the palm can reach them with the arm slightly bent.

Using Two Crutches When the injured leg should bear little or no weight, the doctor or physical therapist will recommend the use of two crutches. To properly use two crutches, support the weight of the body on the uninjured leg and swing both crutches out a step's width in front. The crutches, hands, arms, and shoulders bear the weight of the body as it swings forward to plant the uninjured foot again. Occasionally, two crutches may be necessary for support in walking when both legs are weakened (such as from arthritis, multiple sclerosis, degenerative neuromuscular disorders, or back injury).

Using a Single Crutch One crutch is called for when injury to a lower extremity necessitates limited weight bearing. Place the crutch on the injured side—it is there to take the place of the injured leg or foot. The crutch should swing out in synchrony with the injured leg. Then as the uninjured leg swings forward to complete the step, the crutch should support some of the weight. If there is any doubt about your ability to use a single crutch, use two until your doctor clears you to use one.

Using a Walker Because of its four-point stability, the light-weight aluminum walker may prove to be the best and safest option for assisted weight bearing in the elderly or in those people with impaired balance (for example, following a stroke or other injuries or disorders involving the brain). To use a stationary walker, stand comfortably within its perimeter, grasp the frame on either side, lift it a short distance, place it firmly on its legs, and use it for balance and support to walk the few steps back into it. Some walkers are fitted with wheels so that they can be rolled forward with each step, an especially useful tool for those people unable to lift and place a stationary walker. ■

WRAPPING THE INJURED ANKLE

Following an ankle sprain, support and compression are important. It is always important to keep the pressure of an elastic bandage firm but not tight and evenly distributed. To properly wrap an injured ankle, do the following:

- Use a 3 in. elastic bandage for adults (2 in. in small children).

- Begin at the top of the foot just behind the toes, keeping the bandage rolled neatly and unrolling as you go.

- Wrap once around the foot to secure the end, using a light but firm stretch (never so tight it pinches the skin) to wrap the bandage in smooth and regular overlapping spirals up the foot to the ankle.

- At the ankle, use a figure-eight pattern to go behind and around the ankle, across over the top of the foot, beneath the arch, back across the foot, and around the ankle again.

- Place a few turns up the lower leg—again overlapping in even smooth spirals—and back down.

- If length permits, repeat the figure eight going down the ankle and finish with a few turns on the foot.

- Following injury, an ice bag can be incorporated into the last layer of the bandage. Place a zip-closure bag filled with small cubes or crushed ice on top of the bandage over the injured side, then wrap a few turns of elastic bandage over it to hold it in place. It is recommended that you ice daily until the swelling and pain are diminished.

If the bandage is tightly pinching or uncomfortable at any point, adjust or remove the bandage. ■

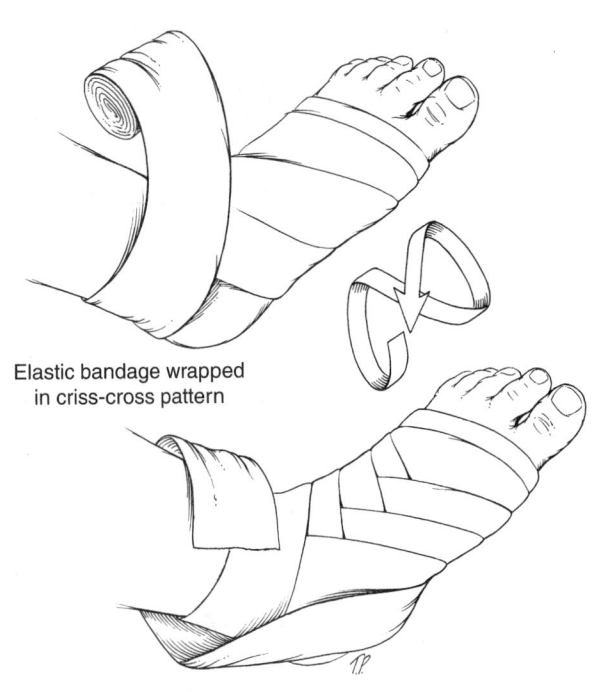

Elastic bandage wrapped in criss-cross pattern

A wide elastic bandage can provide support to a minor injury, such as a sprain or strain. When wrapping a sprained ankle, keep the elastic bandage slightly stretched but not too tight. Starting behind the toes, the bandage is wrapped smoothly, proceeding to the ankle, where a figure eight pattern is used. Cross the top of the foot, beneath the arch, back across the foot, around the ankle again, and around the lower leg.

---

ficiently to return to normal activities within 1 or 2 weeks; grade III injuries may require 8 to 12 weeks or longer.

❖ MALLEOLAR (ANKLE BONE) FRACTURES

Symptoms *(What you may experience)* Significant pain, swelling, bruising (often), and limitation of motion of the ankle following trauma.

Signs and laboratory findings *(What the doctor looks for)* Confirmation of fracture via x-rays.

What is it? On each side of the ankle the bones of the lower leg flare to form prominent bony humps called the malleoli (one is a malleolus). The malleolus on the outer side, formed by the end of the fibula, is termed the lateral malleolus; the other, on the inner side, formed by the end of the tibia, is termed the medial malleolus. While a moderate twisting force might sprain the ligaments of the ankle, a greater force could snap the ends of one of the bones—a malleolar fracture. If the bones on both sides of the ankle break, the injury is termed a bimalleolar fracture; if a third area on the back of the ankle breaks, it is termed a trimalleolar fracture. The more bones broken, the more serious the injury and the more difficult and lengthy the healing.

What you can do Do not bear weight on the foot. Apply ice and stabilize the injured ankle, moving it as little as possible. (See pages 388 and 664 for information on how to make splints.) Elevate the injured leg.

When to call the doctor See the doctor immediately or proceed to the nearest emergency room.

An x-ray showing an ankle fracture indicated by the arrow.

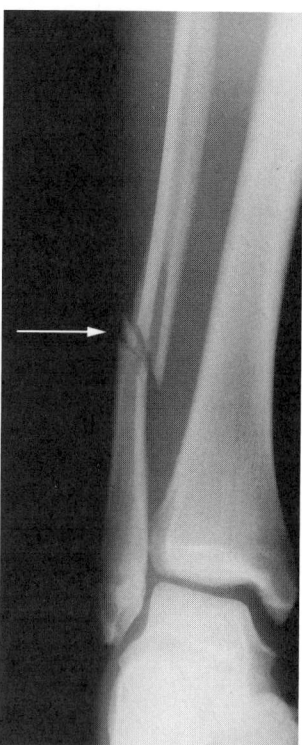

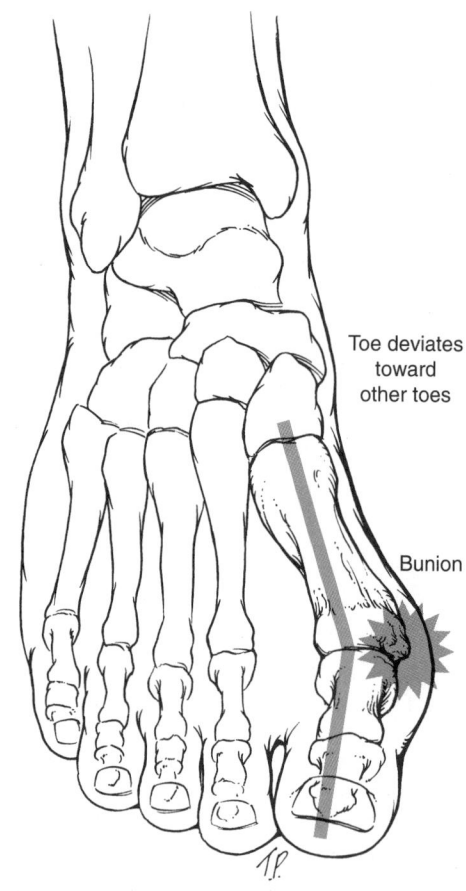

Toe deviates
toward
other toes

Bunion

The large toe can deviate toward the other toes, pushing the base outward and creating a bony hump called a bunion.

Treatment These breaks, when simple, can sometimes be treated by immobilizing the foot and ankle in a cast, but because some malleolar fragments are prone to slip from their proper position, they may need to be surgically fixed with wires or screws to hold them securely in place.

Physical therapy to restore normal mobility to the ankle is important to complete recovery.

Prognosis Good if properly treated. The length of time for the bones to heal depends upon what is broken and whether surgery is done.

The Feet

❖ BUNIONS

Symptoms *(What you may experience)* Bony lump on the inside of the foot at the base of the big toe; tenderness and pain with limited range of motion of the big toe. (See page C-42.)

Signs and laboratory findings *(What the doctor looks for)* Confirmation of diagnosis via x-rays.

What is it? When the big toe deviates toward the other toes it pushes the base outward, creating a bony hump called a bunion. This may occur as a result of arthritis or in some cases an inherited condition called hallux valgus (a deformity in which the big toe rides over or under the other toes). Frequently, the cause is unknown but there may be a genetic basis, since the condition often runs in families. Women are especially predisposed to developing the condition because of mechanical pressure attendant with wearing pointed toe shoes with a high heel, which force the toes into the deviated position. Because the bunion sticks out beyond the normal curve of the foot, it is vulnerable to excess pressure and friction from shoes. This pressure causes thickening of the skin and the development of calluses over the area.

Although a bunion normally causes only a cosmetic deformity with perhaps some minor discomfort, on occasion a more painful inflammation such as osteoarthritis

(OA) or bursitis may arise in the joint or the nearby bursa.

What you can do Wear shoes that fit properly with sufficient room in the toe box to accommodate your feet in a normal position. When the bunion is painful, adhesive felt or foam bunion pads (available at most pharmacies) may offer relief by protecting the bunion from shoe pressure. If inflamed, apply ice and take acetaminophen or ibuprofen.

When to call the doctor If significant pain, redness, or limitation of motion occurs, consult your doctor.

Treatment In extreme cases, surgery to realign the bone of the toe with the foot and to shave away the bony lump may be necessary. The surgery can usually be performed as outpatient surgery, with recovery at home. Fixation wires may be placed during surgery to hold the toe in the realigned position. These wires must remain in place for a few weeks while the bone heals. During the first few days, there may be considerable swelling and discomfort, usually handled easily with ice packs, elevation of the limb, and pain-relieving medication. Return to normal walking may take several weeks.

Prognosis Prognosis is excellent for relief of discomfort with simple conservative maneuvers in most cases. With those cases requiring surgery, prognosis is excellent for relief of both discomfort and deformity.

❖ HAMMER TOE

Symptoms *(What you may experience)* Drawn-up or claw-like deformity of a toe; painful or limited motion of the toe (often).

Signs and laboratory findings *(What the doctor looks for)* Confirmation of diagnosis via x-rays (usually not necessary).

What is it? The condition termed hammer toe occurs when any toe (although it is usually the second toe) draws into a flexed position, tipping the end of the toe downward, like the head of a hammer. In many cases, the cause is unknown, though there may be a genetic basis, since the condition often runs in families. It can also be caused by improperly fitting shoes, too short to allow the toe to fully extend. In people with long-term diabetes, hammer toe can occur as a result of the nerve and muscle damage that often accompanies the disorder.

The condition can sometimes be painful, and the abnormal position and shape of the toe can also cause problems in fitting shoes and may even make walking or running difficult.

What you can do Wear properly fitted shoes having sufficient length to permit full extension of the longest toe.

When to call the doctor If the condition is significantly painful or makes normal daily activities difficult, consult a doctor.

Treatment The doctor may prescribe a special orthotic splint to relieve the pain. In some instances, surgery may be necessary to realign the toe. The procedure can usually be performed on an outpatient basis and involves realigning the bones of the toe and the placement of surgical wires to hold the alignment in position for healing. The wires remain in place for several weeks and then are removed. Pain and swelling that may accompany the procedure usually respond to ice, elevation of the limb, and pain-relieving medications.

Prognosis In most cases, conservative remedies resolve the discomfort. Following surgery, recovery is usually complete.

❖ METATARSALGIA

Symptoms *(What you may experience)* Pain on the underside of the ball of the foot, especially when standing, painful calluses on the ball of the foot.

Signs and laboratory findings *(What the doctor looks for)* Tenderness to pressure applied over the metatarsal heads. X-rays are usually done only to exclude other causes.

What is it? Pain arising in the bones that form the ball of the foot (the ends of the metatarsal bones) can occur for a variety of reasons, including trauma, arthritis, inflammation of the small sesamoid bones under the great toe, foot strain, wearing high-heeled shoes, abnormal patterns of weight bearing or abnormal foot bone structure (particularly hallux valgus or a high arch). With time, these forces flatten the transverse arch and weaken the small muscles within the foot, resulting in uneven distribution of weight across the front portion of the foot and with it, pain and inflammation of this area. Tough calluses form on the sole of the foot over the ball in response to the uneven pressure on the metatarsal heads.

What you can do Wear properly fitted, supportive shoes. A shoe insert that provides padding to the front or a metatarsal bar on the outside of the shoe can be helpful. Some commercial sneakers now have this built in.

When to call the doctor Persistent pain across the ball of the foot or the appearance of calluses should prompt a consultation with the doctor.

Treatment The primary focus of treatment is directed at restoring the normal pattern of weight bearing to alleviate pressure on the metatarsal heads. This relief usually takes the form of specially fitted orthotic supports or pads worn inside the shoe. Rarely is surgery necessary to correct the problem.

Prognosis Prognosis is good if treated properly.

❖ BURNING FEET

Symptoms and signs Burning sensation on the sole of the foot.

What is it? Occasionally, irritation or dysfunction of the nerves supplying the bottoms of the feet causes an abnormal sensation perceived as a hot spot or area of burning on the sole. One of the most common causes of such a sensation is a neuropathy (nerve disorder). The most common cause of neuropathy is diabetes (see page 469). Deficiency of certain B vitamins, most importantly, vitamin B_{12}, exposure to heavy metals and a number of other conditions can lead to neuropathy. Repeated trauma, such as pressure from wearing high-heeled shoes that cramp the toes and feet, can also be a cause. It is occasionally seen in runners due to pounding the feet. Development of a nerve tumor from overuse can also cause

burning pain (see Morton's Neuroma, below.)

What you can do Always wear properly fitting shoes with a flat or sensible heel.

When to call the doctor If despite conservative measures the condition persists, consult your doctor.

Treatment Testing to determine the cause of a neuropathy should be done and appropriate therapy instituted. Specially fitted orthotic supports may redistribute weight and resolve burning irritation caused by overuse.

❖ MORTON'S NEUROMA

Symptoms *(What you may experience)* Numbness, tingling, pain, or burning of the area between the third and fourth toes (usually) or between the second and third toes.

Signs and laboratory findings *(What the doctor looks for)* Pain on squeezing the foot side to side below the toes; tenderness between the involved toes upon pressure (usually).

What is it? The small nerves that supply motion and sensation to the toes pass into them from the body of the foot between the ends of the bones that form the arch (the metatarsal bones). Activities, such as jogging, dancing, or wearing high-heeled or narrow-toed shoes, can cause irritation by entrapping and repetitively rubbing the nerve between the flared ends of adjacent bones. Over time, the nerve builds up a benign swelling, much like a callus, on that section of the bone. This swelling, called a neuroma, is nothing more than a bundle of nerve fibers. This swollen part of the nerve expands within the already tight space between the bones and causes pain, numbness, and burning or tingling sensations in the lower foot and toes. A hallmark of this disorder is that grasping the foot across the ball and squeezing from the sides reproduces the pain by compressing the neuroma between the bone ends.

What you can do Wear properly fitting low-heeled supportive shoes; a special pad, called a metatarsal pad, worn in the shoe may also relieve pressure on the inflamed area.

When to call the doctor If the pain worsens or persists despite the conservative measures outlined on page 716, consult a doctor.

Treatment Injection of corticosteroid medication into the tender area between the third and fourth toes may help reduce inflammation and offer some relief. When the pain persists despite these treatments, surgical removal of the neuroma may prove necessary. Following this surgery, which can usually be performed on an outpatient basis, a period of a few weeks of recovery usually precedes a return to normal activities.

Prognosis Prognosis is excellent if properly and promptly diagnosed and treated.

❖ ACHILLES TENDINITIS

Symptoms *(What you may experience)* Pain, swelling, and tenderness over the Achilles tendon.

Signs and laboratory findings *(What the doctor looks for)* X-rays may be done to exclude other causes.

What is it? Inflammation of the Achilles tendon most commonly results from trauma or overuse; less commonly, this condition may also be associated with other inflammatory conditions, such as ankylosing spondylitis, sarcoidosis, Reiter's syndrome, rheumatoid arthritis, and gout.

What you can do Ice daily or several times a day for 20 to 30 minutes for several weeks. Ice after any sports activity. Rest the tendon and take over-the-counter (OTC) anti-inflammatory medications, such as ibuprofen. Wearing a heel lift may take some of the stretch and stress off the inflamed tendon. Stretching the tendon is usually helpful.

When to call the doctor If the condition persists or worsens despite the conservative remedies outlined above, see the doctor.

Treatment Because the Achilles tendon is vulnerable to rupture, it should *not* be injected with corticosteroid medications. Full doses of a nonsteroidal anti-inflammatory drug (NSAID) and rest usually help.

Physical therapy modalities, such as heat, cold, and ultrasound, may reduce the inflammation and pain.

Prognosis Prognosis is good with prompt and proper treatment.

❖ ACHILLES TENDON RUPTURE

Symptoms *(What you may experience)* Sudden onset of pain with sudden flexion of the foot (moving the toes toward the shin); audible snapping or popping with the flexion; subsequent difficulty walking or standing on the toes.

Signs and laboratory findings *(What the doctor looks for)* Loss of plantar flexion on Thompson test (a squeeze to the calf should make the toes point; rupture of the tendon prevents this action); partial or complete rupture of the tendon as distinguished on examination. MRI may occasionally be needed, but not often.

What is it? This condition usually occurs during athletic activities or in jumps or falls when the foot is sharply forced toward the shin stretching the Achilles tendon beyond its limit. Tearing or rupture of the tendon occurs more commonly in people with Achilles tendon inflammation or in those taking steroid medications.

WHAT IS A HEEL SPUR?

On the sole of the foot, the plantar fascia attaches at the front to the base of the toes and in the back to the heel. Traction along this sheet of tissue (a normal consequence of weight bearing) exerts a force on the bone of the heel. With time, the force deforms the bone, forming a pointed spike or spur. The spur, then, is nothing more than the bone's response to the pulling of the fascia and muscles of the area.

Sometimes, in people with heel pain, an x-ray taken to determine cause will show a heel spur. Although on occasion a large and growing spur may be the cause of significant heel pain, it rarely is the cause of the pain. The spur is a sign of increased stress and not the *cause* of it. Heel spurs occur commonly in people without heel pain, and heel pain often occurs without the presence of a heel spur. ■

What you can do Do not bear weight; stabilize the foot, and seek medical help.

When to call the doctor See your doctor or seek emergency medical attention immediately.

Treatment Treatment may be either with a cast or surgery. You should discuss the pluses and minuses of each approach with your doctor. Surgical repair of the tendon is often necessary, followed by non-weight-bearing immobilization of the foot and ankle in a splint or cast. Recovery may take several months.

Prognosis Prognosis is good if diagnosed promptly and treated appropriately.

❖ PLANTAR FASCIITIS (HEEL OR SOLE PAIN)

Symptoms *(What you may experience)* Gradual (usually) onset of pain over the inner side or bottom side of the heel; pain worse with the first step in the morning or after periods of inactivity; pain worse in bare feet or in shoes with minimally padded soles.

Signs and laboratory findings *(What the doctor looks for)* Pain exacerbated by stretching the arch of the foot by pushing the toes and ball of the foot backward. X-rays are done to exclude other causes.

What is it? This condition, the most common cause of heel pain, results from inflammation of the plantar fascia. The fascia provides support to the arch of the foot and plays an important role in normal foot mechanics during walking. When the foot bears weight or flexes at the ball and toes, the fascia stretches; therefore, such activities as standing, running, or walking place this structure under tension. Excessive, increased, or unaccustomed stress—such as might occur in beginning a walking or running program—can inflame the fascia. With aging, the tissue loses some of its normal elasticity and resilience and could become irritated with routine daily activities. Less commonly, plantar fasciitis can develop in association with general medical conditions such as Reiter's syndrome or rheumatoid arthritis.

What you can do Reduce walking or running duration or switch from these activities to swimming or cycling to reduce stress.

Wear properly fitted shoes, with a flat or very low heel and good sole padding. Sneakers or other soft-soled shoes are preferable to shoes with rigid soles. Heel pads or wedges that are soft are helpful. Avoid wearing rigid or stiff shoe inserts, as these only put added stress on the inflamed fascia.

OTC anti-inflammatory medications, such as ibuprofen, help relieve pain and inflammation. Ice to the heel helps as well, particularly after activity.

Each day, stretch the Achilles tendon and the sole of the foot as follows:

- *Achilles and sole stretch.* Sitting on the floor or the bed, bend the right knee and hip to grasp the ball of the foot and toes with the hands. Gently but firmly pull the toes and ball of the foot backward toward the knee until you feel the stretch or slight discomfort in the sole or heel. Hold the stretch for a count of five. Change feet. Repeat five times for each foot. It is important that stretches become a daily routine, even after recovery to prevent recurrence.

When to call the doctor If the discomfort persists despite 4 to 6 weeks of faithfully following the conservative remedies outlined above, consult your doctor.

Treatment Stronger anti-inflammatory medications available only by prescription may be necessary to reduce the inflammation.

The doctor may prescribe a specially fitted "night splint," which is a device worn during sleep to place constant gentle stretch on the plantar fascia.

In rare persistent cases, injection of the fascia with corticosteroid medication may be necessary. This treatment is reserved only for cases that fail to respond to other means, since steroid injection into this area can in some cases cause wasting of the fatty pad on the bottom of the heel, itself a painful condition difficult to reverse or treat.

Surgery is recommended only in extreme cases and consists of a release of the fascia at the end where it attached to the heel bone, also called the calcaneus.

Prognosis The majority of cases will respond to conservative treatments, provided they are followed faithfully for 6 to 12 months. While sometimes chronic, these almost always go away with time and treatment.

❖ PLANTAR PUNCTURES (STEPPING ON A NAIL)

Symptoms (*What you may experience*) Immediately, pain and bleeding from a puncture to the sole of the foot. Later danger signs: significant pain, redness, and swelling around the puncture and drainage of discolored fluid from the puncture.

Signs and laboratory findings (*What the doctor looks for*) X-rays may be necessary to exclude the presence of foreign material deep in the wound; if there is drainage from the wound, a culture to identify bacterial infection may be needed.

What is it? A common injury to the foot, stepping on a nail, glass shard, large wood splinter, or any other penetrating object can puncture the tough sole of the foot. The puncturing object may carry with it dirt or other contaminants that when driven deep into the foot could pose a risk for infection to develop.

The foot is composed of many compartments formed by fascia (tough fibrous bands) and ligaments that crisscross the interior joining one bone to another. Because of this structure, if an infection develops, the accumulation of blood, pus, or fluid in the area can cause tremendous pressure. The pain from such an infection may be so severe that weight bearing, even tapping or bouncing the foot, becomes unbearable.

What you can do Always cleanse the wound thoroughly with mild antibacterial soap and water or hydrogen peroxide. Keep the wound covered with a dry clean bandage.

When to call the doctor If there is any chance that foreign matter—a piece of glass, metal, or wood—remains in the wound, consult a doctor. If after the injury, the area around the foot becomes significantly more painful, red, warm, or swollen or there is drainage of fluid or pus from the wound, seek medical attention immediately. Failure to do so could allow a potentially severe infection to develop in the foot, necessitating surgical treatment.

Treatment Antibiotic medications may be necessary. Exploration of the depth of the wound under local anesthetic injections (or in some cases, and especially with children, general anesthesia) to remove foreign material or exclude its presence and to thoroughly clean the wound may be required.

A tetanus booster is important for teens and adults if it has been more than 10 years since the last booster. In children (and adults) who have not completed their series of childhood immunizations and may therefore not be completely protected against tetanus, prevention with an injection of tetanus immune globulin may be needed.

Prognosis Prognosis is excellent if promptly and appropriately treated. Although most punctures only cause a few days of discomfort and heal without incident, some become infected. Failure to recognize and aggressively treat an infection within the foot could pose the risk of sepsis (blood poisoning) and threaten the survival of the foot.

❖ FOOT SPRAINS

Symptoms (*What you may experience*) Pain and (sometimes) bruising or swelling of the foot following trauma, usually twisting.

Signs and laboratory findings (*What the doctor looks for*) Localized tenderness to applied pressure; standard x-rays do not contribute except to exclude fracture.

What is it? The tibia and fibula join the foot at the ankle, which itself connects to a series of roughly cube-shaped bones arranged in two rows. These bones—termed the tarsal bones—are analogous to the wrist bones in the upper extremity. They, in turn, connect to the metatarsal bones, which finally terminate in the phalanges or bones that form the toes. All along the length of the foot, these many bones are bound one to another by groups of fibrous ligaments. This structure gives the foot shape, stability, and flexibility.

Any unusual force applied to the foot—such as twisting or excessive bending—can exceed the limits of give in one or more of these ligaments and cause it to tear. Damage to the ligaments of the foot is termed a foot sprain. The injury will usually be quite painful initially and for 1 or 2 days afterward, and then may only hurt with foot motions that specifically stress the injured ligament. That sort of discomfort may remain for several weeks to 1 or 2 months until the ligament finally heals. The amount of swelling is a good indication as to the degree of the injury: A great degree of swelling will usually indicate a more serious injury.

What you can do Immediately apply ice, lightly compress the foot with an elastic bandage to reduce swelling, and elevate the foot. If you have severe pain with weight bearing, you should use crutches.

When to call the doctor If the pain of the injury prevents weight bearing within 48 hours, consult a doctor.

Treatment Use of full doses of an NSAID for short periods are most helpful. Orthotic inserts may help to alter the weight-bearing pattern sufficiently to make walking comfortable during the healing process.

Prognosis Prognosis is excellent; most sprains heal completely with time. More severe injuries may take months.

❖ FRACTURE OF THE BONES OF THE FEET

Symptoms *(What you may experience)* Localized pain and (often) swelling or bruising over the painful area, following trauma (usually a crushing blow or a twisting stress); painful weight bearing.

Signs and laboratory findings *(What the doctor looks for)* Confirmation of the fracture via x-rays.

What is it? Fracture of the bone of the foot can involve the metatarsal bones or the tarsal bones. The former are more likely to break following twisting injuries of the foot and the latter with direct blows, although there is a great deal of overlap.

The most common (and least significant) fracture of a foot bone occurs in conjunction with a lateral ankle sprain—one in which the sole of the foot rolls toward the middle. The anatomy in this region sets up the injury: A tendon of one of the calf muscles runs adjacent to the lateral ankle bone and attaches to the tip of the fifth (little toe) metatarsal bone on the side of the foot. Sharply rolling the ankle over during a spraining injury can put sufficient traction on the tendon to pull it free from the bone, taking the tip of the bone with it. This injury may look like an ankle sprain, but the pain is in a different location.

From this less significant injury, foot bone fractures range in severity to chips and cracks of the squarish bones of the midfoot (which may cause only some bruising and local tenderness to pressure) to the much more serious fractures with dislocation of the midfoot bones. Major, direct high-energy force (usually a motor vehicle accident) is usually necessary to sustain these latter kinds of injuries. When they occur, expert care is required to perfectly realign the bones, since poor alignment of this area could result in a long-term disability.

Equally serious is a fracture of the talus. This bone serves as the pivotal connection between the foot and the leg, jutting upward like a mortise providing the surface on which the tibia rests and rocks securely. Fracture of the talus usually implies a significant and serious ankle fracture, with extreme pain, swelling, and inability to bear weight. Such injuries most often result from forcefully bending the foot back toward the shin, not uncommonly the consequence of the floorboard's being driven up into the foot during a motor vehicle crash. Talar damage requires expert orthopedic surgical care.

Finally, there is the fracture involving the heel bone in the back of the foot. A break of the chunky heel bone usually occurs in a fall or jump from a height or with the high energy force found in a motor vehicle accident. The significant force required to break the heel bone is transmitted up the leg and through the body and may result in associated fractures of the spine in as many as 15 percent of injuries. Tenderness in the back following a jump or fall that seriously injures the heel should always be reported to the treating doctor.

Fracture of the heel usually causes a large amount of swelling, bruising, tenderness, and even blistering of the skin over the heel. Again, expert care is important to the outcome.

What you can do In simple fractures not causing tremendous pain, apply ice, compress the injury lightly with an elastic bandage to reduce swelling, and elevate the injury. In a Jones fracture, or fracture of the fifth metatarsal, wearing a stiff-soled, laced-up shoe to support the fractured bone tip may be all that is needed to keep the foot reasonably comfortable with weight-bearing activities during healing. Sometimes a cast or fracture boot provides more comfort. Rarely, surgery is necessary for fractures of this bone.

For significant injuries causing immediate swelling, bruising, blistering, and pain, do not bear weight. Elevate the limb, apply ice and compress if possible, and proceed to the nearest emergency room for evaluation. See pages 388 and 664 for information regarding splinting the injured foot.

When to call the doctor In minor injuries, if the discomfort worsens or has not significantly subsided within 48 hours, contact a doctor. In serious injuries, consult a doctor immediately or go to the emergency room.

Treatment The simplest foot fractures may require no treatment beyond a stiff-soled shoe. Uncomplicated fractures often require immobilization in a short-leg cast or fracture boot (often one that soon permits walking) for 6 to 8 weeks. Fracture or dislocations of the midfoot, talus, or heel bone may be adequately immobilized in a short-leg cast for 6 to 8 weeks, but if the fracture fragments cannot be kept in proper alignment by casting alone, surgery may be necessary to place fixation wires, pins, or plates to ensure correct healing and the best possible result. In most cases of serious foot fracture involving the talus or heel bone, a period of 10 to 12 weeks without bearing weight may be necessary.

Physical therapy following such injuries plays an important role in a return to normal or near-normal levels of activity. Even very soon after surgery (depending on the type of surgery) physical therapy may be begun to mobilize the injured joint and restore strength to the muscle groups that support it.

Prognosis Simple, uncomplicated foot fractures usually heal without incident in 6 to 8 weeks. Fractures of the midfoot, talus, or heel bone require expert care and perfect anatomic correction for best results. When the heel bone has been broken into multiple pieces, outcome depends upon the location of the pieces and how they heal.

❖ FRACTURED TOES

Symptoms *(What you may experience)* Significant pain and (often) bruising or swelling of the toe and adjacent foot following trauma.

Signs and laboratory findings *(What the doctor looks for)* Confirmation of the fracture via x-rays; deformity of the toenail; bleeding under the nail may indicate a fracture.

What is it? Fractures of the toes commonly occur from tripping, catching a toe on a table leg or door jamb, or dropping a heavy load on the toes. Although fractures can cause significant pain, unless the fracture is combined with a laceration of the overlying skin (an open fracture and therefore more prone to infection) most broken toes are an uncomfortable inconvenience, requiring modest treatment and time to heal. The exception is a significant break of the great toe, which because of its importance to walking and balance may require more sophisticated treatment.

What you can do Immediately apply ice and elevate the foot. If there is bleeding, compress with a clean cloth.

When to call the doctor Open fractures should be seen right away by the doctor for proper cleaning of the damaged tissues and a course of antibiotic medication. Pain that persists at a significant level (sufficient to inhibit normal weight bearing) longer than a few days should prompt a visit to the doctor for x-rays and evaluation. If the toe is sticking out at an angle, you should see the doctor.

THE DIABETIC FOOT AND ITS CARE

Because of its damaging impact on nerves and small blood vessels, diabetes can pose serious risks to the feet. Small traumas and minor foot conditions that would in a nondiabetic person be insignificant can in a diabetic foot rapidly develop into serious medical problems. Nerve damage impairs the ability of the diabetic foot to perceive the discomforts that warn of injury; small injuries may go unnoticed. Tiny cuts around the nails from trimming the toenails too closely, small scratches from walking barefoot, corns, calluses, or blisters from improperly fitting shoes can lead to skin breakdown and infections. Minor infection in a diabetic foot can quickly worsen and spread, sometimes degenerating to a level that if not aggressively treated could become life threatening. In severe cases, the infection may lead to amputation of the toe, foot, or leg.

All people with diabetes should be extremely careful with their feet. General guidelines are as follows:

- *Examine the feet every day.* Because minor traumas may go unnoticed, look carefully at all sides of each foot, between toes, around the toenails, making note of cuts, scrapes, dry skin, calluses, corns, and areas of redness or blisters. Use a mirror if necessary to view the sole and heel of the foot. Report any abnormalities to the doctor.

- *Keep feet clean and dry.* After carefully washing feet with mild soap and warm (not hot) water, dry them completely by patting them (not rubbing) with a soft, absorbent towel or using a handheld hair dryer on the low (warm) setting. Moisturize dry areas. Wear only soft, absorbent, natural fiber socks or hosiery without constricting elastic bands. Change socks as needed to keep the feet dry.

- *Wear the right shoes.* Wear only comfortable, well-padded, supportive shoes that fit. Never exercise or walk in shoes that bind or rub.

- *Avoid extremes of temperature.* Minor degrees of frostbite can occur in diabetic toes without causing perceptible discomfort. Conversely, impaired ability to perceive hot temperatures can result in foot burns in overheated bath water; always test the temperature of bath water with the hand before stepping in.

- *Use extreme caution in care of the toenails.* Instead of clipping nails with clippers or scissors, which could increase the risk of injury; use an emery board instead, carefully filing nails straight across and not too short. In some cases, particularly in an elderly diabetic person, it may be wise to seek the services of a foot professional, such as a podiatrist, for regular routine toenail care. ■

Treatment In most cases, taping the toe to its largest neighbor and wearing a comfortable shoe is sufficient treatment.

Open fractures or displaced fractures of the great toe may require surgical intervention to clean the tissues or immobilize the fracture fragments with a wire or pin.

Prognosis Prognosis is excellent, although the toe may remain somewhat painful for weeks as it heals.

❖ CORNS AND CALLUSES

Symptoms and signs Thickened skin over bony prominences on the foot or toe or between the toes; mild discomfort of the area (rarely). (See page C-43.)

What is it? Corns represent thickening of the outermost layer of skin in response to external pressure over a bony prominence. Usually occurring on the surface of toes where they come into contact with hard shoes, they can also develop between the toes, where one toe exerts pressure on another. Corns on the outer surface are termed hard corns and those between the toes are called soft corns, but the distinction is fairly superficial. The two entities represent the same process, but the added moisture between toes softens corns that form there.

Poorly fitting shoes—usually styles with a pointed toe or flat toe box that leaves insufficient room for the toes in one direction or another—seem to be the primary culprit in the development of corns.

What you can do Wear properly fitted shoes with a roomier toe box (rounded and higher) to reduce the area of pressure. Donut pads, available at most grocery stores, pharmacies, and discount stores, may also offer some relief of pressure directly over the bony area. Relieve pressure points that form corns between the toes by placing soft padding (lamb's wool, mole skin, foam, or felt) between the affected toes. It is not recommended to use OTC razors or medications to shave or dissolve corns, especially if you are diabetic or have any vascular disease.

When to call the doctor If the corn persists despite the measures outlined above, consult a doctor or foot specialist.

Treatment Surgery to shave the underlying bony prominence is the definitive treatment for corns that fail to respond to conservative management.

Prognosis Prognosis is excellent with studious adherence to proper foot wear and foot care.

EIGHTEEN

Lungs and Respiratory System

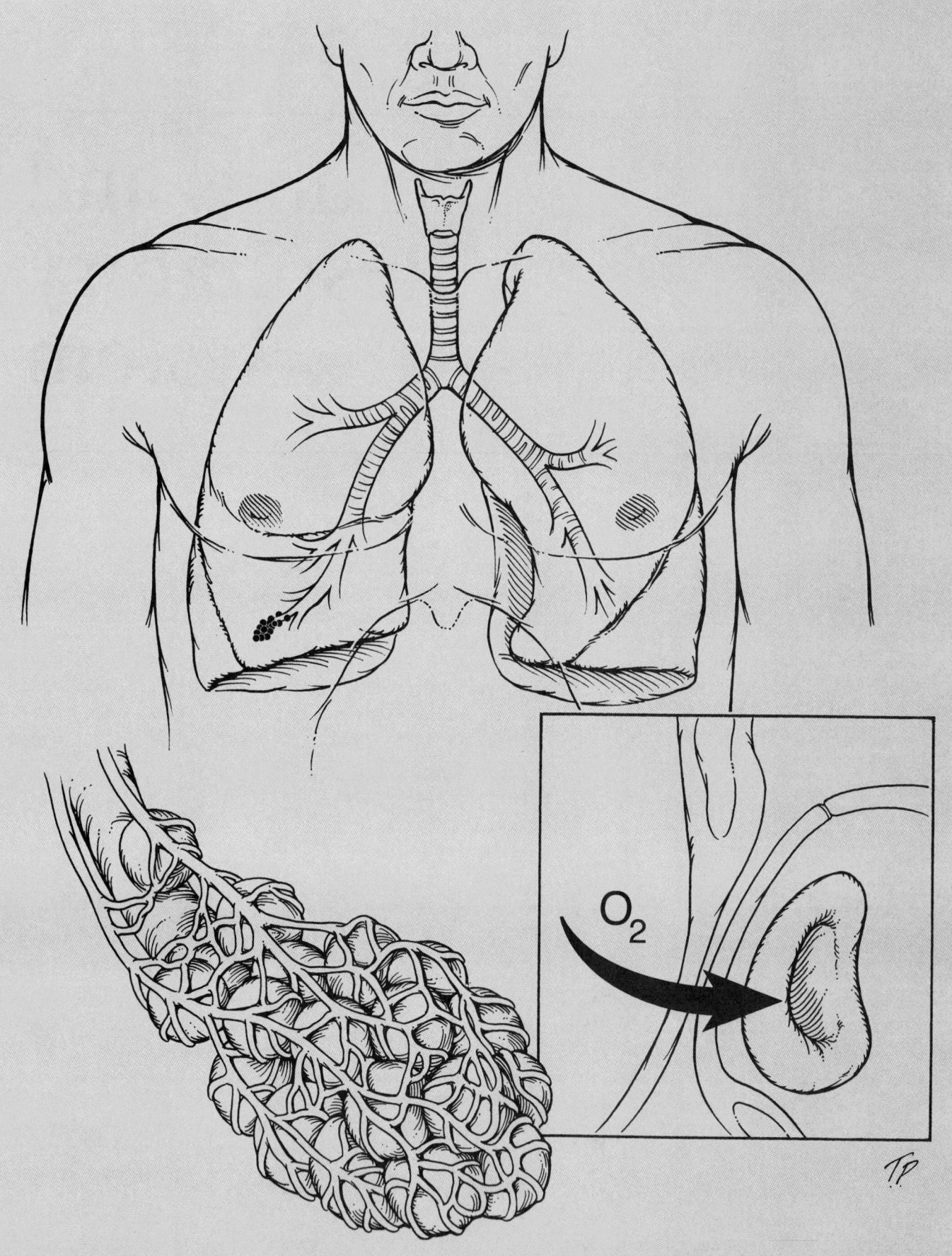

LUNGS AND RESPIRATORY SYSTEM

Understanding the Lungs and Respiratory System

Fifteen times per minute, hour after hour and day after day, the lungs expand and contract, supplying life-sustaining oxygen to red blood cells and removing from them the waste product carbon dioxide.

The act of breathing begins moments after birth. Air enters the nose, where it is warmed and filtered, and passes into the trachea (windpipe). The air molecules then come to a biological fork in the road where the trachea divides into the two bronchi that are the gateways into each of the lungs. As the molecules move deeper and deeper into the lungs, the corridors through which they pass—called bronchioles—subdivide and become progressively smaller. At the tip of each final bronchiole there is a balloon-like structure called an alveolus. This is where the exchange of oxygen for carbon dioxide occurs, and about 300 million alveoli participate.

The alveoli are served by capillaries, which are the tiniest blood vessels. As blood travels through the capillaries, the carbon dioxide it holds passes through the capillary walls and into the alveoli; conversely, oxygen that has entered the alveoli passes through the walls of these respiratory structures and into the red blood cells. The carbon dioxide picked up by the alveoli is exhaled and the oxygenated cells begin their journey to other parts of the body.

But for gas exchange to take place, air has to enter the respiratory system, and it does so through the act of inhalation. During inhalation, the diaphragm—a dome-shaped sheet of muscle that separates the chest and abdominal cavities—contracts. This creates a vacuum around the lungs, causing them to expand. At this point air from the outside rushes into the lungs due to the fact that the air pressure in the chest cavity is lower than that of the outside air. With each normal breath about a pint of air enters the lungs.

The opposite happens during exhalation. The diaphragm relaxes and the expanded lungs deflate. This pushes carbon dioxide-filled air out of the lungs. When this mechanism operates efficiently you will hardly be aware of the act of breathing.

Another component of the respiratory system is mucus. In all of the breathing passages, mucus produced by tiny glands traps impurities. But eventually the mucus and the impurities it traps must be removed. Microscopic hair-like projections called cilia move in a coordinated fashion

Bronchiole and air sac (A) with cross-sectional view (B). Air entering the lungs travels through the trachea, bronchi, and the terminal bronchiole before reaching the air sacs (alveoli). Oxygen is exchanged for carbon dioxide in the alveoli. Red blood cells absorb oxygen from air in the alveoli and transport it throughout the body.

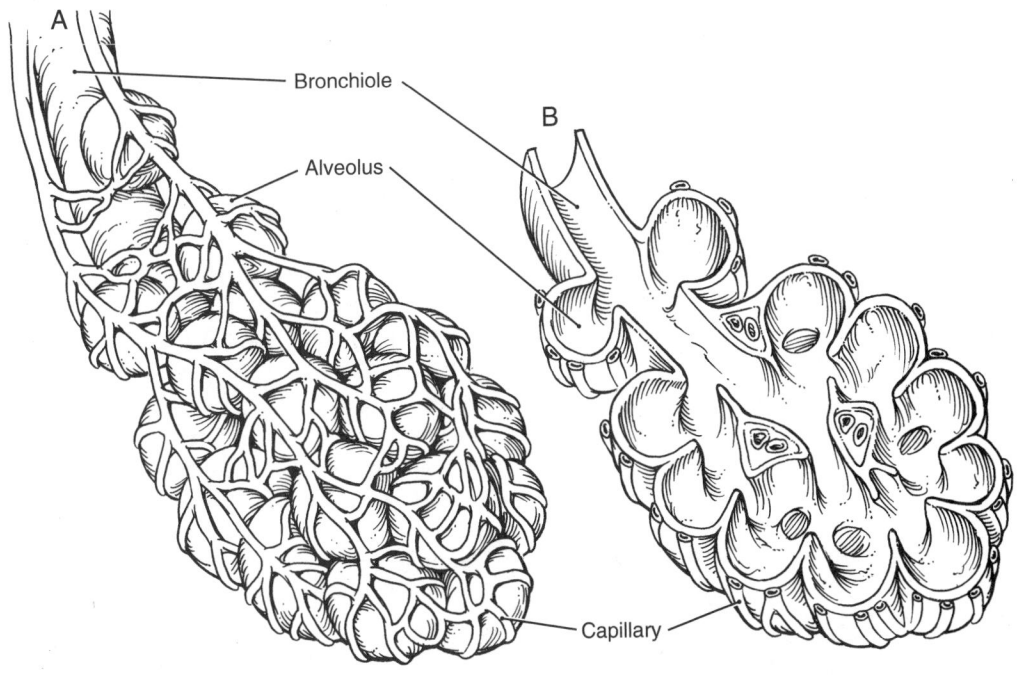

A
Bronchiole
Alveolus
B
Capillary

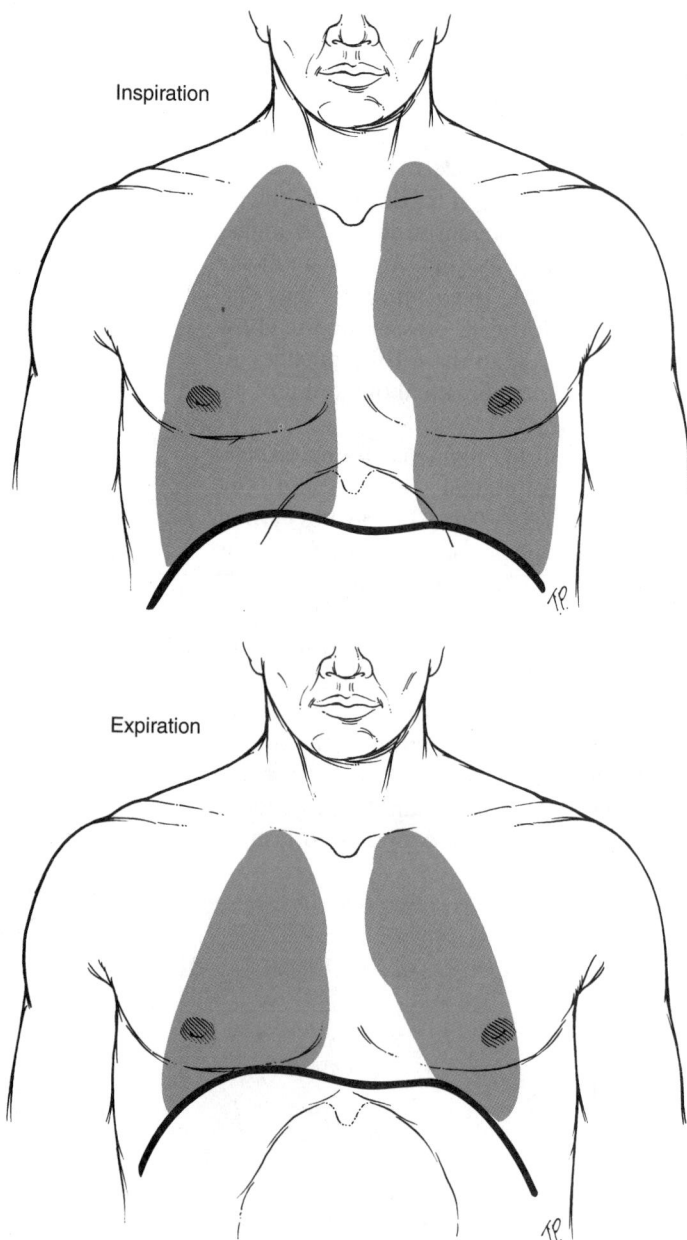

Inspiration

Expiration

The diaphragm is a muscle that separates the lungs from the abdomen. When you take a deep breath (inspiration), you create a vacuum in the chest wall from the combined effects of the flattening of the diaphragm and expansion of the chest wall. This vacuum causes air to flow into the lungs. When you breathe out (expiration) the chest wall and diaphragm relax and air passively leaves the body.

and carry the mucus from the bottom of the lungs toward the throat. Impurities are carried from the deepest recesses of the lungs up to the larger central airways where they can be coughed out or swallowed.

Some of these impurities, primarily bacteria and viruses, can cause infection and lead to illness in some cases. Certain substances can damage the cilia, enabling noxious substances to collect and fester in the lower airways.

Blood flows to the lungs via the pulmonary (pulmonary means relating to the lung) artery, which originates from the heart's right ventricle. Arteries carry blood from the heart to other parts of the body. The pulmonary artery is the only artery that carries deoxygenated blood. In the lungs the deoxygenated blood flows through an intricate network of smaller and smaller blood vessels. When blood enters the capillaries around the alveoli the red blood cells absorb oxygen and the blood releases carbon dioxide. The oxygenated blood then flows back through increasingly larger vessels, eventually reaching the pulmonary veins. Through them, oxygenated blood enters the heart's upper left chamber, the left atrium. From the left atrium blood then flows into the left ventricle, from which it is expelled through the aorta to all other parts of the body.

The soft and spongy lungs, which incompletely surround the heart, are divided into sections called lobes. The left lung has two lobes and the right lung has three. Healthy lungs are a mottled grayish pink; pollutants can cause the lungs to blacken.

The lungs reside in the chest in the upper portion of the trunk. Paired bones called ribs shield the lungs and heart and form a protective umbrella over the upper abdominal organs. But the ribs frame the lungs and do not cover them completely. Consequently the lungs are subject to penetrating wounds. In addition, blunt trauma can cause a rib to break and spear the lung under it.

A thin membranous covering called the pleura covers each lung. It folds back on itself to form a double layer. The inner layer is attached to the lung and the outer layer hangs from the ribcage. Between the layers is a small pocket that is filled with fluid. The pleurae lubricate the lungs so they can expand and contract smoothly and uniformly. If the pleurae become inflamed and roughened due to infection the movement of these layers can be impeded.

Since the lungs—along with skin and the gastrointestinal tract—are the only major organs that are exposed to the outside environment, they are vulnerable to mistreatment and are especially vulnerable to external influences, such as bacteria, fungi, viruses, and airborne irritants, such as tobacco smoke and other chemicals. It is important to provide the best possible conditions for favorable lung function—avoid tobacco smoke and other air pollutants and keep the body fit through proper nutrition and physical activity.

Evaluating the Respiratory Tree

Although your respiratory system contains safeguards to minimize the risk of disease, inflammation, and infection, they do occur. When they strike and you develop the telltale signs of a lung problem—such as coughing, wheezing, or shortness of breath—your doctor has a number of options that can be used to examine the components of the respiratory tree; some of the most commonly used methods are described below. In addition, your doctor can examine respiratory activity to see how well your respiratory system is operating (see Pulmonary Function Tests, this page, and Bronchoscopy, page 729).

CHEST X-RAY

X-rays penetrate the chest and produce black-and-white images on specially treated film. X-rays pass through healthy lung tissue with little or no change, making them appear dark on film. But unhealthy lung tissue is readily visible as a lighter area against the dark background of an x-ray picture.

A chest x-ray is most useful when compared against similar pictures that were taken at an earlier time. Such a comparison is ideal for detecting changes in lung tissue over time.

Chest x-rays can help confirm a diagnosis of pneumonia, a collapsed lung—also called atelectasis—that may be accompanied by pneumothorax (see page 755), or lung cancer. It can help the doctor determine the shape and size of a lung tumor and the extent of infiltration in and around the lung or lungs.

PULMONARY FUNCTION TESTS

Pulmonary function tests are performed to assess how much air a person can breathe in and out of the lungs. Such tests are performed on people with suspected lung problems such as emphysema (see page 756) and pulmonary fibrosis (see page 752).

Pulmonary function tests are done if someone is short of breath, to determine if a lung problem is caused by a process that blocks the airways or hinders lung expansion, to check how effective is therapy in treating a respiratory problem, or to evaluate the degree of efficiency of a person's respiratory system prior to surgery.

A device called a spirometer measures the amount of air entering and leaving the lungs.

You should eat sparingly before the tests. If you smoke, you should refrain from lighting up for 4 to 6 hours before the tests.

The tests can measure the following:

- *Functional residual capacity.* The volume of air that remains in the lungs after a normal breath. To measure this you breathe normally into a spirometer that contains an inert (inactive) gas (usually helium) in a known volume of air. After about 5 minutes the concentration of inert gas in the spirometer and in the lungs reaches equilibrium. The pulmonary function technician records the point of equilibrium and the concentration of gas that remains in the spirometer. Other methods may involve breathing 100 percent oxygen for several minutes to wash out the nitrogen in the lungs, or panting to compress the lung gas while seated in a chamber or body plethysmograph (instrument used to measure change in the volume of the body).

- *Vital capacity.* The volume of air that can be expelled from the lungs after inhaling as much air as possible. To measure it, you inhale as deeply as possible and exhale into the mouthpiece, slowly squeezing out all the air.

- *Residual volume.* The amount of air that remains in the lungs after a maximal exhalation.

- *Forced expiratory volume.* The maximum volume of air that can be expelled from the lungs in a period of time, typically 1 second. You inhale slowly and deeply and exhale as forcefully and quickly as possible.

- *Forced vital capacity.* The greatest amount of air that a person can exhale from his total lung capacity. You inhale slowly and deeply and exhale as quickly as possible.

- *Total lung capacity.* The amount of air your lungs can hold.

Results are interpreted based on a person's age, height, and gender. They usually are expressed as a percentage of the expected value.

Results may be considered abnormal if they are less than 80 percent of normal.

Diffusing capacity tests measure the ability of the lungs to exchange gases. The test is usually performed by taking a deep breath of a gas mixture that contains a small amount of carbon monoxide. After holding your breath for 10 seconds, you blow it out. The technician measures the amount of carbon monoxide that your lungs have absorbed.

Blood gases tests measure the oxygen and carbon dioxide levels in the blood and determine how much acid (pH level) is in the blood. The test is performed by taking a small sample of blood from the wrist or forearm with a needle. After the test the technician will need to apply pressure to the area for 5 minutes. If you are taking anticoagulants (blood thinners) you should tell your doctor or the technician. ∎

You may be asked to stand, sit, or lie down on a table while the x-ray picture is taken. If you are confined to a bed, a portable x-ray machine will be used.

The person taking the picture—either a nurse or a technologist—will tell you to take a deep breath and hold it for a few seconds while the x-ray picture is taken.

There are few risks involved with chest x-rays; they generally are not done if a woman is in the first trimester of pregnancy because there is a very slight risk that the radiation may induce birth defects. If it is essential that such a picture be taken, the fetus can be shielded from the x-rays by the use of a lead apron worn by the mother.

CHEST FLUOROSCOPY

In a chest x-ray, a beam of x-rays passes through the chest for only a few seconds. In chest fluoroscopy a beam of x-rays passes through the chest for about 5 minutes. This allows your doctor to see on a television screen how the lungs, heart, and diaphragm move.

This test may be performed to examine lung expansion and contraction during quiet breathing, deep breathing, and coughing; evaluate possible paralysis of the diaphragm; and detect blockages in the airways (the passages that conduct air into and out of the lungs).

You will be asked during the test to perform certain actions such as coughing. A videotape may be made of the way your respiratory system operates.

If you think that you may be pregnant you should inform your doctor before undergoing fluoroscopy. There is a small risk that prolonged x-ray exposure may be harmful to the fetus.

CHEST COMPUTED TOMOGRAPHY

Computed tomography (CT) scanning can be used to provide cross-sectional views of the interior of the chest. It achieves this by passing an x-ray beam from a computerized scanner through the body at different angles.

The data from a chest CT can be used to create a three-dimensional image of the lungs on a computer screen. This test is especially useful in detecting small differences in tissue density. For example, it can clearly show the presence of tumors or calcified or fatty deposits in lung tissue that cannot be seen on a chest x-ray.

When you have a CT scan you lie face up on a table that slides into the center of the machine, which resembles a large doughnut. You will receive directions from the doctor or technologist on breathing and movement during the 10 to 30 minutes you will be inside the device. You may hear clicking sounds while you are inside. This is the sound of the scanner as it takes pictures.

A dye, also known as a contrast medium, may be injected. This helps enhance the images. If a dye is used you will be asked to fast for 4 hours before the test. The dye may cause you to feel flushed and warm. It also may trigger a brief headache or cause you to experience a salty taste or nausea and vomiting after it is injected.

Like a chest x-ray, a CT scan exposes the subject of the scan to radiation and is rarely used during pregnancy.

PULMONARY ANGIOGRAM

This test allows your doctor to examine blood flow in the lungs. It can help detect a blocked or narrowed blood vessel or a pulmonary embolism (blood clot) in a person who has symptoms but in whom other tests are inconclusive. It also is useful in evaluating blood flow, prior to surgery, in the lungs of a person who was born with a congenital (present at birth) heart defect.

In this test, also known as pulmonary angiography, x-rays are taken after a dye is injected into the pulmonary artery or one of its branches.

The doctor or nurse will determine if you are allergic to anesthetics, dyes, shellfish, or iodine. You will need to fast for about 8 hours before the test.

As you lie on your back, a local anesthetic is injected into your upper thigh area. A heart monitor is attached so that the doctor can check constantly on your well-being during the test. After a small incision is made in your upper thigh, a small tube called a catheter is inserted into your vascular system and is slowly and carefully moved up until it is in the pulmonary artery or one of its branches.

The doctor then injects the dye. This circulates in your lungs' blood vessels while

BRONCHOSCOPY

Bronchoscopy is a diagnostic procedure that enables a doctor to directly view the larynx (speaking chamber of the throat), trachea, and airways through a fiberoptic tube called a bronchoscope. It also creates a passageway through which the doctor can insert a device to withdraw tissue specimens for analysis or foreign bodies that may block one of the air passages.

Direct visual examination of the lungs can help the doctor to diagnose lung cancer, tuberculosis (TB), interstitial lung disease, (see page 752), or a fungal lung infection.

The procedure takes between 45 and 60 minutes. You should fast for 6 to 12 hours before the test. You may receive a sedative to help you relax. If the test is not being performed under general anesthesia, a local anesthetic will be sprayed into your nose and mouth to deaden the gag reflex.

You will lie on an examining table or sit upright in a chair. You should remain still and breathe through your nose.

The doctor then inserts the flexible tube through a nostril, down through the trachea, and into the bronchial tree. The bronchoscope has four channels, two of which provide light. Of the remaining channels, one permits the doctor to see what is in front of the bronchoscope and the other channel is for the passage of medical instruments or additional medication.

After the test you will rest and be encouraged to spit out any saliva that accumulates rather than swallow it. You should not eat or drink until your gag reflex returns, which may take several hours. You may experience temporary hoarseness and a sore throat after the procedure. In addition, you may have a low-grade fever; speak to your doctor if you experience a high fever or chills. If a biopsy (removal and analysis of tissue) is taken you may cough up a small amount of blood for 1 or 2 days. If you develop a shortage of breath or chest pain after the test, it may indicate a collapsed lung and you should contact your doctor.

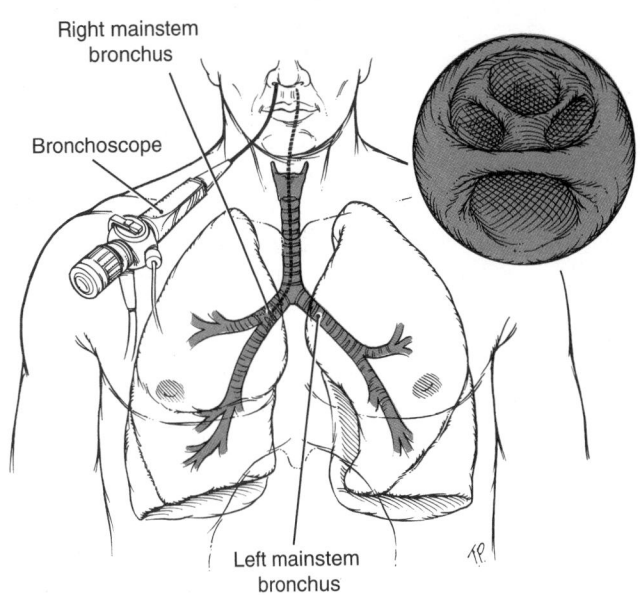

A thin fiberoptic cable attached to a camera is passed into the lungs to visualize the airways and collect tissue and mucus. Hand controls allow the operator to maneuver the tip of the bronchoscope and take specimens.

The flexible fiberoptic bronchoscope is about 5 to 7 mm in diameter, and procedures performed with it are painless and rarely lead to complications. In certain circumstances, however, your doctor may want to use a larger, rigid bronchoscope. The rigid bronchoscope is more difficult to insert and carries certain risks. It is usually employed for the removal of foreign bodies, when a laser is to be used, or when bronchoscopy is performed on children. ■

x-rays are taken. The dye may cause you to feel flushed or nauseated or to experience a salty taste for about 5 minutes following its introduction.

Afterward you will rest in bed for about 6 hours.

Possible complications from this test include tearing of the blood vessel and kidney failure from a severe reaction to the dye. The test should be used during pregnancy only when absolutely necessary.

Viral and Bacterial Infections of the Respiratory System

Several diseases can arise from viral or bacterial invasion of the lungs and other respiratory system components. They can be relatively benign, or dangerous and potentially life-threatening.

❖ VIRAL PNEUMONIA

Symptoms *(What you may experience)* Fever; dry cough; blood in the sputum (a mixture of mucus and discharges from the lungs, bronchi, and trachea); headache; muscle pain; weakness; increasing breathlessness.

Signs and laboratory findings *(What the doctor looks for)* Chest sounds suggestive of a breathing problem; the scope and extent of the infection as detected by chest x-rays; the infectious agent as identified by analysis of sputum or mucus.

What is it? Pneumonia is a general term for several kinds of lung inflammation. About half of all pneumonias are believed to be caused by viruses such as the influenza virus or cytomegalovirus. See Bacterial Pneumonia, page 733, for information on pneumonia caused by bacteria.

The influenza virus can trigger symptoms of pneumonia within hours of infection. It can cause a person's temperature to soar to 104°F or higher.

In pneumonia, the alveoli in your lungs that facilitate the exchange of oxygen for carbon dioxide fill with pus and other liquid. Consequently oxygen is not delivered to the red blood cells, which also cannot release the waste product carbon dioxide. As a result, the cells of your body do not receive the oxygen they need to function.

Until 1936, pneumonia was a leading cause of death in the United States. Even today, pneumonia and influenza combined rank as the sixth leading cause of death in this country. About 15 in 1,000 people have pneumonia each year. In healthy people under age 65, pneumonia rarely poses a serious risk. Mild pneumonia may even be confused with a stubborn cough or cold. In the elderly, however, and those whose immune systems are already weakened by some other disorder, pneumonia can pose a life-threatening risk.

Viral pneumonia never responds to antibiotics because antibiotics have no effect on viruses. Viral pneumonia may be complicated by a secondary bacterial invasion.

What you can do The most important preventive measure is to be alert to any symptoms of respiratory trouble that linger more than a few days. Good health habits—such as proper diet and hygiene, rest, and physical activity—bolster your immune system and increase your resistance to infection. They also help promote a more rapid recovery when illness strikes.

Pneumonia is a common complication of influenza, so getting a flu shot every year is good pneumonia prevention for people who are at increased risk.

When to call the doctor If you become short of breath even when lying down, if you feel pain upon breathing, or if you cough up bloodstained sputum, see your doctor as soon as possible.

Treatment There are no satisfactory medications for most types of viral pneumonia, which usually subside on their own. The best treatment may be a combination of warmth, bed rest, and cough and pain medication, as well as antibiotics to treat any secondary bacterial infection. Depending on your age, symptoms, and general medical condition, your doctor may advise hospitalization. If you are breathless you may need supplemental oxygen, which can be supplied through a face mask or a tube in your nose. In the elderly and those who are immunocompromised, careful monitoring is necessary.

Pain relievers can ease chest pain.

Prognosis Your chances for a rapid recovery are greatest if you are young, if you do not smoke, if your pneumonia is recognized early, if your defenses against disease are working well, and if you do not have any other debilitating illness.

A healthy young person should recover in about 2 to 3 weeks. A heavy smoker may take several months to recover. Following recovery you may feel fatigued for 6 to 8 weeks.

In the elderly and immunocompromised, pneumonia can cause death, sometimes within 24 hours.

❖ INFLUENZA

Symptoms *(What you may experience)* Chills; fever that may be high; muscle pain; sneezing; headache; sore throat; dry, hacking cough; chest pain.

Signs and laboratory findings *(What the doctor looks for)* Sudden appearance of symptoms; severity of symptoms. Your doctor can perform a throat culture to identify the causative agent or a blood test to look for antibodies to the virus, but this is rarely necessary since there is no specific treatment for influenza.

What is it? Influenza, commonly known as the flu, is a respiratory disease caused by the influenza virus, of which there are three types—A, B, and C. Each of the three families of influenza viruses has many different strains. The strains that make up types B and C are relatively stable; however, the ones that comprise type A change constantly. Because of this, new strains of type A influenza appear regularly and cause widespread infection. Antibodies the body can produce that are capable of defending against a previous strain are ineffective against newer strains. Strains are often named after the geographical area in which they first were identified (Hong Kong flu, for example).

About every 10 to 25 years, a strain of influenza virus appears that is dramatically different from the other members of its family. When this happens a pandemic (worldwide epidemic) almost always develops. One particularly virulent strain spread throughout the world in 1918 and caused more than 20 million deaths.

Influenza is thought to be transmitted primarily by airborne particles from an infected person's respiratory tract. During the winter, when groups of people tend to gather in close quarters indoors, the risk of transmission is particularly high.

Outbreaks of influenza tend to occur in winter and early spring when temperatures and humidity are low.

What you can do Immunization against the current strain of influenza virus (see Immunization against Influenza: the Flu Shot, this page) is the best way to prevent the flu.

Certain people are considered to be especially susceptible to influenza and should be immunized each year. Included are those with chronic lung diseases such as asthma (see page 745), tuberculosis, or cystic fibrosis (CF); heart disease; chronic kidney disease; diabetes; or anemia. In addition, anyone who resides in a nursing home or other long-term care facility or who is over age 65 should be immunized annually.

Some people may be allergic to the vaccine. Two antiviral medications—amantadine and rimantadine—may prevent type A influenza, but they must be taken daily for as long as cases of influenza are present in the community.

If you are at high risk you should avoid contact with anyone who shows symptoms of the disease.

When to call the doctor There is no specific treatment for influenza, so a healthy person with the flu should stay in bed and need not see the doctor unless shortness of breath occurs or complications such as acute sinusitis (see page 585) develop. If you are elderly or have a chronic medical condition or a weakened immune system, you should call your doctor as soon as symptoms develop.

IMMUNIZATION AGAINST INFLUENZA: THE FLU SHOT

Some people—those over age 65, residents of long-term care facilities, and people with serious illnesses such as chronic respiratory disease, cardiopulmonary disease, or kidney disease—are highly susceptible to serious complications of the flu. These people, as well as medical and nursing home personnel, should receive a flu vaccination each year.

The vaccine is administered as a single injection in the upper arm. The earlier in the flu season you get immunized the less likely you are to contract the disease. Flu season usually lasts from late fall to early spring.

The flu vaccine is developed according to the assessment of the Centers for Disease Control and Prevention (CDC) against the strain of influenza that is likely to be prevalent every year. If you get immunized there is no guarantee that you will be flu-free; however, if you do develop an illness, it very likely will be mild.

There may be some soreness at the injection site and some people develop low-grade fevers and muscle aches for 1 or 2 days. Because the vaccine uses proteins from eggs, people who are allergic to eggs should not receive the vaccine. If you are allergic to eggs and fall into one of the high-risk groups, you may want to discuss with your doctor the possibility of taking rimantadine or amantadine or a similar antiviral prescription medication during the flu season. A pregnant woman should not receive a flu shot during her first trimester.

People must be immunized every year against the flu because the virus mutates rapidly. Each year a new strain appears that is different enough from previous strains to make the previous immunization ineffective. ■

Treatment Go to bed as soon as symptoms appear and stay there until your temperature returns to normal. Take a fever-reducing medication such as aspirin or acetaminophen and drink fruit juice. Children should not be given aspirin because of the danger of Reye's syndrome (see page 463).

Antibiotics will not work against viruses. However, influenza may lead to a secondary bacterial infection. If you develop complications such as acute sinusitis, bronchitis (see Acute Bronchitis, pag e 732), or pneumonia (see Bacterial Pneumonia, page 733) following influenza your doctor may prescribe an antibiotic.

Two antiviral medications—amantadine and rimantadine—may be useful in treating strains of influenza A. These are most effective if administered as soon as possible after symptoms develop. They are most useful when given to prevent influenza in unimmunized or susceptible people such as nursing home residents and health care workers during an epidemic. A new medication class called neuraminidase inhibitors is effective for both influenza A and B and is expected to be available in 1999 or soon thereafter.

Prognosis In most people the illness is not especially serious and should run its course in about a week. You may feel tired and weak for another week after that.

If a complication such as bacterial pneumonia develops, hospitalization may become necessary.

❖ RESPIRATORY SYNCYTIAL VIRUS

Symptoms *(What you may experience)* Runny nose; low-grade fever; decreased appetite; cough, sometimes with wheezing; lethargy; earache.

Signs and laboratory findings *(What the doctor looks for)* Development of abnormal lung sounds; antibodies to the virus as revealed by laboratory analysis of blood and respiratory secretions.

What is it? Respiratory syncytial virus (RSV) is a contagious virus that infects the lungs and breathing passages. It is a major cause of respiratory illness in people of all ages but young children are at increased risk. In children more than 3 years old and in adults, the virus causes symptoms of a simple upper respiratory tract illness or common cold. But in children less than 3 years old, the virus can affect the lower respiratory tract, causing an illness like pneumonia or bronchiolitis (inflammation of the bronchioles). In such cases, it may lead to respiratory failure.

Epidemics of RSV are common in late fall to early spring and easily spread through households, daycare centers, and schools. Symptoms usually develop within 4 to 6 days after exposure to the virus. Infection usually lasts 7 to 14 days but some cases may last up to 3 weeks. The person still may be contagious for up to a week after symptoms pass.

The highest rates of illness occur in infants 2 to 6 months old.

What you can do No vaccine exists to prevent development of the disease. Since the virus spreads via fluids from the nose and throat of an infected person, it is best to wash your hands after touching someone who has a cold or a known RSV infection. Do not touch your eyes or nose after contact with an RSV-infected person since the virus could enter your body through either portal. In general, it is a good idea to wash your hands frequently during late fall to early spring.

When to call the doctor If you suspect your child has RSV infection, consult your doctor. Call especially if your child has any of these symptoms: a fever over 101°F accompanied by a thick nasal discharge that is yellow, green, or gray; a cough that lasts more than 4 days; difficulty breathing or very rapid breathing; blue lips or nailbeds; or reduced alertness.

Treatment Younger children with RSV pneumonia or bronchiolitis may need to be treated in a hospital where they can be closely monitored and receive oxygen therapy.

Home treatment includes bed rest and plenty of water and fruit juices to drink; use a humidifier, nebulizer, or vaporizer to keep air moist. Remember to clean the device daily so it does not get contaminated with molds.

Prognosis Mild cases usually resolve within 1 to 2 weeks. Children hospitalized with lower respiratory tract infections may spend 5 to 7 days in the hospital.

❖ ACUTE BRONCHITIS

Symptoms *(What you may experience)* Deep cough that brings up gray or yellow phlegm or mucus from your lungs; breathlessness; wheezing; fever; upper chest pain that becomes more severe with coughing.

Signs and laboratory findings *(What the doctor looks for)* Wheezing detected while listening to breathing with a stethoscope; chest x-ray results; bacterial infection as revealed by sputum culture.

What is it? Acute bronchitis is an inflammation of the trachea and the bronchi, which are the main airways of the lungs. It usually results from infection by a virus such as influenza, respiratory syncytial virus, or a member of the family of rhinoviruses responsible for the common cold.

Almost everyone occasionally experiences a case of acute bronchitis. If you do not smoke and you are otherwise healthy you may experience it infrequently. But if you smoke, have a chronic breathing problem such as asthma, or live in a region that has a high degree of air pollution, you may develop it regularly. If your lungs are chronically congested due to heart failure, you also may be more susceptible.

What you can do If you smoke, stop. Avoid cold and damp living or working conditions, which may increase the possibility of developing acute bronchitis.

When to call the doctor If you become breathless, cough up blood, or have a temperature higher than 101°F, contact your doctor. You also should contact your doctor if you have repeated attacks of acute bronchitis.

Treatment There is no specific medical treatment for the viral infection but it is possible to treat the symptoms. Breathing in warm, moist air—using a vaporizer, humidifier, or steam—can temporarily help clear your airways. Bed rest, plenty of liquids, and use of aspirin or another over-the-counter (OTC) remedy to reduce the fever may bring relief and speed recovery. An OTC cough medication can help reduce symptoms; look for products labeled "expectorant," which can help to create a productive (producing sputum or mucus) cough and to clear the lungs. Avoid cough suppressants such as dextromethorphan if you have a productive cough.

Your doctor may prescribe an inhaled bronchodilator medication (a medication used to temporarily open the airways) to help reduce the wheezing. Greenish-yellow

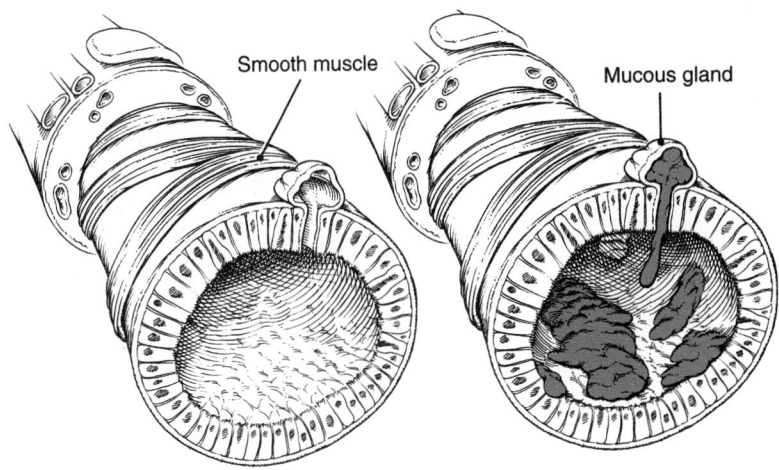

Smooth muscle

Mucous gland

Bronchitis is the result of inflammation of the bronchi, the airways between the trachea (windpipe) and the alveoli. The most typical symptom is a cough that is productive of thick phlegm. Narrowing of the airways due to mucus and inflammation is common but shortness of breath and fever are rare. A productive cough that is accompanied by fever or shortness of breath could be from pneumonia and should prompt a visit to the doctor.

sputum may indicate a secondary bacterial infection that may require antibiotics.

Prognosis Acute bronchitis usually runs its course in a few days. Regular bouts of the disease may be a sign of chronic bronchitis, which is a persistent, worsening inflammation (see Chronic Bronchitis, page 759).

❖ BACTERIAL PNEUMONIA

Symptoms *(What you may experience)* Gradual or sudden onset of symptoms; fever as high as 105°F; cough that produces rust-colored or greenish mucus; chest pain; profuse sweating; increased respiratory and pulse rate; confused or delirious mental state.

Signs and laboratory findings *(What the doctor looks for)* Sounds in your chest suggestive of a breathing problem; the scope and extent of the infection as revealed by chest x-rays; an infectious agent as identified by analysis of sputum or mucus.

What is it? Pneumonia is a general term for several kinds of inflammation of the lungs. About half of all pneumonias are believed to be caused by bacteria.

PNEUMONIA VACCINE: WHO SHOULD RECEIVE IT?

The major types of pneumonia are bacterial pneumonia, viral pneumonia, and mycoplasma pneumonia. Other pneumonias may be caused by *Pneumocystis carinii*, an opportunistic organism that takes advantage of the body's lowered defenses in people with depressed immune systems, such as those with acquired immunodeficiency syndrome (AIDS). Pneumonia also may be due to fungal infections or the inhalation of food, liquid, gases, or dust.

Only pneumonia caused by pneumococcal bacteria can be prevented with a vaccine. This vaccine usually is administered once; children are vaccinated at age 2 and may be revaccinated after 3 to 5 years if they have chronic kidney disease or sickle cell anemia and if they are less than 11 years old at the time of revaccination. Everyone over age 65 also should be immunized. The vaccination does not offer lifelong protection; those under age 66 should be revaccinated every 5 years.

Others who should receive the vaccine are people with diabetes; people with cirrhosis of the liver, congestive heart failure, or chronic pulmonary disease such as emphysema; people who have had their spleens removed; and those who have had organ transplants and take medications to suppress their immune system.

Some people experience minor, short-lived side effects from the shot. In studies, about half of those getting the vaccine experienced swelling and soreness at the site of injection. Less than 1 percent had fever and muscle pain as well as more serious swelling and pain at the site of administration.

The pneumonia vaccine cannot cause pneumonia because it is made from an extract that is not infectious. ∎

ADULT RESPIRATORY DISTRESS SYNDROME

ARDS is a form of pulmonary edema in which fluid accumulates in spaces in the small airways and in the alveoli. The fluid accumulation causes the lungs to stiffen, preventing them from fully expanding. Consequently it becomes difficult to draw a deep breath and the person feels starved for air.

Some causes of ARDS include inhaling stomach contents; sepsis (a systemic infection commonly known as blood poisoning); shock; pneumonia; drug overdose; inhalation of toxic gases; and near-drowning.

ARDS often is associated with the malfunction of other organs due to an inability to absorb oxygen, and the disorders that cause the lung damage. It is a progressive lung problem that develops rapidly. In nearly half of all cases, onset of the condition occurs within 24 hours of the original illness or injury. In nearly all cases it occurs within 3 days.

ARDS produces rapid, shallow breathing and shortness of breath within hours to days of the initial injury. Because less oxygen is being absorbed by red blood cells, there is an increased drive to breathe. Advanced symptoms include mental confusion, weakness, and increased heart rate.

ARDS has a fatality rate of about 50 percent despite assisted-breathing therapy. Treatment consists of mechanical ventilation and removal of the accumulated fluid. These are combined with continuing treatment of the precipitating illness or injury.

Severe ARDS can be fatal. People who recover may have little or no permanent lung damage. ∎

LEGIONNAIRE'S DISEASE

The first identified outbreak of Legionnaire's disease occurred in 1976 in Philadelphia at the Pennsylvania state convention of the American Legion. More than 180 people were affected and 29 of them died. Later studies showed that outbreaks of Legionnaire's disease actually occurred as early as the late 1940s.

Some of its symptoms are similar to those of many other respiratory disorders. They include high fever, a nonproductive (dry) cough, chills, shortness of breath, chest pain, excessive sweating, and headache. Other symptoms include diarrhea, nausea, vomiting, and abdominal pain. Legionnaire's disease may be mistaken for influenza.

The disease is caused by a bacterium that was unknown until the 1976 outbreak. It now bears the name *Legionella pneumophila* and lives principally in water from reservoirs and cooling units of air conditioning systems. Transmission occurs when people inhale contaminated water droplets.

People who smoke cigarettes, the elderly, and people with depressed immune systems—people with AIDS or recipients of organ transplants—are the most likely candidates to develop Legionnaire's disease. People with other chronic diseases also may be at higher risk.

Diagnosis of Legionnaire's disease is based on a person's medical history and physical examination, chest x-rays, and analyses of blood and sputum that show antibodies to the bacteria. If an antibiotic—usually erythromycin—is given early during the course of the disease, the long-term outlook for healthy young people is excellent. However, in people whose immune system is depressed for any reason, the mortality (death rate), even with correct treatment, is 15 to 25 percent.

There is no vaccine for Legionnaire's disease. ∎

In pneumonia, the alveoli in your lungs that facilitate the exchange of oxygen for carbon dioxide fill with pus and other liquid. Consequently oxygen is not delivered to your red blood cells, which also cannot release the waste product carbon dioxide. As a result, the cells of your body do not receive the oxygen they need to function.

A number of bacteria can cause the infection. These include *Streptococcus pneumoniae* (also called pneumococcus), *Haemophilus influenzae, Staphylococcus aureus, Klebsiella pneumoniae, Escherichia coli,* and *Pseudomonas aeruginosa.*

Some cases of pneumonia are caused by the bacterium *Legionella pneumophila.* These pneumonias are often severe and require treatment with high doses of erythromycin. (see Legionnaire's Disease, page 734).

Because pneumonia is a common cause of illness in people whose natural immunity has been compromised, some of these organisms are responsible for what

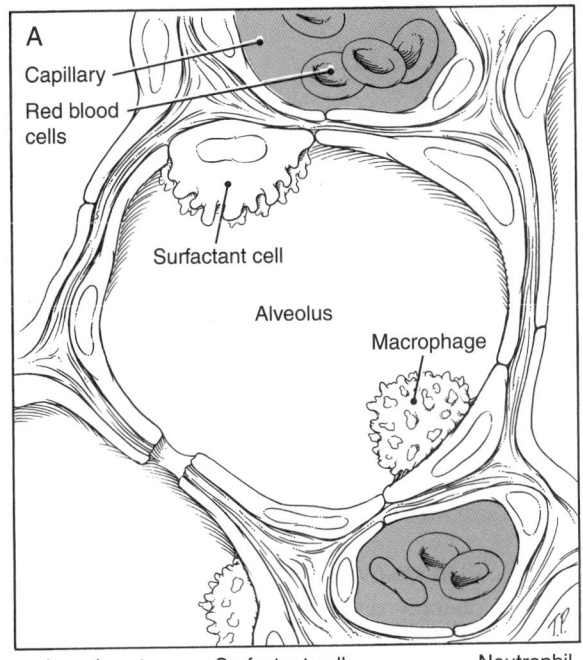

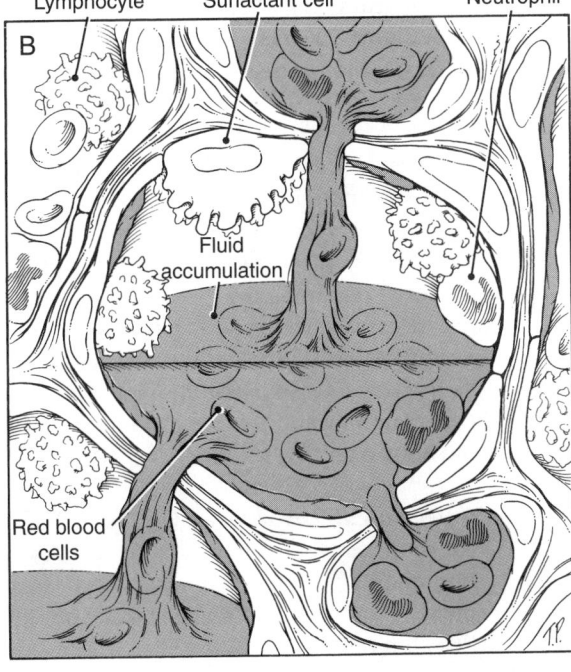

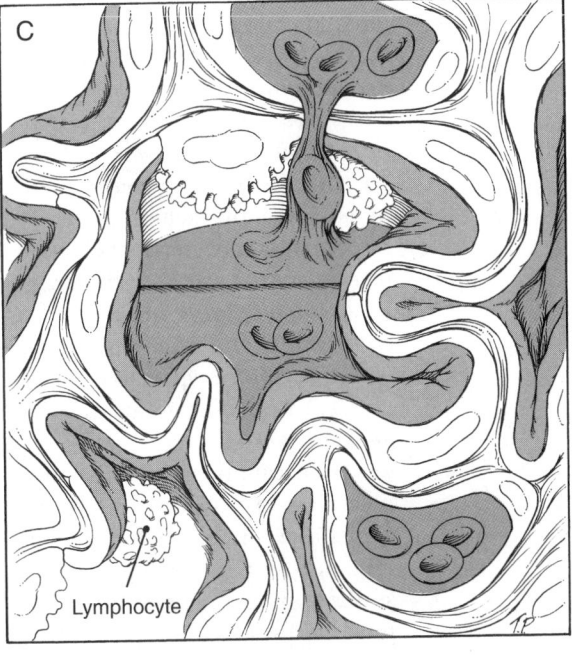

Normal lung cells (A) contain a space for the exchange of oxygen and carbon dioxide (alveolus). Alveoli are lined with two types of cells: Thicker surfactant cells secrete a slippery substance that prevents the lungs from collapsing; oxygen passes through thinner cells in the alveoli into red blood cells in the capillaries. Macrophages engulf foreign particles and infectious agents. Infection of the alveoli is seen in pneumonia (B). Neutrophils and lymphocytes attack the offending organism, which leads to inflammation. Fluid and cells accumulate in the alveoli, often causing shortness of breath. Extensive infection in the lungs can lead to damage of the alveolar walls, leading to leakage of fluid into the alveoli, a condition known as adult respiratory distress syndrome (ARDS). Accumulation of fluid prevents the alveoli from expanding, resulting in severe shortness of breath (C).

COLLAPSED LUNG

Atelectasis is the term used to describe a slow or sudden collapse of a segment of or an entire lung. It occurs when clusters of alveoli collapse or fill with fluid.

The condition often results from occlusion (obstruction) of the airways usually by a plug of mucus. It frequently is seen in people who have chronic obstructive pulmonary disease (COPD) or cystic fibrosis (CF) (see page 752). Individuals who smoke heavily also may be at risk for collapsed lung (smoking increases mucus production and damages the cilia).

Collapsed lung also may be the result of a tumor or inhalation of a foreign body that clogs an airway.

Any condition that makes deep breathing painful or difficult may cause collapsed lung. It also may result from prolonged immobility. Deep breathing exercises and walking as soon as possible after surgery may help prevent collapsed lung.

Prognosis depends on the prompt removal of any airway obstruction and re-expansion of the collapsed lung.

If a small amount of the lung is affected, a chest x-ray will show horizontal lines in the lower portion of the lung. If a segment of the lung is affected, the x-ray will show dense shadows. Shortness of breath may be present.

Treatment consists of removing the cause of the obstruction. Postural drainage, chest percussion (see Postural Drainage and Chest Percussion, page 753), frequent coughing, deep breathing exercises, and medications to thin mucous secretions can help. Sometimes a device called an incentive spirometer is used to encourage deep breathing in order to prevent or treat collapsed lung. If a tumor is the cause of the blockage, it may be

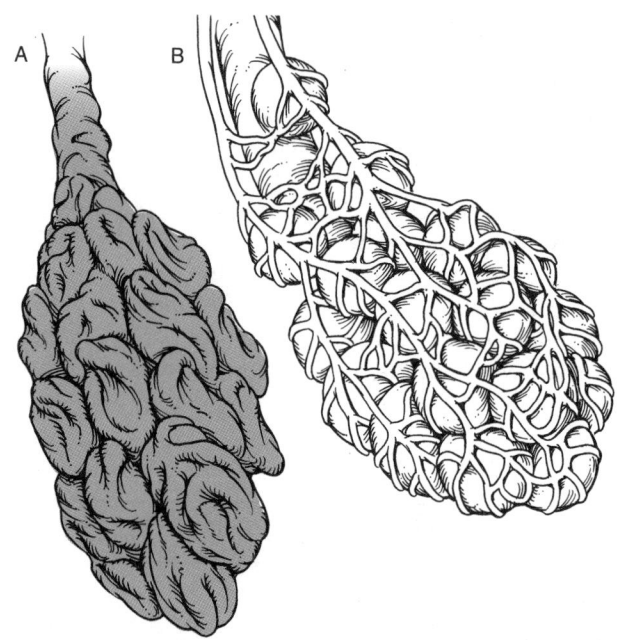

Collapse of a section of lung can occur when an air tube (bronchus) becomes obstructed (A). Compared to a normal air sac (B), the air sacs collapse because all of the oxygen is absorbed and no more air can enter the area. Since this process typically affects only a small portion of the lung it is usually not dangerous.

removed by surgical means or radiation may be employed to shrink it. If only a small part of the lung is affected the problem may resolve on its own. ■

doctors refer to as nosocomial (hospital-based) infections. A hospital-acquired pneumonia generally occurs more than 48 hours after admission. It is the second most common cause of hospital-acquired infection. Organisms commonly involved in this type of bacterial pneumonia are *Pseudomonas aeruginosa, Staphylococcus aureus, Enterobacter, Klebsiella pneumoniae,* and *Escherichia coli.*

Other forms of pneumonia are referred to as community-acquired pneumonia. The most common bacteria involved in this type of pneumonia are *Streptococcus pneumoniae, Haemophilus influenzae, Moraxella catarrhalis,* and *Klebsiella pneumoniae.* Other bacteria responsible for some community-based pneumonias are *Chlamydia* and *Mycoplasma.*

Bacterial pneumonia can attack anyone regardless of age. People who suffer from alcoholism, people with compromised immune systems, people weakened by surgery, and people with other chronic respiratory diseases are at greatest risk.

Pneumonia can lead to adult respiratory distress syndrome (ARDS). This is characterized by fluid accumulation in the small airways and alveoli that prevents the lungs from fully expanding (see Adult Respiratory Distress Syndrome, page 734). It also can cause collapsed lung (see above).

What you can do A vaccine is available against pneumococcal pneumonia (see Pneumonia Vaccine—Who Should Receive It?, page 734, the most common cause of bacterial pneumonia.

Because pneumonia may occur as a complication of the flu, getting a flu shot every year is good pneumonia prevention (see Immunization against Influenza: The Flu Shot, page 731).

When to call the doctor Call your doctor as soon as you recognize symptoms of pneumonia. Early diagnosis and treatment is important; neglect can be life-threatening.

Treatment Many antibiotic medications are available to destroy the bacteria responsible for this type of infection. Supportive measures may include the delivery of humidified oxygen, assisted mechanical ventilation, bed rest, and a pain reliever for chest pain. Hospitalization may be required.

Prognosis Your chances for a rapid recovery are greatest if you are young, if you do not smoke, if your pneumonia is recognized early, if your defenses against disease are working well, and if you do not have any other debilitating illness.

A healthy young person should recover in about 2 to 3 weeks. A heavy smoker may take several months to recover. Following recovery you may feel fatigued for several weeks.

❖ LUNG ABSCESS

Symptoms *(What you may experience)* Cough that may produce blood-tinged or foul-smelling sputum; chest pain on breathing; shortness of breath; sweating, chills, and fever; headache; loss of appetite and weight loss.

Signs and laboratory findings *(What the doctor looks for)* Development of symptoms over several days; diminished sounds of breathing on examination with a stethoscope; area of infection as revealed by a chest x-ray; the organism responsible for infection as identified by analysis of sputum.

What is it? A lung abscess is a contained infected area in the lung that has filled with pus. It may be a complication of pneumonia or it could occur as a result of infectious material being inhaled into the lungs. The material may simply be food or part of a tooth, but if it carries bacteria into the lungs, it could lead to an infection. Such material could be inhaled while you are under anesthesia or while you are unconscious as a result of a head injury or intoxication. Periodontal disease (gum disease) increases the number of bacteria in material that could be inhaled, so it is associated with a greater risk of a lung abscess.

Occasionally a lung abscess also will accompany tuberculosis or infection with parasites or fungi. An abscess also may develop if a tumor blocks one of the airways.

Treatment If the abscess is the result of a bacterial infection, your doctor will treat it with the appropriate antibiotic. If the lung abscess accompanies a fungal infection or tuberculosis, specific medication will be used to treat it.

In some cases it is useful to drain the abscess so the pus can be coughed out. The best body position for doing this depends upon the location of the abscess.

Surgery to drain the abscess may be necessary if it has expanded into the space between the pleural membranes. Sometimes bronchoscopy may be performed to see if the airway is blocked (see Bronchoscopy, page 729).

Prognosis Early treatment with the proper medication improves the prospect for recovery.

Many persons who develop a lung abscess have a chronic illness that predisposes them to develop the abscess. Overall prognosis depends on the type and severity of the underlying illness.

❖ TUBERCULOSIS

Symptoms *(What you may experience)* Cough that brings up blood and pus-filled phlegm; persistent dry cough; fatigue; weakness; weight loss; low-grade fever; chills; night sweats.

Signs and laboratory findings *(What the doctor looks for)* Sounds in the lungs characteristic of a breathing problem as detected by a stethoscope; dullness over the affected area as detected by percussion (tapping) of the chest over the lungs, indicating a collection of fluid; lesions or patchy areas in the lungs as revealed by chest x-rays; the specific agent that causes tuberculosis as identified by the tuberculin skin test or sputum analysis (see Tuberculin Skin Test, page 739).

What is it? Tuberculosis (TB) is a contagious disease that usually attacks the lungs. The bacteria that cause TB, *Mycobacterium tuberculosis*, enter the air when an infected person coughs; other people may then inhale the bacteria. After being inhaled, the bacteria replicate locally and then spread through the body via the blood and lymphatic systems. In about 15 percent of people with active TB, disease caused by TB occurs outside the lungs in parts of the body such as the kidneys and in bone.

Worldwide, TB is a major cause of death, taking 3 million lives each year. About 95 percent of these occur in developing countries. Before the 1940s, when doctors discovered the first of several medications now used to treat the disease, TB was a major health problem in the United States. TB has made a comeback in North America due to the emergence of bacteria that are resistant to one or more of the medications used to treat it, the influx of infected immigrants from developing nations, and the AIDS epidemic with its impact on the immune system, which allows contained TB infections to become reactivated. More than 25,000 cases were reported in this country in 1993.

But infection with the organism does not mean you will actually develop the disease. In 95 percent of those who become infected, a competent immune system will contain the disease. The other 5 percent will develop either a localized or widespread systemic form of the disease. Of those whose immune systems contain the disease, however, 5 percent may develop reactivation disease at some time during their lives. Experts believe that about 10 million Americans are infected but that only about 10 percent will actually become ill. Only people who develop the disease can transmit it.

TB is an equal-opportunity disease, but there are groups of people who have a higher-than-normal risk of contracting it. Included are people whose immune systems are compromised by a disease such as AIDS or diabetes; who are in close physical contact with others known to be infected with TB; who were born in countries with high rates of TB; who are underfed and malnourished; and who abuse alcohol and other substances.

People who are infected usually do not develop the disease for several years. Sometimes TB develops within weeks of infection.

What you can do Avoid contact with people infected with TB. In most cases, extensive exposure is required to become infected. Coughing and sneezing into a tissue can reduce the spread of the disease.

If you are infected with TB but have not yet developed the disease, your doctor may recommend that you take a medication to keep the disease from becoming symptomatic. The medication used in this preventive therapy is called isoniazid, and it kills the TB bacteria that are already in the body. Most people must take the drug for at least 6 months. Children and people infected with human immunodeficiency virus (HIV)—the virus responsible for AIDS—need to take it for a longer period of time. It is essential that you complete the full course of treatment. Partial treatment does not reliably eradicate the organism that causes the disease and makes it more likely that you will develop an antibiotic-resistant form of it.

Because it can cause hepatitis, isoniazid is not appropriate for everyone who has tested positive for TB infection. Your doctor can advise you whether the therapy is advisable in your case.

Preventive therapy sometimes is instituted in people whose infection with TB is questionable. These include people known to be HIV-positive and infants and children who have recently been in close contact with someone with infectious TB.

Vaccines exist and are safe but little is known as to their actual effectiveness. A vaccine is of no value in someone who already is infected.

When to call the doctor If you recently have been in close contact with a person with active TB or if you recently have come from a country in which the disease is common, contact your doctor. If you are a member of a high-risk group your doctor may want to screen you for the disease as a precautionary measure (see Tuberculin Skin Test, page 739).

Treatment The TB bacteria almost always can be killed with medication. The most common drugs used to fight TB are isoniazid, rifampin, pyrazinamide, ethambutol, and streptomycin. Because of the increasing occurrence of antibiotic-resistant organisms, you need to take more than one drug to kill all the bacteria.

For the first 2 weeks that you are taking the medication you will be able to infect others, so you should isolate yourself as much as possible during that time. Afterward, although you are still taking medication, you should no longer be a danger to others.

TUBERCULIN SKIN TEST

To prevent the spread of TB, some states require that children be screened for the disease before entering school. In addition, adults should get tested for TB if any of the following conditions apply:

- You have been in contact with someone who has TB.

- You are infected with HIV or have another condition that weakens your immune system, increasing your risk for contracting TB.

- You are from a country in which TB is very common—for example, most countries in Latin America and the Caribbean, Africa, and Asia (except Japan).

- You use intravenous street drugs.

- You live or work in a high-risk area for TB—for example, migrant farm camps, prisons and jails, nursing homes, and homeless shelters.

The tuberculin skin test—also called the Mantoux PPD (purified protein derivative) test—is a skin test administered at the doctor's office that helps detect TB and distinguish it from other diseases with similar symptoms. In the test, a small amount of PPD tuberculin, which is extracted from dead TB bacteria, is injected via a small needle just under the top layer of skin on the upper forearm. You will be asked to check for a reaction 2 to 3 days later. If you have been infected with *Mycobacterium tuberculosis* a reaction will be evident around the site of the injection. Should any reaction appear, it should be interpreted by a lab technician, nurse, or doctor.

A positive reaction to the test is the appearance of a red, raised, hard area at the injection site. A positive reaction does not necessarily mean that you have an active case of TB. It indicates that the TB bacteria are in your body.

Another cause of a positive reaction to the test is having had a TB vaccination called BCG. This vaccine is not widely used in the United States, but it is often given to infants and children in countries in which the disease is common. But BCG does not always confer protection against TB. A positive reaction to the tuberculin skin test may occur due to the presence of an active TB infection that developed despite a previous vaccination. The BCG reaction weakens over time, so if you were vaccinated many years ago your level of protection may be very low.

On the other hand, a negative result does not necessarily mean you have not been infected with the TB bacteria. You may have been tested too soon after breathing in the bacteria. It takes several weeks after you have been infected for your body to react to the skin test. Because of this, sometimes the test will have to be repeated in about 3 months.

The tuberculin skin test should not be done in people who have had reactions to smallpox vaccinations or who currently have a skin rash or a known case of active TB. ■

Although symptoms of the disease may disappear after several weeks of treatment, you must complete the full course of treatment to be reliably cured. The organism that causes TB goes through prolonged periods of dormancy; antitubercular medications are effective only on actively growing organisms. If medical therapy is to be effective, it must be prolonged. Because it is easy to forget to take TB medication, many communities provide directly observed therapy, a system for giving the medication under the supervision of a nurse or other health care professional.

Antituberculosis medications may cause side effects including nausea and vomiting; yellowish skin or eyes; fever for 3 or more days; abdominal pain; aching joints; dizziness; tingling or numbness around the mouth; easy bruising or bleeding; blurred vision; and ringing in the ears. If you have a serious side effect, call your doctor immediately.

Other more minor side effects are orange urine, saliva, or tears; increased sensitivity to the sun; and interference with chemical means of birth control and some drugs for diabetes, heart, or lung diseases (including theophylline, quinidine, and dilantin).

Prognosis Medical treatment can completely eradicate the disease in many cases. However about half of the people whose disease is caused by bacteria resistant to 2 or more of the antitubercular medications will die. If TB that is resistant to more than one medication infects a person with AIDS, the TB infection is 100 percent lethal.

❖ PLEURISY

Symptoms (*What you may experience*) Pain when breathing deeply; severe, sharp, one-sided chest pain; breathlessness; dry, painful cough.

Signs and laboratory findings (*What the doctor looks for*) Characteristic sounds made by irritated pleurae that are detectable with a stethoscope.

What is it? Pleurisy is a painful disorder in which the pleurae become inflamed.

Under normal conditions the layers of each pleura are wrapped around each lung with a thin lubricating layer of fluid between the two sheets. But infection can cause the pleura to become inflamed or roughened. This can restrict lung movement and cause pain when the lungs expand with breathing, irritating the sensory nerve endings in the pleurae.

Pleurisy can develop as a complication of lung infections such as pneumonia and TB or of the autoimmune disease systemic lupus erythematosus. Pleurisy may also be a symptom of a pulmonary embolism (see page 760).

What you can do Once the condition is diagnosed, you should get as much uninterrupted bed rest as possible.

If you have been prescribed a narcotic medication to reduce pain, avoid overuse because it may lower your ability to cough. To minimize pain when coughing, apply pressure with your hands at the site of pain or hold a pillow across the front of your chest.

Treatment Your doctor will prescribe anti-inflammatory agents to deal with the pleural irritation, but the only way to cure the condition is to treat the underlying disease. If the underlying condition is pneumonia or TB, this would necessitate the use of antibiotics or antitubercular therapy.

Prognosis If treated promptly with anti-inflammatory medications and if any underlying lung infection is treated with the appropriate agents, prognosis is excellent.

❖ EMPYEMA

Symptoms *(What you may experience)* Shortness of breath; dry cough; fever; chest pain on breathing.

Signs and laboratory findings *(What the doctor looks for)* Fluid buildup in the space between the two sheets of the pleural membrane as detected by x-rays; infection as detected by analysis of fluid removed from pleural cavity.

What is it? Empyema is the presence of pus that has accumulated in the space between the two layers of the pleural membrane.

Normally a small amount of fluid lubricates the pleurae, enhancing their ability to move and allow the lungs to expand with breathing. In pleural effusion (see page 740), excess fluid accumulates, inhibiting lung motion and expansion. In empyema, an infection is present, causing the fluid in the pleural space to thicken into pus.

Empyema may occur as a complication of bacterial pneumonia (see page 733) or lung abscess (see page 737) but it is uncommon since the development of antibiotics.

When to call the doctor If you develop pain on deep breathing that goes away and is replaced by breathlessness and fever, consult your doctor. Early diagnosis and treatment of empyema can prevent it from becoming a chronic problem.

Treatment Your doctor will drain the infected fluid by means of a needle and syringe inserted through the chest wall in a procedure called thoracentesis. A regimen of antibiotics will be prescribed to treat the infection. If the empyema is small and caught early, repeated thoracenteses may be sufficient to drain the fluid. But in most cases it will be necessary to perform a thoracostomy using local anesthesia. In this procedure a tube is inserted through a small incision in the chest to allow the thick fluid to drain. Sometimes a thoracotomy (opening of the chest wall) may be necessary to directly remove a section of the pleura that has become thickened and is restricting motion of the lung. The surgery is performed under general anesthesia and will speed recovery from the infection.

Prognosis Prospects for a full recovery depend on the nature of the underlying disorder and how advanced it is at the time of initial treatment.

❖ PLEURAL EFFUSION

Symptoms *(What you may experience)* Shortness of breath; dry cough; fever; sharp chest pain while breathing.

Signs and laboratory findings *(What the doctor looks for)* Sounds of diminished breathing as detected by a stethoscope; fluid accumulation around the lung as shown by chest x-rays; infection as detected by analysis of fluid taken from the area around the lung.

Air entering the space that surrounds the lung (pleural sac) collapses the lung (A). This condition, called pneumothorax, may be due to lung disease, although it usually occurs in younger persons without any apparent cause. Patients often notice chest pain and shortness of breath. A small pneumothorax usually needs no treatment, but a large collapse may require a tube placed in the chest wall to remove the air and expand the lung. Fluid in the pleural sac is called a pleural effusion (B). Common causes of pleural effusion include infection, congestive heart failure, and tumors. Some effusions are small and resolve on their own while others need to be removed to examine the fluid and alleviate any shortness of breath.

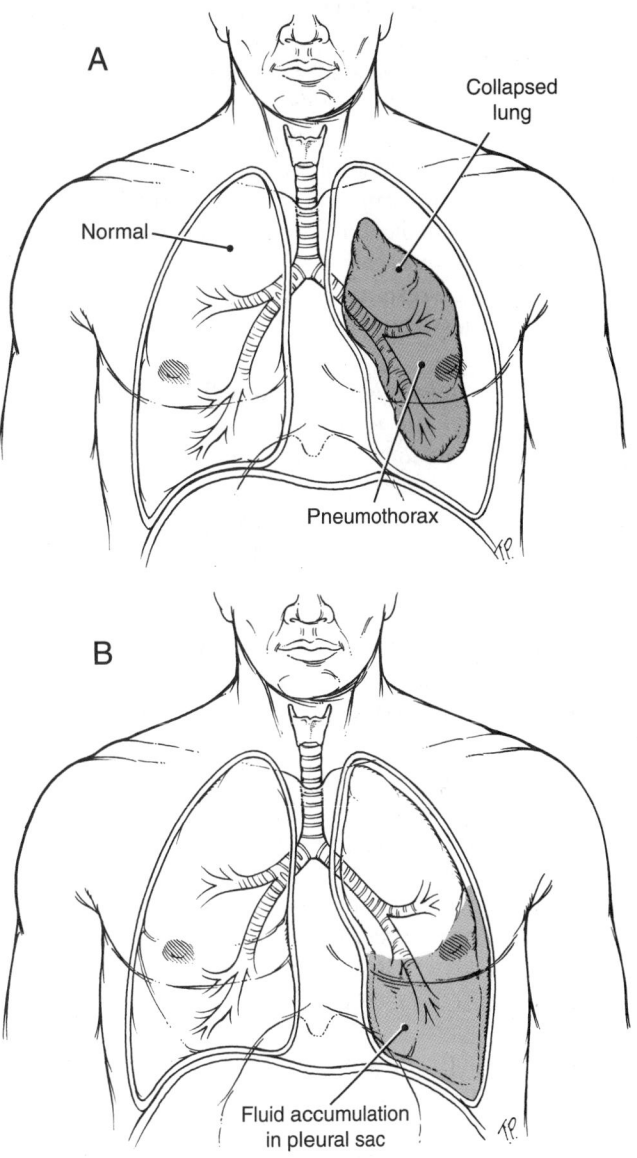

What is it? Pleural effusion is a buildup of excess watery fluid in the space between the pleura that surrounds the lungs. Normally a small amount of fluid lubricates the pleura. An excessive amount of fluid inhibits the lung from completely expanding during breathing and results in breathlessness.

Pleural effusion can occur as a complication of TB, lung abscess, pancreatitis, bacterial or fungal lung infection, congestive heart failure, pulmonary embolism, injury to the chest, cancer, and autoimmune disorders such as systemic lupus erythematosus.

What you can do Seek medical attention if a sense of breathlessness has replaced severe chest pain when breathing. Your doctor may encourage you to do deep breathing exercises to help your lungs expand.

When pleural effusion occurs as a complication of pneumonia, you should seek medical attention promptly for future chest colds.

Treatment Thoracentesis is used to drain the excess fluid. In some cases a thoracostomy is performed to permit fluid drainage. The tube used in this procedure may stay in place for several days. If pleural inflammation accompanies pleural effusion, reabsorption of the pleural fluid may be slow and repeated draining may be necessary.

Effective management of pleural effusion requires that the underlying cause be determined and treated appropriately. For example, if TB is the cause, antituberculosis therapy will be inhibited and cortico-

steroids may be administered to speed resolution of the effusion.

Prognosis Once the fluid is drained, breathing becomes easier. Treating the underlying condition significantly improves the prognosis.

Fungal Lung Infections

Different types of fungi can infect the lungs and cause disease. These diseases occur when people inhale fungus spores that have become airborne.

Fungal diseases often clear up on their own. They also can spread throughout the body via the bloodstream.

❖ HISTOPLASMOSIS

Symptoms *(What you may experience)* Headache; chills; fever; lumps on the leg; cough; chest pain; enlargement of the liver and spleen; ulceration of the tongue, palate (bony roof of the oral cavity), epiglottis (flap-like cover that closes with swallowing to prevent food and liquid from entering the respiratory passages and larynx); breathlessness.

Signs and laboratory findings *(What the doctor looks for)* History of exposure to contaminated soil from areas in which the disease is known to occur; a positive skin test for histoplasmin; fungus as identified by an analysis of sputum; fungal presence as revealed by analysis of tissue from oral ulcerations, lymph nodes, blood, urine, liver, and bone marrow; antibodies to histoplasmosis as detected by a blood test; histoplasma antigens as detected by blood and urine test.

What is it? Histoplasmosis is a fungal infection caused by *Histoplasma capsulatum*, which is found in the feces of birds and bats and in soil contaminated by their feces. In the United States, the disease is most prevalent in the central and eastern states. In the Mississippi and Ohio River Valleys, 80 percent of the inhabitants may have positive skin tests to histoplasmin, indicating prior infection that resolved on its own, as is most commonly the case. Should any of these people subsequently suffer a suppressed immune system, as a result of AIDS or organ transplantation, for example, reactivated disease may occur and quickly progress.

Three forms affect people in the United States—primary acute histoplasmosis, progressive disseminated (widely distributed throughout the body) histoplasmosis, and chronic pulmonary histoplasmosis. A fourth form occurs only in Africa.

Symptoms vary with each form of the disease. The primary form of the disease may feel like a severe cold or flu, is benign, and resolves spontaneously. The progressive disseminated form of the disease, which occurs when the fungus spreads from the lungs through the bloodstream, can involve the liver and spleen and ulcers of the mouth and throat. It also can affect the brain, heart, and adrenal glands. The breathlessness and coughing up of blood-tinged phlegm associated with the chronic form of histoplasmosis resemble TB symptoms.

Histoplasmosis is usually seen in adult men. Fatal disseminated disease is seen more frequently in elderly men and in infants.

Symptoms generally develop 5 to 18 days after exposure to the fungus. However, chronic pulmonary histoplasmosis may progress slowly over many years.

What you can do If your job routinely takes you to places in which the soil or dust may be infected, wear a mask over your mouth and nose to keep from inhaling the fungus.

When to call the doctor If you have developed signs of a respiratory illness after visiting bat-infested caves, chicken coops, or pigeon roosts, see your doctor.

Treatment Treatment is necessary only for those with the progressive disseminated or chronic forms of the disease. Oral antifungal medication such as ketoconazole, amphotericin B, or fluconazole (Diflucan) will be prescribed. For more severe cases, amphotericin B or itraconazole will be prescribed. A person with AIDS will need to take an antifungal medication for life. If oral or throat ulcerations and swallowing problems are present, nutrition may be supplied through a needle inserted into a blood vessel in the arm or hand.

People with chronic pulmonary or progressive disseminated histoplasmosis may require counseling to deal with long-term hospitalization.

Prognosis Prognosis varies with each form of histoplasmosis. The progressive disseminated form kills about 90 percent of people who contract it. Chronic pulmonary histoplasmosis is fatal in 20 percent of people within 5 years of diagnosis.

❖ BLASTOMYCOSIS

Symptoms *(What you may experience)* Cough; chest pain; fever; chills; night sweats; fatigue; loss of appetite; weight loss; a red, measles-like skin rash.

Signs and laboratory findings *(What the doctor looks for)* Identification of the fungus by analysis of sputum from lungs or tissue from skin lesions; accumulation of secretions in the lung as shown by chest x-rays.

What is it? Blastomycosis is caused by the yeast-like fungus *Blastomyces dermatitidis*, which inhabits the soil of the southeastern, south central, and midwestern United States. It usually affects men between the ages of 30 and 50 but no specific occupation is associated with it.

The fungus usually infects the lungs after being inhaled, producing a form of pneumonia. Occasionally the fungus may travel through the bloodstream and affect other areas of the body such as bone, the central nervous system, and the genitourinary system (kidneys).

What you can do Since the fungus is inhaled, people in these parts of the United States who work close to the soil should consider wearing a mask to cover the nose and mouth.

When to call the doctor If you develop pneumonia-like symptoms after inhaling airborne soil and dust, consult your doctor. Symptoms take from weeks to months to develop.

Treatment Not everyone with blastomycosis requires treatment. If symptoms are severe, the fungus responds readily to the antifungal medication amphotericin B. Ketoconazole (Nizoral), itraconazole (Sporanox), or fluconazole also may be effective.

Prognosis With early detection and antifungal treatment, the prognosis is good. But if left untreated, blastomycosis is progressive and often fatal.

❖ CRYPTOCOCCOSIS

Symptoms *(What you may experience)* Weight loss; night sweats; shortness of breath; red, measles-like rash on the face; pain in the bones of the limbs and in the skull, spine, and joints; if the central nervous system is involved, you may experience headache; blurred vision; dizziness; inability to speak; vomiting; noise in your ear when no source of sound is apparent; inappropriate behavior.

Signs and laboratory findings *(What the doctor looks for)* Identification of the fungus by analysis of blood, sputum, urine, prostate secretions, bone marrow, or cerebrospinal fluid; cerebrospinal fluid pressure and glucose levels; lung lesion as shown by a chest x-ray.

What is it? Cryptococcosis is an infection caused by the fungus *Cryptococcus neoformans*. It typically is caused by inhaling the fungus in particles of dust contaminated by pigeon feces. The disease is most often seen in urban settings. In many cases the source of infection is unknown. It most commonly is seen in men ages 30 to 60. It is rare in children.

Cryptococcosis is especially likely to develop in people whose immune systems have been compromised by illnesses such as AIDS, Hodgkin's disease, leukemia, and lymphoma. It also may strike people who take medications to suppress their immune systems, such as people who have undergone organ transplantation.

Symptoms usually are not apparent until the infection spreads from the lungs to other sites such as the central nervous system, skin, bones, prostate gland, liver, or kidneys.

What you can do If you work in an urban setting—especially around sites in which pigeons may congregate or roost—you should consider wearing a mask to cover your mouth and nose so you do not inhale the fungus.

When to call the doctor If you have AIDS or HIV or are taking immunosuppressive medications call your doctor if you experience any symptoms of cryptococcosis.

Treatment Therapy is not necessary unless lung involvement becomes obvious or the disease has spread to other organ systems. In immunocompromised people, *Cryptococcus neoformans* frequently spreads to the brain, causing meningitis (infection of the coverings of the brain). Treatment of disseminated infection involves intravenous administration of amphotericin B or fluconazole. People with AIDS often need long-term therapy to prevent a relapse.

If cryptococcosis has been diagnosed but there are no lung symptoms, close medical observation is required for at least a year to monitor progress of the disease.

Prognosis If the central nervous system becomes involved the disease can be fatal. But treatment with antifungal medications dramatically reduces the risk of death.

❖ ASPERGILLOSIS

Symptoms (*What you may experience*) Wheezing; shortness of breath; cough, possibly with blood-tinged mucus; chest pain; fever.

Signs and laboratory findings (*What the doctor looks for*) A crescent-shaped structure around a circular mass as shown by a chest x-ray; white blood cells in sputum. In some cases, a biopsy of the lung is necessary for diagnosis.

What is it? Members of the fungus *Aspergillus* are just about everywhere on earth, usually in fermenting compost piles and damp hay. It causes infection only in people whose immune systems are weakened, such as people with AIDS, burn victims, people undergoing treatment for cancer, and organ transplant recipients. But the fungus also may produce an asthmatic reaction in people who are allergic or sensitive to it.

Symptoms of disease can appear a few days to a few weeks after infection. Fungal filaments (fibers) can form a ball or plug in a lung cavity left by a previous illness such as TB. This ball is called a mycetoma. *Aspergillus* may also invade the lung tissue, causing a form of pneumonia, or it may infect the airway, causing an allergic reaction in the lung.

Treatment The allergic form of aspergillosis responds well to treatment with corticosteroids, which reduce the inflammation that often accompanies allergic reactions. (See Chapter 29 for more information on allergies.) If the fungus has spread throughout the body you may need a two-week course of treatment with amphotericin B. If lung bleeding is evident, surgery may be necessary to remove the damaged parts of the lung.

Prognosis People with weakened immune systems have a poor prognosis. Otherwise the disease often responds to treatment.

❖ COCCIDIOIDOMYCOSIS

Symptoms (*What you may experience*) Tender, red nodules on the legs, especially on the shins; nasal congestion; cough; fever; headache; sore throat; itchy, red, measles-like rash; joint pain and swelling.

Signs and laboratory findings (*What the doctor looks for*) Presence of the fungus as confirmed by blood tests; fungus spores as identified by examination of sputum; patchy areas in both lungs as shown by a chest x-ray.

What is it? Coccidioidomycosis is caused by inhaling the fungus *Coccidioides immitis*. It is common in the semi-arid climates of the southwestern United States, particularly between the San Joaquin Valley in California and southwestern Texas. It also is known as valley fever or San Joaquin Valley fever, for the place in which it was first discovered.

The disease appears more frequently during warm, dry months. Because of its geography, it generally strikes groups of people who work as migrant farm laborers—Mexican-Americans, Philippine-Americans, and Native Americans. Blacks also are especially susceptible.

Symptoms occur in about 40 percent of people infected after an incubation period of 10 to 30 days.

The rash may appear 1 to 2 days after respiratory or flu-like symptoms develop.

Pregnant women and people with weakened immune systems are at higher risk of developing the disease. In endemic areas, about one-quarter of people infected with HIV also develop coccidioidomycosis.

A secondary form of the disease produces abscesses throughout the body. This form is more common in dark-skinned men, pregnant women, and people with weakened immune systems.

Treatment A mild case of the disease may be treated with bed rest and symptomatic relief. But severe or disseminated disease requires intravenous administration of amphotericin B, ketoconazole, or itraconazole. In some cases, surgery to remove infected areas of the lungs may be necessary.

Prognosis Even with treatment, the progressive, disseminated form of coccidioidomycosis is fatal in 60 percent of people who develop it. The primary form of the disease usually clears up on its own and is rarely fatal.

Chronic Respiratory Diseases

Some pulmonary diseases are not the result of viral, bacterial, or fungal assault. Rather they are the result of processes that inflame the airways and cause the smooth muscle that lines the airways to contract, impeding the flow of air in and out of the lungs, as in asthma; or they may occur as a result of a lifetime of smoking, which damages the respiratory tree and obstructs the flow of air out of the lungs as in chronic bronchitis and emphysema.

❖ ASTHMA

Symptoms *(What you may experience)* Chest tightness; difficulty breathing; wheezing; coughing.

Signs and laboratory findings *(What the doctor looks for)* Functioning of the lungs as determined by pulmonary function tests; a physical abnormality in the lungs as shown by a chest x-ray; sensitivity to various substances as determined by allergy tests.

What is it? Asthma is a respiratory disorder characterized by periods of breathlessness and wheezing. Other common symptoms are cough and chest tightness. The attacks can be mild or severe, can occur at any time, and can be frequent or occasional. They often occur at night. About 14 million Americans—one-third of them children—have asthma.

Although asthma can strike at any age, 50 percent of all cases are first seen in children less than 10 years old. In this age group, boys are affected twice as often as are girls. The disease may fade in many children as they age.

Asthma also appears to have a genetic component. If you have asthma, your children have a greater risk of suffering from the disease. Although 4 to 5 percent of the

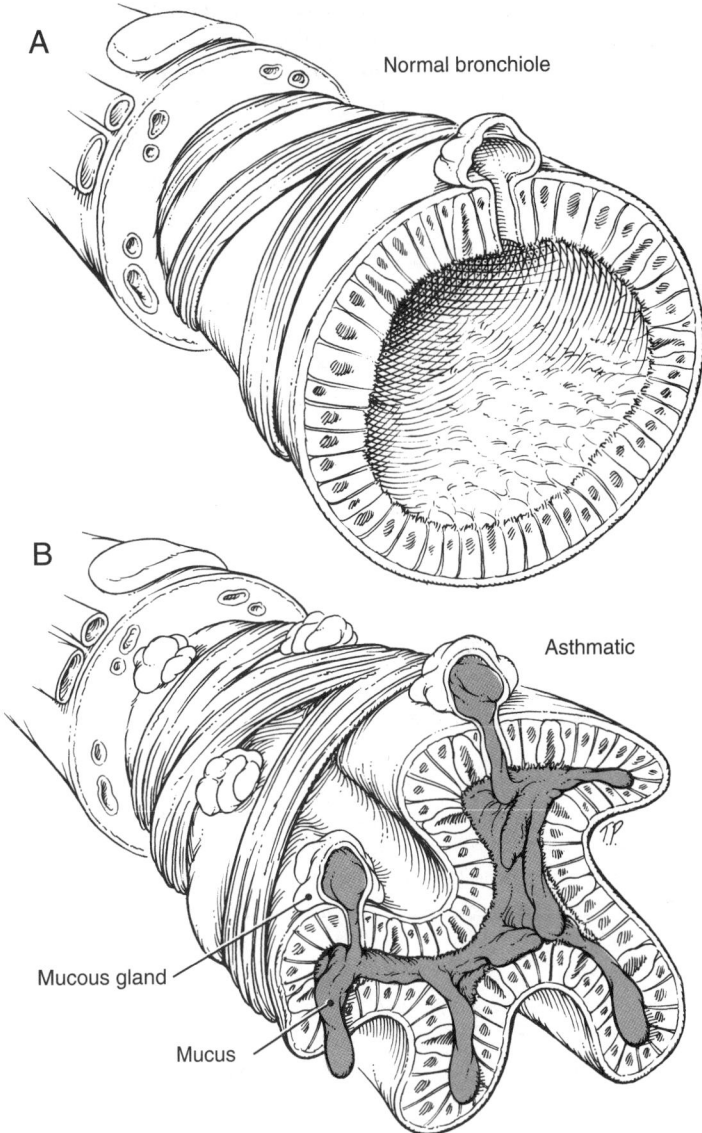

A   Normal bronchiole

B   Asthmatic

Mucous gland

Mucus

Normally, airways are wide open (A). Asthma results from exposure to an allergen or to an environmental agent (B). Exposure leads to inflammation and increased mucus production, causing obstruction of the bronchiole and shortness of breath.

U.S. population has asthma, the incidence of the disease rises to about 20 to 25 percent among those who have a sibling or parent with asthma.

Approximately 85 percent of people with asthma have a form of the disease that is essentially a manifestation of an allergic illness. Once an allergen (an allergy-causing substance) enters the airways it is recognized by a specific antibody (immunoglobulin E, also called IgE) that sits atop mast cells. When the allergen and antibody interact, the mast cell breaks down and releases chemicals—histamine, leukotrienes, and prostaglandins—that trigger the contraction of the smooth muscle that lines the airways. Simultaneously these chemicals cause the airway linings to become inflamed and secrete thick, clogging mucus. When the small bronchioles of the lungs become clogged or are swollen, it is difficult to expel all of the air from the lungs.

White blood cells summoned to the scene 4 to 6 hours after the initial exposure to the allergen contribute to a second wave of inflammation known as the late-phase reaction, and another bout of breathing difficulty occurs.

In nonallergic asthma, more common in adults, the same chemical substances are released with the same effects but the breakdown of the mast cell occurs for an as yet unknown reason.

The National Institutes of Health has defined asthma as having four level of severity: mild intermittent, mild persistent, moderate persistent, and severe persistent. In the mildest form, symptoms appear only briefly and less than twice a week. The severest form consists of continual symptoms, prolonged crises, limitations to physical activity, and lung function that is below 60 per cent of normal.

What you can do Asthma is a chronic disease that may require daily management. The most effective way to control this condition is to form a partnership with your doctor and work to develop specific, written personal plans. Depending upon the stage of the condition, these may involve removing allergens from your environment (see Asthma Triggers, this page), taking daily medication, testing your breathing capacity daily, and learning how to respond to a breathing crisis. Avoid using OTC medication and instead use prescription medication, which is more effective and safer.

Knowing how to spot the early warning signs of an asthma attack is the key to asthma control. Common warning signs include a drop in a peak flow reading (a peak flow meter is a device that, when used twice daily, can assess accurately the degree of airway blockage); a chronic cough, especially at night; rapid breathing; becoming short of breath more easily than usual; chest tightness; itchy, watery eyes; itchy, scratchy, or sore throat; sneezing; a sense of head congestion; runny nose; and headache.

Some air pollutants may be more irritating to sensitive lungs than to normal lungs, so if you can, stay indoors on days when the outside air pollution is especially heavy and avoid dust-raising activities.

ASTHMA TRIGGERS

Asthma episodes can be triggered by allergic or nonallergic mechanisms.

Since most asthma attacks are caused by an allergic mechanism, many factors that trigger asthma can be controlled. Identifying and keeping away from substances you are allergic to can significantly reduce your risk of an asthma attack. Allergies to pollen, animal dander (particles of hair and skin), and insect droppings present in dust are among the most common triggers of asthma. Removing dust and insect remains from the home by cleaning, sweeping, and vacuuming regularly can result in major improvements. (Recently, scientists have discovered that roach droppings may be an important factor in the rising rates of urban asthma.) Covering bedding with airtight plastic covers and avoiding feather pillows may also offer relief (see Creating a Dust-free Room, page 1339). Sulfites, which are used to preserve foods, also may precipitate an asthma attack.

Exposure to environmental pollutants and chemicals can trigger nonallergic asthma. Eliminating cigarette smoke from the environment can help reduce the severity and frequency of asthmatic episodes. Other factors that can trigger nonallergic asthma episodes include smog, natural gas, propane or kerosene used as cooking fuel, wood smoke, and paint fumes.

Viral respiratory infections also can trigger nonallergic asthma. Take precautions to reduce the incidence of respiratory infections.

In 5 percent of people with asthma, sensitivity to aspirin or nonsteroidal anti-inflammatory medications such as ibuprofen may result in an asthma attack. This sensitivity is often associated with nasal polyps, though the cause of aspirin sensitivity is not well understood. Asthma begins within 2 hours of aspirin ingestion and may result in respiratory failure.

Exercise also is known to induce contraction of the muscles that line the airways, also called bronchospasm, in a phenomenon called exercise-induced asthma. A feeling of tightness in the chest and gasping and wheezing generally peak about 10 minutes after the period of activity and can last up to an hour if not treated promptly with inhaled bronchodilators.

Because inhaling cold, dry air also may provoke an asthma attack, running in cold weather is more likely to precipitate an episode of exercise-induced asthma than is swimming in a heated pool, for example. Swimming is one of the most beneficial forms of exercise for people with asthma, apparently because the moisture-saturated air reduces the risk and severity of an asthma attack.

Exercise-induced asthma is not an excuse for avoiding regular physical activity. Despite the fact that it can bring on an asthma attack, exercise is beneficial for most people with asthma. Too often, children with asthma are discouraged from exercising, but it is invaluable in keeping them healthy. With proper care, medication, and your doctor's supervision you or your child theoretically could perform at the same level of excellence as asthmatic Olympian Jackie Joyner-Kersee. ∎

Colds and lung infections can make asthma worse, so take steps to reduce your risk of infection. Be sure to get pneumonia and influenza vaccinations; keep yourself healthy with daily exercise, nourishing foods, and plenty of sleep; and avoid close contact with people who have lung infections.

If you have asthma and are pregnant, consult your doctor about caring for your condition during pregnancy.

In 1997, the National Heart, Lung, and Blood Institute of the National Institutes of Health developed new guidelines to assist people with asthma in managing their conditions. The guides are extensive and detailed and can be ordered from the National Heart, Lung, and Blood Institute Information Center, P.O. Box 10305, Bethesda, MD 20824; Web site: http://www.nhlbi.nih.gov/nhlbi/nhlbi.htm.

When to call the doctor Early diagnosis and treatment of asthma helps preserve lung function later in life, yet too often the symptoms of asthma are misinterpreted or ignored. If you have asthma and notice that your child wheezes or becomes short of breath, your child may have inherited your condition. Make an appointment with a doctor right away so that your child can be diagnosed and treated properly. If you do not have asthma but notice that your child seems to have chronic colds or coughs, consult a doctor regarding whether asthma might be the cause.

Asthma episodes rarely occur without warning. If you pay attention to the signs, you can control a crisis yourself or anticipate the need to consult your doctor. Most people with asthma have warning signs that occur hours before symptoms appear. A peak flow meter can help a person with asthma detect changes in breathing ability before symptoms develop. A peak flow meter can be used like a traffic light. In the green zone, breathing at 80 to 100 percent of maximum, everything is fine. The yellow zone, 50 to 80 percent of maximum, signals caution and medication may need to be increased. If the reading is in the red zone of less than 50 percent of maximum lung capacity, medical attention should be sought.

If emergency symptoms develop—severe breathlessness and difficulty breathing, intense coughing, cyanosis (bluish nailbeds and lips), and racing pulse—seek emergency medical help. Friends and family members should be aware of other emergency signs in people with asthma—sweating, fatigue, lethargy, and difficulty speaking.

Treatment Asthma is a chronic inflammatory disease of the airways, so the first step in treatment is to reduce the inflammation. This can be done by means of the prophylactic (preventive) use of such medications as cromolyn sodium (Intal) and corticosteroids. These are often called controller medications. Acute attacks can be controlled with medications known as bronchodilators, which open the airways. These are often called rescue medications. The earlier such a medication is taken during an attack, the more effective it will be.

Cromolyn sodium can be inhaled from a metered dose inhaler (see How to Use an Inhaler, below), from a device called a nebulizer, or by means of a dry powder inhaler. To prevent asthma symptoms, it should be administered every day. The only side effect of cromolyn sodium is a dry cough. It may

HOW TO USE AN INHALER

Some of the medications used to treat asthma are inhaled beta-adrenergic bronchodilators such as albuterol and terbutaline. These medications are delivered to the lungs via a metered dose inhaler—a portable pressurized container that shoots a specific amount of the medication into the mouth and down the throat to the lungs. The device must be squeezed during inhalation to deliver the medication into the lungs. If these actions are not well coordinated much of the medication will hit the back of the throat and then slide down into the stomach.

- Sit up straight and breathe normally.

- Shake the canister a few times to mix the medication.

- If you have one, attach a spacer to the delivery end of the inhaler. This is a narrow plastic tube that helps collect the medication before you inhale it.

- Put the delivery end of the spacer in your mouth and close your lips around it. If you are not using a spacer, hold the mouthpiece about 2 to 3 in. from your open mouth.

- Squeeze the inhaler and slowly breathe in for about 6 seconds.

- Hold your breath for about 10 seconds. Then exhale through your nose.

- If you are prescribed more than one puff, you may repeat the steps after a few normal breaths.

- If possible, swish some water around in your mouth to remove traces of the medication. ■

take up to 6 weeks for cromolyn sodium to take effect.

Corticosteroids, such as prednisone and methylprednisolone (which are not the kinds of steroids used by some athletes), also can be inhaled through a metered dose inhaler. Common inhaled steroids include beclomethasone, budesonide, flunisolide, fluticasone, and triamcinolone. Alternately, they can be swallowed in pill or liquid form. (In some cases, they can be injected: In this form, corticosteroids are administered in a doctor's office or emergency room for serious episodes.) Like cromolyn, corticosteroids are anti-inflammatory medications that prevent and reduce swelling inside the airways and decrease the amount of mucus in the lungs. Inhaled corticosteroids may cause an oral yeast infection or they may irritate the upper airways and cause coughing. An attachment device on the metered dose inhaler called a spacer can keep these events from happening. Rinsing out your mouth after taking this medication also may keep them from occurring.

Short-term use of oral corticosteroids may increase your appetite and cause fluid retention and weight gain. If you are having problems with side effects, do not stop taking this medication without first consulting your doctor.

When oral corticosteroids are used over a period of years, they may cause hypertension (high blood pressure), bone thinning, cataracts, and muscle weakness. If children take them for a long time, the medications may slow the growth process. Because of these potential side effects, doctors try not to use oral corticosteroids for extended periods.

Bronchodilators are medications used to temporarily open airways that have closed during an acute asthma attack. There are several different classes of bronchodilators including beta-agonists, anticholinergics, and methylxanthines. Bronchodilators cause the muscles around the airways to relax but they do not correct the underlying inflammation. They are a temporary solution and if overused can aggravate asthma by making the airways more sensitive.

Beta-agonists such as albuterol (Proventil, Ventolin), metaproterenol (Alupent, Metaprel), and terbutaline (Brethine, Bricanyl), can be taken in many ways—inhaled with a metered dose inhaler or nebulizer, swallowed as a liquid or tablet, or injected.

Inhaled beta-agonists start working the fastest (usually within 5 minutes) because the medication is delivered straight to the lungs. Oral liquids or tablets take a little longer to start working (about 30 minutes) but their effects last as long as 4 to 6 hours. Injections are used only in a doctor's office or emergency room for severe asthma episodes. They work very quickly but their effects last only about 20 minutes. Nebulizers are a good way for children less than 5 years old to take these medications because children may have trouble coordinating the actions needed to make inhalers efficient.

If you find yourself using a beta-agonist several times a day or more than three times a week, the swelling in your airways may be worsening. You may need another kind of medication, and you should discuss this with your doctor right away.

Some commonly used bronchodilators include albuterol, ipratropium (Atrovent), salmeterol (Serevent), and theophylline (Slo-Phyllin, Theolair, Quibron-T Dividose, Bronkodyl, Elixophyllin). These medications are available as pills, capsules, liquids, or tablets. They can be inhaled in aerosol form.

Theophylline—one of the most popular bronchodilator medications—should not be taken on an empty stomach nor should it be taken with hot food (heat will dissolve it and release too much of the medication at once). It may cause nausea, vomiting, intestinal cramps, diarrhea, headache, muscle cramps, irregular heartbeat, tremor, or restlessness. Call your doctor if you have any of these side effects. Theophylline must be at the right concentration in the bloodstream to have a positive effect, so it is important for you to take it at the time and in the amount that has been prescribed.

A new type of medication, leukotriene inhibitors, is useful in people whose asthma is made worse by aspirin and, in some cases, in those with chronic asthma. Though the role of leukotriene inhibitors is not fully established at present, most authorities believe that they are helpful in a person who has asthma and is sensitive to aspirin.

See Medication Directory, page 1503, for more information on asthma medication.

Prognosis In general, asthma is a disease that can be readily controlled with the proper medication and by taking appropriate steps to avoid substances that can precipitate an asthma attack. Know the warning signs of an asthma attack so you can initiate early treatment. Asthma mortality has been on the rise in recent years, particularly in populations that reside in inner cities. About 5,000 people die from the disease each year.

❖ OCCUPATIONAL LUNG DISEASES

Symptoms *(What you may experience)* Breathlessness; chest tightness; cough.

Signs and laboratory findings *(What the doctor looks for)* Exposure to materials that may be damaging to the lungs as revealed by a complete history of work activities; abnormalities in the lungs, such as scar tissue or fibrosis as detected by chest x-rays; functioning of the lungs as determined by pulmonary function tests.

What is it? Your lungs can be affected by substances present in the air (see Air Pollution and Respiratory Disease, page 750) of some workplace environments. About 65,000 American workers develop a pulmonary disorder related to the workplace each year. About 25,000 deaths due to such respiratory diseases occur each year.

Occupational lung disease is the leading work-related illness in the United States. The lungs of most people can withstand short-term exposure to substances that can be hazardous; long-term exposure can be dangerous.

Sometimes an occupational lung disease can take 20 years or more to develop; others can develop in the short term. Examples of occupational lung diseases are as follows:

- *Asbestosis.* In this disease, long-term exposure to asbestos allows asbestos fibers to accumulate around the terminal bronchioles (the term for the ends of the bronchioles) in the lungs. In its attempt to deal with this invasion, the lung walls off the invasion with scar tissue. This causes thickening of lung tissue and loss of elasticity. Asbestosis may take 30 or more years of exposure to develop. Asbestos workers who smoke are at very high risk of lung cancer. Because of its fire-retardant and sound-proofing properties, asbestos was once used in many common materials such

as pipe and duct insulation, building insulation, roofing materials, brake pads and linings, pot holders, and furnaces. The production of all asbestos-containing materials for home construction and use was banned, in three stages over 7 years, beginning in 1990. But you may have asbestos-containing materials in your home or office, especially if it was built before 1978. City and state agencies can provide information on asbestos and its safe removal.

- *Mesothelioma.* This rare type of cancer, which affects the pleura, is responsible for about 10 percent of deaths among people who work around asbestos (see Mesothelioma, page 765).

- *Byssinosis.* Known more commonly as brown lung disease, this condition is caused by inhaling dust and fibers from hemp, flax, and cotton processing. Peo-

Prolonged exposure to dust containing asbestos fibers can cause lung damage. The small size of asbestos fibers allows them to lodge deep in the lungs, in the air sacs (alveoli) where oxygen is absorbed. Fibers in the lung (asbestos bodies) trigger an inflammatory reaction involving neutrophils and lymphocytes. Prolonged inflammation leads to fibrosis of the walls of the alveoli and of the lining that surrounds the lung (pleura).

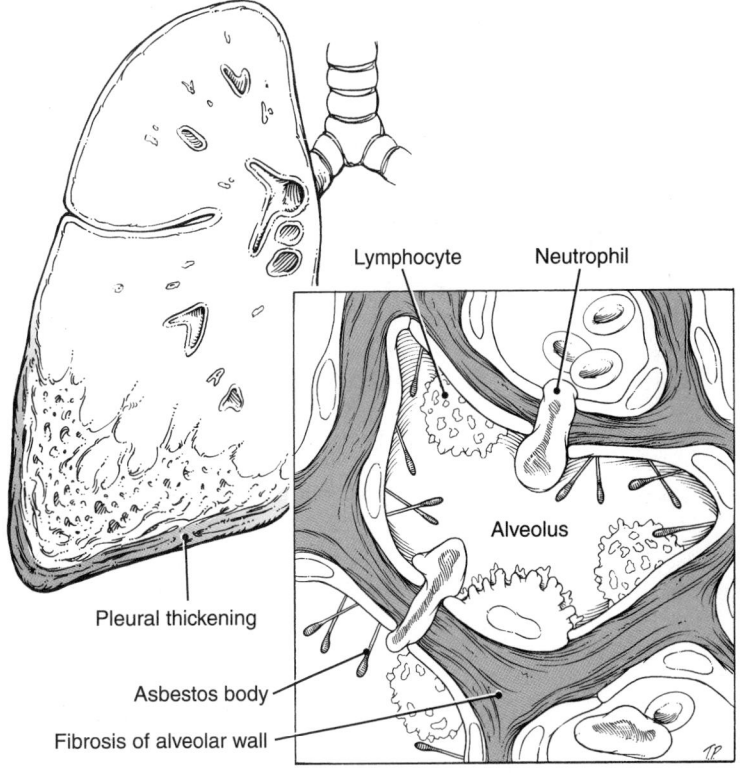

Lymphocyte

Neutrophil

Alveolus

Pleural thickening

Asbestos body

Fibrosis of alveolar wall

ple who work with the fibers during the first cleaning process are at greatest risk. Symptoms, which may mimic those of asthma, generally begin at the start of the work week and dissipate over the weekend. Continued exposure increases the risk of chronic bronchitis and emphysema.

- *Coal workers' pneumoconiosis*. Also referred to as black lung disease, this disease is caused by mineral dust thrown into the closed environment of a coal mine by the industrial processes used to extract the material. In about 3 to 5 percent of miners the dust accumulates in the lung, causing fibrosis (scarring) to develop. In about 5 percent of these people, the area of fibrosis grows over time, causing the lung to be filled with stiff scar tissue that inhibits proper breathing. It takes at least 10 years to develop and is more common in people who mine anthracite coal than those who mine bituminous coal. Consequently it is seen more frequently in eastern U.S. miners.

- *Silicosis*. It is caused by inhalation of particles of crystalline quartz, also known as free silica. Silicosis can affect sandblasters, tunnelers, drillers, and stonecutters. The accumulation of silica

AIR POLLUTION AND RESPIRATORY DISEASE

Air pollution is responsible for increasing the death rate among people with heart and respiratory problems. High levels of air pollution also increase the frequency and severity of asthma attacks.

Do the following if you live in an area in which air pollution is typically heavy or on days when the pollution levels are higher than normal:

- Avoid traffic jams and parking garages.

- Avoid exertion.

- Avoid dust-raising activities.

- Wear a mask or filter over your nose and mouth if you have to go outside.

- Stay inside with the air-conditioning turned on. ■

in the lungs also causes fibrosis. It can take up to 20 years for silicosis to develop, but a person exposed to massive concentrations, such as a tunnel worker, can develop an acute form of the disease; consequently, adult respiratory distress syndrome (ARDS) may develop (see Adult Respiratory Distress Syndrome, page 734).

- *Occupational asthma*. This occurs when someone with asthma is exposed to substances in the workplace that trigger an asthma attack. Up to 5 percent of people with asthma are affected by this problem.

- *Industrial bronchitis*. This inflammation of the airways is seen in coal miners and people subject to brown lung disease. It also may be associated with fumes of certain chemicals. It is unclear whether the lung condition is directly related to the workplace environment or to other irritants the worker may encounter during other times and in other places. Smoking, for example, can exacerbate any lung problem.

What you can do These diseases may not be curable but they are always preventable. Improving ventilation, wearing protective equipment such as masks that cover the nose and mouth, changing work procedures, and educating employees about the dangers associated with the materials with which they come in contact are key factors for preventing these illnesses. Cigarette smoking can aggravate any lung problem, so if you smoke and have been diagnosed or are at risk for developing any of these diseases, you should stop smoking. See Chapter 4 for information on how to stop smoking.

When to call the doctor If you work or have worked in an industry in which you were exposed to any potential lung irritant and have developed symptoms of a breathing problem, see your doctor.

Treatment No effective treatment exists for asbestosis, black lung disease, or silicosis. Bronchodilators are used to treat occupational asthma and byssinosis. Avoiding the substance that causes the symptoms is essential. Rest, drinking plenty of nonalcoholic liquids, and use of a humidifier or vaporizer may offer some relief in the case of industrial bronchitis.

Prognosis Seriousness depends on the nature of the disease and duration of exposure to the offending material. People diagnosed with asbestosis usually die within 15 years of the onset of symptoms. If you have byssinosis, changing your job to one in a different industry can allow the symptoms to clear up before lung problems become chronic. Black lung disease is involved in about 2,000 deaths each year, primarily in Pennsylvania and West Virginia. About 20 to 30 percent of people with silicosis develop crippling respiratory disease and people with acute silicosis may die within 5 years. Any episode of asthma has the potential of causing a fatal respiratory attack, but swift treatment with medication at the first sign of an attack makes the prognosis excellent (see Asthma, page 745). Industrial bronchitis is an acute disease that generally clears up quickly with proper treatment.

❖ SARCOIDOSIS

Symptoms (What you may experience) Shortness of breath; cough; rash; red bumps on the face, arms, or shins; inflamed eyes; weight loss; fatigue; night sweats; fever.

Signs and laboratory findings (What the doctor looks for) Swollen lymph glands between the lungs and patchy areas in the lungs as detected by a chest x-ray; functioning of the lungs as determined by pulmonary function tests; levels of proteins, calcium, and liver enzymes as revealed by blood tests; results of the Kveim test, in which a person is injected under the skin with a small amount of protein from the tissue of a person with known sarcoidosis (this test is not used very often in the United States). In some cases a biopsy of the skin, lung, or other tissue may be required to confirm the diagnosis.

What is it? Sarcoidosis is a mysterious disease that affects many organs and organ systems. It is characterized by the development of granulomas, which are small areas of inflamed cells. These granulomas can look like sores on the face or skin. They also can develop inside the body, such as on the walls of the lung's alveoli or on the walls

of the bronchioles. When this happens the cell overgrowth decreases the ability to absorb oxygen.

Granulomas also may appear in the bones, lymph nodes, liver, eyes, skin, spleen, salivary glands, heart, or nervous system.

Sarcoidosis usually strikes adults ages 20 to 40. It occurs most often and more severely in blacks and affects twice as many women as men. Risk of developing sarcoidosis among whites is higher if you are of Scandinavian, German, Irish, or Puerto Rican descent. It affects about 5 in 100,000 white people in the United States and about 40 in 100,000 blacks.

The disease can be acute, in which case it generally resolves in about 2 to 3 years. It is not a crippling disease and most people with it can conduct their lives as usual. In about 10 to 15 percent of cases it is progressive and chronic.

The cause of sarcoidosis remains unknown. Some doctors believe it is the result of inhaling an infectious or allergic substance such as an uncommon kind of mycobacterium or fungus. Others think it is due to an element such as zirconium or beryllium.

It appears to be a malfunction of the immune system, in which certain white blood cells called T-helper lymphocytes become overactive. This hyper-responsiveness causes the buildup of inflamed cells. Ninety percent of cases involve the lungs.

What you can do You should follow the directions of your doctor, which in many cases results in continuing your normal lifestyle. People with sarcoidosis should not smoke cigarettes and also should avoid exposure to chemicals that can harm the lungs. If you have symptoms of sarcoidosis you should see your doctor regularly. If you have sarcoidosis and plan to become pregnant, discuss the matter with your doctor. Bed rest may be necessary during the last trimester.

Treatment Many people have no symptoms at all and require no treatment. Those with mild symptoms may be observed, since the disease frequently remits (temporarily ceases to cause symptoms) spontaneously. For those who are symptomatic, corticosteroids (such as low doses of prednisone) are usually effective in reducing the inflammation. Such therapy may last 1 or 2 years or for life. Some people, especially those who have high blood levels of calcium, may need to adopt a low-calcium diet, avoid direct exposure to sunlight, and avoid vitamin supplement intake. Regular eye exams are essential because sarcoidosis can damage the eyes with little warning.

Prognosis Most people recover completely within 2 to 3 years. Sarcoidosis appears briefly and heals without intervention in 60 to 70 percent of cases, often without the person knowing or doing anything about it. It is fatal in fewer than 5 percent of people who develop it. Fatalities occur when it affects the function of a vital organ such as the heart, lungs, nervous system, or liver.

❖ PULMONARY FIBROSIS

Symptoms *(What you may experience)* Increasingly severe shortness of breath, which may appear first during exercise; dry cough; chest pain; clubbed (misshapen) fingertips.

Signs and laboratory findings *(What the doctor looks for)* Abnormalities that may be due to fibrous matter as detected by a chest x-ray and computed tomography (CT) scan; results of bronchoalveolar lavage (removal and analysis of cells and fluid from the bronchioles and alveoli); direct examination of the lungs using bronchoscopy; lung tissue biopsy results; lung functioning as assessed by pulmonary function tests.

What is it? Pulmonary fibrosis is a form of, and often is referred to as, interstitial lung disease because it involves the interstitium, which is the tissue between the air sacs of the lungs. A hallmark of the disease is that the alveoli become inflamed, leading to the development of fibrosis in the interstitium. This causes the lungs to become stiff. As the lungs stiffen, breathing becomes more and more difficult. In addition to the alveoli, the disease also may affect the bronchioles and capillaries. When fibrosis of lung tissue occurs, the tissue's ability to carry oxygen is permanently lost.

There are many different causes of pulmonary fibrosis. It may be the result of exposure to environmental irritants such as asbestos, metal or rock dusts, gases, or fumes. Infections such as TB and sarcoidosis also may cause fibrosis of the lung. It also may be related to rheumatoid arthritis or scleroderma (progressive thickening of the skin). There also appears to be a form of the disease that is transmitted from parent to child. In some cases it occurs for no known reason and is referred to as idiopathic (of unknown origin) pulmonary fibrosis.

The idiopathic form of the disease is noninfectious and nonmalignant but is progressive. It can occur at any age but generally is seen in people who are in their 60s or 70s. However, they may have had symptoms for months or even years.

What you can do If you are exposed to materials that might damage your lungs, you should wear a mask that covers your nose and mouth.

If you smoke, stop. If you have been diagnosed with pulmonary fibrosis, take care to avoid lung infections by getting influenza and pneumococcal pneumonia vaccinations.

Treatment See Occupational Lung Diseases, page 749, for information on pulmonary fibrosis related to exposure to environmental irritants. See Tuberculosis, page 737, and Sarcoidosis, page 751, for more information on infectious causes. People with pulmonary fibrosis may be treated with high dosages of corticosteroids and with immunosuppressive agents. Some people benefit from lung transplantation.

Prognosis Once fibrosis and scarring has occurred, the affected tissue has permanently lost the ability to perform the function for which it is designed. Many people live for many years following the onset of symptoms but others die within 5 years.

❖ CYSTIC FIBROSIS

Symptoms *(What you may experience)* Chronic mucous obstruction in the lungs that produces shortness of breath and chronic cough; wheezing; recurring bronchitis and pneumonia; fatigue; intestinal obstruction in newborns; failure to gain weight; large, greasy-looking, foul-smelling bowel movements; salt depletion in hot weather; salty-tasting skin.

Signs and laboratory findings *(What the doctor looks for)* The amount of salt in the sweat (if the sweat test, which is used to measure the amount of salt, is positive, a second test should be done); signs of obstructive lung disease as detected by chest x-rays; stool analysis results (absence of the compound trypsin suggests pancreatic involvement); the gene for cystic fibrosis (CF) as detected by a blood test.

What is it? CF is the most common fatal genetic disease in the United States. It affects an estimated 30,000 children and young adults. It occurs in approximately 1 in 3,300 live births and affects boys and girls equally. Black or Asian children rarely are affected.

CF causes the body to produce an abnormally thick, sticky mucus that can clog the lungs and lead to repeated pulmonary infections. The lungs of babies with CF are normal at birth, but obstruction of the airways causes progressive respiratory diseases. The thick mucus also obstructs the ducts through which enzymes from the pancreas are sent to the small intestine. Without these enzymes, fats cannot be digested, leading to malnutrition and chronic diarrhea. Children with CF often have good appetites and eat large amounts of food but are unable to digest it properly.

The basic defect involves the faulty transport of sodium and chloride (salt) within epithelial cells, which line organs such as the lungs and pancreas, to their outer surfaces. The sweat glands also are affected, causing the child's sweat to be very salty.

The disease occurs when a child inherits a defective gene from each parent. If a child inherits the gene from just one parent then the child will be a carrier. About 4 percent of white Americans—more than 10 million people—are unknowing, symptomless carriers of the defective gene.

Sometimes symptoms of CF occur immediately after birth. Mucus in the intestines makes the first bowel movement too thick and sticky to pass; this is called meconium ileus. But often the disease may not be diagnosed until later in infancy as the baby fails to thrive or has repeated respiratory infections. Two-thirds of people with CF are diagnosed by age 1. The disease sometimes occurs in a mild form and symptoms may not develop until adulthood.

What you can do If CF runs in your family and you are considering having a child, or if

POSTURAL DRAINAGE AND CHEST PERCUSSION

In certain chronic lung diseases, large amounts of mucus can collect in the lungs. Such collections provide breeding grounds for bacteria and resultant infections. It is important to clear the lungs of these unwanted secretions; postural drainage and chest percussion can help to do so.

In postural drainage, the person lies on a bed with the head and chest hanging over the edge, using gravity to drain the mucus into the upper portion of the airway so it can be coughed out.

In chest percussion, the person lies on a smooth surface. The chest is struck gently and repeatedly with cupped hands. The technique also can be applied to the back. These exercises need to be performed one or more times daily; your doctor, nurse, or physical therapist can teach family members how to do this properly.

Coughing during these procedures helps bring the mucus up through the respiratory tree so it can be expelled. ■

you plan to have another child after having one who has the disease, you should consult a doctor, who can advise you about the risk of having another child with CF.

If both parents are carriers, there is a 25 percent chance that any of their children will have CF; if both parents have CF, any child they have will have the disease; if only one parent has it, the child will be a carrier; if one parent has CF and the other is a carrier, there is a 50 percent chance that the child will have the disease and a 50 percent chance that the child will be a carrier. It is difficult, however, for people with CF to have children. In women, too much mucus in the cervix can block the passage of sperm, making conception difficult. Most males with CF are sterile because the mucus plugs up the ducts through which sperm travel.

It is now possible to diagnose CF prenatally, in the second trimester of pregnancy in most cases.

Children with CF may grow up underdeveloped and probably will miss school frequently. Because their immune systems are weak they should be immunized against

THE LUNG TRANSPLANT

Today many people with end-stage lung diseases benefit from the transplantation of one or both lungs. Lung transplantation offers people with pulmonary hypertension (see page 761), emphysema, pulmonary fibrosis, and CF the chance for improved quality of life. But not everyone with end-stage lung disease may be an appropriate candidate for lung transplantation. The risk of the surgery increases with age (adults over age 60 are generally considered to be high risk), obesity, a history of cigarette smoking, and substance abuse.

Healthy lungs removed from a brain-dead donor are chilled and preserved up to 12 hours before being implanted. To be usable, the lungs must be the proper size to fit in a prospective recipient's chest and must conform to the recipient's blood type. The lung or lungs are transported as quickly as possible to the medical center where the surgery will take place. After the organ recipient is anesthetized, an incision is made in the chest and the breastbone is cut and spread apart. A heart-lung machine is used to reroute the blood supply so the operating field is as bloodless as possible. The diseased lungs are cut free of the connecting bronchial tubes and blood vessels and are removed. The donor lungs are then positioned and sewn in place; the chest is then closed. Chest tubes are placed so excess fluid can drain outside the body.

The medical staff keeps a close eye on people who undergo organ transplant procedures. The most common complications are organ rejection and infection.

People who receive organ transplants have to take medication such as cyclosporine, azathioprine, and prednisone that suppress the activity of their immune systems. If a transplant recipient did not take such medications, the immune system would recognize the transplanted tissue as a foreign invader and would attack it. At the same time, because the immune systems of these people are suppressed, they are susceptible to infection by bacteria and viruses.

Doctors must tread a thin line between administering enough immunosuppressive medications to protect a transplanted organ but not so many as to shut down the immune system. To carefully monitor transplant recipients for signs of organ rejection, small pieces of the lung are removed for a biopsy. If the biopsy shows damaged cells, the dosage and type of immunosuppressive medication may be changed.

The average hospital stay for a lung transplant recipient is about 3 weeks. A full recovery from the surgery may take about 6 months. To speed recovery, daily activities should be resumed as soon as possible.

During 1996, surgeons performed 805 lung transplants in the United States. However, three times that number of people needed a lung transplant; as of August 1997, for example, more than 2,500 people were placed on the national registry for a lung transplant. Only a fraction of those who can donate organs do so. The result is that there are not enough organs available for transplant. Because of this, many people have to wait months for their operations. Some die while waiting. ∎

other respiratory, as well as nonrespiratory, infections. Although children with CF are subject to frequent lung infections and steps must be taken to minimize their exposure to people with colds and lung infections, it is important to not overprotect these children. They should be encouraged to be as active as possible and to live as normal a life as possible. Dietary management is very important—individuals with CF should eat nutritious foods with high amounts of essential vitamins and minerals and take a pancreatic enzyme medication to assist in digesting fats.

Family members should seek emotional support to help them face the rigors of caring for a child with an incurable, fatal disease.

Throughout the illness, it is important for the patient and family to learn as much as possible about the disease and its treatment. The Cystic Fibrosis Foundation in Bethesda, MD, Phone: (800)FIGHTCF, can provide educational and emotional support.

Treatment Research into the prevention and treatment of CF has led to many advances, but no cure exists for this disease. Treatment is a lifelong process to relieve the various problems caused by the excess sticky mucus and enzyme deficiencies. A high-protein, low-fat diet can reduce bowel symptoms in children with CF. A pancreatic enzyme medication, made from extracts of animal pancreas and available in powder or granule form, can replace the missing pancreatic enzymes. Postural drainage and chest percussion are exercises that can help clear the lungs of the thick mucus (see Postural Drainage and Chest Percussion, page 753).

Respiratory infections should be treated swiftly and promptly with appropriate dosages of the proper antibiotics. Inhaled tobramycin has recently been approved for use in children with CF. It is useful in the short term (6 months) but it is not yet known whether it will be beneficial in the long-term, as there is concern about the development of antibiotic resistance. Oxygen supplementation also may be prescribed. Progressive damage to the lungs may necessitate a lung transplant (see this page).

Prognosis The disease is almost invariably fatal. The median age of survival is 31.

❖ BRONCHIECTASIS

Symptoms (What you may experience) Cough that produces green or yellow phlegm; blood-tinged mucus; fatigue; loss of appetite; repeated pulmonary infections; bad breath.

Signs and laboratory findings *(What the doctor looks for)* Change in pulmonary structure as revealed by a chest x-ray or CT scan; results of analysis of mucus (it will settle into three distinct layers); and culture for bacteria.

What is it? Bronchiectasis is a chronic condition in which the bronchi become rigid, expanded, and filled with fluid. Because of the loss of tissue elasticity, the fluid cannot drain properly so it becomes stagnant, which can lead to further infection.

Bronchiectasis may be congenital but in most cases it develops during the first 20 years of life after an infectious pulmonary disease such as pneumonia, whooping cough (contagious respiratory tract infection that usually affects children), or TB.

It is a relatively uncommon condition because the illnesses that precede it can be treated effectively with antibiotics or prevented by immunization, but it does occur in almost all children with CF.

What you can do If you have been diagnosed with bronchiectasis, do not smoke, and stay out of smoke-filled rooms. Avoid dust and fumes, which also could provide further irritation.

Treatment An active case of bronchiectasis can be treated by fighting the underlying infection with antibiotics. A person with bronchiectasis can help the fluid to drain from the bronchi by performing postural drainage twice a day (see Postural Drainage and Chest Percussion, page 753).

Inhaling warm mists also can help loosen the thick mucus plugs.

If the infection is confined to a small area of the lung, surgery to remove the affected portion is an option.

Prognosis Prompt treatment with antibiotics—which are sometimes prescribed for prolonged periods—can usually control the underlying infection and prevent the condition from worsening.

❖ PNEUMOTHORAX

Symptoms *(What you may experience)* Breathlessness; sudden, sharp pain on one side of the chest; tightness across the chest.

Signs and laboratory findings *(What the doctor looks for)* Asymmetric movement of the two sides of the chest wall; lung shrinkage and air in the pleural space as shown by a chest x-ray; decreased or absent sounds of breathing over the affected area.

What is it? As air is breathed in and exhaled out of the lungs, each of the two layers of the pleura slips smoothly over the other. A pneumothorax occurs when air accumulates between the two layers, causing them to pull away from each other. This causes part of or all of the lung to collapse.

A pneumothorax may result from a chest injury that allows air from the outside to enter the pleural space or by air escaping from the lung into this cavity (for example, from a puncture wound of the lung). But it also may occur spontaneously without a predisposing trauma. When this happens it may be due to the sudden bursting of an air-containing blister, also called a bleb, on the surface of the lung. This is seen most often in otherwise healthy adults between the ages of 20 and 40. Pneumothorax also can occur as a result of a lung biopsy or a severe asthmatic attack.

Pneumothorax is classified as open (in which air flows between the pleura and the outside environment) or closed (in which air reaches the pleural space from the lung).

If the amount of air that has bled into the pleural cavity is relatively small it may disappear quickly. The seriousness of the problem depends on the size of the injury or on how much air enters the pleura. A large pneumothorax can result in increasing breathlessness and pain as large portions of the lung collapse.

What you can do Penetrating chest wounds should be covered to prevent more air from entering. Seek emergency care.

When to call the doctor Although a small pneumothorax may resolve on its own, the condition should be evaluated by a doctor. Increasing breathlessness and increasing chest pain may indicate that the pneumothorax is increasing in size.

Treatment Therapy depends largely on the size of the pneumothorax and the condition of your lungs. A small pneumothorax (in which less than 25 percent of the lung is collapsed) generally will heal on its own and may require only a few days of bed rest and x-ray evaluation to monitor the amount

THE USE OF HOME OXYGEN

If you have a significant lack of oxygen in your blood as the result of a chronic lung disease, you may need to have supplemental oxygen at home. This can be prescribed by your doctor.

A low level of blood oxygen makes your heart work harder in an effort to supply oxygen to your tissues. Using supplemental oxygen decreases the heart's workload.

If you are homebound and need supplemental oxygen, an electrically powered device called an oxygen concentrator can make oxygen to supply your needs. Once it is plugged in it never needs to be refilled. A backup oxygen cylinder is provided in the event of a power failure.

Oxygen feeds fires so you must be especially careful when you have supplemental oxygen in your home. Anything that can produce intense heat, flames, or sparks should be kept well away from the oxygen source. This means no matches, heaters, or hair dryers. If you have to use a heating pad make sure you do so in another part of the house.

Also, flammable materials such as alcohol and aerosol sprays should not be stored or used around oxygen.

The temperature around the oxygen tank or device should always be lower than 125°F.

If you use oxygen tanks, put them in an out-of-the-way area in which they will not fall. Make sure they are covered tightly when not in use.

Pay close attention to the technician who will instruct you on how to properly use the oxygen tanks or device.

Most oxygen tanks for home use are large and heavy. For those who need oxygen away from home only occasionally, a portable oxygen delivery system, which consists of a small tank of the gas and a wheeled carriage you can push or pull with one hand, may suffice. The cylinder weighs about 15 lbs and supplies about 2 to $3\frac{1}{2}$ hours worth of oxygen.

For those people who regularly need oxygen away from home, an ambulatory unit carried over the shoulder can allow people to participate in the normal activities of daily living outside the home. They weigh as little as 6 to 7 lbs and provide up to about 6 hours of oxygen. Unfortunately these units are more expensive and are not paid for by some medical insurance, Medicaid, or some HMOs.

The supply of oxygen used outside the home can be prolonged by the use of oxygen conservation devices that deliver the oxygen only when the person breathes in.

Oxygen may be delivered either by a nasal catheter, facemask, or a catheter inserted directly into the trachea. The most widely used device, the nasal catheter, also called nasal prongs, is used when low levels of oxygen are needed. The facemask delivers higher oxygen concentrations. Occasionally the transtracheal catheter is employed in people who require high oxygen concentrations but do not want to use a facemask. ■

of air in the pleural cavity and confirm that the lung has regained its normal size and contains air.

A large pneumothorax may require an attempt to suck the excess air out of the pleural cavity. This can be accomplished with a needle and syringe or, more effec-

tively, with a catheter and the application of gentle suction for about 24 hours. Often oxygen is administered by facemask to speed up the absorption of the air. When a pneumothorax occurs more than once, it may be necessary to perform surgery to close off the air-containing blister.

Prognosis Prognosis for a small pneumothorax is excellent. However, if a large pneumothorax is left untreated, death from respiratory failure can result. Spontaneous pneumothorax recurs about 50 percent of the time within 2 years.

CHRONIC OBSTRUCTIVE PULMONARY DISEASE

Also known as chronic obstructive lung disease, this series of illnesses, which includes emphysema and chronic bronchitis, affects an estimated 16 million Americans and claims the lives of approximately 96,000 Americans each year. Chronic obstructive pulmonary disease (COPD) is the fourth leading cause of death in the United States. Men are affected more often than are women, probably because until recently men smoked more heavily. About 80 to 90 percent of cases are caused by smoking (see Smoking and Lung Disease, page 757). A smoker is 10 times more likely than is a nonsmoker to die of COPD. Recurrent or chronic respiratory infections also can cause COPD.

COPD is chronic airway obstruction that worsens gradually over time. Many, if not all, people affected by these diseases will need supplemental oxygen (see The Use of Home Oxygen, this page). However the inflammation that is an early sign of the disease may reverse if the person stops smoking before lung damage is extensive.

❖ EMPHYSEMA

Symptoms (*What you may experience*) Slow, subtle development of increasing breathlessness; chronic cough; weight loss and loss of appetite; barrel-chested appearance; bluish nailbeds; prolonged exhalations with grunting.

Signs and laboratory findings (*What the doctor looks for*) Chest x-ray results; the degree of remaining lung capacity as assessed by pulmonary function tests; signs of right-

SMOKING AND LUNG DISEASE

Smoking is believed to cause 90 percent of all lung cancers and is considered a contributing factor in as many as 30 percent of all cancer deaths. Cigarettes contain at least 43 distinct carcinogens (cancer-causing agents). Smoking is the main cause of COPD.

Smoking by parents also has bad consequences on the health of their children. Smoking during pregnancy accounts for an estimated 20 to 30 percent of low-birth-weight babies and about 10 percent of all infant deaths. Even apparently healthy babies of smokers have been born with narrowed airways and lower lung function.

Children of parents who smoke cigarettes have more colds and ear infections than children of nonsmokers. Children with asthma and parents who smoke have more severe symptoms of their disease. Up to 300,000 cases of lower respiratory tract infections in children less than 18 months old are caused by secondhand smoke.

Secondhand smoke also is believed to cause 3,000 lung cancer deaths each year.

Approximately 23.1 million American women smoke cigarettes. Women over age 34 who currently smoke are 12 times more likely to die prematurely from lung cancer than are nonsmoking women. More American women die annually of lung cancer than of any other type of cancer. In 1996 lung cancer was responsible for an estimated 64,000 female deaths in the United States; breast cancer killed 44,300.

Current estimates are that 26 million American men are cigarette smokers. Current male smokers over age 35 are almost 10 times more likely to die of COPD and are 22 times more likely to die of lung cancer than are nonsmoking males.

About 3.1 million adolescents are current smokers.

The most notorious constituent of tobacco smoke is the addictive chemical nicotine. But cigarette smoke also contains solid particulate matter known as tar. When these particles are inhaled they coat the interior of the lungs. Tar contains thousands of chemicals, a number of which are known to be carcinogens. Some chemicals in tar act in concert with other chemicals in smoke to cause lung cancer.

The smoke from cigarettes also contains carbon monoxide, which attaches to your red blood cells in place of oxygen, decreasing the amount of oxygen your blood delivers to muscle and other tissues. It can make you feel tired and out of breath and cause headache or worsen heart disease symptoms.

In addition, cigarette smoke also paralyzes the cilia present in the airway linings that sweep unwanted debris in the lungs up toward the throat. Smoke also causes your lungs to produce more mucus. When a smoker sleeps the cilia begin to recover and move mucus and impurities out of the lung. This explains the smoker's cough that is present when a smoker awakens.

Smoke also causes deep lung damage by causing the alveoli to stretch and break. This damage is irreparable and eventually leads to emphysema. As more alveoli become damaged, your body puts less and less oxygen into your bloodstream.

In the last few years, more and more evidence has uncovered associations between secondhand, also called sidestream, smoke and heart and lung diseases. It is now clear that you do not have to smoke actively to experience the detrimental effects of tobacco—just inhaling the smoke produced by cigarettes and exhaled by others can increase your risk of developing a dangerous or deadly disease.

Smoking is the single largest preventable cause of premature death and disability in the United States.

So what should you do if you smoke? Simple. You should stop. But only you can make that decision. If you want healthier lungs, talk with your doctor about which smoking cessation program is best for you. See Chapter 4 for more information on how to stop smoking. ■

---

sided heart failure as assessed by an electro-cardiogram (ECG) during the late stages of the disease; the degree of oxygen saturation as gauged by analysis of blood gases.

What is it? In emphysema the millions of alveoli become stretched out of shape or rupture. This destroys the elasticity of the lungs, disrupting their ability to fully contract and expand. Consequently breathing becomes labored and inefficient. People with advanced emphysema expend great amounts of energy to breathe and rid their bodies of excess carbon dioxide. They develop a rounded barrel chest from overinflation of the lungs. The shortness of breath that is the main symptom of emphysema is the result of this inefficient breathing process.

Emphysema is the most common cause of death from respiratory disease in the United States. About 2 million Americans have emphysema; of them, 61 percent are men and 39 percent are women. The disease is increasing among women. Between 1982 and 1994 the prevalence rate in women increased by 11 percent.

Ninety percent of cases of emphysema can be attributed to smoking.

A small percentage of cases of emphysema are caused by an inherited gene mutation that causes a lack of a protective protein called alpha$_1$-antitrypsin (AAT). The protein normally protects the lungs from a natural enzyme that helps fight bacteria and clean up dead lung tissue. However, the enzyme can damage lung tissue if not neutralized by AAT. This can lead to an inherited form of emphysema that can appear when a person is as young as age 30 or 40. Normally emphysema takes decades to develop. About 50,000 to 100,000 Americans alive today (about 1 in 2,500), most of northern European descent, are at risk for developing premature emphysema.

Emphysema increases your susceptibility to life-threatening lung infections such as pneumonia.

As the disease progresses and lung tissue deteriorates, the blood vessels that carry blood to the lungs for oxygen replenishment become narrowed or destroyed. These changes, in turn, make it harder for the right side of the heart to pump blood through the lungs. The right side of the heart ends up working harder and harder, and it eventually weakens and becomes less able to perform this function. The right ventricle distends (enlarges), which causes the pressure to rise in the veins bringing blood from the body to the right side of the heart. The net effect is the development of right-sided heart fail-

ure, also called cor pulmonale. See Pulmonary Hypertension/Cor Pulmonale, page 761, for more information on right-sided heart failure.

What you can do The most important thing you can do to prevent emphysema is to stop smoking; 1 in 7 smokers develops COPD. Many smokers dismiss early symptoms such as smoker's cough. But a simple forced expiration volume test (see Pulmonary Function Tests, page 000) can indicate whether you are at higher risk for COPD. Emphysema develops slowly over decades; if you stop smoking before symptoms develop, you can halt the progression of the disease. See Chapter 4 for information on how to stop smoking.

If you have a family history of emphysema related to AAT deficiency it is important to get screened for the disease as early as possible. Early treatment can slow or halt symptom progression once the disease process has begun.

What you can do If you have emphysema, you should take steps to avoid pulmonary infections. Get yourself immunized against influenza and pneumonia and avoid close contact with people who have colds or lung infections.

You should also take steps to keep yourself as healthy as possible. Eat right and exercise as regularly as you can. While physical activity may cause shortness of breath, this is not dangerous, and prudent exercise can increase your ability to breathe.

When to call the doctor If you smoke and have chronic cough or phlegm or you are experiencing decreased exercise tolerance, see your doctor regularly to be tested for signs of developing COPD.

Treatment Your doctor may prescribe bronchodilators. These include inhaled anticholinergic agents, inhaled selective beta-sympathomimetics, and oral theophylline. Any chest infection that occurs requires prompt treatment with antibiotics.

If emphysema leads to pulmonary hypertension (see page 761) your doctor may prescribe a portable oxygen tank for you (see The Use of Home Oxygen, page 756). The oxygen may not relieve symptoms of breathlessness but it may increase exer-

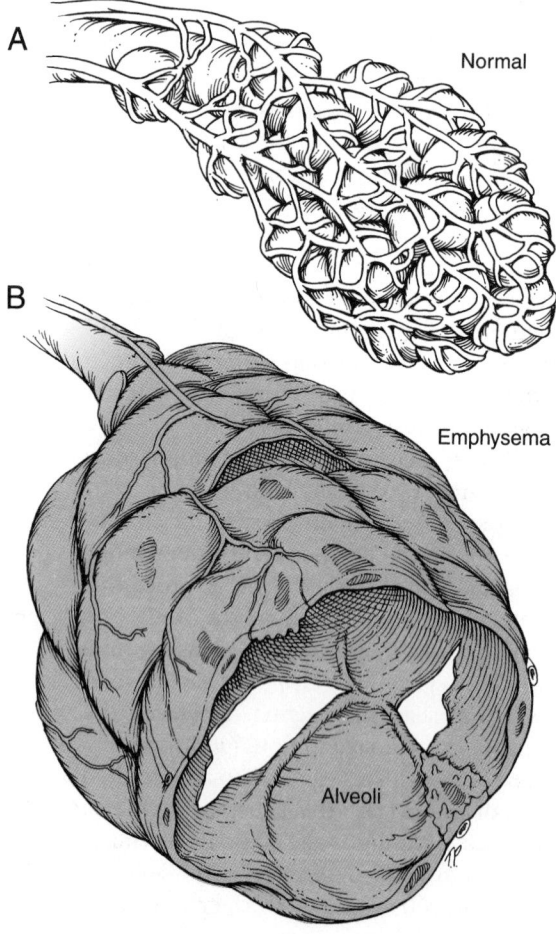

In emphysema (B), prolonged smoking leads to destruction of the walls of the air sacs (alveoli), resulting in larger airspaces. Less oxygen is absorbed into the blood because of the loss of alveoli, leading to shortness of breath.

A Normal

B Emphysema

Alveoli

cise capacity and will prolong survival in people with low oxygen levels.

Lung transplantation may be an option for some people (see The Lung Transplant, page 754). Lung volume reduction surgery is another promising—though unproven—surgical approach for some people.

People who have emphysema related to AAT deficiency should never smoke. Smoking significantly increases the risk and severity of the disease and may cause the lifespan to decrease by 10 years or more. A special drug called alpha$_1$-proteinase inhibitor raises AAT levels in the body and shields the lungs against the destructive enzyme.

Prognosis Emphysema cannot be cured, but if it is caught early, its progression can be halted.

❖ CHRONIC BRONCHITIS

Symptoms *(What you may experience)* A morning cough that produces mucus (over time the amount of mucus increases and coughing lasts well into the day); breathlessness; wheezing.

Signs and laboratory findings *(What the doctor looks for)* History of symptoms and smoking; the degree of lung functioning as determined by lung function tests; signs of infection as detected by a chest x-ray; oxygen level in the blood as determined by blood gases testing.

What is it? Chronic bronchitis is similar to acute bronchitis, but in the chronic form the inflammation of the airways persists and intensifies. It is dangerous because it leads to repeated infections that can thicken and distort the linings of the bronchi and bronchioles. This narrows the airways, and if too much mucus is secreted, they can easily become blocked.

Chronic bronchitis is defined as the presence of a mucus-producing cough that occurs on most days of the month for 3 months a year during 2 successive years without other underlying symptoms to explain the cough. Most people with chronic bronchitis have had daily cough and phlegm throughout the year for many years. It usually is most prominent in the morning. Chronic bronchitis may precede or accompany emphysema.

As much as 5 percent of the general population of the United States may be affected by chronic bronchitis. It is more common in people over age 40. Smokers are more likely than nonsmokers to develop chronic bronchitis. People who work in certain jobs—especially those that involve high concentrations of dust and irritating fumes, such as coal mining, grain handling, and metal working—are at high risk of developing the disease.

Symptoms are exacerbated by high concentrations of atmospheric pollutants such as sulfur dioxide.

If the infections you experience eventually spread into the alveoli, you could develop pneumonia or emphysema. It is important not to ignore the symptoms. Seek treatment at its earliest stages.

If ignored, chronic bronchitis also could lead to pulmonary hypertension and right-sided heart failure (see Pulmonary Hypertension/Cor Pulmonale, page 761).

What you can do Smoking is the leading cause of chronic bronchitis, so the best way to prevent it is to stop smoking. (See Chapter 4 for information on how to stop smoking.) If you work in areas that have high concentration of dust or irritating fumes, you may want to consider wearing a mask that covers your nose and mouth.

If you live in a damp, cold region, you may want to think about moving to a locale that is warmer and drier.

If you have chronic bronchitis, drink lots of water and fruit juice to make your lung secretions less viscous and thick. Stay away from people who have colds and other respiratory infections. Get yourself immunized against influenza and pneumonia.

You should also take steps to keep yourself as healthy as possible. Eat right and exercise as regularly as you can.

When to call the doctor If you continue to cough and produce large amount of mucus after a winter cold seems cured, or if you have a cough that is a constant presence and which is worse in the morning and in damp, cold weather, consult your doctor.

Treatment If you have trouble breathing, your doctor may prescribe an aerosol inhaler that will decrease the inflammation in your breathing passages and widen them, allowing you to breathe more easily. You also may need supplemental oxygen (see The Use of Home Oxygen, page 756). Your doctor also may prescribe antibiotics as a preventive measure against recurring bacterial infections.

Prognosis If the disease is advanced and severe, the long-term outlook is poor. But catching it and treating it early improves the outlook.

Diseases of the Lungs and Cardiovascular System

Your heart and lungs work together to provide oxygen to the body tissues. Deoxygenated blood travels to the right side of the heart, from which it is pumped to the lungs. There, red blood cells absorb oxygen and release carbon dioxide. The oxygenated blood then goes back to the heart—the left side, this time—from which it is sent to deliver oxygen and other nutrients to all other parts of the body.

Sometimes a blood clot may stand in the way of blood on its way to the right side of the heart. If the clot, or a piece of it, breaks off and travels to the lungs, a pulmonary embolism may result. Chronic lung disease may increase the heart's workload and damage it, as in the disease process known as pulmonary hypertension.

❖ PULMONARY EMBOLISM

Symptoms *(What you may experience)* Breathlessness; chest pain; bloody sputum.

Signs and laboratory findings *(What the doctor looks for)* Condition of the lung's blood vessels as revealed by pulmonary angiography (see Pulmonary Angiogram, page 728); chest x-ray results to rule out other causes; ECG results to rule out heart attack; blood clots blocking blood vessels as detected by radionuclide lung scan (V/Q scan).

What is it? An embolus is a clot of blood or other matter that moves through the bloodstream. When it becomes lodged in an artery, blocking blood flow to tissue downstream from the site, it is called an embolism. If an embolus passes through the right side of the heart and into the pulmonary artery and lodges there, it is called a pulmonary embolism. As a cerebral embolism results in the death of brain cells, a pulmonary embolism can prevent a part of the lung from receiving blood and taking up oxygen, so some lung tissue may die.

Pulmonary embolism strikes an estimated 500,000 adults annually in the United States and causes 50,000 deaths. About 10 percent of these deaths occur within an hour of the onset of symptoms. Pulmonary embolism affects three women for every two men.

Most pulmonary emboli result from blood clots, also called thrombi, in the deep veins of the leg or pelvis (see Deep Vein Thrombosis, page 833). An underlying disorder is usually the cause. Most commonly, clot formation may be encouraged by long-term immobility caused by disabling illness. Obesity, atrial fibrillation (a type of heart rhythm irregularity), sickle cell disease, use of oral contraceptives, recent surgery, and

Blood flowing from the heart to the lungs can become obstructed by a clump of material in the blood vessels (pulmonary arteries). This material, or embolus, is usually a blood clot that has broken loose (thromboembolism) but can also be air, tumor, fat, or other substance. Shortness of breath and chest pain are common symptoms of an embolism that is lodged in the lungs.

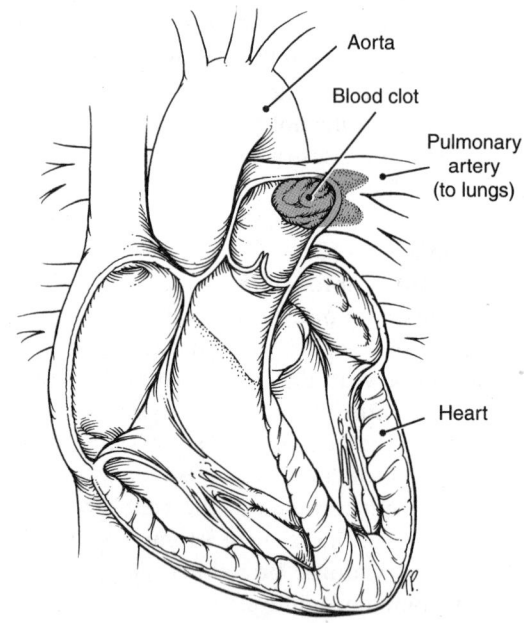

Aorta

Blood clot

Pulmonary artery (to lungs)

Heart

leg fractures also encourage the development of clots and increase the risk of pulmonary embolism. Many people with pulmonary embolism have abnormal clotting factors in the blood that predispose them to blood clots.

What you can do Since immobility and inactivity encourage clots to form in the veins of the leg, being active and moving about helps to keep them from forming. Elastic support stockings may assist blood circulation in the legs. If you are seated for a long time, as on an overseas air flight, get up and move around every once in a while. After surgery it is important to be mobile as soon as your doctor says you may.

If you are a woman over age 35 and are taking oral contraceptives, ask your doctor about other methods of birth control. The risk of thrombosis (blood clot formation) associated with oral contraceptives increases with age.

When to call the doctor Pulmonary embolism is an emergency situation; if you detect any of the symptoms seek medical help immediately.

Treatment As noted above, certain conditions increase the likelihood of embolus formation. But actually making the diagnosis of pulmonary embolism can be difficult, especially if the person being examined already has a disease process that affects the heart and lungs.

Once the diagnosis is established, initial treatment can include the use of painkilling medication if chest pain is severe and oxygen therapy when blood oxygen levels are low.

To prevent further blood clots from forming your doctor may prescribe a blood-thinning medication such as heparin. Heparin therapy, given as an intravenous infusion, may last as long as 10 to 14 days. Warfarin, another blood-thinning agent, is usually then given orally and should overlap with heparin therapy for about 5 to 7 days. In some people anticoagulation therapy can be discontinued after 2 to 3 months; otherwise, treatment may continue for as long as 6 months. If the blood clots are recurrent, anticoagulants may be prescribed indefinitely.

People being treated with medications such as heparin and warfarin may have bleeding complications, so they should be closely monitored. Those who take anticoagulant medications should be careful not to take aspirin—or an over-the-counter (OTC) remedy that may contain aspirin as one of its ingredients—which can further impair blood clotting. Oral anticoagulants also may interact with a number of other medications, so be sure to tell your doctor about any other medications you may be taking. People taking these medications should avoid situations in which they could be injured, such as contact sports or skiing.

Thrombolytic (clot-busting) medications such as tissue plasminogen activator and streptokinase can dissolve clots that have already formed. These medications can be used when a massive pulmonary embolism causes extremely low blood pressure. Thrombolytics should not be used in a person who has had a stroke within 2 months, is pregnant, has uncontrolled hypertension, has active bleeding from any source, or has undergone surgery within the preceding 10 days.

In some cases the blockage must be removed surgically in a procedure called a pulmonary embolectomy (removal of an embolus from a blood vessel).

Prognosis If you have a massive pulmonary embolism—more than a 50 percent obstruction of the pulmonary circulation—and survive the first few days, your chances of a complete recovery are excellent. If the cause leading to the formation of emboli is determined and treated, your risk of having another pulmonary embolism is greatly reduced.

Sometimes a blockage of the pulmonary artery may be partial and so mild as to produce no symptoms.

❖ PULMONARY HYPERTENSION/COR PULMONALE

Symptoms (*What you may experience*) Chronic productive cough; breathlessness upon exertion; wheezing; fatigue and weakness; distended neck veins; enlarged tender liver; fluid retention and swelling in the lower limbs.

Signs and laboratory findings (*What the doctor looks for*) Enlargement of the heart's right ventricle as detected by echocardiography (ultrasound examination of the heart) and a chest x-ray; increased blood pressure in the pulmonary artery as indicated by echocardiography; the degree of oxygen saturation as assessed by analysis of arterial blood gas; heart rhythm as determined by an ECG; functioning of the lungs as detected by pulmonary function tests.

What is it? Cor pulmonale or pulmonary hypertension is a condition that arises from the close interaction between the heart and lungs. (*Cor* means heart; *pulmonale* means related to the lungs.) Under normal conditions the right side of the heart is weaker than the left side because the right side requires relatively little muscle to push the blood through the lungs. Consequently blood pressure in the blood vessels that carry blood to the lungs from the heart is lower than the pressure in the blood vessels that carry blood to the rest of the body from the left side of the heart.

A severe lung disease such as emphysema or other conditions associated with low oxygen levels makes it harder for the heart to pump blood through the lungs. The heart must exert increasing effort and pressure. The heart compensates by distending and thickening the right-sided chambers, but this usually results in right-sided heart failure. Since oxygenation of the blood may decrease, the bone marrow produces more red blood cells, which causes the blood to become thicker and more viscous, further increasing the load on the heart.

About 85 percent of people with cor pulmonale have COPD, and about 25 percent of people with COPD eventually develop cor pulmonale.

Other conditions that could cause the development of cor pulmonale include CF, extensive surgery to remove significant amounts of lung tissue, and chronic altitude sickness. Primary pulmonary hypertension, which often leads to cor pulmonale, is a condition in which the blood vessels in the lung narrow and become blocked without other lung diseases being present. Its cause is unknown but it may occur in association with the use of some diet drugs or with some forms of scleroderma. Secondary pulmonary hypertension may occur when the blood flow to the lungs is elevated—as with atrial septal defect (a congenital heart abnormality)—or the pressure in the left side of the heart is high—as with mitral

stenosis (the narrowing of a specific valve on the left side of the heart).

What you can do Since many cases of cor pulmonale are associated with COPD, which can be caused by smoking, the best way to prevent this disorder is not to smoke (see Chronic Obstructive Pulmonary Disease, page 756).

If you have symptoms suggestive of a serious lung disease such as emphysema, early treatment can slow the progression of the disease and accompanying conditions. Since low oxygen levels are a major contributing factor, the use of oxygen can prevent or delay cor pulmonale.

When to call the doctor If you notice swelling of your ankles and you become winded, weak, and tired upon exercising, contact your doctor. Also contact your doctor if the blood vessels in your neck are bulging.

Treatment Treatment may include medications such as calcium channel blockers to lower increased pulmonary pressure and oxygen to treat low oxygen levels. Your doctor also may put you on a low-salt, restricted-fluid diet to reduce the fluid accumulation in your lower limbs. He also may prescribe a low dosage of an anticoagulant medication to reduce the risk of a blood clot and subsequent pulmonary embolism.

Your doctor also will institute treatment for whatever underlying condition led to the development of cor pulmonale.

In primary pulmonary hypertension, chronic infusion of medications such as prostacyclin to dilate the blood vessels can be helpful. Lung transplantation may be useful in some cases.

Prognosis Since cor pulmonale generally occurs late during the course of COPD and other irreversible diseases, the long-term outlook usually is poor.

Cancers of the Lung and Pleura

Like almost all other parts of the body, the respiratory system is subject to the unrestrained growth of cells commonly referred to as cancer. Cigarette smoking is generally accepted as the major cause of lung cancer.

❖ LUNG CANCER

Symptoms *(What you may experience)* Cough; shortness of breath; wheezing; bloody sputum; weight loss; chest pain; hoarseness. Lung tumors may alter hormone production, leading to such symptoms as gynecomastia (breast enlargement in men) and bone pain. Lung cancer may also cause muscle weakness or difficulty with walking or coordination.

Signs and laboratory findings *(What the doctor looks for)* Abnormal spots on the lungs as detected by a chest x-ray or CT scan; visual inspection of the airways with the aid of bronchoscopy; the presence of abnormal cells as detected by a biopsy, by analysis of sputum coughed up from the lungs, or by thoracentesis.

What is it? Lung cancer is the uncontrolled growth of abnormal cells in the lungs. The abnormal cells may not perform the work of normal cells, and they crowd out and destroy healthy tissue. Some lung tumors are benign, meaning they have a defined border and can be completely excised. Other tumors are malignant—they can invade adjacent tissue and spread to other parts of the body.

Lung cancer kills more men and women than does any other form of cancer. Approximately 160,000 men and women die of lung cancer each year. It was estimated that in 1996 there would be 177,000 new cases of lung cancer.

Given the large air space in the lungs, a tumor located in the outer part of the lung may not produce any symptoms until it is fairly large. Because there are few pain fibers in the lungs, most lung cancers grow silently, without any symptoms, until they are at an advanced stage, which may take 10 to 40 years. Sometimes the first sign is pain from the tumor growing into the lining of the lungs or the ribs and muscles of the chest wall.

As many as 80 percent of all lung cancers are due to tobacco smoke and its many known cancer-causing chemicals. A smoker's risk of developing lung cancer is 8 to 20 times higher than that of a nonsmoker. But stopping smoking decreases the risk of developing lung cancer over time. In 10 years the risk decreases to a level that is 30 to 50 percent of the risk for people who continue to smoke.

Many occupations carry an increased risk of lung cancer. Compared to the general, nonsmoking population, asbestos insulation workers who smoke have 92 times the risk of developing lung cancer, and smelter workers have three to eight times the risk. Risk also is increased for people who work in the manufacturing of industrial gases, drugs, soaps and detergents, paints, plastics, and synthetic rubber.

Radon, a naturally occurring radioactive gas that is formed by the breakdown of radium, is another factor that increases the risk of lung cancer in the United States. Radon problems have been identified in every state. The Environmental Protection Agency estimates that nearly 1 in 15 American homes has indoor radon levels at or above the recommended level of 4 picocuries per liter of air. Radon can be a problem in schools and workplaces, too.

The risk of developing lung cancer is higher for people who live in some urban areas because of their increased exposure to air pollutants. In general, the greater the amount of exposure to a cancer-causing agent, the greater the risk of disease.

Lung cancers are broadly classified as small cell or non–small cell carcinomas. Non-small cell cancers are further divided into large cell, squamous cell, and adenocarcinomas.

- *Small cell carcinomas.* Also known as oat cell carcinomas because the cells resemble oats when seen under a microscope, small cell carcinomas make up 20 percent of all lung cancers. They are the most aggressive form of lung cancer; they tend to grow rapidly and spread early and extensively to other sites in the body. Physically, they are soft and bulky. Small cell carcinomas most commonly cause hormonal disruption. The cells of the tumor may produce adrenocorticotropic hormone, resulting in Cushing's syndrome (see page 1195). Because spread of the tumor may not be apparent, people with small cell carcinomas should be evaluated to see if the cells have spread to the liver, bone, and bone marrow.

- *Large cell carcinomas.* This type of carcinoma accounts for up to 15 percent of all lung cancers. They grow rapidly, spread at an early stage of development, and are strongly associated with smoking. The tumors are soft, bulky masses with large areas of dead tissue. A subtype of this kind of lung cancer is giant cell carcinoma, which is particularly aggressive.

- *Squamous cell carcinomas.* Squamous cell carcinomas account for about 30 percent of all lung cancers and also are associated closely with a history of cigarette smoking. These are bronchogenic tumors, meaning that they originate from the cells that line the main bronchi. About 66 percent involve the main, lobar, and segmental bronchi. The remaining one-third arise in the smaller air passages. The term squamous refers to the flattened appearance of the tumor cells; the tumor cells mimic the appearance of the squamous cells of the skin. Squamous cell carcinoma is associated with excess blood levels of calcium due to a substance the tumor cells produce.

- *Adenocarcinomas.* These are the most common non–small cell cancers. They account for up to 35 percent of all cases of primary lung cancer and are the most common lung cancers seen in women and nonsmokers. Most adenocarcinomas occur deep in the lungs. They often are discovered accidentally on routine chest x-rays. A subtype of adenocarcinoma is bronchoalveolar cell carcinoma. An uncommon type of lung cancer, it affects the alveoli.

Cancer in the lungs also may arise as a metastasis (spreading) of cells from their primary location in another part of the body such as the colon or kidney. Metastases to the lungs from cancers elsewhere in the body usually cause multiple tumors in the lungs.

It is estimated that on average 5 to 10 years elapse between the development of the first lung cancer cell and diagnosis of the disease. Because of this delay, 75 percent of all cancers have spread before diagnosis and cannot be cured by lung resection (surgical removal of part of the lung). Radiation and chemotherapy rarely cure primary lung cancers. Because early diagnosis and treatment of lung cancer is difficult, prevention is paramount.

What you can do If you smoke cigarettes, stop. Talk with your doctor about products and programs that can help you. (See Chapter 4 for information on how to stop smoking.) The sooner you stop, the greater the reduction in your risk for lung cancer. If you do not smoke, make sure your rights to a smoke-free environment are upheld; secondhand smoke has been proven to increase your risk of lung cancer.

Test your home for radon gas if you live in an area in which radon levels are high. See Chapter 3 for more information on testing your home for radon.

Treatment Treatment options depend on the type of cancer, its location, where it occurs in the lung, and whether it has spread to the lymph nodes or other parts of the body outside the lungs.

Although only about one-quarter of lung cancer patients are candidates for surgery, surgery is the only option that holds the possibility of a complete cure. In those cases in which lung cancer is diagnosed while the tumor is still small (less than 3 cm), 75 percent can be removed surgically with a five-year survival rate of 40 to 50 percent. If the cancer is found in the lymph nodes, there is a high probability that it will recur.

Sometimes surgical removal of the tumor is done knowing that it will improve the person's quality of life but not effect a cure. About 25 to 40 percent of all people with lung cancer undergo surgery to remove not just the tumor but the adjacent lymph nodes and a portion of healthy tissue as well. Sometimes it is necessary to remove an entire lung.

If a tumor is obstructing an air passage, air flow may be restored by firing a laser down the airway to obliterate the tissue overgrowth.

Lung cancer can be locally treated by means of radiation therapy in the form of high-energy x-rays. A radiation beam can be tightly controlled so it kills only the cancer cells, leaving healthy tissue relatively untouched. It may be used in conjunction with surgery or chemotherapy.

Chemotherapy, the administration of a combination of powerful anticancer medications, is usually used to treat small cell carcinomas, while surgery is the treatment of choice for squamous cell, large cell, and adenocarcinomas unless the tumor is inaccessible or for some other reason cannot be surgically removed. See Chapter 30 for more information on the treatment of cancer.

Prognosis Only 13 percent of people with lung cancer survive for 5 years after diagnosis.

❖ METASTASIS OF CANCERS TO THE LUNGS

Symptoms *(What you may experience)* Cough; shortness of breath; wheezing; bloody sputum; chest pain.

Signs and laboratory findings *(What the doctor looks for)* Abnormal tissue growth as detected by a chest x-ray, computed tomography (CT) scan, and bronchoscopy; proteins specific to certain forms of cancer (for example, if the tissue is suspected to be a metastasis from prostate cancer, the tissue in the lungs may be tested for the presence of prostate specific antigen).

What is it? Certain cancers have a propensity to spread through the bloodstream. Sometimes malignant cells break off from the main body of a tumor and roam through the bloodstream taking up residence in a far-off organ. Since the lungs have a rich blood supply they are particularly attractive to malignant cells.

What you can do If you detect signs of any abnormality, contact your doctor as soon as possible. Early detection and treatment of cancer may result in a cure and complete eradication of the tumor.

Treatment Metastasis to the lungs may mean that the cancer is at such an advanced stage that its effects can only be mitigated but not reversed. Surgery, radiation therapy, and chemotherapy or any combination of these treatments may be called for depending on the type of cancer, its location, and how advanced it is. See Chapter 30 for more information on the treatment of cancer.

Prognosis Once a cancer has spread to the lungs, the long-term outlook generally is poor.

❖ MESOTHELIOMA

Symptoms *(What you may experience)* Rapid onset of shortness of breath; chest pain; weight loss. The mean age of onset is about age 60.

Signs and laboratory findings *(What the doctor looks for)* Diminished sounds of breathing upon listening with a stethoscope; the extent of fluid accumulation within the pleura and thickening of the pleura as revealed by a chest x-ray and CT scan; results of the examination of fluid in the pleura.

What is it? Mesotheliomas are tumors that arise from the pleura. About 20 percent of cases arise from the peritoneum, which is the membrane that lines other abdominal organs. About 75 percent of mesotheliomas are spread diffusely throughout the pleura or peritoneum (and usually are malignant), while the remainder are localized and usually benign. About three-quarters of all mesotheliomas occur in men.

Many studies have established a relationship between malignant pleural mesothelioma and long-term exposure to asbestos. Only about 8 percent of asbestos workers are at risk for developing the disease. However about 70 to 80 percent of people with malignant pleural mesothelioma report a history of exposure to asbestos. There is no reported association between cigarette smoking and mesothelioma.

Benign mesotheliomas are usually less than an inch in diameter and are confined to the surface of the lung. They are not associated with asbestos but may be associated with hypoglycemia (see page 1182). There is a long latent period between exposure to asbestos and development of a malignant tumor.

What you can do If you are exposed to asbestos through your occupation in mining, milling, or shipyard work or are exposed to insulation, brake linings, or roofing materials, wear a safety mask that reduces your inhalation of asbestos fibers.

Treatment Your doctor may recommend surgery, chemotherapy, or radiation therapy or a combination of these approaches. Pain relievers may be administered by pill, injection, or skin patch. Periodic removal of fluid may be needed to treat breathlessness.

Prognosis Malignant pleural mesothelioma progresses rapidly. Median survival time from the onset of symptoms ranges from 5 to 16 months.

❖ MEDIASTINAL TUMORS

Symptoms *(What you may experience)* Chest pain; trouble swallowing or pain when swallowing; shortness of breath; increased hoarseness. In about half of cases, symptoms are absent.

Signs and laboratory findings *(What the doctor looks for)* Gradual development of symptoms; chest x-ray results; magnetic resonance imaging (MRI) findings to distinguish between blood vessels and tumor masses; potential malignancy as determined by a tissue biopsy.

What is it? The mediastinum is the space in the middle of the chest between the pleurae. Doctors divide the mediastinum into three compartments—anterior (toward the chest), middle, and posterior (toward the spine).

The location of the mass is the chief guide in its diagnosis. Masses in the anterior mediastinum are most commonly thymoma, teratoma, thyroid lesions, or lymphoma. A mass in the middle mediastinum may be an enlargement of the pulmonary artery, it may be an aortic aneurysm (a weakness in the aertic wall), or it may be a fluid-filled cyst. Posterior mediastinal masses may arise from the spinal column or esophagus.

Treatment Most often, such tumors are the result of the spread of a malignant or systemic disease. If caught early, they can usually be removed surgically. See Chapter 30 for more information on the treatment of cancer.

NINETEEN

The Breast

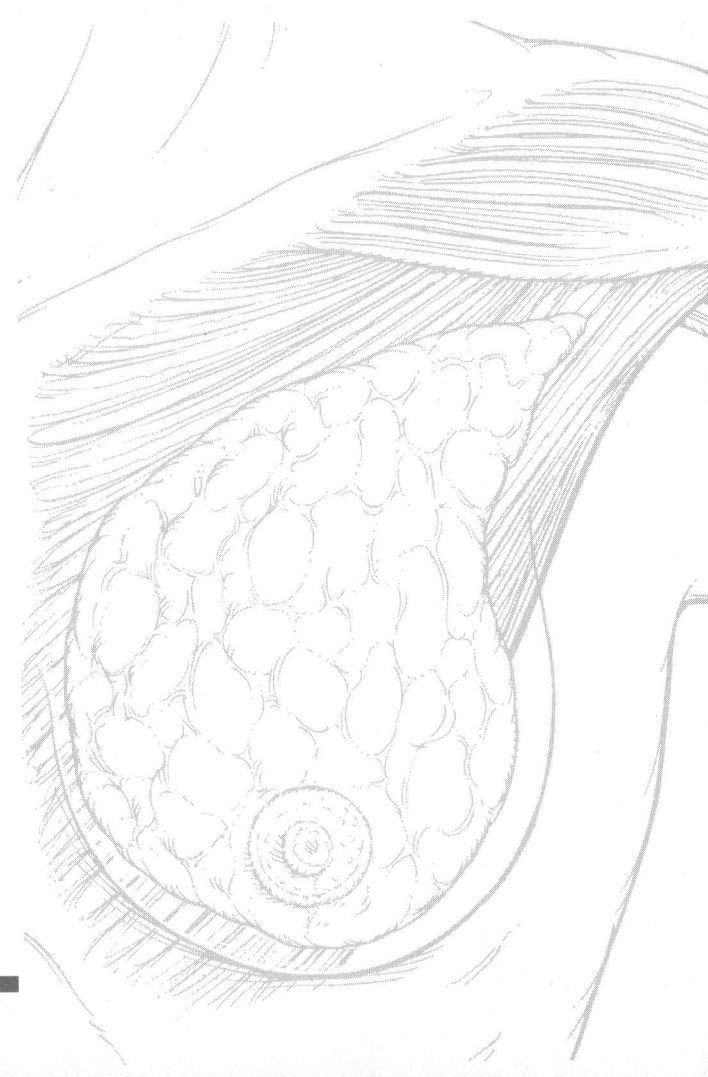

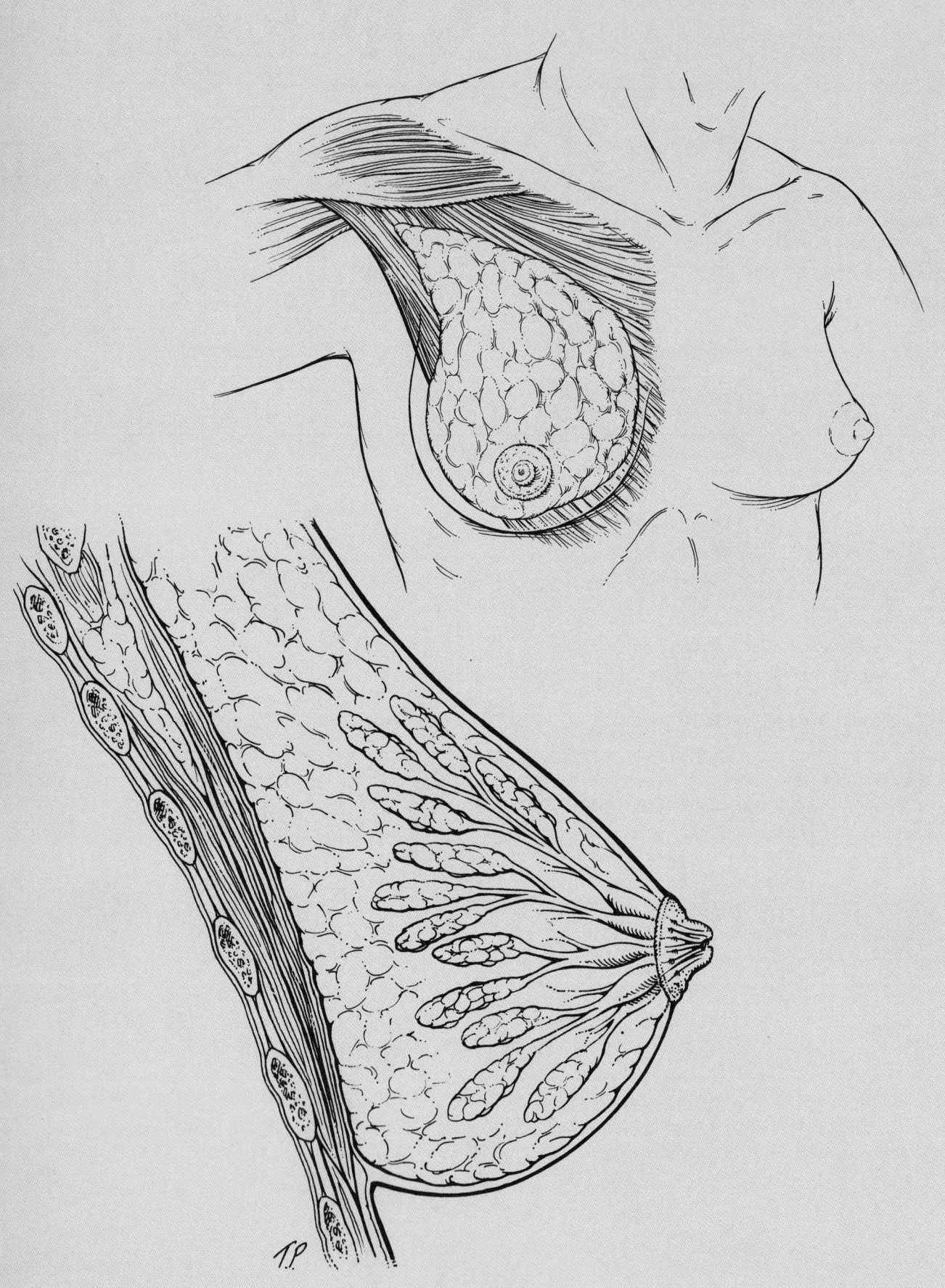

THE BREAST

Breast structure is similar in both genders from birth until before puberty. At puberty in girls, the surge of estrogen hormone drives growth and development of the mammary glands (the milk-producing parts of the breasts) as well as an increase in the fat tissues and supportive fibrous tissues of the breast. These pubertal developments, of course, do not normally occur in boys. In certain unusual circumstances, slight enlargement of breast tissue in men does occur (see page 772).

Disorders of the breast fall into two basic categories: problems originating in the body of the breast (the fat and supportive tissues or the mammary gland itself) and those involving the nipple.

The Mammary Glands

Within the body of each breast, in both men and women, lie specialized glandular tissues for the production of milk; the glands usually remain undeveloped and unproductive in men. Under normal circumstances the mammary glands only become productive in women during pregnancy and afterward, but occasionally males and younger or non-pregnant women may produce milk (see page 782).

The mammary glands consist of 15 to 20 milk ducts that radiate outward from the nipple like the spokes of a wheel toward bundles of glandular tissue embedded in the body of the breast. Problems arise when the ducts or the glandular tissues become infected, form cysts (fluid-filled cavities), or develop tumors.

❖ FIBROCYSTIC BREAST DISEASE

Symptoms (*What you may experience*) Multiple (often) lumps in both breasts (usually), increasing in size and tenderness just prior to menstrual bleeding; nipple discharge (occasionally).

Signs and laboratory findings (*What the doctor looks for*) Multiple breast lumps in women over age 30.

What is it? Fibrocystic breast disease (also often called mammary dysplasia or chronic mastitis) occurs most commonly in women over age 30 but rarely continues after

menopause. The tenderness and lumpiness of the breasts wax and wane with the menstrual cycle, reaching a peak in most women in the days just prior to the onset of menstrual bleeding. The lumps in this case represent areas of growth and dilation of milk duct and surrounding supportive tissues to form cysts. Under hormonal stimulation, the amount of fluid within the cysts can rapidly increase, thus expanding the size of the cysts and stretching their walls, which probably accounts at least in part for the tenderness associated with fibrocystic breast disease.

Your doctor can readily identify a cyst by aspiration, a technique in which the area is numbed with a little anesthetic, a needle is inserted, and the fluid is drawn into a syringe. The cysts also show up well on an ultrasound exam, a procedure in which harmless sound waves are passed through the breast and bounce or echo off tissues within it. A fluid-filled cyst will echo with a

THE PREMENSTRUAL BREAST

At puberty, adolescent girls experience a surge in estrogen hormones that stimulates the development and growth of breast tissues. From this time onward until menopause, the breast responds to the monthly waxing and waning of female reproductive hormones with some degree of swelling and quite often some tenderness in the mildly activated mammary gland—changes that prepare the breast for milk production in the event of pregnancy. The peak of monthly swelling and engorgement of breasts occurs during the week or so before the onset of menstrual bleeding, after which the symptoms subside.

While some women scarcely notice the monthly breast cycle, others experience marked premenstrual swelling and tenderness of breast, particularly those women with fibrocystic breast disease. Premenstrual breast swelling carries no serious medical risk, although it may cause considerable discomfort. Self-care remedies include wearing a supportive bra, taking mild anti-inflammatory medication such as ibuprofen, and applying warm packs. Some women also report that avoiding caffeine, salt, sugar, and alcohol lessens the discomfort. Your doctor may also prescribe a mild diuretic to reduce fluid retention during this time. ■

BREAST SELF-EXAM

The most effective way to fight breast cancer is to detect it early, and the most effective tools to detect early breast cancers are mammography and examination by a skilled doctor or nurse. Although data are insufficient to recommend breast self-exam, women performing breast self-exam find 90 percent of all breast masses. Breast self-exam should not be a replacement for a mammograph or examination by your doctor. Because breast tissue normally has a lumpy, lobular feel, each woman should become familiar with the structure of her breast to be able to recognize the difference between what is normally there and what is not. The breasts change throughout the month, as they respond to the monthly surges of hormones that occur from puberty to menopause, and you should take these charges into account when you are doing a breast self-exam. The best time for women who are premenopausal to examine their breasts is during the hormonally quiet period a few days after the end of monthly menstrual bleeding. After menopause, since the hormonal surges no longer influence breast change, any day will suffice; simply select a day of the month and make that your breast self-exam day.

The following are instructions on how to properly perform a breast self-exam.

1. Lie down comfortably. Raise the left arm over your head, and with the flattened fingers of your right hand, apply massagelike pressure to the left breast beginning with the nipple area and working in a circular pattern or an up-and-down pattern to cover the entire breast, feeling for lumps or tenderness. Do not use the tips of your fingers, which will cause you to feel many lumpy lobules of normal breast tissue. Remember that the breast is shaped like a comma with the tail leading up the side of the body toward the underarm area. Seventy-five percent of all breast cancers arise under the nipple or in the upper outer breast quadrant and in the "tail." If you are thin and you think you feel a lump, be sure what you are feeling is not a rib. A lump will usually move with the breast; a rib, of course, will not. Now repeat this part of the exam with the other breast.

2. Stand in front of a well-lighted mirror with your hands on your hips, and then with your arms raised above your head. Look for symmetry in breast shape, contour, and size. Are there areas of dimpling of the skin? Any change in skin or nipple color or texture? The skin of the breast should flow freely over the underlying tissue much like a sheer curtain in front of an open window on a windy day. Any tethering of the skin or sluggish movement associated with a slight thickening in the same area requires a clinical exam by your doctor.

3. Gently but firmly squeeze the nipple. Is there a discharge of fluid of any kind?

4. Now get into the shower or bath and wet your skin. Repeat the exam on both breasts that you just performed while lying down but now while standing or sitting up in the bath. The wetness enhances the sense of touch and makes it easier for you to feel lumps and the change of position may improve your ability to find a lump.

If you find you have difficulty performing a good exam, contact the local branch of the American Cancer Society or local hospital. They may offer classes in breast self-exam and help you to improve your examination technique. Regardless of whether or not you decide to practice breast self-exam, you should always have an annual clinical breast exam and a mammogram if you are age 50 or older. ■

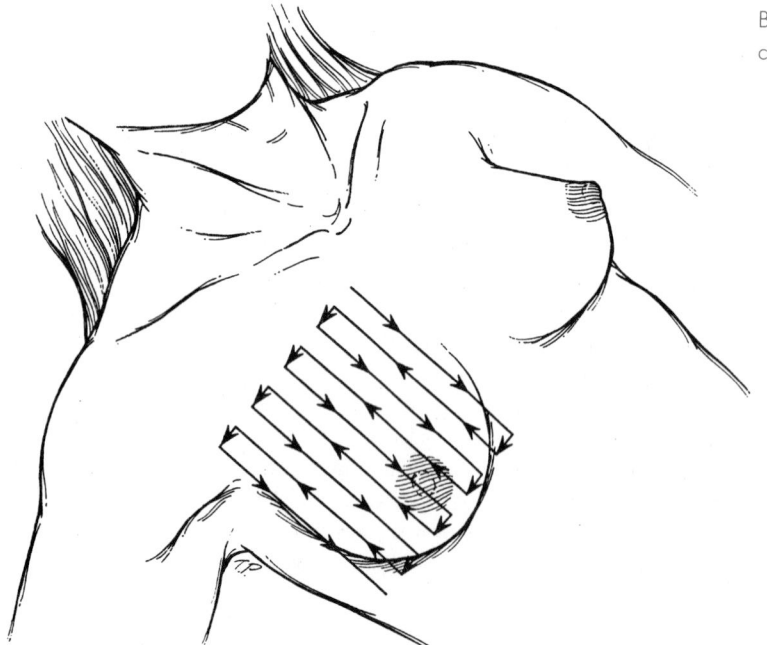

Breast self-exam. Monthly breast self-exams can help to catch a cancer early. The technique is described above.

within it. A fluid-filled cyst will echo with a different pattern than a solid area.

What you can do A number of self-care remedies may prove helpful for some people: reducing intake of caffeine, alcohol, and saturated fats may help; increasing your intake of vitamin E (in supplemental form-200 to 600 IU daily) may also help. Applying warm compresses, wearing a supportive bra, and taking ibuprofen may help to combat the tenderness and discomfort that accompany monthly breast changes. By performing regular monthly breast self-exams you will become familiar with the natural lumpiness of your own breast and will be better able to identify new or changing lumps.

When to call the doctor The appearance of a new lump or a change in the natural lumpiness of your breast should always prompt an evaluation by your doctor.

Treatment Any changing lumpiness or dominant breast mass demands careful evaluation, aspiration of fluid from cysts for examination by a pathologist and, if necessary, removal of the lump. If chronic fibrocystic breast disease causes severe discomfort, your doctor may prescribe danazol or tamoxifen to reduce cyst formation. These medications do occasionally cause adverse side effects, so you will want to discuss their potential benefits with your doctor. Increased supplementation of vitamin E and avoidance of caffeine and related methylxanthines found in coffee, tea, or chocolate may also be recommended, although studies of the effectiveness of these remedies have proven inconclusive.

Prognosis Episodes of pain and cyst formation may continue until menopause, when they subside. Hormonal replacement therapy with estrogens can prolong the disorder.

❖ BENIGN FIBROADENOMA

Symptoms (*What you may experience*) Firm, moveable, nontender breast lump.

Signs and laboratory findings (*What the doctor looks for*) No other specific signs than the lump. Ultrasound will demonstrate no fluid within the mass.

What is it? These harmless breast tumors—typically $\frac{1}{2}$ in. to 2 in. in size—occur in young women, usually before age 30. They form from the supportive fibrous tissues of the breast, as well as the tissues of the mammary glands. Fibroadenomas usually feel rubbery and firm to the touch and are painless. They may enlarge slightly under the stimulation of estrogen during the monthly menstrual cycle surges. During the major hormonal shifts that occur in pregnancy, fibrodenomas can rapidly increase in size, may become a lactating adenoma, and can sometimes be confused with breast cancer.

What you can do Perform regular breast self-exams to become familiar with the natural lumpiness of your own breast at various points in your monthly cycle. If you do discover a lump that you believe to be a fibroadenoma, see your doctor for further evaluation.

When to call the doctor Any persistent breast lump should be evaluated by a doctor as soon as possible.

Treatment In determining the cause of the lump, a surgeon may perform preliminary tests: the ultrasound test to see if the lump has fluid in it (fibroadenomas do not) and possibly a fine needle (sometimes called a skinny needle) biopsy of the lump to identify tissue type. Most doctors, however, will ultimately recommend surgical removal of the lump to allow positive identification of the tissue by the pathologist. In young women—in whom the risk of more serious causes of breast lumps is small—the surgical removal of the lump can be done as an outpatient procedure.

Prognosis Excellent for full recovery after healing of the small surgical incision.

❖ FAT NECROSIS

Symptoms and signs A lump in the breast; tender, bruised skin over the lump (occasionally).

What is it? The term fat necrosis refers to cell death that is limited to those calls in fatty tissue. This slightly unusual condition presumably arises from trauma to the fatty tissues of the breast, although only about half the people who experience fat necrosis recall a specific injury. The disorder usually causes no problems and heals without incident, but because it forms a lump in the breast it may cause alarm.

What you can do All breast lumps demand evaluation by a doctor; however, once the doctor has made the diagnosis of fat necrosis, symptomatic treatment of warm packs and mild over-the-counter pain medication such as acetaminophen may help.

When to call the doctor The discovery of any breast lump should prompt you to call the doctor.

Treatment The lump of fat necrosis usually disappears on its own; however, the safest course is to remove it to be certain the mass is indeed fat necrosis.

Prognosis Excellent for full recovery.

❖ MASTITIS

Symptoms and signs Pain and tenderness; redness and warmth of the skin over that area of the breast; fever (occasionally); tender lymph glands under the arm. (See page C-27.)

What is it? When bacteria invade the milk ducts, the infection they cause occasionally advances up the duct to the gland beyond it, which causes an inflammation of the mammary gland called mastitis. The condition occurs most commonly in breast-feeding mothers, where saliva from the baby's mouth and the mild abrasions that occur from nursing make the introduction of bacteria into the milk duct more likely to occur. Occasionally, however, mastitis arises in other circumstances. The redness and warmth of the tender area of breast tissue help to differentiate mastitis from other causes of breast pain.

What you can do Apply warm packs to the infected breast to help relieve discomfort. Acetaminophen or ibuprofen may also help to relieve pain.

When to call the doctor If the redness, warmth, and tenderness last more than 24 to 48 hours, become rapidly worse, or a fever develops, call the doctor.

Treatment Antibiotic medication to eradicate the infection usually resolves the problem quickly, but the medication may have to be used for many weeks to prevent recurrence.

Prognosis Excellent for full recovery with appropriate treatment, though late recurrence—occurring months to years later—is common.

❖ GYNECOMASTIA

Symptoms *(What you may experience)* Enlargement of one or both breasts (in males); breast tenderness (sometimes).

Signs and laboratory findings *(What the doctor looks for)* Recent use of certain medication (see page 773), indications of underlying conditions that might cause it such as hyperthyroidism or testicular tumors (rarely), and in older men signs of liver disease, kidney disease, or tumors of the lung, liver, or adrenal glands. Laboratory testing to exclude these more serious causes may include: chest x-ray, blood tests to measure function of the thyroid and adrenal glands, and blood tests to detect abnormal levels of certain hormones that may indicate tumors of the testicle, lung, liver, or pituitary gland.

What is it? In its simplest form, the term gynecomastia applies to the swelling of the mammary gland tissue in young men, usually occurring at about the time of puberty. This enlargement occurs quite commonly, usually causes some slight to moderate tenderness in the breast, may involve one or both breasts, and usually resolves on its own within a year.

When gynecomastia occurs in a healthy adolescent at about the time of puberty, it is little cause for concern or extensive investigation. Its appearance in men in their late teens and twenties demands careful examination of the testicles because breast enlargement can occur as a consequence of testicular tumors. In seniors, gynecomastia commonly arises from medication taken for other conditions but can also arise as a consequence of obesity, hyperthyroidism (overactive thyroid gland), andropause (the male equivalent of menopause when production of testos-

COMMON MEDICATION THAT MAY CAUSE GYNECOMASTIA

- Alcohol
- Amphetamines
- Cimetidine (Tagamet)
- Diazepam (Valium)
- Digitalis (Lanoxin, Digoxin)
- Estrogen
- Hydroxyzine (Vistaril)
- Ketoconazole
- Marijuana
- Methyldopa
- Metoclopramide (Reglan)
- Narcotics (codeine, oxycodone, morphine)
- Penicillamine (Cuprimine)
- Progesterone
- Reserpine
- Spironolactone
- Testosterone
- Tricyclic antidepressants (Elavil, Tofranil, Imipramine, Norpramin, Amitriptyline) ■

terone begins to wane), alcoholism, long-standing liver or kidney disease, certain cancers (notably of the lung, liver, and adrenal gland), or male breast cancer.

What you can do In a child entering puberty, the psychological and social stresses that can accompany breast enlargement frequently cause him more discomfort than the disorder itself; as unkind and unfair as it may seem, an enlarged male breast can be the object of locker room ridicule. Reassuring your child that the breast enlargement does not mean he is unmanly and that it will go away soon will help. If the swelling causes discomfort, mild pain medication, such as acetaminophen or ibuprofen and the application of warm packs may help.

When to call the doctor Boys should see the doctor for reassurance when necessary. In men, the appearance of breast enlargement should prompt a visit to the doctor as soon as possible. If drainage of fluid from the nipple occurs, see the doctor right away.

Treatment Stopping the use of any medication that might cause the enlargement, if possible, usually resolves those cases brought on by medication. Cases of pubertal gynecomastia usually require no treatment; occasionally, however, surgery to remove the enlarged gland may offer the only reasonable therapy for enlargement that fails to resolve on its own. Otherwise, therapy for the enlargement involves uncov-

ering and treating any underlying condition that causes it.

Prognosis For simple pubertal gynecomastia and for those cases caused by medication, the prognosis is excellent. In cases where a more serious underlying medical condition has brought on the enlargement, the prognosis will not be as favorable.

❖ BREAST ENLARGEMENT (VIRGINAL HYPERTROPHY)

Symptoms (What you may experience) Rapid and extreme enlargement of one or both breasts, usually at puberty.

Signs and laboratory findings (What the doctor looks for) Excessively large breast(s) in young girls.

What is it? Occasionally the surges of female hormones that occur at puberty and stimulate breast growth and development fail to "turn off" on schedule. The result of this overstimulation—enormous breasts, sometimes weighing 40 lbs or more—can cause some young girls and their families to worry. Unlike the overstimulation of the male breast at puberty—gynecomastia—virginal hypertrophy usually does not spontaneously resolve.

What you can do Reassure your child (or yourself) that the condition is harmless and usually more a cosmetic nuisance than a

BREAST REDUCTION SURGERY

Occasionally, breast development may result in the breasts becoming so large as to become burdensome. Women may choose to have their breasts surgically reduced when breast size causes difficulty in finding clothing that fits properly, causes chronic pain in the back, neck, shoulders, or chest wall from the weight of large breasts, or purely for cosmetic reasons.

Breast reduction surgery, which is routinely performed by skilled plastic surgeons, allows uplifting and tightening of breast structure and removal of a significant amount of fatty and supportive tissue. It is usually performed under a general anesthetic and will require several weeks for the suture wounds and bruising that may occur to heal. In the procedure, the surgeon measures and selects the proper location for the nipple and areola complex, which will be moved to a new, higher location. From this landmark, the surgeon sketches and cuts out a pattern for the smaller breast that will remain, removes the excess skin and breast tissue beneath it, and stitches the new, smaller breast together. In most procedures, the nipple and areola remain attached to a good portion of the mammary gland and its ducts, making it possible in about 50 percent of cases or more for a woman subsequently to breast-feed an infant should she so desire. In some cases, however, repositioning of the nipple requires severing its attachment to the underlying mammary gland and in this event, breast-feeding would not be possible. If you are considering this surgery and may later wish to breast-feed an infant, discuss your concerns with your surgeon.

Healing of the bruises and sutured areas requires a few weeks initially, but as with any cut of the skin, the body will spend the next 2 years remodeling and revising the scar that forms. In most instances the finished breast will show a fine scar from the

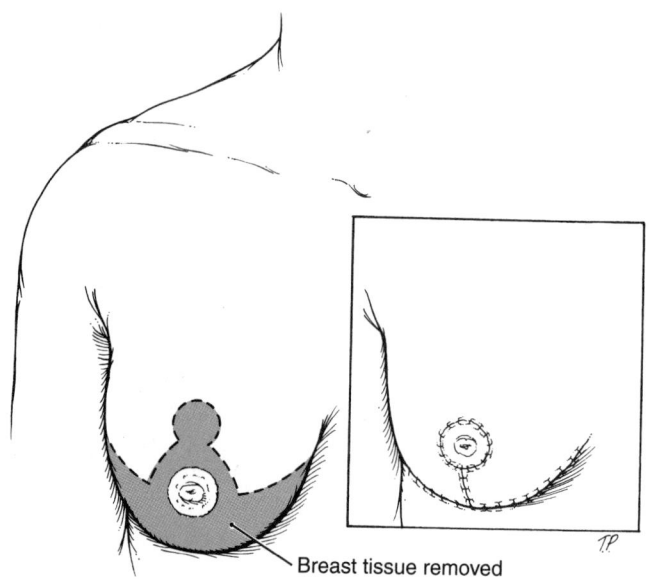

Breast tissue removed

Breast reduction surgery. In order to reduce the size of the breasts, incisions are made on the surface of the breasts, breast tissue and skin are removed, and the breasts are sutured leaving the nipple intact.

nipple downward and a smile-shaped scar in the crease underneath the breast. The scarring around the areola will be less noticeable.

The surgery offers no special risks, and women usually recover without incident. The general risks of this surgery—as with any other—involve the possibility of infection or bleeding and the risk of the anesthetic. ■

BREAST ENLARGEMENT SURGERY

Augmentation mammoplasty (the surgical technique of increasing breast size) became widely available after the development of the artificial breast implant in the 1960s. An estimated 4 million women in the United States have undergone this fairly simple surgical procedure. The surgeon creates a pocket through a small incision under the breast or under the arm, usually under the pectoralis (chest) muscle. Into this pocket the surgeon places the breast implant. Once in place, the implant settles in and the tissues of the pocket are supposed to heal to form a soft capsule around it. In as many as 25 percent of cases, the fibrous tissue of the capsule surrounding the implant becomes overgrown, causing internal scarring and distortion of the breast shape. Occasionally, the capsule scarring may necessitate removal of the implants. ▶

Breast enlargement and reconstruction surgery. For cosmetic breast augmentation, a breast implant is inserted beneath the muscles of the chest wall.

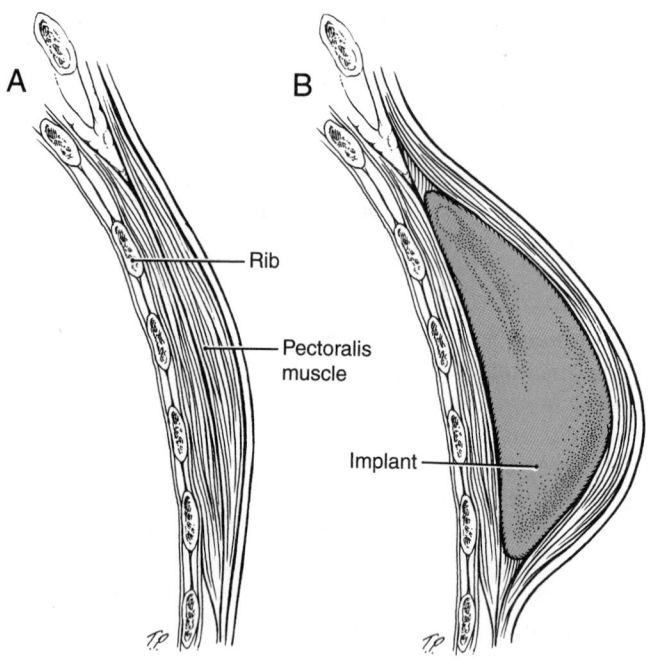

Rib

Pectoralis muscle

Implant

medical dilemma. Wearing a supportive bra will help alleviate the excessive weight.

When to call the doctor If the condition becomes extreme and the weight or size of the breasts cause problems—difficulty finding clothing that fits or back, shoulder, or chest wall pain from the weight—see your doctor for evaluation.

Treatment Plastic surgery to reduce breast size is the only option to correct the problem (see page 774).

Prognosis Excellent with surgical correction. The condition does not predispose to cancer or other breast disorders even if it is left unaltered.

❖ CANCERS OF THE BREAST

Symptoms *(What you may experience)* A single (usually painless) lump in the breast; occasionally, breast pain, nipple discharge, rawness or itching of the nipple, change in breast shape or size, change in breast skin (redness or swelling).

Signs and laboratory findings *(What the doctor looks for)* Aside from the lump, possible signs include swollen lymph nodes under the arm, near the breast bone, or above the collar bone; the appearance of *peau d'orange* (a stippling of the skin that resembles an orange peel).

What is it? Although there are rare variant forms, most cancers of the breast arise from the cells lining the milk ducts; when these cells are abnormal, they are called intraductal carcinomas. The development of cancer in the breast—as in other tissues—occurs when normal cells lose their ability to respond to the growth and development controls that once governed them. Usually, the cause for cancerous change lies in damage to the cell's genetic material. Without the appropriate signals to tell cells when to divide and when to stop, they continue to divide and a growth or tumor forms (see Chapter 30).

The extent of the spread and growth of the cancer is described by an identification system called staging that ranges from stage 0 to stage IV. When the abnormal cells remain confined to the lining of the duct, the cancer is said to be carcinoma in situ, or staying localized to the site, and is classified as stage 0. Treatment that is begun at this in situ stage offers the best chance of cure. As the tumor becomes invasive but still measures less than 2 cm, its classification becomes stage I. As the size of the tumor grows still larger, or if it spreads to the lymph nodes, the classification of stages II and III applies. Treatment at these stages becomes more difficult, which clearly points to the importance of early diagnosis for this disease. When rogue cells break free from the tumor, they can migrate through the bloodstream or the lymphatic channels to distant sites—a process called metastasis. Cancers with proven metastases—termed stage IV—prove the most difficult to treat.

Although we tend to think of breast cancer as a single disease, some stark differences exist between breast cancers that arise before and after menopause. For example, the premenopausal breast cancers follow a much clearer family inheritance pattern than those cancers arising later in life; the risk for development of breast can-

▶ The implant itself consists of a silicone pouch filled with salt water. Previously, silicone gel filled the pouch, but manufacturers have abandoned this material in light of recent controversy and legal wrangling over possible health risks from silicone gel. Some reports suggested an association between leakage of silicone gel from implants and several autoimmune disorders, and in 1992 the Food and Drug Administration (FDA) reached a conclusion that manufacturers had not done sufficient studies demonstrating safety of silicone gel and called for additional study. The FDA further advised all women who had known leakage or rupture of gel implants to consult their surgeon about removal of this type of implant. Women without rupture or leakage need not rush to removal and should weigh the risk of surgery as greater than the risk of the implants. Women who do have symptoms—the most common being joint pain and swelling, unusual rashes and eczemas, or chronic fatigue syndrome (poor physical stamina)—may wish to consult their doctors about the possibility of implant removal even in the absence of known rupture or leakage. However, in spite of the negative publicity surrounding these implants, several large and well-designed clinical studies have failed to demonstrate any causal relationship between the silicone gel implant and an increased incidence of autoimmune disease or breast cancer (another reputed risk to women with implants). ■

EVALUATION OF A BREAST LUMP

Few discoveries frighten a woman more than finding a lump in her breast, but it is important to remember that most breast lumps are not cancers. Their nature is not always evident on clinical breast exam alone, even in skilled hands, and for that reason medical scientists have devised a number of diagnostic tests to sort them out. Mammography should always be done if the lump was detected by clinical breast exam or breast self-exam in women over age 30 (see page 778). The following are other diagnostic tests your doctor may suggest to determine the nature of the lump.

Aspiration of a Cyst A cystic lump is one that is fluid-filled. To better evaluate these kinds of lumps, your doctor may wish to aspirate the cyst (withdraw the fluid with a needle and syringe), both to drain the cyst and to send its contents for evaluation by the laboratory. To perform this procedure, the doctor will cleanse and numb the area to make insertion of the needle relatively painless. Aspiration is usually performed in the doctor's office.

Fine-Needle Biopsy If the lump is solid, your doctor may recommend taking a tiny sample of the lump by inserting a fine nee-

dle into the lump and removing a very slender core of tissue. After cleansing, your doctor will numb the area with a fast-acting anesthetic agent to make this procedure relatively painless.

Core Biopsy A core biopsy is performed with a larger needle or metal tube. The core of breast tissue that is removed may be as slender as a strand of spaghetti or as thick as a pen. Core biopsies are becoming increasingly popular and may soon replace most surgical biopsies. They can be done with palpation, ultrasound, or mammographic direction of the needle. Computerized mammographic core biopsies are sometimes called stereotactic biopsies.

Open Surgical (Excisional) Biopsy In this procedure, your doctor will remove the entire lump through a small incision in the skin. A pathologist will then examine the lump tissue under the microscope to determine its nature. For very small lumps, the procedure may be done by numbing just the area of the lump; larger lumps may require removal under a brief general anesthetic in the operating room. The surgeon will sew or tape the small incision closed, and as is the case for most surgical wounds, it will heal in 7 to 10 days. ■

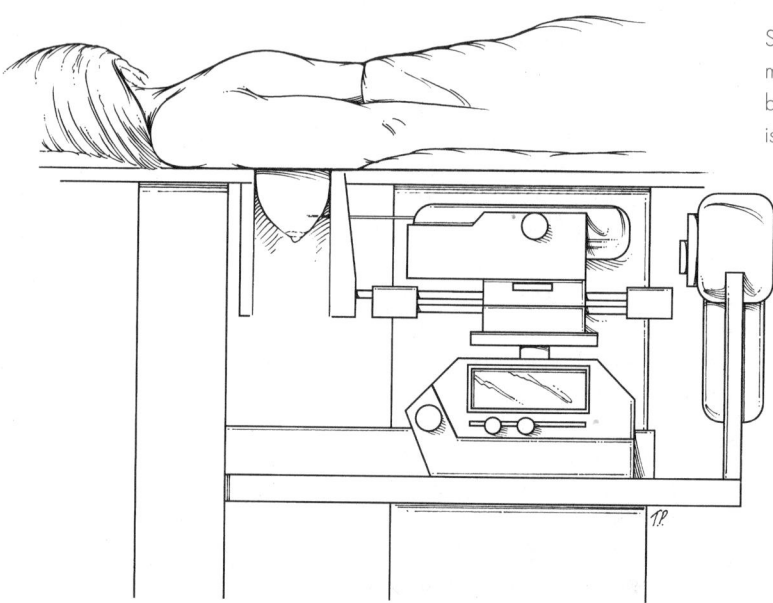

Stereotactic needle biopsy is often used to evaluate breast masses. Mammography or ultrasound is used to direct the biopsy needle to the location of the mass. A core of tissue is then removed for examination.

cer before menopause increases dramatically if a mother or sister has developed it. But most breast cancers develop after menopause, and the role of family inheritance in postmenopausal cancers is less significant. It may be that in the breast cancers arising later in life the cumulative effects of lifestyle choices—drinking alcohol, smoking, poor eating and exercise habits—play a more important role. Well-controlled epidemiologic studies have implicated alcohol intake and obesity with an increased incidence of breast cancer; in contrast, a relationship has been demonstrated between regular exercise and a reduced incidence of breast cancer.

Beyond differences in family risk, however, the premenopausal and postmenopausal cancers differ in their behavior and response to treatment. When breast cancer arises before menopause, it tends to be somewhat more aggressive and fast growing, more likely to spread to distant areas sooner, and more likely to involve both breasts than the type of breast cancer that appears later in life.

The differences in response to treatment occur in part because some breast cancers have a strong response to the female hormone estrogen and others do not. The presence or absence of estrogen receptors indicates whether tumors can respond to

THE MOST COMMONLY DIAGNOSED CANCER IN WOMEN

Each year more than 180,000 women develop breast cancer. The incidence of breast cancer is rising, having increased by 55 percent between 1950 and 1991, and is continuing to climb. After skin cancer it is now the most commonly diagnosed cancer in women, although lung cancer remains the number 1 cause of cancer-related death in women. The chance of developing breast cancer increases with age; the current yearly rates of occurrence in the United States, by age group, are

- 1.27 in 1,000 women aged 40 to 44
- 2.3 in 1,000 women aged 50 to 54
- 3.5 in 1,000 women aged 60 to 64
- 4.5 in 1,000 women aged 70 to 74

You may have heard the frequently quoted American Cancer Society statistic that 1 in 8 American women will develop breast cancer. This figure—which sounds alarming and much higher than the above cited numbers—represents an average lifetime risk and indicates that if the population of American women continues to develop breast cancer at the current annual rate, as many as 1 in 8 of them may develop the disease by the time they are in their 90s. Only a minority of the women who develop breast cancer will die from it. The estimated lifetime risk for women of dying from breast cancer is 3.6 percent; the lifetime risk is based on averages and estimates of future incidence rates and is not particularly meaningful in determining your individual risk, which may be influenced by family history, reproductive history, and lifestyle, such as diet and whether you exercise or smoke cigarettes. While breast cancer occurrence has increased, the breast cancer death rate continues to decline, having fallen about 5 percent in recent years. This decline is most likely due to more women detecting their cancer at an early stage as well as improved treatment (see Five-Year Survival Rate for Breast Cancer Patients, page 781). ■

estrogen and the response may dictate treatment options and to some extent prognosis. Premenopausal cancers tend more often to be estrogen receptor-negative, thus eliminating the use of less toxic antiestrogen medication such as tamoxifen following surgery and leaving chemotherapy with all its attendant side effects as the only additional treatment to combat distant metastases. Later-life cancers are more likely to have estrogen receptors and will usually respond more favorably to antiestrogen therapies.

Although we tend to think of breast cancer as a disease specific only to women—it occurs about 100 times more commonly in women—men also occasionally develop breast cancers. When they do, their cancers tend to be somewhat more aggressive and harder to treat than women's breast cancers, although in general the same principles of treatment apply.

Prevention Be vigilant. Early detection—and improved survival rates—depend on having a clinical breast exam by a doctor or other trained health care provider and a mammography (see page 778). The weight of scientific evidence correlates the increased incidence of breast cancer with obesity, a sedentary lifestyle, and alcohol consumption. Certainly if you have a family risk of breast cancer you should try to make whatever lifestyle modifications you feel you can—such as attaining and maintaining your ideal body weight, exercising regularly, limiting alcohol, and avoiding tobacco—to help reduce the risk of breast cancer.

THE BREAST CANCER GENE

From the moment of our conception, human life depends on the hundreds of thousands of pieces of information stored in the tightly coiled strands of DNA that make our chromosomes. Sometimes the genetic computer code develops a glitch that may cause a disease that can pass from one generation to another (see Chapter 6).

Scientific research has now established methods for and begun the process of identifying, locating, and mapping out the many genes on human chromosomes that may put some of us at risk for particular diseases. A cancer susceptibility gene that passes along a familial risk for breast cancer appears to be one of these. Several years ago, medical researchers reported that "the breast cancer gene" had been found. Many hopes were raised that a cure would soon follow, but the genetic causes of breast cancer have not surprisingly proven to be complex. Two genes on chromosome 17—BRCA1 and BRCA2—have been implicated, but both have multiple mutant forms, making testing difficult and expensive, and researchers suspect that other breast cancer genes will be found. Meanwhile, it is unclear whether BRCA1 and BRCA2 play a role in inherited breast cancer alone, which makes up only 5 to 10 percent of all cases of breast cancer, or whether these genes also play a role in the breast cancer that occurs in women with no family history, a much larger group.

Since there is no certain means of preventing cancer, controversy has arisen over the benefits of testing for the gene. If you have a family history of breast or ovarian cancer, consult with your doctor to learn whether genetic testing can offer you any benefits. Whether or not you are tested for the gene, and whether the results are positive or negative, it is essential that all women with a family history of breast cancer seek appropriate medical counseling and careful monitoring through regular breast exams and mammography. ■

MAMMOGRAPHY

A mammogram test is simply a special kind of x-ray exam. An x-ray beam passes through the breast, which is held flat between two x-ray plates. The beam easily penetrates the fatty tissue of the breast but passes less easily through the denser supportive tissues and glandular tissues, and passes with an even greater degree of difficulty through tougher cancerous tissue. These variations in x-ray penetration produce a shadow picture (very much like an x-ray of your foot, arm, or teeth) delineating the architecture of the breast. Before age 20, the breasts contain so much firm, supportive tissue that mammography will not show much. With age and maturity, the breasts contain progressively less dense tissue and more fatty tissue and taking a good mammographic picture becomes feasible.

Who should have a mammogram and when? Experts agree that women between the ages of 50 and 69 derive benefit from mammographic screening and should receive yearly mammographic exams coupled with a clinical breast exam by a doctor. There is also general agreement that there is little reason to perform routine mammographic exams in women under age 30 because breast cancers rarely occur in this age group. The various authorities do not all agree, however, on recommendations for mammography in women 30 to 49 years old and in women over age 70. Evidence from randomized clinical trials is still lacking regarding the efficacy of mammography in detecting cancers in women in these age groups. Only in studies using extremely high quality mammographic exams has there been any value in using mammography to screen low-risk women between ages 40 and 50, and most studies fail to achieve statistically significant results. While benefits are unclear for low-risk women in their 40s, mammograms may reveal harmless growths, which can lead to unnecessary alarm as well as further diagnostic tests. Some authorities advocate a baseline exam between ages 35 and 40 and then periodic exams for women between the ages of 40 and 49 and in women over age 70 who are otherwise in good health. The US Preventive Services Task Force, the American College of Physicians, and the American Academy of Family Physicians do not recommend routine screening mammograms for women under age 50. The American Cancer Society, The

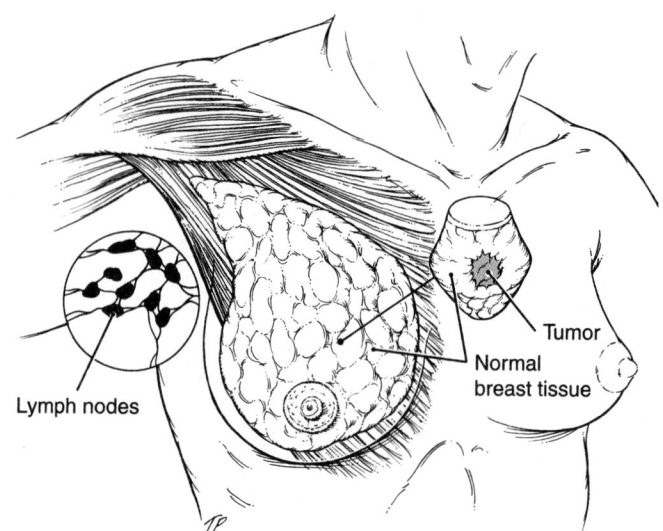

Studies have shown that in stages 0 and I and smaller stage II cancers the cure rate for removing the entire breast and axillary lymph nodes (modified radical mastectomy) is no better than for removing the tumor and a small amount of surrounding normal breast tissue, a procedure called a lumpectomy. Tissue from the lymph nodes is sampled at the time of surgery to look for evidence of tumor spread and a course of radiation therapy is applied to the remaining breast tissue to prevent local recurrence of tumor.

American College of Surgeons, The American College of Radiologists, and most European National Health Services recommend annual mammography for women between the ages of 40 and 50. The National Cancer Institute, under great pressure from the US Congress, revised its position to recommend mammograms every 1 to 2 years for women between ages 40 and 49. A reasonable compromise on this issue has led to a provisional recommendation for mammography for women between ages 40 and 49 who have a strong family history for breast cancer, other factors that increase risk for breast cancer, or women who themselves have a strong desire to have the test done to ease their own worries and fears. ■

When to call the doctor The appearance of a persistent lump in your breast demands a careful evaluation. Although it may certainly prove to be a harmless lump, only thorough investigation will tell. Call your doctor right away.

Treatment Treatment depends on the stage of the cancer at diagnosis and whether the cells are estrogen receptor-positive or -negative. In receptor-positive cancers, the medication tamoxifen (an antiestrogen medication) works well after surgery. In receptor-negative tumors, chemotherapy following surgery offers better results.

Although the mainstay of treatment for many years has been surgical removal of the breast, nipple and areola (the area surrounding the nipple of the breast), and the lymph nodes beneath the arm on that side—a procedure known as a modified radical mastectomy—more women and their doctors are beginning to opt for breast-conserving therapies. In stage 0 and I and some smaller stage II cancers, lumpectomy with axillary node dissection (removal of just the lump and the lymph nodes beneath the arm) followed by radiation treatment to the breast offers cure rates equal to modified radical mastectomy. This approach avoids the trauma of losing the breast, which is a distinct advantage. The downside of lumpectomy is the need for radiation afterward, which commonly causes unpleasant side effects such as fatigue, loss of appetite, and breast swelling and redness that may prove to be permanent. Radiation usually is not necessary following modified radical mastectomy (it is used in only 4 percent of cases), and although modified radical mastectomy is more disfiguring, the majority of women and their surgeons still opt for it, with some women electing to undergo reconstructive breast surgery at the time of surgery or in a second procedure (see below). New techniques are being tested that will enable doctors to determine whether cancer has spread to the underarm lymph nodes without removing them. These procedures will allow doctors to

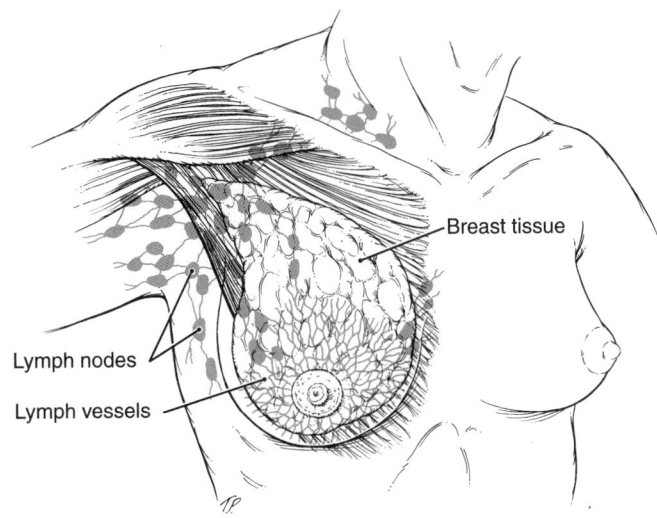

Lymph nodes involved in breast cancer. Breast cancer spreads first by invading the local lymph nodes and later by invading the bloodstream.

BREAST RECONSTRUCTION SURGERY

Women who must undergo surgical removal of the breast— whether a subcutaneous mastectomy (in which only the breast tissue itself is removed, leaving the skin and nipple-areola complex) or a modified radical mastectomy (in which the breast, nipple and areola, and overlying skin and axillary lymph nodes are removed)—may opt for reconstruction either at the time of the mastectomy or in a subsequent procedure later. Reconstruction can recreate the shape of the breast, though there will not be any sensation remaining in the new breast.

There are two common types of reconstruction. First and most common are fat transfer types of reconstruction. Usually, fat and skin are removed via a tummy tuck procedure (in which tissue is removed from the upper abdomen) and moved to the position under the skin where breast tissue was removed. Circulation to this fat and skin is either transferred or reconnected in the new location. Several months later a nipple facsimile is created with surgical movement of local skin, which is tattooed to resemble natural color.

The second and less common reconstruction is with a saline-filled breast implant. Initially, after mastectomy, an expandable pouch is put under the chest wall. Over a period of weeks the pouch is filled with saline to stretch the skin. When the skin is sufficiently large, a final implant is inserted in place of the expandable pouch, and a nipple facsimile is tattooed in place. ■

(A) Modified radical mastectomy for breast cancer involves the removal of the breast, nipple, areola, overlying skin, and axillary lymph nodes on the affected side. (B) By inserting an implant, breast reconstruction surgery—at the time of the mastectomy or later—can restore the shape of the breast.

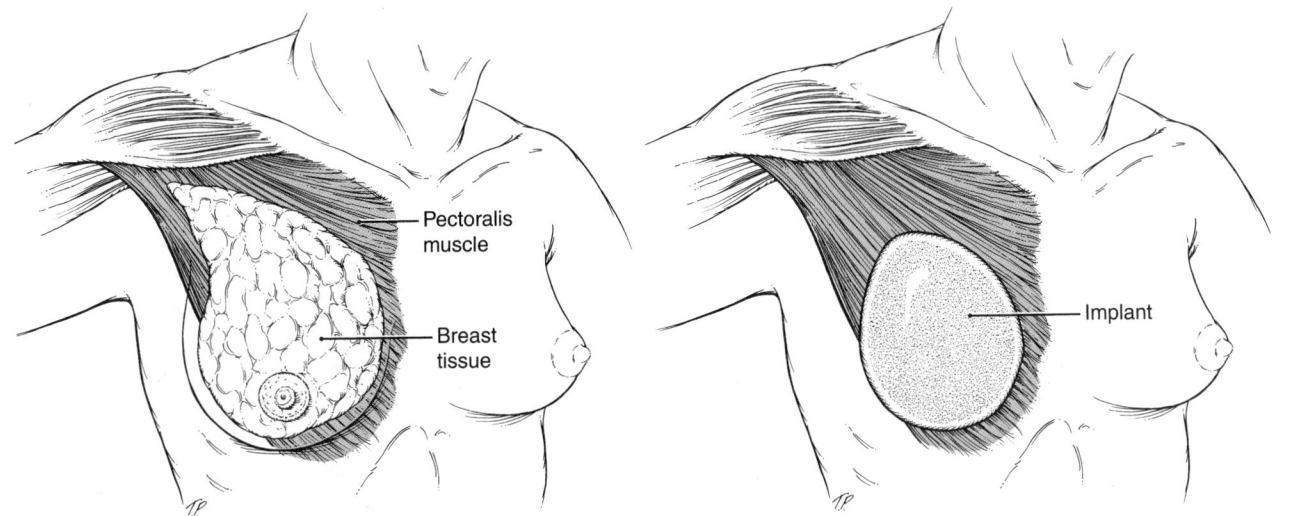

SUPPORT GROUPS FOR BREAST CANCER PATIENTS AND SURVIVORS

While many people are initially reluctant to talk with strangers about what they are going through, joining a cancer support group often becomes invaluable to cancer patients and cancer survivors. Sharing your feelings can alleviate your sense of isolation and help you cope. Your support group can also be a valuable resource for tips on managing your cancer therapy and guidance in choosing specialists as well as advice on coping with the side effects of your treatment.

In addition to the general psychological issues all cancer patients must cope with, breast cancer seems to carry an additional emotional burden for many women. The loss of a breast can affect a woman emotionally long after she has recovered from the loss physically. Some women say, "Fine, save my life. It's not as important as a finger." Others grieve for the breast that nursed their children. Still others feel disfigured and unattractive. Many breast cancer patients and survivors find that discussing their feelings with others who have had breast cancer helps them come to terms with their illness as well as with their fears of a recurrence.

If you have been diagnosed with breast cancer, the following sources may be helpful to you in terms of both treatment and recovery.

- National Alliance of Breast Cancer Organizations (NABCO)
  9 East 37th St., 10th Floor
  New York, NY 10016
  Phone: (800) 719–9154
  The National Alliance of Breast Cancer Organizations is a network that includes many organizations offering help with detection, treatment, and support to breast cancer patients and survivors.

- Reach to Recovery
  c/o American Cancer Society
  1599 Clifton Rd. NE
  Atlanta, GA 30329
  Phone: (404) 320–3333
  Reach to Recovery provides one-on-one help for women who have had breast cancer.

- National Self-Help Clearing House
  25 West 43rd St.
  New York, NY 10036
  Phone: (212) 642–2944
  This organization provides lists of information on cancer organizations, support groups, rehabilitation, and health services.

- Susan B. Komen Foundation
  5005 LBJ Freeway, #370
  Dallas, TX 75244
  Phone: (800) 462–9273 or
  (214) 450–1777
  Web site: http://race4cure.lm.com/
  The Susan B. Komen Foundation provides information on breast cancer treatment.

- The Y-Me National Breast Cancer Organization
  212 W. Van Buren
  Chicago, IL 60607
  Phone: (312) 986–8226 or
  (800) 221–2141
  Y-Me can connect you with other breast cancer survivors and provide information and a support network.

As more and more of those diagnosed with cancer become cancer survivors, coping with survivors' needs has become an issue of growing importance. Many organizations across the country have been created in order to accomodate the needs of this growing number of people. The National Coalition for Cancer Survivorship (NCCS) is one the best examples of such an organization. The NCCS publishes a quarterly newsletter, The Networker, that offers news regarding the concerns of cancer survivors. The NCCS can also help you find a support group in your area, cope with employment problems, resolve insurance issues, and locate other services you may need:

- National Coalition for Cancer Survivorship (NCCS)
  1010 Wayne Ave., Fifth Floor
  Silver Spring, MD 20910
  Phone: (301) 650–8868

In addition, your local hospital has a social service department that is usually able to inform you about the services available to you in your community such as support groups, local supply stores, treatment facilities, and other support services. ■

perform mastectomies but avoid radical underarm surgery in those patients for whom it is unnecessary.

In some stage I and all stage II, III, and IV cancers, follow-up chemotherapy (or hormone therapy in receptor-positive tumors) improves response and survival after surgery (see Chapter 30).

Prognosis Caught early, or at stage 0, 99 percent of women are still surviving at 5 years and 98 percent at 10 years. For women whose cancers are detected at stage I, 95 percent are alive at 5 years. Cancers that are detected and treated later (at more advanced stages) do not respond as well, as shown in the graph on page 781. Early detection and treatment are of paramount importance to survival from this cancer. The percentage of American women who die from breast cancer has been declining due to earlier diagnosis and better treatment. From 1989 to 1993, breast cancer mortality rates fell about 5 percent according to the National Cancer Institute. Still, breast cancer remains the number two

FIVE-YEAR SURVIVAL RATE FOR BREAST CANCER PATIENTS

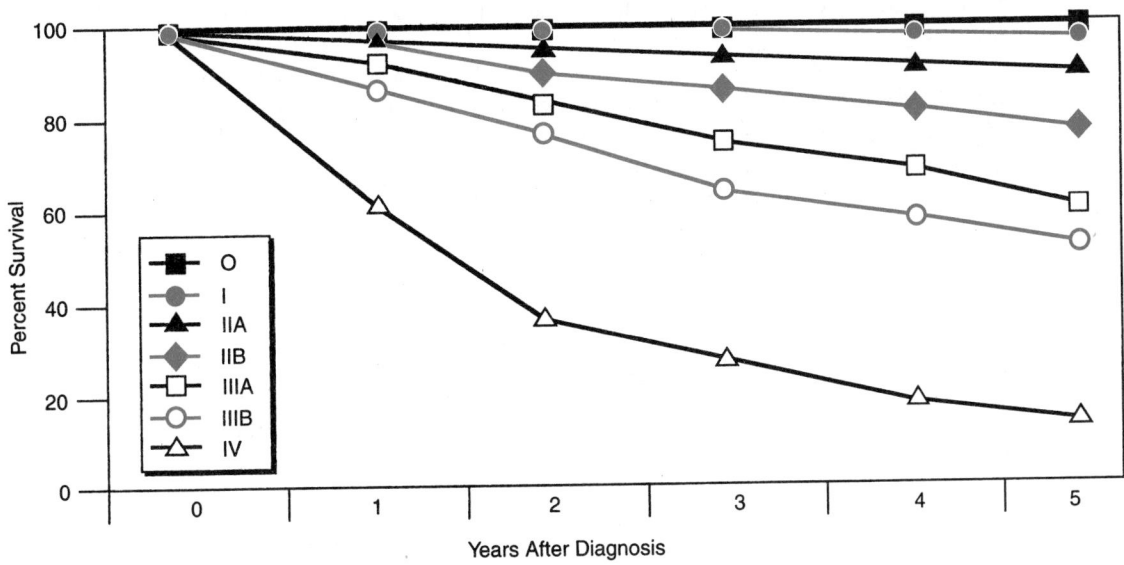

Five-year survival rates for breast cancer patients. Rates are given by stage, referring to how extensively the cancer has spread at time of diagnosis. Stage 0 means the cancer is confined to the lining of the milk duct, while in stage IV, cancer cells have metastasized (migrated to distant sites in the body). Survival rates range from 98 percent for stage 0 patients to 16 percent for stage IV patients. Source: National Cancer Data Base, 1989. Used with the permission of the American Joint Committee on Cancer (AJCC), Chicago. The original source for this illustration is the AJCC Cancer Staging Manual, 5th edition (1997), published by Lippincott-Raven, Philadelphia.

cause of cancer-related death in women (lung cancer is number one). Over 44,000 American women die of breast cancer each year.

The Nipple

The nipple—which can range in color from darker pink to brown—functions in women primarily as the endpoint for breast milk delivery. The 15 to 20 milk ducts empty into the nipple, which contains specialized erectile tissues that stiffen when stimulated by the nursing baby ostensibly to facilitate nursing; however, this reflex occurs in men as well as women. Lighter pink or brown tissue—called the areola—surrounds the nipple. Small glands called Montgomery's glands that are scattered along the perimeter of the areola provide lubricating oil to protect the nipple and keep it supple. Disorders affecting the nipple complex primarily involve infections, abnormal milk production, abnormalities of shape, or scaling of the skin.

❖ INFECTION OF THE MILK DUCTS

Symptoms *(What you may experience)*
Thick, colored (green, yellow, or tan) discharge from one nipple (usually); tenderness of <u>nipple</u> or breast; fever (possibly); swollen or tender lymph glands under the arm.

CAUSES OF NIPPLE DISCHARGE

Except when women breast-feed, the leakage of milky fluid from the breast is abnormal. Any leakage of clear yellow, dark, or slightly bloody fluid from the nipple should prompt a visit to your doctor. Samples of the fluid examined under the microscope may pinpoint the cause. The reasons for nipple discharge run the gamut from harmless to serious and for that reason merit investigation. Slightly colored thin watery discharge may occur in fibrocystic breast disease. Milky fluid can discharge from the nipples (usually it will be both of them) if abnormal secretion of the brain hormone prolactin stimulates milk production; this condition—called galactorrhea—can occur in men, women, and occasionally even children (see page 782). Thick, darker colored discharge may signal infection or a breast abscess (see above). Blood-tinged discharge could indicate a tumor in the milk duct, which could be a harmless growth or a cancerous one, and therefore merits a more extensive evaluation by your doctor. ■

Signs and laboratory findings *(What the doctor looks for)* Growing the suspected bacterium on a culture plate in the laboratory.

What is it? Infection of the milk ducts usually occurs during breast-feeding when the introduction of bacteria from the baby's mouth may occur. During this time the nipple can become cracked, making it more vulnerable to infection.

Occasionally an infected duct can lead to formation of an abscess (boil) within the breast.

What you can do Gentle cleansing of the nipple and the application of warm compresses may offer some relief. You should, of course, cease breast-feeding from the affected breast; however, if possible, continue to express milk to keep production going.

When to call the doctor Persistent colored discharge from the nipple, the appearance of fever, or tender lymph glands under the arm should prompt a visit to your doctor.

Treatment Proven infections will usually require antibiotic treatment, and if an abscess develops, it may require surgical drainage.

Prognosis Excellent with appropriate treatment.

❖ INFECTION OF THE AREOLAR GLANDS (MONTGOMERY'S GLANDS)

Symptoms *(What you may experience)* Redness, tenderness, and swelling of the glands of the areola.

Signs and laboratory findings *(What the doctor looks for)* No specific signs beyond the symptoms.

What is it? The small oil glands scattered along the periphery of the areola function to lubricate and protect the nipple and areolar tissues. Like many other glands opening onto the skin surface, these oil glands appear (under the microscope) as flask-shaped structures that have rounded wells with long slender necks that open onto the surface. The cells lining the inside of the gland produce oil droplets that extrude onto the surface to oil the skin. However, the opening and neck provide a route for bacteria to enter and cause infection. Usually the infection is not serious.

What you can do Gentle, careful cleansing of the affected areas with mild antibacterial soap and water and the application of warm compresses may resolve the problem.

When to call the doctor A persistent infection or one associated with fever, swollen lymph glands near the infection, or spreading of the redness should prompt a visit to your doctor.

Treatment If necessary, treatment with antibiotics (the erythromycins, penicillins, and cephalosporins all work well in skin infections) may be necessary to resolve the infection.

Prognosis Excellent in virtually all cases.

❖ GALACTORRHEA (WITCHES' MILK)

Symptoms *(What you may experience)* Nipple discharge of breast milk (which can be milky white or slightly colored), usually from both nipples.

What is it? When the mammary glands produce a small amount of breast milk in women who have previously had children, it usually is not cause for immediate concern; however, the appearance of significant amounts of milk before pregnancy has ever occurred (or in males or children) merits investigation. The most common cause—abnormal secretion of the brain hormone prolactin, the chief stimulator of milk production—can occur for a variety of reasons ranging from overexercise, unrecognized pregnancy, trauma, and surgery to side effects caused by certain medication (amphetamines, cimetidine, female hormone replacement medication, hydroxyzine, methyldopa, nicotine, narcotics, reserpine, tricyclic antidepressants, verapamil) to more serious causes. The pathologic causes of excess prolactin include pituitary tumors, liver cirrhosis, low levels of thyroid hormone, false pregnancy, renal failure, and disorders of the spinal cord.

Treatment Evaluation begins by looking for causes such as activities or medication and checking the prolactin level. Whatever the cause, the medication bromocriptine can stop the discharge if necessary.

Prognosis Excellent for full recovery in most cases.

❖ PAGET'S DISEASE (CARCINOMA) OF THE NIPPLE

Symptoms *(What you may experience)* Itching or burning of the nipple; rawness or ulceration of the skin of the nipple.

Signs and laboratory findings *(What the doctor looks for)* Special microscopic examination of samples of ulcerated skin demonstrating abnormal (cancerous) cells.

What is it? This rare form of cancer, which accounts for about 1 percent of all breast cancers, usually begins in the milk ducts near the nipple and grows slowly, invading the skin nearby. Usually there is no lump to feel, and the early symptoms—itching or burning of the nipple—may seem unremarkable.

Treatment Lumpectomy and removal of the lymph nodes followed by radiation or mastectomy.

Prognosis Excellent for recovery when the disease is discovered early and treated appropriately. Even when the disease has progressed to the point of causing nipple changes, it rarely spreads to lymph glands or more distant areas of the body.

❖ INVERSION OF THE NIPPLE

Symptoms *(What you may experience)* The nipple points inward or retracts below the level of the areola.

Signs and laboratory findings *(What the doctor looks for)* Mainly signs to exclude more serious causes: lumps; skin changes; dimpling of the breast skin.

What is it? Occasionally, congenital differences in the supportive and erectile tissues of the nipple cause one (usually) nipple to retract inward instead of pointing outward. If the condition arises as the nipples grow and develop at puberty, it should be no cause for alarm. If the nipple begins to retract after puberty, however, it could indicate a growth or swelling within the body of the breast causing pressure on the supportive ligaments.

When to call the doctor Nipple retraction before puberty presents no significant medical risk and can safely be ignored. The appearance of nipple shape changes, such as retraction, after puberty merits evaluation by your doctor right away.

Treatment Retraction before puberty requires no treatment, although plastic surgery can correct appearance if desired. Determining the cause of retraction may involve ultrasound or mammographic tests, and if a lump is responsible for the retraction, surgical removal of the lump should be performed. If the lump proves to be cancerous, more extensive treatment may be necessary (see page 775).

Prognosis Excellent for retraction before puberty or for noncancerous lump removal (see page 775).

TWENTY

Cardiovascular System

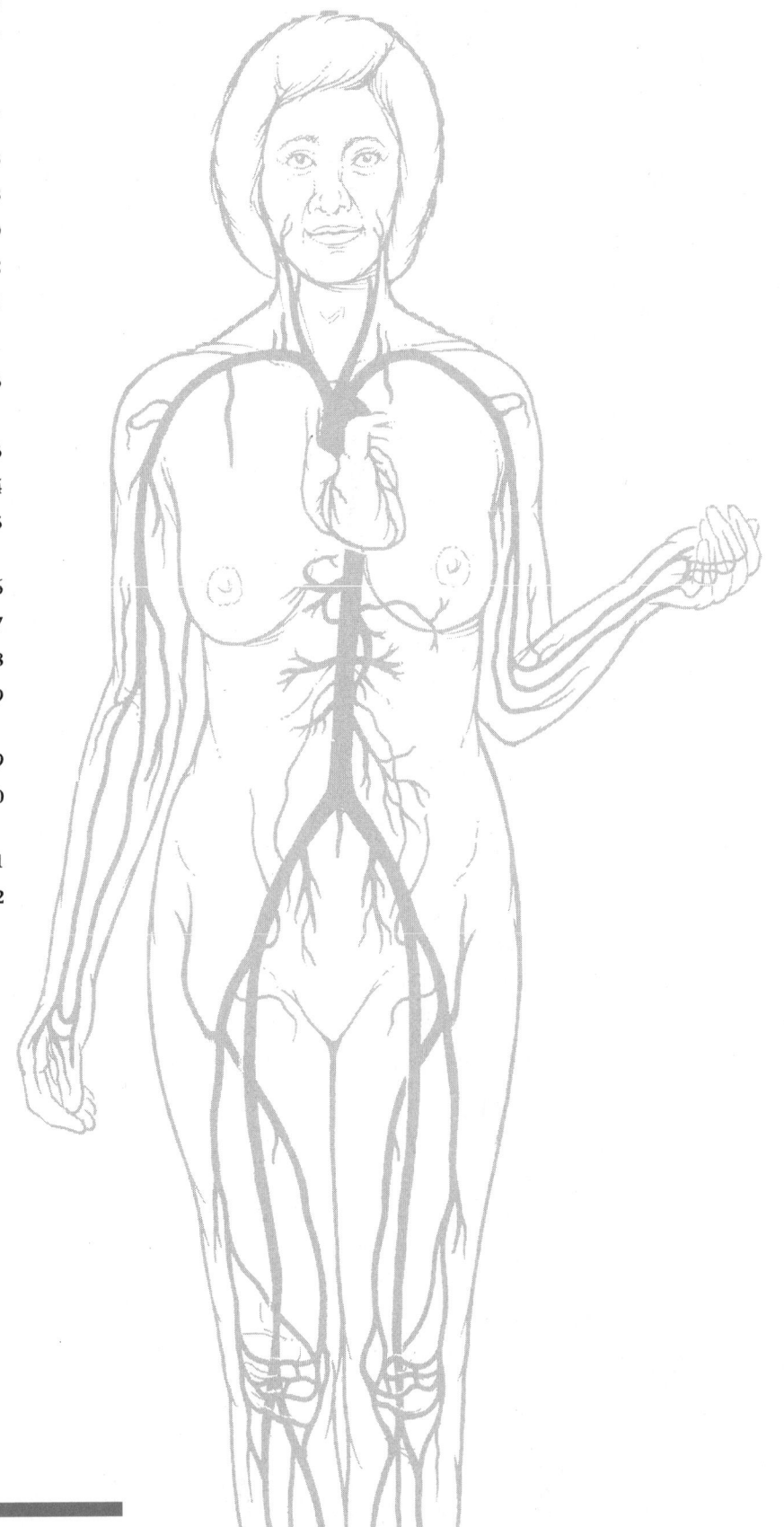

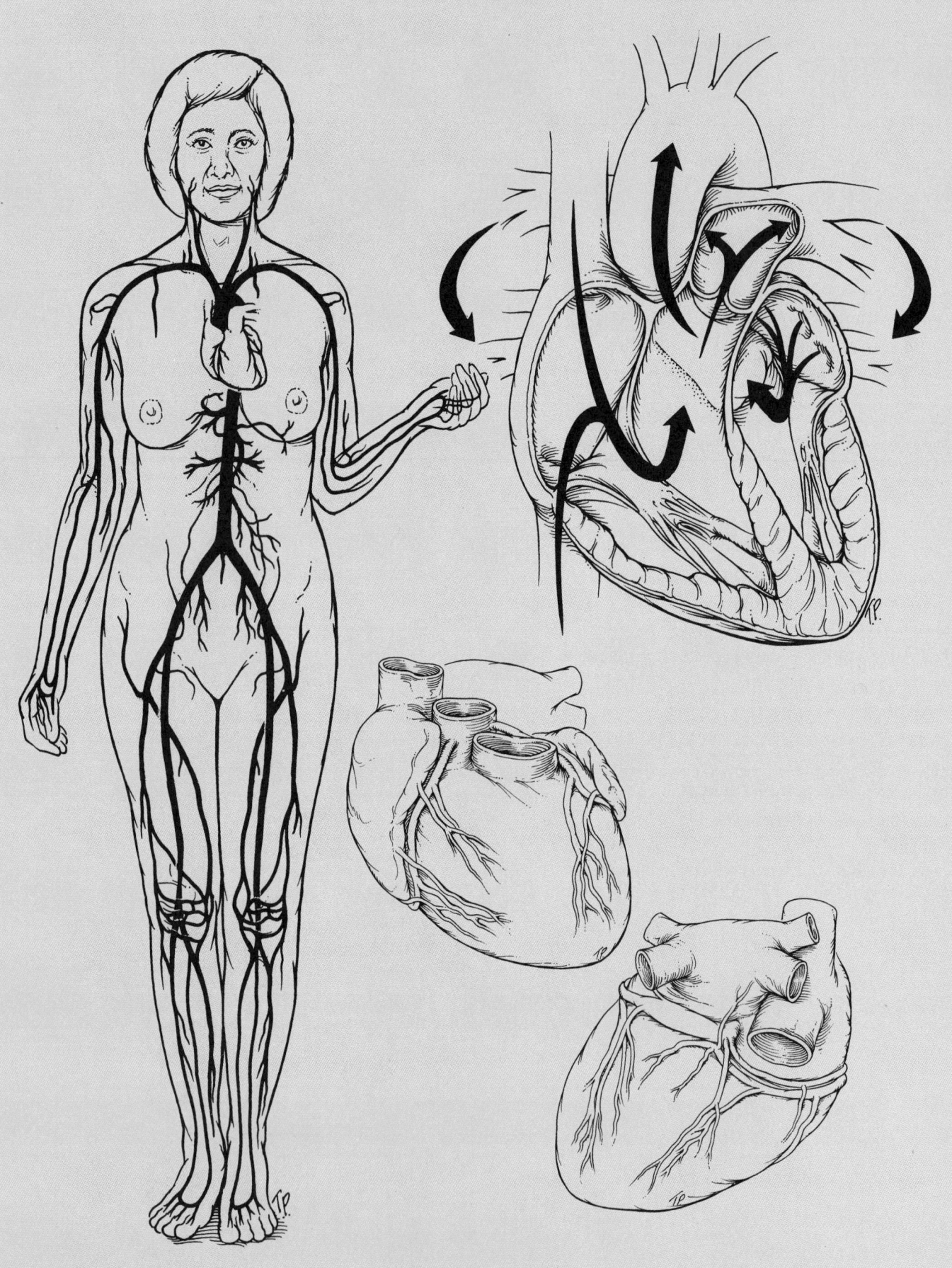

CARDIOVASCULAR SYSTEM

How the Cardiovascular System Works

The heart may not be the site of love and the home of emotion, as it was once thought to be, but this remarkable muscular pump is truly the organ of steadfastness, strength, and endurance. When it stops, we stop.

The size of a fist, the heart contracts rhythmically, on average 72 times a minute (more than once a second) around the clock, year after year, from birth until death. Take a moment to appreciate the miracle of a muscle that pumps about 2,000 gallons of blood through your body every day of your life and never rests for 70, 80, even 100-plus years.

The heart and its blood vessels—a 60,000-mile network of arteries, veins, and capillaries—make up the cardiovascular system. This pulsing system delivers the blood, with its cargo of oxygen and nutrients, to the tissues of the body and then carries off carbon dioxide and other metabolic wastes for disposal.

The heart itself consists of four chambers: the right and left atria (small filling chambers at the top of the heart) and the right and left ventricles (the major pumping chambers, below the atria). To prevent blood from flowing directly from the right to the left side of the heart, the atria are divided by a wall called the atrial septum; the ventricles are separated by the ventricular septum. This ensures that oxygen-poor blood returning to the right chambers of the heart will circulate through the lungs before it can reenter the left chambers and then head out to the body. The heart's network of blood vessels, the circulatory system, has two main divisions: the systemic arterial circulation, which supplies blood to all the organs of the body (including the separate coronary circulation, which supplies the heart); and the venous circulation, which carries blood to the right side of the heart and to the lungs where it unloads waste carbon dioxide and takes on fresh oxygen.

CIRCULATION

Within the heart, a system of four one-way valves regulates the passage of blood between each atrium and its ventricle and between the ventricles and their blood vessel outlets to the lungs or the body. Between contractions when the heart muscle is relaxed (diastole, or the filling phase), blood returning from the body enters the right atrium of the heart from each vena cava (the two large veins that collect blood returning from the lower and upper body). From there, it flows through the tricuspid valve into the right ventricle. After the right ventricle is filled, the ventricle contracts and the valve closes so that the blood cannot flow backward into the atrium. When the right ventricle contracts (systole), blood flows through the pulmonary valve into the pulmonary arteries, which carry it to the blood vessels in the lungs. Once in the lungs, the oxygen-poor blood flows into ever smaller veins and finally into capillaries with walls so thin that gases can pass through them. Here carbon dioxide, the waste product of the body's metabolic processes, passes from the blood into the air sacs of the lungs to be expelled from the body when you breathe.

Fresh oxygen from the air moves from the air sacs and enters the blood across the capillary walls and is brought via the pulmonary veins to the left atrium. Between heartbeats, the blood flows through the mitral valve, filling the powerful left ventricle. Pressure inside the ventricle increases during heart contraction and closes the mitral valve. The contraction pumps the oxygen-rich blood out through the aortic valve into the aorta (the largest artery in the body) for distribution to the entire network of arteries throughout the body. At the point where the aorta leaves the heart, a pair of blood vessels (the coronary arteries) branch off and double back to spread out over the heart itself, sending branches downward to nourish the heart muscle.

CORONARY CIRCULATION

The two main coronary arteries—called the right and left coronary arteries—branch off the aorta just as it leaves the heart. The right coronary artery supplies mainly the smaller right side of the heart, which pumps blood to the lungs for oxygenation as well as to a portion of the septum of the left ventricle. The left main coronary artery divides into several large branches that serve the bigger and more muscular left side of the heart, which pumps blood to the entire body.

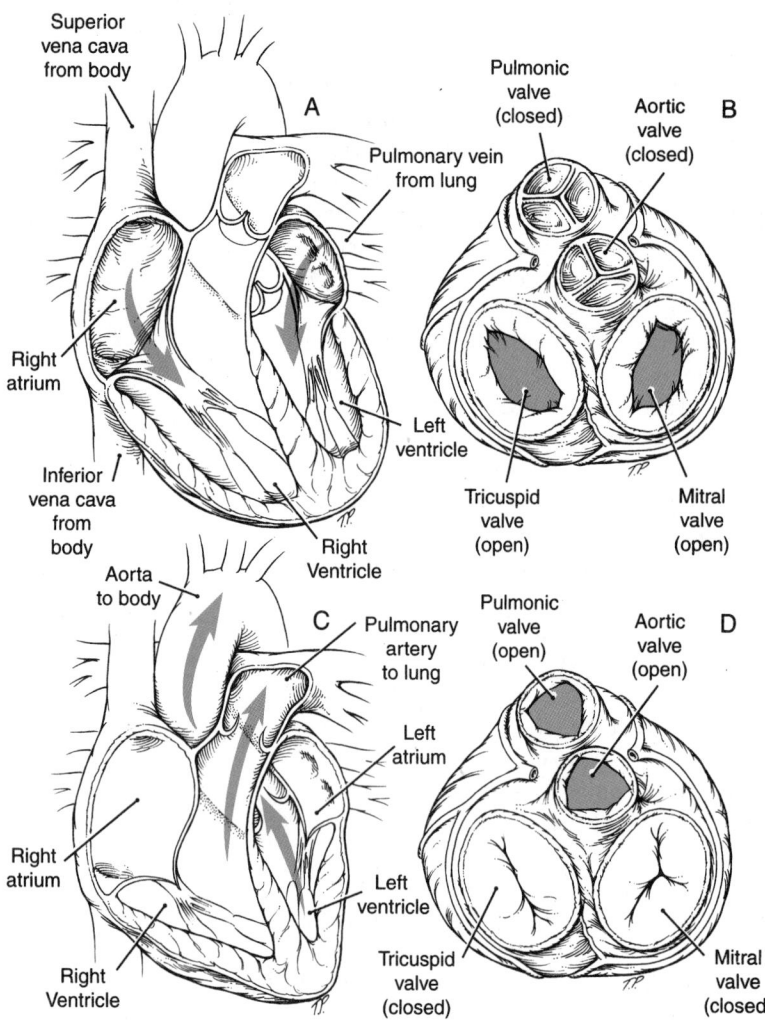

Superior vena cava from body

A

Pulmonary vein from lung

Right atrium

Inferior vena cava from body

Right Ventricle

Left ventricle

Pulmonic valve (closed)

Aortic valve (closed)

B

Tricuspid valve (open)

Mitral valve (open)

Aorta to body

C

Pulmonary artery to lung

Left atrium

Right atrium

Left ventricle

Right Ventricle

Pulmonic valve (open)

Aortic valve (open)

D

Tricuspid valve (closed)

Mitral valve (closed)

(A) In the diastolic part of the pumping cycle, when the heart is relaxed, blood returning from the body enters the right atrium of the heart. It flows through the tricuspid valve, into the right ventricle. (B) Oxygenated blood from the lungs flows into the left atrium, through the mitral valve, and into the left ventricle. The pulmonic and aortic valves are closed. (C) In systole, the active pumping phase, blood flows from the right ventricle through the pulmonary valve into the pulmonary arteries and then into the lungs. (D) Blood in the left ventricle flows through the aortic valve and into the aorta, to the rest of the body. Mitral and tricuspid valves are closed.

Coronary arteries provide the blood supply to the heart. The right and left coronary arteries originate from the aorta and branch out across the surface of the heart. (A) The front surface of the heart contains the left main coronary artery, the left anterior descending artery, branches of the circumflex coronary artery, and part of the right coronary artery. (B) The underside of the heart contains part of the right coronary artery and its main branch, the posterior descending artery, as well as some branches of the circumflex coronary artery.

Heart valves help to ensure that blood flows in only one direction on each side of the heart. On the right side, it flows from the vena cavae to the right atrium, to the right ventricle, to the pulmonary arteries, to the lungs. On the left side, blood flows from the lungs to the pulmonary veins, to the left atrium, to the left ventricle, to the aorta, and to the body.

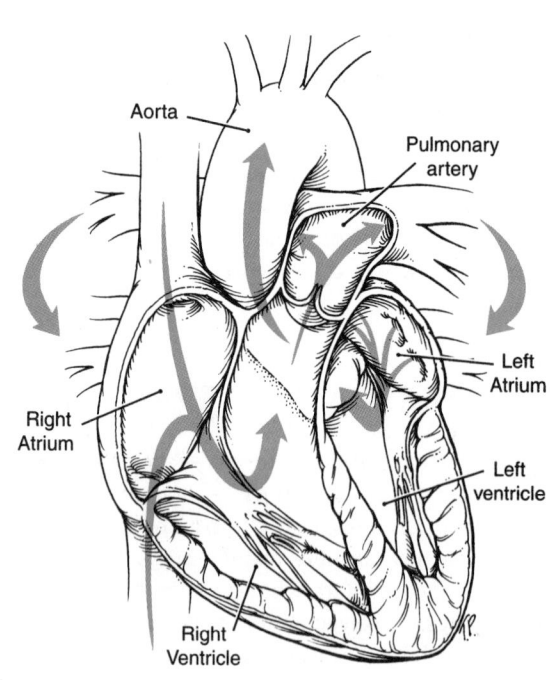

Aorta

Pulmonary artery

Right Atrium

Left Atrium

Left ventricle

Right Ventricle

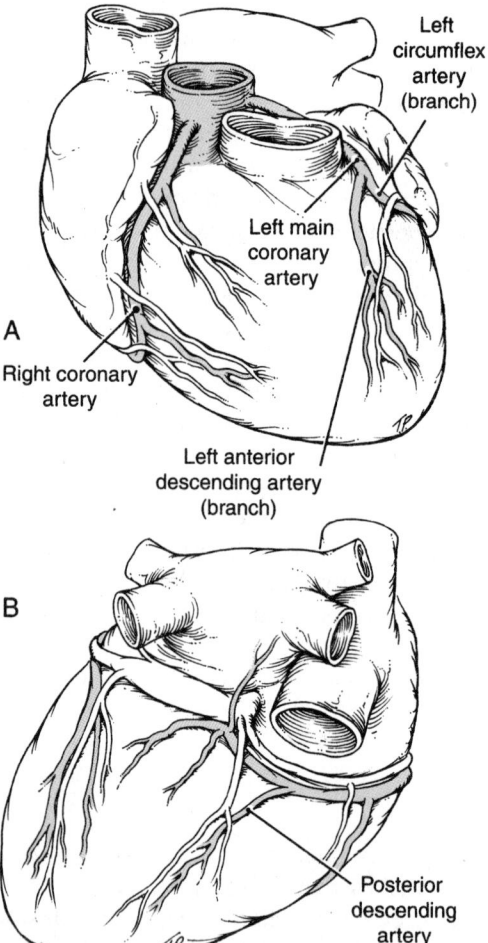

Left circumflex artery (branch)

Left main coronary artery

A

Right coronary artery

Left anterior descending artery (branch)

B

Posterior descending artery

PULMONARY CIRCULATION

Normally, arteries carry oxygen-rich blood, and veins carry oxygen-poor blood. But in the pulmonary circulation, their roles are reversed. The pulmonary arteries bring oxygen-depleted blood to the lungs, while the pulmonary veins return to the heart with freshly oxygenated blood, which is then pumped out to the body.

The heart muscle contracts in a wringing fashion, from apex (the tip) to base, with both right and left chambers contracting at the same time. This cycle of contraction and relaxation, the heartbeat, creates the pulse you can feel in your hand. A built-in electrical signaling center (the sinoatrial node or sinus node), the body's natural cardiac pacemaker in the upper right atrium, originates electrical impulses, which move through the atria to the atrioventricular (AV) node, located between the atrium and ventricle. From here, impulses move through the heart muscle, coordinating the heart's rhythmic contractions. Any disruption of the heart's electrical pacing center can result in changes in the heart rhythm: skipped beats, fluttering, ineffective contraction, racing, or beating so slowly that it fails to generate enough blood flow to the body.

From the aorta, blood moves outward into smaller and smaller arterial branches carrying nutrients and oxygen to the tissues of the body. Just as in the lungs, the size of the arteries diminishes until the tiniest arteries (arterioles) empty into capillaries with walls thin enough to permit nutrients and oxygen to cross. It is here in the capillary beds that cellular wastes are captured by circulating blood, moving from the capillaries to ever larger veins for disposal by the lungs and recirculation, detoxification, or disposal by the liver and kidneys.

Veins lack the strong muscular walls of arteries; they depend on a "milking" effect created by the muscle groups surrounding them to massage the blood along. The effect of gravity tends to make the blood in the veins move down toward the feet (when you stand or sit upright) were it not for a system of valves in the veins that prevent this back-flow of blood. They work much like one-way gates, allowing the blood to pass through, then closing behind it. As long as the valves work properly, the blood progresses through the veins in an orderly manner on its way back to the heart.

PUMPING BLOOD

The percent of blood volume in the ventricle when it is full that is pumped out during contraction is called the ejection fraction. A normal ejection fraction is at least 50 percent, meaning that at least half the blood in the ventricles is pumped out with each beat. In a healthy person, the ejection fraction increases by 5 to 20 percent with exercise. The actual amount of blood pumped by the left ventricle during one contraction is called the stroke volume. The stroke volume and the heart rate determine cardiac output, which is the amount of blood the heart pumps through the entire circulatory system in 1 minute.

BLOOD PRESSURE

Blood pressure is the force exerted against the artery walls. It is determined by the pumping action of the heart and the degree of constriction or dilation of the arteries, including the smallest arteries, the arterioles. Blood pressure varies with activity—lower during sleep and rest, higher during exercise. During exercise, for example, the heart pumps faster to supply more blood while blood vessels constrict, which raises the pressure. Generally, the body makes an immediate adjustment to these changing demands. When you stand up after lying down, blood vessels in your legs and abdomen must quickly constrict to ensure an adequate return of blood to your heart and maintenance of blood supply to your brain. If there is a slight delay in the reflexes that control this adjustment, you may briefly feel dizzy—a not uncommon occurrence in the elderly. When you are at rest, your heart slows and blood vessels relax their walls.

THE REGULATORS

To direct all the instantaneous adjustments the cardiovascular system must make during the course of the day, the body depends on two powerful control systems: the kidneys and the autonomic nervous system, the neural network concerned with automatic control of many basic body functions.

Kidneys When blood passes through the kidneys' filtering system, excess water and the electrolytes, sodium (salt) and potassium, are removed and sent to the bladder to be excreted. By controlling the volume of fluid in the blood, the kidneys can raise or lower blood pressure. If the body becomes dehydrated, for example, the kidneys retain fluid; if sodium and volume levels rise, the kidneys produce more urine to flush out the excess salt.

When blood pressure begins to fall, the kidneys also release an enzyme called renin, which through a complex process, raises blood pressure; renin production halts when blood pressure rises. (For information on managing hypertension, see page 799.)

The Brain and Nervous System   The brain and nervous system also do their part to regulate the heart, blood pressure, the chemical composition of the blood, and a host of other responses needed to keep the cardiovascular system in touch with its internal and external environment. For example, nerve receptors within the blood vessel walls send out signals—via chemicals called neurotransmitters—to the brain about the pressure within the vessels. Other receptors report on the pressure and volume status in the heart's chambers or salt or potassium levels in the blood. The brain then orders the appropriate adjustments. A shortage of oxygen during an exercise workout, for example, will trigger the respiratory center in the brain to speed up breathing in order to deliver more oxygen to the lungs and the blood. When you are frightened or stressed, other neurotransmitters—epinephrine and norepinephrine are the so-called fight-or-flight hormones—are produced by the adrenal glands. These hormones cause the heart to beat faster and blood vessels to constrict. Still others, such as acetylcholine, reverse the response.

EMERGENCY WARNING SIGNS INVOLVING THE HEART

These warning signs could save your life—or the life of a family member or friend—but only if you act promptly. Delaying emergency medical help can prove fatal. Each year, thousands of unnecessary deaths occur because people think their symptoms will pass and refuse to call for help. Become familiar with these classic warning signs and seek immediate emergency medical help if they occur:

- Crushing or squeezing chest pain beneath the breast bone

- Chest pain that goes to the arm, neck, jaw, back, or shoulders

- Chest pain accompanied by a cold sweat or clammy skin

- Chest pain accompanied by fainting or near-fainting, breathlessness, light-headedness, dizziness, or giddiness

- Chest pain associated with nausea and/or vomiting

- Chest pain that aches through to the back

- Chest pain accompanied by blue or pale skin (particularly around the lips)

- Feeling that the heart is not beating properly

- Chest pain accompanied by sense of extreme anxiety—"I think I'm dying"—or overall weakness. ■

Preventing Heart Disease

Although most Americans are aware that prevention and even reversal of some of the most common forms of heart disease are possible with modifications of lifestyle and diet, heart disease remains the major killer of men and women in this country. Clearly, not enough of us are listening.

This section reviews the risk factors that can lead to heart disease and explores those lifestyle changes that can prevent or reverse heart disease. For those individuals whose heart disease is due to congenital or genetic problems, proper medical treatment can in many cases relieve the problem, allowing them to lead normal, active lives. Those heart defects that are likely to be diagnosed and treated at birth or during infancy are covered in Chapter 8. Congenital or genetic heart defects that may not be discovered until adulthood are covered later in this chapter.

UNDERSTANDING ATHEROSCLEROSIS

The destructive mechanism behind many serious cardiovascular disorders is a silent and potentially lethal process called atherosclerosis. Healthy arteries are strong and elastic, and their linings are smooth so that blood can flow freely. With age, these blood vessels become thicker and less elastic, and their calcium content increases. This hardening, called arteriosclerosis, occurs throughout the body's arteries. In atherosclerosis, a form of arteriosclerosis, the inner layers of the artery walls—including the larger arteries and those that supply the heart itself—become thick and irregular. Specialized white blood cells congregate in the artery lining, where they trap oxidized low-density lipoprotein (LDL) cholesterol (the "bad" cholesterol; see page 793). This causes the formation of foam cells that coalesce into fatty streaks and may take up calcium deposits to form a scab-like plaque on the artery lining. These plaque deposits have the potential to rupture and further clog or obstruct the arteries.

Over time, this gradual buildup, which starts early in life as mere streaks of fat, eventually infiltrates the artery wall. This process narrows the channel and reduces the blood supply to the affected area—the heart, brain, legs, or kidneys—increasing the risk of a heart attack, stroke, and other serious arterial diseases. Thus, chest pain (angina), stroke, leg pain, or high blood pressure due to kidney problems may all be caused by insufficient blood flow in arteries narrowed by plaque.

When atherosclerotic plaque sufficiently narrows the arteries supplying blood to the heart, lack of oxygen can cause dysfunction of the muscle or be associated with chest pain. In most cases of heart attack or heart damage, however, a blood clot forms in a site of plaque rupture, suddenly blocking blood flow. The location of the obstruction and the duration of reduced blood flow determine the extent of damage and mechanical complications. Sometimes part or all of an atherosclerotic plaque in the systemic artery circuit breaks off and travels through the blood to distant sites. An embolus, as the moving blood clot is called, may lodge in the brain or arteries supplying the legs, kidneys, or intestines and is potentially life-threatening.

Too often, the first symptom of atherosclerosis you may experience is a serious, potentially fatal one—a heart attack or stroke. That is why it is essential to make lifestyle changes that will prevent, reduce, or eliminate your developing atherosclerosis.

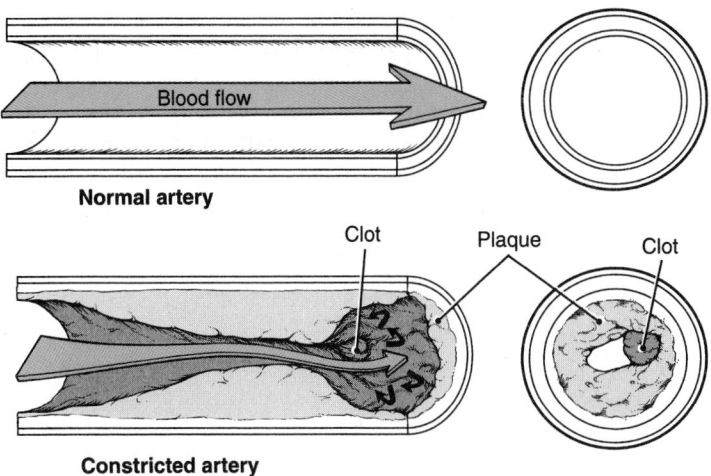

In atherosclerosis, plaque causes the inner layers of the artery walls to become thick and irregular. This narrows the space inside the vessel and can lead to impaired blood flow or plaque rupture, causing blood clots.

Hypertension (high blood pressure) and certain other cardiovascular risk factors can be modified or eliminated; others cannot. So it is important to understand what they are, whether they affect you, and what you can do about them.

RISK FACTORS OUTSIDE YOUR CONTROL

Understanding the risk factors you cannot control—family history, age, gender, and race—can alert you to an impending heart problem and encourage you to remedy those risk factors that you can control.

Age The older you are, the greater your risk of developing and dying from cardiovascular disease. Each year, about 10,000 women and 18,000 men under the age of 45 die from cardiovascular disease. That number climbs dramatically to about 40,000 women and 85,000 men between the ages of 45 and 64 and to nearly 500,000 men and women between the ages of 65 and 84.

Some cardiovascular risk factors, such as diabetes and hypertension, are more common with aging. Atherosclerotic changes are likely to be more advanced in elderly arteries. And as blood vessels age, they become less flexible and less able to respond to the pressure of blood flow. The heart itself may enlarge with age. An enlarged heart is less able to pump blood efficiently than a strong, normal-sized heart.

Gender For many years, heart disease was thought to be primarily a male concern. But now doctors realize that cardiovascular dis-

WOMEN AND HEART DISEASE

Although breast cancer receives a great deal of attention, heart disease is the number one killer of women. It is responsible for half the deaths of women. Yet until recently, heart disease was considered a man's disease. Women were often not screened for heart disease. Coronary artery disease (CAD) was routinely diagnosed later, rather than earlier, in women. In fact, a woman is still more likely than a man to be caught unaware by a myocardial infarction (heart attack) and to die from it.

All this is changing, however, as more and more heart disease studies are including subjects of both sexes in equal numbers. Menopause is now listed as a risk factor for heart disease. Estrogen, a hormone that protects against CAD, is produced in much smaller quantities after menopause, making postmenopausal women more vulnerable to heart disease than younger women.

The risk of heart disease increases for women as they age. Women are usually diagnosed with heart disease a decade later in life than are men. After a myocardial infarction, a woman's prognosis is poorer than a man's. Recent research has also shown that the results of heart disease tests among women differ from those of men, making heart disease harder to diagnose. Even an electrocardiogram (ECG) or exercise stress test (EST) may under- or overdiagnose heart disease in women. These tests, developed on male subjects, may not be as accurate when used to detect heart abnormalities in women, because their hearts are smaller and, in certain situations, react differently.

Fortunately, enormous strides have been made in understanding and treating heart disease in women. Awareness that women are not spared gives a woman at risk a chance to do something about the condition before she becomes another negative statistic. There are lifestyle changes every woman can make to lower her risk. Here are some suggestions.

- If you are approaching or have reached menopause, pay particular attention to the medical care of your heart and the lifestyle changes listed below.

- If you smoke, stop.

- If you lead a sedentary lifestyle, talk to your doctor about gradually making exercise a part of your life. Even walking 20 to 30 minutes a day can lower your risk for heart disease. Almost 90 percent of women do not exercise regularly, and at least 17 percent do not exercise at all (almost twice as many nonexercisers as men).

- If you are obese, begin a weight-loss program—not for vanity's sake, but for the sake of your heart.

- If your diet is high in saturated (mainly animal) fats, cut down on fat and make fresh fruits and vegetables an important part of your diet.

Remember, whether you are a man or a woman, you can help prevent and reverse heart disease and improve your life through dietary and lifestyle changes. ■

ease is not sexist; it simply is slower to arrive in women. (See below for more information.) Men are more likely to have coronary artery disease than are women—but only until women reach menopause. After that the difference between men and women shrinks, so that, overall, about 47 percent of fatal heart attack victims are women.

Family history Perhaps one of the strongest risk factors for heart disease is your family history. Your risk is higher if you have a close relative (mother, father, brother, or sister) who developed the disease before age 55. Your risk is also increased if your parents, grandparents, aunts, or uncles have had episodes of chest pain (angina), a heart attack, or a heart bypass operation.

Other genetic factors passed on from parents to children may promote moderately high cholesterol levels, high blood pressure, diabetes, or obesity. The greatest inherited risk, however, is among people genetically predisposed to dangerously high cholesterol levels, a condition known as familial hypercholesterolemia.

But inheriting a tendency to develop a disorder does not mean you will actually do so. Many diseases—and heart disease is no exception—arise as a complex interplay of inherited tendencies and environment or lifestyle choices. While you have no control over what you inherit from your parents, you do control the kind of life you choose to live. These choices in large measure determine what you make of that inheritance.

Race Cardiovascular disease is the leading cause of death in the United States. Black men have a lower risk for coronary heart disease than white men; however, black men are more likely to suffer a stroke, mainly because of their high risk for hypertension and diabetes. Obesity is an important risk factor for black women, and at the same time contributes to hypertension risk. Compared with whites, blacks develop hypertension at an earlier age—and at any age, the disease is more severe in blacks than in whites. As a result, blacks are 1.8 times more likely than whites to have a nonfatal stroke, 1.3 times more likely to have a fatal stroke, and 1.5 times more likely to die from cardiovascular disease.

A variety of factors may contribute to the increased risk for hypertension among blacks. Lack of access to health care and racial differences in diet, health behaviors, and the ability to excrete sodium from the body may help account for hypertension's heavy toll in this group. Beyond that, more research is needed before the role of race as a genetic entity can be separated from race-linked factors, such as economic status and dietary patterns.

RISK FACTORS YOU CAN MODIFY

Although you cannot alter certain givens in your life, you can do your best to control those risk factors that you *can* modify—for example, high cholesterol levels, smoking, overweight, and a sedentary lifestyle. There are important behavioral and medical measures you can take to help protect your heart and circulatory system. The four major risk factors for coronary heart disease are sedentary lifestyle, high blood cholesterol, high blood pressure (hypertension), and cigarette smoking; each of these can be influenced by lifestyle changes. But there are other risks you can reduce as well, and often when you improve one you will be improving several. For example, if you increase physical activity, you are likely to lose

CHOLESTEROL AND DIETARY FATS

Fats belong to a family known as lipids, which includes triglycerides, sterols (such as cholesterol), several hormones, and waxes.

Triglycerides

Triglycerides (a glycerol molecule attached to three fatty acids) serve the body both as the primary storage form of fat and as a basic fuel for muscle tissue. All dietary fats contain mixtures of fatty acids, although in different proportions: the familiar saturated, polyunsaturated, and monounsaturated fats. The more saturated (with hydrogen atoms) the fat molecule is, the less healthy it is for your heart.

Saturated fats, found primarily in animal foods and dairy products, but also in coconut and palm oil, raise blood cholesterol by slowing the removal of harmful low-density lipoprotein (LDL) cholesterol from the blood. This is why you may develop high blood cholesterol levels even if your diet is low in cholesterol but high in saturated fat.

Polyunsaturated fats, found in vegetable and fish oils, and monounsaturated fats, found in olive and canola oils, lower harmful LDL cholesterol in the blood when substituted for saturated fats in the diet. Most saturated fats are solid at room temperature. When vegetable oils, such as corn or safflower oil, which are high in polyunsaturated fat, are converted into margarine, the oil is hydrogenated to make it firm; thus it becomes more saturated and more of a heart risk.

Although most people understand the correlation between cholesterol and heart disease, they are unaware that triglycerides are also important in determining heart disease risk. New studies show that high triglyceride levels—especially in people with a low level of protective high-density lipoprotein (HDL) cholesterol—increase the risk for heart disease. A ratio of the triglycerides divided by the HDL that exceeds 5 indicates heart disease risk; as the number climbs, so does the risk.

Cholesterol

Cholesterol is a sterol—a waxy, fat-like substance found in animal foods (meat, fish, poultry, eggs, and whole-milk dairy products). Although we have come to view cholesterol as a nutritional demon, it is, in fact, essential for life. Every cell in the body requires cholesterol: It is a critical structural support in cell membranes; it is used to make important hormones, such as estrogen, progesterone, testosterone, aldosterone (helps regulate blood pressure), and cortisol (an adrenal-gland hormone). Cholesterol is also a major component of nerve cells and the brain.

"Good" Cholesterol, "Bad" Cholesterol Only about 20 percent of the cholesterol in your blood comes from food; 80 percent is manufactured by your body, mainly the liver. A balancing mechanism exists so that there is always enough cholesterol for the cells to function properly: The less you eat, the more your body makes, and vice versa. Unfortunately, this mechanism ensures a sufficient supply of cholesterol inside the cells, without regard to levels circulating in the blood. Because cholesterol and triglycerides are fats, they cannot dissolve in the watery fluid of the blood. Instead, they are transported in special proteins called lipoproteins, which typically consist of triglycerides and cholesterol esters in the center of the package and an outer, water-soluble surface containing proteins, cholesterol, and phospholipids.

The names of three of these lipoproteins have become familiar to most Americans: high-density lipoprotein (HDL), low-density lipoprotein (LDL), and very-low-density lipoprotein (VLDL). The density is based on the weight of the lipoprotein molecule: LDLs have relatively little dense protein and high levels of cholesterol; HDLs are high in protein and low in cholesterol; and VLDLs are high in triglycerides. The lipoproteins rate as follows.

HDL cholesterol (average value: 45 mg/dL in men, 55 mg/dL in women), the so-called "good" cholesterol, carries cholesterol from the arterial wall to the liver, where it is recycled for further use or removed from the body. The higher the HDL level, the better. LDL cholesterol (normal value: less than 130 mg/dL), the "bad" cholesterol, transports cholesterol to sites throughout the body where it is used to repair cell membranes and make several hormones. LDLs are associated with a higher risk of heart attack, because as they move through the arteries, they tend to leave accumulations of cholesterol in the blood vessel walls. VLDL cholesterol contains mainly triglycerides (normal triglyceride value: less than 200 mg/dL). ■

UNDERSTANDING YOUR LIPID PROFILE

Screening tests include measurement of total and high-density lipoprotein (HDL) cholesterol. If these values are abnormal or you are at high risk for coronary heart disease, your doctor will request a full profile that includes triglycerides in addition to total and HDL cholesterol. If you are going to have blood drawn for a triglyceride test, be certain not to eat or drink (except water) for at least 12 hours to ensure accuracy. And because the results vary slightly from one laboratory to another, repeat studies to evaluate response to treatment are best done by the same laboratory. Let's consider the different forms.

Total cholesterol (normal: less than 200 mg/dL) measures the sum of all forms of cholesterol. Because total cholesterol is a mixture of "bad" (low-density lipoprotein, or LDL cholesterol) and "good" (HDL) cholesterol, it is important to know the specific lipoprotein fractions if the total cholesterol level is greater than 200 mg/dL.

Ratios comparing these lipid measures help fine-tune heart disease risk. These include:

- Total cholesterol divided by HDL cholesterol (ideally under 5.5, with risk of heart disease climbing as the number increases).

- LDL cholesterol level divided by HDL cholesterol (ideally less than 3.5, with the risk climbing as the ratio rises).

- Triglyceride level divided by HDL cholesterol (ideally under 4, with the risk clearly beginning at 5 and climbing as the number increases). For example, if your triglyceride value is 250 and your HDL is 35, your ratio would be a dangerous 7.

The effects of HDL cholesterol and LDL cholesterol on the risk for heart disease are independent. Thus, if HDL cholesterol levels are very high, this helps to offset the risk associated with LDL cholesterol. On the other hand, in some instances, even when the amount of total or LDL cholesterol is not high, the amount of beneficial HDL cholesterol in the blood is too low (a condition called isolated low HDL cholesterol). Even in the absence of other risk factors for heart disease, this finding alone is enough to warrant concern and a recommendation for lifestyle modification.

The number of blood fat tests continues to increase, with measures now routinely available for separating various kinds of HDL and other lipoproteins. Recent studies have been examining the role of a new suspect, lipoprotein (a) [Lp(a)]. Although there is much we still do not know about the role of Lp(a) in the body, there is evidence that high Lp(a) levels may be an early indicator

of heart disease risk, particularly that of coronary thrombosis.

Making sense of a cholesterol test may be a daunting prospect for even a scientifically astute layman. But your doctor can help you interpret what your lipid profile reveals about your heart disease risk. See below for a summary of lipid levels.

Lipid Levels and Heart Disease Risk

- Total cholesterol

    Desirable: Less than 200 mg/dL

    Borderline: 200–239 mg dL

    Too high: More than 240 mg/dL

- LDL cholesterol

    Desirable: Less than 130 mg/dL

    Borderline: 130–159 mg/dL

    Too high: More than 160 mg/dL

- Triglycerides

    Desirable: Less than 200 mg/dL

    Borderline: 200–400 mg/dL

    High: 400–1,000 mg/dL

    Very high: More than 1,000 mg/dL

- LDL cholesterol/HDL cholesterol ratio

    Desirable: Less than 3.5

    Too high: More than 3.5

- HDL cholesterol

    Desirable:

        For men: More than 45 mg/dL

        For women: More than 55 mg/dL

    Borderline

        For men: 35–45 mg/dL

        For women: 40–55 mg/dL

    Too low

        For men: Less than 35 mg/dL

        For women: Less than 40 mg/dL ■

weight and improve your high-density lipoprotein (HDL) cholesterol and triglycerides—all of which lower your risk for cardiovascular disease. Diabetes is one of the greatest risk factors for coronary heart disease. The diabetes can be controlled, but it is not clear that controlling diabetes per se reduces the risk for coronary heart disease.

A low level of HDL cholesterol is also a major risk factor. HDL levels can be increased somewhat by lifestyle measures and medication. Other risk factors you can modify include the following.

High blood cholesterol and triglyceride levels As blood cholesterol levels rise, the risk for coronary heart disease rises along with it. Elevated triglycerides (blood fats) are clearly a risk factor for coronary heart disease in women and people with diabetes. So it is important to get your cholesterol and triglyceride levels checked by your doctor.

Your cholesterol level is determined by your genetic makeup and the amount of saturated (animal) fat and cholesterol you consume in food. The liver also manufactures cholesterol, so that even if you ate no dietary cholesterol, your liver would supply what your body needs. For individuals with high cholesterol levels, every 1 percent reduction in total blood cholesterol reduces your heart attack risk by 2 percent. Cut your blood cholesterol 15 percent, and your coronary heart disease risk drops by 30 percent. (To learn more about the role of cholesterol and triglycerides in cardiovascular disease, see page 793.)

Hypertension Hypertension (high blood pressure) damages delicate blood vessel linings, especially in the heart, kidneys, and eyes. The complications of untreated hypertension include: enlargement of the heart; congestive heart failure; stroke; scarring of the kidneys, with loss of effective filtering function; aortic dissection (splitting of the wall of the aorta, leaving it weakened and more prone to rupture); thickening of the artery walls; and narrowing or bleeding in blood vessels in the eyes, potentially causing blindness. Elevated blood pressure from any cause that continues unabated and untreated can become rapidly worse (malignant hypertension) and requires urgent medical intervention to prevent serious or even fatal complications.

If you have hypertension, it is extremely important to return to your doctor periodically to get your blood pressure checked, to lose weight if necessary, and to make dietary changes as prescribed by your doctor. If you take medication, take it as prescribed and be certain to get your blood pressure and medication dosage monitored regularly. (See page 799 for more information.)

Smoking Smoking is responsible for 350,000 deaths a year from heart disease, according to a 1990 US Surgeon General report, and is the single most preventable cause of death in the United States. Smoking forces the heart to work harder, while at the same time it compromises its blood supply and damages blood vessels, contributing to atherosclerosis. It also increases the likelihood of a blood clot forming in an already narrowed artery, because nicotine constricts blood vessels, including the coronary arteries. Cigarette smoke also raises fibrinogen levels, which increases the tendency of blood to clot. Carbon monoxide, a poisonous gas in cigarette smoke, reduces the amount of oxygen that red blood cells can carry and also damages blood vessel linings. If you smoke, begin a program to stop (see Chapter 4 for more information on quitting smoking).

Smoke not only damages your lungs and heart, it is a serious hazard to nonsmokers who live with you. A new 10-year study of passive smoke exposure found that regular exposure to second-hand smoke almost doubled the risk of heart disease for both men and women—a far greater risk than previously estimated. Each year, as many as 50,000 Americans may die of heart attacks caused by passive smoking.

Clotting abnormalities The normal clotting process helps seal damaged blood vessels from blood loss. When blood cells called platelets come in contact with a damaged blood vessel, these cells become sticky and tend to clump at the site of the injury. As part of the coagulation process, a chemical called fibrinogen produces filaments of fibrin, which help enmesh platelets and other cells to form a clot. Excessively high levels of fibrinogen increase the risk of developing a blood clot in an artery, leading to a heart attack or stroke. Fibrinogen levels increase with age. You may not be able to alter these levels through your own efforts, but smoking increases fibrinogen—still another reason to quit.

Obesity One of every three or four Americans is overweight; about 34 million adults in this country are obese (20 percent or more above normal weight). If you are overweight, work with a doctor or registered dietitian to set up a nutritional program that will help you lose weight and keep it off. Although excess weight may not directly lead to coronary artery disease, it promotes other risk factors—high cholesterol, hypertension, and diabetes—that do contribute to heart disease. Also, if heart disease is already present, it's further aggravated by extra pounds. (See Chapters 1 and 2 for more information on losing weight.)

Sedentary lifestyle A sedentary lifestyle contributes to obesity and high cholesterol levels. Numerous studies have demonstrated that staying active can help prevent heart disease. Make daily physical activity a part of your life, or include an exercise routine of 20 to 30 minutes in your schedule at least three times a week. Talk to your doctor about an exercise regimen appropriate for your age and condition. If you have risk factors for coronary artery disease you may want to have an exercise stress test before beginning a vigorous exercise program. (See Chapter 2 for more information on maintaining cardiac fitness.)

NEW RISK FACTORS

There is much we do not know about the causes of cardiovascular disease, but researchers are exploring some new risk factors.

Homocysteine

Many researchers are considering adding a new risk factor for cardiovascular disease: high blood levels of homocysteine, an amino acid that may play a role in clogging the arteries that feed the heart, the brain, and the legs. In a recent summary of 18 studies, higher levels of homocysteine were associated with greater risk of both myocardial infarction (heart attack) and stroke, even when other risk factors were taken into account. The increased risk was very similar to the risk associated with higher serum cholesterol.

Fortunately, a relatively simple dietary fix—folic acid—may help cut the risk. Folic acid, recommended for pregnant women and those planning to become pregnant—is found in beans and peas, enriched whole-grain cereals, nuts, orange juice, green leafy vegetables, spinach, and liver. But because folic acid can be destroyed in cooking, food sources may not be sufficient if you are at risk for cardiovascular disease. A folic acid supplement of 400 mcg may be helpful. It is recommended that it be taken with 1 mg of vitamin B_{12}, because a folic acid overdose can hide a deficiency of vitamin B_{12}, which works with folic acid to help the body manufacture red blood cells, and because B_{12} is necessary for homocysteine metabolism.

Lipoprotein (a)

Lipoprotein (a), or Lp(a), is made up of two parts: the "bad" low-density lipoprotein (LDL) molecule and another protein, apo-(a). Lp(a) interrupts the clot-dissolving process, so that if a clot forms in a coronary or carotid artery, the risk of a heart attack or stroke increases. A high level of Lp(a) is a risk factor, just as high cholesterol levels or low levels of "good" HDL cholesterol are (see Cholesterol and Dietary Fats, page 793). The medication nicotinic acid may lower Lp(a), although whether this cuts cardiovascular risk is still not known.

Chlamydia pneumoniae Infection

Chlamydia pneumoniae is not the notorious sexually transmitted bacterium, *Chlamydia trachomatis*, but a widespread microbe that causes a flu-like respiratory condition and sometimes pneumonia. Although the research is preliminary, evidence suggests that this form of *Chlamydia* may infect blood vessel walls and remain there for years, producing inflammation. Here is how it may work: Immune cells called macrophages become infected with *C. pneumoniae* and carry it from the respiratory tract to the arterial wall. The macrophages enter the arterial wall, where they take up LDL cholesterol and thus initiate artery-narrowing plaques. If this theory holds up, someday it may be possible to at least clear up the infection with antibiotic treatment. ■

Uncontrolled Diabetes More than 80 percent of people with diabetes die of some form of cardiovascular disease. Diabetes damages blood vessels, raises LDL cholesterol and triglyceride levels, lowers HDL cholesterol levels, and increases blood pressure. People with adult-onset (type 2) diabetes also tend to be overweight. If you have diabetes, it is extremely important to follow your doctor's instructions and keep your blood sugar levels under control. (See Chapter 26 for more information.)

Menopause When estrogen production declines at menopause, a woman's risk of heart disease increases (see page 792). The availability of estrogen replacement therapy (ERT) now makes menopause a modifiable risk factor. ERT seems to reduce the risk of heart disease and osteoporosis (the bone-thinning disease). But since estrogen may increase the risk of uterine cancer and possibly breast cancer, the decision to use ERT should be made only after you and your doctor evaluate your personal risk factors.

Stress In modern life, stress is everywhere, and it is not necessarily harmful. At present, the connection between stress and heart disease has not been proved. But if you suffer from heart disease, it does appear that your body's reaction to stressful events may increase your risk of having a heart attack. Recent research on stress has singled out the possibly harmful effects of chronic anger and frustration. Blowing up now and then is not harmful, but if your emotional responses get stuck in a constant state of anger and irritation, your physical stress responses may also stall in overdrive, raising blood pressure, constricting blood vessels, and flooding the body with so-called fight-or-flight hormones (cortisol, epinephrine, and norepinephrine) produced by the adrenal glands. These hormones increase heart rate and blood pressure, raise levels of blood sugar, increase the tendency of blood to clot, and may injure the linings of the coronary arteries.

To lower your stress levels, consider learning some relaxation techniques, such as meditation, yoga, or biofeedback. Gardening, exercise, going for a walk, and listening to music are also helpful. Finally, avoid caffeine and cigarettes, which in the long run act as stimulants. (For more information on relieving stress, see Chapter 11.)

Other modifiable risk factors include: illegal drug use (cocaine and amphetamines increase the heart rate, while constricting the coronary arteries and decreasing blood flow to the heart); and certain medications, such as oral contraceptives for women who smoke.

Lifestyle Changes for a Healthy Heart

By now, we have all heard that diet, exercise, and a healthful lifestyle may help prevent or control heart disease; yet, as a nation we are growing fatter and Americans continue to eat high-fat ice cream along with their diet sodas. Here are a few important guidelines to help you cut your heart disease risk. (For more detailed information, see Chapter 1.)

EAT A BALANCED DIET

Eat a wide variety of foods Variety is important—not only for balance, but to provide the vitamins and minerals you need.

Let carbohydrates be 50 to 60 percent of total daily calories Carbohydrate intake should be mainly complex carbohydrates (starches). Try for six servings of grain foods, such as bread, pasta, cereal, and rice; three servings of vegetables; and two servings of fruit.

Limit protein to 15 to 20 percent of total daily calories The average person needs about 50 g of protein a day. Protein is found in meat, poultry, fish, milk and dairy products, eggs, beans, seeds, nuts, grains, and soy products. A 4-oz serving of meat, poultry, or fish supplies 25 to 35 g of protein.

Cut fat to less than 30 percent of total calories If you have heart disease, your

---

GETTING THE FAT OUT

Here are some tips to help you cut back on dietary fat.

- Choose poultry, fish, and lean cuts of meat; remove the skin from chicken and trim all visible fat from meat before cooking.

- Drink skim milk or 1 percent instead of 2 percent milk or whole milk.

- Choose low-fat cottage cheese or low-fat farmer cheese instead of processed, natural, and hard cheeses, such as American, brie, and cheddar.

- Use tub margarine or liquid vegetable oils, which are high in polyunsaturated fat (safflower and corn oils, for example) and monounsaturated fats (olive and canola oils) instead of butter, lard, and hydrogenated vegetable shortenings, which are high in saturated fat. Soft tub margarine is less saturated (hydrogenated) than harder stick margarine.

- Cut down on commercially prepared and processed foods made with saturated fats or oils (palm and coconut). Read food labels to choose those low in saturated fats.

- Avoid organ meats such as liver, brain, and kidney.

- Eat fewer egg yolks; try substituting two egg whites for each whole egg in recipes.

- Avoid mayonnaise and salad dressings, or buy low-fat versions of these products.

- Choose low-fat snacks, such as bagels, air-blown popcorn, fruit, unsalted pretzels, nonfat frozen yogurt or ice milk, and flavored rice cakes.

- Use low-fat cooking techniques, such as broiling, boiling, grilling, roasting, poaching, microwaving, steaming, or stir-frying. ■

---

doctor may wish you to further reduce dietary fat. Studies have shown dramatic benefits from a diet that is severely curtailed in fat. Also, cut saturated fat (animal fat) to less than 10 percent of total calories, and hold cholesterol to no more than 300 mg a day. Read food package labels to help determine how much fat foods contain. According to the National Heart, Lung, and Blood Institute, your total cholesterol and LDL cholesterol levels may begin to drop 2 to 3 weeks after you begin a cholesterol-lowering diet. Over time, you may reduce your cholesterol levels by 30 to 55 mg/dL or even more.

Increase fiber to about 25 to 35 g a day Most Americans consume only about half the amount of fiber they should. Fiber is an indigestible carbohydrate found in the cell walls of plant foods. Fiber plays an important role in helping to prevent cancer, but it also benefits your heart. Fiber-rich foods can help you lose weight or maintain weight loss, because these foods tend to be low in calories, take longer to chew, and make you feel full.

Fiber comes in two forms: soluble and insoluble. Soluble fiber (pectins and gums) may help to lower cholesterol levels. Soluble fiber dissolves in fluids in the large intestine and forms a gel that binds with bile acids in the intestine, which are excreted along with the indigestible fiber. Blood cholesterol levels are lowered, because the liver then converts more cholesterol to bile acids. Good sources of soluble fiber are oat products, dried beans and peas, lentils, apples, and citrus fruits.

Insoluble fiber (found in whole-grain foods, cereals, wheat bran, and many fruits and vegetables) soaks up water like a sponge, adding bulk and preventing constipation by making it easier for the intestine to move waste matter along—including potential carcinogens.

ELEVATED LIPIDS: BEYOND DIET

By cutting back on dietary fats and making other lifestyle changes, you will undoubtedly lower your cholesterol and triglyceride levels. Nevertheless, certain genetic and medical disorders may not respond to these conservative measures. These include:

Inherited Triglyceride Disorders A common inherited disorder is familial hypertriglyceridemia, resulting from either excessive production of very-low density lipoproten (VLDL) by the liver or slowed removal of VLDL triglycerides from the blood. Another genetic disorder can be associated with triglyceride levels greater than 1,000 mg/dL. Individuals who inherit this disorder may suffer bouts of pancreatitis (inflammation of the pancreas) accompanied by abdominal pain, nausea, and vomiting as well as enlargement of the liver and spleen. Because of the possibility of inherited risk, family members should be tested.

Inherited Cholesterol Disorders Familial hypercholesterolemia may cause extreme elevations of LDL cholesterol, with coronary heart disease developing in people in their 30s or 40s. Family members should also be evaluated.

Other Medical Conditions Other disorders can contribute to elevated blood lipid levels, most notably hypothyroidism (underactive thyroid gland). Often, simply correcting this condition with thyroid medication can return elevated cholesterol to normal. People with high cholesterol levels should also be evaluated for other causes, such as a kidney disorder.

Medication Some medications can worsen blood fat levels. They include: beta blockers (such as propranolol and atenolol, but excluding pindolol and acebutolol), diuretics, oral contraceptives, and corticosteroids. ■

As you increase the fiber in your diet, it is important to drink more liquids, because fiber absorbs fluid as it passes through your body. To avoid constipation, drink 8 to 10 glasses of water a day, and add fiber gradually. At the start, too much at once can cause gas, bloating, or diarrhea.

Drink alcohol in moderation only Moderate amounts of alcohol (3 to 5 oz of wine, 8 to 12 oz of beer, or 1 oz of liquor) may help improve HDL cholesterol levels. However, this possible benefit is not a reason to start drinking. Amounts of alcohol in excess of these may raise blood triglycerides.

Make sure your diet includes antioxidants Antioxidants are compounds that prevent the damaging effects of highly reactive oxygen molecules known as free oxygen radicals. These unstable molecules are produced during the normal metabolic process by which the body burns fuel (glucose) to provide cells with energy. Free radical damage to cells has been linked to both cancer and heart disease. In heart disease, these compounds appear to promote the oxidation of LDL which tends to accumulate as fatty plaque in artery walls. The process is similar to the way in which iron rusts.

Animal and population studies suggest that vitamin E, an antioxidant, inhibits LDL oxidation. Although the best way to get your vitamins and minerals is from a balanced diet rich in fresh vegetables and fruit, it is difficult to get large amounts of fat-soluble vitamin E from food (vegetable oils, whole grain cereals, beans, margarine, eggs, fish), especially on a low-fat diet. A vitamin E supplement of 400 IU may help slow atherosclerosis, but proof of this benefit awaits the results of ongoing studies.

On the other hand, supplements of beta-carotene, another antioxidant, did not prove effective in preventing coronary heart disease. In fact, beta-carotene supplements appeared to cause lung cancer in smokers in two clinical trials. Beta-carotene and vitamin C, another antioxidant, are abundantly present in many fresh fruits and vegetables. The best strategy is to include fruits and vegetables as part of a healthful diet. Furthermore, plant foods contain other substances such as phytochemicals that may have disease-fighting properties, perhaps related to their antioxidant effects.

DRUG TREATMENT FOR ELEVATED CHOLESTEROL LEVELS

The first line of therapy should be to change your diet and add an exercise regimen as directed by your doctor (see Lifestyle Changes for a Healthy Heart, page 797). But if blood fat levels fail to respond adequately, your doctor may recommend medication, such as the following:

Statins (Lovastatin [Mevacor], Simvastatin [Zocar], Pravastatin [Pravacbol], Fluvastatin [Lescol], Cerivastatin [Baycol], and Atorvastatin [Lipitor]) The liver cells that produce cholesterol assemble it in a step-wise manner. One crucial step along the way dictates the speed and amount of cholesterol production. It is at this crucial step that a new class of medication comes in: statins, or HMG-CoA reductase inhibitors. Statins slow down cholesterol production, thus reducing the risk of dying from coronary heart disease (CHD). They also reduce overall mortality in men with elevated low-density lipoproten (LDL) cholesterol, whether or not clinical heart disease is present. Recent studies show that statins lower total and LDL cholesterol and significantly reduce deaths from coronary artery disease. They are now the medications of choice for lowering cholesterol. Statins, which are usually taken at dinner or bedtime, are generally well tolerated.

Niacin (Nicotinic Acid) Niacin helps reduce the production of very-low-density lipoproten (VLDL) and LDL and increases the level of the "good" high-density lipoproten (HDL) cholesterol. Some formulations of niacin cause flushing, and the sustained-release varieties have been implicated in liver inflammation (hepatitis).

Bile Acid Binders (Cholestyramine, Colestipol) Cholesterol is converted in the liver to bile acids, which are an important component of bile. Bile acids are released into the intestine, where they aid in digesting dietary fats. Normally, the cells lining the intestine reabsorb bile acids. This process can be blocked by the medications cholestyramine and colestipol, which bind bile acids in the intestine. Preventing reabsorption increases the demand for more bile acids, depleting liver stores of cholesterol. The additional cholesterol to fuel bile production is then drawn from the blood, lowering levels of LDL cholesterol. Unfortunately, triglycerides usually increase with these medications, to some degree offsetting the benefit of reducing LDL cholesterol. The normal dose of bile acid binders can cause gas, bloating, and constipation and may also interfere with the absorption of certain vitamins and medications. ■

STAY PHYSICALLY ACTIVE

Recent studies have shown that even moderate increases in activity level offer substantial health benefits. A brisk, 30-minute walk every other day can help you maintain cardiovascular fitness. Aerobic (the word means "with oxygen") exercise that raises your heart rate (walking, jogging, swimming, biking) and resistance exercise (light weight training) have been shown to reduce elevated blood fat levels and, more important, raise protective HDL cholesterol in the blood. (See Chapter 2 for more information.)

QUIT SMOKING

Cigarette smoke adds to the damage already done by harmful LDL cholesterol levels and promotes atherosclerosis. See Chapter 4 for more information on how to quit smoking.

Managing Hypertension

Hypertension is often called "the silent killer" because it may not cause symptoms for many years, even as sustained high pressure damages delicate blood vessel linings, especially in the heart, kidneys, and eyes. The term hypertension has to do with high pressure of the blood, not with tension or stress in the individual. On the contrary, even the most even-tempered, serene individual may be suffering from this insidious condition.

What is blood pressure? Blood pressure is measured in millimeters of mercury (mm Hg) using a sphygmomanometer attached to a standard blood pressure cuff placed around the upper arm. Sphygmomanometers can be mechanical models that use a gauge for the reading or electronic models that give digital readouts. The measurement refers to how high the pressure inside the artery can raise a column of mercury. The "top number" of a blood pressure reading, the systolic pressure, represents the pressure generated in the blood vessels when the heart contracts and pumps; the "bottom number," the diastolic pressure, represents the resting pressure in the blood vessels when the heart relaxes between contractions. Because blood pressure is affected by strong emotion, activity, temperature, and stress, it should be measured after 10 minutes of rest, in a warm, calm atmosphere; multiple readings on three different occasions should be taken before making a diagnosis, unless blood

BLOOD PRESSURE CLASSIFICATIONS: WHEN TO SEE YOUR DOCTOR

Hypertension is not a black-and-white diagnosis. There are different levels and types of hypertension and, therefore, different degrees of risk. The classifications below may offer some guidance.

Systolic (top number)

- Less than 130 mm Hg: normal blood pressure; recheck within 2 years

- 130 to 139 mm Hg: high normal; recheck within 1 year

- 140 to 159 mm Hg: mild hypertension; recheck within 2 months

- 160 to 179 mm Hg: moderate hypertension; see your doctor within 1 month

- 180 to 209 mm Hg: severe hypertension; see your doctor within 1 week

- 210 mm Hg or higher: very severe hypertension; see your doctor immediately

Note: Isolated systolic hypertension, which occurs mainly in elderly people, is a normal diastolic pressure with an elevated systolic pressure of 140 mm Hg or more.

Diastolic (bottom number)

- Less than 85 mm Hg: normal blood pressure; recheck within 2 years

- 85 to 89 mm Hg: high-normal blood pressure; recheck within 1 year

- 90 to 99 mm Hg: mild hypertension; recheck within 2 months

- 100 to 109 mm Hg: moderate hypertension; see your doctor within 1 month

- 110 to 119 mm Hg: severe hypertension; see your doctor within 1 week

- 120 mm Hg or higher: very severe hypertension; see your doctor immediately ■

pressure is very high. (For more information, see page 800.)

White coat hypertension is when a person's blood pressure is normal when taken at home but is high when taken by a doctor (who may or may not be wearing a white coat!). This phenomenon is thought to be due to the stress of seeing a doctor. Before diagnosing this condition, it is absolutely necessary that measurements taken outside the office be done carefully by someone who has been trained in how to measure blood pressure with a device that is known to be accurate.

The risk associated with an elevated blood pressure and the benefit associated with lowering blood pressure were determined based on blood pressure measured in an office setting. No such information exists for home blood pressure reading. Some experts think that if the stress of going to the doctor raises blood pressure, so must other relatively minor stresses, and that blood pressure–lowering medication should be used based on the office readings. Studies of people with white coat hypertension support this view. These studies demonstrated mildly thickened hearts and other abnormalities in such persons, suggesting that they have been hurt by their higher levels of blood pressure. Other experts have suggested that persons with white coat hypertension may not need to take medications to lower their blood pressure. Everyone agrees, however, that people with white coat hypertension who have evidence of blood pressure–related disease, such as kidney disease or heart enlargement, need to take antihypertensive medication.

WHAT CAUSES HYPERTENSION?

Although about 50 million Americans have hypertension, 95 percent of the time the specific cause remains unclear and the condition is called essential hypertension. In the remaining 5 percent, hypertension is a consequence of some other condition or disorder. Secondary hypertension may be caused by: kidney disease; constriction (coarctation) of the aorta; narrowing of one or both of the arteries that lead to the kidneys (renal artery stenosis); an adrenal gland tumor and other endocrine conditions causing the abnormal release of certain hormones or other body chemicals; a side effect of certain medications; or a consequence of pregnancy.

Significant kidney disease can elevate blood pressure in several ways (see Chapter 26). Kidney disease can lead to faulty stimulation of a protective mechanism within the kidney tissue that governs blood pressure, known as the renin-angiotensin-aldosterone (RAA) system. The RAA system exists to protect us in the event of shock (the sudden catastrophic loss of blood pressure that may occur with uncontrolled bleeding or raging infection). When the flow of blood to the kidneys falls below a critical level—either because blood pressure has dropped dramatically, as it can in serious infection, or because of extreme blood loss—the kidneys sense the drop and release renin, a body chemical that begins a cascade of events that ultimately elevates blood pressure.

Renin stimulates the release of angiotensin, which is converted to angiotensin II. This substance, itself, powerfully constricts the arteries to elevate blood pressure, but also stimulates the release of the hormone aldosterone, which prompts the kidneys to retain sodium and fluid and further elevate blood pressure. The RAA system can become activated mistakenly when constriction in a renal artery impairs blood flow to the kidneys. Problems ensue because the pressure throughout the body is actually normal; it is low only in the artery beyond the crimped or stenosed area leading to the kidneys. This condition, called renal artery stenosis, is most commonly caused by atherosclerosis in the renal arteries that supply blood to the kidneys, but it may also be caused by other conditions like fibromuscular disease; coarctation of the aorta may account for hypertension in early life through the same mechanism. Hypertension results because the kidney releases renin to raise blood pressure. To rule out renal artery constriction as a cause, a dye visible on x-ray is injected into the kidney's arteries. If there is a crimp in the blood vessel, it will be clearly visible. In some centers, the same information can be provided by specialized forms of computed tomography (CT) scans and magnetic resonance imaging (MRI), without the need for catheterization.

The kidneys play a crucial role in regulating water and mineral balance in the body, and in sensing and counteracting an abrupt drop in blood pressure or volume. Therefore, any disease that damages the kidneys can lead to fluid retention that elevates blood pressure. Common offenders include those diseases that damage the filtering units of the kidneys, chemicals or medications that injure kidney tissues (see Chapter 24), autoimmune disorders such as systemic lupus erythematosus (see Chapter 17), and diabetes mellitus (see Chapter 26).

Other hormonal abnormalities may cause hypertension. Occasionally, hypertension results from the abnormal release of aldosterone directly, without first activating the RAA system—a condition termed primary hyperaldosteronism. Another rare cause is the abnormal production of epinephrine (adrenalin) from an adrenal gland tumor (pheochromocytoma). Epinephrine and its cousin norepinephrine (noradrena-

MALIGNANT HYPERTENSION

Emergency symptoms include

- Severe headache

- Irritability

- Confusion

- Loss of consciousness

- Numbness or weakness of an arm or leg

- Loss of vision

- Shortness of breath, chest pain

- Sudden decrease in urine production, blood in the urine

If you, or someone you are with, experience these symptoms, *seek immediate emergency medical attention.*

When blood pressure climbs (sometimes quite abruptly) to high levels, the potential for widespread damage to vital organs demands immediate treatment to bring the pressure down. Because of the danger, doctors refer to the condition of extremely elevated blood pressure, with small amounts of bleeding and leakage of blood vessels in the retina as malignant (extremely high, harmful) hypertension. Usual symptoms are blurred vision, headache, shortness of breath, and, sometimes, chest pain. Diastolic (bottom number) pressures exceeding 130 mm Hg should be reduced within 1 hour to avoid permanent damage or even death.

Such extremely high blood pressure may rapidly trigger serious kidney damage that, if not quickly halted, will result in kidney failure. Signs that the kidneys may be in jeopardy include: sudden onset of gross hematuria (visible blood in the urine); sudden decrease in urinary production (scant amount of urine); sudden increase in fluid retention with swelling of the face, hands, feet, and lower legs. ■

lin)—the hormones mediating the "fight-or-flight" response when we are afraid or angry—exert powerful constricting effects on the arteries, which raises blood pressure. When production of these hormones arises abnormally from a tumor, the release is uncontrolled and erratic and may cause dangerous and unpredictable episodes of hypertension. Elevated blood pressure may also be one of the many symptoms of another adrenal gland disorder, Cushing's syndrome, in which the glands produce abnormally high levels of corticosteroid hormones. Excess production of growth hormone from a pituitary tumor (see Acromegaly, page 1201) also can cause hypertension.

Dangerous elevations of blood pressure can accompany the release of high levels of thyroid hormone, a condition termed thyroid storm or thyrotoxicosis. The condition can also occur in people who inadvertently take too much thyroid medication.

HOW TO TAKE YOUR BLOOD PRESSURE

If you and your doctor have decided that it is important for you to take your own blood pressure regularly, you should enter this stage of your health care feeling that you are exercising some control over your own health.

Keep in mind that blood pressure is not static. It may rise when you are in a stressful situation. It may be lower when you are listening to classical music just before bed time. Be prepared for variations.

Blood pressure is measured with a pressure gauge (sphygmomanometer). Your blood pressure kit will contain a cuff—a strip of fabric to be wrapped tightly around your arm. This strip contains an empty rubber sack (rubber bladder). The strip of fabric should be wrapped around your upper arm so that the rubber sack is over one of the large arteries in the arm. You will then pump air into the rubber bladder until you can no longer hear your heartbeat because the pressure in the cuff is higher than that in the artery. Then you will let the air escape. As soon as the pressure in the rubber bladder equals the pressure in the artery, the blood begins to flow again. Listening with a stethoscope over an artery, you will begin to hear a tapping sound, which is your pulse beat. This first sound indicates your systolic pressure (the top number). When the bladder deflates further and finally no sound can be heard, the reading is called the diastolic pressure (the bottom number).

A good blood pressure reading will depend on having a sphygmomanometer with a cuff that is the proper length and width to fit you. Check with your doctor to determine the size cuff you will need. There is a special cuff for children.

If you are monitoring your own blood pressure, you should take it at a quiet time during the day, not after an argument or after running upstairs to answer the telephone. Your blood pressure is affected by many factors, including stress and activity. It is best to urinate and then sit quietly for a few minutes before beginning the procedure. Remember that activity, a full bladder, caffeine, and smoking may affect blood pressure.

Because your blood pressure rises and falls during the course of the day, you should make a point of not taking your blood pressure so frequently that you upset yourself with varied results. Quite literally, you may end up raising your blood pressure. Choose a particular time of day when you are relaxed, and take your blood pressure at the same time each day.

The Procedure

1. Place your arm at heart level on the arm of a chair or on a table. If you are right-handed, take the pressure in your left arm. If you are left-handed, do the reverse.

2. Wrap the cuff around your bare upper arm approximately 1 in. above the bend in your arm, making sure it fits snugly.

3. If the stethoscope is attached to the cuff, place the flat disc of the stethoscope on your pulse about 2 inches above the bend in your arm. If the stethoscope is not attached, place the stethoscope on the pulse at the bend in your arm.

Squeeze the hand bulb continuously until the number on the gauge is approximately 30 mm Hg above the blood pressure reading you are expecting. Then stop pumping. When you listen through the stethoscope, you should not hear any pulse sound.

Begin to deflate the cuff, slowly, approximately 2 to 3 mm Hg per second. As your pressure falls, listen carefully for the first pulse sound. Note the reading, the moment this occurs. This is your systolic pressure. Continue to deflate the cuff until no pulse sound is heard, and note the reading. This is your diastolic pressure. When you record your blood pressure, the systolic, or higher number, comes first.

Electronic sphygmomanometers for home use have become more affordable; many people prefer them, since the machine does most of the work. Not all brands are equally reliable, however. Consult your doctor or *Consumer Reports* to find out which brand to buy. ■

A number of other medications can also elevate blood pressure: cold and sinus medications containing ephedrine, pseudoephedrine, or phenylpropanolamine; oral contraceptives or estrogen replacement therapy; some newer antidepressant medications such as venlafaxine (Effexor); appetite-suppressant medications; and illegal drugs such as cocaine and methamphetamine. Blood pressure elevations that appear as side effects of medication usually disappear soon after stopping the medication, although return to normal pressure may take several weeks.

The hypertension that sometimes occurs in pregnancy is due to either preeclampsia (see page 160), preexistent renal disease, or preexistent, but previously undiagnosed, essential hypertension. Because blood pressure normally falls in the first trimester of pregnancy, women with hypertension prior to pregnancy often have normal blood pressure when they have their first prenatal visit to the doctor. It is important to remember that angiotensin-converting enzyme inhibitors (ACE-Is) can cause miscarriages and should not be used in pregnancy or by women who may become pregnant.

Hypertension that is caused by other diseases or disorders can often be brought under control by treating the underlying condition. But the cause is unknown for 95 percent of all individuals with hypertension—many of whom may be completely unaware of the problem. Nevertheless, there are many lifestyle changes that can be made—such as increasing physical activity, reducing weight, cutting back on salt—that will lower blood pressure.

WHAT YOU CAN DO TO PREVENT OR REDUCE HYPERTENSION

Because hypertension may cause no symptoms, it is important to be vigilant. Get periodic blood pressure checkups (see the schedule on page 800, Blood Pressure Classifications: When to See Your Doctor). If your blood pressure is elevated, it may be necessary for you to monitor it yourself more often (see page 802, How to Take Your Blood Pressure). Make lifestyle changes that can lower your blood pressure: lose weight if necessary; increase your physical activity; and make dietary changes, such as reducing salt (sodium) intake and following a low-fat diet rich in fruits and vegetables.

Reducing salt The average American consumes about 4,000 mg a day of salt. Because excess sodium encourages the body to retain fluid, blood volume increases, requiring the heart to work harder. Blood pressure response to dietary salt intake varies. However, if pays to cut sodium to 2,500 mg a day if your blood pressure is normal. If you have heart disease, hypertension, or are at risk for these disorders, limit sodium to no more than 2,000 mg a day.

Read food labels to familiarize yourself with sodium levels in food (as well as the levels of fat, cholesterol, carbohydrates, protein, and other nutrients). Try to fit these levels into your daily allotment of sodium. And watch out for hidden salt sources. Table salt (sodium chloride) is the most obvious source of sodium in your diet. Just one teaspoon of salt contains 2,000 mg of sodium, the entire daily allotment of sodium for someone with heart disease. And the salt you add in cooking or at the table may be a mere sprinkling of your total sodium intake. Even natural foods such as milk, meat, and vegetables contain sodium. For example, a cup of milk contains 375 mg of sodium.

To cut down on sodium, read nutrition labels on packaged foods and buy reduced-sodium products; reduce or eliminate salt in cooking, banish the salt shaker from the table; and avoid foods that are high in sodium, such as

- Canned soups
- Most frozen dinners and other convenience foods
- Dehydrated mixes for soups, sauces, and salad dressings
- Soy sauce, catsup, Worcestershire sauce, chili sauce
- Mustard
- Pickles and relishes
- Olives
- Processed cheese and cheese spread
- Baking powder and baking soda
- Canned or frozen vegetables in sauce
- Foods and flavor enhancers containing monosodium glutamate (MSG)
- Frankfurters, cured ham, sausages, and luncheon meats
- Prepared salad dressings
- Salted nuts, chips, and other snack foods
- Any food additive with the word "sodium" (sodium benzoate, a preservative; sodium phosphate, an emulsifier and stabilizer)

Diet The Food Guide Pyramid, established by the US Department of Agriculture, recommends eating five or more servings of

---

ABOUT SALT SUBSTITUTES

If you have been advised to lower your sodium intake, you may wish to use a salt substitute. First check with your doctor.

Some salt substitutes contain a mixture of salt and other compounds. To achieve that familiar salty taste, you may end up using more salt substitute and thus not reducing your sodium intake. Potassium chloride is a common ingredient in salt substitutes. While recent studies have shown that potassium supplements can lower blood pressure, too much potassium can be harmful for people with kidney problems. The kidneys regulate potassium balance; if these organs are impaired, heart and neuromuscular problems may result. Extra potassium may also be hazardous for people with hypertension or heart failure who take angiotensin-converting enzyme (ACE) inhibitors and certain potassium-sparing diuretics. These drugs may cause the kidneys to retain potassium. When combined with extra potassium from salt substitutes, potassium levels may become too high. Before using salt substitutes that contain potassium, consult your doctor.

To enhance the flavor of food while cutting salt, use herbs and spices, flavored vinegars, or lemon juice. ■

MEDICATIONS USED TO TREAT HYPERTENSION

Once elevated blood pressure develops, it is usually a life-long problem that will require treatment with daily medication. These antihypertensive (blood pressure–lowering) medications fall into several broad categories: diuretics, those that lower blood pressure by prompting the kidney to excrete excess fluid volume as urine; beta blockers, designed to slow down the heart rate by blocking the action of the natural blood pressure-elevating substance epinephrine; direct blood vessel dilators that dilate the blood vessels by relaxing the muscle tension in their walls; calcium channel blockers that block entry of calcium into cells; angiotensin-converting enzyme inhibitors and angiotensin II receptor blockers; alpha receptor agonists that decrease outflow of epinephrine by acting on the brain; and alpha blockers that dilate arteries.

Dietary changes and exercise can best lower blood pressure with minimal adverse effects. Unfortunately, many people are unable or unwilling to alter their lifestyle sufficiently, and treatment with medication becomes the only option. The following sections should acquaint you with the major medications used in these categories, their potential side effects, important medication interactions, and warnings. Never stop taking your blood pressure medication on your own! Doing so in some instances can cause dangerous side effects.

Diuretics

Medications to cause the kidney to remove excess fluid (diuretics or "water pills") include such drugs as hydrochlorothiazide. These widely used medications cause the body to eliminate sodium; because water loss accompanies sodium loss, excess fluid is excreted. Diuretics cause the loss through the kidneys of two other important minerals—potassium and magnesium—and these important minerals may need to be replaced. Newer formulations of diuretics have coupled the water-shedding medication with other medications that prevent potassium loss; however, magnesium depletion can still occur. Any of these medications taken over long periods can cause adverse side effects, such as gout, elevated blood fats, mineral losses, impotence, and gynecomastia (enlarged breasts in men) (see page 772). Loss of potassium and magnesium can cause dizziness, fatigue, and muscle cramping. Side effects can be managed by adjusting the dosage. Occasionally, dehydration can occur from too much fluid loss, such as losing extra fluid through sweating with exercise or fever. Your doctor will work with you to select medications that produce the fewest side effects.

Beta Blockers

Slowing down the heart rate and taking some of the work off the heart can also reduce blood pressure. Among the first drugs developed to do this job was a group called beta blockers. The original formulation, a medication called propranolol (Inderal) has now been joined by a host of newer medications—such as metoprolol (Lopressor, Toprol), acebutolol (Sectral), atenolol (Tenormin), labetalol (Normodyne, Trandate), nadolol (Corgard), pindolol (Visken), and timolol (Blocadren). All these medications

act to block the action of epinephrine (adrenalin) and other similar chemical messengers at their site of action—a location called the beta receptor (hence the name, beta blocker). There are three different types of beta receptors—called beta-1, beta-2, and beta-3—each of which prompts different kinds of actions when stimulated. For example, stimulation of one type of beta receptor will speed up the heart rate, of another will dilate the bronchial tubes, opening the breathing passages.

The newer beta blockers can target the individual types of beta receptors, making treatment more specific and reducing the possibility of side effects. Used for blood pressure, these more selective medications act mainly on the heart, slowing its beat; they do not especially affect the beta receptors in the blood vessels or in the airways of the lungs. The early medications of this class commonly caused side effects, including fatigue and wheezing and shortness of breath from constricting the airways in the lungs.

If you are currently taking a beta blocker, you should be aware that with this particular class of blood pressure medication, you *must not* stop taking the medication abruptly. Doing so can sometimes cause a dramatic rise in blood pressure, occasionally to dangerously high levels. Stopping a beta blocker safely requires careful tapering of the dose by your doctor.

Alpha Receptor Agonists (Stimulators)

Blocking the action of the epinephrine system can also be accomplished in the brain by stimulating another type of receptor—termed the alpha receptor—that works to suppress the action of the betas. Just as with a beta-blocking action, alpha stimulators relax the arteries and help to reduce the pressure within them. This class of drugs includes clonidine (Catapres), methyldopa (Aldomet), guanabenz (Wytensin), and guanfacine (Tenex). Use of these medications has declined recently because they tend to cause unpleasant side effects; they are still occasionally used as a second or even third medication in a blood pressure–reducing regimen when other medications cannot do the job alone.

The common side effects encountered with this group of medications include fatigue, dry mouth, sedation (sleepiness), low blood pressure, depression, and impotence in men. Like the beta blockers, these medications must be tapered slowly if they are to be discontinued to avoid the rebound effect of dramatically elevated blood pressure that can occur with abrupt withdrawal.

Alpha Blockers

The alpha blockers, which include prazosin, terazosin, and doxazosin, relax the muscular layer of the arteries, allowing them to dilate, thereby dropping blood pressure. They also have the additional benefits of raising HDL cholesterol (the good cholesterol) and improving urinary function in men with prostate trouble. Although they can prove effective alone in reducing blood pressure, their effectiveness may wane with time; in addition, they commonly tend to cause unpleasant side effects that include severe hypotension (too low a blood pressure), fainting, heart palpitations, headache, and nervous agitation. Their use has been limited primarily to second or third medications in a combination regimen to combat difficult-to-control hypertension. ▶

◆ Direct Blood Vessel Dilators

Other medications directly dilate the tiniest arteries (arterioles) by relaxing their muscle walls. These arteriolar dilators include the medications hydralazine and minoxidil. Because of their side effects—excessive blood pressure reduction, racing heart, headache, and sedation—doctors often turn to this class of antihypertensive medications only when better tolerated ones have proven ineffective.

Angiotensin-Converting Enzyme (ACE) Inhibitors

Keeping the blood vessels open can also be accomplished by interfering with one of the body's blood pressure–elevating mechanisms, called the renin-angiotensin-aldosterone system. (See page 800 for more information about how this mechanism works.) The ACE inhibitors prevent blood vessel constriction by stopping the conversion of the inactive substance, angiotensin I, into the powerful blood vessel constrictor, angiotensin II. Newer still are medications like losartan (Cozaar) that block the action of angiotensin II itself. ACE inhibitors—which include benazepril (Lotensin), captopril (Capoten,) enalapril (Vasotec), fosinopril (Monopril), lisinopril (Prinivil and Zestril), quinapril (Accupril), ramipril (Altace), trandolapril (Mavik), and others—are especially useful in treating the hypertension that occurs with diabetes because they delay loss of kidney function in persons with diabetes who have damaged kidneys. The main and most bothersome side effect is a dry, hacking cough. Other, less common side effects include dizziness, hypotension, swelling, alterations of taste, and occasionally, rash. These medications prevent loss of potassium; you should not take extra potassium (as you might be accustomed to doing with diuretic medications), nor should you combine the ACE inhibitors with the kinds of diuretics that also increase potassium lest the potassium get dangerously high.

High potassium can cause potentially deadly heart rhythm abnormalities.

Calcium Channel Blockers

Another means of relaxing the arteries to reduce blood pressure involves inhibiting the calcium channel, a specialized regulating gate that narrowly defines when the mineral ion calcium can enter the cell. To facilitate proper muscle contraction, the entry of calcium ions into the muscle cells has to be tightly controlled, because calcium inside the cells is toxic. If an excess of calcium floods through the entry portal (the calcium channel) spasm may result, constricting the blood vessel and driving blood pressure up. Medications that block the calcium channel—called calcium channel blockers—prevent the blood vessel constriction caused by this rapid influx of calcium. This class of medications includes such drugs as diltiazem (Cardizem, Cardizem CD, Cardicom SR, Dilacor, Dilacor XL) verapamil (Calan, Calam SR, Isoptin, Isoptin SR, Verelan, Covera HS), amlodipine (Norvasc), felodipine (Plendil), isradipine (DynaCirc, DynaCirc CR), nicardipine (Cardene), and nifedipine, (Adalat, Adalat CC, Procardia, Procardia XL).

Most people tolerate these drugs well, and side effects are relatively mild and few. When side effects do occur, they include: fluid swelling; headache; slow heart rate; gastrointestinal distress (cramping, bloating, stool changes); dizziness; and occasionally heart palpitations. In some persons, calcium channel blockers may worsen the symptoms of congestive heart failure (CHF) (see page 823), although verapamil is used to treat CHF due to diastolic dysfunction. Short-acting forms of nifedipine increase the risk of death in patients with coronary artery disease; thus, short-acting forms of calcium channel blockers should not be used in these patients. ■

---

various fruits and vegetables and six or more servings of grain products (bread, cereals, pasta) every day as part of a balanced diet. Now a new hypertension study goes even further. The Dietary Approaches to Stopping Hypertension (called the DASH diet) found that blood pressure can be lowered significantly by a diet that is low in saturated (animal) fat, very high in fruits and vegetables, and combined with low-fat dairy products. Systolic (top number) pressures dropped an average of 5.5 points in people following the DASH diet, compared to a control group eating a typical American diet.

Potassium supplementation with pills also lowers blood pressure, especially in black men. In a study conducted at Johns Hopkins, potassium supplementation lowered systolic blood 7 mm Hg compared to a group treated with placebo. Persons with kidney disease or on medication need to check with their doctor before taking extra potassium. Dietary sources of potassium include fresh fruits and vegetables, dried fruits, and unprocessed foods.

Exercise Increase your level of physical activity. Regular aerobic exercise (such as walking, jogging, biking, or swimming) also helps lower blood pressure. Sustained elevation of your pulse rate is the key; weight-lifting, for example, does not have this effect. Be sure, however, to work out within your physical abilities. Do not push yourself to extreme fatigue or exercise outdoors in conditions of high heat or humidity, because these factors may drive blood pressure higher. (See Chapter 2 for more information on the benefits of increased physical activity.)

Smoking Cigarette smoking can raise blood pressure and cause complications. If you smoke, make every effort to quit. (See Chapter 4 for more information on quitting smoking.)

Medication   Lowering blood pressure includes reducing the fluid volume of blood by diuresis (shedding excess fluid as urine), dilating the blood vessels by relaxing the muscle tension in their walls (vasodilation), reducing the force with which the heart pumps blood, and slowing the heart rate. Dietary changes and exercise can accomplish these goals. Yet many people are unable or unwilling to alter their lifestyle sufficiently, and treatment with medication becomes the only option. (See page 804, Medications Used to Treat Hypertension, for information on the various medications used to treat the condition.)

Atherosclerotic Disorders

Atherosclerosis, the thickening and narrowing of the inner lining of the arteries, is central to the development of coronary artery disease—the number one cause of fatalities in the United States. Yet atherosclerosis can often be prevented and even reversed by making the lifestyle changes for a healthy heart described on page 797. Cardiovascular disease—along with the dreaded heart attack—is perhaps the major area of health care where your preventive efforts may be richly rewarded.

EVALUATING THE HEART AND BLOOD VESSELS

Doctors use a battery of diagnostic tests to assess the health of the cardiovascular system. The simplest and oldest method of evaluation is to listen to the sounds the heart makes as it pumps and relaxes. Cardiac auscultation (listening to the heart with a stethoscope) provides a wealth of information about the rate and rhythm of the heartbeat: Is it too fast or slow? Are the beats properly and regularly spaced? Are there skips or runs of beats? Auscultation also detects heart murmurs that occur when abnormalities in the valves, or, rarely, the heart muscle, create turbulent blood flow. For example, if the mitral valve sepa-

rating the left atrium and left ventricle fails to seal completely as the ventricle contracts, blood escapes through the space left between the leaflets of the valve, creating a whooshing noise audible through the stethoscope—one kind of heart murmur. Partial occlusion of the arteries in the neck or leg by hard plaque can also disrupt the smooth and silent passage of blood, setting up turbulent blood flow patterns that make the detectable noise called a *bruit* (the French word for noise).

To augment and refine the diagnoses hinted at by auscultation, the doctor has a variety of test methods from which to choose. Abnormalities of the heart valves suggested by the murmur become visible by passing ultrasound waves through the heart—an echocardiogram. As the waves travel through the heart, they bounce off dense tissues, creating an "echo" that forms a shadow picture of the structure of the heart. This test evaluates the size, shape, and function of the valves in a method exactly like that used to allow expectant parents to "see" their unborn child.

Another safe and painless evaluation, the Doppler examination—a test also used in pregnancy to allow expectant parents to "hear" their unborn baby's heartbeat—couples ultrasound waves with a sensitive microphone. The microphone detects the sounds of turbulence or reduced blood flow in occluded arteries, helping to determine both the location and the degree of blockage.

The standard chest x-ray offers the best method for determining overall heart size. Many new methods, however, use x-ray technology in conjunction with various radiopaque (visible on x-ray) dyes and isotope tracers to evaluate the heart and blood vessels. Examination of the coronary arteries using this method—the coronary arteriogram or cardiac catheterization—involves inserting a catheter (a long, slender, flexible hollow tube) into the femoral artery located in the groin. The catheter is advanced until its tip lies at the take-off point of the coronary arteries. Once in place, x-ray dye injected through the catheter fills the artery, producing a silhouette visible on an x-ray. The same kind of examination—arteriography—can delineate the size and shape, as well as detect occlusions or other abnormalities in arteries anywhere in the body.

Doctors evaluate the electrical activity generated by the beating heart most commonly with the electrocardiogram (ECG). In this simple and painless test, 12 electrical sensor pads, placed on the arms, legs, and across the chest, detect the heart's electrical impulses and translate them into characteristic wave patterns on paper. The waves (P, QRS, T, and U) describe the contraction of the small atrial chambers, the larger ventricles, and the period of rest and electrical restabilization between beats. Abnormalities of electrical conduction are caused by events such as damage to the heart muscle and changes in levels of blood hormones, salts, or other chemicals. These episodes make characteristic changes in the wave patterns of the ECG.

The ECG information, which is taken while the patient is resting, may not accurately reflect the presence of coronary artery disease. By adding extra work for the heart, such as walking on a treadmill during the examination, subtle changes that occur with activity may become apparent. This test—the exercise ECG or exercise stress test—provides more complete information about the health and fitness of the heart muscle. Abnormalities on this exam may indicate inadequate blood flow to the heart muscle that could bring about a heart attack under more extreme physical or emotional stress. The exercise evaluation may also include administration of a radioisotope tracer (usually thallium-201; the evaluation is called a thallium stress test) to detect areas of the heart that are damaged or receive insufficient oxygen when stressed. These areas are at higher risk for a future heart attack.

Cardiac magnetic resonance imaging (MRI) enables doctors to evaluate the structure and function of the heart and blood vessels without catheters or exposing the patient to radiation or iodine-containing dyes.

A computed tomography (CT) scan provides cross-sectional images of the heart and great vessels. This technique, however, is not fast enough to avoid blurred images caused by movement in organs such as the beating heart and in the circulatory system. A new technique called ultrafast CT can capture such images, although it is not yet widely available. Ultrafast CT is currently being evaluated for its ability to determine the presence or absence of coronary calcification. If present in large amounts, this implies coronary artery disease.

Positron emission tomography (PET) scans, although not yet widely available, measure heart muscle metabolism—differentiating healthy, well-nourished heart muscle from that deprived of enough oxygen or nutrients for optimal function—again without catheters or dyes.

When fluttering, skipping, or other rhythm abnormalities demand investigation, doctors most often employ the Holter monitor, a small ECG unit patients wear that continuously records cardiac rhythms for 12 to 48 hours. This test correlates symptoms patients feel—a flutter, skip, or flip—with the electrical activity in the heart; to make the correlation, patients press a button on the unit to mark the event as it happens.

Assessment of cardiovascular risk should include laboratory blood tests to determine the levels of blood fats (lipids) and other body chemicals that affect cardiovascular health. These tests include: blood electrolytes (sodium, potassium, calcium, magnesium, and iron); a complete lipid profile to determine triglycerides and the various forms of cholesterol (the so-called "good" HDL cholesterol and the "bad" LDL cholesterol); measures related to blood clotting, such as platelet number; and evaluation of cardiac enzymes, released in large amounts by damaged heart muscle.

❖ CORONARY ARTERY DISEASE: "ATHEROSCLEROSIS OF THE HEART"

Symptoms *(What you may experience)* Sometimes none and sometimes vague symptoms. Chest pain (angina) under the breast bone, worse with stress or physical activity, and relieved with rest; occasionally the pain runs into the neck, throat, jaw, or the arm (see page 808).

Signs and laboratory findings *(What the doctor looks for)* Characteristic changes on ECG at rest or during a stress test (sometimes); blockages in the coronary arteries seen with coronary angiography (x-ray dye studies of the arteries supplying the heart).

What is it? Atherosclerotic plaques—hard blockages of calcium, cholesterol, blood cells, and fibrous tissue—can develop in any artery in the body, rupture, and produce blockage (see Understanding Atherosclero-

WHAT IS ANGINA?

When blood flow to an area of heart muscle diminishes, it impairs the delivery of vital nutrients and oxygen to the cells and the removal of waste products. The lack of oxygen causes problems in the heart's energy production pathways. Its never-ending job requires an enormous amount of energy, which it normally meets by burning fat fuels. That chemical process requires oxygen, which the heart usually has in abundance. In the absence of enough oxygen, however, the heart must turn to an alternative fuel—glucose, or blood sugar. The byproduct of this less efficient combustion is lactic acid, which builds up in the heart muscle and causes chest pain.

In people with coronary artery disease, blood flow within arteries, choked with plaque, may slow to a trickle sufficient to meet the heart's needs at rest, but insufficient to handle the demands of activity. It is for this reason that the classic pains of angina come on with exercise or extreme emotional distress and disappear with rest or calm. Under the stressed conditions, the constricted arteries simply cannot supply enough oxygen to keep up the energy demand, and the heart must burn fuel without it. From that perspective, angina is a signal that the heart is working beyond its capacity, and serves as a vital warning sign to rest.

When angina occurs at rest, during sleep, or on exposure to cold, then the cause may be reduced blood flow, secondary to coronary artery spasm (also called Prinzmetal's angina). Gastroesophageal reflux (heartburn) and other conditions can mimic angina. Your doctor will consider these possibilities.

Angina can also occur—though this is rare—in situations where there is not obstruction of the coronary arteries due to atherosclerosis (for example, aortic stenosis, where the jet of blood through the narrowed orifice of the valve reduces blood flow to the coronary arteries). Other examples include failure to get oxy-

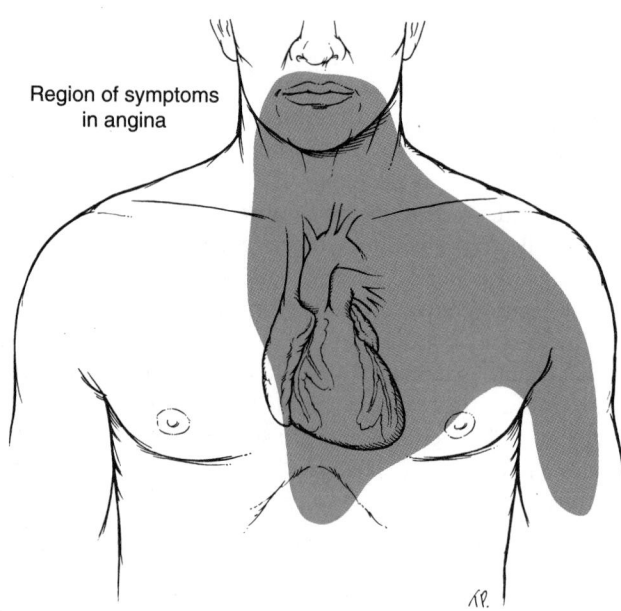

Region of symptoms in angina

Angina is chest pain due to inadequate blood flow to or through the coronary arteries that supply blood to the heart. Symptoms sometimes extend to the neck, jaw, left arm, or upper abdomen.

gen to the heart muscle because of severe anemia or markedly increased oxygen need due to a markedly thickened heart.

Angina can also occur due to spasm of the coronary arteries, a condition called Prinzmetal's angina. It usually occurs at rest and can be precipitated by exposure to cold. Lastly, obstruction of very small vessels supplying blood to the heart can also cause angina, even though blood flows unimpeded through the larger coronary arteries. ■

sis, page 791). When this occurs in the coronary arteries, which supply blood to the heart muscle, it is called coronary artery disease (CAD) or heart disease. CAD is the most common cause of death in America, while lesser degrees cause substantial disability.

When the blockage in an artery becomes extreme, it may permit only a tiny trickle of blood flow, jeopardizing the area supplied by the blocked vessel. Because the powerful left ventricle of the heart, which supplies blood to the entire body, requires a great deal of oxygen, total blockages in the left coronary arteries are more likely to harm the heart muscle (myocardium). This event is commonly known as a heart attack (see Myocardial Infarction (Heart Attack), page 811). Nonetheless, significant blockage in any coronary artery is cause for concern. Limitation of oxygen results in damage that spreads like a wave through

the myocardium. Treatment must be swift, because "time is muscle"—it can take a mere 15 minutes for total blockage and the resulting damage to occur. In as many as one-fourth of people, sudden death may be the first obvious sign of disease in the coronary arteries.

CAD is four times more common in men than women, but the rate changes with age. Under age 40, it strikes eight men for every woman; after age 70 the gender difference vanishes, and men and women develop it at equal rates. The striking difference between the sexes has spurred intense research for the factors that protect younger women from CAD. The female hormone estrogen may offer important protection, since estrogen boosts levels of protective HDL cholesterol. Prostaglandins, hormone-like substances produced by the uterus (they play a role in menstrual

MEDICATIONS USED TO TREAT CORONARY ARTERY DISEASE

Medical therapy to relieve the pain of coronary artery disease must accomplish the goal of improving blood flow to nourish the heart muscle, taking the strain off the heart muscle, and reducing the pressure against which the heart muscle must pump the blood along. Medications that fit this bill fall into several broad categories and may often be prescribed in combination with one another.

Nitroglycerin A single nitroglycerin tablet under the tongue will usually relieve chest pain from coronary artery disease in 1 to 2 minutes. Relief of mild to moderate chest pain may require repeated doses at 3- to 5-minute intervals. If you require repeated doses, however, you need to speak with your doctor because it may signal the need for additional medications or further evaluation. Individuals with coronary artery disease should keep fresh nitroglycerin tablets with them at all times for sublingual (under-the-tongue) use. Nitroglycerin is a potent relaxer of the muscular wall of the arteries, an effect that opens them wider to permit more blood to flow through them. Since the pain of angina (see What Is Angina?, page 808) occurs from lack of blood flow, any remedy that improves blood delivery to the heart muscle will help to keep pain at bay. Longer-lasting medications with action similar to nitroglycerin (isosorbide dinitrate or mononitrate) taken in divided doses throughout the day or the newer sustained-release nitroglycerin work to keep the coronary arteries dilated continually and reduce the strain on the heart muscle. Nitroglycerin can also be applied to the skin, with possible use of sustained release forms as topical creams or self-adhesive patches. Use of the patch makes taking the correct dose of medication easier; after a time, however, some degree of tolerance (meaning the loss of some of its effectiveness) to the long-acting nitrates usually develops. Taking at least an 8-hour break daily from nitrate therapy will reduce the tendency to develop tolerance. Removing the patch from dinnertime until bedtime or from bedtime until morning will create a sufficient daily break. The other common side effects of nitrate therapy include: headache, nausea, dizziness, and hypotension (low blood pressure).

Beta Blockers This class of drugs includes propranolol, metoprolol, acebutolol, atenolol, labetalol, nadolol, pindolol, timolol, and others. These drugs are designed to block the effects of epinephrine and related compounds on the heart and blood vessels, reduce the amount of oxygen the heart needs during times of physical exertion or stress, and lower the blood pressure and heart rate to lessen the work the heart must do. Studies have shown that beta blockers prolong life in people with coronary artery disease after they suffer a myocardial infaction. Virtually all the members of this class of medications will relieve angina and reduce the work the heart must perform; however, one drug, pindolol, has actually increased the occurrence of angina in some cases and has not seemed to be effective in prevention of future attacks.

Beta blockers should be avoided in people with asthma, exceptionally slow heart rate, congestive heart failure, or hard-to-control diabetes, because the medication can worsen these problems—sometimes dangerously. Other side effects that sometimes might occur include: wheezing, fatigue, near-fainting upon arising from lying or sitting, nightmares, disturbances of sleep, slow heart rate, cold hands and feet, impotence, elevation of blood triglycerides, and reduction of "good" HDL cholesterol.

Calcium Channel Blockers This class of drugs includes verapamil, diltiazem, nifedipine, amlodipine, nicardipine, and others. These drugs prevent the entry of the mineral calcium into the muscle cells of the artery wall. Appropriately timed calcium ion entry is necessary for the muscles to contract; therefore, blocking this effect will dilate the coronary arteries, reduce the amount of oxygen needed by the heart as it works, improve blood flow to the heart muscle, and reduce the blood pressure. Side effects that can sometimes occur with taking a calcium channel blocker include swelling of the hands, feet, lower legs, or face; dizziness; too slow a heart rate; constipation; flushing; headache; palpitations; and worsening of the symptoms of congestive heart failure (although verapamil is used to treat congestive heart failure due to diastolic dysfunction). In addition, short-acting forms of nifedipine should not be used for patients with coronary artery disease because it increases the risk of death. The same caveat holds for other, similar, short-acting medications. ■

ASPIRIN THERAPY

Aspirin (acetylsalicylic acid or ASA) could be called the wonder drug of the 20th century. Aspirin relieves pain, stops inflammation, reduces fever, and thins the blood. Studies suggest that it helps people with coronary artery disease reduce the chance of having a heart attack, and that it may even reduce the risk for colon cancer. How can one common, inexpensive medication do all this? Simple. It influences a large system of microhormones involved in hundreds of body functions. These microhormones—called eicosanoids, from the Greek *eicos* (twenty), because they all contain 20 carbon atoms—include such chemical messengers as prostacyclins, leukotrienes, thromboxanes, and the most widely recognized members of this group, prostaglandins.

Among their many actions, some eicosanoids affect blood clotting. For blood to clot inside the body, something has to trigger a complex cascade of special clotting factors. Injury to the tissues can be that trigger. An injury—whether it's a cut to the skin or the trauma of high blood pressure pressing outward and weakening the artery wall—attracts platelets, which are like emergency patches that rush to the site of trauma and coat the area. The platelets produce and release a substance that makes them stick together to make a better seal. Once the seal has formed, the blood-clotting sequence activates. Because most heart attacks result from blood clots forming on a roughened atherosclerotic plaque, preventing the clot will prevent many heart attacks. A small daily dose of aspirin—baby aspirin, half aspirin, or even smaller—can decrease this stickiness and has been proven to decrease the chance of heart attack in people at risk. Bigger doses of aspirin can thin the blood too much or could cause stomach irritation or even ulcers. A single daily dose of the very small coated aspirin tablets now available will usually suffice to prevent platelet stickiness without side effects.

People should consult their doctor before beginning long-term daily aspirin therapy if they have peptic ulcer disease, a history of hemorrhagic (bleeding) stroke, very high blood pressure, liver or kidney disease, or if they take other blood-thinning medications, (such as Coumadin). ■

BYPASS SURGERY

When atherosclerotic plaques block a portion of the coronary arteries supplying blood to the heart muscle, skilled surgeons can bypass that blockage using segments of healthy veins or arteries. In this procedure, the surgeon reuses a piece of a healthy blood vessel (usually the internal mammary artery in the chest near the breast bone or the saphenous vein in the lower leg) and inserts it from the aorta into the coronary artery as a detour for blood to flow around the blocked areas. Most procedures involve creating one to as many as five detours in the coronary arteries.

This major surgical procedure requires opening the chest and transiently rerouting the blood supply through a heart-lung machine to allow the heart and lungs to remain still and quiet during the operation. Symptoms of chest pain, shortness of breath, and dizziness usually abate or at least improve following the surgery, and the need for medications to control symptoms diminishes.

The risk of the surgery, a low 1 to 3 percent in otherwise healthy people, rises in people with weakened ventricles (poor heart muscle pumping function), in the elderly, and among those people with debilitating kidney disease, diabetes, or poor general health. Those people who continue a damaging lifestyle—smoking, poor dietary habits, untreated blood fat elevations, no exercise—typically see blockages form in their newly grafted vessel in time. Preventing platelets (the blood components that instigate clot formation) from clumping together by daily low-dose aspirin therapy improves long-term results.

If the grafted vessels form new blockages, surgery the second time is technically more difficult, less successful, and fraught with greater morbidity than initially.

Heart bypass surgery. A diseased coronary blood vessel can be bypassed using parts of healthy blood vessels from the chest or leg. Blood flow to the heart is then improved.

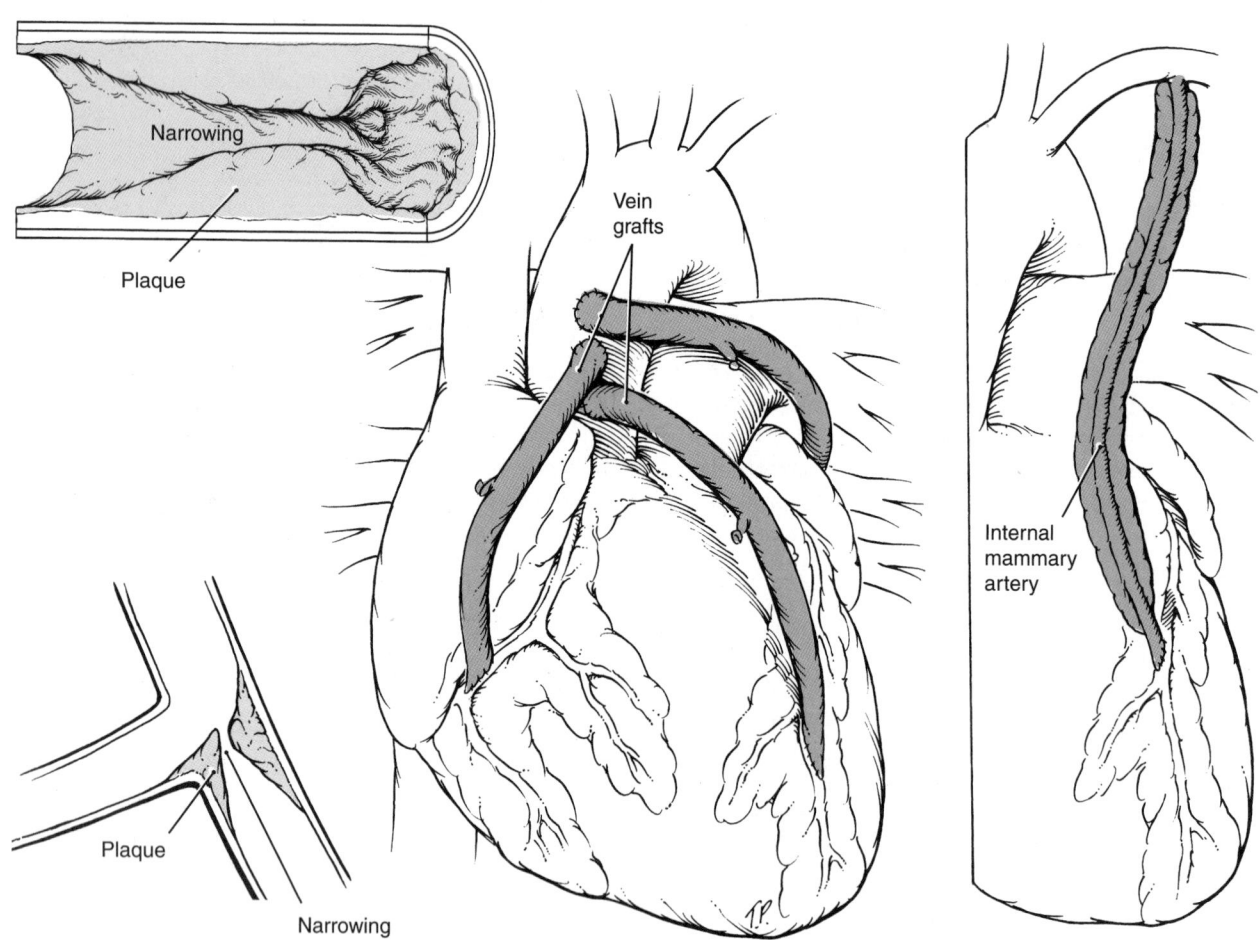

cramps) may also be protective. One of these substances dilates blood vessels and protects against blood clot formation. Giving estrogen to men, however, did not prove useful in reducing their risk. (See Women and Heart Disease, page 792.)

What you can do CAD may be prevented and even reversed in many cases, if you are willing to make the necessary changes in your diet and lifestyle (see Preventing Heart Disease, page 790). First and perhaps foremost: if you smoke, quit. Cigarette smoke is

SUDDEN CARDIAC DEATH

Sudden cardiac death—in which the heart stops beating, breathing halts, and the victim becomes unconscious—should not be confused with a heart attack. When the heart cannot effectively organize the electrical impulses that coordinate pumping, heart muscle contraction becomes erratic, setting up a useless quivering of the muscle called ventricular fibrillation.

Without a working heart to pump oxygenated blood to the brain and the rest of the body, tissues are deprived of vital oxygen. The brain is especially sensitive to lack of oxygen; because the brain also controls breathing, the victim must receive help immediately, or brain death ensues and the event is fatal. A bystander witnessing such an emergency should immediately roll the person onto his or her back and administer a sharp blow with the side of the fist to the breast bone—called a precordial thump—which may restart normal electrical rhythm. Anyone trained to perform cardiopulmonary resuscitation (CPR)—mouth-to-mouth breathing and possibly chest compression—should immediately call for emergency help and begin resuscitation. Timely rescue may be the difference between life and death. (See Cardiopulmonary Resuscitation, page 361.)

Although sudden cardiac death may occur in people not known to have heart disease, it is a serious risk in the first hour or so after a heart attack. Many of these people succumb to a fatal disturbance in heart rhythm brought on by the heart attack even before they reach the hospital. ■

---

a prime promoter of heart disease because it alters LDL cholesterol and makes it more likely to form plaque. (See Understanding Atherosclerosis, page 790, and Risk Factors You Can Modify, page 793; for information on kicking the habit, see Chapter 4.) If you are overweight or lead a sedentary life, talk to your doctor about how to safely lose weight and institute a regular program of exercise. Studies show that improved diet, exercise, and stress-reduction techniques can dramatically improve angina and the quality of life.

When to call the doctor Any episode of symptoms suggesting CAD, particularly chest pain beneath the breast bone or in the left chest or arm—however vague—should prompt an immediate consultation with your doctor. This is especially important advice for men over the age of 40, since CAD is more common in this group. But do not ignore these symptoms in post-menopausal women; by this age, CAD rates for women start to catch up with the rates for men.

Treatment The cornerstone of therapy should always be lifestyle modification—the only therapy that offers an effective means of diminishing risk of recurrence over time. Other, more aggressive therapies with medication and surgery can offer relief of the immediate blockage; but these provide fewer long-term benefits, unless lifestyle changes accompany them. Medical therapy aims to dilate the narrowed coronary arteries to permit better blood flow. A nitroglycerin tablet under the tongue usually relieves angina promptly, but keeping the pain at bay continuously requires regular daily use of one or more of several effective medications (see Medications Used to Treat Coronary Artery Disease, page 809).

Some blockages may be better treated by balloon dilation (see page 814) or by coronary bypass grafting (see page 810). Surgery may be appropriate for the following people: those who still have pain despite medical treatment; those with over 50 percent blockage of the left main coronary artery; those with three coronary arteries partially blocked and a heart whose ability to pump is impaired; and those who still have anginal chest pain after a heart attack.

Prognosis Quite good: 90 percent of people achieve total freedom from the pain of coronary artery disease with treatment, and many achieve an increased lifespan. However, if the disease is untreated it usually progresses relentlessly and often fatally. Over 90 percent of people with CAD are alive at 5 years; prior to modern therapy to prevent and treat this disease, only about 80 percent survived that long. It is important to remember, however, that after a bypass graft the same atherosclerotic process that caused the original blockage will eventually occlude the new blood vessel; therefore, it is important to control the diet and lifestyle risk factors that promote this process.

❖ MYOCARDIAL INFARCTION (HEART ATTACK)

Symptoms *(What you may experience)* Angina is often a precursor of a myocardial infarction, developing years, months, or weeks before. It may also develop after a myocardial infarction. In as many as 25 percent of cases, a heart attack may occur without typical symptoms, or the pattern may range from mild to severe. The classic symptoms are: squeezing or crushing pain beneath the breast bone, in the left side of the chest, running into the arm, neck, jaw, or throat; an unusual feeling of indigestion; cold, clammy sweating; nausea and, occasionally, vomiting; shortness of breath; weakness; a sense of apprehension or impending doom; light-headedness, near-fainting, or loss of consciousness.

Signs and laboratory findings *(What the doctor looks for)* Pallor; profuse sweating; specific and characteristic electrical pattern changes on an ECG; elevations of heart muscle enzymes (chemicals released when the muscle is damaged) demonstrated on blood tests.

What is it? The medical name for a heart attack is myocardial infarction. An infarct is an area of dead tissue resulting from blockage of its blood supply. The term "heart attack," or its medical name, acute myocardial infarction, refers to the death of heart muscle tissue (infarct) resulting from obstructed blood flow; it does not refer to any other acute form of heart disease, such as cardiac arrest caused by malfunction of the heart's electrical system.

A myocardial infarction can be caused either by reduced blood flow to the heart tissue in an artery narrowed by atherosclerotic plaque or, more often, by the rupture of plaque associated with a clot that lodges in a narrowed artery, suddenly blocking blood flow and oxygen supply. The extent of muscle damage and complications is determined by the location of the obstruction and the duration of reduced blood flow. For example, blockage in the coronary artery that supplies the large and powerful left ventricle, the main pumping chamber, and the wall between the chambers could weaken the heart more severely than damage to the right chamber. Blockage of the right coronary artery, however, may cause dangerous disturbances in heart rhythm, because the right artery supplies not only the right ventricle, but usually the sinoatrial node (the heart's natural pacemaker) as well.

If a muscle in your arm or leg began to hurt, you could choose not to use it. But your heart must keep pumping continually and requires a constant supply of fuel. The heart prefers to use fat fuels for energy, but burning fats requires oxygen. When blood cannot reach an area of heart muscle, the muscle must switch to a form of energy production—burning blood sugar, or glucose—that does not require oxygen. Burning glucose for energy creates a waste byproduct—lactic acid—that builds up in the muscle. Lack of blood flow also prevents removal of lactic acid and other waste products, which accounts for the pain of a myocardial infarction. If the blockage threatens a large segment of heart muscle and the blood supply cannot quickly be restored, a large part of the heart muscle may die.

What you can do If there is any question that you may be experiencing heart pain, seek immediate medical help. *Early intervention is the key to saving heart muscle.* Emergency intervention with medications to dissolve a clot or emergency balloon dilation of the blocked artery can be life saving and muscle salvaging.

Every teen and adult should be prepared by taking a course in basic cardiopulmonary resuscitation (CPR) (see page 361). If you develop symptoms suggesting a myocardial infarction, call 911—or ask someone to do it for you—and request immediate emergency medical assistance. Try to remain calm, lie down, and breathe slowly and deeply. If you have nitroglycerin in the form of under-the-tongue tablets or spray, use it at once and repeat every 3 minutes. Chew a regular aspirin to inhibit blood clotting. If you are with a person who may be having a myocardial infarction, call 911 immediately. If the person stops breathing, start emergency rescue breathing (see page 361).

When to call the doctor *Call for help immediately.* The sooner blocked arteries can be opened with so-called clot-busting medication and blood flow restored to the heart muscle, the less the damage. Most of the damage to the heart muscle occurs within the first 2 hours. As cardiologists put it: "Time is muscle." Curtailing the damage and protecting the remaining tissue are major factors in determining a person's survival and future quality of life. Thousands of unnecessary deaths occur each year because people refuse to call for help because they think their symptoms will pass. Any angina that does not respond to nitroglycerin immediately and completely demands medical attention.

IN THE EMERGENCY ROOM

If you suspect you may be having a myocardial infarction (heart attack)—or if you are with someone who may be having one—it is important to get to the emergency room immediately. A myocardial infarction occurs when the blood supply to portions of the heart is cut off. When this happens the portion of the heart muscle that is not receiving blood begins to die almost immediately. The faster you get to the emergency room, the better your chances are of avoiding permanent damage to your heart and of making a full recovery. Treatment for a myocardial infarction is most successful when it is immediate and aggressive.

If you suspect a myocardial infarction, call your doctor or call 911. If you live near a hospital and someone can drive you, this may be faster than waiting for an ambulance. At the emergency room, you will probably be taken to a special room or area for cardiac cases only. Here, the attending physician will examine you, administer a painkiller, and give you an ECG. Morphine is often administered, because it not only relieves pain, but also helps alleviate the tremendous anxiety that usually accompanies a heart attack. Because it is critical to get the blood circulating through the heart again, you will probably be given oxygen immediately, either in the ambulance or at the emergency room. If your ECG shows signs of dangerous arrhythmias, the doctor may give you medication, or he may give your heart an electric shock to attempt to restore a normal heart rhythm. The ECG usually confirms that you are having or have recently had a myocardial infarction, but even in cases where the ECG shows no abnormalities, the doctor will probably keep you for further testing, including blood tests that will determine if a part of the heart muscle has died.

If you arrive at the hospital within 3 hours of the start of your myocardial infarction, the damage to the heart muscle may be stopped or even reversed by administering thrombolytic drugs that work to dissolve the clot that's blocking the blood flow to the heart. These drugs are commonly referred to as clot-dissolving drugs or clot busters. They must be used cautiously because while they may dissolve a clot in one area of the heart, they may also cause bleeding in another, otherwise healthy area of the body, including the brain. One of these drugs, streptokinase, is older and may cause allergic reactions, but it also is much cheaper than t-PA (alteplase). t-PA is tissue-type plasminogen activator that has been genetically engineered from a human protein. Clot-dissolving drugs are given intravenously or they are delivered to the coronary arteries directly, via a catheter.

Clot-dissolving drugs have greatly reduced the death rate from myocardial infarction. But whether these drugs are equally safe for women and whether women receive clot busters when they need them has also been a subject of ongoing debate. Until recently, women were receiving clot-dissolving drugs only half as often as men did, and studies have shown that such drug treatments are not given frequently enough to both men and women.

If you arrive at the hospital within the critical period and a full cardiology team is immediately available, your doctor may decide to perform a balloon angioplasty to open a clogged artery; or, in rarer cases, the doctor may perform emergency bypass surgery to construct a detour around the blocked artery and restore the flow of oxygen to your heart. If your heart attack has been severe, or if you have had emergency bypass surgery, you will spend the initial recovery period in the hospital's cardiac care unit (CCU). Here, you will be monitored continually for further complications. Usually, your stay in the CCU will last somewhere between 24 to 36 hours. In the CCU, you will be monitored by a specially trained cardiac team. A bedside monitor will record your heartbeat, and you may have a catheter inserted into a vein in your neck, then threaded into your right ventricle to record an accurate reading of the pressure in your heart and its output. Your stay will last until you show no signs of heart failure or dangerous arrhythmia—a major cause of death after a myocardial infarction.

The mood of most CCUs is one of continual crisis. Even if your situation is stable, you may witness the patient in the bed next to you going into cardiac arrest and become anxious yourself. The CCU is usually busy 24 hours a day. In the CCU, you can help in your own recovery by asking for pain relief as soon as you need it and by asking your doctor to prescribe something to help you sleep if you cannot sleep. You will want to do all you can do to be discharged from the CCU as soon as possible, so you can continue your recovery at home. Positive steps you can take in this direction include getting enough rest, beginning to move around as soon as possible, and beginning to eat the low-fat diet recommended by your doctor and dietitian. ■

Treatment Emergency treatment with oxygen and medication to relieve pain (morphine) and to dissolve the blood clot. If given promptly, clot-busting drugs, such as tissue plasminogen activator (t-PA), a natural clot-dissolving agent, and streptokinase derivatives that restore blood flow, are powerful weapons in minimizing damage. (For more information, see In The Emergency Room, above, and Recovery After a Myocardial Infarction, page 815.)

Prognosis Depends on the location and extent of the damage, but should be considered "uncertain" in the first few days. More than 20 percent of victims die before reaching the hospital, most within the first hour. Rapid emergency treatment reduces the mortality by as much as 50 percent. During the first 24 hours, the risk of potentially fatal rhythm abnormalities is highest; about 80 percent of the episodes of uncoordinated and ineffective heartbeat occur during this period.

During the first week following a myocardial infarction, there is concern

BALLOON DILATION OF BLOCKAGES

In some instances, when lifestyle changes and medication have failed to resolve angina pain in coronary artery disease, balloon dilation of the blocked artery may offer the best hope for recovery. This procedure—called coronary angioplasty—is done by a doctor who is a cardiologist. It involves inserting a long, slender, hollow catheter tube into an artery in the arm or leg, then passing it along the artery to the heart. There, just as the aorta leaves the heart, lie the two coronary arteries. The doctor guides the tip of the catheter tube into place by a continuous x-ray video that shows the heart and blood vessels. When this catheter tube is in place, the doctor inserts a second, thinner catheter with a deflated balloon at its tip through the hollow one and guides the balloon-tipped catheter forward until its tip is within the narrowed artery. Once it is there, the doctor inflates the balloon; this presses the plaque-filled artery walls outward, dilates the space inside, and makes more room for blood to flow.

Coronary angioplasty requires only local anesthetic (injecting numbing medication only at the spot in the arm or leg where the catheters enter the artery). The procedure usually takes only about an hour and avoids bypass surgery. However, if balloon dilation fails to restore adequate blood flow, bypass surgery is the next step.

The determination of whether coronary angioplasty is a suitable option or bypass surgery is needed depends on four factors: the location of the narrowed area; how accessible it is; whether there are many blockages; and how well the heart works in general. The ideal candidate for coronary angioplasty has a single blockage and has never had a heart attack.

Newer techniques—such as laser atherectomy and stent placement—have expanded the capability of the cardiologist to treat heart disease with these invasive procedures. ∎

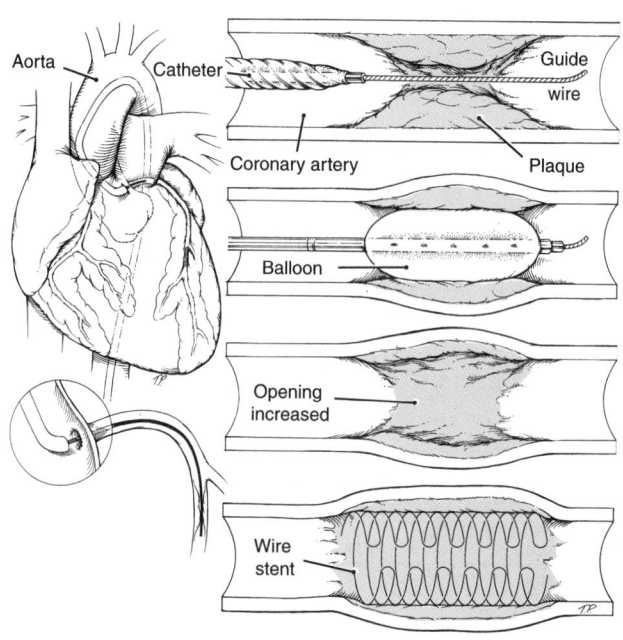

Balloon angioplasty. A small balloon can be inserted into a coronary artery and inflated inside the vessel, physically opening it and pushing aside a plaque. This procedure is sometimes preferred to bypass surgery depending on the function of the heart and the number and location of blockages. Radiologic imaging is used to provide doctors with a picture of the heart and vessels during the procedure. A stent can also be inserted at the time the balloon is inflated and left inside the vessel to help keep it open.

about the risk of weakness in the damaged heart wall (aneurysm) and the possibility of rupture of the wall. Although rupture occurs in only about 1 percent of heart attacks, it is almost immediately fatal. Pericarditis—inflammation of the heart covering (pericardium)—occurs in up to 20 percent of cases and may or may not cause significant discomfort. The possibility of a repeated attack is highest during the first 2 weeks, occurring in about 10 percent of patients. After these initial periods of danger pass, recovery with good medical care is usually the rule (see Recovery After a Myocardial Infarction, page 815).

Before you are discharged from the hospital, you doctor will review the diet and lifestyle changes you must make and the medications you will need. For example, you may take medications to reduce the risk of more clots forming. These may include medications, such as aspirin, to keep platelets from clumping; anticoagulants (warfarin, heparin, dicumarol) to help prevent clotting; other medications, such as beta blockers, to reduce your heart's oxygen requirements; and medications in the digitalis family to enhance a weakened heart's pumping power (see Aspirin Therapy and Medications Used to Treat Coronary Artery Disease, page 809). Angiotensin converting enzyme (ACE) inhibitors (captopril and enalapril, for example) may be prescribed to prevent heart failure and allow the heart to remodel or return to its previous state of contraction (see Medications Used to Treat Hypertension, page 804).

In time, you may also require other procedures, such as cardiac surgery or balloon dilation to bypass or open blocked arteries (see page 814).

RECOVERY AFTER A MYOCARDIAL INFARCTION

When the prognosis is good, recovering from myocardial infarction (heart attack) will, in most cases, take about 6 weeks. If you have been hospitalized, your recovery period will begin in the hospital. Generally, your recovery will be divided into two major phases—early and late recovery—but it will be worth little without the final ongoing phase: maintenance. Maintenance is a life-long project for every heart patient. Your motivation is to avoid ever having to experience a myocardial infarction again.

Years ago, bed rest was recommended for men and women recovering from myocardial infarction. But studies have shown that bed rest probably caused more damage than it prevented, except in cases where complete bed rest is necessary. So do not be surprised when CCU nurses encourage you to sit in a chair as soon as possible and to try to walk slowly up and down the hall. You may even be encouraged to undertake mild calisthenics—moving your arms and legs while you are in bed. As soon as your doctor says it is safe, you should start moving.

Before or soon after you are discharged from the hospital, your doctors will arrange for you to take a limited exercise stress test. This test helps determine your capabilities at home. Some patients refuse this test because they are afraid. If you have been getting up and moving around and sitting in a chair, instead of lying in bed, you will probably have less anxiety about this important test. Studies have shown that heart patients who do not take this test—whether because of anxiety or an accurate reading of their own personal limitations—have the poorest prognosis of all heart patients. All the more reason to get out of bed as soon as you can and get used to moving around. If the results of this test are poor, you will not be released from the hospital until further tests are done and an appropriate therapy treatment is conceived.

As loud and annoying as the hospital environment may be, it is also very protected. Once you leave the hospital to go home, everything changes. For this reason, many heart patients feel vulnerable, rather than elated, when they return home. Once you are at home, you will not see your doctor every day. In fact, your next appointment with your doctor may not be for 2 weeks. Nor will you have nursing care available 24 hours a day, unless your doctor or your family has insisted upon such a precaution. Suddenly, the security of having a trained professional available immediately is gone. In the middle of the night, you may have to go it alone.

The best way to cope with the fear being on your own again may bring and your increased sense of vulnerability is to begin to take control of your situation by making changes in your life that will help you control heart disease and avoid a second heart attack. *If you smoke, you must stop. If you do not exercise, you must start. If you eat a high-fat diet, you must change to a low-fat diet.* Almost everyone knows these are the cardinal rules of preventing heart disease, but having been a heart patient, you can now use your fear to motivate you to follow through on these lifestyle changes and to stick to these positive choices.

During your first 2 weeks back home, you should reassess every aspect of your life to see what you may be able to change to lower your stress level and live a healthier life. With the assistance of your doctor, you will want to plan a diet and exercise regimen that will help lower your blood pressure and your cholesterol level and prevent you from having another heart attack. If you have not exercised before, you can use your recovery period to make exercise a permanent part of your life. Begin by walking or pedaling an exercise bicycle for 10 minutes every day. As you grow stronger, you will be able to increase the time you spend exercising.

A month after your myocardial infarction, it is usually safe to resume driving and other aspects of what constitutes a normal life for you, including going to work, shopping, gardening, and having a social life. By now, you should be doing moderate exercise, such as walking, 30 minutes a day. You should also be eating a low-fat diet. Consult your doctor if you are having trouble breaking old habits, such as smoking or eating a diet high in saturated fat.

By this point in your recovery, it is also usually safe to resume your sex life. Studies have shown that if you have had a myocardial infarction, the odds of having a second one during sex are 1 in 50,000—about the same as they are for having one when you get out of bed in the morning. Despite this reassuring statistic, many myocardial infarction victims and their partners remain anxious about having sex again. If you have had a serious myocardial infarction, your confidence may have been shaken. The best way to resume your sex life is to do it gradually. Most doctors suggest that if you are capable of climbing two flights of stairs without pain or shortness of breath, you are physically ready to resume your sex life.

When you meet with your doctor, it is best to have a frank discussion about sexual activity and how it affects your condition, just as you would any other aspect of your recovery. If you are nervous about having sex, you should talk this over with your partner. Being afraid will only inhibit you from enjoying your reentry into sexual activity. Hearing the facts from your doctor and being reassured by your partner will make you feel more confident. You will want to build up to your former level of sexual activity gradually, and you will be the best judge of when and how this should happen. ■

Disorders of the Heart Valves and Lining

A system of four one-way valves regulates the passage of blood between each of the heart's upper chambers (the atria) and the pumping chamber below (the ventricle) and between each of the ventricles and its outlet to the lungs or the body. The tricuspid valves control blood flow between the right atrium and right ventricle; the pulmonary valve regulates flow between the right ventricle and the outflow to the lungs.

Valves help to ensure one-way flow of blood through the heart. The mitral valve has two cusps, and each of the other valves has three cusps. Contraction of the heart's chambers causes the valves to open and close.

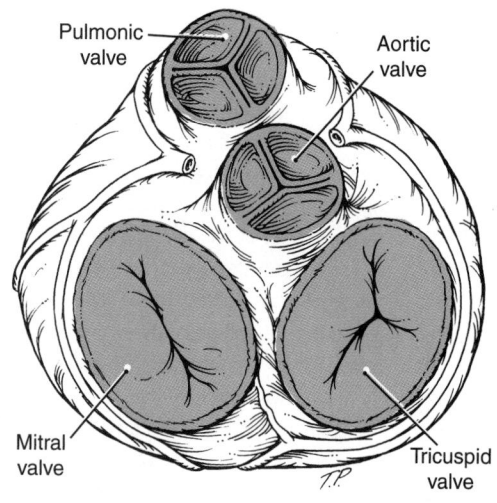

On the left side of the heart, the mitral valve regulates flow between the atrium and ventricle and the aortic valve controls the flow between the left ventricle and the aorta, which delivers blood to the rest of the body. As blood fills the chambers, the valves passively close so that when the heart muscle contracts, the blood cannot go backward.

Three problems may cause valves to malfunction: stenosis (constriction of the opening), regurgitation (failure to close completely), and prolapse (sagging). These disorders can be caused by infection, autoimmune disorders, and congenital (present at birth) abnormalities.

❖ ENDOCARDITIS

Symptoms *(What you may experience)* High fever or persistent, unexplained, low-grade fever; fatigue (usually); night sweats; tender red swellings on fingers, toes, or feet (often); cough and shortness of breath (sometimes); joint pain and swelling (occasionally); stomach or back pain (occasionally).

Signs and laboratory findings *(What the doctor looks for)* Change or new appearance of a heart murmur; tiny hemorrhages (Roth spots) in the retina at the back of the eye; "splinter" hemorrhages under the finger or toenails; laboratory tests showing a high white blood cell count and an elevated sedimentation rate (a nonspecific measure of infection or inflammation), along with a positive blood culture (growing and identifying the bacterial organism from a blood specimen).

What is it? Occasionally, the thin inner membrane (the endocardium) that lines the chambers of the heart and the heart valves becomes infected by bacteria that have invaded the bloodstream. The infection usually occurs in people with preexisting heart disorders, such as an abnormal valve, a septal defect (a small hole in the wall between the pumping chambers), artificial heart valves, or coarctation of the aorta (an abrupt narrowing of the aorta that creates a jet-like, high-pressure stream of blood flow beyond it). These abnormalities make the endocardium more vulnerable to infection if bacteria from another source pour into the bloodstream. This can occur during dental procedures or cleanings; surgical procedures in the upper respiratory tract, urinary tract, or colon; and certain gynecologic procedures. Intravenous drug users are at risk from dirty needles or from improper cleansing of the skin at the injection site.

The subacute form of bacterial endocarditis begins with days to weeks of unexplained fever and vague physical complaints. The fever occurs as blood-borne waves of infecting bacteria stimulate the body's immune defense system. In acute bacterial endocarditis, the onset is sudden and fever is high; in the subacute infection, symptoms may be subtle and the diagnosis harder to make.

Small clots that form along the roughened, infected endocardium may dislodge and travel to distant sites to occlude blood vessels such as the arteries of the heart itself, or those supplying the feet, toes, hands, fingers, lungs, kidneys, or retina. Depending on where they lodge, these traveling emboli, as the clots are called, cause the widely varied symptoms of endocarditis.

Prevention Prevention is the first line of defense if you are at risk for endocarditis. If you know you have a heart or valve abnormality, always notify your doctor, surgeon, dentist, or dental hygienist prior to any surgical procedure (see Antibiotics to Protect the Heart Valves, page 817).

When to call the doctor High fever for more than a day or two without an obvious cause demands investigation by a doctor. The appearance of small hemorrhages beneath the skin or under the nails should prompt an immediate visit to your doctor. However, people who traumatize their fin-

ANTIBIOTICS TO PROTECT THE HEART VALVES

Abnormalities of the structure of a heart valve—whether from scarring after infection or structural abnormalities present since birth—predispose it to infection from bacteria in the bloodstream. Infection of the valve can lead to endocarditis, a more generalized infection of the heart lining (see page 816) and bring with it weakness and recurrent fevers. Endocarditis can ultimately damage the valves to such an extent that they must be replaced. Normally, of course, the blood is free of bacteria that might infect the valves. Such is not the case, however, during and following dental cleaning or repair procedures or surgery (especially of the mouth or intestines) when many bacteria that commonly reside in parts of the body find entry into the bloodstream and pose a danger to abnormally shaped valves.

Because we can usually predict and schedule these kinds of situations, we can protect the valves by killing the bacteria as they enter the bloodstream—before they have a chance to do any mischief to the valve. Doctors have long adopted the routine of giving antibiotics (most commonly erythromycin or penicillin) to patients with valve problems the day before, the day of, and the day following a procedure. If you have a heart murmur, or if you know that you have an abnormally shaped heart valve, you should always alert your doctor or dentist to the situation and take the prescribed antibiotic prior to surgical or dental procedures. ∎

---

gers through work (for example, carpenters) or by excessively vigorous cuticle cleaning may cause traumatic splinter hemorrhages; these hemorrhages should be distinguished from those of endocarditis.

Treatment Hospitalization for large doses of intravenous antibiotic therapy. Medication choice depends on the type of bacteria causing the infection. Oral or home intravenous antibiotic therapy will likely continue after hospital discharge.

Prognosis Fatal if untreated, particularly since it occurs in those who already have heart defects. Good if antibiotic therapy is begun promptly. If the response to medication after 10 days is poor or the damage to the heart valve is severe, it may be necessary to repair or replace the damaged valve or surgically correct the underlying heart abnormality to eradicate the infection.

❖ RHEUMATIC FEVER

Symptoms (*What you may experience*) Recent sore throat; chest discomfort; breathlessness with exertion; fatigue; rash; migrating joint pain and swelling; fever.

Signs and laboratory findings (*What the doctor looks for*) Enlarged heart as shown on ECG or chest x-ray; a pericardial friction rub (abrasive sound audible through a stethoscope); new heart murmur; confirmed recent streptococcal infection (strep throat); antibodies against the streptococcal bacteria as confirmed by blood tests; elevated sedimentation rate.

What is it? Rheumatic fever rarely occurs now in the United States, thanks to antibi-otics that kill the streptococcal organism. Prompt diagnosis and early treatment of strep throat can prevent rheumatic fever. Without prompt treatment of strep throat, the immune system may inadvertently misdirect its assault on the invading bacteria, and instead attack the body's own tissues—usually the heart valves, and primarily the mitral valve. Thus, the damage is not caused by the infection itself. Most cases of rheumatic fever occur in children and adolescents (ages 5 to 15), beginning about 2 to 3 weeks after a bout of strep throat. Left undetected, rheumatic fever can eventually lead to permanent heart damage.

Prevention If you (or your child) develop a painful sore throat accompanied by fever, see your doctor, who may wish to take a throat culture or perform other tests to detect strep infection. Sore throats are common and may be harmless, but rheumatic fever is serious and can be avoided with prompt treatment of strep throat.

When to call the doctor Any severe sore throat accompanied by fever, rash, or pus on the tonsils should prompt a visit to the doctor immediately. Rheumatic fever can be prevented with early treatment of strep infection (see Strep Throat, page 592). If rheumatic fever does develop, early treatment improves outcome.

Treatment The standard therapy for strep throat is a course of oral penicillin or another appropriate antibiotic. Rheumatic fever is treated with antibiotic injections, followed by prophylactic medication for several years to prevent recurrence. People allergic to penicillin can take sulfonamides or erythromycin daily as prophylaxis.

Prognosis After the initial attack subsides (which may be weeks to months), the prognosis depends on the extent of heart damage. Heart failure, cardiomyopathy (heart muscle weakness), and pericarditis (inflammation of the pericardium, the covering of the heart) carry a poorer prognosis. However, 80 percent of children infected with rheumatic fever reach adulthood, and most are not physically limited by the disease. More than 60 percent of patients suffer permanent heart valve damage, which may require surgical repair at a later time.

❖ MITRAL VALVE PROLAPSE

Symptoms (What you may experience) Episodes of vague chest pain; shortness of breath, fatigue, and fluttering or skipping of the heartbeat.

Signs and laboratory findings (What the doctor looks for) Characteristic clicking sound and/or murmur heard through the stethoscope; echocardiogram (heart ultrasound) demonstrates the prolapse.

What is it? Mitral valve prolapse is a condition found in one in 10 people in the general population, and many people have no symptoms. Blood from the small left atrium passes through the mitral valve into the pumping chamber, the powerful left ventricle. The blood rushes into the ventricle and fills it. When the heart contracts, the valve closes forcefully. In mitral valve prolapse, the two halves (or leaflets) of the valve are bigger than necessary, as a consequence, they billow (that is, prolapse) and "flop" to an imperfect closure. The characteristic heart sounds of this condition—the click that is heard with a stethoscope—come from the billowing sound of the blood. Failure to close completely allows blood to flow back through the crack between the leaflets as the heart contracts, causing a whooshing murmur sound.

The cause of the unusual chest pain that sometimes accompanies mitral valve prolapse is uncertain, but medical consensus considers the pain a discomfort rather than a threat to health.

Stress on the billowing valve leaflets over time may snap the cords that stabilize the leaflets during forceful heart muscle contraction. Significant damage to these cords can result in more serious leakage of blood through the valve leaflets (called mitral regurgitation) and may even require surgical repair or replacement of the valve.

What you can do Once it has been diagnosed, become familiar with the symptoms it causes so that you can notify your doctor of changes. You should always notify your doctor, surgeon, dentist, or dental hygienist prior to any surgical procedure (see Antibiotics to Protect the Heart Valves, page 817).

When to call the doctor The appearance of new vague chest pain should always prompt a visit to your doctor (especially true for men over 40 years of age). New shortness of breath at rest or with exertion or persistent fluttering or skipping heartbeat should also prompt a visit to the doctor.

Treatment Persistent disturbances of rhythm may sometimes require medication (the most commonly prescribed being the beta blockers, such as propranolol) to slow and stabilize the heartbeat. Severe valvular dysfunction may require surgical valve repair or replacement.

Prognosis Excellent in most cases. The disorder is often totally innocuous and causes no symptoms. For those people in whom the valvular billowing causes enough damage to impair normal function, valve repair or replacement may become necessary with aging. Although valve replacement is now commonly performed in large hospitals around the country, open-heart surgery has its risks. Following successful valve repair or replacement, however, the prognosis is good.

❖ MITRAL VALVE STENOSIS AND REGURGITATION

Symptoms (What you may experience) Shortness of breath, especially while lying down; awaking after a few hours unable to breathe; rapid heart beat (occasionally); coughing up a little blood (rarely).

Signs and laboratory findings (What the doctor looks for) A "snap" and a rumbling murmur between heart contractions or a blowing murmur with each contraction (abnormal heart sounds heard through the stethoscope); ECG showing typical electrical pattern changes of atrial enlargement or atrial fibrillation (a rapidly quivering beat of the small upper chambers); abnormally shaped valve shown on echocardiogram.

What is it? Stenosis (narrowing or constriction) of the mitral valve, in which the thickened and stiff leaves do not open and close properly, impedes blood flow between the atrium and the ventricle. It usually develops as a consequence of rheumatic heart disease (see Rheumatic Fever, page 817, for more information). In some cases, the symptoms may be so mild that they go unnoticed. As the valve opening narrows, pressure in the atrial chamber rises to maintain normal blood flow through the valve. As the pressure continues to rise, fluid backs up into the lungs (pulmonary congestion and ultimately edema), bringing on breathlessness. Blood vessels in the lungs may burst and produce blood-tinged sputum.

If the mitral valve does not close properly when the heart muscle contracts, some of the blood in the left ventricle can leak back through the partially open mitral valve—a condition called mitral valve regurgitation. The ventricle, which must now pump harder to increase the flow to the rest of the body, enlarges and weakens.

Blood flow in the dilated atrial chamber can become turbulent or stagnant—a condition that favors the formation of small clots that may escape the atrium and lodge at distant sites as emboli in the hands, feet, or more ominously, the brain, causing a stroke. Clots from the right atrium may lodge in the lung.

Prevention As in any heart or valve abnormality, you should always notify your doctor, surgeon, dentist, or dental hygienist prior to any surgical procedure (see Antibiotics to Protect the Heart Valves, page 817). If you have rheumatic heart disease and are at risk for recurrent strep infections, you should take daily prophylactic treatment.

When to call the doctor Coughing up blood or persistent breathlessness of unknown cause should always prompt an immediate visit to your doctor.

Treatment The treatment depends on symptoms; many people go for years with-

HEART VALVE SURGERY

Heart valves that fail to seal effectively because they are stiff and narrow may require surgery to repair them or occasionally even to replace them. Doctors use two opening procedures: balloon valvuloplasty and surgical valvotomy. In a balloon valvuloplasty, the cardiologist inserts a flexible hollow tube (catheter) into an artery, guides it by x-ray to the heart chambers and once in place, inflates a balloon at its tip to stretch open the constricted valve. Although any such procedure carries some risk, this procedure is quite safe. Recovery takes only a few days, and relief of symptoms—particularly shortness of breath—can be almost immediate. Balloon valvuloplasty is of benefit for mitral and pulmonary stenosis.

Open valvotomy involves opening the chest and surgically cutting the constriction of the valve directly, a much more serious and difficult procedure, although it is still done routinely enough to be considered safe. Because it requires opening the chest cavity, recovery takes a few weeks longer than balloon valvuloplasty. But open valvotomy may alleviate symptoms for many years.

More severe valve damage or seriously leaking valves may require removal and valve replacement with artificial or animal graft (pig) valves. This procedure is the most serious of all the valve procedures. It involves opening the chest through the breast bone, connecting the heart to a heart-lung machine (which takes over the circulation and breathing functions of those two vital organs), and surgically removing the damaged valve. In its place, the surgeon will sew in a new valve, either a metal and plastic mechanical one or a natural tissue valve taken from a pig. Surgeons use the pig valve because it is roughly the size of a human valve. It is treated with chemicals to prevent the body from rejecting it.

The choice of which kind of valve to use depends in great measure on the recipient's age, because the natural pig valve wears out more quickly than mechanical valves. Because people under age 65 might expect to live at least another 10 years, a pig valve would most likely require a second valve replacement in the future. In people over the age of 65, however, the natural valve will usually last sufficiently long to avoid reoperation. It has the added benefit of not needing continuous blood-thinning medication to prevent blood clots (a serious problem with artificial metal and plastic valves). The mechanical valve is appropriate for people who must take blood-thinning medications anyway for other reasons, such as heart rhythm problems.

Length of recovery after valve replacement is usually several weeks to a few months, depending on age and state of health prior to the operation. But once recovery is complete, the quality of life is usually excellent.

New techniques using thoracoscopic instruments (flexible lighted tubes through which customized long tools are inserted) are allowing valve surgery to be performed without the need to open the chest completely. Finger-sized ports (tiny cuts into the body) in the chest allow entry of the scope and other instruments. Patients go home in a matter of days, and complete recovery is much quicker. ∎

out symptoms and consequently require no treatment except the precaution of taking antibiotics before dental work or surgery. Those who develop atrial fibrillation may need medication (commonly, digoxin or other newer antiarrhythmic medications) to correct the abnormal rhythm. In addition, because of the risk of forming blood clots, people who develop atrial fibrillation should receive blood-thinning medications, commonly warfarin (Coumadin). In some cases of mitral valve stenosis, doctors recommend surgically separating the scarred, constricted valve leaflets—a procedure called a commissurotomy—to widen the mitral opening. Other doctors favor a newer procedure—balloon valvuloplasty—in which the doctor inserts a thin, flexible catheter (about the thickness of a strand of spaghetti) into the constricted area. A deflated balloon lies at the catheter's tip. Once in place, the balloon is inflated, forcing the leaflets apart and opening the constriction.

More severe cases may require replacing the damaged valve with either an artificial mechanical valve or a pig valve.

Prognosis Good if discovered and treated early. Long-standing mitral valve stenosis can cause pulmonary hypertension (high lung pressure) that may damage the lung permanently. Usually, the prognosis for surgery to open narrowed valves is good. Valve replacement surgery is riskier, but it also has a good prognosis.

❖ AORTIC VALVE STENOSIS AND REGURGITATION

Symptoms *(What you may experience)* Usually, none until middle age or later; then, symptoms include shortness of breath (often), chest pain (occasionally), or fainting with physical exertion (rarely).

Signs and laboratory findings *(What the doctor looks for)* Characteristic harsh murmur during contraction of the heart or blowing, softer murmur in relaxation heard through the stethoscope; weak pulse in the carotid artery; enlarged left heart chamber demonstrated on ECG; abnormally shaped aortic valve shown on echocardiogram or cardiac catheterization (injecting dye into the heart through a hollow tube inserted through a blood vessel in the arm or leg).

What is it? The aortic valve separates the powerful left ventricular pumping chamber of the heart from the aorta, the major artery that supplies blood to the body. The valve can malfunction in two ways: it can become tightly constricted, unable to open fully (stenosis), or the valve leaflets can fail to close completely (causing regurgitation, or backflow of the blood). Calcium deposits in the tissues of the valve stiffen this structure. The hardened leaflets fail to open fully. When the ventricle contracts around the blood within, pressure builds in the pumping chamber, which over time causes the muscle wall to thicken. The disorder may cause no symptoms for many years until the stenosis becomes quite pronounced. When the leaflets fail to open fully, as the heart muscle squeezes, blood is forced through the narrow slit during the entire contraction, preventing effective pumping. During the rest between contractions, the slightly opened valve lets blood flow from the aorta back into the heart. Because getting adequate blood to the body depends on effective function of the left ventricle, damage to the aortic valve sufficient to impair its function usually requires surgical valve replacement.

Constriction of the outflow for blood through the aortic valve can also occur when the muscle wall just beneath the valve thickens, a condition called idiopathic hypertrophic subaortic stenosis, or IHSS. The valve itself may be normal, but the net result is the same: a narrowed opening through which the blood must pass. This particular disorder is common in otherwise healthy young people and may be a cause of sudden death. (For more information, see Cardiomyopathies, page 824).

Prevention There is no self-care remedy for this condition. As with any heart or valve abnormality, you should always notify your doctor, surgeon, dentist, or dental hygienist prior to any surgical procedure (see Antibiotics to Protect the Heart Valves, page 817).

When to call the doctor Any significant new or worsening shortness of breath or persistent chest discomfort (especially in men over 40 years of age) requires prompt medical evaluation. Unexplained fainting, particularly if associated with physical activity, also requires immediate medical care.

Treatment Medications can sometimes help the heart beat more strongly; however, once symptoms begin, valve replacement will usually be the only effective remedy. After replacement, your doctor will prescribe medication to prevent clot formation in the new valve. You may require blood-thinning medication throughout the course of your life after valve replacement, although some tissue valves may require anticoagulants for 6 to 8 weeks after surgery.

Prognosis Once shortness of breath, chest discomfort, or fainting occurs, the prognosis without surgery is poor. With valve replacement, the prognosis is much improved. The risk of the surgery is relatively low (a 2 to 5 percent mortality, meaning 95 to 98 people in 100 will survive the surgery).

❖ PULMONARY AND TRICUSPID VALVE ABNORMALITIES

Symptoms *(What you may experience)* Often none until adulthood, then shortness of breath with physical activity (often), fainting (sometimes), chest pain (often), and, as the condition worsens, swelling of the feet and ankles and tenderness of the upper right abdomen.

Signs and laboratory findings *(What the doctor looks for)* High-pitched murmur (whooshing sound heard through the stethoscope) and a cardiac thrill (vibrating tremor felt along the left side of the breast bone) in pulmonary stenosis radiating to the back. In pulmonary regurgitation, high-pitched murmur between heart contractions. In tricuspid stenosis, rumbling murmur during heart contraction. In tricuspid regurgitation, harsh murmur in systole at the lower sternal border, fluid accumulation in the abdomen, enlarged liver. ECG demonstrating right ventricle enlargement, chest x-ray showing dilated pulmonary artery and right ventricle (in pulmonary stenosis), echocardiogram showing the abnormally shaped valve(s). Diagnosis is confirmed by cardiac catheterization.

What is it? Stenosis of the tricuspid valve (which separates the upper right atrium from the right ventricle) occurs most often following a bout of rheumatic fever. Just as with the mitral valve, stenosis of the opening causes back pressure of blood in the atrium, leading to dilation of the chamber and impaired filling of the ventricle below with blood. Pulmonary stenosis creates the same back pressure strain on the right ventricle, limiting adequate flow of blood into the lung for reoxygenation. Continued stress on the chamber leads to the condition known as right heart failure, in which the liver enlarges and fluid collects in the abdomen (a condition called ascites) and in the feet and legs (edema).

If the valve fails to shut fully, the condition of valvular regurgitation develops. Infection of the tricuspid valve occurs commonly in intravenous drug users, but tricuspid valve regurgitation occurs for several reasons besides a diseased or misshapen valve. For example, it may occur in systemic lupus erythematosus (see page 642).

What you can do There are no self-care remedies for this condition. If you know you have a heart or valve abnormality, you should always notify your doctor, surgeon, dentist, or dental hygienist prior to any surgical procedure (see Antibiotics to Protect the Heart Valves, page 817).

When to call the doctor Any episode of chest pain (especially in men over 40 years of age), breathlessness with or without exertion, and swelling of the feet or abdomen. Liver engorgement may cause pain in the right-upper quadrant of the abdomen and a sense of fullness when eating.

Treatment Medications used sparingly to rid the body of excess fluid (diuretics) may decrease edema and ascites. Surgical correction is the cornerstone of therapy for these valve abnormalities once they begin to cause symptoms. For pulmonary and tricuspid stenosis, balloon valvuloplasty may offer the best results. In this procedure the doctor inserts a thin, flexible catheter about the thickness of a strand of spaghetti into the constricted area. A deflated balloon lies at the catheter's tip. Once in place, the balloon is inflated, forcing the leaflets apart and opening the constriction. More severe cases may require totally replacing the damaged valve with either an artificial valve or a pig's valve. After replacing the valve, the doctor will prescribe long-term medication with warfarin to prevent clots from forming in the new valve. (Valve replacement is seldom done for tricuspid regurgitation.)

Prognosis Many people have the condition for years without symptoms. However, once symptoms begin and progress valve repair or replacement is required. The surgery carries moderate to low risk (2 to 4 percent mortality) with an excellent long-term result.

❖ MARFAN SYNDROME

***Symptoms** (What you may experience)* Few, if any; commonly myopia (nearsightedness); possibly heart palpitations; easy dislocation of joints in some cases.

***Signs and laboratory findings** (What the doctor looks for)* Tall stature with long arms, legs, and very long spidery fingers (arachnodactyly); ectopia lentis (an abnormality of the lens of the eye) may cause severe myopia (nearsightedness) or weak distance vision and detachment of the retina of the eye; mitral valve prolapse (often; see page 818). Sometimes: sunken breast bone (pectus excavatum); loose joints; abnormalities of the aorta and aortic valve.

What is it? Marfan syndrome is an inherited disorder involving the supportive connective tissues, causing abnormalities of the eye, skeletal system, and cardiovascular system. Laxity in the connective tissue support causes most of the problems in Marfan syndrome. Laxity of the support of the first portion of the aorta may cause regurgitation through the aortic valve. Excessive traction and pressure on the aorta may produce small tears in the lining that enlarge and shred the wall, leading to aortic dissection (splitting and weakening of the wall of the aorta). The pressure of the dissection weakens the wall and can cause rupture of the aorta. The supportive laxity can also involve the mitral valve; about 85 percent of people with Marfan syndrome have mitral valve prolapse.

Laxity in the tissues supporting the joints causes them to dislocate easily. Sagging of the lens of the eye can lead to its dislocation and also predisposes to severe nearsightedness and detachment of the retina (the region at the back of the eye containing the visual receptors). Retinal detachment (see Chapter 15) can cause permanent loss of vision and is a medical and surgical emergency.

What you can do There are no self-care remedies for this condition.

When to call the doctor Although Marfan syndrome may be detected early in life, many cases may not be. Early detection is of paramount importance in adolescence to prevent curvature of the spine and other skeletal deformities, as well as to follow the cardiovascular system for signs of ballooning of the aortic root (first portion of the aorta). Because Marfan syndrome is a genetic disorder, children, parents, or siblings of people diagnosed with Marfan syndrome should undergo thorough evaluation by a genetic specialist.

Children with Marfan syndrome should undergo periodic examination by an ophthalmologist, to check for poor vision. During their rapid periods of growth, laxity of connective tissue support of the spine may lead to scoliosis (curvature of the spine), which an orthopedic surgeon can treat with a brace.

People known to have Marfan syndrome who develop sudden symptoms of chest pain, shortness of breath, loss of vision, or fainting should consult their doctor immediately.

Treatment Because of the associated abnormalities of the heart valves that can occur in this syndrome, people with Marfan syndrome and valve abnormalities should take antibiotic medication to prevent valve infection before they have dental cleaning or repair or surgery (see Antibiotics To Protect The Heart Valves, page 817).

Beta blockers can help to slow the dilation of the lax aortic supportive tissues.

Restriction of heavy physical exertion may help to protect the aorta from dissection.

Ongoing evaluation of the diameter of the aorta will signal when the need arises for surgery to replace the worn, dilated aortic root, usually at a diameter of 50 to 55 mm. Life can be prolonged if the aorta is replaced before dissection or rupture occurs.

Prognosis Without treatment, Marfan syndrome commonly causes death by age 40 to 50, usually from complications related to the aorta (dissection, rupture, or heart failure from aortic valve regurgitation). Prompt diagnosis, appropriate treatment, and prophylactic surgical replacement of the dilated aorta prolong life and significantly improve the prognosis.

Disorders of the Heart Muscle and Covering

To move blood throughout the body effectively, the heart muscle must function in peak form. The muscle cannot perform that crucial job if it has been weakened by infection or inflammation or if the tissues that cover the heart are inflamed, infected, or constricted by scarring.

❖ CONGESTIVE HEART FAILURE

Symptoms *(What you may experience)* Shortness of breath with physical activity or when lying flat; awakening short of breath a few hours after going to sleep; dry cough; fatigue; swelling of the feet and legs. Sometimes: vague discomfort in the upper right abdomen; loss of appetite; and nausea.

Signs and laboratory findings *(What the doctor looks for)* Rales (crackling breath sounds heard through a stethoscope); ventricular gallop (a heartbeat heard through a stethoscope that sounds like the three-beat gallop of horses' hooves); enlarged liver; enlarged heart (seen on chest x-ray or demonstrated by characteristic changes on an ECG).

What is it? The heart may fail to pump blood adequately to the lungs or to the body for a variety of reasons—primarily, weakening of the heart muscle from a heart attack or from viral or toxic damage. However, the muscle can also "fail" from working under an excessive burden. Valvular problems, such as constriction of the aortic valve (see Aortic Valve Stenosis and Regurgitation, page 820), may impose an increased workload on the heart. Elevated blood pressure over a long period of time has the same effect: The heart muscle must generate enormous pressure to move the blood along against a "head wind" of blood vessel resistance. Excessive work not only fatigues the heart, but may cause the muscle to hypertrophy (grow larger), which itself causes problems by taking up space within the chambers intended for the blood. Less blood in the chamber means less blood pushed through the valve with each beat, increasing the burden to the heart. Added work leading to heart failure also occurs in disorders that cause the heart to beat exces-

sively fast, such as hyperthyroid disease or various tachycardias (excessively rapid heart rate).

One form of heart dysfunction is diastolic dysfunction, in which impaired heart relaxation and not heart contraction can also lead to congestive heart failure. During the diastolic phase of the heartbeat, the ventricles relax and fill with blood, prior to being pumped out during contraction (systole). But if scarring or fibrosis, for example, stiffen and thicken the heart muscle, the ventricle cannot relax and fill adequately. This raises pressure in the ventricles and causes fluid backup into the lungs. Usually, diuretics are prescribed cautiously for diastolic dysfunction, since reduced blood volume worsens the condition; more often beta blockers or calcium channel blockers are used.

Some medications can contribute to heart muscle failure by reducing the efficiency of the pumping action. Several of these—calcium channel blockers and some medications intended to correct heart rhythm disturbances—may benefit *other* kinds of heart problems, such as angina or hypertension, and yet worsen heart failure by hampering the pumping action. Chronic alcohol abuse can also reduce the heart's pumping effectiveness, and over time may also damage the muscle, causing cardiomyopathy (see Cardiomyopathies, page 824).

A healthy heart can withstand considerable variation in its rate and tolerance for increased work—such as might occur with fever, heavy physical exercise, or heightened emotion. But a heart weakened by coronary artery disease or cardiomyopathy often lacks those reserves, and added demand can tip the balance toward a spiraling cycle of worsening heart muscle failure. Because the heart is really two pumping systems—a right side that sends blood to the lungs for oxygenation and a left side that sends oxygen-rich blood to the whole body—the symptoms of heart failure depend on which of the pumps weakens.

When the left heart fails to function optimally, the symptoms arise because the weak muscle cannot pump enough blood out of the heart chamber with each beat, and the failing heart causes higher pressure between contractions in the heart chamber. The higher pressure during heart relaxation causes fluid to back up in the lungs, causing congestion, and ultimately allows fluid to "leak" from the vessels into the lung tissue and air spaces. This makes the lungs heavier and blocks transfer of oxygen from the air to the blood, causing shortness of breath.

When the right side of the heart fails, the weak muscle pumps less blood into the lungs for oxygenation, and blood backs up into the body. When the backup of blood occurs in the body instead of the lungs, the excess pressure causes fluid to "leak" out of the blood vessels, congesting and enlarging the liver and abdominal cavity, and swelling those areas most affected by gravity—the legs and feet. In most cases, both sides fail to some degree, and the symptoms of heart failure are a combination of these.

What you can do Congestive heart failure (CHF) can be prevented by treatment of high blood pressure, thyroid disease, and underlying diseases, prior to development of CHF. Among those people already diagnosed with the disorder, restricting salt (sodium) intake to no more than 2 g a day and getting gentle, gradually progressive, aerobic exercise under a doctor's direction may help diminish symptoms and improve endurance. Your doctor may limit your fluid intake as well.

When to call the doctor Persistent or progressive shortness of breath or body swelling should prompt an immediate consultation with the doctor. The progression of shortness of breath that happens only with exercise to shortness of breath at rest or lying down also signals a need for a prompt visit to the doctor.

Treatment Avoid alcohol and stop medications that may contribute to heart failure; identify and treat any medical condition (such as thyroid disease or hypertension), valvular abnormality, or rhythm disturbance that may cause or contribute to it.

Medical treatment to improve heart function aims at reducing the pressure against which the heart must work, or to make the muscle pump with more vigor and strength. The mainstay of therapy—diuretics ("water pills")—induces the kidneys to release salt and fluid, reducing the volume of blood and decreasing fluid backup. Another way to ease the heart's workload—reducing the pressure against which it must pump—is best accomplished by a newer class of medications called angiotensin-converting enzyme (ACE) inhibitors. These medications lower blood pressure by dilating the arteries and promoting the release of excess salt by the kidneys, which benefits the struggling heart muscle. Because ACE inhibitors decrease mortality compared with other vasodilators, they have become the front-line medications for heart failure. Recently certain beta-blocking agents have also been shown to improve prognosis. These agents must be used very cautiously as they have the potential to decrease the strength with which the heart contracts.

A third strategy relies on the so-called inotropic medications that strengthen the heart's contractions so that it pumps more effectively. Digitalis (digoxin), the best known in this group, was once the standard therapy for CHF. First used some 200 years ago, the medication still has value for certain people, especially those in atrial fibrillation. People taking digitalis must be carefully monitored because the medication has a very narrow therapeutic range: the difference between the blood level of the medication that is too low to do any good and the level so high it is potentially deadly.

Newer medications in this category include dopamine (Intropin), dobutamine (Dobutrex), and amrinone (Inocor). These medication are usually given intravenously in the hospital to seriously ill patients. These medications have serious risks and complications and may actually worsen the prognosis if used for extended periods.

Because myocardial ischemia due to coronary artery disease may impair the pumping action of the heart and cause CHF, successful surgical measures to alleviate the blockages in the coronary arteries (see Balloon Dilation of Blockages, page 814, and Bypass Surgery, page 810) may improve heart function.

Prognosis Poor to fair, ranging from an annual mortality of 10 percent in people with mild, stable symptoms to a mortality of 50 percent in those with more severe symptoms and progressive disease. As many as 50 percent of people with heart failure may suffer sudden cardiac death (see page 811) most likely from abrupt disturbances in heart rhythm.

❖ CARDIOMYOPATHIES

Symptoms (What you may experience)
Shortness of breath, especially with exercise

(usually); easy fatigability (usually); chest pain (often); "sinking" spells; fainting or near-fainting (sometimes); swelling of the feet and legs (sometimes).

Signs and laboratory findings *(What the doctor looks for)* Enlarged heart and sometimes fluid accumulation in the lungs shown on chest x-ray; a heart murmur (occasionally); galloping heart sounds and crackling sounds when taking a breath, heard through the stethoscope; electrical pattern changes on ECG; dilated or poorly functioning heart muscle shown on echocardiogram.

What is it? A variety of progressive disorders that prevent the heart muscle from pumping effectively. The dysfunction comes from weakness of a muscle made thin from dilation (dilated cardiomyopathy); from excessive muscle thickness narrowing the heart chambers, limiting filling (hypertrophic cardiomyopathy); or, rarely, from infiltration of the heart muscle with fibrous tissue or with certain abnormal materials (restrictive cardiomyopathy).

In the first instance, the heart muscle becomes profoundly weak in the absence of infection or inflammation in the body. A variety of insults can bring about a dilated cardiomyopathy, among them: alcoholism; endocrine disturbances such as thyroid disease, diabetes, acromegaly, and pheochromocytoma (for more information about these disorders, see Chapter 26); viral infection of the heart; and valve abnormalities. When cardiomyopathy occurs, the weak muscle fails to pump the full volume of blood with each contraction, leading to dilation of the chambers and further weakening and thinning of the muscle.

Cardiomyopathy can also occur when the heart muscle becomes overdeveloped. Overgrowth of muscle tissue is often focused in the left ventricle just below the aortic valve. Thickening of the muscle at this point, called idiopathic hypertrophic subaortic stenosis, or IHSS, narrows the outflow of blood leaving the heart for the body. The result—inadequate blood flow to the body and backup of fluid—is the same as in dilated cardiomyopathy. In this case, however, there may be no symptoms for many years. Sudden death during exercise may be the first symptom. In fact, this condition is one of the most common causes of sudden death among athletes under age 35, under-

scoring the need for careful evaluation of young athletes before participation in strenuous physical activity. Because this condition is inherited, family members must be screened once a case is identified. An echocardiogram is usually diagnostic, particularly after puberty, because thickening of the heart muscle often accelerates during puberty.

A restrictive form of cardiomyopathy occurs in amyloidosis (see Chapter 18), a systemic disease in which deposits of thick, starch-like material build up in the tissues. As these deposits continue to form, they crowd the normal heart muscle cells and reduce flexibility and contractility, leading to ineffective pumping of blood to the body and, ultimately, heart failure.

What you can do There are no self-care remedies for cardiomyopathy.

When to call the doctor At the first sign of symptoms suggestive of cardiomyopathy, call your doctor. As a general rule, anyone participating in strenuous athletic activities should have a thorough heart checkup by a doctor. Your doctor will do screening tests to try and identify the cause.

Treatment For most cases of cardiomyopathy, no specific treatment exists. In cardiomyopathy related to alcohol abuse, discontinuing alcohol may result in marked recovery of heart muscle function. Alcohol consumption should be stopped in all people with cardiomyopathy, because it impairs heart function. In those cases related to endocrine disturbances, treatment should be aimed at those disorders (for example, replacing thyroid hormone in thyroid dysfunction). Because blood flow slows in weakened, dilated chambers, sluggish flow may allow small clots to form that can travel to the brain or lungs, plugging small arteries there. Thinning the blood with anticoagulant medications can help to prevent this problem.

In hypertrophic cardiomyopathies, treatment with medications (such as beta blockers and calcium channel blockers) that aim to improve outflow may be beneficial. Newer forms of therapy with pacemakers may be beneficial. In some cases of IHSS, surgery to remove a portion of the overgrown muscle tissue may help. Sometimes, because of poor pumping, blood backs up

HEART TRANSPLANT SURGERY

A heart transplant may prove the only viable option when the heart muscle has sustained damage so severe that it cannot even marginally meet the demands of pumping blood effectively throughout the body and when no combination of medications will work to strengthen its contractions. Doctors can only consider people as suitable candidates for transplantation if replacement of the heart offers a significant chance for quality of life. In general, suitable means reasonably young people suffering from viral, toxic, or ischemic cardiomyopathies (heart muscle weakness), and not beset by other disabling disorders. Successful outcome hinges on finding a suitable donor—one whose tissues "match" the patient's to minimize the possibility of rejection of the donated heart. Rejection occurs because the patient's immune defense system identifies the new heart as "foreign" and sets out to destroy it.

Each of the trillions of cells of which we are made bears markers on its surface that proclaim that it is ours. To protect what is "us" from what is not us, the immune defense system learns to recognize the markers in its own body and to leave tissues bearing those markers alone. Tissues bearing a foreign badge, however, incite the immune defenses to action. The closer the markers match, the less likely the immune system will assault the foreign tissue. Blood relatives offer the best hope for a good match in transplanting tissues that can regrow, such as bone marrow, or those that come in pairs, such as kidneys. But because each of us has only one heart, it is an organ that a living relative cannot donate. So when a heart does become available, it is usually the result of the accidental death of a young, healthy person who is rarely a family member. Therefore, the match will never be a perfect one, and so doctors must rely on suppressing the recipient's immune system with powerful medications to prevent rejection—most often with medication like the immunosuppressant cyclosporine. Even though heart transplantation is fraught with many obstacles, in experienced hands, the success rate of this procedure is quite good; 60 to 75 percent of heart transplant patients survive longer than 5 years. ■

and dilates the chambers, causing transition to a dilated cardiomyopathy; in these cases, treatment with diuretics and afterload-reducing therapy may help.

In restrictive cardiomyopathy, little effective treatment exists, although cautious use of diuretics may sometimes help.

Prognosis Variable with dilated cardiomyopathies; some people remain relatively stable for long periods. Once heart failure symptoms begin, however, they may suffer a steady or rapid decline in heart function. In hypertrophic cases, the disorder may go unnoticed for years, with sudden death being the first indication of a problem.

❖ PERICARDITIS

Symptoms (*What you may experience*)
Pain and tenderness of the chest behind the breast bone, which is worse lying down (almost always); dry cough (common); shortness of breath (common); heart palpitations (sometimes).

Signs and laboratory findings (*What the doctor looks for*) Pericardial friction rub (raspy sound audible on listening to the heart with the stethoscope); electrical pattern changes on the ECG (often); heart enlargement shown on chest x-ray (occasionally).

What is it? The pericardium, two thin leaves of slick, fibrous tissue with a fine layer of fluid between them, covers and cushions the heart and reduces the friction that would otherwise occur with continual beats. Sometimes this covering becomes inflamed from infection by viruses, bacteria, or fungi; from trauma that bruises the heart; as a part of autoimmune inflammatory disorders such as systemic lupus erythematosus, rheumatoid arthritis, or mixed connective tissue diseases; from cancer; or from the toxic insult to the tissues brought on by radiation treatments, after heart attack, after heart surgery, or from certain medications (notably minoxidil and the penicillins). Just as it does in arthritic joints or tendons, the inflammatory process causes pain in the pericardial tissues. However, unlike a painful shoulder you can immobilize to reduce pain, a painful pericardium must sustain the constant irritation of the heart beating. With each beat, the inflamed pericardium is irritated and hurts. Lying down, the heart settles with the effect of gravity and places greater traction on the inflamed tissues, aggravating the pain. Sitting up and leaning slightly forward often relieves the pain by suspending the heart in the middle of the pericardial sack.

The most common cause of pericarditis is also the most innocuous—simple viral infection of the pericardium following an upper respiratory infection, after chickenpox or mumps, or during a bout of influenza. Other more serious pericardial infections also occur, among them: Lyme disease and tuberculosis (TB; once quite rare, but because of increasing rates of TB, becoming more prevalent).

What you can do If the pericardial symptoms follow a cold, flu, or other viral infection, call your doctor. If pain is very mild, treatment (adults only) with aspirin every 4 hours, or ibuprofen every 6 to 8 hours, may help.

When to call the doctor Any time chest pain is present, particularly if associated with cough or shortness of breath, you should consult your doctor.

Treatment Once pericarditis is diagnosed, if aspirin or ibuprofen do not relieve the inflammation, stronger anti-inflammatory medications, such as indomethacin or corticosteroids, are indicated. Severe cases may require hospitalization for intravenous administration of medication, removal of excess fluid that collects between the leaves of pericardial tissue, and, rarely, surgery.

Prognosis Excellent in uncomplicated pericardial inflammation. Cases may not respond as readily if they are caused by underlying autoimmune disorders, cancer, or radiation treatments, or if they follow a myocardial infarction.

❖ MYOCARDITIS

Symptoms *(What you may experience)* Rapid heart beat (commonly); easy fatigability (commonly); breathlessness or shortness of breath with activity (often).

Signs and laboratory findings *(What the doctor looks for)* Ventricular gallop (a heartbeat heard through the stethoscope that sounds like galloping horses); electrical pattern changes on the ECG; heart enlargement and reduced heart muscle pumping power shown on echocardiogram; rise in antibodies (immune defense products) against certain viruses (if the cause is viral) shown on blood tests.

What is it? The heart muscle (myocardium) sometimes becomes inflamed and damaged by infection with viruses (less commonly, bacteria or parasites) or by toxicity from certain medications or illegal drugs. Although the condition itself is rare, when it occurs, it often follows a viral upper respiratory infection, with Coxsackievirus thought to be the most common viral cause. Other infectious causes of myocarditis include: rickettsial bacteria that cause Rocky Mountain spotted fever and parasites that cause toxoplasmosis and trichinosis.

The disorder frequently complicates the health of AIDS victims (see page 858). Noninfectious causes of myocarditis include toxins, such as that produced by diphtheria bacteria, radiation treatments, and drugs, especially cocaine. Lithium (for manic-depressive disorder) and chloroquine (an antimalarial drug) may also damage the myocardium.

Symptoms of myocarditis occur when infection or inflammation attack the heart muscle. When the muscle becomes weak, it cannot pump out the full volume of blood with each contraction, causing weakness and fatigue. As the muscle weakens, the pressure rises in the heart cavity, causing a backup of blood and dilation of the heart. The muscle is strained further by progressive dilation and back pressure.

When to call the doctor At the first appearance of symptoms suggesting myocarditis, call your doctor.

Treatment In rare cases where the cause is infectious, specific antibiotic therapy to eradicate the bacterial invader must come first. Viral etiologies are not usually treatable. Some doctors feel it necessary to treat severe inflammation with corticosteroid medication, although the value of this therapy is not clearly established. Treating the underlying heart failure may require specific medication to improve the force of the heart's pumping, suppress abnormal rhythms, or reduce excess fluid.

Prognosis Depends on the cause: It is very good for spontaneous recovery in many cases, although in patients who develop progressive heart failure, the outlook for recovery is much less positive. The prognosis is not good for myocarditis induced by the medication doxorubicin (Adriamycin) or associated with AIDS.

Disorders of Heart Rate and Rhythm

To function properly, your heart must beat with a steady, continuous, and effective rhythm. It must be able to adjust its rate of beating, minute by minute, to meet the changing demands of going from rest to intense exercise. The mechanism that ensures this constancy and adaptability—an

THE HEART'S OWN PACEMAKER

To enable it to contract in an orderly rhythmic fashion and to pump blood effectively to the lungs and the body, nature has endowed the heart with an electrical system that coordinates the transmission of contraction signals. The central command post—the pacemaker—lies in a cluster of specialized nerve cells in the wall of the upper-right heart chamber. This nerve cluster—called the sinoatrial (or SA) node—generates the electrical impulses that control how quickly the heart beats. At rest, the SA node sends out contraction signals at an average rate of about once a second—or about 60 to 80 times each minute. The pacemaker can sense the need to increase the heart rate in response to fever or other metabolic changes or when the demands of exercise require more oxygen. Electrical impulses generated in the pacemaker move out along bundles of nerve fibers, first in the upper chambers and then to another nerve cluster—the atrioventricular (AV) node—located between the upper and lower heart chambers. This nerve center quickly passes the signal on to the pumping chambers in a sequential manner resulting in a wringing contraction of the heart from tip to top to squeeze the blood from the heart effectively. ∎

internal electrical signaling system spearheaded by a natural pacemaker, the atrial node—can malfunction, resulting in rhythm abnormalities (arrhythmias) (see Sudden Cardiac Death, page 811). The heart may beat too fast (tachycardia), too slowly (bradycardia), ineffectively (fibrillation or flutter), or signals may fail to be conducted properly (heart block).

Rhythm abnormalities can arise from a variety of causes: aging; damage to the heart muscle (heart attack); hormonal alterations (particularly thyroid disorders); or external causes, such as food, alcohol, tobacco, caffeine, and certain medications (both over-the-counter and prescription).

❖ ABNORMAL HEART RHYTHMS

Symptoms *(What you may experience)* Chest sensation of heart racing, fluttering, skipping (palpitations); light-headedness, dizziness (occasionally); fainting (occasionally).

Signs and laboratory findings *(What the doctor looks for)* Irregular pulse or heartbeat heard through the stethoscope; abnormal conduction patterns demonstrated on ECG or by Holter monitor scan.

What is it? Disruption of the heart's normal pacing mechanism can disturb the pattern of impulses stimulating the upper chambers of the heart (the atria) or the lower pumping chambers (the ventricles). Such a disruption interferes with effective contraction, causing symptoms that range from none at all, to dizziness and fainting, to sensations of fluttering in the chest or throat, to sudden death. Ineffective contraction of the ventricles, because of their crucial role in pumping blood throughout the body, poses a far greater threat than ineffective contraction of the atria.

Rhythm disturbances fall into three broad categories: tachycardias (racing beat), bradycardias (sluggish beat), and palpitations (skips, flips, and flutters).

Tachycardia Rapid beating of the heart, at a rate greater than 100 beats per minute, can occur as a normal consequence of exercise, heightened emotion, pain, or fever. It can also accompany certain serious disorders, such a thyrotoxicosis (extreme elevation of thyroid hormone). Tachycardia can be a side effect of some medications, or it can occur as an appropriate response in anemia or shock (cardiovascular collapse and loss of blood pressure). Beating too quickly (usually rates greater than 150 beats per minute) prevents adequate filling of the heart chamber. The smaller volume of blood ejected with each beat can impair blood flow to the brain, bringing on dizziness, light-headedness, and fainting.

Occasionally, episodes of tachycardia lasting several hours occur in the upper chambers, with the heart rate reaching 140 to 240 beats per minute. Because these episodes usually begin and end without warning, they have been dubbed paroxysmal atrial tachycardias, or PATs. A rate this rapid can sometimes cause breathlessness or chest discomfort, but quite often it produces no symptoms at all beyond the awareness of a quick heart beat—which some people have described as feeling a whirlwind inside the chest.

Bradycardia Bradycardia is defined as a heartbeat of less than 60 times per minute. When the heart beats too slowly (fewer than 30 to 40 times per minute), lack of sufficient blood flow to the brain can cause weakness, confusion, and episodes of fainting, particularly in seniors or in people with coronary artery disease. Do not confuse this kind of abnormal sluggish beating with the exceptionally slow (50 to 60 beats per minute), but perfectly normal, resting heart rate that many endurance athletes develop. And be aware that certain medications—most notably the beta blockers used to treat such diverse problems as hypertension, coronary artery disease, and migraine headache—may slow the heart rate, causing the same symptoms as bradycardia from other causes, and may signal the need to reduce the dosage of the medication.

Palpitations (Skips, flips, and flutters)

Extra contractions of the atrial chambers occur when, much like a tic or spasm, one area of the heart short circuits and fires a signal before the scheduled signal to contract. The extra or early signal causes the heart to beat prematurely—a condition called premature atrial contraction (PAC). Some people feel this extra or premature beat as a skip or flip of the heart. This rhythm disturbance occurs in normal healthy hearts and should rarely cause concern. Fluttering of the atrial chambers (atrial flutter) occurs when a regularly spaced electrical signal fires rapidly, causing the upper chamber to contract rapidly (usually 300 times per minute), bringing about a tickling sensation in the throat or chest or shortness of breath and dizziness. The atrioventricular node may block some of these extra beats so that the ventricles continue to pump at a fraction of the atrial rate. For example, if the atria are beating at 300 times per minute, the ventricles may beat at 150 times per minute (called 2:1 block) or 100 beats per minute (3:1 block).

The most common of all rhythm disturbances, however—a condition called atrial fibrillation—can be more threatening. In atrial fibrillation, the upper chambers' electrical signals are totally uncoordinated, resulting in ineffective quivering contractions 400 to even 600 times per minute. The pumping chambers cannot keep up with the rapid beating of the upper chambers and respond with irregularly spaced heart-

beats 80 to 180 times per minute. It occurs in association with a variety of disorders: inflammation of the covering of the heart (pericarditis); injury to the chest; asthma or emphysema (particularly with the use of medications to dilate the breathing passages, such as theophylline); or any cause that raises atrial pressure or causes atrial dilation.

The greatest danger of atrial fibrillation comes from pooling of blood in the upper chambers, which can lead to the formation of small clots. These clots—called emboli—can pass into the bloodstream, travel into small arteries (arterioles) and lodge there, blocking blood flow beyond. In the brain, an embolus can cause a stroke; in the eyes, blindness. The potential seriousness of these consequences—especially among seniors—makes atrial fibrillation a more serious arrhythmia than flutter. The stroke risk is higher among seniors.

When misfiring in the conduction system affects contraction of the lower pumping chambers, a premature ventricular contraction (PVC) results. Many people experience an occasional PVC, a skip or sensation often described as the heart "turning over." In most instances, these isolated PVCs are no cause for alarm. Three or more in a row, however, can cause breathlessness.

Sustained or continuous runs—called ventricular tachycardia—can cause chest discomfort or fainting. With this rhythm disturbance comes an increased risk of developing the most serious arrhythmia of all—the life-threatening arrhythmia called ventricular fibrillation—in which the pumping chamber muscles quiver rapidly but ineffectively in an uncoordinated manner. Occurrence of ventricular tachycardia demands a thorough medical evaluation, whereas ventricular fibrillation is always a medical emergency.

What you can do To slow a racing heart caused by rhythm disturbances in the atria, a few simple measures can sometimes prove effective: pressing on the carotid artery (the major artery to the brain in the neck); coughing; holding the breath; placing the head between the knees; and performing the Valsalva maneuver—taking in a big breath, holding it, and while doing so, bearing down as if to have a bowel movement.

There are no self-care remedies for bradycardia.

Sometimes, fluttering, racing, or palpitations can be made worse by stimulants such as caffeine in coffee or cola drinks, decongestant cold remedies (pseudoephedrine and phenylpropanolamine), or alcohol. Avoiding such substances may help reduce their occurrence.

When to call the doctor A rapid rate causing symptoms that will not stop with the simple remedies outlined above should prompt a visit to the doctor for medical therapy to stop it. Severe breathlessness or fainting demand immediate emergency treatment.

A sluggish heart rate that causes symptoms should prompt a visit to the doctor for evaluation.

Palpitations that occur in repeated runs or that lead to breathlessness, lightheadedness, or loss of consciousness should prompt an emergency visit to a doctor or hospital.

Treatment Daily medications—commonly beta blockers, such as propranolol—may sometimes prove necessary to control tachycardias over the long term.

To break atrial fibrillation, electrical cardioversion—a mild electric shock administered to the heart—reorganizes its electrical patterns and restores normal beating. If cardioversion fails to normalize the rhythm, the heightened risk for stroke (especially in seniors) may require blood-thinning medications, such as warfarin, to prevent clots from forming; medications, such as verapamil, will slow contraction of the pumping chambers, allowing the left ventricle to fill with blood and improve its effectiveness. Most causes of atrial tachycardia can be cured with ablation therapy. This is a form of electrical treatment applied with thin electrical wires placed in the heart to locate and eliminate the rhythm disturbance site.

Sustained ventricular tachycardia demands immediate therapy to suppress the rhythm. Failure to do so puts the person at risk for the onset of the potentially lethal arrhythmia, ventricular fibrillation. The condition requires immediate emergency measures to stabilize the aberrant signals—primarily, the administration of potent antiarrhythmic medications, such as lidocaine. Many antiarrhythmics were formerly used on a daily basis to stabilize the heart, but recent studies have shown that reliance on chemical treatment may worsen the situation.

The type of antiarrhymic a doctor prescribes depends on the cause of the irregular heartbeat and the individual's reaction to the medication. Some medications slow the heart rate; others speed it up; while still others help control abnormal rhythms. People taking antiarrhymics, often used in combination, must be carefully monitored, because in some cases the medications may make rhythm disorders worse. The following list gives a few examples of the different types of antiarrhythmic medications.

- Digitalis slows electrical transmission through the atrioventricular (AV) node, helping to maintain a normal heart rate in persons with atrial fibrillation.

- Beta blockers and calcium channel blockers (verapamil) also slow conduction of rapid atrial beats through the AV node, thereby slowing the ventricular heart rate.

- Adenosine is given intravenously to treat rapid heartbeats originating in the atria or AV node.

WHAT IS HEART BLOCK?

The coordinated beating of the heart depends on the transmission of electrical signals through specialized nerve fiber bundles that course through the walls of the heart chambers. Sometimes, scarring from a previous heart attack, aging, abnormalities in the level of blood minerals (chiefly potassium, sodium, calcium, and magnesium), or certain medications impede or even block the transmission of the pacing signals. A block may cause no obvious symptoms, but an electrocardiogram tracing will demonstrate the delayed signal. Partial blocks usually go undetected, unless an electrocardiogram reveals them. The chief danger of partial blocks is that they may go undetected and progress to full blocks. These complete heart blocks (also called third-degree heart blocks) result when no electrical signals from the natural pacemaker reach the pumping chambers. When this occurs, a backup "emergency" pacing system takes over to signal the heart muscle to contract; however, it does so at a very slow rate, usually fewer than 45 times per minute. Although some people may remain unaware of this slow rate, others perceive symptoms, such as weakness, shortness of breath, or sudden episodes of fainting. Doctors will usually recommend placement of an artificial pacemaker in people who develop complete heart block. (For more information, see Artificial Pacemakers, page 831). ■

ARTIFICIAL PACEMAKERS

The job of a pacemaker is to sustain the beat of a sluggish heart. Pacemakers were first made available in the 1950s, and since then they have allowed at least 2 million people who would otherwise be disabled to pursue normal lives.

Artificial pacemakers are small, battery-powered units that produce electrical impulses when inserted into the chest. A pacemaker usually has two leads. These are attached to the heart so that electrical impulses flow from the wires to the atrium and ventricle, stimulating the heart so that it contracts. Thus, the artificial pacemaker takes the place of the sluggish, natural pacemaker in the heart, helping the heart to work properly once again.

Insertion of a pacemaker is a relatively minor surgical procedure. The patient is given local anesthesia, and the pacemaker is inserted just beneath the chest skin. Whenever the battery wears down (usually after more than 10 years), the unit is changed in a similar manner.

If you have an artificial pacemaker, you should make sure that you write down the year it was inserted and the model that was inserted. Keep this information in a file with your important documents. Most artificial pacemakers have a life span of up to 15 years—which means you may have plenty of time to forget important information, such as the exact date your pacemaker was inserted. In addition, as with any electronic device, your pacemaker may develop problems over the years. If problems occur with your pacemaker, you'll want to have all the information you need at your fingertips.

An artificial pacemaker offers a new lease on life, but this opportunity should not be taken for granted. Routine follow-up with your cardiologist to assess the pacemaker's function is mandatory. You should become aware of symptoms that may indicate that a pacemaker is failing. These include sudden bloating or swelling in your ankles or legs, heart palpitations, difficulty breathing, dizziness, or fainting. If you notice any of these symptoms, you should call your doctor immediately. ■

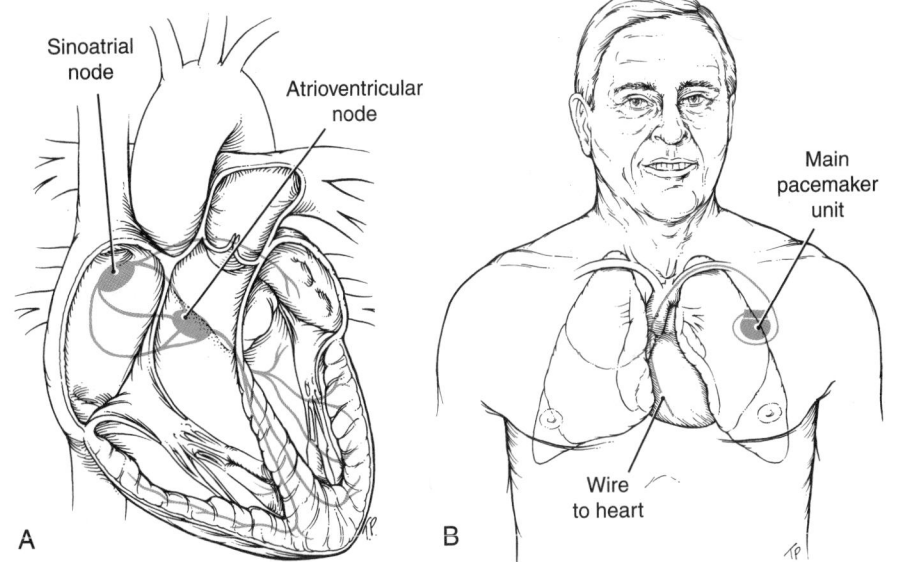

(A) Native pacemaker. The sinoatrial and atrioventricular nodes of the body's nervous system initiate and coordinate the electrical signals that make the heart's chambers contract. Nerve fibers extend from the nodes to other parts of the heart. (B) Artificial pacemaker. If signals are not transmitted properly, a battery-powered artificial pacemaker may help. The device generates and senses electrical signals by means of wires attached to the heart.

Sinoatrial node

Atrioventricular node

Main pacemaker unit

Wire to heart

A

B

- Atropine, which affects nervous system control of the heartbeat, may be used to temporarily speed up a slow heart rate.

- Medications that stabilize heart rhythm by directly affecting the electrical conduction system include: quinidine, procainamide, disopyramide, lidocaine, phenytoin, mexiletine, tocainide, amiodarone (a potent medication with a variety of actions plus serious side effects). The effectiveness of this entire group of medications is being reexamined. Increasingly, cardiologists are controlling life-threatening ventricular arrhythmias with a device called an automatic internal cardioverter defibrillator (AICD). A battery-driven device, similar to a pacemaker, the implanted defibrillator is programmed to stop an arrhythmia with a low-energy shock.

Basically, an AICD consists of a pulse generator (larger than a pacemaker) implanted beneath the skin and muscle of the abdomen or chest. Electrodes that sense the heartbeat and deliver a shock to the heart are inserted through veins to the inside of the heart. The devices vary in sophistication and are constantly being improved. Some internal defibrillators also act as pacemakers, increasing a slow heart rate, as well as keeping a record of any shocks delivered—important information for the doctor.

Prognosis In most cases, rhythm disturbances are mild, carrying a good prognosis for resolution with simple treatments. If the rhythm disturbances produce significant symptoms or degenerate into life-threatening rhythms (such as ventricular tachycardia) the prognosis is poorer.

❖ SICK SINUS SYNDROME

Symptoms *(What you may experience)* Often, no symptoms. In some cases: racing heartbeat, fluttering sensation, fainting, or "sinking" spells; dizziness; confusion; chest pain.

Arterial tree. The long aorta originates from the heart and then curves downward through the chest and abdomen. Many blood vessels originate from parts of the aorta, eventually branching into smaller segments.

Ascending aorta

Heart

Descending aorta

Signs and laboratory findings *(What the doctor looks for)* Abnormal conduction rhythms shown on ECG; rhythm disturbances shown on Holter monitor record that coincide with symptoms (see Evaluating the Heart and Blood Vessels, page 806).

What is it The sinoatrial (SA) node (sometimes called the sinus node) is a bundle of specialized nerve fibers that functions as the heart's primary pacemaker, coordinating its timing and rhythmic contractions. Damage to this node—common in seniors—impairs its function. The damage can be caused by scarring (from a previous heart attack), by sclerosis due to aging, or by infiltration of inflammatory deposits in the diseases sarcoidosis and amyloidosis (see Chapter 18).

When the SA node fails to function properly, another area becomes the pacemaker, so that the heart's contractions are usually slow. Disease of the SA node is often associated with other rhythm disturbances. When contractions are too fast (tachycardia), sick sinus syndrome causes a racing heartbeat and palpitations. When contractions are too slow (bradycardia) the flow of blood to the brain and body is reduced; sluggish circulation to the brain produces confusion, momentary loss of consciousness, dizziness, or fainting. In sick sinus syndrome, the heart rhythm often switches back and forth between too fast and too slow.

When to call the doctor Call your doctor if

- You experience changes in heart rhythm such as fluttering, racing, or a skipping sensation in your chest
- Racing or fluttering leaves you breathless or faint
- You black out or have "sinking" spells

Treatment The treatment for sick sinus syndrome is implantation of an artificial pacemaker (see page 831). Treatment with the medication theophylline may help people who experience bradycardia. Medications that slow the heart (propranolol or digitalis) may worsen the periods of bradycardia and should be avoided unless an artificial pacemaker is in place.

Prognosis Excellent since the advent of the artificial pacemaker.

Disorders of the Peripheral Arteries and Veins

Originating and terminating with the heart, the vascular tree provides an interlacing thoroughfare for metabolic commerce, connecting all parts of the body. Typical disorders in this system disrupt that continuous flow: blood clots, blockage of the channels by hard plaque or structural abnormalities, weakness or rupture of the vessel wall, or damage to the venous valves.

❖ THROMBOPHLEBITIS OF SUPERFICIAL VEINS (INFLAMED BLOOD CLOT)

Symptoms *(What you may experience)* Redness, firm swelling, tenderness, and warmth along a vein (usually of the leg and less commonly the arm).

Signs and laboratory findings *(What the doctor looks for)* No specific signs beyond the listed symptoms.

What is it? The name comes from a combination of *thrombus*, meaning blood clot, and *phlebitis*, meaning inflammatory or infectious process of a vein. Inflammation of a vein may occur for a variety of reasons, but the most common cause is trauma. Injury occurs in the hospital from intravenous (IV) catheters that pierce the vein wall and from solutions and medications that may irritate the blood vessel. The injury can also come from outside, such as a blow that compresses the vein. This kind of trauma might occur in a car accident, or even from something as simple as running into the corner of a table or counter. Trauma to the lining of the vein triggers a local healing and repair response. The process sets up a mild degree of inflammation, which leads to discomfort, local fever or warmth along the course of the vein, redness from increased blood flow, and firm swelling. A blood clot often forms in the inflamed or crushed segment of the vein.

Inflammation in surface veins—such as those used to place intravenous lines in the arm or to draw blood—produces more discomfort than risk. In contrast to blood clots in deeper, larger veins, surface vein clots rarely break loose (become emboli) and travel to lodge in the lung. Occasionally, however, thrombophlebitis arises not simply from an exaggerated healing response, but also from infection in the vein—a condition that can prove dangerous if not recognized and treated with antibiotics. The usual bacterial culprit is *Staphylococcus*, a common bacterium found in the skin.

Sometimes, the inflammation occurs without obvious reason. Such "spontaneous" thrombophlebitis may occur in the leg veins of pregnant and recently pregnant women, in people with varicose veins, and occasionally as a first indication of unrecognized cancer in the abdominal cavity (particularly the pancreas).

What you can do If the inflammation and discomfort are minor, elevate the affected part and apply warm moist packs to it for 15 to 20 minutes at a time intermittently throughout the day. Unlike deep venous thrombosis, people with superficial thrombophlebitis should remain active (that is, continue to walk). You may take an enteric-coated (a coating that prevents the medicine from being released until the pill reaches the intestines) or buffered aspirin unless you are allergic to it or are taking another blood-thinning medication.

When to call the doctor If the condition persists longer than a day or two or if the symptoms are severe or worsening, see your doctor as soon as possible. See a doctor right away if the phlebitis involves a leg vein and the inflammation arises very high in the thigh, near the groin. If you develop shortness of breath, confusion, or fever, see your doctor immediately or seek emergency treatment.

Treatment Simple treatment measures often suffice. For more extensive thrombophlebitis, resolving the problem may require potent blood-thinning medications and hospitalization. Therapy using warfarin (Coumadin), the most frequently used blood-thinning medication, involves stepwise increases in dose individualized to each person. Frequent blood test are used to assess response—easily done on an outpatient basis. This is *rarely* required, however.

In cases of infection of the vein, treatment with antibiotics may not totally eradicate the problem; control of the infection may require surgical removal of the inflamed segment of vein.

Prognosis Excellent in most cases unless a deep vein clot, embolus, or infection complicates the picture. Surgical removal may be required in some severe cases, or when the condition recurs in the same vein.

❖ DEEP VEIN THROMBOSIS (BLOOD CLOT)

Symptoms *(What you may experience)* In as many as 50 percent of cases, no symptoms at all; and in the other 50 percent of cases, the symptoms vary. Symptoms of deep vein thrombosis (DVT) may include a dull, aching tightness in the calf, especially with walking, and occasionally true pain.

Signs and laboratory findings *(What the doctor looks for)* Mild increase in the measured size of the calf; dilation and prominence of the surrounding visible leg veins; low-grade fever and increased heart rate (occasionally); tenderness of the larger thigh veins (sometimes). Diagnosis is confirmed by x-ray using radiopaque dye or by Doppler ultrasound. The Doppler test detects differences in echoes produced by smoothly flowing blood and the turbulence created around a clot in the stream.

What is it? Formation of blood clots in veins deep within the pelvis or legs, often following inactivity due to surgery, stroke, or a major accident. About 80 percent of the time, the clot forms in the deep veins of the calf. It *can* occur in the veins of the thigh or pelvis, and (rarely) in the veins of the shoulder or neck. In most cases, the cause is inactivity. Blood flow in the veins (which have no muscular walls of their own) depends on the contraction of nearby muscle groups (leg, calf, and pelvic muscle). With extended periods of bed rest, the blood will start to pool, which promotes clot formation. For this reason, it is important when forced to full bed rest to move the legs and feet and arms, fill up the lungs with air, breathe deeply, cough, and stretch. When a bedridden person is unconscious, the caregiver must do these things for the person, often by providing antiembolism stockings or a blood thinner to prevent clothing.

Others at risk for blood clots are people with cancer—especially those with cancer of the prostate, pancreas, ovary, or breast—and people with certain rare clotting disorders, called hypercoagulability syndromes.

Most other cases of deep vein clots occur in otherwise healthy women. The use of oral contraceptives increases the tendency to form blood clots in some women; the risk is higher among women over the age of 30 who smoke, or those who have had a history of previous blood clots. Complications from deep vein thrombosis arise either because the clot breaks loose and lodges in a blood vessel in the lung (pulmonary embolus) or because the clot damages the valves in the vein, causing chronic venous stasis.

What you can do If you take birth control pills and smoke, you should stop smoking. To help prevent clots, avoid long periods of immobilization during car trips or air flights. Get out of the car or your plane seat and walk around for a few minutes every hour or so. Elevate your legs above your heart level whenever possible and wear support hose or knee-high support socks.

When to call the doctor Because a deep vein clot may not cause symptoms, the first sign may be related to the clot's having broken loose to travel to the lung (see Pulmonary Embolus, page 760). Emergency treatment is essential if you have a condition that puts you at risk for thrombophlebitis and develop the symptoms of a pulmonary embolus or an embolus elsewhere.

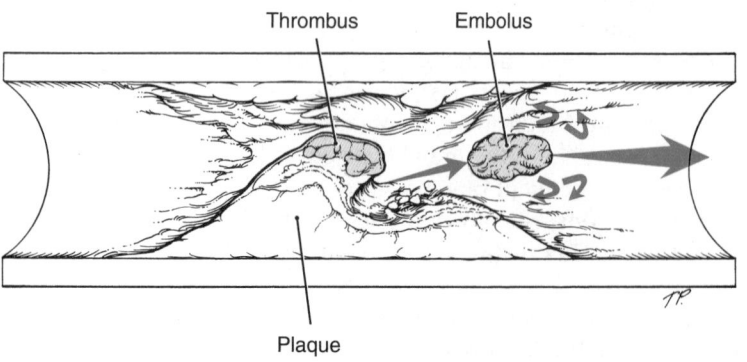

A thrombus (blood clot) can form inside or near a plaque. If part of the plaque or thrombus breaks away from the wall of the artery, it becomes an embolus traveling through the bloodstream. It can then obstruct the blood flow if it becomes lodged at another location such as the brain or heart.

Thrombus   Embolus

Plaque

Treatment The cornerstone of therapy is thinning the blood. This is done to prevent the clot from extending to involve more veins. Frequently, treatment will begin in the hospital. In a week to 10 days, the newly formed clot will adhere firmly to the wall, and there is less risk of the clot fragmenting. Walking will now be encouraged—but not sitting, which puts pressure on the veins of the pelvis and knees, or prolonged standing, which may allow blood to pool in the lower legs.

During this time, blood is thinned with intravenous administration of heparin, an anticoagulant used to prevent the formation of new clots. After heparin is initiated, the doctor will include warfarin, a blood-thinning medication taken orally, so that therapy can continue at home for several months or more. Many doctors feel that thrombolytic therapy with urokinase or streptokinase is the treatment of choice in massive and submassive pulmonary embolism. These agents disintegrate the clot already formed, which may improve blood flow and oxygenation in those with a large blood clot burden.

Prognosis In the absence of complications, the prognosis is excellent for a return to normal activity within a month or two. In most cases, long-term warfarin therapy is used to avoid a recurrence.

❖ VARICOSE VEINS

Symptoms *(What you may experience)* Heaviness or aching fatigue in the legs; itching scaliness of the skin above the ankles. Often, no specific symptoms.

Signs and laboratory findings *(What the doctor looks for)* Dilated twisting blue or purple veins in the legs; spotty brownish discoloration of the skin of the lower leg and ankle; thinning of the skin above the ankle, which may lead to bleeding; non-working valves in the veins shown on Doppler ultrasound exam.

What is it? Blood flowing through the leg veins must in many cases defy gravity on its return journey to the heart. To force the blood along, the veins are equipped with one-way valves that allow the blood to flow past, then close tightly to prevent backward flow. Some people have an inherited tendency for valves to become incompetent over time, which allows the blood in the vein to fall back; backward flow dilates the vein, putting greater pressure on the valve below. It, too, may fail, and the cycle progresses until none of the valves in the segment function well. Veins near the surface of the skin have little tissue to support them; consequently, these veins become dilated and develop varicosities.

Factors that increase pressure in the lower legs—weight gain, pregnancy, occupations requiring prolonged standing or heavy lifting—often contribute to this problem. Up to 15 percent of adults develop varicose leg veins, but the disorder occurs in pregnant women more than in any other group.

Many people simply object to the unsightly appearance of varicose veins. But, cosmetic considerations aside, varicose veins do increase the risk of thrombophlebitis or deep vein thrombosis.

What you can do Wear support stockings to support the veins if you have a family history of deep vein thrombosis, if you have gained substantial weight (whether from pregnancy or not), or if your work requires prolonged standing or heavy lifting. Good-quality support hose for both men and women are available in many colors. Whenever possible, sit with your legs elevated above your heart level. If you are overweight, safely reduce toward your ideal body weight to help relieve pressure on your veins. Regular exercise, such as walking or swimming, is also beneficial.

When to call the doctor Persistent pain, redness, warmth, or swelling should prompt a visit to your doctor. Shortness of breath or other symptoms suggesting pulmonary embolism require immediate medical attention.

Treatment Surgical treatment of larger varicose veins, called vein stripping, involves making one or more incisions in the leg along the course of the affected vein. The vein is tied with a suture to prevent blood flow through it, or tied off in multiple places and clipped to remove the segment of vein between the ties. Interruption of these veins still leaves other, deeper veins intact to accommodate blood flow. Smaller veins can be treated by sclerosis; in this procedure, an irritating solution is injected into the vein.

This causes scarring inside, which effectively seals the vein and prevents it from enlarging.

Prognosis Good with proper self-care to prevent progression of the condition. Good with corrective surgery. The disorder is chronic, however, and usually does not resolve completely—even with treatment.

❖ ATHEROSCLEROSIS OF THE AORTA AND ARTERIES OF THE LEGS

Symptoms *(What you may experience)* Cramping pain in one or both calves, thighs, or buttocks, especially when walking; sense of tiredness or fatigue in the legs, especially with walking; impotence in men (often).

Signs and laboratory findings *(What the doctor looks for)* Weak or absent pulses in the femoral arteries (in the groin, leading to the legs) as well as in the popliteal artery (behind the knee) and the foot arteries; aortic or femoral bruits (whooshing sounds heard through the stethoscope as blood flows through the partially blocked artery); loss of hair on lower legs and feet; reduced blood pressure in the legs compared to the arms; demonstration of blockages on Doppler ultrasound test (measures differences in the sound created by turbulence as blood flows by the blockages); demonstration of blockages on x-ray dye or magnetic resonance angiography studies of the aorta and its branches.

What is it? The aorta—the main artery leading away from the heart—transports blood to the body. From the left ventricle, it courses through the chest and down the center of the abdomen, where it divides into two main branches, the left and right iliac arteries. These further divide into the femoral arteries and others that supply the legs. When atherosclerotic plaque (see Understanding Atherosclerosis, page 790) forms in the aorta, the resulting blockages limit blood flow to the lower part of the body. The muscles of the legs need oxygen and nutrients to operate, especially during exercise. Diminished flow of blood, oxygen, and nutrients to the tissues causes the muscles to turn away from normal metabolic paths that provide energy, to others that operate in conditions of low oxygen. The buildup of waste products from this alternative energy source causes the chief symptom associated with blockages in the leg arteries—claudication, a cramping pain that appears (usually in the calves) with exercise and disappears with rest. The pain may also be felt higher in the leg, in the thigh, or even as high as the buttock. More severe blockages may result in pain in the feet at rest or in the development of skin sores or gangrene (death of tissue).

Reduced blood flow through the aorta can also impair the blood supply to areas fed by branches from it, such as the male reproductive system, resulting in erection difficulties and impotence.

What you can do Lifestyle changes can favorably influence this disorder. Essentially, whether atherosclerosis occurs in the coronary blood vessels or in peripheral arteries, the disease process is the same. Therefore, it's important to treat all cardiovascular disease risk factors: Lower blood pressure if elevated and control diabetes if necessary; limit dietary cholesterol and saturated fat, found mainly in meat and dairy products (see Lifestyle Changes for a Healthy Heart, page 797). Smoking promotes formation of atherosclerotic plaque, and formation of clots on plaque. So, if you smoke, stop (see Chapter 4 for help kicking the habit). Daily walking for a fixed time period (5 minutes, 15 minutes) until calf cramping occurs may help improve blood flow by encouraging development of collateral blood channels around the blocked areas in the leg arteries.

When to call the doctor Abrupt worsening of the pain of cramping, marked reduction in length of walking time until the cramping begins, development of pain at rest, impotence, or sores on the skin from poor circulation require a visit to the doctor right away.

Treatment If the conservative measures of walking and quitting smoking do not give sufficient relief of symptoms, you might get help from medications such as aspirin or pentoxifylline, which allow the blood to flow more easily through narrowed arteries. When symptoms become severe, a vascular surgeon can remove the blocked area of the aorta, iliac, or femoral arteries and replace them with artificial "graft" segments.

Although replacement graft surgery was commonly done in the past, sometimes it is possible to simply remove the occluding plaque—a procedure called endarterectomy. The surgery is done by making an incision in the skin, then surgically opening the artery and scooping out the blockage. In addition, balloon angioplasty (see page 814) can be used to widen the narrowed areas inside the leg arteries. These procedures are not always as successful as the bypass graft method, but the risks are lower.

Prognosis Quite good. Successful removal of plaque or diseased arteries often gives dramatic and impressive elimination of symptoms and return of good circulation to the lower leg.

❖ ABDOMINAL AORTIC ANEURYSM

Symptoms *(What you may experience)* No symptoms in many cases; mild to severe pain in the middle abdomen or low back in 25 to 30 percent of cases.

Signs and laboratory findings *(What the doctor looks for)* Pulsating lump in the middle abdomen; demonstration of the aneurysm on x-ray or ultrasound exam.

What is it? The thick, muscular artery walls are designed to accommodate the higher pressure they must withstand. Occasionally, a weak area develops in the artery wall, allowing the pressure within the artery to push outward to create a bulge or ballooned area—an aneurysm. As the size of the bulge increases, the wall progressively thins until it can rupture, with catastrophic consequences. Aneurysms in the aorta occur most commonly as it runs through the chest (thoracic aortic aneurysm) (see page 838) or as it passes into the middle to low abdomen (abdominal aortic aneurysm). Atherosclerosis (hard plaque deposits) in the wall of the aorta commonly causes the weakness that leads to formation of an aneurysm, but a number of conditions present from birth (congenital) cause weakness or laxity of the muscular, fibrous, and elastic tissues in the arteries. The most common condition is Marfan syndrome (see page 822).

The danger of an aneurysm correlates with its size; a small, stable aneurysm (less than 5 cm wide) poses no immediate threat,

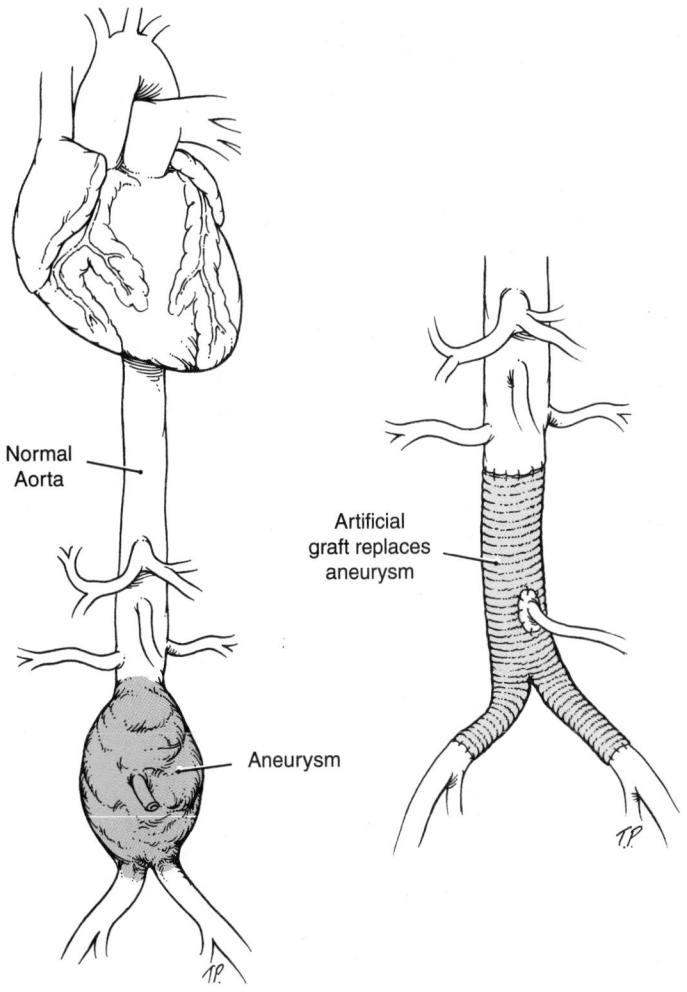

Normal Aorta

Artificial graft replaces aneurysm

Aneurysm

Weakness in the wall of the aorta can lead to a bulge or ballooned area (aneurysm) that can eventually rupture. Large aneurysms are more likely to burst than smaller ones. Surgery can be performed to replace the aneurysm with an artificial graft.

although it must be carefully watched, because it may increase in size. As it does, so does the chance of rupture—which can be sudden and catastrophic, and in many cases lethal, even before a person can reach the hospital or operating room. Unfortunately, aneurysms may cause no symptoms at all; most of them are discovered during physical examinations for other reasons. Pain is the cardinal symptom, but it may be inconsistent: intermittent or constant, mild or severe, or vague. This inconsistency makes diagnosis difficult.

Prevention Persons with hypertension or atherosclerosis elsewhere should be screened for an abdominal aneurysm on physical exam.

When to call the doctor At the first sign of unexplained abdominal pain, seek medical help. If you have a history of atherosclerosis in other areas (coronary artery disease, carotid artery blockage), make regular appointments to see your doctor for physical examinations.

Treatment Small aneurysms can be observed over time, until they become so large that rupture seems imminent. Then, surgery is performed to remove the ballooned segment of aorta and to replace it with an artificial segment of artery. Surgeons will usually recommend this kind of surgery, even in the absence of symptoms, if the aneurysm balloons to 5 to 6 cm in size. For people with symptoms, size is not a consideration; surgery is recommended for all aneurysms. New, noninvasive radiology techniques that provide support for the aorta are in development and may eliminate the need for invasive surgery in many cases.

Prognosis Fair to good. The death rate (mortality) of surgery for repair of abdominal aneurysms ranges from 1 percent at major medical centers up to 8 percent in smaller hospitals (meaning that 1 to 8 in 100 people will not survive surgery). The average risk is about 5 percent. The mortality rate for surgical repair of aneurysms in the chest cavity is considerably higher. However, the risk of ignoring any aortic aneurysm carries an even higher risk: fewer than 20 percent of people survive longer than 5 years without surgery—a result that compares with 60 percent of those treated surgically surviving longer than 5 years.

❖ THORACIC AORTIC ANEURYSM

Symptoms *(What you may experience)* Often, none; sometimes, pain behind the breast bone that goes through to the back. Sometimes: shortness of breath; hoarseness; a brassy cough; difficulty swallowing.

Signs and laboratory findings *(What the doctor looks for)* Aortic valve murmur (regurgitation) audible with a stethoscope; chest x-ray may be suggestive; special x-ray dye studies, CT or MRI scan of the aorta confirm the diagnosis and pinpoint the location.

What is it? Thoracic aneurysms are much less common than abdominal aortic aneurysms (see page 837). In the past, syphilis was a common cause, but today the most common cause is atherosclerosis. As the affected artery hardens with plaque, the pressure of the blood may split the wall, allowing a channel of blood to split the layers of the artery wall—a process called dissection. The outer layers, now thinned, bulge under the pressure of the blood and eventually may rupture.

Most thoracic aneurysms cause no symptoms and are discovered accidentally on chest x-rays taken for other reasons. When they do cause symptoms, the classic one is a sharp pain under the breast bone that seems to go through to the back and may also be felt in the neck. Bulging of the artery can put pressure on adjacent structures, such as the esophagus (making swallowing difficult) or the trachea (causing shortness of breath and cough).

Thoracic aneurysms occur most often in people with severe atherosclerosis and in people with Marfan syndrome, a genetic disorder that makes the artery wall weaker and more elastic. (See page 822 for more information.)

When to call the doctor If symptoms develop suggesting a thoracic aortic aneurysm, get medical evaluation immediately. The aneurysm is likely to worsen and rupture.

Treatment A small aneurysm causing no symptoms can be watched closely. Thoracic aortic dissections are usually treated medically initially. Surgery often can be avoided if the dissection begins beyond the left subclavian artery and the person becomes asymptomatic. If it progresses or is large when discovered, surgery is required to remove the bulging segment and replace it with an artificial aortic graft. If the aneurysm is close to the aortic valve, as it often is, the valve may have to be replaced. In some cases, it may also be necessary to reattach the coronary arteries (which depart from the aorta as it leaves the heart) with small bypass grafts.

Prognosis Surgery is somewhat risky—more so than the 3 to 5 percent mortality rate for the abdominal type. Prognosis depends on the size and location of the aneurysm, as well as the presence of complicating medical conditions, such as hypertension or atherosclerotic disease.

❖ COARCTATION OF THE AORTA

Symptoms *(What you may experience)* Usually none.

Signs and laboratory findings *(What the doctor looks for)* High blood pressure in the arms but not the legs; a harsh systolic murmur (abnormal whooshing sound of the heart when it contracts, heard through the stethoscope, loudest in the back); weak or absent femoral pulses (felt in the groin); enlarged left heart chamber demonstrated on ECG; constriction in the artery shown on Doppler ultrasound exam.

What is it? Branches of the aorta—the large artery that supplies blood to the entire body—go to the head, neck, and arms. The aorta itself makes a U-turn, going down through the chest to bring blood to the abdominal organs and to the lower part of the body. In some people, just after the artery makes this turn and sends off its branches to the arms, it narrows abruptly as though pinched by some unseen force; the pinch is termed a coarctation. Just as happens when a water hose is pinched, the pressure within the hose increases in front of the pinch and diminishes beyond it. Doctors can detect just this kind of pressure difference in people who have a coarctation of the aorta; the pressure will be higher than normal in the arms and lower in the legs. The pulse of the heartbeat arrives weaker and later than it should in the femoral arteries—the large branches of the aorta that feed the legs—because the constriction delays the flow of blood beyond it.

Coarctation, a condition present from birth, can become apparent in infancy if the constriction is severe, causing heart failure. But with a lesser degree of pinch, the defect may remain hidden and silent until later in life, when elevated blood pressure or a heart murmur bring it to the attention of a doctor. However, the lack of obvious symptoms does not mean that the disorder is harmless. The stress of the back pressure created by the narrowing causes a variety of problems: It drastically increases the work of the heart muscle, leading to hypertrophy (overgrowth) of the muscular pumping chamber; it places added stress on the aortic valve (which is often congenitally abnormal as well), leading to aortic valve leakage; and it puts a pressure burden on the wall of the aorta, increasing the risk of weakness, aneurysm, and catastrophic rupture of the aorta. People with unrecognized or untreated coarctation usually die from these kinds of complications before the age of 40.

When to call the doctor Because the disorder usually causes no symptoms, there are no special warning signs to prompt you to seek medical attention. However, if you developed high blood pressure at a young age and have never had the problem fully evaluated for possible causes, including coarctation, you should see a doctor now to have a complete examination.

Treatment The only treatment for this disorder is surgical removal of the pinched segment—a major surgical procedure that carries a mortality of 1 to 4 percent (meaning that 1 to 4 in 100 people will not survive surgery). The risks of the disease, however, far outweigh the surgical risk; therefore, most doctors will recommend surgical repair in all patients under the age of 20 and most patients under the age of 40. After the age of 50, the risk associated with surgery increases, and the chance of preventing complications from long-standing elevated pressure decreases. Recently, balloon angioplasty (see Balloon Dilation of Blockages, page 814) has shown some promise in opening the constriction and may replace open-heart surgery as the treatment of choice.

Prognosis Good if diagnosed and treated early. Poor if left untreated.

❖ PERIPHERAL VASCULAR DISEASE (POOR CIRCULATION)

Symptoms *(What you may experience)* Intermittent calf or foot cramping, especially with activity; aching heaviness during activity; dull, aching pain in the feet at night.

Signs and laboratory findings *(What the doctor looks for)* Weak or absent pedal (foot) pulses; cool, thin, and hairless skin on the lower leg and foot; calcium deposits in arteries of the lower leg visible on x-ray; pressure differences on Doppler ultrasound test (a pressure measure demonstrated by the change in sound of blood rushing through the arteries).

What is it? Atherosclerotic hardening of the arteries that supply blood to the lower legs and feet limits the flow of blood, which brings oxygen and nutrients to the tissues and removes waste products. (See page 807 for more information about atherosclerosis.) The distance a person with peripheral vascular disease (PVD) can walk before cramping begins provides a method of assessing severity. Those able to walk two city blocks or more (about 450 meters) have mild disability; those able to walk only one block, moderate disability; those unable to walk more than half a block, severe disability.

The risk of developing atherosclerotic PVD markedly increases among those who have diabetes or who smoke. The risk is still higher when these factors combine—for example, people with diabetes who smoke. Poorly controlled diabetes is accompanied by high levels of blood sugar, LDL cholesterol, insulin, and triglycerides (see Diabetes Mellitus and Syndrome X in Chapter 26: The Endocrine System for more information). These high levels promote a change in the cholesterol that favors its deposition in the artery wall. Because tobacco smoke also promotes this change, combining the two forces doubles the effect. The condition affects not just the arteries supplying the lower legs and feet, but the hands, fingers, eyes, kidneys, and reproductive organs (especially in men, often leading to impotence).

Persons with diabetes have special foot problems, because poor circulation to the tissues over time will impair the blood supply to nerves as well, producing numbness and loss of sensation. This is an especially dangerous problem in the feet, where trauma from daily wear and tear may go unnoticed because it does not hurt. Infection in a foot with poor circulation causes major problems in healing (see The Diabetic Foot and its Care, page 722, for more information).

What you can do If you smoke, stop immediately. Nothing you can do will help as much (see Chapter 4 for help in kicking the habit). Institute a program of regular walking of a defined distance within the limits of your leg symptoms to encourage the formation of new blood channels to bypass the blocked areas. Wear only well-fitted, supportive shoes, and inspect your feet daily for any visible signs of blistering or pressure. If you have diabetes, stick tightly to your prescribed dietary, medication, and exercise regimen; stick to it as strictly as possible to achieve the best possible control of your blood sugar and fats. Exercise great care in trimming your toenails or seek the aid of a podiatrist to do so safely; ingrown toenails or close trimming may invite infection.

When to call the doctor Development of cramping pain in the foot or calf—or a decrease in the distance you can walk before cramping begins—should prompt a visit to your doctor as soon as possible. Any form of skin break-down—blistering, friction rubs, puncture wound, or cuts, particularly on your feet—should prompt a visit to the doctor.

Treatment Low-dose aspirin therapy may help promote better circulation by preventing microscopic clot formation. Doctors usually recommend a low dose of enteric-coated aspirin daily, unless you are allergic to the medication. Just as in atherosclerotic blockage higher in the leg or aorta, some people may benefit from the medication pentoxifylline. These smaller arteries, unlike those higher in the leg and abdomen, are not amenable to surgical removal and grafting to restore circulation.

Prognosis Fair. Symptoms and circulation will stabilize or improve somewhat with proper care. But the disease will progress if damaging lifestyle habits are not changed.

❖ HYPOTENSION (LOW BLOOD PRESSURE)

Symptoms (*What you may experience*) Dizziness or near-fainting on standing from a crouched, lying, or seated position; fatigue.

Signs and laboratory findings (*What the doctor looks for*) No specific signs; a low blood pressure reading at rest (less than 90/50 mm Hg) or a drop in blood pressure (demonstrated with the blood pressure cuff) of greater than 20 mm Hg upon rising from a reclining or sitting position.

What is it? Hypotension (low blood pressure) afflicts far fewer people and is far less serious than its opposite condition, hypertension. It can develop as a temporary condition—for example, from dehydration due to excessive sweating during exercise or other loss of body salt or water. It sometimes occurs in young women and teens of both genders upon standing up from a reclining or stooped position. In orthostatic hypotension, as the condition is called, blood vessels in the legs fail to respond to the signal to constrict slightly to support the blood in them against the downward pull of gravity. When this happens, a sensation of "browning out" or near-fainting occurs upon rising from a crouch or getting up too quickly after lying down or sitting for a prolonged period.

A similar mechanism accounts for the drop in blood pressure and near-fainting that occur among seniors who take certain medications for hypertension (notably, beta blockers such as propranolol). These medications work by dilating the arteries and slowing the heartbeat; the down-side is that they also prevent sufficient constriction to offset the downward pull of gravity upon standing up and prevent an adequate increase in heart rate. Seniors can also have such symptoms.

Postural hypotension may also be caused by neurologic disorders that affect control of blood pressure by the autonomic nervous system. For example, the body may fail to secrete enough norepinephrine, an adrenal-gland hormone that constricts arteries to maintain blood pressure upon standing up. Two such disorders are idiopathic orthostatic hypotension and Shy-Drager syndrome. A weakened heart may also cause a decrease in blood pressure.

Some people have too little "prime in the pump" when they stand, and the heart may contract so vigorously that it triggers inappropriate signals to decrease heart rate and blood pressure. This is called vasodepressor syncope and may be due to acute or chronic volume deficiency. If chronic, it may be associated with the chronic fatigue syndrome.

If you know you have hypotension as an ongoing condition or as a side effect of medications you take for other conditions, always arise from a reclining position slowly, then sit with your legs dangling for a few moments before standing. Make certain you have support—a chair or table—nearby in case you become dizzy.

When you exercise, replenish needed salts (such as potassium and sodium) in addition to water. Many commercially available sports drinks provide these minerals.

When to call the doctor If you experience repeated near-fainting episodes, persistent dizziness upon standing, or an actual episode of loss of consciousness, see the doctor right away.

Treatment Except for the remedies outlined above in the self-care section, there are no specific therapies for hypotension. If you are already taking medication for blood pressure reduction, your doctor may recommend a change or reduction to avoid the excessive dilation of the leg vessels or heart rate that causes the drop.

Prognosis Hypotension in teens and young women usually improves on its own with age. Hypotension from temporary imbalance of mineral electrolytes readily responds to replenishment of fluids and salts. Hypotension caused by blood pressure medications may persist until the medication is changed.

❖ THROMBOANGIITIS OBLITERANS (BUERGER'S DISEASE)

Symptoms (*What you may experience*) Intermittent cramping in the palm of the hand or arch of the foot; numbness or pins-and-needles sensation in the hands or feet; pain in the hands or feet at rest; painful sores around the nail edges.

Signs and laboratory findings (*What the doctor looks for*) Pallor or coolness of the fingers, toes, or entire end of the foot; intense redness of the feet when hanging down; weak or absent pulses in the feet and wrists.

What is it? Thromboangiitis obliterans (Buerger's Disease) occurs primarily among men aged 20 to 40 who smoke; women account for only 5 percent of people with Buerger's disease. This disorder blocks the arteries—not because of hard plaque buildup as in atherosclerosis, but from inflammation and clotting within the artery. The arteries most affected by this process are the "end" arteries supplying blood to the hands and fingers and the feet and toes; thus the pattern of symptoms, which may come and go, usually with dramatic periods of painful cramping followed by total remission for a time. The blocking of the artery by spasm and blood-clotting can deprive the tissues of needed oxygen and nutrients to the point of tissue death. Loss of fingers and toes to gangrene or amputation is quite common, especially among men who continue to smoke.

The precise cause of Buerger's disease is not known, but the association with smoking is quite clear. Recent research indicates that Buerger's disease may be a reaction to tobacco in persons with a certain genetic makeup, or an autoimmune disorder caused by sensitivity to components of the individual's own blood vessels.

What you can do If you smoke, stop immediately. (See Chapter 4 for help stopping smoking.) Failure to stop smoking will invariably result in progression of the disorder with the subsequent loss of fingers and toes to amputation. Just as with the diabetic foot (see Peripheral Vascular Disease, page 839), diminished sensation in the feet from lack of adequate blood flow increases the likelihood that blisters and wounds will go undetected until infection sets in. Wear well-fitted, supportive shoes and inspect your feet often for signs of injury.

When to call the doctor If symptoms suggesting Buerger's disease develop, see a doctor as soon as possible. Development of coolness or loss of color in a finger or toe calls for immediate medical care because blood flow to the area may be severely impaired. Injury to the skin of the feet should also prompt a visit to the doctor as soon as possible.

Treatment Stop smoking. Protect hands and feet from injury, including heat or burns, chemical injury, poorly fitted shoes, minor surgery on fingers and toes, fungal infections, and cold or medications that cause blood vessel constriction. To promote circulation, elevate the foot of the bed 6 to 8 inches. Newer medications, such as pentoxifylline (Trental), calcium antagonists (diltiazem, for example), and thromboxane inhibitors (anti-inflammatory drugs) may be beneficial.

Prognosis Among those who quit smoking, the prognosis is good. Among those who continue, it is poor.

❖ PRIMARY RAYNAUD'S PHENOMENON

Symptoms (*What you may experience*) Sudden development of whiteness, then blueness, in the fingers of both hands or the toes of both feet; may be followed by redness (uncommon); sharply demarcated skin color changes—usually pale white or blue; throbbing pain (very uncommon); numbness and pins-and-needles sensation (common). (See page C-27.)

Signs and laboratory findings (*What the doctor looks for*) Fingers or toes cool to touch without evidence of large-vessel disease. It is uncommon for the doctor to witness an attack.

What is it? Primary Raynaud's phenomenon occurs primarily in young women (affecting women to men at a ratio of 2:1). It usually first appears between the ages of 15 and 45. In susceptible people, exposure to cold or emotional stress causes an exaggerated constriction in the arteries supplying the fingers. The cause is not clearly known, but it is assumed to be due to an increase in blood vessel alpha-2 nerve receptors, which control arterial constriction in this area. In primary Raynaud's phenomenon, all fingers of both hands (or less commonly, all toes of both feet) are involved equally (the thumbs are usually spared). In secondary Raynaud's phenomenon, major arterial disease may cause asymmetrical attacks in one hand, or just one or two fingers may be involved.

During a Raynaud's attack, the arteries constrict, robbing the fingers of adequate blood flow; the skin of the fingertip becomes white; then, within a few minutes, it takes on a blue cast. There may be associated numbness, stiffness, and aching pain. When the constriction subsequently relaxes—usually spontaneously upon rewarming the fingers—the return of blood flow causes the skin to become very red, and on occasion the fingertips to throb or sting, or rarely to swell. Between attacks, the fingers appear to be normal.

In most cases, the frequency of attacks increases slowly over the years. Rarely, a rapid progression of symptoms occurs with even slight changes in temperature bringing on an attack. Because the frequent bouts of constriction hamper good circulation, wound healing of the hands and feet may be slow. Nonhealing ulcers on the fingertips may occur in secondary Raynaud's phenomenon, but never in primary Raynaud's phenomenon.

What you can do Keep hands (and feet) warm; prevent attacks by always keeping gloves handy in case the weather turns cool. If an attack occurs, warm your hands by rubbing them together, placing them between your thighs or under your arms, or blowing warm breath on them. If warm water is handy, immerse your hands in warm (not hot!) water.

If you smoke, stop; cigarette smoking contributes to constriction of the blood vessels in the hands and feet.

Keep hands and feet moisturized and well lubricated in cold weather to prevent drying and cracking of the skin.

When to call the doctor If you have Raynaud's phenomenon, you should be evaluated by your doctor to rule out an underlying cause. If the constriction fails to respond to rewarming with warm water, and the blue color persists, contact your doctor. If ulcers occur, call your doctor.

Treatment In primary Raynaud's phenomenon, medications are not necessary unless attacks alter quality of life. Medications to dilate the blood vessels may help. Good results have occurred with calcium channel blockers, such as nifedipine. Other vasodilators, like nitroglycerine transdermal patch, have shown some benefit in some cases.

In rapidly progressive symptoms, in complex secondary Raynaud's phenomenon, surgical treatment may be required if all other measures fail. Surgery involves interrupting the sympathetic nerve supply, which offers temporary relief. When the symptoms return, they are usually milder and less frequent.

Prognosis The disorder naturally comes and goes, and although it causes considerable discomfort during episodes, it is generally not a threat to health or tissues of the hand. Primary Raynaud's phenomenon is not associated with other health problems.

TWENTY-ONE

Infectious Diseases

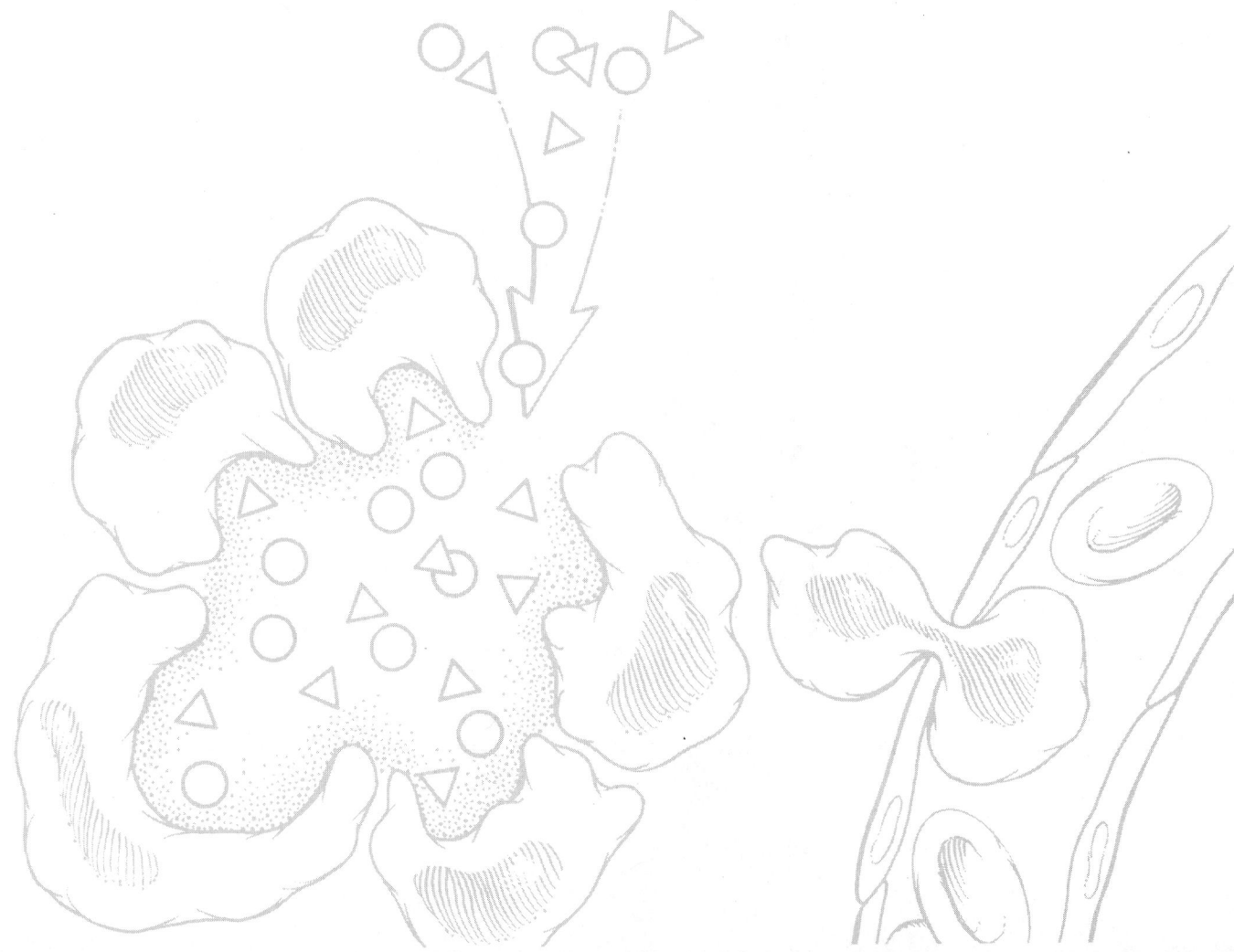

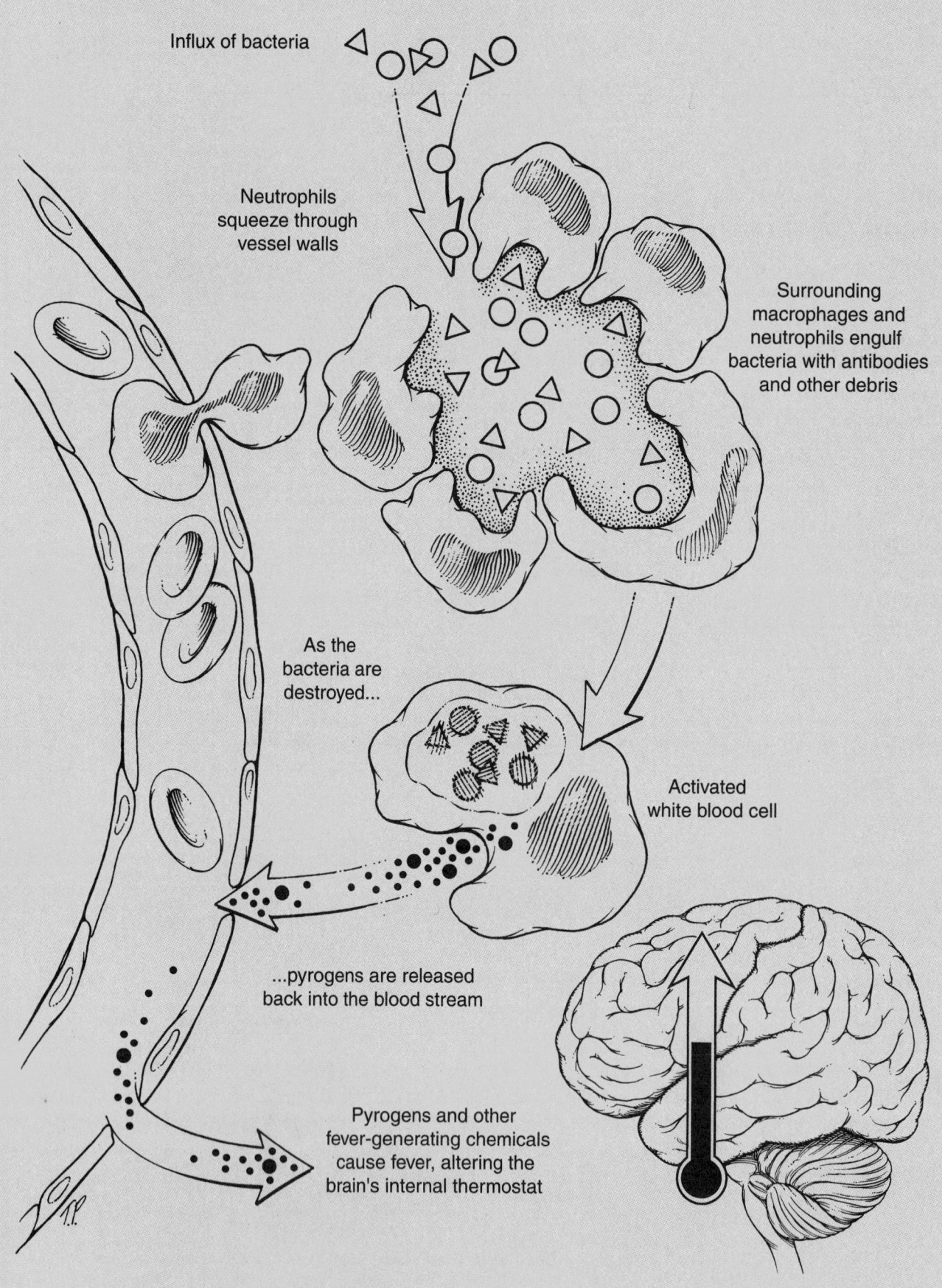

Influx of bacteria

Neutrophils
squeeze through
vessel walls

Surrounding
macrophages and
neutrophils engulf
bacteria with antibodies
and other debris

As the
bacteria are
destroyed...

Activated
white blood cell

...pyrogens are released
back into the blood stream

Pyrogens and other
fever-generating chemicals
cause fever, altering the
brain's internal thermostat

INFECTIOUS DISEASES

What Is Infection?

Infection occurs when a pathogen invades the body, prompting the immune system to mount a defense. Pathogens are microorganisms capable of producing disease—germs, in common language. Pathogens are classified into four basic types: bacteria, viruses, fungi, and parasites although some pathogens defy these classifications. For example, mycobacteria are microscopic life forms with properties of both fungi and bacteria. Other microorganisms are classified as bacteria-like. Protein particles called prions appear to cause some infectious disease, such as mad cow disease (see Bovine Spongiform Encephalopathy, page 461). Although other types of pathogens may yet be discovered, most pathogens fall into one or more of the four main classifications.

The way a pathogen arrives in the human system is highly variable. Pathogens may move from person to person in a variety of ways: by hand contact, which can spread the common cold; cough, which can spread tuberculosis; or kissing, which can spread mononucleosis. Infections also may be spread from animal to person, such as cat-scratch disease, or from insect to person, such as Lyme disease. Pathogens may also come from an environmental source such as food or water and enter the body through ingestion, such as happens in traveler's diarrhea or cryptosporidiosis. Some infections, such as tetanus, are caused by pathogens in dirt that enter the body through a cut or scrape in the skin.

When pathogens invade from outside the body, the resulting infection is referred to as exogenous. Some infections, in contrast, are the result of the migration of microbes from one part of the body to another; these infections are called endogenous. Pelvic inflammatory disease (PID) in women, for example, can result from an exogenous infection, such as a sexually transmitted infection (STI), or from an endogenous infection in which bacteria that are normally present penetrate the uterine wall, such as can happen in childbirth (see Pelvic Inflammatory Disease, page 866). Either way, when the immune system works as it should it recognizes infectious agents as foreign and institutes a search-and-destroy attack against them. Symptoms that result from this battle inside the body can vary widely, but frequently they include reactions such as fever and vomiting. Symptoms can be caused by

the pathogen itself or can result from the fight between the pathogen and the immune system. A healthy immune system constantly protects and defends the body from pathogens. For more information on the immune system, see Chapter 22.

Many infections remain confined to a specific body system and those conditions are in most cases discussed in the chapters devoted to that body system—for example, you will find a discussion of sinusitis in the chapter covering the ears, nose, and throat; you will find meningitis in the chapter devoted to the brain and nervous system; and you will find fungal infections in the chapter covering skin, hair, and nails, where fungal infections most often occur. But those disorders that involve many body systems or simply do not fit well into one, are covered in this chapter on infectious diseases.

THE MICROBIAL WORLD

Many microorganisms naturally inhabit various parts of the body—for example, on top of the tongue or in the intestines—and cause no harm at all. It is only when the body system encounters a microorganism that is a pathogen that the process of infection begins. Most people experience pathogens through common infectious illnesses such as colds and flu—often viral, sore throats—viral or bacterial, athlete's foot—fungal, or pinworm—parasitic.

If you do get an infection, chances are it will clear up on its own with rest and a good supply of liquids to prevent dehydration. In some cases, however, medication may be necessary to fight the infection. The particular medication prescribed depends on the type of pathogen (see page 849).

For the most part, the sickness arises only when the invading microorganism is able to exert its pathogenic capacity. In most cases the immune system overcomes the microorganism immediately, or the microorganism itself may have no pathogenic capacity in a particular part of the body. *Staphylococcus* infection (staph) is an example. *Staphylococcus* bacteria are found on human skin in huge numbers. A blemish on the skin that creates an entrance through which the *Staphylococcus* can pass into the bloodstream can cause a severe infection. However, it only happens when there are other extenuating circumstances, such as a

847

low immune response or a very high number of the bacteria, or both. In general, the ability of a pathogen to cause an infection depends on the pathogenic strength it possesses, the number of microorganisms that have entered the organ system, and the ability of the immune system to ward off the infective process (see The Immune-Fighting Equation, page 849).

Because it is convenient to put all these potential disease-causing microorganisms into the single broad category of pathogens, it is easy to gloss over their differences. However, the various pathogens differ dramatically from each other and their distinguishing features are most important when treatment decisions are made.

Technically, a virus is not an autonomously living thing. It is little more than a clump of genetic material (DNA or RNA) bundled in a protein packet. A virus cannot exist without a host cell to support it. When a virus enters a living cell, whether it is a bacterium, a plant cell, a human cell, or an animal cell, it promptly uses the cell's reproductive machinery to make duplicate copies of itself. It is precisely because a virus is made only of genetic material that killing it can be such a difficult task.

Bacteria are responsible for the overwhelming majority of infections that send people to the hospital, with viruses running a distant second. Viral infections normally result in short-lived illnesses such as colds, flu, or sore throat, and are usually treated in a doctor's office; in fact they are thought to account for the greatest number of visits to the doctor. When viruses infect the body, they invade the cells of the affected tissue and take over the duplicating machinery of those cells to create thousands and thousands of copies of themselves. In the process they usually rupture and destroy the host cells. The resulting cellular debris and free viral particles prompt the immune system to begin to fight the infection. White blood cells rush to the infected area where they turn loose a variety of chemical toxins, fever stimulators, and other agents designed to cripple the intruding viruses. This immune reaction provides defense against the infection but in the process it may also produce symptoms including pain, swelling, heat, redness, rash, and fever.

Bacterial infections are usually more localized, such as an infection in a cut or infection in the sinuses, tonsils, or middle ear. The immune defenses that recognize and counterattack bacteria include a special type of white blood cell that contains tiny packets of caustic chemicals designed to kill and dissolve the bacteria. These white blood cells proceed to the area of infection, surround the bacteria, and quite literally engulf them, in a process called phagocytosis. Once a white blood cell has the bacterial pathogen within its interior, it releases the toxic chemicals into the chamber to kill and dissolve the bacteria. The byproducts of the battle between thousands of white blood cells and bacteria include pus as well as symptoms such as redness, swelling, and pain. Sometimes bacterial infections do not remain limited to one place and spread through the body, causing symptoms such as rash, increased heart rate, a drop in blood pressure, headache, nausea, and diarrhea.

Fungi are a near-constant presence in air, where they float as tiny spores. Generally they are breathed in but sometimes they penetrate through a cut on the skin. In either case the immune system usually stops them from setting up an infection. However, when the air is dense with spores or when the immune system is not functioning strongly, an infection may occur (see The Immune-Fighting Equation, page 849). If many spores are inhaled, some can make their way into the lung and the warm air sacs called alveoli, where they thrive. As the spores multiply they form clusters of yeast. Eventually the entire blood system may be affected by this infection.

In some cases, spores occur in greater concentrations because of an environmental factor. Histoplasmosis, a common American fungal infection, occurs far more often in people who have recently been around a chicken coop or other areas where birds roost, because avian excrement frequently contains *Histoplasma capsulatum* spores.

Parasites literally move into the body. Infections can result from parasites living in your skin, gastrointestinal tract, liver, lungs, and other organs. The smallest parasites, one-celled protozoa, are common residents of the body; however, the immune system keeps their presence under control.

THE IMMUNE-FIGHTING EQUATION

A pathogen invades. An infection occurs. How likely is your immune system to overcome it?

The answer depends on three factors: strength of the microbe, the amount of the microbial invaders, and your body's infection-fighting capacity. These three factors can be expressed in the following equation.

- Pathogenic strength of microbe *times* number of pathogenic microbes, *divided by* infection-fighting ability of the immune system

As the equation illustrates, the success of the immune system in fighting infection does not depend solely on your health. The pathogenic strength of the microorganism is a critical part of the process. A microbe's pathogenic strength, or virulence, reflects its ability to cause illness—its capacity to invade cells and tissue and to elude and resist immune defenses.

Some infectious microbes have pathogenic strength even in low numbers. Rotavirus, a common cause of viral gastroenteritis (see page 875) takes far fewer organisms to wreak havoc on the human system than does cholera, which is a bacterium. Fortu-nately, the gastric illness caused by rotavirus generally involves only a short bout of nausea, diarrhea, and vomiting before the immune system regains the upper hand.

Some infections are so powerful they cannot be overcome by the human immune system alone. Rabies is one example. Rabies is always fatal, even in previously healthy and well-nourished people. However, the incidence of rabies can be drastically reduced by the use of antirabies immunoglobulin and rabies vaccines. Another contributing factor to individual susceptibility or resistance to infectious diseases is genetic background. In animals, it is easy to breed strains that are resistant or susceptible to infections. There are no breeding experiments in people, but there are data suggesting that exposure to a particular disease over generations leads to increased resistance among humans. Survivors of disease were able to mount an immune response to the infections and they passed this ability through these genes to their children. After centuries of natural selection northern Europeans became highly resistant to both tuberculosis and measles. Native Americans had never been exposed to tuberculosis or measles and whole populations were wiped out when America was settled with Europeans. ■

ANTIMICROBIAL MEDICATIONS

In a healthy individual the immune system produces antibodies and takes other countermeasures against infection. These are known as host defense mechanisms. In some cases, however, your immune system will need some help, and your doctor may prescribe a medication. The treatment for an infection varies depending on the pathogen.

Bacterial infections can often be fought effectively with antibiotics. Many antibiotics kill pathogenic bacteria by interfering with their ability to repair the cell wall. The cell wall of bacteria acts as a protective rind, which is continually eroding and under constant need of repair. In fact, the cell wall is an important identifying feature of most bacteria. The cell walls of bacteria are often so distinctive that their detection rests in part on lab tests in which organisms are stained bright blue or red. Some bacteria absorb certain stains more readily than others. In addition, the staining coloration helps highlight unique characteristics of the cell wall.

To divide—to reproduce themselves—bacteria must be able to build more of the cell wall. Any medication that interferes with the bacterium's ability to do this will kill it. There are whole classes of medications that fall into this cell-wall-inhibiting class, most notably, penicillins including ampicillin, amoxicillin, methicillin, and amoxicillin clavulanates and cephalosporins including cefaclor and cefprozil. These medications work by preventing repair of the cell wall but they are not effective against bacteria with no cell walls. Certain bacteria lack a cell wall—for example, mycoplasma, a common cause of upper respiratory, ear, nose, throat, and lung infections. In these cases, medications that affect protein synthesis or other internal bacteria functions are necessary. Antibiotics of the tetracycline group offer this kind of killing power against bacteria.

Other medications work by preventing bacteria access to nutrients they need to live and grow, which ultimately causes the bacteria to die, although not immediately. Medications in this category are called bacteriostatic medications; they hold the infection at bay until the invader finally dies. It is essential to take the full course of these medications because lesser amounts may only slow down or mildly cripple the bacteria and not eradicate it.

Certain viruses and fungi are not nearly as treatable as bacteria, and they require different antimicrobial agents. An antiviral medication, for example, is aimed at damaging the virus without inflicting harm on its host. Because this is difficult to achieve, there are not many effective antiviral medications. One of the outstanding legacies of research into human immunodeficiency virus (HIV), however, has been the development of powerful antiviral compounds.

Some newer antivirals have become standard therapy for viral infections. Some of these are acyclovir, used to treat the herpes virus, and amantadine and its more recent cousin rimantidine, used to treat type A influenza. Treatment for other viruses, however, has remained elusive; there still is no cure for the common cold. For many viral infections, no effective medical treatment exists.

The tough cell walls of fungi can make them difficult to destroy. Because of this strongly protective barrier, eradication of a fungus sometimes requires very potent medications, some of which are similar to cancer chemotherapeutic medications and potentially toxic if a person must take them over a long period of time.

Amphotericin B is the first-line therapy for many serious fungal infections, especially for people who are immunocompromised. However, newer antifungal medications known as azoles offer good alternatives when amphotericin B fails or is inappropriate for treatment. Probably the most popular are fluconazole, which came on the market in 1990, and itraconazole, which was introduced in 1992. Azoles are known for causing fewer side effects than their predecessors.

Parasites have to be fought differently from other kinds of pathogens because they

ANTIBIOTIC RESISTANCE

When an antibiotic is prescribed too often or used inappropriately, some of the target bacteria marshal enough resistance to survive the treatment. These bacteria, in turn, produce a whole new generation with the same resistance. Before long, the intermingling of these select strains results in increasingly resistant generations.

Antibiotics have been overprescribed to meet public demand for treatment during the cold and flu season. Although antibiotics are not appropriate for viral illness, prescriptions often are written for conditions such as bronchitis, which generally is the result of a viral infection. Ironically, inappropriate antibiotic treatment may also make the body susceptible to other infections. Overuse of antibiotics can heighten vulnerability to infections by *Clostridium difficile*, which causes gastrointestinal illness, and *Candida*, a yeast that can cause vaginal discomfort.

Since penicillin's arrival more than 5 decades ago, increasingly powerful resistance to this mold-derived medication has evolved to such a degree that penicillin is now a weak foe against *Streptococcus pneumoniae* in a substantial number of cases. *S. pneumoniae* is the most common cause of pneumonia, as well as many other respiratory infections in the United States that are, in fact, becoming resistant to a variety of medications. In one large study conducted at 30 medical centers, a host of other antibiotics, including erythromycin and tetracycline, encountered substantial resistance from *S. pneumoniae*.

From 1996 to 1997, drug-resistant strains of bacteria causing common maladies, such as otitis media (a middle-ear infection) and pneumonia doubled. In addition, a number of biologic cousins to *Streptococcus*—such as *Staphylococcus aureus*, the bacterium that causes staph infections—have also developed formidable resistance to penicillin, with troubling results. In the summer of 1997, for example, staph infection in a patient hospitalized in the Midwest failed to respond to the antibiotic vancomycin, usually reserved for difficult, resistant staph infections. This opened a potential new chapter in antibiotic resistance; it marked the failure of penicillin's most successful alternative for this illness. Though the staph infection was eventually brought under control through the near-simultaneous administration of several antibiotics, many public health authorities saw the episode as a turning point that signaled a looming rise in vancomycin-resistant staph.

Moreover, some tuberculosis is proving very stubborn to powerful antibiotics. In certain cases, it now costs more than $250,000 to treat, according to the World Health Organization (WHO). In the late 1940s, tuberculosis was thought to be on its way to extinction when sequences of antibiotics were found to cure it in most people. Now, the outlook is clouded by drug-resistant tuberculosis.

All this has meant that treatment for bacterial infection is more expensive than ever and that cure is not always guaranteed. If you or a family member contracts an antibiotic-resistant illness your doctor may well turn to newer medications such as the cephalosporins, which thus far have not ignited the same kind of resistance, or the even newer fluoroquinolones.

Only future years will tell if medical research will be able to keep up with the fast pace of antibiotic resistance. However, historically the development of antibiotics was one of the most important achievements in medical history. The human life span is on average a decade longer since penicillin was introduced more than a half century ago. ∎

actually are animals with similar proteins and enzymes compared to humans. When parasites occur externally, such as ticks and lice on skin and in hair, special creams or shampoos may be used to eradicate them, often without significant threat to the humans they inhabit. However, treatment becomes more complicated for parasites that reside within the body. The goal of therapy is to kill these small animals without hurting the human system in which they live. Many antiparasitic medications do this by interfering with processes specific to the parasite. For example, the microscopic parasites, protozoans, which include *Giardia lamblia*, often are treated with metronidazole (Flagyl), which curtails a critical step in their reproduction process. As a result, organisms die without being replaced by a new generation.

Medications aimed at some of the larger parasites actually paralyze the parasite's body, allowing the pests to be flushed out in waste product. Fortunately, these paralysis-causing medications are specific to the parasitic inhabitants and do not cause the same damage to the human system.

Today, growing resistance by all kinds of pathogens to antimicrobial medication has complicated treatment for many infections. The problem is particularly widespread with the use of antibiotics. In fact, the phenomenon—known as antibiotic resistance—now constitutes a growing health concern. Formerly standard therapies such as penicillin are proving far less effective to new generations of bacteria (see page 850). In the United States, Europe, and elsewhere across the globe, pharmaceutical companies and research scientists are working to formulate new compounds that can overcome this problem. Many scientists believe that the most exciting years in the field of immunology lie ahead, as research into immunization and antimicrobial medications continues and new ways of treating and preventing infectious disease are developed. One of the most promising refinements is expected to come from recombinant DNA technology. In 1997 a new vaccine using genetic engineering was formulated for Lyme disease, a tick-borne condition. It demonstrated 60 to 80 percent effectiveness in protecting most people from tick-borne infection. If this kind of genetic engineering can be perfected, benefits will be reaped by whole populations.

IMMUNIZATION

The discovery of vaccines to prevent disease stands as one of the great landmarks in modern medicine. Thanks to effective vaccines, devastating diseases such as diphtheria and polio largely are confined to the pages of history. In fact, polio should reach global eradication by the year 2000, according to World Health Organization (WHO) estimates.

Vaccines typically contain tiny amounts of dead or severely weakened pathogens that would be capable of causing a specific disease in large and flourishing quantities. A vaccine prompts the body to form a defense system of infection-fighting antibodies before a real encounter occurs, a process called active immunization.

Some vaccines are based on inactivated toxins, which incite immunity against infection despite being inactivated by heat or other forms of sterilization. Some vaccines are based on the pathogens themselves, which have been rendered nonvirulent although they may cause mild inflammation. Booster shots are occasional injections of vaccine that trigger the body's immunologic memory so that it does not lose the ability to produce a full-fledged response to a specific disease.

When a true invader enters the bloodstream after immunization, the body already has the antibodies to respond and ward off the infection. However, not every infection can be prevented in this manner.

Despite the availability of vaccines, nearly every year in the United States more adults die from diseases preventable by immunization than in automobile accidents. Influenza, hepatitis, and pneumonia alone claim more than 60,000 adult lives annually, even though vaccination is the simplest step to prevention. Adults fail to get immunized for reasons ranging from confusion over what is available to poor recognition of risk factors.

The following are some descriptions that may help familiarize you with adult vaccines. Before you decide upon any immunization talk to your doctor about possible side effects. In addition, keep track of whatever shots you may receive in an emergency-room visit so that you and your doctor can keep accurate records. Also be aware that not all vaccines are 100 percent effective.

Influenza (Frequency: every year.) All adults age 65 and over or any person with chronic illness, respiratory impairment, immune system impairment, or at high risk of exposure should be immunized against influenza.

Pneumococcal pneumonia vaccine (Frequency: not precisely determined; about once every 10 years.) All adults age 65 and over (except those with poor immune function because of acquired immunodeficiency syndrome (AIDS), cancer chemotherapy, or organ transplantations should take the vaccine.

LATENCY AND OTHER INFECTIOUS PROCESSES

There is much we do not know about the immune response, but recent research points to the following process. When invading pathogens are recognized, they are taken to a nearby lymph node or to the spleen. Within the lymph nodes or spleen, macrophages surround the pathogen and it is analyzed by the T and B cells. The cells develop a chemical memory of the particular proteins or antigen in the pathogen. These T and B cells recognize the antigen whenever it subsequently reappears in the body and reproduce quickly to subdue it.

If you encounter a virus or bacterium and come down with an infection from which you recover, in some cases you are safe from the same infection forever. However, this is not always the case. Some bacteria have so much variation that even a very specific type, like *Streptococcus pneumoniae*, comes in dozens of slightly different forms known as serotypes. Although your body has previously conquered one serotype, the immunologic memory of your T and B cells may not apply to another serotype.

Lack of natural immunization after exposure to a pathogen may also result from a process called *latency*. This occurs when an infectious agent—a virus, for example—seems to have been eradicated by the body but surfaces again later. This happens when some of the microbes are able to remain in the system undetected, because they are inactive and low in number. When stress or other factors lower immune defenses, they flare up. One example is the herpes simplex virus, which is characterized by recurrence. Another herpes virus that causes chickenpox, herpes zoster, also exhibits this latency. People who have had chickenpox may experience a recurrence of herpes zoster infection in the form of shingles, a painful outbreak of lesions. Because the chance of getting shingles seems to increase with age, it is thought that reactivation of the original infection occurs as a result of age-related decline of the immune system.

In other cases, microorganisms simply seem able to hide out by camouflaging themselves with substances they produce, which tricks the body into accepting them as part of its system. Other microorganisms employ a different strategy to ensure that some of the infection-causing organisms survive; they secrete chemicals that are toxic to the ensuing immune defense, killing cells sent out to battle the infection. Many *Staphylococcus* bacteria are capable of this kind of toxin production. ■

Diphtheria-tetanus (Frequency: booster every 10 to 15 years.) All adults who did not receive a primary series of five injections in childhood should complete a series. All adults and teenagers should update their immunity with a booster shot periodically.

Measles, mumps, and rubella (MMR) (Frequency: one booster for high school/college students.) Adults born after 1956 who do not have blood tests proving immunity, particularly women of childbearing age, should be immunized with MMR. Adults born prior to 1957 in all likelihood developed immunity from natural infection.

Hepatitis B (Frequency: A series of 3 shots consisting of an initial shot, a second after 1 month and a third after 6 months.) All young adults not previously immunized should receive this vaccine, as well as all adults at higher risk, including health care workers, people who receive certain types of transfusions with blood products, hemodialysis patients, homosexual men, bisexual men and their sexual partners, intravenous drug users and their sexual partners, anyone who has had multiple sexual partners within a 6-month period, anyone who has recently contracted another sexually transmitted infection, and people traveling to countries where the risk of contracting hepatitis B is high.

Hepatitis A (Frequency: A 2-shot series consisting of an initial shot and a follow-up booster in 6 to 12 months.) All high-risk adults should receive this vaccine. High-risk groups include travelers to areas where outbreaks of the disease occur frequently, such as underdeveloped nations; people within certain communities or groups where periodic outbreaks occur, such as Alaskan natives, Pacific Islanders, and Native Americans; homosexual and bisexual men; intravenous or street drug users; military personnel, health care workers; daycare workers; and people in prisons or those who live in other institutional settings.

Varicella (Frequency: two doses, given 4 to 8 weeks apart.) All healthy adults with no previous history of varicella (chickenpox) infection, especially health care workers or the family members of people without optimal immune defense such as AIDS and organ transplant patients are candidates for this vaccine.

In addition to those listed previously, your doctor may recommend additional vaccines if you are planning a trip abroad. If you are going to Southeast Asia in the late summer or early fall, your doctor may recommend a vaccine against Japanese encephalitis. There are also shots for cholera and typhoid, diseases which can be a danger for people who travel to certain countries. However, often such travel immunizations are neither fully protective nor long term; discuss them carefully with your doctor.

It is also important to note that sometimes immunization can prevent disease even after exposure to an infectious organism. The classic case is tetanus. The use of a preventive serum of tetanus immune globulin plus a standard dose of tetanus vaccine will provide immediate immunity to people who have either never been immunized against tetanus, or have not been recently immunized and have a contaminated wound (see Do You Need a Tetanus Shot? page 879). Immunization after exposure to illness can also protect against certain types of meningitis and hepatitis.

UNDERSTANDING FEVER

One of nature's infection-fighters is fever. Fever is a defense mechanism that raises the body temperature a few degrees, theoretically hurting the pathogen more than the person, although there is some debate about fever's harmful effects. Some studies show that intervening to reduce fever may indeed prolong the infection; however, letting a fever run its course is by no means a universal recommendation. The most common cause of fever by far is infection, but it also occurs in various autoimmune disorders, such as systemic lupus erythematosus, rheumatic fever, and rheumatoid arthritis; after trauma to the brain, such as stroke or head injury; in cancer; and certain disorders of the blood, gastrointestinal system, and endocrine system.

The common denominator in the many causes for fever is the stimulation of certain members of the white-blood-cell family called monocyte-macrophages. These immune defense cells produce and release hormonal chemical messengers, called cytokines, that travel to the hypothalamus and reset the thermostat there to a higher level. As a

HOW TO BRING A FEVER DOWN SAFELY

When the oral temperature rises above 103°F the discomfort fever causes may outweigh the benefit it brings in combating infection. Discomfort aside, an oral temperature rising beyond 106°F can be dangerous in its own right. Sustained temperatures above this level can exceed the body's capability to cool the vital organs such as the brain, liver, and kidneys. The risk of high fever is far greater in children than in adults; for both children and adults, however, the consequences of sustained elevated temperature can include loss of consciousness, seizures, brain damage, and liver or kidney failure. If you cannot bring a fever of 106° or higher down yourself within an hour, seek emergency medical attention.

To bring down a fever safely:

- Drink plenty of liquids. They can act as an internal coolant. In addition, they help keep electrolytes—the salts and minerals your body constantly needs—replenished and in balance.

- Cover up when cold. Blankets and other bedding can help your body regain a sense of warmth, helping to ward off chills that often accompany fever. When chills diminish, remove excessive layers of blankets or clothing, leaving a light cover.

- Get plenty of rest. Sleep slows body functions, lowering what is known as your core body temperature. It also restores energy.

- Take appropriate over-the-counter medication. Aspirin and other nonsteroidal anti-inflammatory drugs (NSAIDs) help your body return to normal temperature. Aspirin provides an inexpensive, effective remedy for most causes of fever. In some people, however, aspirin can irritate the stomach. Acetaminophen or ibuprofen dosed according to the manufacturer's recommendations are also appropriate. Like aspirin, a dose of either of these medications should be taken at most only every 4 hours. However, if fever responds but returns before the next scheduled dose, you may be able to control the fever by taking one aspirin every 2 hours. If high fever persists despite aspirin therapy, you need medical help. You should also seek medical attention if you have other symptoms as well as fever, or if you continue to feel unwell after the fever is controlled. *Aspirin should never be used in children. Fevers in children should be controlled with acetaminophen (see page 854).* ∎

result, the body suddenly perceives that it is cooler than it is supposed to be, which sets all available means of heat production and conservation in motion, causing shivering—increased muscle work that, much like exercise, produces heat—and the constriction of arteries that supply blood to the limbs; diminished blood flow causes reduced heat loss from these areas.

Body temperature is regulated by a region in the center of the brain called the hypothalamus. Through a complex interplay of hormonal, metabolic, and chemical messages, the hypothalamus keeps body temperature relatively constant—within about

ASPIRIN: AVOID GIVING IT TO CHILDREN AND ADOLESCENTS

Aspirin for fever caused by flu or another viral illness is risky for children and even for adolescents. The combination of a viral illness and salicylate, the main ingredient in aspirin, may lead to Reye's syndrome, a poorly understood but potentially lethal liver disease. Because aspirin may be an ingredient in combination medications, the ingredients of any over-the-counter product given to children should be carefully checked.

The specific cause of Reye's syndrome is not known, but it may occur after a bout of childhood influenza or a viral illness such as chickenpox. Aspirin is thought to increase the risk of Reye's syndrome more than thirty-fold in children under 18 years old. If caught in the early stages, in which a child seems to become lethargic, Reye's syndrome is quite curable. However, even in the early phases when drowsiness sets in, it should be considered a medical emergency. A delay in treatment can lead to coma and even death. In children, particularly those younger than 12 years old, acetaminophen or some other alternative recommended by your doctor should be used in all cases and at all times rather than aspirin. ■

a 2°F variation—despite changes in the warmth or cold of the external environment. Average body temperature falls within the range of 96.8°F to 99.3°F, with the body coolest in the morning and warmest in the late afternoon. Temperature also varies in women with the menstrual cycle—a rise in temperature immediately follows ovulation—and in the first 3 months of pregnancy. Ninety-five percent of people fall within this normal range, which means, of course, that 5 percent do not. Some people's body temperature will be higher than 99.3° or lower than 96.8° and still be normal for them. Fever is a departure from a person's normal temperature range to a new, higher set point. When evaluating a fever, keep in mind that your temperature will vary throughout the day depending on how active you are and the temperature of your surrounding environment, as well as other factors.

Taking your temperature Do you feel hot to the touch? Bear in mind that a hand to the forehead, while generally effective for detecting fever, is really no help in assessing it. If you call your doctor's office to report you have a fever, the first question you are likely to be asked is "What is your temperature?" This is one of the most beneficial pieces of information you can give your doctor over the phone.

An accurate reading can be best made using a standardized thermometer. Currently,

thermometers come in a wide range of types including oral or rectal mercury thermometers, oral or rectal digital thermometers, skin temperature gauges such as bands that change color, and tympanic (eardrum) thermometers. Of these, the most accurate reflection of core body temperature—particularly in young children who may not keep an oral thermometer in place—is a properly taken rectal measurement. Obviously, the difficulty and discomfort of this method make it less attractive to some people. Tympanic temperature offers the easiest and quickest accurate measurement, but it requires the purchase of a special thermometer that looks like the instrument a doctor uses to look into ears. The old standard oral method is probably the most widely used and least expensive measurement; if properly done it is quite accurate.

To properly take an oral temperature, do not eat or drink for at least 20 minutes before making the measurement. Shake down a mercury thermometer or follow the resetting instructions on the newer digital variety. Place the bulb of the thermometer securely to one side of the mouth, under the tongue in the pocket between the back of the tongue and the floor of the mouth. Securely close your lips around the stem. For a mercury thermometer, wait a full 5 minutes by the clock before removing the thermometer. If you find you have difficulty seeing the mercury column to make an accurate reading, it is probably better to use a digital one. A digital thermometer is easier to read and will usually beep to let you know when to remove it.

FEVER OF UNKNOWN ORIGIN

Sometimes when a fever arises an underlying cause cannot be found: no signs of a tick bite or scratch, no history of exposure to an infected person, no contaminated food or water. In short, nothing readily explains the fever's onset. When unexplained fever persists for many days, or even weeks, and hovers at 101°F or higher, it becomes in medical terminology a fever of unknown origin (FUO).

More than a third of all FUOs are caused by an infection, even though the specific pathogen can elude identification. Other causes of FUO range from tumors to skin diseases. FUO can be a complication of human immunodeficiency virus (HIV) infection, particularly among HIV-infected people who have full-blown AIDS. For people who travel outside the United States to a developing country, infections such as malaria are frequently the cause of FUO. To find the pathogenic cause of an FUO, doctors usually perform a variety of tests. Such tests typically detect an infectious agent in one of two ways: by detecting the microorganism's presence in a specimen, such as a throat culture or urine sample, or by visualizing internal organs of the body through an imaging process, such as an x-ray or computed tomography (CT). There are a number of reasons that tests for FUO may not provide definitive answers. First, not all tests aimed at identifying infections work well. Some lack specificity, meaning that they may turn up a probable cause, but the result should not be regarded as confirmatory. Other tests lack sensitivity, meaning they cannot detect the causative agent unless it occurs at relatively high levels. And, finally, some pathogens are so uncommon that there are no reliable ways to test for their presence.

Sometimes, it seems, genes play a role in FUO. A puzzling fever that accompanies a genetic disorder known as familial Mediterranean fever has been attributed to a simple blood protein, pyrin. Pyrin, which helps prevent or modulate fever, may be faulty in some people due to genetic inheritance. Researchers speculate that in these cases pyrin does not work properly.

Most people with FUO have serious diseases: generalized infections such as endocarditis and tuberculosis; localized infections such as liver abscess; tumors such as leukemia, lymphomas, or cancer; or collagen vascular diseases such as periarteritis nodosa. These conditions can be fatal if untreated.

Sometimes the search is unavailing and the fever drags on for a year or more, after which the prognosis improves. The very act of surviving a year without treatment reduces the chance that a person has a serious condition. Sometimes a deep-seated tumor or infection will surface after a year of investigation, but this is rare. Most commonly the fever subsides and no diagnosis is ever established. This kind of recovery, while often baffling and unpredictable, offers physical proof of the power the human body has to heal itself.

HIV and AIDS

The remarkable capacity of the immune system to rid the body of infectious agents allows us to live without worry of disease most of the time. However, in some cases, our immunity can diminish in effectiveness, or even vanish. Certain diseases can cause a partial or complete shutdown of the immune system. Some of these are inherited diseases transmitted through the genes, and some of them are acquired diseases transmitted through direct contact. The most globally widespread of the latter is an infectious disease of recent history, acquired immunodeficiency syndrome, or AIDS. AIDS is caused by the human immunodeficiency virus known as HIV. AIDS attacks the body in several ways. Most significantly, the disease destroys T cells, disarming the body's ability to respond to infectious agents that it would normally easily defeat.

❖ HIV

Symptoms *(What you may experience)* Infection with HIV may be followed by flu-like symptoms as soon as a few days after exposure, but visible or perceptible symptoms may be absent for weeks or even months. This stage, called primary HIV infection, may be marked by swollen glands, fever, and sore throat. Primary HIV infection is followed by early symptomatic HIV infection, which includes yeast infections on the tongue known as thrush, or swollen glands. In many women, severe vaginal yeast infections also surface, or they experience PID (see page 866). Symptoms of these later stages may be the first outward signs of infection. For more information on the stages and symptoms of HIV, see page 859.

Signs and laboratory findings *(What the doctor looks for)* HIV is detectable in blood even at very low concentrations, by testing either for the virus or the antibodies associated with it.

What is it? HIV is a virus, called a retrovirus, which attacks a special kind of white blood cell in the immune system known as

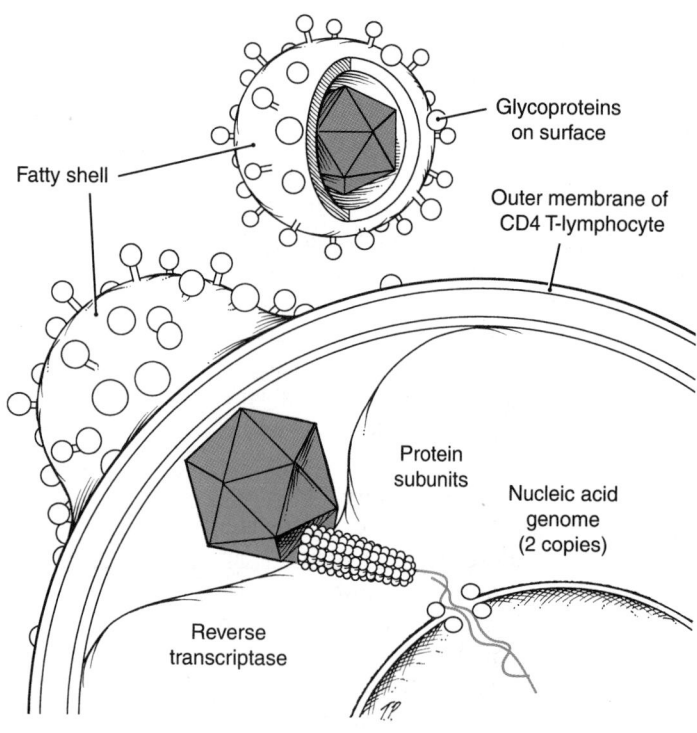

A virus particle, or virion, of human immunodeficiency virus (HIV) is about one ten-thousandth of a millimeter in diameter. To reproduce, viruses use the internal chemical machinery of the cells that they infect. HIV infects and destroys white blood cells known as CD4 T lymphocytes, which normally help to control infections occurring inside other cells. The virion attaches itself to the surface of the T cell and releases its contents (a molecule containing the virus' genetic makeup and proteins that aid in replication) into the cell. Replication of the molecule, or genome, leads to reproduction and spread of the virus. HIV's destruction of T cells impairs the body's ability to respond to other infectious agents that it would normally defeat without difficulty.

a CD4 T lymphocyte. The strength of the immune system is directly related to the circulating numbers of these infection-fighting cells. As they become depleted, so does the overall immune response. Because there is not yet a complete cure for the disease, the aim of treatment is to slow the progress of immune destruction caused by the virus. At present, it usually takes 10 years for an HIV infection to progress to AIDS (see page 858).

An HIV infection generally follows a fairly predictable sequence. After the virus is transmitted, what is called primary infection follows for a brief period of a few weeks. There may be no symptoms of primary HIV

infection. Then the body begins to fight the virus, forming antibodies, which are readily detectable by HIV testing. However, symptoms may still be absent. Often, a period of latency follows in which the virus is present but physical signs of infection are not (see Latency and Other Infectious Processes, page 852). Most people can be infected with HIV for years and have absolutely no symptoms until the immune system becomes suppressed. The full-blown disease caused by the virus—AIDS—eventually results. Technically, AIDS is confirmed by tests that determine the damage to T-cell count, but there are many overlying diseases that are associated with its onset as well. In effect, HIV infection is a continuum; AIDS can be viewed as its final, terminal stage.

People with HIV infection often have concurrent conditions that can be diagnosed before more overt signs surface. Because anemia commonly accompanies HIV infection, a complete blood count (CBC) is often the first test given. The CBC yields red-blood-cell and white-blood-cell counts; a low white-blood-cell count is typical of AIDS. Serologic tests for hepatitis and sexually transmitted infections (STIs) also are done because of the high incidence of concurrent hepatitis and STI, particularly syphilis (see Common Symptoms and Conditions that May Be Caused by STIs, page 861). A serum-chemistry panel to check levels of certain constituents in blood often is also performed—up to 75 percent of HIV-infected people have abnormal liver function.

HIV is transmitted mainly through sexual acts involving exchange of body fluids or through the sharing of needles in intravenous drug use. It can also be transmitted by an infected mother to her infant during fetal development or during childbirth. Although blood transfusions used to be a significant risk factor in people such as hemophiliacs who depend on transfusions, screening of donated blood by serological testing has almost eliminated transfusion-associated HIV.

Despite a decrease in recent years of the spread of the disease in industrialized nations, HIV remains a global health threat. The existence of HIV, the virus that causes AIDS, was unknown little more than a decade ago. Today more than 20 million adults are estimated to be infected. The cumulative total could reach 40 million in the next 5 years, according to the WHO. Some estimates show a new infection of HIV occurs every 30 seconds. The annual transmission rate in the United States is thought to be 60,000 to 70,000.

What you can do HIV infection is a preventable disease in most cases. Abstention from unprotected sex—except in a monogamous relationship—is recommended as the only reliable prevention. If monogamy is not being practiced, the use of a condom along with certain spermicides affords considerable protection (see STI Prevention and Condom Use, page 860). When sex is unprotected, taking the HIV morning-after pill, which contains a potent antiviral combination, may be preventive, but many experts warn that it gives both men and women a false sense of security.

Most doctors advise against kissing a person known to have HIV on the mouth or sharing cups, toothbrushes, razors, or silverware with someone with HIV. Though cases of this kind of HIV transmission are rare, they can occur.

Health care workers are at slightly increased risk due to their contacts with blood and other body fluids from people with HIV. Everyone should take precautions to avoid direct contact with these fluids because generally there is no certain way of knowing who is carrying the virus.

Research continues into development of a vaccine against the virus.

When to call the doctor Call your doctor anytime you have an unexplained flu-like illness. You should be tested periodically if you engage in any of the high-risk behaviors associated with HIV infection or if you learn that a previous sexual partner is infected (see The Ways in Which HIV Is Detected, page 858). To be safe and ensure the earliest diagnosis possible, periodic tests are recommended for persons with sexually transmitted infectious diseases; injection-drug users, homosexual and bisexual men, hemophiliacs, and regular sexual partners of persons in these categories or persons with known HIV infection; prostitutes, persons who received blood products from 1977 to 1985, and heterosexual persons with one or more sex partners in the past 12 months plus noncompliance with condom use in the past 6 months; and persons who consider themselves at risk.

It is recommended that pregnant women be tested; the US Public Health Service has recommended counseling and voluntary testing of all pregnant women. Other people who should also be tested for HIV include people with active tuberculosis and people who may have occupational exposures to body fluids such as blood, semen, vaginal secretions, and cerebrospinal fluid.

Treatment It is critical to discover if you have the HIV virus as early as possible in order to consider initiation of treatment. The past few years have seen not only enormous advances in virus-suppressing therapy for HIV, but also the benefits of adjusting and modifying the treatment regimen because the virus has an uncanny ability to produce new strains that successfully resist even the new, powerful antiretroviral medications.

Symptomatic HIV infection is typified by certain complications, including idiopathic thrombocytopenic purpura (ITP—a severe reduction in platelets that causes blood to spill into tissue) and frequent infections such as pneumonia. Early treatment with antiretrovirals has helped prolong the symptom-free periods of HIV infection.

Protease inhibitors, a special and revolutionary class of antiretroviral drugs, have completely altered the treatment of HIV, enabling doctors to prescribe therapy that significantly slows the replication of the virus and the progression toward AIDS. The following drugs are among those that have proven extremely effective, particularly in combinations that are called cocktail regimens: zidovudine, or AZT (Retrovir); saquinavir mesylate (Invirase or Fortovase); ritonavir (Norvir); indinavir sulfate (Crixivan); and nelfinavir mesylate (Viracept). Treatment with protease inhibitors is generally recommended when the HIV virus levels reach a certain number, or viral load.

However, the HIV virus is proving resistant to some antiretrovirals, in much the same way some bacteria are proving resistant to antibiotics (See Antibiotic Resistance, page 850). Counteracting these drug-resistant HIV strains poses a major challenge. One possible option that is currently being evaluated in clinical trials, is to combine different antiretroviral treatments. Early studies show that multiple combination regimens using different antiretroviral drugs can be quite successful. Studies suggest that by

THE WAYS IN WHICH HIV IS DETECTED

HIV infection is confirmed by detecting antibodies to the virus, the virus with antigens linked to it, or the viral RNA.

The standard HIV test is an assay that screens blood for HIV antibodies by means of a technique known as the ELISA and confirmed by a test called the Western blot. However, there are a number of ways to detect HIV in its early stage.

Home Kits These tests are available in pharmacies or by pharmaceutical catalog for $35 to $50. Blood is obtained by pricking a finger. A drop of blood is then placed on a strip and the strip is mailed in a protected envelope using an anonymous code.

Rapid Tests In-office tests that doctors can use in situations in which immediate results are important in treatment decisions. Positive results require confirmation with a standard test, such as a Western blot.

Saliva Test Available in doctors' offices, the test uses a cotton pad to scrape the inner cheek until wet. The pad is then left to dry for 2 minutes on the swab, after which it is placed in a vial that is submitted to a lab. Results are available by phone or fax within 3 days.

Urine Test This test can be administered only by a doctor and positive results require confirmation with a later blood test.

Viral Detection Other methods to establish HIV infection include new techniques to detect HIV antigens or to detect the viral RNA by the polymerase chain reaction (PCR). This technology has become standard for staging and monitoring the response to retroviral therapy when following the progress of the disease. ∎

using these potent combinations, the chance for resistant strains to emerge and flourish can be significantly reduced. Strict compliance with these complicated medical regimens appears critical to prevent the emergence of resistant virus. Although more work is needed to fully verify the precise way in which this happens, some of the new information gleaned from this combined-therapy approach can already be applied to clinical practice. The emerging problems of viral resistance, the mechanisms by which that process occurs, and the impact of resistance on treatment for HIV infection and AIDS have yet to be fully determined, but the outlook is more hopeful than ever before.

Prognosis Prognosis depends on how the HIV virus responds to early treatment. When treatment fails to limit viral replication adequately, the effects can become life-threatening. The viral load may increase to an extent that renders the body almost incapable of fighting off infection, making it much more vulnerable to devastating illness. Certain lung infections, such as *Mycobacterium tuberculosis* and *Pneumocystis*

carinii infections, as well as certain cancers, such as Kaposi's sarcoma, are characteristic. When such illnesses occur, they may lead to what is called an AIDS-defining diagnosis, meaning that the phase of the disease has moved into such a physically debilitating state that it now constitutes AIDS.

❖ AIDS

Symptoms (*What you may experience*) Extreme vulnerability to infections. As described below, many infectious diseases are associated with AIDS.

Signs and laboratory findings (*What the doctor looks for*) The viral load, which is a measure that reflects the amount of HIV virus in 1 mL of blood serum, and CD4 (a type of T cell) count less than 200. Both viral load and CD4 counts are closely watched as a biological barometer of disease progression.

What is it? AIDS is the final stage of HIV infection. When the T-cell count plummets to a low level, the ability of HIV-infected people to fight off infections is lost. In general, the course of disease is more rapid in people with fairly high viral loads, who require earlier and more aggressive use of antimicrobials to stem opportunistic infections. These infections are called opportunistic because they are caused by a virus or bacterium or other pathogen that usually is not harmful to a person with normal immune function.

Several conditions are so typical of AIDS that their symptoms—such as the dark purple blotches of Kaposi's sarcoma—are considered markers for the disease. In some cases, the first noticeable sign of AIDS is not physical change at all, but a change in mental acuity. People who become fully immunosuppressed by HIV may experience slurred speech, sleepiness or inability to concentrate, or clumsiness in walking or retrieving objects. A recurrent headache may also develop. Both problems of mental ability and headache are frequently caused by the same fungus, *Cryptococcus*, which causes cryptococcal meningitis. Opportunistic infections of the central nervous system like *Cryptococcus neoformans* infection are second only to those affecting the lungs, such as *P. carinii* infection, which causes pneumonia. These types of infections cause the complications and clusters of symptoms known as AIDS, the advanced, terminal stage of HIV. How this process occurs is explained below.

There are six stages in the progression to AIDS: viral transmission, primary HIV infection, seroconversion, latent period, early symptomatic HIV infection, and full-blown AIDS.

1. Viral transmission usually happens through sexual intercourse, exposure to contaminated blood, or perinatal transmission. How soon this virus takes a physical toll is quite variable.

2. Primary HIV infection—also called acute HIV infection or acute seroconversion syndrome—is seen usually about 2 to 4 weeks after the initial infection. A rash may develop on the face and trunk, or on the hands or arms and feet including the palms and soles. Sores may break out on the mouth, esophagus, or genitals. Other symptoms of primary HIV infection include diarrhea, headache, nausea and vomiting, swollen liver, swollen lymph nodes, and muscle ache. However, many infected people never develop any signs of illness following infection.

3. The phenomenon known as seroconversion occurs, in general, at about 6 to 12 weeks after transmission. It is associated with a sharp reduction of virus in the blood, as the body begins to wage war with the infection.

4. The seroconversion stage is followed by the latent period. After seroconversion the level of virus in the blood stabilizes at some value specific for each person. The value may range from less than 1,000 copies per mL to more than 500,000 copies per mL. The CD4 count also stabilizes between 500 and 1,200 per mL, which is appreciably lower than normal but not disablingly immunosuppressive. No symptoms are present, but the CD4 count begins a steady, relentless decline in most people. When the CD4 count reaches 200, the person by definition has early AIDS.

The average time from seroconversion to reaching a CD4 count of 200 or less is about 7 years, but the duration of this period is highly variable. In general the higher the viral load, the more rapid the decline in CD4 count. Some people progress to AIDS in a year, while others do not even after 15 years. A small number of people who were infected 17 to 18 years ago still have no evidence of a decline in CD4 count. These people may have killed or controlled the HIV virus, although no one is certain.

During the latent period, the person may be infected with pathogens that can infect people without HIV, such as the tubercle bacillus, the pneumococcus, and salmonella. Because of the person's immunosuppressed state, these infections can be more severe than they would be in someone who is not infected with HIV.

5. Early symptomatic AIDS is defined by one of the infections above, by a CD4 count of less than 200, or by infection with organisms that almost never infect people with normal immune systems, such as thrush or *Pneumocystis* pneumonia.

6. Late AIDS is defined by a CD4 count of less than 50 and is characterized by infections with pathogens such as toxoplasmosis, cytomegalovirus, and *Mycobacterium avium intracellulare.* Many pathogens involve the nervous system; HIV itself and other pathogens may produce dementia. Severe malnutrition and bone marrow failure is also present at this stage. The prognosis is very poor.

What you can do You can help prolong your health, even when the HIV infection has progressed significantly. Take good care of yourself by insisting on good medical care. Seek a doctor experienced in the care of HIV-infected people, so that whatever infections arise in the course of the disease are likely to be quickly recognized and appropriately treated.

Suppressing HIV to prevent the onset of full-blown AIDS is complicated by several factors. The antiretroviral therapy necessitates adhering to a strict and complex schedule of medication. It requires taking a regimen of drugs that have serious side effects in many people with HIV, ranging from nausea to overwhelming fatigue. Be consistent in your use of prescribed antiretroviral drugs and be prepared for other treatments, such as antibiotic prophylaxis. Prophylactic use of antibiotics for pulmonary infections caused by *Pneumocystis carinii* and *Mycobacterium avium* is known to prolong quality of life.

Treatment Treatment for AIDS involves combating opportunistic infections as they occur. For instance, cytomegalovirus, a specific form of herpesvirus, does not generally cause problems to healthy people, but is a leading cause of blindness in AIDS. *Aspergillus fumigatus*, a mold associated with nuts and grains, can be inhaled without harm by most people, but in people with AIDS, it can cause severe pneumonia or disseminated infection.

Among people with AIDS, such opportunistic infections pose life-threatening and life-altering consequences. Aggressive, preventive treatment of the disease with disease-specific therapies—such as powerful antibiotics—are effective for many. Prophylactic antimicrobials are recommended for infections such as *P. carinii*, toxoplasmosis, tuberculosis, and *M. avium* infection. Sometimes vaccines are recommended to HIV-infected people who lack previous immunization.

Nutrition is of utmost importance. The emaciation that people with AIDS suffer is a complex result of their immunological battle with the viral destroyer of T cells. Local charities and organizations that provide meals on wheels and other supportive services have gone a long way toward preserving the nutritional status of people with AIDS. Some research indicates that stopping smoking and other healthful measures can significantly improve life expectancy. Occasionally, appetite stimulants or anabolic steroids are prescribed.

In addition, group support has been shown to prolong life among the terminally ill. In one study, people who were involved in regular wellness-support meetings survived twice as long as those who did not attend such meetings.

Prognosis Even with antiretroviral therapy, some people seem to naturally experience a more rapid course toward AIDS. Researchers have pondered why some people seem to develop AIDS so suddenly even with good treatment, and others seem to take years to show symptoms of the disease. One reason appears linked to genetic susceptibility. A mutation in two specific genes has been documented to afford carriers some protection. The genes, called CCR5 and CCR2, are not found in the majority of the population. However, they appear to affect the ability to elicit a strong immune response. Although researchers studying this gene-controlled phenomenon are not yet sure just how it works, it is this kind of investigation that many medical experts believe may lead to better control or even cure of the disease.

STI PREVENTION AND CONDOM USE

STI Prevention

Of the three kinds of condoms available today, only one is considered adequate for preventing STIs including HIV. The effective type is the men's latex condom, a latex sheath and prophylactic for contraception. However, the growing number of people who have significant latex allergies is making the use of latex condoms problematic for some; vinyl condoms are an acceptable alternative. The latex condom encloses the penis and collects semen before, during, and after ejaculation, and protects the penis from vaginal secretions, both of which can carry viruses and bacteria. Most experts recommend using a condom that is lubricated with a spermicide, such as nonoxynol-9, which has been shown to kill the HIV virus as well as sperm. However, nonoxynol-9 should be avoided if it causes causes burning and itching. Your doctor can recommend an alternative (see Proper Use of a Condom, page 1162).

Condom Use

- Handle condoms gently and carefully. Fingernails or jewelry that catch on the latex can damage or break it.

- Use a new condom during each act of intercourse.

- Place the condom on an erect penis and unroll it to the base.

- Leave a space at the tip and remove the air pocket in the space prior to intercourse.

- Use a lubricant, but be careful to choose wisely. K-Y jelly, spermicidal foam, or gel are acceptable. Petroleum jelly, baby oil, or cold creams are not; they can damage the condom.

- Hold the condom firmly against the base of the penis during withdrawal. The penis should be withdrawn quickly while still erect, so that the condom remains in place.

If, during intercourse, the condom breaks, both men and women should wash their genitals thoroughly, and follow washing by urinating. Although washing the genitals is not proven to be an effective method for preventing STIs, it can help avoid infection if the condom breaks. ■

Sexually Transmitted Infections

Studies by the US government show that sexually transmitted infections (STIs) are among the most common contagious infections. Worldwide, estimates hold that there are more than 300 million cases of STIs annually; about 20 million new cases occur in the United States alone. These statistics are alarming in light of the fact that STIs are in many cases preventable. The possible consequences of any STI pose a threat to both fertility and quality of life. Pregnant women are at particular risk. The health of the fetus or newborn can be severely impaired if the mother is infected. Early diagnosis and treatment are critical. But so is prevention.

It is important to keep in mind that STIs affect sexually active adults and adolescents from all corners of life. Infected individuals do not necessarily fit the stereotypical profile of a promiscuous person. It is therefore important for potential sexual partners to be as candid as possible with one another about their past histories, including conditions that could be spread by sexual contact, and to practice good preventive techniques in any event.

STIs that previously have been relatively confined to tropical or subtropical areas are becoming more common in the United States. This appears to be due to the explosive growth in international travel, as

COMMON SYMPTOMS AND CONDITIONS THAT MAY BE CAUSED BY STIs

Any itching, burning, or persistent pelvic discomfort should prompt you to see your doctor. However, these four specific symptoms are perhaps the most characteristic of STI. Any one of them is cause for investigation.

Genital Sores

In the United States, genital ulcers or sores generally arise from three STIs: syphilis, herpes simplex virus, or chancroid. Outbreaks of genital ulcers are highly variable; at first they may not look like ulcers at all and may appear as a sudden rash or even a single sore. To determine what caused the ulceration, your doctor may test your blood serum or take a scraping, tissue sample, or fluid from the lesion. In this way, the bacterial or viral agent can be identified so that proper treatment can be undertaken. Antimicrobials may be prescribed, but herpes often clears up on its own. In almost 25 percent of cases, no definitive cause can be pinpointed, which makes determining appropriate therapy more difficult.

Pus-like Discharge

The most prevalent cause of discharge in women is bacterial vaginosis, in which colonies of bacteria known as anaerobes replace normally occurring bacteria within the vagina. The pale white discharge has a fishy scent—the characteristic odor of the chemicals that anaerobic bacteria produce. Though bacterial vaginosis is associated with multiple sex partners, its cause is not fully understood, and many investigators do not consider it an STI. Antibiotics, taken orally or administered intravaginally with an applicator, can clear the infection.

Pelvic Itching

The most common cause of pelvic itching is *Candida albicans*. Many people carry this yeast without symptoms, but it causes vaginitis under certain circumstances that allows its numbers to increase greatly. Common circumstances are pregnancy, diabetes, and antibacterial treatment which removes the normal protective bacteria from the vagina. *Candida* infection is rarely transmitted sexually.

Itch also can be the result of either of two different kinds of minuscule creatures that infest pubic hair: tiny ectoparasites, known as crab lice, that look like tiny sea crabs and are about the diameter of a pinhead, and insect-like creatures known as scabies, which under a powerful microscope look like spiders. Both crab lice and scabies can be transmitted through other ways than just sexual contact—through infested bedding, for example—but they also are linked to multiple sex partners. (Crab lice can possibly be picked up from infestations that manage to survive in bathrooms, although it is not likely.) Generally, both parasites cause intense itching around the pubic area, although in the case of crab lice, tiny splotches of blood on the underwear may be the first sign. In scabies, the initial symptoms may be bumps or a patterned rash that forms curling lines, often on the penis, between fingers, or on buttocks, belly, wrists, and thighs. Symptoms of either can also include low-grade fever and a general feeling of being run down. Both crab lice and scabies can be eradicated with special soaps or shampoo that contain pesticide, and with proper laundering of exposed clothing or bedding.

Burning Urination

One possible cause of burning or stinging during urination is an STI that penetrates the urethra, the tube leading from the bladder. The most common STIs responsible for this condition, known as urethritis, are gonorrhea and chlamydia, but more than a dozen others, including genital herpes, can cause urethritis as well. This symptom, along with sores, often is the first sign of an STI in men. ∎

well as to immigration from those areas. As a result of these and other factors, STIs now know no borders. Pathogens with tongue-twisting names, such as *Lymphogranuloma venereum* and *Granuloma inguinale*—both of which result in genital lesions—have become more commonly diagnosed infections in the United States, even though they previously were rare in temperate climates. The list of STIs has grown from a few familiar names in the era after World War II—syphilis and gonorrhea, among them—to include infections by 19 microbes, several of which are linked to the development of later cancers and to the spread of HIV.

Many experts consider male condoms a good preventive measure because condoms are a barrier to the pathogens that cause STI. Their use by an infected man can prevent transmission to his sexual partner and offer protection to the man who has intercourse with an infected partner.

Though condoms can prevent infection, they are subject to breakage. When a condom ruptures or leaks, intercourse should be halted. Even when the condom does not break, the penis should be withdrawn from the vagina immediately after ejaculation to prevent post-intercourse spillage. Many doctors strongly recommend that all sexual contact that occurs outside of a mutually monogamous relationship include the precaution of using a male condom (see STI Prevention and Condom Use, page 860). In response to the epidemic-like spread of STIs, an international group of physicians and scientists has founded an association to develop affordable means of diagnosing and

limiting STIs, the Sexually Transmitted Disease Diagnostics Initiative. According to this group, and others in the field, the following forecast is likely to become fact unless better intervention takes place.

- More than 300 million new cases of STIs will continue to be documented worldwide annually due to gonorrhea, chlamydia, syphilis, or chancroid.

- Unprotected sexual intercourse will remain the most common reason for serious infection of the genitourinary tract in men and women, from adolescence to middle adulthood, even in developed countries.

- Untreated cases of sexually related diseases, such as syphilis, will result in higher transmission of HIV.

It is critical to seek immediate medical attention if you experience any unusual symptoms in your genitals, and to refrain from sexual activity until you have been examined.

❖ CHANCROID

Symptoms *(What you may experience)* Painful, tender lesions on external genitals (in men, the penis; in women, the vulva); swollen pelvic nodes; formation of an abscess known as a bubo in the groin area.

Signs and laboratory findings *(What the doctor looks for)* Ragged-appearing ulcers (2 to 14 days following exposure) that rupture 1 to 2 days later, leaving a pus-filled discharge; the appearance of a scarlet ring around some lesions; presence of the causative bacterium *Haemophilus ducreyi*, determined through laboratory culture.

What is it? Chancroid, a disease of one or more genital ulcers, was thought for many years to be on the decline in North America. With the advent of HIV, however, the opposite appears to be true. Chancroid shows signs of reemerging as an STI that poses particular dangers. First, it is associated with a heightened risk of HIV transmission. Second, if treatment is delayed, the bubo may become even more inflamed, resulting in severe infection of the urogenital tract. In addition, without proper treatment a phenomenon known as autoinoculation can occur, a process in which the bacteria con-

STI SCREENING IN PREGNANCY

The US Preventive Services Task Force, a panel of physicians and scientists from universities and other institutions, recommends that all pregnant women be tested for herpes simplex virus and for syphilis, that all high-risk pregnant women be tested for gonorrhea and chlamydia, and that HIV testing be done on any pregnant woman with a risk factor for HIV infection, including residence in an area or region with a high infection rate. If these disorders are diagnosed while you are pregnant, your doctor can advise you regarding the precautions necessary to prevent harm to your baby. ■

tinue to infiltrate the body, causing whole new outbreaks of the infection.

What you can do The use of condoms lessens the likelihood of transmission (see page 860).

When to call the doctor The presence of any genital ulcer or sore should prompt an immediate visit to your doctor.

Treatment The antibiotic erythromycin once was standard therapy for this disease. Now, however, increasing resistance to formerly effective antimicrobials requires reliance on multiple drugs, including erythromycin and ceftriaxone (Rocephin) to cure the infection. The bubo often is treated separately with a procedure known as aspiration, in which infected fluid or tissue is withdrawn by means of a syringe and needle.

Tests to exclude other concurrent STIs are usually performed.

Prognosis Good, if treatment is sought early, before autoinoculation occurs or the bubo becomes more enlarged.

❖ CHLAMYDIAL INFECTION

Symptoms *(What you may experience)* Often, none at all. When they do occur symptoms include: pelvic discomfort or abdominal pain; itching around genital area; swollen lymph nodes; fever; fatigue; loss of appetite; pain or aching at the joints, such as knees; pus-like discharge or pain during urination. In men and women, who practice anal sex: rectal bleeding or pain. In women: backache. In men: swelling and tenderness in the penis or prostate.

Signs and laboratory findings *(What the doctor looks for)* Small blister-like formations from which a sample can be extracted, stained, and examined for presence of the bacterium *Chlamydia trachomatis.*

What is it? Chlamydial infection is the most common STI in developed countries. Four million infections occur each year in the United States alone, 10 times the rate of gonorrhea. *Chlamydia* resembles gonorrhea, both in its symptoms and its conse-

quences, which include PID (see page 866) in women and inflammation of the sperm ducts, or epididymitis (see page 1116), in men. Unlike gonorrhea, however, 75 percent of women and 50 percent of men will experience no perceptible symptoms from chlamydial infection.

Chlamydial infections are highly contagious and even people without symptoms are capable of transmitting the disease to a sexual partner. Indeed, the absence of symptoms contributes to its spread because people who are unaware that they are infected pass it to others through vaginal or anal intercourse. Typically, this is how it is spread, although *Chlamydia* can also enter through other parts of the body, particularly the eyes, when touched or rubbed by hands that have come in direct contact with the bacteria.

Chlamydial infection is common among adolescents and young adults in the United States; for this reason, many gynecologists advocate screening for the infection among all women in their early 20s. However, one study has shown that about 25 percent of infected women who take standard *Chlamydia* tests never follow up on their results. Because chlamydial infection can cause acute salpingitis (inflammation of the fallopian tubes) and infertility in women, and urethritis and epididymitis in men, early diagnosis and treatment is essential (for more information on salpingitis and epididymitis, see pages 1116 and 1138; for more information on urethritis, see page 1070). In developing countries, so many infected pregnant women pass the organism to their babies during childbirth that it has become a leading cause of blindness in some parts of the world (see STI Screening in Pregnancy, page 862).

What you can do Male condoms during sexual intercourse can help prevent exposure (see page 860). Infected people who are under treatment should refrain from sexual intercourse, even with the protection of condoms, for at least 7 to 10 days after antibiotics are started.

When to call the doctor Sexually active people who experience any flu-like illness, including swollen lymph nodes or fever, should notify their doctors and include an explanation of their sexual history. Because chlamydial infection often occurs in the absence of symptoms, all partners who have had sexual contact with a single infected person within the previous 2 months should be evaluated.

Treatment   Your doctor will probably prescribe one or more of several antibiotics. Treatment that includes azithromycin (Zithromax) or doxycycline is the most common approach, but an alternate regimen of erythromycin or ofloxacin (Floxin) is also often used. As with other STIs, your sexual partners should be tested for the disease and treated, if necessary, to prevent reinfection.

Prognosis   Good. Treatment usually clears the system of the infection within a week. If symptoms persist, your doctor should be notified—antibiotic resistance may occur (see page 850).

❖ GENITAL HERPES

Symptoms (*What you may experience*) Itchy, painful, or tingly bumps that become small flesh-colored or slightly discolored sores that may occur at any number of sites including on the vulva, in the vagina and cervix, on the penis, in and around the mouth, anus, and buttocks. Flu-like symptoms may be present in the initial outbreak, even before any bumps are noticed: fever; tiredness; headache. Within a few days, the small bumps typically become larger, burst into blisters or open sores, and cause pain, itching, and a burning sensation during urination (possible).

Signs and laboratory findings (*What the doctor looks for*) Confirmation of infection with herpes simplex virus-2 (HSV-2) through laboratory tests on fluid from the sores. If the outbreak occurs without visible sores, your doctor may check for ulcers internally, examining areas of the urinary and genital tract, such as the cervix in women or the urethra in men.

What is it?   Genital herpes, one of the most common STIs, affects more than 1 of every 10 young adults. Reliable estimates are between 500,000 to 1 million new cases of genital herpes diagnosed each year in the United States. Genital herpes is caused by HSV-2, although herpes simplex virus-1

(HSV-1), the virus responsible for cold sores, may occasionally be implicated. There is some evidence that HSV-1 may be a milder form of the disease, and that it diminishes the effect of a HSV-2 infection. But both viruses have a similar course of disease and both usually incubate for about 5 days in the body before outward symptoms surface.

Genital herpes usually is transmitted through intercourse, but it can be passed through other sexual acts as well, such as oral and anal sex. There is a strong association between genital ulcers like those caused by herpes and transmission of HIV. Genital herpes can also be transmitted to newborns through the birth process if the mother has an active infection.

The initial attack generally lasts only 2 to 3 weeks, but subsequent bouts may arise any time after the first infection, even years later. Some people may experience only a single outbreak; others may experience occasional outbreaks throughout their entire lives, often associated with periods of stress. Recurrence sometimes is preceded by a burning sensation or tingling in the genital area.

What you can do   There is no cure for genital herpes and it is a highly contagious infection, so prevention is crucial. The use of condoms for sexually active adults somewhat lessens the likelihood of transmission, but HSV-2 can infect skin of the vulva or the groin, areas which are not covered by the usual condoms. The only truly effective preventative is abstinence, but since that does not appeal to most people, it is wise to use condoms for all sexual contacts, even when there is no evidence of infection (see page 860). Symptoms are not always apparent and the virus can be passed during acts of sexual intimacy even after the eruptions have healed completely. Vaccines against the herpes viruses have been under development for some time, and they remain a future possibility.

When to call the doctor   Consult your doctor if you see any evidence of skin eruptions near genitals or if a sexual partner has revealed a history of the disease. Because genital herpes can affect an infant severely, any pregnant woman who suspects she may have the disease should call her doctor immediately for consultation.

Treatment   Your doctor can prescribe the

antiviral medication acyclovir for a first attack of genital herpes, which helps sores heal. You may also be advised to take sitz baths and over-the-counter painkillers to ease the discomfort. Your doctor may recommend testing for other common STIs, since many people have a concurrent infection. If recurrences are frequent, your doctor may prescribe acyclovir, valacyclovir (Valtrex), or famciclovir (Famvir) to suppress them.

Prognosis The toll inflicted by herpes is emotional, as well as physical. The unpredictable nature of recurrence makes the infection frustrating to people with the infection. To date, no cure has been found for the disease.

Complications can occur, but they are relatively rare in adults. Generally, with proper treatment, the disease runs its course in less than a month and remains in remission for relatively long periods.

❖ GENITAL WARTS

Symptoms *(What you may experience)* Pink or brown cauliflower-like lesions—tiny raised bumps or blisters—on or near the genitals, the anal area, or any other moist skin surface, which may be either isolated or in dense patches. (See page C-35.)

Signs and laboratory findings *(What the doctor looks for)* Genital warts growing in the vaginal or anal area that may not be visible except on internal inspection during a rectal or cervical exam.

What is it? Genital warts, known scientifically as condylomata acuminata, are small, benign protrusions that appear 1 to 2 months following exposure to a viral infection that was passed through sexual contact. Since the 1960s, cases of genital warts have multiplied ninefold, making it an STI of increasing concern. While the warts themselves are benign, the virus that causes genital warts, the human papillomavirus (HPV), has been linked to several cancers, most significantly cervical cancer. HPVs are responsible for most of the 529,000 cases of cervical cancer diagnosed each year representing 65 percent of the cases in industrialized countries and 87 percent of those in developing countries,

according to the WHO. As the virus infiltrates skin cells, it multiplies and forms small, wart-like sores on the penis, labia, cervix, anal region, or within the vagina. These sores tend to be softer and smoother than other types of warts. Infection with HPV is transmitted by direct contact with the skin of an infected person, usually during sexual activity.

What you can do The use of condoms and limiting the number of sexual partners helps prevent the spread of genital warts (see page 860) Condoms are not foolproof, however, since they may not cover all areas that can become infected. A person with genital warts should have them removed to help prevent spread of the disease. Beyond that, certain cautionary measures, such as declining to share towels or grooming aids in a gym or fitness center, can prevent the less common forms of transmission. Frequent hand washing in such settings also has been shown to reduce the spread from touch. The fetus can become infected if the mother carries HPV, so early diagnosis is important.

When to call the doctor Any time you see an outbreak or rash in the genital area that is not easily attributed to an allergic reaction, consult your doctor. Do not scrub the area. Instead, keep it as dry as possible and avoid tight clothing. Do not try to self-treat this problem. Do not use an over-the-counter wart ointment to treat genital warts. If you are diagnosed with this condition, your sexual partner should also be checked by a doctor.

Treatment Several over-the-counter preparations purport to remove warts, but genital warts are best treated by a doctor. Generally, a medication called podophyllum (Podocon-25 or Podofin) is applied topically, then rinsed off several hours later. If warts persist, your doctor may recommend other means of removing the warts, such as cryotherapy (surface freezing) or laser treatment.

Prognosis No one treatment works for everyone and sometimes genital warts prove resistant to several different therapies, so it is important to keep in mind that they are benign. However, even when the warts disappear, an outbreak should not be forgotten. Anyone who has had an infection should notify their doctor of this past history so that regular check-ups can be part of the health care routine. Women with warts in the cervical area should be sure to undergo regular pap-smear testing because the virus has been linked to cervical cancer.

❖ GONORRHEA

Symptoms (*What you may experience*) In men: painful urination that includes white or light-colored discharge, occurring 2 to 14 days after infection. In women: urgent, frequent urination and vaginal discharge about 21 days after infection, but often symptoms are so mild that they escape notice.

Signs (*What the doctor looks for*) Presence of the bacteria through microscopic examination of urethral or vaginal discharge; the sample is placed in a special broth or gel known to spur growth of *Neisseria gonorrhoeae*. A culture to detect chlamydia infection also may be taken, since chlamydia often mimics gonorrhea and vice versa (see Chlamydial Infection, page 863).

What is it? Gonorrhea is an STI caused by the bacterium *Neisseria gonorrhoeae*. More than 400,000 cases are reported in the United States each year. Gonorrhea is a major health problem worldwide, and no group is more affected than adolescents. The disease affects more than 1 percent of young women before they reach age 20. Gonorrhea is more common and severe in women, although in many women symptoms are mild or absent. In addition, the complications of gonorrhea in women—PID, infertility, and premature delivery—occur more commonly and are more serious than the complications that may affect men.

Because gonorrhea may be asymptomatic, it often leads to complications before it is diagnosed. Sterility can occur because the infection can spread into the fallopian tubes, causing PID (see below). In men, symptoms are usually more apparent, but if the infection is not treated, complications such as epididymitis (see page 1138) can occur, causing pain, tenderness, and possible long-term damage. Pregnant women

with gonorrhea can pass the infection to the eyes of the baby during childbirth, which is why hospitals always use special eyedrops in newborns. If untreated, gonorrhea can cause a form of arthritis, as well as severe heart complications.

Although long associated with sexual intercourse, transmission through oral-genital contact has been reported with increasing frequency. This form of the disease is known as gonococcal pharyngitis.

What you can do Condoms help limit the spread of gonorrhea (see page 860). Gonorrhea can be prevented by abstaining from sexual contact with anyone known to have had the disease in the recent past. If you know that you have the disease, abstain from sexual contact until the infection has been completely eradicated. Nonsexual transmission is very rare; casual contact usually poses no health threat. However, the disease can be passed to eyes by rubbing them after touching an infected area.

When to call the doctor Any discharge or unexplained pelvic pain merits evaluation by a doctor. Although pelvic pain has many causes other than an STI, no persistent discomfort should be ignored.

Treatment Because of the growing problem of antibiotic resistance, gonorrhea is difficult to treat and control (see Antibiotic Resistance, page 850). Your doctor will put you on antibiotics, such as ceftriaxone (Rocephin) or ciprofloxacin (Cipro, Cipro IV), until symptoms disappear and the bacteria is gone from your system. People with complications such as PID (see below) may be hospitalized and treated with intravenous antibiotics.

Prognosis If gonorrhea is treated promptly, complications can be prevented and the infection eradicated. Since symptoms, particularly in women, can be mild enough to escape notice, complications may occur before the disease is diagnosed.

❖ PELVIC INFLAMMATORY DISEASE

Symptoms (*What you may experience*) Lower abdominal pain; pain during intercourse; nausea, vomiting, and fever; menstrual periods that are painful and/or lengthy; abnormal vaginal discharge; pain between menstrual periods; painful urination; spotting between menstrual periods (possible).

Signs and laboratory findings *(What the doctor looks for)* Cervical discharge; tenderness of the tubes, ovaries, and cervix on pelvic examination; cervical infection with *Neisseria gonorrhea* or *Chlamydiatrachomatis*; abscess of the tube or ovary shown through ultrasound test.

What is it? Pelvic inflammatory disease, or PID, is one of the most serious complications of STI in women; it is also the chief preventable cause of infertility. Both *Neisseria gonorrhea* and *Chlamydia trachomatis* infection (see Gonorrhea, page 866 and Chlamydial Infection, page 863) can lead to PID. Even with proper antibiotic therapy, about one of every four women who has PID will have lingering problems, such as internal scarring. When PID occurs from an STI or other bacterial invader, it is an exogenous infection. But sometimes naturally occurring bacterial inhabitants of the body can cause PID. The reason for this kind of invasion, known as an endogenous infection, remains somewhat elusive. However, it is important to recognize that PID is not exclusively caused by STIs.

PID occurs as infection spreads from the vagina and the cervix to the upper part of the reproductive tract: the uterus, fallopian tubes, and ovaries. When it involves the uterus, it is called endometritis; when it involves the tubes, salpingitis. Occasionally, the infection involves the tube and ovary, developing a localized abscess, called a tubo-ovarian abscess (see page 1124).

PID can also occur from infection with naturally occurring bacterial inhabitants of the reproductive tract, and from streptococcal and anaerobic bacteria, gram-negative rods (usual invaders of the urinary tract), and *Haemophilus influenzae* bacteria.

The symptoms, particularly lower abdominal pain, can mimic a wide variety of other conditions from which PID must be differentiated by x-ray and laboratory tests. These possibilities include ectopic pregnancy, appendicitis, hemorrhage, rupture or torsion (twisting) of an ovarian cyst, endometriosis, septic (infected) abortion, urinary tract infection, and gastrointestinal infection.

The disorder most commonly strikes young, sexually active women, especially those who have had multiple sex partners, who have never borne children. Smoking, frequent douching, and the use of an intrauterine contraceptive device (IUD) also may increase the risk for PID.

What you can do PID is one of the most serious complications of STI and major cause of infertility in women. Yet in many cases the disease is preventable, if you follow the precautions necessary to prevent STIs. If you are sexually active—particularly with multiple sexual partners—prevent infection by safe-sex practices, such as using barrier contraception (see STI Prevention and Condom Use, page 860). If you are diagnosed with PID, your sexual partner should be tested as well, even if he shows no symptoms, to prevent reinfection.

When to call the doctor If you suspect that you may have been exposed to an STI, see your doctor for testing. In addition, anytime you develop persistent abdominal discomfort, especially if associated with vaginal discharge, fever, or a rash, consult your doctor. Although abdominal pain has many causes other than PID, none of them should be ignored.

Treatment Treatment with antibiotic medication to eradicate the infection is the cornerstone of therapy. The choice of medication should be tailored to the infecting organisms. Common choices include cefoxitin (Mefoxin), cefotetan (Cefotan) plus doxycycline (Doxy or Vibramycin), and clindamycin (Cleocin) plus gentamicin (Garamycin). PID that causes severe pain or fever usually requires hospitalization for intravenous antibiotic therapy and to rule out any other possible reason for the symptoms, which could include ectopic pregnancy, appendicitis, and pelvic abscess. Pregnant women, adolescents, or women who are HIV positive may require hospitalization if they develop PID.

In cases where PID has advanced, surgery may be indicated to remove or repair damaged tissues, including the reproductive organs (uterus, ovaries, and fallopian tubes). As a result, PID can lead to infertility in women. For more information on PID, see page 1116.

Prognosis Even with appropriate treatment, 25 percent of women with PID develop long-term problems, such as recurrent episodes of infection, painful intercourse (due to scarring), chronic pelvic pain, and greatly increased risk for ectopic pregnancy. Recurrent episodes and associated problems can in rare cases lead to the need for a hysterectomy. With each successive episode of infection, a progressively increased risk of infertility occurs; 20 percent of women develop infertility from a single episode of PID, 35 percent after a second, and 75 percent after a third.

❖ SYPHILIS

Symptoms *(What you may experience)* One or more chancre sores that resemble large bug bites, often hard and painless, on the genitals or in and around the mouth; swollen lymph nodes in the pelvic area; unexplained rash, often on the palms of the hands and soles of the feet; patchy hair loss; fatigue; tender joints.

Signs and laboratory findings *(What the doctor looks for)* The bacterial microorganism responsible for the infection, *Treponema pallidum*, which looks like a tightly coiled bedspring under the microscope. Diagnosis usually is made by examining swabbings or scrapings from the chancre, or if sores are absent, by tests on blood serum.

What is it? Syphilis is a highly contagious disease that is spread primarily by sexual activity, including oral and anal intercourse, but occasionally is transmitted by prolonged kissing or close body contact with an infected person. Even touching a sore that occurs from syphilis can result in disease transmission because the bacteria are capable of invading skin that appears unbroken but that may have minute abrasions. Pregnant women who have the disease may pass it to the fetus; this form of the infection, called congenital syphilis, can cause abnormalities or even fetal death. The incidence of syphilis has been rising steadily in the United States since the mid-1980s due in part to the HIV epidemic.

In the early stages, the symptoms are so variable that syphilis often is called "the great imitator" because it can be mistaken for many other conditions. Typically, the disease occurs in distinct stages. The primary stage occurs within 10 to 90 days after exposure, when the chancre sores or other symptoms occur. The chancre heals without leaving a scar within 2 to 6 weeks. Because the lesion is painless, the primary stage may go unrecognized by the infected person. The secondary stage may overlap with the primary stage. It begins within 6 weeks to 6 months after exposure and may last 1 to 3 months. The characteristic symptom is a rosy rash. It may appear anywhere on the body, but a rash on the palms and soles is characteristic of syphilis. During the secondary stage, symptoms may become systemic and include weight loss, fever, and patchy hair loss. After the secondary stage comes the latent stage in which the infection lies dormant in the body without outward symptoms. If the syphilis is not treated, a person may progress to the tertiary stage, characterized by serious disorders such as heart and brain dysfunction. If the diagnosis is not made, syphilis can remain undetected for decades until severe health problems arise.

What you can do Avoid close or intimate contact with an infected person. During the primary and secondary stages in particular, all skin lesions are highly infectious. Since people with syphilis may be unaware they are infected, be sure to use a condom during sexual activity (see page 860). If you have been diagnosed with syphilis and are undergoing treatment, do not engage in sexual contact until follow-up tests have confirmed its eradication.

When to call the doctor If syphilis is diagnosed early and treated, it can be completely cured. Sexually active people who fail to use condoms and who are not in a monogamous relationship should seek medical treatment for any unexplained illness, no matter how mild.

Treatment Your doctor is likely to prescribe penicillin or, if you are allergic to penicillin, doxycycline or tetracycline instead. After administration of any of these antibiotics, tests on blood serum are conducted at 1, 3, 6, and 12 months, until the complete absence of disease is confirmed. Many people treated for syphilis will develop fever, headache, chills, and inflammation after treatment, which can be treated with antihistamines.

Prognosis Syphilis is curable. With prompt diagnosis and treatment, all that is usually required are strong doses of oral or injectable antibiotics. However, if treated in the last stage of the disease, there may be lingering damage to internal organs and to the central nervous system, even after the infection is eradicated.

❖ TRICHOMONIASIS

Symptoms (What you may experience) In women: profuse green or yellow vaginal discharge that may have a foul odor; extreme itchiness. In men: no symptoms. In both sexes: mild irritation or slight burning sensation on urination.

Signs and laboratory findings (What the doctor looks for) In women: vaginal discharge that may be evident only on examination of the cervix, in men: epididymitis or prostatitis (inflammation of the prostate). In both sexes: diagnosis is confirmed by mucus samples taken by direct swab of the genitals or by special testing of a urine sample.

What is it? Trichomonas vaginalis is a tiny parasite, known as a protozoan, that moves by waving wand-like tentacles. Trichomoniasis often accompanies gonorrhea and it is a fairly common STI even in developed countries, due to a high prevalence in prostitutes. In women, it is one of the most common causes of vaginitis (see page 1109).

What you can do Condom usage in nonmonogamous relationships has proven effective in diminishing transmission of the disease (see page 860). However, trichomoniasis infection rates cannot be explained solely by sexual intercourse, so some of the transmission remains ill defined. However, the same preventative measures that apply to STIs also apply to trichomoniasis.

When to call the doctor If you experience an unusual discharge, particularly one accompanied by pain on urination or during intercourse, consult your doctor.

Treatment A course of metronidazole can cure the disease.

Prognosis Good; relapses are rare, although reinfection is common.

Food-Borne and Water-Borne Infections

In terms of public health, food-borne and water-borne illnesses deserve special attention. Of all the routes of transmission a pathogen can take, food and water provide the potentially quickest way for infection to spread. Other infections, such as widespread flu, may have more morbid consequences, but because the travel of the microorganisms that cause them requires direct exposure to a carrier or infected person, they typically take longer to develop into actual epidemics.

In addition to food poisoning, traveler's diarrhea, and viral gastroenteritis discussed at the end of this section, parasitic infections may also be spread through food and water. Parasitic infections are discussed on page 892.

WATER-BORNE INFECTIONS

Each year, swimmers and surfers on American coasts from Southern California to South Florida suffer what some beach goers have dubbed the Malibu flu, a name derived from one of the first places it was described. Bacterial and viral illnesses picked up in the Pacific Ocean remain a source of summertime illness. But it is not ocean swimming alone that has been traced to outbreaks of "swimmer's flu." In Oregon several years ago a nonfatal epidemic of *Escherichia coli* 0157:H7—the same bacterium implicated in infecting children through undercooked beef—was traced to a recreational swimming area where it had contaminated the water. In one case in Great Britain, 30 people became ill after using a pool that a sick swimmer had vomited in during the opening day of the facility. Inadequate chlorination was blamed for the outbreak. The best prevention in these situations, say experts, is to make sure you do not swallow water and thoroughly wash after swimming.

For people who go camping or hiking, the urge to quench one's thirst at a cool stream or spring should be resisted. Even

WHAT TO LOOK FOR IN A WATER PURIFIER

If you wish to put your water through several extra filtration steps to be on the safe side, water purifiers are helpful devices. Keep in mind, however, that most medical experts advise against relying solely on such a system if you are severely immunocompromised. For individuals with impaired immune function, bringing water to a vigorous boil for 10 minutes is safer than using a purifier. High temperature kills most microbial pathogens. Check the label or attached information for the following before you purchase a water-purifying system.

Certification National Sanitation Foundation certification means that contaminant-reduction claims are considered true by that organization, and also that the system is found to be structurally sound.

Bacteriostatic measures This is a statistic based on how much the system limits the passage or growth of certain bacteria. If you have an illness that has weakened your immune system, this measure should be checked with your doctor after a vendor has explained the numbers to you.

Chlorine class Chlorine is widely used for water disinfection. But it can produce taste and odor changes that may make you think twice about drinking water that is not flavored. A class-1 rating aims to reduce chlorine by 75 percent or more; a class-2 refers to 50 to 74 percent reduction of chlorine; a class-3 a 25 to 49 percent reduction.

Particulate classification This refers to the removal of tiny particles from the water, according to their size. Class-1 systems remove the tiniest particles; class 6 guarantees removal only of particles more than 50 times larger than particles removed by a class-1 purifier. Such sediments are minute, but, if they are not filtered out, cloudy water is likelier to result.

VOC claim This acronym stands for volatile organic chemicals and refers to a long list of compounds and chemicals that the system purports to reduce. ■

---

died after an outbreak of *E. coli* was linked to unpasteurized apple juice.

Even the usually safe drinking water of towns and cities can cause illness on occasion. In 1993 in Milwaukee more than 400,000 cases of cryptosporidiosis, which can cause flu-like symptoms, were reported. *Cryptosporidium* infection, a common parasitic cause of diarrhea, can be spread through food or person-to-person contact, but water is the most common route. The infection causes nausea, watery diarrhea, fever, and abdominal cramping. The organism, *Cryptosporidium parvum*, has been found in some beverages, as well as in wells and springs. The Milwaukee outbreak eventually was attributed to contamination of the city's water supply.

In some parts of the country, boiling water is recommended during seasonal variations in the water table. This is particularly true for people who are immunocompromised, which means they have weakened immune systems that make them more vulnerable to pathogens. In other areas, many residents purchase home filtration systems, which can be bought at home-improvement centers (see What to Look for In a Water Purifier, above). Keep in mind that municipal water supplies are required to meet federal disinfection standards and benign sediments can give water a cloudy, tainted appearance, even when it is perfectly safe to drink.

crystal-clear water can harbor harmful parasites, bacteria, and viruses. If you believe that the drinking water wherever you are is not pure, use bottled water for drinking. If you need to purify water yourself, see above.

Boiling water also may be necessary after a weather-related catastrophe such as flooding, when your area's drinking water may have become tainted.

The process of sterilization by heating is termed pasteurization. Named for Louis Pasteur, the French scientist who discovered that high temperatures could kill harmful bacteria, pasteurization is a process the US government requires for milk and many other foods. Many fruit drinks have been a long-time exception. However, federal officials now ask juice producers to indicate on labels that their products are unpasteurized. In 1996 several children became ill and one

FOOD-BORNE INFECTIONS

A number of pathogens are transmitted by food; poor hygiene in handling food and inadequate cooking or refrigeration are responsible for the majority of contamination cases. Simple, common-sense precautions can prevent this transmission (see page 61).

Perhaps the most widely reported food-borne pathogen has been *E. coli*, a bacterium that makes its home within many living creatures—including you. It has been found to occur in a potentially deadly strain known as 0157:H7. *E. coli* 0157:H7 has contaminated meat on several occasions in the United States, as well as in Japan. Less than a decade ago on the US West Coast, several children developed hemolytic uremia syndrome, a potentially fatal form of kidney failure, from undercooked beef patties at a fast-food chain. In 1997 similar events unfolded when tainted hamburger patties turned up in Colorado.

The *E. coli* 0157:H7 organism makes a toxin that is similar to toxins made by other bacteria, such as *Shigella*. It kills cells, causing the symptoms of abdominal pain and blood in the stools. It may also enter the bloodstream and cause destruction of red blood cells and kidney failure. This combination is called the hemolytic-uremic syndrome, which usually affects children under 10 years old. Adults are less likely to develop toxic symptoms, but if they do they may also develop blood clots and coma due to brain damage. This combination of the destruction of red blood cells, kidney failure, formation of blood clots, and coma is a condition called thrombotic thrombocytopenic purpura and has a very high mortality rate. It is because of these severe consequences that *E. coli* 0157:H7 has attracted so much public notice and governmental regulation.

Although *E. coli* 0157:H7 has made headlines, another bacterium, *Salmonella*, is far more common. All known forms of salmonella are pathogenic to humans but their effect varies depending on the species. One form causes short-lived food poisoning, another typhoid fever. People frequently pick this up while traveling (see Traveler's Diarrhea, page 874 and Sources of Infectious Disease During Travel, page 899), but they can get it from their own kitchen counters. Salmonellosis can be contracted from cutting boards and table tops that have been used to slice contaminated poultry or other food. Chicken is more commonly associated with salmonella contamination than any other animal and undercooked eggs often are implicated in outbreaks. The bacterium is sometimes colloquially referred to as the "picnic pestilence" because it often affects several people who have ingested a food, such as mayonnaise-laden salad, that has been growing the bacteria.

Thanks to Americans' growing preference for fresh fruits and vegetables, more fresh produce is being imported than ever before. In some cases, there are infectious consequences. Many off-season fruit and vegetables, such as Guatemalan raspberries and Mexican strawberries, are becoming available year-round. But as outbreaks of *Cyclospora* and hepatitis A have shown, these fruits can pack more than fresh flavor. Federal and state health officials have reported picking up potentially pathogenic bacteria even in the florets of cauliflower and the stalks of broccoli; the problem may lie with pathogens in the water used to hydrate the plants. Since these foods are often eaten raw, it is particularly difficult to protect oneself from infection.

In 1997, the US Food and Drug Administration (FDA) approved meat irradiation, a process in which fresh and frozen meat are exposed to levels of radiation that kill disease-causing microbes. The decision to allow irradiation of beef, lamb, and pork followed earlier approval by the FDA of the same control measures for poultry. Before issuing approval, the FDA conducted a scientific review to make certain that irradiation does not affect food in any way except to sterilize it. Agency officials concluded that neither the nutritional value nor the taste and appearance of the food is altered through irradiation.

Irradiation procedures have been used for decades, but not on a widespread basis in the food industry, although the process has been endorsed by both the American Medical Association and the WHO. The FDA's approval, it is hoped, will significantly reduce the possibility that Americans will be exposed to potentially harmful food-borne microbes. However, irradiation only is an additional tool for eradicating meat contaminants, not a replacement for other safety measures. Consumers still need to be careful about choosing, preparing, and cooking poultry, meat, and fresh vegetables or fruit.

Nonetheless, federal authorities have begun to survey some food-borne pathogens more intensely, as part of a collaborative effort with state public-health officials. Their list of priorities includes *E. coli* 0157:H7 and *Salmonella*, along with other organisms that have also come under closer scrutiny. All typically cause gastrointestinal problems, such as diarrhea, and all are transmitted by food. The list includes:

Campylobacter Transmission typically is by the fecal-oral route and results from inadequate hand washing by food handlers. It has also been found to contaminate 70 to 90 percent of chicken, and so can be spread by

MEAT CONTAMINATION

In August 1997, an estimated 25 million tons of processed beef were pulled from freezer shelves at restaurants and supermarkets—the largest meat recall in this country's history. Federal officials traced the contamination, from *E. coli 0157*, to a Nebraska meat-processing plant. But by the time the beef was being discarded by food outlets, more than a dozen people had reported symptoms. Although the precise way the potentially lethal *E. coli* got into the meat remains open to debate, the original site was tracked to a slaughter facility. Generally, *E. coli* is associated with fecal matter, so contamination could have occurred at one of several points in the processing or packaging.

How did it happen? The US Department of Agriculture tries to enforce the government's stringent controls on the processing of meat; it conducts inspections of facilities that butcher, package, store, and sell meat. However, sometimes the system fails to detect contamination along the chain of events that takes livestock from pasture lands to serving platters. After such incidents, the FDA approved meat irradiation, a process in which meat is exposed to disease-killing levels of radiation to rid meat and poultry of infectious microbes. Also, the USDA is shifting from older "sniff and poke" forms of inspection to more modern culture-based methods.

One way that you can protect yourself is to always thoroughly cook beef, poultry, and fish at a high temperature. Meat that would be considered very well-done is thought to pose little threat. If you are at a restaurant and receive a steak that is pink or reddish when you cut into it, you may be running a risk of contamination. In your own home, cooking steak to 145°F on a meat thermometer will ensure that your meat is safe. ∎

improper food preparation. This organism causes diarrhea, cramping, and abdominal pain. In recent years, this bacterium has been responsible for significant outbreaks of infection, particularly on the west coast. It causes such severe, sharp pain that it can be initially mistaken for appendicitis.

THE WISH LIST

History has shown that the best formula for avoiding infection is to take the straightforward, preventive steps that are summed up in the acronym WISH.

- *Wash* hands, food, clothing, bedding, and launderable household items routinely, as well as fresh food products.

- *Immunize* yourself against all vaccine-preventable diseases if possible.

- *Seek* medical advice from your doctor when appropriate and, in the meantime, follow recommendations of a medically reviewed source book, like this one, that stresses preventive measures such as condom use to prevent STIs and precautions to avoid food-borne and water-borne infections.

- *Heat* water and food appropriately, particularly when in areas where sterilization is not assured. ∎

Listeria This bacteria is found in soil and feces. Transmission usually occurs through dairy products. Unfortunately, pasteurization does not always kill all the *Listeria* contaminants in tainted dairy products. Pregnant women and their developing fetuses are at particular risk from listeriosis. In adults, the infection can result in bacterial meningitis, sepsis or gastroenteritis.

Salmonella As mentioned on page 871, transmission occurs most often through contaminated poultry and eggs. However, some outbreaks have occurred where this link was not apparent, at least initially. For example, one brief epidemic was traced to ice cream, another to alfalfa sprouts imported from Finland. *Salmonella* bacteria often have a penicillin-destroying enzyme, so other strong antibiotics are required to kill them.

Shigella Transmission occurs from exposure to what doctors refer to as the "Four Fs"—fingers, flies, food, and feces. *Shigella* bacteria cause sickness that closely resemble salmonellosis, for which it is sometimes mistaken, but bloody diarrhea is more common in *Shigella* infection. Fortunately, the treatment regimen is the same.

Vibrio Transmission most often occurs through tainted seafood or seawater exposure (see Safety Hints for Buying Seafood, page 875). Though this organism can cause cholera, in the United States it is associated with a form of food poisoning. The diarrhea can be explosive and painful, but generally is short-lived.

Yersinia Transmission is through contaminated food or by contact with animal feces. The diarrhea closely matches the kind caused by *Salmonella* and *Shigella*.

All of these organisms invade and irritate the lining of the intestine, which causes the intestinal tract to secrete copious amounts of mucus to help fight off the invaders. This, in turn, makes stools runny and interferes with the entire digestive process, particularly food absorption. Because the bacteria actually invade the body and grow inside the tissues, this kind of food poisoning is associated with fever, abdominal pain, and sometimes blood in the stools. In children or seniors, these bacteria can invade the bloodstream, and may cause either sepsis or infections of distant organs such as the heart (see Endocarditis, page 816) or a joint (see Infectious Arthritis, page 650).

What should you do if you come down with a case of food-related diarrhea? See a doctor, but in the meantime, drink plenty of fluids. If you experience symptoms of dehydration, such as less-frequent urination, your doctor may recommend a commercial rehydration solution, such as the electrolyte mixtures available for children. In an emergency, you can make your own rehydration solution by mixing $1^1/_2$ tsp of salt and $1^1/_2$ tbs of sugar in 1 pt of boiled water.

❖ FOOD POISONING DUE TO BACTERIAL TOXINS

Symptoms (*What you may experience*) Abrupt, generally violent onset of vomiting or diarrhea; cramps; abdominal pain; general weakness; malaise.

Signs and laboratory findings (*What the doctor looks for*) Food poisoning due to bacterial toxins is not a real infection (see below), so fever and high white blood cell count do not occur. There is no bacterial invasion of the bowel wall, so abdominal pain is mild or absent. The person may show signs of dehydration such as pallor, cold extremities, low blood pressure, tachycardia (rapid heartbeat), and confusion or coma.

What is it? Bacteria grow in food and make toxins which are absorbed when the food is eaten. The bacteria do not invade the body and may even be dead before the food is eaten. Reheating food often kills bacteria, but does not always inactivate toxins. The most common cause is a toxin made by *Staphylococcus aureus*. This organism comes from skin and may pass from the hands of kitchen staff into food. Another common cause of toxic food poisoning is *Bacillus cereus*, which is almost completely incapable of causing invasive disease.

Sometimes food is contaminated before cooking and the bacteria are hardy enough to survive the cooking process, or the food is not thoroughly cooked. Commonly, food becomes contaminated by a food handler after the dish is prepared, or by a cutting board. This form of food poi-

soning, although physically wrenching, usually lasts no longer than 24 to 36 hours. Some people may experience vomiting only, or diarrhea only; others may be afflicted with both at about the same time. This condition often begins with nausea followed by vomiting that may include what are known as dry heaves, meaning that the stomach has been emptied of food but its spasms persist, and may be accompanied by diarrhea. Fevers are extremely rare with bacterial toxin food poisoning. If you have a fever, this suggests an invasive bacterial infection.

What you can do Cook food thoroughly. It is equally important to maintain food at 4°C storage temperature, particularly egg salad, mayonnaise, rice pudding, cream, tartar sauce, and fried rice.

For bacteria to make toxins, food must become a good "culture dish" and must sit at room temperature for several hours or at warm temperatures outdoors as can happen at a picnic. Avoid vats of mayonnaise sitting out at dubious temperatures at fast food restaurants; choose mustard or catsup instead. Before eating in any restaurant, check for the restaurant's Health Department Grade, which, by law, should be posted for public viewing somewhere in the restaurant; in many restaurants, the certificate hangs on the wall near the rest rooms. If the grade is anything below an "A," do not eat there. If you become sick after eating at a restaurant, find out immediately if anyone else in your party has also become sick. If so, report it to the health department as soon as possible, so that the restaurant's food-handling procedures can be reviewed.

Most cases of food poisoning resolve on their own after 1 or 2 miserable days. It is essential to avoid dehydration. Keep drinking fluids. Even very small amounts of fluid taken regularly can help prevent dehydration. Store-bought or homemade oral rehydration fluid is the best thing to drink if dehydration is severe (see above).

When to call the doctor If you cannot stop vomiting or having diarrhea, if you have a high fever—which may suggest a different diagnosis—or if you faint or become weak and light-headed after prolonged vomiting or diarrhea.

Treatment If the diarrhea is severe, your doctor may recommend an intestine-slowing drug such as loperamide (Imodium), if you can keep it down. If you cannot stop vomiting, you may need intravenous fluids or, if your symptoms are severe, a prescription suppository such as prochlorperazine (Compazine) or promethazine (Phenergan).

Prognosis Excellent. This is a short-lived disease. Believe it or not, your appetite will return in a few days.

❖ TRAVELER'S DIARRHEA

Symptoms (What you may experience) Abrupt onset of three or more episodes of diarrhea in 24 hours, or one or two episodes of diarrhea accompanied by nausea, vomiting, weakness and/or fever; painful, explosive gas; fatigue; cramps; appetite loss.

Signs and laboratory findings (What the doctor looks for) The presence of white blood cells, called fecal leukocytes, in the stool, suggesting an invasive bacterial infection. Less commonly: evidence of parasites or amoebae in a stool culture. The most compelling aid to diagnosis is your recent whereabouts; if you have recently traveled out of the country, be sure to tell your doctor.

What is it? In most cases, traveler's diarrhea is a bacterial infection caused by unsanitary handling of food. The infection is transmitted by the fecal-oral route; it is mainly caused when food handlers do not adequately wash their hands after they use the bathroom. The most common culprit—in an estimated 40 to 70 percent of cases—is *E. coli* bacteria. Less common are parasitic infections, such as giardiasis, caused by a protozoan, or amebiasis, caused by an amoeba. Traveler's diarrhea is most common among visitors to Mexico, Morocco, El Salvador, Kenya, Bangladesh, and other parts of Central and South America, Africa, and Asia. Mercifully, this disease, although it can be severe, is usually of limited duration. In 80 percent of cases, it lasts less than a week; in most people, it lasts 3 or 4 days.

What you can do Traveler's diarrhea is preventable, although for thousands of conscientious tourists each year, one lapse is all it takes. For instance, many travelers remember to drink bottled water, but brush their teeth with tap water or drink a bottled cola with ice cubes made from tap water. If you are traveling in an area where this problem commonly afflicts tourists, your motto should be: "Boil it, cook it, peel it, or forget it." Avoid ice, tap water, vegetables, salads, foods sold by street vendors, and caffeinated beverages from soda fountains. Drink bottled water, sodas, wines, beer, tea, and coffee; brush your teeth with bottled water. If you wear contact lenses, use bottled water to rinse them. To be on the safe side, you might want to take your own supply of bottled water from home; estimate at least one quart-sized bottle per person per day. Limit your fruits to foods you can peel, such as oranges or bananas; grapes, for instance, are probably not safe. Talk to your doctor about treating traveler's diarrhea prophylactically. There are several medications that are proving effective in preventing this disease including bismuth subsalicylate (Pepto Bismol) or antibiotics. Other treatments are based on introducing beneficial microbes into the intestinal tract to prevent colonization by bad bugs during travel. These formulations are known as "probiotics." The most common one may be right in your own refrigerator; some studies have shown that the *Lactobacillus* bacteria in yogurt can prevent diarrhea. Medications that contain these infection-fighting microorganisms are not yet widely available in the United States, however, so your best strategy may be prevention.

When to call the doctor Call your doctor if you have a high fever—over 101°F—bloody diarrhea, or are unable to stop vomiting.

Treatment It is essential not to become dehydrated. Keep drinking fluids, if you can keep them down. If you are unable to drink, you may need intravenous fluids. If your fever is less than 101°F and the diarrhea is not bloody, your doctor may prescribe an antimotility drug such as Lomotil to slow down the intestine and combat the diarrhea. You also may need a round of antibiotics. If you have a parasitic infection, you will need an antiparasitic; the particular medication will depend on which parasite is involved.

Prognosis Excellent. Although symptoms can be intense, traveler's diarrhea is almost always a short-lived disease.

❖ VIRAL GASTROENTERITIS

Symptoms *(What you may experience)* Diarrhea; nausea; abdominal cramps; vomiting; muscle ache; low grade fever; loss of appetite; weakness; malaise. Symptoms may persist for 7 to 10 days.

Signs and laboratory findings *(What the doctor looks for)* One of the common pathogens that cause viral gastroenteritis in children, the rotavirus, determined by a specific stool test called Rotazyme which your doctor may decide to give you. However, for most causes of viral gastroenteritis there is no specific diagnostic test and no specific treatment.

What is it? Viral gastroenteritis is a viral infection of the intestine. Like traveler's diarrhea, it is most commonly transmitted by the fecal-oral route and may be caused when food handlers do not adequately wash their hands after they use the bathroom. Viral gastroenteritis can also be spread through a contaminated water supply, including through shellfish that inhabit water contaminated by raw sewage.

The causative pathogen in food or water in this case is a virus, not bacteria. Viral gastroenteritis can be caused by several viruses, but the two most important causes of viral gastroenteritis are rotavirus and the Norwalk virus. Rotavirus is widespread, with three different viral forms that can infect people. It may be the most common cause of infectious diarrhea in the world. Procedures that satisfactorily prevent the spread of bacteria and parasites do not keep rotavirus out of the food supply. It is found worldwide. It can be spread through physical contact, such as a handshake, as well as by utensils or objects, such as silverware. The Norwalk virus commonly is found in bodies of water, and can infect swimmers who frequent lakes and pools, though shellfish and salad ingredients are the most common causes of actual outbreaks.

What you can do Rotavirus tends to be endemic in daycare centers. If your children are in daycare or play with other children, or even with other children's toys, urge them to wash their hands—and wash your

own—as often as possible. The rotavirus vaccine is approved; over time, its use in children can be expected to reduce the incidence of disease in adults.

In addition, avoid raw shellfish.

When to call the doctor Most adults with viral gastroenteritis are merely inconvenienced for a day or two. The presence of high fever, abdominal pain, or incessant vomiting suggests a different diagnosis and should prompt a call to your doctor. People who are truly at risk of death from rotavirus infection are children under the age of 1 year and older seniors.

Treatment To treat the diarrhea your doctor will probably recommend an antimotility agent, which slows down intestinal function, such as loperamide (Imodium). If your symptoms are severe and dehydration is a worry, you may need intravenous fluids or a prescription suppository such as prochlorperazine or promethazine to ease the nausea and vomiting. Like other intestinal infections, viral gastroenteritis tends to run its course fairly quickly.

Prognosis Excellent.

SAFETY HINTS FOR BUYING SEAFOOD

Never buy or prepare fish without observing the following recommendations from the US Food and Drug Administration.

- Make sure that the fish has a salt-and-sea odor—a smell reminiscent of the ocean. This helps guard against buying one with any spoilage.

- Examine the fish. In a fresh catch, gills should be rosy and eyes should be shiny, not cloudy or enlarged. Flesh should retain much of its original color.

- Look at how the fish are laid out by the vendor. Are they on a bed of cold, clear-colored ice? Are the fish spread adequately apart? If they are fresh and unfrozen, they should not be touching, even if they are displayed dockside.

- If you buy a fish that has been frozen, cook and eat it as soon as it is thawed. Fish that are bought fresh can be stored in your freezer for weeks without worry.

- Make sure shellfish, such as oysters and clams, have shells that are clamped shut. If they are not closed, do not buy them. During cooking the shells should unclasp as they are heated. If shells do not open during cooking, do not eat the contents. ■

Multisystem Infectious Diseases

Many disorders caused by viruses, bacteria, and fungi involve more than one body system and cause varied symptoms. Within this book we have generally discussed disorders according to the body part or system most affected by them. Thus, pneumonia is covered in Chapter 18, Lungs and Respiratory System, and strep throat in Chapter 16, Ear, Nose, and Throat. The following multisystem infections, however, simply do not fit into a single category as defined by body parts and systems.

❖ INFECTIOUS MONONUCLEOSIS

Symptoms *(What you may experience)* Fever; swollen lymph nodes in the neck; heavy white-purplish patches on the tonsils and throat; tenderness in the left or right upper abdomen; a red measles-like rash (occasionally); fatigue; malaise, or loss of sense of well-being.

Signs and laboratory findings *(What the doctor looks for)* Tender lymph nodes in the neck; enlarged and tender spleen or liver; elevation of liver enzymes detected by the "mono spot" blood test (a rapid test to detect antibodies), elevation of lymphocyte numbers, a kind of white blood cell. In some cases abnormalities of the heart's electrical activity, as shown by an electrocardiogram, may develop.

What is it? Mononucleosis derives its name from the presence of increased numbers of monocytes, or atypical lymphocytes, found in the blood samples of infected people. The disorder arises from infection by the Epstein-Barr virus, a member of the family of herpes viruses. Infection can occur at any age, but the incidence peaks in late adolescence and early adulthood, between ages 10 and 35. The virus first causes fever, sore throat, and a rash (in about 15 percent of cases) and can seem much like streptococcal pharyngitis, or strep throat. In fact, about a third of people who develop mononucleosis also have strep throat. The viral infection persists much longer than a typical sore throat, however, and after a time, other symptoms may occur, such as hepatitis (liver inflammation), neuritis (nerve inflammation), meningitis or encephalitis (inflammation of the brain or its covering tissues), and myocarditis (inflammation of the heart muscle).

What you can do Rest, particularly if you have fever. Drink plenty of fluids. If you have any pain or discomfort in either side of the upper abdomen, but especially the left side, avoid heavy physical contact, whether through work or sports, because this symptom suggests enlargement of the liver or spleen. These organs, when enlarged, can be bruised or damaged—and can even rupture—from a hard blow to the side. Once the diagnosis of mononucleosis is made, you can prevent the spread to other susceptible people by avoiding intimate oral contact; the virus passes in saliva and upper respiratory secretions—hence its common name, "the kissing disease."

When to call the doctor When sore throat or fever persists for more than 48 hours, especially if accompanied by a rash and swollen lymph glands, you should visit your doctor right away. Without testing, there is no way to be sure that the symptoms are not caused by *Streptococcus* or some other treatable bacterial pathogen.

SEPTIC SHOCK

Septic shock is not in itself an infection; it is the body's response to the presence of large numbers of bacteria in the bloodstream. Rarely, shock can be produced by overwhelming viral or fungal infection, by malaria, or even by noninfectious immunological events such as incompatible blood transfusions. But at least 90 percent of septic shock of cases are due to bacteria.

Septic shock is initially characterized by fever; low blood pressure; quick, rapid breathing; and lethargy. Untreated, it leads to multiple organ failure. If three or more organs fail, the mortality rate is over 90 percent. Sepsis alone is fatal in 30 to 40 percent of cases.

The source of the bacteria varies. There may be an obvious portal of entry such as a wound. The person may have a disease associated with bacteria in the blood, such as meningococcal meningitis; in some cases the source may not be apparent. Septic shock is the major cause of death in people who suffer severe burns. The burned flesh serves as a culture for certain sepsis-associated bacteria, known as gram-negative bacteria for their capacity to absorb a particular kind of tissue-staining chemical. Septic shock is thought to be on the rise because of the longer lives many Americans now enjoy. Treatments and conditions associated with elderly care, such as catheterization and bed sores, have increased the incidence of this condition. ■

Treatment No specific treatment has been developed yet to eradicate the Epstein-Barr virus. For now, time and your immune system do the job. However, treatment may include eradication of a simultaneous strep infection with antibiotics. The doctor must take care in choosing this antibiotic; the administration of amoxicillin, an antibiotic in the penicillin family, brings out a fiery, measles-like rash in 90 percent of people with mononucleosis.

Prognosis Excellent in most cases. Fever and sore throat usually disappear in 7 to 10 days, swollen lymph glands and enlarged liver or spleen in a month. All symptoms may not completely resolve right away; weakness and fatigue linger for several months. The prognosis can be poor if rupture of the spleen or encephalitis occurs.

❖ CHRONIC FATIGUE SYNDROME

Symptoms *(What you may experience)* Overwhelming fatigue; relentless tiredness; muscle weakness or ache; loss of vigor; chronic, flu-like symptoms; inability to concentrate; tender lymph nodes.

Signs and laboratory findings *(What the doctor looks for)* History of acute infection, such as a cold, bronchitis, or mononucleosis (see page 876); or high stress, although many people report no initial trigger event.

What is it? Chronic Fatigue Syndrome (CFS) is nothing new. The syndrome was first described in the 1800s, and pronounced a neurosis. Similar illnesses, known by different names, date back 2 centuries, according to the National Institutes of Health. In the early 1980s, when the disease first surfaced in American news reports, most of those affected were women in their 30s and 40s with good educations and socioeconomic standing. Since then, doctors have documented the syndrome in people of all ages, races, and financial classes, and from different countries around the world. The cause is uncertain but an infectious explanation is thought probable. Despite considerable evidence, some members of the medical community remain suspicious about the legitimacy of CFS as a clinical disease.

More than twice as many women as men are diagnosed with CFS. A true gender difference may exist, as it does with lupus and multiple sclerosis, diseases that affect more women than men. Another explanation is that more women than men consistently seek regular medical care. People diagnosed with CFS often describe its onset as sudden but not terribly worrisome because many of the symptoms—headache, tender lymph nodes, fatigue and weakness, muscle and joint aches, inability to concentrate—mimic those of the flu. Although flu symptoms usually go away in a few weeks, CFS symptoms either persist or recur frequently for more than 6 months, and people with CFS feel increasingly drained.

There appears to be an overlap between CFS and neurally mediated hypotension, a form of low blood pressure. Neurally mediated hypotension results when the autonomic nervous system, which controls heart rate and blood pressure, misinterprets the body's needs during upright posture and sends a message to the heart to slow down and lower blood pressure. This low blood pressure results in fatigue.

What you can do Learning how to manage the feelings of fatigue can enable you to improve daily quality of life. A healthy diet, adequate rest, and light exercise are helpful in controlling symptoms. Individuals with CFS who learn to pace themselves—both physically and emotionally—do much better because stress has been found to exacerbate the disease.

When to call the doctor Anytime there is a lingering sense of fatigue following a bout of flu, a cold, or any mild infection, consult your doctor. In some people CFS is characterized by a feeling of tiredness that simply will not go away. In others, it takes on a kind of recurrent physical backlash; you may feel well enough to go on a picnic or other outing, for example, but feel overcome with exhaustion midway through or immediately afterward.

Treatment Diagnosing and treating CFS is difficult because many other diseases share its symptoms. Diagnosis becomes, in effect, a process of elimination. Different explanations including anemia (iron-poor blood), hypoglycemia (low blood sugar), environmental allergy, or candidiasis (a body-wide yeast infection) have been submitted as explanations for the disorder.

Some physicians have reported success with treatments including antivirals, antidepressants, and drugs that boost the immune system, although few of these specific treatments have undergone FDA-sanctioned testing. The antiviral drug acyclovir (Zovirax) has been tested in a scientific trial but results were not impressive because as many people with CFS reported feeling better when taking a placebo as when taking acyclovir.

In the 1980s, the illness was known as chronic EBV because it was once linked to the Epstein-Barr virus. However, high levels of those antibodies have since been found in healthy people as well as in people with CFS. Now CFS is considered to be part of a continuum of illnesses that has fatigue as its major symptom.

According to the National Institutes of Health, doctors often prescribe antidepressants for people with CFS, with generally good results. In addition, some people with CFS benefit from the benzodiazepines, a class of drugs used to treat acute anxiety and sleep problems. And, even though no specific CFS treatments exist, symptomatic treatment still can be quite helpful. Nonsteroidal anti-inflammatory drugs (NSAIDs) may benefit the body aches or fever associated with the illness and antihistamines may help relieve some allergic symptoms. Treatment to raise blood pressure in some people with neurally mediated hypotension and chronic fatigue may improve symptoms of fatigue.

Prognosis Variable, although many people seem to get over CFS with time. No single therapy has proven effective for CFS.

❖ TETANUS

Symptoms (What you may experience) A recent dirty wound, which may be quite small; tingling or discomfort at the site of the wound; tightness in the muscles of the jaw, face, abdomen, neck, and back; difficulty swallowing; difficulty breathing; difficulty passing urine or stool (occasionally).

Signs and laboratory findings (What the doctor looks for) Hyperreflexia (overactive reflexes); muscle contractions; slight fever.

What is it? Tetanus results from an exotoxin secreted by the anaerobic bacteria *Clostridium tetanii*. It normally finds its way into the body through a puncture wound contaminated with soil, dust, or animal feces carrying the bacteria. These bacteria produce a toxic substance that interferes with the electrical nerve signals. This toxic nerve disruption may first produce symptoms of slight numbness, tingling, or discomfort around the area of a puncture wound or cut. As the toxin spreads it may extend to the nerves supplying the muscles. Frequently, the toxin strikes the nerves supplying facial and jaw muscles, causing strong spasms in them, which gives this disease its common name, lockjaw. As tetanus progresses, spasm of other muscles, including the neck, back, respiratory, and throat muscles, leads to difficulties in swallowing and breathing. Untreated, the disease is fatal. It is more prevalent in agricultural regions and developing countries that lack mass immunization programs.

What you can do This illness need never occur; immunization against tetanus completely protects from disease. In the United States, there are fewer than 100 cases a year. Keep your immunization up to date with regular (every 10 to 15 years) booster shots. If you are traveling to an underdeveloped country, check with your doctor about the need for a booster shot. In addition, you should clean all wounds—no matter how insignificant—with soap and water. Keep open wounds clean and covered, especially if you are gardening, engaging in outdoor activities, or for any other reason in contact with manure or dirt. If you sustain a dirty puncture wound, immediate administration of tetanus immune globulin (TIG) into a muscle will provide protection against the subsequent development of tetanus.

When to call the doctor If you have a puncture wound and are unsure about your immunization status, consult your doctor. The appearance of any of the signs of tetanus should prompt a call to the doctor right away. Be alert for these symptoms following cuts or puncture wounds in seniors, especially because this group is the one most likely never to have been immunized against tetanus.

DO YOU NEED A TETANUS SHOT?

The question of whether or not to get a tetanus shot usually arises in adolescents and adults after they have stepped on a nail, cut a finger, scraped a shin, been bitten by an animal, or sustained any wound that prompts a need for medical treatment. The tetanus bacterium is microscopic and does not require a large wound to make its entrance into the body. Even tiny cuts, scrapes, or punctures could admit these microscopic invaders if they happen to be in the vicinity, and tetanus can result in people without immunity to the infection.

Several factors contribute to a higher risk for the development of tetanus:

- The conditions of injury. Where did it occur? How likely would it be for the tetanus bacteria to be present? A puncture to the foot in a cow pasture carries greater risk than a knife cut in your home. The more the chance of dirt in the wound, the higher the risk for tetanus.

- Speed of wound cleaning. Wounds should be thoroughly cleaned with soap and water immediately. Delay in wound cleaning for more than a few hours increases the risk of tetanus.

- The depth of the wound. Punctures and cuts that penetrate deeper into the tissues make proper cleaning difficult and increase the chances for tetanus bacteria to find their way to a deep location where there is less oxygen. *Clostridium tetanii* bacteria thrive in an anaerobic (lacking oxygen) environment. The deeper the wound, the higher the risk for tetanus.

In addition to proper and prompt cleaning of wounds, prevention of tetanus rests on immunization against it. Everyone should receive the complete series of tetanus toxoid vaccine injections, which most children now receive as a part of their baby shots, and should maintain immunity with booster vaccines every 10 to 15 years throughout life. If you have not had the initial series, you should begin now to complete them. If you have suffered a high-risk wound, you may also need immediate protection through tetanus immune globulin (TIG) until you can complete your series of tetanus immunizations. If you have had a series in years gone by, but no booster in 10 to 15 years, you need a tetanus shot.

On the other hand, frequent tetanus shots—commonly in small boys who are always injuring themselves—can lead to severe soreness in the arms because of the immune response to the vaccine. There is no point in giving tetanus toxoid if the person was fully immunized and the last booster was less than 5 years ago. ■

Treatment Although people with established clinical tetanus are always given antibiotics and TIG, these treatments have never been shown to be of value. People with tetanus are admitted to an intensive care unit, and once the muscle spasms interfere with respiration, the patient is given medications, intubated, and put onto a respirator. Artificial respiration is maintained until the muscle spasms stop, which may take weeks. However, during this time the patient may die of complications of ventilation (such as pneumonia) or of unstable pulse and blood pressure induced by the effects of the toxin on the circulatory center in the brain. Once the symptoms have subsided, a susceptible person will require a full course of tetanus immunization shots for future protection. Unlike many infectious diseases, having this disease does not grant immunity to it.

Prognosis Tetanus is fatal within 10 days of the onset of symptoms in about 30 to 40 percent of unimmunized persons. Age appears to play a role in outcome; mortality rates among people over age 50 are far greater than for those under age 50. If symptoms develop within 3 days of exposure the prognosis is poor.

Childhood Diseases Beyond Childhood

❖ RUBEOLA (RED MEASLES)

Symptoms *(What you may experience)* Fever; stuffy nose; sore throat; sneezing; coughing; eye symptoms including redness, watering, irritation, and sensitivity to light. Initial symptoms followed by a red, spotty rash. (See page C-31.)

Signs and laboratory findings *(What the doctor looks for)* Typical rash; Koplik's spots (small red spots with bluish-white centers on the lining of the mouth or gums that appear before the rash); redness of the throat; yellowish patches on tonsils; low white-blood-cell count determined through blood tests.

What is it? Measles results from infection with a virus transmitted by breathing in infectious droplets of respiratory fluids that are released into the air when people with the disease cough and sneeze nearby. Development of symptoms in a susceptible person—a person who never had the disease or a vaccination against it—usually occurs 10 to 14 days following exposure to the infected person. It begins much like a cold with several days of nasal stuffiness, sneezing, coughing, watery and irritated eyes, and a sore throat. Unlike a cold, however, a profound malaise, which includes discomfort and a sense of not feeling well, may occur along with a fever that can reach moderately high levels of 103°F to 104°F and can last up to a week. The Koplik spots in the mouth occur about 2 days before the typical rash of measles and may vanish when the rash appears. About 4 days after the initial onset of the cold-like symptoms, a blotchy, brick-red rash that feels slightly raised to the touch begins on the face and behind the ears. The rash moves down the torso, then to the arms and legs, and finally to the palms and soles of the feet. The disease is most infectious during the first 4 days but remains so until the rash fully clears.

What you can do Rest in bed and drink plenty of fluids. If fever becomes too high or symptoms cause too much discomfort, treat them. For pain and fever, take acetaminophen in a dose appropriate to age, weight, and manufacturer's listed recommendations. For cough, over-the-counter (OTC) cough suppressants containing dextromethorphan may help. For stuffy nose, try OTC medications containing pseudoephedrine or commercially available plain saline (salt-water) nasal sprays. Breathing moist air from a steam kettle or steam vaporizer helps moisturize the dry, irritated respiratory tract. This illness is entirely preventable by appropriate immunization.

When to call the doctor Call your doctor right away if any symptoms arise that might suggest the development of complications, including fever that rises above 103°F and fails to break with treatment, severe headache or neck stiffness, a cough that produces colored phlegm, breathing difficulties, swollen lymph glands in the neck, and severe or throbbing ear pain.

Treatment As with many viral illnesses, no specific medication eradicates the virus; that job falls to your immune system. A person with measles should be isolated from susceptible people and take plenty of fluids, bed rest, and symptomatic treatment.

Prognosis Usually quite good, with full recovery in a few weeks. However some complications are possible including measles pneumonia, which occurs in 1 to 7 percent of cases, bacterial infections such as pneumonia or middle ear infections, which occur in 15 percent of cases, and, rarely, encephalitis, a viral infection involving the coverings over the brain, which occurs in about 1 in 2,000 cases. Infection grants lifelong immunity to the disease.

❖ MUMPS

Symptoms *(What you may experience)* Fever (usually low grade); malaise, or an irritable uneasy discomfort; painful swelling of one or both cheeks. Symptoms suggesting possible complications: headache or neck stiffness; high fever; extreme fatigue and sleepiness; abdominal pain; nausea and vomiting; pain in the testicles. (See page C-30.)

Signs and laboratory findings *(What the doctor looks for)* Tenderness and swelling of the parotid gland in either cheek; redness and swelling of Stenson's duct (the opening of the parotid-gland saliva duct on the inside of the cheek). Mumps virus in saliva, which can be detected by laboratory tests if the diagnosis is in doubt.

What is it? Mumps, like many of the so-called childhood infections, occurs when susceptible people come into contact with droplets of infected saliva or respiratory secretions from people with the disease. Susceptible people include those who have had neither the disease nor a vaccination against it. The onset of illness usually occurs 2 to 3 weeks from the time of exposure. Unfortunately, an infected person can pass the disease to others during the 24 hours before symptoms appear, and for about 3 to 7 days afterward. Slight fever and loss of sense of well-being herald the onset, followed quickly by discomfort and swelling in one or both of the large saliva glands in the cheeks, (the parotid glands), or in the saliva glands under the tongue on the floor of the mouth. Eating sour foods such as pickles and citrus fruits or juices strongly stimulates saliva production and may magnify parotid gland pain.

Infection by the mumps virus of tissues other than the salivary glands—commonly, the pancreas, meningeal tissue (thin tissue covering the brain and spinal cord), and the ovaries and testicles—can complicate the illness. Rarely, deafness may develop if the virus infects the auditory nerve.

In men, mumps virus tends to infect the testicles, causing a disorder called mumps orchitis. Twenty-five percent of adult men who contract mumps virus develop orchitis. In spite of potentially considerable discomfort, mumps orchitis rarely causes sterility.

What you can do Rest in bed as long as you have fever. Drink plenty of fluids. Remain isolated from any susceptible person. If fever or discomfort become a problem, treat with acetaminophen according to manufacturer's package recommendations. Apply warm, not hot, compresses to the cheek or cheeks to help relieve discomfort. Avoid sour foods and beverages. Be alert to the development of any new symptom that may suggest a more serious course.

If you are a man and your testicles hurt, supporting their weight on a towel bridge and applying ice packs offers considerable relief. To build the bridge, fold a soft bath towel lengthwise twice. Lie down and place one end of the towel under your right thigh near the buttock, bring the towel across the front of your thigh, pass it under the scrotal sack so that the towel gently supports the testicles, and then pass it over the front of the left thigh and under the left thigh near the buttock.

When to call the doctor Call your doctor right away if symptoms arise that suggest the development of complications, including high fever, nausea and vomiting, abdominal pain, pain or swelling in the testicles, ringing of the ears, drainage of pus from the parotid or salivary ducts into the mouth, and severe headache or neck stiffness.

Treatment As is the case with many viral infections, there is no medication that specifically eradicates the mumps virus; the immune system will handle the infection. Simply supporting the body with nutrition, fluid, and bed rest may be all that is necessary in the absence of complications. However, some cases of testicular infection become so painful that they require such measures as the injection of anesthetic (numbing) medication or the intravenous administration of hydrocortisone, a potent anti-inflammatory steroid medication, to reduce swelling.

Development of meningitis or pancreatitis may require hospitalization to provide intravenous fluid and medications for headache or to stop the vomiting.

Prognosis Excellent. In the absence of complications the disease usually runs it course in about 10 to 14 days. Infection usually grants lifelong immunity to the disease.

❖ RUBELLA (GERMAN MEASLES)

Symptoms *(What you may experience)* Mild fever, sore throat, and stuffy nose (sometimes); tender lymph glands at the back of the neck or behind the ears (usually); joint ache (sometimes, especially in young women); light pink rash (sometimes). (See page C-31.)

Signs and laboratory findings *(What the doctor looks for)* Characteristic pattern of lymph gland enlargement—behind the ears and at the base of the skull; patchy redness of the roof of the mouth and the throat; blood tests demonstrating a low white-blood-cell count and low platelet count demonstrated through blood tests; platelets are necessary for normal blood clotting. Presence of the virus through laboratory test of respiratory secretions.

What is it? Unlike rubeola, the onset of rubella frequently causes few symptoms, although there may be occasionally a low-grade fever, a mild sore throat, or a little nasal stuffiness. The most characteristic symptom is the appearance of tender, swollen lymph nodes at the base of the skull and behind the ears. The onset of symptoms usually occurs 2 to 3 weeks after exposure. Although most people think that the hallmark of a measles infection is a rash, as many as half of rubella infections cause no rash to appear. When it does, a very fine pink rash develops over the course of 2 to 3 days, showing first on the face, then on the trunk, and finally on the arms and legs. In each area, it fades after about a day. About one in four people—more commonly young women—develop aching joints that may persist for a week or more. Spread of the disease occurs when susceptible people come in contact with respiratory-fluid droplets released into the air with a cough or a sneeze. Those people at risk to contract rubella include anyone who has never had the disease or who has not received vaccination against it. The disease itself is of minor consequence in the vast majority of cases, with the important exception of pregnant women. Rubella infection during pregnancy can cause serious birth defects in the fetus.

What you can do The best strategy is prevention: take the MMR series if you have never had it to prevent the possibility of contracting measles, mumps, and rubella. Women must practice birth control for 3 months following immunization to insure no pregnancy occurs during this time. It is now clear that one vaccination does not provide lifelong immunity against these diseases. There have been epidemics of all three diseases in college students who were vaccinated in infancy. Current regulations require that all college students show proof of revaccination before entry. There are no current regulations regarding MMR vaccination in adults. However, revaccination every 20 years is wise if exposure to any of these diseases is likely.

If you get infected, take acetaminophen for fever or pain if the symptoms are bothersome. As always, drink plenty of fluid and rest if fever develops. Isolate yourself from any susceptible person, as the disease is contagious to others from about 1 week before noticeable symptoms develop and for about 2 weeks afterward.

When to call the doctor Symptoms usually are quite mild. See your doctor if headache or neck stiffness develop; these symptoms may signal mild encephalitis (viral infection of the brain). Significant joint aching, especially if accompanied by swelling or warmth in the joint, should be evaluated by your doctor immediately. The development of bleeding, which can include easy bruising, bleeding of gums, and prolonged bleeding after cuts or dental work, may signal a serious drop in the number of platelets in the blood. See your doctor right away if any of these symptoms occur.

Treatment Like many viruses, there is no specific medication that kills the rubella-causing virus. Treatment is symptomatic for pain such as headache and joint pain.

Prognosis Excellent for full recovery in most instances in 3 or 4 days. Rarely, in about 1 in 6,000 cases, a syndrome of encephalopathy (abnormal brain function) occurs within 1 week of the rash, although the cause has yet to be clearly understood. One in five cases of this postinfection syndrome proves fatal.

❖ ERYTHEMA INFECTIOSUM (FIFTH DISEASE)

Symptoms *(What you may experience)* A slightly bumpy rash on the chest and back that may itch; headache; loss of sense of well-being (sometimes); joint ache (occasionally); low-grade fever (rarely). (See page C-30.)

Signs and laboratory findings *(What the doctor looks for)* Identification of the virus through blood tests.

What is it? This viral disease occurs most commonly in children 4 to 10 years old, but can occur in adolescents and adults as well. Its common name, fifth disease, comes from its being the fifth of the common childhood diseases that cause a rash. The onset of infection is unmistakable in children; the cheeks appear fiery red as if they had been slapped. A few days later, a lacy red rash that comes and goes appears on the body. In adults, especially women, aching or swelling of the joints of the hands is a more common symptom. The arthritic symptoms may last one to several months before it completely resolves. Rarely, the virus causes encephalitis (an inflammatory condition of the brain), for which the warning signs are powerful and persistent headache and sensitivity to light. Contracting the virus during pregnancy may cause disturbances in pregnancy, including miscarriage. Also rarely, the virus can cause a very serious condition called aplastic anemia, which occurs when something damages the bone marrow, which produces blood cells and prevents the body from replacing its red blood cells. Aplastic anemia occurs most frequently in people who have sickle cell disease, an inherited type of anemia seen primarily in blacks.

What you can do There are no specific remedies except symptomatic treatment for this illness. Headache or joint pain may respond to acetaminophen dosed according to manufacturer's recommendations. Cool baths, moisturizing skin lotions, and over-the-counter antihistamine preparations (Benadryl or Tavist) may help to relieve the itching of the rash.

When to call the doctor Call your doctor right away if you develop severe headache or high fever, or extreme fatigue, easy bruising, or severe joint pain. Pregnant women should notify their doctor right away.

Treatment As with many viral diseases, no specific medications exist to eradicate the virus. In most cases no treatment beyond that for mild discomfort is needed.

Prognosis Excellent for full recovery, although the viral symptoms may linger for 1 month or longer before completely disappearing.

❖ ROSEOLA INFANTUM (SIXTH DISEASE)

Symptoms *(What you may experience)* Several days of high fever followed by a pink rash on the chest and back as the fever breaks. (See page C-31.)

Signs and laboratory findings *(What the doctor looks for)* Low white-blood-cell count demonstrated through blood tests; tenderness of the area around the liver (occasionally); changes in liver function determined through blood tests (occasionally).

What is it? Roseola infantum—also known as exanthema subitum and sixth disease—primarily strikes children under 2 years old; however, older children and adults can also contract this disease. It is caused by human herpes virus 6, which is a virus in the herpes family but is not the herpes simplex virus 1 or 2 that can cause sexually transmitted herpes. The illness usually begins with 3 to 4 days of high fever; when it breaks, a pale pink, slightly bumpy rash appears on the chest and the back. The rash usually fades in a few days, with no further complications. However, some evidence suggests that the virus may rarely cause a kind of hepatitis (liver inflammation) and a syndrome much like infectious mononucleosis caused by the

Epstein-Barr virus, which is also in the herpes family.

What you can do Rest and increase your fluid intake. If fever rises above 103°F, you may wish to treat with acetaminophen dosed according to manufacturer's recommendations.

When to call the doctor Persistent high fever that lasts longer than 48 to 72 hours or a fever that fails to respond to measures to bring it down should prompt a call to the doctor. Dark-colored urine, yellow-tingeing of the skin or whites of the eyes, or discomfort in lymph glands or the upper right abdomen could signal complications; call your doctor right away. Persistent inability to recover strength and vigor lasting longer than a couple of weeks may suggest chronic fatigue and merits a visit to the doctor.

Treatment No specific medication eradicates this virus; the immune system must do that job.

Prognosis Excellent for full recovery in the vast majority of cases.

❖ VARICELLA (CHICKENPOX)

Symptoms *(What you may experience)* Fever and malaise, or loss of sense of well-being; the eruption of itchy red bumps that quickly develop into blisters, then rupture to become crusty sores. Rarely: headache; difficulty maintaining balance when walking; respiratory symptoms such as painful or difficult breathing. (See page C-30.)

Signs and laboratory findings *(What the doctor looks for)* The typical rash; low white-blood-cell count demonstrated by blood tests.

What is it? Chickenpox, the name by which most people know varicella, passes easily from person to susceptible person through breathing in droplets of respiratory secretions or by contact with the pox sores. The onset of symptoms occurs 10 to 20 days after exposure to the illness. The rash begins first on the face, scalp, neck, and body, and spreads outward with new bumps appearing last on the areas farthest from the center, the legs, arms, hands, and feet. The rash proceeds through predictable stages. First itchy red bumps appear; within a few hours a clear blister forms on top, which soon becomes a pustule, with yellow-white pus replacing the clear watery fluid. The pustule then ruptures and a crusty sore forms. This cycle repeats in each new area until finally—usually after about 1 to 2 weeks—all the crusty sores have healed. Up until the last spot has healed the disease can be transmitted to a susceptible person through contact with the sores.

Although, except for the misery of itching, the symptoms may be mild, bacterial secondary infection of the open sores can sometimes occur. Streptococci can invade and cause cellulitis (locally spreading skin infection). In adults more commonly than children, viral pneumonia may occur. Encephalitis (viral brain infection) occurs rarely, in about 1 in 1,000 cases.

What you can do Rest in bed when feverish and increase intake of clear fluids. Treat symptoms of high fever or discomfort with acetaminophen dosed according to manufacturer's recommendations. *WARNING: Do not use aspirin. Aspirin products given to children or teenagers with chickenpox may cause Reye's syndrome, a potentially deadly liver disorder (see pages 463 and 854).*

Isolate the infected person from contact with any susceptible person, especially those people with immune system problems. Shower with mild antibacterial soap (Dial or Lever 2000) to reduce the chance of complicating infection of the sores. Cool baths with oatmeal soap (Aveeno or similar mild soap) may offer some relief. If the blisters weep fluid, you can apply an astringent solution (Domeboro's soak solution) to dry the fluid.

When to call the doctor Fever lasting more than 1 or 2 days or the return of fever once it has disappeared may signal secondary bacterial infection and should prompt a call to the doctor. Development of painful or difficult breathing or of excessive sleepiness and fatigue suggest the possibility of pneumonia or even of Reye's syndrome. A severe headache suggests the chance of encephalitis. Any of these complicating symptoms should prompt a call to the doctor right away.

Treatment Most cases of chickenpox require little treatment beyond symptomatic care. One medication currently available, Acyclovir, specifically kills the chickenpox virus; its administration will reduce the severity of symptoms, shorten the duration of the illness, and decrease the number of days the virus can pass to a susceptible person. Acyclovir must be given within 48 hours of onset of illness to be effective. Some doctors recommend the medication to adults who contract the virus because the symptoms are often more severe in adults and because a 2-week absence from work because of contagiousness may create financial hardship. Acyclovir is not routinely used in children. Bacterial infections that occur, such as cellulitis and pneumonia, require antibiotic medications, in either topical or oral form.

Prognosis Excellent in the absence of complications, with complete resolution usually within 2 weeks. Chickenpox only occurs once in a lifetime, but the virus can remain latent for decades reactivating as shingles (herpes zoster) later in life.

❖ STREPTOCOCCAL ERYTHEMA (SCARLET FEVER)

Symptoms *(What you may experience)* Sudden development of a bad sore throat; painful swallowing; fever, headache; nausea; tender swollen lymph glands in the neck; spotty rash on the upper torso that spreads over the body, excluding face, palms, and soles.

Signs and laboratory findings *(What the doctor looks for)* Characteristic rash; strawberry tongue, or coated tongue dotted with enlarged red papillae (taste buds); pus on the tonsils; presence of strep bacteria verified by throat-swab by culture or rapid strep test.

What is it? The diagnosis of scarlet fever struck terror into the hearts of parents a generation ago, because of the risk of serious complications involving the heart and kidney. Today, with antibiotic treatment of strep-related throat infections, scarlet fever and acute rheumatic fever occur rarely. The term scarlet comes from the appearance of the rash that accompanies the infection; it is bright red and looks almost like a sunburn that seems more intense in the large skin creases, such as the groin, axillae (arm pits), bend of the arms, and neck. You can usually see red, slightly raised bumps scattered throughout the affected areas as well. The rash may last for 2 to 5 days, may take on a kind of brownish spotty appearance as it fades, and may peel. The illness runs its course in a few days, but treatment should continue for at least 10 days to reduce the chance of complications.

The strep infection can cause complications within the throat and respiratory tract, such as sinusitis, middle ear infection, or the formation of abscesses (large, pus-filled pockets, much like boils on the skin) in the tissues around the tonsils themselves.

The most serious possible complications from scarlet fever, or any streptococcal infection, appear a week or more after the infection and are not caused by the bacterium, per se. These complications involve the heart—rheumatic fever—and the kidney—glomerulonephritis, and occur because the body's own immune defenders accidentally attack the tissues of the heart or kidney. This case of mistaken identity comes about because the means by which the immune cells recognize the foreign nature of the bacteria depends on special markers on the bacterial surface. Unfortunately, certain body tissues may have similar markers on their surfaces. As the immune defenders go after the bacteria, heart or kidney tissues get accidentally caught in the cross fire. The most important reason to thoroughly treat all streptococcal infections is to prevent these serious complications.

What you can do Scarlet fever is not a disorder to attempt to treat on your own. Once the diagnosis has been made by a doctor, however, self-care includes maintaining adequate fluid intake. Throat pain may make drinking uncomfortable. Stick to water or weak tea instead of fruit juices, especially citrus juices which can burn. Gargle frequently, hourly or more often, with warm salt water—1 tsp of salt dissolved in 1 cup of warm water—to make a hostile environment for the bacteria. Use OTC numbing throat lozenges or sprays to help relieve pain, especially before trying to eat. Eat soft foods that are easy to swallow such as soft cooked eggs, soups, milk toast, and Jell-O. If vomiting is present, use clear liquids only.

When to call the doctor At the first sign of severe sore throat accompanied by fever and a rash, you should contact your doctor (see Septic Shock, page 876). After receiving the diagnosis of scarlet fever, call your doctor right away if you develop renewed symptoms of fever, change in urinary frequency or color of urine, extreme fatigue, or painful joints. These symptoms may suggest the development of complications.

Treatment Many doctors treat suspected cases of streptococcal infection immediately with long-acting penicillin shots. A single shot of benzathine penicillin G adequately treats the infection. Oral antibiotic therapies must continue uninterrupted for 10 days even if symptoms disappear, as they usually do in 2 to 4 days. People who cannot take penicillin can take erythromycin 3 to 4 times daily for 10 days. A quick but expensive alternative is the new medication azithromycin that can effectively treat the disease with a single tablet taken daily for 3 days. Antibiotics only shorten symptoms by about a day, so they are primarily prescribed to abort complications such as acute rheumatic fever.

Prognosis Excellent for full recovery in the vast majority of cases, with adequate treatment.

❖ DIPHTHERIA

Symptoms *(What you may experience)* Sore throat; runny nose; fever; hoarseness; malaise, or loss of sense of well-being.

Signs and laboratory findings *(What the doctor looks for)* Characteristic tightly adherent gray discharge on the throat. Presence of the pathogen confirmed by actually growing the bacterium on a culture plate in the lab.

What is it? Diphtheria rarely occurs today, thanks in large measure to the effective vaccine against it that is a part of the routine series of shots that infants and children can, and should, receive before starting school. Diphtheria immunization is given along with pertussis (whooping cough) and tetanus vaccines in a series of five DPT injections between birth and age 5 years. Because immunity to tetanus and diphtheria begin to wane, and because whooping cough is not a problem after early childhood, at about age 15 the tetanus and diphtheria portions require booster vaccinations, which should be received about every 10 years to maintain immunity. In most instances, when adults receive a tetanus shot following a cut, bite, or puncture wound, they receive diphtheria vaccination too. If immunity to diphtheria wanes, susceptibility to infection returns.

Diphtheria, caused by a bacterium called *Corynebacterium diphtheriae*, can infect the respiratory passages or the skin around wounds. The symptoms of respiratory infection may be mild at first and may include sore throat, runny nose, and fever. These symptoms are then followed by the development of severe exhaustion, a sense of extreme fatigue so severe that getting out of bed is more than you can do, which may be accompanied by high fever. In some cases, the infection involves the heart muscle, causing disturbances of heart rhythm and heart muscle weakness, and nerves, causing difficulty swallowing, double vision, and slurring of speech.

What you can do   The diagnosis of diphtheria is an emergency; you should not attempt to treat this illness yourself. The best self-care is prevention. If you have not received diphtheria toxoid immunization in the last 10 years, update your immunization.

When to call the doctor   If you develop any symptoms suggestive of diphtheria, and have never been vaccinated against it or have not had a booster vaccination in over 10 years, see your doctor immediately.

Treatment   Antitoxin (immune serum produced in horses against the diphtheria bacterium) available from the Centers for Disease Control and Prevention (CDC) must be given immediately, in varying amounts depending on the severity of the symptoms and how long they have been present. Antibiotics help—both penicillin and erythromycin are effective—but do not replace the antitoxin.

Prognosis   Poor, unless appropriate medical therapy is begun right away.

Animal-Borne Infections

❖ LYME DISEASE

Symptoms *(What you may experience)* A recent tick bite and, in many cases, a rash. (See page C-47.) Later: flu-like aches with fever and chills (in about 50 percent of cases). Still later: persistent joint and muscle aches; headache and neck stiffness; Bell's palsy (weakness of nerves on one side of the face).

Signs and laboratory findings *(What the doctor looks for)* A specific rash called erythema migrans that is red and ring-like and spreads outward from the site of a tick bite (also called a bull's-eye rash); antibodies against the bacterium causing Lyme disease, demonstrated through the enzyme-linked immunosorbent assay (ELISA)—positive in about 90 percent of people soon after infection.

What is it?   Lyme disease, named for the town in Connecticut where the disorder was originally described, occurs from infection with the bacterium *Borrelia burgdorferi* passed by the bite of a tick. Lyme disease occurs widely throughout all areas of the United States—although most cases arise in the northeastern, Pacific coastal, and midwestern areas—as well as in Europe, Asia, and Australia. Ticks carrying the disease pass it to humans or other animals during feeding cycles; larval ticks feed in late summer, nymphs the following spring and early summer, and adult ticks during the fall. Most infections occur during the late spring and summer when the small size of the ticks in the larval and nymph stages makes their detection difficult. It is easier to spot an adult tick, which is 2 to 3 mm in size, and remove it before it can feed sufficiently long to transmit the disease, which appears to take at least 48 hours. The specific type of tick that carries the Lyme bacterium is the *Ixodes* tick, which has a red body and black legs.

Symptoms of Lyme disease usually begin within 1 week after the bite, although in some cases they may take up to 1 month to develop. Initial symptoms include flu-like fever, chills, and body aches, and the typical red, ring-like rash that spreads over a several-day period outward from the site of the

Ticks live in grassy and wooded areas. Infections transmitted by deer ticks can cause Lyme disease; those transmitted by wood ticks can cause Rocky Mountain spotted fever. If untreated, these infections can cause serious disease. Most cases of Lyme disease occur during late spring or summer. Untreated Lyme disease may become dormant and reveal itself at a later time. Rocky Mountain spotted fever is not confined to the Rocky Mountain region. When spending time in wooded or brushy areas, use tick repellent, minimize exposure of skin, and inspect yourself and your children regularly.

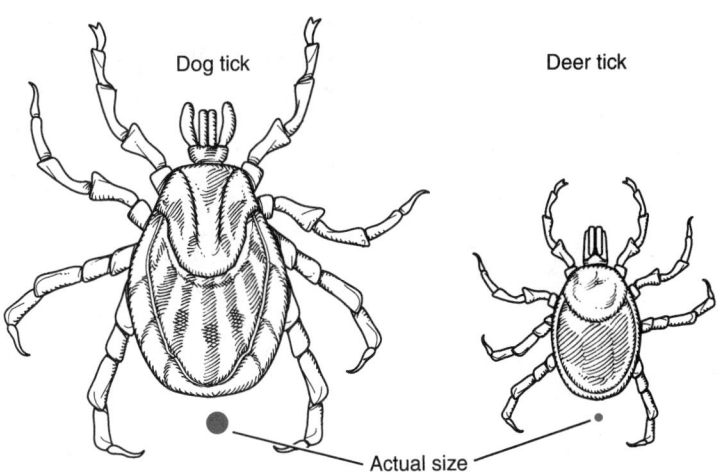

Dog tick

Deer tick

Actual size

tick bite, as an enlarging circle with a clear center. Be aware, however, that the rash may not occur in as many as 20 percent of cases and the flu-like symptoms may not occur in 50 percent of cases. These early symptoms resolve in about 1 month with or without treatment.

The bacterium can then spread by way of the bloodstream to cause symptoms involving the skin, nerves, heart, muscles, and joints. Fatigue and malaise occur commonly at this stage. A specific infection of the nerve that supplies the facial and eye muscles can cause a weakness of these muscles leading to difficulty smiling or drooping of the eyelid on one side (see Bell's palsy, page 469).

If untreated the infection may become dormant; months to years later mild to severe symptoms may appear that involve many organ systems. These include arthritis; neurologic manifestations such as headache, hearing loss, and inflammation of the optic nerve (see Optic Neuritis, page 529); and cardiac abnormalities.

What you can do Prevention of the disease is your best approach. When spending time outdoors in wooded or brushy areas, use tick repellent on exposed skin. When possible, wear long-sleeved shirts with long pants tucked into socks to reduce the chances of tick attachment. Immediately upon returning home, inspect yourself—and your children—for ticks, looking especially carefully in the groin, scalp, and arm pits, where ticks may escape casual detection. Remove all ticks promptly (see How To Remove a Tick, page 1306).

When to call the doctor If you develop flu-like symptoms or the ring-like rash, especially within a month of having been bitten by a tick or having been in wooded or brushy areas, see your doctor right away and be cer-

tain to mention the bite or exposure. However, many people with Lyme disease have no recollection of a tick bite.

Treatment Treatment with antibiotics such as tetracycline, doxycycline, amoxicillin, or cefuroxime (Ceftin) for 10 days (for the disease in the early stages) to 3 to 4 weeks (for later stages) works well to eradicate the bacterium. If the infection has caused severe neurologic or cardiac complications, 2 to 4 weeks of treatment with ceftriaxone, administered by injection, may be recommended.

Prognosis Good results in most cases with appropriate treatment. The earlier therapy

Petroleum jelly, mineral oil, or any cooking oil can be used to smother a tick and make it fall away from the skin. If this method is unsuccessful after 30 minutes, tweezers can be used gently to lift off the tick, which should then be crushed on a hard surface. The affected skin should then be washed carefully. Do not use a lit match, a cigarette, or a cigarette lighter to remove a tick.

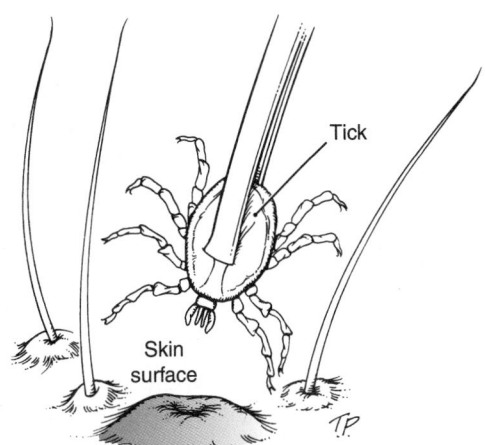

Tick

Skin surface

occurs, the better the result. In cases not diagnosed for years, some residual nerve, joint, and muscle symptoms may remain.

❖ ROCKY MOUNTAIN SPOTTED FEVER

Symptoms *(What you may experience)* A recent tick bite; fever; body aches; chills; severe headache; nausea and vomiting; extreme fatigue. After several days: a red, spotty rash (in 90 percent of cases).

Signs and laboratory findings *(What the doctor looks for)* The typical red, spotty rash appearing first at wrists and ankles then spreading to the body; the presence of antibodies to the organism that causes the disease, demonstrated through blood tests.

What is it? Rocky Mountain spotted fever (RMSF) passes to humans through the bite of a wood tick or dog tick infected with the organism *Rickettsia rickettsii*. Rickettsial organisms are not free-living bacteria, but rather bacterial parasites that are unable to exist on their own and must live inside another cell or perish. Despite its name, the disorder occurs throughout the United States, in fact, most commonly in the eastern third and not the Rocky Mountains.

Within 3 to 10 days after a tick bite, the disease sets in with severe flu-like symptoms including fever, chills, nausea, vomiting, headache, muscle aches, and sometimes cough. A few days later, a rash begins in most cases. It first appears faintly at the wrists and ankles and then becomes more pronounced as it spreads over the next 2 to 3 days to the limbs and trunk. Inflammation of the heart muscle, damage to the kidneys, enlargement of the spleen and liver, and jaundice (yellowing of the skin and whites of the eyes) can occur in some cases.

What you can do When spending time in wooded or brushy areas, wear protective clothing, use tick repellents, carefully inspect the body for ticks afterwards, and properly remove all ticks promptly upon discovery (see How to Remove a Tick, page 1306).

When to call the doctor At the first sign of flu-like symptoms or rash following a tick bite, contact your doctor immediately.

Treatment In most cases the infection responds promptly to treatment with antibiotics for 7 to 10 days. Doxycycline eradicates the infection, but may need to be administered intravenously in severely affected individuals. Chloramphenicol (Chloromycetin) may be preferred for pregnant women and children.

Prognosis With early detection and antibiotic treatment, the prognosis is quite good for full recovery. In seniors, however, mortality rates from RMSF can be as high as 70 percent, and in the very young, as high as 20 percent.

❖ HUMAN EHRLICHIOSIS

Symptoms *(What you may experience)* Fever; tick bite from the deer, dog or lone-star tick; flu-like symptoms including headache, muscle aches, chills, nausea, and vomiting.

Signs and laboratory findings *(What the doctor looks for)* History of tick bite 1 to 3 weeks prior to symptoms; low white-blood-cell count or low platelet count revealed through blood tests; bacterial evidence of organism in blood; liver function abnormalities.

What is it? Human ehrlichiosis is caused by the bacterium from the genus *Ehrlichia*, but it really represents two distinct diseases. Human monocytic ehrlichiosis (HME) can be picked up from a tick-carrying dog or from an area of infestation by ticks that carry the organism. Human granulocytic ehrlichiosis (HGE) is carried by the same deer tick as Lyme disease. Both are new diseases, although HME preceded HGE by a few years. HME first was detected in the late 1980s in a man who was clearing brush at a vacation home and whose serologic tests proved negative for all other likely causes. Both infections can be life-threatening but respond well to a range of antibiotics.

What you can do Wear long-sleeved shirts and protective clothing and use insect repellent when hiking. Avoid known areas of infestation, such as brush and shrubbery.

When to call the doctor Flu-like symptoms associated with a tick bite or a recent visit to a wooded area or camp site merit evaluation by your doctor. Most cases have been found in New York and surrounding states.

Treatment The antibiotics doxycycline and tetracycline have proven effective.

Prognosis Excellent, with prompt and proper treatment.

❖ TULAREMIA

Symptoms *(What you may experience)* Headache; fever; nausea; muscle ache; fatigue (sometimes extreme); cough and chest pain (sometimes); a sore on the skin or the eye; swollen lymph glands. Occasionally: tenderness in the left upper abdomen (where the spleen lies); rash.

Signs and laboratory findings *(What the doctor looks for)* History of recent exposure to small mammals such as rabbits or muskrats, or tick bite; ulcerated skin sore accompanied by swollen lymph glands; pneumonia indicated by crackling breath sounds; rise in the production of antibodies against the disease, demonstrated through blood tests; positive blood cultures for *Francisella.*

What is it? Tularemia—sometimes called rabbit fever by hunters—usually occurs when people come into contact with the meat of infected rodents, which can happen when skinning or cleaning wild rabbits or muskrats. The bite of ticks infected with the bacterium, *Francisella tularensis*, can also pass the disease to people. A few days to a week or so after exposure, a sore develops at the site where the bacteria entered the skin through a small scratch, cut, or tick bite. Soon after, lymph glands in the vicinity of the sore become swollen. Occasionally, the bacteria enter the body through the lungs, when the infectious matter is breathed in during skinning or cleaning of rodents, or via the bloodstream from an infected sore, and tularemia pneumonia develops. Passage of tularemia from one person to another can occur at this stage from infectious droplets of respiratory secretions released with coughing.

Complications of the disease arise when the bacteria spread through the blood to infect the coverings of the brain, causing meningitis, the covering of the heart, causing pericarditis, or the bones, causing osteomyelitis.

What you can do When you skin and dress rabbits or other rodents, you should take the precaution of wearing protective clothing, gloves, goggles, and a mask that covers your nose and mouth. Wear protective clothing and tick repellent while hunting in wooded or brushy areas. Wash, or otherwise disinfect, the clothing and equipment afterward. Thoroughly cook wild rabbit you intend to eat.

When to call the doctor At the first signs of fever, severe fatigue, and a newly erupted sore on the skin following exposure to wild rodents or their habitat, see your doctor and relate your history of contact with the animals.

Treatment Antibiotic therapy eradicates the bacterium. Streptomycin by injection into the muscle combined with tetracycline by mouth every 6 hours works well. Medication must be continued until the fever subsides and for 4 to 5 days afterward.

Prognosis Excellent for full recovery, with prompt and appropriate antibiotic therapy in the absence of complications.

❖ CAT-SCRATCH DISEASE

Symptoms *(What you may experience)* A crusting sore or blister-like protrusion at the site of a scratch inflicted by a cat; chronic swollen lymph nodes which can persist for weeks or months.

Signs and laboratory findings *(What the doctor looks for)* History of recent cat encounter, including a bite; if no telltale scratches or bite marks can be found or recalled, the presence of the bacterium usually responsible, *Bartonella henselae*, determined through blood-culture or serum tests.

What is it? Cat-scratch disease is a bacterial infection named for the event that most commonly causes the illness, although dog scratches or bites can also be responsible. The bacterium has been found in fleas, which is how it is believed to pass among populations of cats. The scratch or bite characteristic of cat-scratch disease can cause infection wherever the wound is infected, but the disease most often results from scratches along the arms, hands, and face.

Half of all individuals who are infected experience no symptoms other than swollen glands. Most others have a low-grade fever and flu-like symptoms. A few grow much sicker with a variety of complications that

PET-RELATED INFECTIONS

Pets can be a great source of joy, but precautions need to be taken to ensure that they are not also a source of infection. Many pet stores distribute disease-prevention guides when a pet is purchased and it is a good idea to ask for one if it is not provided. Pamphlets on preventing exposure to *Salmonella*, for example, are standard hand-outs for new owners of lizards or turtles.

Dogs and cats are the most common source of animal-borne transmission. Cats and dogs typically pick up fleas and ticks and cats also pick up mites. You or your children may feel the unwelcome presence of these pests. Some people have a particularly pronounced reaction to flea bites, known as a flea allergy. Lyme disease (see page 886) can also be transmitted by family pets. Cats that contract mites can impart a form of scabies during a simple act of petting.

Dogs and cats can be more direct sources of infection, too. Bacteria that cause gastrointestinal disorders can be passed on through dog or cat excrement. The preventive measure is simple: Wash immediately with soap and water following any kind of contact with animal waste and do not let feces accumulate in yards or litter boxes where it can attract even more pests, such as flies.

Dog and cat bites can transmit infectious disease. Cultures taken from bite sites show that *Staphylococcus* and *Streptococcus* occur fairly commonly at the wound, although transmission of these two organisms through a bite from a domestic animal is rare. Two other organisms that can cause severe infections, *Capnocytophaga canimorsus* and *Pasteurella multocida*, are found in the oral cavity of both dogs and cats. In general, cat bites are associated with a much higher infection rate. This is because a dog bite tends to result in a wound that bleeds and is more easily cleaned, while a cat bite tends to puncture the flesh and create a deep wound that is harder to clean. Cats also harbor higher rates of some potentially infectious agents.

There are no truly accurate figures on how many dog or cat bites occur annually, but the number is probably close to 2 million. Children are bitten most frequently both because they are smaller and more vulnerable, and because they often fail to read animals' warning cues. ■

may include high fever, pneumonia, and other disorders.

What you can do Careful, protected play with cats, particularly kittens, can help prevent infection. Be sure to wash scratched or bitten areas with antiseptic soap immediately. Keep all pets free of fleas.

Treatment In most cases, no treatment is needed and the disorder resolves on its own. If treatment is necessary, your doctor may prescribe any one of a number of antibiotics.

❖ TOXOPLASMOSIS

Symptoms (*What you may experience*) Swollen lymph nodes; muscle aches; low-grade fever lasting weeks or months.

Signs and laboratory findings (*What the doctor looks for*) Stippling (change in the eyes characterized by the formation of very tiny dark spots that resemble pin pricks) detected by eye exam; confirmation of the infection through blood-serum tests.

What is it? Toxoplasmosis is the result of an infection by an intracellular parasite, *Toxoplasma gondii*, that is usually found in one of two places: the intestines of cats and undercooked meat. Many people carry the organism without feeling its effects, but some people are at higher risk of complications. It can be a threat to pregnant women because the infection may cross the placenta to the fetus and cause miscarriage or stillbirth.

What you can do Keep away from soil used by cats for defecation; litter boxes should be emptied and disposed of with care. Pregnant women should refrain from this chore. Do not eat undercooked meat, particularly steak tartare.

When to call the doctor People who may be immunocompromised or pregnant should see their doctors if they experience symptoms consistent with toxoplasmosis.

Treatment Therapy varies depending on the individual. Antibiotics are the treatment of choice, but children, adults, pregnant women, and infants may all be treated with different medications.

Prognosis Excellent for otherwise healthy adults; variable for infants who contract the infection during fetal development.

❖ RABIES

Symptoms (*What you may experience*) Recent animal bite; pain followed by numbness or tingling at the site of the bite along with sensitivity to temperature changes of the surrounding skin; painful throat spasm when swallowing fluids; bizarre behavior and mood swings; muscle spasm; spasm of the vocal cords indicated by whistling sounds with breathing; seizures; weakness or loss of function of body parts.

Signs and laboratory findings (*What the doctor looks for*) No specific signs in the affected person beyond the symptoms complex; the presence of antibodies to rabies in the potentially rabid animal, determined by examination of the animal's brain; presence of antibodies in human blood or skin biopsy.

What is it? Rabies is a very rare disease in the United States, although travelers outside the United States may find themselves in an area where the disease is endemic. Rabies occurs when the rabies virus passes from infected animals to humans, usually through a bite wound. Dogs, cats, raccoons, skunks, and bats are the most frequently implicated animals. The virus, found in saliva, passes from infected animals through a bite. Development of symptoms of the disease may not occur for 10 days to as much as 7 weeks later. Occasionally, rabies is acquired by inhalation, usually after exposure to bat guano in caves or attics.

The disease of rabies occurs when the virus infects the nerves in the area of the bite, travels to the brain where it causes encephalitis, and finally migrates back to the salivary glands.

What you can do Make sure all household pets are regularly inoculated for rabies. Never approach, pet, or handle a wild or unknown animal. Veterinarians, spelunkers, and others with occupational or recreational exposure to potentially rabid animals should be vaccinated against rabies.

When to call the doctor Any bite by a high-risk animal demands immediate evaluation by a doctor. Any bite by a suspicious animal or a domestic animal that does not have a current rabies vaccination requires quarantine of an animal to determine whether it develops symptoms of rabies, or sacrifice of a sick animal to examine the brain for rabies. If the animal escapes, you should operate on the assumption that it had rabies and seek treatment accordingly.

Treatment Because of the slow nature of the rabies virus, vaccination after the bite prevents the development of rabies. The current recommendations include careful cleaning of the bite wound, administration of a shot of human rabies immune globulin (HRIG) into the site of the bite and into the buttock muscle to grant immediate transient immunity, followed by a series of three

to five vaccinations with rabies vaccine given into the arm muscle. Adverse reactions to the vaccine occur rarely, but they can include allergic reactions.

Prognosis Excellent, with prompt and complete antirabies therapy with correct vaccines, which may not necessarily be the case in third world countries. The disease is uniformly fatal without treatment.

❖ PLAGUE

Symptoms (*What you may experience*) High fever; muscle pain; malaise, or loss of sense of well-being; extreme fatigue; swollen lymph glands in the neck, groin, or under the arms. Sometimes: coughing up of blood-tinged phlegm; neck stiffness. Ultimately: profound illness, even to the point of delirium.

Signs and laboratory findings (*What the doctor looks for*) History of recent contact with wild rodents, such as rats, ground squirrels, or prairie dogs, in areas where plague occurs; presence of the plague-causing bacterium determined by microscopic inspection of pus taken from swollen lymph nodes or by growing the bacterium on a culture plate in the laboratory from samples of blood or pus.

What is it? Plague—the infamous disease known throughout history, responsible for wiping out huge segments of the population of Europe for 300 or more years after its introduction in the late 14th century—occurs from infection by the bacterium *Yersinia pestis*. It is extremely rare in the United States. Rats or other rodents carrying fleas infected with the bacterium transmit the disease to humans. The bacterium enters the body of a human or a rat through the flea bite. A pustule (pus-topped sore) usually forms at the site of the infected bite. Once inside, the bacteria spread throughout the body via the blood stream. The lymph glands swell, become quite tender, and may even drain pus and form what historically were called buboes, giving rise to the name bubonic plague. The bacteria can also infect the lung, causing a highly contagious pneumonia, pneumonic plague, in which the infection spreads person-to-person through infectious droplets of respiratory secretions released into the air with coughing. Left untreated, hemorrhaging under the skin turns it dark purple to black, giving rise to yet another name, black plague.

What you can do In areas known to harbor plague-carrying fleas, do not pet or handle rodents, living or dead. Spray to repel or kill fleas when in endemic areas; in the United States these areas include most prominently New Mexico, but also California, Nevada, and Arizona.

When to call the doctor If you have been in an area where plague is endemic and you develop any of the listed symptoms, especially if you have sustained bites or had contact with rodents, call your doctor immediately and relate your history. Delay of treatment can be fatal.

Treatment Treatment with antibiotic therapy to kill the infecting bacteria must begin promptly. An initial dose of the antibiotic streptomycin injected into the muscle, followed by repeated injections of streptomycin, plus oral tetracycline every 6 hours offers the best treatment currently available. To reduce the likelihood of transmission to others, hospitals strictly isolate people with pneumonia from plague.

Prognosis Fair to good if treatment begins early; quite poor if it is delayed.

Parasitic Infections

The incidence of illnesses attributed to intestinal parasites has risen in recent years, probably as a result of the AIDS epidemic, which has meant a rise in opportunistic infections by parasites. Parasites of the intestines may either be single-celled protozoa, such as *Giardia lamblia* or *Cryptosporidium*, or helminths (worms), such as pinworm or hookworm.

Most worms enter the body through what is known as the fecal-oral route; they are transmitted by improper sanitation practices, usually when food preparers and handlers do not adequately wash their hands. Parasites can, however, enter the body from the soil or water—when you are fishing knee-deep in a stream, for example, or standing barefoot on a sandy bank. To prevent tapeworm and trichinosis, thoroughly cook pork and beef. To avoid hookworm and strongyloides, parasites that enter the body through bare skin, do not go barefoot in unpaved areas.

Parasites have different life cycles and medications are designed differently for each one. Depending on the specific parasite involved, you will need to take antiparasite medication for days to weeks. However, just because your symptoms match those of some of the parasitic diseases described below is no reason to conclude that you have a parasite. There are numerous accounts in the medical literature of people who falsely believed that they had become infected with parasites and became fearful and concerned about it, only to learn no parasite was responsible for their discomfort.

❖ TAPEWORM

Symptoms *(What you may experience)* Vague (often) nausea; diarrhea; abdominal discomfort; fatigue; hunger.

Signs and laboratory findings *(What the doctor looks for)* The presence of macro-

AMEBIC DYSENTERY

One of the most serious forms of diarrhea is amebic dysentery, caused by the protozoan *Entamoeba histolytica*. *E. histolytica* chews large holes in the lining of the colon. Symptoms include abdominal pain, fever, and stools containing blood and mucus. Through the holes in the colon, the protozoa may spread to internal organs, usually the liver. Amebic dysentery is not unknown in the United States, but is usually acquired in underdeveloped countries.

Giardia lamblia is a protozoa that attaches to and infects the small intestine. *G. lamblia* does not cause ulcers or spread internally; its main effect is to interfere with food absorption, which leads to mild diarrhea and severe intestinal gas. The parasite is passed through the fecal-oral route and occurs most often in people who travel to countries with polluted water and people who engage in anal sex.

Cryptosporidium parasites in healthy people cause a short, sharp watery diarrhea which is self-curing within 2 to 3 weeks. In people with AIDS, there is no mechanism available to eliminate the parasite, so profuse watery diarrhea persists indefinitely and may even be fatal. Cryptosporidia survive the usual chlorination procedures for municipal water, and epidemics have occurred. ■

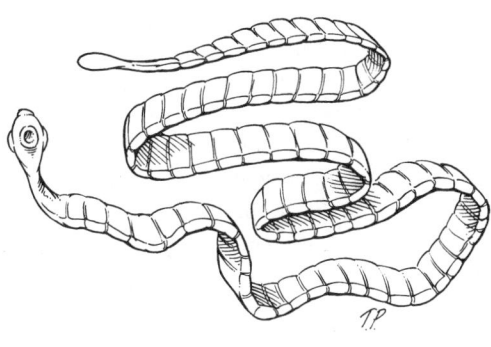

Tapeworms can be transmitted to people directly or indirectly from beef, pork, fish, dogs, rodents, human feces, and contaminated water. Some tapeworms can grow to a length of up to 25 ft inside the human body. Wash your hands carefully before eating or preparing meals. When you cook pork, beef, or fish, make sure the food is cooked thoroughly.

cytic, megaloblastic anemia, in which red blood cells, are large, pale, and scarce, suggesting B$_{12}$ deficiency, shown through blood tests; an elevation in the number of certain white blood cells called eosinophils that suggest a parasitic infestation or allergy, shown through blood tests; a detached segment of the tapeworm in the bowel movement; tapeworm segments and eggs in the stool, discovered through microscopic examination.

What is it? Tapeworms that infest humans come in six types identified in most cases by their source: beef, pork, fish, dog, rodent, and dwarf—so called because it is small and because there is no other source than humans. Except for pork tapeworm, all these parasites occur regularly in the United States, although incidents of infection are rare (see Meat Contamination, page 872).

Pork tapeworm occurs most commonly in Latin America, Spain, Africa, India, China, Southeast Asia, the Slavic countries, and Mexico, but rarely elsewhere in North America. Humans pick up this parasite when they eat undercooked pork containing the tapeworm cysts or by eating food or water contaminated by human feces. The parasite can also pass person-to-person from hand to mouth if the hands come in contact with contaminated water or surfaces. Once in the intestine, the worm grows to a length of up to 21 ft.

Infection of fish tapeworm, found in Europe, Canada, Japan, the United States, and the southern parts of Africa and South America, occurs from eating raw or poorly cooked freshwater fish, salmon included. Once in the intestine, the worm can reach a length of 25 ft.

Beef tapeworm occurs anywhere cattle farming exists. Humans pick up the worm from eating undercooked meat of infected cattle, which contains the worm cysts. The worm grows quite large in the human intestine, reaching a length of up to 25 ft.

The rodent tapeworm passes to humans through an intermediate carrier. Fleas, beetles, and cockroaches pick up the cysts and people may unwittingly eat them in foods such as cereals, meals, or other dry-storage products. The adult worm that develops in the human intestine is fairly small, usually under 20 in. long.

Dog tapeworm occurs most commonly in children who may inadvertently swallow the intermediate carrier, an infected flea or louse. This parasite, also small, reaches a length of 6 to 24 in.

The dwarf tapeworm exists only in humans and passes person-to-person in feces and rarely in contaminated food or water. It grows to a length of about 12 in. in the human intestinal tract.

What you can do Cleanliness in food preparation and careful hand washing help prevent infection. If traveling or dining out, take care to eat food properly cooked. In endemic areas, avoid raw foods, including peeled fruits, salads, and ice, that may be contaminated.

When to call the doctor Unless the abdominal discomfort becomes severe, there would be little to prompt you to call the doctor. Discovery of a tapeworm segment in the stool, undergarments, or bedding should immediately prompt a visit to your doctor. Bring the segment with you.

Treatment Specific medications to kill the worm, called antihelminthics, will eradicate the infestation. The most commonly used medications are niclosamide and praziquantel (Biltricide), which work quite well, with cure rates over 95 percent. Some doctors recommend a purge (laxative medication) afterward to rapidly eliminate segments of the worm from the intestine. Careful hand washing and disposal of the feces for about 4 days following therapy will insure that no living scolex (a head segment capable of regenerating a new worm) passes to someone else.

Prognosis Excellent. Usually the segments of the worm pass out in the feces within 48 hours. Follow-up examination of the stool finding no newly regenerated segments at 3 or 4 months proves the cure.

❖ PINWORM

Symptoms *(What you may experience)* Intense nighttime itching of the rectal area and, in women, the external genital area; a sensation of something crawling in the anal area; poor quality sleep; restlessness; mild abdominal discomfort (occasionally).

Signs and laboratory findings *(What the doctor looks for)* The worm or eggs on the skin near the anal opening.

What is it? The pinworm, *Enterobius vermicularis*, thrives all over the world. Infestation by pinworms occurs most often in children, but older siblings or adults in the household can easily become infested as well. Humans are the pinworm's only host, with the parasite passing from one person to another in a hand-to-mouth fashion through contaminated food or drink, on hands, or on clothing or bedding. From the time a person swallows a pinworm egg until an adult pinworm begins to make its own eggs takes about 4 weeks. Eggs can live 2 to 3 weeks outside the intestinal tract. Infestation causes intense itching of the area near the anus, especially at night when the adult female worm comes to the surface to lay eggs. You might occasionally spot an adult worm, which is only about $1/2$ in. long, in the bowel movement in heavy infestations.

What you can do Careful cleansing of the area around the rectum followed by hand washing with soap and water after bowel movements, especially in children, helps to reduce transmission. Because scratching increases the likelihood of infection, trim nails close and keep them clean. Launder bedding regularly.

When to call the doctor If a child, or an adult, in your household demonstrates or complains of anal itching, contact your doctor as soon as reasonably possible. The doctor will likely ask you to collect a special tape sample to assist in the diagnosis.

Treatment All members of the household should probably receive simultaneous treatment with medication to eradicate the pinworm, because it can easily bounce back and forth throughout the family. The antihelminthic used most often is mebendazole (vermox) a chewable tablet given as a single dose immediately and repeated at 2 and 4 weeks; however, pregnant women should not take this medication.

Prognosis Excellent, once treated.

❖ HOOKWORM

Symptoms *(What you may experience)* An itchy, red rash that may form blisters on hands or feet, where the worm larvae usually enter. Subsequent symptoms: episodes of coughing up blood-tinged phlegm; asthmatic wheezing. Later symptoms: loss of appetite; abdominal discomfort; diarrhea; fatigue; shortness of breath with activity; pale complexion.

Signs and laboratory findings *(What the doctor looks for)* Anemia, low iron level,

A child who has itching around the anus may have an infection with pinworm. At night, the worms deposit eggs in the anal area. To detect them, a piece of standard, transparent, adhesive cellophane tape can be swabbed around the anus when a child first gets up in the morning. A doctor can then search the tape for eggs under a microscope. This infection can spread within families, but effective medical treatments are available.

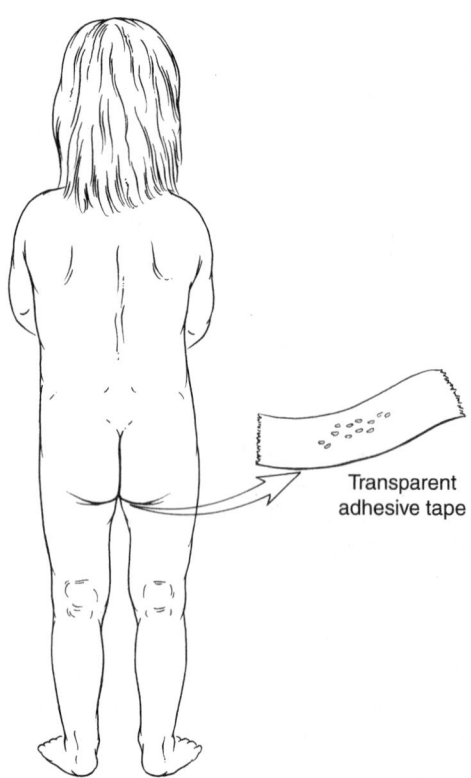

Transparent adhesive tape

marked increase in the number of eosinophils (white blood cells that fight parasites), demonstrated through blood tests; hidden blood loss and hookworm eggs, demonstrated through stool specimens.

What is it? Hookworm infestations occur in areas with warm, moist soil—the tropical and subtropical regions of the world—and in the southeastern United States. The human intestine is potentially vunerable to the two species of worms called hookworms, *Ancylostoma duodenale* and *Necator americanus*. The eggs, shed into the intestine, pass out in the stool; if they fall onto warm, moist soil, they will hatch into larvae. The tiny larvae are infective for up to a week and can penetrate the bare skin of feet and hands, where they cause an intensely itchy, red dermatitis. The larvae then enter the bloodstream and migrate to the lung where they cause coughing, asthmatic symptoms, and bloody phlegm. The tiny hair-like projections in the airways of the lung brush the larvae along with the respiratory secretions up the respiratory tree and toward the mouth where they are swallowed, finally reaching their destination in the intestine. They attach there and mature to adult worms about 1/2 in. long, begin to shed their eggs, and the cycle begins again.

Anemia occurs in hookworm infestation because the adult worms attach onto the lining of the intestine and suck blood, causing significant losses of iron. Symptoms of iron-deficiency anemia, such as pale complexion, fatigue, shortness of breath with activity, and altered nail growth, occur only after significant depletion. In heavy infestations, gastrointestinal symptoms, such as loss of appetite, diarrhea, and abdominal pain may occur.

What you can do Avoiding contact in the first place is your best defense. Wearing sturdy shoes when walking in endemic areas where the soil is warm and moist, and wearing gloves when working in such soils can help prevent the larval penetration that begins the disease. After diagnosis and treatment, a diet rich in lean protein and iron will help recovery.

When to call the doctor If you develop an itchy, red rash, particularly on the hands or feet, consult your doctor immediately. Stopping the hookworm infestation early prevents the later complicating symptoms. The appearance of any of the later symptoms merits investigation by a doctor right away. Examination of the stool specimen for eggs confirms the diagnosis.

Treatment Once the doctor establishes the diagnosis of hookworm, treatment consists of antihelminthic medications, such as mebendazole, that result in cure rates of 35 to 95 percent. Repeated treatments about 2 weeks apart may be needed in heavier infestations. Pregnant women should not take this medication. If severe anemia has occurred, your doctor may recommend taking prescription-strength iron supplements for 2 months, such as ferrous sulfate or chelated iron. Either form should be sufficient to correct the anemia, although ferrous sulfate, the less expensive of the two, can cause some stomach upset and constipation. Chelated iron causes fever side effects.

Prognosis Excellent, if discovered early and treated. Poor, and potentially deadly in children, if left to progress untreated.

❖ TRICHINOSIS

Symptoms *(What you may experience)* Early symptoms: loss of sense of well-being; abdominal cramping; diarrhea. Later—after about 1 week and lasting up to 2 months: tenderness in the muscles; conjunctivitis (redness and irritation of the thin membrane covering the eyes); swelling of the face and around the eyes; fever.

Signs and laboratory findings *(What the doctor looks for)* Elevation of muscle enzymes and elevation of white blood cell numbers, especially eosinophils, demonstrated through blood tests. Increase in the number of antibodies the body produces to defend against the parasite, also demonstrated through blood tests; presence of larvae in muscle tissue, determined by biopsy and microscopic examination, to confirm the diagnosis.

What is it? Trichinosis, caused by the parasite *Trichinella spiralis*, occurs when people eat raw or undercooked pork, boar, or bear meat infested with *Trichinella* cysts. Other food sources, more common outside the United States, also can harbor the parasite. These include the meat of the dog, frequently eaten in east or southeast Asia; horse, not uncommonly eaten in France; and wild game such as bear, walrus, or wild pig. Commercially available pork in the United States rarely poses a problem, and cases of trichinosis are rare.

The worm larvae reside in cysts in the muscle meat of the animal. When eaten, human stomach juices break the cysts apart and release the larvae, which quickly mature and embed in the lining of the intestine. It is during this stage that the early intestinal symptoms, cramping and diarrhea, occur. Within about a week mature female worms begin to release their larvae into the bloodstream and tissue fluids, which carry them to most parts of the body. Larvae reaching the muscles form cysts and hibernate there for months to years; the body destroys larvae that wind up elsewhere. The migration and embedding of the larvae in the muscle sets up a pronounced inflammatory reaction that includes fever, muscle ache, swelling, muscle spasm, weakness, and extreme fatigue. Symptoms at this stage may also include hoarseness, coughing, and difficulty breathing. Rarely, if the larvae migrate to other areas before the body destroys them, they can incite such symptoms as headache and neck stiffness, from inflammation of the brain and its coverings; heart pain, from invasion of the heart muscle or lining; and kidney pain.

What you can do   Never eat undercooked pork or wild game.

When to call the doctor   If you think you may have eaten poorly cooked meat, particularly outside the United States, and you develop diarrhea and cramping, see your doctor right away. If you develop muscle tenderness and other symptoms, even if you are not sure of having eaten poorly cooked meats, see your doctor for evaluation as soon as possible.

Treatment   Early, intestinal symptoms respond to treatment with antihelminthic medications such as mebendazole. Pregnant women should not take this medication. Once muscle invasion has occurred, mebendazole and similar drugs do not reliably eradicate the infestation. Severe muscle symptoms may require hospitalization and the use of potent corticosteroids to subdue the inflammatory reaction.

Prognosis   Good for full recovery in most cases; rarely, overwhelming infestations or complications such as heart failure or pneumonia can prove fatal.

❖ ASCARIASIS

Symptoms *(What you may experience)*   Mild abdominal swelling and vague discomfort; vomiting (occasionally); transient episodes of coughing, wheezing, and shortness of breath; passing an adult ascaris worm in the stool or vomit (rarely); intestinal obstruction.

Signs and laboratory findings *(What the doctor looks for)*   When respiratory symptoms are present, large numbers of eosinophils (the white blood cells responsible for fighting parasites), demonstrated through blood tests; presence of eggs, demonstrated through examination of the stool; presence of larvae, demonstrated through microscopic examination of respiratory phlegm.

What is it?   Infestation with the worm *Ascaris lumbricoides* occurs in an estimated 1 billion people around the world. It is the most common intestinal round worm, aside from hookworm. It occurs regularly in areas with inadequate sanitation, where personal hygiene is poor, or areas that use human feces as fertilizer. The infestation passes to another person from the inadvertent consumption of fecally contaminated soil or water containing *Ascaris* eggs. Eggs can remain infective in soil for years.

Once ingested, the eggs hatch in the intestine and release larvae that can migrate through the walls of the intestine into the bloodstream, and finally into the heart and lung. Once in the lung, they burrow into the air sacs, get coughed up into the throat and swallowed, and wind up back in the small intestine to mature into adult worms, which reach about 16 in. in length, to begin the cycle of egg production anew. During the migration to the lung, the respiratory symptoms predominate with coughing, wheezing, and shortness of breath. Occasionally hives appear during this phase. During this migratory phase, the larvae can wander and wind up in a wide variety of body tissues, such as brain, kidney, eye, or spinal cord, and cause symptoms that affect these areas. Although most persons infected with

Ascaris have no symptoms, complications that can result from wandering *Ascaris* larvae make it imperative that the parasite be eradicated fully when first discovered.

Prevention Protect yourself from contracting an infestation by avoiding food and drink, except if sealed, bottled, and prepackaged, in areas of questionable sanitation.

When to call the doctor If you develop symptoms suggestive of *Ascaris* infestation or see an adult worm in stool or vomit, call your doctor immediately.

Treatment The medication of choice, pyrantel pamoate, cures the infestation with a single dose 85 to 100 percent of the time. Mebendazole also works quite effectively; pregnant women should not take this medication. Reexamination of the stool for eggs at 2-week intervals confirms cure or indicates the need for repeated treatment.

Prognosis Very good, if treated before complications develop.

❖ STRONGYLOIDIASIS

Symptoms *(What you may experience)* Itchy (sometimes intensely) rash, usually on the feet; stomach pain; nausea; diarrhea (sometimes with blood and mucus); weight loss; dry cough; loss of sense of well-being.

Signs and laboratory findings *(What the doctor looks for)* Changes in the chest x-ray (transient); elevations in eosinophils, the white blood cells responsible for fighting parasites, and specific antibodies the body produces against the parasite, demonstrated through blood tests; presence of worm larvae determined by examination of stool, urine, or phlegm specimens.

What is it? Strongyloidiasis is caused by infestation with the parasite *Strongyloides stercoralis*. It occurs commonly in tropical and subtropical regions, in the southeastern United States where the climate is humid and hot, and in Appalachia. The infestation usually begins when the active larvae in warm soil burrow into the bare skin of the feet and migrate from there through the bloodstream and into the lung. Once the larvae enter the air sacs of the lung, they are coughed up into the throat with respiratory secretions and swallowed, and thus find their way into the intestine where they mature into adult worms that reach 1 to 2 in. in length. The cycle from initial infestation to maturity may be as short as 3 to 4 weeks. Adult worms can live for up to 5 years in the intestine, with females releasing eggs that hatch into larvae and leave the intestine with the feces to begin the cycle anew.

The larvae can incite pronounced inflammation during their migration, with the immune system attempting to fight the invaders along the way. Migration through the lung produces such symptoms as low-grade fever, cough, wheezing, and shortness of breath. In the intestine, the adult worms can produce symptoms ranging from mild diarrhea, abdominal pain, and gas to severe symptoms, including vomiting, and fever.

What you can do After diagnosis, proper nutrition with plenty of good-quality protein and all essential vitamins and minerals can help speed recovery.

When to call the doctor Any time diarrhea persists longer than a couple of days, you should notify your doctor. The appearance of bloody diarrhea, especially, requires investigation. A cough that persists for more than a week or produces blood-tinged phlegm demands evaluation by a doctor.

Treatment The antihelminthic thiabendazole (Mintezol) causes side effects in about 30 percent of people who take it. These include headache, vomiting, dizziness, weakness, and fuzzy thinking. Pregnant women should consult their doctor before taking any medication. Follow-up examination of the feces to prove eradication of the parasite is important, because any remaining worms will multiply and reestablish the infestation. A second medication also used to treat strongyloidiasis, ivermectin (stromeotol), seems to cause fewer side effects.

Prognosis Good, when discovered and treated early.

❖ TRICHURIASIS (WHIPWORM)

Symptoms *(What you may experience)* Few, in light infestations. Abdominal cramping; diarrhea; gas; nausea; vomiting; rectal spasm and pain; passage of blood from the rectum; weight loss.

Signs and laboratory findings *(What the doctor looks for)* Anemia from chronic blood loss and elevation of eosinophils (the white blood cells responsible for fighting parasites), demonstrated through blood tests; presence of eggs or occasionally, even adult worms, demonstrated through examination of the stool.

What is it? Whipworm, the parasite *Trichuris trichiura*, infects people of all ages worldwide, especially in hot, humid regions such as the tropics and subtropics. The infestation occurs when a person eats food, water, or soil contaminated with the parasite eggs. Once eaten, the eggs hatch in the intestine and the thin, whip-like worms, which reach about 2 in. in length, attach to the lining of the colon (large intestine) and remain there. Adult females produce more eggs that pass out with the feces to begin the cycle again. The infestation occurs most readily in areas without proper sanitation systems to dispose of human waste or in regions in which human feces may be used as fertilizer. Because the eggs require a period of 2 to 4 weeks in soil to become active and infective, passage from person to person cannot occur.

What you can do Wash hands well and often when living or traveling in hot, humid areas. Avoid eating raw fresh fruits, vegetables, unprocessed juices, water, or ice in areas where sanitation might be a problem because these foods might reasonably retain contaminated soil on their surfaces. Sealed beverages, canned foods, and well-cooked foods are probably safe.

When to call the doctor Any time diarrhea persists for more than 48 hours, especially if it contains blood, you should call your doctor right away. Persistence of any of the listed symptoms for more than a few days should prompt a visit to your doctor.

Treatment Mebendazole, an antihelminthic, cures 80 percent of cases with the first round of medication. Heavier infestations may require a repeated treatment. Pregnant women should not take this medication.

Prognosis Excellent, with proper treatment.

Traveler's Infections

Although there are many infectious dangers right in your own back yard, when you leave your own home, environment, food, and water, you may encounter unusual bacterial, viral, or parasitic invaders. Some of these infectious organisms produce mild or merely bothersome symptoms, while others can prove serious. But thanks to preventative immunizations and medications, travel to foreign or exotic areas need not be fraught with the worry of becoming ill.

Depending upon your destination, guidelines exist for preventive vaccines and treatments for such diverse disorders as malaria, yellow fever, cholera, hepatitis, and traveler's diarrhea. You will find more information about these and other traveler's infections in the entries that follow. For more information on health precautions to take when traveling, see page 74.

❖ TYPHOID FEVER

Symptoms *(What you may experience)* Vague, gradual (usually) development of malaise, or loss of sense of well-being; headache; cough; sore throat; bowel changes, most often constipation, but sometimes thick, green diarrhea; rosy-colored blotches on the skin; abdominal bloating and tenderness; spiking (up and down) fever.

Signs and laboratory findings *(What the doctor looks for)* Enlarged spleen; low white-blood-cell count demonstrated through blood tests; presence of the causative bacterium on a culture plate grown from samples of the blood, stool, or urine.

What is it? People contract typhoid, or as it is often called, typhoid fever, by consuming food or drink contaminated with bacteria of the *Salmonella* genus. The name originates from infection by one specific member of this group, *Salmonella typhi*. The condition occurred commonly in the United States prior to the routine safe handling of sewage. Today, it occurs rarely in the United States but is a major disease in regions of the world that lack proper sanitation.

The symptoms of typhoid begin about a week or two after consuming contaminated food or drink, with the gradual and increasing onset of headache, cough, sore throat, malaise, abdominal pain, and constipation, although in some cases, a person may suffer the passage of thick, green loose stools, termed "pea soup" diarrhea. The fever goes up in a stair-step fashion—in which it spikes, comes down, spikes higher, comes down less, etc.—for about a week, during which time the person becomes sicker and sicker. During the second week, a rosy-colored, blotchy rash appears on the trunk in many cases, lasting 3 to 4 days. The individual spots tend to be small, about $3/4$ to $1^1/_2$ in. in size. Barring the development of complications, which can be quite serious, even fatal, the illness runs its course in another week or so. Relapse may occur as much as 2 weeks later. In some cases, the bacteria find a hiding place, often the gall bladder, where they remain quietly infective bringing about a typhoid carrier state. The carrier does not appear to be ill, but continues to shed infectious bacteria in the stool, unwittingly exposing others to the disease.

Complications such as gastrointestinal bleeding or rupture and, less often, blood clots, pneumonia, or infection of the bone, kidney, heart muscle, or brain coverings, may occur in as many as one-third of cases that do not receive proper treatment.

What you can do Avoid contaminated food and drink in areas without proper sanitation. Suspect foods include any uncooked or undercooked food; foods not kept properly hot or chilled, especially those which contain eggs; fresh fruits and vegetables that may have been washed in contaminated water or handled with contaminated hands; water from unsealed bottles; and ice. Carefully and properly handle raw chicken and eggs because these foods can be sources of the bacteria. Wash hands, utensils, and countertops with soap and water after using them.

When to call the doctor Early symptoms of typhoid may appear much like a simple virus or stomach flu; however, if these symptoms last more than 48 hours, see your doctor.

Treatment Effective treatment with antibiotic medications for two weeks, such as

SOURCES OF INFECTIOUS DISEASE DURING TRAVEL

SOURCE	DISEASE
Undercooked Meat	Toxoplasmosis, trichinosis, salmonellosis
Drinking Water	Hepatitis A, giardiasis, amebiasis, travelers' diarrhea
Fleas	Plague
Sandflies	Leishmaniasis
Mosquitoes	Dengue, malaria, yellow fever
Unpasteurized milk, goat cheese, or dairy products	Brucellosis, salmonellosis, campylobacteriosis, listeriosis
Undercooked fish or shellfish	Hepatitis A, tapeworm, salmonellosis, cholera and cholera-like illnesses

ampicillin, double-strength trimethoprim/sulfamethoxazole (Bactrim or Septra), or ciprofloxacin, should eradicate the infection. If the bacteria hide and a person becomes a typhoid carrier, antibiotics may not be able to eradicate the infection. Eradication may require removing the gall bladder, where the bacteria hide out.

Prognosis Quite good for full recovery, in 98 percent of cases with prompt and effective treatment. Poor in older seniors or the very ill, particularly if complications arise; relapse occurs in as many as 15 percent of these cases.

❖ MALARIA

Symptoms *(What you may experience)* Recurring bouts of fever, chills, and sweats; headache; muscle and joint aches; fatigue; dizziness. Occasionally: dry cough; abdominal symptoms including nausea, vomiting, cramping, diarrhea, and loss of appetite.

Signs and laboratory findings *(What the doctor looks for)* History of travel to a malaria-hazardous area; reduced numbers of white blood cells and anemia, shown through blood tests; presence of the parasite in red blood cells, identified by microscopic examination of blood; occasionally: jaundice (yellowing of skin and whites of the eyes).

What is it? Malaria occurs when parasites of the *Plasmodium* genus enter the bloodstream, through the bite of an infected mosquito of a specific type, called the *Anopheles* mosquito. Although transmission usually occurs via mosquito bite, passage from infected mother to child or by transfusion of infected blood can also occur.

Worldwide, *Plasmodium* strains of four types—*P. falciparum, P. vivax, P. malariae,* and *P. ovale*—cause malaria, with some types more common in certain areas, making your travel destination an important consideration in preventive treatment against malaria. For the most part, the disease poses no danger in temperate climates, but occurs in tropical and subtropical zones, including Haiti, South and Central America, Africa, India, countries of the Middle East, parts of Mexico, Southeast Asia, China, and Oceania. Of the more than 100 million cases of malaria worldwide, most arise in tropical regions of Africa. Although the disease kills about 1 million adults and children each year, only about four people die annually in the United States; all known US fatalities resulted from malaria acquired outside the country, mainly in tropical Africa.

The disease passes from infected people to others when the female *Anopheles* mosquito bites an infected person, picking up the parasite gametocytes (akin to eggs and sperm) in the blood she consumes. Once in the mosquito, these gametocytes develop into more mature forms called sporozoites that reside in the mosquito salivary gland. Now when the infected mosquito bites, she will inject these malarial forms into another person, where they will develop, multiply, and invade the liver and blood. This maturation cycle occurs in waves, destroying red blood cells and resulting in the recurring bouts of fever, chills, and sweats, and ultimately in anemia. Symptoms usually appear within 2 weeks after the bite of the infected mosquito, but in some instances can take as long as 1 to 2 months. Untreated, the bouts of illness can persist for 8 months to several years. Persistent infection for 50 years can occur after infection by the *P. malariae* strain.

Prevention When planning travel to areas with a high risk of malaria, ask your doctor if you should take preventive medication. If the answer is yes, begin before you depart, continue during your stay, and do not end treatment until a month after you return home. In the malarious area, protect yourself from mosquito bites. Wear clothing to cover most of your body and apply mosquito repellents such as DEET to the remaining exposed skin, especially during the hours of peak mosquito activity, dusk to dawn. Treat living quarters to kill mosquitoes with pyrethrum sprays, powders, or burned coils. Bar entry of mosquitoes to living areas with screens or mosquito netting.

When to call the doctor Before you depart for your trip, see your doctor for appropriate preventative medication. The regimen will vary depending on where you travel; certain areas tend to harbor mosquitoes that carry malarial parasites resistant to some medications. At the first appearance of fever, shaking, chills, and sweats, seek medical attention.

Treatment The regimen designed to eradicate the malarial parasite depends on which of the four types of *Plasmodium* has caused the infection. Some strains of malaria no longer respond to the standard antimalarial medication chloroquine (Aralen) and will require alternative treatments. The standard regimen for treatment with chloroquine works for sensitive strains. Resistant strains usually respond to mefloquine, doxycycline, proguanil, or quinine. The medication pyrimethamine/sulfadoxine (Fansidar) taken as a single dose of three tablets can also augment chloroquine treatment or can be used as a one-time, self-treatment regimen in suspected cases where no medical facilities exist; however, only *P. falciparum* responds.

Upon return to safe areas, a 2-week course of the drug primaquine will eradicate the parasite from the liver if needed.

Prognosis Generally very good for full recovery in uncomplicated infections, with appropriate treatment. The most potentially serious complication is infection of the brain by the parasite, which has a 25 percent mortality rate even with treatment, another reason why prevention is so important.

❖ YELLOW FEVER

Symptoms (*What you may experience*) Mild to severe onset of fever; headache; body ache; malaise; pain behind the eyes; sensitivity to light. In severe cases: wracking body aches; decreased production of urine; jaundice (yellowing of the skin and whites of the eyes); bruising; bleeding from the nose, mouth, kidney, or stomach.

Signs and laboratory findings *(What the doctor looks for)* Initially: rapid heartbeat; flushed face; bloodshot eyes; absence of fever. Then: slow heartbeat; fever; low blood pressure; jaundice; signs of hemorrhage. Low white-blood-cell count, elevations of bilirubin (a yellowish liver pigment), and elevations of infection-fighting antibodies produced by the body against the virus, shown through blood tests.

What is it? Yellow fever, caused by a virus, occurs after the bite of an infected *Aedes* mosquito. For the most part, the disease occurs in the tropical and subtropical regions of Africa and South America, but occasionally during the hot seasons, may extend into the more temperate zones of these countries. Symptoms begin a few days to a week after the infecting bite, and may be mild or quite severe.

What you can do If you intend to travel into areas where yellow fever exists, you must protect yourself with vaccination against yellow fever. Pregnant women cannot take the vaccine, and if possible should not travel to these areas. While in the area, protect yourself from mosquito bites. Wear clothing to cover most of your body and apply mosquito repellents such as DEET to the remaining exposed skin, especially during the hours of peak mosquito activity, dusk to dawn. Treat living quarters to kill mosquitoes with pyrethrum sprays, powders, or burned coils. Bar entry of mosquitoes to living areas with intact screens or mosquito netting.

When to call the doctor Consult your doctor regarding preventive vaccination prior to your trip. At the first sign of fever, body ache, headache, and pain behind the eyes, seek medical attention.

Treatment There is no treatment to eradicate this viral illness.

Prognosis Good in mild cases, poor in severe cases. Recuperation to regain strength takes several weeks. Mortality rates run high in severe infections, again pointing to the importance of preventive vaccination.

❖ CHOLERA

Symptoms *(What you may experience)* Grey, watery, frequent stools of enormous quantity; profound thirst, from dehydration due to fluid lost in the diarrhea.

Signs and laboratory findings *(What the doctor looks for)* History of travel to areas where cholera occurs; presence of the organisms determined through laboratory cultures; signs of dehydration including low blood pressure, rapid heartbeat, dry skin, and decreased production of urine or tears.

What is it? Cholera is caused by consuming food or drink contaminated with the bacterium *Vibrio cholerae*. People with the disease develop massive diarrhea, sometimes losing more than 15 qt of water each day in the stool. Cholera is not, in the truest sense of the word, an infection. The symptoms of cholera arise not from the bacterium per se, but rather from a toxin produced by it that causes the lining of the intestine to secrete copious amounts of water.

The disease occurs where people are forced together under crowded conditions with inadequate sanitation and hygiene, for example, during war, in refugee camps, or in famine. It occurred very rarely in the Western hemisphere prior to 1991, when a localized outbreak arose in Peru and spread to other parts of South and Central America, Mexico, and the United States.

The disease begins, sometimes quite rapidly, with the development of severe, watery diarrhea, with fluid losses in the stool not uncommonly reaching more than a quart an hour. At that rate, dehydration and shock can develop quickly. The stool appears gray, but has no unpleasant fecal smell, and usually does not have blood in it. Untreated, the disease is commonly fatal.

What you can do Cholera infection is deadly. If you intend to travel into areas where cholera occurs—those areas previously mentioned, as well as portions of India, Asia, and Africa—you can try preventive measures by receiving the cholera vaccine, but many authorities consider the vaccine ineffective. The immunization, given in two shots, an initial shot and a second in 1 to 4 weeks, may provide immunity for a limited time. If you remain in an area where outbreaks occur, you need a booster vaccination every 6 months. Also, in areas where cholera exists, you should take great care not to eat fresh fruits or vegetables, undercooked foods, ice, or drink any water except bottled water or water from known disinfected sources.

When to call the doctor If you develop diarrhea characteristic of cholera and have been in a cholera-hazardous area, seek medical attention immediately.

Treatment Fluid replacement formed the cornerstone of cholera therapy—replenishing the amount of fluid lost in diarrhea volume for volume—and reduced the mortality of cholera victims long before the advent of antibiotic medications. It still should be considered the cornerstone, although antibiotic medications do shorten the course of the disease. In most cases, antibiotics such as those in the tetracycline family including doxycycline (Vibra-Tabs), ampicillin, trimethoprim/sulfamethoxazole, or the fluoroquinolones (Floxin or Cipro) will eradicate the toxin-producing bacteria. Strains of *Vibrio cholerae* resistant to antibiotics do occur; where possible, the laboratory can test to see if the bacterium will respond to treatment.

❖ LEISHMANIASIS

Symptoms (*What you may experience*) Fever that occurs irregularly after travel to any one of the several countries where the disease is endemic. An ulcerating skin lesion, usually 1 to 2 cm in diameter, which persists for months.

Signs and laboratory findings (*What the doctor looks for*) Evidence of the parasite in blood or in a skin biopsy; overproduction of an immune globulin, gamma globulin, found through blood-serum tests; enlarged liver.

What is it? Leishmaniasis is caused by a microscopic parasite of the genus *Leishmania* that is transmitted by sandflies. Some medical experts divide leishmaniasis into categories based on geographic areas and the appearance of the ulcers. Leishmaniasis is a global disease that affects more than 1 million people annually. There are two forms: visceral, which occurs internally, and cutaneous, which occurs on the skin. Cutaneous leishmaniasis largely is confined to

the South American countries of Brazil and Peru, and the Middle Eastern countries of Saudi Arabia, Iran, and Syria. Visceral leishmaniasis occurs in Bangladesh, the Sudan, India, and Nepal. Visceral leishmaniasis, also known as kala-azar, is fatal unless treated. Like several other emerging pathogens, *Leishmania* is now being linked more and more to HIV infection. In some developing countries, 70 percent of adults who have visceral leishmaniasis also have a concurrent HIV infection. The World Health Organization (WHO) has endorsed a global plan for containing leishmaniasis, so serious is the threat. The plan calls for close cooperation among the 88 countries in which the disease occurs.

What you can do When traveling to areas where leishmaniasis is endemic, protect yourself from insect bites. Wear clothing to cover most of your body and use insect repellents such as DEET on all exposed skin. Stay away from areas of known infestation of the insects. Because sandflies flourish in the desert and are active during the day, they are harder to avoid than mosquitoes, although protective bed netting does help protect against their bite.

When to call the doctor If you have symptoms, unwise use of antibiotics should be avoided. If your doctor has given you antibiotics for your travels or if you have some in your medicine cabinet, refrain from using them until you seek adequate medical attention. All people who have traveled to a foreign country and return with a fever of unknown origin (see page 854) should explain their histories and itineraries to their doctors. Leishmaniasis is a condition that can surface weeks or months after the initial infection.

Treatment Treatment depends on the form of leishmaniasis infection. Cutaneous disease is often not treated. If you have visceral disease, your doctor probably will prescribe a special salt solution that kills these protozoans, which may be injected or given intravenously. An alternative is the antibiotic amphotericin B (Fungizone).

Prognosis Good, with appropriate treatment and adequate bed rest. However, the recovery period is dependent on the type of leishmaniasis and the person's general health.

Emerging Infectious Diseases

In 1993, a mystery illness with flu-like symptoms began striking down people in the American Southwest. Within 6 months, 27 people had died of the disease, which was eventually traced to a virus carried by deer mice (see Hantavirus, below). Just a few years later, in the summer of 1996, vacationers on Maryland's shore were warned that a microorganism known as *Pfisteria piscicida* had filled the waters of the Chesapeake Bay coastline with a chemical toxic to humans as well as to fish. Sometimes it seems as if every week a new and devastating infectious disease is appearing to threaten our health.

These two situations illustrate how quickly a pathogen can surface; when such incidents capture the public's imagination they leave the impression that new infections arise spontaneously. Actually, however, a variety of factors and circumstances must coincide for new pathogens to emerge suddenly. The threat is usually transient and limited, particularly with proper intervention. In 1992, for example, a form of encephalopathy found in cows, bovine spongiform encephalopathy (BSE), was linked to a human brain disorder, Creutzfeldt-Jakob disease. In response, the US Department of Agriculture banned importation of cattle from BSE-infected countries. Mad cow disease, as it has been called, is just one of many alarming diseases to surface in the last few years. Necrotizing fasciitis, for instance, was dubbed a new form of flesh-eating strep in news reports when some unusual cases surfaced a few years ago but, actually, it is not a new disease and has been limited to a fairly well-defined set of circumstances. The image may conjure up a portrait of flesh-ingesting microbes that infect whole populations like a science-fiction creation, but typically, the bacterium, *Streptococcus pyogenes*, afflicts people predisposed to infection, such as a person with diabetes or a senior. The strep invades an area of skin that has been traumatized in some way. The infection, which is subcutaneous, turns skin red and, in certain areas, hot and swollen. Once an infection is established, gangrene can develop, often with fatal results. Necrotizing fasciitis is one of several devastating infections to have made the news in recent years. A few others are discussed below.

TOXIC SHOCK SYNDROME

Toxic shock syndrome causes a serious, severe illness characterized by sudden high fever and a drop in blood pressure. It is a complication of infection by *Staphylococcus aureus* or *Streptococcus pyogenes.* Staph, commonly found in the nose and on the skin, can become deadly if allowed to penetrate the body through the circulatory system. Toxic shock syndrom is not directly due to the bacteria but to an elaborated toxin. Toxic shock syndrome is most often linked to the postsurgical period, when toxins produced by staph can infiltrate wounds and make their way into the body's blood supply, causing life-threatening blood poisoning. Toxic shock syndrome became a household word in the early 1980s when some menstruating women who used a particular kind of tampon came down with a mysterious, sometimes fatal, infection. The infection was diagnosed as toxic shock syndrome and it was assumed that the staph in the mucous membranes of the vagina proliferated, penetrating the vaginal walls and leaching into the blood supply (see Toxic Shock Syndrome, page 1110).

The symptoms—muscle ache, weakness, and liver or kidney failure—can end in death, despite treatment. Gangrene is one complication; in some older medical texts, gangrene is used synonymously with toxic shock.

Symptoms also include a high fever, a scarlet rash on the extremities that looks like a bad sunburn, a drop in blood pressure, and decreased urination. Intravenous antibiotics are recommended, although there is no evidence that they affect the outcome. Aggressive supportive therapy in an intensive care unit can lower the mortality to below 3 percent but not to zero. Recent reports suggest that gamma globulin infusions may be beneficial.

HANTAVIRUS

Hantavirus causes severe respiratory distress. It also is characterized by headache, backache, chills, muscle ache, and a sunburn-like rash on the face. The severity of the illness is variable. It is carried to humans by rodents and has been found in rats in different parts of the United States, as well as throughout the world. The deer mouse is its primary source of infection. In 1993, an outbreak of hantavirus occurred in the southwestern United States, which led to identification of the syndrome. Treatment options are limited because the agent is a virus and unresponsive to antibiotic treatment.

MENINGOCOCCAL INFECTIONS

Meningococcal infections include meningococcal sepsis and meningococcal meningitis, which typically are characterized by a cluster of symptoms that can include fever, headache, drowsiness, and confused thinking. Sometimes the onset is so rapid that the first perceptible sign that the condition is more than a flu is diminished mental acuity, or mental fuzziness. It also causes a striking purple rash. Meningococcal infection is a serious condition, and requires immediate treatment, usually with penicillin, but due to increasing problems of antibiotic resistance, other antimicrobials may be used. Even after the medical emergency has passed, there may be residual damage to the central nervous system.

The bacteria has caused epidemics in groups of people sharing close quarters, such as military barracks. A vaccine is available which prevents group A and group C meningococcal disease plus some minor types, but unfortunately does not protect against group B meningococci, which can account for 40 percent of cases. The vaccine is used in military recruits and during epidemics in schools and colleges. Meningococcal sepsis is infectious, but only about 1 in 100 persons infected with meningococci in the nose develop the sepsis syndrome. By far the most susceptible group is children; 82 percent of all cases of meningococcal meningitis occur in children under 2 years old. If a case of meningococcal meningitis occurs in a household, children should be given rifampin or minocycline to protect them from meningococcal disease that may be incubating. Adults are also often given medication, although there is little evidence that they need it.

EMERGING INFECTIONS

At least 30 new infectious diseases worldwide have been identified in the last 20 years, according to the WHO. Some infections are actually "new" while some have been around but have only recently been identified. An estimated 100 million people now are chronically infected with hepatitis C, a virus that was unknown only a few years ago. Millions of others have been affected by any of several newly recognized infectious diseases, such as Lyme disease and *E. coli* 0157:H7. Moreover, several serious medical conditions have been linked in recent years to infections, such as peptic ulcers to *Helicobacter pylori* infection. In addition, diseases such as malaria, cholera, and tuberculosis—once considered to either be under control or diminishing—are on the upswing.

Newly identified or reemerging infectious diseases pose a significant health threat. Increasing drug resistance has complicated treatment and control, and many tests for some of these organisms, such as those for group B *Streptococcus*, lack the sensitivity to detect some cases of infection. Lack of a concrete diagnosis makes doctors hesitant to prescribe antibiotics due to the growing problem of antibiotic resistance (see page 850).

Emerging infectious diseases that could affect you tend to fall into three categories: newly identified pathogens, long-recognized pathogens that are making a comeback, and known pathogens that are now being linked to illnesses that earlier were mistakenly attributed to other causes.

More than 2 dozen newly identified pathogens have been found in the last quarter of this century. They include such diseases as infection with Ebola, a virus not even known to exist 2 decades ago and whose natural host remains a mystery. In Zaire in the early 1990s, an Ebola outbreak that caused hemorrhaging, fever, and death to most people who contracted it captured world attention, but was contained and affected relatively few. A greater danger, in the minds of many in the medical community, lies with viruses that elude early detection, such as hepatitis viral infections. Hepatitis C, for example, now is considered to be the underlying reason for most liver disease in the United States. For more information on hepatitis, see the section on acute viral hepatitis in Chapter 23.

Some established pathogens have been reemerging, posing a new threat across the world. Among them, health authorities are concerned with *Campylobacter*, now thought to be carried by most chickens in the United States. Though only one of many causes of gastroenteritis, the effects of *Campylobacter* on the population have only recently been appreciated because *Salmonella* was presumed to be the country's major poultry contaminant. Like *Salmonella* and other bacteria, there seems to be mounting resistance by *Campylobacter* to standard antibiotic therapies. In addition, it now is being linked to inexplicable and sudden paralysis, known as Guillain-Barré syndrome, which, although usually not permanent, causes people to become disabled and often bedridden.

In addition, there are pathogens whose virulence was mistakenly assumed to be on the wane. Cholera, gone for decades, reached epidemic proportions in South America in the early 1990s. Diphtheria has risen like a returning tide in several European nations because of declining immunization rates. The dreaded dengue fever, a malaria-like syndrome that also is transmitted by mosquito, has proliferated, leaving 2 billion people worldwide at risk of catching it.

Other diseases that medical science seemed to have curtailed have been associated with emerging infections as well, for a different reason. These are diseases that occur in the aftermath of an infection, a situation described as clinical sequelae. What this means is that while the first, or primary, symptoms of the disease have been overcome, health problems surface later that may be even more serious than the initial ones. This is why prompt medical treatment can be so important. Lyme disease, for example, now is linked to a serious illness called carditis, which can cause severe cardiac abnormalities, including dangerous changes in heartbeat. Facial nerve paralysis, known as Bell's palsy, also has been linked to Lyme disease and now is recognized as one of the disease's unusual but significant aftereffects. Only a few years ago such disruptions in heartbeat and facial paralysis probably would have been characterized as a separate and distinct disease. But there has been much progress in finding and confirming associations of certain symptoms with previous infection, which has led some scientists to tentatively conclude that many more conditions may be infectious than previously assumed.

Also, it is important to keep in mind that some diseases are disappearing completely, a result of effort and innovation in infectious disease research. Leprosy, polio, smallpox, and many other diseases have been defeated or soon will be.

You have only to look at a schoolyard or retirement center to see the huge difference vaccines and other forms of prevention have made. American children and adults no longer face the real possibility of death from infectious disease as did earlier generations. In the United States, both men and women typically now live about 25 years longer than people did early in this century. Early prevention and treatment of infectious disease is one of the primary reasons for these additional years. Research promises to keep such advances in health intact and perhaps even extend longevity significantly within your lifetime.

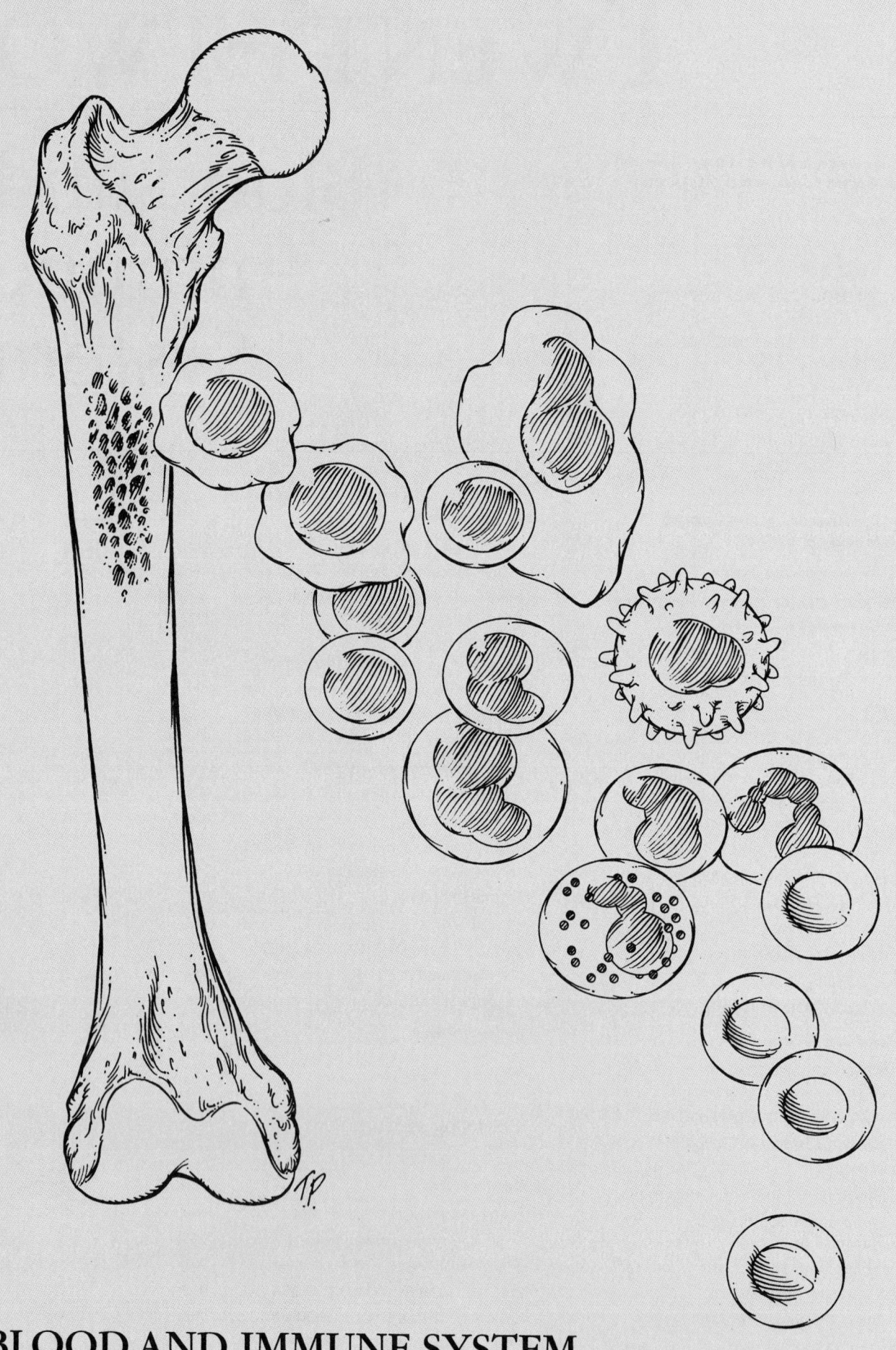

BLOOD AND IMMUNE SYSTEM

Understanding Your Blood: Its Function and Makeup

It may be impossible to discuss blood without starting with the popular associations the word itself conjures up. Mention "blood" and images of that red, gooey stuff that seeps, trickles, oozes, spurts, and flows may stream through your mind. You may think in terms of movie or television images that make you grimace, squirm, or turn away. In one way or another, the idea of blood makes most people a bit squeamish.

But let's look closer. In terms of your body and your health, blood is a complex and essential fluid. At the same time, it is not merely a liquid, but a tissue—that is, a group of cells acting together to perform highly specialized functions. The very thickness of the blood is actually due to the concentration of the millions of cells laboring within it.

Blood is the body's vehicle for those substances that sustain life and promote health. Without blood and the functions it performs, the body itself would not be able to operate. Moreover, the blood acts as one of your body's most telling barometers, testifying to your biologic health and balance. In numerous instances, a close reading of the blood's elements and the equilibrium among those elements will reflect the overall health of the larger system.

Blood is composed of a fluid called plasma. Suspended within the plasma are red and white corpuscles (blood cells), platelets, and fat globules. In addition, a great variety of other chemical substances and gases, including carbohydrates, proteins, hormones, oxygen, carbon dioxide, and nitrogen, are swept along by the blood as it streams through your blood vessels.

Blood is pumped by the heart throughout the body by means of a system of arteries, arterioles, capillaries, venules, and veins. (For a complete discussion of the cardiovascular system, see Chapter 20.) Moreover, the blood system is part of two parallel circulatory systems: the *circulatory system* handles blood, and the *lymphatic system* contains lymphatic fluid and many of the blood cells associated with immunity.

As the blood circulates away from the heart and lungs, it passes through the arteries, transporting to the body's tissues oxygen from the lungs and nutrients from the gastrointestinal system. Blood that leaves the heart is referred to as arterial blood. Bright red or scarlet, arterial blood usually will pulsate as it flows from a cut artery.

Having deposited the oxygen and nutrients, the blood returns to the heart through veins, carrying carbon dioxide to the lungs and other waste products to the kidneys. Blood that is returning to the heart is referred to as venous blood; it is usually dark red or crimson and flows steadily as it issues from a cut vein. Blood moves in the aorta at an average speed of 30 cm per second. The entire trip around the vascular system takes about 20 seconds.

The blood has a myriad of functions. It transports nutrients, oxygen, and other indispensable substances to body tissues. At the same time it extracts carbon dioxide and other waste products that would otherwise poison the system. It regulates body temperature. It distributes hormones and other agents that regulate cell function. The blood operates as a medium for the immune system, carrying molecules called antibodies. These help your body guard against infections by counteracting with foreign substances (antigens).

Blood consists of approximately 22 percent solids and 78 percent water. The average volume of blood in a man's body is 10 to 12 pints; in a woman's body, it is 8 to 9 pints. The blood itself is made up of red blood cells (erythrocytes), white blood cells (leukocytes), and platelets (thrombocytes), which are suspended in plasma. In normal circumstances, the total blood volume circulating within the body makes up approximately 8 percent of the body weight.

PLASMA

In the blood, the blood cells and platelets float around in a thin, colorless or faintly yellow liquid called plasma. Plasma consists mostly of water. In addition, each quart of plasma contains about 2 ½ oz of protein. One type of protein, albumin, is manufactured in the liver. Not only does albumin furnish food for the body's tissue, but it also provides pressure that keeps your blood from seeping out of the vessels and flooding your body's tissues.

Another important group of plasma proteins is called globulin. Some of these proteins work to destroy potentially disease-producing microorganisms; others are active in the formation of blood clots.

909

Blood plasma also consists of electrolytes, sugar, glucose, and fats, which fuel your body's fundamental operations. It transports iron, which is essential for hemoglobin production, the oxygen-laden protein found in your red blood cells. It conveys a number of important hormones, such as thyroid hormone, and serves as a vehicle for numerous clotting factors that facilitate blood flow, prevent blood loss, and repair injuries to blood vessels. In addition, plasma is both the medium for circulating minerals, vitamins, bilirubin (a pigment found especially in blood and bile), and gases, among other substances, throughout the body and the means of chemical communication between different parts of the body.

One last note on plasma: when the clotting agents are removed from plasma, the fluid that remains is called serum.

RED BLOOD CELLS: WHAT THEY ARE AND WHAT THEY DO

Red blood cells, or erythrocytes, make up the majority of blood cells in the blood system. Manufactured from stem cells mostly in the bone marrow, red blood cells act as your body's transport system, shuttling oxygen from the lungs through the bloodstream, out through capillaries, and delivering it to the tissues. Once the delivery is made, the red blood cells gather up carbon dioxide, a waste product of cell activity, and return it to the lungs where it is breathed out. The key to this elaborate transit system is the presence within your red blood cells of countless molecules of hemoglobin, the oxygen-carrying pigment of the red blood cells (see page 920).

Once in the lungs, hemoglobin combines almost immediately with oxygen. The blood cells become bright red and deeply oxygenated. They move out through the arteries to deliver their load to the tissues. Enzymes then help the red cells draw out carbon dioxide and water (waste products of cell function), which are then taken back through the veins to the lungs.

The body of a red blood cell consists of a sponge-like frame that holds the hemoglobin in a protein membrane. The rest of the cell is made up of a fatty substance.

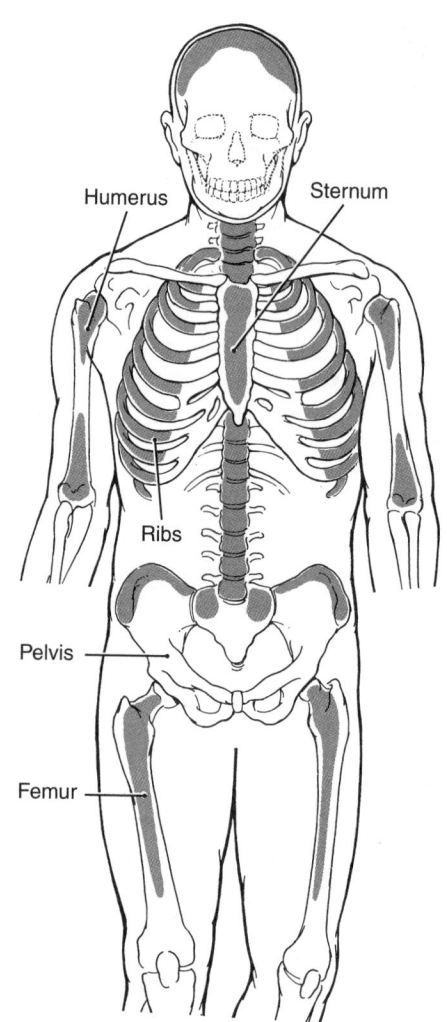

Bone marrow, the site of red blood cell production in adults, is primarily located in the skull, sternum, vertebrae, ribs, pelvis, hips, and in part of the humerus and femur.

While red blood cells transport oxygen to the body's tissues and carbon dioxide away from the tissues, they also play an important role in the regulation of the acid-base balance of the blood and the formation of bile (part of the digestive juice secreted by the liver and gallbladder).

In traveling through the circulatory system, red blood cells are subject to tremendous wear and tear. These cells are continuously dying, disintegrating, and being replaced. The average life of a red blood cell is 120 days. As the red blood cells break down, cells of the spleen, liver, and bone marrow pick up the debris. The proteins and iron are then stored and used in the formation of new red blood cells.

In adults, red blood cells are produced in the bone marrow, principally in the spinal vertebrae, ribs, breastbone, skull, and at the ends of the thigh and upper arm bones. Proper formation of red blood cells depends on healthy conditions in the marrow, which are promoted most importantly by sufficient dietary iron, but also by sufficient amounts of cobalt, copper, amino acids, vitamin B_{12}, and folic acid.

The body naturally regulates the total mass of red blood cells in the circulatory system within narrow limits. In a healthy system, there are enough red blood cells to ensure proper oxygenation, yet they are not packed tightly enough to hinder blood flow.

WHITE BLOOD CELLS: WHAT THEY ARE AND WHAT THEY DO

Like red blood cells, most white blood cells, or leukocytes, are produced in the bone marrow, although some are produced in the lymph nodes, thymus, and spleen as well. White blood cells play a crucial role in the body's defense system. Larger than red blood cells, white blood cells are actually a mixed assortment of cells differing in size, shape, activity, and function. Together, they ward off and combat foreign particles that threaten the body's health and integrity.

White blood cells travel like scavengers, seeking out the presence of pathogens (microorganisms or substances capable of causing disease). Whenever disease-causing bacteria or viruses attack the body, chemicals are released that beckon the white blood cells, which then penetrate tissue and sift through debris. Drawn and directed by injured cells, some white blood cells are capable of moving between the circulatory and lymph systems. Some ingest and destroy the invading substances. Afterwards, white blood cells return to the bloodstream, except for the most common ones (neutrophils) (see page 918 for a more detailed discussion of the immune system).

There are two basic types of white blood cells that collectively guard the body against such potentially infectious foreign agents as bacteria, viruses, fungi, and parasites. Granulocytes—so named because of the *granules* (small particles or grains) in their cytoplasm—are the most numerous type. Formed in the bone marrow, granulocytes include functionally distinct cells called neutrophils, eosinophils, and baso-

phils. Neutrophils are the most common white blood cells; eosinophils and basophils are far less numerous but perform essential functions nonetheless.

The other type of white blood cells, agranulocytes or mononuclear leukocytes, lack granules. Included in this type of white blood cell are lymphocytes and monocytes. Lymphocytes are formed in the lymph nodes, thymus, spleen, and bone marrow. Lymphocytes are responsible for promoting the body's immunity against disease. They include B cells, which produce antibodies, and T cells, which attack foreign and virus-infected cells. Monocytes are formed from the cells lining the capillaries in various organs, primarily the spleen and bone marrow. They assist the granulocytes in defending against disease-carrying microorganisms.

Thus, the various white blood cells work together to fight infection and repair injury. Neutrophils ingest bacteria and small particles; they also produce chemicals that destroy the bacteria. Monocytes, which make up around 8 percent of the body's white cells, ingest larger particles and pick up cell debris that results from bacterial attack. Their actions make up the *inflammatory response*; the inflammation, swelling, and pus you may notice around infected areas of the skin are partly a result of the outpouring of neutrophils at the site.

Lymphocytes make up about a quarter of the body's white cells. While they do not have the ability to ingest and destroy particles, they form the body's immune response. This crucial function of providing the body with its natural immunity to disease involves B cell lymphocytes and T cell lymphocytes. B cell lymphocytes produce antibodies that guard your body against bacterial invasion. T cell lymphocytes produce cellular immunity. By generating substances that act as antitoxins, they can offset much of the damage that bacterial toxins and chemicals can cause.

Eosinophils, which make up between 1 and 4 percent of your white blood cells, are capable of eliminating foreign particles. They also perform the vital task of modulating the effects of certain immunologic situations to prevent the body from harming itself. When foreign proteins, called antigens, invade the blood, your body responds by manufacturing antibodies to counteract

HOW BLOOD CLOTS

Each day, numerous holes and tears appear within the vessels of the blood system. Some of these injuries are minor in size and consequence; some are large and more serious. Whenever a blood vessel is severed or ruptured, an elaborate biologic process, called hemostasis, is set in motion to prevent blood loss and repair the injury.

Immediately after a blood vessel is ruptured or cut, the wall of the vessel contracts. This contraction or spasm slows down blood flow; it is caused in part by the release of certain factors from the tissues and blood platelets. As the vessel contracts and constricts, platelet plugging and blood coagulation begin to take place.

Platelets repair vascular openings in several ways. When platelets come into contact with a damaged vascular surface, they immediately swell, assume irregular forms, become sticky, and release granules and other substances. These substances (factors) are instrumental in forming the plug and promoting coagulation. As platelets congregate at the injury site, they form a platelet plug, a fairly loose mat that blocks blood loss.

When the tear in the blood vessel is very small, platelet plugs are sufficient to seal them off. When the injury is large or the trauma somewhat severe, the next step is blood coagulation, or clotting. Clotting is the process by which blood changes into a jelly-like, nonfluid mass. More than 50 substances present in the blood are necessary for coagulation to run smoothly. Some of these substances, called procoagulants, promote coagulation; others, which inhibit coagulation are called anticoagulants. Whether or not the blood will coagulate when it should, but *only* when it should, depends on the balance between the two.

Clotting takes place in three steps. First, in response to a rupture in the vessel or damage to the blood itself, a complex cascade of chemical reactions occurs in the blood involving numerous blood coagulation factors. The result is the formation of prothrombin activator. Second, prothrombin activator prompts the conversion of prothrombin into thrombin, which is formed when elements in the blood are exposed to air, foreign substances, juices from injured tissues, or prothrombin activator. Third, the thrombin acts to convert a blood plasma protein, fibrinogen, into fibrin fibers. This insoluble, elastic, stringy substance forms a meshwork in which the corpuscles are entangled. Thus, a clot is formed.

Blood clots are composed, then, of a mesh-like structure of fibrin fibers, running in all directions and entrapping blood cells, platelets, and plasma. The fibrin fibers also adhere to damaged surfaces. Once the clot forms, it begins to contract. Most of the fluid is extracted from the site. This process of clot retraction pulls together the edges of the broken blood vessel. The damaged cells and protein fragments then stimulate the healing of the wound by repair and scar formation.

Clotting involves a number of substances that are termed variously by names as well as numbers. Some of the most common are:

- Factor I: fibrinogen

- Factor II: prothrombin

- Factor III: tissue factor

- Factor IV: calcium

- Factor V: proaccelerin; labile factor

- Factor VII: proconvertin; serum prothrombin conversion accelerator

- Factor VIII: antihemophilic factor

- Factor IX: plasma thromboplastin component; Christmas factor; antihemophilic factor B

- Factor X: Stuart or Proctor factor

- Factor XI: plasma thromboplastin antecedent

- Factor XII: Hageman or glass factor

- Factor XIII: fibrin stabilizing factor; Laki-Lorand factor

- Prekallikrein: Fletcher factor

- High-molecular-weight kininogen: Fitzgerald factor; HMWK

Clotting and bleeding disorders arise when there is a deficiency or defect in a specific factor (for example, factors VIII and IX in hemophilia). Treatment for those disorders often involves replacing those factors by infusion. ■

The first stage in wound repair is the formation of a platelet plug. As platelets discover a vascular break, they gather and swell, becoming sticky, and release substances necessary to form a plug and promote coagulation (clot formation).

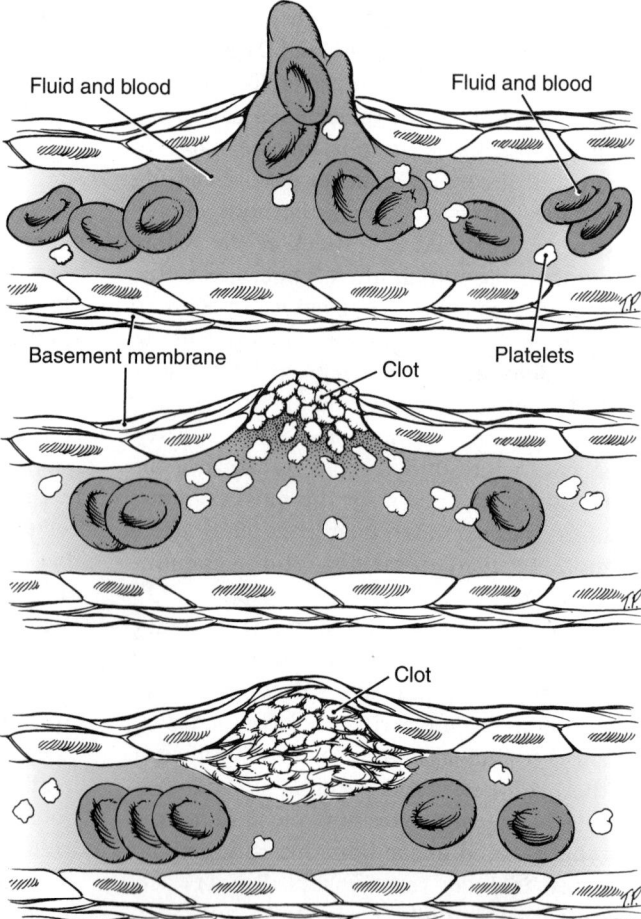

BLOOD GROUP TYPING

Years ago, medical professionals noticed that some transfusions were successful but most were not. Whether immediately or days after, many individuals would develop fierce, and sometimes deadly reactions to the transfused blood. This observation led to important discoveries about blood and blood groups.

The type of blood you have is genetically determined and is defined by whether or not you have certain protein molecules or antigens in your blood. Based on the presence or absence of these antigens, your blood is classified according to two systems, the ABO and the Rhesus (Rh) systems. The ABO system, discovered in 1901 by Landsteiner, is of prime importance in blood transfusions. The Rhesus (Rh) system is especially important in obstetrics.

The population is divided into four ABO blood groups—A, B, AB, and O. These groups correspond to the presence or absence of two antigens, A and B, on the surface of the red blood cells. Also called agglutinogens because they provoke the blood cells to become stuck to one another, these antigens are inherited. Consequently, you may have neither A nor B on your cells, or you may have one, or you may have both simultaneously. Your blood type would be categorized accordingly. If you are in the A group, you have the A antigen on the surface of your red blood cells. Those in the B group have the B antigen on red cells. AB has both A and B antigens. O has neither A nor B antigens.

In addition, individuals in each group have in their blood serum the antibody that corresponds to the red cell antigens. These antibodies are called agglutinin. Thus, if you have type A blood, your red blood cells are coated with A antigens, and antibodies against B are present in your blood serum. If you have type B blood, you have anti-A antibodies. People with AB blood have both A and B antigen, and no antibodies. Those who have group O blood have no antigens and both anti-A and anti-B antibodies.

Because each person spontaneously forms antibodies against antigens that his own red blood cells lack, blood collected for transfusions is compatible for some recipients but not for others. Should a person receive blood that contains blood group antigens different from his own, antibodies in his blood would attack these foreign cells within the transfused blood. In order to make transfusions safe, blood groups are matched (see page 914).

Since type O blood can interact with any other type without provoking an antibody reaction (see page 914), people with type O blood are considered universal donors. People with AB blood are considered *universal recipients* because they can receive any type without developing a strong reaction to the blood.

The exact makeup of a person's blood—which antigens it carries—is determined genetically. Because blood composition is inherited in a consistent manner, knowledge of one's blood type can be used to exclude paternity. Serious medical complications can result from the way in which antigens and antibodies interact during transfusions, transplantation, or other surgical procedures. Therefore, being aware of your blood group is important.

In addition to classifying blood groups according to the ABO system, each of these categories is divided into two Rh types. The Rh classification indicates whether you have an antigen, called Rhesus component or factor, in your blood. If you are Rh-positive, you have the component; if you are Rh-negative, you do not. Knowing that Rh factor is present or absent in your blood is of particular importance during pregnancy.

The human body does not spontaneously produce antibodies to fend off Rh factor. However, a woman can develop antibodies after she is exposed to Rh-positive blood during her first pregnancy. Specifically, problems can arise when a mother is Rh-negative and the father is Rh-positive. Should the fetus inherit the father's Rh-positive blood, it becomes incompatible with that of the mother. This initial incompatibility sensitizes the woman, and she begins to produce the antibodies that will react to and attack the incompatible blood in her body. Thus, any subsequent exposure to Rh-positive blood, such as with a second pregnancy, can lead to serious complications. The antibodies can pass through the placenta and attack the developing fetus. There is a very real chance that the fetus will develop severe anemia as a result. With each pregnancy, the risk of such complications increases.

However, Rh disease is not the problem it once was. Through prenatal screening, serum used to prevent Rh-negative women from developing antibodies, and effective therapy for an affected fetus and infant, Rh incompatibility makes a pregnancy a high-risk condition, but not a tragic one.

Eighty-five percent of white Americans are Rh-positive. Among African-Americans, the percentage is slightly higher. Virtually all Asian-Americans and Native Americans have Rh-positive blood.

In the United States, approximately 47 percent of the population has type O blood; 41 percent has type A; 9 percent has type B; and 3 percent has AB. Overall, O positive blood is the most common group; then A positive, B positive, O negative, A negative, AB positive, B negative, and AB negative. ∎

the antigens. During this process, specialized cells known as mast cells release the chemical histamine (which acts at the site of injury), and eosinophils work to temper its effects. Otherwise, too much histamine can trigger an allergic reaction.

Basophils comprise less than 1 percent of all white blood cells. They are not only involved in the body's immunologic reactions, but also produce heparin, an anticoagulant that prevents the blood from clotting at random sites within the blood vessels.

PLATELETS: WHAT THEY ARE AND WHAT THEY DO

Platelets, or thrombocytes, are small, colorless, granular cells that contain several clotting factors, various enzymes, and other

BLOOD TRANSFUSIONS

There are many medical emergencies and conditions that necessitate blood transfusions. Most transfusions are done to replace blood when a great deal has been lost in some type of injury. Approximately 14 percent of people undergoing surgery require blood transfusions. Transfusions are also used to treat certain blood disorders.

Today, blood transfusions are safer than ever, but like all medical procedures, they are not risk-free. In all cases, the possible risks of transfusion must be weighed against the possible benefits. To reduce the likelihood of complications, blood banks crossmatch the recipient's and the donor's blood. A sample of your blood will be matched with some of the donor blood to confirm that they are compatible.

There are many antigen systems in the body. Antigens are the substances that stimulate the formation of antibodies; the antigen-antibody reaction forms the basis for immunity (see page 918). Yet, only the blood types (ABO system) and Rh system are specifically tested before most transfusions (see page 913). The A and B antigens are most important, because if you lack one or both of these, your plasma contains antibodies against them. These antibodies can cause rapid destruction of blood cells (hemolysis) if you are given mismatched blood. In an emergency, type O blood can be given to any recipient, although only concentrated red blood cells should be given. Otherwise, there is a chance that the recipient will receive plasma from a donor that may contain the anti-A or anti-B antibodies (see page 940).

The other important antigen routinely screened for is the D antigen of the Rh system. Approximately 15 percent of the population lacks this antigen. If you lack the D antigen and receive D-positive blood, you will likely develop anti-D antibodies that can complicate future transfusions.

Despite such testing, there are a number of transfusion-related complications that, however infrequent, present an important consideration when weighing the risks and benefits of transfusions.

Hemolytic Transfusion Reactions

Hemolytic transfusion reactions are the most potentially serious complications of transfusion. Such reactions can be fatal. These reactions are most severe when, for some reason, there is a mismatch in blood types. Upon receiving incompatible blood, the individual's natural antibodies attack the foreign blood, causing hemolysis (the rapid breakdown within the vascular system of red blood cells which it releases). The severity of these reactions depends on the amount of red blood cells given. This reaction is most dangerous when a person is under anesthesia. Because an anesthetized patient cannot respond to such early warning symptoms as chills or muscle tenderness and pain, the reaction may not be noted until it is well advanced.

Other symptoms of a hemolytic reaction include fever, shaking, chest pain, low back pain, pain along the vein in which the transfusion was given, nausea, hives, or pink urine. Symptoms that signal more serious reactions include labored, difficult breathing; a precipitant drop in blood pressure; shock; vascular collapse; and renal failure. When these symptoms are recognized during the transfusion, the transfusion should be stopped immediately.

Sometimes, hemolytic reactions are less severe and develop gradually. You may not notice a reaction until 5 to 10 days after the transfusion; then you may notice fever, chills, backache, and headache. If you do experience any of these symptoms soon after receiving a transfusion, contact your doctor.

Leukoagglutinin Reactions

Leukoagglutinin reactions are immune reactions to the proteins present in white blood cells or platelets. Usually, these types of reactions happen only after an individual has been sensitized through previous transfusions or pregnancy. Leukoagglutinin reactions are most often signaled by fever and chills within 12 hours of the transfusion. In more severe reactions, a serious cough or labored breathing may result. Leukoagglutinin reactions tend to respond well to acetaminophen and diphenhydramine. In severe cases, corticosteroids can help.

Anaphylactic Reactions

Anaphylactic reactions are rare immune reactions, marked by hives or bronchospasm during a transfusion. These reactions almost always occur in people who are deficient in plasma protein—most frequently, immunoglobulin A (IgA)—and who have consequently developed antibodies to them. Transfusions of washed or frozen red blood cells may be necessary to avoid future reactions.

The risk of such immunologic reactions increases with each blood transfusion. If you are exposed to different blood antigens from different donors, you may develop greater sensitivity to foreign blood groups as time goes on.

Communicable Disease

Another complication associated with transfusions is the possibility of contracting a *communicable disease* through the transfused blood. All blood products (red blood cells, platelets, plasma, cryoprecipitate) can transmit viral infection. Despite the use of routine blood screening, transfusion-related hepatitis remains a problem. Hepatitis viruses cause problems that range from mild chronic infections to liver failure (see page 1046).

Blood transfusions can spread other communicable diseases, such as cytomegalovirus infection, syphilis, malaria, toxoplasmosis, and acquired immunodeficiency syndrome (AIDS). The risk of contracting such diseases through transfusion has significantly decreased, because hospitals and blood banks have adopted more rigorous screening procedures.

Increased Blood Volume and Iron Overload

Finally, people with heart problems can have difficulties handling the increased blood volume that transfusions can introduce into the system. Repeated transfusions of red blood cells can result in iron overload. In extreme cases, too much iron can lead to liver damage, heart failure, arrhythmia (irregular heartbeat), arthritis, or bronze diabetes (in which the skin takes on a bronze tint). Iron overload can also cause impotence or sterility.

THE COMPLETE BLOOD COUNT AND OTHER COMMON BLOOD TESTS

A blood test is often conducted as part of any routine medical examination. Assessment of the presence and amount of electrolytes (chloride, potassium, sodium, phosphorus), sugar, creatinine (a substance found in urine that can be used to measure kidney function), fats and cholesterol, uric acid (another substance found in urine), proteins, hormones, and gases, to name a small fraction of substances measured, provide a window on how your body is functioning. This information is used to rule out certain disorders and to help make accurate diagnoses.

When your doctor wants to measure blood fats and glucose levels, you will be instructed to fast overnight. Otherwise, blood tests can often be conducted without regard to when you last ate. Usually, the blood will be taken from a vein in the arm. After the area is cleansed with alcohol, a thin needle will be inserted, and blood drawn into a syringe. When only a few drops are necessary, a small sample of blood will be taken from your fingertip. Your fingertip will be pricked, and the blood will be drawn up from capillaries into a small vial called a capillary pipette.

The complete blood count, or CBC, enumerates the blood cells within the bloodstream. The number of each type of blood cell—red blood cells (erythrocytes), the various white blood cells (leukocytes), and platelets (thrombocytes)—is counted, and any abnormality in shape or size is noted. The percentage of total blood volume occupied by red blood cells (hematocrit value) is also measured as is the amount of hemoglobin (the iron-rich molecules that carry oxygen to the body's tissues) within the red blood cells.

Usually the blood count is calculated per cubic millimeter (mm^3) of whole blood. The normal count in each cubic millimeter of blood is on average 5 million red blood cells in males and 4.5 million in women. The white blood cell count averages 5,000 to 10,000/mm^3, whereas platelets average 150,000 to 450,000/mm^3. In healthy blood, the hematocrit value is around 42 percent in women and 47 percent in men.

A differential blood count tells the percentage of various white blood cells in each 100 cells counted. In order to arrive at a detailed white blood cell count, a very thin layer of blood on a glass slide is stained and examined under a microscope. The shape and structure of the various types of white blood cells are identified and studied as are the overall number of proportions. In healthy blood, neutrophils usually represent 40 to 60 percent of the white blood cell count; lymphocytes, 20 to 40 percent;

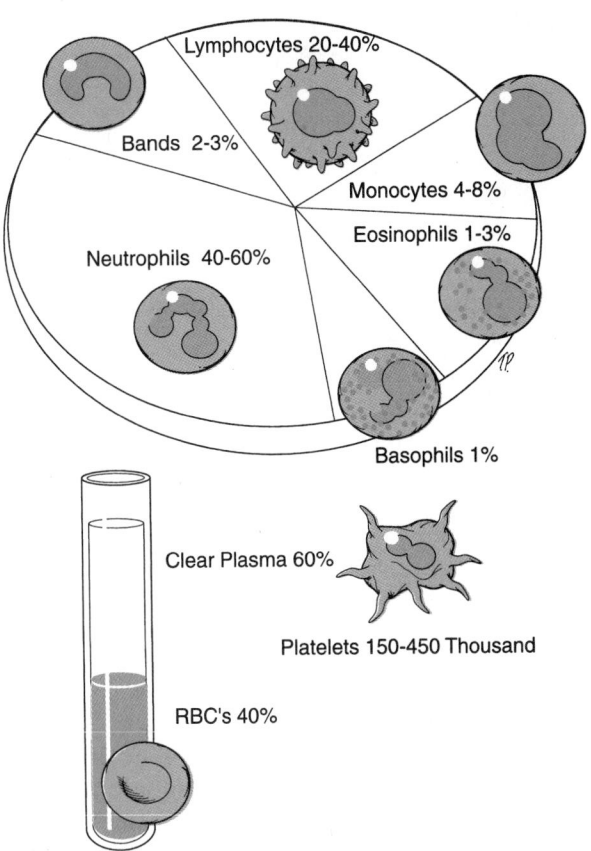

Blood is made up of fluid (plasma) and cells (red blood cells, white blood cells, and platelets). The most common kind of blood cell is the red cell. Red blood cells play a central role in exchanging oxygen for carbon monoxide in the lungs. Neutrophils (40 to 60 percent of all white blood cells) fight infection by destroying bacteria. Bands (2 to 3 percent) are newly produced young neutrophils. Lymphocytes (20 to 40 percent) make antibodies and help identify foreign tissues and invaders. Monocytes (4 to 8 percent) are present in many organs and remove foreign elements and microorganisms. Eosinophils (1 to 3 percent) fight parasitic infections and are involved in allergic reactions. Basophils (1 percent) deliver antibodies that remove foreign particles. Platelets play a major role in blood clotting. Normal blood cell counts are red blood cells 4 to 5 million/mm^3, white blood cells 5,000 to 10,000/mm^3, and platelets 150,000/mm^3 to 450,000/mm^3.

monocytes, 4 to 8 percent; eosinophils, 1 to 3 percent; and basophils, around 1 percent. ▸

active substances, including the neurotransmitter serotonin. Most platelets originate in the bone marrow cells. They are the tiniest cells in your body. Since each milliliter of blood contains approximately 250 million platelets, they are always nearby to perform their basic function—to make the blood clot.

Platelets work to promote vascular constriction, stem bleeding, and repair injured blood vessels. Normally, the walls of your blood vessels, the endothelium, are lined with a smooth layer of cells, called endothelial cells. Whenever blood vessel walls are damaged, platelets congregate to form plugs at the site. This process of coagulation or clot formation is completed when certain proteins that further clotting are released by the platelets and plasma (see page 912).

▶ Red blood cells are not counted in the differential blood count, but their shape, size, and color are evaluated.

Some of the other tests run to assess the blood system and diagnose blood disorders include the following:

- *Erythrocyte sedimentation rate (ESR)* measures the time it takes for red blood cells to settle to the bottom of a container. When cells settle faster than expected, this suggests that other factors are at work such as anemia, infection, inflammation, or cancer.

- *Coombs' antiglobulin tests* form the basis for diagnosing immune hemolytic disorders by detecting the presence of certain antiglobulins on the surface of red blood cells. These abnormal antibodies (immunoglobulin [IgG] antibodies) interact with the hemoglobin molecules in such a way as to make the cells fragile. When the body produces these antibodies, the result is often autoimmune hemolytic anemia, the type of anemia that arises when red blood cells are broken down (hemolyzed) faster than the bone marrow can produce replacement cells (see page 925). In a Coombs' test, a rabbit antibody is mixed with the person's red blood cells. If IgG antibodies are present on the surface of red blood cells, the rabbit antibodies make the cells clump together (agglutination). The indirect Coombs' test is performed by mixing the person's serum with type O red blood cells. After a period of incubation, Coombs' reagent is added. In this procedure, agglutination indicates the presence of free antibody in the individual's serum.

- *Coagulation tests* assess how long it takes the blood to clot and are used to diagnose or rule out the existence of clotting disorders. Numerous coagulation tests are available to assess different parts of the complicated process of coagulation. The most commonly used are the prothrombin time and activated partial thromboplastin time. The prothrombin time test is used to monitor the effects of coumadin (an anticoagulant medication) therapy, and the activated partial thromboplastin time test is used to gauge the correct dose of another anticoagulant medication, heparin. ■

In addition to being instrumental in blood coagulation, platelets carry a number of proteins, hormones, enzymes, growth factors, and other substances that are essential to the body's balance and health. Platelets are active in the system for anywhere between 8 and 12 days, after which time they are eliminated through the spleen, liver, and lungs.

Understanding the Lymph System and Spleen

Most people regard the body's circulatory system as a system of blood vessels, stretching out into rivers and tributaries that spread all the way to the fingers and toes. While this is true, the perception is incomplete. There are actually two circulatory systems: one for blood, the other for lymphatic fluid.

Just as blood circulates through the blood vessels, lymphatic fluid circulates between the cells that make up the different tissues. While blood circulates exclusively through blood vessels, lymphatic fluid, also called lymph, passes through the tissues themselves and fills the spaces between cells. Derived from blood plasma, this clear, watery tissue fluid seeps out through the porous walls, bathes the cells, and carries oxygen, nutrients, and water from the bloodstream to them. Cell waste products, such as carbon dioxide and water, are picked up by the lymph and transported back to the blood system. In this way, lymph acts as the conductor between the blood and the tissue cells.

The lymphatic system is made up of lymphatic vessels and capillaries that lie close to veins and arteries in most tissues, with the exception of the nervous system. Lymphatic vessels float like fine hairs among the cells, gathering up excess fluid from the tissues. Because the walls of lymphatic capillaries are porous, substances of various sizes can pass through their walls. Like blood vessels, lymphatic vessels have valves that prevent the lymph from flowing in the wrong direction.

Along the vessels lie lymphatic nodes or glands. These small bodies vary in size: the smallest are the size of a pinhead and the larger ones resemble grapes. They function primarily to filter out bacteria and other toxic substances that are flushed out from the tissues by the fluid. Lymph nodes bunch together at various sites in the body. The axillary nodes are located under the armpits; they filter the lymph from the upper limb and chest wall. The cervical nodes are found under your chin and in your neck; they filter the fluid from the head, mouth, and tongue. Lymph nodes in the groin (inguinal nodes) filter lymph from

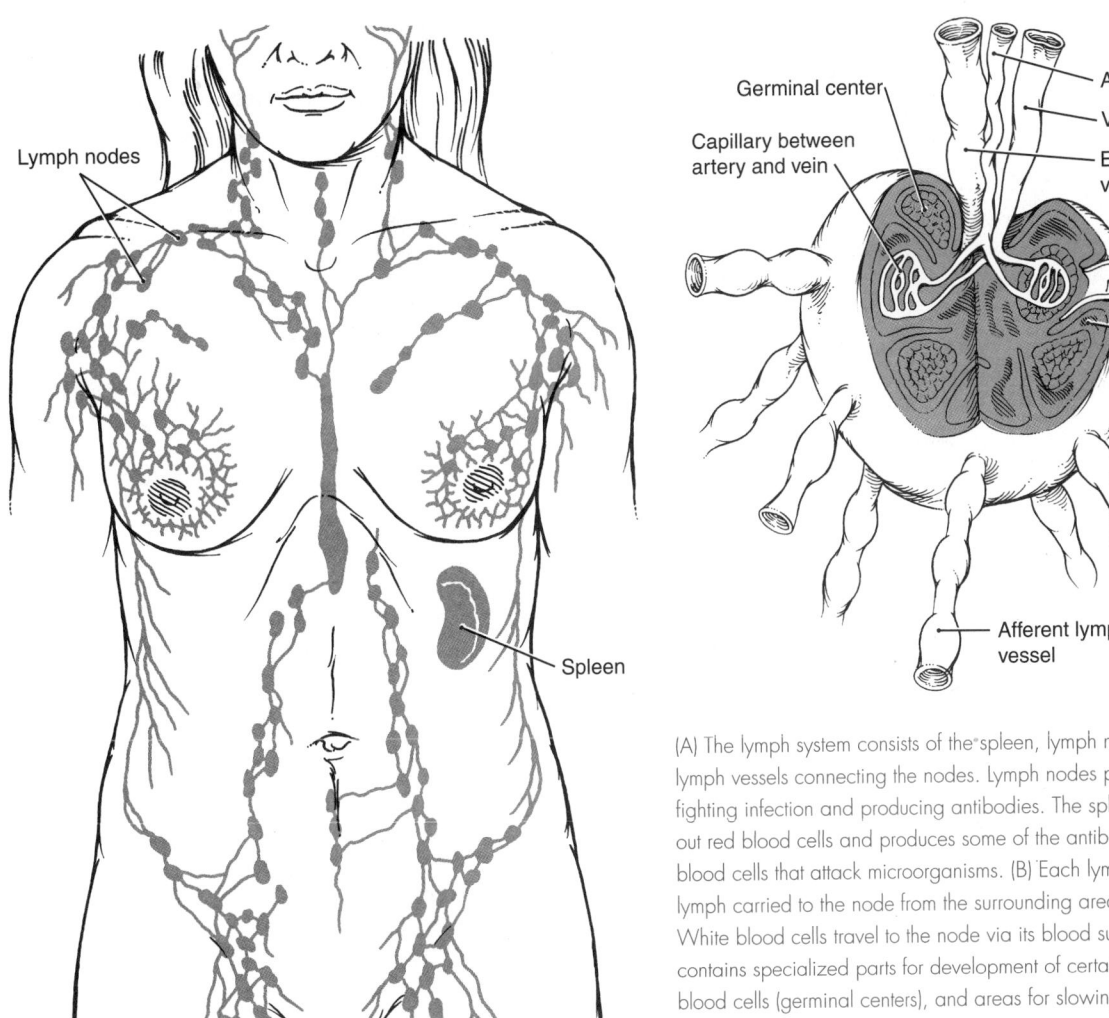

Lymph nodes

Spleen

Germinal center

Capillary between artery and vein

Artery

Vein

Efferent lymph vessel

Sinus

Afferent lymph vessel

(A) The lymph system consists of the spleen, lymph nodes, and the lymph vessels connecting the nodes. Lymph nodes play a key role in fighting infection and producing antibodies. The spleen removes worn-out red blood cells and produces some of the antibodies and white blood cells that attack microorganisms. (B) Each lymph node filters lymph carried to the node from the surrounding area of the body. White blood cells travel to the node via its blood supply. The node contains specialized parts for development of certain types of white blood cells (germinal centers), and areas for slowing lymph to allow debris and microorganisms to be consumed (sinuses).

the lower abdomen and lower limbs. The lymph from the internal organs passes through clusters in the abdomen and chest, called abdominal and mediastinal nodes.

Lymph travels to the nodes through the lymph vessels. As harmful substances are filtered out, you may notice a swelling around your lymph nodes—in your neck, for example, especially when there is an infection. The fluid is then emptied into two lymphatic ducts—the right lymphatic duct and the thoracic duct—and moved on to the heart through the main vein, the superior vena cava. In that way, lymph is recycled, put back into the bloodstream to start its journey again.

Sometimes, an infection is apparent only when lymph nodes swell as they fill with infection-fighting cells. This is why your doctor may feel your jaw or neck if you complain of feeling ill, to check for evidence of swollen lymph nodes. The tonsils and adenoids, for example, are similar to lymph glands, and serve the same immune-protective function. Because they are positioned strategically at the entrance to the breathing and swallowing passages, tonsils and adenoids can screen bacteria and viruses that enter the nose and mouth. As a result, low-level infection of the tonsils may occur, helping the immune system form antibodies to defend against future infections. Sometimes, the response is not minor, but the tonsil swells rather dramatically (see page 592).

A certain type of lymphocyte, the T lymphocyte, is produced in the lymph nodes.

HOW THE IMMUNE SYSTEM WORKS

When all is working the way it should, the immune system rids our bodies of infectious agents, allowing us to live without worry of disease most of the time. When faced with foreign invaders, the body marshals its army of white blood cells. Together, these cells act as guardian and active agent against infection. It is this complicated cellular activity that constitutes the body's immune response.

The body's white blood cells (leukocytes) are a very mixed lot. They are principally responsible for guarding the body against such potentially infectious foreign agents as bacteria, viruses, fungi, and parasites. There are cells called *granulocytes* that have granules in their nucleus; this type includes distinct cells called *neutrophils, eosinophils,* and *basophils.* Those white blood cells that lack granules are called *agranulocytes*; these include *lymphocytes* and *monocytes.*

While the body's white blood cells work together to ward off infection and to repair damage done by foreign agents, each has a slightly different function. Neutrophils ingest bacteria and small particles and produce chemicals that destroy the bacteria. Monocytes ingest larger particles and gather up cell debris from bacterial attack. Eosinophils are capable of eliminating foreign particles; together with basophils, they are involved in the body's immunologic reactions.

While all leukocytes have a role in the body's immune response, lymphocytes play the largest part in providing the body with its natural immunity to disease. There are two main types of lymphocytes: *B cells*, which produce antibodies, and *T cells*, which attack foreign and virus-infected cells. Yet, the precise workings of the body's immune system are not wholly understood. We do know that B lymphocytes generate antibodies, clusters of molecules that form in response to the antigen, the foreign substance (usually a protein) produced by an invading organism. The antigen alerts the immune system to the invader's presence.

There are five general classes of antibodies: IgG, IgM, IgA, IgE, IgD. Also referred to as the gamma globulins, these antibodies target the infectious agent and signal other white blood cells to approach and destroy. This kind of immune reaction is called a humoral response. ▶

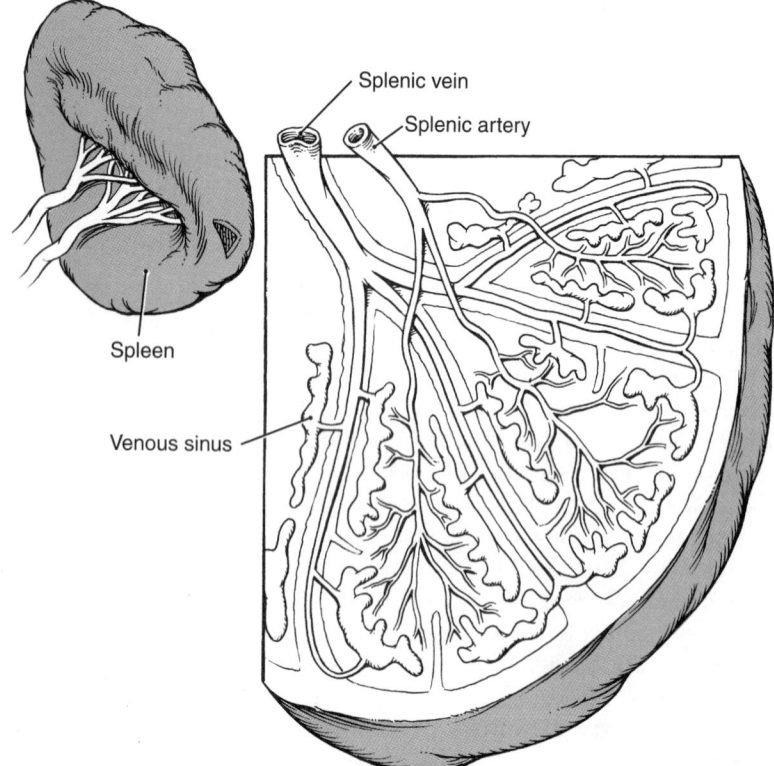

Anatomy of the spleen. The spleen is a fist-sized organ in the upper left part of the abdomen. Blood enters via the splenic artery. In the venous sinuses of the spleen lie lymphocytes and phagocytes, which are white blood cells that consume foreign particles and other cells. A primary function of the spleen is the removal of red blood cells that are no longer functional. Blood leaves via the splenic vein.

Splenic vein

Splenic artery

Spleen

Venous sinus

(The other type, B lymphocytes, are formed in the bone marrow; they make antibodies, also called gamma globulins, in response to foreign substances found in the system.) T cells play a vital role in the body's defense. As these cells mature, they are poured into the bloodstream by which they travel in search of pathogens (see page 918). Many are transported through the lymphatic fluid as well.

In addition to cleansing the body's tissue fluids and aiding in the body's immunity processes, the lymphatic system serves a number of other functions. Lymph nodes help the body absorb digested food, especially fat, in the abdomen. And they filter out any malignant cells that may enter the lymphatic system. (That is why swelling in the armpit may be a sign of breast cancer.)

Another important organ related to the lymph system is the spleen. A long, dark-red tissue located in the upper-rear-left section of the abdomen, the spleen consists of cells that ingest small particles (worn-out cells, bacteria, fungi, and viruses). The spleen is actually sponge-like lymphatic tissue, differentiated into white and red blood cells.

In the human embryo, the spleen produces all types of blood cells. In adults, only lymphocytes and monocytes are produced in the spleen. If, however, the bone marrow is damaged, the spleen can function to manufacture other cells. The smooth muscles

▶ T lymphocytes, manufactured in the thymus gland, make chemicals that foster antibody production. These lymphocytes are involved in the body's allergic response to foreign particles. T cells generate antibodies that neutralize proteins carried in invading microorganisms, thus guarding the body against potential damage from them. T cells also provide the chemicals to guard against an exaggerated reaction after immunization and vaccination.

In addition, T cells aid in the actual destruction of pathogens, either by digesting the invading agents or by sending out toxic compounds to destroy them—an act described in the scientific community as "delivery of the lethal hit" or a cell-mediated response. Different types of T cells operate in the direct assault, including *helper T cells*, which provide the toxins responsible for the lethal hit, and *memory T cells*, which retain the capability to recall and initiate an immune response when reexposure occurs.

Despite rigorous research, just how these processes operate from this point is mostly a matter of educated conjecture. It is highly likely that when the presence of pathogens is detected, they are taken to a nearby lymph node or to the spleen, where macrophages (wandering cells) surround them. Here, T and B cells perform a kind of analysis. Because T cells retain chemical memory of the particular protein (antigen) in the pathogen, they may be able to recognize it whenever it reappears in the body. B cells can then reproduce quickly to subdue it.

Thus, the immune response takes two forms: adaptive and innate. Adaptive, or "active," immunity occurs when the body responds to pathogens it perceives as new and foreign. Once these antigens are sensed and identified, a cascade of events that make up the immune response is set in motion. Innate immunity refers to the human system's remarkable ability to defeat infection before it truly gets under way by recognizing and quickly subduing pathogens it had previously encountered.

Most of the time, the immune system works wonderfully well to rid our bodies of disease-producing agents. Sometimes, however, our adaptive immunity can diminish, occasionally to the point of being almost ineffective. When lymphocyte production is curtailed or weakened, the body suffers what is called an immunodeficiency, leaving it vulnerable to serious infection (see page 944). Certain diseases can cause a partial or complete shutdown of the immune system. Some of these are inherited diseases transmitted through genes, and some of them are acquired diseases transmitted through direct contact.

The most widespread, and most widely publicized acquired immune disease in recent history is acquired immunodeficiency syndrome, or AIDS. AIDS is caused by the human immunodeficiency virus, HIV, which attacks the body in several ways. Most significantly, it destroys the body's T cells and disarms their ability to respond to infectious agents that normally would be easily defeated and inconsequential. For more information see AIDS in Chapter 21.

Other diseases are inborn and prevent the immune system from acting as it normally would to prevent infection (see The "Boy in the Bubble" Disease, page 944). Still other illnesses cause immunodeficiency that is treatment related. In the case of organ transplantation, for example, immunosuppressive therapy—use of drugs that intentionally suppress the immune response—is necessary; otherwise the body would recognize the transplanted organ as foreign and begin to mount an immune response against it (see Immunodeficiency, page 944). In all of these situations, pathogens (disease-producing organisms) that ordinarily would not actually cause serious disease can result in life-threatening infection, because the immune system is impaired. ■

and elastic tissue of the spleen enable it to contract and discharge blood cells into circulation. The spleen also functions to store and filter blood. Small particles such as bacteria and spent red blood cells are removed from circulation through the spleen.

Finally, T cell lymphocytes mature from simple white blood cells in the thymus, an organ located near the heart. Because T cells serve such an important role in the body's cellular immune response, the thymus is an essential part of the lymph system.

The Red Blood Cell System and Its Disorders

An exacting process of checks and balances regulates the red blood cell system. When all goes well, the bone marrow works to produce sufficient numbers of red blood cells to compensate, because those in circulation naturally die off and disintegrate. Whenever there is a condition or circumstance that causes a drop in the amount of oxygen transported to the tissues by the red blood cells, the body will ordinarily increase its production of these cells. Whenever something compromises the ability of your bone marrow to keep up with your body's demand for red blood cells, production at other sites in the bone marrow will normally kick up its supply.

In other words, at all times, your body needs a sufficient number of red blood cells in circulation to ensure that the tissues, even those at the tips of your fingers and your toes, get enough oxygen. A significant drop or deficiency in the number of red blood cells in your bloodstream—and thus, in the amount of oxygen making its way through your body—constitutes the blood disorder anemia. At the same time, if too many red blood cells are produced, the flow of your blood can become impeded and sluggish, in which case you may have a disorder called polycythemia.

Both anemia and polycythemia can be caused by a multitude of conditions. In addition, how severe the anemia or polycythemia is and how well it responds to treatment varies greatly, often depending on what caused it to arise in the first place.

ANEMIAS

Anemia is the most common type of blood disorder. It can result either because red blood cells are being lost too rapidly or because they are being produced too slowly. Anemia also arises when the supply of hemoglobin is diminished. Typically, anemias are classified according to whether the condition is related to diminished production, accelerated loss of red blood cells, or distorted cell size or shape.

The most common cause of anemia is a shortage of iron in people's diets. Iron is used to make up hemoglobin; whenever it is lacking, each red blood cell will have an insufficient amount of hemoglobin. In the vast majority of cases, iron-deficiency anemia is easily corrected by increasing your consumption of iron (for a more detailed discussion, see page 921). Iron deficiency can also be a sign of an occult (hidden) bleeding and should cause you and your doctor to investigate.

It is possible for someone to become anemic, for example, after losing a lot of blood rapidly. Usually, though, assuming there is no subsequent hemorrhage, the person's body will be able to compensate for the loss within a few weeks. Thus, the anemia is transient.

When the blood loss is chronic, however, the body may not be able to make up for the hemoglobin that is being rapidly lost. Red blood cells are then produced with too little hemoglobin.

In some cases, the body produces red blood cells that are so fragile that they rupture easily as they pass through the capillaries. This is often due to genetic abnormalities. When this happens, red blood cells die off much too quickly for them to be replaced. This type of accelerated loss and destruction of red blood cells is referred to as hemolytic anemia (see page 925).

Whenever something—for example, excessive x-rays, nuclear exposure, certain industrial chemicals, and some drugs—damages bone marrow and interferes with its function, to the point that it cannot keep up with the body's demand for red blood cells, the condition is called aplastic anemia (see page 947).

If your diet is deficient in vitamin B_{12} or folic acid, or if for some reason your body cannot absorb these nutrients, the production of red blood cells in the bone marrow slows down. The resulting disorders are called megaloblastic anemia (see page 924).

Symptoms of anemia—including fatigue, an ashen pallor, weakness, faintness, listlessness, languor, weariness—usually appear gradually, so that at first, the condition is easy

WHAT IS HEMOGLOBIN?

Hemoglobin, the protein-iron compound transported by red blood cells, carries oxygen from the lungs to the tissues. Each red blood cell contains millions of molecules of hemoglobin, which consists of heme (the pigmented, iron-rich component) and globin (a simple protein). In the lungs, each molecule of heme combines with one molecule of oxygen, through a process called oxygenation, forming the compound oxyhemoglobin. As the blood travels to tissues where oxygen is low and carbon dioxide is high, oxyhemoglobin liberates oxygen in exchange for carbon dioxide. Whenever hemoglobin is liberated from disintegrating red blood cells, it is removed from circulation by cells that have the power to ingest such matter. The cells of the liver and spleen are especially active in this process. The globin is converted to amino acids and reused; iron is stored in the liver and reused; and non-iron–containing pigment is converted to bilirubin, which is then excreted.

As with the other blood components, hemoglobin is present in the blood in carefully regulated amounts. The average amount of hemoglobin in the blood averages 14 to 18 g per 100 ml of blood in adult males; 12 to 16 in females; and somewhat less in children. Low hemoglobin levels indicate anemia. If a person inherits mutated hemoglobin, the abnormal forms can cause a number of diseases. The most common forms are as follows:

- *Hemoglobin S*, which causes sickle cell anemia (see page 927) by altering the cells' physical structure.

- *Hemoglobin C* and *hemoglobin E*, which cause chronic hemolytic anemia (see page 925).

- *Hemoglobin S-C*, which causes a usually mild disease in the fourth decade of life.

- *Hemoglobin M*, in which the iron bonds abnormally (too tightly) to oxygen, is associated with congenital cyanosis, a disease with a benign course and symptoms that include slightly bluish, gray, or purple skin discoloration. Hemoglobin M should be distinguished from acquired methemoglobinemia, which affects normal people when they are exposed to toxins, such as nitrites and certain drugs, that cause the normal hemoglobin to bind to oxygen abnormally. Acquired methemoglobinemia can cause a serious or even fatal problem in oxygen delivery to the heart and brain.

- *Thalassemia*, in which not enough of the globin part of hemoglobin is made. ■

to overlook or dismiss. However, if left untreated, exhaustion, breathlessness, and sallowness can get worse. After a while, severe or prolonged anemia can increase the workload of the heart dramatically. Over time, if the anemia is not corrected, normal exercise and exertion, which greatly increase the demands for oxygen in the tissues, can result in acute cardiac failure.

POLYCYTHEMIC DISORDERS

Whenever your body's tissues lack oxygen because there is too little oxygen in the atmosphere—such as at high altitudes, or because some illness or condition interferes with the amount of oxygen that gets delivered—the blood-forming organs automatically produce larger quantities of red blood cells. The increased concentration of red cells makes the blood fluid thicker (also known as increased viscosity), causing the flow of blood through the vessels to become sluggish. Blood viscosity can also be increased by disorders that increase the amount of proteins in the blood, even though the red blood cell count is normal. At the same time, the rate of blood through the veins back to the heart usually increases. Consequently, if you suffer from polycythemia, you may experience weakness, blurred vision, ringing in your ears, itchy skin, dizziness, head congestion, and headaches. Your skin may take on a red or ruddy tint. You may feel tenderness or fullness around your stomach, and have frequent nosebleeds and engorged veins. In rare, severe forms, polycythemia can lead to a stroke.

Polycythemia and anemia may each occur as a disorder in and of itself, or as a secondary symptom of another, underlying illness.

❖ IRON-DEFICIENCY ANEMIA

Symptoms (*What you may experience*) At first, no notable symptoms; as condition progresses: ashen pallor; fatigue; breathlessness; palpitations; paleness around nails, gums, and eyes; rarely, a condition called pica (craving for non-food substances such as ice, clay, or soil).

Signs and laboratory findings (*What the doctor looks for*) In slight to moderate cases (early stages), a nearly normal count of red blood cells, in severely advanced cases (late stages), a reduced count of red blood cells. Other signs include individual red cells that are pale and diminished in size and reduced amounts of hemoglobin within individual cells.

What is it? Most people who have anemia do not have enough iron in their blood. Without sufficient dietary iron, the body simply cannot produce adequate hemoglobin, the substance within the red blood cells that carries oxygen from the lungs to the tissues.

Iron-deficiency anemia is usually a chronic condition that results if a person's diet does not contain enough iron or if the body does not absorb iron efficiently enough. In adults, iron-deficiency anemia is almost always caused by steady or severe blood loss.

Iron deficiency is among the most common biologic disorders. It occurs most commonly in children, poor people, and women of all ages. Because bleeding often causes this form of anemia, menstruating women are especially at risk for the condition. It is estimated that at least one-fifth of all women in the United States suffer from iron-poor blood. Most doctors recommend an iron supplement to guard against iron-deficiency anemia during pregnancy, because a woman's blood volume naturally increases during pregnancy and the growing fetus needs additional hemoglobin.

Both men and women may develop iron-deficiency anemia as a result of chronic blood loss, such as can occur with peptic ulcers or colon cancer. People who donate blood regularly can become iron-depleted unless they take iron supplements. Moreover, iron-deficiency anemia is common in the elderly as a result of chronic gastrointestinal bleeding. Gastrointestinal bleeding can be triggered by ulcers, hemorrhoids, large hiatus hernias, polyps, colitis, colon cancer, the inflammatory bowel disease known as Crohn's disease (see Chapter 23), vascular irregularities, and angiodysplasia (see Chapter 20). Chronic aspirin use can also cause diffuse bleeding from the stomach.

Iron-deficiency anemia is seen in infants, children, and adolescents, especially during growth spurts. When children are undergoing rapid growth, they need a great deal of iron for the development of new muscle and hemoglobin. Moreover, children who are exposed to lead poisoning are at high risk for iron-poor blood.

In addition to the more common anemic-related symptoms—including fatigue, paleness, and labored breathing, especially during exercising and exertion—iron deficiency can interfere with the body's natural defenses against infection.

VITAMIN SUPPLEMENTS AND BLOOD BUILDING: FACTS AND MYTHS

In our modern quest for quick fixes and easy solutions, there seems to be a pill for everything, including building and securing healthy blood. Whether it's a vitamin to enhance immunity or a mineral to build strong blood, there is a bottle claiming to address the need. And too often we reach for it, without appreciating the complexity of our body and its chemistry.

There is no question that vitamins and minerals are needed to ensure that the content of your blood is healthy and balanced. Too little iron can lead to iron-deficiency anemia. Too little folic acid can cause folate deficiency anemia. Too little B_{12} can cause pernicious anemia. Vitamin K promotes coagulation. Vitamin A builds healthy red blood cells and fortifies the immune system. Vitamin C is needed to help heal cuts and bruises, and to assist in the body's absorption of iron; it also protects against cancer-causing cell damage. Vitamin E is needed for healthy blood cells. Vitamin B_6 (pyridoxine) is essential for immune functions and for the synthesis of red blood cells. Calcium fosters healthy blood coagulation.

In most cases, adequate amounts of all vitamins and minerals can be derived from a healthy, balanced, diverse diet. When consumed in foods, vitamins and minerals are almost invariably good for you. In pill form, though, especially in high doses, they can cause trouble, or even be fatal.

This is not to say that vitamin supplements are never helpful. Supplementary iron or folic acid can indeed prevent or reverse certain forms of anemia. However, when you purchase these supplements without consulting your doctor, it may not be clear to you how much you need. The ideal dosage will depend on your age, your weight, your gender, and your stage of life.

What is more, some supplements are simply ineffective. In some instances, they can actually be harmful. Currently the government does not test dietary supplements for safety or usefulness. There are no regulations that attest to the fact that they are what they say they are or do what they claim to do. Nor is there clear and consistent information about how much of which vitamin is needed to perform what function.

In recent years, there have been links drawn in the popular press between the use of antioxidants—minerals such as selenium and chromium—and healthier blood. According to new studies, these substances do seem capable of defusing the agents that injure cell membranes. Yet the problems associated with high doses of these minerals include neurologic and gastrointestinal problems as well as impaired immune functioning. And other, unseen or unknown risks may only become apparent after the damage is done. We all must recognize that, short of eating a varied, healthy diet, there is no simple, sure way—and no miracle pill—for building strong blood. ■

What you can do Although there is a great deal of iron available to us, our food is generally iron-poor. Foods that are relatively rich in iron include liver, oysters, and legumes (peas and beans). Fair sources of iron include beef, poultry, pork, lamb, and fish. Even though cereals and breads are iron-fortified, they actually provide little iron that our bodies can readily absorb. Having said that, the best way to address anemia is to prevent it through a healthy, varied diet. If you have any doubts about the sufficiency of iron in your diet, talk to your doctor. Particularly at times when iron deficiency is likely—during pregnancy or nursing, in childhood—ask your doctor to recommend an iron supplement.

When to call the doctor In the early stages of anemia, there may be no symptoms, or few that you will notice. You may be able to ignore that fact that you tire easily, look pale, and find yourself occasionally breathless, or you may chalk it up to lack of sleep, stress, the holiday season, or simply the aging process. However, if you are experiencing fatigue and the other symptoms just described, it may be worthwhile to check it out with your doctor.

When the exhaustion becomes severe enough that it interferes with your day-to-day functioning, or when you tire so quickly that you are unable to complete tasks or engage in activities that normally give you pleasure, contact your doctor immediately.

Even when the symptoms are mild, it is important to have the condition diagnosed, just in case there is some other, more severe cause underlying the anemia.

Treatment If your doctor suspects that you have anemia, she will order blood tests to verify the diagnosis. In order to treat iron-deficiency anemia, the source needs to be determined. When your anemia is induced by blood loss, your doctor will likely run other tests to find out if there is an underlying condition. A HemoQuant test that measures blood in the stool, for example, can tell if your anemia is due to blood loss in the digestive tract, which could point to such conditions as colon cancer or peptic ulcer.

In children, iron-deficiency anemia can be caused by inadequate diet, but this is exceptionally rare in adults. When that is the case, treatment will involve reviewing and modifying your diet. The amount of absorbable iron varies in different foods, but the most useful is found in meats (especially liver), fish, poultry, eggs, legumes, leeks, potatoes, and rice. Although many wheat products, including breads and cereals, are fortified with iron, the body cannot readily absorb it in this form. Iron supplements may be helpful for children, pregnant women, and others whose diets may be low in natural iron, such as vegetarians or people on weight-reducing diets. Drinking citrus juice while eating iron-rich foods or taking an iron supplement will increase your body's ability to use the iron. Iron supplements should be taken with caution—in small doses and only to correct a proven deficiency—as supplements can be harmful when not needed.

Your doctor will almost certainly recommend medications, such as iron salts (ferrous sulfate). These are usually taken orally, but if a patient cannot absorb iron, they may be administered by intramuscular injection. Diagnostic tests or surgery may be advised if the underlying cause is blood loss from the digestive tract—such as with colon cancer, hemorrhoids, or polyps. If you have severe anemia that needs immediate correction, your doctor may consider giving you a transfusion of packed red blood cells (see page 940). Transfusion is used only when blood replacement is needed faster than can be obtained by iron replacement, or when it is difficult to keep up with blood loss.

Prognosis Excellent. Although iron-deficiency anemia can be a serious condition, especially when it goes untreated for a long period of time, once diagnosed, it almost always responds to iron therapy, and its effects can usually be quickly reversed. The underlying cause of the iron deficiency is more important than anemia itself.

❖ FOLIC ACID-DEFICIENCY ANEMIA

Symptoms (*What you may experience*) Few obvious symptoms in the early stages; as the disorder progresses, low endurance and easy exhaustion; fatigue; rapid heartbeat; weight loss; diarrhea; sore tongue.

Signs and laboratory findings (*What the doctor looks for*) Anemia associated with increased size of red cells; low levels of folic acid in red blood cells.

What is it? Folic acid, also known as folate, is a member of the vitamin B group. It is found in raw fruits and vegetables—especially citrus fruits and green leafy vegetables—and in organ meats such as liver and kidney. Because folic acid is necessary for the production of red blood cells, if your diet is deficient, you are at increased risk for a type of anemia called megaloblastic anemia.

Folic acid-deficiency anemia is relatively common. Because absorption occurs along the entire gastrointestinal tract, though, it rarely results from the inability of the system to absorb the nutrient. By far, the most common reason for folate deficiency is alcoholism. Because alcoholics typically derive most of their calories from drinking, many are seriously malnourished and anemic. When people consume large amounts of alcohol over time, they lose the ability to absorb folic acid, among other nutrients, in their digestive tract. People are also at risk for developing folic acid deficiency if they overcook vegetables or do not consume enough fruit. People with anorexia are at risk for this type of anemia because any kind of systematic starvation frequently results in malnutrition. The elderly are frequently at risk, because they tend not to eat enough fresh fruit and vegetables. Certain anticonvulsant medications can also induce folic acid anemia.

Women who are pregnant or breast-feeding and children who are experiencing natural developmental growth spurts (during infancy and adolescence, for example) need additional folic acid. Unless the supply increases to meet the need, anemia can arise.

Folic acid deficiency can also occur as a result of an underlying illness. For instance, the body's need for folic acid increases sharply whenever red blood cells are consumed faster than they can be produced (see Hemolytic Anemias, page 925). Any form of hemolytic anemia could (but is not very likely to) result in significant folic acid deficiency: sickle cell anemia, severe thalassemia syndromes, and hereditary spherocytosis (a condition in which the red blood cells are small, spherical, and fragile). If you have certain dermatitis disorders such as psoriasis (see Chapter 28) and certain cancers such as metastatic tumors and acute leukemia, a blood test may turn up folic acid deficiency as well.

The symptoms of folic acid anemia are similar to those of other forms of anemia.

Consequently, it can be accurately diagnosed only through a complete blood workup (see page 915). Tests will include a blood count that will measure the level of folic acid in the blood. Your doctor will also want to determine, if possible, the reason for the deficiency. Depending on the underlying cause, the condition may be chronic, requiring long-term management, or acute, requiring a short period of treatment.

Prevention You can guard against folic acid deficiency by making sure that your diet is balanced. Avoiding alcohol will lower your risk for the condition. So will taking supplements—but only with a doctor's supervision. If you are pregnant, your doctor will likely prescribe a vitamin supplement complete with folic acid.

Treatment In most cases, oral folic acid prescribed daily will be sufficient to correct the anemia. In rare cases, your doctor may recommend injections if there is an underlying disorder of the intestinal tract that interferes with absorption.

Prognosis In most cases, folic acid–deficiency anemia responds well to treatment. Where the anemia is secondary to another condition, prognosis depends on the seriousness of the underlying illness.

❖ VITAMIN B$_{12}$ DEFICIENCY AND PERNICIOUS ANEMIA

Symptoms (*What you may experience*) In early stages there are usually no obvious symptoms. As the condition worsens, symptoms include reduced endurance during exercise; rapid heartbeat; diarrhea, diminished appetite and weight loss; disturbed balance and gait; sore tongue; numb hands and feet; memory loss; depression; dementia.

Signs and laboratory findings (*What the doctor looks for*) Blood tests showing a deficiency of vitamin B$_{12}$ in the blood, as well as fewer and enlarged red blood cells; blood tests showing the presence of antibodies to intrinsic factor or parietal cells, the stomach cells that make intrinsic factor; and abnormal Schilling test, which measures your body's ability to absorb vitamin B$_{12}$.

What is it? One of the megaloblastic anemias, pernicious anemia is a chronic, progressive anemia caused by the inability of the body to absorb vitamin B$_{12}$. Vitamin B$_{12}$ is needed to produce sufficient numbers of normal red blood cells.

After being ingested, vitamin B$_{12}$ binds with a protein called intrinsic factor (IF), which is secreted by the cells lining part of the stomach. Intrinsic factor is needed so that vitamin B$_{12}$ can be absorbed in the small intestine. The vitamin B$_{12}$–intrinsic factor complex that forms travels through the intestine and is absorbed in the lowest portion of the bowel (the ileum).

Since vitamin B$_{12}$ is present in all foods of animal origin, including meat, fish, and dairy products, dietary deficiencies are extremely rare. Only the strictest of vegetarians—particularly vegans, who avoid eggs and dairy products as well as meat and fish—stand at risk for pernicious anemia because of their diets. In those cases, a vitamin supplement usually provides adequate amounts of vitamin B$_{12}$ to make up for their dietary shortage.

In the vast majority of cases, vitamin B$_{12}$ deficiency arises when a defect in the digestive tract interferes with the body's ability to absorb the nutrient. These cases of pernicious anemia are caused by an autoimmune disorder. This type of congenital condition fosters the production of antibodies that interfere with B$_{12}$ absorption. Pernicious anemia is most often a consequence of long-standing gastritis (inflammation of the stomach), which is generally characterized by gas pains, tenderness, nausea, and vomiting. Intestinal disorders such as ileitis or chronic pancreatic insufficiency can also account for B$_{12}$ deficiency. Furthermore, abdominal or intestinal surgery that eliminates the site at which intrinsic factor is produced can lead to vitamin B$_{12}$ deficiency. A condition called blind loop syndrome frequently causes an overgrowth of bacteria in the intestine that makes absorption more problematic. Occasionally, severe Crohn's disease results in sufficient destruction of the ileum to retard vitamin B$_{12}$ absorption (see Chapter 23). In rare cases, vitamin B$_{12}$ deficiency is caused by a parasite called fish tapeworm (see page 892).

Pernicious anemia is somewhat rare. There is a hereditary component to the disease that indicates a predisposition to develop pernicious anemia, not direct inheritance of the disease. The presence of a hereditary component makes it sometimes possible to predict who is *at risk* for developing this disorder.

If your doctor suspects that you have pernicious anemia, or if you show some of the risk factors, including a family history of the disorder, your doctor will order blood tests to measure the amounts of vitamin B_{12} in your blood. A Schilling test may also be done.

Pernicious anemia is a chronic, slowly progressing disorder that requires treatment. In addition, medical treatment is necessary to determine if there is another serious condition causing the problem in B_{12} absorption.

Treatment People with pernicious anemia cannot absorb oral vitamin B_{12}; therefore, treatment involves regular injections of vitamin B_{12}. In general, replacement is usually given daily at first. After the first week, injections are given weekly for the first month, then monthly for an indefinite length of time. Neither oral supplements nor dietary changes are useful because the underlying problem is the inability of the digestive tract to absorb the vitamin.

In severe cases, especially with elderly people, transfusions of packed red blood cells—usually given over 10 to 12 hours—will be recommended. Because urinary tract and pulmonary infections are common in elderly people with pernicious anemia and there is an increased risk of having stomach cancer, these conditions will be monitored closely.

Prognosis Excellent. At one time fatal—thus the name—pernicious anemia now responds well to treatment. In fact, patients tend to respond to therapy immediately, usually reporting a greater sense of well-being shortly after the first few injections. However, if the condition goes untreated or has progressed for some time before treatment is begun, there can be some residual damage to the nervous and digestive systems.

❖ ANEMIA OF CHRONIC DISEASE

Symptoms (*What you may experience*) Fatigue; exhaustion and breathlessness following exertion; weight loss; loss of appetite; fever; chills; muscle tenderness or pain; joint tenderness and pain.

Signs and laboratory findings (*What the doctor looks for*) Blood tests showing anemia abnormalities in iron metabolism as well as signs and symptoms of a chronic, underlying condition.

What is it? Anemia of chronic disease (ACD) is a common condition that develops as a result of another chronic disease. Usually, this type of anemia is hard to distinguish from iron-deficiency anemia. Yet, in most cases, your medical history will point to the possibility that a chronic disease has caused the anemia.

Conditions that are often at the root of this type of anemia include inflammatory disease, such as rheumatoid arthritis; kidney failure; endocrine failure or hormone deficiency, such as hypothyroidism (underactive thyroid gland); chronic liver disease; trauma; or tumors.

As a rule, the anemia associated with chronic disease is itself mild and stable. The symptoms tend to appear insidiously over a period of 3 to 4 weeks.

If your doctor suspects that you have anemia of chronic disease, a bone marrow biopsy may be ordered to make a precise diagnosis (see page 948).

Treatment Addressing iron deficiency and other anemic symptoms is unnecessary. Anemia of chronic disease can be cured only if the underlying condition is cured or brought under control. Occasionally, transfusions may be advisable.

Prognosis Prognosis depends on the primary disease.

❖ HEMOLYTIC ANEMIAS

Symptoms (*What you may experience*) Weakness; fatigue; lightheadedness; dizziness; palpitations; sore throat.

Signs and laboratory findings (*What the doctor looks for*) Deformed red cells and elevated number of young red blood cells, called reticulocytes, revealed on microscopic examination; jaundice; enlarged spleen or liver.

What is it? Hemolytic anemias are a group of disorders that arise when red blood cell survival is reduced, either episodically or continuously. The term *hemolysis* means destruction of red blood cells; accordingly, hemolytic anemias arise when red blood cells are broken down (hemolyzed) faster or earlier in their life spans than usual, such that the bone marrow cannot produce enough new replacement cells. As the red blood cells break down, hemoglobin is released and diffused into the surrounding fluid. When hemolysis happens within the blood vessels, the body cannot retain the hemoglobin. Instead, the hemoglobin is lost through the kidneys.

Bone marrow works naturally to increase red blood cell production in response to reduced cell survival; therefore, anemia will occur only when the ability of the marrow to compensate is outpaced, either because red blood cell survival is extremely short or because bone marrow function is impaired.

Hemolytic anemias can be both acquired and inherited, and they are generally classified according to whether the defect is intrinsic to the red blood cells or triggered by some external factor.

The most well known type of inherited hemolytic disorder is sickle cell anemia (see page 927), but there are may other types of inherited hemolytic anemias (see page 925). For some people, hemolytic anemia can be triggered by environmental factors. Infections, certain drugs, and exposure to certain chemicals can cause red blood cells to break down faster than they can be replaced.

From time to time, intense physical exertion—for example, marching or running for a long stretch of time—can actually cause physical trauma to red blood cells. Certain heart problems, such as valve narrowing or mechanical heart valves, can cause turbulent blood flow, which in turn can induce fragmentation of the red blood cells. Hemolysis can also result when blood flow through the small vessels is impeded by the presence of clots or disease along the walls.

Hemolytic anemias also can stem from an immune response against your own red blood cells, in which case, they are called autoimmune hemolytic anemias. Autoimmune hemolytic anemia is an acquired disorder in which an antibody (an autoantibody) binds to the red blood cell membrane and causes the cell to take on a spherical shape. Consequently, the red blood cells lose strength and malleability. Thus compromised, the red blood cells cannot withstand the stress of circulation, nor can they pass easily through the capillaries. Many become trapped and destroyed in the spleen. The spleen especially plays a predominant role in the destruction of red blood cells. In patients with autoimmune hemolytic anemias, the spleen is the principal site of red blood cell destruction.

The majority of autoimmune hemolytic anemias arise in association with such conditions as systemic lupus erythematosus (SLE, or lupus) chronic lymphocytic leukemia, or lymphoma. Other cases of autoimmune hemolytic anemias are drug-induced.

With autoimmune hemolytic anemia, the symptoms can come on so rapidly that they can be extremely severe. At the same time, in all forms of hemolytic anemia, symptoms can range from relatively mild to quite severe. In early stages the person may be able to dismiss or ignore the fatigue, weakness, and breathlessness, but over time, hemolytic anemia can cause significant medical problems. The spleen and liver may become swollen and tender as they work overtime to collect, filter, and destroy the compromised red blood cells.

Similarly, long-term anemia can cause serious heart problems. Your heart will work harder in an attempt to push adequate oxygen out to the tissues, and in severe cases, angina and congestive heart failure can occur (see Chapter 20).

Treatment If some medication is at root of your anemia, your doctor will advise you to discontinue the drug. If your condition arises from autoimmunity, the doctor will prescribe corticosteroid medications, such as prednisone; these will often slow down the destruction (hemolysis) of red blood cells. However, if you have not responded well to corticosteroids, your doctor may recommend a splenectomy (surgical removal of the spleen) thus eliminating the major site of red blood cell destruction. When steroids or splenectomy are not adequate to control hemolysis, drugs that suppress the immune system are commonly used, such as intravenous immunoglobulin azathioprine (Imuran), or cyclophosphamide (Cytoxan).

In regard to inherited forms of hemolytic anemia, treatment depends on the specific form; therefore, descriptions of treatment options will be included in the entries that follow.

Whenever anemia is life-threatening, blood transfusions will be given. The transfused blood cells may still have a shortened survival rate, but they can nevertheless bridge the crisis and be life-saving.

Prognosis Some hemolytic anemias are difficult to bring under control, but they are rarely fatal. When hemolytic anemia has an identifiable root and that condition can be treated successfully, the prognosis for the anemia is quite good. Treatment for autoimmune hemolytic anemia has a high success rate. Between 50 and 75 percent of patients show marked improvement or have a complete remission after splenectomy.

❖ SICKLE CELL ANEMIA

Symptoms *(What you may experience)* Fatigue; rapid heartbeat (palpitations); breathlessness; lightheadedness; susceptibility to infections; skin ulcers on the lower legs; susceptibility to vision and retina problems; in children, delayed growth and development. Crisis symptoms: blocked blood vessels and damage to organs leading to acute pain (hemolytic crisis); a precipitant drop in the number of circulating red blood cells (aplastic crisis).

Signs and laboratory findings *(What the doctor looks for)* Tests show an abnormal type of hemoglobin, called hemoglobin S, within rigid, crescent-shaped erythrocytes.

What is it? Sickle cell anemia is a family of inherited blood disorders that cause the body to produce defective hemoglobin. This type of defect leads to chronic hemolytic anemia (see page 925), with a variety of severe consequences. Individuals who have the disease typically enjoy periods of relative health that are interrupted by episodes of severe illness, called crises. Furthermore, they are always anemic and vulnerable to infections.

Normally, red blood cells are round and flexible, but those individuals who inherit sickle cell disease have red blood cells that carry hemoglobin S. When exposed to low levels of oxygen in the capillaries and elsewhere, molecules of hemoglobin S stick together, making blood cells rigid. Instead of having the flexibility that would allow them to squeeze through tiny blood vessels and carry needed oxygen to the tissues, red blood cells take on the shape of crescents or sickles and plug up the blood supply. As the cells change their shape, or *sickle*, they also become fragile.

Cells that are fragile then tend to break up, or *hemolyze*, prematurely. Many of the diseased cells are sequestered and destroyed in the spleen. At the same time, the bone marrow is sometimes unable to pro-

Normal red blood cells (RBCs) are shaped like a doughnut with a depression instead of a hole. They contain hemoglobin that serves to transport oxygen from the lungs to the cells of the body. In sickle cell anemia, hemoglobin polymerizes, or gels, inside the red blood cell. This distorts the red blood cells into a sickle shape, causing them to be brittle and easily destroyed. The shape also causes the red blood cells to lodge in small blood vessels, which blocks the flow of blood, and leads to a sickle cell crisis.

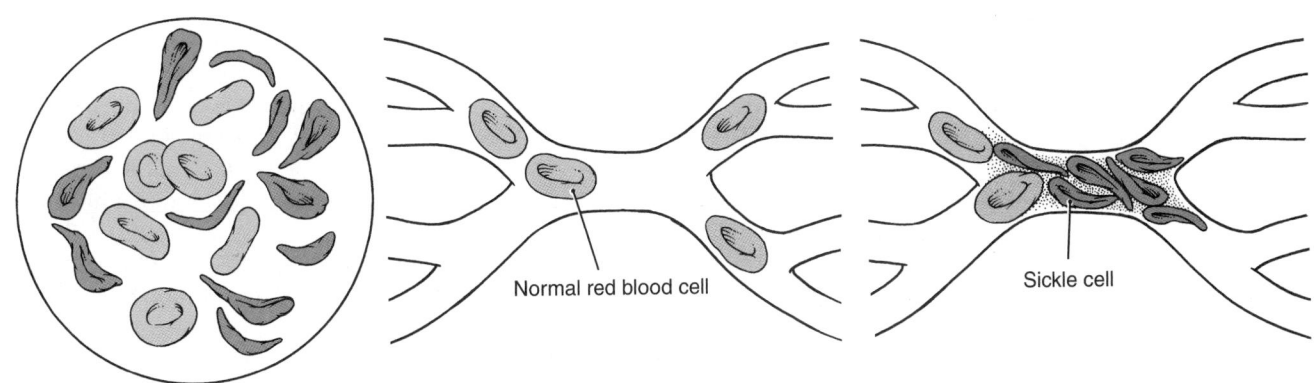

Normal red blood cell

Sickle cell

duce enough replacement cells to compensate for the loss. The damaged cells kill tissue by blocking their blood supply—at times quietly, at other times with great pain.

Sickle cell disease afflicts several million people around the world—particularly those whose ancestors came from Africa, the Middle East, the Mediterranean, and India. It is believed that the sickle cell mutation provided some protection against malaria, which is why the mutation is most common in those areas where malaria is prevalent. In the United States, sickle cell disease affects approximately 80,000 African-Americans. Each year, one in 12 African-American babies is born with a genetic tendency to pass sickle cell disease on to their children. One birth out of 400 in African-Americans will produce a child with the disease.

A child inherits the disease when both parents pass on the recessive hemoglobin S gene. Children who receive only one such gene become carriers of sickle cell trait. This means that although red blood cells are malformed, there are no symptoms. Yet, if a person carries one copy of the gene, that person is not anemic but may experience breathlessness, lightheadedness, and palpitations at high altitudes or in an unpressurized airplane. This is because whenever oxygen is thin, sickling may occur.

Sickle cell anemia usually appears in the first year of life. Children with the disorder usually reach puberty later than their peers. They can have painful swelling in the hands and feet. Adults with the condition often have a condition called acute chest syndrome, which causes fever and chest pain. Chronic hemolytic anemia produces jaundice, gallstones, an enlarged spleen, and ulcers over the lower leg that do not heal. Infections are often the most serious complications associated with sickle cell disease—including pneumonia, meningitis (inflammation of the membrane surrounding the brain and spinal cord), blood infections, and inflammation of the bone marrow.

The other serious complication related to sickle cell disease is susceptibility to periodic acute sickling crises, which are debilitating and at times life-threatening. When acute sickling occurs, small blood vessels may become obstructed and severe pain results. The sickled red cells break down (hemolyze) at a greatly increased rate. The tissue throughout the body can be damaged or destroyed. Crises can occur spontaneously, but they are usually prompted by such factors as infection, dehydration, hypoxia (decrease of oxygen in the air), pregnancy, cold, emotional stress, or surgery.

In addition, temporary failure of red blood cell production in the bone marrow is associated with this disease. These aplastic crises happen when the ability of the bone marrow to compensate for reduced cell survival is severely compromised. Lasting hours or days, these episodes cause acute pain in the bones, back, chest, abdomen, and spleen. Other symptoms include breathing difficulties, fever, abnormal heart rate, and an increase in the number of white blood cells in circulation (see page 946). Over time, these episodes can lead to stroke and priapism (painful, prolonged erection without sexual stimulation). Repeated episodes can affect the central nervous system, liver, spleen, kidney, and other organs. The heart can become enlarged, and damage to the kidney can lead to blindness. In its most severe form, strokes and early death can occur.

Prevention Various blood tests, including hemoglobin electrophoresis, a laboratory procedure that isolates and identifies the presence of hemoglobin S, will reveal if you carry the sickle cell trait, which will be of concern if you are considering marriage and children. If you know that sickle cell anemia runs in your family, consult a genetic counselor. If both you and your partner carry the trait, there is a one in four chance for each of your children to inherit sickle cell disease. Prenatal testing now makes it possible to determine whether you are carrying a child with sickle cell disease.

What you can do If you or a family member has the disorder, there are steps you can take to ensure a healthier life. In most cases, sickle cell anemia is a chronic, multisystem disease. As a result, if you have the disease, you will need to be involved in comprehensive medical management. On the whole, a close working relationship with your doctor, attention to general medical care, and good nutrition will translate into a healthier existence.

If you have sickle cell disease, your body will be particularly vulnerable to infection. Sometimes, these infections can be life-threatening. Avoid exposure whenever possible. When you do contract an infection, seek treatment immediately. Your doctor may recommend pneumonia and flu vaccines to help ward off infection. Conditions such as eye problems, surgery, and pregnancy can cause special problems, and treatment should involve specialists.

There is no question that managing the demands of a chronic illness along with the normal demands of everyday living is simply not easy. Understanding the nature of the illness can ease some of the difficulty. To that end, many community hospitals and health centers offer support groups and educational workshops. The Sickle Cell Disease Association of America provides information and support and has chapters in many cities. You can contact the national headquarters at 3460 Wilshire Boulevard, Suite 1012, Los Angeles, CA 90010. The phone number is (800) 421–8453.

Treatment Up until recently, treatment for sickle cell anemia aimed only at controlling the symptoms. The disease itself had been incurable. Historically, if you had the disease, you would have been maintained on folic acid supplements, your pain would have been managed with medication, and routinely, you might have received transfusions. While this type of palliative treatment is still a matter of course in most cases of sickle cell disease, recent studies have found new, promising ways of treating and perhaps curing the condition.

In severe cases, the use of the drug hydroxyurea (Hydrea) has been shown to decrease sickle cell disease's disabling attacks by at least half. Daily doses of hydroxyurea, a drug traditionally used to treat cancer, seem to reduce the frequency of painful crises as well as decrease the number of hospitalizations and transfusions.

A second series of studies have shown bone marrow transplants to be highly successful in curing children with advanced symptoms. Most of the research has been conducted on children under 14 years of age using marrow transplants from matched sibling donors (see page 960). New tests will likely extend the application of treatment.

At the same time that these new procedures are being developed and used, palliative treatments—measures to relieve symptoms—may still be necessary. Blood transfusions may be used to prevent crises. Folic acid supplements will likely be prescribed, because the disease increases the body's need for this vitamin. Antibiotics will be given, either to treat an infection as it happens or to prevent one from happening. During a crisis, medications to relieve the pain and prevent dehydration will be recommended. When there is not enough oxygen in the bloodstream, oxygen will be administered.

Prognosis Despite current research, there is no clear cure for sickle cell disease. The manifestation and severity of the disorder vary from individual to individual. Therefore, so does the prognosis. Nevertheless, with comprehensive medical care, many people with sickle cell disease can live relatively healthy, full lives.

OTHER INHERITED ANEMIAS

In addition to sickle cell disease, there are a number of rare forms of anemias that are passed on genetically. These include glucose-6-phosphemolytic anemia, thalassemias, and spherocytosis.

❖ GLUCOSE-6-PHOSPHATE DEHYDROGENASE (G-6-PD)-DEFICIENCY ANEMIA

Symptoms *(What you may experience)* Fatigue; heartaches; dizziness; fever; chills; jaundice.

Signs and laboratory findings *(What the doctor looks for)* Blood tests reveal G-6-PD deficiency.

What is it? Glucose-6-phosphemolytic anemia occurs when a hereditary enzyme defect causes red blood cells to be broken down faster than they are produced, thus causing hemolytic anemia (see page 925). In the most common form, patients seem normal until they encounter a drug, infection, or food that destroys red blood cells that are vulnerable because of a weakened G-6-PD enzyme. This disorder appears most frequently in people of Mediterranean and African descent. Symptoms range from mild to severe, depending on which type of defective gene for the enzyme is present. In people of African descent, symptoms tend to be milder than in people whose ancestors came from the Mediterranean. Hemolysis (rapid loss of red blood cells) and related anemic symptoms tend to be episodic; certain foods, drugs, or infections may stimulate these episodes.

The gene for the enzyme is sex-linked; because it is carried on the X chromosome, this disease almost always affects boys and men (who have only one X chromosome), rather than girls and women (whose second X chromosome tends to mitigate the power of the abnormal gene).

What you can do Avoid those foods and drugs that trigger hemolytic episodes. Your doctor can perform tests to help determine which foods or drugs cause problems. These may include such drugs as the antimalarial primaquine, the antiarrhythmic quinidine, and the antibiotics sulfonamide and nitrofurantoin. Also, if you have a susceptibility to hemolytic reactions, you may hemolyze during infections. You will want to avoid exposure to infection whenever possible. Your doctor may recommend flu and pneumonia vaccines.

Treatment Usually no treatment is necessary. If you develop an infection, seek treatment immediately.

❖ THALASSEMIA

Symptoms *(What you may experience)* Fatigue; breathlessness; dizziness; and other symptoms of anemia; jaundice; retarded growth.

Signs and laboratory findings *(What the doctor looks for)* Anemia associated with very small red cells. Genetic screening shows gene mutations or a deletion of specific gene loci.

What is it? Thalassemia is caused by inherited defects in hemoglobin. It can induce symptoms common to anemia, including fatigue, dizziness, and breathlessness, as well as poor growth, enlarged spleen, and in some instances, heart failure. The severity of the disease varies, depending on the type of defects involved.

In its mildest and most common form, thalassemia minor or thalassemia trait, the body produces blood cells that resemble those in iron-poor blood, but there are no symptoms. Because those who have thalassemia trait carry only one recessive gene,

the disorder is not active. Yet at high altitudes where oxygen is scarce or after vigorous activity, they may tire easily, feel weak, and appear pale. These people also act as carriers and can pass the gene to their offspring.

When a child inherits two matching genes for the disorder, thalassemia can be manifest in two somewhat distinct defects. The first type is called alpha-thalassemia and arises when hemoglobin lacks sufficient amounts of the protein alpha-globin. This form occurs most frequently in people of Southeast Asian descent. Usually, it produces very mild, occasional symptoms. However, in rare instances, it can cause a fetus that has inherited the disorder to be stillborn.

In the second form, called beta-thalassemia or Cooley's anemia, the hemoglobin lacks sufficient amounts of the protein beta-globin. This form is seen mostly in people coming from Mediterranean regions—Italians, Greeks—and to a lesser extent, in Asians and blacks. Beta-thalassemia tends to be more uniformly severe. Children born with this disorder tend to be normal at birth but show signs of severe anemia in the first year of life. Numerous clinical problems can result, including jaundice, failure to grow, and bony deformities, including abnormal facial structure.

Because the gene for thalassemia is recessive, both parents must pass on the genes before an offspring manifests the disease. If you have only one gene, you carry the trait—and occasionally have mild symptoms. If your partner also has the recessive gene, the chances are one in four that you will likely pass the disease to any child you conceive together.

What you can do If there is a history of thalassemia in your family or if prenatal testing reveals the genetic malformation or deficiency, consult with a genetic counselor. Any pregnancy will have to be closely monitored.

If you have thalassemia trait, the mild form of the disease, treatment will probably not be necessary; however, it is essential that you avoid unnecessary consumption of iron, because there is a high risk for iron overload.

Treatment There is no cure for thalassemia. When thalassemia is mild, treatment may not be warranted. Transfusions are necessary only if you are battling acute infections.

When thalassemia is more severe, treatment is necessary to prolong life. Treatment usually involves repeated blood transfusions of packed red blood cells. While these types of transfusions are necessary to control the disease, the cells carry a large amount of iron that can overload the body's vital organs. To counteract this risk, the drug deferoxamine may be given to flush iron out of the body through the urine.

Prognosis While severe, the course of this disease has been significantly modified recently with the use of transfusion therapy. However, years of transfusion and iron overload can cause heart problems and hormonal dysfunctions. In its most severe form, thalassemia can lead to death from cardiac failure between the ages of 20 and 30 years.

❖ HEREDITARY SPHEROCYTOSIS

Symptoms *(What you may experience)* Fatigue and other symptoms of anemia; jaundice; gallstones; abdominal tenderness. In children, retarded growth.

Signs and laboratory findings *(What the doctor looks for)* Examination of blood samples reveals small, spherical, fragile erythrocytes and elevated hemoglobin levels.

What is it? Normal red blood cells are biconcave disks, strong enough to withstand the stress of circulating for 120 days and malleable enough to pass through smaller capillaries. Hereditary spherocytosis is a condition passed on genetically in which red blood cells are small, spherical, and fragile. These spherocytes are prone to break down prematurely, usually in the spleen, causing chronic hemolytic anemia (see page 925).

Hereditary spherocytosis is often diagnosed in childhood, but milder cases are sometimes discovered late in adult life. Severity varies from person to person. Symptoms of anemia may or may not be present, because, in many cases, the bone marrow is able to compensate for the loss of red blood cells. Aplastic crises—in which the bone marrow is unable to compensate for the shortened cell survival—may be prompted by infection, folate deficiency (see page 923), or other factors, resulting in severe anemia.

Prevention Whenever you are at risk of passing on a serious genetic condition to your offspring, you may want to consult with a genetic counselor before conceiving a child.

Treatment If it is discovered that you have hereditary spherocytosis, your doctor will recommend folic acid supplements. At times, surgical removal of the spleen (splenectomy), while not correcting the defect, can eliminate the primary site of blood cell destruction.

POLYCYTHEMIA VERA AND SECONDARY POLYCYTHEMIA

In both of these disorders there is an overproduction of red blood cells (see also Polycythemic Disorders, page 921).

❖ POLYCYTHEMIA VERA

Symptoms *(What you may experience)* Weakness; headaches; blurred vision and ringing in the ears; itchy skin; dizziness; red hands and face; fullness in the upper abdomen; constant feeling of head congestion; nosebleeds; in severe cases, blood in vomit or stool.

Signs and laboratory findings *(What the doctor looks for)* Engorged veins; enlarged spleen and liver; blood tests that show increased red blood mass; elevated white blood and platelet count; unusually high values of vitamin B_{12} and the enzyme leukocyte alkaline phosphatase in the blood; increased blood volume without increase in volume of plasma.

What is it? Polycythemia vera, also known as primary polycythemia, is a bone marrow disorder characterized by autonomous overproduction of red blood cells. It is a relatively common disorder. Typically surfacing in late middle age—it rarely occurs in adults under the age of 40—polycythemia vera is slightly more common in men than in women. In most cases, the cause is unknown.

Symptoms appear gradually. Most patients present with symptoms related to expanded blood volume and increased blood viscosity. Common complaints include headache, fatigue, blurred vision, dizziness, and ringing in the ear (tinnitus). Severe itching, especially following a warm shower or bath, and frequent nosebleeds may also be present. Some people experience episodes of gouty arthritis (see Chapter 17).

The most serious complication of polycythemia vera is thrombosis—the formation of blood clots within the vascular system. The formation of such clots can lead to heart attack or stroke. There is also a high incidence of peptic ulcers as well as gastrointestinal bleeding related to this disorder. There is a high risk (10 to 30 percent) that patients with polycythemia vera will eventually develop acute leukemia.

Treatment Treatment is necessary in all cases of polycythemia, because the high concentration of blood cells makes blood thicker and blood flow more sluggish. Without treatment, symptoms will worsen and the risk of stroke or heart attack will increase.

The treatment of choice for polycythemia vera is a procedure called phlebotomy. In this procedure, blood is systematically withdrawn from the vein in order to lessen circulating red cells. Initially, about a pint of blood is taken every few days; then, depending on the individual, a pint is withdrawn every few weeks or months. The goal is to maintain blood hemoglobin level within the range of low to normal values.

Because repeated phlebotomy produces iron deficiency, the frequency of this procedure is gradually decreased. Iron supplements are *not* recommended, because they tend to thwart the goals of therapy; iron deficiency helps to keep the red blood cell count down to normal levels.

If your blood also has high white blood cell and platelet counts, medications such as radioactive phosphorus may be prescribed. Usually, one round of such treatment is all that is necessary. However, when radioactive phosphorus therapy is used over a period of years, there is some link with the transformation of normal white blood cells to leukemia cells.

The role of aspirin in preventing thrombotic complications is still being debated.

High doses can cause increased gastrointestinal bleeding. In some cases, though, one tablet daily may be effective (see page 943).

In rare cases where the spleen has become enlarged, the doctor may consider splenectomy (surgical removal of the spleen).

Prognosis There is no cure for polycythemia vera. However, with proper treatment, a person generally feels normal and the risk of heart attack or stroke decreases. A small percentage of people with polycythemia vera develop acute leukemia after a period of years.

❖ SECONDARY POLYCYTHEMIA

Symptoms (*What you may experience*) Weakness; headaches; blurred vision and ringing in the ears; itchy skin; dizziness; red hands and face; sensation of fullness in the upper abdomen; constant feeling of head congestion; nosebleeds.

Signs and laboratory findings (*What the doctor looks for*) Engorged veins; enlarged spleen and liver. Blood tests show increased red blood mass; elevated white blood and platelet count; increased blood volume without increase in volume of plasma.

What is it? Whenever the tissues become oxygen deprived, the bone marrow will automatically produce large quantities of red blood cells. This often happens at high altitudes, where there is too little oxygen in the atmosphere. It can also happen when another condition interferes with the amount of oxygen that gets delivered to the body's tissues. A high concentration of red blood cells then begins to build up and move through the blood. The overall effect is to increase blood viscosity. In other words, the flow of blood through the vessels becomes sluggish.

Secondary polycythemia can develop in response to low blood oxygen concentration that has resulted, for example, from smoking, severe lung disease, abnormal hemoglobin, congenital heart disease, certain cysts, or tumors. It commonly occurs in people who live in high-altitude areas, where the air they breathe has less oxygen. Because there is insufficient oxygen in the blood, the body attempts to overcome the deficiency by boosting its production of red blood cells—sometimes to the point of putting too many into circulation.

Once you see your doctor, blood tests may reveal an increased count of red blood cells. Further tests and examinations may uncover a serious underlying illness.

What you can do If you are diagnosed with secondary polycythemia, there are certain lifestyle changes you can make to eliminate those things that cause or aggravate increased red blood cell levels. If you smoke, you should stop. If you are using diuretics, these may intensify viscosity by reducing the plasma volume. Losing weight, if you are overweight, can also help.

Treatment In cases where polycythemia is a secondary condition, treatment depends on diagnosing and treating the underlying illness. Treatment will involve determining the cause and eliminating aggravating factors. In some cases, a doctor may consider phlebotomy, the systematic withdrawal of blood from the vein in order to lessen circulation volume.

Bleeding Disorders

Each day, the body is subject to injury and insult, however mild or imperceptible. Blood vessels too are torn, cut, or injured many times a day and at many sites, often without our even realizing it. The body relies on an elaborate system to repair injuries, cuts, and tears in blood vessels—both minor and significant—and to prevent excessive bleeding.

Platelets are instrumental in this process of repair and coagulation. As they circulate in the bloodstream, these round or oval disks adhere to each other and to the edges of an injured vessel wall, forming a plug or promoting clotting to stop the loss of blood.

The normal circulating platelet count is maintained within relatively narrow, limits. Because a platelet has a life span of approximately 10 days, about 25 million platelets (25,000 per microliter of blood) must be produced each day to maintain a steady state. When injury, infection, or other conditions draw and consume platelets, the bone marrow naturally responds by increasing production to compensate for the destruction.

Bleeding disorders result from a disruption in the body's elaborate repair and blood-clotting process. Clotting or coagulation—the process by which the body repairs injury, cuts, or tears in the vascular system and prevents blood loss—relies on numerous substances, or factors, that are released by platelets or are present in plasma. Some of these factors, called procoagulants, promote coagulation. Others, called anticoagulants, inhibit coagulation. Whether or not blood will coagulate depends on the balance between the two.

Whenever there is an injury, platelets stick to a blood vessel. By releasing certain factors, they stimulate enzyme reactions and produce a web-like protein network that in return encircles and contains the platelets. Then, if necessary, a clot can form to seal off the broken ends of the injured vessel, and stem bleeding (see page 912). For this process to work completely, each clotting factor must be transformed from an inactive to an active state.

Bleeding disorders occur when there is a problem at specific locations within the clotting operation. If, for example, there is a defect or deficiency in any of the many blood-clotting factors, excessive bleeding and related complications can result. If for some reason there is a deficiency in the number of circulating platelets (thrombocytopenia), or an abnormal increase in the platelet level (thrombocytosis), clotting and vessel repair become disordered, and the body's health becomes disrupted.

❖ THROMBOCYTOPENIA— LOW PLATELETS

Symptoms *(What you may experience)* Easy and excessive bruising; measles-like rash, usually on the lower legs; nosebleeds; blood in vomit or stool; unusually heavy menstrual flow.

Signs and laboratory findings *(What the doctor looks for)* Blood tests show abnormal decrease in platelet count.

What is it? Thrombocytopenia is a condition in which the number of platelets in the blood is abnormally low. There may be reduced production of platelets, decreased survival of platelets, or increased consumption of platelets within the body. For the blood to operate normally, there needs to be an adequate number of well-functioning platelets in circulation at all times (see How Blood Clots, page 912). As the platelet count falls, the risk of bleeding rises.

In most cases, thrombocytopenia will produce no or few physical symptoms. Usually, the bone marrow automatically compensates for the platelets' shortened life span by producing a higher percentage of new ones. Because young platelets are especially active in clotting, bleeding problems may not occur even though the total concentration of platelets is low.

In more severe instances or when there is some other platelet dysfunction, patients with thrombocytopenia may bleed from a number of sites, including the nose, mucous membranes, gastrointestinal tract, skin, and vessel puncture sites. There may be excessive bleeding after surgery or dental work. Often, a measles-like rash will appear on the skin, usually around the feet and hands.

In many cases, the reason for the low platelet count can be traced to another condition. Then the disorder is considered secondary. When a low concentration of platelets cannot be traced to other precipitating factors such as a particular drug, or a specific disease, the disorder is referred to as immune thrombocytopenic purpura. Named because of the purplish cluster of small marks (petechiae) that appears on the surface of the skin when there is bleeding into the lower layers of skin, immune thrombocytopenic purpura often arises as an autoimmune response. For unknown reasons, antibodies produced within the spleen and lymph tissue attack and destroy the body's own healthy platelets.

Immune thrombocytopenia occurs in two forms: acute and chronic. Acute immune thrombocytopenic purpura occurs most often in children. It is often preceded by a viral (or sometimes bacterial) respiratory infection. Most children (between 80 and 90 percent) recover without treatment in 2 to 6 weeks. Chronic immune thrombocytopenic purpura (CITP) can occur at any age, but it is most common in women between the ages of 20 and 45. This diagnosis can be made only when all other causes of platelet destruction have been ruled out. About 10 percent of adults with CITP will have a spontaneous remission within 1 to 2

years after diagnosis, but others will need treatment. The most serious complications—bleeding into the brain or digestive tract—occur only rarely.

Mild thrombocytopenia can occur during pregnancy, for example, which is considered normal. Other causes of secondary thrombocytopenia are less benign. Sometimes, the bone marrow is unable to produce sufficient replacement cells, perhaps because it has been damaged or destroyed by radiation, cancer chemotherapy, or exposure to toxic chemicals, such as benzene and insecticides. Thrombocytopenia can be a complication of infection with human immunodeficiency virus (HIV) or viral hepatitis. Drugs such as thiazide diuretics, alcohol, and estrogen can also interfere with platelet production. Certain malignancies, such as multiple myeloma, acute leukemia, and lymphoma, can infiltrate the bone marrow and interfere with platelet production.

Reduced platelet production can also result from hereditary abnormalities of the platelet-producing cells in the bone marrow. These genetic disorders include Wiskott Aldrich syndrome and May-Hegglin anomaly.

Accelerated platelet destruction is a common secondary manifestation of autoimmune disease. Conditions associated with autoimmune destruction of platelets include lupus, lymphoma, leukemia, thyroiditis, colitis, ileitis, HIV infection, rubeola (measles), rubella (German measles), chickenpox, viral hepatitis, and Lyme disease.

A blood test and complete platelet count will confirm whether you have thrombocytopenia. If the results of such tests are positive, a bone marrow examination and more detailed blood work-up may point to the cause of low concentration of platelets.

Treatment In general, therapy for thrombocytopenia is planned according to the specific defect involved—whether it is an abnormality in platelet production, in the rate of consumption, or in the length of platelet survival.

For secondary thrombocytopenia, your doctor will treat the underlying condition. If your platelet count is severely diminished as a result of some medication you are taking, your doctor will likely modify or discontinue that particular form of treatment.

Frequently, when thrombocytopenia cannot be corrected directly, because either the source is unknown or the underlying illness cannot be cured, treatment involves long-term management. Therapy may aim at improving platelet production or at decreasing the rate of destruction. Treatment of CITP may include, for example, the use of corticosteroids, intravenous gamma globulin, and immunosuppressive medications. Platelet transfusions can be helpful in managing the disorder when it arises from production defects. Regardless of the type of defect, you will probably be advised not to use aspirin or other medications that tend to impair the clotting function of platelets.

Sometimes, surgical removal of the spleen is recommended to relieve the symptoms or modify the condition if you are not otherwise responsive to medication. When bleeding is severe, the blood that has been lost may need to be replaced through transfusions of packed red blood cells, whole blood, or occasionally, platelet concentrates (see Blood and Blood Products Transfusions, page 940). Platelet transfusions can be useful in both preventing and stopping bleeding caused by thrombocytopenia.

Prognosis Prognosis for thrombocytopenia depends on the root of the problem. Prognosis is quite good when the cause of the disorder can be identified and corrected; in other cases, management can be reasonably effective.

❖ DISSEMINATED INTRAVASCULAR COAGULATION AND RELATED CONDITIONS

Symptoms (*What you may experience*) Fatigue, ashen pallor, and other symptoms of anemia; fever in the absence of infection; severe bleeding from numerous sites in the body following trauma or surgery.

Signs and laboratory findings (*What the doctor looks for*) Low platelet count or high fibrinogen concentration in the blood; formation of blood clots.

What is it? Disseminated intravascular coagulation (DIC) is a clinical condition that involves altered blood coagulation. Usually arising as a complication of another disease or condition, this disorder is also referred to as intravascular coagulation and defibrination syndrome.

There are certain medical conditions that almost inevitably involve the consumption of a large number of platelets—for example, viral infections, bacteria in the blood, inflammation of a blood or lymph vessel, pregnancy, or cancer. With these and other conditions, it is always possible that there will be sufficient cell damage to cause a dramatic increase in the rate of platelet use and the amount of clotting factor in circulation. In most cases, normal repair will occur in time, and balance will restore itself. However, in rare instances, the process can consume platelets to the degree that the coagulation process becomes disordered (see page 912).

In normal circumstances, coagulation is confined to a localized site by a combination of blood flow and circulating clotting inhibitors. Whenever the stimulus to coagulate is too great, the body's control mechanisms can become overwhelmed, leading to excessive clotting. Instead of being limited to injury sites, activated clotting factors begin to move throughout the bloodstream, causing platelets to clot in small blood vessels. This unnecessary coagulation uses up the body's supply of the plasma protein, fibrinogen, clotting factors, and platelets. This depletes the amount available to attend to actual injury sites. The body also reacts by stepping up the system to dissolve the clots, thus promoting generalized bleeding. Depending on how transient such altered coagulation is, the bleeding and clotting that result can be either mild and transient or severe and risky.

DIC is the condition that arises when the entire coagulation pathway is affected. It can result in spontaneous bleeding. Oozing around even minor punctures and wounds may be an indication of DIC. Blood clots can cause bits of tissue to die, which then appear as gangrenous sites on the skin.

DIC can be caused by a number of serious conditions or illnesses. Conditions that might trigger random or disordered coagulation include sepsis (which results from toxic products in the bloodstream); widespread bacterial or fungal infection; severe burns; head injuries; cancer; and major hemolytic transfusion reactions. DIC can cause or result from certain obstetric complications, such as amniotic fluid embolus, septic abortion, or retention of a dead fetus.

There are other related conditions that involve intravascular coagulation and bleeding: thrombotic thrombocytopenic purpura (TTP), hemolytic-uremic syndrome (HUS), and HELLP syndrome (see below). With these disorders, though, the platelet consumption is concentrated at particular sites.

TTP is a rare, potentially fatal condition arising from a defect in platelets that results in the development of blood clots (thrombi) along the walls of the blood and lymph vessels. TTP primarily affects young adults between the ages of 20 and 50. Women manifest the disorder slightly more often than men. It appears that estrogen use or pregnancy (see HELLP, below) occasionally precipitates the syndrome. There is also a link between TTP and HIV infection.

Symptoms and signs, which vary according to the severity of the condition, reflecting hemolytic anemia (see page 925), are fatigue, breathlessness, palpitations, ashen or yellow cast to complexion, dark urine, and enlarged spleen—as well as the deficiency in platelet count, sudden pain in the upper abdomen, fever in the absence of infection, and bleeding into the skin and around the gums.

Occasionally, intermittent neurologic problems are associated with TTP. Such neurologic complaints include headaches, confusion, language impairment, and lethargy or stupor. In its most severe form, TTP can cause coma, seizures, and paralysis on one side of the body (hemiparesis).

A similar disorder is HUS. An uncommon defect, HUS affects the platelet function within the small blood vessels. HUS occasionally appears in children after an infection that has caused diarrhea. In adults, estrogen use or pregnancy often precipitates the condition. Every so often it occurs during the postpartum period, or as a complication of kidney transplantation or malignant hypertension (severe high blood pressure with swelling of the brain). Patients taking the anticancer drug mitomycin seem to be at higher risk for the syndrome. There may also be a genetic component involved. Individuals affected with mild forms will experience fatigue, breathlessness, ashen pallor, rapid heartbeat, and bleeding. In more severe cases, individuals may experience kidney failure, heart failure, and stroke.

Another related condition, HELLP syndrome, is a frequent complication in pregnancy. As many as 50 percent of women who have preeclampsia (toxemia of late pregnancy) will develop thrombocytopenia at the time of delivery. Usually, blood tests show red blood cell loss or hemolysis, elevated liver enzymes, and low platelet count in association with the preeclampsia (hence the *HELLP* acronym).

A doctor will confirm any suspicions about intravascular coagulation by arranging for the patient to undergo various blood tests, including a platelet count and assessment of the concentration of the coagulation factor fibrinogen.

Treatment DIC is treated only by addressing the underlying condition. Transfusions may be necessary to replace the clotting factors depleted by widespread coagulation. Rarely, the anticoagulant heparin is given intravenously to prevent clotting.

TTP is usually treated on an emergency basis with a procedure called plasmapheresis. In this type of transfusion procedure, the patient's blood is removed from her body, its elements separated by means of a centrifuge device. The plasma is discarded before the blood is injected back into the patient. The patient is then injected with normal plasma. Plasmapheresis is usually repeated daily until the patient is in complete remission. The procedure has been shown to be quite effective in correcting TTP. The transfusion may be supplemented with prednisone and antiplatelet agents, such as aspirin and dipyridamole.

In children, HUS is in most cases self-limiting and requires only conservative management to avoid kidney failure. In adults, there is a risk of permanent kidney damage and, in rare cases, death; therefore, treatment tends to be more aggressive. As with TTP, the most effective treatment is plasmapheresis, repeated daily until remission is achieved.

In most cases of HELLP, the condition may disappear when the pregnant woman's hypertension is controlled and the baby is delivered, but platelet transfusion and plasmapheresis may be needed.

Prognosis DIC is often not a serious condition in and of itself, unless the coagulation component is severe. In that case, blood clots can cause damage to major organs as well as painful sores on fingers and toes.

However, the underlying condition often is severe. The success with which DIC can be corrected depends on the co-existing condition. When, for example, DIC occurs with cancer, it can be chronic. More often, though, the episodes are acute, and can be corrected.

Once almost invariably fatal, TTP can now be treated with remarkable results through plasmapheresis. Today, between 80 and 90 percent of patients recover completely. Of these, only 10 to 20 percent relapse. Neurologic symptoms are almost always reversed.

The prognosis for children with HUS is excellent. In adults, when plasmapheresis is undertaken early in the course of the illness, survival, correction of the blood abnormality, and restoration of normal kidney function are highly likely.

❖ THROMBOCYTOSIS— HIGH PLATELETS

Symptoms *(What you may experience)* Burning, throbbing, or painful sensations in hands and feet.

Signs and laboratory findings *(What the doctor looks for)* Random clotting (thrombosis) in both veins and arteries; high platelet count, which can be accompanied by major changes in white or red blood cell counts (for example, in polycythemia vera).

What is it? Thrombocytosis (sometimes referred to as thrombocythemia) is a condition characterized by a high concentration of platelets circulating in the bloodstream. If your platelet count reaches very high levels, you may experience symptoms that are associated with bleeding or a hypercoagulable state: occasional tingling, burning, or throbbing sensations in your feet or hands, which, at times, can be quite painful. In its most severe form, this random clotting in both veins and arteries can lead to stroke, coronary artery occlusions (clots blocking the flow of blood), and damage or death of tissue.

In many cases, an elevated level of platelets is an indication or symptom of another illness. Secondary thrombocytosis may result from malignancies, including carcinoma, agnogenic myeloid metaplasia (see page 953), and chronic myelogenous leukemia (see page 962), as well as from chronic inflammatory conditions, including rheumatoid arthritis. In some cases, an elevated platelet count may indicate iron deficiency, an enlarged or compromised spleen, or polycythemia vera (see page 931).

On the other hand, an elevated platelet count may indicate a discrete disorder in which there are intermittent or permanent blockings (occlusions) of the small blood vessels. In essential thrombocytosis, obstructions can cause temporary deficiencies in the blood supply. Over time, these interruptions in blood flow can result in the destruction of brain or optical tissues. The most severe cases can lead to stroke, coronary artery obstructions, and damage or death to tissue.

Patients with primary or essential thrombocytosis are almost always asymptomatic; therefore, the condition is usually detected first by a routine blood count. Whenever a complete blood count (CBC) indicates the presence of a markedly elevated platelet count, further tests will be ordered to determine if the condition is an illness or a symptom of underlying illness.

Treatment The choice of treatment for thrombocytosis will depend on the full diagnosis. Usually, there is no treatment when there are no symptoms. Patients with essential thrombocytosis and related symptoms may take an aspirin on a daily basis. When that does not seem to work, therapy that aims to repress bone marrow production may be considered. Drugs such as busulfan, hydroxyurea (Hydrea), and alpha-interferon have been shown to decrease clotting formation in the bloodstream. However, such treatment can lead to gastrointestinal bleeding or excessive bleeding during surgery.

Secondary thrombocytosis usually clears up whenever the underlying condition is corrected.

Prognosis Many times, thrombocytosis responds dramatically to aspirin. In other cases, the use of drugs to repress bone marrow production is able to bring the condition under control; however, there is some concern that over the long run, such treatment can cause cancer. For those whose elevated platelet count is due to another condition, prognosis depends on that condition.

❖ HEMOPHILIA

Symptoms *(What you may experience)*
Large and deep bruises; pain, swelling, and warmth in knees, elbows, hips, and shoulders, and in arm and leg muscles; blood in urine; black or tar-like stool; excessive and protracted bleeding from cuts, injuries, or after surgery or dental work.

Signs and laboratory findings *(What the doctor looks for)* Deficient or defective clotting factors VIII or IX; in extreme cases, bleeding into the head, neck, or digestive tract.

What is it? Many people are familiar with what is popularly called the royal disease, hemophilia, at least by reputation. Hemophilia—a bleeding disorder inherited by Queen Victoria's descendants who, through marriage, introduced it into the 19th century royal houses of Germany, Spain, and most notoriously, Russia—is romantically imputed to be the curse and downfall of the Romanov tsars in prerevolutionary Russia.

Notwithstanding the romance, hemophilia is a very real and troublesome family of inherited disorders that compromises specific clotting factors. The result is disruptions and disorders in the body's normal coagulation processes, manifested by excessive and abnormal bleeding. While surface bleeding and bruising may occur and be visible, the greater threat lies with internal bleeding, most commonly at the joints—knees, ankles, elbows—but also into the muscles and gastrointestinal tract. The severity of bleeding varies from person to person.

In its mildest forms, hemophilia may not become apparent until later in life; troublesome bleeding may happen only after surgery, tooth extraction, or a major injury. More severe forms are usually apparent during infancy when, for example, a newborn is circumcised or when an infant begins to crawl or walk. Young children who have the disease may bruise easily or bleed spontaneously after minor mishaps or for no obvious reason.

There are two basic types of hemophilia. The most common type is classic hemophilia or hemophilia A. In this form, there is an insufficient or deficient supply of the coagulation factor VIII within the blood. Factor VIII may be quantitatively reduced, or present but defective. In the second type, hemophilia B, or Christmas disease, coagulation factor IX is lacking or functionally abnormal.

Both hemophilia A and hemophilia B are X-linked recessive diseases. This means that as a rule, females who inherit the gene are symptomless carriers; males who inherit the gene have the disease. Approximately 1 in 10,000 males in this country is affected with hemophilia. In rare instances, female carriers are affected when their normal X chromosomes are inactive and unable to prevail over the hemophilic X chromosomes. A female child can also inherit the disease when her mother is a carrier and her father has hemophilia. Most often, hemophilia occurs in families that have histories of the disease. However, new cases sometimes occur in families with no apparent history (see page 939).

Hemophilia is a lifelong condition and, as such, requires careful management and comprehensive treatment. Internal bleeding into the muscles and soft tissue strains the nerves, causing pain, interfering with flexibility, and deadening sensation. In some instances, when this type of bleeding is not curbed, it can bring about permanent nerve damage and muscle deterioration. When blood collects in the joints, it not only causes chronic pain, but over time, a joint disorder called osteoarthritis can develop; as the cushioning cartilage begins to deteriorate, the joints can be damaged.

In the most severe cases, bleeding into the head, neck, or digestive system can be extremely serious. As a result, any head injuries should be treated as an emergency, because there is a possibility that major bleeding is occurring.

What you can do With good medical treatment, education, and careful planning, most people with hemophilia live full lives. There is no question that if you or someone you love has hemophilia, carrying on normally can be challenging; from time to time, the disorder will inevitably interfere with school, work, and social involvements. However, by and large, if you understand the disorder and involve yourself responsibly in managing it, you can live a relatively normal life.

Besides a good working relationship with your doctor, support groups and such other assistance are the best ways of navi-

INHERITANCE PATTERNS FOR HEMOPHILIA

The disease that we now call hemophilia was noted in writing as early as 2,000 years ago. By the fifth century AD, it was recognized as an inherited disease that affects mostly boys. The transmission of hemophilia from unaffected mothers to their sons was first described in the United States in the first years of the 19th century.

Hemophilia is a disorder that arises when there is a defect or deficiency in clotting factor VIII (antihemophilic factor—AHF) or in factor IX (plasma thromboplastin component). The genes that contain the instructions for manufacturing these factors are carried on the X chromosome. Hemophilia arises when an abnormality or error in the gene is inherited in such a specific way as to cause the factor to be made incorrectly or not at all.

As you may remember from your basic high school biology class, when conception brings together a sperm cell and an egg cell, it also brings together 23 pairs of chromosomes. The female contributes one of her two X chromosomes to the egg. Some of the male's sperm cells carry his X and some his Y chromosomes. It is always the sperm that determines the child's gender: XX is a girl; XY is a boy. If a Y-bearing sperm reaches the egg, the child will be a boy.

The abnormality that causes hemophilia originally arises from a mutation, a change that occurs by chance in the DNA code of the gene. Occasionally, the mutation is new and hemophilia appears in a family that has no history of the disorder. In most families, though, the mutant gene has been around for generations and is passed down through the females of the family on the X chromosome. If a daughter receives the defective gene on one X chromosome, the chances are high that she will also receive a normal gene on the other X chromosome. Her body is then able to produce the appropriate factors. But because a boy receives only one X chromosome, there is no other to instruct his body to manufacture the necessary clotting factor. The Y chromosome will not have the gene to trigger the production of factor VIII or factor IX. Therefore, when a girl inherits the defective gene, she is a carrier; when a boy inherits a hemophilia gene, he will likely have hemophilia.

Women rarely have the disease; they may have reduced levels of factor VIII or IX, but seldom have symptoms. In very rare cases, a woman can have hemophilia if she has only one functioning chromosome, or hemophilia genes on both her X chromosomes. This happens when she develops a new mutation on her normal X chromosome, or if her father has hemophilia and her mother is a carrier.

Approximately one-third of boys who have hemophilia are born to women with no known family history of hemophilia. However, tests show that, rather than being produced by random mutation within the child's gene, most times the disease is passed on by mothers who are hemophilia carriers without being aware of a family history of the disease. These women may have received the recessive, abnormal gene through females in their families, even though the disease itself had not been apparent in male family members. Perhaps no males were born in a previous generation, or affected males were never diagnosed or died in infancy. Studies suggest that fewer than 10 percent of cases of hemophilia occur as a result of new mutations. ■

gating this demanding condition. Especially during particularly difficult times, knowing where to turn for extra help and support can spell the difference between managing well and just hanging on. In many cities, hemophilia treatment centers offer comprehensive care to persons with hemophilia and their families. Through information, educational materials, psychological and social supports, and referrals to other agencies, these centers can help you get through the most complicated times. The National Hemophilia Foundation and its information center—Hemophilia and AIDS/HIV Network for the Dissemination of Information—collect and disseminate information. In addition, there are local chapters that can provide advocacy, financial assistance, and other direct services. You can write the Hemophilia Foundation at The SoHo Building, 110 Greene Street, Suite 303, New York, NY 10012, or call (800) 42-HANDI.

As much as possible, it will help if you engage in appropriate physical activities. You should avoid activities that entail a high risk of injury, such as contact sports. Moderate exercise, such as walking, swimming, and bicycle riding, can help damaged joints function because it strengthens your muscles and this in turn protects your joints. Your doctor may recommend physical therapy as a way of improving joint and muscle functioning.

There will be times when you need pain relief. Talk about this with your doctor, because aspirin, which can cause internal bleeding, should never be used.

Treatment Depending on the severity of the condition or the situation, hemophilia is regularly treated with either medication or infusions of clotting factor concentrates.

For mild hemophilia A, a medicine called desmopression (DDAVP), which is slowly infused into the vein, can stimulate the release of factor VII, prompting blood vessels to contract. Desmopressin may also be useful in preparing individuals with mild hemophilia for surgery or dental proce-

BLOOD AND BLOOD PRODUCTS TRANSFUSIONS

Up until relatively recently, blood transfusion meant transfusing whole blood. While whole blood is still transfused today, it is transfused much less often. Instead, there are various ways in which transfusions are prepared and administered. Mostly, blood and blood products are prepared in ways that address an individual's distinct health needs.

Whole blood is used sometimes if an individual has lost a large quantity of blood through major surgery, trauma, or recent bleeding from the digestive tract. Fresh whole blood provides all the blood's components: red blood cells, plasma, and fresh platelets. Whole blood may occasionally be preferable during cardiac surgery or following a massive hemorrhage when more than 10 units of blood are required in a 24-hour period. However, transfusing whole blood puts demands on the body, especially the heart, as it must accommodate the additional volume of fluid. Fortunately, whole blood is seldom necessary.

These days, donated blood is separated into its various components—packed red blood cells, fresh-frozen plasma, cryoprecipitate, coagulation factor concentrate, granulocytes (a type of white blood cell), and platelets—and each is given as needed.

Red Blood Cells

Red blood cells will be transfused when someone is deficient in red blood cells but does not need either the other components or the additional volume. Red blood cells are generally stored in the form of *packed red blood cells* or *packed frozen red blood cells*.

Packed Frozen Red Blood Cells Packed frozen red blood cells are prepared by removing white blood cells and plasma from blood before freezing. Red blood cells are frozen in a preservative solution and can be stored up to 3 years. However, the technique is cumbersome and expensive and is used mainly to maintain supplies of very rare blood types. The cells are thawed just before transfusion.

Packed Red Blood Cells Packed red blood cells are used most commonly to raise the concentration of red blood cells in individuals with anemia or to replace those lost after acute bleeding. Each unit (volume of about 300 ml) is usually sufficient to raise the concentration of red blood cells by 4 percent. Packed red blood cell transfusion may be recommended during a crisis of sickle cell anemia (see page 927) or other inherited anemias, or to treat such conditions as thalassemia and glucose-6-phosphate dehydrogenase deficiency (see Other Inherited Anemias, page 929). Packed red blood cells are usually preferable to whole blood because they do not increase circulating blood volume much above normal. In addition, because white blood cells are mostly absent, this type of transfusion reduces the risk of undesired antigenic reactions to the infused blood (see page 914).

Plasma Components

Up until 1965, people with hemophilia were treated in the hospital with transfusions of whole blood or fresh-frozen plasma. Either form contained normal levels of coagulation factors. However, the body is incapable of holding the large amounts of fluid needed to provide sufficient clotting factor. As a result, the fluid would flow into the confined space of a knee, ankle, or elbow, causing joint damage and considerable pain. Clearly, this method was only partially effective. Today, plasma components can be transfused in the form of purified factors to correct clotting disorders.

- *Cryoprecipitate* and *purified factors* can be stored frozen or in freeze-dried form. With a number of the factors now available in more easily used forms, people with hemophilia, von ➧

dures. However, bleeding episodes, even minor ones, may need to be treated promptly by infusion (slow injection into a vein) of clotting factor replacement.

Standard treatment for hemophilia B or more severe hemophilia A is based on infusion of factor concentrates, which replaces the missing or deficient clotting factor. For hemophilia A, factor VIII is used; for hemophilia B, factor IX is necessary. (Desmopressin is not useful in hemophilia B.)

Clotting factor is derived from donated human blood or manufactured through genetic engineering (in which case it is called recombinant factor VIII). It is supplied as purified concentrates, as fresh-frozen plasma, or as cryoprecipitate, a clotting factor concentrate derived from donated human blood (see above). The dose of the factor is carefully calculated to raise the level of factor according to the patient's specific need. Clotting factor concentrates are now heat-treated to prevent transmission of HIV. Unlike factor VIII concentrates, factor IX concentrates contain a number of other proteins that may increase the risk of thrombosis (blood clots). Patients should discuss this risk with their doctor.

Whether DDAVP or some other blood product is used, the doctor can help the patient learn to infuse himself at the first signs of bleeding. This will mean that patients can travel and in general have greater freedom of movement. Persons with hemophilia should not use medications that might worsen bleeding, such as aspirin. Aspirin is often a "hidden" ingredient in over-the-counter medications, so it is important to read labels carefully and consult with the doctor about which medications are appropriate for use (see page 943).

Willebrand's disease, and other clotting deficiencies can treat themselves at home, work, or school. It takes very little time to reconstitute the concentrate before it is self-infused. Cryoprecipitate can also supplement fibrinogen in cases of disseminated intravascular coagulation (see page 935) or bleeding due to the lack of this protein in the blood (hypofibrinogenemia).

- *Plasma concentrate* can be used to treat thrombotic thrombocytopenic purpura (see page 935).

- *Plasma protein fraction* is a solution made up of the proteins from human plasma and is used to treat shock caused by bleeding, trauma, infections, burns, or surgery.

White Blood Cells

Transfusions of white blood cells are seldom necessary, because antibiotics are widely available. However, white blood cells may be infused in some cases of severe leukopenia (see page 944). White blood cells can be stored for only about 12 hours.

Platelet Transfusions

Platelet transfusions can be used to treat specific cases of thrombocytopenia (see page 933) that arise when leukemia (see page 958), radiation therapy, or chemotherapy has suppressed or interfered with platelet production. Since transfused platelets will not last longer than the person's own platelets, such transfusions are not useful in cases of immune thrombocytopenia. In addition, when an individual has immune thrombocytopenia, transfusions can stimulate destructive antibodies against these cells, and therefore are used only in the most dramatic cases. More often, platelet transfusions are used to control bleeding in people who have lost blood through injury or after prolonged surgery; the process is called massive blood replacement.

Using Your Own Blood

The safest source of blood is an autologous transfusion—one in which you use your own blood. Your immune system will not react to your blood as though it were foreign. Nor can you contract an infection that you do not already have.

In many circumstances, such as emergencies or if you have a disorder that affects your blood, you will have to use blood from random donors. But when you and your doctor have scheduled elective surgery, you can donate your own blood ahead of time (see Chapter 32). Usually, blood is taken over a period of a few weeks. It will be stored and used whenever necessary during the procedure. It may be more costly to use autologous transfusions, because more work is required to label, store, and deliver your own blood. However, for many people, the peace of mind is well worth the cost.

When it is not possible or practical to use your own blood, you may elect to use blood from a designated donor—perhaps a relative or friend who has the same blood group. However, personally knowing the person does not ensure that the blood is completely compatible or safe. In fact, properly tested blood from unknown donors can be a safer source. Recent data indicates that the rate of infection is about the same for designated donors as it is for random donors. ■

Most of the time, it will be necessary to coordinate care with an orthopedic surgeon to help manage chronic joint problems that commonly arise from hemophilia. Should recurrent internal bleeding result in joint destruction, the doctor may suggest having the affected joints surgically replaced. For more information on joint replacement, see Chapter 17.

Prognosis With comprehensive management, life can be full for a person with hemophilia. It may be necessary to take extra care to minimize bleeding that can result from physical activity, surgery, or dental procedures. In some cases, if the patient's body develops antibodies to the infused clotting factor, hemophilia becomes more difficult to treat. On rare occasions, patients develop inhibitors to the factor, in which case they may not be adequately protected against bleeding.

Today, the major problems for persons with hemophilia are recurrent joint bleeding and transfusion-acquired viral infections, such as hepatitis B and acquired

HEMOPHILIA, HIV INFECTION, AND AIDS

People with hemophilia use blood products and clotting factor concentrates extracted from human plasma derived from thousands of donors. There is always a chance that they will be exposed to blood-borne viruses. No doubt, the most devastating exposure involves HIV, which causes AIDS.

In the late 1970s and early 1980s, the nation's blood supply—and thus the clotting factor concentrates—became contaminated with HIV. Tragically, almost 90 percent of the 8,000 to 10,000 persons with severe hemophilia who were living in the United States at that time became infected with HIV. An ever-increasing number of those infected have since been diagnosed with AIDS. So far, more than 4,500 persons with hemophilia have died from AIDS.

HIV has also been transmitted to sexual partners of people with hemophilia and to their newborns. HIV infection has added a profound new weight to the financial and emotional burdens that people with hemophilia already bear.

Beginning in the mid-1980s, new screening and processing procedures have made the blood supply safer. Concentrates are now heat treated, which kills most of the HIV. Many concentrates are pasteurized or treated with solvent detergents. In addition, new factor products are in development that will be produced artificially without using blood products. ■

immunodeficiency syndrome (AIDS) (see page 941).

❖ VON WILLEBRAND'S DISEASE

Symptoms *(What you may experience)* Nosebleeds; excessive menstrual bleeding; easy bruising; tar-like stool.

Signs and laboratory findings *(What the doctor looks for)* Blood tests show normal levels of platelet number and development, but a reduction in von Willebrand's factor (vWF) and sometimes of factor VIII.

OTHER CLOTTING DISORDERS

With few exceptions, the liver forms almost all blood-clotting factors. Therefore, diseases of the liver—such as hepatitis, cirrhosis, and acute yellow atrophy—can depress the clotting system so greatly that the individual develops a severe tendency to bleed. Only when these conditions are corrected will the bleeding problems clear up. In the meantime, iron and folic acid supplements may be recommended.

Another cause of depressed formation of clotting factors within the liver is *vitamin K deficiency*. Vitamin K is needed to form five important clotting factors: prothrombin, factor VII, factor IX, factor X, and protein C. A deficiency of vitamin K can cause an insufficiency of these coagulation factors, which in turn can lead to a serious bleeding tendency.

Because vitamin K is continuously synthesized by bacteria in the intestinal tract, deficiency seldom arises from low dietary intake. Instead, it usually stems from gastrointestinal disease that in turn causes poor absorption. In many cases, this inability to absorb and synthesize vitamin K is caused by liver disease or blocked bile ducts.

Because the problem usually lies in the body's ability to absorb vitamin K, treatment involves injecting or infusing the nutrient. In preparation for surgery or dental procedures, your physician may advise prophylactic (preventive) injections of vitamin K. This is especially true for individuals with liver disease or obstructions of the bile ducts. Such treatment is administered 4 to 8 hours before the procedure and stimulates the production of enough clotting factor to prevent excessive bleeding during the procedure. ■

What is it? Named after the early 20th century Finnish doctor who first described it, this group of chronic, congenital bleeding disorders is caused by defective or deficient von Willebrand clotting factor, a protein that facilitates platelet adhesion.

In many cases of von Willebrand's disease, there is also a deficiency of factor VIII. These two factors usually blend to form the active substance that the body needs so that platelets cluster around blood vessel injuries. Although the platelet count is normal in von Willebrand's disease, there is a defect in the way in which platelets gather and the way in which clots develop.

Von Willebrand's disease is the most common hereditary bleeding disorder, and it has several different types. Most forms of von Willebrand's disease are associated with mild to moderate bleeding. It affects both men and women equally. Only in very rare cases are the symptoms severe. The most telling symptom, in children and adults alike, is frequent nosebleeds. In fact, nosebleeds can be so alarming that they warrant visits to the doctor or the hospital emergency room. Other symptoms include a tendency towards bruising, blood in urine or stool (characterized by a black or tar-like appearance), and excessive bleeding during surgery or dental work. Typically, bleeding is exacerbated by aspirin use, and generally, the tendency to bleed decreases during pregnancy or estrogen use.

What you can do If you have von Willebrand's disease, avoid using aspirin (see page 943). Be sure to consult a doctor who is an expert in the disease, especially if you are contemplating surgery or thinking about conceiving a child.

Treatment Because von Willebrand's disease is usually mild, most cases do not require treatment. Before surgical or dental procedures, though, it may be necessary to use the drug desmopressin (DDAVP) or transfusion of blood products to reduce the risk of excessive bleeding.

DDAVP, which is administered through infusion, raises the level of both von Willebrand factor and factor VII in the blood. It is used most frequently following more serious injuries or to manage severe cases. Transfusions of plasma, cryoprecipitate, or platelets also may be used when DDAVP is ineffective or harmful (in some rare forms of von Wille-

ABOUT BLOOD-THINNING MEDICATIONS AND ASPIRIN

For a number of medical reasons, your doctor may recommend medications that delay the blood's coagulation process. The most commonly used anticoagulants, or blood-thinning medications, are heparin and coumarin. These anticlotting medications, as well as aspirin, may be given to high-risk individuals to reduce the possibility of stroke, heart attacks, or other serious blood clots.

Heparin is used to prevent or treat blood clots. It is frequently used after surgery to prevent clotting, and slows clotting time instantaneously. Heparin is usually administered by injection in relatively small amounts. When heparin is injected, the time it takes for blood to clot generally increases from a normal time of about 6 minutes to 30 or more minutes. If, however, serious bleeding results, certain drugs like protamine immediately counteract the effects.

Coumarin (Coumadin, warfarin) is used to prevent or treat blood clots, pulmonary embolism (blood clot in the lung artery) or atrial fibrillation (rapid heart contractions). This medication is often prescribed in persons with atrial fibrillation and in those with serious blood clots in the leg (see Deep Venous Thrombosis, page 833). Coumarin antagonizes the action of vitamin K. It causes the blood's normal coagulant activities to decrease gradually by acting on the plasma levels of prothrombin and factors VII, IX, and X, all of which are formed in the liver. As these elements fall, the blood "thins." Unlike heparin, the coagulation process is not blocked immediately with coumarin. Normal coagulation returns 1 to 3 days after discontinuing the medication. Coumarin is usually administered orally. If you take coumarin, you must be scrupulous about reporting for tests—usually weekly—of your blood's ability to coagulate. That way your doctor will know if you are maintaining the correct balance between having your blood thinned just right and too much. Too much means you are at risk for bleeding.

Aspirin deters the body's clotting processes by neutralizing certain enzymes involved in platelet clustering. Recently, daily use of aspirin has been much touted as a preventative measure against heart attacks and strokes—especially for people who have already had one heart attack or stroke, or who have a personal or family history of heart disease or high blood pressure. In addition, aspirin may be a useful counterbalance if you have thrombocytosis (a high platelet count that causes random coagulation and puts you at risk for obstructions to the blood supply—see page 937).

Aspirin's effects last for the life of the platelet. The effects may reverberate throughout the system for 7 to 10 days, although the major effects last for only 3 to 5 days.

Other medications that are used to treat specific blood disorders can naturally, as a side reaction, decrease clotting formation in the bloodstream. These include busulfan (Myleran), hydroxyurea (Hydrea), and alpha-interferon.

While blood-thinning medications serve very important functions in regulating blood flow, they can at the same time cause serious excessive bleeding during surgery or dental procedures. More serious bleeding problems can surface in occasional or chronic gastrointestinal bleeding and in hemorrhaging at other sites in the body. Furthermore, using these medications can lead to anemia. When the internal bleeding is serious enough, you may be directed to discontinue the medication. Otherwise, the doctor may recommend an iron supplement.

Blood-thinning medications can also unmask other mild forms of bleeding disorders, such as von Willebrand's disease or thrombocytopenia, or exacerbate more severe bleeding tendencies. If you already have a bleeding disorder, not even aspirin should be used—for any reason. Aspirin can be a "hidden" ingredient in many over-the-counter remedies, so read labels carefully and consult your doctor.

One last word on medications and bleeding: Certain antibiotics such as ticarcillin and some cephalosporins can also cause mild bleeding tendencies, presumably because they coat the surface of platelets. Nonsteroidal anti-inflammatory drugs can cause transient bleeding as well. If you already have bleeding tendencies, discuss these with your doctor before any medications are prescribed. ■

---

brand's disease). An expert physician is needed to make this determination. You will be warned to avoid aspirin or other medications that can worsen bleeding.

Von Willebrand's disease can occur either as a spontaneous mutation or be inherited. If you are considering pregnancy, genetic counseling will help you determine your risks of having a child with the disorder and the options available. If a close relative has von Willebrand's disease, you should consider being tested for the disorder.

Prognosis Excellent. Ordinarily, the disorder is mild. Even in more serious cases, replacement therapy is generally effective.

The White Blood Cell System and Its Disorders

Just as with the red blood cell system and the blood's coagulation system, a healthy balance among the body's complex systems is often reflected in the balance of the cells in the white blood cell system. But here, among the white blood cells (leukocytes), it is not always easy to judge when an imbalance is a sign of trouble and when it is a sign that the system is functioning as it should. Many times, if all things are going well, there will be an increase in the number of white blood cells in circulation. Unusually high or

IMMUNODEFICIENCY

Immunodeficiency occurs when the body's immune defenses are not acting in the way they normally would be expected to function; that is, the response to infection is absent or impaired. Mild immunodeficiency often is due to the general physical stresses that we endure from day to day. Our system simply becomes depleted—too taxed to respond adequately to stimulation from antigens. Perhaps no setting so adequately illustrates the effects of mild immunodeficiency as a college campus around final-exam time. The immune changes that occur during academic exam periods have been well documented, right down to changes in blood chemistry. Colds and sore throats can become rampant, sending nurses and doctors at university clinics scrambling to meet a higher-than-normal caseload. Why? The combination of stressors—psychological duress, "all nighters" of study, and poor nutrition from snack-food "fuel"—causes a well-known result: reduced resistance to infection.

Generally, however, these periods of immunodeficiency—marked by heightened susceptibility to infection—are transient. Not always, however. Sometimes immunodeficiency can result from a chronic illness, in which the body becomes so worn down fighting the disorder that it becomes vulnerable to infection. Seriously ill individuals may become vulnerable to infection by bacteria nestled in the soil of a houseplant, for instance, or to the spores that float from a moldy piece of bread. The medical community has a special term for such a state: "immunocompromised." Doctors also have a particular phrase to describe such illnesses: they are called "opportunistic infections," and they are a growing problem across the world.

Some of the recent medical advances that have made it possible for populations worldwide to survive once life-threatening disorders have at the same time cleared the way for opportunistic infections. Sometimes, treatment aimed at wiping out an invader will leave the body in an immunologically weakened state. When this happens, it is called treatment-related immunodeficiency. Bone marrow transplants for leukemia, chemotherapy for cancer, and corticosteroid treatment for severe asthma leave many beneficiaries of these successful therapies far less able to battle microbes that otherwise would be benign. The challenge facing patients and doctors alike is to see to it that the patient stays healthy, with a resistance that will be fortified during vulnerable periods of treatment. Once treatment is complete, the immune system will be restored and resume its duties. ■

THE "BOY IN THE BUBBLE" DISEASE

Until fairly recently, certain inherited disorders that impaired immune function sentenced many children to early death or to living in completely sterile surroundings. Born without the ability to ward off infection, these children were forced to live in an antiseptic world of isolation. The most famous of these was a boy named David, who lived his life inside a protective, barren enclosure reminiscent of a space module. Hence, he became known as the "boy in the bubble."

Several years after David's death, a research team from the National Institutes of Health—Drs. French Anderson, David Blaese, and Ken Culver—developed a revolutionary treatment for children who suffer from inherited immunodeficiency disorders. Using new, recombinant DNA techniques, the trio genetically altered white blood cells to render them capable infection fighters. They reasoned that when the revised cells were injected into the children's systems, new cells would multiply, and, eventually, there would be sufficient cells to fight off many infections successfully. That effort is widely perceived to constitute a cure. Around the same time, other treatments were being developed to help such children ward off pathogens (microorganisms that produce disease). Today, both approaches are used to ensure the greatest possible chance of a healthy childhood.

David, the "boy in the bubble," did not live long enough to benefit from this radical feat of genetic engineering. Wanting to lead a more normal life, he left his "bubble" and died shortly thereafter. However, he lives on in medical texts as an example of the genetic disorder his life came to typify, and as an inspiration for the medical battle against it. ■

low white blood cell counts are seen frequently in laboratory tests, yet such variations seldom reflect a blood disorder in and of itself. An acute increase in the number of mature or immature leukocytes (white blood cells)—leukocytosis—*is* part of the normal response to infection, allergy, or inflammatory conditions. A drop in white blood cells—leukopenia—is either a reaction to drug use or chemotherapy, or a transient sign of a very early viral infection.

Yet, there are times when, rather than being a symptom of a problem elsewhere in the body, an elevated or reduced level of white blood cells points to a disorder within the blood system itself.

❖ LEUKOPENIA—LOW WHITE BLOOD CELL COUNT

Symptoms (*What you may experience*) Fatigue; decreased appetite; fever; mouth ulcers; swollen lymph glands; abdominal tenderness; skin infections; rashes on the face; gum disease.

Signs and laboratory finding (*What the doctor looks for*) Examination and tests may reveal a swollen spleen and enlarged liver, as well as a significant decrease in white blood cell count.

PRECAUTIONS FOR IMMUNO-COMPROMISED INDIVIDUALS

Individuals with compromised immune systems are advised to take extra precautions to minimize the possibility of infection. Below are some suggestions that can help reduce your risk of exposure. It is important to keep in mind, however, that the common cold, influenza, and most common infections actually pose little threat. It is wise to be careful, but it is not necessary to carry caution to extremes.

1. Keep in frequent touch with your doctor and let her know of any possible exposure to infectious disease. For some transmittable illnesses, postexposure injections to aid the immune system may be recommended. Also, though live-virus vaccines usually are not considered appropriate for immunocompromised persons, immunizations derived from killed pathogens may be advised.

2. Do not smoke. Cigarette smoking, in particular, has been linked to diminished immune function. Consult your doctor about drinking alcoholic beverages in any amount. Some research shows that even moderate liquor intake can reduce the infection-fighting capacity of the immunocompromised.

3. Get adequate sleep. Studies show that when you do not get enough rest, you increase your risk of infection; for those whose immunity is compromised, the risk is even greater.

4. Eat a healthy diet. Good nutrition, particularly fresh fruits and vegetables, supplies the body with necessary nutrients, in ways that cannot be duplicated simply by taking over-the-counter supplements.

5. Consider boiling your drinking water. Check with your local public health department or water sanitation agency on the purity of the water in your community and find out how consistently it meets national standards. You also need to know if there is a way to stay informed when those standards have not been met, such as a "warning line" you can call. You

may also want to consider using bottled water rather than water from the tap.

6. Wash hands frequently, particularly as you prepare food, and after being touched or embraced. Some health authorities also recommend wearing gloves in social situations in which you will be shaking a number of hands.

7. Avoid crowded situations where you could be exposed to infection. During the winter, when people stay inside, infections are more likely to spread. In addition, close contact with children, who often are exposed to a variety of childhood diseases in group settings, such as school classes or day care, can increase the likelihood of exposure.

8. Limit travel. Planes, in particular, recirculate air breathed by passengers, which tends to spread colds and flu.

9. Use caution when following an exercise regimen. Low- to moderate-level exercise often is encouraged, even in the immunocompromised, to prevent excessive loss of body strength. However, too much exertion can have the opposite effect.

10. Take medications appropriately. Make sure to follow the instructions on your prescription medications, including the designated times. Several helpers, from "pill calendars" to alarm-clock "reminders," are available to help prevent incorrect dosing.

11. Cultivate a good support system. Social support, particularly wellness communities and other groups, seem to bolster the immune system in ways that are not fully understood.

12. Do not share eating utensils. Check with your doctor; usually this prohibition includes religious rituals in which liquid is shared as a part of a communion or other ceremony.

13. Avoid musty places, damp spaces, and dust in general. Sometimes an attic or garage is the perfect breeding ground for molds and other pathogens that could be inhaled, causing illness. ■

What is it? Leukopenia is a marked drop in white blood cells. Typically, it occurs in response to other conditions. A mild case of leukopenia may indicate a low-grade viral infection, in which there are no symptoms or only mild symptoms, such as mouth ulcers, fatigue, and a decreased appetite. At the other extreme, leukopenia could be a symptom—along with mouth sores, fever, weight loss, and bone pain—of acute leukemia or other bone marrow malignancies. One of the more ominous, but uncommon, causes of leukopenia is aplastic anemia. In addition, leukopenia can result from HIV infection, lymphoma, lupus, rheumatoid arthritis, or folic acid or B_{12} deficiency.

Chronic symptoms of leukopenia in children may indicate a congenital condition. If severe leukopenia is combined with specific deficiencies of the immune system, the condition can be quite serious. It may be associated with certain hereditary skin disorders, or with other genetic disorders.

A drop in white blood cells may occur as a reaction to certain drugs or cancer chemotherapy that interferes with production in the bone marrow. High doses of the antibiotics penicillin, cephalosporins, and sulfonamides are also associated with leukopenia. Clozapine, which is used to treat schizophrenia, can reduce the level of white blood cells in circulation.

When to call your doctor If you have a chronic form of leukopenia, your susceptibility to infection increases. It is therefore important to avoid infections whenever possible (see above). If it appears that you

AUTOIMMUNITY

The body's immune system can react in ways that seem puzzling, even to the most knowledgeable medical experts. Such is the case with many autoimmune diseases, in which the immune system seems to become confused, mistaking naturally occurring proteins within the body as enemy invaders, and waging a devastating war that is tantamount to friendly fire.

Autoimmune disease is, in essence, a subversion of the immune function. Instead of protecting the body, the immune system reacts against the body's own tissues, developing antibodies against proteins produced by internal cells. As antibodies attack, the reactions are felt not only in the immediate area, but throughout the body as well, especially in the connective tissues and skin.

Autoimmune diseases are divided into two general categories: the autoimmune hemolytic disorders, such as autoimmune leukopenia and acquired hemolytic anemia (which are covered in this chapter), and the collagen diseases, such as systemic lupus erythematosus (lupus, or SLE), rheumatoid arthritis, and scleroderma (which are covered in Chapter 17). The list of autoimmune diseases is growing as research identifies autoimmune processes at the root of more illnesses; for instance, type I diabetes has been linked to autoimmunity.

Sometimes the mechanism for the autoimmune reaction is relatively well understood, even though the reason the disease surfaces in the first place remains elusive. It is believed, for example, that in arthritis the cartilage cells within the joints produce a protein that prompts the immune system to attack the joint tissue. Generally, the sequence of events is as follows: The body begins to identify certain proteins, expressed in the cells of cartilage tissues, as foreign antigens. The immune system then responds by destroying as many cells as possible. This may manifest itself in physical deformity—swollen joints and gnarled fingers. At this time, there is no treatment that effectively stops the encroaching destruction—only therapy aimed at alleviating symptoms and slowing the progression.

Yet, scientists hope soon to unlock the mystery of such autoimmune responses. When they do, powerful treatments, even cures, are expected to follow. ■

have an infection or related symptoms, such as fever or inflammation, for an extended period of time, contact your doctor.

Treatment In most cases, your doctor will begin by seeking the cause of the leukopenia. Whenever possible, the cause will be addressed, and if that is successfully treated, your white blood cell count will probably return to normal.

When it appears that the leukopenia is not related to any underlying condition, your doctor will order a bone marrow biopsy to determine if there are fungi or bacteria in the marrow cells or if the problem lies in white blood cell production.

When the condition is chronic, your doctor will likely attempt to prevent infections and treat them immediately should they occur. Sometimes a mild antibiotic, trimetho-prim-sulfamethoxazole (Bactrim-DS), will be used prophylactically.

Corticosteroids, such as prednisone, can be effective in raising the leukocyte count.

❖ LEUKOCYTOSIS—HIGH WHITE BLOOD CELL COUNT

Symptoms (*What you may experience*) In mild cases, fever, infection, and abscesses. In severe cases: abdominal tenderness; breathing difficulties.

Signs and laboratory findings (*What the doctor looks for*) High white blood cell count.

What is it? Leukocytosis, a very high white blood cell count, may occur for several reasons. Ordinarily it is caused by the presence of infection as the bone marrow steps up production of leukocytes in response to infections or inflammatory conditions. When this is the case, leukocytosis is usually transient and will be diagnosed through a complete blood count.

While most cases of leukocytosis are related to infection, very high white blood cell counts can occasionally arise when bone marrow production increases in response to excessive bleeding, extensive operations, coronary occlusion (the closing off of an artery), malignant growth (tumor), pregnancy, certain intoxications, and toxemias (bacterial toxins in the blood). People who take lithium and chronic smokers frequently have mild leukocytosis.

An increase in the number of a particular type of white blood cell, eosinophils (eosinophilic leukocytosis), occurs in some allergies, asthma, animal parasite infestation, chlamydia, eczema, psoriasis, lupus, and Hodgkin's disease, among other disorders.

In leukocytosis, the number of white blood cells may vary from a 50 percent increase to many times more than normal. Leukocytosis is early and marked in severe infections when the patient's resistance is good. If infection and resistance are less marked, it appears later to a lesser degree and disappears more quickly.

Treatment In most cases, leukocytosis itself requires no treatment. Once the underlying condition is cleared up or managed, the white blood cell count will return to normal. However, when the eosinophil count is extremely high, there is a risk of tissue damage and fibrous growths around the heart. Because this can lead to widespread organ dysfunction and progressive heart disease, aggressive treatment is necessary, usually with both corticosteroids and hydroxyurea.

Bone Marrow Disorders

Bone marrow is the soft tissue that resides within the bones. It is responsible for the production (hematopoiesis) of red blood cells, platelets, and most white blood cells. When something goes wrong with the bone marrow, the consequences are serious: the production of cells is no longer orderly, causing deficiencies or excesses, or the outpouring of the wrong cells into the blood, as in leukemia. Deficiencies usually manifest in anemia, bleeding disorders, and vulnerability to infections.

During childhood, all the bones in the body contain active marrow that contributes to hematopoiesis. As the body matures, the bones of the spine, skull, ribs, and pelvis are most active in forming blood cells and hemoglobin. However, whenever an increased level of blood cells is needed, the bone marrow in the arms and legs may be stimulated to resume active production.

❖ APLASTIC ANEMIA

Symptoms *(What you may experience)* Fatigue and weakness that worsen progressively; lightheadedness; pallor; easy bruising and bleeding; susceptibility to infection.

Signs and laboratory findings *(What the doctor looks for)* A complete blood count showing severe anemia with a reduction in immature forms of red blood cells (reticulocytes), the neutrophil type of white blood cells, and platelets. Bone marrow examination showing a defect or deficiency in blood cell production. In more severe cases, spontaneous hemorrhaging into skin, mucous membranes, internal organs, and other tissues.

What is it? An unusual and serious disease, aplastic anemia is caused by a dramatic decrease in the production of all types of blood cells within the bone marrow. The word *aplastic* refers to the lack of development of anorgan or tissue or of the cells that originate in an organ or tissue. Aplastic

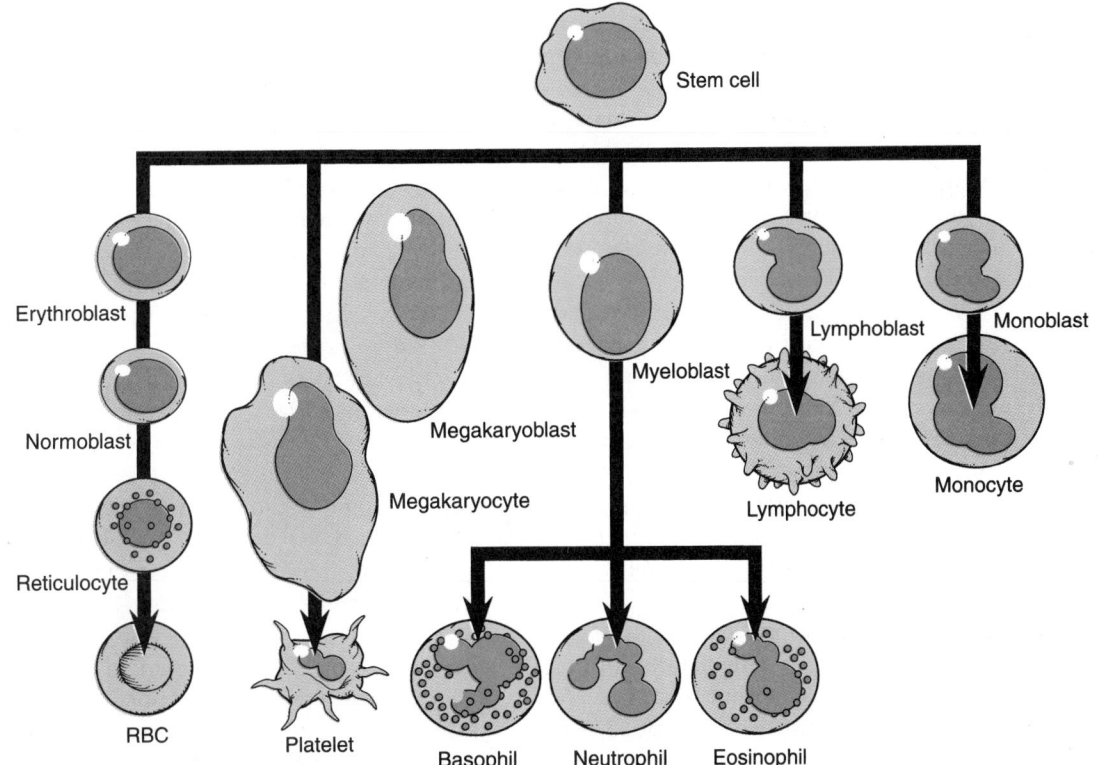

Blood cell development. Stem cells are the precursors of all blood cells. In the bone marrow, a stem cell differentiates into an immature red blood cell (erythroblast), white blood cell (myeloblast, lymphoblast, monoblast), or platelet (megakaryoblast). Immature cells develop into full-grown red blood cells (RBCs), platelets, basophils, neutrophils, eosinophils, lymphocytes, and monocytes before being released into the bloodstream.

BONE MARROW ASPIRATION AND BIOPSY

In order to diagnose specific blood disorders and to determine their source, your doctor may order a bone marrow examination. Marrow examination will allow a technician to assess how smoothly blood cell production is going. In the lab, a hematologist or pathologist will evaluate cell production in the marrow, the overall balance and makeup of blood cells, as well as their shape and proportion.

A sample of marrow can be obtained easily by needle aspiration and biopsy; usually both are done. *Aspiration* is the process by which a small sample of marrow is drawn out through a long needle. A *biopsy* involves cutting and removing a small piece of tissue for microscopic examination.

Usually, these tests are done in the doctor's office, a hospital, or a special laboratory. If this type of test is part of your diagnostic process, you will receive a local anesthetic around the area from which the bone marrow sample will be taken. In most instances, the sample is taken from the large pelvic bone in the back or the breastbone. After the skin is sterilized with antiseptic, a long aspirating needle is inserted into the spongy marrow in the bone. Because the needle must penetrate thin bone, it is strong and sharp. Once the needle is firmly in the marrow cavity, a few drops of marrow are drawn. The marrow is then placed on a piece of glass and studied under a microscope. A bone marrow biopsy should also be performed, because it yields additional important information. The biopsy can be performed on its own or at the same time as the aspiration. After the site of the biopsy is infiltrated with an anesthetic, a needle is inserted into the bone and a small, solid piece of marrow is removed. During the process, you may feel pressure or a slight dull pain as the needle

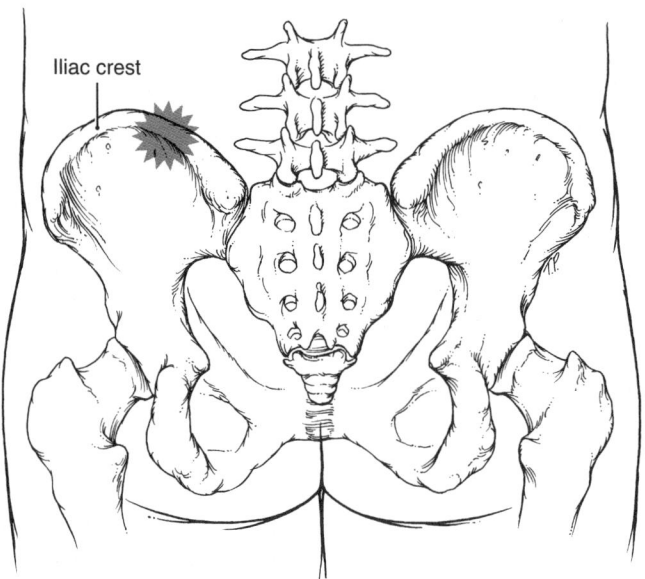

Iliac crest

The crest of the pelvic iliac bone is the most common location for performing a bone marrow aspirate and biopsy. During the procedure, a sample of liquid marrow and a thin core of bone are removed for microscopic examination.

is inserted and the marrow removed. Your doctor will bandage the area. The discomfort only lasts a few minutes, although the area may be tender for several days. The area may appear bruised, and in a few instances, the puncture site may bleed. If the area does not heal in a couple of weeks, contact your doctor. ■

anemia is generally prompted by injury to or abnormal suppression of the marrow; this condition prevents blood cells from developing and maturing normally. Aplastic anemia may be acute or chronic, but it is, as a rule, progressive. It is most commonly diagnosed in older children, adolescents, and the elderly.

Almost half of all cases of aplastic anemia are idiopathic—that is, they have no clear cause, but rather appear to occur spontaneously. In other cases, the condition seems to be triggered by certain medications (chloramphenicol, phenylbutazone, sulfonamides, and anticonvulsants), toxic substances (benzene, arsenic, nitrogen mustards, certain insecticides), chemotherapy, or radiation.

Viral hepatitis may also be associated with aplastic anemia. The majority of cases develop in males within the first few months after hepatitis has surfaced. Pregnant women are at higher risk for developing milder forms of aplastic anemia, although the condition tends to subside after delivery. In some instances, the condition is related to lupus or other autoimmune conditions in which the body's immune mechanisms are unable to distinguish clearly what are normal substances and what are foreign. Accordingly, antibodies are produced against normal parts of the body, causing marrow injury. In some instances of aplastic anemia, there appears to be a family history and genetic predisposition.

As with all anemias, this condition leaves you feeling constantly and increasingly fatigued. At times you may feel weak, lightheaded, and dizzy. Because the platelet count is also low, clotting problems develop. Therefore, you may bruise easily or bleed excessively. The low number of white blood cells leaves you vulnerable to bacterial and fungal infections, the most common of which are upper respiratory infections, gum disease, blood poisoning, and inflammation around the rectum and anus.

What you can do If you are diagnosed with aplastic anemia, you will be advised to use antiseptic soaps to reduce the risk of skin infection, to shave with electric razors instead of blades to avoid unnecessary bleeding, and to use stool softeners to avoid irritating your rectal area.

Treatment Whenever the condition underneath the anemia is known, treatment will address it. Mild cases of aplastic anemia are treated with supportive care. Your doctor will advise you on ways of avoiding infections and will treat those you contract aggressively with antibiotics. Women who have aplastic anemia may be put on medications such as oral contraceptives to inhibit ovulation so that their menstrual flow is not excessive.

In some cases of aplastic anemia, transfusions of red blood cells or platelets will be helpful. However, transfusions must be performed sparingly to prevent the occurrence of immune reactions that can cause problems if bone marrow transplantation becomes necessary at a later date. Bone marrow transplantation will be considered in severe cases of aplastic anemia, especially in those under the age of 40 with siblings who can provide allogenic bone marrow (see page 960). When marrow transplantation is not the right treatment, therapy may involve attempts to suppress the immune system with such products as antithymocyte globulin (ATG). Treatment with ATG is generally administered in the hospital over a period of 5 to 8 days in conjunction with transfusion and antibiotic support. Other medications, such as cyclosporine, androgens, and occasionally corticosteroids (prednisone), may be given in combination with ATG. Usually, an individual's blood count will increase within 4 to 12 weeks after treatment.

Prognosis The prognosis of patients with aplastic anemia varies, depending on the cause. The prognosis is good when the condition is transient from exposure to drugs or toxins, unless the agent has totally destroyed the marrow. The outlook is less favorable when aplastic anemia is associated with hepatitis or constitutional factors. In any case, when the illness is severe and left untreated, it can be rapidly fatal.

At the same time, even in the most complicated forms of aplastic anemia, allogenic bone marrow transplantation can be highly successful—with an 80 percent survival rate—in young adults when marrow is donated by siblings. In older adults or those who have previously been exposed to blood products, survival rate following marrow transplantation runs between 40 and 70 percent. Over half of those who receive immunosuppressive therapy in conjunction with ATG or other medications respond well to treatment.

There are some long-term complications that arise from aplastic anemia: an increased risk for developing malignancy, acute leukemia, and tumors, especially as a result of immunosuppressive treatment.

❖ REFRACTORY ANEMIAS (MYELODYSPLASIA)

Symptoms *(What you may experience)* Fatigue; weakness; pallor; labored breathing; bruising and bleeding problems; infection and fever.

Signs and laboratory findings *(What the doctor looks for)* Significant drop in erythrocyte, leukocyte, and platelet count.

What is it? Refractory or dysplastic anemias originate in disorders of the blood-forming cells within the bone marrow. These rare disorders tend to have a lengthy clinical course and present with a wide range of cell abnormalities. Like aplastic anemia, these disorders reflect a significant drop in the level of white blood cells and platelets as well as red blood cells. In many cases, the complexity of the disorder makes managing the condition difficult.

Because these anemias affect production of red blood cells, white blood cells, and platelets in the bone marrow, symptoms arise in all areas of blood functioning. Fatigue, weakness, and congestive heart failure can be provoked by chronic anemia; tendency to bruise easily signals thrombocytopenia (reduced platelet count), while recurrent infection reflects a significant leukopenia. Usually, the onset of symptoms is so gradual that you may have difficulty identifying an actual illness.

Dysplastic refractory anemias can be seen in younger patients as a result of exposure to radiation, certain drugs, or toxic chemicals. Exposure to alcohol, lead, and certain antibiotics can also lead to the condition. However, in many of these instances, the condition is reversible.

Your doctor may discover that you have refractory anemia through a complete blood count. One form of the condition seems to surface in men around the age of 50 after a long, latent course. Initially there is a tendency to miss the diagnosis, because the anemia is mild and the symptoms are vague. Many times, patients are treated unsuccessfully for other forms of anemia, with iron, folic acid, or B_{12} supplements, yet over time, the anemia worsens and other symptoms emerge.

Some forms of refractory anemias are associated with chromosomal abnormalities. These disorders, myelodysplasia (or myelodysplastic syndrome) and preleukemic syndromes, occur most frequently in adults over the age of 60. In many cases, these conditions progress to acute leukemia. With myelodysplasia and preleukemic syndromes, symptoms include anemia, infections, and bleeding problems.

Another such condition, sideroblastic anemia, occurs in both inherited and acquired forms. Generally, the acquired form is a disease of older adults. Both forms result in the manufacture of ineffective red blood cells, which then gives rise to iron overload. Iron overload is the condition caused when the body stores iron in levels that greatly exceed normal. Iron overload can lead to damage to tissues, glands, and organs. Most significantly, it can cause liver damage and heart dysfunction. It increases a person's susceptibility to infection and may eventually lead to diabetes and cancer.

Treatment Managing dysplastic anemias requires support and treatment over the prolonged course of the disease. Individuals may remain stable for years with only mild levels of anemia. However, treating the anemia with vitamin B_{12} or folic acid is not especially effective. Iron should not be used, because there is a tendency towards iron overload. With more severe conditions, treatment usually involves regular support with red blood cell and platelet transfusions.

When the condition has progressed and complications seem life-threatening, chemotherapy and bone marrow transplantation, specifically with younger patients, have been proven effective.

Prognosis Fair. Certain types of refractory anemia may slowly become more severe or evolve into acute leukemia. For people with sideroblastic anemia, the greatest risk comes from iron overload as a result of either excessive dietary iron absorption or the regular transfusions needed to maintain adequate hemoglobin levels.

In cases where acute leukemia develops, prognosis depends on the effectiveness of treatment for that condition (see page 961).

❖ MONOCLONAL GAMMOPATHIES

Symptoms (What you may experience) In most cases, there are no symptoms. In severe cases, mental confusion, sluggishness, visual defects.

Signs and laboratory findings (What the doctor looks for) Lab tests show abnormalities of plasma cells and increase of monoclonal protein level.

What is it? Most commonly found in older people, monoclonal gammopathies are the result of monoclonal proteins in the blood. These abnormal proteins mimic antibodies formed in the bone marrow. Monoclonal gammopathies are usually detected through routine blood tests. Some studies show that they occur in 10 percent of people over the age of 60. In 75 percent of these cases, there are no symptoms of any significance and the condition remains stable; this is called monoclonal gammopathy of undetermined significance. In about 25 percent, however, the amount of monoclonal protein in the blood increases, and within 15 years, these individuals prove to have a malignant disorder such as multiple myeloma (see page 951), amyloidosis (see page 952), and lymphoma (see page 954).

Treatment In the vast majority of cases, monoclonal gammopathy has little medical significance in and of itself, and there is usually no need for treatment. Your doctor will, however, want to observe that monoclonal protein levels remain stable. In those cases where the levels increase, the existence of such proteins points to a more serious disease that will need to be assessed and treated.

❖ MULTIPLE MYELOMA

Symptoms *(What you may experience)*
Fatigue and other signs of anemia; nosebleeds and bleeding gums; susceptibility to infection; progressive pain in bones, chest, and back; spontaneous bone fractures, especially in the vertebrae or ribs. In severe cases, constipation; profuse or decreased urination; excessive sleepiness; fluctuating levels of consciousness; kidney failure; incontinence; numbness or loss of strength in extremities.

Signs and laboratory findings *(What the doctor looks for)* A physical examination revealing bone tenderness, soft lumps, neurologic signs related to spinal cord compression; enlarged spleen, liver, and tongue. Various blood tests showing abnormal levels of calcium, uric acid, creatinine, and blood proteins. Bone marrow examination showing myeloma cells; skeletal x-ray showing significant thinning of bones, or punched-out spots indicating tumor invasion.

What is it? Multiple myeloma is a malignancy of plasma cells, a type of white blood cell in the bone marrow. Also called Kahler's disease or myelomatosis, this cancer produces uncontrolled proliferation of the plasma cells; as the cells grow, they manufacture substances that cause the bones to become weak, fragile, and painful. Bone deterioration happens most frequently in the ribs and back. Eventually, the growth of plasma cells interferes with the production in the marrow of normal red blood cells, white blood cells, and platelets. Anemia, susceptibility to infection, and bleeding problems typically result.

Ordinarily, plasma cells produce antibodies to fight infection. In multiple myeloma, mutation of one such cell gives rise to a new line of abnormal cells. The new line of cells increases the amount of proteins in the blood. These paraproteins secreted by the malignant plasma cells cause physical problems, including hyperviscosity syndrome (which impedes blood flow) and kidney failure.

This cancer is usually first noted by anemia or by back pain that increases with activity and gets progressively worse over time. Related pain may also be felt in the hips, ribs, and neck. Also, early on, you may experience symptoms of anemia—fatigue, pallor—and be subject to recurrent infections.

The cause of multiple myeloma is unknown, although there may be some relation to radiation, exposure to industrial or agricultural toxins, or genetic predisposition. These blood marrow tumors affect mostly older people. It is a disease that most commonly strikes people in their 70s; only 3 percent of patients are younger than 40. It occurs more often in men and is twice as common among blacks.

What you can do Although there is no cure for multiple myeloma, there are things you can do to help you tolerate the disease. Drinking plenty of fluids can prevent dehydration and ward off kidney failure. Stay active. Exercise, but do not overdo it. Moderate exercise can help your bones retain calcium and strengthen them. If pain is severe, orthopedic support devices such as a back brace or cane can help you stay involved in reasonable activities. By maintaining mobility, you may be able to forestall bone loss.

Treatment During early stages or with mild cases of the disease, your doctor may choose to observe rather than treat. Most commonly, treatment is required for bone pain or other symptoms of the illness. For more advanced cases, corticosteroids (for example, prednisone) may be prescribed, coupled with melphalan (Alkeran). Combination chemotherapy with alkylating agents is also commonly used. Individuals who do not respond to standard therapy may do better with low-dose continuous-infusion therapy with vincristine, doxorubicin (Adriamycin), and dexamethasone.

Analgesics can alleviate bone pain. Surgical repairs may be necessary to strengthen unstable bones. Radiation directed at specific sites, such as neck and back, can control severe pain and disease in that area. Allogenic bone marrow transplantation can offer some hope for cure; however, because this disease usually affects older adults, transplantation is not a realistic option for many myeloma patients.

Prognosis There is no cure for multiple myeloma—apart from bone marrow transplantation, which has benefited a small number of individuals with this condition. Treatment can prolong life for several years and offer relief of symptoms.

❖ AMYLOIDOSIS

Symptoms *(What you may experience)* Fatigue and weakness; breathlessness; numbness and swelling in hands and feet; weight loss; bruising, especially around the eyes (raccoon face).

Signs and laboratory findings *(What the doctor looks for)* Anemia may not be apparent, although tests may show the presence of monoclonal protein in blood serum or urine; amyloid deposits are revealed by biopsy of the gums, rectum, stomach, kidneys, liver, or bone marrow.

What is it? In amyloidosis, a complex protein mixture called amyloid is deposited throughout the body, affecting specific sites and organs in the body. The condition is rare, and its severity depends on the organs affected by amyloid deposits. If amyloid accumulates only on less crucial sites, the symptoms tend to be mild. On the other hand, in its most serious form, amyloidosis can cause kidney failure and congestive heart failure.

Amyloidosis is rare in individuals under age 40; it is most common in men in their mid-60s. Weakness and fatigue are the dominant symptoms. Weight loss can be striking. Labored breathing, swelling in the hands and feet, numbness, tingling, or prickling sensations, and lightheadedness may occur. Rashes on the neck, face, and upper eyelids are not uncommon. In some cases, voice changes occur.

Amyloidosis can cause carpal tunnel syndrome (a painful disorder of the wrist and hand), orthostatic hypotension (rapid drop in blood pressure upon sudden standing or moving), and congestive heart failure.

In 8 to 16 percent of cases, amyloidosis is associated with another condition such as a malignancy, myeloma, Hodgkin's disease, lymphoma, or rheumatoid arthritis. Secondary amyloidosis is also sometimes seen in relation to cystic fibrosis, tuberculosis, or other inflammatory processes.

What you can do If you have this condition, you are at risk for kidney disease and heart failure; therefore, you will be advised to restrict your dietary consumption of salt and your use of diuretics.

Treatment In secondary amyloidosis, management depends on the treatment of the underlying disease. If the underlying condition can be resolved, the amyloidosis can be stabilized. When it is the primary disease, treatment will aim at easing and correcting the symptoms. If the condition is limited to specific organs and deposits are obstructing the lungs, bladder, or urethra, for example, surgery may be needed to alleviate the obstructions.

Your doctor may prescribe certain medications such as melphalan, which has led to remission in some individuals. In addition, other anti-inflammatory medications (methotrexate, chlorambucil, or cyclophosphamide) may be prescribed to address the specific areas or organs that are affected, and analgesics may be prescribed to relieve the pain. Because you may be susceptible to infection, antibiotics are often prescribed. If amyloidosis leads to kidney failure, the doctor may recommend dialysis or, in some cases, kidney transplantation.

Prognosis Primary amyloidosis is usually chronic. Generally, it progresses gradually, but long-term prognosis is poor, because it can lead to general malnutrition and heart and kidney failure.

❖ WALDENSTRÖM'S MACROGLOBULINEMIA

Symptoms *(What you may experience)* Fatigue; weakness; headaches; weight loss; ashen pallor; nosebleeds; blood in urine or tar-like stool; rashes caused by bleeding into the skin (purpura); vertigo; nausea, and visual disturbances; mild lethargy; stupor.

Signs and laboratory findings *(What the doctor looks for)* Physical examination revealing enlarged spleen and engorged blood vessels; complete blood count showing abnormal, rapid blood viscosity, and presence of immunoglobulin M (IgM) paraprotein; bone marrow biopsy showing infiltration of abnormal plasmacytic lymphocytes.

What is it? Waldenström's macroglobulinemia is a malignant disease of the lymphocytes and plasma B cells. As abnormal cells proliferate in the marrow, they characteristically secrete an abnormal protein, the IgM monoclonal protein, which causes a myriad of physical symptoms. This relatively rare disorder is most commonly diagnosed in individuals in their 60s and 70s and is twice as common in men as in women.

Symptoms usually appear insidiously in the form of continuous fatigue, lightheadedness, lethargy, and nausea. As the condition progresses, blood flow is compromised, causing bleeding into the body's tissues. Disturbances of vision can occur because of bleeding within the eye. The heart's workload is greatly increased by the high blood viscosity (hyperviscosity syndrome) associated with the condition. When severe, it can lead to life-threatening complications, such as coma, convulsions, and stroke. The condition can also manifest itself in certain sensory and motor symptoms: sudden deafness, stiffness in the spine, vertigo, and alterations in consciousness.

Treatment Patients who have developed hyperviscosity syndrome (stupor or coma) will be treated on an emergency basis with plasmapheresis, a process by which blood is removed from the body and centrifuged (separated into its various components). The packed red cells are then suspended in a solution and reinjected into the patient. Usually, this rapidly reduces the level of IgM protein and can provide dramatic relief of heart and brain symptoms. Other treatments include intermittent chemotherapy with chlorambucil or cyclophosphamide, which tend to be quite effective. New drugs such as fludarabine and cladribine have produced encouraging results.

Prognosis Waldenström's macroglobulinemia is a slowly developing disease. Most people live at least 3 to 5 years after diagnosis. The survival rate beyond 10 years is reasonably good, with the condition reaching a plateau.

❖ SYSTEMIC MASTOCYTOSIS

Symptoms *(What you may experience)* Patchy or widespread brownish, flat or raised skin nodules; fever; flushing; severe itching; swelling; abdominal pain.

Signs and laboratory findings *(What the doctor looks for)* Decreased blood pressure; blood tests showing an increased level of mast cells.

What is it? Mastocytosis is a condition in which there is an increased level of mast cells, the cells that originate in the bone marrow and then migrate to the body's connective tissue. Mast cells contain heparin (which inhibits coagulation) and histamine (which exerts pharmacologic action at the site of injury) and play an important role in the cells' defense against foreign substances and in blood coagulation during injury and infection.

Mastocytosis is most commonly noted in itchy, widespread patches on the skin. Densely infiltrated with mast cells, these brown patches can be flat or raised. Almost any irritation to the area can exacerbate the condition, causing swelling and itching at the site, as histamines are released.

Frequently, mastocytosis is a mild and passing childhood condition. In some cases, though, it can be a systemic condition that becomes progressively worse, with mast cells infiltrating the body's organs, tissues, and bones. It then gives rise to fibroids (clumps of fibrous tissue).

Treatment Histamine-related symptoms—itching and swelling in particular—may respond to cromolyn or low-dose prednisone. In more severe cases, chemotherapy and radiation may be effective in relieving symptoms.

❖ MYELOID METAPLASIA

Symptoms *(What you may experience)* Breathlessness on exertion; progressively worsening fatigue; rapid heartbeat; paleness; abdominal pain or tenderness; night sweats; weight loss; bloated feeling; abnormal bleeding.

Signs and laboratory findings *(What the doctor looks for)* Enlarged spleen; blood tests and bone marrow biopsy reveal anemia; increased numbers of immature leukocytes; abnormally shaped red blood cells; excessively large platelets; progressive bone marrow fibrosis.

What is it? Also known as agnogenic (of unknown origin) myeloid metaplasia and idiopathic myelofibrosis, myeloid metaplasia can arise when there is a deranged proliferation of red blood cells, white blood cells, and platelets in the bone marrow. This proliferation can cause the marrow to become gradually scarred. Fibroids (clumps of fibrous tissue) develop, rendering the marrow less capable of producing blood cells. Thus, this disease is characterized by a varied pattern in cell growth: excessive production, inadequate production, and abnormalities in cell maturation and function. Whenever there is inadequate cell production, other organs, such as the spleen and liver, work to compensate for the drop. As a result, these organs can become enlarged and tender.

Although myeloid metaplasia is usually a disease of late middle age or old age, it can occur in young adults and in infants. Many times, myeloid metaplasia is a secondary condition. It can be caused by exposure to chemotherapy, benzene, or radiation, or it can stem from other such illness as leukemia, carcinoma, or tuberculosis.

The course of the illness varies from person to person. Sometimes, the disease will progress to leukemia. Sometimes, it will prompt cardiac disease, gastrointestinal hemorrhage, strokes or other obstructive blood clots, or rather serious infections.

What you can do If you have myeloid metaplasia, you will be more susceptible to infection. Therefore, it is important that you avoid infection whenever possible and contact your doctor if you have symptoms of infection—fever or inflammation—for any length of time so that it can be treated immediately.

Treatment Myeloid metaplasia is treated with medications including melphalan, hydroxyurea, and corticosteroids (for example, prednisone). The anemia may be treated with transfusions, folic acid, or corticosteroids. The spleen may be removed surgically (splenectomy) when it becomes so enlarged that it traps the platelets or causes considerable pain. Sometimes, small doses of radiation of the spleen may lessen the symptoms.

Prognosis Although myeloid metaplasia cannot be cured, it can be managed effectively for several years.

Lymphomas

Lymphomas are a diverse group of cancers that affect the lymphatic system, including the spleen and lymph nodes or lymph glands. Connected by small vessels called lymphatics, lymph nodes are located throughout the body (see page 916).

Often the first symptom of lymphoma is a prolonged swelling around the lymph nodes behind the ears and in the groin and armpits. Transient swelling of the lymph nodes is not uncommon. Many of us are familiar with swollen glands at the neck that accompany infection; however, prolonged swelling that persists for several weeks should always be evaluated by a doctor.

Lymphomas are commonly divided into Hodgkin's disease and non-Hodgkin's lymphoma. The latter category embraces a varied group of malignancies that are widely diverse in their symptoms and progression. Lymphoma is also a fairly common complication of HIV and AIDS. In this setting, it is usually an aggressive large cell form that requires the immediate attention of an oncologist.

❖ HODGKIN'S DISEASE

Symptoms (What you may experience) Painless swelling of lymph nodes in the armpits, neck, or groin; persistent fatigue; fever and chills; night sweats; weight loss and loss of appetite; severe itching; loss of bladder or bowel control; numbness or loss of strength in the arms and legs.

Signs and laboratory findings (What the doctor looks for) Abnormalities in white blood cells and anemia shown on a complete blood cell count. Large cells called Reed-Sternberg cells shown on lymph node biopsy.

What is it? Named after the 19th century physician Thomas Hodgkin, Hodgkin's disease is a group of cancers that usually arise within lymph node areas and spread in an orderly fashion to surrounding areas. Hodgkin's disease is distinct from the other types of lymphomas by virtue of its mode of spreading as well as the remarkable curability of some types. Although the cause of Hodgkin's disease is unknown, presence of the Epstein-Barr virus in some tumors leads to the speculation that such viral factors may be involved in the disease's development. In addition, there is a slight increase in the incidence of the disease in people who have had infectious mononucleosis or HIV infection.

Hodgkin's disease, along with the other types of lymphomas, is the third most common form of cancer in children. The rate of occurrence of the disease rises with age; young adults in the 20- to 29-year age group are particularly prone to developing it. Hodgkin's disease was once thought to also occur in people over age 50, but this was due to confusion with non-Hodgkin's disease. Most patients seek medical attention because they discover a painless mass, usually in the neck. Others contact their doctor because of fevers, drenching night sweats, weight loss, or severe itching.

If these problems do not disappear within a few weeks, or if they persist even after a doctor prescribes antibiotics, further medical attention is called for. To determine whether you have Hodgkin's disease, your doctor will conduct a thorough physical exam, attending closely to the areas around the lymph nodes. First he will check the nodes close to the body's surface—in the neck, groin, armpits, legs, and arms. In some cases, the doctor may be able to tell if there is an abnormal mass merely by feeling it. Yet there are other nodes that lie deeper in the body and cannot be so easily felt. Therefore, a lymph node biopsy (the removal and analysis of node tissue) will be needed to diagnose Hodgkin's disease (see page 956).

Also it is likely that the doctor will order complete blood and urine tests as well as magnetic resonance imaging (MRI) and computed tomography (CT) scans. Further tests may be required to evaluate the condition of the spleen, liver, and abdominal lymph nodes. A CT scan of the chest and abdomen may be ordered to determine whether the disease is localized or has spread throughout the system. In addition, to discover the full extent of the malignancy, a surgical procedure called laparotomy (exploratory surgery of the abdomen) may be necessary; this is typically done while the patient is under general anesthesia.

All of these tests are part of an overall diagnostic procedure called staging the tumor, designed to specify the extent of the disease. Staging is crucial for determining how advanced the cancer is and for planning the most effective treatment for each individual. There are four stages of Hodgkin's disease: stage I is localized, or confined to the original lymph region; stage II means that the cancer has spread to adjacent lymph areas, but is restricted to either below or above the diaphragm; stage III indicates that the cancer has spread to regions both below and above the diaphragm; and stage IV means that it has spread beyond the lymph regions to lungs, liver, bone marrow, or other tissue. Once the stage of the tumor has been determined, treatment will begin immediately.

When to call the doctor Many times, especially in children, painless enlargements in the lymph node region are the only symptom of Hodgkin's disease. Therefore, if such swelling does not decrease in 2 to 3 weeks, or if antibiotics that may have been prescribed to treat a suspected infection fail to reduce the swelling, contact your doctor immediately.

What you can do Dealing with any type of cancer—from the moment the diagnosis is suspected through the actual process of diagnosis and treatment—requires not only responsible medical attention, but abundant emotional and practical support as well. Because many people who have Hodgkin's disease are children, the ordeal can be profoundly distressing for both parent and child alike. Support, in the form of information and educational resources, is available, usually through your doctor, the local hospital, or national cancer organizations. Sources of support and information include The National Cancer Institute (NCI), Office of Cancer Communications, NCI Building 31, Room 10A24, Bethesda, MD 20892, (800) 4-CANCER; and the American Cancer Society (ACS), 90 Park Avenue, New York, NY 10016, (212) 586-8700. Finally, your doctor, the hospital, or local chapter of ACS may be able to refer you to a support group in your community to help you and your family cope with this often frightening, always complicated illness. Many people find support groups to be extremely helpful in helping them deal with Hodgkin's disease.

Treatment Treating Hodgkin's disease aims at bringing about remission—the total absence of any detectable signs or symptoms of the disease. Once all traces of cancer are gone, treatment will likely continue for 1 or 2 years in order to avert any recurrence.

When the spread of the cancer is limited in stage I or II, radiation therapy is usually the primary treatment (see Chapter 30

LYMPH NODE BIOPSY

Lymph nodes are round masses of tissue found at intervals along the lymphatic vessels in your body. Lymph nodes cluster at various sites, but principally in the neck, armpit, and groin. They produce lymphocytes and monocytes—two types of white blood cells that act as filters, keeping bacteria from entering the blood cells. While they trap cancer cells as well, they may in turn become sites of metastatic cancer (that is, cancer that metastasizes, or spreads to a different area of the body).

If your doctor suspects that you have Hodgkin's disease or another form of lymphoma, she will want to have your lymph nodes evaluated. Many times, a doctor will be able to make a relatively reliable conjecture about the presence of lymphoma by feeling the lymph nodes closest to the body's surface with her fingertips. However, many other lymph nodes reside deeper inside the body, making it impossible for a doctor to make any type of analysis based on touch. Therefore, the doctor will most likely order a lymph node biopsy, a procedure by which one or more nodes or a piece of the node tumor will be removed and studied under a microscope.

The process by which Hodgkin's disease is diagnosed involves a very specific type of lymph node biopsy and evaluation, called staging. Staging a tumor is part of a comprehensive series of tests that usually includes blood and urine analyses, computed tomography (CT) imaging, and skeletal x-rays. Staging helps determine the extent of the disease and often directs treatment. While staging may be used in developing a precise diagnosis in other lymphomas, it is especially important when dealing with Hodgkin's disease, because the disease progresses in such an orderly fashion. Stage I of the disease involves one lymph node region and indicates that the disease is quite restricted. Stage II involves two lymph node areas on one side of the diaphragm. Stage III means that lymph node regions on both sides of the diaphragm are involved. Stage IV means that the disease has spread and infiltrated the bone marrow or liver. If the disease is localized, treatment with radiation may be sufficient. If it has spread, systemic chemotherapy must be given. ■

for more detailed information on cancer treatment). Affected regions are radiated over several weeks or months. In addition to radiation of the lymph nodes that are clearly involved, radiation may be administered to other lymph nodes that are likely to be affected if the disease spreads. In some cases, radiation is used in conjunction with chemotherapy (the administration of a combination of powerful anticancer medications).

For advanced Hodgkin's disease (stages III and IV), the primary treatment is aggressive chemotherapy. Usually administered for 6 to 12 months, chemotherapy can not only bring about remission, it can also produce a number of side effects of varying discomfort and severity.

In general, anticancer medications work by disrupting a cancer cell's ability to grow and duplicate. However, chemotherapy will destroy healthy cells along with diseased cells. As a result, chemotherapy can suppress a person's immune response because there may not be sufficient numbers of normal, disease-engulfing granulocytes (a type of white blood cell) and antibody-producing lymphocytes to fight off infection. Often, then, infections become persistent problems during and following treatment. Some people can go on to develop leukemia or other cancers as a relatively rare, but potential long-term effect of certain radiation and chemotherapies. At the same time, chemotherapy can cause sterility in both men and women. As with any treatment, it is important to weigh the possible side effects of combined treatments against the likely benefits and to understand that complications can arise with any type of aggressive treatment.

The chemotherapy combination—or cocktail, as it is popularly called—most commonly used in treating Hodgkin's disease is the ABVD regimen: doxorubicin (Adriamycin), bleomycin, vincristine, and dacarbazine. This combination seems to produce the least problematic side effects while effectively treating the cancer. The ABVD regimen tends to cause less toxicity than other combinations. In the long run, the chance of sterility is lower, as is the risk of developing leukemia over time.

When relapse follows chemotherapy, treatment will likely be repeated—at a higher dose, and possibly with radiation therapy. Usually, in these cases, autologous bone marrow transplantation—in which bone marrow is removed before chemotherapy and replaced afterwards—is also recommended so that the body can tolerate larger doses of anticancer drugs (see page 960).

Moreover, since infertility is a very real consequence of such treatment, some doctors recommend that young men freeze their own sperm to be used later in artificial insemination should they wish to father a child.

Prognosis When Hodgkin's disease is detected early and treated promptly, as many as 90 percent of the cases are cured. Eighty to 90 percent of children who are diagnosed with the disease and treated promptly survive at least 5 years. When one lymph node region is affected, 90 percent of Hodgkin's patients are disease-free after 10 years. When two lymph node regions are affected, the cure rate after 10 years is 70 percent.

❖ NON-HODGKIN'S LYMPHOMA

Symptoms (*What you may experience*) Painless enlargement of lymph nodes with or without swelling of the abdomen; persistent fatigue; fevers; chills; night sweats; loss of appetite; nagging cough or wheezing. In more severe cases, sudden onset of high fever; severe constipation or profuse urination; involuntary loss of urine or stool; numbness or loss of strength in the arms and legs; mental confusion; drowsiness.

Signs and laboratory findings (*What the doctor looks for*) Biopsy and blood test revealing preponderance of small, nodular, or abnormally shaped lymphocytes, mixed with large cells; elevated levels of the enzyme lactate dehydrogenase.

What is it? Non-Hodgkin's lymphoma is the name given to a varied group of malignancies of the lymphocyte (a type of white blood cell). Unlike Hodgkin's disease, whose cellular origin is unresolved, about 90 percent of non-Hodgkin's lymphomas are derived from B lymphocytes and 10 percent from T lymphocytes (both of which play a role in the body's immune response; see page 918). Nonetheless, as a group, these lymphomas are so varied that some are "indolent" and slow-growing while others are aggressive and immediately life-threatening. Yet even some slow-growing lymphomas are difficult to cure and in time may become aggressive, while some aggressive lymphomas are completely curable.

Non-Hodgkin's lymphoma is one of the most rapidly increasing cancers. Its incidence seems to be increasing at an annual rate of 4 percent in men and 3 percent in women. Although the reasons for this are not clear, there is some speculation that exposure to viruses, radiation, pesticides, solvents, fuels, and animal viruses may play a role. Nutrition is also thought to play a possible role. Individuals suffering from immunodeficiency diseases, such as HIV infection, severe combined immunodeficiency syndrome, and Wiskott-Aldrich syndrome, run a higher risk for developing non-Hodgkin's lymphoma.

More common than Hodgkin's disease, non-Hodgkin's lymphomas also occur more frequently among people who have received organ transplants or whose immune mechanisms are inhibited by immunosuppressive therapy (usually given to transplant recipients to prevent rejection of the foreign tissue or organ). Non-Hodgkin's lymphoma is typically diagnosed in middle age, although it can develop in older people.

People suffering from non-Hodgkin's lymphoma typically contact their doctors because they have a painless lump at the site of the lymph node, around the pelvis, abdomen, throat, and neck glands. They may have fevers, drenching night sweats, or weight loss.

These types of lymphomas usually begin to spread before they are detected. Any organ can be affected by an aggressive lymphoma. The most common sites, aside from lymph nodes themselves, are the gastrointestinal tract (representing 40 percent of all other primary lymphomas), skin, and bone and bone marrow. The sinuses, lungs, spinal cord, brain, and the membranes surrounding the heart all may be involved.

The procedure used to diagnose non-Hodgkin's lymphomas is similar to that used in detecting Hodgkin's disease. If a doctor suspects lymphoma, she will order blood tests, x-rays, and biopsies of the lymph nodes, bone marrow, and any other tissue masses that may be tumors to determine if in fact there is malignancy involved. A spinal tap may be ordered to check for abnormal cells in the fluid of the spine. If these tests indicate that cancer has spread into the liver, bones, or spleen, a CT scan may be ordered to examine other organs. Then precise staging of the tumor—classifying it according to the extent of the disease—will determine the most effective treatment. Based on all the test results, the doctor will identify the malignancy according to its stage: stage I is localized, or confined to the original region; stage II means that the cancer has spread to adjacent areas, but is restricted to either below or above the diaphragm; stage III indicates that the cancer has spread to regions both below and above the diaphragm; and stage IV means that it has spread to many areas in the body, including the lungs, liver, spleen, bone marrow, or other tissue.

Recently, the National Cancer Institute sponsored a formulation that also identifies lymphomas (lymphatic tumors) according to their cell size. They are also characterized

OTHER LYMPHOMAS

There are many lymphomas—cancerous tumors that begin in lymphatic tissue. Each variety looks different under the microscope. After Hodgkin's disease and non-Hodgkin's lymphoma, the following are among the more common (though they are relatively rare).

Burkitt's Lymphoma

Burkitt's lymphoma is a cancer involving the immature lymph cells. It also affects sites other than the lymph nodes, liver, kidney, and spleen. Somewhat rare in the United States, it is most common in children of African descent. There is a strong association between this disease and the Epstein-Barr virus. In the United States, Burkitt's lymphoma is seen most commonly in individuals with HIV infection.

Central Nervous System Lymphoma

Central nervous system lymphoma, a form of lymphatic cancer commonly found in individuals infected with HIV, affects the brain and spine. This is a serious disease; however, a person's chances of responding to treatment are greatly increased if treatment combines radiation and chemotherapy

Gastric Lymphoma

Gastric lymphoma initially mimics ulcers and gastritis, with pain, loss of appetite, and gastrointestinal bleeding. Because the diagnosis is frequently made at the time of exploratory surgery, the majority of cases are treated by removing part or all of the stomach. However, recent studies have suggested that the use of chemotherapy and radiation may be as effective as surgery, without the risks. Some "gastric" lymphomas are actually deranged reactions of lymph tissue to a bacterium, *Helicobacter pylori*; these will respond to antibiotics. These lymphomas are often called MALT (mucosa-associated lymphoid tissue) lymphomas by doctors.

Testicular Lymphoma

Testicular lymphoma often appears in lumps within a man's testicle. In young men, such testicular mass usually indicates testicular cancer, but in men over age 45, lymphoma is more likely. Testicular lymphoma frequently occurs with bone marrow or central nervous system disease. ■

by their level of cell activity—whether they are slow developing or aggressive. Thus lymphatic tumors are classified into three broad categories: low-grade, intermediate-grade, and high-grade.

Treatment If you have been diagnosed with low-grade non-Hodgkin's lymphoma but have no active symptoms, your doctor may take a watch-and-wait course. In contrast, some intermediate- and high-grade non-Hodgkin's lymphomas need to be treated aggressively. Treatment usually involves a combination of anticancer drugs, such as chlorambucil, cyclophosphamide, doxorubicin, vincristine, and prednisone.

In some cases of low- and intermediate-grade lymphoma, radiation therapy is used, supplemented by brief intensive chemotherapy (see Chapter 30 for more information on the treatment of cancer). When the cancer has spread into the stomach or abdominal cavity, surgery may be needed to remove all or most of the tumors; after that, one or more courses of chemotherapy will be used. For patients with high-risk aggressive lymphomas, bone marrow transplantation may increase the likelihood of cure (see page 960).

Prognosis Although radiation therapy may cure localized, slow-growing lymphomas, most are no longer localized when first diagnosed, and are essentially incurable. Nonetheless, these lymphomas are responsive to initial treatment and allow for long survival after diagnosis. The 5-year survival rate is greater than 80 percent; the 10-year survival rate is approximately 75 percent. With some aggressive non-Hodgkin's lymphomas, the prognosis depends on their response to combination chemotherapy, with almost one-third proving curable. The prognosis tends to be more favorable for young, healthy patients who are in a less advanced stage of the disease. Autologous bone marrow transplantation is effective in about half the cases for which it is recommended (see page 960).

Leukemias

Leukemias are serious blood disorders that are classified as cancers because they involve the uncontrolled proliferation of abnormal blood cells that spread through the body. Over time, the cancer affects various organs of the body. Depending on how swiftly the condition is diagnosed and treated, these disorders have varying degrees of severity.

Beginning in the body's blood-forming tissues, including the bone marrow and lymph system, these cancers arise when large amounts of abnormal white blood cells and both mature and immature white blood cells—called blasts—develop and accumulate. Just what causes abnormally large number of blast cells to proliferate and stagnate in their development is largely unknown. Yet, when this happens, they suppress the bone marrow's production of normal red blood cells, other white blood cells, and platelets. As these abnormal white blood cells rapidly multiply, they spill over into the bloodstream and lymph system.

Because the production of other, healthy cells is hindered, the body's tissues and organs are at risk for damage. When the number of healthy white blood cells is insufficient, the body's ability to fight invading microorganisms becomes severely impaired. With the body's natural immune response compromised, damage can arise from infections that take advantage of the body's weakened state (opportunistic infections). The deficiency in platelet production means that the blood's clotting capability is diminished. Spontaneous internal bleeding—especially into tissues and organs—often results in damage. Anemia, prompted by the reduced number of red blood cells, also occurs as a secondary condition in leukemia. Consequently, the body's organs and tissues can suffer from a shortage of oxygen. Rarely, the high numbers of blasts can cause blockage of blood vessels, depriving vital tissues of normal blood flow.

Leukemias are classified according to the type and maturity of white blood cell affected as well as the pace at which the disease progresses. When the cancer affects granulocytes, a type of white blood cells formed in the bone marrow, it is called myelogenous leukemia. As the name implies, monocytic leukemia affects the monocytes, white cells also produced in the bone marrow. Lymphocytic leukemia affects lymphocytes that are produced in the lymph system as well as in the marrow. Typically, acute leukemia comes on suddenly and progresses quickly with proliferation of blasts. Unless treated promptly, these types of leukemia can be fatal in a matter of weeks. Chronic leukemia, characterized by an overproduction of both blasts and mature blood cells, progresses slowly and is resistant to cure. Survival for 1 to 10 years is typical.

Researchers speculate as to the cause of leukemia. It is possible that exposure to radiation, some toxic chemicals, and certain viruses plays a role in the development of the disease. In some cases, there may be a genetic vulnerability involved. Yet the exact cause has not been determined.

❖ ACUTE LYMPHOCYTIC LEUKEMIA

Symptoms *(What you may experience)* Fatigue and other symptoms of anemia;

bruising and small hemorrhages into the skin; bleeding from mucous membranes; fever; pain in the bones.

Signs and laboratory findings *(What the doctor looks for)* Enlarged liver, spleen, or lymph nodes; bone marrow biopsy and blood tests showing high concentration of immature blood cells that would otherwise develop into lymphocytes.

What is it? Also known as childhood leukemia and acute lymphoblastic leukemia, acute lymphocytic leukemia (ALL) is a malignancy of the lymphoblasts (an immature form of lymphocyte). These malignant lymphoblasts lose their ability to mature and differentiate. They proliferate uncontrollably, eventually replacing normal bone marrow elements and infiltrating other organs.

Acute leukemias are the most common malignancies in children and ALL comprises 80 percent of acute leukemias in children. The peak incidence is in children between 3 and 7 years old. However, ALL is also seen in adults and comprises almost 20 percent of adult acute leukemias. There is no clear cause for ALL. However, some toxins (such as benzene), chemicals, and radiation have been linked to this as well as other forms of leukemias.

Symptoms—such as bleeding in the skin, gums, and mucous membranes; infections; bone and joint pain; headaches; confusion; and labored breathing—may arise abruptly, or they may be present for some time before a doctor is consulted.

What you can do Living with cancer, whether it involves you directly or someone in your family, can be profoundly stressful. In those instances when it touches a child, it becomes perhaps even more important that family members avail themselves of emotional support as they care for their child. The Leukemia Society of America offers counseling and other forms of help to families of children with leukemia. You can find the number of the nearest chapter in your phone book, or contact the national office at 733 Third Avenue, New York, NY 10017, phone: (212) 573-8484.

Treatment Acute leukemia was once invariably fatal. Today it is treatable and potentially curable through chemotherapy. After diagnosis, treatment will likely involve a com-

BONE MARROW TRANSPLANTS

A bone marrow transplant is a complicated procedure in which bone marrow is removed from a donor and injected into a recipient's vein. Once the donor marrow is injected into one of the recipient's veins, it travels through the bloodstream and eventually occupies the bone marrow space. Within a very short time, the new marrow begins to manufacture new blood cells.

Bone marrow transplants are the preferred treatment when, for a number of reasons, the marrow ceases to produce the three types of blood cells (red, white, and platelets). Bone marrow transplantation is most commonly used in severe cases of aplastic anemia, leukemia, and lymphoma. Sometimes, bone marrow transplantation is used for treating individuals whose conditions may otherwise be fatal in a very short time or where remission has been achieved but serious relapse is probable. Bone marrow transplant is also being used with more frequency to treat certain genetic diseases such as thalassemia, sickle cell anemia, or severe combined immunodeficiency disease.

In addition, bone marrow transplants offer the opportunity to use aggressive, often toxic drugs (usually anticancer drugs) in the high amounts that are often necessary to achieve cure; these toxic drugs can permanently harm the bone marrow and its functioning, and a successful transplant following such chemotherapy provides an infusion of healthy marrow.

The likelihood that transplantation will be successful is largely dependent on the match between donor and recipient. The donor is either a close relative—brother, sister, or parent—or an unrelated donor. Sometimes, the marrow is taken from the patient.

The ideal source for donor marrow is an identical twin. When an individual has an identical twin who is willing to donate marrow, the procedure is called *syngeneic transplantation*. Because identical twins have the same genetic makeup, the recipient is at lower risk for *graft-versus-host disease* (GVHD)—the severe reaction to or rejection of the transplant.

When the donor is a brother, sister, parent, or, rarely, an unrelated person (see below) it is called *allogeneic* transplantation. In order to measure the compatibility of the donor marrow to the host, the doctor will conduct a test for human lymphocyte antigens (HLA test). This test examines six proteins found on the surface of the white blood cells as well as on most other cells in the body. The odds of finding an HLA donor/recipient match increase proportionately with the number of siblings in a family.

In some cases, bone marrow is taken from an ailing person, who is then subjected to high doses of chemotherapy and, in some cases, irradiation. The marrow is subsequently reinjected into the patient. This is called an *autologous* transplant, and it presents no risk of graft-versus-host disease. This, however, is not suitable when the person's own bone marrow contains malignant cells. Nevertheless, research is progressing into ways of purging cancer cells from the person's marrow before reinjecting it.

Occasionally marrow is taken from someone who is unrelated to the recipient. A National Bone Marrow Registry exists to help locate donors whose HLA system is matched or nearly matched to that of the recipient. This is referred to as a matched unrelated donor transplant allogeneic procedure.

In allogeneic and syngeneic bone marrow transplantation, the bone marrow is generally removed from the donor and injected into the recipient on the same day. For the donor, the procedure is usually done in the hospital under general anesthesia. In most cases, the bone marrow is removed from the donor's hipbone. In autologous transplantation, the bone marrow is stored frozen until the person has completed the high-dose chemotherapy. Then, the stored marrow is thawed and injected back into the body.

Unless there is some major complication, a patient typically stays in the hospital for less than 4 weeks during this process. Generally, the room is set up to guard against infection. This is essential, because the individual's own immune system is compromised. So, for example, it is likely that the room will be ventilated with filtered air to minimize the risk of infection. Intravenous antibiotic treatments are also routine.

The major risk of bone marrow transplants is GVHD. When the recipient has a severe reaction to the donor marrow or rejects it completely, the result can be disease or even death.

When GVHD occurs, donor T lymphocytes injure the recipient's tissue, particularly in the skin, liver, and gastrointestinal tract. The second most serious complication resulting from bone marrow transplantation is the recurrence of infection. All bone marrow transplant patients receive immunosuppressive therapy in order to reduce the possibility of GVHD. This, unfortunately, leaves them vulnerable to infection (see page 945).

In addition to the importance of the compatibility between the donor marrow and the recipient, the success of bone marrow transplantation involves other factors. First, there is the age of the individual at the time of the transplant. The younger the patient, the better chance there is of a successful transplant. The incidence of GVHD (the major cause of transplant failure) and infection increases with age. With children, teenagers, and young adults, the chance of long-term survival after marrow transplantation is more than 80 percent.

Second, a history of transfusions increases the chance of transplant rejection and GVHD. Even a single transfusion can make the prognosis less favorable. Often, the same condition that makes transplantation desirable is the same condition that made transfusions necessary in the patient's past. If these transfusions included white blood cells—also referred to as transplantation antigens (or antibodies)—the individual may have become sensitized and is then at risk for rejecting the donor marrow. It is especially important to avoid, whenever possible, transfusions during the time it takes to find a suitable donor. As soon as one is available, the marrow transplant should be performed.

Finally, the patient's health and medical status at the time of the transplant also make a difference. People who harbor infections tend to do less well. Nevertheless, in many situations, bone marrow transplantation offers the most promising path for a return to health. ■

bination of anticancer drugs, including daunorubicin, vincristine, and sometimes asparaginase. Often, the corticosteroid prednisone is also used. In some cases, a chemotherapeutic drug such as methotrexate or other drugs will be injected into the spinal fluid. See Chapter 30 for more information on the treatment of cancer.

At the same time as these drugs work to kill the cancer cells, they may also interfere with the normal functioning of the bone marrow, the immune system, and some organs. During this period, intensive supportive care may be necessary, including transfusion and antibiotic therapy. For children, treatment may slow their growth; however, the child usually catches up when treatment is discontinued.

The initial goal of therapy is remission—the state in which there are no abnormal cells or malignancies present, and all symptoms abate. However, remission is not the same thing as cure. Once remission is achieved, methotrexate or other drugs may be continued as preventive treatment to reduce the possibility of relapse. Also, radiation to the central nervous system may be recommended to kill cancer cells that may linger outside the reach of other medications.

Treatment involving low-dose chemotherapy may continue well past the early signs of remission to guard against relapse. In rare cases where a person relapses or seems at high risk for relapse, a bone marrow transplant may be recommended.

Prognosis Without treatment, bleeding and infection can lead to death within months. With treatment, this type of leukemia can be cured in many cases. The younger the individual is and the lower the white blood cell count at the time of diagnosis, the higher the chances of cure. Between 50 and 70 percent of all children treated for ALL achieve complete remission at 5 years after initial diagnosis, and most go on to live a disease-free life. In general, treatment for adults must be more aggressive than for children; the prognosis for adults is not as favorable, with about 20 percent achieving long-term remission.

❖ ACUTE NONLYMPHOCYTIC LEUKEMIA

Symptoms (*What you may experience*) Fatigue; breathlessness; weakness; pale complexion; fevers; recurrent infections; bruising and bleeding; rash or small red marks on the skin; lack of appetite; weight loss; puffy gums; blurred vision or loss of vision; headaches; seizures; lightheadedness; loss of speech; partial paralysis.

Signs and laboratory findings (*What the doctor looks for*) Bleeding from the small or large intestine; bleeding in the brain; signs of infection; blood tests reveal overproduction of immature white blood cells (blasts).

What is it? The most common form of leukemia, acute nonlymphocytic leukemia (AML) is characterized by a malignancy of immature white blood cells, called blasts. These cells lose their ability to mature and differentiate into granulocytes, proliferate in an uncontrolled fashion, accumulate in the blood system, and ultimately replace normal elements of bone marrow. Because in AML the cells of the bone marrow are affected, but not the lymphocytes and lymph system, this disease is also referred to as myelogenous, myelogenic, or myelocytic leukemia, from the Greek *myelos* for marrow (hence, the *M* in AML).

Most people with AML seek treatment after they have been acutely ill for only a few days or weeks. Yet, at that time, the anemia is usually profound. Generally, there is bleeding in the skin, gums, and mucous membranes. If you have this type of leukemia, you are more susceptible to infection, such as cellulitis (an infection of the skin and underlying connective tissues), pneumonia, and inflammation around the rectum. You may experience frequent bone and joint pain, headaches, confusion, and labored breathing.

The cause of AML is not clear. However, some toxins (such as benzene) and radiation have been linked to leukemia. In addition, a number of chemicals may have some connection to the cancer's development.

AML appears chiefly in adults. While it can occur in young adults and children, the average age at diagnosis is 50. The rate of occurrence, while low, rises with age.

Treatment Treatment most commonly consists of chemotherapy—using an anthracycline such as daunorubicin or mitoxantrone in combination with cytosine arabinoside. In people over the age of 60, treatment frequently aims at relieving the symptoms. However, in many cases, aggressive chemotherapy will be used with older people as well. See Chapter 30 for more information on the treatment of cancer. After a patient has entered a complete remission, further chemotherapy or a bone marrow transplant—either allogenic or autologous—will be needed to prevent relapse (see Bone Marrow Transplants, page 960).

Prognosis As with many blood-related cancers, the younger a person is at detection, the better are his chances of remission. The overall remission rate in response to chemotherapy is 65 percent, with most people under the age of 40 achieving complete remissions. In terms of postremission treatment with chemotherapy or bone marrow transplant, 50 percent of patients younger than 45 achieve long-term, disease-free survival. In general, the majority of patients who achieve remission and receive postremission treatment have a reasonable prognosis of longer-term survival.

❖ CHRONIC LYMPHOCYTIC LEUKEMIA

Symptoms *(What you may experience)* Swollen lymph nodes; fatigue and other symptoms of anemia; infection; weight loss; bleeding; night sweats.

Signs and laboratory findings *(What the doctor looks for)* Enlarged spleen causing tenderness under left ribs; blood tests showing high proportion of lymphocytes (a type of white blood cell).

What is it? Chronic lymphocytic leukemia (CLL) is the most common type of leukemia in the Western world and accounts for approximately 30 percent of all leukemias. As the name suggests, CLL occurs when there is a slowly progressing cancerous propagation of lymphocytes over time. These small, long-lived lymphocytes accumulate to the point that they interfere with immune system and bone marrow production. If left unchecked, they infiltrate the body's organs.

This form of blood cancer is most commonly seen in older adults; in fact, 90 percent of all cases involve people over 50. CLL occurs in men two to three times more often than in women. Unlike other leukemias, CLL is not linked with exposure to drugs, chemicals, or radiation. A hereditary component is suspected, since the disease sometimes runs in families.

Symptoms of CLL develop gradually. Most cases are detected by chance during routine blood tests. A person may seek treatment because of chronic feelings of fatigue or tenderness around the spleen or liver.

The course of the disease varies from person to person. Because CLL results in the overproduction of mature, functional lymphocytes, it is not uncommon for someone with the disease to survive for many years without treatment. For others, the cancer progresses rapidly, and treatment is required early in the course of the disease.

In approximately 10 percent of all cases, CLL will transform into another malignancy. In rare cases, CLL itself remains stable, but an isolated lymph node will evolve into an aggressive large-cell lymphoma (Richter's syndrome)—in others, multiple myeloma develops (see page 951).

Treatment In the early stages of the disease, many doctors choose to follow the condition through regular blood counts. In fact, treatment in the early phase has not been shown to improve long-term survival. Only when it appears that the cancer is progressing will chemotherapy be recommended. Indications for treatment include progressive fatigue, a severe decrease in the number of platelets (see page 933), or the development of anemia. Initial therapy usually includes chlorambucil, prednisone, and fludarabine or other drugs to correct anemia and to reverse the decrease of platelets.

In rare instances, when the spleen has become enlarged, it may be removed surgically.

Prognosis As with the course of the disease, the prognosis varies from patient to patient. Mostly, it depends on the stage of the disease at the time it is diagnosed. The average length of survival is 7 years or longer if the diagnosis is made during an early stage of the disease. The disease often proceeds slowly but is resistant to cure. Patients with advanced stage disease may live 4 or more years.

❖ CHRONIC MYELOGENOUS LEUKEMIA

Symptoms *(What you may experience)* Fatigue, ashen pallor, and other symptoms of anemia; weight loss; night sweats; abdominal fullness; swollen lymph nodes; moderate to severe bleeding and bruising; frequent fever and infections; pain in the bones; sudden appearance of small, red marks (purpura) on the skin.

Signs and laboratory findings *(What the doctor looks for)* Enlarged spleen, which can cause pressure under the left ribs; blood tests reveal an overproduction of cancerous versions of granulocytes; a low presence of the enzyme leukocyte alkaline phosphatase; in about 90 percent of cases, an abnormal chromosome translocation, called the Philadelphia chromosome, is also uncovered through DNA testing for the *bcr/abl* fusion gene.

What is it? Myelogenous means produced or originating in the bone marrow. Chronic myelogenous leukemia (CML), also called chronic myeloid, myelocytic, or granulocytic leukemia, is marked by the proliferation of cancerous granulocytes within the marrow.

The typical course of chronic myelogenous leukemia begins with a stable, chronic phase in which there are few active symptoms. Normal bone marrow function continues, and white blood cells continue to carry out their immunologic function as usual. In this phase, the disease is usually detected only through routine blood tests. The disease can remain stable for years.

Ultimately, however, CML can suddenly progress and accelerate at an alarming rate. The accelerated phase may last for 1 year or longer. Virtually all cases then evolve into an acute or blast phase. Called a blast crisis, this acute phase is particularly resistant to treatment. Immature blood cells begin to accumulate in the bloodstream. At this stage, the person may notice a red rash called petechiae on the skin, which signals thrombocytopenia (see page 933). With platelet production compromised, bleeding into the skin, as well as in other organs, becomes more likely. At this point, the disease can be fatal.

CML accounts for approximately 20 percent of all cases of leukemia in Western countries. It most often appears in young to middle-aged adults, with a slightly higher incidence in men. There is some evidence that indicates better survival in women than men.

In most cases, it is not clear what caused CML to develop. However, there seems to be an increased incidence in people who have been exposed to excessive amounts of radiation or certain chemicals. CML is associated with a characteristic chromosomal abnormality, the Philadelphia chromosome, a spontaneous mutation.

Treatment Treatment during the chronic phase usually consists of chemotherapy administered orally. The focus is on controlling the white blood cell count and reducing swelling of the spleen. Busulfan, hydroxyurea, and alpha-interferon seem to maintain stability. Sometimes, allopurinol is included to suppress gouty symptoms caused by the death of the cancer cells (see Chapter 30 for more information on the treatment of cancer). During the chronic phase, if a suitable donor can be found (preferably a sibling) whose human leukocyte antigen (HLA) matches that of the patient, an allogenic bone marrow transplant provides the best chance for survival (see page 960).

Once the disease reaches the acute phase, its course can be altered only by high-dose chemotherapy, coupled with total-body irradiation, then followed by allogenic bone marrow transplantation. Therapy with daunorubicin, vincristine, and prednisone will often lead to remission, but remission can be short-lived.

If your spleen has become seriously enlarged and painful, your doctor may recommend having it removed (splenectomy) to relieve the pain and reduce the risk of bleeding.

Prognosis While many of the chemotherapeutic approaches to CML may address the symptoms successfully, the disease itself can be fatal. Only bone marrow transplantation seems to offer the possibility of cure. However, more evidence is accumulating that long-term remissions may be achieved with alpha-interferon; it is thus becoming front-line therapy. With those under age 55 who have HLA-matched siblings, a bone marrow transplant has a success rate of approximately 60 percent. The best results are with those under age 40 who are transplanted within one year of the initial diagnosis.

TWENTY-THREE

Digestive System

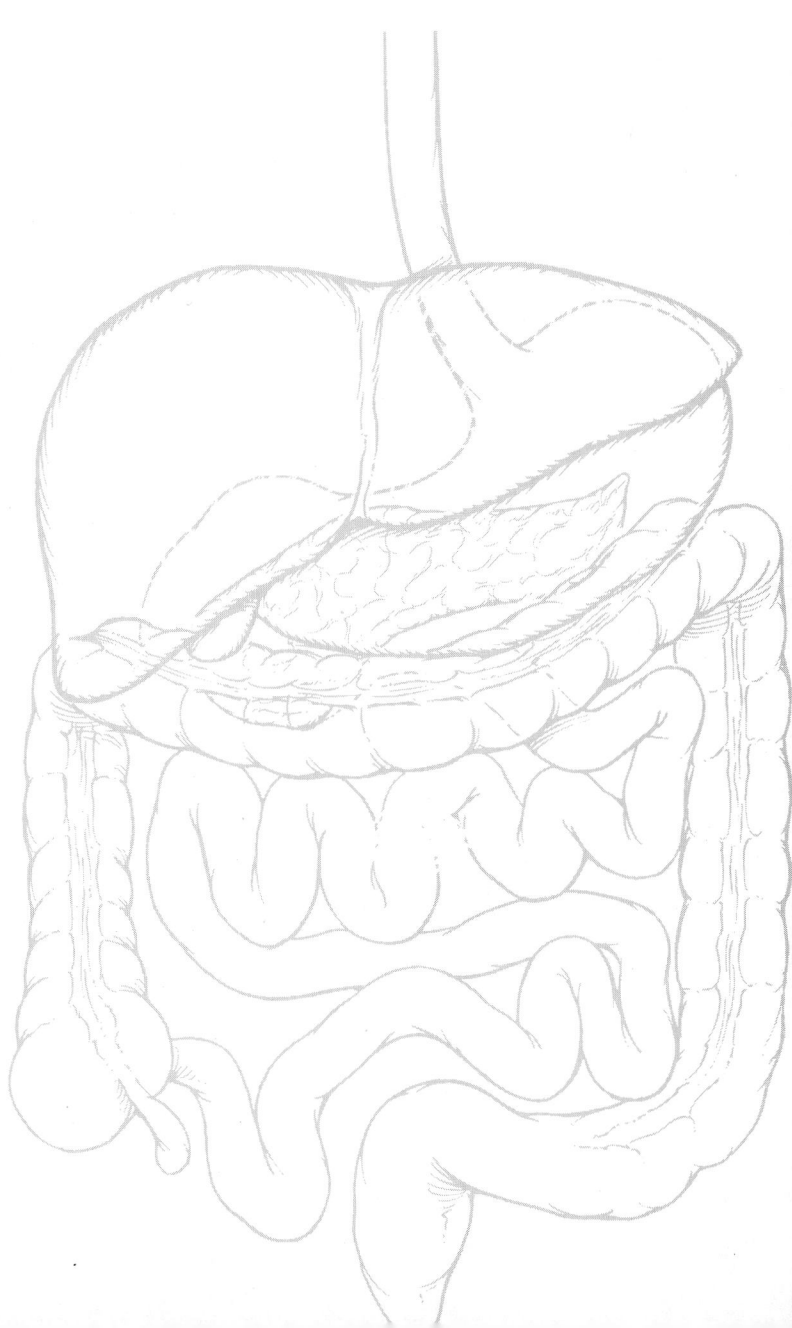

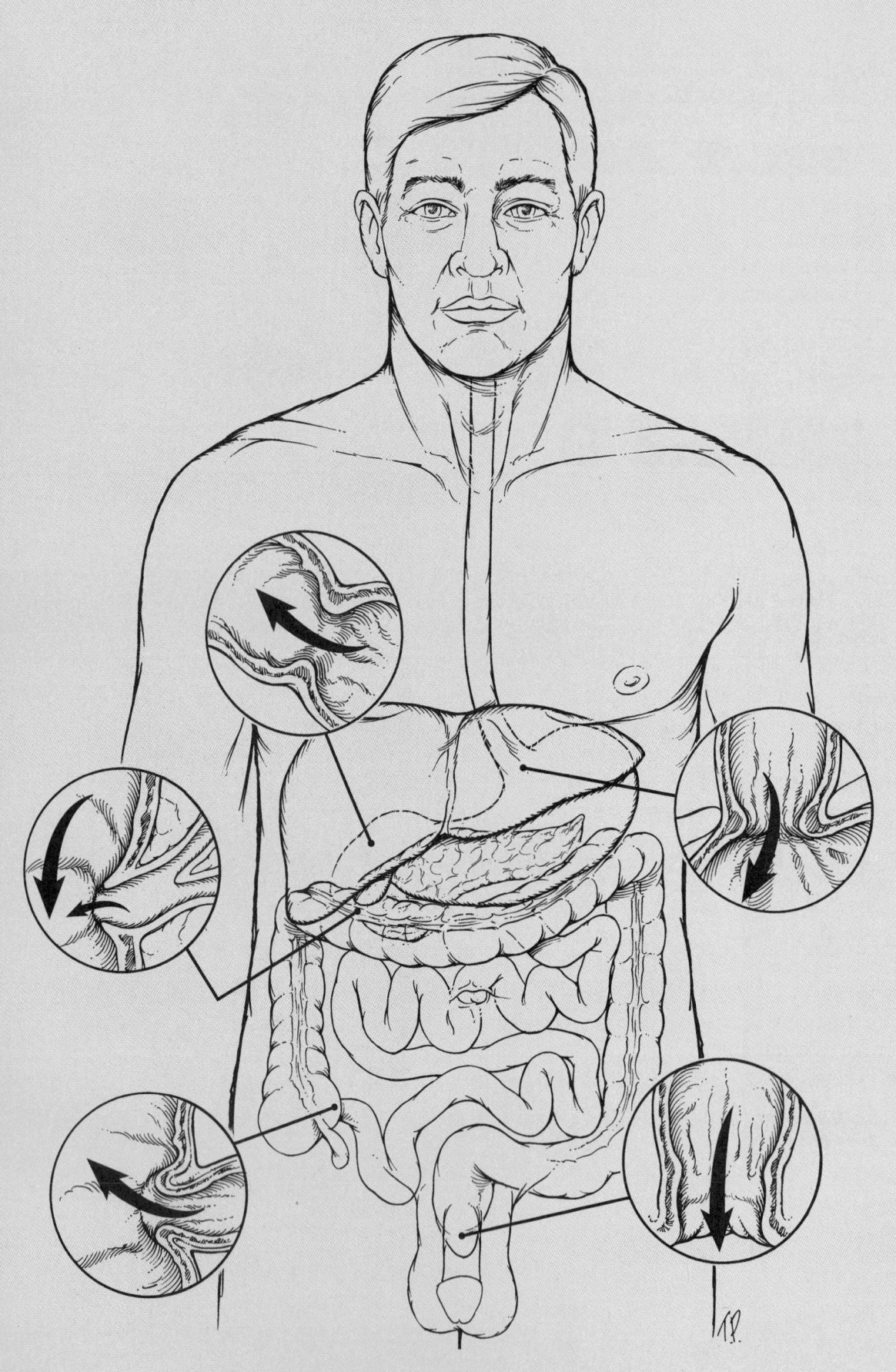

DIGESTIVE SYSTEM

Digestion begins in the mouth. With each bite, as your teeth crunch food into pieces small enough to swallow, a powerful enzyme in the saliva called amylase begins breaking down complex carbohydrates. Saliva also lubricates the food (this helps you swallow without choking) and contains some protective antibacterial agents.

When food is adequately chewed and moistened, it is pushed by the tongue to the back of your throat. Swallowing is more complicated and dynamic than it sounds: Food does not simply slide into the esophagus. The muscles in the pharynx at the back of the throat move up, wrap themselves around the food, and pull it down into the esophagus. At the same time, the epiglottis and vocal cords cover the windpipe (trachea) to direct food away from the airway and lungs—a critical maneuver that helps prevent choking. With a series of rhythmic contractions, the food is squeezed down the muscular esophagus much like toothpaste through a tube.

Next, food enters the stomach, a muscular sac that can hold 1½ L of food in most adults. The chemical breakdown of what has just been eaten continues here, as hydrochloric acid, the potent main ingredi-

ent in the gastric juices, activates an enzyme called pepsin, which digests protein. The harsh stomach acid is similar in strength to that in a car battery, but it usually leaves the stomach and small intestines unscathed: These organs are armed with several effective defenses, including a thick layer of mucus (which sits on top of the mucosal lining) plus acid-buffering bicarbonate in the small intestine. As the stomach churns food into ever-tinier bits, the pylorus, a valve between the stomach and the duodenum, slowly releases these refined particles (by now, smaller than 1 mm in diameter) into the small intestine.

The small intestine is vascular (containing many blood vessels) and tortuous. About 1 in. in diameter, it coils loosely in the abdomen; spread out, it would be more than 20 feet long. It has three parts: the

(A) During normal breathing, air passes into the nose or mouth, to the back of the oral cavity, and down the trachea (windpipe) and into the lungs. (B) During eating, muscles in the back of the throat pull food down into the esophagus (food pipe). The epiglottis closes over the trachea to direct food away from the airway and to prevent choking.

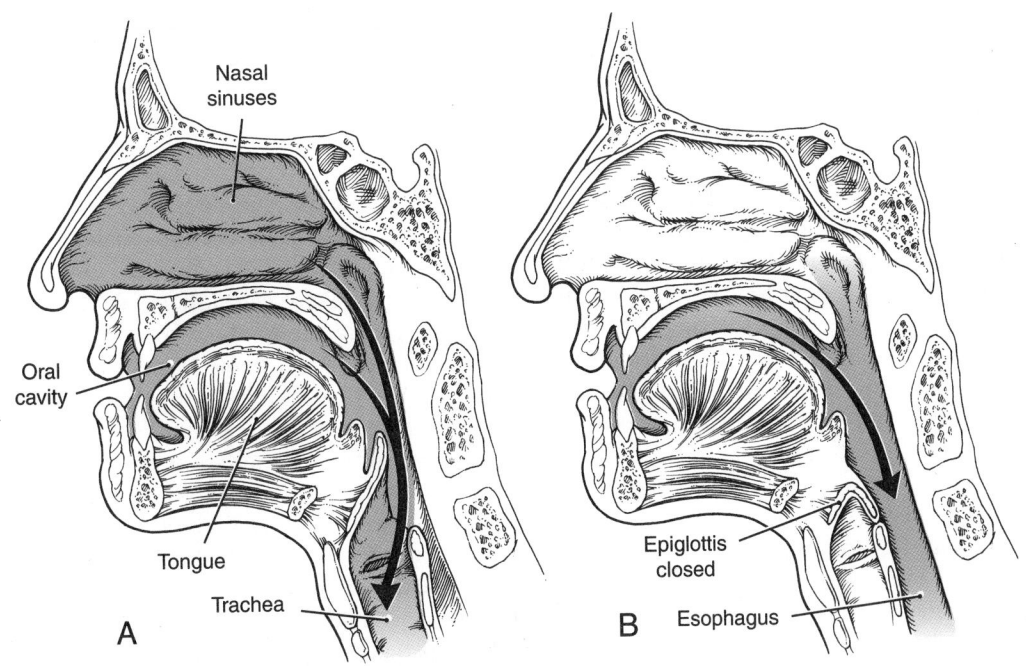

A

Nasal sinuses

Oral cavity

Tongue

Trachea

B

Epiglottis closed

Esophagus

967

UPPER ENDOSCOPY

In upper endoscopy, a gastroenterologist passes an endoscope, a long flexible tube equipped with a tiny headlight and video camera, through your mouth and throat into the upper digestive tract—the esophagus, stomach, and duodenum (the top part of the small intestine). This procedure, done with you lying on your left side, allows the doctor to see the linings of these organs and spot disease. Some problems that cannot be detected with x-rays can be seen clearly through an endoscope. Some gastroenterologists refer to this procedure, and other forms of endoscopy, as EGD, for the tongue-twisting term esophagogastroduodenoscopy, which means "examination with a tube."

Upper endoscopy is the main test for upper gastrointestinal bleeding. It can also detect inflammation (found in esophagitis, gastritis, and other "itises"); mucosal tumors; ulcers and erosions; abnormal narrowings or blockages such as strictures or stenoses; and infections (such as *Candida* esophagitis or *Helicobacter pylori*) of the lining of the upper gastrointestinal tract.

During endoscopy, your gastroenterologist may perform a biopsy, threading a cutting tool through the endoscope to take a small sample of tissue. A biopsy can be performed for many reasons; having a biopsy does not mean that you have cancer. If you have a polyp, an abnormal growth of tissue, your doctor will pass a wire loop through the endoscope to snare and remove it. The endoscope can also be used to cauterize any bleeding areas; dilate a stricture; inject medication (using extra-long needles, threaded through the endoscope); place a rubber band over an abnormal blood vessel to stop bleeding; guide placement of a feeding tube; and photograph any abnormal findings.

Upper endoscopy, which generally takes less than 30 minutes, is very safe, with a low risk—about 1 in 1,000—of complications. It is done with informed consent, which means you should have a full understanding of the risks involved. Potential complications include a tear or tiny hole (called a perforation) in the lining of the esophagus, stomach, or duodenum that may heal on its own, or may require surgery to repair; aspiration of gastric fluids into the lungs, which could develop into pneumonia; bleeding, if a biopsy is done or a polyp is removed (usually, bleeding is minimal; rarely, it may require surgery or a blood transfusion); a reaction to the sedative given before the procedure (thus, tell the doctor if you are allergic to any medications). Also, many people experience a sore throat for several hours afterward. There is a minimal risk of infection with any procedure. If you have valvular heart disease, you may need to take prophylactic antibiotics.

Because your doctor needs to see every part of the upper gastrointestinal tract, upper endoscopy cannot be performed on a full stomach. You will be asked not to eat or drink anything after midnight the night before and, to minimize the risk of bleeding, to stop taking aspirin for at least 2 days beforehand. If you are taking aspirin or any medication regularly, do not skip a scheduled dose without talking to your doctor first.

Shortly before the procedure begins, you will be asked to remove eyeglasses and dentures; you may want to remove contact lenses, as well. You will be given an intravenous, short-term sedative such as diazepam (Valium) or midazolam (Versed) and/or narcotic such as meperidine (Demerol) or Sublimaze (Fentanyl) to help you relax and make you feel drowsy during the procedure. Also, your doctor will probably spray the back of your throat or ask you to gargle with a numbing medication to prevent you from gagging as you swallow the endoscope. You should not feel any pain or discomfort from the procedure itself.

Finally, because the sedative or narcotic can impair your judgment and reflexes (and may cause you to forget what happened during the procedure itself), plan on having someone drive you home after the endoscopy. At some hospitals, the procedure will be canceled or performed without sedation if you do not have an escort home. ■

duodenum, which is short (only about 1 foot long); the jejunum (about 8 feet long), which absorbs most nutrients, and the ileum (about 12 feet long), where vitamin B$_{12}$ and bile salts (fat-dissolving detergents made by the liver, released into the duodenum and then recycled) are absorbed. The pancreas and liver secrete their own enzyme-rich, food-dissolving fluids into the mix of digesting food and intestinal juices. All the while, the muscles in the intestine knead and push the food along toward the colon until all of the digested nutrients are absorbed through the intestinal walls.

The ileum joins the colon, also called the large intestine, at the cecum (pronounced "sea-come"), its widest part. The colon is responsible for removing salt and water from what is left of the food—which, until now, has remained largely liquid. With its nutrients and most of its water absorbed, food now begins to resemble stool; the digested mass becomes more solid here, as well. In its final, digested form, the food travels through the sigmoid (so named because of its "S" shape; the Greek letter S is called *sigma*), the last part of the colon, to the rectum, where the mass, now called feces, remains until it can be expelled through defecation.

THE ESOPHAGUS

The esophagus is a muscular tube about 9½ in. long. It moves food (by a series of rhythmic contractions, in a process called peristalsis) from the back of the mouth to the stomach, first by voluntary muscles (over which you have some control), and then by involuntary muscles. In the process, it must also protect the airway and lungs—by making sure food does not stray down the trachea (windpipe)—and prevent any backup of food and harsh acid from the stomach. Food travels in a one-way path down the esophagus, which has an entrance and an exit: The upper esophageal sphincter, at the very top, relaxes to let food enter the esophagus, and the lower esophageal sphincter, a strong ring of muscles at the bottom, near the diaphragm, also relaxes temporarily so food can pass into the stomach. Failure of the lower esophageal sphincter can lead to gastroesophageal reflux disease (GERD), a common ailment, better known as chronic heartburn. Other disorders associated with the esophagus include swallowing problems, infection, and cancer.

❖ GASTROESOPHAGEAL REFLUX DISEASE

Symptoms *(What you may experience)* Heartburn; pain in the chest or upper abdomen, particularly, pain that wakes you up in the middle of the night; regurgitation (vomiting, belching acid); difficulty swallowing; chronic sour or bitter taste in the mouth; frequent bursts of salty-tasting saliva (water brash); hoarseness; sore throat; coughing; wheezing; repeatedly needing to clear your throat. All of these symptoms may be worse or more common at night, or when you are lying down or bending over.

Signs *(What the doctor looks for)* Evidence of mucosal damage, as seen on upper endoscopy (see Upper Endoscopy, page 968); esophagitis (inflammation of the lining of the esophagus, which can range from mild redness to erosions or ulcers); stricture (an abnormal narrowing of the esophagus; see Stricture, page 975); bronchitis; aspiration pneumonia (caused when stomach acid travels up the esophagus and seeps down the airway, into the lungs, usually during sleep).

What is it? In GERD, the stomach's juices (hydrochloric acid and pepsin) back up, or reflux, into the esophagus, which, lacking the stomach's powerful defenses, is poorly equipped to handle this onslaught of acid. As a result, the esophagus can become inflamed or even permanently damaged.

Everyone suffers from occasional heartburn, particularly after eating too much or too rich a diet. But for an estimated 17 million Americans, heartburn and the other symptoms of GERD are a frequent—even daily—ordeal. The primary trouble is caused by the lower esophageal sphincter (LES) the muscular door at the base of the esophagus, near the diaphragm. This sphincter is designed to keep the stomach's contents from straying upward by opening only when you are eating or swallowing and by remaining tightly shut the rest of the time. In GERD, this valve often fails by relaxing spontaneously, allowing the digestive juices to irritate the esophageal lining. Prolonged exposure to this acid can cause esophagitis (inflammation), stricture (an abnormal narrowing of the esophagus, see page 975), or an esophageal ulcer. For most people with GERD, the problem is chronic; many sufferers require long-term treatment with acid-buffering or acid-reducing medicine and lifestyle changes. A few may need surgery to help protect the esophagus.

One possible cause of heartburn is hiatal hernia, a very common condition (found in an estimated 40 percent of Americans) in which the stomach pokes through the diaphragm, preventing the LES from closing completely, and allowing acid to travel more freely back into the esophagus (see Hiatal Hernia, page 970). The good news is that, for millions of people, a hiatal hernia is often silent, never causes the bothersome symptoms of GERD, and never needs to be treated.

GERD can lead to a condition called Barrett's esophagus, in which chronic acid exposure causes changes in the lower esophageal lining. Usually gray-pink in color, it is replaced by inflamed salmon-colored tissue. This is a premalignant condi-

HIATAL HERNIA

In hiatal hernia, the stomach pokes through the hiatus, a teardrop-shaped hole in the diaphragm where the esophagus meets the stomach. This creates a faulty seal, preventing the LES from closing completely and allowing acid to travel more freely back into the esophagus, producing heartburn and other symptoms of GERD.

The exact causes of this extremely common condition—hiatal hernia is found in an estimated 40 percent of all Americans, and the majority of people over age 60—are not known. Some people are born with it; others develop it, often as a consequence of obesity (due to prolonged pressure on the diaphragm), or after a traumatic event—a bout of violent vomiting or coughing, severe straining during a bowel movement, or sudden physical exertion.

Fortunately, for millions of people, a hiatal hernia is silent, never causing bothersome symptoms and never needing treatment. However, if you have a large hiatal hernia, if a significant portion of your stomach is pushed above the diaphragm, you may need surgery to repair this problem. People with a large hiatal hernia are more likely to develop complications including iron-deficiency anemia (if this pressure causes bleeding over time) and, rarely, a shutoff of blood supply to the stomach, which, in turn, may cause chronic chest pain and swallowing difficulty, may result in severe tissue damage to the stomach, and can be a medical emergency. ■

A hiatal hernia occurs when the stomach protrudes upwards through the opening in the diaphragm where the esophagus usually meets the stomach. The lower esophageal sphincter can then have difficulty closing, a problem that can lead to gastroesophageal reflux. Surgery can be helpful in severe cases.

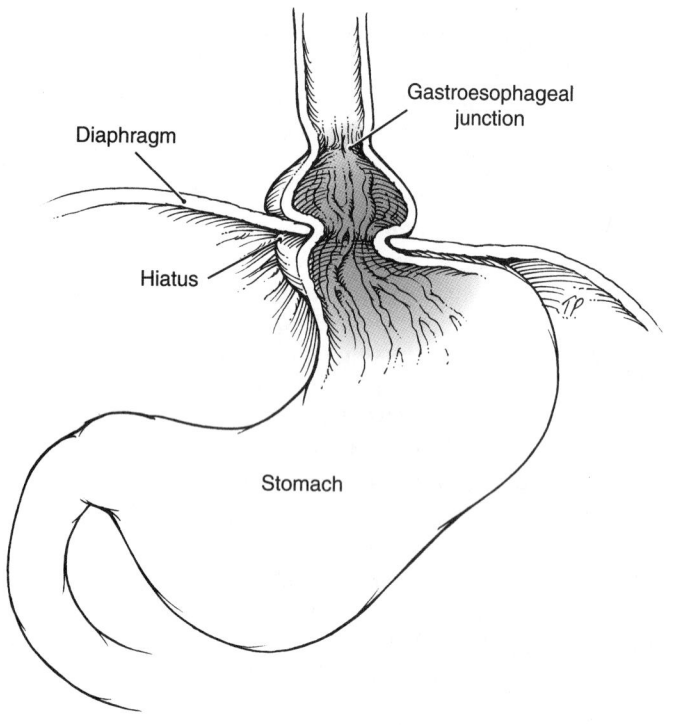

Diaphragm

Gastroesophageal junction

Hiatus

Stomach

tion; it can lead to esophageal cancer (see Cancer of the Esophagus, page 983). If you are diagnosed with Barrett's esophagus, you will need ongoing surveillance with endoscopy (see Upper Endoscopy, page 968), probably every other year, to check for the development of cancerous cells.

What you can do There is much you can do to ease the symptoms of GERD. One simple and effective change you can make immediately is to elevate the head of your bed at least 6 in. If possible, with concrete blocks, boards, or bricks under the bed frame. Raising your head with pillows alone will not be as effective, because bending at the waist increases pressure in the abdomen and stomach, and this increases reflux.

Changing your diet You may have found that certain foods add to the problem. Reflux-encouraging foods (which can cause the LES to relax, allowing acid to reflux into the esophagus) include coffee, chocolate, fatty or spicy foods (such as pizza), carbonated beverages, peppermint, spearmint, citrus fruits, tomatoes, whole milk, and onions. All of these may not cause heartburn; simply avoid foods that worsen your symptoms, once you determine what those are. Also, eating smaller, more frequent meals, with light snacks in mid-morning and mid-afternoon, may be helpful. Avoid eating for at least 3 to 4 hours before going to bed.

Other things you can do If you are overweight, lose weight; obesity can make it harder for the LES to stay closed. (For more information on losing weight, see Chapter 1.) Stop smoking (which also relaxes the LES; see Chapter 4 for information on how to stop smoking). Avoid drinking alcohol (see Chapter 5 for information on cutting down alcohol use). Also, if you are taking any medications, mention them to your doctor. Medications that can make reflux worse (by decreasing LES pressure) include theophylline, calcium channel blockers, nitrates, anticholinergics, antidepressants, and progesterone. Other drugs can irritate the esophagus directly. These include doxycycline (Doryx), tetracycline, quinidine, potassium chloride, iron supplements, and most nonsteroidal anti-inflammatory drugs (NSAIDs). NSAIDs are common painkillers such as aspirin and ibuprofen, found in Advil and Nuprin; however, acetaminophen, which is not an NSAID and is found in Tylenol, does not cause this irritation.

When to call the doctor If your symptoms are mild or intermittent—occasional heartburn after a spicy meal—over-the-counter remedies may be sufficient. But if the problem is chronic or frequent, or if over-the-counter remedies have not helped, call your doctor. If your symptoms are dramatic—such as vomiting or regurgitating blood, inhaling stomach contents while you sleep, or having severe chest pain that lasts more than 15 minutes and does not respond to treatment—call immediately. Severe chest pain may also be a sign of heart disease or a heart attack—(see Chapter 20).

Treatment For many people, the first step is lifestyle modification (see What You Can Do, page 970). Beyond that, drug therapy includes over-the-counter antacids and acid-blocking medications and prescription-strength medications that target symptoms in different ways. If symptoms persist, surgery may be needed.

Over-the-counter antacids These include simethicone (Mylanta), Maalox, Tums, Rolaids, and Gaviscon. The liquid forms of these medications work faster, although the tablets are more convenient. These medications neutralize acid; they do not heal the inflammation of esophagitis. Because they do not buffer all the acid all the time, they are better for symptomatic relief—easing heartburn in people who overeat, for instance, and in pregnant women. If you are pregnant, check with your doctor before taking any antacid.

Side effects: Magnesium-containing antacids can cause diarrhea; aluminum-containing antacids can cause constipation. Your doctor may advise you to alternate antacids to avoid these problems.

Over-the-counter histamine H_2 receptor blockers Famotidine (Pepcid-AC), cimetidine (Tagamet HB), and ranitidine (Zantac 75) among others. H_2 receptor is the abbreviation for the histamine (a substance in our body's tissues) receptor that stimulates gastic acid secretion. By blocking H_2 receptors these drugs cause the stomach to make less

acid and are effective in people with mild-to-moderate symptoms.

Prescription medications Prescription medications include H_2 blockers at higher doses and proton pump inhibitors, including Omeprazole (Prilosec) and lansoprazole (Prevacid). These medications selectively block the pump mechanism in the acid-making cells, shutting off acid production in the stomach. Stomach acid is not necessary for the body to digest food, and taking these medications will not cause malnutrition. Proton pump inhibitors are very effective.

Prokinetic medications, including bethanechol, metoclopramide, and cisapride, are good for long-term use, and they help heal painful inflammation and work in a variety of ways: Some strengthen the muscle tone of the LES, keeping acid from refluxing into the esophagus. Some speed up digestion by causing the stomach to empty faster—which, in turn, narrows the window of time that reflux can occur. Cisapride (Propulsid), the most commonly used of these medications, is often used in combination with other therapies, such as H_2 blockers or proton pump inhibitors.

Mucosal protectors, such as sucralfate, protect the irritated mucosa, the lining of the esophagus. Sucralfate contains aluminum, which coats and soothes the irritated lining; this medication is helpful for people with severe esophagitis. Because of the aluminum, constipation is the main side effect of this medication. To be effective, the tablets must be crushed and drunk as a slurry.

Surgery If your doctor is confident that GERD is the problem, if your symptoms are debilitating, and if medical therapy has failed to control the problem, you may need surgical treatment. The most common procedure is called a Nissen fundoplication, in which the top of the stomach is wrapped around the esophagus, creating an envelope that acts as a valve. This procedure usually produces effective results immediately; after surgery, many people find that they never again need an antacid. However, complications of surgery can include difficulty burping, increased abdominal bloating, and flatulence. Also, if you ever experience severe vomiting—from food poisoning, for example—this may rip the sutures, causing the wrap to slip and reflux symptoms to return.

❖ NEUROGENIC DYSPHAGIA

Symptoms *(What you may experience)* Difficulty swallowing food, or feeling that it becomes lodged in your throat on the way down; coughing, sputtering, or choking when you try to eat; having food or liquid back up through your nose; drooling (because of inability to swallow saliva). These symptoms may be silent for weeks or even months. Many people automatically compensate for increased difficulty—by chewing their food into ever-finer portions before swallowing or eating in certain positions to make swallowing easier—without realizing that there is a problem.

Signs and laboratory findings *(What the doctor looks for)* Decreased ability to cough or a disabled gag reflex, which protects the airway and lungs from food or liquid; evidence of malnutrition or dehydration; unexplained fevers, which may suggest infection of the lungs from food in the airway. Your doctor will probably want you to undergo a cine-esophagram (videofluoroscopy), an imaging test that studies the muscular sequence of events involved in swallowing. A routine barium swallow test alone is considered inadequate, because swallowing is such a complicated and rapid process (see Other Diagnostic Tests of the Gastrointestinal Tract, page 984).

What is it? Neurogenic dysphagia (also called preesophageal dysphagia, because, technically, the trouble happens in the oropharynx at the back of the throat, just before food reaches the esophagus) is a neurologic problem, caused by a disease or impairment involving the nervous system. Most commonly appearing after a stroke, it can also develop in people with neurologic disorders including Parkinson's disease, Alzheimer's disease, multiple sclerosis, Huntington's disease, amyotrophic lateral sclerosis (ALS, also known as Lou Gehrig's disease), poliomyelitis, chronic meningitis, Guillain-Barré syndrome, or myasthenia gravis, or as a result of traumatic head injury. *Note.* Neurogenic dysphagia is often accompanied by depression (see page 1224, and talk to your doctor if you are experiencing any of the warning signs discussed there), which may need to be treated, as well.

When to call the doctor See your doctor if you have any prolonged difficulty in swallowing. If you can no longer eat a normal diet or are unable to take in adequate nutrition, you are at serious risk of becoming dehydrated or malnourished. If you cannot protect your airway and lungs by coughing or gagging, you are also at risk of choking or developing an aspiration pneumonia. In fact, any prolonged difficulty in swallowing should prompt a medical evaluation. Thus, if this problem persists for more than a couple of days, do not wait for it to get better on its own, particularly if you have a neurologic disease.

Treatment Treatment depends on the severity of the problem and the underlying medical condition. Sometimes, neurogenic dysphagia is the first signal of a neurologic disorder—Parkinson's disease, perhaps, or multiple sclerosis. In this case, medication that treats the symptoms for these diseases may improve your ability to swallow, as well. You will probably need to work with a swallowing therapist (usually a speech-language pathologist or occupational therapist), who can help you develop postures and strategies that make eating easier. For instance, if you have muscle weakness on one side because of stroke, it may help to turn your head or sit in a certain position. The therapist can also teach you how to swallow in a way that protects your lungs. You may also need to modify your diet by consuming thick liquids or pastes, which are easier to swallow than liquids or solids.

Some people with cognitive impairment who cannot learn or remember these techniques or who have a greater risk of respiratory complications—because they are unable to cough or gag and thereby protect the airway and lungs—may need to have a feeding tube (see Nutritional Supplementation and Feeding Tubes, page 1000) placed in the nose or stomach, temporarily or permanently.

Tell your doctor about any other medications you may be taking: Many medications including sedatives, anticonvulsants, neuroleptic agents, corticosteroids, lipid-lowering medications and topical anesthetics, can make this problem worse.

❖ ACHALASIA

Symptoms *(What you may experience)* Trouble swallowing both liquids and solid food, regurgitation of saliva or undigested food. Many people wake up to find undigested food on the pillow. Choking (particularly during the night); belching; weight loss; halitosis (bad breath); chest pain or heartburn not necessarily related to mealtime.

Signs and laboratory findings *(What the doctor looks for)* Dilation, poor muscle contraction, and incomplete emptying of the esophagus as seen in barium swallow x-ray images (see Barium Studies, page 976). The diagnosis is also made by ruling out other disorders by endoscopy (see Upper Endoscopy, page 968) and esophageal manometry, a series of tests to measure the muscle contractions in the esophagus. Among other disorders, scleroderma, esophageal spasm, and cancer of the esophagus can produce similar symptoms.

What is it? In achalasia, the LES loses its ability to relax; it stays closed. The result is that food and liquid collect in the esophagus, sometimes causing regurgitation. If not treated, achalasia can (rarely) lead to esophageal cancer. Occasionally, cancer at the gastroesophageal junction—where the stomach meets the esophagus—involves the nerves that affect the LES, causing a secondary achalasia.

When to call the doctor If symptoms persist more than 1 or 2 day, contact your doctor. Waiting longer can lead to malnourishment or dehydration.

Treatment Conventional therapy for achalasia is to unlock the sphincter muscles, using a pneumatic dilator: A stiff balloon is expanded until it rips open the LES. This is usually done on an outpatient basis in a clinic or doctor's office, with a sedative, while you are conscious. The risk of perforation with this procedure is about 2 percent. If the dilator perforates the esophagus, intravenous antibiotics or surgery may be required to repair the injury. For some people with achalasia, even multiple dilation attempts are unsuccessful, and surgical myotomy—in which the muscle is cut, rather than torn apart—may be necessary. This procedure, which requires general anesthesia and several days of hospitalization, may result in problems with gastroesophageal reflux, because cutting the LES

partially disables the LES and hinders its ability to prevent reflux of stomach acid into the esophagus.

A promising new treatment involves a compound called botulinum toxin type A (Botox). Injected directly into the esophagus, botulinum toxin acts on the nerves that regulate the LES, causing the LES to relax. Although its long-term results are not yet known, botulinum toxin has proven effective for several months at a time. Its main drawback is that—although successfully used at hospitals such as Johns Hopkins and elsewhere—this treatment is not yet permanent; repeat treatment will be needed several months later. Given its effectiveness, however, most patients choose to return for further treatment.

Prognosis Good, although more than one session of esophageal dilation may be needed over the course of several weeks to adequately lower LES pressure to prevent blockage of the passage of food and liquids at the lower esophagus. Usually, dilation brings a permanent cure. However, the effect of botulinum toxin may wear off after several months; the medication's long-term success has not yet been determined, and the problem may return as the medication wears off.

❖ ESOPHAGEAL SPASM

Symptoms *(What you may experience)* Chest pain, usually under the breast bone, which may be dull or intense. Pain, which can last several hours, may also radiate up to the jaw, around the back, down the arm, and may—like pain from heart disease—be relieved by nitroglycerin. You may also experience swallowing difficulty and regurgitation.

Signs and laboratory findings *(What the doctor looks for)* Tissue damage in the lower esophagus, seen in a biopsy (performed during endoscopy; see Upper Endoscopy, page 968), that suggests chronic gastroesophageal reflux.

Because these symptoms are similar to those of heart attack or angina, the doctor's immediate goal is to rule out a cardiac cause, with tests to detect a heart attack (see Chapter 20). If, however, there is reason to suspect that your heart is not the problem—a history of swallowing trouble, perhaps—your doctor may omit the cardiac workup and begin gastrointestinal testing.

What is it? Esophageal spasm is a severe, abnormal clenching of the muscles in the esophagus. It can occur secondary to severe gastroesophogeal reflux but also for unknown reasons. A major difficulty in diagnosing esophageal spasm is that—like any other muscle spasm—when the clenching stops, the esophagus may appear normal. For your doctor to make the diagnosis of esophageal spasm, you may need en-

doscopy and a pH probe (see Other Diagnostic Tests of the Gastrointestinal Tract, page 984) to rule out reflux as the cause, or esophageal manometry, a series of tests to measure the muscle contractions in the esophagus.

What you can do Chew food well; large pieces of food can provoke spasm. Avoid cold or hot foods or liquids. If you have gastroesophageal reflux, treating those symptoms can reduce the likelihood of spasm. Make every effort to reduce stress (see Recognizing Stress, page 305), which is known to trigger esophageal spasm in some people.

When to call the doctor If you are having intense chest pain that lasts for more than 10 to 15 minutes, call your doctor or go to the emergency room.

Treatment Finding the right treatment for esophageal spasm can be challenging or even a bit frustrating for both you and your doctor. Some medications work better for some types of spasm; unfortunately, no medication is completely effective. Medical treatment may include the following:

Nitrates Nitroglycerin or isosorbide dinitrate, commonly used to treat angina. Nitrates cause a significant drop in blood pressure. Always take nitroglycerin when you are sitting or lying down, preferably with your feet elevated, to minimize your risk of becoming dizzy or light-headed or fainting. These medications also may cause a headache.

Calcium channel antagonists Diltiazem, (Cardizem) and nifedipine (Procardia), commonly used to treat high blood pressure. Side effects may include constipation, dizziness or light-headedness and low blood pressure. These medications may also exacerbate symptoms of congestive heart failure (see Chapter 20).

Anticholinergic medications Hyoscyamine sulfate (Donnatal), dicyclomine (Bentyl), or propantheline bromide, medications that relax smooth muscle. Side effects can include dry mouth, dizziness or light-headedness, blurred vision, nausea, drowsiness, weakness, and a feeling of nervousness.

HICCUPS

Everyone gets the hiccups: sudden, involuntary contractions of the muscles you use to breath. These brief spasms, which usually involve only one side of the diaphragm, are sparked by irritation to the nerves that control these muscles. The result is dramatic: The glottis (the voice box) slams shut, cutting off air flow and making the characteristic sound.

Most of the time, hiccups are a temporary annoyance, cured by such time-tested methods as swallowing a spoonful of sugar or holding your breath and counting to 10. Hiccups can be caused by a host of activities, most of them benign. Some of these include sudden excitement, strong emotion, eating too much, even drinking too much water too fast. Drinking too much alcohol can also bring on a case of the hiccups; so can excessive smoking, stress, or reflux.

Chronic hiccups, on the other hand, can be debilitating and may result in an inability to eat, weight loss, exhaustion, insomnia, severe reflux esophagitis, and even arrhythmias of the heart. These can be caused by many conditions, including pregnancy, diabetes, hyperventilation, gout, uremia, pneumonia, lung cancer, asthma, general anesthesia, pericarditis, myocardial infarction, esophagitis, diaphragmatic hernia or irritation, gastric ulcer, stomach cancer, liver disease, pancreatic disease, inflammatory bowel disease, bowel obstruction, and trauma. Some hiccups have psychological causes. Certain medications including barbiturates, steroids, benzodiazepines, and alpha methyldopa may also cause hiccups. If you have chronic hiccups, in addition to a thorough history and physical exam, you may need to undergo other tests, including endoscopy, chest radiography and fluoroscopy, abdominal ultrasound, and a computed tomography (CT) scan of the head, to determine the cause.

Treatment may begin with physical attempts to break the reflex arc that causes the hiccups. Simple activities such as holding your breath and breathing into a paper bag raise the level of carbon dioxide in the blood; this often inhibits hiccups. Pulling your knees up to your chest can change the pressure on the diaphragm; this is sometimes successful, as well. Some people are helped when a plastic or rubber catheter is threaded several inches through the nose and moved back and forth, swabbing the pharynx. In people with persistent hiccups, medications including baclofen (Lioresal), chlorpromazine (Thorazine), metoclopramide (Reglan), phenytoin (Dilantin), and quinidine sulfate may solve the problem. Acupuncture and hypnosis also may help. In extreme cases, the phrenic nerve (which supplies the diaphragm) can be blocked with medication or surgery. ■

Other treatment Medications to eliminate gastroesophageal reflux (see Gastroesophageal Reflux Disease, page 969). Dilating the esophagus with a bougie or pneumatic dilator (see Stricture, below). The risk of perforating the esophagus during pneumatic dilation is 3 to 5 percent, and fewer than half of the people who undergo this therapy find lasting relief of symptoms. Some people are treated with a surgical procedure called esophagomyotomy: A surgeon makes a lengthwise incision along the esophagus, so the muscles can no longer contract completely; this procedure requires general anesthesia and several days of hospitalization. However, the main complication of this treatment is reflux; because the LES can no longer close completely, acid is able to flow from the stomach into the esophagus. Treatment of certain psychiatric problems—most commonly, panic attacks or depression—also may help ease symptoms.

Prognosis Good. Despite its frightening onset, esophageal spasm is not life-threatening. However, for reasons that are poorly understood, it can be a recurrent problem, with medication and/or other therapy bringing only limited relief.

❖ STRICTURE

Symptoms (What you may experience) Feeling that solid food gets stuck on the way down, particularly, pieces of meat, apple, or bread; discomfort, but usually not pain, in swallowing; frequent heartburn or reflux. Here, as in other swallowing disorders, symptoms often develop silently and insidiously, as individuals—not immediately realizing they have a problem—simply compensate for any increased difficulty by chewing their food into extra-fine pieces before swallowing or by choosing not to eat foods they find hard to digest.

Signs and laboratory findings (What the doctor looks for) Any narrowing of the esophagus seen during endoscopy (see Upper Endoscopy, page 968) or a barium swallow test (see Barium Studies, page 976); a meat impaction, a piece of meat that becomes lodged in the esophagus, is diagnosed (and removed) during endoscopy, or is seen in a barium swallow test; abnormal tissue that suggests chronic reflux. Your doctor may also want you to

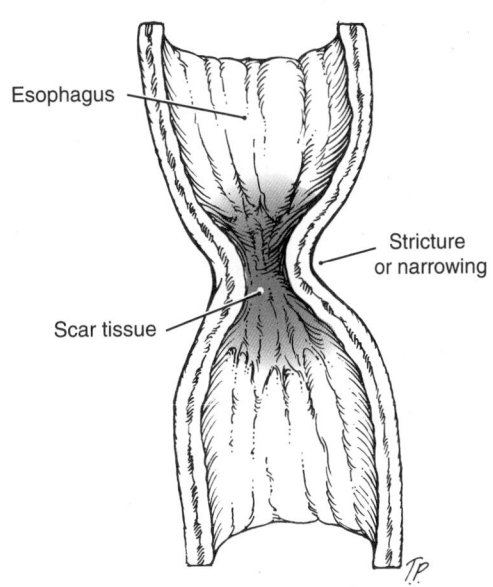

An abnormal stricture, or narrowing, sometimes develops in the esophagus. A stricture can occur from gastroesophageal reflux disease, scar tissue, esophageal cancer, or other causes. Strictures can lead to discomfort with swallowing, and persistent difficulty with swallowing should prompt a medical evaluation. Strictures can often be dilated, or widened, through an endoscope.

undergo a barium swallow x-ray test, to evaluate the length and contour of the narrowing, and an esophageal biopsy, performed during endoscopy.

What is it? An esophageal stricture (also called esophageal stenosis) is a narrowing of the esophagus caused by fibrous scar tissue or the growth of cancerous tissue in the esophagus. Most commonly, it occurs as a result of GERD, developing after weeks to months of tissue damage caused by the chronic injury of reflux (see Gastroesophageal Reflux Disease, page 969), an abnormal amount of acid in the esophagus. Other causes include the swallowing of a toxic substance (see Caustic Injury of the Esophagus, page 979), complications of medical treatment (see Medication-Induced Esophagitis, page 980, and Radiation-Induced Esophagitis, page 981), sclerotherapy (see Bleeding Varices, page 982), severe or prolonged infection (see *Candida* Esophagitis, page 978), and even previous surgery. Esophageal cancer (see Cancer of the Esophagus, page 983) often mimics benign stricture. Thus, an impor-

BARIUM STUDIES

Barium, like the opaque material used in angiography, is a dye that is visible on an x-ray. Often, this test is used in addition to or instead of EGD colonoscopy, or flexible sigmoidoscopy. In some instances, a barium series is better than endoscopic tests. On a barium x-ray, defects in the lining of the gastrointestinal tract show up as silhouettes. The distinction between this test and a procedure involving a scope (such as an endoscope) is akin to the difference between looking at a bird directly and seeing its shadow on the ground.

In an upper gastrointestinal (GI) series, (involving the esophagus, stomach, and duodenum), barium is swallowed in a solution that resembles a chalky milkshake. Like thick paint, this viscous liquid slowly creeps down the GI tract, coating the stomach and intestine. The radiologist watches barium's downward path on a fluoroscope (an x-ray machine). An upper GI series usually takes less than 30 minutes.

In a barium swallow test, still photographs are made as barium makes its way through the esophagus.

In a cine-esophagram (also called dynamic radiographic studies), moving pictures are taken of the dynamic swallowing process in real time, so the doctor can see how all the muscles involved in the complicated process of swallowing work together and separately; the difference here is that of a snapshot versus a videotape. Swallowing cannot be seen during endoscopy, in part because the patient is sedated but also because the endoscope itself prohibits a good look.

In the stomach, barium's effectiveness may be augmented with the help of a gas-releasing pill, which expands the stomach, revealing more detail. Upper GI barium studies are helpful in finding obstruction, narrowing (from causes including a benign stricture, and a tumor). Barium is also helpful in spotting problems in the jejunum and ileum; most endoscopes do not reach far enough into the small bowel for a physician to see these areas. If the barium studies involve your small intestine, the examination

may last several hours, because pictures are made at 15-minute or half-hour intervals.

In a barium enema, barium enters the digestive tract from the other end, injected through the rectum and pumped into the colon; this will probably make you feel that you need to have a bowel movement. In preparation for the barium enema, you will probably be asked to take a laxative the night before, and a cleansing enema the morning of the procedure. During the procedure, you will be asked to change your position from time to time as the barium travels through your colon. The doctor may push on your abdomen in an attempt to propel the barium higher into the bowel. As in barium studies of the stomach, extra air (this time, pumped into the colon through the rectum) can provide clearer, more detailed pictures. A barium enema can show polyps, colon cancer, and changes indicative of Crohn's disease or ulcerative colitis. One problem with this test is that any vestiges of stool can sometimes resemble polyps; also, because the S-shaped sigmoid colon overlaps itself and the enema tip is in the rectum, it is often difficult to see everything here. Thus, most doctors feel that a barium enema is not complete without an accompanying flexible sigmoidoscopy. The barium will pass harmlessly from the body in the stool (which may be much lighter in color for the next few days). Your doctor may suggest that you take a laxative to hasten this process.

Barium studies are very safe, with a low risk—less than 1 in 1,000—of complications. It is done with informed consent, which means you should have a full understanding of the risks involved. Potential complications include a tear or tiny hole (called a perforation) in the lining of the gastrointestinal tract, which may heal on its own or may require surgery to repair it; aspiration (for an upper GI series) of gastric fluids into the lungs, which could develop into pneumonia; bleeding (usually bleeding is minimal; rarely, it may require surgery or a blood transfusion). There is a minimal risk of infection with any procedure. ∎

tant part of diagnosis is determining whether the narrowing in your esophagus is benign scar tissue or a malignant growth; this can be done by biopsy, performed during endoscopy (see Upper Endoscopy, page 968).

When to call the doctor If you have persistent trouble swallowing, experience a progressive or recurring change in your ability to swallow over several days, or have a strong feeling that food is stuck in your esophagus, consult your doctor. Difficulty swallowing can occur from benign or malignant disorders, so get these symptoms checked out promptly.

If you feel that a piece of food has become lodged in your esophagus, call your

doctor immediately; you may need to go to the emergency room.

Treatment The goal is to enlarge, or dilate, the obstructed opening and, thus, relieve discomfort and improve swallowing. This can be done during endoscopy, with a lubricated, thermoplastic dilator threaded like a long, tapered bead over a flexible-tip guide wire. Or, it may be done with a weighted, tapered rubber device called a bougie (pronounced "boojie"), which steadily pushes its way into the esophagus, flattening tissue and widening the opening as it goes. A third approach uses a balloon, threaded into the endoscope and filled with air (called a pneumatic dilator) or water (this is similar to the balloon dilation used to treat people with heart disease). Treatments can often be performed on an outpatient basis, with mild anesthesia or sedation if needed; as with endoscopy, you will be asked not to eat or drink anything for several hours ahead of time. In all of these techniques, the risk of complication—primarily, esophageal perforation—is low. However, to minimize the odds of infection after esophageal dilation, people with heart valve problems, endocarditis, or accumulation of fluid in the abdomen (also called ascites) may be given antibiotics.

Which method is best for you? This depends on the underlying cause; for example, if a stricture that appears to be caused by reflux is complicated by Barrett's esophagus (see Gastroesophageal Reflux Disease, page 969), dilation alone may not be sufficient. Esophageal stricture does not develop overnight; neither can it be cured quickly. Scar tissue is tough and usually requires several dilating sessions in which the stricture is stretched or torn apart, because it tends to close as it heals. For more complicated or tortuous strictures, your doctor may use fluoroscopy, a radiographic procedure in which a swallowed, radio-opaque dye is used to illuminate the stricture and surrounding tissue, for greater precision in placing the guide wire.

Esophageal strictures, particularly those caused by reflux, tend to recur and often need to be reopened. Some people with recurrent strictures learn to keep symptoms at bay by dilating themselves at home, using a bougie (described on page 976) as needed. If your doctor prescribes medicine for reflux, take it regularly to minimize the likelihood of recurrence.

If your stricture involves Barrett's esophagus (see Gastroesophageal Reflux Disease, page 969), you will probably need periodic esophageal endoscopy with biopsy to check for the presence of cancer or abnormal cells.

❖ ESOPHAGEAL RINGS AND WEBS

Symptoms *(What you may experience)* Intermittent problems with choking, or having food become stuck on its way down. For example, during a meal, a piece of meat or bread may become lodged in the esophagus; you may be able to dislodge the chunk of food by coughing or regurgitating and continue eating without further trouble. This may happen occasionally for years. If it is occurring every day, the problem is probably not a ring or web and may be a stricture, an abnormal narrowing of the esophagus (see page 975).

Signs and laboratory findings *(What the doctor looks for)* A meat impaction, a lodged piece of meat (visible on a barium swallow test or endoscopy; see Barium Studies, page 976, and Upper Endoscopy, page 968) that causes sudden, total obstruction of the esophagus, is the classic presentation of a lower esophageal ring, signs of iron-deficiency anemia (a cause of some esophageal webs); spooning of the fingernails and toenails (in which the nails appear concave, or sunken).

What is it? An esophageal ring, commonly referred to as a Schatzki's ring, is a thin, restrictive band of tissue, that bulges the lining of the esophagus (like a narrow belt that is several sizes too tight). A web is thicker and more fibrous than a ring but much narrower and less significant than a stricture (an abnormal narrowing of the esophagus; see page 975). Webs can be caused by iron-deficiency anemia; they are sometimes associated with postcricoid cancer (a rare form of cancer located high in the esophagus, near the Adam's apple). They also can be a consequence of graft-versus-host disease (a result of bone marrow transplantation).

What you can do Changing your eating habits—eating more slowly and chewing your food thoroughly—can make food easier to swallow.

Be sure to tell your doctor if you have previously experienced a meat impaction, even if you were able to cough or regurgitate and dislodge the meat by yourself. Because they can be thin, rings in the lower esophagus are sometimes hard to detect and may be missed or misinterpreted on a barium swallow test or endoscopy. Thus, your medical history may be a key factor in diagnosis.

Treatment Rings and webs are much simpler to treat than strictures; they usually respond well to dilation (either with the guide wire technique during endoscopy, or with a bougie, described in Stricture, page

975), often after a single treatment. If a web is caused by anemia, treating the underlying problem with iron replacement will help prevent recurrence and may minimize your odds of developing postcricoid cancer. Sometimes, however (especially with lower esophageal rings that cause only occasional trouble), simply changing your eating habits, as described on page 977, can bring complete relief and eliminate the need for further treatment.

❖ *CANDIDA* ESOPHAGITIS

Symptoms *(What you may experience)* Difficulty, mild discomfort, or severe pain during swallowing; a feeling that food gets stuck on its way down after you swallow; nausea; loss of appetite.

Signs and laboratory findings *(What the doctor looks for)* Oral thrush, a yeast infection that may be visible in an examination of your throat; or the telltale white, cheesy patches of *Candida* plaques (splotches of yeast infection in your esophagus), visible during endoscopy; positive results of a biopsy of the cells lining your esophagus (see Upper Endoscopy, page 968).

What is it? *Candida* esophagitis is a yeast infection in the esophagus, caused by the same troublesome fungus that produces oral thrush and vaginal yeast infections. A classic opportunistic infection (so named because it tends to develop when the body's defenses are already weakened by illness), it is almost always a complication of another disease—most commonly, infection with human immunodeficiency virus (HIV); the immune system-compromising virus that causes acquired immunodeficiency syndrome (AIDS). A diagnosis of *Candida* esophagitis does not mean that you have HIV or that you are going to develop AIDS. Cancer (and chemotherapy to treat it), poorly controlled diabetes, inadequate nutrition, a chronic illness, and even drug or alcohol abuse can also hamper the body's immune system and allow *Candida* esophagitis to develop. Some people are prone to recurrent *Candida* infections.

What you can do Be sure to give your doctor a detailed medical history. Often, when the history suggests that *Candida* esophagitis is a likely possibility, doctors prefer to take the less invasive approach by treating with antifungal medications (see below) for a week to 10 days and performing endoscopy only if the symptoms persist.

When to call the doctor If you have trouble or pain on swallowing that lasts more than 1 or 2 days; call your doctor. The risks in waiting are becoming dehydrated and malnourished and—equally serious—developing a systemic (spread throughout the body) infection.

Treatment The goal is to kill the fungus, and the drugs that do this are called antifungal agents. Depending on the severity of your symptoms, you may receive treatment orally—in the form of a pill, if you are able to swallow it; or in a medicated, nonabsorbable wafer (which, like a cough drop, stays in the mouth until it dissolves); or intravenously (which may require hospitalization). The mainstay of treatment is oral nystatin (Mycostatin) in wafer form, taken four times a day; clotrimazole (Mycelex) is also used in this manner. Medications in pill form include ketoconazole (Nizoral) and fluconazole (Diflucan). Intravenous antifungal agents include amphotericin B.

Prognosis This depends on the underlying condition. If, for example, *Candida* esophagitis is caused by poorly regulated diabetes, it will likely improve as the diabetes is brought under control. If it is the result of a temporary breach in the immune system—by chemotherapy to treat cancer, perhaps—here again, as the body's defenses grow stronger, the infection's foothold should diminish. If, however, the fungal infection results from HIV, *Candida* esophagitis may be a recurrent—although treatable—problem.

❖ HERPES ESOPHAGITIS

Symptoms *(What you may experience)* Difficulty, mild discomfort, or severe pain during swallowing; a feeling that food gets stuck on its way down after you swallow; nausea; loss of appetite.

Signs and laboratory findings *(What the doctor looks for)* Blisters, seen during endoscopy, and/or shallow ulcers in the esophageal lining. Positive results of a biopsy or brushing of the cells lining the esophagus (see Upper Endoscopy, page 968).

What is it? As with *Candida* esophagitis, herpes simplex esophagitis is an opportunistic infection that tends to develop when the body's defenses are weakened by illness. It is usually a symptom of a larger problem—most commonly, a consequence of a disease that suppresses the immune system.

When to call the doctor If you are unable to eat or drink properly, consult your doctor. Becoming malnourished or dehydrated is a major danger—especially if your immune system is already hampered by a serious infection.

Treatment The most common and effective medication is acyclovir, which may be given either by mouth or intravenously. If you are experiencing severe difficulty swallowing, have a high fever, or are vomiting blood, you will probably need the intravenous treatment, which lasts a week (and may be done on an outpatient basis). Acyclovir works by inhibiting the virus's ability to reproduce. It does not kill the virus outright, but shortens its duration, giving the body time to heal. Some people are infected with acyclovir-resistant strains of herpes and may be given other medications, including vidarabine or foscarnet. During your illness, be sure to get plenty of fluids and nourishment, to sustain your body and boost your immune system.

Prognosis This depends on the underlying condition. (For more information on herpes, see Fever Blisters/Cold Sores, page 1283.)

❖ CYTOMEGALOVIRUS ESOPHAGITIS

Symptoms *(What you may experience)* Difficulty, mild discomfort, or severe pain during swallowing; a feeling that food gets stuck on its way down after you swallow; nausea; loss of appetite.

Signs and laboratory findings *(What the doctor looks for)* Erosions or ulcers in the tissue lining the esophagus, as seen in endoscopy. Positive results on a biopsy or brushing of the cells in the esophageal lining (see Upper Endoscopy, page 968).

What is it? Cytomegalovirus (CMV) esophagitis is an infection of the blood vessels underneath the lining of the esophagus. Generally, it is an opportunistic infection that occurs when the body's defenses are weakened by illness (most commonly, in AIDS, or during chemotherapy for cancer).

When to call the doctor If you are unable to eat or drink properly, call your doctor. Becoming malnourished or dehydrated is a major danger—especially if your immune system is already hampered by a serious infection.

Treatment The mainstay of treatment is the medication ganciclovir, given intravenously for 2 to 3 weeks; another medication that has proven helpful is foscarnet (Foscavir). Both medications slow the viral infection, giving the body a chance to heal. Be sure to get plenty of fluids and nourishment, to sustain your body and boost your immune system.

❖ CAUSTIC INJURY OF THE ESOPHAGUS

Symptoms *(What you may experience)* Symptoms vary, depending on the toxic substance that has been swallowed: Acids cause

The esophagus can be damaged if a toxic substance (such as lye) is swallowed. (A) Superficial injuries affect only the inner lining of the esophagus. (B) Deeper injuries can lead to strictures (see illustration, page 975). (C) The most severe injuries cause perforation through the entire wall of the esophagus, requiring surgical treatment.

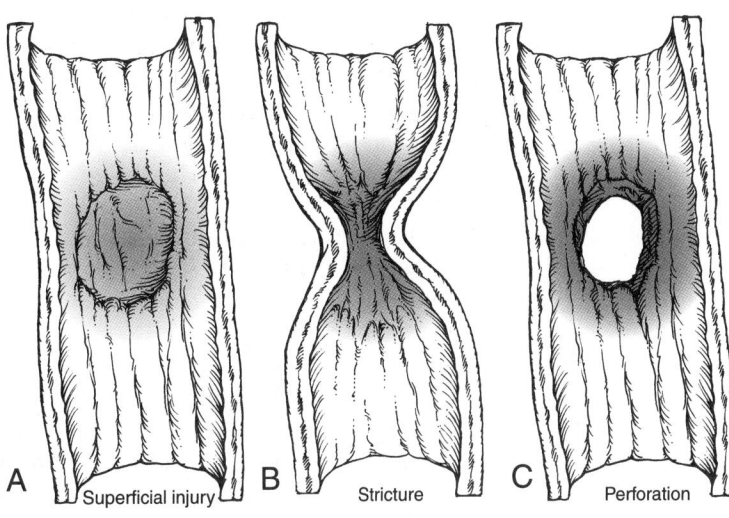

A Superficial injury   B Stricture   C Perforation

immediate pain and usually are vomited quickly. Unfortunately, caustic agents (the most common is lye, found in such household products as Drano)—which can cause severe damage to the lining of the esophagus—often do not produce immediate pain, have no peculiar taste, and may not be expelled right away.

Signs and laboratory findings *(What the doctor looks for)* Esophageal injury, seen in endoscopy (see Upper Endoscopy, page 968). An x-ray may be needed to determine the extent of injury.

What is it? Caustic injury is damage to the tissue of the esophagus, caused by swallowing a toxic substance. A superficial injury involves only the lining of the esophagus; injury that extends deeper into the wall produces intense inflammation and, with time, can cause a stricture (an abnormal narrowing of the esophagus; see page 975) to form as it heals. Deeper injuries perforate or rupture the esophagus and require surgery.

What you can do If possible, bring the container of the hazardous agent to the doctor. Do not try to neutralize the acid (with baking soda) without consulting your doctor first. For caustic injury (from swallowing lye), do not drink anything. Call your doctor or go to the emergency room immediately.

When to call the doctor If you have swallowed anything that could injure you, call your doctor immediately. Do not wait to see if it hurts.

Treatment Treatment may include corticosteroids, to help prevent a stricture from forming; intravenous antibiotics, to prevent infection; intravenous nutrition (to give the esophagus a chance to heal, avoid additional injury from eating or drinking, and prevent you from becoming malnourished or dehydrated); and intravenous drugs to reduce gastric secretions and minimize acid in the esophagus. If you have a third-degree injury, you will probably need surgery to remove the damaged tissue and minimize your risk of infection.

Prognosis This depends on the extent of the injury. Your chances of a complete recovery are very good with a superficial injury. Injuries of the esophageal wall may lead to formation of a stricture, which may eventually need to be dilated. Cancer may be a complication of deep injury; if you have damage of this severity, you will need regular follow-up exams with a gastroenterologist.

❖ MEDICATION-INDUCED ESOPHAGITIS

Symptoms *(What you may experience)* Swallowing difficulty, which may get worse over time, pain under the breastbone on swallowing (this may occur days to weeks after taking pills), vomiting blood, or blood in the stool.

Signs and laboratory findings *(What the doctor looks for)* An ulcer, stricture (abnormal narrowing), or mass—sometimes containing visible pill fragments—as seen on a barium swallow test or endoscopy. Because the abnormal appearance of medication-induced esophagitis can sometimes mimic other conditions (such as cancer or a stricture), a biopsy (taken during endoscopy; see Upper Endoscopy, page 968) may be needed to make the diagnosis.

What is it? This problem develops when medication designed to treat one problem causes another. Simply put, one or more pills get stuck in the esophagus and dissolve there—usually just above the LES—instead of their intended destination, the stomach. This can cause intense injury. This occurs with large pills, taken with too little water, or taken just before bedtime. These can include tetracycline, doxycycline, clindamycin (Cleocin), alendronate sodium (Fosamax), potassium chloride, iron preparations, quinidine, and analgesics such as aspirin or other nonsteroidal anti-inflammatory drugs. Pills containing high concentrations of iron or potassium can be particularly irritating to the tissue lining the esophagus.

What you can do Take pills with at least a full glass of water. Do not take pills immediately (less than 15 minutes) before bedtime or before lying down. If you feel that a pill had trouble going down, drink one or two more glasses of water. Take extra care if you have other esophagus problems: Ask your doctor to prescribe smaller pills or a liquid form of the medication. Do not break pills in half without consulting your doctor first;

this may change the way the medication is absorbed.

Treatment It may be necessary for a gastroenterologist, during endoscopy (see Upper Endoscopy, page 968), to remove pill fragments that have become embedded in the esophageal lining, or to push them downward into the stomach. The best treatment is prevention—to use smaller or different medications, or change the way you take them (see page 980).

Prognosis Excellent, if you stop taking the pills that have caused the problem; your esophagus should heal within 1 to 6 weeks. However, if you continue taking these same pills, and continue having trouble, you may develop a stricture (an abnormal narrowing of the esophagus; see page 975), which may require dilation, or even a perforation, or hole, in the esophagus, which may need surgery.

❖ RADIATION-INDUCED ESOPHAGITIS

Symptoms *(What you may experience)* After undergoing radiation therapy for cancer: difficult or painful swallowing; regurgitation of blood; inability to eat or drink; chest pain below the breastbone.

Signs and laboratory findings *(What the doctor looks for)* Inflammation, as seen on endoscopy or a barium swallow test (see Upper Endoscopy, page 968, and Barium Studies, page 976).

What is it? Radiation-induced esophagitis is an example of treatment doing harm as well as good. It is a complication of radiation therapy, usually for cancer in the chest, where the esophagus is included in the radiation field. High-dose radiation can lead to a stricture (an abnormal narrowing of the esophagus; see page 975), perforation, or even a fistula (a large hole in the esophagus).

Treatment If you are unable to swallow, you may need intravenous nutrition or even a temporary feeding tube in your stomach until the acute injury heals. If a stricture develops, you may need dilation; if there is a perforation or fistula, you will probably need surgery. Some chemotherapeutic agents, called radiation-sensitizing drugs, designed to make cancer more responsive to radiation, can make the damage even worse. Healing may be delayed until the chemotherapy and radiation treatments are stopped. Your doctor also may prescribe medication for pain.

Prognosis This depends on the dose of radiation that your esophagus received and whether you developed a stricture, perforation, or fistula. In most cases, it takes a few weeks for the inflammation to heal completely and for the esophagus to return to normal.

❖ SWALLOWED FOREIGN BODIES

Symptoms *(What you may experience)* Difficulty swallowing (usually immediately after swallowing the foreign body), choking, pain in the esophagus or chest. Nausea, vomiting, abdominal pain, gastrointestinal bleeding (blood in the stool), and fever may develop a few hours later, if the object becomes caught lower in the intestinal tract. If a foreign body is obstructing the air passage, the Heimlich maneuver and other emergency measures to clear the passage must be taken immediately (see page 358 for directions).

Signs and laboratory findings *(What the doctor looks for)* A foreign body lodged in the esophagus, as seen in upper endoscopy or an x-ray (or lower endoscopy, if your doctor suspects that the object is lower in the intestinal tract; see Upper Endoscopy, page 968, Flexible Sigmoidoscopy, page 1006, and Colonoscopy, page 1011).

What is it? This problem occurs when an item that is not supposed to be ingested is swallowed. Small children are particularly prone to this; coins, small toys or parts of games, broken crayons, and ballpoint pen caps rank among the most commonly swallowed objects. In adults, it is not uncommon for denture wearers to ingest (inadvertently) a foreign object, such as a fish bone or toothpick. Dentures eliminate most of the tactile sensitivity of the palate, and wearers simply may not feel the foreign body in the mouth when they swallow. People with mental impairment caused by alcohol or drug use, or by stroke or neurologic or psychiatric illness, also are susceptible.

In some cases, foreign bodies can completely block the airway, requiring emergency care (see page 358). In most cases—an estimated 80 percent—the foreign object passes on its own through the body. Sometimes, although breathing is not obstructed, the object either poses a danger or becomes lodged in the intestinal tract. About 20 percent of the people who ingest a foreign object need to have it removed endoscopically; fewer than 1 percent require surgery to remove the object.

What you can do If you have small children, child-proof your home by conducting a sweep of every room in which your child is allowed to roam freely. Remove all objects smaller than a quarter. Place toxic chemicals—the contents are harmful if swallowed, and even the lids of the bottles can be a choking hazard—out of reach, remove breakable items, and cover all electrical outlets. See Chapter 3 for more detailed information on child-proofing your home.

If you wear dentures, take extra care when eating fish, and do not leave a toothpick in your mouth for prolonged periods.

When to call the doctor If you know that an object has been swallowed or have reason to suspect (from the symptoms listed on page 981) that this has happened, call your doctor. *Swallowed batteries must be removed immediately.* They can corrode the esophagus and cause major damage quickly. Button-sized batteries, often used in toys and watches, are an increasingly common hazard. A child who has swallowed a battery must be taken to the emergency room immediately.

If the object is not sharp or corrosive, and your doctor advises you to watch and wait, call your doctor again if it has not passed from the body within a week. You may need additional x-ray tests to see if the object is making progress through the body.

Treatment Treatment depends on what has been swallowed: The risk of perforation or development of a fistula (a large hole in the esophagus) is high with sharp objects such as toothpicks, pins, nails, bones, paper clips, wire, razor blades, and (particularly in children) coins that become lodged in the esophagus. These objects are usually extracted in endoscopy; in rare cases, however, surgery may be necessary to remove the object. With batteries, the risk of damage to the esophagus and digestive tract is so high that this is considered a medical emergency.

❖ BLEEDING VARICES

Symptoms *(What you may experience)* Vomiting blood; passing blood in the stool; dizziness; fainting; or symptoms of cirrhosis (see page 1043).

Signs and laboratory findings *(What the doctor looks for)* Varices are varicose veins inside the esophagus, visible on endoscopy or in an upper gastrointestinal (GI) series. Similar veins may be visible in the skin, near the navel; in some cases, hemorrhoids may also indicate a problem with varices (however, hemorrhoids are so common that this is not a definitive sign). Some people have encephalopathy (an inability to think clearly); in conversation, they may sound unclear or even incoherent. This is probably a result of toxins, which normally are filtered by the liver, entering the bloodstream.

What is it? Although varices appear in the esophagus, they are caused by disease in the liver. A condition called portal hypertension develops over months or years as the liver becomes so severely scarred (usually from cirrhosis) that blood coursing from the abdominal organs can no longer filter through it. But the blood must go somewhere, and over time, the body develops an abnormal bypass around the liver—varicose veins in the gastroesophageal junction, the point where the stomach meets the esophagus. The pressure in these irregular veins is great; if they rupture, they may bleed profusely. (see Cirrhosis, page 1043, for more information.)

When to call the doctor Because the bleeding can be so heavy, this is a life-threatening problem. If you are vomiting blood—particularly if you have a history of liver disease—call the doctor right away. If you cannot reach your doctor, go to an emergency room immediately.

Treatment Treatment of bleeding varices begins with intravenous blood and fluids, followed by endoscopy (see Upper Endoscopy, page 968) to identify the true source of bleeding (as many as half of patients with portal hypertension experience internal bleeding from a source other than varices). Treatment may include the following:

Medication The first step is to stabilize the blood volume, by controlling blood pressure with medications including vasopressin (given intravenously) and nitrates, or somatostatin (Sandostatin), which decreases blood flow to the GI tract. The medication propranolol (Inderal, Inderide), which lowers blood pressure, may also be given to reduce your risk of further bleeding; you may need to take this medication for life.

Other treatments The most effective treatment strategy is simply to eliminate the ruptured vein. This is often accomplished with a procedure called banding—literally, using a rubber band to tie off the varices, a procedure similar to that used to treat some hemorrhoids—or with sclerotherapy, injecting a chemical that causes the vein to form a clot and wither away. Complications of sclerotherapy include having a clot form in the large portal vein; fever, chest pain, or inflammation; esophageal perforation (which also may necessitate surgery) and esophageal stricture (an abnormal narrowing of the esophagus; see page 975). Banding may have similar, but probably fewer, complications. With both banding and sclerotherapy, about five sessions—one every week or so—are needed before the varices disappear.

Some patients undergo a procedure called transjugular intrahepatic portosystemic shunt, in which an interventional radiologist creates a bypass for blood by tunneling through the scarred liver and inserting a tube, or shunt, as a makeshift passageway; this takes pressure off the esophageal varices. Other patients are treated with a device called a Sengstaken-Blakemore tube, an inflated balloon that pushes against the wall of the esophagus, compressing the varices and stopping bleeding. Patients must be sedated to minimize the risk of pulling out the tube, which could cause major damage.

❖ SCLERODERMA OF THE ESOPHAGUS

Symptoms *(What you may experience)* Heartburn; difficulty swallowing or feeling that food becomes stuck on its way down; chest pain; weight loss.

Signs and laboratory findings *(What the doctor looks for)* Abnormal tone and function of the smooth muscle region in the lower esophagus, poor tone and weakened contractions in the lower sphincter, visible on manometry testing (a series of tests to determine the muscle contractions in the esophagus). You may also need radionuclide transit studies, which can help determine the stage of the disease.

What is it? Many people who suffer from the connective tissue disorder scleroderma (see page 643) also experience problems in the esophagus—particularly, reflux. This is what happens: Over time, the smooth muscle tissue in the lower esophagus loses its tone and ability to contract; the nerves in this area often become impaired, as well, and the lower esophageal sphincter (LES) is unable to keep the stomach's harsh juices out of the esophagus.

What you can do People with scleroderma are more likely than most to develop complications (particularly, an esophageal stricture, or abnormal narrowing, see page 975) if the level of acid in the esophagus is not controlled. Thus, it is important to work with your doctor to get reflux under control.

When to call the doctor If you are experiencing severe pain, or if you are unable to eat and are losing weight, contact your doctor. Waiting to seek help can lead to malnourishment or dehydration.

Treatment Unfortunately, there currently is no way to treat the underlying problem— the scleroderma affecting your whole body—and reverse the muscle deterioration in the esophagus. Thus, therapy is aimed at easing the symptoms by treating reflux (see Gastroesophageal Reflux Disease, page 969).

❖ CANCER OF THE ESOPHAGUS

Symptoms *(What you may experience)* Difficult or painful swallowing; weight loss; a feeling that food is becoming stuck on the way down (particularly in the area between

OTHER DIAGNOSTIC TESTS OF THE GASTROINTESTINAL TRACT

Because the symptoms for many conditions involving the gastrointestinal tract are similar, several diagnostic tests may be necessary to determine the cause. Some commonly performed tests are covered here (see also Upper Endoscopy, page 968, Flexible Sigmoidoscopy, page 1006, Colonoscopy, page 1011, and Barium Studies, page 976).

Often, the starting point is the blood—tests, for example, to determine whether anemia (caused by internal bleeding) is present. (For more information, see The Complete Blood Count, page 915).

Stool Blood Tests There are many tests (such as Hemoccult) designed to detect the presence of hidden blood in the stool, including some for home use. In the most commonly used tests, you or a doctor place a thin smear of stool on a chemically treated card, which is then sent to a laboratory for chemical analysis. Many physicians recommend beginning yearly blood stool testing in people at normal risk of developing colon cancer (those without a personal or family history of polyps or cancer; see Colorectal Cancer, page 1022) at age 50. These tests can be valuable; but keep in mind that having blood in your stool does not necessarily mean that you have cancer. Many people have gastrointestinal bleeding, caused by a host of problems including hemorrhoids and ulcers. However, any blood in the stool should be investigated with flexible sigmoidoscopy, colonoscopy, anoscopy, or barium enema studies to determine the cause.

Anoscopy The purpose of this brief procedure, which may be performed by a family practitioner, internist, gastroenterologist, or proctologist, is to examine the anus. The doctor inserts a lubricated, funnel-shaped tool into the anus, and then removes the tool's core, called an obturator, leaving the tubular shell in place for a few minutes. Anoscopy is helpful in diagnosing conditions of the anus and rectum, including hemorrhoids, fistulas, and fissures.

X-ray Fistulography In this brief procedure, a radiologist injects dye, using a needle or catheter, into a fistula (see Anal Abscess and Fistula, page 1027) and uses x-ray pictures to determine its exact path.

Anorectal Manometry This test uses balloons, inserted into the anus, to measure pressures in the internal and external anal sphincters and in the rectum. Anorectal manometry, performed by a gastroenterologist, can be useful in diagnosing irritable bowel syndrome and in determining the cause of fecal incontinence.

Angiography An angiogram, performed by a radiologist, involves a dye that x-rays cannot penetrate; thus, the passage of dye through the body can be seen on an x-ray. The dye, usually injected through a catheter threaded into the groin, is guided into the arteries that feed the gastrointestinal tract: the celiac artery, the superior mesenteric artery, and the inferior mesenteric artery. Some people have an allergic reaction to this dye; if you are allergic to iodine or shellfish, tell your doctor. This test can help determine the cause and course of gastrointestinal bleeding; it may also be used to show ischemia—an area where blood flow is shut off—in the bowel; and it can be helpful in staging pancreatic cancer.

Computed Tomography Scan A computed tomography (CT) scan is a painless, noninvasive series of circular x-ray pictures, done with you lying on your back, photographed by a machine that encircles the body like a giant tube. Individually, these images are thin slices of anatomy; but together—in a computer-generated compilation—they create a comprehensive view of the body. These pictures are usually enhanced by the use of a high-contrast dye, which may be given orally, rectally, or intravenously. Some people have an allergic reaction to this dye; if ▶

the middle of the chest and stomach); regurgitation (including spitting up or vomiting blood); choking (coughing or gagging because food goes down the wrong pipe); hoarseness, frequent or lengthy bouts of hiccups. Another symptom is chest pain, which may be chronic, may occur during eating or drinking, or may be more noticeable when you eat certain foods (particularly, citrus juices or alcohol). Unfortunately, for many people, early symptoms are silent, masked by excellent compensatory techniques: Someone may simply chew food more completely before swallowing, for example, or drink more water with meals to wash food down, or change the diet to avoid such hard-to-digest foods as breads, meats, raw apples, and carrots.

Signs and laboratory findings (*What the doctor looks for*) Evidence of any irregular tissue, mass, or obstruction, as seen on a barium swallow test (see Barium Studies, page 976) or endoscopy and confirmed by a biopsy, taken during endoscopy (see Upper Endoscopy, page 968).

What is it? Esophageal cancer is malignant cell growth of the lining of the esophagus. It can be caused by many factors including tobacco, alcohol, or a diet rich in nitrates (found in hot dogs, pepperoni, and other meats); ingesting a caustic agent such as lye; or radiation therapy for another disease. Achalasia (see page 972) and Barrett's esophagus (see Gastroesophageal Reflux Disease, page 969) are also associated with the development of esophageal cancer. There also may be a genetic component; rarely, cancer of the esophagus can run in families.

you are allergic to iodine or shellfish, tell your doctor. The scan can still be done, but it may not be as sensitive. CT scans of the gastrointestinal tract and abdominal organs may be helpful in diagnosing unexplained weight loss or pain, or palpable masses detected during a physical exam that cannot be seen with a scope (such as a colonoscope). The CT tube is not as small as the magnetic resonance imaging (MRI) machine, and claustrophobia is usually not a problem. The CT scan is also faster, lasting around 15 to 30 minutes; newer models only take several minutes.

Magnetic Resonance Imaging Like a CT scan, an MRI is a painless, noninvasive series of circular pictures that produces a comprehensive image of the body. These images—thin slices of anatomy assembled by a computer into cohesive pictures—may be helpful in diagnosing unexplained weight loss or pain, or palpable masses detected during a physical exam that cannot be seen with a scope (such as a colonoscope). The MRI procedure takes an average of 45 minutes and is done with you lying completely still, on your back. One drawback for many patients is the machine itself; the tube is small, and this can produce claustrophobia. Some hospitals offer sedatives, play soothing music, or even show videos in an attempt to help patients relax.

Ultrasound Ultrasound, also a painless, noninvasive process, makes pictures using high-frequency sound waves, like sonar on a submarine. It may be performed from the outside, through the abdomen, or from inside the body, using a probe inserted in the rectum (this is called transrectal ultrasound) or attached to an endoscope. Ultrasound can be helpful in diagnosing gallstones, pancreatitis, and gynecologic problems, and in guiding a biopsy of the liver and/or pancreas.

Esophageal Motility Test Usually performed by a gastroenterologist, this test is designed to detect abnormal muscle contractions in the esophagus. A doctor threads pressure-measuring tubes (usually via the nose) down the throat and into the esophagus and then measures the pressures in the esophagus and lower esophageal sphincter while you swallow. An esophageal motility test is useful in diagnosing or evaluating chest pain that is not caused by the heart (called noncardiac chest pain), such as that produced by esophageal spasm or reflux.

pH Probe In this test, a tiny electrode is threaded through the nose into the esophagus, and you wear a special recorder (about the size of a Sony Walkman), usually for 24 hours. The monitor records the number and duration of episodes in which the pH level in the esophagus is abnormal (when it drops lower than 4), reflecting a reflux of acid into your esophagus. Your job is to push a button whenever you feel pain; your doctor will examine the data and correlate your symptoms with the rise and fall of acid.

Bleeding Scan This abdominal scan, performed by a radiologist, is used when someone has bleeding somewhere within the gastrointestinal tract, but doctors are unable to pinpoint its source. A small amount of your blood is removed, mixed with a radioactive tracer—which causes your red blood cells to make an image that glows on an x-ray—and then injected back into your body. This test requires a certain minimal amount of bleeding; otherwise, the tracer cannot be seen. If your gastrointestinal bleeding is a slow trickle or an ooze, this test might be negative.

Bernstein Test This test is used to determine whether chest pain is originating in the esophagus. A gastroenterologist threads a thin tube through your nose, drips solution through it, and asks if you feel any pain. The key is that two kinds of solution are used: One is a benign saline solution, a placebo; the other contains acid, and you are not told which is which. If your pain corresponds to the presence of the acid-containing solution, you may have esophagitis, usually from gastroesophageal reflux disease. ■

What you can do You can help minimize your chances of developing esophageal cancer—or having a recurrence of it—by removing as many risk factors as you can find in your diet and lifestyle. If you smoke or drink alcohol excessively, now is the time to stop. See Chapter 4 for information on quitting smoking; see Chapter 5 for information on cutting down alcohol use.

When to call the doctor If you are vomiting or spitting up blood, call your doctor immediately. Also call if you have noticed persistent or recurrent trouble swallowing—even if you are able to dislodge any food that gets stuck in the esophagus by yourself. Too often, people ignore swallowing difficulties, and the cancer is diagnosed after it has spread beyond the esophagus. Successful treatment depends on early diagnosis.

Treatment This depends largely on the stage at which the cancer is diagnosed. If it is localized, you will probably undergo surgery to remove the tumor; you may undergo radiation therapy, as well. If it is considered inoperable, your doctor may recommend chemotherapy or radiation, and/or laser therapy or a stent (a tube inserted in the esophagus) to keep the esophagus open, so food can get down. These procedures may relieve your symptoms but, unfortunately, will not cure the cancer. (For more information on the treatment of cancer, see Chapter 30.)

Prognosis Because advanced esophageal cancer is usually not curable, early detection is critical. Thus, it is essential to have any swallowing difficulties investigated promptly by a doctor.

THE STOMACH

The stomach, hollow and muscle-bound, is a huge reservoir, a storehouse where food and liquid—in most adults, about 1½ L at a time—can linger for several hours. Fat and protein content help determine how long food stays in the stomach; movement of food is also orchestrated by an elaborate network of nerves, triggered when the stomach stretches to make room for food.

When food, squeezed through the esophagus by waves of muscle contractions, reaches the stomach, its powerful walls begin to churn. Mixing in its own harsh gastric juices, the stomach grinds the food from bite-sized chunks into a mushy pulp (called chyme) that can trickle through a gate of muscle called the pylorus into the small intestine, where most of the nutrients are absorbed into the body.

The stomach is in some ways a misunderstood organ. Many people believe food is entirely digested here and that the intestine's job is simply to handle excretion. Not so; in fact, the stomach is not essential to life. In the process of digestion, it is the intestines that do the lion's share of the work. However, the stomach does make eating much more comfortable: Its holding capacity makes it possible for you to eat meal-sized portions. Without it—if food traveled directly from the esophagus to the intestine—you could digest only tiny amounts at a time.

The stomach's wrinkled mucous membrane lining—pitted with openings so the gastric, or digestive, juices can seep through—resembles the surface of a sponge. Most of the time, this lining is remarkably resistant to the formidable components of these juices, particularly, to hydrochloric acid, toxic as the acid in a car battery, which ultimately involves an enzyme called pepsin. Pepsin, in turn, begins digesting protein. The most common disorders of the stomach, including gastritis and peptic ulcer disease, occur when stomach acid succeeds in penetrating the lining, causing painful craters and erosions that may bleed.

The stomach, like other organs in the digestive system, also manufactures its own chemical regulators: One of the most important of these is the hormone gastrin (made in the antrum, or curved base of the stomach), which stimulates acid production. In Zollinger-Ellison syndrome, the regulation process goes awry as a tumor mass-produces gastrin in uncontrolled amounts, stimulating excessive production of hydrochloric acid, which overwhelms the stomach lining and causes devastating ulcers and erosions.

❖ PEPTIC ULCER DISEASE

Symptoms *(What you may experience)* Stomach pain, burning, or a gnawing feeling, usually in the middle of the night or between meals (when your stomach is empty), which may be relieved when you take antacids or eat something (however, in some people, these symptoms may become worse with food); pain in the chest or upper abdomen—particularly, pain that wakes you up in the middle of the night; blood in the stool; black, tarlike stool (melena), or maroon-colored stool; nausea; vomiting (this may appear as a bland, mucousy liquid, may have blood or digested blood, and may resemble coffee grounds).

Signs and laboratory findings *(What the doctor looks for)* Tenderness or extreme

The stomach is a large reservoir for food, which can remain in the stomach and be digested for several hours. Food then passes through the pylorus into the small intestine, where many nutrients are absorbed into the body. Food travels from the small intestine into the large intestine (colon), where it is concentrated. Finally, the processed material exits the body through the rectum and anus.

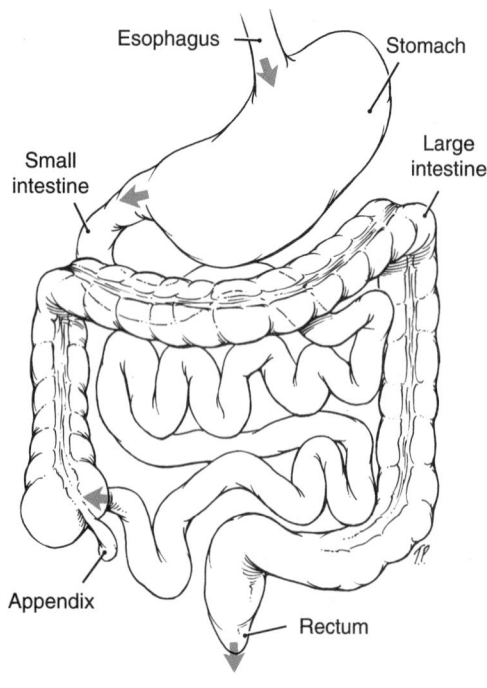

Esophagus

Stomach

Small intestine

Large intestine

Appendix

Rectum

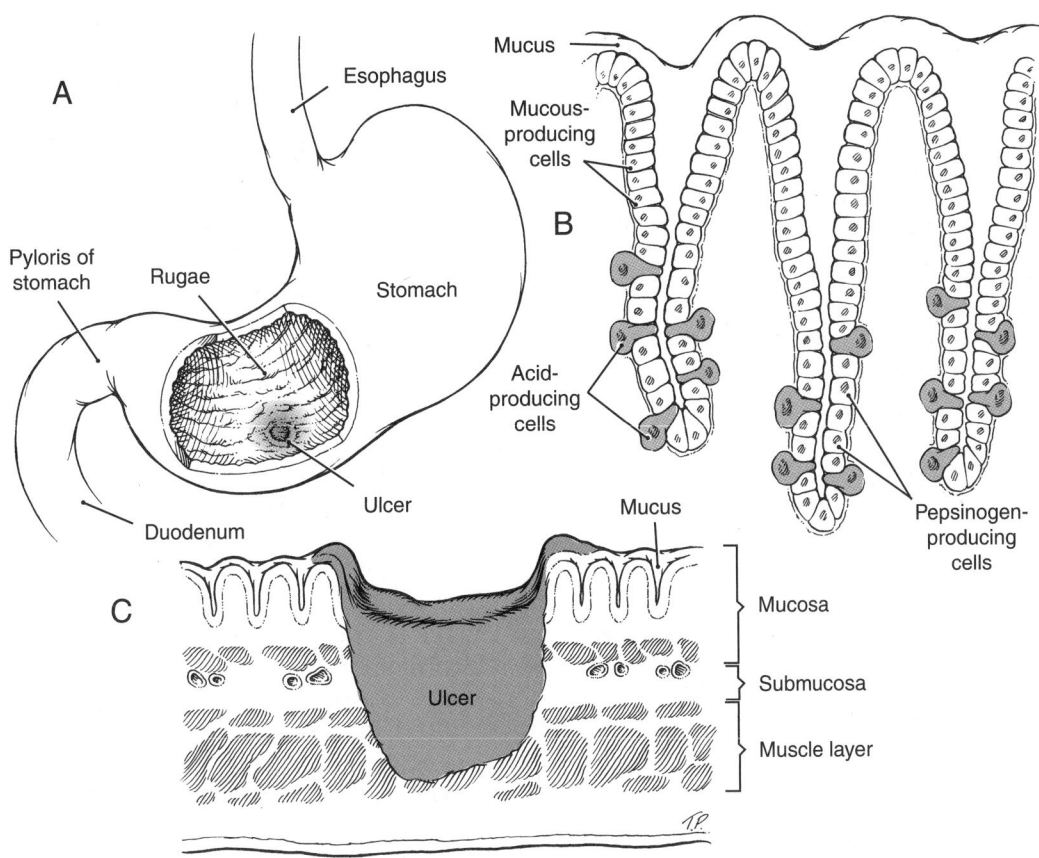

A peptic ulcer is a crater in the lining of the stomach or duodenum (the first part of the small intestine). Ulcers cannot form or be maintained without an acidic environment. (A) A typical site of a gastric (stomach) ulcer is shown. Rugae are folds that normally exist in the stomach's mucous membrane. (B) There are three main types of gastric glands: mucus-secreting cells, hydrochloric acid-secreting cells, and pepsin-secreting cells. Pepsin cleaves proteins from food into smaller pieces. (C) Breakdown of the mucus lining produced by the mucus-secreting cells can lead to ulcers; this type of damage may be caused by the presence of *Helicobacter pylori* bacteria or by nonsteroidal anti-inflammatory drugs, such as ibuprofen, naproxen, and aspirin. An ulcer that extends completely through the mucosa, submucosa, and muscle layers can perforate the stomach and cause its contents to leak into the abdominal cavity.

tenderness of the abdomen or stomach in a physical exam; rebound tenderness (when a doctor presses on the stomach, and pain comes immediately afterward, as the doctor's hand is lifted). Extreme or rebound tenderness could be a sign of a perforated ulcer, which could mean peritonitis and is a surgical emergency. Microscopic or visible blood in the stool (which could suggest that the ulcer is bleeding); whitish craters, which may have blood or blood clots in the center, in the normally pink lining of the stomach, as seen in endoscopy; or the shadow of a crater in an upper GI series. If your doctor suspects that you may have a bleeding ulcer, you will probably need an endoscopy; if you have pain alone, with no blood in the stool, an upper GI series may be sufficient for diagnosis (see Upper Endoscopy, page 968, and Barium Studies, page 976). Your doctor will also check for the presence of *Helicobacter pylori* (see page 988), either with a biopsy done during endoscopy, or a blood test. If you have recurrent ulcers, your doctor may check your blood for elevated gastrin levels, which may suggest Zollinger-Ellison syndrome, also known as gastrinoma (see Zollinger-Ellison Syndrome (Gastrinoma), page 991).

What is it? A peptic ulcer is a painful crater in the lining of the stomach or duodenum. Stomach acid plays a crucial role in its development: Without acid, ulcers cannot form or be sustained. Normally, thick, buffering layers of mucus cover the mucosal lining of the stomach, making it impervious to its own acid. But nonsteroidal anti-inflammatory drugs (NSAIDs, common pain relievers such as aspirin, ibuprofen [Advil], or naproxen [Naprosyn] can disrupt these natural defenses; so can a form of bacteria called *Helicobacter pylori* (*H. pylori*, also called HP). These two culprits—not stress or dietary indiscretions, which for decades were widely considered to be the major instigators—are the main risk factors for peptic ulcer. Peptic ulcers are extremely common: An estimated 4 million Americans have an ulcer in the stomach (called a gastric ulcer) or duodenum; duodenal ulcers, which are almost always benign, are four times as common as gastric ulcers. This year alone, about 350,000 new cases will be diagnosed—mostly in people between age 55 and 65.

If a gastric ulcer is found, your gastroenterologist should perform a biopsy during endoscopy (see Upper Endoscopy, page 968); gastric cancer often appears indistinguishable from a benign ulcer. If a duodenal ulcer is diagnosed, you probably will not need a biopsy; ulcers that form here are rarely cancerous.

What you can do Avoid or limit your use of most NSAIDs; you may want to use acetaminophen, which is not an NSAID, for pain. If you are taking a daily aspirin, make sure that it is the kind that dissolves in the intestine, not the stomach (enteric coated). Talk to your doctor about switching to baby aspirin, or taking it with meals. Avoid alcoholic beverages and cigarettes, which can make symptoms worse, delay or prevent healing, and even cause recurrent ulcers. If you are taking potassium or iron supplements—which may irritate the stomach's lining—ask your doctor if you can take these pills differently, or take a different form of the medication (one that dissolves in the small intestine, rather than the stomach).

When to call the doctor Call your doctor immediately if you are vomiting blood or material that resembles coffee grounds (this is blood coagulated by stomach acid); if you have black, tarlike stool, maroon stool, or bright red blood coming from your rectum; if you have severe abdominal pain, if you cannot keep down food or drink and are at risk of becoming dehydrated or malnourished.

Some medications, including iron-rich vitamins, prenatal vitamins, bismuth subsalicylate (Pepto-Bismol), and charcoal, can result in black stool that is otherwise normal and does not require medical attention.

Treatment Medication If you are diagnosed with *H. pylori* infection, you will probably be given several medications: a regimen of bacteria-killing antibiotics, plus H_2 blockers or proton pump inhibitors—many of the same medications used to block acid in gastroesophageal reflux disease (GERD)—to reduce or stop acid production and help the ulcer heal.

Antibiotics for *H. pylori* may include a combination of metronidazole (Flagyl), clarithromycin (Biaxin), and Pepto-Bismol. As with any antibiotic, take every pill; do not stop when your symptoms get better, because you risk creating a drug-resistant strain of bacteria, having a prolonged or recurrent illness, and making this problem harder to treat.

H_2 blockers cause the stomach to make less acid by blocking histamine receptors and may include prescription-strength doses of cimetidine (Tagamet), ranitidine (Zantac), famotidine (Pepcid), or nizatidine (Axid). Proton pump inhibitors, which selectively disable the pump in acid-making cells—thus stopping acid production completely—are more powerful and include omeprazole (Prilosec) and lansoprazole (Prevacid). You may also be given sucralfate (Carafate), a modified, prescription-strength antacid that coats the stomach, binds to the ulcer crater, and promotes healing.

About 8 weeks after your course of therapy, your doctor should perform a repeat endoscopy, to make sure the gastric ulcer has healed (and to confirm that gastric cancer is not present). If you have a duodenal ulcer, a repeat endoscopy is not necessary unless your symptoms persist. It is possible, although generally not recommended, to use over-the-counter antacids to fight peptic ulcer disease. Because huge doses are needed in order to match the prescription-strength versions of these medications and the treatment of accompanying *H. pylori* infection is essential to prevent recurrence, this is not a practical option for most people.

Surgery Fortunately, current medical therapy is so effective that ulcer surgery is increasingly rare. However, depending on the location and extent of the ulcer, you

ULCERS AND THE *H. PYLORI* REVOLUTION

Don't worry too much—you'll get an ulcer.

Even as late as the 1980s, common knowledge held that ulcers were caused by stress. This view was so entrenched that when Barry Marshall, a young Australian doctor, put forth a radical new idea—that most ulcers were instead caused by a simple, whirlygig-shaped bacterium—the medical establishment ridiculed him. Few believed that bacteria could survive in the inhospitable, acid-soaked environment of the stomach.

The notion was dismissed as absurd until Marshall, fed up with the naysaying and convinced that the bacterium—which he named *Helicobacter pylori* after the helicopter shape—was to blame, tested his theory on himself. He swallowed a walloping dose of *H. pylori*, got sick, and, just as he had expected, developed an ulcer. Then he cured himself with a regimen of antibiotics and bismuth (found in Pepto-Bismol) and changed the course of ulcer treatment worldwide.

Now, thanks to Marshall, most people with duodenal and gastric ulcers can be cured by one of several multidrug regimens, including omeprazole and clarithromycin; ranitidine bismuth citrate plus clarithromycin; or bismuth, metronidazole, tetracycline, and an H_2 blocker. Some newly tested drug combinations, involving two antibiotics and omeprazole, lansoprazole, or ranitidine bismuth citrate (all taken for 2 weeks), may be even more effective and may also lower the risk of developing antibiotic resistance. *H. pylori* cannot be eradicated in a few days, and some strains of it are more virulent than others. To avoid a chronic or recurrent infection, it is necessary to take every last pill of the drugs prescribed.

Scientists now believe that half of the world's population is colonized with *H. pylori* and that infection with this bacteria probably happens in childhood. However, why ulcers eventually develop in only some of these people remains unknown. ∎

---

may need surgery—elective or emergent—in addition to the medications listed on page 988. Your doctor may remove the ulcer altogether, or oversew it with a patch of tissue taken from another part of the intestine. If your ulcer is bleeding, it may be necessary to stop blood loss by tying off the bleeding artery. Another surgical option involves cutting the nerve supply to the antrum (the base of the stomach). This procedure lowers gastrin production and lowers acid production but does not affect your body's ability to absorb or digest food. Sometimes, it is necessary to remove the antrum entirely and connect the main body of the stomach directly to the small intestine.

Prognosis Excellent, thanks to better medications—particularly, therapy for *H. pylori*, along with proton pump inhibitors and H_2 blockers, for protection from further acid injury and healing. Not so long ago, peptic ulcer was a recurrent disease that could plague someone for years or even a lifetime. Now, for most people, eradicating *H. pylori* is sufficient to cure the ulcer disease.

GASTRITIS

Gastritis is irritation, inflammation, or erosion of the lining of the stomach. (Most medical terms ending in *itis* indicate inflammation.) It may be caused by many factors, including medications such as NSAIDs; severe injury elsewhere (for reasons not entirely understood, trauma, such as a bad burn, or serious illness can affect the digestive tract); *H. pylori* infection; an autoimmune disease (such as pernicious anemia); Crohn's disease; and even some allergies. In general, gastritis is divided into two categories: erosive, in which the stomach's lining is abraded—like a skinned knee—and perhaps also bleeding, and nonerosive, in which the stomach can appear deceptively normal in endoscopy and biopsy is needed to help pinpoint the source of the problem.

❖ EROSIVE GASTRITIS

Symptoms *(What you may experience)* Stomach pain; recurrent upset stomach; burning, or a gnawing feeling, usually in the middle of the night or between meals, when your stomach is empty (which may be relieved when you eat something, or—as with peptic ulcer disease—these symptoms could become worse with food); blood in the stool (rarely). In some people, however, erosive gastritis is silent, producing no symptoms.

Signs and laboratory findings *(What the doctor looks for)* Erosions, tiny hemorrhages—about as big as the head of a pin—which may give the stomach's lining a moth-eaten appearance on upper endoscopy (see Upper Endoscopy, page 968). An upper GI series, which shows only shadows, is not as sensitive a test for erosive gastritis and may miss this condition.

What is it? Erosive gastritis is usually less severe than peptic ulcer disease, even though it shares many symptoms and responds to many of the same medications.

The distinction between an erosion and an ulcer is the depth of tissue invasion. Although the symptoms can be markedly similar, erosions are more superficial and do not tend to involve the deeper big blood vessels that can cause significant bleeding. Gastritis can be a chronic problem or, depending on its cause, can last only a few days. As with peptic ulcer disease, stomach acid can cause these erosions and prevent healing. Gastritis can, in fact, be a precursor to ulcer in some people.

What you can do   These are the same steps as for preventing peptic ulcers: Avoid or limit your use of most NSAIDs. Acetaminophen (Tylenol), which is not an NSAID, does not harm the stomach. If you are taking a daily aspirin, talk to your doctor about switching to baby aspirin, enteric-coated aspirin, or taking it with meals. Avoid alcoholic beverages and cigarettes, which can make symptoms worse, delay or prevent healing, and even cause new ulcers. If you are taking potassium or iron supplements—which may irritate the stomach's lining—ask your doctor if you can take these pills differently or take a different form of the medication (one that dissolves in the small intestine, rather than the stomach).

When to call the doctor   If the symptoms last more than a few days, call your doctor.

Treatment   If *H. pylori* is the cause, the first step will be a regimen of antibiotics to eradicate the bacterium, taken together with antacid medications. As with any antibiotic, take every pill; do not stop when your symptoms get better, because you risk creating a drug-resistant strain of bacteria, having a prolonged or recurrent illness, and making this problem harder to treat.

You will probably be given several antibiotics, which may include metronidazole and clarithromycin, and bismuth subsalicylate (Pepto-Bismol)—plus an H_2 blocker or proton pump inhibitor. These are the same medications used to block acid in peptic ulcer disease and GERD; they work by reducing or eliminating acid production, protecting the inflamed lining from further injury and promoting healing. H_2 blockers,

which cause the stomach to make less acid by blocking histamine receptors, may include prescription-strength doses of cimetidine, ranitidine, famotidine, or nizatidine. Proton pump inhibitors, which selectively disable the pump in acid-making cells— thus stopping acid production completely—are more powerful and include omeprazole and lansoprazole. You may also be given sucralfate, a modified antacid that coats and soothes the lining and promotes healing.

Prognosis   With treatment, excellent.

❖ NONEROSIVE GASTRITIS

Symptoms (What you may experience)   Stomach pain; recurrent upset stomach; burning or a gnawing feeling, usually in the middle of the night or between meals, when your stomach is empty (which may be relieved when you eat something or—as with peptic ulcer disease—these symptoms could become worse with food); blood in the stool (rarely). In some people, however, nonerosive gastritis is silent, producing no symptoms.

Signs and laboratory findings (*What the doctor looks for*)   Redness, irritation, or inflammation, but no erosions visible in endoscopy (see Upper Endoscopy, page 968). However, in many people with nonerosive gastritis, the lining of the stomach appears perfectly normal, and a biopsy is needed to make the diagnosis. The presence of *H. pylori*, as seen on biopsy or found on an antibody blood test; evidence of pernicious anemia elsewhere in the body (vitamin B_{12} deficiency, suggested by a blood smear, or measured directly in a blood test). Lack of stomach acid in the gastric secretions, as measured in endoscopy (in pernicious anemia, the acid-producing cells atrophy).

What is it?   Nonerosive gastritis is irritation or inflammation of the lining of the stomach, but here, the damage to the lining is microscopic, as compared to the more obvious, moth-eaten appearance of erosive gastritis. In fact, the hallmark of this problem is the lack of erosion or any visible break in the lining of the stomach, even though the symptoms may be the same as those of erosive gastritis. Microscopic examination of a tissue sample (a biopsy taken during endoscopy, see Upper Endoscopy, page 968) reveals the presence of inflammatory cells, showing an immune system response to something: The range of causes may include Crohn's disease, syphilis, pernicious anemia, or even a reaction to certain medications.

Treatment If the problem is caused by *H. pylori* infection, you will need a regimen of antibiotics, probably accompanied by an H_2 blocker or proton pump inhibitor to limit or stop acid production and give the irritation a chance to heal (see Treatment for Erosive Gastritis, page 989). If the underlying trouble is pernicious anemia, you will need a lifetime of vitamin B_{12} injections for replacement therapy (see Pernicious Anemia, page 924).

Prognosis This, too, depends on the underlying cause of gastritis: If it is *H. pylori*, symptoms should go away as the infection is eradicated. If the cause is pernicious anemia, you will need vitamin B_{12} replacement therapy throughout the course of your life.

❖ ZOLLINGER-ELLISON SYNDROME (GASTRINOMA)

Symptoms *(What you may experience)* Diarrhea, which may persist for years. The symptoms of acid hypersecretion, or too much acid in the stomach and esophagus, which may include stomach pain, burning, or a gnawing feeling, usually in the middle of the night or between meals (when your stomach is empty), which may be relieved when you eat something (however, in some people, these symptoms may become worse with food); diarrhea, blood in the stool; black, tarlike stool, or maroon-colored stool; nausea; vomiting (this may appear as a bland, mucousy liquid, it may be bloody or have digested blood, which resembles coffee grounds). Heartburn, pain in the chest or upper abdomen, regurgitation (vomiting, belching acid), difficulty swallowing, chronic sour or bitter taste, frequent bursts of salty-tasting saliva, hoarseness, sore throat, cough, wheezing.

Signs and laboratory findings *(What the doctor looks for)* Evidence of malabsorption (see Malabsorption Syndromes, page 995); history of recurrent ulcers, ulcers that are resistant to treatment, ulcers in unusual combinations—in both the duodenum and stomach, as seen on endoscopy (see Upper Endoscopy, page 968)—or in unusual locations, such as in the distal duodenum. Elevated levels of gastrin in the blood and acid in the stomach (tested after you have fasted overnight). Your doctor may perform a secretin stimulation test, with an intravenous or intramuscular injection of the hormone secretin (which stimulates gastrin production in patients with Zollinger-Ellison syndrome), followed by a blood test.

What is it? Zollinger-Ellison syndrome, a rare condition, may incorporate symptoms of ulcers (see Peptic Ulcer Disease, page 986), malabsorption (see Malabsorption Syndromes, page 995), or GERD (see Gastroesophageal Reflux Disease, page 969). It is caused by a tumor that produces the hormone gastrin, which normally controls acid production. This tumor (called gastrinoma) or tumors usually appears in the pancreas but may also be seen in the stomach, liver, duodenum, or ovaries. Finding the tumor is an important first step in treatment. Equally important is determining—through imaging studies that may include computed tomography (CT) scan and magnetic resonance imaging (MRI)—whether the tumor is a primary tumor, secondary tumor, or metastasis—an offshoot or satellite of a tumor that originated elsewhere. Complicating the diagnosis is that Zollinger-Ellison syndrome itself may be part of a larger disorder called multiple endocrine neoplasia-I, an inherited condition involving additional tumors of the pituitary gland and parathyroid (see Multiple Endocrine Neoplasia Syndrome, page 1199). It is unclear what causes Zollinger-Ellison syndrome, although a genetic link is suspected, and a strong family history of peptic ulcer, or a personal or family history of parathyroid or pituitary tumors may increase the risk. There is no means of prevention, though early diagnosis and treatment may prevent metastatic spread of the gastrinoma.

What you can do For more than one-third of patients, unexplained chronic or recurrent diarrhea is the sole symptom and may precede ulcer symptoms *by as much as 8 years*. This is an important, early window of opportunity for cure. If you have persistent diarrhea, discuss the possibility of Zollinger-

Ellison syndrome with your doctor at once. In this serious disease, early diagnosis is critical. Also, familiarize yourself with your family history (see page 991), and tell your doctor about a family history of peptic ulcer disease, parathyroid cancer, or pituitary cancer. Finally, it is essential to find the most skillful, experienced surgeon available (see Choosing a Surgeon, page 1429).

Treatment This may vary considerably, depending on the nature and extent of the problem. First, thanks to proton pump inhibitors (see discussion in Treatment of Peptic Ulcer Disease, page 988), there is excellent medical therapy to relieve symptoms and heal ulcers. You will probably need to take this medication throughout the course of your life if the gastrinoma cannot be surgically removed; patients with Zollinger-Ellison syndrome who discontinue treatment tend to suffer severe complications from the rebound of acid production, including aggressive recurrence of ulcers, hemorrhage, or even perforation—when an ulcer is so deep that it creates a hole in the stomach. By eliminating stomach acid, proton pump inhibitors allow the ulcers to heal and prevent new ones from forming.

However, these medications treat only the symptoms and do not address the cause of the ulcers: the gastrin-making tumor or tumors. The definitive treatment is surgery: Finding and removing this tumor—as early as possible, before it has a chance to spread—can cure Zollinger-Ellison syndrome. Unfortunately, a very small tumor can make a large amount of gastrin, and even with the latest technology, these tumors can be difficult to locate. Thus, an experienced surgeon at a major medical center is the best hope for cure. Afterward, your blood gastrin level will be monitored to gauge the success of the surgery.

Total gastrectomy, or removal of the stomach, can prevent complications by ending acid secretion but is rarely necessary these days, because of proton pump inhibitors. It may be necessary to remove part of the pancreas, intestines, liver, or duodenum to cure the disease. Surgery is not recommended for people with multiple endocrine neoplasia-I, with extensive metastases, or whose general health is considered too frail to endure the rigors of a major procedure. If you have metastatic disease, you may also be given chemotherapy, which has been found to shrink tumor size, improve symptoms, and prolong life.

❖ GASTRIC (STOMACH) CANCER

Symptoms *(What you may experience)* Loss of appetite; weight loss; feeling full after eating very little; experiencing pain when you eat; recurrent indigestion; blood in the stool; black, tarlike stool; vomiting or vomiting blood; fatigue; malaise. Many people with stomach cancer experience no symptoms at all.

Signs and laboratory findings *(What the doctor looks for)* Blood in the stool, unexplained iron-deficiency anemia; the presence of an ulcer (which can appear indistinguishable from stomach cancer) in endoscopy or an upper GI series; an ulcer that does not heal after 8 weeks of treatment (with the medications discussed in Peptic Ulcer Disease, page 986). Malignant cells, found in a biopsy and/or brushing of tissue during endoscopy (see Upper Endoscopy, page 968). If cancer is found, you may also need a CT scan to check for metastases (cancer cells that have spread elsewhere) and/or fluid in the abdomen.

What is it? Gastric cancer is a malignant tumor arising from the lining of the stomach; like an ulcer, it may bleed. An estimated 20,000 to 25,000 new cases are diagnosed in the United States each year; the disease is more common in men than women. Fortunately, there has been a fourfold decrease in the incidence of stomach cancer over the last 50 years—probably attributable to better diet.

There is an environmental component to stomach cancer: In Japan, it is the most common cancer, affecting 1 of every 1,000 people. Interestingly, when Japanese people move to the United States, their risk of developing stomach cancer drops significantly. Also, it occurs more commonly in countries with a high consumption of smoked fish and meat. A number of conditions can increase the risk of stomach cancer, including gastritis, pernicious anemia, gastric polyps, and gastric ulcer. The triggering factor in many cases seems to be an initial injury to the stomach's mucosal lining, either from illness; repeated exposure to aspirin, alcohol, nitrates in food (excessive exposure to such foods as hot dogs and lunch meat); infection (with bacteria including *H. pylori*); and ironically, even previous stomach surgery.

Treatment Surgery—gastrectomy, removal of part or all of the stomach—can cure the disease, if caught in time. If the disease is diagnosed early, before it reaches the lymph nodes, and before it invades the layer of muscle beneath the lining of the stomach—or spreads elsewhere—the disease is curable in as many as 90 percent of people. Depending on the location and extent of the tumor, your surgeon may need to remove at least half of your stomach. In some patients, the lymph nodes adjacent to the stomach are removed, as well.

If you have a more advanced tumor or metastatic cancer, you may need radiation therapy to provide symptomatic relief. If the tumor is hampering your ability to eat and drink, you may also need a feeding tube to prevent malnutrition and dehydration (see Nutritional Supplementation and Feeding Tubes, page 1000). Currently, the idea of neoadjuvant chemotherapy—given at the time of surgery, as it is in breast cancer—is being investigated as a promising means of treatment. See Chapter 30 for more information on the treatment of cancer.

Prognosis This depends on the stage at which the cancer is diagnosed. The likelihood of a cure is best (see above) when the cancer is diagnosed early, before penetrating beneath the lining of the stomach, reaching the lymph nodes, or spreading elsewhere. Unfortunately, most people with gastric cancer are diagnosed with positive lymph nodes, distant metastases, and local extension of the tumor. At that stage, the 5-year survival rate is less than 20 percent. Thus, early diagnosis is essential. If you have any of the symptoms or any of the risk factors discussed in What Is It?, page 992, contact your doctor for a complete physical.

THE BOWEL: SMALL INTESTINE AND COLON

The small intestine is a loosely coiled tube, about 1 in. in diameter, and stretching to more than 20 feet. The small intestine absorbs nutrients, including vitamins and minerals, from all you eat and drink. The small intestine is remarkably efficient. Its absorbing powers are maximized by countless fingerlike projections, called villi, which carpet the intestinal lining. Each of these undulating villi, in turn, has its own microvilli, giving the small intestine, in effect, functional space the size of a tennis court.

The small bowel (doctors tend to use the words *bowel* and *intestine* interchangeably) has three segments: the duodenum, jejunum, and ileum.

The duodenum is short, only about a foot long (the name is Latin for "twelve fingers"). It secretes bicarbonate, the active ingredient in baking soda, which buffers the stomach's harsh acids. Iron and other minerals are absorbed in the duodenum. In addition, bile, made by the liver, plays its role here: Like a powerful detergent, bile renders fats into digestible, microscopic fragments. The pancreas also secretes its enzyme-rich fluid into the duodenum, to help the body absorb these fats. The jejunum, about 8 feet long, handles the main business of absorbing most nutrients. Proteins, sugars, vitamins, and minerals are absorbed here. In the ileum, about 12 feet long, vitamin B_{12} and bile salts (fat-attacking detergents made by the liver, released into the duodenum, and then recycled to be used again) are absorbed. The ileum joins the colon at the cecum (pronounced "sea-come"), its widest part. Thus, with the aid of the food-dissolving juices from the liver and pancreas mixed with its own secretions, the intestine kneads and pushes food onward, until all of the digested nutrients are absorbed through its walls.

The colon, also called the large intestine or large bowel, is about 6 feet long; it connects the small intestine with the rectum and anus. It's major job is to remove salts and water, a process that may take several days, from what is left of the food—which,

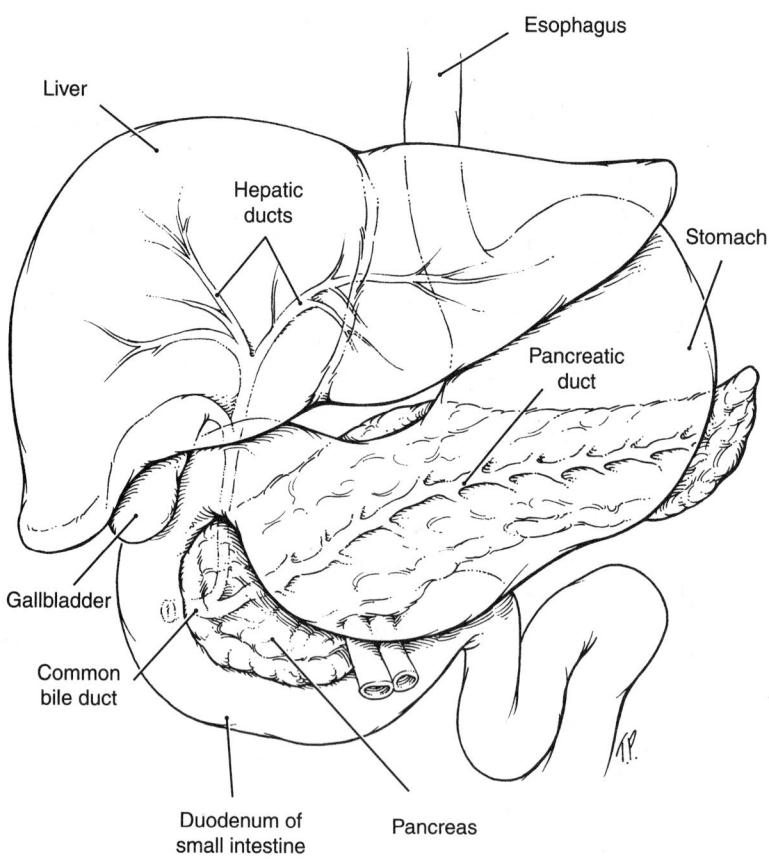

Liver

Esophagus

Hepatic
ducts

Stomach

Pancreatic
duct

Gallbladder

Common
bile duct

Duodenum of
small intestine

Pancreas

The coiled small intestine has three parts—the duodenum, the jejunum, and the ileum—and its function is to absorb nutrients from food. Bile made by the liver and stored in the gallbladder renders fats into soluble fragments. The pancreas secretes fluids that assist in fat absorption. Ducts from the liver, gallbladder, and pancreas connect to the duodenum.

until now, has remained largely liquid. With its nutrients harvested and most of its water drained, food here—including fiber, which cannot be digested—begins to resemble stool. The colon's job is to dry out stool, make it solid, and absorb most of the remaining water. In its final, digested form, the stool travels through the sigmoid (so named because of its "S" shape), the last part of the colon, to the rectum, where it is stored until it can be conveniently expelled through defecation. Bowel function varies greatly from person to person; normal bowel movements can range from as many as three stools a day to as few as three a week. A normal movement is formed but is not hard, contains no blood, and is passed without cramps or pain.

The small intestine is about 1 in. in diameter and 20 feet long. (A) It contains numerous projections called plicae circulares, each containing numerous villi and microvilli that increase the surface area for absorption of nutrients from food. The villi's two main cell types are the enterocyte, which digests and absorbs food, and the goblet cell, which secretes mucus. (B) A cross-section of the small intestine is shown.

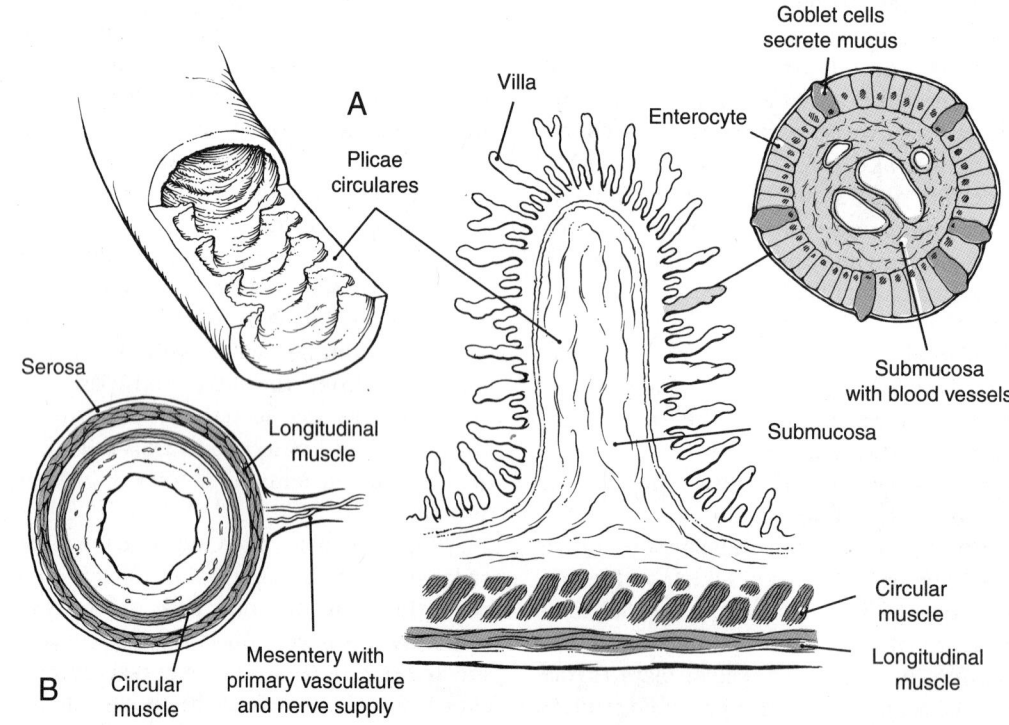

A

Villa

Goblet cells
secrete mucus

Plicae
circulares

Enterocyte

Submucosa
with blood vessels

Submucosa

Serosa

Longitudinal
muscle

Circular
muscle

Longitudinal
muscle

B   Circular
muscle

Mesentery with
primary vasculature
and nerve supply

The Small Intestine

MALABSORPTION SYNDROMES

Although a host of problems can cause malabsorption syndrome, the symptoms are confusingly similar. The most common symptom is steatorrhea: stool that is characterized by excess fat and is frothy, oily, and particularly foul-smelling. Whatever the cause of malabsorption, it causes calories and nutrients delivered into the small intestine with every meal to be squandered. Instead of being absorbed, they pass through to the colon and beyond. Consequently, your body is robbed of the protein, fat, carbohydrates, vitamins, and minerals in the food you are eating. Deficiencies of vitamins A, D, E, and K, folic acid, and calcium occur because these nutrients are excreted with the stool. If not treated, you will become malnourished. Some common causes of malabsorption are discussed here (see also Chronic Pancreatitis, page 1061).

❖ CELIAC DISEASE (NONTROPICAL SPRUE)

Symptoms (*What you may experience*) In children: diarrhea, weight loss, failure to thrive. In adults: chronic, foul-smelling diarrhea that does not respond to treatment; flatulence; weight loss; and chronic fatigue. You also may develop problems associated with vitamin deficiency: scaling skin (also called hyperkeratosis, a result of vitamin A deficiency); bruising (a result of vitamin K deficiency); blood in the urine (also from lack of vitamin K); numbness and tingling (from lack of vitamin D and calcium); muscle spasms or bone pain (also from vitamin D and calcium deficiency).

Signs and laboratory findings (*What the doctor looks for*) Characteristic blunting or flattening of the villi (which normally resemble fingers) lining the small intestine, as seen microscopically in biopsies taken during endoscopy (see Upper Endoscopy, page 968). The presence of numerous inflammatory cells, detected by a biopsy, underneath where the villi used to be.

What is it? Celiac disease is a reaction by certain immune system cells (called T-lymphocytes) to gluten, a protein that is found in many grains, especially in wheat, rye, barley, and oats. Normally, these cells are designed to protect the body against invaders; but in celiac disease, the body mistakenly perceives gluten as the enemy and attacks it. In the process, the lining of the small intestine becomes inflamed and inefficient in absorbing nutrients. Although the exact causes are not known, celiac disease seems to have a genetic component: Susceptibility seems to be inherited, and this disease is particularly common in people of western Irish descent, affecting an estimated 1 in 300. Half of all individuals with celiac disease are diagnosed during childhood, as early as 8 months of age. In adults, the disease is most commonly diagnosed between the 20s and 50s.

What you can do Because some people (see above) inherit a genetic susceptibility to celiac disease, familiarize yourself with your family medical history, and tell your doctor if anyone else in your family has experienced trouble eating grains, particularly, wheat, rye, barley, and oats. If there is a family history of celiac disease, or if you are a woman of western Irish descent, breastfeeding and postponing the introduction of foods with gluten may offer some protection to your children.

If you are diagnosed with celiac disease, gluten must be totally excluded from your diet. Because gluten is a hidden component of many prepared foods—canned soups, peanut butter, tomato, mustard, chip and dip mixes, lunch meats, candy bars, yogurt, and hot dogs, to name just a few—you will need to become a diligent checker of ingredients on every food item you buy. If you are not certain whether a food contains gluten, try restricting your diet, testing foods one by one to see which disagree with you. You also may find it worthwhile to enlist a dietitian's help in developing a gluten-free diet.

Treatment The goal is simple—removing gluten from the diet—but this can be a difficult task, because gluten is a frequent ingredient of prepared foods (see above). Your doctor can advise you on ways to achieve a gluten-free diet; also, specialized, gluten-free cookbooks can provide tremendous practical help. Once your diet is gluten-free, your symptoms should improve within a few weeks. If there is significant inflammation in the intestinal lining, your doctor may also prescribe a short course of corticosteroids. For unknown reasons—even if gluten is successfully removed from the diet—a few people with celiac disease develop lymphoma (see Lymphomas, page 954) or small bowel cancer (see Small Bowel Cancer, page 1009).

Prognosis Celiac disease sometimes goes into spontaneous remission in children around age 5, causing only occasional symptoms. In others, strict adherence to a gluten-free diet can lead to healing of the small intestine.

❖ TROPICAL SPRUE

Symptoms *(What you may experience)* Chronic diarrhea, which does not respond to treatment; flatulence; weight loss; and weakness. You also may develop problems associated with vitamin deficiency: scaling skin (also called hyperkeratosis, a result of vitamin A deficiency); bruising (a result of vitamin K deficiency); blood in the urine (also from lack of vitamin K); numbness and tingling (from lack of vitamin D and calcium); muscle spasms and/or bone pain (also from vitamin D and calcium deficiency).

Signs and laboratory findings *(What the doctor looks for)* Obvious blunting or flattening of the villi (which normally resemble fingers) lining the small intestine, as seen microscopically in biopsies taken during endoscopy (see Upper Endoscopy, page 968). The presence of numerous inflammatory cells, detected by a biopsy, infiltrating the intestinal lining. The main diagnostic help is your recent history—namely, whether you have visited an endemic tropical area, such as Central and South America, Cuba, Puerto Rico, certain parts of Africa, India, and Asia.

What is it? This infection, which causes inflammation in the intestinal lining, and malabsorption as a result, is a consequence of visiting tropical regions. The exact pathogen or cause—whether bacteria, amoeba, or something else—is unknown but is probably present in drinking water.

What you can do Although the exact cause is not known, if you are traveling in an area where this problem commonly afflicts tourists, your motto should be: "Boil it, cook it, peel it, or forget it." Avoid ice, tap water, vegetables, salads, foods sold by street vendors, and caffeinated beverages from soda fountains. Drink bottled water, sodas, wines, beer, tea, and coffee; brush your teeth with bottled water. If you wear contact lenses, use bottled water to rinse them. To be on the safe side, you might want to take your own supply of bottled water from home; estimate at least 1 quart-sized bottle per person per day. Limit your fruits to foods you can peel, such as oranges or bananas; grapes, for instance, are probably not safe.

Treatment To treat the inflammation, your doctor will probably prescribe an antibiotic such as tetracycline, or a combination sulfa drug such as trimethoprim and sulfamethoxazole (Bactrim), which, depending on the severity of the disease, may be continued for as long as 6 months. To combat any vitamin deficiency or anemia, you also may be given supplemental folic acid, vitamin B_{12}, and other vitamins.

Prognosis Excellent.

❖ BACTERIAL OVERGROWTH

Symptoms *(What you may experience)* Chronic diarrhea, which does not respond to treatment; flatulence; weight loss; and weakness. You also may develop problems associated with vitamin deficiency: scaling skin (also called hyperkeratosis, a result of vitamin A deficiency); bruising (a result of vitamin K deficiency); blood in the urine (also from lack of vitamin K); numbness and tingling (from lack of vitamin D and calcium); muscle spasms and/or bone pain (also from vitamin D and calcium deficiency).

Signs and laboratory findings *(What the doctor looks for)* The presence of undigested fat in a stool sample; signs of anemia (also detected by a blood test for vitamin B_{12} deficiency); low protein in the blood. During endoscopy (see Upper Endoscopy, page 968), your doctor may want to obtain some intestinal secretions to culture for the presence of bacteria; diagnosis is most commonly made using a simple breath test, which detects certain gases produced by bacterial overgrowth.

What is it? Normally, despite the food and liquid that pass through it every day, the small intestine is relatively sterile. But here, a breakdown in the intestine's normal defenses—designed to minimize gut bacteria—allows bacteria to colonize. If unchecked, these bacteria eventually compete with normal digestive functions. Enzymes made by these bacteria attack bile salts (made by the liver, these salts help the body absorb fat) and vitamin B_{12}. Scavenging bacteria snatch the food that should rightfully be absorbed by your body.

Bacterial overgrowth is the intestinal equivalent of algae flourishing in a stagnant pond. This may be caused by a mechanical problem, such as a fistula, stricture, or scar tissue from previous surgery—anything that impedes the intestine's ability to empty—that keeps food trapped in, or moving sluggishly through, the intestine. Also known as the blind loop syndrome, this can occur after surgery, if a surgeon inadvertently creates a cul-de-sac—a loop of bowel where bacteria can grow. Sometimes, the culprit is another illness: For example, in conditions such as diabetic neuropathy, scleroderma, and amyloidosis, poorly functioning intestinal muscles can cause food and stool to stagnate, with the same result.

What you can do Although most causes of bacterial overgrowth are unavoidable, if you have diabetes, keeping your blood sugar under control will considerably lower your risk of developing this problem. Laxatives, which can speed the progress of food through the gut, do not cure bacterial overgrowth. One reason is that laxatives primarily affect the colon; also, they do not address the underlying cause of this disorder.

Treatment The initial treatment is a course of antibiotics for 1 to 2 weeks. Subsequently, most people remain symptom-free for months; however, some people require either a repeat dose or a different antibiotic weeks to months later.

Depending on the underlying problem, you may need further treatment. If the cause is mechanical—a dead-end loop of bowel created during previous surgery—you may need further surgery to fix it. If the trouble is caused by a disease that affects the intestinal muscles, treating the underlying disease may ease symptoms. For instance, better control of blood sugar if you have diabetes should help. If you have scleroderma, your doctor may prescribe a medication such as octreotide (Sandostatin), which reduces the amount of secretions in the gut and helps prevent bacteria from developing.

Prognosis The prognosis depends on the underlying problem. If your situation is amenable to surgery, it is highly likely that this can be cured.

❖ AMYLOIDOSIS

Symptoms *(What you may experience)* Chronic diarrhea, which does not respond to treatment; constipation; blood in the stool; flatulence; weight loss; weakness; vomiting after meals; jaw pain; drooling; difficulty chewing; an enlarged tongue. You also may develop problems associated with vitamin deficiency: scaling skin (also called hyperkeratosis, a result of vitamin A deficiency); bruising (a result of vitamin K deficiency); blood in the urine (also from lack of vitamin K); numbness and tingling (from lack of vitamin D and calcium); muscle spasms or bone pain (also from vitamin D and calcium deficiency).

Signs and laboratory findings *(What the doctor looks for)* Abnormal buildup of protein, seen in a biopsy (usually of the rectum); evidence of arthritis in the temporomandibular (jaw) joint; evidence of gastrointestinal bleeding, detected in a blood stool test or during endoscopy (see Upper Endoscopy, page 968); evidence of gastric outlet obstruction or bowel obstruction; rectal prolapse; palpable enlargement of liver and spleen; evidence of cardiomyopathy (which can be another ramification of amyloidosis), including fluid swelling in the ankles, shortness of breath, and sounds of fluid in the lungs; muscle weakness; numbness or tingling in the hands and feet.

What is it? Amyloidosis (see also page 952) is a disease in which deposits of a protein mixture called amyloid accumulate throughout the body, eventually affecting organs, nerves, and muscles. The condition is rare, and its severity depends on the organs affected by amyloid deposits. Amyloidosis can have ramifications in the intestine, hindering the ability of muscles to squeeze food through to the colon. For reasons not fully understood (perhaps due to bacterial overgrowth, see above), malabsorption occurs in about 5 percent of people with amyloidosis.

Treatment Unfortunately, because there is no treatment for the underlying problem of amyloidosis, the goal here is to relieve symptoms. Your doctor may prescribe a regimen of antibiotics, if bacterial overgrowth is a component of the problem. If you are unable to eat, or if you are at risk of becoming malnourished or dehydrated, you may need temporary intravenous feeding or liquid nutrition supplements (such as Ensure or Sustacal).

❖ WHIPPLE'S DISEASE

Symptoms *(What you may experience)* First, joint pain; fever; chronic cough; abdominal pain. Later, chronic diarrhea, which does not respond to treatment; flatulence; weight loss; and a general feeling of weakness. Neurologic problems, which may include personality changes; confusion; seizures; headache; visual disturbances; numbness, weakness, and tingling in the hands and feet; stiffness in the neck. You also may develop problems associated with vitamin deficiency (from prolonged malabsorption): scaling skin (also called hyperkeratosis, a result of vitamin A deficiency); bruising (a result of vitamin K deficiency); blood in the urine (also from lack of vitamin K); numbness and tingling (from lack of vitamin D and calcium); muscle spasms and/or bone pain (also from vitamin D and calcium deficiency).

Signs and laboratory findings *(What the doctor looks for)* The presence of many characteristic macrophages, which are immune system cells that scavenge foreign invaders (signaling infection), seen in a biopsy of the small intestine, taken during endoscopy (see Upper Endoscopy, page 968); whitish-looking villi, seen in endoscopy; unabsorbed fat in the stool; swollen lymph nodes throughout the body (felt in a physical exam); changes in the appearance of your skin; low-grade fever; a heart murmur; abdominal tenderness or a palpable mass in the abdomen; fluid in the belly; swollen feet, enlarged spleen; anemia, detected in a blood test.

What is it? This is a very rare condition whose cause, long unexplained, is now known to be a systemic infection by the bacterium *Tropheryma whippelii*. This organism is commonly found in soil, which is why most of the people infected are farmers. It most often affects white men in their 40s.

When to call the doctor If you cannot eat, or are at risk of becoming malnourished or dehydrated, of if you have a seizure or any of the neurologic problems listed above, call your doctor.

Treatment Your doctor will prescribe a year-long regimen of antibiotics, which may include a combination sulfa drug such as trimethoprim and sulfamethoxazole.

Prognosis Your symptoms will probably improve gradually: After antibiotics begin, fever and diarrhea should disappear within a couple of weeks, and you should be able to regain weight soon thereafter.

FOOD (LACTOSE, SUCROSE, FRUCTOSE) INTOLERANCE

Symptoms *(What you may experience)* Painful gas; bloating; diarrhea; flatulence. With lactose intolerance, these symptoms tend to develop 2 to 6 hours after you drink one or two glasses of milk or eat a large amount of dairy products, especially on an empty stomach.

Signs and laboratory findings *(What the doctor looks for)* Positive results on a hydrogen breath test after you drink a sample of lactose, sucrose, or fructose. Positive results on a lactose tolerance blood test (see Treatment, page 999).

What is it? Lactose, fructose, and sucrose intolerance arise from the body's inability to absorb one or more basic sugars. If the body is unable to absorb these sugars, the bacteria in the digestive tract ferment them into gasses that can cause diarrhea, abdominal discomfort, and other distressing symptoms.

Intolerance of lactose, the sugar in cow's milk (found in all dairy products), is extremely common—affecting nearly 50 million American adults. The cause is a deficiency of the enzyme lactase, normally produced by cells in the intestinal lining. Lactase breaks down milk sugar (a combination of two sugars) into single sugars that can be absorbed into the bloodstream. Lactose intolerance is more prevalent in some racial and ethnic groups than others: For example, an estimated 75 percent of all African American, Jewish, Native American, and Mexican American adults have some degree of lactose intolerance, and 90 percent of Asian American adults have the condition; Americans of northern European descent are least likely affected. In rare cases, children are born lacking the ability to produce lactase; however, most often, the deficiency develops over years or decades.

Fructose is most common in grapes, nuts, figs, dates, honey, and apple or pear juice; many commercial soft drinks and cola drinks contain 55 percent fructose as a sweetener. An estimated 70 percent of healthy people cannot completely absorb the amount of fructose in a pound of grapes. (Diarrhea is more common in the summer, when people tend to eat more fresh fruit.) Sucrose is present in sugar cane, table sugar, candy bars, and many unprocessed fruits. Although sucrose intolerance is rare in the United States, 10 percent of people of Inuit descent lack sucrose-isomaltase, the enzyme necessary to digest sucrose.

It is very common, after an infection or illness, such as viral gastroenteritis or food poisoning, to have temporary food intolerance. If you have never before had this kind of trouble, you will almost certainly be able to eat your normal diet again within several weeks.

What you can do If you have lactose intolerance and symptoms are mild, you can take an over-the-counter enzyme replacement medication before eating a dairy product. Also, you might be able to tolerate special milk—available in most grocery stores—in which 70 percent of lactose is removed. Become a diligent checker of food labels: Lactose is a hidden ingredient in many prepared foods, including breads; breakfast cereals; instant potatoes; soups; mixes for pancakes, biscuits, cakes, and cookies; salad dressings; lunch meats and hot dogs (except kosher); margarine; and even some nondairy products, such as powdered coffee creamer and whipped desert topping. Milk products also produce symptoms; thus, it is important to look for these words on food labels: whey, curds, dry milk solids, sodium caseinate, and nonfat dry milk powder.

Because milk and dairy products contain calcium and other essential nutrients, if your meals are largely dairy-free, it will be important to eat calcium-rich foods to meet daily nutritional needs. Many green vegetables, including broccoli, kale, and some greens, are high in calcium and low in lactose, so are seafood, including oysters, salmon, sardines, and shrimp; certain forms of tofu; and molasses. Ask your doctor for a list of recommended foods.

For fructose and sucrose intolerance, the only treatment is avoidance: Determine which foods contain these sugars, and do not eat them; or, if you can tolerate mild amounts of these sugars, eat them sparingly. Read the labels on packaged foods and beverages. Ask your doctor for a list of foods to avoid. You may also need to consult a nutritionist or dietitian for help in planning a balanced diet.

Lactose, sucrose, and fructose are found in many prescription medications and over-the-counter medicines; consult your doctor or pharmacist if you have questions.

When to call the doctor Your doctor can help you determine if your symptoms are due to food intolerance or another condition. If your symptoms are mild, however, following the suggestions above should relieve the problem.

Treatment Your doctor can use various tests to determine lactose intolerance. One is a hydrogen breath test: Normally, hydrogen is undetectable in the breath; however, when sugars such as lactose are not digested, bacteria in the colon can produce various gases, including hydrogen, which is absorbed into the bloodstream, carried to the lungs, and exhaled. Another is a lactose tolerance blood test: In this test, given on an empty stomach, a baseline blood sample is drawn to measure your fasting blood glucose level; then you drink a lactose-containing beverage, and more blood samples are taken over the next 2 hours to determine whether this glucose level rises. If your body is unable to digest the lactose, it will not be broken into simpler sugars, and your glucose level remains unchanged.

The lactose tolerance and hydrogen breath tests should not be given to infants or young children, who are more likely to become dehydrated from the diarrhea caused by the large dose of lactose. Most

NUTRITIONAL SUPPLEMENTATION AND FEEDING TUBES

Good nutrition—getting enough calories, vitamins, and minerals every day—is essential. Without it, your body is more vulnerable to illness. Many ailments can hamper the body's ability to get the fuel it needs. Some diminish the appetite; others make it difficult for you to swallow food, keep it down, or absorb its nutrients.

If your problem is poor appetite, or if you are unable to eat large meals, try eating small, nutritious meals several times a day, and make every calorie count. A glass of juice, for instance, will do your body more good than the same amount of soda. If you are unable to take vitamins in pill form, drink them: A calorie-packed liquid supplement, such as Ensure or Sustacal, can meet all of your daily nutritional needs.

If, for whatever reason, you cannot eat or drink enough and are at risk of becoming malnourished, you may need extra help, in the form of a feeding tube.

Tubes Through the Nose

A nasogastric (NG) tube, a small rubber tube inserted through the nose into the stomach, is an excellent temporary solution to this problem. Depending on your condition, you may have a nasoduodenal tube, which empties into the duodenum instead of the stomach. NG tubes are most often used in people who will likely recover the ability to eat on their own within a few weeks or who are too ill to receive a gastrostomy tube (see below). Several times a day, you, a family member, or a nurse will simply pour a nutritionally complete liquid meal (such as Ensure or Sustacal) down the tube, directly into the stomach or small bowel. Because these tubes are prone to becoming clogged, especially with pills, make sure that whatever you pass through it is soluble or small enough to be easily flushed from the tube. Also, to avoid hardening of any residue in the tube, be sure to flush the tube with water after each use.

As with any form of treatment, there are complications: In some people, the tube can cause nasal and throat irritation (although this is now less of a problem, because the tubes are smaller and softer); there is also a slight risk of aspiration (if liquid is inadvertently inhaled into the lungs), which may lead to pneumonia. Also, because this food is concentrated, some people experience diarrhea; if this is a problem, talk with your doctor or dietitian. It may help to try stretching out or dividing the feedings, allowing your body to digest smaller portions at a time. To minimize the risk of aspiration, make sure that your head is elevated for at least 2 hours after each feeding. If you are receiving continuous feeding, your head should be perpetually elevated.

Percutaneous Endoscopic Gastrostomy

Percutaneous endoscopic gastrostomy (PEG) tubes are placed during esophogastroduodenoscopy. Working first from the inside, a gastroenterologist passes an endoscope through the throat into the stomach and shines a light through the abdominal wall. At that precise circle of light, the doctor sterilizes and numbs the skin, and then inserts a needle through the abdominal wall to meet the endoscope in the stomach. Through that needle, the doctor threads a flexible guide wire, then uses the endoscope to snare the guide wire and pull it out through your mouth. For the next few minutes, you will have a wire extending through your mouth and out through your abdominal wall; the procedure is almost over. Then, the doctor threads the tube—a long, thin straw, with a mushroom-shaped bottom end—through the wire in your mouth, back down your esophagus, and into your stomach, until the tapered end pops out through the abdominal wall, leaving the mushroom-shaped part behind. Last, the doctor pulls the straw until there is resistance—when the bottom part is snugly tucked against the abdominal wall. The same kind of liquid meals used with an NG tube (Ensure or Sustacal) are used here, administered with a syringe or pump.

With any opening in the skin, there is the potential for infection. Thus, you will need to clean the skin around the area periodically with hydrogen peroxide and allow it to get plenty of air; avoid tight-fitting waistbands and plastic bandages that prevent the skin from breathing (use gauze instead).

Because these tubes are prone to becoming clogged, especially with pills, make sure that whatever you pass through it is soluble or small enough to be easily flushed from the tube. Also, to avoid having any residue in the tube hardening, be sure to flush the tube with water after each use. Because this food is concentrated, some people experience diarrhea; if this is a problem, talk with your doctor or dietitian. It may help to try stretching out or dividing the feedings, allowing your body to digest smaller portions at a time.

Over time, a PEG can be replaced with a button, a port (like the opening on a beach ball) with a cap that is flush with the skin. With a button, food is injected directly into the opening; there is no unsightly tube extending from the body, and no risk of it pulling out.

Surgically Implanted Tubes

The jejunostomy tube itself (and its use and maintenance, see above) is similar to that used in a PEG, but it is usually placed in the jejunum (and thus is called a jejunostomy tube)—where most nutrients are absorbed—by a surgeon through an abdominal incision, under general anesthesia. A surgically implanted tube is a better option for some people who are not candidates for PEG, including people with previous abdominal surgery and people who are very obese or whose stomach does not empty (the PEG procedure cannot take place if the gastroenterologist is unable to see the light shining through the abdominal wall). ■

---

pediatricians recommend changing from cow's milk to soy formula and watching for an improvement in symptoms in very young children. If necessary, the doctor may also perform a stool acidity test, which measures the amount of lactic acid—produced when undigested lactose is fermented by colon bacteria—in the stool.

SHORT BOWEL SYNDROME

Symptoms *(What you may experience)*
These depend on the underlying condition (see below) and may include diarrhea, stool that is very sticky or oily; abdominal pain; indigestion; pain under the right ribcage; severe weight loss; fatigue; weakness; involuntary muscle contractions; bone pain; excess bleeding and easy bruising; symptoms of peptic ulcer disease (see Peptic Ulcer Disease, page 986).

Signs and laboratory findings *(What the doctor looks for)* Anemia; bone thinning, visible on x-ray; loss of muscle mass and other signs of wasting; diminished sensation in the hands and feet; elevated liver enzymes and/or disrupted electrolytes (detected in a blood test); abnormal levels of potassium (seen in a blood test); jaundice; evidence of cirrhosis.

What is it? Short bowel syndrome is an extreme loss of small intestine, to the extent that you no longer have the minimal amount—at least 6 feet—required to absorb the body's nutrients. Different nutrients are absorbed in different parts of the small intestine; particularly important are the ileum and duodenum. Short bowel syndrome can be caused by several events, including trauma; a small bowel tumor; bypass surgery for morbid obesity; and extensive surgery for Crohn's disease. Small bowel syndrome also may occur spontaneously, if the bowel somehow becomes twisted or tangled (creating a situation called a volvulus), shutting off blood supply, and killing healthy intestinal tissue.

Treatment If short bowel syndrome is caused by intestinal bypass surgery for morbid obesity, the syndrome may be reversible with further surgery.

In other situations, your doctor will want to stop the chronic diarrhea and address the risk of vitamin deficiency and malnourishment: Your doctor may prescribe an antimotility agent, such as diphenoxylate and atropine (Lomotil), to slow down the intestinal processes and combat the diarrhea. If the diarrhea is severe, you may need temporary intravenous hydration or nutrition. For long-term treatment, you may need water-soluble forms of vitamins such as A, D, E, and K, which are easier to absorb, and you

may need supplemental liquid nutrition and protein (such as Ensure or Sustacal). Because you are now functionally lactose-intolerant (the enzymes needed to digest lactose are in the small intestine), your doctor will probably tell you to avoid dairy products and other lactose-containing foods, which can worsen the diarrhea.

The symptoms of peptic ulcer disease occur because peptides in the small intestine, which normally inhibit stomach acid, are missing. These symptoms can be effectively remedied with drugs including H_2 blockers, which cause the stomach to make less acid by blocking histamine receptors, and may include prescription-strength doses of cimetidine (Tagamet), ranitidine (Zantac), famotidine (Pepcid), or nizatidine (Axid). Proton pump inhibitors, which selectively disable the pump in acid-making cells, thus stopping acid production completely, are more powerful and include omeprazole (Prilosec) and lansoprazole (Prevacid). Sucralfate (Carafate), a modified, prescription-strength antacid that coats the stomach, binds to the ulcer crater, and promotes healing, also may help.

INTESTINE INFECTIONS

Infections of the intestines include traveler's diarrhea, food poisoning, viral gastroenteritis, and parasitic infections.

❖ TRAVELER'S DIARRHEA

Symptoms *(What you may experience)*
Abrupt onset of diarrhea accompanied by nausea, vomiting, weakness, or fever; painful, explosive gas; fatigue; cramps; loss of appetite.

Signs and laboratory findings *(What the doctor looks for)* The presence of white blood cells in the stool (called fecal leukocytes), suggesting an invasive bacterial infection—or, less commonly, evidence of parasites or amoebae—found in a stool culture. The most compelling aid to diagnosis is your recent whereabouts: If you have recently traveled out of the country, tell your doctor.

What is it? In most cases, traveler's diarrhea is a bacterial infection caused by unsanitary handling of food. The infection is transmitted by the fecal–oral route: It is mainly caused when food handlers do not adequately wash their hands after they use the bathroom. The most common culprit (in an estimated 40 to 70 percent of cases) is *Escherichia coli* bacteria; less common are parasitic infections, such as giardiasis (caused by a protozoan) or amebiasis (caused by amoebae). Traveler's diarrhea is most common among visitors to Mexico, Morocco, El Salvador, Kenya, Bangladesh, and other parts of Central and South America, Africa, and Asia. Of the 3 million tourists who travel to Mexico each year, an estimated 25 to 50 percent return with diarrhea. Fortunately, this disease, although severe, is usually of limited duration: In 80 percent of cases, symptoms last less than a week; in most people, 3 or 4 days. For more information on traveler's diarrhea, see Chapter 21. See also Chapter 3 for precautions to take when traveling.

What you can do Traveler's diarrhea is preventable, although for thousands of conscientious tourists each year, one lapse is all it takes: For instance, many travelers remember to drink bottled water, but brush their teeth with tap water, or drink a bottled cola—with ice cubes made from tap water. If you are traveling in an area where this problem commonly afflicts tourists, your motto should be "Boil it, cook it, peel it, or forget it." Avoid ice, tap water, vegetables, salads, foods sold by street vendors, and caffeinated beverages from soda fountains. Drink bottled water, sodas, wines, beer, tea, and coffee; brush your teeth with bottled water. If you wear contact lenses, use bottled water to rinse them. To be on the safe side, you might want to take your own supply of bottled water from home; estimate at least 1 quart-sized bottle per person per day. Limit your fruits to foods you can peel, such as oranges or bananas; grapes, for instance, are probably not safe. Talk to your doctor about treating traveler's diarrhea with Pepto-Bismol or prescription antibiotics, which you will need to take for the duration of your stay.

When to call the doctor Call your doctor if you have a high fever (over 101°F), have bloody diarrhea, or are unable to stop vomiting.

Treatment It is essential not to become dehydrated: Keep drinking fluids. If you are unable to drink, you may need intravenous fluids. If your fever is less than 101°F and the diarrhea is not bloody, your doctor may prescribe an antimotility medication such as diphenoxylate and atropine to slow down the intestine and combat the diarrhea; you also may need antibiotics. If you have a parasitic infection, you will need an antiparasitic medication.

Prognosis Excellent; although symptoms can be intense, traveler's diarrhea is almost always a short-lived disease.

❖ FOOD POISONING

Symptoms *(What you may experience)* Abrupt, generally violent onset of vomiting and diarrhea, cramps, abdominal pain, general weakness and malaise.

Signs and laboratory findings *(What the doctor looks for)* Because this problem usually resolves after the organism clears from the body, the actual toxin that caused the poisoning is rarely identified and, thus, hardly ever treated specifically. Fevers are extremely rare with food poisoning. If you have a fever, this suggests a different diagnosis, such as gastroenteritis (see page 1003).

What is it? Food poisoning is caused by extremely potent toxins, made by bacteria such as *Staphylococcus* or *Salmonella*. Sometimes, the food is contaminated before it is prepared, and the bacteria are hardy enough to survive inadequate cooking. Other times, food is contaminated by a food handler after the dish is prepared: When someone handling raw chicken, for instance, fails to wash her hands before touching other food. Food poisoning, although miserable and sometimes violent, usually lasts no longer than 24 to 36 hours. Some people may have vomiting or diarrhea only; others may be afflicted with both, sometimes simultaneously. Other bacterial infections, such as shigella and cholera, are usually transmitted by the fecal–oral route; this mainly happens when food handlers do not adequately wash their hands after using the bathroom.

What you can do Cook food thoroughly. Equally important: Maintain food at correct temperatures, particularly, egg salad, mayonnaise, rice pudding, cream, tartar sauce, and fried rice.

For the bacteria to make these toxins, food must become a good culture dish and must sit at room temperature for several hours (at a picnic, for example). Avoid vats of mayonnaise at fast-food restaurants; choose mustard or catsup instead. Before eating in any restaurant, check for the restaurant's Health Department Grade, which, by law, should be posted for public viewing (in many restaurants, the certificate hangs on the wall near the rest rooms). If the grade is anything below an "A," leave. If you become ill after eating at a restaurant, find out immediately if anyone else in your party has also become sick. If so, you should report this to the health department promptly, so the restaurant's food-handling procedures can be reviewed.

When to call the doctor If you cannot stop vomiting or having diarrhea, if you have a high fever (which may suggest a different diagnosis), if you faint or become weak and light-headed after prolonged vomiting or diarrhea, call your doctor immediately.

Treatment It is essential not to become dehydrated: Keep drinking fluids. If you cannot stop vomiting, you may need intravenous fluids or, if your symptoms are severe, a prescription suppository, such as prochlorperazine (Compazine) or promethazine (Phenergan).

Prognosis For most people, excellent. This is a short-lived disease. Believe it or not, your appetite will return in a few days. However, in very young children, the elderly, and people with a compromised immune system, food poisoning (particularly with *E. coli*) can be deadly. If you or a family member is in one of these high-risk groups, and you suspect severe food poisoning, call your doctor or go to the emergency room immediately.

❖ VIRAL GASTROENTERITIS

Symptoms *(What you may experience)* Diarrhea, nausea, abdominal cramps, vomiting, muscle aches, low-grade fever, loss of appetite, weakness, malaise. Symptoms may persist for a week to 10 days.

Signs and laboratory findings *(What the doctor looks for)* If a rotavirus is suspected, your doctor may give you a specific stool test, called Rotazyme. For most causes of viral gastroenteritis, however, there is no specific diagnostic test and no specific treatment.

What is it? Viral gastroenteritis is a viral infection of the intestine. Like traveler's diarrhea, this is most commonly transmitted by the fecal–oral route—mainly caused when food handlers do not adequately wash their hands after using the bathroom—except here, the unwelcome addition to your food is a virus, not bacteria. Viral gastroenteritis may also be present in shellfish that inhabit water contaminated by raw sewage.

What you can do Avoid raw shellfish. Rotavirus also tends to be endemic in daycare centers. If your children are in daycare, or whenever they play with other children—or even other children's toys—encourage hand washing (and wash your own) as often as possible. See Chapter 9 for more information. See also Chapter 21 for more information on viral gastrointestinal infection.

Treatment To treat the diarrhea, your doctor will probably recommend an antimotility agent, which slows down intestinal function, such as loperamide (Imodium). If your symptoms are severe and dehydration is a concern, you may need intravenous fluids, or a prescription suppository such as prochlorperazine or promethazine to ease nausea and vomiting. Like other intestinal infections, viral gastroenteritis tends to subside fairly quickly.

Prognosis Excellent.

❖ PARASITIC INFECTION

Symptoms *(What you may experience)* Acute or chronic (daily or intermittent) diarrhea; weight loss, loss of appetite, abdominal cramps, low-grade fever.

Signs and laboratory findings *(What the doctor looks for)* Presence of cysts or worms in the stool; the presence of Giardia (a common parasite) on antigen tests of stool; the presence of eosinophils (specific white blood cells, which fight parasitic infection) in the blood. Also, swelling, also called edema, in the face, hands, and feet—an allergic reaction to certain toxins made by parasitic worms.

What is it? Invasion of microorganisms such as protozoa or amoebae, or of worms, such as roundworm or tapeworm. Parasitic worms may be microscopic or grow to reach amazing lengths: A single tapeworm, for instance, may become 30 feet long. As with other types of infections, most of these are contracted by the fecal-oral route; they are transmitted by improper sanitary conditions, usually when food handlers do not adequately wash their hands after using the bathroom. Other parasites, however, may enter the body from the ground, burrowing into your skin when you are standing barefoot in a river, for instance. Parasitic infections are most common in countries lacking strict water safety standards. For example, in St. Petersburg, Russia, the water has been notoriously contaminated with Giardia cysts. In the United States, cryptosporidia and microsporidia have been found in well water, rivers, lakes, and streams, and even drinking water in some cities. See Parasitic Infections, page 892, for more information.

What you can do If you go camping or backpacking, resist the urge to drink from lakes and streams without first filtering or boiling the water (portable water filters are available in most camping supply stores). To prevent tapeworm and trichinosis, avoid undercooked pork and beef; do not eat steak tartare. To avoid hookworm and strongyloides, parasites that enter the body through bare skin, do not walk barefoot in a pasture or in an infected area. If you believe your own drinking water is contaminated, use bottled water for drinking, purchase a filter for your faucet (varieties range from on-the-faucet, to under-the-sink, to whole-house filters), boil water, or add a tiny amount of bleach (following the instructions on the bleach container). Boiling water or adding bleach may be necessary after a weather emergency such as a hurricane, when your area's drinking water may be contaminated.

Treatment Depending on the specific parasite (various parasites have differing life cycles, and medications target each one differently), you will need an antiparasite medication for days to weeks.

VASCULAR/MESENTERIC BOWEL DISORDERS (ACUTE AND CHRONIC MESENTERIC ISCHEMIA)

Symptoms *(What you may experience)* *Acute:* Severe abdominal pain, cramps, blood in the stool, nausea, vomiting, diarrhea or constipation. *Chronic:* Symptoms are less dramatic than the acute form and may include chronic abdominal pain after eating, fear of eating (sitophobia) because pain follows each meal, weight loss, diarrhea, constipation, and upset stomach.

Signs and laboratory findings *(What the doctor looks for)* Extreme tenderness suggesting diffuse peritonitis (inflammation within the abdomen); shock (when the blood pressure is dangerously low and unstable, a medical emergency); severe metabolic abnormalities on a blood test; damaged or dead tissue suggesting loss of blood flow to the gut, as shown by an angiogram, abdominal x-rays, ultrasound tests, and/or a computed tomography (CT) scan.

What is it? Mesenteric ischemia is the intestinal equivalent of a heart attack or angina: *Ischemia* means there is an inadequate blood supply, and acute or recurrent obstruction of blood flow to the bowel causes intermittent or permanent tissue damage. Ischemia may be caused by atherosclerosis or a blood clot in one of the three major intraabdominal arteries. Although the events leading to atherosclerosis and clot formation are complex, the result is impediment to blood flow: Plaque or a clot becomes lodged in the artery, shutting off blood flow downstream. Starved of oxygen, the affected tissue sends out an emergency distress signal—severe pain. Depending on the cause, and whether blood flow is restored in time to save the tissue, this pain could be transient (like angina) or could last hours. If blood flow does not return, bowel tissue may die.

What you can do As with a heart attack, the best prevention is a lifetime of healthy eating, to avoid plaque buildup in your arteries (see Lifestyle Changes for a Healthy Heart, page 797). However, next best is to limit the damage with prompt medical attention.

When to call the doctor If you believe mesenteric ischemia is happening—particularly if you have a personal or family history of heart disease, stroke, or atherosclerosis—call your doctor or go at once to the emergency room. Here, as with heart attack and stroke, time is of the essence.

Treatment Treatment for mesenteric ischemia depends on the results of the angiogram, which also shows the state of the artery in question. If the angiogram shows a distinct blockage, you will probably need emergency surgery. However, if your general health is considered too frail to withstand a major operation, surgery may not be a reasonable option. At some major medical centers, angioplasty (inserting a balloon into the artery, and expanding it to flatten the blockage, restore blood flow, and save tissue) has been used successfully. Another option is the intravenous administration of a vasodilator, an artery-dilating drug such as papaverine, in an attempt to open the blocked vessel. If studies reveal that it is too late to save the ischemic bowel, you may need surgery to remove the damaged section of intestine. If there is extensive tissue loss, you may need total parenteral nutrition (see Nutritional Supplementation and Feeding Tubes, page 1000) or permanent intravenous feeding.

BOWEL OBSTRUCTION

Symptoms *(What you may experience)* Abdominal pain; vomiting; inability to move your bowels (but unlike constipation, there is no normal sensation that you need to have a bowel movement); inability to pass gas; abdominal distension.

Signs and laboratory findings *(What the doctor looks for)* A medical history of previous abdominal surgery (suggesting the possibility of a surgery-caused adhesion in the intestine); a palpable mass in the abdomen; abdominal tenderness; lack of bowel sounds, or abnormal bowel sounds. An intestinal obstruction, as seen on x-ray. In making the diagnosis, your doctor will probably check for the presence of blood in the stool, which may indicate cancer or another problem in the intestinal lining, during a rectal exam.

What is it? Obstruction of the bowel is a serious problem that occurs when mechanical impediment or functional obstruction blocks the progress of stool. Often, this is due to a twisted bowel or an adhesion (caused by previous abdominal surgery) that squeezes the opening of the bowel. But bowel obstruction also may result from other disorders, including ileus, a condition that may result from intestinal surgery or from metabolic disruption (after an infection, for example), in which the bowel temporarily stops working; a bowel hernia (in which a loop of bowel pushes through an abnormal opening and becomes trapped); intussusception in very small children (in which one segment of the intestine slides into another segment, creating a kink or blockage); cancer; inflammatory bowel disease; Crohn's disease; ulcerative colitis; and gallstone ileus, in which a large gallstone (greater than 1 in. in diameter) erodes through the gallbladder into the intestine and becomes stuck, usually in the ileum. In toxic megacolon, the bowel can become massively dilated, with muscle function severely impaired. The result of bowel obstruction is that blood supply to the bowel is hindered or shut off entirely, and the bowel is at risk of dying. If not treated, this can lead to perforation, sepsis, or shock, and possibly death.

When to call the doctor This is an emergency. If you experience any of the symptoms mentioned above (particularly if you have ever had abdominal surgery), call your doctor at once. If you have a bowel obstruction, the sooner you receive treatment, the better your chances of survival.

Treatment Because time is of the essence, treatment often means emergency surgery to remove the obstruction. The extent of surgery will depend on the underlying cause and severity of damage. You may need a temporary or permanent colostomy (see Ileostomy, Kock Pouch, Ileoanal Pouch, and Colostomy, page 1012); if the entire small intestine is damaged, the surgery itself may cause short bowel syndrome (see Short Bowel Syndrome, page 1001). An exception to surgery is when the blockage is caused

FLEXIBLE SIGMOIDOSCOPY

The sigmoidoscope is a flexible tube, about 2 feet long and the width of your forefinger. Equipped with a miniature video camera and headlight, lubricated and inserted through your rectum, it allows the doctor to see the lining of your sigmoid colon and spot any abnormalities. Some problems that cannot be detected with x-rays can be seen clearly through a sigmoidoscope.

Flexible sigmoidoscopy (also called proctosigmoidoscopy), a procedure that is done with you lying on your left side, may be performed by an internist, family doctor, or gastroenterologist. For most Americans, it is the main screening test for colon cancer. The American Cancer society recommends that people at average risk—people without a family or personal history of colon cancer—undergo a baseline flexible sigmoidoscopy at age 50, and then a follow-up procedure every 5 years.

During flexible sigmoidoscopy, your doctor may perform a biopsy, threading a cutting tool through the sigmoidoscope to take a small sample of tissue. A biopsy can be performed for many reasons; having a biopsy does not mean that you have cancer. The sigmoidoscope can also be used to photograph any abnormal findings. If you have a polyp, an abnormal growth of tissue, your doctor will take a biopsy, so that a pathologist can examine the tissue for the presence of cancer. If one polyp is found, it is very important for your doctor to determine if this is an isolated growth or one of several (see Colon Polyps, page 1021). You will need to undergo colonoscopy—a similar procedure, done by a gastroenterologist, that allows a deeper and more through exploration of the colon.

Flexible sigmoidoscopy, which generally takes less than 30 minutes, is very safe, with an extremely low risk—about 1 in 20,000—of complications. It is done with informed consent, which means you should have a full understanding of the risks involved. Potential complications include a tear or tiny hole (called a perforation) in the lining of the colon, which may heal on its own or may require surgery to repair it, and bleeding, if a biopsy is done (usually, bleeding is minimal; rarely, it may require surgery or a blood transfusion). There is a minimal risk of infection with any procedure. Because air is pumped into your colon—making the area larger, and maximizing the doctor's field of vision—you may feel discomfort from cramps or distension during the procedure. This will get better immediately after the procedure, as soon as you pass the excess air, although your abdomen may feel tender for the next few hours. The presence of the sigmoidoscope may also give you a mild sensation that you need to have a bowel movement.

For your doctor to see as much as possible, your colon must be clean before the procedure. This means you will need to use laxatives or two enemas (this varies, according to your doctor's instructions and your own situation); you may also be asked not to eat or drink anything after midnight the night before and (to minimize the risk of bleeding) to stop taking aspirin for at least 2 days beforehand. If you are taking aspirin or any medication regularly, do not skip a scheduled dose without talking to your doctor first.

One key difference between flexible sigmoidoscopy and colonoscopy is the degree to which you have cleaned the colon. Although enemas and laxatives help remove stool before flexible sigmoidoscopy, some vestiges of fecal matter, along with some gas, may remain. Thus, most doctors do not attempt to cauterize any bleeding areas found during sigmoidoscopy; there is a risk that any lingering traces of stool or pockets of gas may ignite, causing a miniexplosion and injuring tissue. If further work or exploration is needed, this will probably be done during colonoscopy. ■

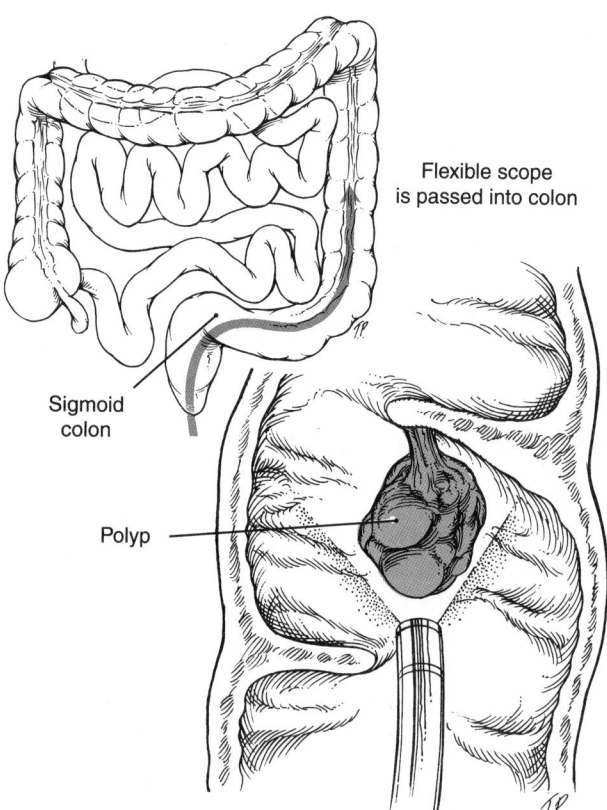

Flexible scope
is passed into colon

Sigmoid
colon

Polyp

The flexible sigmoidoscopy, which is a safe procedure and takes less than 30 minutes to perform, allows a doctor to see into the colon nearest the anus. It is used as a main screening test for colon cancer. A flexible tube with a video camera and headlight is inserted into the rectum and advanced through part of the colon. A biopsy may be taken to examine a small sample of tissue for the presence of cancer or other disease. Polyps, which are small, distinct growths that may lead to cancer, can also be found.

by a volvulus (a twist or knot) in the sigmoid colon: It is often possible to undo or reduce the volvulus with a barium-guided enema or endoscopy. Similarly, in the case of intussusception in young children, a barium x-ray (see Barium Studies, page 976) can push the intestine back into its proper shape. This is best done in a large hospital that has experience performing the procedure on very small children. For functional obstruction (in ileus, for example), the first step is to rest the bowel, which means you can have nothing by mouth (not even water) and you must have intravenous fluids. You may also need nasogastric suction to remove any stomach contents, and you may need endoscopy to decompress the dilated colon.

CROHN'S DISEASE

Symptoms *(What you may experience)* Diarrhea, abdominal pain, blood in the stool or black, tarlike stool (another indication of intestinal bleeding); unexplained fever; anal fissures and fistulas; weight loss; in children, failure to grow. Less commonly, aches and pains in the joints; light hurting the eyes (rarely) (the result of a disrupted immune system); persistent mouth ulcers.

Signs and laboratory findings *(What the doctor looks for)* On endoscopy or barium studies (see Upper Endoscopy, page 968, and Barium Studies, page 976), abnormalities in the intestine and colon including swelling, also called edema; stricture (constriction caused by scar tissue); fistula formation (an abnormal connection, or passageway, that develops between loops of bowel, or between loops of bowel and other organs or the skin); cobblestone inflammation (tiny bumps) in the intestine; ulcers or erosions; anemia (because of decreased vitamin B_{12} absorption or because of blood loss); abnormal electrolyte levels, seen in a blood test. In making the diagnosis, your doctor will want to rule out infectious causes (such as *Clostridium difficile* or other infections that can mimic Crohn's disease; see *C. Difficile* Colitis and Antibiotic-Associated Diarrhea, page 1015) of your symptoms by culturing your stool for the presence of bacteria and parasites. If the area of inflammation can be reached with the endoscope, your doctor may take a biopsy, or sample of tissue, to look for a distinctive type of inflammation found in most patients with Crohn's disease.

What is it? No one knows what causes Crohn's disease, but it is believed to be an abnormal immune response, characterized by inflammation in the gut, to something in the digestive tract—to the food or bacteria

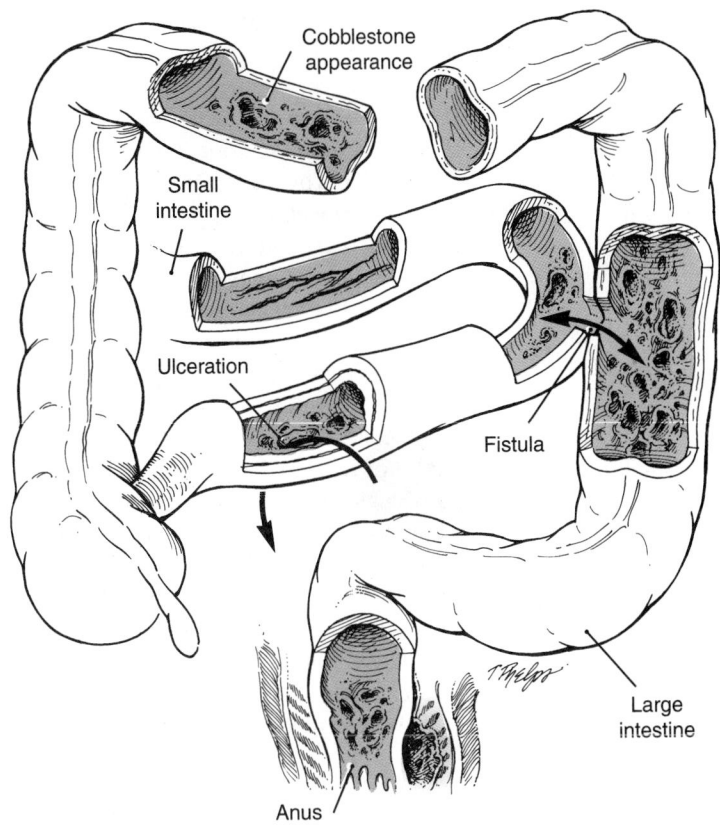

There is an inherited tendency to Crohn's disease, an inflammatory bowel disease that appears to be caused by an abnormal immune response to something in the digestive tract. Crohn's disease primarily involves the small intestine but can also involve the large intestine and anus, and it typically occurs in patchy regions that are interspersed among normal segments of bowel. Swelling and inflammation lead to the appearance of cobblestone. The disease may affect all layers of the intestinal wall, leading to ulceration and fistulae. Medications that fight inflammation or infection or that suppress the immune system may be used as treatments, although nearly 50 percent of people with Crohn's disease may eventually need surgery.

in the intestines or even to the lining of the bowel itself. This illness itself is not simply inherited; scientists believe that more than one faulty gene is needed for this disease to develop. However, there is an inherited tendency to Crohn's disease. From 10 to 15 percent of people with Crohn's disease have a family history of this disorder; an additional 5 to 7 percent of these people have a family history of ulcerative colitis. For those with a family history of inflammatory bowel disease (both Crohn's and ulcerative colitis), early onset in the teens and 20s is more likely; but 90 percent of people with Crohn's disease develop symptoms before age 40.

What you can do Because chronic diarrhea can deplete your body of essential nutrients, if you have Crohn's disease, it is doubly important that you eat a balanced diet and maintain a high fluid intake, to avoid becoming dehydrated. Instead of eating three big meals a day (which can be harder for your body to digest), eat small meals five or six times a day. Bananas, which replace potassium lost through diarrhea, are an excellent snack. Avoid or limit your intake of hard-to-digest foods such as popcorn, small seeds, and nuts; spicy foods; caffeine; alcohol; and lactose-containing foods—all of these may irritate the intestine. Also, in some people, exercise causes diarrhea or makes it worse; if you are interested in keeping fit, ask your doctor about developing a mild exercise program.

Because its cause is poorly understood, there is no known means of preventing Crohn's disease, a disorder that can be frustrating and even debilitating at times. For teens and young adults with severe disease, both the disease and its treatment can exact a heavy toll. Many people are greatly helped by taking charge of their symptoms—by learning as much as possible about the latest research and treatment—and by talking to others experiencing the same problems. For more information, or to find out about a support group near you, write The Crohn's and Colitis Foundation of America, Inc., National Headquarters, 444 Park Avenue South, 11th Floor, New York, NY, 10016-7374, or call (212) 685-3440 or (800) 343-3637.

When to call the doctor Call your doctor if you have chronic diarrhea that does not respond to over-the-counter medications; blood in the stool, or black, tarlike stool; if you are unable to eat or drink; if you have intense abdominal pain; or if you have unexplained fever that lasts more than 1 or 2 days.

Treatment There is no cure for this chronic condition; the aim of treatment is to suppress the inflammatory symptoms and preserve the bowel. Crohn's disease comes in many degrees of severity; some people are easily treated with medication, while others have intractable disease that may

require—as last resort—surgery.

Medication Depending on the severity of your disease, you may need one or more of these medications:

- *Anti-inflammatory drugs:* Sulfasalazine, mesalamine (5-ASA), olsalazine (Dipentum), prednisone, mercaptopurine (6-MP, Purinethol), azathioprine (Imuran)

- *Antibiotics:* Metronidazole (Flagyl), ciprofloxacin (Cipro)

If you are being treated at a university research center, and if your disease is severe, your doctor may also prescribe methotrexate or cyclosporine (Sandimmune)—two powerful medications that suppress the immune system. As yet, these medications are considered experimental for treatment of Crohn's disease, and they are used mainly when other medications have failed. Prednisone, mercaptopurine, methotrexate, and cyclosporine, although effective, like many medications, can have long-term side effects; for instance, they can lower the body's resistance to opportunistic infections. Thus, the goal is to get your disease under control, and then to cut back the medications as much as possible.

Nutritional treatment If the inflammation is severe, your doctor may want to give your bowel a chance to rest for several weeks, either by enteric feeding (a liquid diet) or total parenteral nutrition (see Nutritional Supplementation and Feeding Tubes, page 1000).

Surgery In some cases—particularly in people who have recurrent bowel obstruction, fistulas, intraabdominal abscesses, strictures, or symptoms not responsive to medication—surgery is needed to remove or open a segment of the bowel. Nearly half of all people with Crohn's disease may need surgery at some point, usually around 8 to 10 years after symptoms begin. Because intestinal surgery itself can cause many problems—scar tissue, bowel obstruction, stricture, infection—this is not a primary therapy. Because Crohn's disease tends to recur, it is impractical and unfeasible to keep removing segments of bowel with each bout of symptoms. If your gastroenterologist wants you to undergo repeat surgery, seek a second opinion: More aggressive medication therapy (described on page 1008) could be sufficient to treat the problem.

Prognosis Although there is no cure for Crohn's disease, new medications and nutritional and surgical therapies can allow excellent management of the disease.

MECKEL'S DIVERTICULUM

Symptoms *(What you may experience)* Abdominal pain, rectal bleeding, bloody stool. However, many people never experience symptoms.

Signs and laboratory findings *(What the doctor looks for)* Evidence of rectal bleeding, detected in a stool blood test (see Other Diagnostic Tests of the Gastrointestinal Tract, page 984). An outpouching, about 2 in long, in the lower part of the small intestine, seen during a small bowel series (see Barium Studies, page 976).

What is it? Meckel's diverticulum is a congenital abnormality, in which a small pouch grows in part of the wall of the small intestine. Unlike the pouches seen in diverticulosis, this pouch contains stomach mucosa; in effect, stomach tissue is growing in the bowel. Although many people live for years or even a lifetime without experiencing symptoms, this tissue may become inflamed, and an ulcer (similar to a gastric ulcer) may develop. In severe cases, this inflammation may cause intestinal blockage or may even result in perforation, which could lead to peritonitis.

Treatment The standard form of treatment for symptomatic Meckel's diverticulum is surgery to remove the diverticulum, or pouch. This procedure requires hospitalization and is performed under general anesthesia.

Prognosis Excellent.

SMALL BOWEL CANCER

Symptoms *(What you may experience)* Black, tarlike stool (melena), blood in the stool, rectal bleeding; vomiting; abdominal pain or cramps, especially after eating; abdominal distension; weight loss; fatigue; general weakness or malaise. However, in some people, small bowel cancer is silent, producing no symptoms.

Signs and laboratory findings *(What the doctor looks for)* A palpable abdominal mass, felt in a physical examination; evidence of a tumor or mass, as seen in endoscopy of the small bowel, a CT scan, or a small bowel barium series; jaundice (caused if a tumor is blocking a bile duct); signs of iron-deficiency anemia. (See Upper Endoscopy, page 968, Other Diagnostic Tests of the Gastrointestinal Tract, page 984, and Barium Studies, page 976).

What is it? Small bowel cancer is a rare—fewer than 3,000 new cases are diagnosed every year in this country—malignant tumor of the ileum, jejunum, or duodenum. The tumor can be constricting, narrowing the channel, or may be polypoid, protruding into the intestine. Sometimes, small bowel cancer is linked to other diseases. For reasons that are poorly understood, it may be a complication of celiac disease (see Malabsorption Syndromes, page 995); also, cancer in the duodenum is associated with familial adenomatous polyposis (FAP) and hereditary nonpolyposis colon cancer (HNPCC; see Hereditary Forms of Colorectal Cancer, page 1023). Benign tumors in the small bowel are extremely rare, tend not to produce symptoms, and usually are found incidentally.

What you can do Be sure to tell your doctor if you have a family history of celiac disease, FAP, or HNPCC; more frequent screening for cancer may be recommended.

Treatment If your cancer is in the jejunum or ileum, the main form of treatment is surgery to remove the cancerous part of the small intestine and reconnect the remaining intestine. If your cancer is in the duodenum, because of its proximity to other organs, you may need a more extensive operation called a Whipple procedure (see page 1064). Radiation therapy and chemotherapy are not effective in curing small bowel cancer. Benign tumors are usually removed surgically. Many of these tumors, although harmless, tend to grow in the lower small bowel—out of reach of the endoscope and thus are difficult or impossible to biopsy without surgery. Only after their removal are they determined to be benign.

The Colon

❖ ULCERATIVE COLITIS

Symptoms *(What you may experience)*
Blood in the stool or black, tarlike stool
(which suggests intestinal bleeding);
chronic diarrhea; abdominal pain; weight
loss; joint aches or pains; unexplained fever;
eye pain when you look at bright light; persistent canker sores in the mouth.

Signs and laboratory findings *(What the
doctor looks for)* Edema, ulcerations, or
erosions in the intestine, seen in endoscopy
(see Upper Endoscopy, page 968); an intestinal lining that bleeds easily when touched
during endoscopy; characteristic skin
lesions; evidence of arthritis in the spine or
joints; jaundice (due to inflammation of the
bile ducts); inflammation in the eye.

What is it? Ulcerative colitis is an unexplained inflammatory disorder of the colon
and rectum that is due to damage caused by
the body's immune system and that cannot
be attributed to any other pathogen. There
appears to be a genetic component: Fifteen
percent of people with ulcerative colitis
have a family history of the diseases, and
another 2 to 3 percent have a family history
of Crohn's disease. Although diagnosed most
commonly in early adulthood, ulcerative colitis can develop at any age.

Ulcerative colitis is a medical diagnosis
of exclusion: A doctor pinpoints the problem by first determining what it is not.
(Ulcerative colitis is *not* linked to psychological stress.) Thus, the first step is to investigate infectious causes of symptoms, such
as *Salmonella* and *Shigella* organisms,
amoebae, and gonorrhea, and to rule out
Crohn's disease, which can be hard to distinguish from ulcerative colitis. Ulcerative
colitis can also be accompanied by other
problems, such as biliary disease, in which
the bile ducts become scarred.

During colonoscopy (see page 1011),
the damage from ulcerative colitis appears
contiguous: Your doctor will see disease
beginning in the rectum, continuing into
the colon, and sometimes reaching all the
way to the ileum. Ulcerative colitis is linked
to colon cancer, and you should undergo a
full colonoscopy (which allows doctors to
see much more of the large bowel) instead

of a flexible sigmoidoscopy for surveillance
of colon cancer.

Ulcerative proctitis This is a form of ulcerative colitis, limited to the rectum only. There
are other causes of proctitis, including temporary irritation and inflammation that can
develop from rectal intercourse or infection.

Toxic megacolon In severe ulcerative colitis, the colon becomes enlarged and dilated
and does not contract well. This serious
condition, known as toxic megacolon, is
usually associated with fever and abdominal
pain. The concern is that the colon will perforate—a medical emergency that could
result in peritonitis and death.

What you can do Because chronic diarrhea can strip your body of essential nutrients, it is very important to eat a balanced
diet and maintain a high fluid intake, to
avoid becoming dehydrated. Instead of eating three big meals a day (which can be
harder for your body to digest), eat small
meals five or six times a day. Bananas, which
replace potassium lost through diarrhea, are
an excellent snack. Avoid or limit your
intake of hard-to-digest foods such as popcorn, small seeds, and nuts; spicy foods; caffeine; alcohol; and chocolate—all of these
may irritate the intestine.

Finally, ulcerative colitis can be frustrating and even debilitating at times. However,
many people are greatly helped by taking
charge of their symptoms—by learning as
much as possible about the latest research
and treatment—and by talking to others
experiencing the same problems. For more
information, or to find out about a support
group near you, write The Crohn's and Colitis Foundation of America, Inc., National
Headquarters, 444 Park Avenue South, 11th
Floor, New York, NY, 10016-7374, or call
(212) 685-3440 or (800) 343-3637.

When to call the doctor Call your doctor if
you have chronic diarrhea that does not
respond to over-the-counter medications; if
you have blood in the stool, or black, tarlike
stool; if you are unable to eat or drink; if you
have intense abdominal pain; or if you have
unexplained fever that lasts more than 1 or
2 days.

Treatment Ulcerative colitis comes in many
degrees of severity; some people are easily

COLONOSCOPY

Colonoscopy is a more extensive version of flexible sigmoidoscopy (see page 1006). The colonoscope is about 5 feet long—more than twice the length of the sigmoidoscope—and the procedure is done with sedation. Because of the length of the colonoscope and the greater risk of complications—1 in 1,000—colonoscopy should be performed by a board-certified or board-eligible gastroenterologist.

The colonoscope is a lighted, flexible tube equipped with a tiny video camera. It is lubricated and inserted through your rectum and allows a doctor to explore the lining of the bowel thoroughly, all the way to the cecum, and to search for any abnormalities. Some problems that cannot be detected with x-rays, or reached with a sigmoidoscope, can be seen clearly with a colonoscope.

During the procedure, done with you lying on your left side, the gastroenterologist may perform a biopsy, threading a cutting tool through the colonoscope to take a small sample of tissue. A biopsy can be performed for many reasons; having a biopsy does not mean that you have cancer. If you have a polyp, an abnormal growth of tissue, your doctor may use electrocautery to snare it with a wire loop, passed through the colonoscope. The colonoscope can also be used to cauterize any bleeding areas; dilate a stricture; inject medication (using extra-long needles, threaded through the endoscope); and photograph any abnormal findings.

Colonoscopy, which generally takes about 45 minutes, is a safe procedure, with a low risk—about 1 in 1,000—of complications. The risk increases if other procedures (such as a polypectomy, or polyp removal) are performed. It is done with informed consent, which means you should have a full understanding of the risks involved. Potential complications include a tear or tiny hole (called a perforation) in the lining of the bowel, which may heal on its own or may require surgery to repair it; bleeding, if a biopsy is done or a polyp is removed (usually bleeding is minimal; rarely, it may require surgery or a blood transfusion); a reaction to the sedative given before the procedure (thus, be sure to tell the doctor if you are allergic to any medications). Also, many people experience abdominal tenderness for several hours afterward. There is a minimal risk of infection with any procedure.

The bowel must be as clean as possible before colonoscopy, for two reasons: One is so that the doctor can see every part of the lining. The other is that, if you need electrocautery to stop bleeding or remove a polyp, any vestige of stool or pocket of gas can ignite, causing a miniexplosion and injuring tissue. Thus, the night before, you will have the unappealing but necessary task of drinking a 4-quart jug of a solution (such as Go-Lytely or Colyte), that flushes out the gastrointestinal tract, from the top down. You will also be asked not to eat any solid food at least 2 hours before you start drinking this solution, not to eat or drink anything at all after midnight, and (to minimize the risk of bleeding) to stop taking aspirin for at least 2 days beforehand. If you are taking aspirin or any medication regularly, do not skip a scheduled dose without talking to your doctor first. Also, any medication taken within 1 hour before you start drinking the solution may be flushed from the body and not absorbed.

As many as half of all people who drink one of these solutions—despite the makers' attempts to make them more palatable with such flavors as pineapple—feel nauseated during the process. Many patients find it extremely helpful to drink this solution when it is very cold.

Shortly before the procedure begins, you will be given an intravenous, short-term sedative such as diazepam (Valium) or midazolam (Versed) or a narcotic such as meperidine (Demerol) or fentanyl (Sublimaze) to help you relax and make you feel drowsy. Because air is pumped into your bowel—making the area larger to maximize the doctor's field of vision—you may feel discomfort from cramps or distension during the procedure. This will get better immediately afterward, as soon as you expel the air, although your abdomen may still feel tender for the next few hours. The presence of the colonoscope may also give you a mild sensation that you need to have a bowel movement (do not worry—this is impossible; your bowels are empty). During the procedure, you may be asked to change positions as the colonoscope moves through your intestine. Sometimes, fluoroscopy (x-ray testing) is also performed during colonoscopy. You should not feel any pain or discomfort from the procedure itself.

About 1 percent of people experience gastrointestinal bleeding after a polypectomy. This may occur immediately, or blood may appear several days or even a week after the colonoscopy. It is very common to have trace amounts of blood in your stool. But if you notice a significant amount of blood, call your doctor immediately.

Finally, because the sedative or narcotic can impair your judgment and reflexes (and may cause you to forget what happened during the procedure itself), plan on having someone drive you home after the colonoscopy. At some hospitals, the procedure will be canceled or performed without sedation if you do not have an escort home. ∎

---

treated with medication, while others seem to have intractable disease that may require surgery. In 70 percent of people with the condition, symptoms occur intermittently; in others, symptoms may be continuously active.

Medication Depending on the severity of your disease, you may need one or more of these medications:

- *Anti-inflammatory drugs:* Sulfasalazine, mesalamine, olsalazine, prednisone, mercaptopurine, azathioprine

- *Antibiotics:* Metronidazole

If you are being treated at a university research center, or if your disease is severe, your doctor may also prescribe methotrexate or cyclosporine—two powerful medications that also suppress the immune system. As yet, these drugs are considered experimental for treatment of ulcerative colitis, and they are used mainly when other medications have failed. Because prednisone, mercaptopurine, methotrexate, and cyclosporine, although effective, can have long-term side

ILEOSTOMY, KOCK POUCH, ILEOANAL POUCH, AND COLOSTOMY

An ostomy—an ileostomy or colostomy—is a surgically made opening in the abdominal wall that creates a new exit route for stool, which then collects in a small plastic bag, firmly affixed to the skin. The United Ostomy Association estimates that more than 15,000 Americans are "ostomates," people with ostomies. Ileostomies are most often performed on people with Crohn's disease or ulcerative colitis; colostomies are most common in people with rectal cancer. Both procedures may be used as temporary solutions, as well, for people whose intestines need time to recover from illness or injury. Over the last few years, however, fewer ileostomies and continent ileostomies, known as the Kock pouch have been performed—thanks to a breakthrough operation known as the ileoanal pouch procedure: The colon is removed, and the end of the small intestine is made into a pouch and connected directly to the anus (an ileoanal pull-through procedure), allowing people to defecate normally. In all of these procedures, your ability to urinate normally will not be affected.

For many people, an ostomy does not mean the end of normal life; instead, it is an end to pain, weight loss, the side effects of medications, and debilitating symptoms. It is not uncommon

for doctors to hear, "I wish I'd done this sooner" from people who, except for the ostomy, feel otherwise normal for the first time in years. Depending on your body shape, physical condition, lifestyle, and clothing preferences, you may even get to have some say in where the ostomy is placed.

You can do almost anything with an ostomy (except wear a bikini): get pregnant and have a baby, ride a bicycle, ski, even play professional football, like one record-setting National Football League place-kicker, who refused to let his ileostomy slow him down. Talk to your doctor before beginning any strenuous exercise program. If you do engage in contact sports, you will need special protection; also, you should avoid heavy lifting, which may cause a hernia to develop around the ostomy site. ◗

Intestinal diseases that require time for recovery or surgical removal of a portion of the intestines may result in a temporary or permanent ileostomy (A) or colostomy (B), which are surgically created openings in the abdominal wall. Stool then collects in a small, disposable, plastic bag that can be attached to the skin. The presence of an ostomy generally does not prevent a person from carrying out functions such as getting pregnant or engaging in physical activity.

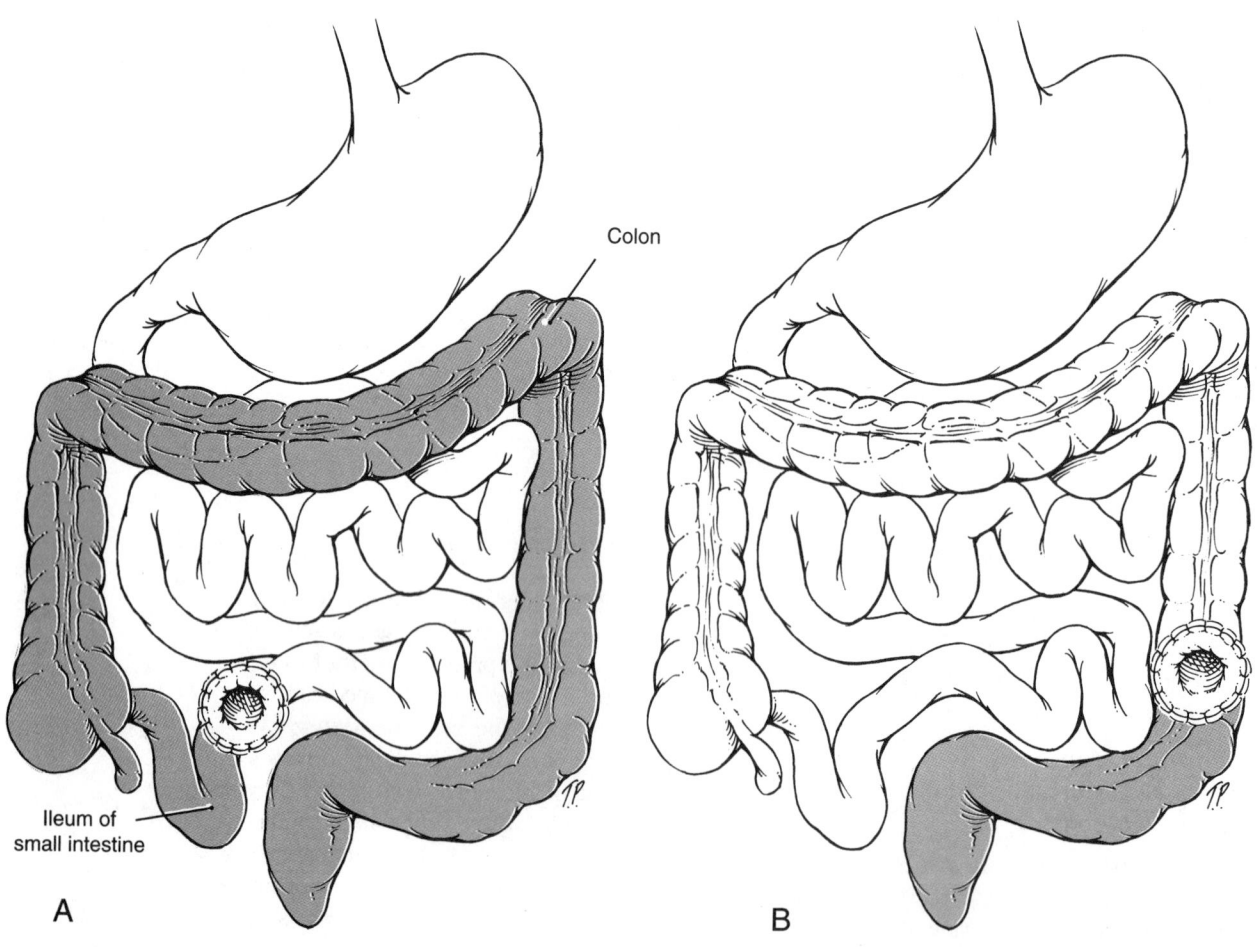

Colon

Ileum of small intestine

A

B

▶ But this return of confidence often takes time. At first, most people who undergo an ostomy procedure feel overwhelmed with worries about body image, sexuality, the ability to work, and the day-to-day management of the bag (also called the appliance). These are very important concerns, and before undergoing any form of ostomy, you should discuss all of them with your doctor and ileostomy nurse. At some hospitals, an enterostomal therapist, trained to help people face such quality-of-life issues, is also available. Ask your doctor for the names of other patients who have gone through this procedure, and for information about local support groups. After surgery, it may be very helpful for a home nurse to visit, to make sure you are properly caring for the ostomy and, equally important, to make sure you are coping adequately with this change. Many insurance companies pay for a home health nurse; find out if you are eligible to receive this service.

Ileostomy

In an ileostomy, part of the ileum (the last part of the small intestine) is brought outside the abdominal wall through the surgical opening. This procedure requires several days of hospitalization and is done with general anesthesia. The material that passes through this opening will be much more liquid than normal stool, because it never reaches the colon, where most of the water is removed before defecation. Immediately after surgery, there will be some edema (fluid swelling) around the area. The stoma, the band of intestine sewn in place at the opening, should be pink or dark red; your doctor may need to check this opening (to make sure the tissue is healthy, or to check for a stricture, an abnormal narrowing caused by scar tissue) by shining a light or gently threading an endoscope through this opening. It may take several days for your intestine to begin functioning normally—for peristalsis, the rhythmic muscle contractions that move food through the digestive tract, to commence. You will not be allowed to eat or drink anything until bowel sounds and other signs (such as your ability to pass gas) indicate that your gut is working again. For the first few weeks after surgery, you will probably be on a restricted diet. Even after you have healed, you may want to steer clear of certain high-residue foods including popcorn, nuts, corn, cabbage, and mushrooms; ask your doctor for dietary guidelines. During the 6 to 8 weeks afterward, as your body recovers from this major surgery, you will need to take it easy. Walking is the best exercise for now. Avoid lifting anything heavier than 10 lb, and ease back into your normal physical activities, including sexual intercourse. Almost everyone who undergoes an ostomy operation experiences some difficulty in resuming sexual activity, including impotence. This is normal. Some people are helped by changing positions; most people find that the best medicine here is time, with generous helpings of patience and understanding from your partner. If you are having persistent trouble, seek help from your doctor, your ostomy nurse, or enterostomal therapist. Do not be discouraged. It will get better.

It is essential that you keep the area around any form of ostomy meticulously clean and that the appliance fits properly; otherwise, an annoying cycle may develop: The bag does not adhere well to irritated skin; in turn, leakage of stool may aggravate this irritation. Complications from inadequate hygiene or leakage of stool—which contains many irritants, including bile acids, harsh pancreatic enzymes, and a high concentration of alkali—may include contact dermatitis (redness or irritation), ulcers, or raised nodules in the skin. Skin irritation may also be caused by an allergic reaction to the appliance; (changing brands should fix this problem) or by irritation of the hair follicles (shaving the area with an electric razor or clipping with scissors can help here). Some people develop a skin infection (with tiny pustules), which usually gets better with a thin layer of nystatin powder, applied each time you change the bag. An estimated 15 to 25 percent of people with ostomies—usually, those with a recurrence of Crohn's disease—eventually need additional surgery; this may be because of a prolapse or shrinkage of the stoma (the opening) or may be due to scar tissue, adhesions, or development of a fistula. Some people experience blockage of the stoma (usually caused by difficult-to-digest foods such as the ones mentioned above), with symptoms including nausea, vomiting, abdominal cramps, and an absence of stool in the bag. This form of obstruction is usually removed by flushing the opening with a catheter, and administering intravenous fluids to prevent dehydration.

Kock Pouch

This procedure is similar to an ileostomy, except there is no external bag. Instead, a surgeon creates a nipple valve with a cap, similar to the kind on an inflatable beach ball, small enough to be covered with a band-aid or gauze patch. Stool remains in a reservoir, or pouch, made in the small intestine. Your job is to intubate the pouch several times a day, by inserting a catheter inside it; stool flows through this directly into the toilet. Immediately after surgery, and for several weeks thereafter, you will wear a catheter, which extends from the stoma and empties into a bag, which must be irrigated frequently. The catheter is temporary—a respite that allows the stoma to heal and gives the valve time to settle in.

Problems related to the stoma itself are usually minor, and include a discharge of mucus (which means that you will need to change the gauze more frequently), and difficulty emptying the pouch because of thick stool; this will probably improve if you drink prune juice and additional fluids throughout the day. The major source of trouble with a Kock pouch is the nipple valve: In as many as 15 percent of patients, it tends to slip or prolapse, causing incontinence (leakage of stool) and difficulty inserting the catheter; in severe cases, surgery may be needed to repair the valve. A more common complication is called pouchitis: inflammation (seen through the endoscope as bright red, with swelling, tiny areas of bleeding, and small ulcers) within the pouch itself. The cause of pouchitis is not completely understood; it may be related to the inflammatory bowel disease that caused you to need surgery in the first place. Or it may be a form of bacterial overgrowth (see Malabsorption Syndromes, page 995). Pouchitis typically has a sudden onset; symptoms may include nausea and vomiting, fever, cramps and tenderness, and diarrhea and malaise; some people experience joint pain, as well. Fortunately, although it can be dramatic, pouchitis responds fairly quickly (within a few days) to treatment with broad-spectrum antibiotics, which must be taken for 10 to 14 days. ▶

◆ Ileoanal Anastomosis (Pouch)

This breakthrough operation, also known as pelvic pouch, or the ileoanal pull-through procedure, has become the procedure of choice for the majority of people with ulcerative colitis or FAP who require surgery. This procedure is not ideal for some people, however, including people with Crohn's disease, people who have fecal incontinence or poor sphincter muscle tone, or people who have had part of the small bowel removed in previous surgery. Its great advantages: no bag, no catheter, no ostomy. You can have bowel movements in the normal way. In a variation on this procedure, an ileorectal anastomosis is created, linking the end of the small intestine to the rectum.

This is major surgery, like the procedures discussed above, with general anesthesia and similar hospitalization time—the better part of a week. The idea here is that the small intestine is made to do the work of the entire bowel: A surgeon removes the diseased colon, rectum, and anal canal, and stretches out the small intestine, using its end (the ileum) to create a new rectum, a pouch or reservoir where stool is stored until normal defecation. There are three types of reservoirs, shaped like a "J," "S," or "W"; the surgeon will determine which type is right for you during surgery, based on the length and configuration of your small intestine. In rare cases, despite surgeons' extensive attempts to connect the ileum to the anal canal, the small bowel simply will not reach, and a permanent ileostomy is made instead.

For about 2 months after surgery, you will have a temporary ileostomy; its purpose is to give the anastomosis (the surgical connection of tissue) a chance to heal. When this is removed (in a procedure called an ileostomy takedown), the pouch will begin working on its own. Be patient: For the first weeks or even months, expect erratic, frequent bowel movements—as many as 15 a day. Within a year, as the reservoir adapts, you will probably be having only five or six bowel movements a day. For those first few months, bulking agents such as psyllium, or an anti-diarrheal medication such as loperamide, may help produce fewer bowel movements. Certain foods, such as cheese, peanut butter, applesauce, rice, bananas, and mashed potatoes, can also help decrease the frequency of bowel movements. Complications include pouchitis (see page 1013) and small bowel obstruction (a risk of any form of abdominal surgery; see Bowel Obstruction, page 1005); stricture, which may need to be treated with dilatation (see Anal Stricture, page 1027); or development of a small leak in the anastomosis (which may be caused by a fistula or abscess; see Anal Abscess and Fistula, page 1027).

Colostomy

In a colostomy, a procedure similar to ileostomy in hospitalization and recovery, the stoma is made using part of the large intestine. One difference: people who have had an ileostomy cannot begin eating normal food until there is evidence that the bowel is working; people who have had a colostomy usually need to eat food before the colostomy begins to function. The nature of the stool that passes from this opening—unlike the irritating material that emerges through an ileostomy—is basically normal; it has made it through the normal digestive process. Constipation and even fecal impaction can occur (particularly in people who have been troubled by constipation before); bulk fiber may help regulate your bowel movements. Complications include problems with blood flow (the colon, in general, has a less well-developed blood supply than the small intestine); some people develop a stricture, which may eventually need treatment. Your gastroenterologist will check for problems by shining a light or gently threading an endoscope through this opening. There are variations on the colostomy procedure: Instead of a bag, there is an option called a continent colostomy ring (such as the Erlangen magnetic colostomy device); like the Kock pouch (see page 1013), it is emptied several times a day. Or, some people with end-sigmoid colostomies opt for colostomy irrigation: flushing the intestine with lukewarm water. These people, too, have a cap, instead of a bag, and need to cleanse the bowel only once a day. However, irrigation is a time-consuming procedure, taking 1 to 2 hours a day; also, it must be performed regularly, at the same time each day. Thus, if you have a hectic or erratic schedule, this is probably not an ideal option. ∎

effects (for instance, they can lower the body's resistance to opportunistic infections), the goal is to get your disease under control and then cut back on these medications as much as possible.

Nutritional treatment If the inflammation is severe, your doctor may want to give your bowel a chance to rest for several weeks, either by enteric feeding (a liquid diet) or total parenteral nutrition (see Nutritional Supplementation and Feeding Tubes, page 1000).

Surgery In some cases—particularly in people who have toxic megacolon, perforation, or evidence of cancer or abnormal cells, or symptoms not responsive to medication—surgery is needed to remove the colon, a procedure called a *colectomy.* Surgery can cure ulcerative colitis.

If you have ulcerative proctitis, your doctor may recommend a topical treatment (probably anti-inflammatory enemas) in addition to the medications discussed on page 1011.

If you have toxic megacolon, your doctor's first goal will be to rest your bowel. For several days, you will receive intravenous fluid, steroids (to fight the inflammation), antibiotics (to combat infection), and absolutely nothing—not even water—by mouth. If your symptoms do not improve within several days, it will probably be necessary for your colon to be removed.

Prognosis With proper medication, 70 percent of individuals with ulcerative colitis can be kept in remission. For those in whom the disease is progressive, removal of the colon provides a cure.

❖ *C. DIFFICILE* COLITIS AND ANTIBIOTIC-ASSOCIATED DIARRHEA

Symptoms *(What you may experience)* Diarrhea; fever; severe cramps; spasm in the rectum; dehydration; weight loss. These symptoms may last days or weeks.

Signs and laboratory findings *(What the doctor looks for)* Positive results of a *C. difficile* toxin test in a stool sample; pseudomembranes, yellow, raised plaques in the colon, seen in colonoscopy (see page 1011); also, the presence of fecal leukocytes (suggesting inflammation of the colon) in the stool; elevated levels of white blood cells in a blood sample. If the toxin test is negative for *C. difficile* but you have recently taken an antibiotic for another ailment, you may be diagnosed as having antibiotic-associated diarrhea.

What is it? *C. difficile* colitis is an infection caused by *Clostridium difficile*, a form of bacteria normally present in about 3 percent of adults. It usually develops after an antibiotic has wiped out the normal gut bacteria that keep it under control. Unchecked, *C. difficile* proliferates rapidly, making a toxin that damages the colonic mucosa, allowing diarrhea to occur.

When to call the doctor Call your doctor if you are severely ill and at risk of becoming dehydrated; if you have a high fever or severe cramps; or if you have diarrhea that persists longer than a few days.

Treatment The first step is to stop the original antibiotic, if you are still taking it. If symptoms do not improve, your doctor will probably prescribe a oral metronidazole. Alternatively, a resin (a prescription cholesterol-lowering medication such as cholestyramine [Questran] or colestipol [Colestid]) can be used to absorb the toxin in the stool and keep it from reaching the intestinal cells; however, this treatment is usually not as effective as oral metronidazole.

Antibiotic-associated diarrhea usually responds to stopping the offending antibiotic. Your doctor may also recommend that you eat active yogurt cultures, in an attempt to repopulate the normal gut bacteria.

Prognosis Good; however, relapses with *C. difficile* colitis are very common and tend to occur 3 to 10 days after you stop taking the antibiotics. You may need several rounds of treatment to eradicate this infection.

❖ ACUTE APPENDICITIS

Symptoms *(What you may experience)* Severe cramps; abdominal pain (at first, near or above the navel); inability to eat; fever; nausea; vomiting. After several hours, as the appendix becomes more inflamed, the pain shifts to the lower right abdomen.

Signs and laboratory findings *(What the doctor looks for)* Extreme tenderness, either when the doctor touches your abdomen or when pressure from the doctor's hand is released (this is called rebound tenderness); abnormally high levels of white blood cells (showing significant infection); obstruction, abscess, or rupture of the appendix, seen on CT scan or ultrasound.

What is it? The appendix, called the vermiform appendix (because this appendage is shaped like a worm) is a 3- to 6-in. long cul-de-sac attached to the cecum, part of the colon. Acute appendicitis develops when the opening of the appendix becomes blocked. This obstruction can be caused by several problems, including lymphoid hyperplasia, an abnormal buildup of immune tissue; a little stone of stool, called a fecalith, that finds its way into the appendix and plugs it; an intestinal stricture or tumor; and, rarely, a swallowed foreign body. Infection begins behind the obstruction; as it builds, the pressure in the appendix—and the pain this causes—escalates. If untreated, an abscess can develop, the appendix may rupture, and peritonitis—a surgical emergency, in which the infection spreads throughout the lining of the abdomen—may follow.

Treatment Acute appendicitis is a surgical emergency; the operation to remove the appendix, called an appendectomy, will probably be done as soon as the diagnosis is made. Your doctor may perform this procedure traditionally, via an abdominal incision, or laparoscopically, using a tiny telescope equipped with a video camera (so the surgeon can see your internal organs on a television screen in the operating room) and special instruments that allow the appendix to be removed through the much smaller incision. The appendix has no known function in humans, and its removal does not affect digestion in any way.

Prognosis Excellent, especially with early diagnosis. When the appendix is removed, the problem is solved. If, however, there is a complication such as peritonitis or an abscess, your recovery period will probably take longer.

❖ DIVERTICULAR DISEASE: DIVERTICULOSIS AND DIVERTICULITIS

Symptoms *(What you may experience)* Diverticulosis usually has no symptoms but may cause rectal bleeding. Diverticulitis

Diverticulosis occurs when an area of the colon balloons outward, forming a small pocket (diverticula). This common condition leads to complications in up to 20 percent of people who have it. These include inflammation (diverticulitis) and rectal bleeding. Diverticulitis can lead to a hole or abscess in the intestine, which allows intestinal material to leak into the abdominal cavity. This condition, called peritonitis, is a medical emergency.

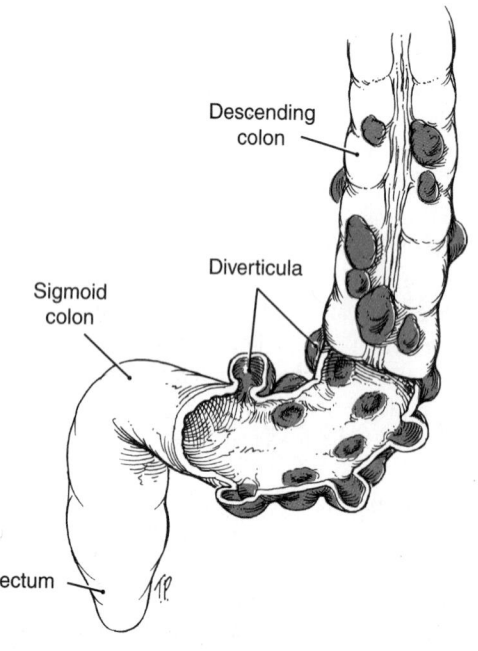

Descending colon

Diverticula

Sigmoid colon

Rectum

may cause significant rectal bleeding (bright red blood); fever, abdominal pain; a change in bowel habits; (rarely) passing air during urination or the presence of stool in the urine or vagina.

Signs and laboratory findings *(What the doctor looks for)* Extreme tenderness of the abdomen or stomach in a physical exam; rebound tenderness—when the doctor presses on the stomach, and pain comes immediately afterward, as the doctor's hand is lifted. *Note:* Extreme or rebound tenderness could be a sign of a perforated diverticulum, which could lead to peritonitis—a surgical emergency, in which infection spreads throughout the lining of the abdomen. Evidence of shock (dangerously low blood pressure, a medical emergency).

What is it? Diverticulosis is the development of numerous tiny pockets, called diverticula, in the colon (generally in the sigmoid). It is the most common condition affecting the colon. By age 80, an estimated half of all Americans have at least some degree of diverticulosis. The problem seems to originate when two or more of the muscular bands that encircle the colon begin to contract at the same time, hindering the colon's ability to move its contents—a mixture of gas, liquid, and waste—along to the rectum. When this material becomes trapped, it tends to press against the wall of the colon, creating diverticula.

For most people, this condition never produces any troublesome symptoms. However, complications from diverticulosis develop in as many as 20 percent of people. One of these is rectal bleeding; the other is diverticulitis, inflammation caused when one or more of these diverticula become infected. In severe cases, diverticulitis can lead to a hole or abscess in the intestine, causing peritonitis, in which intestinal material spills into the abdominal cavity—a medical emergency. There is no definite cause of diverticulosis, which can take years to develop; however, some evidence suggests that the disease is more likely to develop in people who eat very little fiber.

What you can do There is no proven strategy for preventing diverticulosis. However, because the disease may be linked to a lack of dietary fiber (see above), a diet high in fiber (found in beans, whole grains, certain fruits and vegetables) may lower your likelihood of developing this condition. Your doctor may also recommend a fiber supplement. It may take your body several weeks to adjust to a high-fiber diet. Adding too much dietary fiber too soon can cause gas and abdominal pain from distension.

Some doctors believe that patients who already have diverticulitis can minimize their risk of recurrent infections by avoiding such hard-to-digest foods as popcorn and seeds, which may become lodged in the colon.

Treatment *For rectal bleeding* In most people, episodes of rectal bleeding from diverticulosis resolve on their own. However, as many as 25 percent of patients with diverticulosis experience at least two bouts of rectal bleeding. If the bleeding returns or does not stop, an interventional radiologist, guided by an angiogram, may infuse a vasoconstrictor (an artery-constricting drug such as vasopressin) directly into the area of bleeding. If this does not stop the bleeding, you may need surgery to remove the diseased section of the colon.

For diverticulitis If your symptoms are severe, your doctor will want to start by giving your bowel a chance to rest—which means ingesting nothing by mouth and receiving nutrition and antibiotics intravenously. This may last a minimum of several days, or—depending on the degree of inflammation—up to 2 weeks. If your symptoms do not improve with medical therapy, or if you have a complication such as an abscess or fistula, you may need surgery.

Surgery Depending on the severity of the inflammation, it may be necessary for a surgeon to remove part of your colon. In some people, this is a two-stage procedure: The first part is a temporary colostomy (see Ileostomy, Kock Pouch, Ileoanal Pouch, and Colostomy, page 1012), to give the bowel a chance to heal. After a period of convalescence (lasting several weeks or months), this colostomy is usually removed, and the remaining colon is reconnected.

❖ IRRITABLE BOWEL SYNDROME (SPASTIC COLON)

Symptoms *(What you may experience)* Diarrhea; constipation; constipation alternating with diarrhea; abdominal pain; bloating; gas pain; excessive flatulence; increased belching; mucus in the stool; small stools (rabbitlike pellets) or flat, ribbon stools. Symptoms tend to worsen during times of stress.

Signs and laboratory findings *(What the doctor looks for)* A palpable, tender sigmoid colon (suggesting spasm) on physical exam; hypersensitive bowel reaction to distension in a test called anorectal manometry (in which a balloon is inflated in the rectum, causing distension). In addition to your medical history, note any recent or current stressful events or situations.

Because irritable bowel syndrome (IBS) is often a diagnosis of exclusion, your doctor should make a meticulous effort to rule out all other disorders. This may require a detailed history to detect food intolerance; blood tests including a complete blood count; stool analysis for parasites; and flexible sigmoidoscopy with biopsy, to make sure there is no structural abnormality or other disease such as ulcerative colitis.

Diagnosis is supported by your answers to one or more of the following questions: Are your symptoms aggravated by meals? Are they relieved by moving the bowels? Do you experience looser stools or more frequent bowel movements with the onset of pain? Do your symptoms wake you up at night?

What is it? IBS, also known as spastic colon, is a motility problem (involving intestinal muscle contractions and movement of stool) with no known cause. In IBS, the bowel is hypersensitive; it overreacts to mild stimulation by going into spasms—perhaps in response to eating, or to distension caused by gas, or to the presence of stool itself.

Because no evidence of disease can be seen when the colon is examined, IBS is known as a functional disorder. IBS causes no permanent harm to the intestines and does not lead to more serious conditions, such as intestinal bleeding or cancer. While stress and depression may contribute to flare-ups, IBS is not the result of a personality disorder.

In some people, IBS is a mild annoyance; in others, it can be debilitating—affecting the ability to socialize, work, or travel. Unlike many intestinal disorders, IBS can be greatly affected by stressful circumstances.

At some time or another, almost everyone has a change in bowel habits, particularly during periods of stress. One of every nine schoolchildren is estimated to suffer a painful episode of IBS-like symptoms once every 3 months. With IBS, the colon not only is more sensitive, but its reactions are stronger than in most people. Certain medications and foods may trigger spasms; also, women with IBS may experience more symptoms during their menstrual periods—perhaps because reproductive hormones somehow increase the colon's susceptibility to spasm.

What you can do People with IBS have a hyperreactive bowel, one prone to spasms. The most likely triggers to spasm seem to be diet and emotional stress.

Eating a proper diet—and removing items in your diet that make this problem worse (see below)—can do much to ease your symptoms. When you eat, your colon begins contracting—a response that normally may cause the urge to have a bowel movement within 30 minutes to an hour. If you have IBS, this urge may come sooner, and you may have crampy diarrhea. Contractions may be stronger or more violent if your diet is high in fat (found in such foods as whole milk, cheese, butter, margarine, meats, and vegetable oil). Dietary fiber tends to keep the colon mildly distended, which, in some people, helps prevent spasms. Some forms of fiber keep water in the stool (and help prevent stools from becoming hard and painful). Your goal should be to eat enough fiber so that you have soft, painless, easy-to-pass bowel movements. (For more information on increasing fiber, see Water, Fiber, and Exercise, page 1019). Eating too much fiber too soon can cause painful gas and bloating. It will take your body a few weeks to adjust to your new diet.

Stress can worsen the spastic contractions of the colon. Although the exact link between stress and IBS is unclear, it is known that the colon is controlled in part by the nervous system. Talk to your doctor about stress reduction and relaxation techniques (see Chapter 11 for more information on relieving stress). Exercise also may help; however, in some people, it actually worsens diarrhea.

When to call the doctor If the symptoms of IBS—or the fear of pain and diarrhea—are disrupting your life, causing you to withdraw from normal activities, consult your doctor. Also, any symptoms that are not usually associated with IBS, like fever, weight loss, rectal bleeding, or persistent, severe pain, should be investigated.

Treatment This varies greatly, depending on your doctor and the degree of symptoms. First, many people are greatly helped simply knowing that this disorder has a name, that it is benign, and that it is not a manifestation of a personality disorder. IBS symptoms often improve with a high-fiber diet (see above) and fiber supplements that contain psyllium, although at first, the increase in fiber can cause more bloating and distension. Also, your doctor will probably recommend that you screen your diet to identify and avoid foods that aggravate your symptoms. These may include coffee, fruit sugars, legumes, cruciferous vegetables (cabbage, broccoli, brussels sprouts, cauliflower). Your doctor may prescribe an antispasmodic medication such as dicyclomine (Bentyl) or hyoscyamine (Levsin). Your doctor may give a mild laxative or a mild antidiarrheal agent, but this is not primary therapy. Other treatments may include a tricyclic antidepressant, for depression and pain control, or a sedative drug for patients with anxiety. Your doctor also may want you to try biofeedback (see Fecal Incontinence, page 1028). Of concern is that some people, in an attempt to control their bowels or reduce stress, can become dependent on laxatives or tranquilizers. Although these may help for limited periods, neither of these is a good long-term option for relieving your symptoms.

Prognosis IBS can be a lifetime condition, either continuous or intermittent, but it does not affect the health of your digestive system or lead to more serious conditions.

CONSTIPATION AND IMPACTION

Symptoms (*What you may experience*) Infrequent (fewer than three a week) bowel movements; dry, hard, or rough stools that are painful and difficult to pass; a feeling that your rectum is full, even after you have had a bowel movement.

Signs and laboratory findings *(What the doctor looks for)* The presence of stool on a barium x-ray test, colonoscopy, or proctoscopy; hard stool, felt during a rectal exam.

What is it? Most people think they need to have a bowel movement every day. However, regularity varies from person to person and even changes in the course of the normal life span. Some people have two or three bowel movements every day, but others may have one bowel movement every 2 or 3 days. In some people, constipation is sudden and is a manifestation of another abdominal problem, such as bowel obstruction (see page 1005) or diverticulitis (see Diverticular Disease: Diverticulosis and Diverticulitis, page 1016). Constipation also may be caused by general anesthesia or by many medications, including (to name just a few) anticholinergic medications, iron, opiates, tranquilizers, and sedatives. It can be a chronic problem for pregnant women (particularly those taking iron-rich prenatal vitamins); for people who are bedridden, particularly the elderly; and for people who have head or spinal injuries. In some people, the function of the colon is disrupted by other problems, including thyroid disease, or a neurologic illness such as Parkinson's disease.

But for millions of Americans, constipation is the result of a poor diet with inadequate fiber, lack of exercise, stress and anxiety, and pain from hemorrhoids or fissures (see Hemorrhoids [Piles], page 1025, and Anal Fissures, page 1024).

What you can do See Water, Fiber, and Exercise, above.

When to call the doctor Call your doctor if you have a sudden, unexplained onset of constipation (see Bowel Obstruction, page 1005); if constipation persists despite your efforts to solve the problem (see Water, Fiber, and Exercise, above); if constipation alternates with diarrhea; if you have blood in the stool; or if you have severe abdominal pain.

Treatment It may be that some simple changes in your diet and lifestyle will be enough to solve this problem (see Water, Fiber, and Exercise, above). Millions of Americans, however, require a little help, at first,

WATER, FIBER, AND EXERCISE

Normal bowel movements are soft, easy to pass, and contain fiber, the material in vegetables, fruits, and whole grains that cannot be digested. Fiber adds bulk to stool, keeps it moving through the digestive tract, and retains water—which, in turn, helps prevent the stool from becoming hard or rough.

Fiber is good for the body. A high-fiber diet promotes peristalsis, the rhythmic muscle contractions by which the intestine moves food. It can relieve or cure constipation, can help treat diarrhea, can ease many of the factors that cause hemorrhoids or lead to an anal fissure, and—because high-fiber foods tend to be healthier—may even help prevent many intestinal problems, including colon cancer and diverticulosis. If you are not used to it, eating too much fiber can cause uncomfortable abdominal bloating and gas as the body adjusts to the increase in bulk. It is best to begin increasing your daily fiber intake gradually, by making a few changes. Try broccoli or carrots instead of french fries with your dinner; eat apples, pears, and potatoes with the peels on (much of the fiber is found in the skin of fruits and vegetables and is lost when peeled).

Fiber also comes in concentrated form: Bran, psyllium, and methylcellulose help the body produce softer, bulkier stool. These forms of fiber, called bulking agents, are, in effect, natural and are not addictive. Psyllium fiber, in fact, can help people with diarrhea, as well, by minimizing the number of watery stools.

Water is an essential part of a good diet. Ideally, you should drink the equivalent of eight glasses a day; keeping in mind that water is in many other healthful beverages, such as juice and milk.

And finally, exercise can work wonders on the inside of the body as well as the outside. It can promote healthier, more regular bowel movements (it also may lead you to drink more water). Again, it may be more helpful if you worry less about how much you exercise than how often. Walking is a fine form of exercise. Start taking the stairs instead of the elevator, for instance. Work in the garden. Put your child in the stroller and walk around the block. Every little bit helps. ■

in surmounting constipation and achieving regularity. Bulking agents (discussed in Water, Fiber, and Exercise) are gentle, act slowly, and have a natural effect. Laxatives and enemas, on the other hand, should be considered temporary solutions only and should be used with great care (see Laxatives and Enemas: Dangers of Overuse, page 1020).

Your doctor may prescribe a stool softener (such as mineral oil), which allows the stool to absorb more water and thus become softer and easier to pass; or an osmotic agent, which keeps water in the intestine (and makes stool easier to pass), such as lactulose sorbitol, magnesium oxide, or magnesium citrate.

If you have an impaction, you may need several enemas, with phosphate solutions (such as Fleet), given once or twice a day

LAXATIVES AND ENEMAS: DANGERS OF OVERUSE

Bulking agents—bran, psyllium, and methyl-cellulose fiber supplements—are not laxatives. They work slowly—a high-fiber diet, administered a few spoonfuls at a time—and their effect is natural. They are not addictive.

Laxatives and enemas, on the other hand, can be harmful if overused. They may interfere with the body's normal digestive functions, irritate the intestinal lining, disrupt normal peristalsis (the series of muscle contractions by which food is moved through the bowel), cause cramps, and disturb the balance of fluid and electrolytes. Chronic use of an over-the-counter laxative, or a home remedy such as castor oil, can result in lazy bowel syndrome, in which—without the use of a laxative—constipation is worse than it was before.

Many laxatives bind chemically with other drugs you may be taking, decreasing their effectiveness. Thus, although laxatives and enemas can be very helpful occasionally, they should never be considered anything but a temporary solution for constipation. ∎

until there is no more stool; or, if the impaction is hard, with mineral oil, which softens stool. Although you may need more than one mineral oil enema, for most people this is preferable to digital removal, a procedure done in a doctor's office or outpatient clinic, in which the doctor's finger is used to excavate the impaction. Though unpleasant, the procedure is not painful, and no anesthesia is needed.

❖ FLATULENCE

Symptoms (*What you may experience*) Abdominal bloating; voluntary or involuntary passage of gas.

Signs and laboratory findings (*What the doctor looks for*) Evidence of abdominal distension, seen during a physical exam; a hollow sound (indicating the presence of gas in the abdomen), heard during abdominal percussion (in which the doctor's finger taps on the abdomen).

What is it? Gas is present in everyone. It finds its way into the digestive tract when you swallow air, which happens to some extent with every swallow of food or drink you take but also may occur unconsciously, particularly when you are nervous. Some disorders, such as peptic ulcer disease, which involve excessive salivation, may also result in increased air swallowing. Much of this air goes back out the way it came in—through the mouth, by belching. But some of it is propelled into the intestine. Carbonated beverages also can increase belching.

Gas is also made in the intestine. Methane, hydrogen, and carbon dioxide are produced when gut bacteria ferment carbohydrates and amino acids. Certain high-fiber fruits and vegetables (including the notorious baked bean), which are not entirely digested—and which thus constitute important bulk in the stool—produce hydrogen; hydrogen is also produced in great quantities in people with lactose (and other forms of sugar) intolerance. Some medications, such as cholestyramine, can cause or worsen flatulence.

Occasional flatulence, although it can be socially embarrassing, is generally not considered a problem. People pass gas dozens of times a day—often in increments so tiny that they are not even aware of it. Excessive flatulence, however, may be a symptom of another problem, such as food intolerance (see page 998) or IBS (see page 1017).

What you can do In addition to altering your diet (see below), you can strengthen your anal sphincter muscles to help delay flatulence by doing Kegel exercises: Lie on your back, with your knees bent, and your feet about 12 in. apart. Clench, as tightly as you can, the muscles around your anus (the ones you use when trying not to pass gas), and hold for as long as you can—working up to 20 seconds. Relax the muscles slowly, take a deep breath, and repeat. These exercises can also be done when you are standing (in the shower, for instance), sitting (even driving a car), and urinating.

When to call the doctor If you feel that excessive flatulence is interfering with the quality of your life or if you have pain from abdominal distension, consult your doctor.

Treatment Your doctor will probably recommend that you screen your diet to identify and avoid foods that exacerbate your symptoms. These may include coffee, fruit sugars, legumes, cruciferous vegetables (cabbage, broccoli, brussels sprouts, cauliflower). If your symptoms are linked to a high-fiber diet or fiber supplement, try cutting back to smaller amounts and building your fiber intake slowly. Too much fiber, in a body that is not accustomed to it, can cause flatulence and abdominal distension. An over-the-counter product (such as Beano) containing an enzyme that breaks down the sugars in beans may be helpful. Avoid medications that may be worsening your symptoms or use alternatives.

Some people are helped by products containing simethicone, a medication that dissolves gas bubbles, or charcoal-containing compounds. Anticholinergic medications such as dicyclomine, have been helpful in some people. Some people with upset stomach and a feeling of uncomfortable fullness after meals find it helpful to take an antacid about 30 minutes before eating.

Prognosis Excellent, if your symptoms are found to be exacerbated by certain foods and you are able to change your diet. However, in some people, flatulence is a chronic problem. Fortunately, although it can be annoying, it is not harmful to your health.

❖ COLON POLYPS

Symptoms (*What you may experience*) Usually, none. Nearly all polyps are silent, causing no symptoms, or rarely, such nonspecific symptoms as rectal bleeding or diarrhea.

Signs and laboratory findings (*What the doctor looks for*) One or more protuberances in the lining of the colon, seen in colonoscopy, barium enema, or flexible sigmoidoscopy. Positive results on a Hemoccult test, to detect hidden blood in the stool.

What is it? A polyp is an abnormal, mushroom-shaped growth sprouting from the lining of the colon. Some polyps have stalks; others are bumps that resemble the cap of the mushroom. Some polyps are benign; called hyperplastic polyps, these are usually small, without stalks, and do not progress to become cancerous. Others,

called adenomatous polyps, are known as premalignant, or precancerous; if these continue to grow, it is likely that they will contain cancerous cells. Adenomatous polyps are believed to result from mutations in the DNA (the genetic material) of the lining of the colon in response to a lifetime of exposure to a low-fiber, high-fat Western diet or other environmental influences. Only the largest polyps (greater than $\frac{1}{2}$ in. in diameter) tend to bleed (thus, one drawback of the Hemoccult stool test is that it does not detect potentially cancerous polyps at their earliest). In some families, there is a genetic predisposition to develop numerous adenomatous polyps and colorectal cancer (see Hereditary Forms of Colorectal Cancer, page 1023).

What you can do The primary means of preventing polyps is dietary: eating a diet that is low-fat, low in red meat, rich in fruits and vegetables, and high in soluble fiber. Secondary prevention is vigilant screening: The American Cancer Society recommends that beginning at age 50, you should have a baseline flexible sigmoidoscopy, to be repeated every 5 years afterward for life. Also at age 50, you should begin a yearly stool blood test. If anything abnormal is found, you will need more frequent monitoring or colonoscopy. If you have a family history of colon cancer, you should begin screening sooner—perhaps as early as your teens or 20s (see Hereditary Forms of Colorectal Cancer, page 1023).

When to call the doctor If you have blood in the stool, a change in bowel habits, or chronic diarrhea that does not respond to over-the-counter treatment, consult your doctor.

Treatment Treatment depends on the extent and nature of your polyps. If you have hyperplastic polyps (as determined by a biopsy), no further evaluation is needed. However, if you are found to have one or more adenomatous polyps, this suggests that your whole colon is at risk, and you will need a full colonoscopy to detect and treat any other growths. Polyps can be removed by cauterization during colonoscopy, or they may be removed during the biopsy itself (also during colonoscopy). Because there are no nerve endings in the lining of the colon (the nerves that control the colon are in the muscles surrounding it), this is a painless procedure. Occasionally, polyps cannot be removed by colonoscopy, and surgery is necessary.

If you have FAP, and hundreds of polyps are found in endoscopy (see Hereditary Forms of Colorectal Cancer, page 1023), the treatment is to remove the colon. The more adenomatous polyps you have, or the bigger the adenomatous polyps, the higher your risk of getting colon cancer.

Prognosis Your prognosis depends on the nature and number of polyps you have. If the polyps are hyperplastic, your prognosis is excellent. If they are adenomatous, you will need regular follow-up colonoscopy (see page 1011) at least every 3 years. If hundreds of adenomatous polyps are found, you probably have FAP (see Hereditary Forms of Colorectal Cancer, page 1023), and you will probably need to have your colon removed to prevent colon cancer. If colon cancer is suspected, you may need further treatment (see below).

❖ COLORECTAL CANCER

Symptoms *(What you may experience)* Usually, colorectal cancer is silent, producing no symptoms. Some people experience painless rectal bleeding, or microscopic blood in the stool; in some people, cancer forms a ring around the colon, causing a change in bowel habits—either constipation or difficulty having a complete bowel movement, or diarrhea.

Signs and laboratory findings *(What the doctor looks for)* Polypoid mass, detected on flexible sigmoidoscopy, colonoscopy, or air-contrast barium enema (see Flexible Sigmoidoscopy, page 1006, Colonoscopy, page 1011, and Barium Studies, page 976); the presence of cancer cells on samples of these masses, taken for biopsy. It should also be noted that because many people have more than one cancerous polyp, if your cancer was detected during a routine flexible sigmoidoscopy, you should have a full evaluation of the colon with colonoscopy or barium enema with air contrast to detect abnormalities of the lining of the colon.

What is it? Colorectal cancer, a tumor that arises from the lining of the colon, is the second leading cause of cancer death in

the United States; this year, nearly 140,000 people will be diagnosed with it, and more than 50,000 will die from the disease. Some people inherit a form of colon cancer (see Hereditary Forms of Colorectal Cancer, page 1023); however, for most people who develop colon cancer, the high-fat, low-fiber Western diet is almost certainly a component. Colon cancer is much less common, for instance, in Asia and Africa. Most cases of colon cancer occur after the age of 50. But if you have a family history of colorectal cancer or polyps in the colon, or if you have ever had a cancerous polyp, ulcerative colitis, or Crohn's disease, your risk of developing colon cancer is higher; you should be checked more frequently and at a younger age.

What you can do The primary means of preventing colon cancer is dietary: eating a low-fat diet, low in red meat, rich in fruits and vegetables, and high in soluble fiber. Secondary prevention is vigilant screening: The American Cancer Society recommends that beginning at age 50, you should have a baseline flexible sigmoidoscopy (see Flexible Sigmoidoscopy, page 1006), to be repeated every 5 years afterward for life. Also at age 50, you should begin a yearly stool blood test. If anything abnormal is found, you will need more frequent monitoring or colonoscopy. If you have a family history of colon cancer, you should begin screening sooner—perhaps as early as your teens or 20s if you have FAP or HNPCC (see Hereditary Forms of Colorectal Cancer, page 1023).

When to call the doctor If you have any of the symptoms listed above—particularly if you have a family history of polyps or colon cancer—call your doctor. Too often, people ignore warning signs such as rectal bleeding, attributing them to harmless causes. Early diagnosis can save your life.

Treatment This depends on the extent and severity of your cancer. It may be that only the cancerous polyp or polyps will need to be removed; this will be done during colonoscopy. Or, it may be necessary for your colon to be removed, an operation known as a colectomy. You also may need external-beam radiation treatment. Although receiving the radiation is itself a painless procedure, it may produce side effects

HEREDITARY FORMS OF COLORECTAL CANCER

In almost all cases of colorectal cancer—as many as 90 percent—there is a mutation in a gene called adenomatous polyposis coli (APC), which normally acts as a regulator, a genetic brake that halts cell growth. When APC goes awry, it affects at least two other genes and interrupts the normal cycle of cell life and death, causing unchecked cell growth—in other words, cancer. In most people, this mutation is believed to develop over time, brought about by environmental factors such as a diet too rich in fat and too skimpy in cancer-fighting fruits and vegetables. In some people, this genetic chain of events happens sporadically, for no known reason. And some people—in families prone to colorectal cancer—are born with the APC mutation already in place. The many forms of inherited colorectal cancer include the following:

Familial Adenomatous Polyposis

Familial adenomatous polyposis (FAP), in which hundreds or even thousands of adenomatous polyps (see Colon Polyps, page 1021) carpet the colon and rectum, manifests itself as early as childhood. Diagnosis is made when a gastroenterologist finds at least 100 adenomatous polyps (determining the type of polyp is crucial—see Colon Polyps, page 1021; there are many types of familial polyposis syndromes). If the colon is not removed, cancer is inevitable. Although cancer may have started years or even decades earlier, most people who are not screened for the presence of cancer are diagnosed in their late 30s and early 40s. Many people with FAP also develop polyps elsewhere, such as in the small intestine and stomach; these growths may be benign or malignant. The development of FAP manifestations outside the colon used to be called Gardner's syndrome; this distinction has become less important in recent years, as scientists have learned that most people with FAP develop problems elsewhere. Abnormalities and lesions may also appear in the form of subcutaneous cysts in the scalp, face, and extremities; benign growths in the skull and bones, lesions in the jaw; and tumors in the nasopharynx, thyroid, and pancreas. Hepatoblastoma, cancer in the liver that can be cured if caught early (see Liver Cancer, page 1052), occurs in about 1 in 300 at-risk people under the age of 5. Because of these other problems, if you have FAP—even if you have undergone treatment for colorectal cancer—you should have thorough physical examinations yearly, beginning in childhood. Children in families with FAP should begin screening with yearly flexible sigmoidoscopy at age 12; at age 25, this can be reduced to every other year, and at age 35, to every 3 years. After age 50, the risk drops to that of the average American (see Colorectal Cancer, page 1022). Genetic testing, looking for mutation of the APC gene, is also recommended. Treatment involves surgery to remove the colon, and one of several procedures including an ileoanal anastomosis, ileorectal anastomosis, or ileostomy (see Ileostomy, Kock Pouch, Ileoanal Pouch, and Colostomy, page 1012). You will need regular follow-up monitoring, which may include endoscopic evaluation, with biopsy or brushing of tissue, of the remaining rectum, the stomach, and duodenum.

An anti-inflammatory drug called sulindac (Clinoril), tested in FAP patients at Johns Hopkins, has been found to shrink polyps and decrease their number. One day, it may be possible to prevent colorectal cancer in people with FAP. The drug also may be useful in preventing some of the other growths associated with this disorder.

Hereditary Nonpolyposis Colorectal Cancer

Hereditary nonpolyposis colorectal cancer (HNPCC) is an autosomal dominant syndrome—meaning it can be inherited from either parent—in which colorectal cancer arises from a single malignant lesion in the colon. As many as 6 percent of all cases of colon cancer are caused by HNPCC. Affected individuals tend to develop cancer at a younger age than most Americans—in their 40s—and the cancers tend to arise on the right side of the colon. Families with HNPCC are also at risk of developing cancer in other areas, including the endometrium, stomach, small intestine, liver, kidney, ureters, or ovaries. Scientists believe the genetic permutations involved in HNPCC include a breakdown in repair genes (the DNA mismatch repair genes)—whose job, normally, is to fix genetic mutations before they can cause trouble. If colorectal cancer is found and HNPCC is suspected, you will be advised to reduce your risk of future cancer by having your colon removed. Women should also undergo annual screening for endometrial cancer, which may include testing of endometrial cells or abdominal or transvaginal ultrasound, beginning at age 25. ■

---

including diarrhea and anemia. Some people also need adjuvant chemotherapy, a regimen of powerful drugs such as 5-fluorouracil and levamisole (Ergamisole), designed to kill any other colon cancer cells before they create another tumor. If the cancer has spread to the liver, you may need abdominal surgery to remove cancerous tissue there, as well. See Chapter 30, for more information on the treatment of cancer.

Prognosis This depends on the extent of your cancer. Fortunately, when detected and treated early, this is one of the most curable forms of cancer. More than 75 percent of people with colorectal cancer detected early can be completely cured of the disease and can return to a normal life. With increasing early detection, fewer people need major surgery to remove cancerous tissue each year. Today, only a small percentage of patients treated for colon cancer need a permanent colostomy.

THE RECTUM AND ANUS

Now, after its long journey through the esophagus, stomach, small intestine, and colon, what entered the body as food has become waste material. Muscles in the sigmoid colon slowly propel this matter into the rectum, where it collects as stool. Further muscle contractions in the rectum push stool through to the anal canal, its last stop before exiting the anus in a bowel movement.

Encircling the anal canal are two rings of muscle, powerful valves called the anal sphincters. One of these sphincters, the external, is a voluntary muscle; you can control it. The internal sphincter is involuntary; it relaxes when stool reaches it. Both of these sphincters control the exodus of stool, in the form of a bowel movement, and the passage of gas (flatulence); however, the external sphincter is the door in charge of fecal control.

At the juncture where the rectum meets the anal canal are about a dozen tiny recesses in the folds of the anal lining, called crypts, and a handful of tiny projections, called papillae. Abscesses and fistulas can develop in these crypts. The anus, rich with nerves, is particularly sensitive to pain; even a tiny tear, called an anal fissure, can be excruciating.

During a bowel movement, the muscles around the anal sphincter relax. Internal hemorrhoid veins swell slightly, helping ease the stool out of the body; the moist cushion of mucus that lines the rectum also helps smooth the way. Normally, stool is soft, contains no blood, and is easily passed without straining. If a bowel movement is difficult and the stool is hard or rough, it can scrape against these veins, causing irritation.

❖ ANAL FISSURES

Symptoms *(What you may experience)* Sharp pain, hypersensitivity, and a tearing feeling in the anus, especially during a bowel movement; pink blood when you wipe; traces of pink blood in the stool.

Signs and laboratory findings *(What the doctor looks for)* A visible tear, laceration, or ulcer near the anus; spasm of the anal sphincter (a reaction to the pain of the fissure upon being touched) during a rectal exam; an external skin tag (a small flap of skin, which sometimes develops near the lower end of a fissure).

What is it? An anal fissure is a longitudinal tear, caused by some form of trauma, or a small ulcer that develops as a result of chronic infection, in the tissue near the anus. Although generally tiny (less than $1/2$ in.), fissures can be excruciating, particularly during a bowel movement, due to the abundant supply of nerve endings lining the rectum and anus. Several events can cause a fissure: the passage of large, hard or rough stools; the trauma of childbirth; severe diarrhea; infection, including syphilis or gonorrhea; and rectal intercourse.

What you can do Many fissures are caused or made worse by the same factors that produce hemorrhoids and constipation, including lack of fiber in the diet, lack of exercise, stress and anxiety, and irregular bowel habits (for example, ignoring the urge to have a bowel movement can cause extra stress on the anus). Thus, eating more fiber—found in whole grains and bulk fiber supplements—and more fruits and vegetables should do much to produce softer, more regular bowel movements and minimize your chance of having anal fissures (see Water, Fiber, and Exercise, page 1019). These steps are particularly important during traveling, which can challenge even the best of diets and most regular of bowel habits. Laxatives are not a good long-term solution for anal fissure (see Laxatives and Enemas: Dangers of Overuse, page 1020).

When to call the doctor If you are in intense pain, to the point where you cannot defecate, or if you have rectal bleeding, you should consult your doctor.

Treatment Fortunately, the torment of an anal fissure often responds fairly quickly—within a few days—to treatment. The first step is to halt the cycle of pain: An anal fissure, itself painful, causes a spasm of the anal sphincter, which brings on more pain. For immediate pain relief, your doctor will probably recommend a local anesthetic ointment (a solution containing lidocaine or phenol) or spray, to be applied several times a day; and warm (but not hot) sitz baths, for 10 to 15 minutes after each bowel movement or as often as needed. Keeping the stool soft—and bowel movements as painless as possible—is also critical. Your doctor will probably recommend that you use a stool softener such as docusate sodium (Senokot-S) for at least a week. Do not strain when making a bowel movement. If you are having difficulty, wait a while and try again.

Most fissures heal on their own. As a last resort, if your fissure is chronic or deep, the result of infection or repeat trauma, you may need surgery to cut the internal sphincter; this changes the angle at which stool approaches the anal canal and eases some of the pressure that stool places on the rectum. The internal sphincter is not necessary for fecal continence. You can still maintain control with an external sphincter. This simple procedure can be done on an outpatient basis, with local anesthetic.

Prognosis Excellent. However, if the fissure is a result of repeat trauma (from chronic straining during bowel movements, for instance), it may return if you do not change your bowel habits. See Water, Fiber, and Exercise, page 1019, and ask your doctor for help in preventing a recurrence of symptoms.

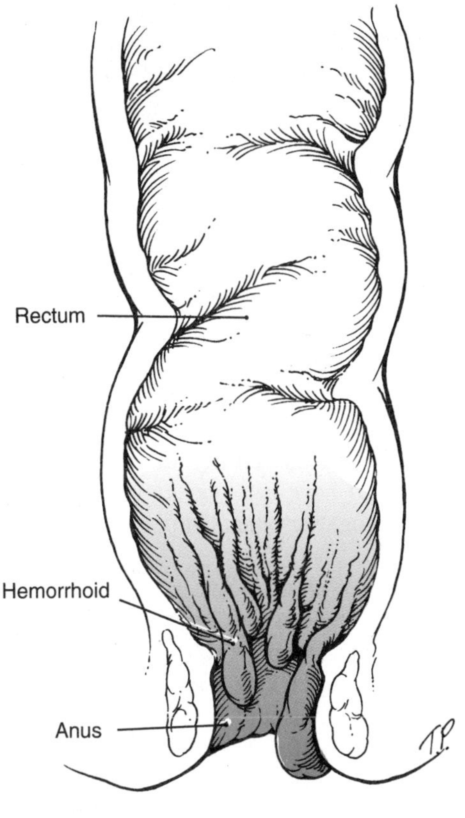

Hemorrhoids are large varicose veins in the anal canal. Childbirth, chronic constipation, or heavy lifting can cause the veins to bulge, clot, become irritated, or bleed. Increasing fiber intake can help to minimize symptoms. Medications may help to decrease inflammation, and surgery is available for severe cases.

❖ HEMORRHOIDS (PILES)

Symptoms *(What you may experience)* Bright red blood, not mixed with stool, during a bowel movement; rectal bleeding (which may continue long after the stool has passed); rectal burning, itching, or discomfort during a bowel movement; a feeling of prolapse—that the inside of your rectum is swelling or poking outside—during or after a bowel movement.

Signs and laboratory findings *(What the doctor looks for)* Discharge of blood (from irritation in the lining); skin irritation (caused by inadequate hygiene) immediately outside the anus; inflammation or edema (fluid swelling) in the rectal lining; prolapse of hemorrhoids, which may appear red, blue, or black, if the blood supply has been damaged; presence of internal hemorrhoids on anoscopy (see Other Diagnostic Tests of the Gastrointestinal Tract, page 984). If an external hemorrhoid has thrombosed, or clotted: an engorged, blue, smooth lesion beneath the skin immediately outside the anus.

What is it? Internal hemorrhoids are large varicose veins that lie just beneath the layer of cells that lines the anal canal. Although these swell slightly during a bowel movement, they normally pose no problem. However, certain events or conditions—the trauma of childbirth, the extra weight and pressure of pregnancy or obesity, chronic constipation (with straining), prolonged standing or sitting, heavy lifting, rectal intercourse—can cause these veins to bulge or prolapse, become irritated, and bleed. If the prolapse is severe, thrombosis—a blood clot or blockage of blood flow—may occur, causing the vein and surrounding mucus to become black and appear dead. Sometimes, the cause appears to be hemorrhoids but is actually further inside the rectum; if your doctor suspects this, you may need flexible sigmoidoscopy (see Flexible Sigmoidoscopy, page 1006) to check for inflammation or cancer. If you are over age 40 and have rectal bleeding, you should also have a complete exam of the colon.

A thrombosed external hemorrhoid is a painful blood clot that develops in a hemorrhoid that has been pushed outside the anus. Thrombosed external hemorrhoids tend to occur at a younger age and usually follow certain traumatic events, including childbirth, heavy lifting, exercise, severe straining to have a bowel movement, even violent coughing or sneezing.

What you can do Some hemorrhoids are caused or made worse by the same factors that produce hemorrhoids and constipation, including lack of fiber in the diet, lack of exercise, stress and anxiety, and irregular bowel habits (for example, ignoring the urge to have a bowel movement can cause extra stress on the anus). Thus, eating more fiber—found in whole grains and bulk fiber supplements—and more fruits and vegetables a day should do much to produce softer, more regular bowel movements and minimize your symptoms (see Water, Fiber, and Exercise, page 1019). These steps are particularly important during traveling, which can challenge even the best of diets and most regular of bowel habits. Laxatives are not a good long-term solution for preventing hemorrhoids (see Laxatives and Enemas: Dangers of Overuse, page 1020).

When to call the doctor If you have rectal bleeding, or if you are in severe pain, consult your doctor.

Treatment There is much you can do on your own to ease symptoms and cause the hemorrhoids to recede (see Care of Hemorrhoids, below). But if your hemorrhoids are more severe, or if they are inflamed, prolapsed, or thrombosed, you may need immediate treatment, including the following:

- *Sclerotherapy:* As with sclerotherapy of varicose veins in the leg, this treatment, performed on an outpatient basis and requiring only mild local anesthesia, consists of injecting an irritating chemical solution directly into the vein or into the tissue surrounding it. This causes a harmless blood clot to form. Starved of its life-sustaining blood supply, over the next few weeks, the hemorrhoid gradually shrinks and fades away.

- *Banding:* Placing a rubber band around the base of the hemorrhoid cuts off its circulation. Within a few weeks of this procedure, also done on an outpatient basis (in a doctor's office or clinic) and usually requiring no anesthesia, the dead vein shrinks and falls off.

- *Cryosurgery:* Liquid nitrogen or carbon dioxide can be used to kill the hemorrhoid by freezing it instantly. In this painless procedure, which requires no anesthesia or hospitalization, a surgeon, gastroenterologist, or proctologist applies a probe directly to the hemorrhoid. However, because this procedure is not as precise as the ones

CARE OF HEMORRHOIDS

An acute flare-up of hemorrhoids can be agonizing. Fortunately, with care and plenty of rest, most people's symptoms improve noticeably within a few days. Here are some tips to help speed your recovery:

Relieve the Pain and Ease the Swelling For immediate comfort, you may want to begin with an anesthetic spray containing a numbing benzocaine solution (such as Dermoplast) and a series of disposable ice packs (available at pharmacies). Narrow enough to be worn inside your underwear (preferably when you are lying in bed), these small icepacks release cold crystals when you activate them. You can also use medicated, witch hazel-containing pads (such as Tuck's) for wiping as well as for cold compresses, or you may prefer a rectal ointment (such as Preparation H). Take warm sitz baths—either sitting in a warm tub or using a portable unit that fits over the toilet—several times a day or as often as needed. For additional pain relief, your doctor may also recommend a nonsteroidal anti-inflammatory drug, such as ibuprofen (Advil) or naproxen (Naprosyn).

Keep Clean The presence of hemorrhoids can make it harder to clean the area immediately outside the anus. But now more than ever, good hygiene is essential to avoid irritation and promote healing. Use a soothing, medicated pad (such as Tuck's) or a baby wipe with aloe; another bonus of frequent sitz baths is that these will help maintain cleanliness, as well.

Ease Pressure on the Area During an acute flare-up, lie down as much as possible, to ease pressure on the anus. Do not linger on the toilet (to read, for instance); this can make hemorrhoids worse. Finally, never strain during a bowel movement. If the stool does not pass easily, stop, and try again later. ■

mentioned on page 1026, and because the dead tissue may drain or bleed for days or weeks, cryosurgery generally ranks third of the outpatient procedures.

- *Surgical excision:* Once considered standard therapy for severe hemorrhoids, this procedure is generally reserved for the worst cases, because it can produce scar tissue, which, in turn, can make bowel movements difficult, and rarely, cause an anal stricture.

Prognosis Good, particularly if your hemorrhoids are the result of a dramatic event such as childbirth. However, if they have been caused by repeat trauma (from chronic straining during a bowel movement, for instance), you run the risk of further trouble if you do not change your bowel habits (see Water, Fiber, and Exercise, page 1019, and ask your doctor for help in preventing a recurrence of symptoms).

❖ ANAL ABSCESS AND FISTULA

Symptoms *(What you may experience)* Anal swelling, redness, tenderness; fever; abdominal pain.

Signs and laboratory findings *(What the doctor looks for)* Tenderness on a digital rectal exam; inflammation in the anus; an elevated white blood cell count, suggesting infection; discharge from the anus; a tube-like opening between the rectum or anal canal and surrounding tissue, as seen during a physical exam, or during anoscopy or sigmoidoscopy or x-ray fistulography (see Other Diagnostic Tests of the Gastrointestinal Tract, page 984); a palpable, cord-like expanse in the anus, felt during a physical exam.

What is it? An anorectal abscess is an infection, usually beginning in the anal crypts, recesses in the folds of the anal lining; however, abscesses may originate deeper, underneath the skin or within the muscles surrounding the rectum and anal canal. Because of the abundance of nerve endings lining the anal canal, the most painful abscesses are the ones nearest the surface; deeper lesions tend to produce duller, more diffuse pain. If an abscess is high, in the rec-

tum or pelvis, the pain may even be felt in the lower abdomen. An anorectal abscess can be associated with inflammatory bowel disease, such as Crohn's disease.

A fistula is an improper opening between two normally closed spaces. An anal fistula is a tube-like passageway from the anal canal to the external skin around the anus. Anal fistulas can be caused by drainage of an abscess (either spontaneous or surgical drainage); they may be caused by trauma, particularly, childbirth, but also radiation therapy or pelvic surgery; or they may be the result of other diseases, including tuberculosis, intestinal cancer, and Crohn's disease. Some infants are born with congenital fistulas.

When to call the doctor If you have a fever that persists more than 2 days or if you have severe pain in the abdomen or rectum, consult your doctor.

Treatment The treatment for an abscess is surgical removal and drainage. If the abscess is in the anus, this can be done as an outpatient procedure. If it is higher in the rectum, or near the sigmoid colon, you may need open surgery. Because an abscess near the colon carries the risk of peritonitis (the spread of infection within the lining of the abdomen), it must be treated immediately.

Sometimes, drainage itself can cause another problem—a fistula—if, instead of closing over, the drained lesion heals to form a tube. Most fistulas also are treated with surgery—a procedure called a fistulotomy, in which the main opening and tubelike tract are unroofed, leaving behind a ditch. If this operation involves part of the anal sphincter, fecal incontinence may result.

❖ ANAL STRICTURE

Symptoms *(What you may experience)* Difficulty or pain in passing a bowel movement.

Signs and laboratory findings *(What the doctor looks for)* Scar tissue, a narrowing in the opening or lining of the anal canal, as seen in anoscopy (see Other Diagnostic Tests of the Gastrointestinal Tract, page 984) or during a physical exam.

What is it? An anal stricture is a tight ring of scar tissue that encircles and constricts the anus, hindering your ability to have a bowel movement. The tissue of the rectum and anus is fragile and injures easily. Stricture can be caused by radiation therapy for prostate cancer; by chlamydia or herpes simplex infection of the anus (see Sexually Transmitted Infections, page 861); or by trauma to the anus, such as that caused by rectal intercourse or insertion of a foreign object.

What you can do Avoid rectal intercourse or inserting any foreign object into the rectum.

When to call the doctor If you are unable to have a bowel movement, call your doctor.

Treatment Treatment is based on the underlying condition and severity of the stricture. If it is moderate, a stool softener such as docusate sodium and a bulk fiber supplement (see Water, Fiber, and Exercise, page 1019) may be sufficient to allow normal bowel movements. If it is severe, you may need to have it dilated, or opened, surgically with one or more tiny cuts in the scar tissue. This can be done as an outpatient procedure by a surgeon.

❖ ANAL ITCH

Symptoms (*What you may experience*) Persistent itching around the anus.

Signs and laboratory findings (*What the doctor looks for*) Redness and inflammation, seen during a physical exam.

What is it? Anal itch, as its name suggests, is persistent, annoying itchiness around the anus. It can be caused by several factors, including the following:

- Allergic reaction, or contact dermatitis, a skin reaction to local anesthetics (especially solutions or sprays ending in *caine*), soaps, ointments, antibiotics (such as tetracycline), or even certain foods

- Dermatologic problems, skin disorders such as psoriasis or atopic dermatitis

- Infection by microbes (such as candidiasis), bacteria (which can be caused by excessive scratching) or parasites, such as pinworms and scabies

- Diseases including diabetes mellitus or liver disease

- Proctologic disorders, such as skin tags, or irritation from a draining fistula

- Poor or overzealous hygiene—either as a result of residual feces, which can irritate the skin, or too much soap and scrubbing

- Excessive warmth, caused by too-tight leggings, tights, or underwear; overly warm bed clothing; or obesity

- Psychological response to anxiety. There is a recognized cycle of anxiety, which causes itching, which in turn produces more anxiety. Excessive scratching can worsen the condition.

Treatment Treatment varies, depending on the cause of the problem. If a food cause is suspected, steer clear of spicy foods—particularly peppers—and citrus fruits, such as grapefruit. Minimize the warmth around the area by switching to boxer shorts and loose-fitting, lightweight clothes and bedclothes. After a bowel movement, your goal should be to clean the area as gently and efficiently as possible with soft, moistened toilet paper (avoid scratching or rubbing harshly with dry or rough paper), a washcloth or medicated pad soaked with witch hazel (such as Tuck's), or a premoistened baby wipe. Sitz baths in warm (but not hot) water, several times a day, also may help relieve symptoms and keep the area clean. Do not apply soap or anesthetic ointments (which make the problem worse in some people) directly to the anal or perianal area. Some people are helped by applying baby talcum power, to keep the area dry. Hydrocortisone acetate (1 percent solution) may help reduce symptoms. Your doctor may also prescribe a fungicide (such as a 3 percent odochlorhydroxyquin solution). You may also require treatment for any underlying disease or parasite infection.

❖ FECAL INCONTINENCE

Symptoms (*What you may experience*) Chronic fecal soiling; inability to stop a bowel movement from occurring.

Signs and laboratory findings (*What the doctor looks for*) Diminished rectal sensation, muscle tone, and motor function of the internal and external anal sphincters, as seen in anorectal manometry; muscle weakness, as seen in cinefluoroscopic studies performed during proctography; diminished muscle function, measured during rectal retention and defecation studies (which measure the muscles' ability to retain objects and liquids); diminished pelvic floor function, or prolapse of the pelvic floor (which could interfere with the muscular ability to retain stool), as seen in dynamic radiographic studies of the anus and rectum; diminished anorectal reflexes, evident in an anal wink test, a test of the anal reflex upon being touched (equivalent to the knee reflex test in a normal physical exam), and in neurophysiologic testing of the pelvic floor and anal sphincters. Signs of chronic diarrhea. Also, evidence of any underlying medical condition or neurologic disease, such as diabetes, myasthenia gravis, syphilis, multiple sclerosis, or spina bifida (a common cause in children), from a careful medical history and physical exam.

What is it? Fecal incontinence is, at best, embarrassing and, at worst, socially devastating. It can happen in any age group and for a variety of reasons, including diseases that affect the nervous system (a few examples are noted above) or mental impairment. Some people, as a result of surgery, have a smaller than normal amount of space to hold stool in the rectum; other people develop problems with the reflexes or muscle tone in the anus, rectum, and pelvic floor. Some people, particularly the elderly, can have overflow incontinence, in which liquid stool seeps around an impaction (see Constipation and Impaction, page 1018). Although the anal muscles become less efficient as you age, incontinence is not an inevitable part of aging. See Chapter 12 for more information on incontinence.

People who are prone to chronic diarrhea may have trouble perceiving liquid stool or difficulty retaining it (as opposed to solid stool, which is often easier to control). Anyone experiencing severe or violent bouts of diarrhea—associated with food poisoning, for example—can have isolated episodes of fecal incontinence. But that is a temporary problem, not associated with the chronic loss of fecal control discussed here.

When to call the doctor Many people, embarrassed by this problem, delay treatment and suffer these symptoms for months or even years longer than necessary. Fecal incontinence is nothing to be ashamed of, and there are many good treatments that can help solve this problem. If you are unable to control bowel movements, consult your doctor.

Treatment The first step is for your doctor to determine the cause and ascertain which nerves or muscles are not working properly and whether any other disease is involved. Treatment is based on these findings and may involve the following:

Kegel exercises In addition to altering your diet, you can strengthen your anal sphincter muscles to help delay flatulence by doing Kegel exercises: Lie on your back, with your knees bent, and your feet about 12 in. apart. Clench, as tightly as you can, the muscles around your anus (the ones you use when trying not to pass gas), and hold for as long as you can—working up to 20 seconds. Relax the muscles slowly, take a deep breath, and repeat. These exercises can also be done when you are standing (in the shower, for instance), sitting (even driving a car), and urinating.

Biofeedback This simple technique is effective in more than 70 percent of people who are able to contract their external anal sphincter or gluteal muscles and who have normal ability to sense rectal distension (to feel when stool is in the rectum). Briefly, this is how it works: Working with a monitor that measures the contractions of your external sphincter, your doctor will help you learn to associate and coordinate these contractions with rectal distension. Practice is essential: You will need to practice sphincter contraction exercises at least three times a day and to contract the sphincter at any sensation of rectal urgency or distension. This is a trial-and-error process that takes time to learn, so do not be discouraged if you have setbacks.

Surgery As a last resort, surgery to repair a poorly functioning anal sphincter, by tightening the anal canal and improving the angle of anal muscles, can be helpful in some people. However, it is not terribly successful in helping control diarrhea. Ultimately, your doctor may suggest a colostomy (see Ileostomy, Kock Pouch, Ileoanal Pouch, and Colostomy, page 1012).

Medication If incontinence is associated with diarrhea, your doctor may also prescribe bulk laxatives, fiber psyllium supplements such as Metamucil or Citrucel; an antidiarrheal medication such as diphenoxylate and atropine (Lomotil), which slows the motility, or movement, of the intestine; an anticholinergic drug such as loperamide (Imodium), which slows the motility in the colon; or a bile acid-binding resin such as cholestyramine (Questran), which causes mild constipation.

Prognosis This depends on the underlying cause of the incontinence. However, an estimated 70 to 80 percent of people with fecal incontinence—regardless of the cause—are helped by treatment.

THE LIVER, GALLBLADDER, AND PANCREAS

Technically, the liver, gallbladder, and pancreas are not part of the gastrointestinal system; yet their function is crucial to the body's ability to digest food, absorb its contents, and dispose of harmful substances.

Of these, the most important is the liver. Bile, which renders fats into digestible bits, is made here and sent into the duodenum via a series of channels called bile ducts. Blood clotting factors and other important proteins, including glycogen, a storage form of glucose, are made in this football-sized factory and shipped through-

(A) Bile is made in the liver, stored in the gallbladder, and transported via ducts to the duodenum, where it renders fats into soluble fragments. The liver also produces blood-clotting factors and other important proteins and processes toxins such as alcohol. (B) Liver cells are arranged into hexagonal lobules, which maximize cellular contacts with blood vessels in the liver. Each lobule has a central vein that connects to the hepatic vein. Bile is secreted into tiny canaliculi that lead to the common bile duct. Kupffer cells, which line the blood canals within the liver, help to remove old red blood cells and other particles from the blood.

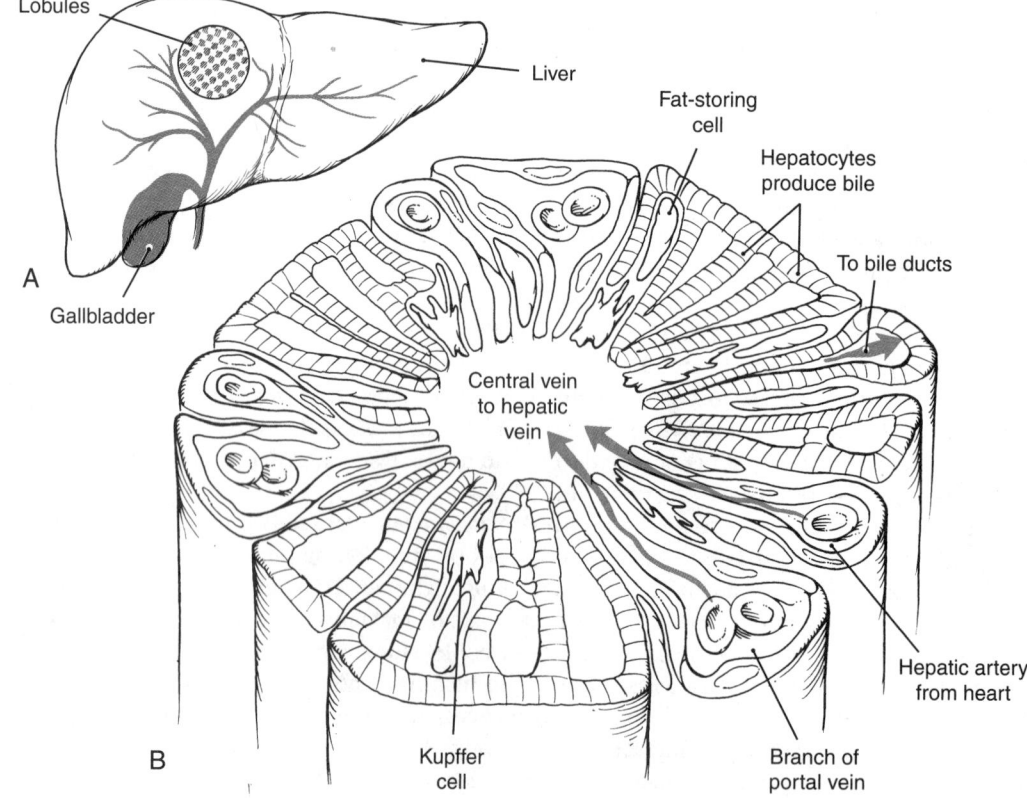

Lobules

Liver

Fat-storing cell

Hepatocytes produce bile

To bile ducts

A

Gallbladder

Central vein to hepatic vein

Hepatic artery from heart

B

Kupffer cell

Branch of portal vein

DIAGNOSTIC TESTS OF THE LIVER, GALLBLADDER, AND PANCREAS

Because the symptoms for many conditions involving the abdominal organs are similar, several diagnostic tests may be necessary to determine the cause. Some commonly performed tests are covered here (see also Blood Tests to Monitor the Liver, page 1035, Laparoscopy, page 1032, Endoscopic Retrograde Cholangeopancreatography, page 1033, Liver Biopsy, page 1036, A Word on Jaundice, page 1036, and Pancreas Function Tests, page 1060).

Percutaneous Transhepatic Cholangiogram

Percutaneous transhepatic cholangiogram (PTHC, also abbreviated as PTC) is an x-ray test that can show blockages in the bile ducts (from a stone or bile duct disease). In this test, usually performed by a radiologist, contrast dye—visible on an x-ray—is injected with a long, thin needle through the chest or abdominal wall into the liver and bile ducts.

PTHC, which generally takes less than an hour, is a very safe procedure, with a low risk—about 1 in 1,000—of complications. It is done with informed consent, which means you should have a full understanding of the risks involved. The main risk is of minor internal bleeding.

You will be asked not to eat or drink anything after midnight the night before and (to minimize the risk of bleeding) to stop taking aspirin for at least 2 days beforehand. *Note:* If you are taking aspirin or any medication regularly, do not skip a scheduled dose without talking to your doctor first.

Shortly before the procedure begins, you will be given an intravenous, short-term sedative such as diazepam (Valium) or a narcotic such as meperidine (Demerol) or fentanyl (Sublimaze) to help you relax and make you feel drowsy. You may also be given an antibiotic to minimize the risk of infection. You will receive a local anesthetic, injected in the skin over the liver, that will make part of your abdomen feel numb. Thus, when the long needle is injected, and as it makes its way through your liver to the bile duct—with the help of x-ray imaging for guidance—you should feel no pain or discomfort (or, at worst, only a fleeting sensation of pain or fullness). When the needle is safely nestled in the bile duct, the radiologist threads a guide wire over the needle, removes the needle, and then threads a thin plastic tube over the guide wire (which is also removed). The dye is then injected through this tube.

PTHC is done on a movable table. When the dye is in place, the radiologist takes a series of x-ray pictures, with you tilted at various angles, so every aspect of your liver and bile ducts may be seen. Afterward, you will be asked to lie on your right side for several hours in a recovery room, where you will be monitored for any sign of complications. Do not be surprised if you do not remember anything after the procedure; this amnestic effect of the medication is very common. Finally, because the sedative or narcotic can impair your judgment and reflexes, plan on having someone drive you home after the procedure. At many hospitals, PTHC is only performed as an inpatient procedure.

Oral Cholecystogram

This test, which has largely been supplanted by more sophisticated diagnostic tests, also involves dye, but instead of being injected—as in endoscopic retrograde cholangiopancreatography and PTHC—it is swallowed. The dye is absorbed by the intestines and excreted by the liver into bile. The dye-coated bile amasses in the gallbladder, and an x-ray is taken. If the gallbladder does not fill with bile, this can suggest the presence of gallstones.

TC-IDA Scan

The TC (pronounced "tek") -IDA (technetium-labelled iminodiacetic acid) scan is a sophisticated nuclear medicine test, involving a radioactive compound injected into a vein in your arm. This compound, called a radionuclide, is specifically programmed; it heads directly to the liver, where it is absorbed and secreted into the bile—making the liver, gallbladder, and bile ducts visible on a special camera (similar to an x-ray machine). A TC-IDA scan is often used to look for bile duct and gallbladder disease. ■

out the body as needed. Perhaps most important, the liver—the only internal organ capable of regenerating itself when injured—acts as a filter, screening and culling potentially toxic ingredients from food, medications, and alcoholic beverages. The liver is resilient but not impervious to damage from alcohol, drugs, or a virus; this damage, called hepatitis, may be temporary inflammation, or it can be chronic, sometimes resulting in severe scarring, called cirrhosis.

The pear-shaped gallbladder, a reservoir that sits just under the liver, stores bile, which passes from the liver through the cystic duct. During a meal, the gallbladder contracts, sending bile acids back through the cystic and common bile duct into the small bowel. Although bile's job is to dissolve fats, bile itself is laden with a fatty-like substance called cholesterol. In many people, gallstones form in the gallbladder; if one of these stones becomes too large or is unfortunately placed and blocks a bile duct, the gallbladder can become inflamed.

The oblong pancreas, larger than the gallbladder but less than a third the size of the liver, makes many potent digestive enzymes. These, too, flow through ducts to the small intestine, where they attack fats, proteins, and carbohydrates, breaking them into digestible molecules. Two hormones

LAPAROSCOPY

The concept behind laparoscopy is that of the endoscope: A tiny tube, with a headlight and video camera is inserted into the body. The main difference is that the laparoscope does not enter the body through the mouth or anus but through a peephole, a tiny (usually less than 1/2 in.) incision made in the abdominal wall. To move the internal organs out of the way and maximize visibility, the surgeon or gastroenterologist pipes gas into the abdomen. This procedure is performed under general anesthesia. Surgical instruments, including a thin needle for biopsy, may be passed through the laparoscope, or may be introduced through separate puncture sites. Laparoscopy generally requires hospital admission. The main advantage of laparoscopic surgery is its comparatively minor toll on the body—smaller incision, reduced rate of complications, and minimal recovery time—as compared to open surgery. Laparoscopic removal of the gallbladder, called a laparoscopic cholecystectomy, is performed in more than 400,000 Americans each year (see Treatment Options for Gallstones, page 1056).

Laparoscopy, which generally takes less than 1 hour, is a very safe procedure, with a low risk—about 1 in 300—of complications. It is done with informed consent, which means you should have a full understanding of the risks involved. The main risks are of internal bleeding, infection, perforation, or bile duct injury.

You will be asked not to eat or drink anything after midnight the night before and (to minimize the risk of bleeding) to stop taking aspirin for at least 2 days beforehand. If you are taking aspirin or any medication regularly, do not skip a scheduled dose without talking to your doctor first.

You will receive general anesthesia so that you will be asleep during the procedure. Afterward, you will be asked to lie down for several hours in a recovery room, where you will be monitored for any sign of complications. You will most likely be admitted to the hospital at this time. ∎

Abdominal surgery can sometimes be performed through a laparoscope, which is a tiny tube with a video camera and headlight that is inserted directly into the abdomen through a small hole in the skin. This generally requires hospital admission and general anesthesia but has fewer complications and less recovery time than an open abdominal operation. Laparoscopic removal of the gallbladder (cholecystectomy) is performed in more than 400,000 Americans each year.

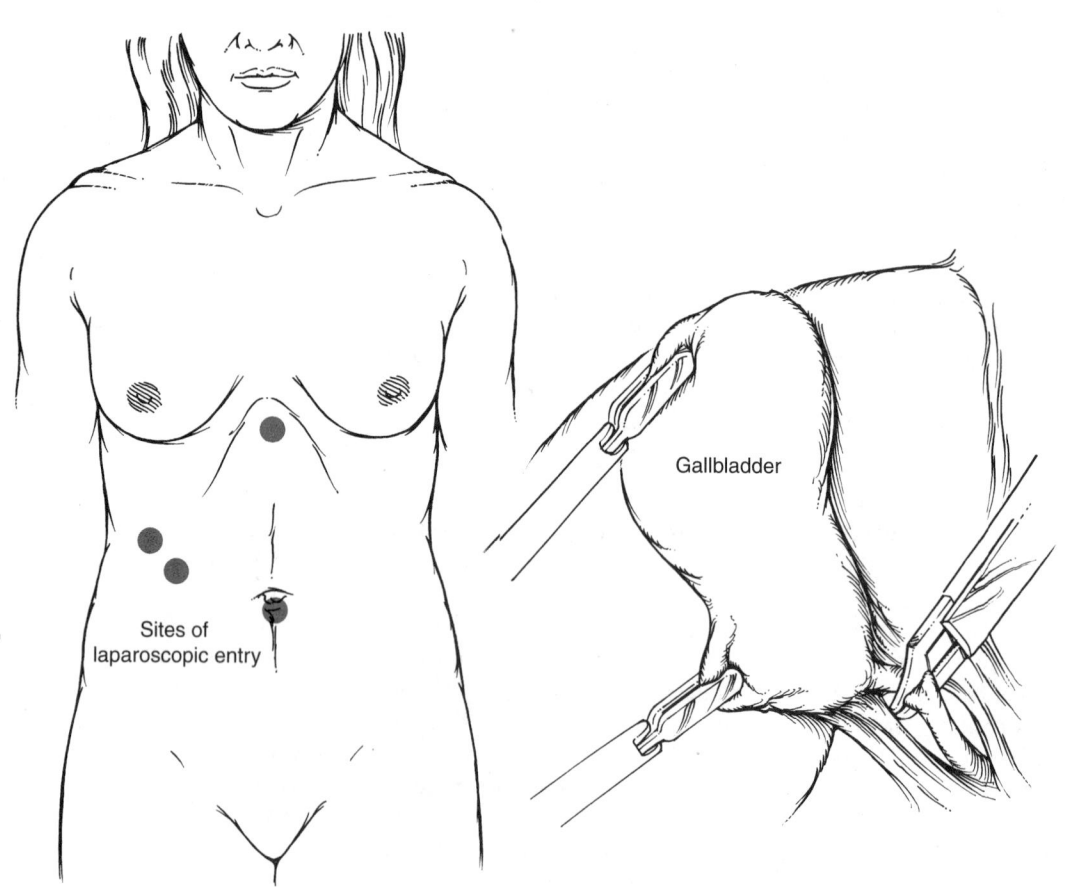

Sites of laparoscopic entry

Gallbladder

ENDOSCOPIC RETROGRADE CHOLANGIOPANCREATOGRAPHY

Endoscopic retrograde cholangiopancreatography (ERCP) is a sophisticated procedure that combines two kinds of technology: the endoscope and the x-ray. Performed by a gastroenterologist, ERCP allows the doctor to examine the pancreas, bile ducts, liver, and gallbladder. Some problems that cannot be detected with other imaging techniques can be seen clearly with ERCP. As with other procedures involving a scope (such as esophagogastroduodenoscopy, flexible sigmoidoscopy, and colonoscopy), it allows the doctor to perform some therapeutic procedures, as well. With ERCP, a doctor can dislodge a gallstone stuck in the bile duct and pull it into the intestine (so it then may pass normally from the body); reopen a clogged bile duct (or create a new opening); insert a tube, called a stent, to help the duct stay open, allowing bile to drain more freely; and photograph any abnormal findings. During the procedure, your doctor may also perform a biopsy, removing a small sample of tissue for study under a microscope. A biopsy can be performed for many reasons; having a biopsy does not mean that you have cancer.

In ERCP, done with you lying on your left side most of the time (although you will be asked to shift positions several times during the procedure), the doctor passes a duodenoscope, a flexible, lighted tube equipped with a video camera, through your mouth and throat into the upper digestive tract: the esophagus, stomach, and duodenum, the top part of the small intestine. The duodenoscope is similar to an endoscope, but the angle is different; the duodenoscope is side-viewing—the opening difference between looking out of the windshield of a car and looking out of the driver's side window. Then, using the duodenoscope's camera to find the ampulla (the opening where the bile and pancreatic ducts drain into the duodenum), the doctor threads a smaller tube, called cannula, through the duodenoscope. Through this tube, in turn, the doctor injects opaque dye, which makes the bile ducts and pancreatic ducts visible on an x-ray. You may feel some discomfort when the dye is injected, but no pain.

ERCP, which generally takes less than 1 hour, is very safe, with a low risk of complications. It is done with informed consent, which means you should have a full understanding of the risks involved. The most common complication, which develops in an estimated 1 to 3 percent of people—is temporary pancreatitis (inflammation of the pancreas, see Acute Pancreatitis, page 1060), caused by injection of the dye. Although this damage is not permanent, the pain may be severe. If you experience any abdominal pain after ERCP, call your doctor. Other potential complications include a tear or tiny hole (called a perforation) in the lining of the esophagus, stomach, or duodenum, which may heal on its own or may require surgery to repair; aspiration, which could develop into pneumonia; bleeding, if a biopsy or other procedure is done, or a polyp is removed, or a sphincterotomy is performed (usually bleeding is minimal; rarely, it may require surgery or a blood transfusion); a reaction to the sedative given before the procedure (thus, be sure to tell the doctor if you are allergic to any medications). Also, many people experience a

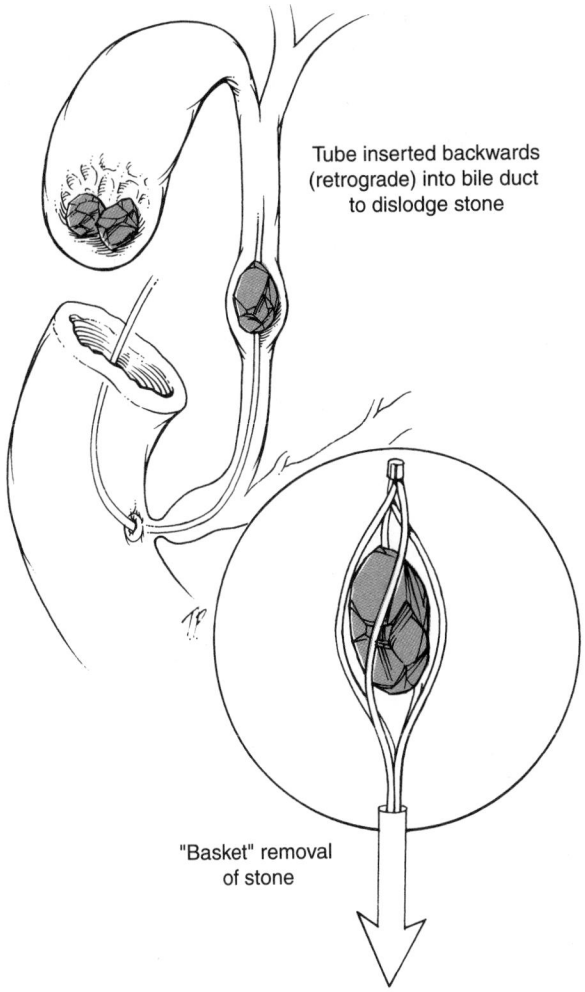

Tube inserted backwards (retrograde) into bile duct to dislodge stone

"Basket" removal of stone

Endoscopic retrograde cholangiopancreatography (ERCP) allows a doctor to examine the pancreas, bile ducts, liver, and gallbladder. A narrow tube is passed into the mouth, down the throat, and into the upper digestive tract. This procedure also provides capabilities for dislodging a gallstone from the bile duct, opening a clogged bile duct, inserting a stent to help a duct stay open, photographing abnormal findings, and taking biopsies for laboratory examination. Dye is injected through the tube to make the ducts visible on radiologic images. The procedure is safe and takes less than 1 hour.

sore throat for several hours afterward. There is a minimal risk of infection with any procedure.

Because your doctor needs to see every part of the upper gastrointestinal tract, ERCP cannot be performed on a full stomach; you will be asked not to eat or drink anything after midnight the night before, and (to minimize the risk of bleeding) to stop taking aspirin for at least 2 days beforehand. If you are taking aspirin or any medication regularly, do not skip a scheduled dose of medication without talking to your doctor first.

Shortly before the procedure begins, you will be asked to remove eyeglasses and dentures; you may want to remove ▶

contact lenses, as well. You will be given an intravenous, short-term sedative (such as diazepam) or a narcotic (such as meperidine or fentanyl) to help you relax and make you feel drowsy during the procedure. Also, your doctor will probably spray the back of your throat or ask you to gargle with a numbing medication to prevent you from gagging as you swallow the duodenoscope. You should not feel any pain or discomfort from the procedure itself. Although you will be conscious throughout the procedure, and able to answer questions and follow instructions, you may not remember anything about it afterward; this is very common.

Finally, because the sedative or narcotic can impair your judgment and reflexes, plan on having someone drive you home afterward. At many hospitals, the procedure will not be performed if you do not have an escort home. ■

made by the pancreas—called insulin and glucagon—are critical to the body's ability to metabolize sugar. The pancreas, too, can become inflamed, usually from alcohol abuse, and its digestive enzymes can go awry and begin attacking the gland itself. Because these abdominal organs share such close quarters, a problem in one organ—gallstones, for example, or cancer—can have serious ramifications in neighboring organs, as well.

The Liver

The liver—at about 3 lb, the body's largest solid organ—is a remarkable, intricate machine. All of the blood that passes through the intestines, rich with absorbed nutrients, can only reach the heart and lungs by first passing through the liver. Unlike other internal organs, such as the stomach, the liver is essential to life. However, because its cells are so efficient, you do not need the entire organ to survive; you can get by with less than half of a liver.

About the size of a football and located in your upper right abdomen, the liver plays two major roles: It neutralizes toxins and wastes and synthesizes new chemicals essential for blood clotting and other functions.

As it fulfills these main functions, it performs other vital tasks. Among other things, it serves as a factory where important substances, including most of the proteins in the blood, are made and exported throughout the body. Blood clotting is regulated here; the liver makes most of the factors that clot blood and begin to heal a wound. When the liver's function is hampered by disease, the body's ability to recover from injury is severely impaired.

Raw proteins, delivered in the food we eat, are converted into amino acids and other basic components here. Medications, absorbed from the stomach and bowel, are converted into forms the body can use, or they are broken down and excreted from the body. When you need quick energy and get a surge of glucose, it comes from your liver. The liver stores glycogen, the starch form of glucose.

Among the liver's largest exports is bile, a detergent the liver makes to dissolve fat in the digestive tract, so the body may absorb it more easily. The bile flows through several channels, called bile ducts, into the intestine.

The liver acts as a massive filter, which detoxifies harmful substances—including potentially dangerous ingredients in the food we eat—and excretes the worst offenders. Finally, the liver is the only solid organ in the body able to regenerate itself. When part—even as much as 70 percent—of its tissue is damaged, by alcohol, drugs, or a virus, such as hepatitis A, B, or C—all of which cause the liver to become inflamed—the liver manages its own recovery by creating new replacement cells and tissue.

Yet, as powerful and resilient as the liver is, it is particularly vulnerable to alcohol, which is a toxin. To the liver, even a wine cooler or a can of beer is poison, although for most people, one drink has no lasting, harmful effects on the body. However, if you are also taking any form of medication, or if you drink heavily, then the effect of alcohol can be additive. Over time, the liver can become inflamed and enlarged, a condition called alcoholic hepatitis. Then, fatty liver—a condition in which globules of fat infiltrate the liver and harm its ability to function—may develop. With further damage, the liver becomes scarred, cirrhotic. When too much tissue is destroyed, the liver can no longer handle the burden of toxins that constantly wash through it and can no longer make its important substances, and liver failure results. Liver damage from alcohol or other toxins is often insidious; because the liver is

BLOOD TESTS TO MONITOR THE LIVER

Blood tests can tell your doctor much about the state of your liver and help pinpoint the cause of liver disease. These include the following.

Liver Function Tests Liver function tests (LFTs) are liver enzyme tests that measure specific liver enzymes in the blood. Elevated levels of alanine aminotransferase (ALT) and aspirate aminotransferase (AST), enzymes made by liver cells, can suggest liver damage. (These enzymes used to be called SGPT and SGOT; most doctors now adopt the current terms.) When liver cells are injured or inflamed, these enzymes seep into the bloodstream. In acute viral hepatitis, they may skyrocket; but in chronic hepatitis, they may be only moderately elevated. The normal range varies, depending on the laboratory your doctor uses. In many liver disorders, these enzymes may be only mildly higher than normal, and not conclusive on their own. Because AST may also be elevated in heart and muscle disease, it is not considered as specific a test as ALT.

Elevated levels of the liver enzymes alkaline phosphatase and gamma-glutamyltranspeptidase (GGTP) can indicate trouble with bile drainage—either in the liver itself or in a bile duct. Gallstones are common causes of elevated alkaline phosphatase and GGTP; the flow of bile can also be obstructed or hindered by a tumor, cyst, some forms of hepatitis, and cirrhosis. Like AST, alkaline phosphatase is not terribly specific to the liver; it can also be elevated in other diseases. If only alkaline phosphatase is elevated, the trouble may not lie in the liver.

Serum Albumin and Prothrombin Time When the liver is seriously damaged, in cirrhosis, it is unable to make normal amounts of a major protein called albumin. Blood levels of albumin that are less than 3.5 mg/dL can suggest significant liver disease. Prothrombin time (PT, or protime) is a test that measures, in seconds, the blood's ability to coagulate. Among the liver's many products are important factors involved in blood clotting; when the liver is seriously compromised and unable to maintain its normal manufacturing load, there is a shortage of these factors, and it takes much longer for blood to begin to clot.

Bilirubin Test Bilirubin is the pigment that gives bile its distinctive color. It is a by-product of heme, an ingredient in red blood cells. Normally, only a modest amount of bilirubin—less than 1.2 mg/dL—circulates in the blood. But when red blood cells are destroyed, or when bilirubin is not processed as quickly as usual by the liver, its levels rise in the bloodstream. Jaundice—yellowing of the skin and whites of the eyes—is usually visible when bilirubin levels are greater than 3 mg/dL. Because bilirubin can be elevated in many liver and biliary tract disorders, this alone is not a definitive liver function test, it does not tell doctors why the bilirubin is elevated.

Serum Iron and Ferritin Tests Technically, these are not liver function tests, because they do not reveal specific information about the liver. But in hemochromatosis, a liver disease in which the body is overloaded with iron, the percentages of iron and ferritin in the blood are much higher than normal.

Serum Ceruloplasmin and Copper Urine Tests In Wilson's disease (see Inherited Liver Disorders, page 1049), characterized by deposits of the mineral copper throughout the body, the blood (serum) level of ceruloplasmin, a copper-containing transport protein, is much lower than normal. There is also an excessive amount of copper in the urine.

Serum Alpha$_1$-Antitrypsin This is an inhibitor of certain enzymes, called proteolytic enzymes, which break down protein, and it is lacking in the blood of people with alpha$_1$-antitrypsin deficiency (see Inherited Liver Disorders page 1049).

Antimitochondrial Antibodies A positive result of this test is a strong suggestion of primary biliary cirrhosis, a rare autoimmune disease that attacks the bile ductules (small ducts inside the liver).

Serum Globulin, Antinuclear Antibodies, and Antismooth Muscle Antibodies These factors, involved in the body's immune system, are elevated in autoimmune hepatitis.

Viral Hepatitis Antibodies Specific antibodies, elevated in hepatitis A, B, C, and D, allow your doctor to determine the exact form of viral hepatitis you have. ■

---

so resilient, someone can be diagnosed with cirrhosis who has never experienced jaundice or suffered any other symptoms of liver damage. Although the liver can be damaged by many substances, the symptoms of liver trouble are often similar. For example, a host of problems can result in jaundice. Thus, sophisticated diagnostic testing is often necessary to determine the particular cause of damage.

❖ ACUTE VIRAL HEPATITIS

Symptoms *(What you may experience)* Jaundice (yellowing of the skin or whites of your eyes, and/or a brownish or orange tint in the urine—see A Word on Jaundice, page 1036); unusually light-colored stool; unexplained fatigue that persists for weeks or even months; flulike symptoms, such as fever, loss of appetite, nausea, and vomiting; abdominal pain.

Signs and laboratory findings *(What the doctor looks for)* Elevated liver enzymes on liver function tests (see Blood Tests to Monitor the Liver, page 1035); positive results of a specific antibody test to hepatitis A, B, C, or D (the hepatitis E test is not universally available in this country) performed as part of a blood test or in routine blood donation; recent exposure (reported in your medical

LIVER BIOPSY

In a liver biopsy, usually performed by a gastroenterologist, a thin needle is inserted into the liver, and a tiny sample of tissue is removed, to be examined under a microscope by a pathologist. This test is done to find the cause of suspected liver disease (if someone has an enlarged liver, or elevated results of liver function tests, for example) or to ascertain its stage (that is, to learn how advanced the disease is) and to help determine the best course of treatment. Liver biopsy is also needed, often, in the first months after a liver transplant, to make sure the new liver is functioning properly.

The procedure itself, usually done in a hospital on an outpatient basis, takes very little time—less than 1 minute. The gastroenterologist performs a physical exam and may also use an imaging technique, such as ultrasound or computed tomography (CT), to pinpoint the best site for the biopsy and guide the needle there. Before the procedure, your skin and the area just beneath it will be numbed with an injected local anesthetic. About half of all patients who undergo a liver biopsy feel no pain; the rest feel brief discomfort in the area of the biopsy and occasionally in the right shoulder. Afterward, you will be sent to a recovery room, where you will be monitored to make sure there are no complications.

Complications Liver biopsy is an extremely safe procedure; the risk of complications is less than 1 percent. The main complication is bleeding from the site where the needle enters the liver; other potential problems include inadvertent puncture of other organs on the way to the liver—the kidney, lung, or colon—or biopsy of the gallbladder instead of the liver (which may result in bile leaking into the abdominal cavity, resulting in peritonitis). But again, the risk is very low; the risk of dying from a liver biopsy is less than 0.1 percent.

Variations on the Procedure Liver biopsy can also be performed during laparoscopy (see Laparoscopy, page 1032) or before open surgery. A less common form of biopsy—mainly done in people with blood clotting disorders or in people with significant ascites (fluid swelling in the abdomen)—is transvenous or transjugular liver biopsy. This procedure, performed by an interventional radiologist, involves a tiny tube, inserted into the internal jugular vein in the neck, and guided with fluoroscopy (see Other Diagnostic Tests of the Gastrointestinal Tract, page 984), into the hepatic vein, which runs through the liver. When the tube is in place, the doctor guides a biopsy needle through it, into the liver. ■

history) to someone with hepatitis. It may take 4 weeks or longer for the body to produce antibodies to a hepatitis virus. Thus, even if a blood test is negative, you may still develop hepatitis. If symptoms persist, return to your doctor for another blood test. And if you believe you have been exposed to hepatitis, ask your doctor for immunization at once.

What is it? Five contagious viruses are known to cause inflammation of the liver: hepatitis A, B, C, D and E. The first three are the most serious in the United States. Hepatitis D cannot take hold in the body unless a person is already infected with hepatitis B; thus, if you are not infected with hepatitis B, you are not at risk for hepatitis D. Hepatitis E, a health problem in India and Asia, is extremely rare in this country.

A WORD ON JAUNDICE

Jaundice develops when infection or inflammation blocks bile ductules in the liver, causing bile—a detergent that dissolves fats so the body can digest them more easily—to back up into the bloodstream. The yellow color is caused as bile pigment accumulates in the skin. Although it is an important warning sign of acute viral hepatitis, and its color may be frightening, it is not in itself a life-threatening condition. ■

Although their impact on the liver can vary greatly, hepatitis viruses B and C have the potential to develop into chronic hepatitis (see Chronic Hepatitis, page 1041) and to cause permanent liver damage.

Hepatitis A Hepatitis A is responsible for about one-quarter of all cases of hepatitis in the United States. Unlike other forms of hepatitis, hepatitis A is most commonly transmitted in drinking water or food contaminated with fecal matter that contains the virus; high concentrations of the virus live in feces from an infected person. Like many forms of food poisoning, this disease could be largely prevented by proper hygiene. Hepatitis A can also be transmitted by deep kissing, by anal sex, and by using contaminated needles to administer intravenous drugs. This virus is tenacious: At normal room temperature, it can survive for up to 4 hours in a speck of contaminated fecal material on someone's hand, the outside of a diaper, or—a common problem in daycare settings—on a hard surface such as a ball, cup, or spoon. When contaminated sewage is dumped into fishing waters, shellfish can contract the virus. People who eat the tainted shellfish raw, or even swim in polluted waters, can contract the virus, as well. Some beaches, particularly those in urban areas, post health warnings when the water is hazardous; others allow you to swim at your own risk. If you are worried about this risk, contact the local health department or stay in a boat or on the beach. Hepatitis A is especially common in the Middle East, South and Central America, Eastern Europe, Africa, and Southeast Asia.

Each year, according to estimates by the Centers for Disease Control and Prevention, some 150,000 Americans are infected with hepatitis A. Because the incubation period is 2 to 6 weeks, it is easy for the infection to be spread before any symptoms have developed. In a daycare center, for example, if proper hygiene is not scrupulously observed, the infection can spread rapidly. Fortunately, the virus is seldom life-threatening. In most people, it produces temporary flu-like symptoms and jaundice (see A Word on Jaundice, page 1036), runs its course—there is no specific treatment—and the body recovers within 6 months. The disease hardly ever results in serious complications to pregnant women or their unborn children. However, in a small percentage of cases—particularly in the elderly, and in people already suffering from such liver problems as alcoholic hepatitis or cirrhosis—hepatitis A can produce complications. For reasons that are unclear, some people seem to get better, with improvements in symptoms and liver function tests and then suffer a relapse after about 4 weeks. Some people have more than one relapse. Sometimes, jaundice persists longer than 2 months; however, chronic liver disease does not occur. Very rarely, acute infection with hepatitis A can result in rapid liver failure (see Liver Failure, page 1046).

Hepatitis B Nearly 300,000 Americans contract hepatitis B every year; it is the most common cause of viral hepatitis. Hepatitis B is spread in infected blood and other bodily fluids (semen, vaginal secretions, saliva, open sores, and breast milk). Hepatitis B is not spread by casual contact. You cannot get it from holding hands, having someone cough or sneeze on you, playing with an infected child, dry kissing on the lips, or eating food prepared by someone who has the virus. An estimated 40 percent of those infected do not know how they acquired hepatitis B. Because the incubation period can be 1 to 6 months, it can be difficult to pinpoint the source of exposure. Like hepatitis A, hepatitis B may be present in

contaminated beaches and raw shellfish. As many as 10 percent of all people infected with hepatitis B develop chronic hepatitis (see Chronic Hepatitis, page 1041); young children and infants are particularly at risk of becoming chronically infected or of becoming carriers of the disease (see below). Most people manage to fight off the infection successfully within a few months, developing an immunity that lasts a lifetime. Thus, once your body has cleared itself of the virus, you will never again develop hepatitis B (although you could still develop another form of hepatitis). Immunity can be checked by a test called anti-HBs (antibody to hepatitis B surface antigen). The anti-HBs test registers the presence in the blood of an antibody to the outside of the hepatitis B virus. If you have ever had hepatitis B, antibodies to the virus will always be present in your blood, and because there is a tiny risk that the anti-HBs test showed a false-positive, and that you could still pass on the virus, you will not be allowed to donate blood, plasma, tissue, body organs, or sperm.

An estimated 1 million Americans are lifelong carriers of hepatitis B. If you are infected with hepatitis B for more than 6 months, then you are considered a carrier— even if you feel fine and are free of symptoms. This means that you can transmit the virus to others by having unprotected sex, sharing needles, deep kissing, sharing food or drinks, or engaging in any of the risky behavior described in What You Can Do, page 1038. (Because hepatitis B can be a sexually transmitted disease, it is particularly prevalent in young adults.) Being a carrier also means that your liver is more vulnerable than normal to injury (for steps you should take, see Treatment, page 1039). If you are a carrier of hepatitis B and are pregnant, you have an estimated 90 percent likelihood of passing on the virus to your unborn baby. Thus, all pregnant women should be tested for hepatitis B, and all babies should be given immunoglobin and should be vaccinated at birth (see Vaccines to Prevent Hepatitis, page 1038) to protect them from getting the virus. For reasons not understood, the hepatitis B virus spontaneously goes away in a very small percentage of carriers. Some people who are carriers develop chronic hepatitis (see Chronic Hepatitis, page 1041). According to the American Liver Foundation, in the United States, hepati-

VACCINES TO PREVENT HEPATITIS

Two forms of viral hepatitis—A and B—are preventable with vaccines. By far, the more serious and common infection is with hepatitis B. In the United States, more than 300,000 people are infected with the hepatitis B virus every year, and more than 5,000 people die from illnesses related to the virus. Those most likely to get hepatitis B, which is transmitted through contaminated blood and body fluids, are sexually active young adults. However, millions of Americans—whether because of their occupation, habits, or because a family member or close friend is infected—are also at risk. You may be at risk of contracting hepatitis B if your job causes you to come in contact with other people's blood: if you are a doctor, nurse, or emergency technician (or even if you are simply giving first aid to an injured person, for example, on a school playground or at an office picnic), dentist or dental hygienist, rescue or hospital worker, or if you work at a funeral home or prison.

Before traveling to regions such as the Pacific Islands and Asia, where hepatitis B is prevalent, you should be immunized for the disease. Be sure to schedule your immunization more than 2 weeks before you are leaving, and do not neglect to get the follow-up booster shots.

In an attempt to eliminate hepatitis B, the Centers for Disease Control and Prevention and the American Academy of Pediatrics have recommended that all infants be vaccinated for hepatitis B shortly after birth, with the second dose at between 1 and 2 months, and the third between 6 and 18 months.

The vaccine is given in three parts. *In order for the vaccine to be completely effective, you must have all three shots.* The vaccine may be given to anyone at any age. For children, the vaccine is likely to provide immunity for at least 9 years, but perhaps much longer. For adults, the vaccine provides immunity for at least 5 years.

Hepatitis A is not as common in the United States and is mainly recommended for US military personnel and for individuals with underlying liver disease. However, two vaccines, both using inactive hepatitis A particles, are available: The body, fooled by the inactive virus, makes antibodies to it, and these antibodies, in turn, protect the body against the real virus. With both vaccines, the main reported side effect is soreness at the injection site, which should go away in 1 or 2 days. The vaccines provide effective immunity in an estimated 90 percent of those who receive them; a test that checks for the presence of antibodies in the blood can determine whether the vaccine has indeed provided immunity. ■

tis B is responsible for 5,000 deaths each year—from hepatitis itself and from other damage to the liver, including liver cancer, cirrhosis, and liver failure (all of which can be triggered by chronic hepatitis).

Hepatitis C About 4 million Americans have hepatitis C; most of these people have never experienced any symptoms, and few realize that they even have this virus, which used to be identified by what it was not; in fact, until the late 1980s, it was called "non-A, non-B hepatitis." A large number of Americans contracted hepatitis C from blood transfusions until the 1980s, when new purity tests dramatically lowered the risk of becoming infected from donated blood. Now, about 170,000 Americans become infected with this virus each year; and, although it is usually silent, some scientists believe the annual death rate from hepatitis C will triple—to 24,000—over the next 20 years. Although a small percentage of people infected with hepatitis C manage to clear the virus on their own, the majority develop a chronic infection (see Chronic Hepatitis, page 1041). Most of these people have no symptoms and live normal, healthy lives. Fewer than one-quarter of people with chronic infections eventually develop complications, including cirrhosis, liver cancer, and liver failure. Chronic infection with hepatitis C is the leading cause for liver transplants. Hepatitis C, like hepatitis B, is a blood-borne virus that can be transmitted through blood transfusions. Since 1990, however, screening tests have dramatically reduced this risk. It is most commonly spread through infected needles, shared by intravenous drug users and, much less often, through unprotected sex (in which a condom is not used). Most people are diagnosed when a routine blood test reveals elevated liver enzymes, or when a hepatitis C virus antibody (anti-HCV) test, given at the time of blood donation, is positive. This test can remain positive even several years after someone has recovered from acute hepatitis C—even if the body is no longer infected with the virus. Currently, there is no vaccine to prevent hepatitis C.

What you can do There is much you can do to prevent viral hepatitis. The rules have become familiar because the efforts to prevent acquired immunodeficiency syndrome (AIDS) apply to hepatitis, as well: Do not use intravenous drugs or share needles; avoid unprotected sex, that is, sex without a condom, and, because condoms can break, make sure to change condoms with each sexual act (see Chapter 25 for more information on the proper use of a condom). Do not share chewing gum, drinks, razors, toothbrushes, or pierced earrings with anyone; and if you have your ear or any other part of your body pierced, or if you get a tattoo, make sure the needle is properly sterilized. If you must touch or clean up blood (or items with blood on them, such as tissues or tampons), wear disposable gloves.

To clean an area with blood on it, use bleach (one part bleach to ten parts water). To prevent hepatitis A, in addition to the steps listed on page 1038, wash your hands frequently, particularly after using the bathroom or changing a baby's diaper. Also, avoid raw shellfish, which may be contaminated with hepatitis A or B.

Vaccines are available for hepatitis A and B. If you are exposed to the blood or body fluids of an infected person, you need this protection immediately (see Vaccines to Prevent Hepatitis, page 1038). Because most forms of viral hepatitis have an incubation period that lasts several weeks to months, you still have an opportunity to protect yourself from infection. To boost your immune system and help your body ward off the virus, you should also get an immunoglobulin shot (see Treatment, below).

When to call the doctor If you have been exposed to anyone with hepatitis, talk to your doctor about immunization. Even if this exposure was days or weeks ago, it is probably not too late to take steps to prevent infection. If you have any of the symptoms of hepatitis noted above, particularly jaundice, see your doctor.

Treatment Treatment begins with steps to prevent infection, including immediate immunization (see Vaccines to Prevent Hepatitis, page 1038) if you have been exposed to hepatitis A or B (there is no vaccine for hepatitis C). You can also receive temporary immunization with an immune-boosting shot called immune serum globulin, which should be given within 2 weeks of your exposure to the virus.

Bed rest—as much as possible—is necessary to speed recovery. Make every effort to eat a high-calorie, high-protein diet. If you are experiencing nausea, it can be difficult to get the calories you need to recover. Try eating as much as you can in the morning, when nausea tends to be lightest. Also, take extra care of your liver, which is now vulnerable to further injury. Do not drink alcohol; never mix alcohol with acetaminophen (found in Tylenol) because the combination can harm the liver; and check with your doctor before taking any medication. Six months is the mile marker for hepatitis B or C; if viral hepatitis lasts longer than this, it is then considered to be chronic hepatitis, and you may need more aggressive treatment (see Chronic Hepatitis, page 1041).

Prognosis If you are able to clear the virus from your body within 6 months, your prognosis is excellent. If the virus persists, you may develop chronic hepatitis (see Chronic Hepatitis, page 1041)—which may well be silent, producing no symptoms—for years, or even a lifetime.

❖ ALCOHOLIC AND DRUG-INDUCED HEPATITIS

Symptoms *(What you may experience)* Jaundice (yellowing of the skin or whites of your eyes, and/or a brownish or orange tint in the urine (see A Word on Jaundice, page 1036); unusually light-colored stool; unexplained fatigue that persists for weeks or even months; flulike symptoms, such as fever, loss of appetite, nausea, and vomiting; abdominal pain, and sometimes confusion or disorientation. Some people have no symptoms.

Signs and laboratory findings *(What the doctor looks for)* Evidence of inflammation, found in a liver biopsy; recent or recurrent consumption of drugs, prescription or over-the-counter medications, and/or alcoholic beverages (reported in your medical history); elevated liver enzymes on liver function tests; an enlarged, palpable liver (felt during a physical exam); evidence of fluid retention in the abdomen; signs of mental impairment or difficulty concentrating (which may signal liver failure); evidence of malnutrition (another possible signal of long-term alcoholism or drug use). Because it may take weeks or months for some drugs to produce symptoms of hepatitis, be sure to list in your medical history every medication—including over-the-counter drugs—you have taken within the last 2 months.

What is it? Hepatitis is inflammation of the liver, and it can be caused by exposure to alcohol, drugs—even over-the-counter medications and health food store products—and toxic chemicals such as chloroform and carbon tetrachloride (once commonly used in industrial cleaning fluids). Alcoholic hepatitis is not limited to people who drink excessively, although significant, long-term alcohol consumption (more than two drinks a day) is the major cause of this condition. Everyone's body tolerates alcohol differently; many factors, including a person's size, metabolism, sex, and fat content, play a role here. Thus, moderate or even occasional drinkers can develop an enlarged, inflamed liver; sometimes, a single bout of heavy drinking can bring on this inflammation. Fatty liver, a symptomless condition, in which fat infiltrates the liver (see Fatty Liver, below), may develop before this inflammation begins. Because the damage can continue even after alcohol has passed from the body, symptoms may worsen even after someone stops drinking. Over time, with further drinking, the initial inflammation can become more severe, developing into serious conditions including cirrhosis (see page 1043) and liver failure (see page 1046). The liver damage may also be accompanied by fluid retention and confusion (probably a result of toxic chemicals not being cleared from the body). Conversely, the livers of some of the heaviest drinkers, for reasons no one understands, remain remarkably unscathed from serious liver damage.

Many medications can damage the liver, but some tend to cause more harm than others. These include prescription medications, such as hydrocarbons and high-dose intravenous tetracycline, especially in pregnant women; some anticonvulsants, including phenytoin (Dilantin) and valproic acid (Depakene); methyldopa; tranquilizers including chlorpromazine (Thorazine); medications used to treat tuberculosis including isoniazid and rifampin; and even vitamins, including vitamin A and niacin. A general anesthetic called halothane, commonly inhaled during surgery, can produce symptoms of hepatitis within a few days to 2 weeks after an operation. Taking more than the recommended dose of acetaminophen (found in Tylenol), or mixing even small amounts of acetaminophen with alcohol can cause serious liver problems and may even result in liver failure. In massive doses, acetaminophen robs the liver of glutathione, a potent chemical whose job is to detoxify such drugs on a molecular level by sopping up poisonous agents called toxic free radicals. With one of its main defenses disabled, the liver becomes more vulnerable to toxins and particularly susceptible to injury.

What you can do If you drink alcohol, do not have more than two drinks a day; a drink is a glass of wine or 12-oz can of beer, or $1\frac{1}{2}$-oz portion of hard liquor. Never mix any drug—not even over-the-counter medications, and particularly not acetaminophen—with alcohol. Take all medications, even vitamins, in their recommended dosages. If you have any questions, do not guess; ask your doctor. If you have ever had any liver problems or gallstones, be sure to mention this to your doctor before you take any form of medication.

When to call the doctor If you have any of the symptoms listed above, see your doctor as soon as possible.

Treatment For alcoholic hepatitis, the main treatment is simply to stop consuming alcohol and give the liver a chance to heal itself. For more information on alcohol addiction, see Chapter 5. If your doctor suspects that you are also malnourished, you may be given nutritional supplements. For drug-induced hepatitis, as well, the main treatment is to stop the offending drugs. If your symptoms were caused by too much acetaminophen, your doctor will try to restore glutathione levels in the body—and detoxify the acetaminophen—with similar drugs, including *N*-acetylcysteine or *l*-methionine.

Prognosis In a few cases, especially in people who have already experienced liver damage, alcoholic hepatitis and drug-induced hepatitis can be fatal. For most people, however, the inflammation lasts about 2 weeks. If you stop drinking alcohol or taking the medications that caused this problem, the liver will begin to heal itself, and your prognosis is excellent.

❖ FATTY LIVER

Symptoms *(What you may experience)* There are no specific symptoms associated with fatty liver (also called steatohepatitis), which is not usually a disease in and of itself. Instead, fatty liver is associated with other conditions, including heavy drinking of alcohol, obesity, diabetes, poor diet, tuberculosis, and the use of corticosteroids.

Signs and laboratory findings *(What the doctor looks for)* An enlarged, palpable liver, felt during a physical exam, or seen in ultrasound, magnetic resonance imaging (MRI), or computed tomography (CT) scan; mildly elevated liver enzymes, seen in liver function tests; infiltration of fat in the liver, determined by a needle biopsy or suggested by ultrasound, MRI, or CT scan.

What is it? Fatty liver (also called fatty infiltration of the liver), as its name suggests, is the buildup of fat deposits in the liver—enough to increase the organ's weight by at least 5 percent. Although it is not known exactly what causes fat to accumulate in the liver, scientists speculate that a liver damaged by alcohol or illness simply becomes less efficient at breaking down fat, causing it to stockpile. Taking estrogen may contribute to fatty liver, although this has not been shown conclusively. You cannot get fatty liver by eating a high-fat diet, although such a diet may lead to other health problems, including coronary artery disease. Fatty liver does not cause the inflammation of hepatitis or the scarring of cirrhosis. However, a related condition called nonalcoholic steatohepatitis (NASH), inflammation of the liver associated with fat deposits in the liver, tends to affect middle-aged adults—particularly those with diabetes—who are overweight. The American Liver Foundation estimates that NASH develops in between 20 and 40 percent of very obese Americans. In this disease, the liver can become scarred, leading to cirrhosis (see page 1043).

What you can do If you have diabetes, work with your doctor to get your blood sugar level under control with diet, drugs, or insulin. If you are seriously obese, talk to your doctor about medications and the prospects for surgery helping you to lose weight (see Chapter 1). If you are a heavy drinker, see Chapter 5 for information on stopping drinking.

Treatment Treatment of fatty liver—which, unless you have NASH, is not itself a serious disease and does not harm the liver—is aimed at controlling the underlying condition that has caused it. This is a reversible condition: If you have fatty liver because of excess alcohol consumption or obesity, you will begin to lose fat in the liver as soon as you stop drinking or lose weight, respectively. Getting your blood sugar under control, if your diabetes has caused fatty liver,

will also produce an immediate improvement.

Prognosis The prognosis depends on the underlying condition and whether or not you can change that. Uncontrolled diabetes, for example, can produce many serious health problems and may even be fatal. Untreated alcoholism may result in hepatitis, cirrhosis, or liver failure. And unchecked obesity may cause many health problems as well and raises your likelihood of developing diabetes, heart attack, or stroke. NASH may lead to cirrhosis; however, if NASH is associated with obesity, the prognosis improves with significant weight loss.

❖ CHRONIC HEPATITIS

Symptoms *(What you may experience)* Malaise; loss of appetite; fatigue that lasts for months and may be severe; jaundice (yellowing of the skin or whites of your eyes, and/or a brownish or orange tint in the urine); unusually light-colored stool; flulike symptoms, including fever, loss of appetite, nausea, and vomiting; abdominal pain; confusion or disorientation. Some people have no symptoms.

Signs and laboratory findings *(What the doctor looks for)* Inflammation of the liver, as seen on a needle biopsy of the liver; elevated liver enzymes, detected in liver function tests; palpable, enlarged spleen and/or liver felt during a physical exam; abdominal swelling, swollen extremities, or other evidence of fluid retention, as seen in a physical exam; manifestations of a disordered immune system, including acne, absence of menstruation; anemia, detected in a blood test; high blood levels of gamma globulin (especially immunoglobulin G), antinuclear antibody, LE cells, antimitochondrial antibodies, and smooth-muscle antibodies (these are associated with autoimmune hepatitis); signs of impaired mental function or encephalopathy (caused by a buildup of toxins in the brain), evident during the physical exam and patient interview, including unresponsiveness or inappropriate responses to questions, difficulty concentrating or remembering, and neglect of personal appearance; previous diagnosis of hepatitis B or C; prolonged use of medications (reported in your medical history) including the hypertension medication methyldopa, isoniazid (used to treat tuberculosis), the seizure-suppressing medication phenytoin, and nitrofurantoin (Macrodantin, Macrobid) (used to treat urinary tract infections); evidence of malnutrition.

What is it? Chronic hepatitis is a term used to describe two distinct conditions, one fairly benign, the other much more serious: chronic persistent hepatitis and chronic active hepatitis. Note: Jaundice develops when infection or inflammation damages bile ductules in the liver, causing bile—a detergent that dissolves fats so the body can digest them more easily—to back up into the bloodstream. The yellow color is caused as bile pigment accumulates in the skin. Although it is an important symptom of chronic hepatitis (and its color can be frightening), it is not in itself a life-threatening condition.

Chronic persistent hepatitis In an estimated 75 percent of cases, chronic persistent hepatitis is simply acute viral hepatitis (B or C) that has lingered for longer than 6 months. Fatty liver, a symptomless condition in which fat infiltrates the liver, may also be present (see Fatty Liver, page 1040). In their chronic forms, both hepatitis B and C can lead to cirrhosis (see page 1043), liver failure (see page 1046), and/or liver cancer (see page 1052). People who are infected with hepatitis D (which needs prior infection with the hepatitis B virus to take hold in the body) are more likely to develop problems than those with hepatitis B alone. Most individuals with chronic persistent hepatitis, however, have mild symptoms (fatigue, which can be debilitating, is often the worst), which may flare and then recede for months or even years. Sometimes, for reasons not understood, the disease simply vanishes after years or even decades.

Chronic active hepatitis This serious disease may be caused by viral hepatitis, although no one knows why some people with viral hepatitis progress to this form of the disease. Chronic active hepatitis also can—for reasons not understood—be triggered by an immune system gone awry (this is sometimes called autoimmune chronic hepatitis). Here, liver tissue is not simply inflamed; it can be systematically destroyed, along with tissue elsewhere in

the body, by your own antibodies and lymphocytes (white blood cells) which—in a misguided attempt to protect the body—mistakenly recognize it as a foreign invader. Women are more prone to autoimmune hepatitis, often developing it in adolescence or early adulthood. On blood tests, people with this disorder are found to have elevated levels of antinuclear antibodies and/or smooth muscle antibodies. Unfortunately, because the immune system is affected, some people develop other autoimmune disorders, including thyroid problems (see Chapter 26), diabetes mellitus (see Chapter 26), vitiligo (patchy areas in which skin pigmentation is lost, see Chapter 28), or Sjogren's syndrome (see page 645). If not treated, chronic active hepatitis may lead to many complications, including cirrhosis (see page 1043) and liver failure (see page 1046).

Treatment If you have chronic persistent hepatitis, you will probably receive no specific treatment; however, you should be followed closely, with repeat liver biopsies as needed, to detect changes in liver function that can affect your general health.

Treatment for chronic active hepatitis depends on the form you have. For autoimmune hepatitis, treatment with corticosteroids (particularly prednisone) has been shown to control the disease, reducing symptoms, improving liver function tests, and prolonging life in most people. Long-term use of prednisone causes its own set of side effects, however, including bone and joint thinning, weight gain, and the development of hypertension and diabetes. Thus, in recent years, many doctors have given prednisone in lower doses, in combination with an immunosuppressive medication called azathioprine (Imuran). Unfortunately, prednisone does not prevent deterioration in about 15 percent of people (particularly, those diagnosed with serious liver damage). In these individuals, liver transplantation may be considered (see page 1047).

If you have chronic hepatitis B or C, you may be given thrice-weekly injections of an immune-boosting medication such as interferon alpha 2-b (Intron) for at least 6 months. Although this medication does not eradicate the virus in everyone, it has produced major improvement—reducing liver inflammation and bringing liver enzyme levels back to normal—in about 20 percent of those infected with hepatitis B and in about 40 percent of people with hepatitis C. However, some people seem to get better and then experience a relapse of symptoms, which may improve again, with repeat treatment. Interferon often causes complications of its own, including depression, headache, malaise, loss of appetite, and flu-like symptoms. The medication also can suppress bone marrow and lower your number of white blood cells and platelets. Thus, you may not be eligible for this medication if you have a history of depression, an autoimmune disease such as diabetes, a diminished white blood cell or platelet count, or a kidney transplant. Once you begin interferon therapy, you should have regular blood tests to monitor your liver enzymes, white blood cells, and platelets. Although interferon alpha 2-b may not cure hepatitis B and C, doctors believe that its long-term use may deter or prevent worsening of symptoms, including the development of cirrhosis. Currently, many antiviral medications including ribavirin (Virazole), are being tested in combination with interferon.

Prognosis This varies tremendously, depending on the form of chronic hepatitis you have and your symptoms. Chronic persistent hepatitis may vanish on its own after many years, or it may last a lifetime, producing few symptoms, or occasional flare-ups of symptoms. Chronic active hepatitis, if not treated, unusually leads to cirrhosis, liver failure, and death. The 10-year survival rate in untreated patients is about 10 percent.

❖ CIRRHOSIS

Symptoms (*What you may experience*) Persistent fatigue, which may be debilitating at times; jaundice (yellowing of the skin or whites of your eyes, and/or a brownish or orange tint in the urine—see A Word on Jaundice, page 1036); usually light-colored stool; flulike symptoms, such as fever, loss of appetite, nausea, and vomiting; abdominal pain; swelling in the legs or abdomen; intense itching; confusion, disorientation, changes in sleeping habits, or personality changes; increased sensitivity to medications or alcohol; vomiting blood or blood in the stool.

Signs and laboratory findings (*What the doctor looks for*) A palpable, enlarged liver, felt during a physical exam; evidence of fluid swelling in the legs and/or abdomen (fluid in the abdominal cavity is called ascites), found during a physical exam; signs of impaired mental function or encephalopathy (caused by a buildup of toxins in the brain), evident during the physical exam and patient interview, including unresponsiveness or inappropriate responses to questions, difficulty concentrating or remembering, and neglect of personal appearance; the presence of varices, large blood vessels, in the esophagus and/or stomach, seen during endoscopy (see Bleeding Varices, page 982); scarring of the liver, seen during a CT scan, ultrasound, a radioisotope liver/spleen scan, or exploratory laparoscopy; the presence of scar tissue in a needle biopsy of the liver; the presence of characteristic, tiny, expanded blood vessels (telangiectasia, also called spider dilations of blood vessels) in the skin, especially in the face and upper chest.

What is it? Cirrhosis is the product of severe liver damage or chronic liver disease. Scar tissue permeates the liver, obstructing blood flow and hampering its ability to do its main jobs: to cleanse the body of toxins; to process nutrients, hormones, and medications; and to make crucial proteins and clotting factors. Although cirrhosis may be stopped or slowed down, its damage is permanent and often fatal. Cirrhosis is the seventh leading cause of death by disease in the United States. The National Institute of Diabetes and Digestive and Kidney Diseases, of the National Institutes of Health, estimates that 25,000 people die from it each year.

Its earliest signs are often subtle; in many people, the disease progresses silently for years or even decades, until the scarring becomes extensive. As the liver loses functioning cells, it also loses ability to make vital proteins: Diminished production of the protein albumin, for instance, causes swelling in the abdomen and feet. A growing inability to meet the body's demand for clotting factors causes someone with cirrhosis to bruise and bleed easily. Jaundice is common (see A Word on Jaundice, page 1036). Bile products or other factors in the bloodstream can cause extreme itching. Also, there is a greater chance for gallstones to form (see page 1054). Over time, the inflamed, scarred liver also fails as a detoxifier. A healthy liver protects the body from

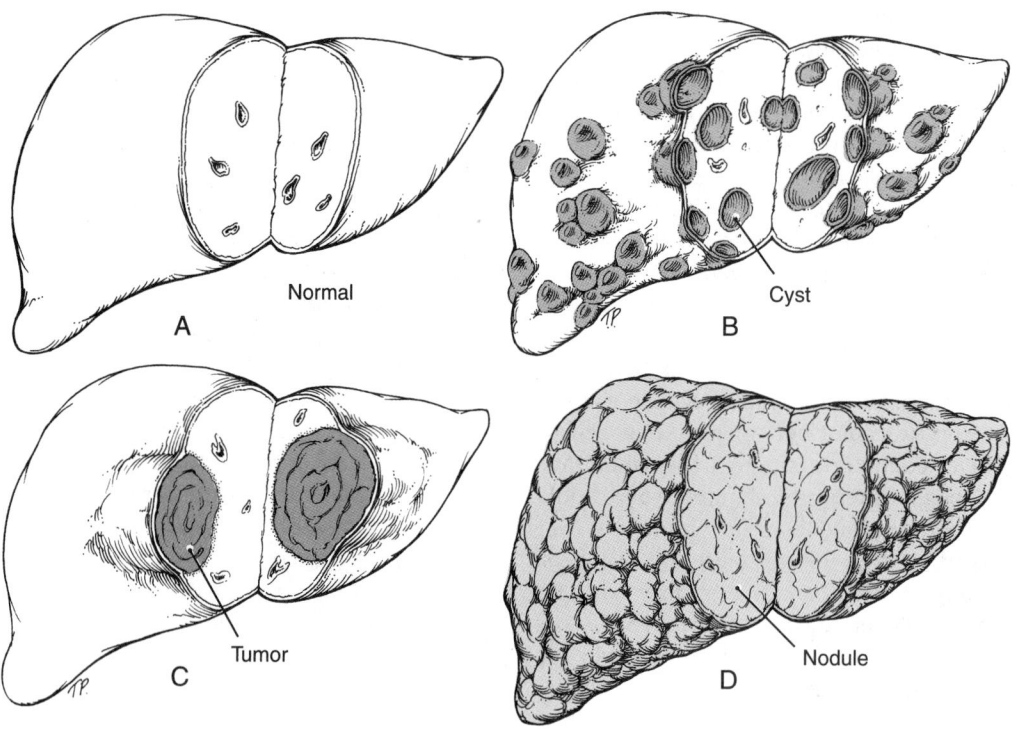

A Normal

B Cyst

C Tumor

D Nodule

(A) The normal liver is shown along with a cross-section. (B) Benign or cancerous tumors can arise in the liver or occur as secondary tumors from other primary locations in the body. In Africa and Asia, primary liver cancer accounts for up to half of all cancers. Liver cancer can develop after years of cirrhosis. (C) Hepatic cysts occur in about 30 percent of people with polycystic renal disease. The cysts may become infected or cause abdominal discomfort. (D) Cirrhosis, a major cause of death in the US, is characterized by permanent scarring and multiple nodules. Cirrhosis impairs the natural functions of the liver, obstructs blood flow, and can lead to the backup of blood in other parts of the body, such as the spleen and esophageal vessels. Many diseases, including alcoholism and infections, can cause cirrhosis.

potential toxins and impurities. But cirrhosis-scarred tissue makes an inefficient, and ultimately ineffective, cleanser: Drugs, alcohol, and other toxins stay in the system and circulate in the blood longer than they normally would; instead of wearing off at their usual rate, they can build up, magnifying the drugs' effect and also their side effects. In its late stages, cirrhosis produces a characteristic musty breath odor; this is called fetor hepaticus, and it is caused when waste products are not properly metabolized and excreted. The burden of toxins causes mental problems, including confusion, personal-ity changes, and unresponsiveness (at worst, coma).

One of the most serious complications of cirrhosis is its effect on abdominal blood vessels. Normally, blood in the massive portal vein flows from the intestines and spleen through the liver. Cirrhosis impedes this blood flow, causing a condition called portal hypertension to develop. Pressure builds as in a clogged pipe. The backup of blood causes the spleen to swell, and the body makes a valiant attempt to divert blood, by creating new outlets that bypass the liver. Some of these are huge, tortuous blood vessels, called varices, that emerge in the esophagus and stomach (see Bleeding Varices, page 982). Despite their size, these new vessels are not strong enough for the workload. Their walls are dangerously thin and, if the tremendous pressure continues, highly prone to breakage. This is a medical emergency; unchecked bleeding varices can be fatal in a matter of hours. *If you are vomiting blood, go to the emergency room at once.*

Many people believe cirrhosis is the end result of a lifetime of drinking too much alcohol. It can be; chronic alcohol abuse is the most common cause of the disease in the United States. However, even social drinkers can develop alcoholic cirrhosis;

women tolerate alcohol less well than men and, even if they drink less, are more likely to develop cirrhosis. But there are many other causes, and cirrhosis may strike at any age. Chronic viral hepatitis (B, C, and D) can lead to cirrhosis (although drug therapy may forestall or prevent continued liver damage in many people, see Chronic Hepatitis, page 1041), as can, rarely, a severe reaction to a prescription medication or extensive exposure to an environmental toxin, such as carbon tetrachloride. A number of diseases can also result in cirrhosis; these include Wilson's disease and alpha$_1$-antitrypsin deficiency (see Inherited Liver Disorders, page 1049), cystic fibrosis, hemochromatosis (abnormal buildups of iron in the liver and other organs, see Inherited Liver Disorders, page 1049), galactosemia (a congenital metabolic defect), congestive heart failure, glycogen storage diseases (in which the body cannot use sugars properly), and schistosomiasis (a parasitic infection). A blockage in a bile duct—the drain through which bile flows to the intestines—may cause biliary cirrhosis. For reasons not understood, primary biliary cirrhosis—characterized by microscopic inflammation and scarring of the bile ducts—is more common in women in their late 30s, 40s, and 50s. The most common form of cirrhosis in babies is biliary atresia, a disease in which the bile ducts are injured or nonexistent, causing bile to amass in the liver. If this disease, characterized by jaundice, is diagnosed in time, a surgeon can create a new bile duct, and prevent further damage. Even gallbladder surgery, to remove a gallstone, for instance, can result in bile duct blockage and lead to cirrhosis.

What you can do The easiest way to prevent alcoholic cirrhosis is simply to drink in moderation. This means, do not have more than two drinks a day; a drink is a glass of wine or a 12-oz can of beer, or a 1½-oz portion of hard liquor. (See Chapter 5 for more information on overcoming alcohol addiction.) If you have ever had alcohol-related liver problems, such as alcoholic hepatitis, avoid alcohol altogether. Poor nutrition, particularly associated with alcohol or drug abuse, is believed to play a role in the development of cirrhosis, although this is not completely understood. Thus, eat a well-balanced diet, and take a daily fat-soluble vitamin supplement.

If you have hepatitis or other liver problems contact your doctor before taking any vitamin or form of medication. Because cirrhosis can also be caused by exposure to environmental toxins, take care when using chemicals at work, in your garden, or around the house. Wear gloves and protective clothing to prevent absorption into the skin, and if any chemical splashes on your skin, wash immediately. Avoid inhaling chemicals, and open a window or use a fan to promote good ventilation; wear a mask, if needed. Preventing other forms of cirrhosis is more difficult; sadly, many people never realize they are at risk of developing this disease. However, if you have been diagnosed with another condition, such as hemochromatosis, you may be able to prevent extensive liver damage by meticulous management of the primary condition, for example, regularly removing excess iron by phlebotomy (drawing 1 pint of blood per week). For more information, see Treatment, below.

When to call the doctor If you have any of the symptoms on page 1043, call your doctor. If you are vomiting blood, go to the emergency room immediately.

Treatment Treatment of cirrhosis depends on the stage at which your disease was diagnosed and its underlying cause. The immediate goal is to prevent or delay further damage to the liver, minimize the complications, and treat specific symptoms. If you have alcoholic cirrhosis, you must stop drinking now. If your cirrhosis is caused by autoimmune hepatitis, you may need a regimen of corticosteroids or other immunosuppressive medications, such as azathioprine, for life (see Chronic Hepatitis, page 1041). If viral hepatitis is the underlying cause, you may not receive further medication treatment with interferon. If you have Wilson's disease, characterized by a buildup of copper (see Inherited Liver Disorders, page 1049), your doctor may prescribe medications, such as penicillamine, that deplete the body's copper supply. For hemochromatosis (see Inherited Liver Disorders, page 1049), removing 1 pint of blood per week can help bring iron levels under control. It may be possible to treat a blocked bile duct—determined by tests including endoscopic retrograde cholangiopancreatography (ERCP, see page 1033) and ultrasound—with surgery.

Fluid accumulation in the abdomen can be eased by eliminating salt (which causes your body to retain water) from your diet; your doctor also may prescribe a diuretic to help you excrete salt and water. If you have extreme swelling, it may be necessary for your doctor to insert a catheter directly through the abdominal wall (in a procedure called large volume paracentesis which can be done on an outpatient basis) to drain excess fluid. Some people with cirrhosis suffer severe itching; the prescription medication cholestyramine (Questran) is often helpful. Portal hypertension can be lessened with blood pressure medications including beta blockers. Esophageal varices should be treated promptly (see Bleeding Varices, page 982). Dietary changes, as well as prescription medications such as lactulose, which causes a mild diarrhea (which traps toxins in the gastrointestinal tract and removes them), may also help relieve confusion and other mental changes brought on by cirrhosis. Decreasing your daily ingestion of protein can lessen the amount of toxins that form in the digestive tract. Also, fat-soluble vitamins may help provide good nutrition and strengthen the body's reserves.

If you have severe cirrhosis and are at risk of liver failure, you may be a candidate for a liver transplant (see Liver Failure, page 1046, and Liver Transplant, page 1047).

Prognosis Prognosis depends on the stage and cause of cirrhosis. There are many things you can do to prevent further damage (see Treatment, above). Also, much hope comes from the liver itself: This remarkable organ can tolerate extreme adversity and, if damage is not too severe, can even regenerate. Many people live for years with cirrhosis. If the damage is too great, you may need a liver transplant. Although this procedure is generally reserved as a last resort, liver transplantation has been successful in saving the lives of many people with cirrhosis. New techniques to prevent the body from rejecting the donor organ may make this operation even more successful in the future.

❖ LIVER FAILURE

Symptoms *(What you may experience)* Symptoms of advanced cirrhosis: persistent fatigue, which may be debilitating at times; jaundice (yellowing of the skin or whites of your eyes, and/or a brownish or orange tint in the urine—see A Word on Jaundice, page 1036); unusually light-colored stool; flulike symptoms, such as fever, loss of appetite, nausea, and vomiting; abdominal pain; fluid swelling in the legs or abdomen; intense itching; confusion, disorientation, changes in sleeping habits, or personality changes; increased sensitivity to medications or alcohol; vomiting blood or blood in the stool.

Signs and laboratory findings *(What the doctor looks for)* A palpable, enlarged spleen and liver, felt during a physical exam; evidence of fluid swelling in the legs or abdomen, found during a physical exam; signs of impaired mental function or encephalopathy (caused by a buildup of toxins in the brain), evident during the physical exam and patient interview, including unresponsiveness or inappropriate responses to questions, difficulty concentrating or remembering, and neglect of personal appearance; the presence of varices (enlarged blood vessels) in the esophagus and/or stomach, seen during endoscopy (see Bleeding Varices, page 982); scarring of the liver, seen during a CT scan, MRI, ultrasound, a radioisotope liver/spleen scan, and/or exploratory laparoscopy; the presence of scar tissue in a needle biopsy of the liver; the presence of characteristic, tiny, broken blood vessels (telangiectasia, also called spider veins) in the skin, especially in the face; a characteristic tremor, called asterixis liver flap, of the hands.

What is it? Liver failure is the last stage of cirrhosis. Over time, as scarring continues, the liver becomes less able to do its job. Toxins accumulate in the body, because the liver can no longer filter them; the body is highly sensitive to drugs and alcohol, because their effect becomes cumulative. The kidneys begin to fail. Huge, tortuous blood vessels, called varices, develop in the esophagus and stomach (see Bleeding Varices, page 982) as the body makes an effort to reroute blood flow around the blocked liver; these alone may be fatal, because they break easily and can cause hemorrhage. Fluid buildup in the brain can cause serious swelling, which may result in a coma and death.

When to call the doctor Go to the emergency room immediately if you are vomiting blood or if you have significant amounts of

LIVER TRANSPLANT

Even as recently as a decade ago, a diagnosis of liver failure—the end stage of diseases such as advanced cirrhosis in adults, or, in children, biliary atresia or alpha₁-antitrypsin deficiency—was a death sentence. Today, with the advent of liver transplant, more sophisticated surgical techniques, improved means of preserving the donor organ, and new medications to help the body fight rejection of the donor organ, the prognosis is much more hopeful.

Who is eligible? The requirements vary, depending on many factors, including the hospital and surgeon; your general state of health (that is, whether you have any other potentially life-threatening health problems); the stage of your disease (at some hospitals, the sickest patients are at the top of the waiting list; however, patients who are less sick may be better able to withstand the rigors of the operation); and your age (adults younger than age 65 and children are considered better candidates than the elderly, although, again, there are no iron-clad rules). Some hospitals refuse to perform a liver transplant on someone with alcoholic liver disease unless there is clear evidence that the person has abstained from alcohol for at least 6 months and is taking part in a counseling program. There is also much debate over whether someone with liver cancer should receive a liver transplant, because, among other reasons, the immune-suppressing medications that must be taken to keep the body from rejecting the new liver might result in a recurrence of cancer.

Promising results from a study at the Naval Medical Research Institute in Bethesda, MD, suggest that a new, combined drug therapy might prevent the body from rejecting a donated organ and may free transplant patients from a lifetime of medication, which can have its own serious side effects. The new medications, given in a single injection—which, in animal studies, has had no side effects—teach the body to recognize the transplanted organ as a friend, rather than an enemy that needs to be attacked. The doctors hope to begin testing this new approach in people soon.

Currently, liver transplant recipients must take antirejection, or immunosuppressant, medications such as cyclosporine and corticosteroids throughout the course of their lives. The main problem with these drugs is that they disable the body's ability to fight any enemy—including bacteria and viruses. Thus, with a compromised immune system, transplant recipients are more susceptible to illness. Most postoperative deaths are caused by infection and occur within the first 6 months after surgery. Still, the survival rates of people who have received a liver transplant are extremely encouraging. An estimated 90 percent of liver transplant recipients are alive 1 year afterward, and nearly 85 percent are alive in 5 years. These survival rates are expected to improve as techniques for fighting rejection become even better. The main drawback to liver transplantation is the sheer scarcity of donor organs. Although this year more than 25,000 people in the United States will die of cirrhosis alone, fewer than 4,000 Americans will receive a transplant. Many people, adults and children, will die on the waiting list.

Fortunately, the body does not need an entire liver—which means that two people may benefit from each donated organ. Also, as with kidneys, it is possible for a living person to be a donor: A parent may donate one lobe of the liver to a child. The procedure itself, usually performed at major medical centers, is complicated and grueling, lasting several hours. ■

---

blood in the stool, if you have significant abdominal swelling or pain, if you are confused or have other mental problems, or if you are unable to urinate.

Treatment Until recently, liver failure was universally fatal. Even now, most people who have liver failure do not recover, and treatment is mainly palliative, aimed at reducing specific symptoms and easing discomfort. Currently, the only hope of treatment is liver transplantation (see Liver Transplant, above).

❖ LIVER ABSCESS

Symptoms *(What you may experience)* Unexplained fever, which lasts for days or even weeks; chills; weight loss; loss of appetite; nausea; weakness; abdominal pain; occasionally, pain in the right side of the chest; some people also experience jaundice (yellowing of the skin or whites of your eyes, and/or a brownish or orange tint in the urine—see A Word on Jaundice, page 1036). Recent diarrhea, which may have been bloody, reported in your medical history.

Signs and laboratory findings *(What the doctor looks for)* Abnormalities on blood tests, including anemia, an increase in the number of white blood cells (leukocytosis) and elevated bilirubin; positive results of a blood culture for bacteria (not all people with liver abscess show positive culture results); elevated levels of enzymes that are abundant in liver cells, such as alkaline phosphatase; the presence of a fluid-filled mass on a radionuclide liver scan, ultrasound examination, and/or CT scan; the presence of an amoeba, such as *Entamoeba histolytica*, in the stool. In some cases, a liver abscess is associated with recent foreign travel.

What is it? A liver abscess is a pus-filled lesion in the liver, caused by infection, either from bacteria or an amoeba. Amebic infections, transmitted by drinking contaminated water or coming in contact with infected fecal matter (from a food handler with poor hygiene, for instance), tend to develop more slowly than bacterial infections, which may have a dramatic onset. Several conditions can give rise to bacterial (usually streptococci or staphylococci) infection in the liver. An obstructed bile duct—blocked by a gallstone, perhaps, or a tumor, or stricture (abnormal narrowing, usually caused by scar tissue)—can become infected. Infection elsewhere in the abdomen, such as in diverticulitis or appendicitis, or even from some distant site in the body, may spread to the liver. Trauma also may result in infection. Some abscesses, however, have no apparent cause. Some people have a lone abscess; others have several.

What you can do Use caution in foreign travel. If you are traveling in a tropical region, or in an area where the water may be unsafe, your motto should be "Boil it, cook it, peel it, or forget it." Avoid ice, tap water, vegetables, salads, foods sold by street vendors, and caffeinated beverages from soda fountains. Drink bottled water, sodas, wines, beer, tea, and coffee; brush your teeth with bottled water. If you wear contact lenses, use bottled water to rinse them. To be on the safe side, you might want to take your own supply of bottled water from home: Estimate at least 1 quart-sized bottle per person per day. Limit your fruits to foods you can peel, such as oranges or bananas; grapes, for instance, are probably not safe.

When to call the doctor If you have a fever that persists for more than a few days, jaundice, or unexplained abdominal pain, call your doctor.

Treatment Treatment depends on whether the abscess has been caused by bacteria or an amoeba. If an amebic infection is to blame, you may be treated with medication alone; your doctor may prescribe one or several medications including metronidazole (Flagyl) or chloroquine (Aralen). If the infection is bacterial, you will probably need surgery to drain the abscess and open any blocked bile ducts (or create a new drain, so bile can flow unimpeded from the liver to the intestine). Then, depending on the spe-

cific form of bacteria, you will need to take one or more antibiotics, such as chloramphenicol (Chloromycetin), clindamycin (Cleocin) and/or tobramycin (Nibcin), or gentamicin (Garamycin), for at least several weeks.

Prognosis Liver abscess is a serious and potentially fatal condition; if not treated, infection may spread into the abdomen, chest, or lungs. Even when the problem is correctly diagnosed and treated, at least 20 percent of people with a liver abscess do not survive; the risk of dying is higher in people with more than one abscess.

❖ BENIGN LIVER CYSTS

Symptoms *(What you may experience)* Pain and tenderness in the upper right abdomen; occasionally, fever and jaundice (yellowing of the skin or whites of your eyes, and/or a brownish or orange tint in the urine—see A Word on Jaundice, page 1036). Some people experience no symptoms.

Signs and laboratory findings *(What the doctor looks for)* The presence of one or more fluid- or gas-filled masses or calcified lesions in the liver, as seen by CT scan, ultrasound, and/or sulfur colloid scintigraphy (a nuclear medicine scan of the liver, using a radioactive dye); peripheral blood eosinophilia (elevated levels of a certain white blood cell known to be activated in allergic reactions and parasitic infection); positive results of blood tests for echinococcal antibodies (which can determine the presence of this parasite); a history of cysts in the kidney, pancreas, or spleen; travel (even many years ago) to, or immigration to the United States from, a region where echinococcosis or amebiasis (forms of parasites) are endemic, including Mexico, South America, Africa, Australia, Mediterranean countries, the Middle East, Northern Canada, and Alaska, as reported in your medical history; a previous history of amebic infection.

What is it? Benign, that is, not cancerous, cysts may develop in the liver for several reasons. Some people have polycystic disease, in which many cysts form in the kidneys, pancreas, liver, and even spleen. These cysts may never cause any harm, unless they happen to block a bile duct; however, cystadenomas (rare tumors, which usually affect women in their 40s) and choledochal (in the common bile duct) cysts have the potential to become cancerous and should be removed. Cysts may also form in the liver, as they can elsewhere in the body, in someone with a parasitic infection. Although such infections are rare in the United States, they are common in many places in the world (listed on page 1048). If you have ever traveled there, you might have been exposed to amoebae in drinking water or contaminated food. Echinococcal (hydatid) cysts are tapeworm larvae that tend to live in the intestines of dogs (mainly in the Middle East) and are spread via the dogs' stool. Some cysts, caused by gas-forming bacteria, are filled with gas and pus. If you have one or more liver cysts—unless an amebic infection is obvious—your doctor will probably want to perform a fine-needle aspiration of the cyst, in which the fluid inside is drawn out, examined, and cultured.

What you can do Use caution in foreign travel. If you are traveling in a tropical region, or in an area where the water may be unsafe, your motto should be "Boil it, cook it, peel it, or forget it." Avoid ice, tap water, vegetables, salads, foods sold by street vendors, and caffeinated beverages from soda fountains. Drink bottled water, sodas, wines, beer, tea, and coffee; brush your teeth with bottled water. If you wear contact lenses, use bottled water to rinse them. To be on the safe side, you might want to take your own supply of bottled water from home: Estimate at least 1 quart-sized bottle per person per day. Limit your fruits to foods you can peel, such as oranges or bananas; grapes, for instance, are probably not safe.

When to call the doctor If you have persistent abdominal pain or tenderness, an unexplained fever, or if you have ever traveled to a country where amebic infection is common, call your doctor.

Treatment Treatment depends on the underlying cause and location of the cyst. If a benign cyst is blocking a bile duct, you will need surgery to remove the cyst and reopen the duct. If you have a cystadenoma or choledochal cyst, surgical removal will be necessary, because these have the potential to become malignant (cancerous). If you

have an echinococcal cyst, you will probably need to have this drained by a surgeon with a needle; afterward, a parasite-killing solution (probably saline, silver nitrate, or ethanol) will be injected into the cyst. At some medical centers, this is done under CT guidance, for extra precision. Draining an echinococcal cyst is a delicate procedure; if any of the cystic fluid is inadvertently spilled into the abdominal cavity, an anaphylactic reaction can occur; also, this spillage could sow the seeds for future cysts and ongoing infection. If this happens, or if you are not a candidate for surgery (if you are elderly or if your health is considered too frail to withstand the rigors of an operation), you may need systemic medication to eradicate the parasite, such as mebendazole (Vermox) or albendazole (Albenza).

❖ INHERITED LIVER DISORDERS

Symptoms *(What you may experience)* Most inherited liver disorders can—but do not necessarily—cause jaundice (yellowing of the skin or whites of your eyes, and/or a brownish or orange tint in the urine—see A Word on Jaundice, page 1036). Other symptoms may vary, depending on the specific disorder:

- *Alpha₁-antitrypsin deficiency:* Swelling of the abdomen and/or legs; loss of appetite; fatigue; in later stages, constant itching; nosebleeds, bruising; extreme fatigue after eating protein; difficulty breathing.

- *Wilson's disease:* Malaise; loss of appetite; fatigue that lasts for months and may be severe; unusually light-colored stool; flulike symptoms, including fever, loss of appetite, nausea, and vomiting; abdominal pain; confusion or disorientation; difficulty with speech; trembling, which may affect your ability to write; unsteadiness and difficulty walking; depression; suicidal impulses; personality changes.

- *Hemochromatosis:* A bronze tint to the skin; joint pain; heart irregularities; impotence; malaise; loss of appetite; fatigue that lasts for months and may be severe; unusually light-colored stool; flulike symptoms, including fever, loss of appetite, nausea, and vomiting; abdominal pain; frequent urination, excessive thirst and other symptoms of diabetes.

- *Gilbert syndrome:* Mild jaundice.

Signs and laboratory findings *(What the doctor looks for)*

- *Alpha₁-antitrypsin deficiency:* Low blood levels of alpha₁-antitrypsin, found in a blood test; abnormal liver function tests; liver injury, detected in a needle biopsy; enlargement and scarring of the liver, found in ultrasound and/or x-ray scans; evidence of lung disease.

- *Wilson's disease:* Excess copper in the blood, found in a serum ceruloplasmin blood test (which looks for a protein involved in copper binding); excess copper excreted in the urine, found in a urine test; characteristic patterns of copper pigments in the eyes, called Kayser-Fleischer rings (seen on slit-lamp examination performed by an ophthalmologist); the presence of copper in the liver, as detected in a needle biopsy; hemolytic anemia (a loss of red blood cells), seen in a blood test; elevated liver enzymes, seen in liver function tests.

- *Hemochromatosis:* Irregular heartbeat; evidence of diabetes mellitus (resulting from damage to the pancreas); iron overload in the blood, as confirmed by blood tests including a percent saturation of iron test (which evaluates the ratio of iron to a chemical called transferrin); a positive result of a serum ferritin (also elevated in hemochromatosis) test; the presence of iron deposits in a needle biopsy of the liver.

- *Gilbert syndrome:* A fluctuating increase in blood levels of bilirubin (a yellow pigment, made by the liver and excreted into bile); other liver function tests and cholangiography are normal.

What is it? *Alpha₁-antitrypsin deficiency*
This is the most common genetic cause of liver problems in children, affecting about 1 in every 2,000 people, according to the American Liver Foundation. Alpha₁-antitrypsin is a substance made by the liver whose main job is to suppress enzymes that break down proteins. Too-low levels of alpha₁-antitrypsin may lead to hepatitis (see Chronic Hepatitis, page 1041), cirrhosis (see page 1043), and liver failure (see page 1046);

this deficiency can also cause lung problems, including emphysema. It is an autosomal recessive disorder, in other words, both parents must pass on the genetic trait in order for a child to be born with alpha₁-antitrypsin deficiency. However, for reasons no one understands, only about 10 to 20 percent of those born with this deficiency actually develop liver disease. It is possible to be a carrier of the deficiency but have a normal life, with no evidence of the disease. The diagnosis is often made in newborns, who have jaundice, abdominal swelling, and poor appetite. However, its symptoms may also appear in late childhood, adolescence, or early adulthood. This disease is highly variable: In about 25 percent of affected individuals, alpha₁-antitrypsin deficiency is a debilitating illness, leading to cirrhosis and liver failure. But about 75 percent of the people with this deficiency have no significant liver disease after infancy. Even among those who develop cirrhosis, there is a variability: Many people with cirrhosis live for years without significant symptoms.

Wilson's disease This is a rare inherited disorder that affects about 1 of every 30,000 people and is characterized by deposits of copper throughout the body. Like alpha₁-antitrypsin deficiency, this is an autosomal recessive disorder; that is, you can only develop Wilson's disease if you receive the genetic defect from both parents. In Wilson's disease, from birth onward, the liver has difficulty in a key aspect as a cleanser: Because of a defective protein, the liver is unable to rid the body of copper. With no means of exiting from the body, copper stockpiles in the liver, brain, and other organs. The signs of Wilson's disease, particularly jaundice, can occur as early as childhood, but the disease is most commonly diagnosed during teenage years. If not treated, copper buildup can be devastating: It may hamper kidney function, cause severe bone disease and osteoporosis, affect mental function, impair speech and gait, and cause severe trembling and depression. In the liver, it can produce symptoms of severe hepatitis (see Chronic Hepatitis, page 1041) or even cirrhosis (see page 1043), with accompanying complications. Fifty years ago, a diagnosis of Wilson's disease carried a terrible prognosis, with symptoms progressively worsening, and death usually before age 30. Now, however, medications that deplete the body's copper have revolution-ized the prognosis and dramatically improved life span.

Hemochromatosis In this common inher-ited disorder, (also known as iron overload disease), affecting about 1 in every 250 peo-ple, the body is overwhelmed by iron. Unable to process and dispose of it in the normal way, iron accumulates throughout the body. In the pancreas, this can result in severe diabetes mellitus. In other organs, it can lead to arthritis, heart problems, chronic fatigue, and impotence. In the liver, it can cause cirrhosis and, in 25 percent of affected individuals, liver cancer. Early detection is very important because if hemochromatosis is detected in time, it can be treated successfully, and organ damage can be prevented. A genetic test is available for the gene responsible for 85 percent of cases of hemochromatosis. Anyone with a family history of this condition should undergo genetic testing or blood tests for iron overload (see What You Can Do, below). Hemochromatosis is most com-monly diagnosed in middle age—between ages 40 and 60. It is usually diagnosed later in women, who are protected somewhat until menopause. In their child bearing years, most women generally lose signifi-cant amounts of iron during menstruation, pregnancy, and lactation.

Gilbert syndrome Gilbert (with the French pronunciation, "zheel-bear") syndrome is a common but benign liver disorder that affects an estimated 5 percent of the adult population. It is congenital (that is, present from birth) and probably inherited. Its main symptom is mild jaundice, with yellowing of the whites of the eyes. This is due to an increase in bilirubin, a product of hemoglo-bin (the red pigment in red blood cells). Made in the spleen, bone marrow, and else-where in the body, bilirubin journeys in the blood to the liver, where it is changed chem-ically and then excreted into bile, which then travels to the intestines. Normally, small quantities of bilirubin are present in the blood; in Gilbert syndrome, this level increases with starvation or stress such as the presence of another illness such as the flu. Many people with Gilbert syndrome are initially misdiagnosed. Although the syn-drome is benign, correct diagnosis is criti-cal, mainly, to make sure that jaundice is not being caused by something far more seri-ous.

What you can do *Alpha$_1$-antitrypsin deficiency* If you have any relatives with this disease, even if you have no symptoms of liver trouble, you should find out if you are a carrier, by having a blood test. Chil-dren can inherit the deficiency only if both parents are carriers.

Wilson's disease Avoid alcohol, which can make symptoms worse, and foods high in copper, including shellfish, nuts, liver, chocolate, and mushrooms. Talk with your doctor before taking any medication.

Hemochromatosis If you have been diag-nosed with this disorder, avoid alcohol, which can make your symptoms worse. Avoid iron-containing vitamins as well as foods such as red meat that are rich in iron, and talk to your doctor before taking any medication. If you have not been diagnosed with hemochromatosis—even if you have no symptoms—but any member of your family has this condition, you should undergo blood tests for iron overload, and/or a genetic test for hemochromatosis. Even if you have anemia, this does not rule out the possibility of hemochromatosis; it is possible to have both conditions at the same time.

Gilbert syndrome Eat a balanced diet, and eat small snacks throughout the day to keep food in your stomach. In people with this disorder, bilirubin levels tend to rise during fasting.

Treatment *Alpha$_1$-antitrypsin deficiency* Because the symptoms can range from severe to mild to nonexistent, treatment varies. Treatment is designed to relieve spe-cific symptoms: For example, severe itching can be treated with phenobarbital or cholestyramine. Fluid retention can be treated with a diuretic, which helps rid your body of excess salt and water. To avoid nutri-tion problems, you may need supplemental vitamins, such as vitamins E, D, and K. One of the most serious complications in people with cirrhosis (see page 1043) is the devel-opment of large veins in the esophagus and stomach (see Bleeding Varices, page 982). These veins are the body's attempt to shunt blood around the scarred liver; they are large, tortuous, and their walls are dangerously thin and prone to rupture. If you vomit blood or have significant bleeding in the stool, go to the emergency room at once. If the cirrhosis progresses, and the liver begins to fail (see Liver Failure, page 1046), you may need a liver transplant (see Liver Transplant, page 1047). Many people with alpha₁-antitrypsin deficiency have been successfully treated with a liver transplant.

Wilson's disease The problem is excess copper, and the goal of treatment is to clear copper from your body. Medications called chelating agents including D-penicillamine and trientine (Syprine), have revolutionized treatment for Wilson's disease. These medications, administered in combination with vitamin B₆ (pyridoxine), thwart organ damage by removing excess copper from the body. Chelating agents are not cures; Wilson's disease is a chronic problem, and these medications must be taken throughout the course of your life.

Hemochromatosis The goal is to lower skyrocketing iron accumulations in your body. This is done by removing 1 to 2 pints of blood (phlebotomy)—which is loaded with iron—once a week, until you achieve a reasonable level of body iron. Depending on original blood iron levels, it may take months or even years to accomplish this. Then, to avoid reaccumulating iron, you will need a long-term maintenance plan with regular withdrawals of blood (every 2 to 4 months) for the rest of your life.

Gilbert syndrome There is no specific treatment.

Prognosis Prognosis depends on when these diseases are diagnosed, and the extent or lack of organ damage they have caused. The prognosis for alpha₁-antitrypsin deficiency depends entirely on the severity of the disease. Many people with this deficiency live normal lives. However, if you develop cirrhosis, this may lead to liver failure, and you may need a liver transplant. The prognoses for Wilson's disease and hemachromatosis, if caught early, are excellent with lifelong treatment. The prognosis for Gilbert syndrome, which is benign and requires no treatment, is also excellent.

❖ LIVER CANCER

Symptoms *(What you may experience)* Jaundice (yellowing of the skin or whites of your eyes, and/or a brownish or orange tint in the urine); fluid swelling in the legs and/or abdomen; abdominal pain; loss of appetite; weight loss; malaise; nausea and vomiting. Some people have no symptoms.

Signs and laboratory findings *(What the doctor looks for)* A medical history reporting certain illnesses (previous or current), including hepatitis (in any form), hemochromatosis, alpha₁-antitrypsin disease, cirrhosis, alcoholism, or any form of cancer. The use of birth control pills or hormone therapy (taken during menopause), reported in your medical history. These hormones do not cause liver cancer but can make benign tumors grow bigger. The presence of a benign tumor or malignant cells in a needle biopsy of the liver; abnormal results on liver function tests; the presence of a mass in the liver, seen in ultrasound, x-ray, MRI, or CT scans; a palpable, enlarged liver, felt during a physical exam; positive results of an alpha-fetoprotein blood test.

What is it? Tumors in the liver may be benign or cancerous. They may originate in the liver (these are called primary tumors), or because the liver is the body's major filter, cancer cells from tumors elsewhere in the body may been carried into the liver by the bloodstream and become lodged inside it, taking root and growing as satellites (these are called secondary tumors or liver metastases).

Benign tumors Most benign tumors in the liver are found inadvertently, during an x-ray, MRI, CT scan, or ultrasound test for another condition. The most common of these is called cavernous hemangioma, a blood-filled growth that tends to get bigger in women who take replacement hormones or birth control pills. Other benign tumors include hepatocellular adenoma and focal nodular hyperplasia, which also are sensitive to birth control pills and hormone replacement therapy. Hepatocellular adenoma may rupture if it becomes too large, causing abdominal bleeding.

Malignant tumors Most cancers that affect the liver originate elsewhere in the body; often, an enlarged liver (caused by metastatic, or secondary, liver cancer) is the first sign that someone has cancer in another organ. Primary liver cancer makes up less than 1 percent of all cancers in the United States. However, in Africa and Asia, it accounts for as many as half of all cancers. This may be because those regions have a much higher incidence of hepatitis B (see Acute Viral Hepatitis, page 1035), which can cause a form of liver cancer called hepatocellular carcinoma. Hepatocellular carcinoma can also occur in other forms of chronic liver disease, including chronic hepatitis, cirrhosis, hemochromatosis, and tyrosinemia (a genetic disease of abnormal acid metabolism). Some environmental factors are also known to cause cancer. Aflatoxin, a product made by a mold found in rotting peanuts, is responsible for many cases of liver cancer in Africa; lengthy exposure to polyvinyl chloride, a chemical used in making plastics, can cause a rare form of liver cancer called angiosarcoma.

What you can do Most primary liver cancer develops after years of cirrhosis, from any cause. When possible, treating the underlying disease may forestall or prevent the development of liver cancer. Treatment includes blood withdrawal, for hemochromatosis, and drug therapy for hepatitis, or stopping alcohol consumption, for alcoholic hepatitis or alcoholic cirrhosis. Antihepatitis vaccines can also eliminate the development of many liver problems (see Vaccines to Prevent Hepatitis, page 1038).

Treatment *Benign tumors* Cavernous hemangioma and focal nodular hyperplasia usually are not treated, unless they become large enough to interfere with liver function or cause discomfort. Hepatocellular adenoma, however, because of its risk of bleeding, may need to be removed surgically if it becomes too large. This requires open surgery, general anesthesia, and hospitalization for several days. You may not be a candidate for surgery if you are over age 70, or if your general health is considered too frail to withstand the rigors of a major procedure. All of these growths should shrink considerably in women who stop taking birth control pills or replacement hormones.

Malignant tumors Metastatic cancer in the liver—from colon cancer, for example—

can be removed surgically if there is only one area of metastasis. Primary liver tumors that are small and limited to one lobe of the liver may be treated successfully with surgery to remove the tumor. New therapies, currently being studied, include using a tiny needle to inject alcohol directly into the tumor and chemically clotting off the blood supply to a tumor with a chemotherapeutic drug (this is called chemoembolization). Many new, promising chemotherapeutic drugs are being studied at academic medical centers around the country. Talk to your doctor about enrolling in a study testing one of these drugs, or call the National Cancer Institute Cancer Information Services at (800) 4-CANCER, or write to Public Inquiries, Office of Cancer Communications, National Cancer Institute, 9000 Rockville Pike, Bethesda, MD, 20892.

Prognosis This depends on the type of tumor, the stage at which it was diagnosed, the state of the liver (the prognosis is better in people with little or no cirrhosis), and the presence or absence of cancer elsewhere in the body. The prognosis for benign tumors is excellent. Unfortunately, for most primary liver cancers, treatment may not lead to cure. The cure rate for tumors treated with surgery or liver transplantation is currently, on average, less than 30 percent. However, better therapies and techniques for treating hepatocellular carcinoma, particularly when chemotherapy is combined with liver transplantation, have resulted in prolonged survival. The prognosis for cancers metastatic to the liver depends not only on the tumor in the liver (which may be successfully removed with surgery) but also on the state of the cancer elsewhere and its potential for treatment and cure. If there are multiple metastases in the liver, surgery is probably not an option.

The Gallbladder and Bile Ducts

The gallbladder, about the size and shape of a pear, is a holding tank for bile, the main fluid made by the liver. Its name describes its function: *Gall* is another word for bile, and a bladder is a reservoir. The gallbladder, situated on your right side just under the liver, is an integral part of the biliary system.

Through this network of ducts, or drainage tubes, the liver, gallbladder, and pancreas are all connected: Bile flows from the liver and gallbladder into the small intestine, where it plays a major role in digestion (see How the Digestive System Works, page 967).

Two channels extending from the liver come together to form the common hepatic duct, which later becomes the common bile duct—which, in turn, runs into the duodenum. The gallbladder is connected to the common bile duct by another conduit, called the cystic duct. The common bile duct also joins the pancreatic duct. Any blockage in the common bile duct may cause inflammation and other problems in the pancreas.

Bile is a complex liquid, rich in cholesterol. It contains fats (called lipids), bile salts (which help bile dissolve fat into more easily digestible molecules), and dark brown bile pigment, called bilirubin. It is bilirubin, a waste product, that gives bile its distinctive yellow-brown color (and makes stool brown) and is responsible for jaundice, in which the body and whites of the eyes are tinged with yellow. The gallbladder can hold about a cup of concentrated bile at a time; the adult liver makes up to 3 cups of bile in a day.

When you eat, the gallbladder contracts to send bile through the common bile duct into the duodenum to help your body break down food. When bile is no longer needed, the gallbladder relaxes and begins storing bile again. Normally, the body conserves bile—recycling it by absorbing it from the intestines into the bloodstream, through which it is taken back to the liver. In many people—particularly women, individuals who are obese, and those over age 60—bile crystallizes inside the gallbladder, forming crystals, or stones. These crystals may be silent, producing no symptoms and requiring no treatment. Or, if they block a gallbladder duct or migrate into the bile duct or pancreas, they can cause excruciating pain and need to be removed immediately.

❖ GALLSTONES

Symptoms *(What you may experience)* Severe, steady (not fluctuating) pain in the upper right abdomen, which may spread to include the chest, back (between the shoulder blades), and shoulders; this pain may last as little as 15 minutes or as long as several hours; you may feel a repeat episode of pain a few hours later, or it may take weeks, months, or even years for another attack to occur. Also, nausea; vomiting; sweating; and jaundice (yellowing of the skin and whites of the eyes). Many people have silent gallstones and may experience no symptoms for months or years, or even a lifetime.

Signs and laboratory findings *(What the doctor looks for)* The presence of gallstones on ultrasound, abdominal x-ray, oral cholecystogram, or a CT scan; elevated liver function tests (suggesting a blocked bile duct, with bile backing up into the liver); obstruction in the gallbladder, seen in a TC-hIDA scan (see Diagnostic Tests of the Liver, Gallbladder, and Pancreas, page 1031); the presence of gallstones in the bile duct, determined by ERCP (see page 1033) or percutancous transhopatic cholangiogram (PTHC) (see Diagnostic Tests of the Liver, Gallbladder, and Pancreas). The presence of Murphy's sign—a surge in pain felt when the doctor places a hand under your right rib cage and asks you to take a deep breath.

What is it? Gallstones are extremely common: This year, more than 1 million Americans will be diagnosed with them and will join the ranks of the estimated 20 million Americans (10 percent of the population) who already have them. Fortunately, the majority of those with gallstones never need treatment: Fewer than 20 percent of people with gallstones will actually develop symptoms or complications in their lifetime. Although no one knows exactly why, some people are more likely to develop gallstones than others. These include women between ages 20 and 60 (who are twice as likely to develop gallstones as men); pregnant women or women who have taken birth control pills or replacement estrogen therapy for menopause; men and women who are overweight; people who go on crash diets and lose weight very rapidly; men and women over age 60; Mexican American men and women; Native Americans (who have the highest prevalence of gallstones of all ethnic groups in the country; most Native American men have gallstones by the time they are 60), particularly the Pima Indians of Arizona (who, incidentally, are also prone to diabetes, an estimated 70 percent of Pima Indian women have gallstones by age 30). Other contributing factors may include a diet high in fat and cholesterol and low in fiber an improperly functioning gallbladder muscles (so the gallbladder does not contract well and thus does not empty completely).

Gallstones are crystals, small deposits created when the main components of bile—cholesterol and bilirubin—precipitate out of solution, as sugar on a string hardens to make rock candy. Some gallstones are tiny—as small as a grain of sand; others reach the size of a golf ball. Some people have only one stone; others develop thousands. When the gallbladder has a thick, soupy accumulation of tiny crystals, but no obvious larger stones, this is called biliary sludge. For unknown reasons, gallstones are made up of either one main ingredient or the other—either cholesterol or bilirubin, but not both. In the United States, of the people with the risk factors mentioned on page 1054, most—nearly 80 percent—develop cholesterol stones. Bilirubin, or pigment, gallstones are more likely to develop in people with severe liver disease (in which the makeup of bile may change and contribute more readily to crystal formation) and in people with blood disorders including sickle cell anemia.

In millions of people, gallstones are silent, never causing symptoms. Many people may not be aware that they have gallstones; gallstones are often discovered incidentally, during diagnostic tests for other conditions. But about 20 percent of all people with gallstones eventually do need treatment, for symptoms that usually begin with a dramatic attack of pain, called acute cholecystitis—believed to result when a gallstone becomes lodged in the cystic duct. Gallstones may also make their way through the cystic duct to become lodged in the common bile duct. This obstruction may resolve on its own; some people experience relief of pain after as little as 15 minutes. Or, it may be prolonged, lasting for hours without relief. The longer the blockage and the accompanying pain last, the greater the likelihood that the gallbladder will become inflamed—and this, in turn, usually leads to fever and infection of the gallbladder. Gallstone-caused blockages—which may cause severe pain, inflammation, and infection—are extremely serious, potentially life-threatening, and in need of immediate treatment. Gallstone-produced inflammation in the pancreas is the most

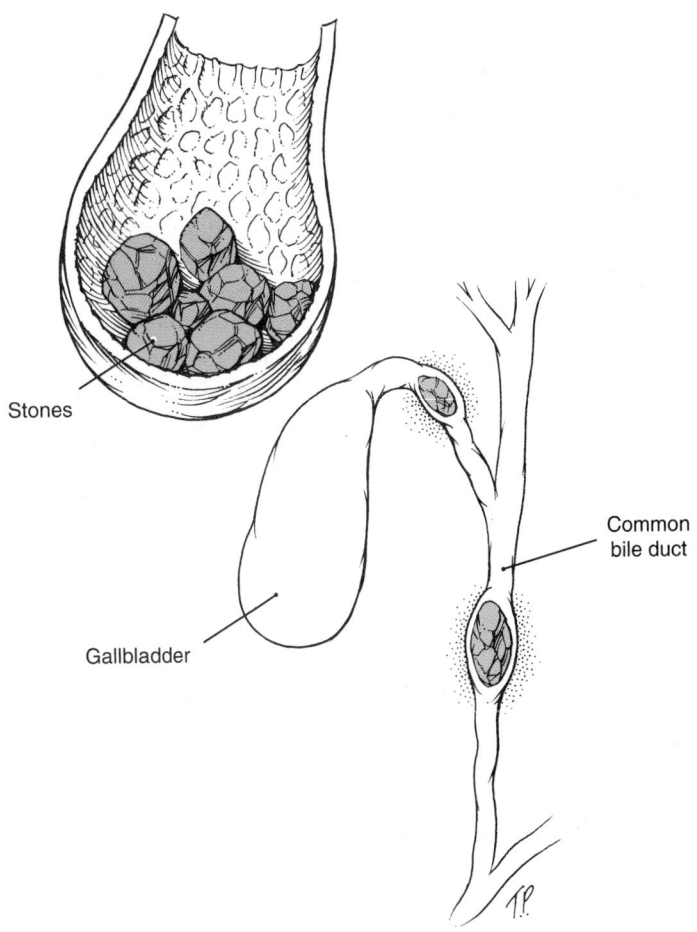

Stones

Common bile duct

Gallbladder

Gallstones (crystals of cholesterol or bilirubin pigment in the gallbladder or its ducts) are very common and often create no symptoms and require no treatment. Nevertheless, about 20 percent of people with gallstones develop pain when a stone becomes lodged in a duct. An obstruction may disappear spontaneously or lead to a life-threatening infection or bowel obstruction.

common cause of pancreatitis (see Acute Pancreatitis, page 1060). In rare cases, a gallstone may erode through the wall of the gallbladder, enter the intestine, and migrate to the wall of the ileocecal valve (the point at which the small and large intestines meet); this is called a gallstone ileus, and it may result in bowel obstruction—another very serious and potentially life-threatening event (see Bowel Obstruction, page 1005) requiring emergency treatment.

What you can do Although it may not be possible to prevent gallstones entirely, controlling your weight by following a sensible, low-fat, low-cholesterol, high-fiber diet may

TREATMENT OPTIONS FOR GALLSTONES

Although the gallbladder plays an important role in digestion, as a storehouse for bile, it is not an essential organ: You can live without it, and millions of Americans do (see Prognosis, below). Until recent years, most people with troublesome gallstones had only one main treatment option: An operation called the cholecystectomy, open surgery to remove the gallbladder. This procedure, which has been used successfully for more than a century, is very safe, but it takes its toll on the body: It involves a 5- to 8-inch incision through muscle, fat and abdominal tissue, 4 or 5 days of hospitalization, and several weeks of recovery time.

In the last decade, a new procedure, called laparoscopic cholecystectomy (belly-button surgery) has surpassed the standard cholecystectomy and now is performed in 80 percent of Americans who require gallbladder surgery. The procedure, which takes a little more than 1 hour and is performed under general anesthesia, has many advantages: For one thing, although it requires several incisions, instead of one large one, these are tiny, each less than $1/2$ in. long. The laparoscope is a long, thin, flexible tube with a headlight and video camera, through which surgical instruments can be passed. To enlarge the surgical arena and maximize visibility, the surgeon pipes air into the abdomen. (This causes temporary distension, which should go away when the air passes naturally from the body.) The smaller incisions mean quicker recovery time, shorter hospital stays (at some institutions, this is done as an outpatient procedure), and a return to normal activities—including work—within a few days. As a bonus, there is no large, unsightly scar, as in the open procedure. Laparoscopic cholecystectomy is especially helpful as a means of treatment in people who might not be considered good candidates for open surgery: the elderly or people whose general health is frail. However, it is not for everybody. Someone with an acutely inflamed gallbladder, for instance, should probably have open surgery. Acute inflammation increases the likelihood of complications. A particularly large stone, lodged in the bile duct, may also be difficult to extract through a $1/2$ in. opening.

Although the gallbladder—essentially just a holding tank for bile—is not a vital organ, the common bile duct, which transports bile from the liver to the small intestine, is a crucial conduit that must be preserved. However, some stones may be left behind in the common bile duct and removed by other means, including a cutting device used during ERCP (see page 1033); remaining stones may also be chemically dissolved with medication (see below). Injury to the bile duct is more common with laparoscopic cholecystectomy than with the standard procedure.

Nonsurgical Approaches Gallstones can be dissolved chemically, by pills such as ursodiol (Actigall) or chenodiol (Chenix) that dilute bile, or by an injected chemical, called methyltertbutyl ether (however, this can cause adverse effects such as nausea and vomiting). But these approaches tend to work best in small cholesterol (as opposed to biliary) stones. People with one or two large stones may be candidates for a technique called shock wave lithotripsy, which uses sound waves to crush stones into tiny fragments that can then be dissolved by the bile-thinning pills. The main problem with the nonsurgical approaches is that few people are true candidates, and in half the people who try them—because the gallbladder is still present, and presumably the factors that created the gallstones still exist—gallstones return within a few years. ■

lower your risk (see Chapter 1 for more information on losing weight).

When to call the doctor If you have severe pain in the upper back or abdomen that lasts longer than 15 minutes, go to the emergency room immediately; serious pain means that something is wrong. Among other things, this pain could be caused by a heart attack or bowel obstruction.

Treatment The first step is to determine (with ultrasound and the other diagnostic tests mentioned on page 1054) the exact cause of the pain and site of blockage: the gallbladder, common bile duct, or pancreas. You will be given broad-spectrum antibiotics, such as ampicillin (Omnipen), gentamicin, and metronidazole, to treat infection, and pain medications and analgesics for pain and fever. You will probably need to hospitalized, at least overnight, for observation. Although on some occasions doctors opt for watchful waiting (if diagnostic tests show few gallstones and suggest that this blockage was an isolated or rare incident), in most cases, the next step is to remove the gallstones. See Treatment Options for Gallstones, above.

Prognosis For most people treated for gallstones, the prognosis is excellent. The gallbladder is simply a storehouse for bile; without it, bile still travels from the liver to the duodenum via the common bile duct, and digestion continues normally. Rarely, for unexplained reasons, some individuals experience a complication called postcholecystectomy syndrome, in which they feel pain in the right upper abdomen, where the gallbladder used to be. If this persists, you may need to undergo ERCP (see page 1033), during which a gastroenterologist performs a procedure called a sphincterotomy—cutting the valve that keeps bile contained within the common bile duct. This procedure relieves the pain, and although, as a result, the bile flows unceasingly into the duodenum, most people experience no further complications.

If you opt for a nonsurgical approach (see Treatment Options for Gallstones, page 1056), you run the risk of having new gallstones form, particularly—if obesity is a risk factor in your case—if you do not adopt a more healthful diet and lose weight. About half of the people treated with nonsurgical approaches experience a recurrence of complications of gallstones within a few years. Gallstones may be linked to the development of cancer in the gallbladder or bile duct; some doctors speculate that early removal of a troublesome gallbladder may help prevent this.

❖ BILE DUCT DISEASE

Symptoms *(What you may experience)* Pain under the right rib cage; nausea; vomiting; fever; chills; jaundice (yellowing of the skin and whites of the eyes), which may be intermittent; dark urine, unusually light-colored stool. Some people experience no symptoms. In others, symptoms are severe, requiring emergency treatment.

Signs and laboratory findings *(What the doctor looks for)* Tenderness in the right upper abdomen, felt during a physical exam; dilation in the common bile duct (just above an obstruction such as a gallstone), and/or the presence of a stone in the bile duct, visible in ultrasound, a CT scan, or PTHC; elevated results of serum bilirubin and alkaline phosphatase tests; the presence of bacteria and inflammatory cells in blood cultures; elevated results of pancreas function tests (see Diagnostic Tests of the Liver, Gallbladder, and Pancreas, page 1031); the presence of abnormal bile ducts (if the obstruction is caused by primary sclerosing cholangitis), seen in ERCP (see page 1033); positive results of an antimitochondrial antibody blood test (if the cause is primary biliary sclerosis; see Diagnostic Tests of the Liver, Gallbladder, and Pancreas, page 1031).

What is it? Bile duct disease—obstruction or inflammation in the common bile duct, which may block or hinder the flow of bile—is most commonly caused by gallstones (see page 1054), stones that form in the gallbladder. Even after open or laparoscopic surgery to remove the gallbladder, a gallstone may be left behind in the common bile duct (which is preserved during gallbladder surgery), where it may or may not produce troublesome symptoms. Many people with bile duct stones live for years without symptoms; some never need treatment. In most, however, the stones can cause an acute obstruction—characterized by fever, chills, and severe pain—and require emergency treatment. Obstruction may also be caused by trauma (scar tissue from gallbladder surgery, for example), cancer (see Cancer of the Gallbladder and Bile Ducts, page 1058), cysts, or a disease such as primary sclerosing cholangitis (see below). Cysts in the bile duct, called choledochal bile duct cysts, are usually congenital and should be surgically removed because they may lead to cancer (see Cancer of the Gallbladder and Bile Ducts). Another cause of bile duct disease is a rare autoimmune disorder called primary biliary cirrhosis. This is a microscopic disease of the bile ductules, tiny ducts inside the liver; it is not apparent in most imaging and diagnostic tests. The main test for this is an antimitochondrial antibody blood test (see Diagnostic Tests of the Liver, Gallbladder, and Pancreas, page 1031).

Primary sclerosing cholangitis This disease is characterized by scarring and narrowing of the bile ducts in and out of the liver, resulting in a backup of bile in the liver. The exact cause of primary sclerosing cholangitis is not clear, although the disease is known to be more common in men than women, and it is often (in as many as 80 percent of the people who have it) associated with ulcerative colitis (see page 1010). It is usually diagnosed in adults between ages 30 and 60. The disease can be stable for many years but tends to be slowly progressive. Over time, it may lead to cirrhosis (see page 1043), liver failure (see page 1046), or cancer of the bile ducts, called cholangiocarcinoma (see Cancer of the Gallbladder and Bile Ducts, page 1058).

Ascending cholangitis Ascending cholangitis is infection, usually with *Escherichia coli* bacteria, and inflammation in the main bile duct or branch ducts. It is usually a secondary problem, caused by obstruction. (If there were nothing blocking the bile duct, there would be no foothold for infection.) Ascending cholangitis is characterized by Charcot's triad of symptoms: right upper abdominal pain, jaundice, and fever with chills. These symptoms may wax and wane, because the bile duct may not be totally blocked; when bile flow is better, symptoms improve temporarily.

When to call the doctor If you have severe abdominal pain and fever, with or without jaundice, call your doctor at once.

Treatment The main form of treatment for bile duct obstruction is to remove the offending stone or cyst, widen the bile duct, or create a new opening in the bile duct with ERCP (see page 1033) or surgery.

- *Primary biliary cirrhosis:* Like most autoimmune diseases, primary biliary cirrhosis is not well understood; if the disease progresses, it may lead to liver failure (see page 1046) and the need for a liver transplant (see page 1047).

- *Primary sclerosing cholangitis:* There is no specific treatment for this disease; instead, treatment is aimed at its symptoms. If you have significant bile duct obstruction, you may need ERCP to enlarge or reopen a blocked duct. Itching can be treated with cholestyramine; infection is usually treated with antibiotics. You may also need supplemental vitamins.

- *Ascending cholangitis:* The first step is to treat the infection with antibiotics and administer intravenous fluids, if you are dehydrated. However, if the obstruction that is the underlying cause of the infection is not treated, the infection will likely return.

Prognosis Prognosis depends on several factors, including the severity of your symptoms and the presence of localized infection or sepsis. Overall, however, the prognosis for bile duct disease is good. About 20 percent of people with stones in the bile duct pass them spontaneously, on their own, and no further treatment is needed. If you are not one of these lucky few, you may need surgery or ERCP to remove the stone. The prognosis for primary sclerosing cholangitis varies. Some people have the disease for years without symptoms. Others, however, develop cirrhosis (see page 1043) or liver

failure (see page 1046) after several years of symptoms. Over time, about 10 percent of people with this disease develop a tumor of the bile ducts, called cholangiocarcinoma (see Cancer of the Gallbladder and Bile Ducts, below).

❖ CANCER OF THE GALLBLADDER AND BILE DUCTS

Symptoms *(What you may experience)* Jaundice (yellowing of the skin and whites of the eyes), which may be intermittent; dark urine; usually light-colored stool; pain in the upper right abdomen, under the right rib cage (however, nearly half of people with cancer of the bile ducts do not experience pain); loss of appetite; weight loss; nausea and vomiting; fever with or without chills; diarrhea; constipation.

Signs and laboratory findings *(What the doctor looks for)* The presence of one or more masses in the gallbladder or bile ducts, seen in ERCP (see page 1033), ultrasound, CT (see Other Diagnostic Tests of the Gastrointestinal Tract, page 984), and/or PTHC (see Diagnostic Tests of the Liver, Gallbladder, and Pancreas, page 1031); tenderness in the right upper abdomen, felt during a physical exam; dilation in the common bile duct (just above an obstruction or mass); elevated results of serum bilirubin and alkaline phosphatase tests; the presence of bacteria and inflammatory cells in blood cultures; a medical history of gallstones, choledochal cyst, primary sclerosing cholangitis, or ulcerative colitis.

What is it? Tumors in the gallbladder and bile ducts are rare; each year, fewer than 4,000 Americans are diagnosed with bile duct cancer, and about 6,000 develop gallbladder cancer. Tumors may also be benign; of these, papilloma and adenoma are the most common. Half of all cancerous bile duct tumors develop in the upper third of the biliary tract, often involving the liver. Tumors may also develop in the middle part, near the portal vein and hepatic artery, and the lower third, often involving the pancreas and duodenum.

Cholangiocarcinoma is a known complication of several diseases: Choledochal bile duct cysts, if not removed, are likely to lead to cancer; cancer also develops in about 10 percent of people with primary sclerosing cholangitis. Cholangiocarcinoma is linked to ulcerative colitis. Cholangiocarcinoma and gallbladder cancer have also been linked to gallstones; whether or not they are linked to the same risk factors is not clear. A rare form of bile duct cancer in the United States (although it is more common in Asia) is caused by Clonorchis sinensis, a form of roundworm found in raw freshwater fish.

What you can do Several conditions have been linked to one form of bile duct cancer, called cholangiocarcinoma, including choledochal bile duct cysts, primary sclerosing cholangitis, gallstones, and ulcerative colitis. There is no known cure for primary sclerosing cholangitis; however, if you have this disease, be aware of the risk and discuss with your doctor the need for vigilant follow-up care. If you travel in Asia, avoid raw freshwater fish; a form of roundworm called *C. sinensis* is known to cause bile duct cancer (as well as other health problems, including infections in the bile duct and cirrhosis).

When to call the doctor If you have any of the symptoms listed above, call your doctor immediately. If you have a choledochal cyst, seeking treatment right away may prevent cancer. Also, some doctors believe that prompt removal of the gallbladder after a gallstone attack may reduce the likelihood of developing cancer of the gallbladder.

Treatment Treatment depends on the nature of the tumor and its location. Benign tumors are usually removed surgically. Cancerous tumors in the gallbladder and in the middle and lower third of the bile duct are also treated with surgery. Tumors in the upper third of the bile duct may be removed surgically; although they are often unresectable (in other words, unable to be removed with surgery), they may respond to radiation therapy. Radiation therapy may also be used in addition to surgery in tumors lower in the bile duct. (See Chapter 30 for more information on cancer treatment.) Other treatment is mainly palliative, for example, inserting a stent, using ERCP or during surgery, to keep the bile duct open.

Prognosis Prognosis, too, depends on the nature and location of the tumor. The prognosis for benign tumors is excellent. Most cancerous gallbladder tumors are diagnosed when it is too late for cure. If you have any of the risk factors listed in What is it?, page 1058, talk to your doctor. The prognosis of bile duct tumors depends greatly on where they sit in the bile duct. Tumors in the upper third have the worst prognosis; tumors in the middle and lower third may be cured with surgery and radiation.

The Pancreas

The oblong pancreas stretches like a finger pointing toward the spleen, behind the stomach and within a loop of the duodenum tend curves around the head of the pancreas. Longer in size than the gallbladder but much smaller than the liver, it plays two main roles. First, as an exocrine gland, it is crucial to the digestive process: Its potent enzymes and an alkaline substance called sodium bicarbonate (the same ingredient in baking soda) flow through ducts to the duodenum, where they attack fats, proteins, and

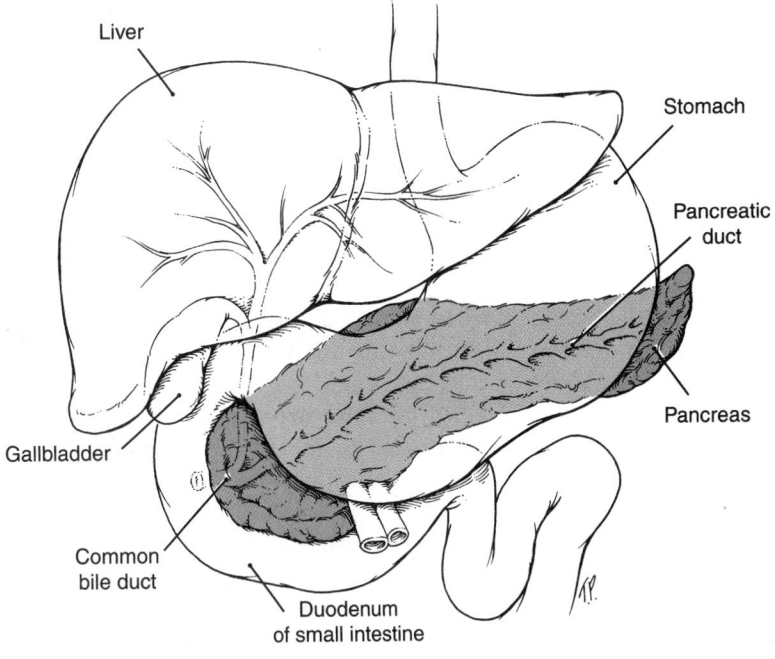

The pancreas secretes proteins and sodium bicarbonate, which break down fats, proteins, and carbohydrates to aid in digestion. The pancreas also makes several hormones, including insulin and glucagon, for the metabolism of sugar. Diabetes mellitus occurs if the pancreas loses its ability to make insulin. Alcohol abuse is a common cause of pancreatic inflammation.

Liver

Stomach

Pancreatic duct

Pancreas

Gallbladder

Common bile duct

Duodenum of small intestine

PANCREAS FUNCTION TESTS

Pancreas enzyme tests measure specific enzymes made by the pancreas: amylase and lipase. Elevated levels of these enzymes can suggest damage in the pancreas. When pancreatic cells are injured or inflamed, these enzymes seep into the bloodstream. Of the two, lipase is the more specific; amylase is also made elsewhere in the body (in the salivary glands, for example). A stool test, called a fecal fat collection test, can also be a good indicator of pancreatic function. In this test, you will be asked to eat a high-fat diet for a certain period (usually 24 or 72 hours) and to save your stool in a special container. Afterward, your stool will be checked for the presence of excess fat. Malabsorption, particularly of fat, is a major problem in chronic pancreatitis, because the pancreas is unable to produce the enzymes needed to help the body digest fat. ■

carbohydrates, splitting them into digestible molecules. Second, as part of the endocrine system (see Chapter 26), the pancreas makes many hormones, two of which—insulin and glucagon—are critical to the body's ability to metabolize sugar. When the pancreas loses its ability to make insulin, diabetes mellitus results (see Chapter 26). For a discussion of cystic fibrosis, another disease that can affect the pancreas, see Chapter 18.

Like the liver, the pancreas can become injured with alcohol abuse; like the biliary system, it may also be affected by stones. When the pancreas becomes inflamed, in a condition called pancreatitis, its digestive enzymes can go awry and begin attacking the gland itself. Cancer of the pancreas is not often curable, although a surgical procedure offers some hope (see The Whipple Procedure, page 1064) and is the fifth-deadliest form of cancer in the United States.

❖ ACUTE PANCREATITIS

Symptoms *(What you may experience)*
Pain in the upper abdomen, which may be severe or even debilitating and may extend to the back; this may strike suddenly or may begin as mild discomfort that gets worse when you eat and slowly builds to a steady pain. Also, nausea; vomiting; fever, weakness.

Signs and laboratory findings *(What the doctor looks for)* A very tender upper abdomen, on physical exam; a rapid pulse; low blood pressure; evidence of dehydration; elevated levels of amylase and lipase (digestive enzymes made by the pancreas) in the blood; abnormal blood levels of minerals and electrolytes, including calcium, magnesium, sodium, potassium, and bicarbonate; elevated levels of sugar and fats in the blood. All of these abnormalities in the blood should return to normal after the attack is over.

What is it? Acute pancreatitis is a sudden inflammation of the pancreas, which affects as many as 80,000 Americans each year. Although the disease has several known causes (see below), exactly why the pancreas reacts to these triggers—and precisely what happens during an attack—is unclear. In a process that probably requires several "on" switches to be mistakenly activated, the digestive enzymes of the pancreas (normally harmless within the gland) begin to digest the pancreas itself. This process is called autodigestion. Some of these enzymes, such as trypsin, initiate a chain reaction by activating other enzymes, resulting in tissue damage, rampant swelling of cells and blood vessels, and bleeding.

Acute pancreatitis usually lasts several days, and it usually gets better on its own (although this may be of little comfort to someone in the throes of an attack). Even if you have more than one attack, chances are good that you will recover fully. However, in about 20 percent of cases, acute pancreatitis may be severe, involving other organs. Rarely, acute pancreatitis may result in widespread bleeding, severe tissue damage, and cyst formation within the pancreas, which if not treated may even be fatal.

The overwhelming majority of cases of acute pancreatitis are caused either by alcohol abuse or gallstones. Other possible causes include abdominal trauma, abdominal surgery, prescription medications, or rarely, other diseases (such as mumps); about 15 percent of all attacks of acute pancreatitis have no identifiable cause. If the underlying cause is not treated, a chronic form of the disease may result (see Chronic Pancreatitis, page 1061).

What you can do Most cases of acute pancreatitis are caused either by alcohol abuse or by gallstones. If you drink alcohol, do not have more than two drinks a day; a drink is a glass of wine or a 12-oz can of beer, or a 1½-oz portion of hard liquor. Take all medications, even vitamins, in their recommended dosages. If you have any questions, do not guess; ask your doctor. Although it may not be possible to prevent gallstones entirely, controlling your weight by following a sensible, low-fat, low-cholesterol, high-fiber diet may lower your risk (for the major risk factors, see Gallstones, page 1054). Also, eating several small meals throughout the day, instead of two or three large ones, may help ease some of the burden on the pancreas.

When to call the doctor If you have severe abdominal pain that lasts for more than 20 minutes, call your doctor or go to the emergency room.

Treatment Because, in most cases, acute pancreatitis goes away on its own, treatment is aimed at relieving specific symptoms. If you are at risk of becoming dehydrated, you may need intravenous fluids; this will also help restore normal blood pressure. If you cannot control vomiting, you may need a suppository such as promethazine (Phenergan) or trimethobenzamide (Tigan) or, if your symptoms are severe, a nasogastric tube, inserted through the nose, to remove gastric juices from the stomach; this can help relieve nausea and vomiting. If the damage to the pancreas is severe, you may need to be fed intravenously for several weeks to give the pancreas a chance to heal. You may also need antibiotics, if any infection develops. If the damage has been caused by drinking alcohol, you must stop drinking immediately or risk causing chronic damage to the pancreas. If the underlying cause of the pancreatitis is gallstones, you may need surgery to remove the gallbladder (see Treatment Options for Gallstones, page 1056) or ERCP (see page 1033) to reopen a blocked bile duct. If the inflammation is severe, these additional treatments may be done a month or so after the initial attack, to give the pancreas time to heal.

Prognosis Prognosis depends on the underlying condition, which is usually either gallstones or alcohol abuse. In most cases, once the initial inflammation has healed and the underlying cause has been treated, the prognosis is excellent.

❖ CHRONIC PANCREATITIS

Symptoms *(What you may experience)* Initially, the symptoms of acute pancreatitis: pain in the upper abdomen, which may be severe or even debilitating and may extend to the back; pain may strike suddenly, or may begin as mild discomfort that gets worse when you eat and slowly builds to a steady, persistent pain; nausea; vomiting; fever, weakness. Over time, you may also experience weight loss, even if your appetite and eating habits are normal. Also, symptoms of diabetes mellitus (see Diabetes Type I, page 1174).

Signs and laboratory findings *(What the doctor looks for)* A history of heavy drinking or, rarely, gallstones; loss of pancreatic enzymes, suggested by pancreas function tests; evidence of malabsorption, confirmed by a fecal fat collection test (see Diagnostic Tests of the Liver, Gallbladder, and Pancreas, page 1031); damage in the pancreas, seen on ERCP (see page 1033) ultrasound, or CT scan; evidence of diabetes (see Chapter 26).

What is it? Chronic pancreatitis is usually a miserable condition, involving repeat attacks of acute pancreatitis along with chronic or recurrent pain that may last for hours, days, or even months. The events happening within the pancreas are probably the same as with acute pancreatitis (see Acute Pancreatitis, page 1060): The pancreas's potent digestive enzymes (normally harmless within the gland) attack the very tissue that produced them. Some of these, such as trypsin, involve other enzymes, creating tissue damage, rampant swelling of cells and blood vessels, and bleeding. As the disease continues, the pancreas loses its ability to generate vital enzymes needed for digestion and absorption of nutrients (this problem is called exocrine insufficiency).

In more than 90 percent of cases, chronic pancreatitis is the result of years of excessive alcohol consumption. However, it may also develop after one bout of acute pancreatitis, if the ducts within the pancreas are severely damaged. Many people live for years with damage to the pancreas from alcohol abuse but have no symptoms. At first, if your major symptom is severe pain, it may be difficult for your doctor to tell whether the problem is acute or chronic pancreatitis. But with chronic pancreatitis, in addition to the pain, there is usually more evidence of long-term damage: malabsorption, from a lack of digestive enzymes made by the pancreas; weight loss (due to the malabsorption, your body is not getting the nutrients and calories it needs);

and diabetes mellitus (see Chapter 26) from damage to the islet cells in the pancreas, which make insulin. Chronic pancreatitis is more common in men than women.

What you can do Because nearly all cases of chronic pancreatitis are caused by alcohol abuse, the best way to prevent this disease is to avoid alcohol. If you have ever had an episode of acute pancreatitis, the pancreas is already vulnerable to damage, and you should stop drinking immediately.

When to call the doctor If you have an episode of abdominal pain that lasts more than 20 minutes, call your doctor or go to the emergency room. If you have unexplained weight loss that lasts more than a few weeks, call your doctor. This is also a warning sign of pancreatic cancer, which is nearly always fatal if not treated early.

Treatment Treatment is directed at managing your nutritional and metabolic needs and relieving pain. Minor pain is usually treated with analgesics. If you have an enlarged pancreatic duct, you may need ERCP to drain it (see page 1033), or in severe cases, surgery may also be needed to drain or remove part or most of the pancreas. You will probably be given fairly strict dietary guidelines, which will help you limit your intake of fat and protein (which the body now has trouble digesting). You may also need to take supplemental pancreatic enzymes, which will help your body absorb food and may help you regain some or all of the lost weight.

Prognosis Many people with chronic pancreatitis, with dietary changes, medications, and nutritional supplements, have fewer, milder attacks, and a good prognosis. However, if you do not stop drinking, none of the other treatments will provide help in the long term.

❖ CONGENITAL ABNORMALITIES OF THE PANCREAS

Symptoms *(What you may experience)*

- *Annular pancreas.* Feeling extremely full, even after small meals; stomach pain; nausea; vomiting; because these symptoms may be mild, many people

experience them for years without realizing there is a problem.

- *Pancreas divisum.* Many people never experience symptoms; however, when symptoms do occur, they are usually those of acute pancreatitis: pain in the upper abdomen, which may be severe or even debilitating and may extend to the back; pain may strike suddenly or may begin as mild discomfort that gets worse when you eat and slowly builds to a steady pain. Also, nausea; vomiting; fever, weakness.

Signs and laboratory findings *(What the doctor looks for)*

- *Annular pancreas.* A ring of tissue surrounding the pancreas, seen in ultrasound, a CT scan, or ERCP; a history of acute pancreatis (which may be a complication of annular pancreas).

- *Pancreas divisum.* Abnormalities in the pancreatic ducts, seen in ERCP; a tender upper abdomen, on physical exam; a rapid pulse; low blood pressure; evidence of dehydration. Elevated levels of amylase (a digestive enzyme made by the pancreas) in the blood; abnormal blood levels of minerals and electrolytes, including calcium, magnesium, sodium, potassium, and bicarbonate; elevated levels of sugar and fats in the blood. Some people have no other risk factors for chronic or acute pancreatitis, as suggested by their medical histories—a red flag suggesting that this may be a congenital abnormality.

What is it?

- *Annular pancreas.* In this congenital disorder, which may be diagnosed in childhood or adulthood, a ring of pancreatic tissue grows around the duodenum. Many people live for years with no symptoms, but over time, this ring can choke the duodenum, causing a blockage.

- *Pancreas divisum.* Pancreas divisum may be the pancreatic equivalent of cleft palate: The pancreatic duct is divided, with its halves unable to grow or function together, and this affects drainage of the pancreas. Here, too, many people live for years—or even all their lives—without symptoms. But in some people, for unclear reasons, one of these ducts becomes stenosed, or closed, by scar tissue. The pancreas becomes overloaded; its juices back up, and inflammation—identical in symptoms to an episode of acute pancreatitis—results. The key to diagnosis is watching the anatomy of the pancreatic ducts during ERCP (see page 1033).

Treatment

- *Annular pancreas.* The treatment is not to cut the pancreas, but to reroute the food around the duodenum during abdominal surgery, a procedure that requires hospitalization and general anesthesia.

- *Pancreas divisum.* The main form of treatment, done during ERCP (see page 1033), is to reopen a blocked pancreatic duct and restore normal flow within the pancreas.

Prognosis With treatment, the prognosis for both disorders is excellent.

❖ CANCER OF THE PANCREAS

Symptoms *(What you may experience)* Unexplained weight loss, which may be significant (more than 20 lb); jaundice (yellowing of the skin and whites of the eyes); dark urine; unusually light-colored stool; abdominal pain, which may spread to the lower back; nausea and vomiting; itching; unexplained depression.

Signs and laboratory findings *(What the doctor looks for)* An enlarged, palpable gallbladder or abdominal mass, felt during a physical exam; the presence of a mass, found in CT scan or ultrasound; a blocked pancreatic and bile duct (double duct sign) on ERCP; cancerous cells on a needle biopsy of the pancreas (which may be done during ultrasound or CT).

What is it? Cancer of the pancreas—mainly because it produces no early symptoms and is rarely diagnosed before it has spread to the liver, intestine, stomach, or elsewhere—is often fatal. About 27,000 people in the United States are diagnosed with

it each year; about 26,000 people die from it every year, making it the fifth-deadliest form of cancer in this country. There may be a genetic component; pancreatic cancer seems to run in some families (a famous example is the family of former President Jimmy Carter, whose mother, brother, and sister all died of the disease). Scientists at Johns Hopkins are working on understanding the genes involved in pancreatic cancer, work that may one day lead to an early screening test. Also, the National Familial Pancreas Tumor Registry, based at Johns Hopkins, a nationwide database on pancreatic cancer patients and their families, is actively searching blood and tissue samples for the genetic origins of the disease. For more information, write the National Familial Pancreas Tumor Registry, Attn: Dr. Ralph Hruban, 600 N. Wolfe St., Meyer 7-181, Baltimore, MD 21287.

When to call the doctor If you have unexplained weight loss, jaundice, or abdominal pain, especially if anyone in your family has died of pancreatic cancer, call your doctor immediately. Do not wait to see if these symptoms get better on their own.

Treatment For many people, treatment is palliative, aimed at treating specific symptoms. If the flow of bile is blocked by the tumor, for example, you may need ERCP to have a draining tube, called a stent, placed in the bile duct between the duodenum and the liver. For pain, you will probably be given narcotics. For weight loss caused by malabsorption—when a lack of pancreatic enzymes is interfering with your body's ability to digest the nutrients in food—you may be given supplemental pancreatic enzymes. Some surgeons only remove small pancreatic tumors. At Johns Hopkins, however, in a complicated operation called the Whipple procedure, surgeons resect a considerably larger amount of tissue (see The Whipple Procedure, page 1064), with some promising results.

Prognosis If the cancer has spread massively, or if it has metastasized to distant sites that cannot be reached with surgery, the prognosis is poor. Unfortunately, for most people, diagnosed after months of weight loss, jaundice, or abdominal pain, the average survival is less than a year. This is why, if you have unexplained weight loss or

THE WHIPPLE PROCEDURE

The pancreaticoduodenectomy, also called the Whipple procedure is removal of part of the pancreas, all of the duodenum, gallbladder, bile duct, and sometimes part of the stomach. It is a dramatic solution to a desperate problem: usually, advanced pancreatic cancer, which is almost always fatal within a few months.

Because it is an arduous procedure, one that requires extreme precision and expertise, the Whipple procedure is not performed at many medical centers. Twenty years ago, one in four people who had the operation never made it home from the hospital. But at Johns Hopkins, where surgeons have made many refinements in the operation—and performed more Whipple procedures than surgeons at any other medical center—fewer than 2 percent of

people die from the procedure itself. As recently as 20 years ago, no one with cancer of the head of the pancreas who underwent the procedure lived for 5 years; today, Johns Hopkins surgeons report a survival rate of 26 percent for these patients. Patients of any age—even in their 80s—are eligible for the procedure, which offers hope where there used to be none.

The pancreaticoduodenectomy, in which the gallbladder, bile duct, duodenum, part of the pancreas, and sometimes part of the stomach are removed, is known as the Whipple procedure. The Whipple procedure is performed to treat pancreatic cancer at an early stage. Advanced pancreatic cancer is usually fatal within a few months. Surgeons at The Johns Hopkins Hospital have performed more Whipple procedures than surgeons at any other medical center.

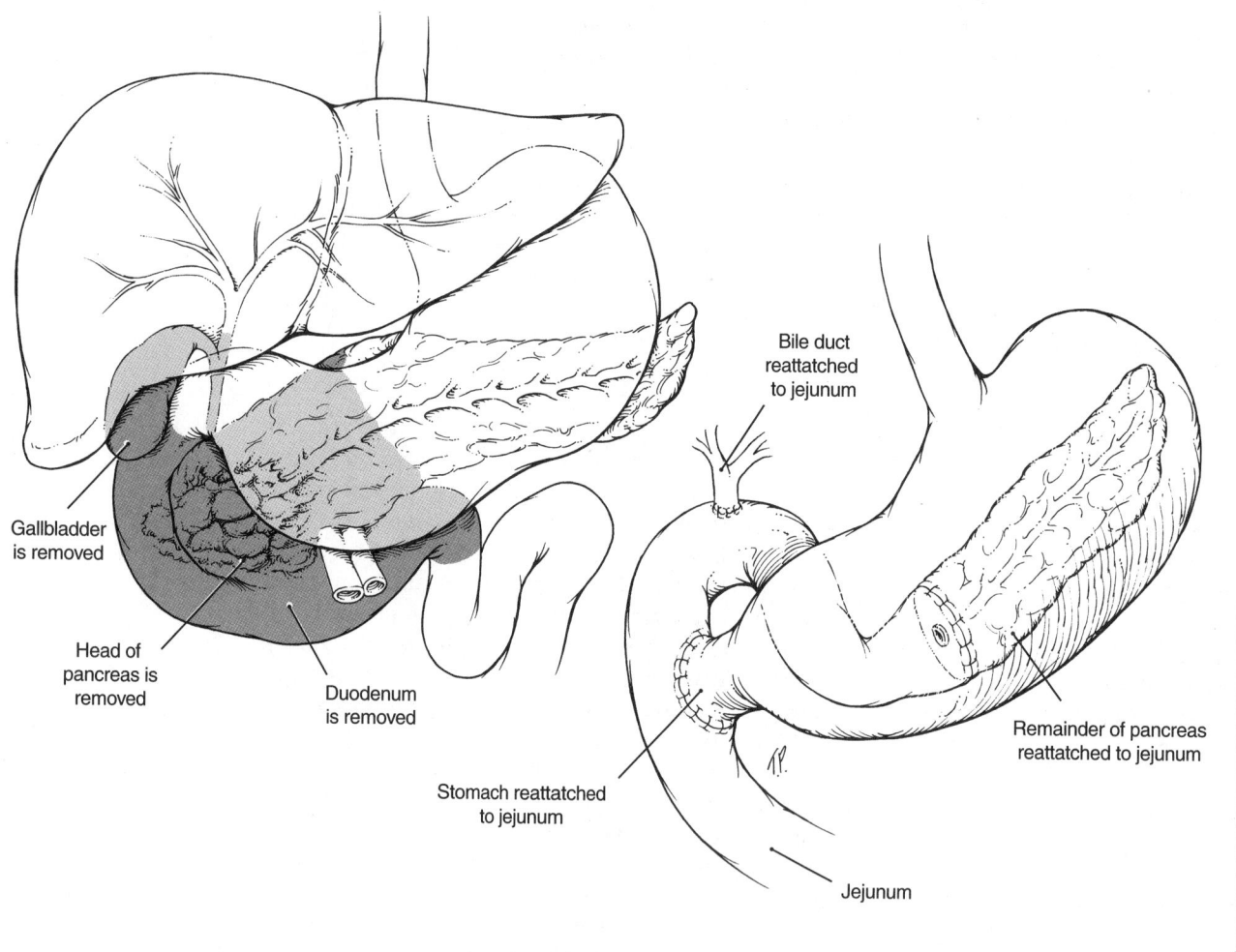

Gallbladder is removed

Head of pancreas is removed

Duodenum is removed

Stomach reattatched to jejunum

Bile duct reattatched to jejunum

Remainder of pancreas reattatched to jejunum

Jejunum

jaundice—*especially if anyone in your family has died of pancreatic cancer*—get these symptoms checked out by a doctor as soon as possible. Time is of the essence. If the cancer can be resected surgically, there is a chance for cure. At Johns Hopkins, the 5-year survival rate for people who have undergone the Whipple procedure is as high as 26 percent.

TWENTY-FOUR

Urinary Tract

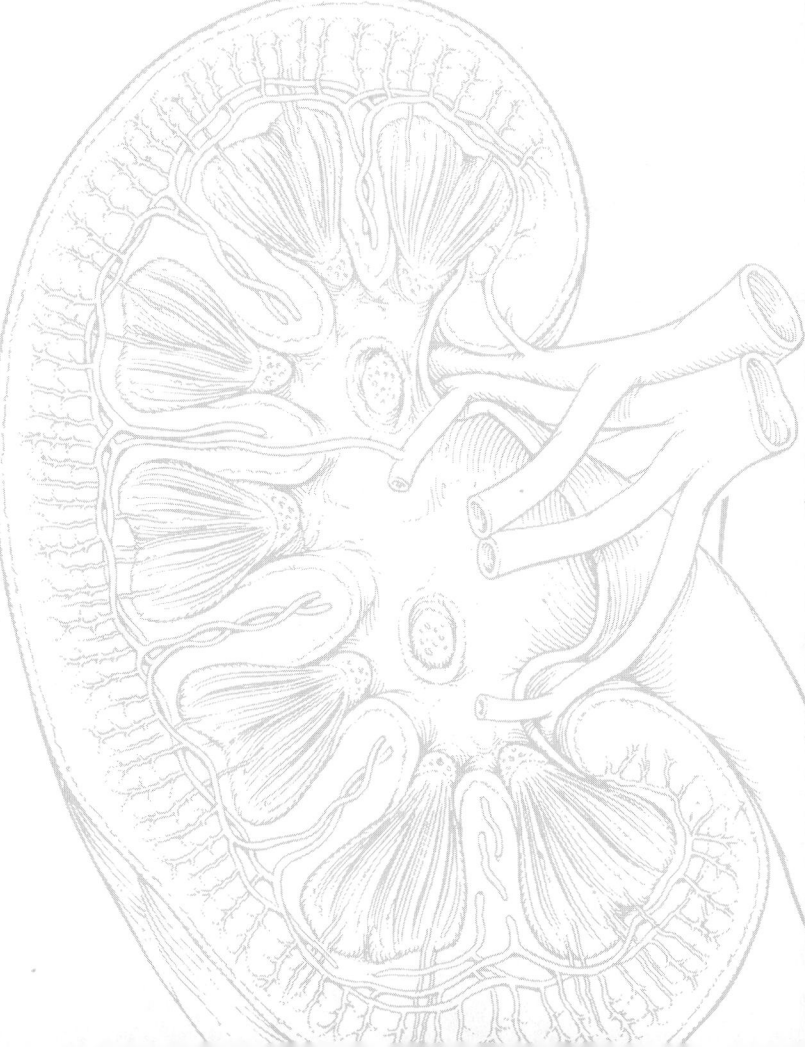

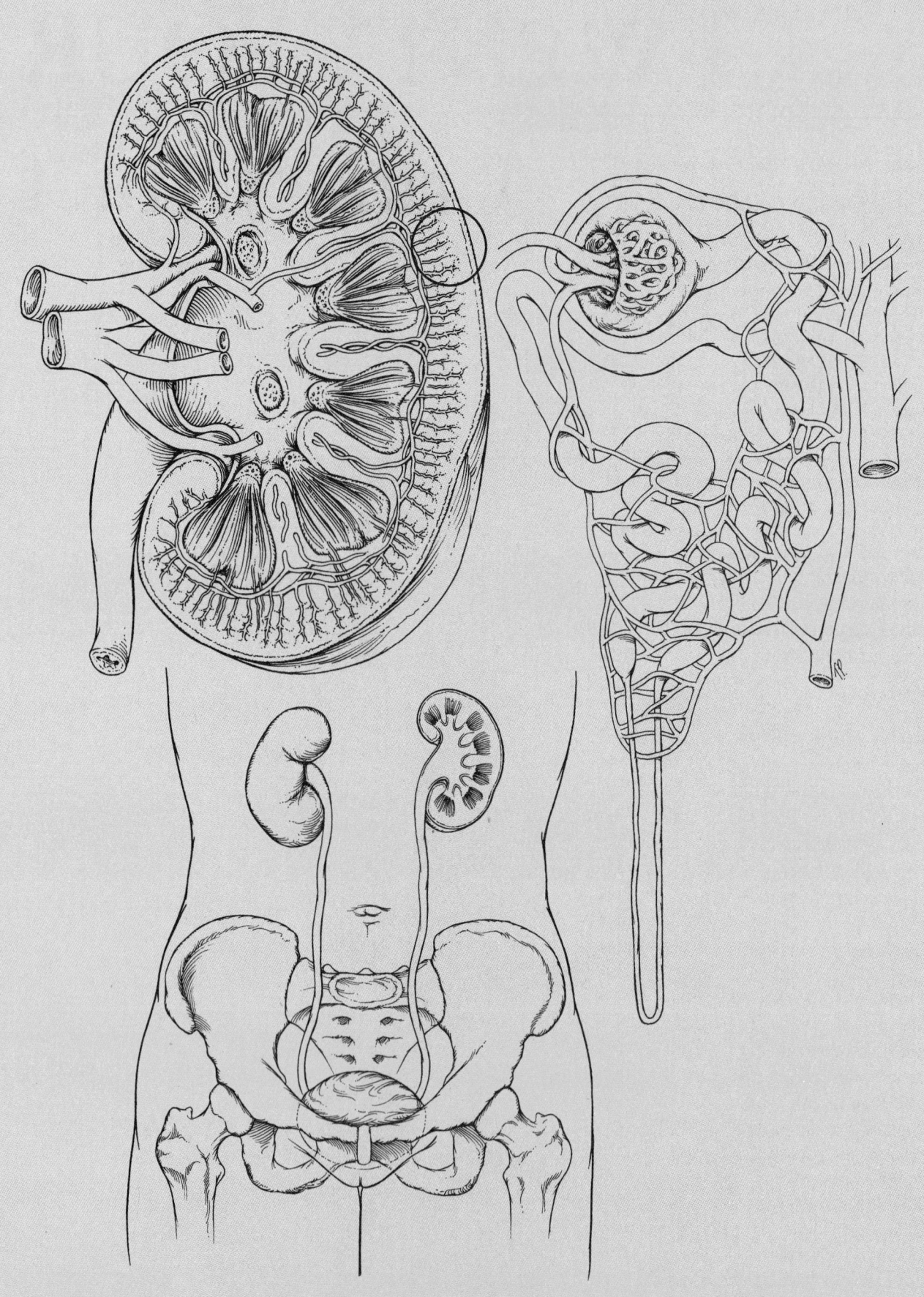

URINARY TRACT

How the Urinary Tract Works

The urinary tract normally consists of a pair of bean-shaped kidneys, each about 12 cm (4³/₄ in.) long in adults, attached by its ureter (urine tube) to the urinary bladder, a reservoir that empties to the outside through another tube, the urethra. The reproductive organs lie adjacent to the urinary tract, and in the case of men, in particular, problems in the urinary tract may be caused by abnormalities of the reproductive organs (and vice versa). See Chaper 25 for information about disorders involving the reproductive organs.

The urinary tract is part of the body's excretory machinery, which serves to eliminate waste material from the body. Most of the cells in the body use protein to perform their various functions, and when protein is broken down, nitrogen-containing waste products are produced, the most common of which is urea. Wastes, fluid, and chemicals in the blood are filtered by the kidneys (see How the Kidneys Work, page 1078). Approximately 1 million filtering units, called nephrons, compose each kidney. Small pores allow the blood to be filtered and this filtered material makes up the urine, which is collected by tubules (tiny tubes). These tubules combine together to eventually form one ureter, which drains the urine from each kidney to the bladder and finally is excreted through the urethra and out of the body.

The Bladder and Urethra

The bladder is a sac with muscular walls that contract to force the urine from the body through the urethra. As the bladder fills with urine, nerve fibers within its walls detect stretching and, when full, signal the need to empty the bladder. As children, we learn to correctly interpret this signal, and if all is working as it should, can suppress the urge to release the urine until we choose to. Sometimes, whether because of infection, injury, disease, or age, the system malfunctions.

❖ CYSTITIS

Symptoms *(What you may experience)* Abrupt onset of the following: frequent uri-

nation, sudden and urgent need to urinate, and pain or burning on urination; sensation of pressure or pain in the lower abdomen or back (often). Sometimes: strong or foul-smelling urine; bloody urine; low-grade fever.

Signs and laboratory findings *(What the doctor looks for)* Blood, pus, and bacteria on microscopic examination of the urine.

What is it? Infection of the urinary bladder is experienced by 20 percent of all women at least once. It occurs more commonly in women and girls than in males possibly because the female anatomy makes it easier for infection to occur. The urethra is short in

WHAT DOES THE URINALYSIS TELL?

The standard urinalysis, performed in doctors' offices, hospitals, and labs across the country countless times every day, involves examination of the urine specimen by chemical analysis and under the microscope. The chemical analysis relies on the urine dipstick, a plastic strip of chemically treated pads, each designed to detect or measure various components of the specimen. Typically, the dipstick measures the acidity of the urine, detects the presence of glucose (sugar), blood, protein, infection-fighting white blood cells and related markers of infection, and certain indicators of diabetes and liver abnormalities. Spinning a tube of urine at high speed in a centrifuge will cause any solid material in the urine to collect at the bottom of the tube. A drop of this collected material examined under the microscope will detect bacteria, red blood cells, infection-fighting white blood cells, yeast, certain parasites (particularly trichomonas), chemical crystals, and casts. Casts represent proteins made within the kidney that can trap inflammatory cells, red blood cells, or debris. An instrument measures urine concentration.

With this simple and inexpensive test, a doctor can detect a variety of problems—not only infections, but diabetes, kidney stones, and liver disorders as well as less common conditions that alter the urine acidity or the ability of the kidneys to concentrate the urine properly.

Properly Collecting a Urine Specimen

Collecting the specimen properly will ensure an accurate report. Differences in anatomy make collection of a clean specimen easier in men than in women. The urethra in women opens into the upper area between the labia (lips) of the vulva (the female external genital tissues) above the vagina. Because this area stays moist, it is a haven for bacterial growth. Urine passing by the hair and skin of this region can pick up these bacteria and contaminate the specimen, giving false-positive results. To guard against contamination, women need to carefully cleanse the genital area before collecting the specimen. Most doctors will provide premoistened cleansing pads for this purpose. Use one hand to spread the lips of the vulva apart, then using four sterile pads in succession, wipe from the front of the genital area to the back of the area. Uncircumcised men should retract the foreskin and use one sterile gauze pad to clean the glans (head). Both men and women should release the initial urine flow into the toilet, then collect the specimen from the middle of the urine stream. ■

WHAT CAUSES DISCOLORED OR FOUL-SMELLING URINE?

Abnormalities in appearance or smell of urine can indicate a variety of disorders. Here are some of the more common causes associated with urine changes.

- Bright red color usually indicates fresh blood from trauma or infection.

- Bright yellow color is commonly seen after taking multivitamins containing riboflavin (vitamin B_2).

- Dark red-orange color occurs after taking Pyridium, a urinary analgesic (pain reliever) often prescribed for urgency associated with urinary tract infection. The color comes from a pigment in the medication.

- Green color occurs after taking over-the-counter (OTC) urinary analgesic medications such as Azo-Natural. The color comes from a pigment in the medication.

- Smoky brown or gray color (also described as cola or tea color) usually indicates ruptured red blood cells, seen in glomerulonephritis (see page 1084) following streptococcal infection. The urine may also be foamy like the head of poured beer.

- Murky or cloudy appearance may indicate infection.

- Foul smell usually means infection.

- Pungent asparagus smell occurs only in certain people after eating asparagus or foods prepared with asparagus. Some people are unable to metabolize (the chemical conversion process that provides energy for vital bodily functions) asparagine, an amino acid in the vegetable, which passes into the urine, imparting a characteristic smell. The smell will appear quickly after eating the asparagus, persist a few hours, and dissipate. ■

SELF-CARE TIPS TO REDUCE RISK OF CYSTITIS IN WOMEN

- Keep fluid intake up.

- Avoid long intervals between urinations—4 to 5 hours during the day and 8 hours at night should be the maximum.

- Urination immediately after sexual intercourse has been shown to reduce urinary tract infection rates.

- Use of diaphragms and spermicidal agents for contraception has been linked with urinary tract infections. If you have trouble with urinary tract infections, consider a change in contraceptive method. ■

CYSTITIS IN PREGNANCY

Bacterial contamination of the urine during pregnancy occurs quite commonly. As many as 7 percent of pregnant women will be found to have bacteria present on examination of a urine specimen. Hormonal changes that occur during pregnancy—causing dilation of the ureters—as well as the weight of the pregnant uterus pressing on the bladder may be factors.

Often the presence of bacteria causes no symptoms, but that does not preclude its causing potentially serious problems. As many as one-third of pregnant women with untreated bacteria in the urine (even when their presence causes no symptoms) will develop kidney infection by the third trimester. Treatment with antibiotics can reduce this risk to less than 5 percent. Because the development of this kind of severe kidney infection can put the baby at risk by predisposing the mother to early labor and premature delivery, all urinary infections should be treated regardless of whether or not they cause symptoms.

Many women fear that taking antibiotics might harm the fetus, but except for certain classes of medications this is not a concern. Your doctor will discuss with you those antibiotics that are generally safe during pregnancy. Pencillins and cephalosporins are generally regarded as safe in pregnancy, and while they are less effective than the medications used in nonpregnant women, they are the preferred therapy in this situation. ■

females—a mere $2\frac{1}{2}$ to $5\frac{1}{4}$ cm (1 to $2\frac{1}{8}$ in.) long—and it opens very close to the anus, an area colonized with bacteria from the vagina, rectum, and skin. Normally, if these bacteria find their way into the urethra, urinating washes them away. In addition, the body secretes protective antibodies (molecules that attack foreign substances—antigens—in the body) into the urethra to create a hostile environment against bacteria. If something disrupts these normal defenses, bacteria can enter the bladder, multiply, and gain a foothold; the resulting infection causes the symptoms you feel.

Cystitis can arise from a variety of factors. Among sexually active females, the introduction of bacteria—the usual culprit is *Escherichia coli*, a normal inhabitant of the nearby colorectal area—into the urethra during sex is the most common cause. In fact, the first episode of cystitis for many women occurs soon after they become sexually active, giving rise to the term "honeymoon cystitis."

Other causes of cystitis in women are unrelated to sexual activity, occurring instead during times of physical or emotional stress—times coinciding with brief lapses in immune defense strength. Some women are more prone to infections because bacteria are better able to adhere to the cells that line the vagina, urethra, bladder, and ureter.

Because the bladder is a reservoir for urine, infection limited to the bladder is usually more painful than serious. However, it is important to treat an infection promptly

EVALUATION OF CHRONIC URINARY INFECTIONS

Repeated infections signal a need for your doctor to fully evaluate the urinary tract in search of stones or predisposing structural abnormalities such as pelvic kidneys, horseshoe kidneys, duplication of the collecting system (double ureters on one side), or incompetent bladder valves (see Other Congenital Kidney Disorders, page 1092). Searching for these and other abnormalities requires several specific tests.

Intravenous Pyelogram

In this x-ray examination, the technician injects a dye (visible only on x-ray) into a vein. This dyed blood then makes its way to the kidney which filters it out, illuminating on the x-ray the general shape of the kidney as well as the urine-collecting system all the way from the kidney to the bladder. The dye usually contains iodine. If you are sensitive to iodine, be certain to alert the technician before this test. If kidney function, also called renal function (renal means relating to the kidney), is not normal, there is a risk the dye could cause acute kidney failure. The doctors will discuss this with you.

You will remain awake during the intravenous pyelogram (IVP), which should take about 30 minutes. The technician will insert an IV (catheter—tube—into the vein) through which to administer the dye. Although there is usually only a little discomfort associated with placing the IV, when the dye enters the vein you may feel slightly flushed, a little woozy, and experience some slight burning along the vein. The sensation should pass right away. When the technician finishes taking the x-ray pictures, the IV can usually come out. It sometimes happens, though infrequently, that the dye irritates the vein and causes mild inflammation and tenderness in the vein for a few days afterward.

Voiding Cystourethrogram

In this x-ray study, the technician instills a dye visible on x-ray into the bladder through a thin flexible tube. You will then be asked to urinate forcefully to expel the dyed urine during the taking of the x-ray pictures. If the valves that separate the bladder from the ureters do not close properly (see Vesico-ureteral Reflux, page 1091), the pressure of urination will force some urine backward (up the ureter) toward the kidney.

Filling the bladder with dye for the voiding cystourethrogram (VCUG) can cause a feeling of uncomfortable fullness and swelling, and since you will be awake for the procedure, you will have to put up with a short period of discomfort. It is not significantly painful and will not last long; you will soon be able to get some relief by urinating. Once you have completed the VCUG, you should feel fine.

Magnetic Resonance Imaging and Computed Tomography

These specialized tests are used to investigate many health problems. Magnetic resonance imaging (MRI) relies on computer integration of magnetic images to generate an almost three-dimensional picture of the structures under examination. Computed tomography (CT) scan uses x-rays to the same effect. (Before undergoing an MRI, you will be asked if there is metal in your body, such as a pacemaker. If so, the test will not be performed.) In the urinary tract, these tests work especially well to evaluate the kidneys, to detect cysts (fluid-filled cavities), stones, and tumors (tissue masses).

You will remain awake for an MRI or CT scan, and apart from placing an IV, the test is not painful. You will lie on a movable table that will slide into a tunnel-like cylinder for the test. If the test requires your head and neck to be inside the tunnel, you will have mirrors that allow you to see out and this will lessen the claustrophobic feeling. The machine makes whirring, tapping, and drumming noises intermittently; the MRI machine can be particularly loud. There is no pain associated with these tests. If the CT scan requires dye, you may feel some flushing or wooziness or a sensation of burning along the vein as the dye flows into it. These sensations pass quickly and once the test is complete, you should feel fine. Dye may be associated with temporary kidney failure if the kidneys are not working normally. This will be explained to you before the test.

Cystoscopy

The doctor directly examines the inner wall of the urinary bladder and openings to the ureters by passing a lighted rigid or flexible viewing scope into the bladder. The cystoscope lets the operator view the walls, take samples of abnormal tissue, and burn away small areas of abnormal tissue.

Although you will usually be awake for this test, because inserting the cystoscope can sometimes be uncomfortable most doctors will numb the area with local anesthetic medication to block the pain. (In children, the doctor may request that general anesthesia be used during the test.) With the local anesthetic to block the pain, you should tolerate the test without difficulty. If the purpose of the test was just to look, you should have minimal discomfort following the test. If the doctor removed a stone or tissue, you might experience a little discomfort or some irritation from blood in the urine afterward. ■

because the bladder is connected to the kidneys through the ureters, making it possible for infection to ascend from the bladder and cause kidney infection. See Acute Pyelonephritis, page 1082, for information on this type of kidney infection.

Although cystitis is common in sexually active women, repeated infections in this group as well as cystitis in prepubescent girls and males of any age merit evaluation by a doctor (see Evaluation of Chronic Urinary Infections, above). In men over age 50, urinary tract infections become more common and are often associated with incomplete emptying of the bladder due to benign prostate hypertrophy (see page 1146).

Repeated infection may signal abnormalities in the anatomy of the urinary tract that could, if undiagnosed, increase the risk of kidney damage.

What you can do At the first sign of possible infection, increase your intake of water and fluids such as cranberry juice (which contains hippuric acid, thought to have some slight added value in preventing infection). For a short period (1 or 2 days), the frequent and urgent need-to-go symptoms can be relieved by taking an over-the-counter (OTC) urinary tract antispasmodic medication containing pyridium in low dosages. These remedies should not be taken for more than a few days because the medication masks the pain and might allow a serious infection to go untreated and gain a foothold. Do not take antibiotics without checking with your doctor. This can make a serious infection harder to treat.

When to call the doctor A urinary tract infection should always be evaluated by a doctor. If symptoms develop—particularly if bloody urine or significant fever (over 100° F) develops—call your doctor right away.

Treatment Identifying and killing the invading bacteria with antibiotics is the cornerstone of therapy. Depending on the severity of symptoms and the choice of medication, your doctor may prescribe a course of treatment lasting 3 days, 7 days, or 10 days or may prescribe a single dose. Be certain to take all the medication that is prescribed. Although symptoms should disappear in 1 to 2 days, more time is needed to completely eliminate the bacteria. Taking only a portion of the antibiotics may make the infection harder to treat later. For frequently recurring infections, daily long-term, low-dosage antibiotic therapy to suppress infection, taking hygienic precautions, or even taking antibiotics at the time of sexual relations may be necessary.

Prognosis When identified and treated properly, the prognosis is excellent for rapid, full recovery.

❖ URETHRITIS

Symptoms (*What you may experience*)

Gradual onset of the following: burning or stinging on urination; discharge of fluid from the urethral opening (the discharge may be watery or thick; cloudy, clear, or discolored).

Signs and laboratory findings (*What the doctor looks for*) Bacteria- and infection-fighting white blood cells on microscopic examination of the discharge fluid; growth of bacteria in the lab from samples of the discharge fluid; common bacterial causes (*Chlamydia trachomatis* or *Neisseria gonorrhea*) as detected by rapid office tests.

What is it? Bacterial infection of the urethra occurs commonly, especially in men, usually causing symptoms of burning or stinging on urination. It probably represents the most common type of urinary tract infection in men. Almost always, men contract the infection through sexual contact with an infected partner. (Although in men urethritis usually causes considerable discomfort, the vaginal infection may cause no detectable symptoms in women, leading to the unwitting spread of infection.)

What you can do Prevent contracting an infection of the urethra by safe sexual practices (use a protective barrier, such as a condom, during intercourse).

When to call the doctor Intense discomfort with urination, particularly if it is accompanied by fever, severe pain, or discharge, should prompt a visit to the doctor as soon as possible. Also, any sexual contact with a person at risk for a sexually transmitted disease, even if you are asymptomatic, should prompt a visit to the doctor.

Treatment Antibiotics to eradicate the infecting bacteria form the cornerstone of therapy for urethritis. Effective medications include a single dose of a long-acting cephalosporin, such as ceftriaxone, followed by a 7-day course of fluoroquinolones such as floxacin, a 7-day course of doxycycline, or a single dose of the antibiotic azithromycin (a form of erythromycin). Erythromycin is the best choice in pregnant women.

Because the infection can pass from person to person through sexual contact, both the infected person and any sexual partners should receive treatment.

Prognosis Excellent if diagnosed promptly and fully treated. Failure to treat could result in the infection's progression, with the possibility of infection of deeper tissues or scarring of the reproductive tissues.

❖ HEMATURIA (BLOOD IN THE URINE)

Symptoms (What you may experience) Pain upon urination; urinary urgency; pain in the lower abdomen over the bladder (sometimes); pain in the side (sometimes). It is possible to have hematuria and experience no other symptoms.

Signs and laboratory findings (What the doctor looks for) Blood in the urine on dipstick test or visible with the microscope. Protein in the urine may indicate a problem within the kidney itself.

What is it? Hematuria, meaning blood in the urine, occurs for a wide variety of reasons. Common causes include infection, passage of a kidney stone (see page 1088), the side effect of certain medications (anticancer medication and some antibiotics), damage from toxic substances (such as occurs during abuse of the pain medications propoxyphene, acetaminophen, and nonsteroidal anti-inflammatories), trauma (see Kidney Injury, page 1074), and benign prostatic hypertrophy (see page 1146). Hematuria also may occur as a complication of other major diseases such as glomerulonephritis (see page 1084), sickle cell anemia (see page 927), diabetes mellitus (see page 1174), and cancers of the urinary tract (see Cancer of the Bladder, page 1075, and Cancer of the Kidney, page 1094).

When urinary bleeding occurs in an amount sufficient to see with the naked eye, it can be both painful and frightening—even a small amount of blood in the urine looks like a lot. Take note of any other symptoms that occur along with the bleeding; this information will give your doctor important clues to the cause. For example, does pain accompany the bleeding? If so, note how severe it is, where you feel it (at the site of urine passage, in the lower abdomen, or in your back), and when (unrelated to passing urine, only at the start of passing the urine, only at the end, or throughout urination). Note whether the urine smells strong or foul (indicators of infection) and whether you have fever, feel nauseated, or vomit. Because so many disorders can cause the bleeding, it is essential that a doctor evaluate you.

Initial evaluation of bleeding is simple—a urinalysis in the office to determine if infection is the cause. More elaborate tests and procedures such as urine cytology (a test to look for cancerous cells in the urine specimen), x-ray procedures, or cystoscopy (see Evaluation of Chronic Urinary Infections, page 1069) are used to rule out other disorders. A 24-hour urine test for protein excretion may be ordered to determine if the kidneys' filtering units are damaged.

When to call the doctor Any passage of blood in the urine demands a visit to your doctor as soon as possible.

Treatment The best mode of therapy depends upon the cause of the bleeding. See specific disorders mentioned above for treatment.

Prognosis If infection is the cause of hematuria, the prognosis is excellent with prompt diagnosis and treatment; however, the prognosis for other causes, such as diseases of the kidneys or bladder, depends on the extent of the disease. Even in these cases, early diagnosis and prompt treatment improves prognosis, again underscoring the importance of never ignoring blood in the urine.

❖ URINARY INCONTINENCE (LEAKY BLADDER)

Symptoms (What you may experience) Involuntary loss or leakage of urine.

Signs and laboratory findings (What the doctor looks for) Sometimes: evidence of blood or infection in the urinalysis; evidence of uterine, bladder, or urethral prolapse (displacement) or enlarged prostate; weakness of the muscles of the pelvis or rectum. Associated signs depend on the underlying cause.

What is it? Incontinence occurs commonly in the older population, affecting as many as 25 percent of seniors. The problem occurs often in middle-aged women who have borne multiple children and suffer from pelvic relaxation (see page 1120). Loss of urine can occur for several reasons relating to the bladder muscle or the bladder sphincter (the thick muscle layer controlling the outlet between the bladder and the urethra). There are four types of incontinence.

- *Stress incontinence* occurs when coughing, sneezing, straining, physical activity, or laughing causes urine to leak, often in a sudden spurt; these activities abruptly increase the pressure in the abdomen (and therefore the bladder) and place an added stress on the muscular bladder wall and bladder sphincter. This form commonly afflicts women with uterine prolapse and pelvic relaxation because stretching of the liga-

ments that support the uterus and bladder prevents the normal continence mechanism from working. In menopausal women, loss of estrogen can lead to weakness of the pelvic support tissues, as well.

- *Overflow incontinence* occurs when the bladder fills beyond its capacity to hold; urine dribbles out as the kidneys continue to produce more urine. This form of incontinence often occurs in elderly men who suffer from an enlarged prostate (see Benign Prostatic Hypertrophy, page 1146) The large prostate gland compresses the urethra, preventing adequate outflow of urine and leading to excessive filling and bladder distention (see Urinary Retention, page 1073).

- *Urge incontinence* occurs most commonly when the bladder muscle becomes spastic (characterized by spasms) with excessive stimulation from infection, inflammation, prostatic enlargement, or problems with bladder control. In this form of incontinence, the leakage usually follows an urgent need to urinate, hence the name.

- *Total incontinence* occurs when the bladder sphincter completely fails, usually because of damage to the nerve supply (spinal cord injury, for example), to the nerves or muscle during surgery, from cancer spreading to the area, or when a fistula develops (an abnormal connection between the bladder and the surface of the skin or the vagina). Fistulas can arise due to childbirth, surgery, pelvic irradiation, cancer, chronic indwelling catheter (used in people who have lost function of the bladder and must wear a catheter to drain urine), or chronic infection or occur as a congenital (present at birth) defect.

What you can do   If you suffer from incontinence (or care for someone who does) you can provide protection from accidents with special absorbent shields (in cases of mild to moderate amounts of leakage) designed slightly differently for men and women; in cases of large-volume incontinence, fully protecting and absorbent disposable undergarments designed for adults of either gender can be used.

KEGEL EXERCISES TO IMPROVE BLADDER CONTROL

Dr. Arnold Kegel developed this set of exercises to strengthen the muscles of the pelvic floor. Contraction and relaxation of these muscles allows voluntary control of urination. When the muscles weaken, as they sometimes do after bearing the added weight of multiple pregnancies, control over urine flow may fail and leakage or loss of urine can result. By exercising the muscles, you can strengthen them and in many cases regain or improve bladder control.

You must first locate the muscles you are trying to exercise. Here is an easy way to locate them: Allow the urine to flow, then try to slow or stop the stream without using the muscles of your abdomen, legs, or buttocks. Think of tensing the muscles around the opening of the vagina, pulling them inward and upward. Once the urine slows or stops, become aware of the muscles that are doing the work. Notice how the pull of those muscles feels. Another method is to contract the rectal area as though you were attempting to stop the passage of gas. This action also tenses the correct muscles. Now begin to exercise the muscles regularly, three or four times each day as follows:

- Tighten the muscles by squeezing them slowly to a count of four and then relaxing them slowly to a count of four. (If the muscles are extremely weak, begin by contracting and relaxing to a slow two count and then work up to more.)

- Repeat the cycle of tightening and relaxation nine more times for a total of 10 sets.

- Do these sets of 10 cycles morning, noon, evening, and at bedtime.

Be sure to check your technique in the mirror now and then to be certain you are not using your stomach or buttock muscles by placing your hand on your abdomen or buttocks as you tighten. Your hand should not feel your abdomen or buttocks tighten if you are doing the exercises correctly. You should see some improvement in bladder control within 3 or 4 weeks. ■

In cases related to pelvic relaxation, strengthening the muscle tone of the pelvic support muscles may reduce episodes of stress incontinence (see Kegel Exercises to Improve Bladder Control, page 1072).

When to call the doctor The development of recurrent or persistent episodes of urine leakage should prompt a visit to the doctor.

Treatment The treatment approach depends on the type of incontinence and the cause.

- *Stress incontinence* therapies include surgical and nonsurgical options. If low estrogen has weakened or thinned the surrounding tissues, application of estrogen creams to the vaginal and urethral openings may be all that is needed. Medications to improve the strength of the urethral muscle tone, such as phenylpropanolamine, may also help. When the pelvic support has relaxed, bladder resuspension (surgery to pull the bladder back up to its proper location) will usually correct the problem.

- *Overflow incontinence* therapy is directed at the underlying cause of the obstruction to bladder emptying (see Urinary Retention, below). In cases in which the cause is spasm of the urethra or a noncontracting bladder, such as may occur in association with diabetes mellitus, the best course may be to train the patient in the technique of self-catheterization (insertion of a sterile catheter through the urethra and into the bladder to drain the urine) to prevent the overflow.

- *Urge incontinence* treatment relies on making the muscular wall of the bladder or urethra less irritated and spastic by treating the underlying problem—infection—or treating the symptoms with medications such as oxybutynin (Ditropan), propantheline (Pro-Banthine), or tricyclic antidepressant medications such as imipramine.

- *Total incontinence* usually requires a surgical remedy; for example, a bladder damaged by trauma, surgery, or cancer may be reconstructed or a new bladder may be constructed and an access port created that can be catheterized.

Prognosis In most cases the prognosis is good with appropriate surgical or nonsurgical treatment.

❖ URINARY RETENTION

Symptoms *(What you may experience)* Dribbling of urine after urination; urine leakage following urgent need to urinate; inability to urinate even with painful bladder fullness; urine infections.

Signs and laboratory findings *(What the doctor looks for)* Incomplete emptying of the bladder (more than 100 mL of urine left in bladder after urination).

What is it? The term urinary retention means that the voluntary act of urination fails to empty all the urine from the bladder. This situation occurs most commonly in men and in the majority of cases is the result of enlargement of the prostate gland (see Benign Prostatic Hypertrophy, page 1146). Since the prostate gland surrounds the urethra, enlargement of the gland can prevent urine outflow. Urethral stricture (scarring or narrowing of the tube leading from the bladder to the outside) or meatal stenosis (narrowing of the opening of the urethra) can also obstruct urine release. Stricture usually occurs due to scarring from previous urethral infections (such as gonorrhea), surgery, or trauma. Radiation (x-ray) therapy for cancer in nearby areas (the prostate gland in men or the reproductive organs in women, for example) can occasionally cause damage to the urethra and result in stricture formation. A stricture can also occur as a congenital defect. Another structural cause that can obstruct the free outflow of urine is cancer (see Cancer of the Bladder, page 1075, and Prostate Cancer, pages 1147 and 1360). Any of these structural causes of obstruction can bring about retention of urine.

Certain medications—cold remedies such as decongestants, narcotic analgesics, calcium channel blockers used in treating hypertension (high pressure), spinal and general anesthetics, and the anticancer medication vincristine—can cause temporary urinary retention. In people taking any of these medications, the sudden development of painful bladder fullness accompanied by an inability to pass urine should raise suspicion about the medication. Discontinuing the medication will usually resolve the disorder in time; however, relief of pain may require immediate medical attention to drain the bladder of urine. As the bladder has a finite capacity for storage (the average bladder holding about 500 mL without discomfort), prompt relief of the retention is important.

In some cases, weakness of the bladder muscle may prevent the bladder from emptying fully, sometimes leaving as much as 450 mL of urine or more. This may occur as a result of diabetes mellitus, which can damage the nerves that control bladder emptying.

What you can do Middle-aged men known or suspected to have enlargement of the prostate gland should be cautious in taking OTC cold and allergy remedies. These medications may cause the muscle in the prostate gland to contract and suddenly obstruct the outflow of urine, causing extreme discomfort.

When to call the doctor Any time you experience significant pain from bladder fullness and you cannot urinate, seek immediate medical help. This condition must be remedied by placement of a catheter to drain the urine from the bladder. Failure to relieve the obstruction could result in kidney failure and acute azotemia (the retention in the blood of excessive amounts of waste product).

The persistence of dribbling, difficulty in getting the urine stream started, or a change in the force or volume of the urine stream warrants a prompt visit to the doctor. These symptoms, while not as urgently dangerous as a complete inability to urinate, indicate partial obstruction of the flow. The precise cause and management must be sought.

Treatment Complete blockage of the flow of urine is an emergency that requires placement of a catheter to drain the bladder of urine. If greater than 500 mL of urine drains during this catheterization procedure, the bladder has been overfilled and stretched. This will fatigue the muscle of the bladder wall, preventing normal contraction and urine release. The bladder may need a rest and the doctor must leave the catheter in place until the muscle can recover its ability to contract normally (sometimes for as little as 8 hours, other times for a day or

more). Alternately, patients can learn to catheterize themselves until bladder function returns.

Retention caused by stricture or meatal stenosis requires dilation (widening) of the narrowed area. In this procedure, the doctor inserts a small, blunt metal rod into the urethral opening to slightly stretch the narrowed area. Then one after another, progressively wider rods will follow, each only a tiny bit wider than the last, and each gently stretching the narrowed area a bit more.

Occasionally, the stricture or stenosis is narrowed severely enough to require surgery to adequately enlarge the area. See Cancer of the Bladder, page 1075, for information about therapies employed to relieve obstruction caused by cancer. See Prostate Cancer, pages 1147 and 1360, and Benign Prostatic Hypertrophy, page 1146, for information about therapies employed to relieve obstructions related to the prostate gland.

When urine pools and stagnates in the bladder, gravel or sediment can form. Most bladder stones pass on their own, but because the bladder is a large holding bag, a small stone within it may go undetected for some time. As layer upon layer of sediment encrusts the small stone, it may become too large to easily pass through the outflow opening to the outside. Your doctor can determine whether it can be dissolved through medication or removed with a cystoscope passed through the urethra into the bladder.

Prognosis Meatal stenosis and strictures respond well to treatment, but they tend to tighten again, and in time usually require repeated dilation or surgical correction. The prognosis for other causes varies. See specific entries as referenced above.

❖ KIDNEY/BLADDER/ URETHRAL INJURY

Symptoms *(What you may experience)* History of trauma to the abdomen or back; blood in the urine; pain in the side (from kidney trauma); pain in the lower abdomen or lower back; nausea; swelling of the abdomen.

Signs and laboratory findings *(What the doctor looks for)* Blood in the urine and abdominal swelling and tenderness; bruising over the flank or lower abdomen; fever (occasionally); significant hypotension (low blood pressure).

What is it? Injury to the kidney and connecting ureters rarely occurs by virtue of their position deep within the body. The rib cage and a thick surrounding fat pad confer protection from external trauma, and the ureters run their course safely deep within the abdomen. The bladder, cradled within the pelvis, is sheltered from external trauma. A penetrating injury, such as a stabbing or shooting, a blunt trauma, a fall from great height, or a motor vehicle accident, may cause injury to the vital urinary tract structures.

Bruising of the kidney with resultant bleeding may resolve itself without special treatment; however, hospitalization and careful observation are usually in order to watch for such complications as infection, hemorrhage (bleeding), or shock from damage to the blood supply. (Shock in a medical sense does not imply emotional trauma but rather a potentially serious fall in blood pressure.) Damage to the blood supply of the kidney can quickly bring about severe impairment of kidney function. Laceration (tearing) of the kidney or ureter, rupture of the bladder, or laceration of the urethra will usually require surgery.

When to call the doctor Do not ignore symptoms of urinary bleeding, bruising of the back or abdomen, or pain following a fall or motor vehicle accident. Immediate medical evaluation is necessary.

Treatment An injury to the bladder or urinary tubes will often require surgical repair—in effect, sewing the torn area back together, followed by drainage of the area in and around the injured organs.

Following surgery, since the kidneys continue to produce urine, a catheter is left in the bladder to drain the urine or to keep the injured urethra open.

If infection occurs, intravenous antibiotics to eradicate the bacteria will be necessary.

Lacerated kidneys will often heal themselves. Severe lacerations may sometimes respond to simple repair by sewing the torn area back together; however, the injury may

be sufficiently severe to require kidney removal.

Shock requires the administration of intravenous fluids. Blood transfusion may be necessary to stabilize blood pressure.

Prognosis Good, depending on the extent of injury. A good portion of a single kidney can prove sufficient to preserve kidney function, so even if the injury results in loss of one kidney the prognosis is favorable for a full and normal life. The most common and potentially serious complication following injury to the ureters or urethra is scarring (which may cause narrowing) following the repair of the tear.

❖ CANCER OF THE BLADDER

Symptoms *(What you may experience)* Sometimes: increased frequency of urination; urgent need to urinate; discomfort during urination; visible blood in the urine.

Signs and laboratory findings *(What the doctor looks for)* Blood in the urine (visible or detectable by chemical or microscopic examination in 90 percent of cases); cancerous cells as detected by cytology of the urine (usually); cancerous cells as revealed by biopsy of abnormal tissue seen through the cystoscope.

What is it? Bladder cancer, like cancer of the skin, begins superficially, with 98 percent of cases arising in the epithelium (the thin protective layer of skin) lining the inside of the bladder. Most fall under the rubric transitional cell carcinoma, denoting their origin in the special surface cells of the bladder called transitional epithelial cells. Only about 2 percent arise from other types of cells within the bladder.

The disease usually strikes people ages 60 to 70 and occurs almost three times more commonly in men than in women. Cigarette smoking is responsible for 50 percent of all cases of bladder cancer; if you are a smoker, your risk of bladder cancer increases fourfold. Stopping smoking decreases, but does not eliminate, the increased risk. Chronic exposure to industrial dyes or solvents also increases the risk, accounting for 10 to 15 percent of all cases of bladder cancer.

Because the problem begins in the surface of the bladder, unless it happens to

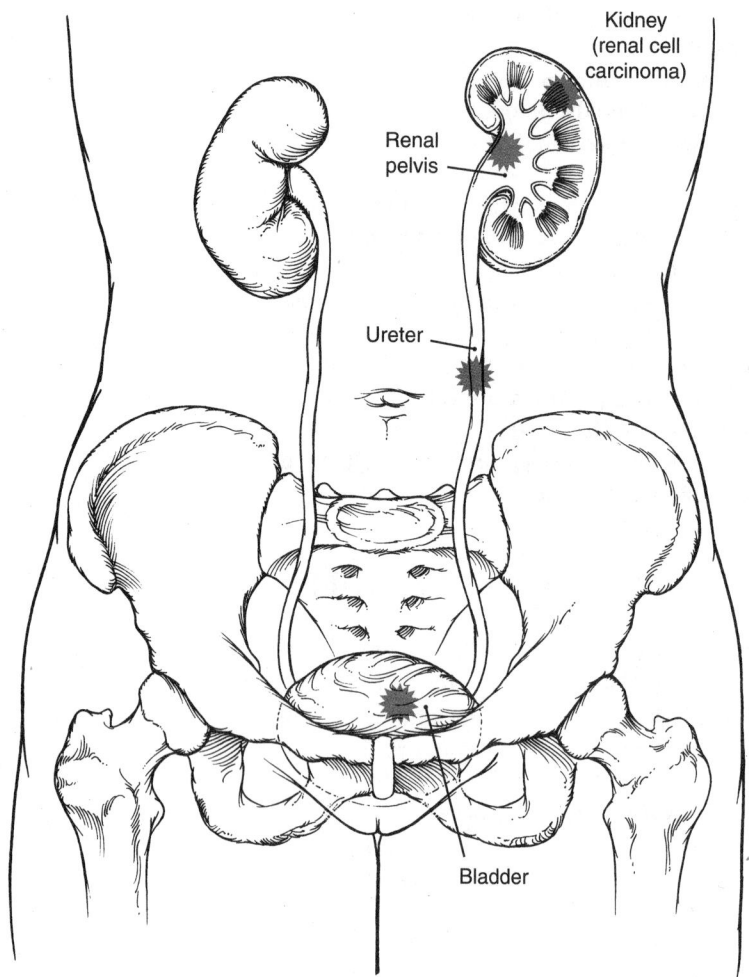

Kidney
(renal cell
carcinoma)

Renal
pelvis

Ureter

Bladder

Urinary cancer may cause bloody urine, discomfort during urination, or increased frequency of urination. Most cancers that arise in the kidney are renal cell carcinomas, which originate in the proximal, or central, tubule. Bladder cancer is the most common cancer of the collecting system in adults. Cancer can also occur in the renal pelvis or, more rarely, in the ureter or urethra. Other types of urinary system tumors are more common in children.

develop in a location near the bladder opening where it might cause irritation during urination, it may go undetected for a substantial period of time. Bladder cancer almost always causes some degree of bleeding; amounts invisible to the naked eye can be detected by chemical or microscopic examination of the urine specimen. Since blood in the urine represents the first detectable sign of cancer for 85 to 90 percent of people, those people at highest risk should have their urine examined regularly for blood.

The natural course of bladder cancer and the optimum treatment for it depend on the stage of the tumor (how deeply it has penetrated the surrounding and underlying areas) and whether it has metastasized (spread) to areas such as lymph nodes or other organs. In about 50 percent to 75 percent of bladder cancers, discovery occurs in the least invasive stages (when the cancer is completely localized within the epithelial layer without invasion into deeper layers). Spread to lymph nodes or other organs rarely occurs with these superficial tumors. Once the tumor has penetrated more deeply into the muscular wall of the bladder or surrounding fat layer, the tendency for metastases to lymph nodes or distant sites increases. As with most cancers, early detection and treatment dramatically improve prognosis. See Chapter 30 for more information on cancer diagnosis and treatment.

What you can do If you smoke, stop, because smoking clearly raises the risk for this cancer.

When to call the doctor Anytime you note the appearance of blood in the urine, you should see the doctor. Painless passage of blood is especially characteristic of cancers of the urinary tract, although other causes can account for it.

Treatment Treatment usually involves removal and examination of the cancerous tissue by means of the cystoscope. The staging of the tumor will then be identified and the type of cell that became cancerous will be determined.

Tumors that show no invasion to layers beyond the epithelium may require no further treatment except frequent surveillance for recurrence. For aggressive or recurrent early stage cancers, the doctor may recommend intravesical chemotherapy (cancer-destroying medications instilled directly into the bladder through a catheter). The usual regimen involves weekly administration of the chemotherapeutic medication for 6 weeks. Discomfort and bleeding with urination frequently occur as side effects of this kind of therapy.

Tumors that have invaded into the muscle of the bladder wall may require more aggressive treatment, usually with an exended field of surgery including the following:

- *Radical cystectomy* involves removal of the bladder, surrounding fat and support ligaments, and the prostate and the seminal vesicles (glands that contribute secretions to the ejaculate) in men or, in women, the uterus, cervix, urethra, ovaries, and a portion of the wall of the vagina adjacent to the bladder. If control of the disease demands that the surgeon remove the bladder entirely, an artificial reservoir may be created to hold urine. The ileal conduit—the most common and successful method used to achieve this goal—uses a small section of intestine to function as the bladder into which the doctor sews the ureter from each kidney. This artificial bladder is sewn to the inside of the abdominal wall and empties through a small hole on the front of the abdomen into a plastic pouch. As the pouch fills with urine, the patient can easily empty it. In some cases, the surgeon may be able to construct a new bladder from the intestine; this procedure, called a continent diversion, does not require a drainage bag.

- *Radiation therapy* X-rays are used to destroy tumor cells. Although tolerated fairly well, radiation therapy is fraught with unpleasant gastrointestinal complications. Used alone, the risk of recurrence of the cancer can be as high as 30 to 70 percent.

- *Systemic chemotherapy* The use of cancer-destroying medications administered by mouth or vein can improve survival in cases in which the cancer has spread to lymph nodes or to distant organs. Usually a combination of chemotherapeutic medications is used, often including cisplatin.

Prognosis Survival is excellent for bladder cancers detected early (while still involving only the epithelial layer) and treated promptly and properly. The prognosis, as for most cancers, declines with delay in discovery or treatment, underscoring the importance of never ignoring blood in the urine.

The Kidneys

The kidneys lie in the right and left sides of the back at the bottom of the ribcage where they are protected by the ribs and a cushioning fat pad. This pair of vital organs has many functions. They serve as the body's fil-

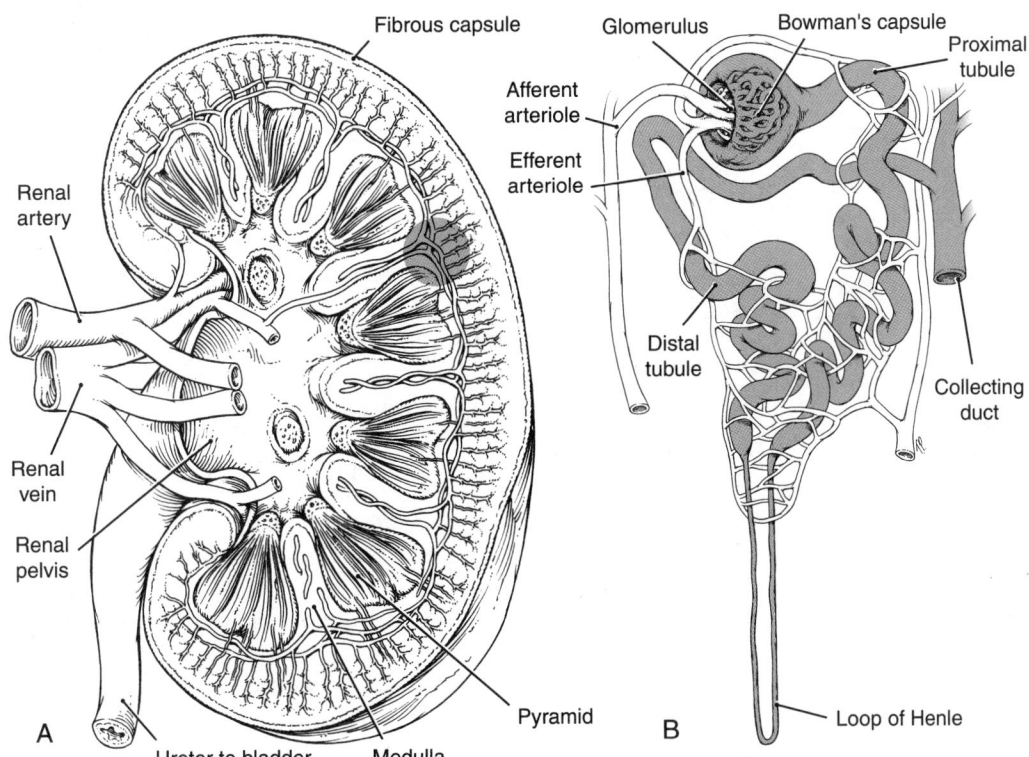

Renal artery

Renal vein

Renal pelvis

A — Ureter to bladder — Medulla — Pyramid

Fibrous capsule

Glomerulus — **Bowman's capsule** — **Proximal tubule**

Afferent arteriole

Efferent arteriole

Distal tubule

Collecting duct

B — Loop of Henle

(A) Two kidneys, each about 10 to 12 cm long, rid the body of nitrogen-containing waste products and regulate the body's balance of fluid, acid, and electrolytes such as potassium. Kidneys take in blood, filter it, and produce urine for excretion. (B) Each kidney contains a million or more tiny filtering units called nephrons that are located in the cortex or near the medulla. Blood is filtered in the glomerulus and then passes through a series of tubules, where water and various chemicals such as sodium, chloride, glucose, amino acids, and hydrogen may flow across the tubules' membranes. The collecting duct then returns the processed urine to the renal pelvis for transport to the urinary bladder.

ters to cleanse the blood of waste products. They regulate the amount of fluid in the body and of vital chemicals such as sodium, potassium, acid, and calcium. In addition to their vital role in cleansing the blood, the kidneys function as glands, producing a hormone called renin that regulates blood pressure and another called erythropoietin which regulates blood count. The kidneys are also responsible for making the active form of vitamin D, which helps regulate calcium in the body. Although nature normally endows us with two kidneys, one healthy one (or even a part of one in reasonably good working order) can suffice if needed.

How the Kidneys Work

Almost 2 pints of blood laden with waste products arrive at the kidneys via the renal

The glomerulus consists of a mass of convoluted, or coiled, capillaries containing tiny pores. Waste products, other chemicals, and some water crosses into the tubules. Filtered fluid must pass through the capillary endothelium (lining), capillary basement membrane, and the podocyte, which envelops the glomerular capillaries. An inflamed kidney may allow larger particles, such as proteins or blood cells, to pass into the urine, and these particles may be detectable through laboratory testing.

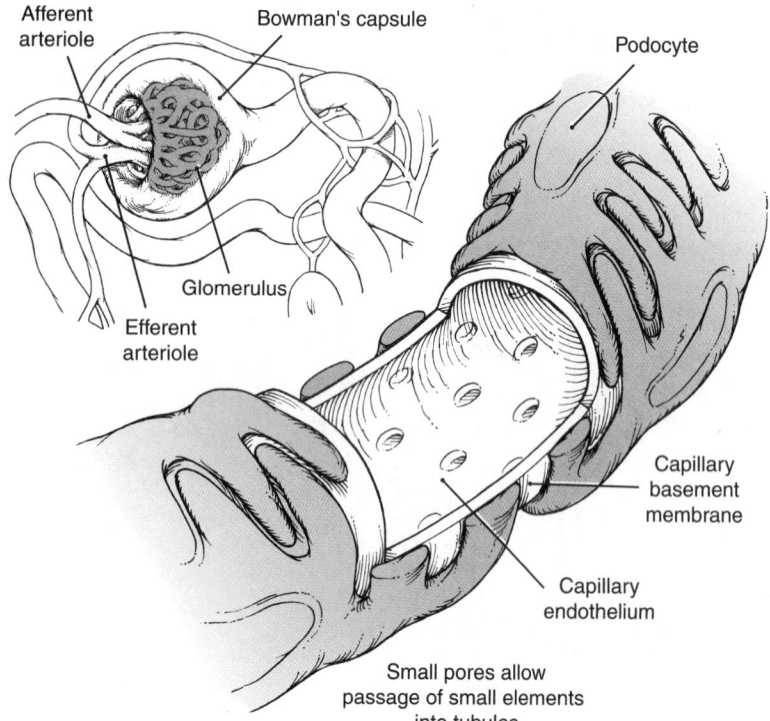

Afferent arteriole

Bowman's capsule

Podocyte

Glomerulus

Efferent arteriole

Capillary basement membrane

Capillary endothelium

Small pores allow passage of small elements into tubules

arteries (one going to each kidney) every minute. This blood is carried through ever smaller renal arteries into the specialized filtering structures.

The kidneys contain millions of nephrons, tiny filtering units that have two parts. The glomerulus filters waste and fluid from the blood to create urine, and the tubule concentrates and excretes the waste products into the urine while allowing water and essential salts, minerals, and nutrients to be reabsorbed back into the bloodstream. The glomerulus consists of a twisted mass of convoluted capillaries (the tiniest blood vessels) with sieve-like walls perforated by tiny filtration pores. Large particles, including blood cells and proteins, remain in the bloodstream while waste products, electrolytes, nutrients, and some of the water cross into the tubule. When the kidneys become infected or inflamed, the glomeruli allow larger molecules to pass into the urine. That is why doctors test urine for protein, an indication that the kidneys are not functioning properly. Blood cells may also pass through if the holes are large enough.

In the tubule, several sophisticated hormonal processes occur that determine which substances will be excreted and which will be reabsorbed into the bloodstream. In the tubules, the kidneys adjust the acidity of the blood as well as the water, salt, and mineral content. Once the blood has been filtered, it leaves the kidney through the renal vein. The collected waste fluid passes as urine through ever larger collecting tubes. The collecting tubes coalesce in the kidney's core and drain via the ureter to the bladder. The kidneys produce urine continually, day and night, passing about $3^{1}/_{2}$ pints daily, though this can vary considerably depending upon how much you drink.

❖ KIDNEY FAILURE

Symptoms *(What you may experience)*

- *Acute failure:* Rarely, none; in other cases, loss of appetite; nausea; vomiting; malaise (loss of sense of well-being); sudden decrease in urine production; headache; muscle cramps or spastic twitches; drowsiness.

- *Chronic failure:* progressive worsening of the above symptoms; metallic taste in the mouth; hiccups; itching; bronze color to the skin; mental dullness.

Signs and laboratory findings (What the doctor looks for)

- *Acute failure:* Blood tests demonstrating a sudden elevation of blood urea nitrogen (BUN) and creatinine (substances in the blood that serve as indicators of kidney function), high levels of potassium and acid, low levels of calcium, and high levels of phosphorus; elevation of blood pressure (sometimes); a pericardial friction rub (scratchy heart noise heard through the stethoscope), seizures, coma (occasionally).

- *Chronic failure:* Progression of the signs listed above; anemia; asterixis (flapping movements in the hands if held out straight as if stopping traffic).

What is it? As a consequence of certain medical problems, the function of the kidneys can decline sharply, a condition termed acute kidney failure. Conditions that block the flow of urine—enlarged prostate, meatal stenosis, or cancers—can cause back pressure on the kidney's filtering tissues, which may lead to varying degrees of kidney failure. Sometimes, not enough blood is able to reach the kidney, which causes irreversible kidney failure. This may occur with severe dehydration from nausea, vomiting, or diarrhea. Other causes include severe heart failure and infections, which lower blood pressure and therefore blood flow to the kidneys. Certain medications (such as angiotensin-converting enzyme inhibitors and nonsteroidal anti-inflammatory drugs) may change blood flow to the kidney's glomerulus and cause irreversible kidney damage. These medications should be used with caution if there is underlying kidney disease. If blood flow is restored, kidney functions should improve to normal within a few days.

Kidney tubule damage from a toxin brings on the acute failure. Such damage can come from outside the body—such as a reaction to antibiotics, x-ray dye, or other medications.

The damaging agent can arise from within the body. For example, natural body substances such as the pigments that give color to blood or muscle, can damage the

NUTRITION IN KIDNEY DISEASE

The nutritional management of kidney disease is complex; each person is different and dietary guidelines must be tailored to fit. You will work closely with a dietitian or nutritionist to construct a diet regimen that meets your needs. Some basic tenets exist, however.

Protein Intake Sufficient protein intake is needed to repair the wear and tear of living; however, for people with damaged kidneys, protein is a two-edged sword. Too much of it can cause an elevation of BUN and place an added burden on the already damaged kidney. Too little of it, and the body begins to consume its own protein stores—muscle mass—to harvest a supply of critical protein building blocks necessary for the business of living. This harvest will also elevate BUN. The patient with limited kidney function must walk a fine line between getting enough protein to meet daily needs and not overdoing it. A protein-restricted diet may be prescribed by your doctor.

Salt and Water Restriction This is necessary in people with kidney disease who have hypertension or edema of the feet, lower legs, or abdomen.

Potassium Restriction Potassium restriction is a consideration when kidney function has fallen to low levels or if the tubules of the nephrons have been damaged as in some forms of interstitial nephritis (see page 1084). Foods rich in potassium include garbanzo beans, soy beans, and papaya. Other dried beans, apricots, bananas, melons, oranges, pears, prunes, artichokes, avocado, brussels sprouts, carrots, potatoes, pumpkin, spinach, and tomatoes also contain considerable amounts of potassium.

Phosphorus Restriction This is important in preventing damage to bones that can occur in kidney failure. Limiting foods high in phosphorus—eggs, dairy products, and meat—may be necessary. This can make finding enough protein difficult because all these foods also are excellent sources of protein.

Magnesium Restriction Restricting magnesium should always be a consideration because the failing kidney cannot eliminate it. Do not use any magnesium-containing antacids or laxative medications. ■

kidney if they reach it. Any injury that crushes muscle or any disorder that destroys muscle may liberate large quantities of the muscle pigment myoglobin into the blood.

Rarely, a condition that causes the widespread destruction of red blood cells (such as a reaction to transfused blood or a snake bite) liberates huge amounts of the red blood cell pigment hemoglobin into the blood. When blood containing these free pigments arrives at the kidneys to be filtered, the pigments damage and overwhelm the filtering units and escape into the urine. The urine may appear dark brown.

Sometimes during chemotherapy for leukemia the medication can cause the formation of extremely high levels of uric acid

DIALYSIS

We depend on our kidneys to cleanse our blood of waste, regulate chemicals, and remove fluid. If they cannot adequately perform these crucial jobs, the toxic compounds build up in the blood and, in effect, poison us. Fluid may fill the lungs and potassium and acid buildup can be fatal.

Kidney failure was a death sentence until the development of dialysis about 35 years ago. This medical breakthrough—which entails the use of a filtering machine (hemodialysis) or filtering fluids (peritoneal dialysis) to remove the toxins—allows people with temporary kidney failure to survive until their kidneys heal. It also enables an estimated 100,000 people with chronic and irreversible kidney damage to live reasonably normal and productive lives—keeping them going for years after their kidneys have failed them. Dialysis also can give some people with kidney failure the chance to remain healthy while awaiting a suitable donor for a kidney transplant.

As with any serious medical procedure, the benefits of dialysis must be carefully weighed against its risks. Complications associated with it include infection of the area of dialysis access, peritonitis, hypotension, and death (extremely rare).

How do doctors decide who should receive dialysis? In general, the decision makes itself. For example, the doctor will usually recommend dialysis when the kidneys can no longer put out enough urine to keep the body's fluid level in balance even with diuretic medications, or when they cannot remove enough acid, potassium, or magnesium from the blood. Doctors will also recommend dialysis if other medical problems such as pericarditis (inflammation of the covering over the heart), seizures, or coma develop because of kidney failure. Symptoms of kidney failure such as nausea, vomiting, or mental dullness also may prompt starting dialysis. Doctors routinely rely on two simple blood tests to help them make the determination of when to begin dialysis: blood creatinine and BUN. When the creatinine rises above 8 mg/dL or the BUN climbs to 100 mg/dL, the benefits of dialysis begin to outweigh the risks. Once kidney function is less than 10 percent of normal—or less than 15 percent of normal in diabetics—symptoms or signs occur which call for the start of dialysis. (These are rough guidelines; a doctor evaluates each person's condition in making the decision about when to start dialysis.) There are two methods of dialysis currently in use.

Hemodialysis

A dialysis machine filters the wastes directly from the blood through an access port. This point of access can be created by making a fistula, surgically joining an artery and a vein, almost always in the arm. Alternately, the doctor can gain reliable access to the bloodstream by means of a shunt, using a section of synthetic blood vessel to join the artery and vein. Occasionally, because a shunt or fistula may take time to be ready for use (a shunt, 2 to 4 weeks; a fistula, 4 to 8 weeks), a large tube called a hemodialysis catheter will be used at the start of hemodialysis. The catheter will be inserted underneath the collarbone, usually into a vein in the neck. This will be removed once the shunt or fistula is ready to use.

In emergencies, short-term catheters may be placed in large veins in the neck (underneath the collarbone) or in the leg. The technician will connect the tubing of the dialysis machine to the access port. The dirty blood leaves from the shunt or fistula through a tube and passes through the dialysis machine where artificial membranes function like the filtering units of the kidney, cleansing the blood of the toxic wastes and returning it into the port. Special fluids in the machine serve to balance the body's water level and chemicals. The process takes 3 to 4 hours on average to complete, and most patients will require three treatments each week, either at the dialysis center or in some cases at home.

Peritoneal Dialysis

Peritoneal dialysis takes advantage of the ease with which fluids can pass through the walls of the many capillaries (the tiniest blood vessels) within the abdominal cavity. In this procedure, the patient performs the dialysis at home, placing a volume of dialysis fluid into the abdominal cavity through an access port in the abdomen. The fluid is left in long enough to allow the toxic wastes to leave the blood and pass into the fluid within the cavity, then drained out. This is usually done 4 times per day. Continuous ambulatory peritoneal dialysis is the name of this method. Alternately, a machine can automatically do the exchanges at night while a person is sleeping, leaving some fluid in the abdomen during the day. This is called continuous cycler-assisted peritoneal dialysis. Providing an access port requires a doctor, who implants a permanent peritoneal dialysis catheter into the abdominal cavity. Because this method uses the tissues of the abdominal cavity lining—the peritoneal tissues—as the filtering membrane, peritonitis (the infection or inflammation of the peritoneal tissue) can complicate the process and is a serious concern. Peritoneal dialysis has been a boon to patients in whom blood vessel access is difficult—children with poor veins. Because this type of dialysis is performed at home, eliminating the need to go to a dialysis center three times a week, some people prefer it to hemodialysis. ■

in the blood. At high levels, uric acid can form into crystals and block urine flow in the nephrons, causing acute renal failure.

Severe infections that spread through the blood and some antibiotics used for treatment are common causes of acute kidney failure. Acute renal failure may develop postoperatively due to severe blood loss or decreased blood flow to the kidney (as sometimes occurs in aortic surgery or heart surgery).

Effects on the kidney such as those listed above typically cause a marked reduction of urine production within 1 or 2 days

KIDNEY TRANSPLANTATION

When the kidneys stop working, replacing them may be an option; however, not everyone with kidney failure is a candidate for transplantation. People with serious medical problems involving other organ systems—coronary artery disease, cancer, widespread active infection—are not generally considered healthy enough to undergo such a major operation. Age is not necessarily a prohibitive factor.

Once the transplant team has determined a person to be a good candidate for transplant, the next (and often most difficult) hurdle is to find a suitable donor. Because the body's vigilant immune defense system functions to attack and destroy any foreign substance that enters the body, the more similar the donated kidney is to the recipient's own tissues, the less likely that the body will reject it. The determination of a good match relies on tissue-typing studies that compare the identifying markers on the tissues of the recipient with those on the tissues of a potential donor. Usually, the best matches will be found from among the person's family members—in general, the closer the relation, the better the match. Because kidneys come in pairs and each of us can live quite nicely with just one healthy kidney, a willing donor can spare one kidney for a relative without compromising the donor's health. It is essential, however, to make certain that both of the donor's kidneys are healthy before removing one.

The idea of donating a kidney can be a daunting prospect even when willing. A new technique called laparoscopic nephrectomy, pioneered by doctors at Johns Hopkins, may revolutionize the removal of donor kidneys. The standard operation of the past entailed a major surgery to remove the donated kidney, an incision halfway around the donor's side, a 6-day hospital stay, and a recuperation lasting 3 months. In the new operation, the kidney is removed through an incision slightly larger than a silver dollar. After a 2-day hospital stay, the donor can more quickly return to a normal routine. The results of this new procedure are being evaluated.

When no kidneys are available from blood relations, transplant of closely matched cadaver kidneys (those donated after death) can be performed. Although transplants from living well-matched donors are statistically the most successful—more than 90 percent work well at the 1-year mark—good matches of cadaver kidneys work nearly as well at 1 year. Unfortunately, the wait for a cadaver kidney may last as long as 2 to 3 years.

In either event, the kidney transplant team must neutralize the recipient's immune defense system (with powerful inflammation-suppressing medications such as cyclosporine, prednisone, or Imuran) to give the body a chance to accept the new kidney. If the immune system brings its defenses to bear on the foreign organ, it will fail. If circumstances permit and another suitable kidney can be found, a second or rarely even a third transplant may be done, but the risk of rejection increases in these subsequent operations.

The chief ongoing hurdles for organ-transplant recipients include the ever-present risk of rejecting the organ and an increased susceptibility to infection, because the immune defenses must be continually suppressed with drugs. ∎

---

of the causative event. This period of reduced urine output can last from a few hours to several weeks, after which a period of increased urine output may begin. Usually the kidneys resume their functioning and the levels of the BUN and creatinine in the blood slowly begin to normalize. These are both good signs that recovery of kidney function has begun.

Other parts of the kidney can be affected such as the glomerulus. Infections and other diseases such as vasculitis can affect the glomerulus, causing acute glomerulonephritis (see page 1084). Areas between the tubules (interstitium) can also be affected.

Chronic damage to the kidney can result from a variety of medical disorders such as polycystic kidney disease (see page 1090), chronic hypertension, and chronic kidney infections. Glomerulonephritis causes more chronic kidney failure than any other cause. Diabetes mellitus is the most common cause of glomerulonephritis, causing kidney failure and requiring dialysis. Diabetes may lead to damage of the nephrons. The progression of kidney damage can go unnoticed for a prolonged period because symptoms may be mild until kidney function has dropped to less than 15 percent of normal. The damage from poorly controlled diabetes mellitus typically occurs gradually, progressing to chronic kidney failure and finally to total loss of kidney function in some patients with diabetes.

When the damage is extreme the kidneys usually become so scarred that they virtually cease to function. Survival in this condition—termed end-stage kidney disease—demands ongoing dialysis (see page 1080) or kidney transplantation (see above). Without dialysis, end-stage kidney disease is invariably fatal.

What you can do You *may* be able to minimize the damage, prolong kidney function, and withstand the rigors of ongoing dialysis by careful attention to diet (see Nutrition in Kidney Disease, page 1079) and use of medications, in some cases.

When to call the doctor Any sudden decrease in urine production or change in urine color, particularly if it follows a serious illness or injury, should prompt a call to the doctor right away.

Treatment Therapy for acute kidney failure must first address the underlying problem that caused the failure—for example, if a medication caused it, the medication must be stopped immediately, a blockage of urine flow should be relieved, or intravenous fluids should be given if the problem is severe dehydration. When the kidneys fail to produce urine, the initial therapy may be aimed at increasing production with diuretics (agents that increase urination) such as furosemide. If the kidney fails to respond by increasing production or if toxins or potassium build up, dialysis should begin, at least temporarily until the kidneys recover.

In chronic kidney failure, controlling hypertension and fluid balance with diuretics or antihypertensive medications may help preserve function. Great care must be taken not to use medications that prevent the loss of potassium (already a problem for the damaged kidney). These medications include triamterene, amiloride, spironolactone, and certain beta blockers. Even nonsteroidal anti-inflammatory drugs (NSAIDs), such as ibuprofen and others, can cause an increase in potassium. People with kidney disease should avoid these medications whenever possible. Angiotension-converting enzyme inhibitors can also increase blood potassium levels but are helpful in treating some kidney diseases such as chronic glomerulonephritis before severe damage has occurred; this will require careful monitoring of potassium.

When diet and medications are no longer effective in maintaining adequate kidney function, dialysis or transplantation must be performed.

Prognosis Those cases of acute kidney failure that are going to resolve will usually do so within 6 to 8 weeks, although it may take 6 months to a year to maximally recover function.

With appropriate dietary and medical management, patients with mild to moderate chronic kidney failure may live reasonably normal and productive lives for many, many years.

End-stage kidney disease is fatal unless dialysis is begun promptly or a kidney transplant is possible.

❖ ACUTE PYELONEPHRITIS

Symptoms (*What you may experience*) High fever, sometimes 102°F or higher; shaking chills (often); pain in the side (on either side at the junction of the ribcage and the low back) and discomfort with urination or the need to urinate urgently (commonly); nausea, vomiting, and diarrhea fairly often; malaise and weakness.

Signs and laboratory findings (*What the doctor looks for*) Tenderness to side percussion (tapping over the kidney); positive culture (growth of infecting bacteria) from a urine specimen; an elevation of white blood cells on blood count; white blood cells and perhaps white-blood-cell casts in the urinalysis. (Casts are formed by proteins made within the nephron, and represent damage within the kidney rather than in the bladder.) If a structural anomaly is suspected, an ultrasound, computed tomography (CT) scan, or intravenous pyelogram (IVP) may be performed.

What is it? Acute pyelonephritis (bacterial infection of the kidney) is more serious than cystitis. Infection reaches the kidney most often by ascending the ureter from the origin of the infection in the urinary bladder. Because a kidney infection implies a threat to the working tissues of a vital organ, it should be treated aggressively and thoroughly by a doctor.

Infections involve the kidney more commonly when a structural abnormality exists—for example, when a stone obstructs a portion of the urine-collecting system, when the kidney lies in an abnormal position, or when the urine-collecting system develops abnormally (see Other Congenital Kidney Disorders, page 1092).

What you can do Because most infections reach the kidney via an infected bladder, techniques to help prevent bladder infection will help reduce the risk of kidney infection (see Self-Care Tips to Reduce Risk of Cystitis in Women, page 1068).

When to call the doctor At the first sign of

urinary tract discomfort—painful urination, blood in the urine, or pain in the side or bladder area—consult your doctor. If you develop high fever with urinary tract symptoms, call the doctor right away.

Treatment The cornerstone of therapy for pyelonephritis is the use of antibiotic medications to eradicate the offending bacteria. The choice of antibiotic depends on which bacterium has caused the infection, which is identified by culturing the organism in the laboratory. (In 80 percent of cases, *E. coli* is the offending organism.) Because the infection involves a solid vital organ, the course of treatment with the antibiotic will usually last at least 2 weeks to ensure a complete eradication of the bacterial invader. Commonly prescribed medications for urinary infection include ampicillin, cephalexin, trimethoprim-sulfamethoxazole, ciprofloxacin, and ofloxacin.

Once treatment has begun and the medication starts to kill the bacteria in the kidney, fever may persist for up to 3 days. Fever that continues longer may signal that the antibiotic is not killing the bacteria as expected and warrants a call to the doctor.

In many cases of severe infection, with high fever, nausea, and vomiting, admission to the hospital and intravenous (IV) antibiotic therapy may be necessary for 1 or 2 days.

Repeating the urine culture after treatment to ensure complete eradication of the bacterial infection is essential.

Prognosis Most women (80 to 90 percent) treated for pyelonephritis make a swift and complete recovery. In 10 to 20 percent of patients, one course of antibiotics does not eradicate the infection, and in 5 to 10 percent of patients no antibiotic regimen is able to permanently clear the urine of bacteria. Persistent bacteriuria is much more common in elderly women than in young ones.

❖ CHRONIC INTERSTITIAL NEPHRITIS

Symptoms *(What you may experience)* Polyuria (passage of more than 3 liters of urine a day); nocturia (frequent nocturnal urination). Later: edema of the feet and ankles and hypertension. (Note: Polyuria and nocturia are nonspecific symptoms seen in many disorders ranging from diabetes mellitus to enlarged prostate to congestive heart failure.)

Signs and laboratory findings *(What the doctor looks for)* High levels of protein and glucose as detected by urinalysis; elevated potassium or low sodium, phosphate, bicarbonate, and uric acid levels as detected by blood tests.

What is it? The nephrons are composed of the glomeruli (which do the initial filtering of the blood) and tubules (which gather and regulate chemicals in the urine). The space in between these structures is called the interstitium. This space mainly contains fibrous connective and supportive tissues, but also plays an important hormonal role, producing and releasing renin (important in blood pressure control) and erythropoietin (important in stimulating red-blood-cell production). The interstitium and the tubules are closely interrelated; disorders of the tubules and interstitium will with time disrupt normal glomerular function, as well. Disease in these related systems is the instigating cause for an estimated 20 percent of all people undergoing treatment for end-stage kidney disease.

The functions of the tubules and interstitium are to concentrate or to dilute the urine and to maintain mineral balance. Consequently, when these areas of the kidney malfunction, the kidney may fail to adequately reabsorb glucose, phosphate, proteins, and sodium. Levels of these substances may fall in the blood, bringing on symptoms characteristic of the disorder. Acid is normally removed by the kidney tubules. Damage to the interstitium, which surrounds the tubules, can cause acid buildup in the body. Potassium is also regulated by the kidney tubules. Damage in the interstitium can cause both too much or too little potassium in the body, both of which can be fatal.

A wide variety of conditions can slowly damage and impair the tubules and interstitium, including toxicity from heavy metals, medications, or analgesics, immunologic diseases, urinary tract obstruction, chronic infection, diabetes mellitus, radiation damage, amyloidosis (see page 997), certain congenital (present at birth) abnormalities of the kidney and metabolic disorders, and sickle cell disease.

The clinical course of chronic interstitial nephritis depends in large measure on the underlying cause and how severely it has damaged the kidney. In general, if the insult to the kidney tissues is massive and sudden, kidney function will rapidly deteriorate (see Acute Interstitial Nephritis, below). More often, sporadic or continuous lower-level exposure occurs, resulting in a more gradual and progressive loss of function.

When to call the doctor Symptoms are often gradual, and you may not be aware of having this problem. You should see a doctor if you experience persistent output of high volumes of urine or awaken multiple times during sleep to urinate (without other reasonable explanation such as enlargement of the prostate gland or heart failure).

Treatment Appropriate treatment of the underlying cause is the cornerstone of treatment—for example, stopping further damage created by substances toxic to the kidney. Once impairment develops to a severe degree, as in all worsening kidney conditions, dialysis or transplantation may be the last options available.

Prognosis Prognosis is good only if the underlying cause can be identified promptly and the damage halted before severe changes have occurred.

❖ ACUTE INTERSTITIAL NEPHRITIS

Symptoms *(What you may experience)* Fever (usually); pain in the side; slightly raised rash that comes and goes (sometimes if secondary to a medication allergy); blood in the urine (occasionally).

Signs and laboratory findings *(What the doctor looks for)* White blood cells, white-blood-cell casts, and red blood cells under microscopic exam of the urine; sudden loss of kidney function as demonstrated by blood tests showing an elevation of BUN and creatinine; elevation in the number of eosinophils (specialized white blood cells that respond in allergic reactions) as detected by a complete blood count.

What is it? Acute interstitial nephritis is an inflammation in the areas between the tubules of the nephrons. This suddenly occurring disorder commonly arises as an allergic response to medication. It is often caused by the beta lactam antibiotics such as methicillin, ampicillin, or the cephalosporins. It can develop with NSAIDs, other antibiotics (such as erythromycin, sulfonamides, tetracycline, ciprofloxacin, or trimethoprim/sulfamethoxazole), diuretics (such as thiazides or furosemide), cimetidine (an ulcer medication), allopurinol (used to treat gout), and phenytoin (a seizure medication). In addition, a number of infections (such as streptococcus, Legionnaire's disease, Epstein-Barr virus, diphtheria, and mycoplasma) and immunologic diseases may also stimulate the reaction.

There may be pain with acute interstitial nephritis, which occurs because the kidneys swell, stretching their nerve-rich covering. This disorder may lead to kidney failure within a few days to several weeks. Chronic interstitial nephritis may do its damage gradually over years.

When to call the doctor The sudden appearance of blood in the urine, pain in the side, or a rash during or following a course of any medication listed above should prompt an immediate visit to the doctor.

Treatment If the condition has arisen because of an allergic reaction to medication, stop the medication. Doing so may prove sufficient to resolve the condition. However, the most immediate and serious concern involves addressing kidney failure if it occurs.

Steroid medications in high dosages (such as prednisone) may help to speed the return of kidney function.

Prognosis Complete recovery of kidney function occurs in many cases. The longer the duration of kidney failure, the poorer the prognosis for complete recovery of kidney function.

❖ ACUTE GLOMERULONEPHRITIS

Symptoms *(What you may experience)* Sudden passing of cola-colored urine in small amounts; edema of the feet, lower legs, and sometimes hands and face; foamy urine, like the head of a poured beer.

Signs and laboratory findings *(What the doctor looks for)* Red blood cells and red-blood-cell casts and elevated protein levels in the urine; hypertension; kidney biopsy (tissue sample) demonstrating characteristic patterns on microscopic examination.

What is it? This inflammatory process of the kidney affects the glomeruli. The inflammatory process itself occurs for a variety of reasons but sometimes results from the irritation caused by deposits of antigen-antibody complexes. (Antigens are substances that trigger an antibody reaction. Antigen-antibody complexes are the immune defense clusters that result from fighting infection or from a reaction against an antigen in the body). These complexes form along the glomerulus and set in motion a series of processes that may call forth stimulants to inflammation, inflammatory cells, and destructive enzymes to attack both the complex and, unfortunately, the tissue to which it has attached. The resultant battle damages the glomerulus, making it more porous, and allows protein and sometimes red blood cells to leak into the urine. The loss of protein from the blood circulation into the urine contributes to edema. The kidney may also abnormally reabsorb sodium, which also contributes to the swelling.

The instigating cause for the glomerulonephritis may be a recent infection elsewhere in the body, commonly a streptococcal infection such as strep throat (see page 592) or impetigo (see Chapter 28). This type of glomerulonephritis, which may follow streptococcal illnesses by 1 to 3 weeks, is named poststreptococcal glomerulonephritis. Another common type of glomerulonephritis is called IgA (immunoglobulin A type) nephropathy (see page 1085). Damage to the glomerulus can also occur as a part of a more generalized disorder such as systemic lupus erythematosus (SLE, lupus), Wegener's granulomatosis, polyarteritis nodosa (see page 640), or Goodpasture's syndrome (see page 1086). In these cases the damage to the glomeruli may follow a rapidly progressive course requiring medical intervention to halt or retard the inflammatory process.

Unchecked damage to a significant percentage of the glomeruli can result in kidney failure, making early diagnosis and therapy crucial.

When to call the doctor The appearance of cola-colored urine, foamy urine (like the head of a beer), or edema following strep throat, impetigo, or a viral cold or flu should prompt an immediate visit to the doctor.

Treatment Appropriate treatment depends on the underlying cause but, in general, therapy is initially aimed at treating the hypertension with medications, encouraging the body to eliminate the excess fluid with diuretics, restricting salt and fluid intake to further reduce the demand on the kidneys, and when necessary, suppressing the inflammatory process with corticosteroids or, in more severe cases, inflammation-cell-destroying medications. There are many side effects associated with these medications, including predisposition to life-threatening infections. When these measures fail to halt kidney failure, which could result in fluid in the lungs, buildup of poisonous wastes, or dangerous levels of potassium or acid, dialysis may be necessary.

In a few instances (especially in Goodpasture's syndrome), removing damaging antibodies or immune complexes from the blood by a process called plasma exchange is beneficial.

Prognosis Prognosis depends on the cause of the glomerulonephritis. Poststreptococcal infections usually resolve with antibiotics alone. Other types of glomerulonephritis may respond to inflammatory-cell-suppressor medications. In some cases, the disorder causes progressive damage that can lead to kidney failure and necessitate dialysis or kidney transplantation.

❖ IgA NEPHROPATHY (BERGER'S DISEASE AND HENOCH-SCHÖNLEIN PURPURA)

Symptoms *(What you may experience)* Blood in the urine; in Henoch-Schönlein purpura (HSP), blotchy rash, joint pain, abdominal discomfort.

Signs and laboratory findings *(What the doctor looks for)* Microscopic blood in the urine; characteristic IgA antibodies visible on microscopic examination of kidney biopsy; previous viral illness.

What is it? In 1968 Jean Berger described this acquired kidney disorder now regarded as the most common form of glomerulonephritis in the world. The name IgA nephropathy derives from the deposit of immune complexes of the immunoglobulin A type in the glomeruli. In its milder form, the disorder may cause only episodes of microscopic bleeding in the urine, and for many years was thought not to pose significant health risk. But the disease is more aggressive than originally thought, with estimates of as many as 25 to 40 percent of cases progressing to end-stage kidney failure.

The origins of the disease are not clearly understood. It may be caused by an abnormality in the immune system.

A second type of IgA-related disease is called Henoch-Schönlein purpura, and has probably been known since as early as 1806. Unlike Berger's disease, in HSP other organs are involved; people with HSP appear much more acutely ill, suffering purpura (blotchy purple rashes), swelling, painful arthritic joints, blood in the urine, and gastrointestinal complaints. Its origins are also unclear.

Although the clinical picture varies between Berger's disease and HSP, the effect on the kidney (at least at the microscopic level) is much the same, giving rise to the current view that they may be two ends of the spectrum of a single disease.

When to call the doctor Persistent blood in the urine should always merit investigation by a doctor. The sudden development (especially following a viral, throat, or respiratory illness) of purpura accompanied by joint swelling, abdominal complaints, and urinary bleeding warrants immediate medical attention.

Treatment Treatment with steroid medications to arrest the autoimmune process may help to limit the damage in some cases, although this is controversial. If blood pressure is significantly elevated, antihypertensive medications may be needed, at least in the short term.

Dialysis may become necessary if kidney function declines.

Prognosis The majority (about 70 percent) of people have a good prognosis for recovery, with perhaps an increased risk for hypertension and possibly mild kidney function impairment. In the minority (about 30 percent), the kidney damage will progress to chronic kidney failure, necessitating dialysis.

The passage of significant amounts of protein in the urine, hypertension, and abnormal kidney function are associated with a less positive prognosis.

❖ GOODPASTURE'S SYNDROME

Symptoms *(What you may experience)* Sudden passing of cola-colored urine of small volume; edema of the feet, lower legs, and sometimes hands and face; coughing up of blood; easy fatigability.

Signs and laboratory findings *(What the doctor looks for)* Iron deficiency anemia; blood and protein in the urine as demonstrated by urinalysis; specific antibodies designed to attack a portion of the glomerulus, as detected by blood tests.

What is it? This disorder occurs only rarely, but when it does, it afflicts males six times more commonly than it does females. Most often it occurs in young white men who smoke. The reasons why it affects men more commonly than it does women are not entirely clear.

Goodpasture's syndrome, like other forms of acute glomerulonephritis, arises when antibodies settle in the kidneys (see Acute Glomerulonephritis, page 1084) and in the lungs.

When to call the doctor The first sign of bleeding in the urine or coughing up of blood should prompt a visit to the doctor right away. The kidney damage will be far more likely to be reversed when identified and treated early.

Treatment Removing the antibody from the blood by a procedure called plasma exchange, along with suppressing the formation of new antibodies using steroid medications or cytotoxic (inflammatory-cell-destroying) medications offers the best course of therapy.

Prognosis Prompt diagnosis and treatment substantially improves the prognosis for recovery of kidney function in Goodpasture's syndrome. Once the damage has become severe, the prognosis worsens for kidney recovery, and dialysis or transplantation may be required. Bleeding in the lung is life threatening and must be treated.

❖ NEPHROTIC SYNDROME

Symptoms *(What you may experience)* Edema of the hands, feet, lower legs, and face; shortness of breath (sometimes); abdominal bloating or tightness (sometimes); weight gain (from fluid retention); foamy urine.

Signs and laboratory findings *(What the doctor looks for)* Protein in the urine; low blood albumin (a protein in the blood); elevated cholesterol; kidney biopsy findings consistent with this syndrome.

What is it? One major job of the kidneys' millions of nephrons is to cleanse the blood of toxic wastes. The polluted blood arrives at the kidney, and the nephrons discharge the toxins, excess fluid, and chemicals as urine, returning clean blood to the circulation. The glomerulus prevents other components in the blood—particularly the protein molecules and the blood cells—from escaping during the filtering process.

To achieve the dual goal of letting some things out and keeping others in, nature designed the nephrons with lining cells precisely spaced with small pores between them. These pores are large enough to allow those toxic substances to pass into the urine, but small enough to retain circulating blood components and most of the protein. (*Note:* A small amount of urinary protein is normal.) In nephrotic syndrome, these pore spaces enlarge due to damage to the glomerulus, and abnormal amounts of protein leak from the blood into the urine; the albumin (a major protein) level in the blood becomes low. As the amount of protein in the blood falls, edema develops in the legs, hands, face, and feet, and fluid builds up in the abdomen (causing the bloated tightness) and the lungs (causing shortness of breath). The liver tries to make proteins to compensate for this protein loss and sometimes makes too much lipoprotein, which leads to high cholesterol levels. One severe complication is the formation of blood clots (in the lungs and in the veins of the kidney), because the balance between proteins that help blood clot and proteins that prevent blood clots is altered to favor blood clot formation.

About one-third of cases of nephrotic syndrome arise when other diseases—such as diabetes mellitus, lupus, or amyloidosis—damage the kidney. The remainder of cases usually develop as a consequence of primary glomerulonephritis, minimal change disease, membranous nephropathy, focal and segmental glomerulosclerosis (see also Acute Glomerulonephritis, page 1084).

What you can do Restriction of dietary sodium (salt) to under 2 g per day may prove helpful in controlling the swelling.

When to call the doctor Particularly when you suffer from diabetes, lupus, or amyloidosis and you develop symptoms suggestive of nephrotic syndrome, you should notify your doctor right away.

Treatment Treatment begins with reducing the loss of protein to the urine, whatever the cause. Steroid medications such as prednisone taken for several months bring about remission in certain cases. Diabetes mellitus is an important exception where steroids are of no benefit. Relapse may occur within the first year, but may respond to yet another round of steroids. A nephrologist (kidney specialist) will discuss whether steroids will be beneficial. Factors include the specific disease and the findings of the kidney biopsy.

Long courses of steroid medications, while sometimes effective, are not without serious side effects: increased susceptibility to infections, weight gain, heightened appetite, diabetes mellitus, hypertension, bone abnormalities, mood changes, and a characteristic and peculiar distribution of increased body fat as round, puffy swelling of the cheeks (referred to as a moon face) and accumulation of fat at the base of the neck (referred to as a buffalo hump).

When prednisone fails to allay the protein leakage, potent cytotoxic medications such as cyclophosphamide may prove effective. Cyclophosphamide can cause damage to the bone marrow, bladder cancer, blood in the urine, and infertility. Other immuno-suppressive medications may also be used.

Prognosis In many cases the disease follows a mild intermittent course, waxing and waning without ever progressing to kidney failure. In some cases, when episodes of protein leakage in the urine appear more frequently and persist longer, the prognosis worsens. In the most severe cases, long-term dialysis or transplantation may be required because of kidney failure.

❖ KIDNEY STONES

Symptoms *(What you may experience)* Sudden onset of intermittent spasms of pain, often severe, in the right and left sides of the middle back; pain in the testicles or labia, particularly pain that radiates from the side or groin; nausea and vomiting (often); painful sense of urgent need to urinate (sometimes); visible blood in the urine (occasionally).

Signs and laboratory findings *(What the doctor looks for)* Blood in the urine as detected by chemical or microscopic evaluation; presence of the stone as detected by x-ray or ultrasound tests.

What is it? As many as half a million Americans suffer each year with the pain of kidney stones, and that pain can be considerable—it is frequently compared to the pain of childbirth for women, and men often describe it as the worst pain they have ever experienced.

Although the development can occur at any age, it most often happens during middle age (between ages 30 and 50) and afflicts men four times as often as it does women. By age 60 and beyond, this gender disparity disappears, perhaps because stones become less common after age 60. The tendency to develop certain kinds of stones may be inherited. Diet, occupation, geography, weather, and season of the year may play a role in the development of kidney stones. They occur more commonly in people with sedentary jobs, during the summer months, and especially in hot, humid regions (probably due to relative dehydration in this kind of climate). The converse of that relationship is also true: one of the most important measures to reduce the development of kidney stones is to regularly drink plenty of water. Chronic urinary tract infections may also contribute to the formation of stones, affecting up to 15 percent of people with stones.

The stones form as tiny crystals in the urine, building up layer by layer (like a pearl forming around a grain of sand in an oyster). Most stones are quite small, but even 1-mm stones can cause severe symptoms. As long as a stone remains in the kidney, it causes no symptoms; it is when it begins to move down the ureters toward the bladder that it causes agonizing pain. Imagine a pebble the

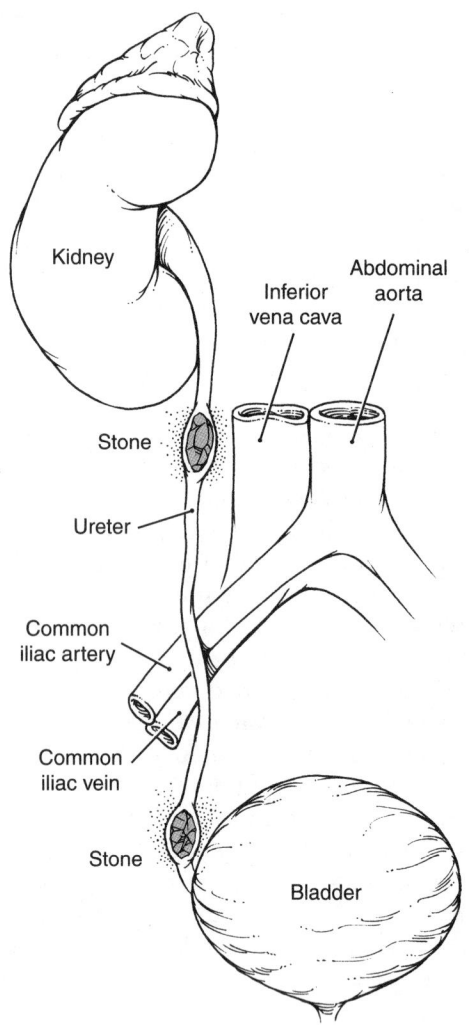

Kidney stones, which typically cause pain in the right and left sides of the middle back or in the groin, nausea, or bloody urine, are more common in men than in women. Kidney stones may occur in the ureter near the bladder or they may be located closer to the kidney. A stone that becomes lodged in the ureter on its way to the bladder may need to be surgically removed. Stones can also be associated with infections, which require medical therapy.

size of a green pea attempting to travel through a tube the width of a match stick—it is easy to see why a moving kidney stone causes not only pain but bleeding. There are several narrowed areas along the route from the kidney to the bladder that will impede a stone's passage. At these locations the stone causes the most pain or may prove to be so large that it simply cannot go further and will become lodged.

The compositions of stones vary—most contain blends of calcium (such as calcium oxalate) and a minority contain crystals of uric acid or a combination of uric acid and calcium oxalate. Infectious stones are always caused by bacteria. Cystine stones are extremely rare. Those stones made of calcium will show up on x-rays, making the diagnosis easier. Uric acid stones (which account for about 15 percent of stones) may not show up on x-ray studies without an injection of x-ray dye (see Intravenous Pyelogram, in Evaluation of Chronic Urinary Tract Infections, page 1069) to make them visible in the x-ray picture or computed tomography (CT) scan.

What you can do In nearly all cases, some measures may be taken to prevent recurrence of kidney stones. The types of measures depend on the type of stone and the metabolic abnormality that contributed to the formation of the stone. In all cases, drinking a lot of water is one of the best ways to prevent stones. In some cases dietary modifications may prove beneficial. In people who repeatedly form uric acid stones, reduced intake of foods containing amino acids of the purine family (present in shellfish and organ meats such as liver, kidney, and pancreas) may diminish the production of uric acid and thereby inhibit stone formation. Restricting calcium intake severely is not advised because it can actually increase stone formation. In addition, calcium is an important part of your diet.

When to call the doctor The first appearance of the kind of pain described above should warrant an immediate visit to the doctor or to the emergency room.

Treatment Pain control takes first priority and may require the use of potent analgesics administered by IV or injected into muscle. In many cases, the stone migrates downward and finally into the bladder,

STONE REMOVAL METHODS

Ureteroscopy

Doctors can retrieve stones in the ureter that have failed to pass on their own. The doctor guides a rigid or flexible, slender, lighted scope through the urethra, through the bladder, and up into the ureter. The scope allows the surgeon to see the stone lodged in the tube, to pass a basket-like device through the scope, grasp the stone, and extract it. Alternatively, the surgeon may break up the stone with shock waves or a laser. The same technique can retrieve fragments of stones broken up by lithotripsy. The longer the wait to retrieve a lodged stone with the stone basket, the greater the risk for complications.

Lithotripsy

Stones smaller than 2 cm (slightly less than an inch) that lie in the ureter or within the kidney itself can be safely removed without surgery in many cases by a process called extracorporeal shock wave lithotripsy or simply lithotripsy. In this procedure, the patient is sedated and a machine outside the body delivers a shock wave directed at the stone. The energy of the wave breaks the stone into small fragments that usually pass on their own down the ureter over a period of weeks; if necessary the doctor can retrieve with the scope those fragments that have failed to pass within 3 months.

Percutaneous Nephrolithotomy

Large stones in the kidney cannot be effectively broken up with lithotripsy or ureteroscopy. Doctors remove such a stone via a scope placed through a small hole that penetrates the skin, muscle, and kidney. Through these nephroscopes, stones are broken up and the pieces removed. At the end of the procedure, a small tube is left in the tract to drain the kidney while healing occurs (usual a few days to a few weeks).

Surgical Removal (Lithotomy)

Although it once offered the only means to retrieve a lodged stone, surgery is today needed in fewer than 5 percent of all people with kidney stones. Doctors usually reserve open surgical removal methods for large stones lodged within the kidney itself. Surgical removal requires an incision through the left or right side of the mid-back and then into the kidney. The risk of the surgery is higher than that associated with other methods of stone removal but surgery is still routine enough to be considered safe. ■

where it does not cause further pain. If the stone becomes lodged along the way, the doctor may have to retrieve it (see Stone Removal Methods, above).

Half of all people who experience a kidney stone for the first time will pass another stone within the next 5 to 10 years, so you will need to work with your doctor to prevent this from becoming a chronic problem. Several steps can help prevent recurrence. Most important is complete removal of all stones. If stone formation is associated with infection, the infection must be eradicated. Any anatomical abnormalities that lead urine to pool must also be corrected—usually surgically. If you pass a stone, save it for the doctor to examine. Your doctor will analyze the content of your stone if available and determine by blood and urine tests (a 24-hour collection may be performed) if a metabolic disorder led to the formation of the stone, to help prevent additional stones in the future through diet modification or medications.

Prognosis Excellent if identified and treated promptly and if the stone fails to pass quickly. Failure to retrieve a stone lodged in the urine tube can lead to massive dilation of the tube above the stone and back pressure that will ultimately damage the filtering tissues of the kidney.

❖ POLYCYSTIC KIDNEY DISEASE

Symptoms *(What you may experience)* Pain in the abdomen or side; blood in the urine; urgent and frequent need to urinate or burning upon urination.

Signs and laboratory findings *(What the doctor looks for)* Medical history demonstrating frequent urinary infections or kidney stones; family history of polycystic kidney disease or kidney failure; hypertension (often); blood or protein in the urine as detected by urinalysis; enlarged kidneys (on physical examination or demonstrated by x-ray); multiple cysts on the kidneys as detected by ultrasound examination or CT scan.

What is it? This kidney disorder occurs in 1 in 1,000 people, arising because of a genetic defect that can be identified on chromosome studies. As many as 1 in 10 people requiring dialysis have developed kidney failure because of polycystic kidney disease; it represents one of the five most common causes of kidney failure.

The autosomal dominant form of this disorder passes from an affected parent to child, and any child who receives a copy of the defective gene will develop the disease. Because the gene is a dominant one (meaning that inheriting even one copy from one parent will cause the disease), those children without the disorder can rest easy that they do not carry the defect and cannot pass it along to their own children. The vari-

ability of this disorder involves not whether the disorder will develop in those who inherit the gene, but when. In some cases, the disorder becomes symptomatic in a person by age 20, in other people symptoms appear much later in life. But 45 percent of all people who inherit the disease will develop kidney failure by age 60, requiring dialysis or transplantation.

In this disorder, when blood appears in the urine, it is usually the result of rupture of a cyst (fluid-filled cavity), and this rupture in most instances also causes significant pain in either the abdomen or the side. These symptoms can also occur if a kidney stone has formed and is trying to move through the ureter or because of infection, both of which occur quite often in this disease. As many as 20 percent of people with this disorder develop kidney stones—a rate much higher than in the general population. Sometimes cancer develops in the cysts. The kidneys can become so large that breathing becomes difficult. If so, they may need to be removed.

Because of the kidney's important role in blood pressure regulation, polycystic kidney disease often affects blood pressure. Most people with this disorder ultimately develop hypertension; one-half have developed it by the time their disorder has been diagnosed.

People who inherit polycystic kidney disease may develop aneurysms. These dilations commonly occur in the arteries supplying a portion of the brain and sometimes in the aorta (the main artery supplying blood to organs), placing people with this disorder at heightened risk for stroke or death due to blood vessel rupture. Other features of this disorder are cyst formation elsewhere in the body (liver, ovary, pancreas, or spleen), heart valve abnormalities, and diverticula (weakness in the walls) of the colon. For more information on aneurysms see Chapters 14 and 20.

See Other Cystic Disorders of the Kidneys, page 1091, for more information about other disorders causing kidney cyst development.

What you can do If you have a family history of polycystic disease, make sure you have your blood pressure and kidney function checked regularly. Your doctor may order an ultrasound or CT scan for diagnosis of these kidney cysts.

OTHER CYSTIC DISORDERS OF THE KIDNEYS

Simple Solitary Cysts

Simple solitary cysts occur commonly and usually increase in incidence with age. They generally cause no trouble. Often their presence is uncovered incidentally on x-ray examinations done for unrelated reasons. In most cases, they present no threat to health, although their discovery warrants some investigation— usually with ultrasound tests or a CT scan—to confirm their benign nature. Occasionally, a kidney cancer could contain some cystic fluid-filled areas, so the appearance of a cyst demands evaluation. Once the doctor is assured that no cancer lurks within the cyst, the normal recommendation is to watch the cyst with periodic reevaluation.

Acquired Cystic Kidney Disease

Acquired cystic kidney disease usually occurs in people who have had kidney failure and have been on dialysis therapy. Many dialysis patients (more than 80 percent of people who have been on dialysis for longer than 5 years) develop multiple cysts on their already-damaged kidneys. Why this happens is not clear, but the development of this kind of cystic disease demands careful investigation because, about 5 percent of the time, the cysts harbor cancer. Discovery of such a cancerous cyst greater than 3 cm or causing symptoms may require removal of that kidney.

Medullary Cystic Disease

Medullary cystic disease is a very rare inherited disorder that resembles polycystic kidney disease in many respects. However, while virtually all people who inherit medullary cystic disease progress to kidney failure, they rarely exhibit blood in the urine and do not develop hypertension. On the contrary, their kidneys waste salt and water, forcing them to dramatically increase their intake of these substances to prevent dehydration. Unfortunately, there are no effective medical therapies to prevent progression to end-stage kidney failure that requires dialysis or kidney transplantation.

Medullary Sponge Kidney

Medullary sponge kidney is caused by the development of dilated (expanded) outpouchings (not true cysts) of the collecting ducts. The many outpouchings give the kidney a Swiss cheese or spongy appearance—hence the name. It occurs in about 1 in 5,000 people and, although congenital, usually does not cause symptoms that would result in its discovery until late middle life (between ages 40 and 60). When it does, the symptoms include visible blood in the urine, recurrent bouts of kidney infection, and the frequent development of kidney stones. The main thrust of treatment is to prevent stone formation and treat infection. It is very uncommon for medullary sponge kidney to cause significant kidney failure. ■

When to call the doctor Blood in the urine, significant or persistent abdominal or side pain, or frequent infections should prompt you to see the doctor for a complete urologic evaluation.

Treatment There are no clearly effective therapies available to prevent the development of kidney failure; treatment of hypertension with medications may slow the rate of kidney damage.

Infections demand antibiotics. Treatment may involve 2 weeks or more of IV therapy followed by long-term daily antibiotics taken by mouth. If the infection is not severe, antibiotics can be taken by mouth.

Episodes of pain or bleeding (from cyst rupture or stone passage) usually respond to bed rest, sedative or analgesic medications, and increased fluid intake.

Once kidney function declines sufficiently to threaten life, dialysis or transplantation is needed.

Prognosis Virtually all people who inherit this disease will develop hypertension and ultimately some degree of reduced kidney function, often culminating in kidney failure. As many as 10 to 15 percent of people will develop aneurysms of the brain arteries or, more rarely, of the aorta.

❖ VESICO-URETERAL REFLUX

Symptoms *(What you may experience)* Frequent bouts of urinary infection. Symptoms of urinary infection include frequent or urgent need to urinate; burning on urination; fever (occasionally); blood in the urine (occasionally). Often vesico-ureteral reflux has resolved in childhood and no symptoms can be felt in adults, although long-term damage may exist.

Signs and laboratory findings *(What the doctor looks for)* Evidence of blood, bacteria, protein, or pus in the urine; stunted growth or scarring of the kidney as detected by kidney x-ray studies; backflow of urine from the bladder up the ureters as demonstrated by voiding cystourethrogram (VCUG).

What is it? Normally urine flows from the kidney down into the ureters and then into

OTHER CONGENITAL KIDNEY DISORDERS

Sometimes inborn abnormalities of the urinary tract are apparent at birth and diagnosed by the doctor at that time (see page 226 for information on these congenital urinary abnormalities). The conditions described here are those that may escape notice until later in childhood or in adulthood.

Uretero-Pelvic Junction Obstruction

Uretero-pelvic junction obstruction is a congenital abnormality of the collecting system that occurs more commonly than does any other. Along with polycystic kidney, this condition is the most common reason for the development of a kidney mass in newborn infants.

The collecting system of the kidney is composed of millions of tubules; a single tubule is connected to each nephron. Tubules merge into larger tubes, which merge repeatedly until coalescing into one large common area called the pelvis of the kidney. The area where the pelvis of the kidney meets the ureter is called the uretero-pelvic junction. Occasionally, urine cannot pass freely from the pelvis of the kidney into the ureter, either because of blockage (such as a kink in the ureter, narrowing of the opening, or a kidney blood vessel that crosses the path) or because scarring or fibrous tissue disrupts the effective generation of peristalsis (rhythmic waves of muscle contraction) that helps to direct the urine to the ureter.

In this condition, the kidney initially works normally, filtering blood and making urine, but it cannot drain at an adequate rate. The urine backs up, dilating the ureters and the collecting tubes within the kidney itself—a condition called hydronephrosis. Ultimately, the dilated tubes cause pressure on the nephrons, crowding them and, if left untreated, permanently damaging them.

Its presence can be suspected even before birth by a characteristic appearance on prenatal ultrasound. Specific x-ray studies, such as ultrasound and voiding cystourethrogram (VCUG) will be necessary after birth to confirm the diagnosis.

Treatment of the disorder involves surgery to relieve the obstruction and often to reshape the pelvis of the kidney to permit more effective drainage. Significant improvement in kidney function usually follows relief of the obstruction, especially in infants.

Solitary Kidney

Occasionally, people are born missing one of their kidneys. Usually, this abnormality causes no significant problems, since a single normally functioning kidney can carry the load of cleansing the blood and adequately perform the many regulating functions of the kidney without difficulty. The condition proves a threat only if something—severe infection, disease, or injury—damages the kidney.

Pelvic Kidney

In their normal location, the kidneys lie cushioned in fat within the bony protection of the rib cage. Occasionally, one kidney (very rarely both) may develop in an unusual location, resting in the pelvic cavity. Although a kidney in this position usually works just as it should, its location puts it at greater risk of injury. The abnormality may be discovered incidentally on x-ray or scan studies done for other reasons.

Horseshoe Kidney

Occasionally, the two kidneys develop joined or fused at their lower ends, no longer resembling two bean shapes, but a single horseshoe shape. As with pelvic kidney, this abnormality can make the organ more vulnerable to injury. Horseshoe kidney is also associated with more frequent urinary tract infections and kidney stones as well as a greater risk of obstruction of the collecting tubes. The condition may escape detection until investigation of frequent infection or stone formation by intravenous pyelogram (IVP) brings it to light. See Evaluation of Chronic Urinary Infections, page 1069, for information on IVP.

Duplication of the Ureter

Occasionally, some people develop an extra kidney, pelvis, and ureter on one side. This duplication may go unnoticed, causing no problems for years. More commonly, however, the extra system does not drain properly, creating an increased risk of infection, especially in children. The abnormality can be easily seen on IVP studies of the kidney. ■

the bladder. A set of one-way valves guards the opening where the ureters enter the bladder to prevent urine reflux (abnormal backward flow) into the ureters when the bladder contracts during urination. In some people, the valves do not function properly and backflow occurs, creating abnormal pressure on the tubes and carrying the risk of bacteria making their way to the kidneys. This disorder usually becomes evident in childhood and represents the most common cause of urinary tract infection of this age group. Diagnosis of the problem relies on the VCUG (see Evaluation Of Chronic Urinary Infections, page 1069). In many cases, reflux is detected on prenatal ultrasound examinations.

When to call the doctor Development of a urinary tract infection in a child of either sex or recurrent infections in an adult should prompt investigation by a doctor for possible abnormalities. Although infections occur more commonly in teenage and adult women, repeated infections (more than one or two a year) should prompt investigation by a doctor.

Treatment Treatment depends on the severity of the backflow. Children should be given preventive antibiotic therapy until the reflux resolves or is surgically corrected. Recurrent infections in children can cause irreversible damage. In women who are of childbearing age, surgery may also be prudent. In men and older women, no more than vigilant observation and prompt treatment of infection with prophylactic antibiotics may be needed. In severe cases, surgery is required to correct the problem. If surgery becomes necessary, the procedure, which is performed under general anesthesia, involves moving and repositioning the ureter on the affected side.

Prognosis Surgery is quite successful, stopping the backflow 95 percent of the time. If undiscovered and left untreated, vesico-ureteral reflux is the most common cause among children or young adults of severe hypertension and kidney failure.

❖ RENAL ARTERY STENOSIS

Symptoms *(What you may experience)* None (often); headache or dizziness (occasionally).

Signs and laboratory findings *(What the doctor looks for)* Sudden worsening of blood pressure readings; abdominal bruit (an abnormal whooshing sound audible through the stethoscope); narrowing of one or both kidney arteries as detected by x-ray dye studies; worsening kidney failure.

What is it? Nature has endowed the kidneys with a specialized ability to sense when blood pressure falls and to release artery constricting substances to elevate the pressure. This protective mechanism becomes important, for example, in injury accompanied by loss of large amounts of blood, in severe infection when blood pressure may fall critically low, or in heart attack.

These sensors interpret reduced blood flow to the kidney as a drop in blood pressure. Occasionally, blood flow to the kidney is reduced by a narrowing of the arteries while the blood flow to the rest of the body is perfectly normal or may be too high already. The sensors, unaware of what is going on in the body, raise the pressure anyway and hypertension results. Renal artery stenosis accounts for 1 or 2 in 100 cases of hypertension.

Several conditions that narrow the arteries of the kidneys can result in reduced blood flow to one or both kidneys. One is the buildup of plaque associated with atherosclerosis (hardening of the arteries) within the arteries of the kidneys, which occurs more commonly among older people and smokers and may be found in as many as 40 percent of people with atherosclerosis of the legs. An abnormality of the artery called fibromuscular dysplasia occurs more commonly in young people, especially in young women. To investigate the possibility that narrowing of the arteries of the kidneys may be the cause of hypertension, doctors rely on the renal arteriogram, a test in which x-ray dye is injected into the arteries, making them—and any narrowing along their lengths—visible on the x-ray picture. The dye may have side effects: Some people have allergic responses to the dye; some people with moderate kidney damage are prone to worsening kidney function as a result. The doctor will explain the risks before doing the procedure.

Treatment In some cases, the hypertension will respond to therapy with medication designed to lower blood pressure (see Medications Used to Treat High Blood Pressure, page 804). This approach usually works best in older people with atherosclerotic narrowing of the arteries who are too ill to undergo surgery or angioplasty; however, a word of caution: Use of angiotensin-converting enzyme inhibitor medications in people with narrowing of both arteries can cause significant reduction of blood pressure and precipitate kidney failure, so careful monitoring is required. Correction of the narrowing with surgery or with angioplasty (balloon dilation) provides more definitive therapy, especially if the kidneys already show damage.

In young, otherwise healthy people, correction of the defect by angioplasty of the narrowed segment or by redirecting blood flow around the narrowing with surgical bypass grafts offers the best treatment option.

Prognosis Discovered early and treated promptly, the prognosis can be good for maintaining good kidney function and improving or stabilizing the blood pressure. Unrecognized or left untreated, the hypertension will ultimately affect the eyes, blood vessels, and the kidneys. Permanent damage to kidneys, ultimately leading to kidney failure, can result.

❖ BLOOD CLOTS IN THE KIDNEY VESSELS

Symptoms *(What you may experience)* Sudden onset of pain in the abdomen or side and blood in the urine (following trauma to the abdomen or back).

Signs and laboratory findings *(What the doctor looks for)* Blood in the urine, presence of the clot as detected by x-ray dye studies of the arteries or veins.

What is it? Clots in the blood vessels of the kidneys, also called renal vein thrombosis, are seen most commonly in newborn infants as a result of prolonged delivery and dehydration. In adults, they are often seen with nephrotic syndrome (see page 1087) or following severe injury to the abdomen or back (such as might occur in a serious fall, crushing injury, or major car accident) that may directly traumatize the blood vessels supplying the kidneys or cause swelling within the abdomen sufficient to put pressure on them. In either event, the rate of blood flow within the vessel may slow, allowing the blood to clot. (Occasionally, a clot that forms elsewhere, such as the heart, can travel through the blood to lodge in the main artery of the kidney.) A clot within the artery prevents blood flow to the kidney, with the potential danger of tissue death. A clot in the vein prevents blood from leaving the kidney, causing a buildup of pressure within the kidney and the potential for damage.

The sudden appearance of pain in the abdomen or side and blood in the urine following a severe injury to those areas raises suspicion that a clot has formed.

The doctor will usually recommend x-ray dye studies of the blood vessels (arteriography or venography). In these tests, dye injected directly into the artery or vein makes the vessel visible on x-ray. The clot is visible as a dark area within the illuminated vessel, because it prevents the dye from going beyond it. There are risks associated with the administration of dye (some people experience allergic reactions); your doctor will explain the risks before the procedure.

When to call the doctor If you experience pain in the back, side, or abdomen after an injury to that area or you have bloody urine after the injury, see the doctor immediately.

Treatment The chief aim is to dissolve the clot, most often through the administration of blood-thinning medications such as heparin or warfarin (Coumadin) or blood-clot-dissolving medications such as urokinase or streptokinase. On rare occasions both renal arteries are blocked and emergency surgery is needed.

Prognosis Promptly treated, the prognosis is good for recovery. Undetected, especially in clots involving the artery, the affected kidney may die. However, one functioning kidney can effectively perform the work of cleansing the blood and regulating fluid and mineral balance. If the clot occurs in a person with a single kidney, its failure requires long-term dialysis or kidney transplantation.

❖ CANCER OF THE KIDNEY

Symptoms *(What you may experience)* Blood in the urine (usually); pain in the side; unexplained weight loss (sometimes); unexplained fever; pain in the bones (occasionally).

Signs and laboratory findings *(What the doctor looks for)* Blood in the urine visible on microscopic examination; a solid lump in the kidney as detected by x-ray studies; an elevation of calcium in the blood (about 10 percent of the time) or an increase in the number of red blood cells (about 5 percent of the time) as demonstrated by blood tests. (The symptoms of kidney cancer are variable and may make the diagnosis difficult.)

What is it? The majority of cancers of the kidney—termed renal cell carcinomas—arise in the cells of the proximal tubule. They account for a little over 3 percent of cancers in adults. Of about 24,000 adults who develop cancer of the kidney each year, about 10,000 die of the disease. Caught early, before the tumor has broken through the capsule (outer covering) of the kidney, it is often curable. (See illustration on page 1076.)

This cancer most often strikes men between the ages of 60 and 70—occurring about twice as commonly in men as in women. While no clear cause is known, the only significant lifestyle risk yet implicated is cigarette smoking, though obesity and exposure to certain chemicals may also play a role. Some inherited syndromes are associated with cancer of the kidney, but these account for a minority of cases. Most often the cancer arises with no family history.

The investigation of symptoms suggestive of cancer will usually include x-ray dye studies, CT scan (the most reliable and useful method for detecting the tumors and determining the extent of their spread), and chest x-rays and bone scans to detect metastasis to the lung or bone.

What you can do If you have a family history of this type of cancer and you smoke cigarettes, stop.

When to call the doctor If you pass bloody urine, call the doctor right away.

Treatment The cornerstone of treatment involves surgery to remove the diseased kidney. If the remaining kidney is healthy, it can easily cleanse the blood and perform all the vital functions that kidneys perform.

The surgery is successful if the cancer has not spread beyond the bounds of the kidney itself. Once it has metastasized to distant areas, no regimen of chemotherapy or radiation therapy has yet emerged that effectively treats the disease, although promising research in immunotherapy and other areas is being pursued.

Prognosis Prognosis depends on the surgical stage of the tumor. In people whose can-

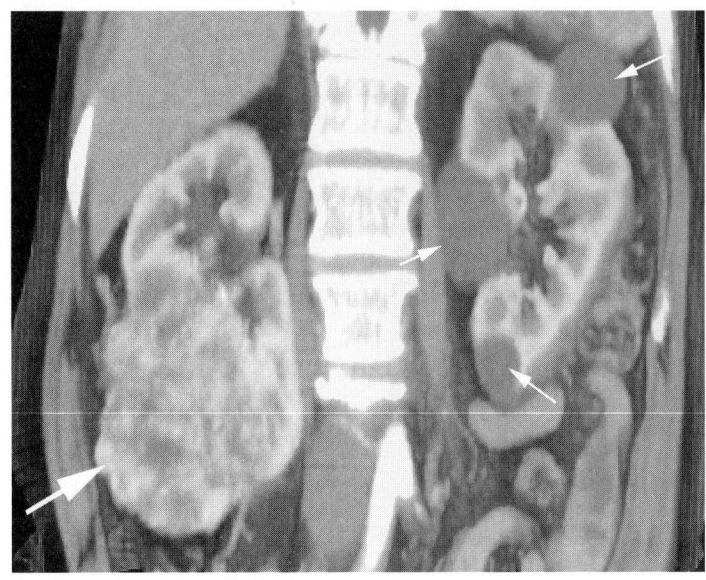

Kidney tumor. Arrow indicates a large benign tumor at the bottom of the right kidney (left side of picture). Caught early, before the tumor has broken through the outer covering of the kidney, a cancerous tumor in the kidney is often curable. The left kidney (right side of the picture) has several cysts seen as large gray masses on CT scan (arrows).

cer is surgically removed—and if surrounding areas are free of cancer cells at the time of surgery—the 5-year survival rate is 50 to 70 percent. Five-year survival rates decline to 15 to 35 percent in those whose cancer involves lymph nodes and the circulatory system; it declines to 5 percent or less in people with distant metastases.

TWENTY-FIVE

Reproductive System

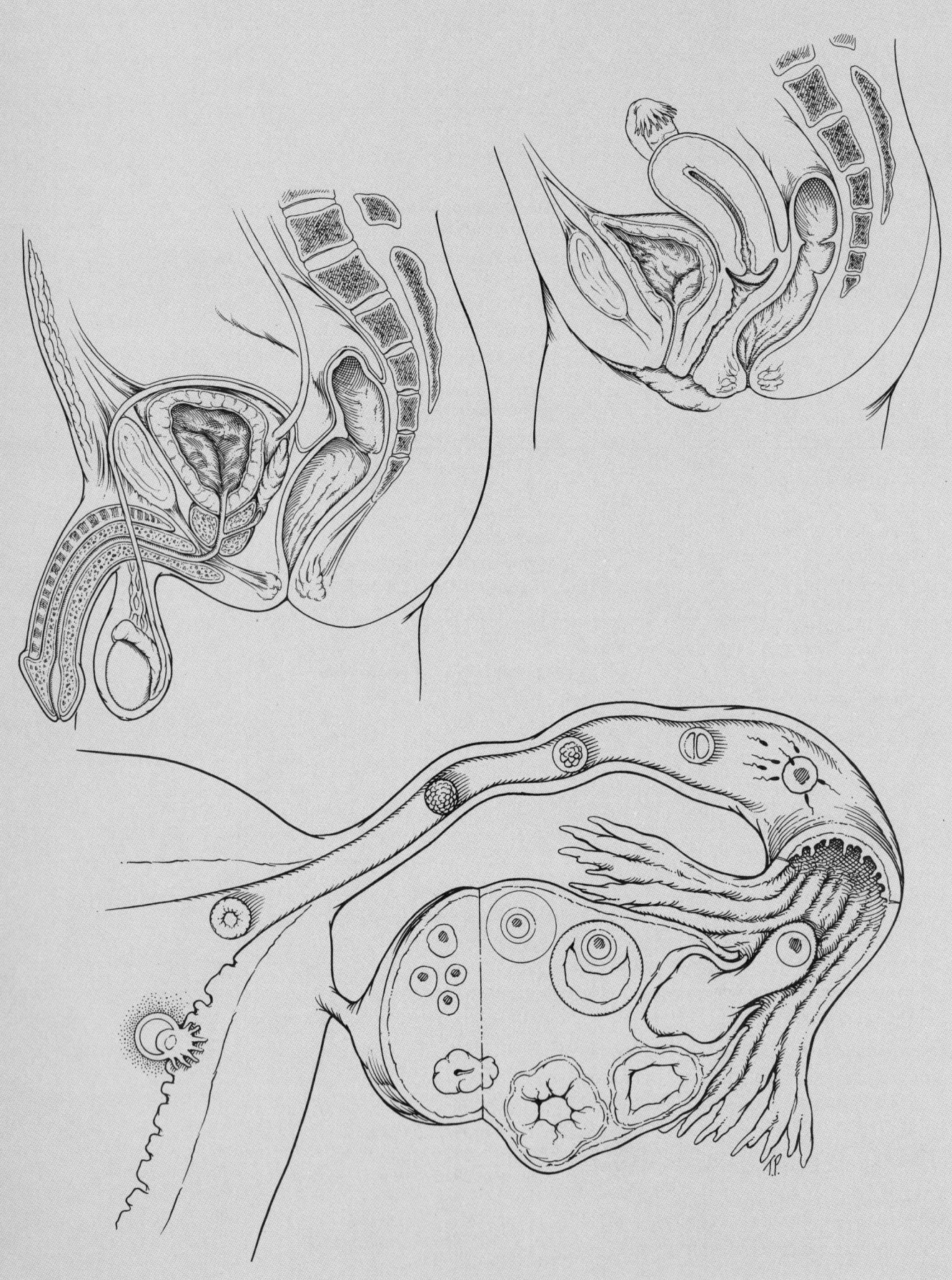

THE REPRODUCTIVE SYSTEM

While the primary function of the reproductive system in men and women is the creation of offspring, the sex hormones play crucial roles in one's overall health. This chapter discovers first the female reproductive system, then the male reproductive system, and lastly fertility and infertility. Information about the normal functioning of the reproductive systems as well as how best to maintain reproductive health through regular check-ups and screenings is presented. Disorders of the reproductive system that arise from infection with viruses, fungi, or bacteria; absence or abnormal structure of one of the organs; disruption of normal function; trauma; and cancer are all discussed here. For information on sexually transmitted diseases, see Chapter 21: Infectious Diseases.

THE FEMALE REPRODUCTIVE SYSTEM

The female reproductive system consists of the uterus, fallopian tubes, ovaries, and external genitalia. Although the reproductive system's primary function is the bearing of children, the sex hormones produced by the ovaries also play crucial roles in maintaining bone density and in the growth, maintenance, and repair of the reproductive tissues.

The visible external portion of the reproductive system in women consists of two fleshy outer folds of skin (the labia majora or greater lips) and within those, two smaller, thinner folds (the labia minora or lesser lips). These structures offer some protection to the delicate and sensitive tissues beyond them. Most sensitive of all is the clitoris, a small node of erectile tissue that stiffens during sexual arousal much as the penis does in males. The clitoris is situated where the folds of the labia meet in the front. The labia guard the opening of the urinary tract (the urethral meatus, the entrance to the urethra, which leads to the bladder) as well as the vagina, a canal approximately 5 in. long with muscular walls. The uterus lies at the inner most recess of the vagina. The lower end of the uterus, the cervix, protrudes into the vaginal vault.

The uterus is a small (about 2.5 to 3 in. in the nonpregnant state), hollow organ shaped like an upside-down pear. Its thick muscular walls are powerful enough to expel the fetus during childbirth.

On either side of the uterus, the fallopian tubes, a pair of slender hollow tubes, extend outward, draping their fringe-like ends near the ovaries to gather in the eggs released with each monthly reproductive cycle. Despite their tiny size, only about 1 in. long, the ovaries at birth contain about 1 million dormant eggs, a number sufficient to last a reproductive lifetime.

Maintaining Reproductive Health

In women, maintaining reproductive health involves having periodic pelvic exams complete with Pap smear (see The Periodic Pelvic Exam and Pap Smear, page 1100) usually performed by a family practitioner, gynecologist, or nurse practitioner. These simple and inexpensive check-ups can detect not only infection of the vagina, cervix, uterus, or fallopian tubes but also cysts or tumors of the ovary and cancer of the cervix.

MENSTRUATION AND OVULATION

The menstrual cycle occurs during a woman's reproductive years, from puberty until menopause. In the first years following the onset of puberty, the menstrual cycle may be irregular, but most women's cycles become predictable, occurring at regular intervals that are spaced an average of 28 days (a range of 24 to 31 days) apart. Day 1 of the menstrual cycle is by convention considered the first day of bleeding, which commonly lasts for 5 to 7 days. During the subsequent week or two of the cycle, the chosen egg for the next ovulation undergoes its maturation process. The ovaries usually alternate in releasing a single egg per monthly cycle. In some cases of multiple births, the ovaries release more than one egg. The chosen egg matures under the influence of rising and falling reproductive hormone levels, is released

THE PERIODIC PELVIC EXAM AND PAP SMEAR

Regular pelvic exams performed by a family practitioner or gynecologist will help ensure a woman's reproductive health. An initial pelvic exam should be performed at age 18, or earlier if a woman is sexually active. Subsequently, exams should occur regularly, preferably every year.

Before the pelvic exam begins, the woman's weight and blood pressure are taken. The doctor may also ask the woman to provide a urine sample. After undressing, the woman lies flat on an exam table with knees bent and feet supported by stirrups. The doctor will first examine the woman's external genitals for any signs of abnormality and then proceed to the internal exam. To examine the interior of the vagina and cervix, the doctor uses a speculum, a duck-bill shaped instrument that holds the walls of the vagina apart, enabling the doctor to inspect the tissues for discoloration, abnormal growths, and to obtain a sample of the cells of the cervix for the Papanicolaou (Pap) smear to detect cancer. At the same time, any abnormal cervical secretions can be sampled if necessary to detect infection.

The doctor will also perform a bimanual (two-handed) exam to feel the uterus, cervix, fallopian tubes, and ovaries, searching for abnormalities in size or shape that could indicate tumors of those structures, or an unusual degree of tenderness that could indicate infection. The doctor will insert two lubricated and gloved fingers into the vagina while pressing on the abdomen with the other hand. Then the doctor will insert a finger into your rectum, evaluating the interior organs from a different angle. Abnormalities in size, shape, or tenderness may necessitate further evaluation by ultrasound, computed tomography (CT), or magnetic resonance imaging (MRI).

Routine screening for cancer of the cervix using the Pap smear should be done in all women who are or have been sexually active and still have a cervix. The screenings should begin at the onset of sexual activity and should be repeated at least every 3 years. The Pap smear is one of the most helpful screening tests available, because it allows for early diagnosis of cervical cancer, which if caught early is often curable. If the results of your Pap smear are abnormal, the test will usually be repeated for verification of results. Those tests found to be abnormal a second time may necessitate specialized sampling procedures such as colposcopy (see Procedures for the Diagnosis and Treatment of Cervical Disorders, page 1113). The doctor can then biopsy these areas for microscopic exam by a pathologist. ∎

A plastic or metal speculum is inserted into the vagina to hold apart the vaginal walls. A spatula and then a brush is inserted and rubbed against part of the cervix to obtain a small sample for the Papanicolaou (Pap) smear. A rectal exam may be performed as well as a combined vaginal/abdominal exam to assess the uterrus and ovarian structures.

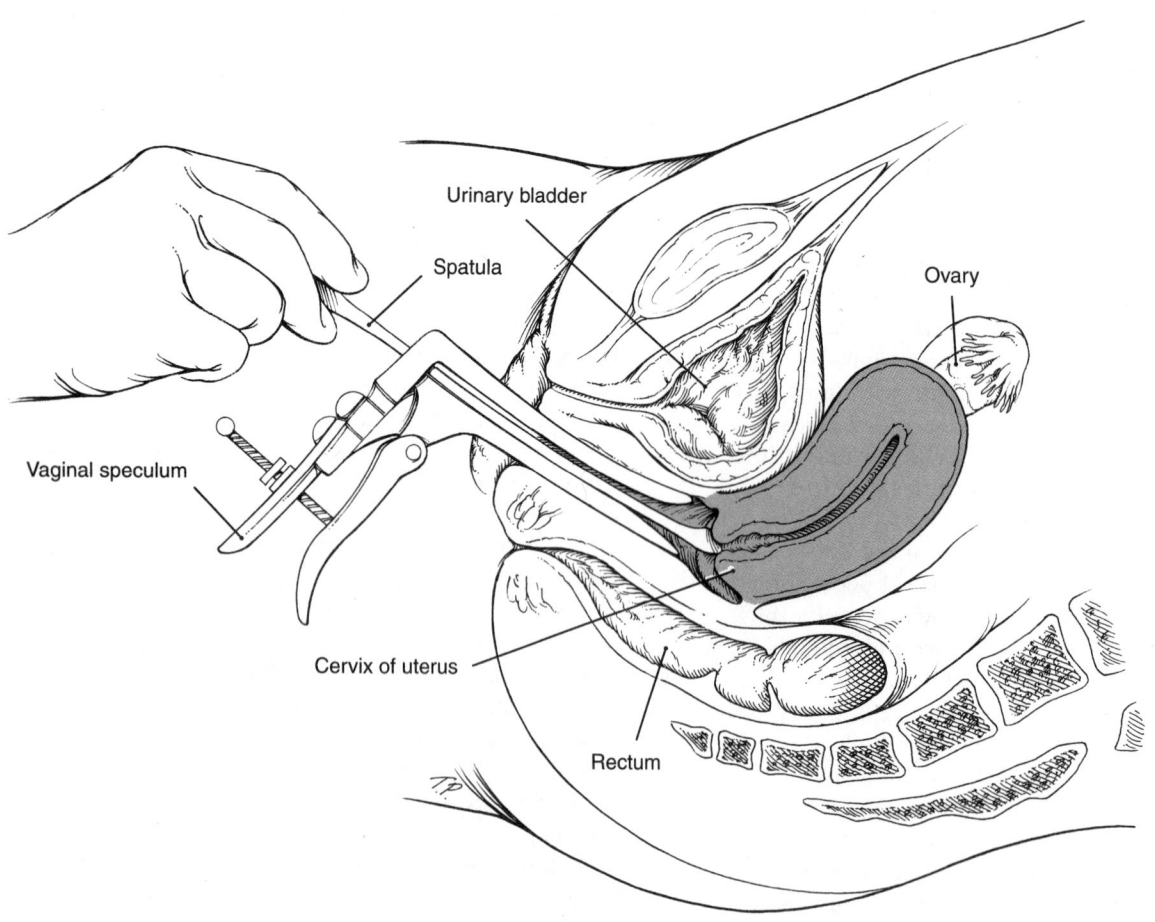

Urinary bladder

Spatula

Ovary

Vaginal speculum

Cervix of uterus

Rectum

The menstrual cycle occurs from puberty to menopause for an average of 28 days each month. Day 1 of the cycle is defined by the first day of bleeding. Follicle-stimulating hormone (FSH) from the brain's pituitary gland prompts an ovarian follicle to develop (follicular phase). The egg (or eggs) that will ovulate matures in the next week or two. Hormone levels rise and fall throughout the cycle. Estrogen released from developing follicles causes the uterine lining (endometrium) to proliferate. The egg is released from the ovary (ovulation) about the 14th day of the cycle, after which the luteal phase begins. The egg develops inside the follicle, which passes through primary and secondary stages. A corpus luteum gland forms from the ruptured follicle. Regulated by luteinizing hormone (LH) from the pituitary gland, the corpus luteum begins to secrete progesterone, which promotes secretions from the endometrium. If fertilization occurs, the menstrual cycle is interrupted. If not, unfertilized eggs degenerate after a few days. During pregnancy, the corpus luteum remains active for many weeks, but it eventually becomes an inactive corpus albicans.

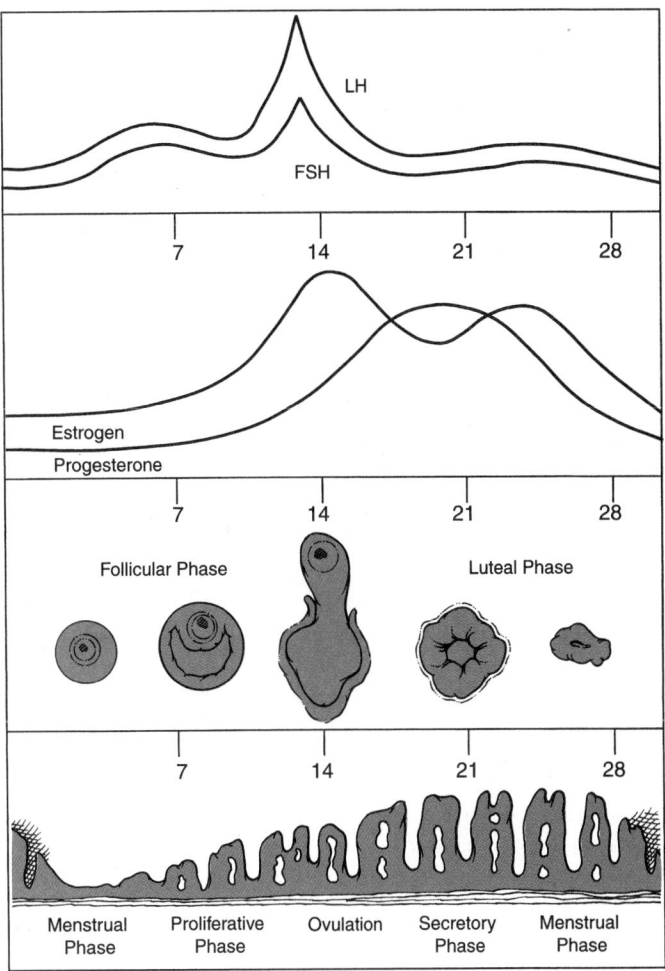

from the ovary, and is gathered in by the fringed ends of the fallopian tube. The egg then travels down the fallopian tube where it may or may not be fertilized by the male sperm. It drops into the uterine cavity where, if it has been fertilized, it will burrow into the thick lining of the uterine wall that has been prepared to receive it and begin to develop and grow. If it has not been fertilized, it will degenerate in a few days, and under the influence of changing levels of reproductive hormones, the thick lining of the uterus will slough as menstrual blood flow.

In the "textbook" 28-day cycle, ovulation occurs on day 14, although it is during the first half of the cycle that variability occurs from that norm. For women with a shorter monthly cycle, ovulation will occur as early as day 10, for those with a cycle longer than 28 days, it may occur on day 17 or even later. Once ovulation does occur,

PREMENSTRUAL SYNDROME

One to 2 weeks preceding the onset of the menstrual period, as many as one-third of premenopausal women suffer some of the numerous symptoms attributed to premenstrual syndrome (PMS). These symptoms include breast tenderness and swelling, bloating, weight gain, swelling of the feet and ankles, acne outbreaks, irritability, depression, food cravings, difficulty concentrating, aggressiveness, lethargy, and changes in libido. In most women, the symptoms are an intermittent, mildly troublesome nuisance, but in about 10 percent of cases, symptoms may recur frequently and be severe enough to disrupt normal activities. The disorder most commonly afflicts women ages 25 to 40.

Although many possible factors have been espoused, a specific cause remains unclear. As a result, most current therapies may work in some cases, but have not necessarily been proven effective in specifically designed clinical studies. Some doctors have reported danazol to be helpful in some cases. Others have tried natural progesterone (orally or as intravaginal suppositories) given daily during the premenstrual phase of the cycle, but studies have not confirmed its safety or efficacy. A woman should consult her doctor to learn if there is a therapy that can relieve her individualized symptoms.

Restricting sugar and alcohol consumption may help to control hypoglycemia (which may complicate the syndrome) and restricting salt intake may help to reduce fluid retention. A program of regular exercise may also help reduce anxiety and depression. ■

DYSMENORRHEA (PAINFUL PERIODS)

Painful periods occur in two distinct patterns: primary dysmenorrhea and secondary dysmenorrhea.

Primary Dysmenorrhea

Primary dysmenorrhea usually begins within 1 to 2 years of the onset of menstruation, with 50 to 75 percent of all young women affected with it to some degree at some time. Symptoms of cramping, nausea, diarrhea, feeling flushed or faint, headache, and back or inner thigh pain may last up to several days. Pelvic exam usually does not reveal any identifiable structural cause; the cramps occur because excessive constriction of the blood vessels of the uterus causes lack of oxygen to the uterine muscle, and with that, release of prostaglandins (specific microhormones) that control contraction of the muscular uterine wall. For a minority (about 5 percent) of women, the symptoms are severe and incapacitating. Endometriosis sometimes proves to be the cause, but diagnosis of the condition is not possible until it has progressed over many years (see Adenomyosis and Endometriosis, page 1117). Treatment with ibuprofen, ketoprofen, mefanamic acid, or naproxen generally helps relieve symptoms. Suppressing ovulation with oral contraceptive agents (birth control pills) may also prove helpful.

Secondary Dysmenorrhea

Secondary dysmenorrhea begins later, often as late as age 30 to 40. Examination will usually uncover a cause, such as an intrauterine device (IUD), endometriosis, pelvic inflammatory disease (PID), benign tumor (myoma) in the uterine wall, cervical stenosis with obstruction to menstrual flow, or rarely some other structural abnormality. Diagnosing which of these conditions is causing the pain may require a more extensive investigation. A laparoscopic exam, performed using an illuminated optic instrument that is inserted through the abdominal wall, can differentiate between such causes as endometriosis and PID. Specialized x-ray studies, for example, MRI scan or hysterogram and direct viewing with the hysteroscope can detect myomas in the uterine wall. Once the problem has been identified, treatment is tailored to the specific cause. ∎

however, it almost uniformly will be 14 days until the next onset of bleeding.

To gauge the length of a cycle, keep an accurate menstrual diary. Designate the first day of any significant show of blood as day 1 and mark that on your calendar. When the first show of blood occurs in the next month, mark that day. Do the same for several months to determine a pattern of average length. Doing this will enable you not only to know when to expect your monthly flow, but will make it easier for you to spot abnormalities in your cycle that could be caused by pregnancy, infection, or other disorders.

❖ MITTELSCHMERZ

Symptoms and signs *(What you may experience)* Lower abdominal pain at ovulation; occasionally spotting or mild bleeding with the pain.

What is it? At the midpoint of the menstrual cycle (about day 12 to 14), when ovulation occurs, many women experience abdominal pain called mittelschmerz, from the German, meaning middle pain. It is not known what causes mittelschmerz, but researchers theorize that when the follicle ruptures, and the egg is released, fluid and sometimes a small amount of blood may be released into the abdominal cavity with the egg, causing mild irritation and pain. Although in most women, the event passes without notice, occasionally, it may be accompanied by dull pain in the lower abdomen, lasting from a few minutes to several hours. Mittelschmerz can be helpful for women trying to get pregnant because it can help pinpoint ovulation, but for some women, the pain may cause concern and may even be severe enough to be confused with appendicitis.

What you can do Mild over-the-counter analgesic medications usually will control the pain.

Treatment Occasionally, to relieve the pain a woman may require more potent medications such as prescription-strength anti-inflammatory agents (for example, naproxen or aspirin) or small doses of acetaminophen with codeine. Severe, recurrent ovulation pain may respond to the administration of birth control pills.

IRREGULAR OVULATION AND MENSES

Symptoms *(What you may experience)* Missed periods; spotting between periods; difficulty conceiving a pregnancy.

Signs and laboratory tests *(What the doctor looks for)* Imbalances in reproductive hormone levels as revealed by blood tests or endometrial biopsy.

What is it? Although it is normal at the beginning and at the end of reproductive life for women to menstruate less frequently and to experience a somewhat unpredictable cycle, some women experience infrequent menses throughout their reproductive years. The exact nature of the disturbance is unclear, and in most cases no treatment is necessary, unless irregular ovulation is preventing a desired pregnancy. Irregular ovulation may sometimes relate to an overproduction of the androgen (male) hormones relative to the estrogen (female) hormones. The excess production may be from overactive adrenal glands or occasionally from an ovarian tumor. Ultrasound, computed tomography (CT), or magnetic resonance imaging (MRI) scans can usually identify these causes. In some cases, the overproduction can be traced to excessive amounts of exercise or rarely to the illicit use of anabolic steroids in female body builders or elite athletes.

What you can do Keep a careful menstrual diary. Although doing so will not prevent or cure the problem, it will provide valuable information for the doctor.

When to call the doctor If you routinely have fewer than the usual 11 to 13 menstrual cycles per year, consult your doctor.

Treatment If the cause is too little estrogen, administration of extra estrogen will usually compensate, restoring menses frequency, improving fertility, and reducing the risk of osteoporosis. If the problem is too much androgen, the treatment will depend on the cause of the excess. The recommendation may be as simple as reduction of excessive exercise or discontinuance of illicit steroid preparations, but could also mean surgery to remove an ovarian or adrenal tumor.

Infertility caused by infrequent ovulation generally responds well to administration of drugs such as clomiphene (Clomid). For more information, see Causes of and Treatments for Infertility, page 1160 in this chapter.

Prognosis In general, good, with treatment appropriate to the cause.

❖ AMENORRHEA (ABSENT PERIODS)

Symptoms *(What you may experience)* No menses by age 16 (primary amenorrhea) or absence of menstrual periods for longer than 6 months (secondary amenorrhea).

Signs and laboratory findings *(What the doctor looks for)* Abnormalities in the uterus or cervix shown by pelvic exam; hormonal imbalances revealed by blood or urine tests; negative pregnancy test.

What is it? Amenorrhea simply means absence of menstrual bleeding that can occur for a variety of reasons. The term applies both to a failure to begin menstruation (primary amenorrhea) or to cessation of menstruation for longer than 6 months in the absence of pregnancy (secondary amenorrhea).

In the primary form, menstrual cycling has not yet begun by age 16. Most of the time, these young women are developing normally, just a little more slowly than their peers who have begun to menstrate by age 12 or 13. They may be very thin or in some cases very athletic, and lack sufficient weight and the slight rise in body fat necessary to trigger the onset of menses. The delay should cause no alarm if other sexual characteristics such as breasts and hair in the pubic area or under the arms have begun to develop. If by age 16 these characteristics have failed to appear, developmental or hormonal abnormalities may be responsible.

Once menstrual cycling has become regular, its sudden disappearance should be evaluated. Secondary amenorrhea almost always results from disruption of the estrogen balance, which can be caused by several conditions. The common possible causes include pregnancy, rapid weight loss, extreme physical or emotional stress, obesity, frequent strenuous exercise, medications that suppress ovulation, and discontinuance of birth control pills. Failure to resume cycling after childbirth is commonly due to breastfeeding. It may also occur because of damage to the pituitary gland, however, which is responsible for stimulating hormonal release. This type of damage, termed postpartum pituitary necrosis, can occur on rare occasions during delivery. Other pituitary disorders, such as benign tumors, can also be responsible. (For more information, see page 1200.)

What you can do If you are absolutely certain that you are not pregnant, try first to remedy lifestyle contributors: eat a weight-maintaining balanced diet, exercise moderately, and try to reduce stress. In most instances, it is safe to wait up to 6 months before becoming concerned.

When to call the doctor If you miss a period, check with your doctor to be certain you are not pregnant. If your cycle fails to resume within 6 months, consult your gynecologist.

Young women who fail to menstruate by age 16 should consult a doctor.

Treatment Treatment is very often unnecessary, although because lack of estrogen can contribute to osteoporosis, many doctors will recommend low-dose birth control pills or estrogen pills and calcium supplements to reduce this risk. The doctor also may prescribe various combinations of hormones to determine that the ovaries are indeed functioning. A course of progesterone, for example, is often used to stimulate a cycle of bleeding, which would indicate that estrogen levels are normal.

Persistent amenorrhea in women hoping to conceive may require referral to a fertility specialist.

Prognosis Excellent with appropriate treatment. In many cases of primary amenorrhea, the condition resolves on its own with time.

MENOPAUSE

Menopause is a time of transition, as a woman's reproductive period draws to a close. In Western cultures, women reach menopause at an average age of 51, although it may occur as early as 40 or may not occur until later in the fifth decade. The timing of this process may in part be hereditary. The climacteric, the period during which there is gradual loss of ovarian function, may last from 1 to several years, culminating in menopause, the cessation of menstrual periods. Although menstruation ceases, a woman's ovaries do not stop producing hormones; they continue to produce low levels of hormones for the next three to four decades of a woman's life.

Changes in the body can be unsettling, and indeed many women find that as the hormonal production from the ovaries begins to wane, unpleasant symptoms can result. Among the most common and often troublesome symptoms of this stage of reproductive life are hot flashes—sudden intense sensations of heat sweeping over the face and trunk, accompanied by red flushing of the skin and sometimes profuse sweating. As many as 80 percent of women experience hot flashes during the climacteric period. The flashes occur more commonly at the end of the day, during sleep, or during periods of tension and stress. Hot weather and the consumption of hot foods or beverages may also cause them to be more severe. Hot flashes will cease when the body finds a new hormonal balance. Until then, it is important to remember that hot flashes are a normal response by the body to the hormonal changes. Avoidance of alcohol and caffeine, a program of regular exercise, and stress reduction or relaxation techniques may help to reduce the severity and discomfort of hot flashes. If the hot flashes are particularly frequent and uncomfortable, consult your doctor about available remedies. Hormonal replacement therapy with medications containing estrogen or a combined regimen of estrogen and progesterone, taken by mouth or given by injection, can offer relief, but carry other benefits and risks (for more information see Hormone Replacement Therapy, page 1105). The prescription medication, clonidine, usually used in the treatment of high blood pressure, has also shown benefit in reducing hot flashes. It can be given orally or in transdermal patches.

During the climacteric period, menstrual periods may become erratic in timing and fluctuate from light or absent to heavy and prolonged, reflecting the ups and downs of hormonal production. Women who do not wish to become pregnant may wish to continue using contraceptive protection until they have not had a period for one year or until blood tests indicate that the ovary is no longer producing estrogen.

POSTMENOPAUSAL BLEEDING

Once menstrual cycling ceases, it should not resume. Any instance of vaginal bleeding that occurs 6 months or more following the menopause merits investigation by a doctor. Although the causes (polyps, erosions of the cervix from prolapse of the uterus, atrophic vaginitis, dysfunctional uterine bleeding, or use of estrogen without progesterone) are most often not serious, no episode of postmenopausal bleeding should ever be ignored because women in this stage of life have a greater risk of endometrial and cervical cancers.

Treatment options depend upon the cause. See the specific entries in this chapter for more information about each disorder. ■

HORMONE REPLACEMENT THERAPY

The decision whether or not to replace hormones after menopause is a complex one that every woman should discuss with her doctor, taking into account both the risks and the benefits of therapy. Little doubt exists that replacing female hormone can mitigate most of the unpleasant symptoms of age-related or surgically-caused menopause. Disturbances of mood, hot flashes, and discomfort with intercourse that can occur with thinning of the vaginal tissues all seem to respond well, and short-term hormonal therapy that offers relief until a new hormonal balance is achieved is appropriate in many cases. However, we still do not know all we need to know about the serious health benefits versus the risks of long-term hormonal therapy.

Replacement therapy has been employed since the 1970s when the prescribing of estrogen gained great popularity. The subsequent finding of a substantially increased risk of uterine cancer in those women who took it led to its falling somewhat out of favor. In addition, there is concern that hormone replacement leads to an increased risk of breast cancer, though the various studies have had inconsistent findings. On the other hand, without sufficient estrogen, the risk for osteoporosis rises, bringing with it an entirely different set of problems. More importantly, menopausal women who take estrogen significantly reduce their risk of cardiovascular disease and possibly reduce the risk of stroke. Thus, a woman and her doctor will need to consider the woman's personal and family history before determining that the benefits of hormone therapy outweigh the risks. Recent studies also suggest that estrogen replacement may slow the development of Alzheimer's dementia.

Current recommendations for replacement therapy advise taking the lowest possible dose of estrogen hormone that will control menopausal symptoms. For most women, a dose of oral estrogen (Premarin) of 0.3 to 0.625 mg will suffice, although some women require substantially more. Taking a dose that exceeds the minimum necessary amount can result in weight gain, fluid retention, and changes in blood lipid (cholesterol) levels.

The hormone, which can be absorbed through the skin, can be administered in a transdermal gel or patch. This route of administration allows lower doses of the hormone to be administered because the oral version must be digested, absorbed, and make a pass through the liver to become effective. There is some indication that topical administration causes fewer adverse changes in blood lipid (cholesterol) levels because it does not require the first pass through the liver.

In women who still have their uterus, the administration of a progestin compound (Provera), usually taken during the last week to 10 days of the month, along with the estrogen lessens the risk of developing endometrial (uterine) cancer. It will allow the uterine lining to build up and regularly slough, mimicking the natural monthly shedding cycle. Estrogen alone should not be used in women who still have a uterus.

Since a part of the normal female hormone milieu includes a small amount of testosterone as well, some doctors will recommend the addition of a small dose of it along with the estrogen. This regimen is especially helpful to offset the loss of muscle and bone mass that many women experience as they age, as well as to restore the loss of libido that may accompany menopause.

The choice to undertake hormone replacement therapy brings with it the need for careful, regular health screening of the breast, uterus, and ovaries. Make and keep appointments for regular mammograms, breast and pelvic exams, and Pap smears. ■

Because reproductive hormones also function in maintaining the suppleness and lubrication of the vaginal tissues, their lack can cause vaginal dryness and thinning of the vaginal lining, both of which can make sexual intercourse uncomfortable. Vaginal dryness can usually be overcome by the use of either vaginal lubricant products or estrogen or testosterone creams.

Some women are at risk for the development of osteoporosis (thinning of bone density) during this period of their reproductive lives. For additional information see page 654.

External Genitalia (Vulva)

The opening of the vagina, called the vestibule, is protected by the external genitalia. These structures, collectively called the vulva, consist of the mons pubis, the mound-shaped tissues covering the pubic bone that become covered with hair at puberty, the labia minora and majora, and the clitoris. Just within the vestibule of the vagina lie several important glands (Bartholin's glands) that secrete fluids to lubricate the vaginal opening. Although cancer of the vulva occasionally occurs, infection by bacteria, viruses, or fungi causes the majority of problems in the external genitalia.

❖ CANDIDA VULVOVAGINITIS

Symptoms *(What you may experience)* Itching of vulva and vaginal vault; discharge, usually white, curd-like, and without significant odor; pain during intercourse.

Signs and laboratory findings *(What the doctor looks for)* Yeast organisms visible

OTHER CAUSES OF EXTERNAL ITCHING

Although vulvovaginal yeast infection (*Candida albicans*) most commonly causes itching of the external genitalia, other factors both infectious and noninfectious, can do so. Among these are the following:

Trichomonas Vaginalis

Infection by this organism (a sexually transmitted protozoan, not a bacterium) causes intense itching of the vulvovaginal area and usually a malodorous, frothy, pale yellow to greenish discharge.

Tinea Cruris (Jock Itch)

Not limited to male athletes, this fungal infection can occur in anyone subject to wearing damp/sweaty, tight-fitting clothing for prolonged periods. It appears as a scaly, red, itchy rash in the creases and folds of the groin area (see page 1288).

Pediculosis Pubis (Crab Lice)

Infestation with this human louse can cause intense itching in the genital areas covered with pubic hair. The live adult lice look like small transparent ticks (see page 1305).

Allergic Dermatitis

Use of fragrant or deodorant sprays, powders, pads, or tampons can sometimes cause an allergic reaction of the vulvar area, complete with rash and itching (see page 1290). ■

on microscopic examination of discharge specimen.

What is it? Candida albicans is the yeast fungus usually responsible for vulvar itching and discharge. It is commonly the offender that women often refer to any vulvovaginal itching as a "yeast infection," but be aware that all itches are not necessarily caused by yeast. A number of other infectious organisms could cause these symptoms, and it may require microscopic examination of the discharge to be certain of the diagnosis (see Other Vaginal Discharges, page 1109 for more information on other causes of vaginitis).

Certain conditions and treatments, including pregnancy, diabetes mellitus,

acquired immunodeficiency syndrome (AIDS), treatment with corticosteroid medications, and the use of the birth control pill or certain antibiotics, which can disrupt the normal ecology of the vaginal canal by destroying the so-called friendly bacteria that populate the vaginal canal and keep the yeast fungus in check, give the yeast fungus the opportunity to flourish. Heat, moisture, and clothing that does not permit sufficient air circulation to allow the area to dry may increase the risk for *C. albicans* vulvovaginitis. Women who test positive for the human immunodeficiency virus (HIV) may suffer recurring yeast infections that cannot readily be explained by these other factors.

What you can do To prevent a yeast infection, wear cotton underwear to allow air to circulate. Although a number of medications to treat yeast infections have recently become available over-the-counter, be cautious in making a hasty self-diagnosis.

When to call the doctor See your doctor about any vulvar or vaginal itch or discharge that is recurring or that fails to respond promptly to over-the-counter medications.

Treatment In the past, women with yeast infections would consult their doctors, who would prescribe an appropriate antifungal medication. But many antifungal medications are now available over-the-counter, and women who have been diagnosed with yeast infections in the past may feel comfortable using the over-the-counter medication to treat the condition. Products containing antifungal medications such as butoconazole 2 percent, terconazole 0.8 percent, clotrimazole 1 percent, or miconazole 2 percent, are available in creams or tablets that are applied intravaginally at bedtime for 1 to 7 days, depending upon the type of medication purchased. Generally, the shorter the course of treatment, the more expensive the medication. The shorter course of treatment is more convenient but occasionally less effective. In some cases, oral antifungal medications, such as ketoconazole or fluconazole may be needed to eradicate the infection. Consult your doctor if the condition fails to respond to over-the-counter remedies or promptly recurs.

Prognosis Excellent with proper treatment.

❖ BARTHOLIN'S GLAND CYST

Symptoms *(What you may experience)* Recurring tender swelling on either side of the entrance to the vaginal canal; occasionally, drainage of pus from the tender lump.

Signs and laboratory findings *(What the doctor looks for)* A tender lump in the lower portion of either of the labia minora.

What is it? The Bartholin's glands that lie just inside the entrance to the vaginal canal produce a lubricating fluid to protect these tender tissues as well as to facilitate penetration during intercourse. Occasionally, trauma or infection in the area can lead to obstruction of one of the Bartholin's glands. Buildup of secretions or infection within the obstructed gland will cause it to swell, sometimes to as large as 4 cm (about 2 in.); pressure caused by stretching the tissues can lead to considerable discomfort. Sometimes pus from infection within the gland can leak from the neck of the gland.

What you can do Apply warm, not hot, wet compresses to the area and take an over-the-counter analgesic/anti-inflammatory medication such as ibuprofen to help relieve pain.

When to call the doctor If you develop fever or a rash, note drainage of pus, or the swelling fails to respond to the simple measures described above, get medical attention.

Treatment If there is drainage of pus, your doctor may collect a sample of it for culture and testing to identify the infectious organism; the result will help to guide proper antibiotic choice. To relieve the pressure, the doctor will either aspirate (withdrawing the pus with a needle and syringe) or perform an incision and drainage ("lancing" the abscess with a scalpel). Relief is almost immediate. In cases of repeated recurrence of cyst infection, the doctor may recommend a procedure called marsupialization in which the gland and its duct are opened surgically and a flexible catheter is sewn in and left in place until a "new" duct can form around it. This more extensive procedure will usually be performed under general or spinal anesthesia in an outpatient surgery center.

INFECTIOUS SORES ON THE EXTERNAL GENITALS

A number of disparate infectious organisms can cause lesions or sores on the vulva. Refer to the descriptions and photographs of typical examples of common infections to aid in identification. Most of these disorders are spread by sexual contact; they and their treatments are fully covered in Chapter 21 under the heading Sexually Transmitted Infections, page 861. Do not attempt self-treatment for any of these disorders; instead, see a doctor any time a lesion develops in this area. Prompt proper treatment may prevent the development of later complications.

- Herpes simplex virus II appears as a cluster of clear to white blisters on a red, tender base. The appearance is usually preceded by an abnormal sensation (tenderness, itching, or burning) in the area. The blisters usually recur in the same or a nearby location.

- Lymphogranuloma venereum (LGV) may briefly appear as a blister or ulcer on the labia or anus, but disappears quickly and may go unnoticed. Subsequently (1 to 4 weeks) tender lymph nodes appear sometimes in the groin, but in women more often in the rectal area. Rectal pain and bloody rectal discharge may be the first signs.

- Condyloma acuminata (veneral warts) appear as lacy, cauliflower-like growths, usually on the labia minora, but can extend up into the vaginal canal to the cervix or all the way to the rectal area. They grow quickly and usually itch.

- Syphilis appears usually as a painless, white to yellow ulcer (called a chancre) most often on the labia or region of the anus and rectum (although it can also appear on the cervix) usually within 3 to 4 weeks after sexual contact with an infected person. ■

Prognosis Excellent with prompt and proper treatment.

❖ VULVAR INJURY (BRUISES AND LACERATIONS)

Symptoms and signs *(What you may experience)* Pain; swelling; discoloration following trauma.

What is it? Trauma to the vulva most often occurs from straddle injuries, landing on the crossbar of a bicycle for example. This crushing type injury can result in simple bruises, but can also rupture blood vessels in the labia that can cause bleeding within the tissues and the development of a hematoma (clotted blood that forms a mass). Occasionally, the swelling may be sufficient to require drainage of the accumulated blood. Lacerations may require repair by a doctor. It is possible, although rare, that the blow could be so placed as to crush or tear the urethra (the urine outflow tube). Be alert for any sign of blood in the urine that could signal such an occurrence.

What you can do For simple bruises and swelling, apply a cold pack to the area. Take acetaminophen or ibuprofen for discomfort.

When to call the doctor Swelling that causes significant pain, blood in the urine, or an open laceration of the tissues requires prompt medical attention.

Treatment Lacerations must be cleaned and closed with sutures. Some hematomas must be opened and drained. Open wounds may require antibiotics to prevent infection. Laceration of the urethra will require referral to a urologist.

Prognosis Excellent with proper treatment.

❖ CANCER OF THE VULVA

Symptoms *(What you may experience)* Chronic irritation or itching of an area of the vulva; persistent white patch or scaly area on the vulva; later, a firm lump or growth on the vulva; persistent ulcerated area on the vulva.

Signs and laboratory findings *(What the doctor looks for)* Biopsy (removal of a piece of tissue) examined under the microscope is needed to confirm the diagnosis of cancer.

What is it? Cancer of the vulva rarely occurs in women under age 50. It involves the squamous (most superficial layer) cells of the skin. Some connection has been made by researchers to previous infection with the human papillomavirus, which is known to cause damage and cancerous transformation in cervical cells (see page 865), and a history of genital warts may predispose women to this cancer (see Infectious Sores on the External Genitals, page 1107). Transformation from a normal cell to a cancerous one does not occur overnight, but rather over a continuum ranging from mildly dysplastic (abnormally changed) to cancerous, a process that may take many months to years.

What you can do Perform a self-exam regularly. If the area seems persistently abnor-

mal, visit your doctor to have the area examined.

Treatment

- Medical therapy. Topically applied medicated creams such as a mixture of betamethasone and crotamiton may help to relieve the itching; testosterone propionate in petrolatum jelly is used to treat certain types of precancerous lesions.

- Surgical therapy. Selection of appropriate surgical treatment depends on whether the biopsy of tissue demonstrates that the cancer remains confined to the superficial layer (carcinoma *in situ*) or has spread to deeper layers or adjacent organs or lymph nodes (invasive cancer). In carcinoma *in situ*, the lesion and a wide margin of surrounding normal tissue should be removed. Sometimes, laser therapy or superficial removal of all vulvar skin, with subsequent skin grafting, may be necessary. Invasive cancer will necessitate radical vulvectomy and removal of the lymph nodes in the region. In patients too weak to withstand this extensive surgery, radiation (x-ray) therapy to the area may help.

Prognosis Early diagnosis and prompt appropriate treatment greatly improves the odds. Surgical removal of small lesions (under 3 cm) that have not spread to other areas results in 90 percent of patients cancer free at 5 years. Larger cancers or cancers that have spread to distant areas have a poorer prognosis, with 25 percent of patients surviving 5 years.

The Vagina

The vagina is a canal about 5 in. long with ridged, muscular walls that normally touch but can relax to open the size of the canal sufficiently to accommodate the passage of an infant during childbirth.

THE HYMEN

In young girls, a thin membrane (called the hymen) spans the vaginal canal, fully or, more often, partially blocking the opening.

This membrane will usually be stretched or broken either by athletic activities or failing that, by first intercourse. Rarely, the hymen completely spans the vaginal opening (a condition called *imperforate hymen),* obstructing the outflow of menstrual blood and causing considerable pain once cycling begins. In these instances, a doctor must make an incision to open the hymen to relieve the obstruction.

❖ CANDIDA VAGINITIS (YEAST INFECTION)

For information on candida vaginitis see the section on Candida Vulvovaginitis, page 1105.

❖ OTHER VAGINAL DISCHARGES

***Symptoms** (What you may experience)* Vaginal discharge, sometimes with a fishy or rotten odor.

***Signs and laboratory findings** (What the doctor looks for)* Specific testing by microscopic analysis, culture, or rapid identification kit to determine which organism is responsible.

What is it?

- *Trichomonas vaginitis.* The causative organism in this infection is the *Trichomonas vaginalis* protozoan, a single-cell microbe with four whipping "tails" or flagellae. Infection with it usually causes a thin, frothy, yellow to green discharge and intense itching. It is usually passed from person-to-person by sexual contact. Although women have easily discernible symptoms from the infection, men often do not, and can unwittingly pass it to another sexual partner.

- *Bacterial vaginosis.* Also known as *Gardnerella* vaginitis, infection with this bacterium causes a grayish, sometimes frothy discharge with a characteristic fishy odor. The odor becomes especially prominent when a drop of potassium hydroxide solution is added to it for microscopic evaluation. This infection does not generally cause itching or irritation. It is not passed by sexual contact.

- *Doerderland's vaginitis.* This infection

actually represents an "overgrowth" of the *Lactobacillus* bacteria that normally inhabit the vaginal canal and help to maintain its acid balance. Occasionally, when this occurs, women develop a heavy, sometimes curd-like discharge that looks, and to some extent behaves, like a candidal yeast infection. When the doctor examines or cultures the discharge, no yeast are found, only an overabundance of the rod-shaped "friendly" inhabitants.

- *Retained tampon.* Occasionally, a woman may inadvertently fail to remove a tampon before inserting a new one. When this happens, the soiled tampon may become lodged in the recess of the vaginal vault where it may remain for some time before a watery brownish foul-smelling discharge draws attention to it. The danger of retained tampons is, of course, infection, and most specifically, of the staphylococcal variety that could lead to Toxic Shock Syndrome (see page 1110).

TOXIC SHOCK SYNDROME

Toxic shock syndrome is a very rare condition. Although toxic shock syndrome can occur in children or in men, more than 90 percent of cases occur in women of childbearing age who use tampons. Symptoms often begin within the first 5 days of the onset of the menstrual period. They include the sudden onset of high fever, vomiting, and watery diarrhea; occasionally, the syndrome may also result in sore throat, muscle aches, headache, a red rash (usually not raised bumps but red discoloration that often peels on the palms and soles as it heals), and sometimes conjunctivitis (pinkeye). In severe cases, extremely low blood pressure and heart and kidney failure can occur.

Toxic shock syndrome is not technically an infectious disease. Although it occurs because of a specific strain of staphylococcus bacterium, it is a toxin produced by the bacterium that causes the illness and not the bacteria themselves. Treatment involves replacement of fluids to combat dehydration from the high fever, antibiotics to eradicate the toxin producing bacteria, and removal of the cause of the accumulation of toxin (such as a tampon).

One common source of staphlococcal infection that can lead to toxic shock is the improper use of tampons during menstruation. Researchers theorize that super-absorbent tampons provide a breeding ground for the normally harmless bacteria that produce the toxin. For this reason, women who choose to use tampons should be careful to change them frequently, never leaving the same tampon in place for more than 8 hours. ■

DOUCHING: PRO AND CON

In most cases, women should not douche because the female reproductive tract produces mucus to cleanse itself, and the population of friendly bacteria serve to maintain the correct level of acidity. Routine douching can upset that normal balance.

Resist the temptation to douche, particularly before seeing a doctor, if a vaginal discharge develops. Douching can wash away the clues to the cause of the vaginal discharge. The characteristics of a discharge may be the chief means of identifying an infection; douching the discharge away will only make it more difficult for the doctor to make a correct diagnosis.

Occasionally, the doctor may recommend douching to combat a specific type of infection, for example, a vinegar or iodine (Betadine) solution to combat certain bacterial or chronic yeast infections or a baking soda solution in cases of bacterial vaginosis. But unless a woman is specifically instructed by her doctor to do so, douching is neither a necessary nor appropriate means of maintaining reproductive tract health. ■

What you can do Do not be too hasty to declare any vaginal discharge "yeast" and treat with over-the-counter yeast medications.

When to call the doctor With any discharge that causes discolored discharge, significant discomfort, spotting of blood, fever, or strong odor.

Treatment Trichomonas responds to the medication metronidazole taken orally as a single 2,000-mg dose or as two 1,000-mg doses taken 12 hours apart. If this method fails, resorting to treatment with doses of 500 mg twice a day for 7 days usually eradicates the microbe. Because the infection passes sexually, both the infected person and all sexual partners must be treated simultaneously. This drug is chemically related to the medication disulfiram (Antabuse), which is used to prevent alcohol use by causing extreme nausea and even death. Do not drink alcohol when taking metronidazol. It is also unsafe to take this medication during pregnancy.

Bacterial vaginosis also responds to treatment with metronidazole taken orally in doses of 500 mg twice daily for 7 days or as a single 2,000 mg dose. Intravaginal application of metronidazole gel twice daily for 5 days or clindamycin cream once daily for 7 days will also eradicate the infection.

Doerderland's vaginitis responds to measures that curb the overgrowth of the *Lactobacillus* organisms. The easiest measure is to gently douche the vaginal canal with a dilute solution of baking soda and water to make the vaginal tract slightly less acid and the environment less hospitable to the bacterium. There are several commercial preparations, or you can make your own with 1 tbs baking soda in 1 qt warm water, instilled with a bulb syringe. Avoid overusing baking soda because maintaining the proper acid balance is important to vaginal health.

Retained tampons must be removed as soon as possible and the vaginal canal gently irrigated with a weakly acidic solution, such as vinegar and water.

Prognosis Excellent in all cases if promptly identified and appropriately treated.

❖ VAGINAL TEARS AND LACERATIONS

Symptoms (What you may experience)
Vaginal bleeding after trauma.

Signs and laboratory findings (What the doctor looks for) Tears or cuts in the vaginal tissue; pelvic fracture as demonstrated by x-rays.

What is it? Trauma to the vagina is most often the result of sexual assault, although occasionally may occur during consensual sexual intercourse (for information about sexual assault, see page 315). Vaginal tears that result from causes other than rape generally occur from accidental penetrating injuries, (for example, straddle falls onto jagged or pointed surfaces) or from blunt or crushing pelvic trauma, such as a major motor vehicle accident.

Bleeding and the possibility of infection, particularly if there is also a pelvic fracture, are the major risks complicating vaginal lacerations. Rupture of the large pudendal artery or vein can cause significant bleeding that will require surgical repair.

Even with major trauma to the pelvis, the uterus, fallopian tubes, and ovaries rarely sustain significant damage owing to their protected position deep in the pelvis, their small size, and their relative mobility.

What you can do If possible, apply pressure with a clean cloth dressing and cold pack to the area and seek medical help immediately.

Treatment The doctor will need to examine the vaginal canal with a lighted speculum, as is done in a routine pelvic exam, to assess the size and nature of the tear. In the case of crushing or blunt pelvic trauma, x-rays will be needed to search for pelvic bone fractures.

Uncomplicated tears can be repaired in the office or emergency room under a local anesthetic. Those tears associated with a significant amount of bleeding and swelling may require general anesthesia in the operating room to be adequately examined and repaired. Antibiotics to prevent infection may also be necessary.

Prognosis Excellent if promptly and properly treated.

❖ VAGINAL ATROPHY (ATROPHIC VAGINITIS)

Symptoms (What you may experience)
Vaginal irritation and dryness; painful sexual intercourse; incontinence of urine.

Signs and laboratory findings (What the doctor looks for) Red, thin, fragile vaginal mucosa (lining).

What is it? The female reproductive hormones, particularly estrogens, play a critical role in keeping the vaginal tissues supple, lubricated, and healthy. When the levels of these hormones wane with menopause, the vaginal lining begins to atrophy, becoming thin and losing its elasticity and lubrication. The tissues tear and abrade more easily, sometimes making sexual intercourse quite painful and unpleasant. Because of the intimate association of the vaginal canal with the urethra (urine outflow tube) symptoms of urethral atrophy may also occur, primarily incontinence or dribbling of urine.

When to call the doctor Speak to your doctor about these troubling conditions when they arise.

DYSPAREUNIA (PAINFUL INTERCOURSE)

Sexual intercourse should not be painful. When it is, a specific cause can usually be found. Among the common causes for painful intercourse (dyspareunia) are the following:

- Vulvovaginitis (infection of the external genitalia).

- Remnant of the vaginal hymen. This membrane that spans the vaginal opening usually stretches or ruptures in adolescence with athletic endeavors, but sometimes persists, causing pain with first intercourse and possibly several episodes thereafter.

- Vaginismus (voluntary or involuntary contraction of the muscles around the vaginal opening often the result of fear, pain, previous sexual trauma, or extreme negative attitudes regarding sex learned in childhood) (see Vaginismus, page 1128).

- Vaginal atrophy with insufficient lubrication. The pain can usually be overcome with use of a water-soluble lubricant during intercourse.

- Infection and tumors can also cause pain. For more information, see Cervicitis, page 1113; Pelvic Inflammatory Disease, page 1116; Adenomyosis and Endometriosis, page 1117; Other Ovarian Cysts, page 1125 and Tubo-Ovarian Abscess, page 1124; and the sections on cervical, page 1114, vaginal, page 1112, uterine, page 1123, and ovarian cancer, pages 1125 and 1363. ■

Treatment Use of a water-soluble lubricant will usually provide symptomatic relief of the pain that may occur during intercourse.

The condition usually responds well to low doses (0.3 to 0.6 mg) of estrogen, taken by mouth, or estrogen creams applied locally to the vaginal tissues.

Prognosis Excellent with proper treatment.

❖ VAGINAL CANCER

Symptoms (What you may experience) Often: Watery discharge; painful intercourse; bleeding following intercourse. Occasionally and later in the disease: Frequent or urgent need to urinate; painful bowel movement. *Note:* There are many more common and less ominous reasons for these symptoms.

Signs and laboratory findings (What the doctor looks for) Visual exam and staining may demonstrate abnormal areas; biopsy confirms the suspected diagnosis.

What is it? Cancers of the vagina are extremely rare. They fall into the following two categories: clear cell adenocarcinoma and squamous cell carcinoma.

Clear cell adenocarcinoma occurs in women whose mothers took the drug diethylstilbestrol (DES) during pregnancy. An estimated 2 million fetuses were exposed between 1947 and 1971 when DES was administered to expectant mothers to control diabetes or to prevent threatened miscarriage. Current estimates suggest a range from 1 in 700 to 1 in 7,000 women exposed in the womb to this drug could develop clear cell cancer. The time of peak incidence in developing this cancer occurs between ages 15 and 22 .

Diagnosis depends on an initial evaluation with staining of the vaginal lining, magnified examination and biopsy of any nonstaining areas. Each year, continued vigilance through regular screening with both a Pap smear of the cervix *and* the vaginal walls is imperative.

Squamous cell carcinoma, seen in women ages 45 to 65, arises from the most superficial layer of cells lining the vagina. It grows quite slowly, but undetected, may invade nearby areas such as the bladder or rectum causing discomfort in passage of bowel movements or an urgent or frequent need to urinate. The periodic pelvic exam with Pap smear of the vaginal lining will aid in early discovery of these rare cancers.

What you can do If you were exposed to DES in the womb or if you are uncertain but were born between 1947 and 1971 you should have an annual gynecologic evaluation. Be sure to advise your gynecologist or doctor of your risk. Older women, ages 45 to 65, who may have become lax in having regular pelvic examinations after the need for contraception has waned should not neglect this important health screen.

When to call the doctor The development of a bloody discharge following intercourse or of persistent watery vaginal discharge, urgent urination, or painful bowel movement in women of this age group should prompt a visit to the doctor.

Treatment The cornerstone of therapy is surgical removal of all or part of the reproductive system. The extent of removal depends on the age and health of the woman, the size of the cancer, and whether the cancer has spread to adjacent areas or to lymph nodes in the region. Large or invasive cancers may require removal of the uterus, ovaries, part of the vagina, and some of the pelvic lymph nodes. Small, localized cancers may be adequately treated with a less extensive surgery, followed by radiation treatments.

Prognosis Good in clear cell adenocarcinoma, detected early and treated promptly. These cancers have a 5-year survival rate of 80 to 85 percent. The overall 5-year survival for the squamous cell carcinoma is only about 30 percent, pointing out the need to find these tumors very early, before invasion can occur.

The Cervix

The cervix is actually the narrow neck of the inverted pear-shaped uterus that protrudes into the vaginal canal. Because the cervix must withstand exposure to a greater degree of trauma, during sexual intercourse, for example, than the remainder of the uterus, its surface within the vaginal canal is covered with a layer of tougher more skin-like cells. This layer of epithelium gives way to a different kind of cell, one capable of producing mucus. When cervical cancers arise, it is often in this zone of transition between these two kinds of cells. To receive accurate Papanicolaou (Pap) smear results it is important that the doctor collects sample cells from this critical area. Occasionally, another sample may need to be taken to be certain the specimen includes these cells.

Disorders involving the cervix include infection, the formation of benign cysts (fluid-filled cavities) or polyps, and cancer.

❖ CERVICITIS (CERVICAL INFECTION)

Symptoms *(What you may experience)* Pain during intercourse with deep thrusting; colored or blood tinged vaginal discharge.

Signs and laboratory findings *(What the doctor looks for)* Red, swollen, tender cervix on pelvic exam; excessive or discolored cervical mucus or pus.

What is it? Infection of the cervix commonly occurs in sexually transmitted diseases caused by herpesvirus or such bacteria as *Neisseria gonorrhoeae* or *Chlamydia* species. Not all cervicitis is sexually related; these infections commonly occur following tears in the cervix that may occur during childbirth or abortion or in women with intrauterine devices (IUDs).

When to call the doctor See your doctor as soon as possible if you develop symptoms suggestive of cervicitis, particularly if accompanied by a rash or fever.

Treatment Initial herpesvirus infections should be treated promptly and aggressively with acyclovir (Zovirax) for at least 10 days to minimize the risk of establishing a cycle of recurrent herpes outbreaks. Long-term suppressive therapy with this drug may also be an option in cases of significant discomfort from frequent recurrences.

Neisseria gonorrhoeae responds to a variety of antimicrobial medications: ceftriaxone, cefixime, ciprofloxacin, ofloxacin, spectinomycin, and trimethoprim-sulfamethoxazole.

PROCEDURES FOR THE DIAGNOSIS AND TREATMENT OF CERVICAL DISORDERS

Various new methods and technologic advances now allow doctors to better examine and more specifically treat cervical disorders. These methods include the following:

Colposcopy The colposcope allows the doctor to magnify the cervical tissues by 10 to 20 times their normal size. Under magnification, the doctor can better assess the size and extent of abnormal areas of the cervical epithelium (covering) and can see whether the abnormality extends past the transformation zone and into the endocervical canal. The application of a weak acetic acid solution (vinegar) helps to clear away cervical mucus and to make the altered areas more visible. Iodine-based stain swabbed across the cervix will clearly delineate these abnormal areas, which do not take up the stain and appear as white patches, pointing out the areas to biopsy for microscopic exam. Colposcopy can be performed in the doctor's office without anesthetic.

Cryosurgery Application of extremely cold solutions (such as liquid nitrogen) to the areas of abnormal cervical epithelium destroys the cells by freezing. The frozen tissue will slough away as the normal cervical tissue heals from below. At the opposite end of the spectrum, the same result, destruction, sloughing, and healing, can be obtained by using extreme heat (cauterization) to burn away the abnormal cells. Cryosurgery can be performed in the doctor's office without anesthetic.

Loop Electrosurgical Excision Procedure (LEEP) In the case of cervical intraepithelial neoplasia (CIN), when the cervical lesion is entirely visible, the doctor can remove it in the office under local anesthesia; LEEP is a simple, quick procedure that involves using a wire loop charged with a low-voltage electric current to scoop out the abnormal area.

Laser The CO_2 laser, along with the magnification of the colposcope, can be used to treat large visible cervical lesions; its destructive power can be more tightly controlled and thereby minimize damage to surrounding normal tissue. Use of the CO_2 laser requires special training.

Conization Using either a scalpel or the CO_2 laser, the doctor removes most of the cervix, which in most cases will completely remove the lesion. The entire specimen can then be sent to the pathologist, allowing for a more thorough microscopic assessment of the extent of the lesion. Its use should be limited to cases where there is evidence of CIN III on Pap smear, severe dysplasia, or carcinoma *in situ*. ■

Chlamydia species respond best to doxycycline or azithromycin, but ofloxacin or sulfisoxazole are also effective choices.

See page 861 for more information on the treatment of sexually transmitted infections.

Cervicitis that is not sexually related should be treated with an antibiotic that will be selected based on the type of bacteria causing the infection.

CERVICAL EROSIONS AND ABRASIONS

Occasionally, women may develop erosions or abrasions on the cervix. These red, inflamed patches on the cervix, visible only during pelvic exam, usually occur from irritation by an intrauterine device (IUD) or from trauma sustained during sexual intercourse. Like an abrasion on the skin, these cervical erosions represent a break in the protective surface that may make the underlying, exposed tissue more vulnerable to infection. The erosions can have an ominous appearance and cause some concern on the part of the doctor who must make certain (by Pap smear, colposcopy, or biopsy) that they are simple abrasions and not early cervical cancers. Occasionally, they may persist and the doctor may recommend cautery or cryosurgery to slough the damaged tissue and permit more rapid healing. ■

Prognosis Excellent if detected promptly and treated appropriately. Left untreated, cervical infections can ascend in the reproductive tract. Infections of the uterus, fallopian tubes, or ovaries could permanently impair fertility by scarring or by leading to the necessity of hysterectomy to eradicate the infection.

❖ NABOTHIAN (INCLUSION) CYSTS

Symptoms (What you may experience) Usually none.

Signs and laboratory findings (What the doctor looks for) Fluid-filled cavities on the cervix.

What is it? These benign cysts form when one of the mucous glands in the cervix becomes obstructed. The obstruction may arise as new tissue grows over the gland following the trauma of childbirth, for example, or when the cervical tissues begin to thin with age, trapping pockets of normal secretions.

Treatment Usually no treatment is necessary. Occasionally, the doctor may elect to remove a Nabothian cyst by cryotherapy (the application of extreme cold to freeze

the tissue) see Procedures for the Diagnosis and Treatment of Cervical Disorders, page 1113 for more information.

Prognosis Excellent.

❖ CERVICAL POLYPS

Symptoms (What you may experience) Vaginal discharge; abnormal spotting or bleeding. *Note:* these symptoms are not specific to this disorder, but occur in many disorders in the female reproductive tract.

Signs and laboratory findings (What the doctor looks for) Small mushroom like growths on the cervix, visible on speculum examination.

What is it? These small benign growths on the cervix occur commonly after the onset of menstruation. Although the cause of cervical popyps is not clearly understood, cervical inflammation may play a role in their development. The symptoms are usually quite mild, but they should not be ignored because the cause of the polyps should be investigated. Abnormal vaginal bleeding and discharge may be caused by benign polyps, but your doctor will want to perform a careful examination to rule out other causes, such as uterine myomas or polyps, or more ominous possibilities, such as endometrial cancer. Cervical polyps rarely become cancerous.

When to call the doctor Abnormal vaginal bleeding or a persistent discharge should always prompt a visit to your doctor.

Treatment Treatment can often be carried out in the doctor's office, by removing the polyp(s) and sending the specimen to the pathologist for microscopic analysis. Large polyps or evidence of a dilated soft cervix may necessitate surgical D&C (dilation and curettage) to reach the stalk of the polyp and to explore the upper reaches of the uterine cavity, sampling those tissues as well to exclude endometrial cancer as a cause.

Prognosis Excellent.

❖ CANCER OF THE CERVIX

Symptoms (What you may experience) Blood-tinged or discolored nonitching vaginal discharge, spotting after intercourse, or bleeding. *Note:* These symptoms are not specific to this disorder, but may occur in many disorders in the female reproductive tract.

Signs and laboratory findings *(What the doctor looks for)* Abnormal area of cervix may be visible on speculum examination; Pap smear and biopsy confirming cancerous cells in the cervix.

What is it? Cancer of the cervix occurs when previously normal epithelial (superficial covering) cells undergo a process termed "malignant transformation." Damage to normal cells can make them grow unchecked and change their appearance. These changes, known as dysplasia, can be detected by a Pap smear. Additional changes in these dysplastic cells may culminate in cancer, which may invade nearby normal tissues and spread to other sites in the body. Among the causes of dysplasia and cervical cancer are infection with the human papilloma virus (HPV), cigarette smoking, multiple sexual partners, long-term use of oral contraceptive agents, and intrauterine exposure to DES. Women who are HIV positive are also at higher risk for developing cervical dysplasia.

Dysplasia of the cervix, also called cervical intraepithelial neoplasia (CIN) can be detected prior to becoming cancerous with the Pap smear (see The Periodic Pelvic Exam and Pap Smear, page 1100).

Once cancerous change has occurred, it may remain confined to the most superficial layer of the cervical covering (at this stage termed carcinoma *in situ*) for 2 to 10 years before it invades to deeper layers. Once the cancer has progressed beyond the boundary of the superficial layer, it can slowly invade nearby structures, such as the ureters, bladder, and rectum if untreated.

At the time of surgery, the progression of the cancer will be staged according to the following guidelines: stage 0, confined to the superficial layer; stage I, confined to the cervix; stage II, extends beyond the cervix, but not to the pelvic wall or into the lower portion of the vagina; stage III, extends into the pelvic wall, the lower portion of the vagina, or ureter; stage IV, extends beyond the pelvis to the bladder and/or adjacent or distant organs.

Prevention Prevention and early detection is paramount. When cervical cancer is discovered and treated early, 99 women in 100 survive the disease; when the disease is not diagnosed before it is in the most advanced stage, only 7 women in 100 survive it. To prevent this disease, you should:

- Undergo regular pelvic exam and Pap smear screening to detect abnormalities
- Limit the number of sexual partners to reduce exposure to HPV
- Stop smoking
- Use a diaphragm or condom to protect the cervix during intercourse

When to call the doctor In women known to have advanced cervical cancer, the development of significant vaginal bleeding could signal erosion of an artery. Seek immediate medical attention at the hospital.

Treatment

- Carcinoma *in situ* (stage 0). In women who have already borne their children, total hysterectomy is the treatment of choice. In women still desirous of having children, cervical conization or loop electrosurgical excision procedure (LEEP) are acceptable alternative treatments. Pap smears every 4 months for 1 year and every 6 months for a second year are advisable.

- Invasive Cancers. Simple hysterectomy is an adequate treatment for stage I cancers smaller than 7 mm in size. Larger stage I and stage II cancers may respond to either radical hysterectomy or radiation therapy. The choice of which depends to some degree on the age and health of the woman; younger women may opt for radical surgery, because it causes fewer long-term complications and may preserve ovarian function. Stage III and stage IV must be treated with radiation.

Prognosis Survival depends on the stage at which the cancer is discovered and treated. At Stage 0, appropriate treatment results in 99 to 100 percent survival; at stage I, 76 percent; at stage II, 55 percent; at stage III, 31 percent; and at stage IV, 7 percent.

The Uterus

The uterus, or womb, a hollow organ with thick muscular walls, is shaped like an upside down pear and is positioned in the low middle of the abdomen. Only about 2.5 to 3 in. in length (prior to pregnancy), the uterus is capable of expanding sufficiently to carry a 20 in. or longer fetus and its muscular walls are powerful enough to push the fetus out during the birth process.

Each month, in response to timed fluctuations of female reproductive hormones, the lining of the uterus expands dramatically, building up a rich cushion of blood and endometrium (the lining cells of the uterus) to receive a fertilized egg. If fertilization of the egg fails to occur, the lining sheds as the monthly menstrual cycle (see Menstruation and Ovulation, page 1099).

The major disorders affecting the uterus include infection of the lining, abnormally located pockets of lining tissue, abnormalities of the menstrual cycle, growths of the muscular wall, relaxation of uterine support, disorders of development and structure, and cancer.

❖ PELVIC INFLAMMATORY DISEASE, ENDOMETRITIS, SALPINGITIS

Symptoms *(What you may experience)* Lower abdominal tenderness; abdominal pain; vaginal discharge. Sometimes: vaginal bleeding, nausea, vomiting, fever. *Note*: these symptoms are not specific to this disorder.

Signs and laboratory findings *(What the doctor looks for)* Cervical discharge; tenderness of the tubes, ovaries, and cervix on pelvic exam; cervical infection with *Neisseria gonorrhea* or *Chlamydia trachomatis* identified by laboratory tests; an abscess of

CONGENITAL ABNORMALITIES OF THE REPRODUCTIVE TRACT

As the reproductive tract develops during gestation, abnormalities can sometimes occur in the position or shape of the uterus; occasionally, the uterus may not develop at all. These alterations from the norm can cause problems in menstruating, conceiving a pregnancy, or carrying a baby to term. Identification of these abnormalities can usually be made by ultrasound or MRI studies or by an x-ray study called a hysterosalpingogram in which a dye visible on x-ray is infused into the uterus to illuminate its internal shape. The dye will also outline the shape, size, and patency (whether they are open) of the fallopian tubes.

Retroverted Uterus Instead of the normal position in which the uterus lies tilted forward over the bladder, a retroverted uterus tilts backward, pressing instead against the rectum and sacral bones. In general this change will not prevent conception or successful delivery of a healthy baby, but it may cause some back discomfort as the expanding uterus presses against the sacrum.

Bicornuate Uterus Occasionally the uterus develops in a split configuration with a wall down the center of the uterine cavity. The term bicornuate implies two horns or two cavities. This configuration can cause some difficulty in conceiving or in carrying a baby to term because of space constraints, and surgical repair may be recommended.

Absence of Uterus As the name implies, in rare instances the reproductive tract forms without a uterus. In this case, of course, there would be no menstrual cycling at puberty and conception would be impossible.

Androgen Insensitivity Syndrome Rarely, when normal menstruation fails to occur, the doctor investigating this abnormality discovers that the cause is androgen (testosterone) insensitivity syndrome. In certain rare instances, a male infant is born whose cells are unable to respond to the male sex hormone, testosterone. As a consequence, those structures that require this hormone for their development, in particular those physical characteristics that we associate with "maleness," fail to develop. When this occurs, the baby will appear to be female from birth onward, and will develop female sexual characteristics, such as breasts, that are under estrogenic influence. What cannot develop, however, are the female reproductive organs, a uterus, fallopian tubes, and ovaries. The testicles, which would descend from the abdominal cavity into the scrotal sac (see The Male Reproductive System, page 1130) under androgenic stimulation by testosterone, will remain within the abdomen. There is an increased risk for the development of testicular cancer if they do, and for this reason, the doctor will recommend their surgical removal.

In virtually all cases, androgen insensitivity syndrome will not be recognized until after puberty when menstrual cycling fails to occur, at a time long after the child has made personal and psychosocial identification as a female. Only chromosomal (genetic) analysis can confirm this suspected diagnosis when exam of the genetic material reveals the presence of the male "Y" chromosome, which genetically female cells do not possess. How to convey this information to the adolescent and her parents is a delicate matter of medical ethics, best determined on an individual basis by the doctor in charge of the person's care. Little is served by disrupting a person's life or confusing a stable psychosocial identity; people with androgen insensitivity syndrome are in appearance infertile females, and counseling toward that end is what is usually important, not the nature of their chromosomes. ■

the tube or ovary shown by ultrasound scan.

What is it? Pelvic inflammatory disease (PID) occurs as infection spreads from the vagina and the cervix to the upper part of the reproductive tract: the uterus, fallopian tubes, and ovaries. When it involves the uterus, it is called endometritis; when it involves the tubes, salpingitis. Occasionally, the infection involves the tube and ovary, developing a localized abscess, called a tubo-ovarian abscess (see Tubo-Ovarian Abscess, page 1124).

Pelvic inflammatory disease is the most common serious infection in women of child-bearing age. Often, the causative bacteria are sexually transmitted ones, such as *Neisseria gonorrhoeae* or *C. trachomatis* (see page 867), but PID can also occur from infection with "naturally occurring" bacterial inhabitants of the reproductive tract, and from streptococcal and anaerobic bacteria, and gram-negative rods (usual invaders of the urinary tract).

The symptoms, particularly lower abdominal pain, can mimic a wide variety of other conditions from which PID must be differentiated by laboratory and x-ray studies. These possibilities include ectopic pregnancy, appendicitis, hemorrhage, rupture, or torsion (twisting) of an ovarian cyst, endometriosis, septic (infected) abortion, urinary tract infection, or gastrointestinal infection.

The disorder most commonly strikes young, sexually active women (especially those who have had multiple sex partners) who have never borne children. Smoking and frequent douching also may increase risk for PID.

What you can do PID is one of the most serious complication of sexually transmitted infections (STIs) and a major cause of infertility in woman. Yet in many cases the disease is preventable, if you follow the precautions necessary to prevent sexually transmitted diseases. If you are sexually active, particularly with multiple sexual partners, prevent infection by safe sex practices, such as using barrier contraception (see page 860 for more information on preventing sexually transmitted diseases). The sexual partner of anyone diagnosed with PID should be tested as well to prevent rein-

fection, even if your partner shows no symptoms.

When to call the doctor Anytime persistent abdominal discomfort develops, especially if associated with a vaginal discharge, fever, or a rash, consult your doctor. Although abdominal pain has many causes besides PID, none of them should be ignored.

Treatment Treatment with antibiotics to eradicate the infection is the cornerstone of therapy. The choice of medication should be tailored to the infecting organism, but common choices include cefoxitin, or cefotetan plus doxycycline, and clindamycin plus gentamicin. PID that causes severe pain or fever usually requires hospitalization for intravenous antibiotic therapy and to be certain that there is no other reason for the symptoms, for example, ectopic pregnancy, appendicitis, or pelvic abscess. Pregnant women, adolescents, or women who are HIV positive should also be hospitalized if they develop PID.

Prognosis Even with appropriate treatment, 25 percent of women with PID develop long-term problems, such as recurrent episodes of infection, painful intercourse (from scarring), chronic pelvic pain, and greatly increased risk for ectopic pregnancy. Recurrent episodes and associated problems can in rare cases lead to the need for a hysterectomy. With each successive episode of infection, a progressively increased risk of infertility occurs. One in five women develop infertility from a single episode of PID, one in three after a second, and three in four after a third occurrence of PID.

❖ ADENOMYOSIS AND ENDOMETRIOSIS

Symptoms *(What you may experience)* Constant aching abdominal pain 2 to 7 days prior to menses; severe menstrual cramps. Occasionally: Painful intercourse (dyspareunia) or rectal pain and bleeding; premenstrual syndrome (see Premenstrual Syndrome, page 1101).

Signs and laboratory findings *(What the doctor looks for)* In endometriosis, the presence of tender, firm lumps behind the

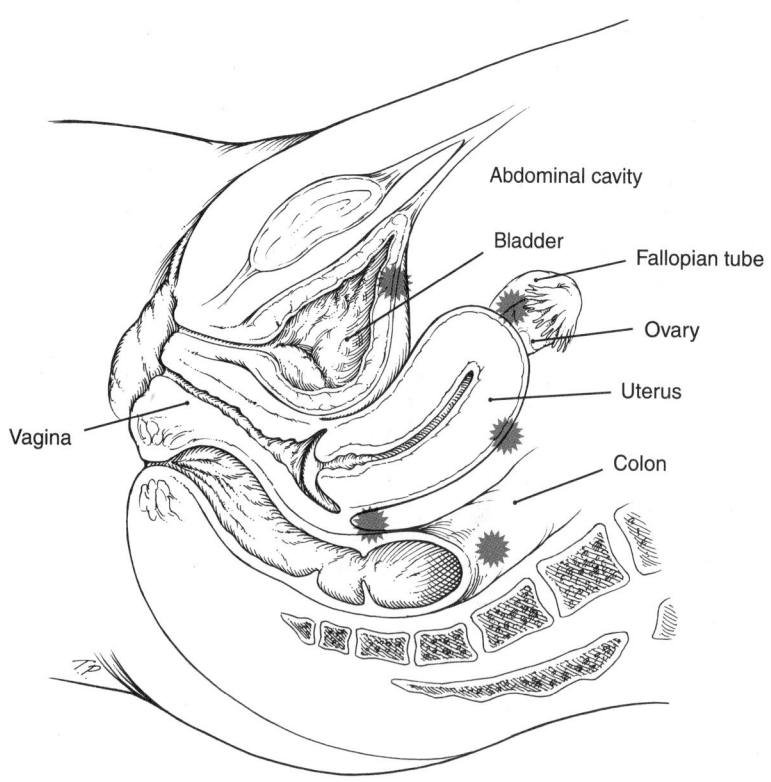

Cells of the inner lining of the uterus (endometrium) sometimes grow in abnormal sites outside the uterus in the fallopian tubes or on the ovaries. Other possible sites of abnormal cell development include the gastrointestinal tract, bladder, vagina, or elsewhere inside the abdominal cavity. Symptoms depend on location, and both medical and surgical treatments are available.

cervix on pelvic exam. In adenomyosis, a tender enlarged uterus on pelvic exam. Laparoscopic examination may be necessary to confirm the diagnosis.

What is it? The lining layer of the uterus (called the endometrium) sometimes grows in an abnormal location invading into the muscular uterine wall or completely outside the uterus. When it occurs within the myometrium, the muscle wall of the uterus, it is termed adenomyosis; when these growths develop outside the uterus in the fallopian tubes or on the ovaries, or in areas outside the reproductive tract entirely, such as the gastrointestinal tract, the bladder, or scattered inside the abdominal cavity, it is termed endometriosis.

The symptoms caused by adenomyosis generally become more prominent with age. They include worsening menstrual cramping, lasting throughout the entire menstrual period, and associated with prolonged or excessive blood flow. The symptoms of endometriosis depend on where the ectopic (out-of-place) endometrial tissue develops. Because the endometrial tissue usually responds to monthly hormonal fluctuations, it may build up, break down, and bleed each month along with the normal endometrium lining the uterus. But unlike the endometrium inside the uterus, which is sloughed off with each menstrual cycle, endometriosis has no way of leaving the body. With each menstrual cycle, the condition worsens. If this aberrant menstrual bleeding occurs into the abdominal cavity or the fallopian tube, it may cause aching abdominal discomfort or painful intercourse; into the gastrointestinal tract, pain and rectal bleeding; into the bladder, painful urination and the passage of urinary blood. Ectopic endometrial tissue in the fallopian tubes can cause scarring and infertility. Specialized testing, such as MRI, proctosigmoidoscopy, laparoscopy, or laparotomy and biopsy, may be necessary to differentiate adenomyosis or endometriosis from other conditions, such as PID, or ovarian or uterine tumors, that may cause similar symptoms and may even appear similar on ultrasound scans.

When to call the doctor Persistent abdominal discomfort or other symptoms suggestive of adenomyosis or endometriosis should not be ignored.

Treatment Analgesic medications, sometimes with mild narcotic pain relievers such as codeine, or nonsteroidal anti-inflammatory medications, such as ibuprofen, may prove helpful in alleviating symptoms of both adenomyosis and endometriosis.

The treatment for adenomyosis is most commonly hysterectomy, usually followed by long-term estrogen therapy (see Hysterectomy, page 1121). If a woman with adenomyosis wishes to have a child, treatment with danazol and leuprolide acetate (Lupron) may reduce symptoms long enough to allow her to conceive and give birth, but this therapy cannot be continued long-term.

Both medical and surgical measures are used to treat endometriosis.

- *Medical Therapy.* The goal of medical therapies is to inhibit ovulation and reduce the cyclic hormonal stimulation of the endometrial tissues. They include combination oral contraceptive medications (birth control pills) or injections of progesterone or estrogen; nafarelin nasal spray or leuprolide injections (both gonadotropin releasing hormone inhibiting medications); and danazol.

- *Surgical therapy.* Surgical treatment in women under age 35 and those still desirous of having children is usually to remove the growths and break apart any scar tissue by cauterizing the abnormal areas or vaporizing them through the use of a laparoscope and laser surgery. These surgeries can often be performed through "button hole" incisions made just below the navel using the laparoscope (a pencil-sized illuminated optical instrument) and laser. Cases of extensive disease may require a full laparotomy in which a "bikini" incision is made and the endometriosis is removed using meticulous microsurgical techniques. In women who no longer desire to become pregnant, or in women disabled by the discomfort, total hysterectomy (removal of the uterus, both ovaries, and tubes) may be necessary.

Prognosis If the disorder is detected early, the chance that it will respond to laser or electrocautery surgery and that reproductive function will be preserved is good. Total hysterectomy is curative of symptoms.

❖ ENDOMETRIAL HYPERPLASIA

Symptoms *(What you may experience)* Heavy, prolonged menstrual flow; bleeding between menstrual periods.

Signs and laboratory findings *(What the doctor looks for)* Confirmation by endometrial biopsy.

What is it? Occasionally, especially at the extremes of reproductive life, teens and women nearing menopause, the lining layer of the uterus becomes too thick. Between periods, it may in a sense collapse under its own weight and "shed" resulting in midcy-

D&C AND ENDOMETRIAL BIOPSY

When it becomes necessary to obtain a sample of the lining of the uterus (an endometrial biopsy) or to scrape it away when it is overgrown (curettage), the gynecologic surgeon will recommend a D&C (dilation and curettage). Because the opening of the cervix (neck of the uterus) is narrow, the doctor must first relax and enlarge (dilate) the cervical opening to pass the necessary instruments into the uterine cavity. The dilation procedure could cause some discomfort without either a local anesthetic to numb the cervix or, often, a general anesthetic. The uterine lining, itself, feels little pain.

A D&C involving endometrial biopsy or endometrial sampling is usually performed in the doctor's office under local anesthesia or no anesthesia at all. A small-caliber sampling device is used so that the cervix does not need to be dilated (widened). If a more thorough procedure is needed, the D&C is usually performed in a hospital operating room, under local anesthesia with sedation. Generally, the patient can return home that same day.

Following the procedure it is normal for a woman to experience a few days of brown vaginal spotting. A doctor should be contacted if there is significant passage of fresh, red blood. ■

cle bleeding, or the period may occur on schedule, but with an excessively large volume of menstrual blood flow. When the problem occurs in older women, the doctor must always obtain a biopsy (tissue sample) for microscopic analysis to be certain that the condition is benign.

When to call the doctor Unusually large volume menstrual periods or bleeding between cycles (that persists more than one or two cycles) should prompt a visit to your doctor.

Treatment In young women, oral contraceptive agents can help to suppress the exuberant growth of the lining and may solve the problem. Any bleeding that fails to respond to oral contraceptives warrants a surgical scraping away of the uterine lining (dilation and curettage, or D&C) to be certain the process is benign. The discovery of precancerous cells in the uterine lining warrants a hysterectomy. Although hormone therapy may reduce the bleeding, it will not reduce the risk of future endometrial cancer in these cases.

Prognosis Excellent with prompt diagnosis and appropriate treatment.

❖ PELVIC RELAXATION AND UTERINE PROLAPSE

Symptoms *(What you may experience)* A sense of fullness in the vagina; bladder pressure or urinary dribbling. Occasionally: Cervix protruding from the vaginal opening.

Signs and laboratory *(What the doctor looks for)* Sagging of the uterus into the vagina.

What is it? Support of the female reproductive organs rests on several ligaments that connect the uterus to the bony pelvis. During pregnancy, the weight of the fetus, placenta, and amniotic fluid can dramatically increase the load these ligaments must bear, weakening and stretching them. Each successive pregnancy worsens the damage. As the uterus loses its support, it begins to sag, putting pressure on the bladder.

In mild cases, the uterus may sag minimally, but with time, it may slip progressively farther down into the vaginal canal, until in extreme cases, the entire cervix and even uterus may drop out of the vaginal opening.

Often when the pelvic support fails, herniation of one or more of the adjacent structures into the vaginal canal can complicate the prolapse. Herniation of the bladder (a cystocele) may cause dribbling, incontinence, or a sense of frequent need to urinate (see page 1071). Herniation of the lower rectum (a rectocele) may produce a sensation of rectal fullness and the need to move the bowels. Herniation of a portion of the small intestine (an enterocele) may also occur, although it may cause few symptoms unless the bowel were to become entrapped within the vaginal hernia.

What you can do Strengthen the pelvic musculature by regularly performing the Kegel Exercises (see page 1072).

When to call the doctor If you can see or feel the cervix near the opening of the vaginal canal or if you suffer persistent discomfort from urinary dribbling or rectal urgency, notify your doctor.

Treatment General supportive measures include

- Weight reduction in overweight women
- A high fiber diet to keep the stool soft and reduce straining, which increases pressure in the abdomen
- Use of a pessary, a supportive device worn in the vaginal canal to temporarily support the falling uterus in women who either cannot or will not consider surgical options
- Hysterectomy or a pelvic resuspension procedure (surgical correction in which the uterine ligaments are shortened, strengthened, or more securely affixed to properly support the uterus)

Prognosis Good with appropriate management.

SURGERY TO CORRECT PELVIC RELAXATION

The ligaments designed to support the uterus and other pelvic structures sometimes stretch and sag with aging, as a consequence of the extra weight caused by pregnancy, or following hysterectomy. If the uterus is still present, it will sag into the vaginal canal, sometimes even protruding from the vaginal opening. Loss of pelvic support puts added stress on the bladder or the rectum, creating the additional problems of urinary continence and bowel habits. Even though the added weight of the sagging uterus may seem the more obvious cause of symptoms, its removal alone will not cure the problem. Relief of symptoms associated with pelvic relaxation depends upon carefully elevating the vaginal tissues. The surgery to correct this problem, called a pelvic resuspension, involves elevating the vaginal canal and tacking it securely to the bones or other structures higher in the pelvis to restore it to its normal position. Many women may opt to undergo removal of the uterus at this time, while others may elect to keep the uterus. In such cases, returning the uterus to its normal position will usually mean shortening and strengthening the support ligaments.

If the weakness and sag of tissues has allowed adjacent hollow structures, the urinary bladder, bowel, or rectum, to herniate into the vaginal canal (creating a cystocele, enterocele, or rectocele) these protrusions should be repaired at the same time.

In most cases, the surgery will be performed through the vaginal canal, not requiring an incision in the abdominal wall; the typical hospital stay lasts 5 to 7 days. Recovery at home will usually last an additional 1 to 2 weeks followed by another month to 6 weeks of limited physical and sexual activity as well as no lifting and no driving. ■

❖ FIBROID TUMORS

Symptoms *(What you may experience)*
No symptoms whatsoever; frequent need to urinate; heavy menstrual bleeding and dysmenorrhea. Occasionally: abdominal pain.

Signs and laboratory findings *(What the doctor looks for)* Irregular enlargement of the uterus on pelvic exam; possibly low-red-blood cell count (anemia) from bleeding.

What is it? These common, benign tumors (also called myomas or fibromyomas) arise from the muscle and connective tissues of the uterine wall. They are usually round, and may occur in multiples giving the uterus an irregular, lumpy feel. They may develop virtually anywhere in the uterus, that is, the wall, just below the lining or outer covering, near the cervix, within the support ligaments, sometimes even attaching to and "robbing" blood supply from neighboring organs.

Although the tumors may remain relatively small and may cause no symptoms whatsoever, occasionally they grow quite large and especially under the influence of hormonal stimulation during pregnancy may enlarge and complicate the delivery.

When to call the doctor Any unusual, prolonged vaginal bleeding should prompt a visit to your doctor.

Treatment If bleeding is heavy or prolonged enough to cause anemia, menstrual flow can be stopped with injections of 150 mg medroxyprogesterone (given every 28 days) or oral doses of danazol (400 to 800 mg) daily.

In some cases, surgery may become necessary. For women of childbearing age who desire to have children, a myomectomy (surgical removal of the fibroids alone) may be recommended. For other women, partial or total hysterectomy is more often the treatment of choice (see Hysterectomy, this page). A myomectomy is more difficult to perform, is not recommended for certain types of fibroids, and cannot prevent recurrence as hysterectomy can.

Prognosis Surgery cures the problem. Myomectomy does not pose a risk to later pregnancies. However, some obstetricians may recommend that future babies be deliv-

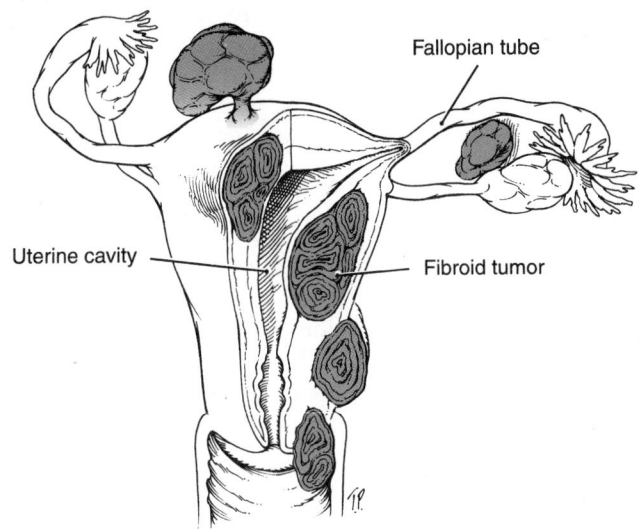

Fibroid tumors are common, benign tumors that can occur virtually anywhere in or around the uterus. They occasionally become large, cause abdominal pain or heavy menstrual bleeding, or complicate delivery of a child. Hormone therapy may reduce the size of tumors or surgical removal of the fibroids or of the uterus may be necessary.

ered by cesarean section. There is some concern that the surgical scar that remains in the uterine wall following myomectomy may be vulnerable to rupture during labor contractions. Such rupture is no longer considered likely if the surgical excision of the myoma was done properly.

HYSTERECTOMY

Removal of the uterus may be the optimal treatment for a variety of gynecologic disorders, including uterine cancer, severe dysfunctional bleeding with anemia, severe endometriosis, large or bleeding fibroid tumors, or prolapse. In most instances, removal of the uterus can be done either through an incision in the abdominal wall or through the vaginal canal. The extent of a hysterectomy depends upon the woman's age and health and the nature of the disorder being treated.

Partial hysterectomy implies that the doctor removes most of the uterus, leaving the cervix and a portion of the base of the uterus.

In a total hysterectomy, the doctor removes the entire uterus and cervix. In some cases, the procedure must also include removal of one or both fallopian tubes and ovaries (a salpingo-oophorectomy).

A radical hysterectomy is necessary only in cases of advanced spread of cancer. In addition to those tissues removed in a total hysterectomy, the radical procedure also implies removal of the upper part of the vagina and usually some of the lymph nodes in the area.

All these procedures must be performed in the hospital, under a general anesthetic. The operation itself usually takes 1 to 2 hours; recuperation in the hospital is usually less than 1 week. The woman has limited activity for the following 6 to 8 weeks which usually means no heavy lifting, driving a car, sexual intercourse, or vigorous sports. ■

❖ DYSFUNCTIONAL UTERINE BLEEDING

Symptoms and signs (What you may experience) Unpredictable vaginal bleeding in amount or duration.

What is it? At the beginning and the end of the reproductive stage of a woman's life, when the production of hormones may be erratic, the endometrial lining may build up excessively, failing to shed on time and when it does, flooding heavily. Occasionally, the hormonal abnormalities arise from stress or illness, but may also be the consequence of other reproductive system disorders (see Polycystic Ovarian Syndrome, page 1124) or excessive doses of estrogen. During the childbearing years, dysfunctional bleeding can be the result of ectopic pregnancy or miscarriage, and these possible causes must always be ruled out by your doctor.

What you can do Usually, this disorder is not serious, but, if persistent, should not be ignored. It is helpful if you can provide the doctor with an accurate estimate of the loss of blood you have experienced. The easiest way to assess loss is to keep track of the number and absorbency of pads or tampons you use per day.

When to call the doctor Bleeding that occurs at unexpected times or in unusually large amounts should prompt you to consult your doctor.

Treatment In most cases, even moderately severe bleeding can be stopped by a short course of hormonal therapy (oral contraceptive agents containing estrogen). When more severe bleeding occurs, hospitalization, with bed rest and injections of hormone may be necessary, followed by several months of oral contraceptive agents to prevent recurrence. If anemia has resulted from blood loss, supplementation with iron may also be recommended.

When hormone therapy fails to stop the bleeding, your doctor will recommend a surgical remedy, usually a D&C procedure to scrape away the excess tissue lining the uterus. This procedure usually prevents further bleeding. Some of this tissue will go to the pathologist for microscopic examination to help determine the cause of bleeding.

Prognosis Excellent after appropriate treatment.

HYDATIDIFORM MOLE (MOLAR PREGNANCY)

Symptoms (What you may experience) Rapid, excessive uterine growth during pregnancy; vaginal bleeding; absence of fetal movements; severe nausea and vomiting; passage of tissue resembling a cluster of grapes from the vagina.

Signs and laboratory findings (What the doctor looks for) Larger than expected uterus. Occasionally: hypertension; absent fetal heart tones; ultrasound confirmation of molar pregnancy.

What is it? In about 1 pregnancy in 2,000, a benign growth called a hydatidiform mole arises around the fertilized egg in the tissues that would normally become the placenta. Occasionally, such a growth develops from a small piece of placenta left from a previous pregnancy or miscarriage. As these tissues grow, they destroy the developing embryo and expand rapidly within the uterus, increasing its size much more quickly than expected. Although 80 percent of these tumors are benign, they should still be removed quickly because in about 15 percent of cases, the tumor makes a change and aggressively invades the uterine wall, potentially causing serious problems such as hemorrhage. In a minority of cases (about 2 percent), a fast-growing cancer, termed "choriocarcinoma," develops following the hydatidiform mole. The cancer quickly spreads to other parts of the body. Persistently elevated blood levels of the pregnancy hormone, human chorionic gonadotropin (HCG), following treatment for a benign hydatidiform mole could indicate the presence of such a cancer. Ultrasound scans can usually detect these problems immediately.

When to call the doctor Development during pregnancy of the symptoms listed above should prompt an immediate call to the obstetrician, particularly the symptoms of excessive bleeding or the passage of tissue.

Treatment Benign moles can be removed easily in surgery. The suction procedure, much like a D&C, will leave the uterus and ovaries intact and make future conception possible. Invasive moles and cancers may sometimes require hysterectomy, but in most instances can be managed with chemotherapy.

Prognosis Good with prompt diagnosis and appropriate treatment. Except when hysterectomy is necessary, future pregnancy is usually still possible following treatment for benign or invasive moles or even choriocarcinoma.

❖ UTERINE CANCER

Symptoms *(What you may experience)* Abnormal bleeding. Later stage discovery: Low abdominal pain. *Note*: The symptoms occur commonly in disorders of the female reproductive system and are not specific to this condition.

Signs and laboratory findings *(What the doctor looks for)* Endometrial biopsy showing cancerous cells on microscopic examination.

What is it? Cancer of the uterus, the second most common cancer of the female reproductive system, strikes women at or past menopause (ages 50 to 70). Risks for this cancer increase in obese women, women who have type 2 diabetes mellitus or polycystic ovary syndrome, women who have never had children, who use unopposed estrogen hormones (those without any progesterone hormone), or who have had long-term therapy with the drug tamoxifen for breast cancer.

When to call the doctor If you develop abnormal vaginal bleeding that persists or is of significant amount, consult your doctor.

Treatment Preliminary evaluation with endometrial biopsy, x-rays of the chest, kidneys, and ureters, and an endoscopic exam of the bladder and colon will help to determine the appropriate course of treatment based on whether the cancer has spread.

The surgical treatment is total hysterectomy (removal of uterus, both fallopian tubes, and both ovaries) and if samples taken at surgery from the tissues inside the abdomen indicate extension of the cancer beyond the uterus, radiation treatments or radium implants before and possibly after surgery may be in order.

Prognosis Five-year survival rate with prompt diagnosis and appropriate treatment is 80 to 85 percent.

The Ovaries and Fallopian Tubes

A pair of ovaries, tiny oval structures about the size of an almond, lies suspended deep in the middle of the pelvic cavity. At birth, the ovaries contain all the eggs they will

CHRONIC PELVIC PAIN

Although pain in the pelvic area is not unusual, it can be cause for concern. A host of disorders can be the source of pelvic pain, which may be why it is one of the most commonly reported symptoms for which women seek relief. A woman who experiences pain for longer than a few hours in the pelvic area, or a woman whose pelvic pain recurs or is accompanied by other symptoms such as vaginal bleeding or fever, should consult her doctor.

To determine the cause of the pain, the doctor will ask the following about the type of pain the woman is experiencing: Is it acute, a sudden attack of severe pain, possibly with accompanying symptoms? Or is it chronic, that is, pain and discomfort you have been experiencing over a longer period? If it is chronic, does the pain come and go, or do you experience the discomfort most of the time?

The information that the woman provides describing the nature of the pain can help the doctor diagnose the problem. For example, does anything make it better or worse? Does it occur with intercourse or with orgasm? Is it better or worse with your menstrual period? Does it nauseate you or make you feel faint? Is it worse with lifting or with straining to urinate or when having a bowel movement? Does it cause you to avoid certain activities? Has it disrupted your family life or your work?

Recurrent bouts of pain occur with dysmenorrhea (painful periods), with dyspareunia (painful intercourse), with mittelschmerz (midcycle ovulation pain), or with endometriosis. More information can be found about these disorders under these headings.

Continuous pain may occur with scarring (adhesions) from chronic pelvic inflammatory disease, abdominal surgery, or endometriosis. Disorders such as uterine prolapse, benign tumors or cancers involving the uterus, ovary, bowel, or bladder, or irritable bowel syndrome (see page 1017) can also contribute to constant pelvic pain.

Psychosomatic chronic pelvic pain can arise as a consequence of sexual or physical abuse, or can accompany other emotional and psychological disorders, such as depression and schizophrenia. The emotional and psychological overlay does not rule out the possibility of serious associated physical disease, which should always be excluded.

In the United States, chronic pelvic pain accounts for 40 percent of the laparoscopies performed and more than 10 percent of the hysterectomies. Severe symptoms lead to strain in family and marital relationships, job stress, and numerous medical and surgical procedures. Chronic pelvic pain should not be ignored. A doctor needs to properly diagnose and recommend appropriate treatment for the condition. ■

TUBO-OVARIAN ABSCESS

Sometimes pelvic infection results in the formation of an abscess in and around the tube and ovary. An abscess is a localized pocket of infection surrounded by a thick protective wall. The body forms the wall in an attempt to prevent the infection from spreading widely (keep it contained). When a tubo-ovarian abscess (TOA) develops, eradication of the infecting bacteria, thriving deep within the infected pocket, can rarely be accomplished simply by administration of antibiotics by mouth, or even by the intravenous route. Surgical removal of the affected tube and ovary is usually necessary. Less extensive treatment will very often leave a smoldering infection that will recur at a later time, perhaps more widely disseminated. Removal of one tube and ovary will not render the woman sterile and will preserve the possibility of bearing children in the future. If the abscess involves both tubes and ovaries, however, the usual course of treatment will be total hysterectomy. ■

ever have, usually about a million between them, and certainly more than enough to last through a reproductive lifetime of ovulations.

Each ovary lies in close proximity, although not directly attached, to the open end of one of the pair of fallopian tubes. The tubes are slender hollow passageways about 4 in. in length, no larger inside than the diameter of a needle. Their open ends are flared and fringed to better help gather the egg, which bursts free from the ovary into the tube and toward the uterus at the time of ovulation.

Disorders affecting the ovaries and tubes primarily include infections, cystic disorders, and ovarian cancer.

❖ POLYCYSTIC OVARIAN SYNDROME

Symptoms *(What you may experience)* Menstrual disturbances; difficulty or inability to conceive; obesity. Often: excessive body hair growth (hirsutism).

Signs and laboratory findings *(What the doctor looks for)* Elevated testosterone and luteinizing hormone (LH) levels as shown by blood tests; multiple cysts in the ovaries demonstrated by ultrasound studies.

What is it? Polycystic ovarian syndrome, also called Stein-Leventhal syndrome, affects as many as 5 percent of women of reproductive age. Although little is understood about what causes it to develop, it is an endocrine (hormonal) disorder in which the levels of estrogen, androgen (testosterone), and LH

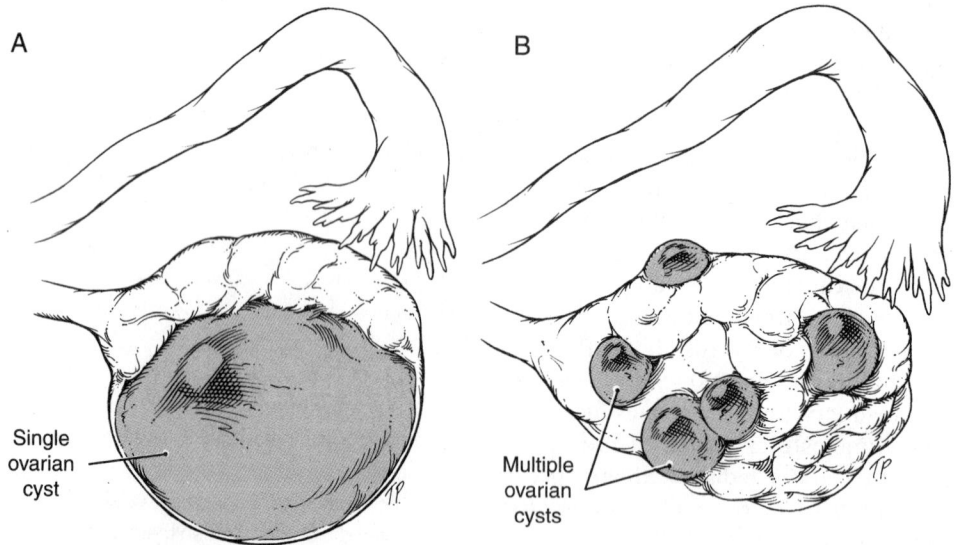

(A) A fluid-filled ovarian cyst may develop from an unruptured follicle or other ovarian tissue. Cysts can cause abdominal pain, menstrual spotting, or irregularity. (B) In polycystic ovarian syndrome, multiple cysts are associated with obesity, hirsutism, insulin resistance, and elevated levels of certain hormones.

A

Single ovarian cyst

B

Multiple ovarian cysts

remain at constant relatively elevated levels rather than the normally fluctuating surges and ebbs of these hormones that characterize the female menstrual cycle. Elevation of the estrogen hormone, estrone, contributes to obesity, a common problem for women with this syndrome. Excessive androgen (male) hormone levels result in hirsutism. Constant high levels of LH lead to suppression of the follicle stimulating hormone (FSH), preventing normal maturation of the egg and ovulation, and consequently, disrupt normal menstrual cycling and encourage the formation of cysts.

Women with polycystic ovarian syndrome often have insulin resistance syndrome (see Insulin Resistance and Syndrome X, page 1178) and are also at higher risk for the development of breast and uterine cancer because of the prolonged elevation of estrogen, unopposed by progesterone.

When to call the doctor Young women with excessive body and facial hair, who are obese, have menstrual disturbances or have not menstruated should be evaluated for this syndrome.

Treatment Weight reduction is helpful in obese women with this syndrome. Androgen hormones are converted to estrone in body fat, and the greater the amount of body fat the higher the levels of estrone may be.

Women with polycystic ovarian syndrome who do not wish to become pregnant can be treated with medroxyprogesterone acetate (10 mg/day for 12 days a month) to encourage regular shedding of the uterine lining. This shedding will normalize menstrual periods and prevent excessive growth of the endometrium. A low-dose birth control pill may also help and may even be effective in reducing the thickness of body and facial hair after 6 months to 1 year. Heavy growth of body hair may also respond to doses of dexamethasone (0.5 mg at bedtime) or spironolactone, a drug commonly used for high blood pressure, 25 mg three times daily.

Women who desire to become pregnant may need to stimulate ovulation using fertility medications such as clomiphene, although in some cases, dexamethasone may accomplish the same thing. Wedge resection of the ovary, in which a wedge shaped piece of the ovary is surgically

OTHER OVARIAN CYSTS

Each month during a woman's reproductive lifetime, one (usually) of the million or so eggs resting dormant within the ovaries begins to develop in response to the surges and ebbs of the reproductive hormones. As it does, the tissues surrounding the maturing egg, called the follicle, enlarge and begin to produce hormones that support its development. When the time for ovulation arrives, the enlarged follicle, now bulging at the surface of the ovary, ruptures, propelling the mature egg into the abdominal cavity.

Occasionally, the follicle fails to rupture, remaining instead as a tense, fluid-filled cyst at the ovarian surface. Although these cysts may cause no symptoms at all, sometimes, they will cause spotting, menstrual irregularity, vague abdominal/pelvic discomfort, and occasionally pain with deep thrusting during sexual intercourse. Most of these follicular cysts resolve spontaneously, left alone or with a course of treatment with oral contraceptive pills. Any cyst that has not resolved after 2 months on birth control pills should be investigated further by ultrasound or laparoscopy with biopsy.

Dermoid cysts, also called benign teratomas, occur in women of all ages from childhood until beyond menopause. They arise from deposits of skin precursor cells, such as those destined to become hair, skin, teeth, and nails, left within the ovary during the earliest stages of fetal development. These precursor cells, if they begin to divide and develop, can result in the production of a cyst, filled with fluid and with remnants of skin or related structures. The cysts can reach a size of up to 15 cm (about 3 to 4 in.) and are almost always benign, only very rarely ever degenerating to develop cancerous cells. In about 15 percent of cases, they occur in both ovaries.

Dermoid cysts can twist (because of their rather large size relative to the tiny ovary) and cause intense and considerable abdominal pain. Most doctors will recommend removal of the affected ovary, if the woman's health and age allow it. ■

removed, has been used for many years to stimulate ovulation and fertility, although the procedure is rarely used today.

Prognosis Good for improvement of symptoms and the possibility of conception with appropriate treatment.

❖ CANCER OF THE OVARY

Symptoms *(What you may experience)* No symptoms. Sometimes: Vague sense of abdominal/intestinal discomfort; pelvic pressure or pain.

Signs and laboratory findings *(What the doctor looks for)* Firm enlarged ovary on pelvic exam; elevated blood level of CA-125 (an antigen marker not exclusive to ovarian cancer); irregular enlargement of the ovary shown by ultrasound or MRI.

What is it? Tumors, or growths, on the ovary occur quite commonly and most of them are benign. Malignant tumors of the ovary, ovarian cancer, represent the most common and deadliest of the reproductive tract cancers, diagnosed in over 25,000 women annually (in 1998). It primarily strikes women around the time of menopause or after (ages 40 to 65). Ovarian cancer is the cause of death for more than 14,000 women annually (in 1998), making it the fifth most common cause of death from cancer among women in the United States.

Ovarian cancer has been shown to have a strong genetic predisposition. Women with no family history of ovarian cancer have the lowest risk for developing it; those in which one or more first-degree relatives (parents or siblings) have had it carry a much higher risk. Approximately 3 in 100 women with such a risk will have hereditary ovarian cancer syndrome and a 40 percent lifetime risk for developing ovarian cancer. For this reason, women with a strong genetic predisposition for this cancer should undergo removal of both ovaries before age 35 or as soon as they have borne their children. Until that time, they should be carefully screened every year.

Ovarian cancer is difficult to detect in the early stages, which accounts in part for its deadliness. As important as it is for all women to undergo periodic pelvic exam, especially women with a family history of ovarian or other reproductive cancers, this method alone does not lead to early detection of ovarian cancer because cancers that can be felt by the gynecologist during a bimanual pelvic exam are generally larger and more advanced. Recommendations for how and when to screen for this cancer vary, but there does not seem to be sufficient benefit from screening women of low risk (no family history) without symptoms. A combination of available screening tools, including pelvic exam, ultrasound, and color Doppler imaging of the ovaries and sequential measurements of CA-125 tumor antigen, seems to offer the best chance of early detection of the cancer in the high-risk population.

If on pelvic exam, one or both ovaries seem to be enlarged or a growth is felt, the age, reproductive stage, and family risk of the woman must be considered in evaluating the mass because most ovarian masses prove to be benign. Any mass that is found to be solid on ultrasound examination, that is, not a fluid-filled cyst, or a cyst that persists longer than 4 to 6 weeks should be investigated. Such masses in women near the time of menopause or after should be evaluated; an exploratory laparotomy with biopsy of the mass will determine whether it is an ovarian cancer. The laparotomy procedure, in which the gynecologic surgeon opens the abdomen with an incision, is usually preferred over the less extensive laparoscopy (viewing and taking the biopsy specimen of the mass through a small "stab" incision using the flexible lighted scope) because it offers the opportunity to examine and sample lymph nodes in the region if necessary to better assess the extent of spread of the tumor if it proves to be cancerous.

What you can do If you have a known significant family risk for ovarian cancer, you should be vigilant in making and keeping annual screening visits with your doctor. Discuss the benefits of early removal of the ovaries with your doctor.

Long-term use of oral contraceptive agents appears to reduce the risk of ovarian cancer.

Treatment Standard therapy for this disorder is complete abdominal hysterectomy with removal of both ovaries, the fallopian tubes, and the omentum (a fibrous and fatty apron-like tissue that covers the abdominal contents). A sample of lymph nodes in the area should also be removed. In all cases, except very early cancers localized to the ovary without evidence of spread, chemotherapy should follow the surgery.

Prognosis Because the cancer rarely causes early symptoms, in as many as 75 percent of women the ovarian cancer has extended into neighboring tissues or lymph nodes by the time the diagnosis is made. Late treatment accounts for the poor overall prognosis. Although the 5-year survival for early disease detection is fairly good at approximately 89 percent, with spread to adjacent tissues it drops to 36 percent; spread to distant areas or lymph nodes reduces 5-year survival to only 17 percent, pointing up the extreme importance of early diagnosis in this disease.

Sexual Dysfunction

Intensity of sexual response varies from woman to woman, and appears to be governed by a vast number of disparate factors including hormonal levels, age, sexual experience or lack of it, upbringing (including family and religious training), the past experience of sexual trauma, emotional response to a partner, and fear of potential pregnancy.

The majority of women enjoy normal, satisfying sexual lives, uncomplicated by anything more than transient dysfunction. Many women, like many men, do experience some level of sexual dysfunction from time to time. Most are relatively easy to treat and pose no great threat to a woman's ability to procreate or enjoy a rewarding relationship.

❖ FEMALE SEXUAL AROUSAL DISORDER

Symptoms *(What you may experience)* An inability to maintain arousal sufficient to complete sexual activity; an absence or inadequate lubrication; a lack of emotional and physical response to the sexual stimulation of your partner.

Signs and laboratory findings *(What the doctor looks for)* A determination of whether your lack of arousal occurs only with your partner, only in certain circumstances, or if you have never experienced any sort of sexual arousal. Diseases, such as diabetes mellitus, need to be ruled out as possible causes. A woman's sexual and medical history, upbringing, possible emotional or physical trauma related to sex, or teachings that could result in guilt or withholding of sexual feelings, as well as the woman's present experiences may offer clues to the cause of dysfunction.

What is it? Female sexual arousal disorder (FSAD) is roughly equivalent to male erectile dysfunction (impotence). Normal sexual arousal in both sexes involves an engorgement of the genitals with blood. In males, this results in erection; in females, it results in the secretion of vaginal lubrication, enlargement or (erection) of the clitoris and surrounding tissues, and a widening of the vaginal opening. On a physiologic level, FSAD involves a failure of the genitals to become sufficiently engorged with blood to cause adequate lubrication or relaxing of the vagina to permit intercourse.

An underlying medical condition, such as hypertension or diabetes, can lead to FSAD, but most often, the cause is psychological. It may be related to past personal history or recent changes, experiences, or crises, for example, interpersonal distress with her partner.

What you can do If a woman occasionally fails to become aroused or if a woman's partner desires sex more often than she, the woman is perfectly normal. If, however, the problem persists and is becoming distressful to either partner, it should be acknowledged and discussed openly. Denying the problem can lead to the breakup of a relationship or marriage.

When to call the doctor If a woman suspects her lack of arousal is due to an illness or physical condition, she should call her doctor and find out what to do. If you do not have an existing medical condition and if emotional or psychological stress may be contributing to your lack of arousal, your doctor may recommend counseling to help you understand your feelings. If your lack of arousal has caused a rift in your marriage or contributed to an already existing rift, consult your doctor and seek couples therapy in order to resolve the conflicts.

Treatment Like treatment for impotence, treatment for FSAD may be as simple as switching medications, or it may involve counseling to resolve some underlying conflict either within yourself or hostility or anger toward your partner.

Prognosis Excellent. With the proper medical attention or counseling and an empathetic and cooperative partner, FSAD should be resolved.

❖ FEMALE ORGASMIC DISORDER

Symptoms *(What you may experience)* An inability to have an orgasm despite adequate stimulation.

Signs and laboratory findings *(What the doctor looks for)* Assessment of a number of different factors including age, relative sexual experience, a woman's attitudes toward sex and her partner, past or present experiences that may have influenced a woman's attitude toward sex.

What is it? Female orgasmic disorder is distinct from FSAD in that you may be highly aroused but cannot cross the threshold from arousal to climax. It is not just failure to have an orgasm during intercourse. Many women who have orgasms with their partners regularly through manual or oral stimulation may not do so during intercourse. In contrast to men, women learn how to orgasm, typically in the context of a trusting relationship. This learning curve increases until the fifth decade when it plateaus.

Orgasmic disorder can be lifelong or it can occur in women who have previously had little difficulty climaxing. For the 10 percent of women who have never experienced orgasm, the causes most often have to do with sexual inexperience, performance anxiety, or past experiences, such as religious upbringing or sexual trauma, that have led to inhibited sexual response. For a woman who has experienced orgasm in the past but can no longer do so, anger, resentment, or hostility toward her partner can also be the cause, as can anxiety, personal crises, and other stress factors. Certain medications may affect response as well, especially the newer antidepressants called selective serotonin reuptake inhibitors (SSRIs) such as fluoxetine (Prozac).

When to call the doctor   Call your doctor if you suspect your problem is due to medication. You should consider counseling and contact your doctor or a counselor if you feel that your disorder has begun significantly to affect your sex life and your relationship, particularly if it may be a result of the dynamics of the relationship, or if it has left you depressed.

Treatment   Counseling will be the most effective treatment. A qualified sex therapist should be able to get to the root of your problem and help you resolve it. Depending on how deeply rooted your disorder is this may take a few weeks, months, or longer.

Prognosis   Excellent to very good. Although it is estimated that a certain percentage of women never have orgasms, most women can and do. Seeking treatment will significantly improve the likelihood of resolving your disorder.

❖ VAGINISMUS

Symptoms *(What you may experience)* Difficult and uncomfortable or impossible penetration of the vagina.

Signs and laboratory findings *(What the doctor looks for)* Involuntary contraction of the muscles of the outer third of the vagina, making the opening too narrow to permit intercourse.

What is it?   Long defined as an involuntary spasm of the muscles surrounding the vagina making intercourse impossible, vaginismus is a relatively rare condition. As such, it is a reflex response, not a willed "closing off" by the woman. It may, however, actually be more common, if the definition is expanded to include involuntary muscle spasms that cause a narrowing of the vaginal opening, which still permits intercourse, but causes it to be painful or uncomfortable. Often the source of vaginismus is rooted in trauma: sexual assault, painful, perhaps immature intercourse, difficult pelvic exam, and emotional trauma regarding sex (feeling that it is "dirty" to enjoy sex). It can also be caused by a medical condition such as PID (see page 1116).

What you can do   Acknowledge the problem before it damages your relationship or marriage.

When to call the doctor   Call the doctor if you suspect your vaginismus is related to a pelvic disorder. If you believe that your condition is emotional in origin, seek counseling from a therapist trained in dealing with sexual disorders.

Treatment   Vaginismus is most commonly treated with progressive vaginal dilation and, if necessary, a combination of counseling or couples therapy. Progressive vaginal dilation involves the use of vaginal inserts, each progressively larger than the last, which help condition the vaginal opening. As one becomes comfortable, the next larger size is inserted in the vagina and worn until it is comfortable. This continues until the vagina has been dilated sufficiently for intercourse to take place painlessly.

In some cases, simultaneous counseling will assist a woman in uncovering the basis of the disorder. The counseling will aim to alleviate anxiety or guilt or other factors that may exacerbate vaginismus.

❖ INHIBITED SEXUAL DESIRE

Symptoms *(What you may experience)* A persistent and encompassing absence of sexual desire or appetite; absence of sexual fantasies; persistent lack of interest in sexual contact with a sexual partner or an avoidance of sexual contact with a sexual partner.

Signs and laboratory findings *(What the doctor looks for)* Underlying conditions. Most prominently: relationship problems; sexual trauma; depression; stress; and family crisis. Possibily: hormone deficiencies; alcoholism; kidney failure; or other chronic illness, such as diabetes, as well as certain medications.

What is it? Sometimes called loss of desire, inhibited sexual desire is more accurately the diminishment of desire by one of several psychological or biologic mechanisms. It is usually the result of some other dysfunction, illness, sexually-related emotional trauma, or depression. Far too often, it is the result of a breakdown of communication and understanding in a long-term sexual relationship, and its underlying grief, hostility, anger, depression, or sense of misunderstanding.

Treatment Self-treatment is possible, but fraught with difficulty. The various factors that build up to inhibition of desire tend to accumulate over long periods and can take considerable time to resolve. Although partners may spend a great deal of time at the beginning of a relationship having sex, they may not actually talk about it much, which may lay the groundwork for considerable future misunderstanding. Two individuals are almost guaranteed to have differing ideas about what lovemaking means, what it should entail, and the place it should have in a relationship. While passion and romance at the beginning of a relationship may compensate for or at least cover up some of the differences couples have, major life changes, such as the arrival of a child, can uncover those differences and throw a wedge between partners (see Communication Strategies for Couples, page 311, and Couples Counseling Before and During Marriage, page 310). Many people think of having an affair, "just to make sure the equipment is working." Such a solution will only worsen the trouble and increases the risk of a sexually transmitted infection. A skilled counselor can help keep people from engaging in behavior that can potentially worsen their situation.

Prognosis Good, if the underlying problems are addressed. If the problems are ignored or denied, they can lead to the breakup of a family.

❖ GENDER DYSPHORIA

Symptoms and signs *(What you may experience)* A recurrent or pervasive sense that you should have been born a male; the desire to adopt a male gender identity; the desire to dress as a male to pass as a male.

What is it? Gender identity dysphoria (GID) is rare, though it may be underreported by those for whom the disorder is either mild, transient, or simply unacknowledgeable for reasons of socialization or upbringing. It is not known what causes the disorder.

What you can do Seek the help of a Gender Identity Program or one who is an expert in the treatment of this disorder. Academic medical centers may assist in referrals. Support groups will tend to reinforce the cross-gender identity and behaviors.

When to call the doctor Living with gender dysphoria is not easy, and individuals with this condition can benefit from the help of a therapist. If you are depressed or have considered or attempted suicide, you should contact a doctor or mental health professional who specializes in such issues as soon as possible.

Treatment Psychiatric counseling is the best method of treatment. It enables a woman to feel more comfortable with her conflicting urges and provides ways of resolving emotional conflicts. Sex change operations have been performed, but experts no longer regard this as an effective way of helping people cope with GID.

THE MALE REPRODUCTIVE SYSTEM

The male reproductive and urinary systems are more intimately related than the female systems. Problems affecting one system tend to affect the other. In fact, the same medical/surgical specialist, the urologist, cares for both urinary and reproductive system problems in men.

The male genital organs include the testicles, vas deferens, seminal vesicles, prostate gland, and the penis, which is both a sexual organ and a urinary tract organ because the urethra (urine tube) runs lengthwise through its center.

The scrotum, which hangs from the groin, contains the testicles and keeps them at optimal temperature for sperm production. After puberty, sperm mature inside the epididymis after being produced in tubes just outside the testicles. The spermatic cord carries sperm in the ductus (vas) deferens and also contains blood vessels, nerves, and muscles. The urethra carries urine or sperm through the penis. The prostate secretes fluid that helps to maintain the liquid consistency of sperm-containing semen.

The testicles, a pair of spherical structures about 2 in. in length, hang suspended in a sack of skin (the scrotum) just behind the penis. During development inside the womb, the testicles migrate from their starting position in the abdominal cavity through an opening in the abdominal wall near the groin and into the scrotum. The migration occurs to keep the testicles at optimal temperature for sperm production; internal body temperature is too high. The spermatic cord contains the arteries and veins that supply blood to the testicles and the tubes to carry the sperm from them. The cord also contains small muscles that can contract to pull the testicles closer to the body in cold weather or relax to drop them further from the body when temperatures rise.

Within the protective capsule covering each testicle are tightly coiled tubes. It is here, under the influence of rising levels of male reproductive hormone at puberty, that continuous, lifelong sperm production takes place. As they are produced, the sperm are sent to the *epididymis*, a long, coiled tube along the top and back of the testes, where they mature into motile sperm.

A single ejaculation of semen, a mixture of sperm with fluid secreted by the prostate gland and seminal vesicles, may contain 500 million sperm. The seminal fluid provides not only volume but protection; without the prostatic secretions, the sperm would not easily survive the acid environment of the vaginal canal.

Disorders of the male reproductive system discussed in this section include infection, cysts, trauma, developmental abnormalities, erectile and sexual dysfunction, and cancers. Fertility issues are discussed in the next section of this chapter, and a more detailed discussion of STIs appears in Chapter 21.

The Penis

The penis consists of a body or shaft of erectile tissue, and an expanded head, called the glans penis, covered at birth with a redundancy of skin, called the foreskin, from which it emerges when erect and into which

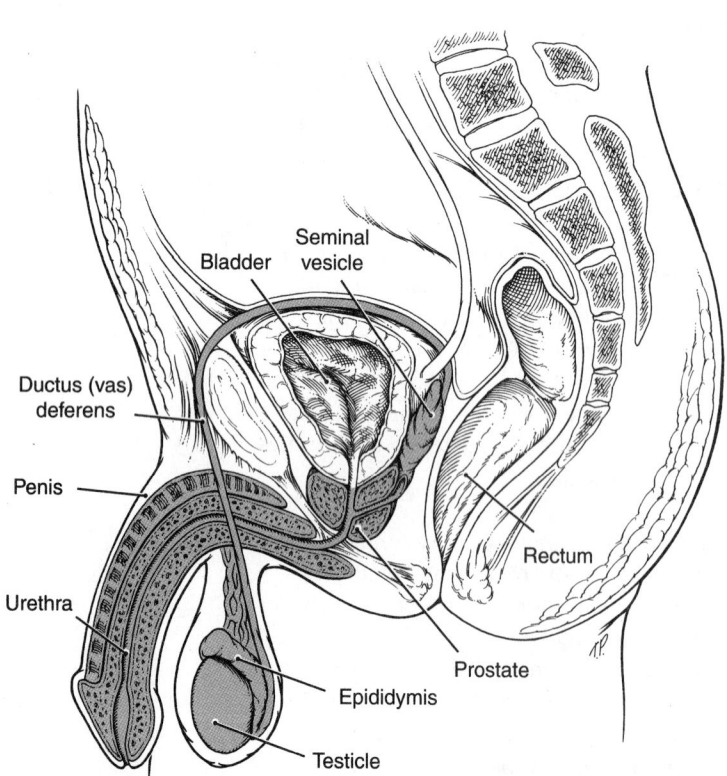

Bladder

Seminal vesicle

Ductus (vas) deferens

Penis

Urethra

Rectum

Prostate

Epididymis

Testicle

it retracts when flaccid (soft). The urethra runs along the underside of the penis, providing a passageway for both urine from the bladder and for semen during ejaculation.

The body of the penis is composed of three rod-shaped structures made of a spongy network of interconnected blood vessels with some smooth muscle tissue.

The ability to have and maintain a penile erection requires normally functioning nerves to the area, an unobstructed blood supply, and normal male hormonal levels. Penile erection occurs primarily as a result of psychological and emotional factors accompanying sexual arousal, although direct stimulation of the penis can cause or contribute to the erection through local reflexes. As a result of sexual arousal, the brain and central nervous system cause the release of several neurotransmitters in the penis. The most important neurotransmitter is nitric oxide, a substance closely related to nitrous oxide (laughing gas). In response to these neurotransmitters, blood vessels in the penis dilate so that the spongy tissue of the erectile bodies becomes engorged, causing the penis to straighten and stiffen.

❖ BALANITIS

Symptoms (What you may experience) Redness and discomfort of the head (glans) of the penis; white clumpy discharge beneath the foreskin (occasionally).

Signs and labortory findings (What the doctor looks for) Occasionally: Microscopic analysis of specimen of discharge demonstrating bacteria or yeast infection. Sometimes: Laboratory tests showing elevated blood sugar or urine sugar (signs of diabetes mellitus).

What is it? The glans penis sometimes becomes irritated or inflamed. The condition occurs more commonly in men with diabetes mellitus and almost exclusively in uncircumcised men, particularly if the foreskin is tight and constricting around the penis. A variety of causes may be responsible, including the following:

- Urethral infection (such as with the STI, *Neisseria gonorrhea*)

- Allergic or irritant reaction to chemicals such as soaps, detergents, chemicals used in clothing manufacture, and contraceptive creams

- Yeast infection, especially common in men with diabetes mellitus, owing in part to the high sugar content of their urine

- Inadequate hygiene

What you can do Uncircumcised men should make every effort to keep the glans penis clean and dry by pulling back the foreskin each day when bathing to carefully wash the area with mild soapy water and then rinse well. Afterward, retract the foreskin and thoroughly dry the head of the penis.

When to call the doctor If you have diabetes mellitus, the development of balanitis can signal some degree of loss of good blood sugar control.

Any irritation, swelling, redness, or discharge, particularly if the discharge is bloody, merits a visit to your doctor.

Treatment Treatment depends on the cause. If any irritants such as chemicals can be identified, their use should be stopped. Very mild topical anti-inflammatory creams containing cortisone, such as those intended for use in the rectal area or with children, can help to relieve discomfort from the irritation. Applying a cortisone cream to a yeast or fungal infection can cause it to worsen.

Infections with bacteria may respond to frequent cleansing with antibacterial soaps or antiseptic solutions. Yeast infections will often respond to over-the-counter topical creams designed to treat women's vaginal yeast infections or may require stronger prescription antifungal remedies.

If the foreskin (in uncircumcised men) is so tight that proper hygiene is not possible, circumcision may be necessary to prevent recurrent episodes of infection.

Prognosis Good with prompt diagnosis and appropriate treatment.

❖ PHIMOSIS AND PARAPHIMOSIS

Symptoms and signs Inability to retract foreskin over glans penis.

What is it? Phimosis is a constriction of the opening of the foreskin such that the foreskin cannot be retracted over the glans penis. Phimosis may arise from balanitis or it may arise on its own. It is particularly common in men with diabetes mellitus.

Occasionally, a tight foreskin may become lodged in the retracted position. This condition, known as paraphimosis, constitutes a medical emergency. The tight foreskin may restrict blood flow to the penis and cause permanent damage.

Prevention To prevent phimosis, men, particularly those with diabetes, must practice good genital hygiene (see Balanitis, page 1131).

Treatment Circumcision will treat phimosis and prevent the occurrence of paraphimosis.

❖ HYPOSPADIAS

What is it? The opening of the urine tube (urethra) usually develops in the center of the tip of the penis. When the opening of the urethra develops in an abnormal location, farther down the shaft of the penis, it is termed hypospadias. Usually, the problem is discovered in infancy, unless it is only very minimally displaced. Further discussion of this condition can be found in on page 219.

❖ PEYRONIE'S DISEASE (CURVATURE OF THE PENIS)

Symptoms *(What you may experience)* Bending of the penis with erection (sometimes causing pain); difficulty performing intercourse.

Signs and laboratory findings *(What the doctor looks for)* Curved erect penis; palpable plaque or scar in shaft of penis.

What is it? This disorder, first described by a French doctor named Peyronie, develops when tough scar-like tissue forms within the rod-like erectile bodies within the length of the penis. In the flaccid (soft) state, no deformity is apparent. During erection, the scar tissue cannot stretch and expand, so the penis bows or curves toward the side of the Peyronie's plaque. The bend is sometimes quite painful, but even when it

is not, it makes penetration during intercourse difficult or impossible. Why the scar develops is not clearly understood. Occasionally the problem may even disappear on its own.

When to call the doctor If the curvature causes significant pain or disruption of normal sexual activity, consult a urologist.

Treatment Although various treatments have been tried throughout the years, none has proven singularly effective. Initially, the best approach may be to allow the condition to resolve itself. Vitamin E supplements may help in a minority of cases. Surgery involving correction of the curvature, a removal of the plaque, or both may be necessary.

Prognosis Approximately more than half of the cases resolve spontaneously. Surgical correction is quite successful at restoring sexual function.

❖ PRIAPISM

Symptoms *(What you may experience)* Prolonged, painful erection.

What is it? Priapism is a prolonged, often painful erection which is not associated with sexual stimulation. The name of this syndrome is derived from Priapus, a Greek god of fertility. Priapism can occur during use of medications that affect the central nervous system, such as trazodone (Desyrel), carbidopa-levodopa (Sinemet), or respiradone (Respirdal). It may also occur as a result of certain diseases, such as sickle cell disease or leukemia. Rarely, priapism results from spinal cord injury or tumor. Often priapism is due to penile injection therapy for impotence. In many cases, the cause of priapism is unknown.

When to call the doctor One should notify the doctor immediately when prolonged or painful erection occurs, particularly if the condition is not associated with sexual stimulation. Failure to correct priapism within a few hours can cause permanent damage to the erectile tissue of the penis, leading to impotence.

Treatment Initial treatment usually involves relieving the engorgement of the penis. After giving an anesthetic, the doctor will drain the blood from the penis and may inject medications to slow blood flow to the organ. After the erection has subsided, the doctor will attempt to determine the underlying cause.

Prognosis In nearly all cases, the erection can be relieved and potency can be preserved. In many cases the cause of priapism can be identified and future episodes can be prevented.

❖ CANCER OF THE PENIS

Symptoms *(What you may experience)* Persistent, usually painless, scaly, sore or wart-like growth on the penis, usually on or near the head; bloody discharge from beneath the foreskin.

Signs and laboratory findings *(What the doctor looks for)* Excisional biopsy demonstrating cancerous cells in the growth.

What is it? This very rare form of cancer almost always occurs in men who have not undergone circumcision. Without biopsy, it can be difficult to differentiate cancerous growths from other types of penile warts and sores. As with any cancer, left untreated, the cancer can invade deeper and surrounding tissues and can even spread to distant sites.

What you can do Regularly examine the penis for growths, scaly areas, or sores. Do not ignore any unusual growth or eruption. If uncircumcised, clean under the foreskin daily with soap and water.

When to call the doctor Any growth or lesion that develops on the penis should prompt a visit to the doctor. Even though most will be benign or infectious and can be readily treated, none should be ignored.

Treatment Removal of the growth is the definitive treatment. If at surgery, the growth proves cancerous, removal of some surrounding tissue, a clear margin around the cancer, will be necessary including, in many cases, a portion of the penis. The more advanced the cancer, the greater the amount of tissue that will need to be removed to eradicate the cancerous cells, pointing up, once again, to the need for

WHAT CAUSES A BLOODY EJACULATE?

Occasionally, semen will be streaked or tinged with blood. Although the appearance of blood can be quite alarming, its cause is almost never a dangerous one. If the appearance of blood persists or is large in volume, consult a doctor so that appropriate microscopic exam of the seminal fluid and exam of the prostate and testicles can be done. ∎

PENILE SORES

Most sores on the penis arise as a part of sexually transmitted infections (STIs). A complete discussion of these diseases can be found on page 861. A brief description of the types of sores these diseases cause has been listed here to better help identify any eruptions that are seen. A doctor should be consulted about any skin erosion, sore, or growth that appears on the penis. Many may appear to resolve on their own without treatment, only to cause serious problems later in life.

- Syphilis usually first appears as a single eroded or ulcerated area on the shaft or tip of the penis. It will usually have a mildly raised red rim surrounding a shallow crater filled with creamy or yellow-green debris. This is called the primary chancre. The syphilis bacterium (*Treponema pallidum*) will be visible under special microscopic analysis of specimens taken from the ulcer.

- Lymphogranuloma venereum causes a small sore not unlike the chancre of syphilis in appearance: a crater filled with cream to yellow-green debris. It will usually appear on the shaft of the penis, near the base, or even in the groin. The hallmark is the development of painful, swollen lymph nodes in the groin.

- Condyloma (penile venereal warts) will appear as lacy exuberant cauliflower-like growths, rapidly increasing in size, usually causing itching. They may range from the tip of the penis to the base of the shaft.

- Herpes simplex virus appears as clusters of clear or white blisters with a red rim. The painful blisters rupture, forming a crater that then crusts over and heals. The condition tends to recur in the same general location. Recurrence may be heralded by tingling, itching, or pain at the site.

- Cancer of the penis or scrotum usually appears as a scaly, red patch that is occasionally painful. It does not respond to simple remedies and persists. It may later erode the skin, leaving a chronic "sore" that does not heal. ∎

RASHES OF THE SCROTUM AND GROIN

Rashes occur quite commonly on the skin of the scrotum and in the groin area. Most rashes are benign and easy to treat, but the appearance of a persistent rash warrants checking by a doctor. Infection with bacteria, fungi, or viruses causes the majority of rashes in this area, but occasionally, skin cancers do arise in the skin of the scrotum or on the penis and may appear as a scaly patch (see Cancer of the Penis, page 1133). Among the common rashes of the scrotum and groin are the following:

Candida albicans (Yeast Infection)

The rash caused by this fungus develops in the warm, moist areas of folds of skin. It commonly causes diaper rash in infants, but can occur in adults, particularly in those who are obese. The rash is red, itches or burns, and has an advancing fiery red margin with "satellite" spots beyond the advancing boundary.

Tinea Inguinalis (Jock Itch)

Occurs in the skin creases of the groin. Its cause is also fungal, and it blossoms in areas of skin constricted for protracted periods by tight, sweaty clothing, hence its association with athletes. This rash tends to be itchy, scaly, and to have a raised, light red-brown margin. It may begin as a small scaly patch, but with time, the infection spreads outward, leaving the area behind the margin clear and the skin apparently unaffected.

Herpes Simplex Virus

Causes redness and clusters of blisters, much like a rash, in the groin or on the scrotum. For more information, see Penile Sores, page 1133. ■

early diagnosis in many cancers. Even in relatively advanced cases, sufficient penile tissue can often be saved to permit normal sexual activity and urination.

Prognosis Good if diagnosed promptly, while still localized, and treated appropriately.

❖ ERECTILE DYSFUNCTION OR IMPOTENCE

Symptoms *(What you may experience)*
Chronic inability to maintain penile erection sufficient to complete intercourse or achieve sexual satisfaction.

Signs and laboratory findings *(What the doctor looks for)* Hormonal inbalances such as testosterone deficiency; vascular dysfunction that impairs blood circulation; impairment of nerve reactions; loss or impairment of desire, such as that which may accompany stress, depression or other potential emotional difficulties; physical trauma to the pelvic region that may have caused nerve damage.

In order to diagnose and treat the condition properly, the doctor will need a detailed medical history (including any medications being taken); a sexual history (which should include emotional expectations, techniques and practices, and, ideally, a discussion with the partner); a physical exam; laboratory evaluation of levels of testosterone and other hormones.

It may be necessary for the doctor to refer the patient for a psychological evaluation. A referral for endocrine evaluation may also be needed to evaluate hormone function.

What is it? Most doctors have over the last several years begun to abandon the term "impotence" as outdated and not useful clinically. Most men lose their ability to achieve an erection from time to time. Frequently the problem is associated with alcohol intake, illicit drug use, or use of medication. If such episodes occur infrequently and do not last long, they are no cause for concern. A serious erectile dysfunction is one that affects the person for a continuous period of time.

A significant portion of the population suffers from a chronic inability to maintain sufficient erection to complete intercourse or achieve sexual satisfaction. The National Institutes of Health (NIH) estimates that approximately 7 million American men suffer from erectile dysfunction. If partial erectile dysfunction is included in the definition, the numbers increase dramatically, to approximately 30 million. The frequency of the disorder increases with age. At age 40, approximately 5 percent of the population is affected; by 65, 15 to 25 percent are affected. Fifty percent of men over age 75 are affected by erectile dysfunction. Medical causes of erectile dysfunction in older men include atherosclerosis, diabetes, and pelvic surgery.

Psychological factors such as stress, depression, and performance anxiety are another important cause of erectile dysfunction. Job loss, worries over family, finances, or other personal issues can cause loss of desire, or loss of ability to lose oneself in sexual communication. For most men, arousal begins almost automatically, but when they begin to think about it, it draws attention to itself, potentially causing the man to become anxious and worried thinking about erection. The erection can then fail because of anxiety. Psychologically-based erectile dysfunction can become a self-sustaining phenomenon.

What you can do Excessive consumption of alcohol or the use of illicit drugs can cause many health problems as well as affecting sexual function including erectile dysfunction. If use of these substances may be the source of erectile dysfunction, an effort should be made to stop using them. Help can be provided by entering a program such as Alcoholics Anonymous (AA) (see Chapter 5).

Communication between partners should be evaluated. Relationship difficulties may be affecting the man's sex life. Certain emotional situations, such as depression, performance anxiety, and even anger, can lead to difficulty maintaining erections. Consider couples therapy in order to work out differences and establish healthy lines of communication.

When to call the doctor If your difficulty in achieving or maintaining an erection lasts for several weeks and has you worried, consult your doctor. If you have chronic difficulty maintaining an erection in sexual situations, but regularly experience night and morning erections, you should also consult your doctor.

Treatment Treatment will depend on the etiology, or biologic and psychological origins, of your dysfunction. Erectile function depends upon normal testosterone levels, adequate penile blood supply, intact nerve function, and the absence of psychological problems that inhibit sexual performance. Treatment will depend upon which of these areas is causing the problem.

The doctor will first evaluate any medication being used (including illegal drugs) and alter or discontinue them, if possible.

Two commonly prescribed medications, cimetidine and spironolactone, may cause impotence, as may some antihypertensives, tranquilizers, and antidepressants. If the dysfunction is caused by taking medication for an ongoing medical condition, treatment may be as simple as switching medications. However, the medical condition could also be the root of the dysfunction. More often than not, erectile dysfunction is the result of the combination of two or three factors.

VIAGRA

The release of the prescription medication Viagra (sildenafil) onto the market marked the first oral treatment for erectile dysfunction, commonly known as impotence. Erection occurs when a chemical message within the penis causes the smooth muscle cells that normally hold back the flow of blood into the penis to relax and allow blood into the erectile chambers. These chemical messages can be broken down over time by enzymes in the penile tissues. Viagra works by preventing the breakdown of these chemical messages through the suppression of the enzymes.

Other treatments for erectile dysfunction include an injection in the side of the penis prior to intercourse that directly relaxes the smooth muscle cells; a vacuum pump used to remove air from around the penis, drawing blood into it; and, used as a last resort, penile implants. Injection therapy was accidentally discovered in 1982, and the first medications designed specifically for this purpose were approved by the FDA in 1995. Injections and suppository insertions can be painful and in some rare cases cause priapism, a nonstop erection that destroys penile tissue unless an antidote is administered. Therefore the excitement generated by an oral treatment with few side effects has been understandably phenomenal.

Viagra will not work for all men with erectile dysfunction but considering the ease of taking a pill compared to the other available therapies, it is being used as a first line of treatment, with other therapies being employed after a trial of Viagra has failed. Only 10 percent of men taking the medication reported side effects of headache, dizziness, facial flushing, indigestion, and visual disturbances. The only medications it should not be used with are nitrate medications, commonly used to treat heart disease. It should be used with caution in men taking medication for liver or kidney disease and those with bleeding disorders or retinitis pigmentosa, a disease of the eye marked by progressive loss of retinal response.

Some doctors are worried about the potential for abuse of Viagra and its social implications. Men not suffering from erectile dysfunction who have heard of the effects of Viagra may be asking for it to increase their sexual abilities without concern for their partners. In older marriages that have settled into a life that does not include sexual intercourse, Viagra may lead to an inequality of desire, possibly leading to an imbalance in the relationship. But the social side effects of Viagra pale in comparison to the relief it offers to couples who have suffered with impotence.

Viagra may also help women who experience sexual dysfunction, and studies are currently being conducted to determine its effects. ■

Information as to whether nocturnal and morning erections are being experienced needs to be provided to the doctor. If night and morning erections are being experienced, but there is no erection during sexual contact, this may indicate that the difficulty is primarily psychological in origin. The doctor will recommend ways to relieve or divert stress or a referral to a doctor (psychologist, psychiatrist, or social worker) who works with sexual dysfunction will be made.

If night or morning erections are not being experienced, this likely indicates that there is a physical reason, such as poor blood supply to the penis, nerve damage, diabetes mellitus, or hormone disturbance, preventing an erection.

Several effective therapies have been developed for erectile dysfunction. If stress, depression, performance anxiety, or relationship difficulties are thought to contribute to the problem, your doctor may recommend counseling in which you, and ideally your partner, work with a therapist to resolve the underlying issues.

If insufficient male hormone is the cause of your difficulties, testosterone therapy can restore erectile function. Testosterone can be given by injection or by a patch placed on the skin. Other medications may relieve erectile dysfunction caused by some psychological problems, such as depression.

Erectile dysfunction is often treated with injection therapy. While men are often initially apprehensive about injecting medication into their penis, most eventually decide that this is the best treatment for them.

For erectile dysfunction not responsive to more conservative treatments, a penile implant may be indicated. These surgically implanted devices replace the spongy erectile tissues on either side of the penis that normally fill will blood and cause erection. One type keeps the penis in a constant state of erection, but it can be bent in order for it to lie flat next to the body. The other type uses a squeeze pump and implants that can be pumped up with liquid. Discussion with a doctor will determine the right choice of implant.

Erectile dysfunction associated with vascular abnormalities can be treated with surgery. Surgery for erectile dysfunction is successful, however, only in carefully selected persons, such as those who are young or who have erectile dysfunction due to trauma.

Penile implants can provide penile erection when other treatments do not help erectile dysfunction. (A) One type contains a pump that is squeezed by hand to inflate the implants with liquid. (B) The other type consists of erect implants that can be bent during times of no sexual activity.

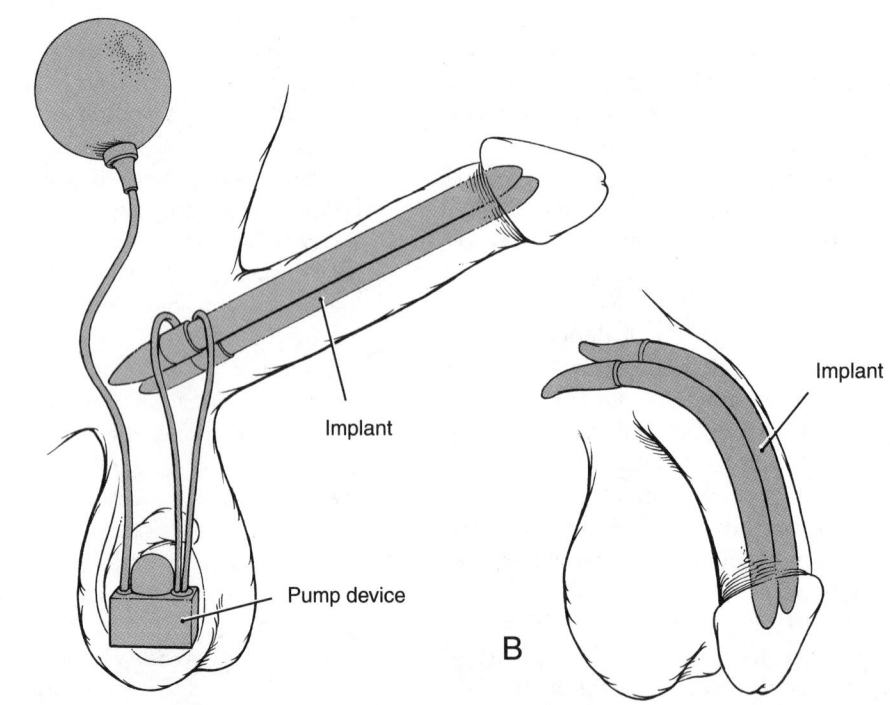

Implant

Pump device

A

Implant

B

Prognosis Dependent upon the cause of the problem. Erectile dysfunction that has no physical cause can often be resolved through psychiatric or sex therapy. Given the number of effective therapies currently available, almost all physical causes of erectile dysfunction can now be treated noninvasively. Surgery remains an effective option for the uncommon patient whose erectile dysfunction is not responsive to conservative measures.

❖ PREMATURE EJACULATION

Symptoms and signs *(What you may experience)* Ejaculation before penetration; the inability to prolong erection and hold off orgasm until you or your partner is satisfied.

What is it? Premature ejaculation occurs most commonly in young men. The problem is related to the physiologic differences between male and female sexual response. The average time it takes for a man to become stimulated to orgasm is approximately 2 to 3 minutes; a woman's average time is approximately 10 to 15 minutes. This difference is at the root of most cases of premature ejaculation. Many men who masturbated as youngsters wanted to reach climax rapidly in order to minimize guilt or the chances of getting caught. This behavior is not something that is unlearned rapidly, and may contribute to premature ejaculation. Premature ejaculation is the single most common sexual dysfunction of men and between couples.

What you can do Talk to your partner. Openness is of considerable importance in preventing or averting premature ejaculation. Do not have sex with someone you do not know well or with someone with whom you have not yet addressed issues of contraception and disease prevention. Do not have sex if you feel coerced, guilty, or otherwise anxious.

Talk to your partner. Find out how her body works, and how you can stimulate her. Talking can go a long way toward alleviating performance anxiety and other factors that can be a detriment to your sex life. Generally, penile penetration alone does not provide enough stimulation for most women to achieve orgasm. By talking and experimenting, you can discover what works for your partner.

Do what you can to alleviate guilt or anxiety. For example, if you are worried about STIs or the possibility of pregnancy, use condoms (see Proper Use of a Condom, page 1162), which may also help prevent premature ejaculation in that they affect penile sensation. Together couples can learn ways to prevent premature ejaculation.

When to call the doctor Generally, premature ejaculation is not serious enough, and is easily enough resolved, that it is not usually necessary to consult your doctor. If, however, it is creating a problem in your relationship, do not hesitate to ask for a doctor's help.

Treatment Although there are mild, local-anesthetic creams and gels available for use directly on the penis to deaden sensation and medications that prolong time to orgasm, behavior modification is usually the best way to treat premature ejaculation.

The most effective treatment is practice holding off orgasm. As you are having sexual intercourse, stop when you feel that you are on the threshold of orgasm. Withdraw from your partner and allow about 30 seconds to elapse, until the sensation of impending orgasm subsides. Resume intercourse. As you feel again on the threshold of orgasm, again withdraw and allow another 30 seconds or so to elapse. Repeat as often as necessary to provide adequate time for your partner's stimulation.

Also effective is the "squeeze" method, which is another way of postponing orgasm, in this case involving your partner. Again, you withdraw as you feel orgasm approaching, but upon your withdrawal, your partner squeezes your penis at the junction of head and shaft for about 30 seconds, withholding any other stimulation. Repeat as often as necessary in order to allow your partner time for stimulation.

Eventually, by repeating one of the above methods, you will learn to hold off orgasm until it is appropriate. If these methods fail, your doctor can prescribe medications that may help but, unfortunately, not without effects.

Prognosis Excellent. Ninety-five percent of men whose early ejaculations cause a detriment to their sex life can learn to prolong their erections and hold off ejaculation. Those who cannot learn to hold off ejaculation can learn other techniques to reduce anxiety and enhance their enjoyment of sex, and their ability to please their partner.

❖ RETROGRADE EJACULATION

Symptoms *(What you may experience)* Little or no ejaculate is released from the penis at orgasm.

Signs and laboratory findings *(What the doctor looks for)* Presence of sperm in your urine following orgasm.

What is it? Retrograde (or backward) ejaculation is a harmless condition in which semen is ejaculated back into the bladder rather than out through the urethra and penis. Semen is then discharged when you urinate. It is most often associated with diabetes, use of certain medications such as antihypertensives, and as a side effect of surgery that involves the prostate or nerves that go to the prostate and bladder.

Treatment If the condition is a side effect of medication, discontinuing or changing the medication may be possible. There are also medications that are available to counteract the condition, though these are not always effective.

Prognosis If everything else is normal, there is no reason for retrograde ejaculation to interfere with a man's sex life unless he is trying to initiate a pregnancy. In these situations a woman can be inseminated with sperm obtained through catheterization immediately following intercourse.

The Testes and Scrotum

The testicles, a pair of egg-shaped structures about 2 in. in size, are the male gonads, responsible for producing not only sperm cells, but male reproductive hormones (primarily testosterone) as well. The testes hang suspended within the scrotal sac. While their exposed location is important in temperature control (sperm cannot be produced effectively at body temperature), it also makes them highly vulnerable to injury.

Unlike the female gonads (the ovaries), which are carefully padded and protected within the pelvis, the testicles hang unprotected and vulnerable. Disorders commonly affecting them include injury, infection, cyst formation, diminished function, and cancer. The issues of infertility are dealt with later in this chapter, page 1151.

❖ EPIDIDYMITIS AND ORCHITIS

Symptoms *(What you may experience)* Common: Painful swelling of the testicle/scrotum; fever; painful urination.

Signs and laboratory findings *(What the doctor looks for)* Extreme tenderness and swelling (and sometimes redness and warmth) of the epididymis or testicle on physical exam. Sometimes: redness and warmth of the epididymis or testicle.

What is it?

- *Epididymitis.* After sperm are produced, they travel out the top of the testicle into a long coiled tube that runs down the back of the testicle where they acquire the ability to swim. This tubular structure, the epididymis, can sometimes become infected by bacteria. When this occurs, the structure becomes extremely tender and even warm to the touch over the course of a few hours (much like the warmth and tenderness of a boil on the skin).

  Sexually transmitted bacteria commonly cause the disorder in younger men (those under age 40); often urethral infection with a penile discharge and discomfort with urination will accompany epididymitis. The nonsexually transmitted forms typically occur in older men and may be associated with infections of nearby urinary tract structures, such as the bladder or the prostate gland.

- *Orchitis.* When infection extends to involve the entire testicle, it is termed an orchitis. Although this disorder can arise as an extension of infection elsewhere in the urinary/reproductive tract, such as the epididymis or prostate, it can also occur as a complication of certain viral infections, most notably mumps (see page 880).

SCROTAL LUMPS

Lumps in the scrotum can arise from a variety of structures. Their discovery can cause concern. Although most of the causes are benign, every lump found in the testicle or scrotum merits evaluation by a doctor. Among the common benign causes for lumps in the scrotum are the following:

Hydrocele The testicle is surrounded by a thin layer of fluid to reduce the friction that occurs as the body moves. Occasionally, an excess amount of fluid accumulates beneath the sheath surrounding the testicle. It will appear as a soft, usually painless, swelling in the scrotal sac. To aid in its identification, the doctor will shine a light through the swelling, a procedure termed "transillumination" because light will pass through the fluid in a hydrocele. Ultrasound may also be used to evaluate the lump.

Spermatocele This painless fluid-filled cyst develops at the top of the testicle, near the epididymis. It too will feel soft and "give" when lightly squeezed. It originates in the loose supportive tissues of the spermatic cord that tethers the testicle to the interior of the pelvis.

Varicocele This generally painless swelling occurs more commonly on the left side of the scrotum. While standing up, this scrotal mass feels like a bag of worms, a sensation that diminishes when lying down. The mass is made up of enlarged, twisted varicose veins that fill and engorge with standing and drain when lying down. Light during transillumination will not pass through the blood in the varicocele; therefore, ultrasound may be of more value in evaluating this condition.

Hernia Herniation of the intestine into the scrotal sack can also cause a lump. See Hernia and Hernia Repair, page 1141 for more information.

Testicular Cancer Cancers of the testicle are relatively uncommon and occur in men in their 20s and 30s. Testicular cancers are characteristically firm and nontender. Any suspicious lump in the testicle should be evaluated using ultrasound.

With the exception of hernia and cancer, these scrotal masses cause no problems, and can usually be left alone without worry. Occasionally, a urologist may recommend their surgical repair to improve fertility. But all scrotal lumps should be examined by a doctor to eliminate the possibility of testicular cancer. ■

Scrotal masses should always receive medical evaluation. There are several causes of benign masses. (A) A hydrocele, which is soft and usually painless, has excess fluid beneath the sheath surrounding the testicle. (B) A spermatocele is a painless cyst that develops from the spermatic cord and rests at the top of the testicle. (C) A varicocele is a mass of enlarged veins that feels like a bag of worms and diminishes when lying down.

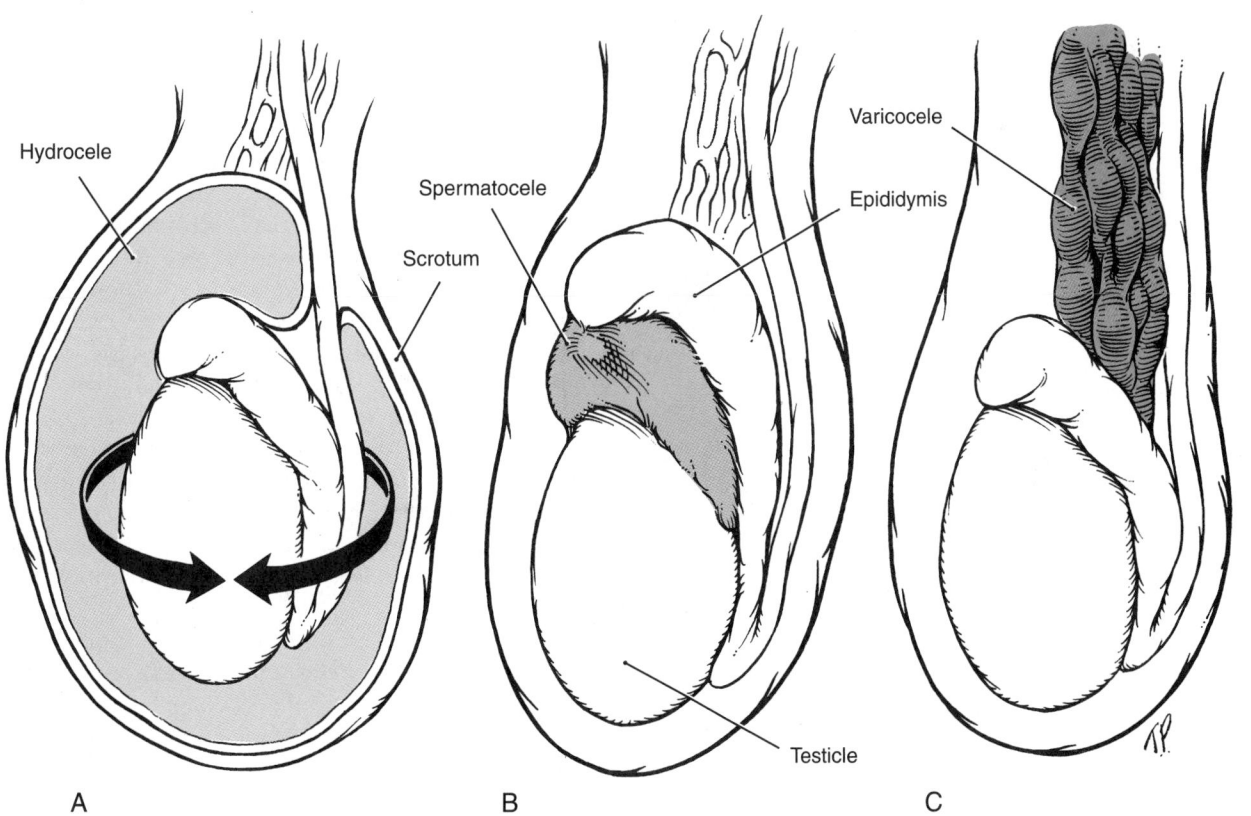

Hydrocele

Spermatocele

Scrotum

Varicocele

Epididymis

Testicle

A   B   C

TESTICULAR SELF-EXAM

Every male from the time of high school onward should examine his testicles each month. Cancer of the testicles, which mainly strikes younger men, can be deadly, but if found early it is usually curable. Learning to correctly perform this exam can be lifesaving. Follow the simple steps listed below once a month, after bath or shower. The warmth helps to loosen and relax the tissues, and moist skin enhances the ability to feel any lumps.

1. Examine one testicle at a time.

2. Gently grasp the testicle between your thumb and first finger, rolling it between them to feel for any lumps on its surface. Be sure to feel the entire surface, top to bottom.

3. Be aware that a small soft structure, the epididymis, is attached to the top and back of the testicle. Soft blood vessels and a firm cord-like structure, the vas deferens, also may be felt behind and above the testicle. Become familiar with the normal shape and feel of your own testicles; in that way changes from the norm will be more apparent to you.

If a new lump is found, do not panic. Remember that most lumps are benign, but that all of them merit investigation and evaluation by an experienced doctor. Resist the temptation to repeatedly check the lump, since doing so might make it more swollen or tender and hamper the doctor's evaluation. ∎

All men should examine their testicles monthly to screen for signs of testicular cancer. Roll the testicle carefully between the thumb and first finger, checking the entire surface for lumps. Blood vessels, the epididymis, and the ductus (vas) deferens can normally be found at the top and back ends of the testicle. Be sure to examine each testicle individually.

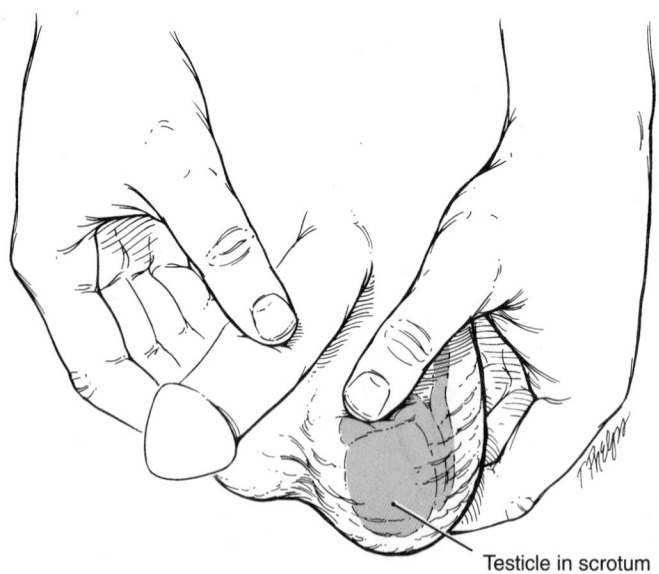

Testicle in scrotum

What you can do Bed rest with support of the testicles/scrotum can be helpful to relieve pain (see The Bellevue Bridge for Testicular/Scrotal Swelling, page 1142).

When to call the doctor Pain and swelling of the testicles is not normal; any such occurrence should prompt immediate evaluation by a doctor.

Treatment Infectious causes require an extended course of antibiotic therapy: 10 to 21 days in most cases of sexually transmitted infection, along with treatment of sexual partners; nonsexually transmitted cases require 3 to 4 weeks of antibiotic therapy to eradicate the infection.

Prognosis Good with prompt diagnosis and appropriate and sufficient treatment. With delay in diagnosis or inadequate courses of therapy, the infection may persist, extend to involve deeper tissues or form abscesses, or may cause decreased fertility.

❖ TRAUMA TO THE TESTES AND SCROTUM

Symptoms *(What you may experience)* Swelling; bruising; bleeding; pain.

What is it? The testicles hang in a vulnerable position outside the protection of the bony pelvis, covered only by skin and a thin layer of fluid. Their location puts them at increased risk for injury from a direct blow or a fall. The pain that follows trauma to the testicles is deep and severe, causing nausea, light-headedness, and sweating, an unpleasant experience well known to virtually all males. But despite the pain associated with it, a blow to the scrotum rarely causes permanent injury to the testicles. Their structure is spongy and resilient, and their loose attachment to the body helps to absorb and lessen the shock that might occur from being struck by a blunt object or in a straddle fall. In most cases, the pain will pass in a few moments, and the testicles will not swell, bruise, or suffer serious harm.

What you can do Gently support the injured testicles and scrotum and apply a cold pack for mild swelling (see The Bellevue Bridge for Testicular/Scrotal Swelling, page 1142).

When to call the doctor In general, you should seek medical help right away if the pain that follows trauma to the scrotum lasts longer than an hour or is associated

HERNIA AND HERNIA REPAIR

The term hernia simply means an outpouching or projection of an organ or a part of an organ through the wall that normally contains it. That definition could apply to the disk between the vertebral bones of the spine (a herniated disk) or the herniation of a part of the intestine through a weak area of the abdominal wall. Sometimes this kind of hernia occurs at the site of previous abdominal surgery and is called an incisional hernia. But by far the most common kind of hernia occurs in the inguinal or groin region in men. That is not to say that women cannot develop them, but the occurrence in women is far less common.

In males, the testicles develop within the abdominal cavity and prior to birth, migrate through an opening in the abdominal wall in the groin to their final position in the scrotal sac. The opening, called the inguinal canal, persists as a passageway for the spermatic cord that tethers the testicles to their blood supply within the abdominal/pelvic cavity. Occasionally, the diameter of the opening ruptures or stretches, often from heavy lifting or other forms of straining that increase the pressure within the abdominal cavity, creating sufficient room around the spermatic cord to permit a loop of intestine to work its way through. An inguinal hernia is the loop of bowel that protrudes through the ring, and is usually felt as a soft swelling or lump in the groin. Early on, the outpouching may only be felt by a doctor checking for a hernia. In this exam, one familiar to most young men involved in athletic endeavors, the doctor evaluates the strength and laxity of the inguinal ring, by pushing a finger along the spermatic cord within the scrotal sac up to the ring where the cord dips into the abdominal cavity. A herniated loop of bowel can be felt sometimes, but an increase in abdominal pressure, such as occurs with coughing, will cause the hernia to bulge against the tip of the doctor's finger, making it more obvious.

At this time, the doctor can also check to see if the hernia can be pushed back into the abdominal cavity easily (a reducible hernia) or is entrapped outside the cavity (an incarcerated hernia). An easily reducible hernia does not require immediate repair; however, once it has become entrapped, surgery to release it and repair the ring should be performed as soon as possible. Not doing so raises the risk of strangulation of the bowel, with compromise of its blood supply and tissue death. When this condition arises, the surgery becomes urgent and more difficult.

There have been a number of methods devised by surgeons to repair the lax ring. Some of them involve simply anchoring and tightening the existing ligamentous tissues. Occasionally, especially if the hernia is large and has been present for a long time, the supportive tissues have frayed and thinned to the point that

Heavy straining or increased abdominal pressure can cause the intestines to herniate (protrude) abnormally through the abdominal wall and into the scrotum. Correcting a hernia requires surgery, and the need for surgical correction becomes more urgent if the intestines become irreversibly trapped outside the abdominal cavity.

there is no strong anchoring tissue available. In these instances, the surgeon may elect to sew a tough, synthetic fabric graft across the opening to provide a stronger, longer lasting repair.

Successful, uncomplicated hernia repair is usually performed on an outpatient basis and requires a recuperative period of 1 to 2 months without driving or lifting. After the healing period, most people can return to their normal level of activity. ■

---

with significant swelling, discoloration, or a puncture of the skin.

Treatment In the majority of cases, bed rest, support of the scrotum with a bridge, cold packs, and medication to relieve pain are sufficient treatment.

In more severe cases, surgery to relieve the pressure caused by bleeding and swelling

on the testicle and its blood vessels may be necessary. Severe crushing injury to the testicle could necessitate its removal.

Prognosis Excellent if promptly diagnosed and appropriately treated. Failure to do so could result in infection, the formation of blood clots, future infertility, or loss of a testicle that prompt action could have saved. It

THE BELLEVUE BRIDGE FOR TESTICULAR/SCROTAL SWELLING

When the testicles or scrotum become injured, inflamed, or infected, the pain can be considerable. Even the pull of gravity on the weight of the testicles can be uncomfortable. The Bellevue Bridge is a simple device that can be easily constructed to give support to these tender tissues. Here are two easy methods:

Using 2-in. wide sports or adhesive tape, tear two lengths of tape, one 18 to 24 in. long and another about 3 to 4 in. shorter. The length of tape should match the size of the individual. Lay the adhesive sides together, the shorter piece centered over the longer, and stick the two together. This will leave about 2 in. of sticky tape at either end. Now stick one end of the bridge to one thigh, slip the length of tape gently beneath the testicles and scrotum, and up over the other thigh. Put just enough tension on the tape to give support to the testicles. Stick the other end to that thigh.

A second method is to use a thin bath towel, folded lengthwise. Tuck one end under one thigh, bring the towel over the front of the thigh and gently beneath the testicles and scrotum, then up and over the other thigh to finally tuck in under that thigh. ■

is important to note, however, that the loss of one testicle does not impair fertility, diminish sexual drive, or result in deficient testosterone production. A single functioning testicle can suffice.

❖ TESTICULAR TORSION

Symptoms *(What you may experience)* Sudden onset of swelling and severe pain of one testicle, without injury or abdominal pain. Often: nausea; vomiting; faintness.

Signs and laboratory findings *(What the doctor looks for)* Testicular tenderness; sometimes: "high lie" or exaggerated elevation of the affected testicle in relation to the other testicle.

What is it? Although the testicles hang suspended in the scrotal sack, they are normally securely anchored at either end. Occasionally, the mooring allows too much slack and the testicle can twist, crimping the spermatic cord and the blood vessels that run within it. The condition, termed testicular torsion, occurs more frequently in infants and young men, typically between ages 10 and 20. It can cause infants to be inconsolable. Unfortunately, the condition is often silent in this age group. In older men, significant testicular pain without preceding injury should raise the possibility of torsion (although there could be other explanations, such as infection). Twisting of the cord cuts off the blood supply to the testicle and causes the pain. If not promptly recognized and corrected, torsion endangers the testicle.

When to call the doctor Because of the risk that inadequate blood supply could destroy the testicle, do not attempt to treat sudden onset testicular pain on your own or adopt a wait-and-see attitude. Seek medical help immediately.

ANDROPAUSE (MALE MENOPAUSE) AND TESTOSTERONE REPLACEMENT

Although both genders make some testosterone throughout life, at puberty, the testicles begin to produce increasing amounts of this potent male reproductive hormone, giving rise to the development of adult male sexual characteristics: deepening of the voice and increasing muscularity, body hair, genital growth, and the activity of oil glands in the skin. The level of testosterone production declines in men as they age and with this drop, some effects of the hormone wane. Wasting of muscle mass, especially in the shoulder girdle and chest, loss of sexual drive or interest, reduction of body hair, thinning of the skin, and some degree of depression may indicate the onset of this decline, termed andropause, or "male menopause." Very rarely, the condition is treated using hormone therapy.

Although this diminishment commonly occurs in senior men, its occasional appearance in younger men should prompt an inves-

tigation for cause. Genetic disorders, such as Klinefelter's syndrome (the presence of three sex chromosomes—two female "X" chromosomes as well as a single "Y"—instead of the normal one "X" and one "Y") may not become readily apparent until adulthood and may be a cause for low levels of testosterone activity. Tumors, such as lymphoma, may invade the testicle and reduce testosterone production. Pituitary tumors, such as prolactinomas, can alter the normal brain regulation of testosterone production and thereby diminish its effect.

Testosterone is usually administered in a form absorbable through the skin, usually as a patch or topical gel applied daily to a shaved area of scrotal skin or on the back. Most doctors avoid the use of oral preparations of testosterone, because they do not seem to work as well, and their long term use has been associated with liver damage.

Side effects of replacement can include oiliness of the skin, eruptions of acne, and a decrease in high-density lipoprotein (HDL) cholesterol (the "good" cholesterol) in some men, and a possible increased risk of prostate cancer. ■

Treatment The torsion (twist) must be relieved immediately, often by surgery. After returning the testicle to its proper position, the urologic surgeon will also anchor it into place as a precaution against future episodes of twisting.

Prognosis Good if identified and treated promptly. If not corrected within a few hours, the testicle may die from lack of blood supply and will have to be removed.

❖ CRYPTORCHIDISM (UNDESCENDED TESTICLE)

Symptoms (*What you may experience*) Usually none.

Signs and laboratory findings (*What the doctor looks for*) Absence of one or both testicles from the scrotum.

What is it? The name, cryptorchidism, comes from the Greek roots cryptos, meaning hidden, and orchis, which refers to the testicle. The testicles normally develop within the abdominal/pelvic cavity and in most instances (94 to 97 percent of the time) during the month before birth complete their migration through an opening in the wall of the abdomen/groin and are firmly in place within the scrotal sac at birth. In as many as one in three premature infants, and in a much smaller percentage of full-term baby boys, one or both of the testicles have not yet completed the descent and remain "undescended." Curiously, it is slightly more common for the right testicle to fail to descend. The condition persists in less than 1 percent of male infants by 1 year of age. If by that time the testicle(s) remain within the abdominal cavity, surgical correction is in order. Ideally this procedure should be done before 2 years of age, both to reduce the risk of infertility (production of healthy sperm cannot occur at normal body temperature) and to reduce the risk for testicular cancer, which is slightly higher for men with cryptorchidism, occurring in 5 percent of patients whose testicle(s) remain within the abdominal cavity. The risk is not actually reduced by the surgery, but since cancer of a hidden testicle is harder to diagnose at an early stage, the surgery allows for early diagnosis of cancer should it occur.

Sometimes, the testicle has descended, but is not tethered firmly and is able at times to retract completely into the abdominal cavity (called a retractile testicle). This condition does not carry the same risk for infertility or cancer (see Testicular Torsion, page 1142).

When to call the doctor If you or your child has one or both testicles that cannot be felt within the scrotal sac, consult your doctor for a thorough evaluation.

Treatment In some cases, administration of the pregnancy hormone HCG can induce the testicle(s) to drop into their normal position. If hormonal therapy fails to correct the condition, surgery is necessary.

In the surgical correction procedure, termed an orchiopexy, the testicle is brought through the normal abdominal opening at the groin, tunneled down into the scrotal sac, and stitched into place. In cases in which the undescended testicle has gone unrecognized until past puberty, the choice may be made to perform orchiopexy, but often removal is recommended. When cryptorchidism persists past puberty, the excess heat will likely have rendered the testicle incapable of sperm production, and removal eliminates the risk of testicular cancer. Once men reach middle age, the risks associated with surgery may outweigh the risk of cancer. In this case, your doctor may not recommend surgery.

Prognosis Good if recognized early and corrected before 2 years of age, although sometimes this condition is associated with hypogonadism (see Hypopituitarism, page 1203) and simply returning the testicle to its proper location will not ensure fertility. Unfortunatley, the "descended" testicle on the other side also does not function normally. Up to 75 percent of men may be infertile if both testicles failed to descend and up to 50 percent may be infertile if only one remained undescended.

❖ CANCER OF THE TESTICLE

Symptoms (*What you may experience*) A painless lump in the testicle.

Signs and laboratory findings (*What the doctor looks for*) Microscopic examina-

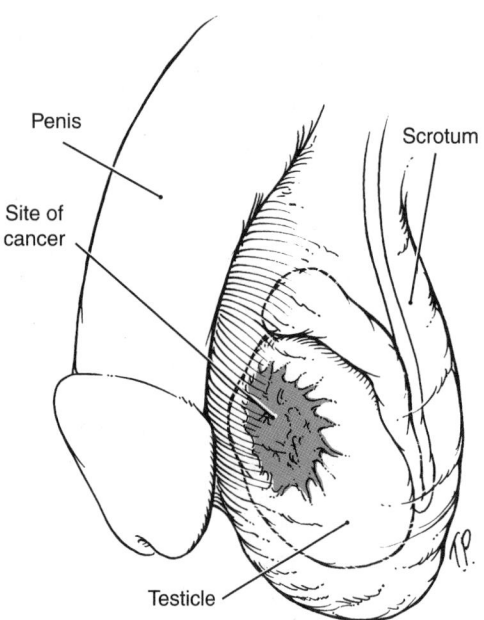

Rarely, cancer develops directly on or inside the testicle, most often in men between ages 20 and 35. If examination and imaging techniques suggest a solid mass in the testicle, the entire testicle should be removed, because a biopsy without testicular removal can spread the cancer and complicate treatment. Men should examine their own testicles regularly.

tion of tissue from the testicle (after its complete removal) will show cancerous cells.

What is it? Cancer of the testicle occurs rarely; only 2 or 3 men in 100,000 develop it annually. In the course of a lifetime, a man's risk is 2 in 1,000. When it does develop, it usually strikes younger men, generally between ages 20 and 35, and is slightly more common in the right testicle than in the left. The latter association parallels the slight increased tendency for the right testicle to fail to descend into the scrotum at birth, a condition that increases the risk of cancer development.

The cause of this cancer is unknown but seems to be associated with both genetic as well as environmental influences. For example, the undescended testicle, remaining exposed to the higher temperature of the abdominal cavity, could be seen as responding to an abnormal environmental insult; however, in as many as 10 percent of the people with an undescended testicle, the cancer develops in the other normally descended testicle, suggesting a genetic

potential, not an environmental one. Exposure to maternal doses of exogenous estrogen or diethylstilbestrol (DES) while in the womb has also been associated with an increased development in testicular cancer. Precisely why these factors seem to influence the development of cancer is unclear; no specific cause and effect relationship has ever been established.

Most cancers of the testicle develop from the germ cells. These tumors are called seminomas and nonseminomas. Less commonly (representing less than 5 percent of testicular cancers) are cancers derived from the supportive tissues. These are called Leydig cell tumors and Sertoli cell tumors.

Left undetected, the cancer has a tendency to spread to the liver, lung, and lymph glands. Whether the cancer has spread will determine the proper treatment and predict the survival of the disease. It is imperative that the testicular lump not be simply biopsied if cancer is suspected. To do so can spread the cancer and make treatment much more difficult. When such noninvasive studies as ultrasound imaging, transillumination, and physical examination suggest a solid mass in the testicle, the proper course is to remove the testicle intact for pathologic examination. The kind of testicular cancer and the extent of spread of the tumor will be assessed at this time.

Tumors that remain confined to the testicle are designated as stage I, those that have spread to lymph gland in the back of the pelvic cavity are stage II, and those that have spread to distant sites are termed stage III. Staging is carried out near the time of diagnosis and involves obtaining a CT scan of the abdomen and pelvis and chest x-rays. Proteins in the blood, such as alphafetoprotein and beta-HCG, serve as markers of testicular cancers; the doctor will measure these levels before and after surgery.

What you can do Regularly examine the testicles (see Testicular Self-Exam, page 1140) and immediately report any unusual enlargement to your doctor.

Treatment Removal of the affected testicle and its cord is the initial treatment. If staging by x-ray, CT scan, and serum markers indicates the cancer has spread, additional treatment may be necessary. Early-stage seminomas usually are treated by radiation to the region of the lymph nodes. Nonseminomas may require surgery to remove the lymph nodes (a retroperitoneal lymph node dissection). Advanced tumors of either type should receive chemotherapy.

Prognosis The 5-year survival of men with stage I cancers treated with surgery and radiation is 98 percent, which underscores the powerful life-saving impact of early detection. Effective chemotherapies have also improved survival of patients whose tumors have spread, even among those who have extensive disease. Survival for all stages of testicular cancer is over 95 percent.

The Prostate Gland

The prostate gland sits just beneath the urinary bladder and surrounds the urethra (urine tube). It produces a glandular fluid that makes up one-third of the volume of semen, releasing these secretions into multiple ducts that empty into the urethra. The prostatic secretions provide a more hospitable environment for the sperm cells and help to improve their survival in the acidic environment of the vaginal canal.

The gland commonly enlarges with age (see Benign Prostatic Hypertrophy Enlarged Prostate, page 1146) and because of its location, surrounding the urethra, can cause constriction of the urine passageway and difficulty urinating. Other problems commonly affecting the gland are infections and cancer.

❖ PROSTATITIS (ACUTE)

Symptoms *(What you may experience)* Common: Painful urination; fever; pain over the bladder, in the low back, and in the perineal area (between the testicles and rectum).

Signs and laboratory findings *(What the doctor looks for)* Bacteria grown in cultures of urine; extreme tenderness of prostate on rectal exam.

What is it? Because of its proximity to the urinary system, bacterial infections of the bladder or urethra can sometimes migrate up the prostatic ducts to infect the prostate gland. The onset of the infection, like most acute infections, is often sudden and dra-

matic, with the abrupt development of painful, urgent, and frequent urination as the infection swells the gland. Fever and chills often accompany the infection as well.

When to call the doctor If symptoms suggesting acute prostatitis develop, particularly high fever and chills, seek medical help right away. Fever and chills can indicate that the bacteria have entered the blood stream, a potentially serious result.

Treatment Hospitalization and administration of intravenous antibiotics is usually necessary until the fever breaks. Once it has, therapy should continue with the administration of oral antibiotics for 4 to 6 weeks longer.

In cases in which the prostate has swollen enough to obstruct the normal flow of urine, placement of a catheter (a flexible tube inserted through the urethra and into the bladder) will be necessary to empty the urine.

Prognosis Excellent with prompt and appropriate therapy. Chronic prostate infection develops only rarely.

❖ PROSTATITIS (CHRONIC)

Symptoms *(What you may experience)* Vague, persistent, low back or perineal pain. Often: discomfort with urination. Sometimes: no symptoms.

Signs and laboratory *(What the doctor looks for)* Growth of bacteria from prostatic secretions; an enlarged, mushy prostate on rectal exam.

What is it? Migration of bacteria from an infected urinary bladder or urethra into the prostatic ducts and into the prostate gland sometimes does not cause the explosive development of symptoms of acute prostate infection, but rather pursues a slower course. When infection in the prostate gland persists chronically at this lesser intensity, it may cause varying degrees of low back and perineal pain, but may cause no directly obvious symptoms, such as burning or urgency with urination. Because it does not incite the intense response of the immune system seen in acute prostatitis, a reaction that causes swelling and increased blood flow that carries antibiotics to the site of infection, the chronic form is much more difficult to eradicate.

Occasionally, chronic prostatitis results from infection with the kinds of bacteria that commonly invade the urinary tract, such as *Escherichia coli, Pseudomonas,* and *Enterococcus.* More commonly, culture turns up none of these microorganisms. In the past doctors have termed this condition nonbacterial prostatitis, although recent medical speculation indicates that even these cases may result from infection with atypical bacterial organisms, such as chlamydia, mycoplasma, ureaplasmas, or viruses that do not readily grow in the laboratory with standard culture techniques. At present, however, the consensus holds that nonbacterial prostatitis is a noninfectious inflammatory disorder of the prostate.

What you can do Warm sitz baths may offer some relief of the low back and perineal discomfort, as may over-the-counter anti-inflammatory medications, such as ibuprofen or aspirin.

When to call the doctor The development of chronic urinary discomfort should always prompt evaluation by a doctor. Persistent low back pain, which can result from a wide variety of causes besides the prostate should also prompt a visit to your doctor.

Treatment Because it concentrates better in the prostate gland, the antibiotic trimethoprim-sulfamethoxazole works well. Also effective are the newer antibiotics of the quinolone class (Floxin, Cipro) as well as cephalexin, carbenicillin, minocycline, and erythromycin. The duration of therapy should be 2 to 3 months.

Prognosis This disorder is difficult to cure, but can be controlled with suppressive antibiotics.

❖ BENIGN PROSTATIC HYPERTROPHY (ENLARGED PROSTATE)

Symptoms *(What you may experience)* Reduced caliber and force of urine stream; awakening frequently to urinate at night; urgent need to urinate. Occasionally: inability to pass urine (urinary retention).

Signs and laboratory findings *(What the doctor looks for)* Enlarged prostate on rectal exam; increased residual (postvoiding) urine volume. Occasionally: elevated level of blood urea nitrogen and creatinine.

What is it? With age, the prostate gland tends to increase in size for reasons that are poorly understood at present, although it appears that the endocrine system plays a role. The incidence of this disorder, which afflicts only about 1 out of 5 men in their 40s, rises to 1 in 4 men by age 55, 1 in 2 by age 75, and 4 out of every 5 men over the age of 80.

(A) A finger can be used to examine the rectum for masses. At the same time, the prostate can be checked for masses or enlargement. (B) The normal prostate rests at the neck of the bladder, surrounding the urethra. (C) In benign prostatic hypertrophy (BPH), the normal tissue of a man's prostate gland gradually increases in mass, causing prostatic enlargement. This can compress the urethra and cause problems with urination, such as dribbling or difficulty starting the stream. Medications or surgery are treatment options.

Urethra   Normal prostate   BPH

The gland's location, beneath the bladder and around the urethra, coupled with the fact that benign hypertrophy particularly affects the prostate tissues immediately surrounding the urethra, accounts for the hallmark and often most troubling symptom of the disorder: diminished force and caliber of the urinary stream. The more significant the overgrowth of the tissue becomes, the more difficulty men will have in getting a urine stream started, maintaining a strong and forceful flow, and stopping the flow without dribbles and spurts of urine. With time, the enlarged gland can protrude into the bladder, often partially blocking the opening to the urethra within the bladder and making it difficult for the bladder to completely empty. Urine remaining in the bladder after urination (called postvoiding residual urine) forms an hospitable environment for bacterial growth as well as for the formation of sediment that could lead to bladder gravel or stones.

Occasionally, the enlarged gland suddenly swells and occludes the outflow of urine. The enlargement of the prostate usually involves both the secretory glands and the muscle of the prostate. Certain antihistamine preparations commonly found in both prescription and over-the-counter cold remedies can cause the muscle of the prostate to contract, resulting in urinary retention (see Urinary Retention, page 1073).

When to call the doctor Progressive diminishment of the urine stream or the appearance of blood in the urine should prompt evaluation by a doctor. Seek medical attention right away for sudden inability to pass a normal amount of urine, particularly if associated with a need to urinate or lower abdominal discomfort.

Treatment Medical treatment is aimed at reducing the influence of testosterone (the male reproductive hormone) on the gland or relaxing the muscle of the prostate gland. The medication finasteride (Proscar) offers the benefit of decreasing testosterone influence without diminishing sexual drive, and in general should be used in men with very large prostate glands. Medications such as alpha blockers, which relax the muscle of the prostate, offer relief of symptoms and improved urinary flow regardless of prostate size.

TURP—PROSTATE RESECTION SURGERY

TURP, an acronym for transurethral resection of the prostate, is the second most commonly performed surgery in men over age 60 in the United States. In this operating room procedure, under a general or spinal anesthetic, the urologist inserts a thin instrument, called an operating cystoscope, into the urethra, passing it up the urine tube to the site of obstruction. The cystoscope has a miniature telescopic camera lens with a lighted tip that allows the surgeon to view the interior of the urethra (and bladder) as he brings a tiny cutting device to the area. With this device, the surgeon cuts away the enlarged portion of the gland where it hinders the urine outflow, boring an open channel through it. The removed pieces will be sent to the pathologist for microscopic exam to determine if any cancerous cells lurk within the enlarged area.

Afterward, a flexible catheter will be placed through the open channel into the bladder to drain urine for a few days as the urethra heals. A short hospital stay, usually only overnight, follows the procedure.

Although the surgery generally relieves the symptoms of enlarged prostate, often it may cause a condition known as retrograde ejaculation. When this occurs, semen released with ejaculation flows backward into the bladder rather than forward out the urethra. This condition causes no harm, but will impair fertility in a man still desirous of fathering children. Rarely, the procedure results in more serious and persistent difficulties, such as impotence or urinary incontinence.

Men with a lesser degree of enlargement may benefit from a less invasive operation, called a transurethral incision procedure (TUIP). This procedure, usually performed as an outpatient surgery, uses the same instrument, the operating cystoscope, to relieve the symptoms by simply incising (cutting open or splitting) the obstruction without removing any tissue. It carries a risk of fewer complications and often can maintain normal forward ejaculation. ■

As the gland grows larger or the symptoms more severe, surgery becomes necessary to relieve the obstruction. The surgery can be performed through an abdominal incision, or more commonly, through the urethra (see TURP—Prostate Resection Surgery, above for more information about this procedure).

Prognosis Good for relief of symptoms with medical or surgical treatment. Surgery has a slightly higher probability of improving symptoms.

❖ PROSTATE CANCER

Symptoms (*What you may experience*) Common (early stage): no symptoms. Less common (later stages): weight loss; bone pain; urinary retention.

Signs and laboratory findings (*What the doctor looks for*) Firm or lumpy prostate

Prostate cancer is common in men. (A) Stage A cannot be detected on rectal examination, but can be seen in surgical specimens (after surgery for prostate enlargement, for example). (B) Stage B can be felt on examination, but the prostate itself remains the only affected area. (C) In stage C, the tumor begins to extend outside the prostate gland. (D) In stage D, spread occurs to distant sites. Advanced stages are more difficult to treat.

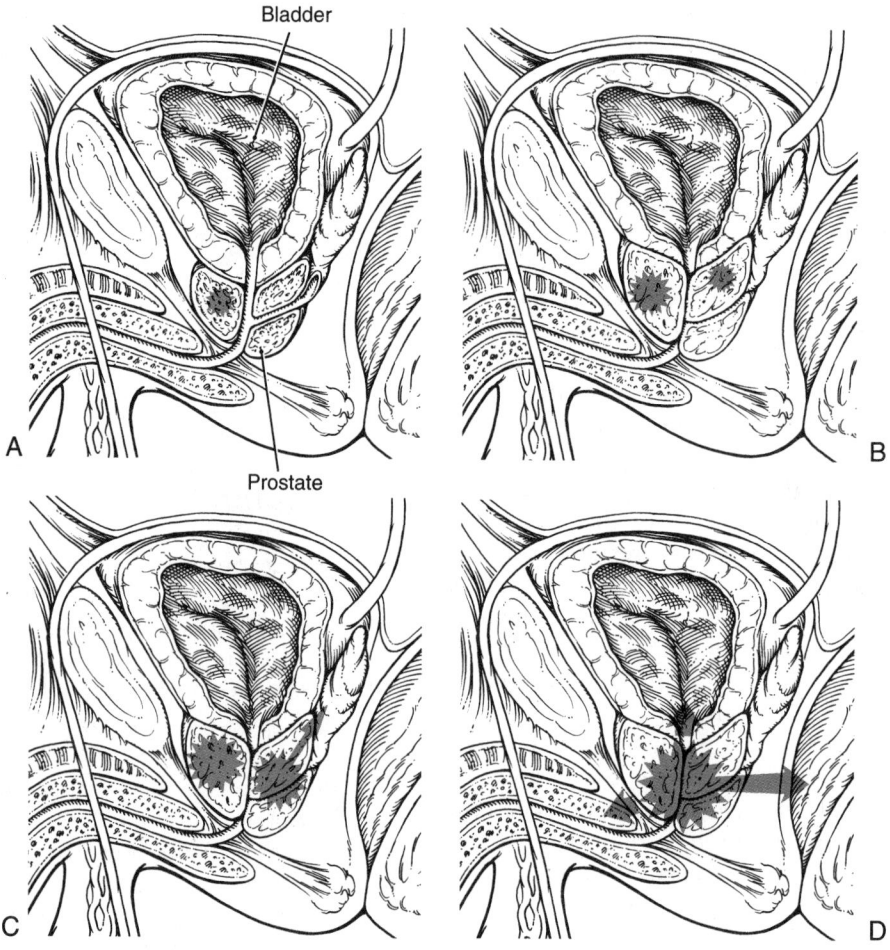

Bladder

Prostate

A   B   C   D

on rectal exam; usually, elevated blood level of prostate specific antigen (PSA).

What is it? Cancer of the prostate is the second most common cancer (after skin cancer) found in American men. About 184,500 new cases will be detected in 1998. The incidence of this cancer appears to be on the rise, but the statistics reflect not so much an increase in occurrence as an increase in early discovery through the more common use of screening tests. The cancer is age related, with risk increasing from age 50 onward. It occurs more commonly among African American men than those of other ethnic groups. It is estimated that in 1998, prostatic cancer will claim 39,200 lives in the United States.

Cancerous cells usually arise in the outer regions (peripheral zone) of the gland, where they can often be felt on digital rectal exam by a doctor. Both normal and cancerous prostate tissues produce PSA that passes into the blood. When the amounts of

this prostate marker increase in the blood, it can signal the presence of a cancer (see PSA Testing: Pros and Cons, page 1149).

Aggressiveness of the cancer can be estimated by its size, the degree of abnormality of the cells that make it up, termed "differentiation," and the extent of spread. Tumors that are small and well-differentiated (less abnormal in appearance under the microscope) usually remain confined to the prostate gland. Larger poorly-differentiated tumors (those with very abnormal appearing cells) tend to spread aggressively. The latter should be treated aggressively, and immediately.

What you can do PSA screening, a blood test for the detection of prostate cancer, may be recommended, depending upon personal and family history (see PSA Testing: Pros and Cons, page 1149).

Treatment If the doctor suspects prostate cancer, because of elevated levels of PSA in the blood or an abnormal digital rectal exam, the next step in evaluation is often the transrectal ultrasound and biopsy of the abnormal area to verify the presence of cancerous cells and to grade the cancer. If the biopsy is positive, a radionuclide bone scan may be performed to detect spread of the cancer to the bones. If your doctor suspects that the disease has spread elsewhere, additional imaging studies, such as a CT scan or MRI, may be used to stage the tumor. The extent of spread will guide treatment recommendations.

Potential treatments include the following:

- *Radical prostatectomy.* In this procedure, the prostate gland, seminal vesicles, and part of the vas deferens are completely removed. Urinary incontinence and inability to achieve an erection once routinely complicated this surgery, but refinements to the procedure now allow most men to maintain urinary continence after surgery and to preserve erection for many. Ideal candidates for this surgery are those with cancer confined to the prostate gland, that is, not yet broken through the outer capsule. Once the tumor has invaded beyond this boundary, the chance that the cancer has spread to lymph nodes, bone, or other distant sites is higher and other methods should be employed in addition to or in place of prostatectomy.

- *Radiation (x-ray) therapy.* Delivery of radiation to the prostate gland to kill cancerous cells can be achieved either by an x-ray beam directed from the outside or by radioactive "seeds" implanted into the gland. The chief advantage to this approach is that it minimizes the risk of incontinence and may lessen erection difficulties.

- *Hormonal therapy* involves blocking or antagonizing the action of testosterone. As listed below, the method employed can interfere at various spots in the endocrine control system:

  - At the level of the brain (pituitary gland or hypothalamus), *therapy with estrogens* (female hormones) or medications that mimic LH releasing hormone can reduce testosterone stimulation, but can also cause such side effects as breast enlargement, hot flashes, blood clots, and impotence.

PSA TESTING: PROS AND CONS

The advent of an easily performed and widely available blood test for detection of prostate cancer has made early diagnosis of this disease possible. Although the availability of such a test would seem to be unequivocally good, there is considerable disagreement among experts in the field about whether this test should be included in the routine laboratory evaluation of adult males. The test presents levels of false-positive and false-negative results. A low reading does not always mean a clean bill of prostate health, and elevations do not always mean cancer. Disagreement arises in how to interpret the results of the test, how to proceed on the basis of that interpretation, and whether routine screening should be done.

The problem is that both normal and cancerous prostate tissues produce a substance called prostate specific antigen (PSA) that passes into the blood where it is detected during laboratory analysis of a blood sample. When the amounts of PSA increase in the blood, the increase can indicate, but does not always indicate, the presence of cancer. PSA levels below 4 ng/mL generally correlate with a low likelihood of cancer; readings above 10 ng/mL strongly suggest cancer. As many as two-thirds of men with PSA levels of 10 ng/mL will prove at biopsy not to have prostate cancer. Because prostate cancer occurs in some men who have normal or even low PSA levels, a digital rectal examination should always accompany PSA testing.

Since it is not known whether small tumors are likely to spread quickly or cause significant harm, their detection as reflected in a slight elevation of PSA can expose patients to the risk of treatment, associated potential complications, and expense. For this reason, although most urologists agree with the use of PSA as a screening tool, the US Preventive Services Task Force does not recommend routine PSA screening as beneficial because there are insufficient data to inform us whether early detection of prostate cancer by screening for elevated PSA, followed by early treatment, actually reduces death rates from prostate cancer. The Task Force further recommends that people who require a PSA test should be given objective information about the potential benefits and harms of early detection and treatment.

The American Cancer Society and the National Cancer Institute recommend yearly PSA testing combined with a digital rectal exam beginning at age 50. For men at high risk for prostate cancer, for instance, African American men or men with a strong family history of prostate cancer, these organizations recommend that screening begin at age 40.

Before undergoing PSA testing to screen for prostate cancer, however, it should be understood that a positive test will lead the doctor to suggest further testing, involving a prostate biopsy and possibly surgery, with its attendant risks. While surgery and radiation therapy appear effective in prostate cancer, treatment may not be appropriate for all men, particularly those too old or too ill to live at least 10 to 15 years.

A valuable use of PSA testing is in identifying recurrence after the diagnosis of prostate cancer has been established and the disease has been treated, that is, a stable or undetectable level that begins to rise again can signal local recurrence or metastatic progression of the disease. ■

- At the level of the adrenal glands, treatment options include *ketoconazole, aminoglutethimide*, and *prednisone.* The drawbacks of this kind

RADICAL PROSTATECTOMY

Damage to critical nerves during removal of the prostate gland by traditional surgical approaches often results in difficulty achieving and maintaining an erection. This complication is minimized by a procedure pioneered and perfected by Dr. Patrick Walsh, Urologist in Chief of the Brady Urological Institute at Johns Hopkins. The radical retropubic prostatectomy, sometimes referred to as the "nerve-sparing technique," allows the surgeon better access to the prostate and a more accurate approach to the urethra (urine tube). With better exposure of these structures, the surgeon can preserve the penile nerve bundles that are attached to either side of the prostate gland. It is damage to these nerves that results in impotence following surgery. If both bundles of nerves are unharmed, potency returns to 90 percent of men in their 40s, 75 percent of men in their 50s, and 60 percent of men in their 60s.

Radical retropubic prostatectomy is a procedure wherein an incision is made in the abdomen that extends from the navel (umbillicus) to the pubic area. The lymph nodes surrounding the prostate are first removed and examined for signs that the cancer has spread. If prostate cancer is found, the operation is usually stopped at this point because no benefit is derived from removing the prostate once the cancer has spread. If no cancer is found in the lymph nodes, the bladder is pulled back to reveal the prostate. Then the prostate, seminal vesicles, and a portion of the vas deferens are removed. The bladder is reattached directly to the urethra at the sphincter, a muscle that is responsible for continence (urinary control). After the operation, a catheter is left in the urethra and bladder for approximately 3 weeks. Most men go home after 3 to 4 days in the hospital with the catheter in place; they return later as outpatients to have the catheter removed. ■

of therapy mainly involve the development of adrenal insufficiency (see Disorders of the Adrenal Glands, page 1195, for more information.)

- Interference at the testicular level generally means *removal of the testicles* (orchiectomy), which may be necessary in some cases; the main side effects are hot flashes and impotence.

- At the level of the prostate gland, testosterone influence can be diminished by the use of anti-androgen medications, such as flutamide, that preserve potency, but can cause some nausea or diarrhea.

Prognosis After radical prostatectomy for clinically localized cancers, 30 percent recur by 10 years. If the cancer has broken through the capsule, recurrence rates are higher.

Recurrence rates for localized cancers treated with radiation alone is 56 percent at 10 years and are higher with more advanced stages.

Sexual Dysfunction in Men

From time to time during adulthood, most men, indeed, most people, experience what is known as sexual dysfunction, or the emotional or physical loss of ability, desire, or interest in sexual activity. Transient interference with sexual desire or ability is normal, but an interruption that continues for days or weeks or months can be the signal of some deep-seated medical or emotional problem and should be analyzed. There are few reliable studies available to show exactly how many people may be afflicted by a long-term sexual dysfunction, but almost everyone is affected by at least transient sexual dysfunction, most of which will not be cause for intervention.

❖ INHIBITED SEXUAL DESIRE

Symptoms *(What you may experience)* A persistent and encompassing absence of sexual desire or appetite; absence of sexual fantasies; persistent lack of interest in sexual contact with a sexual partner; or an avoidance of sexual contact with a sexual partner.

Signs and laboratory findings *(What the doctor looks for)* Your doctor will look for underlying conditions. Most prominently relationship problems; sexual trauma; depression; stress; and family crisis. Other possibilities are hormone deficiencies, alcoholism, kidney failure, or other chronic illness, such as diabetes, as well as certain medications.

What is it? Sometimes called loss of desire, inhibited sexual desire is more accurately the diminishment of desire by one of several psychological or biologic mechanisms. It is usually the result of some other dysfunction, for example, illness, sexually-related emotional trauma, or depression. Far too often, it is the result of a breakdown of communication and understanding in a long-term sexual relationship, and the underlying grief, hostility, anger, depression, or sense of misunderstanding.

Treatment Self-treatment is possible, but fraught with difficulty. The various factors that build up to inhibition of desire tend to accumulate over long periods and can take considerable time to resolve. Although partners may spend a great deal of time at the beginning of a relationship having sex, they may not actually talk about it much, which may lay the groundwork for considerable future misunderstanding. Two individuals are almost guaranteed to have differing ideas about what lovemaking means, what it should entail, and the place it should have in a relationship. While passion and romance at the beginning of a relationship may compensate for or at least cover up some of the differences couples have, major life changes, such as the arrival of a child, can uncover those differences and throw a wedge between partners (see Communication Strategies for Couples, page 311, and Couples Counseling Before and During Marriage, page 310). Many people think of having an affair, "just to make sure the equipment is working," but this is not a solution, and will only worsen the trouble—in addition to risking a sexually transmitted infection. A skilled counselor can help keep people from engaging in behavior that can potentially worsen their situation.

Prognosis Good, if the underlying problems are addressed. If the problems are ignored or denied, it can lead to the breakup of a family.

❖ GENDER DYSPHORIA

Symptoms and signs *(What you may experience)* A recurrent or pervasive sense that you should have been born female; the desire to adopt a female gender identity role; the desire to dress as a woman to pass as a woman.

What is it? Gender identity dysphoria (GID) is rare, though it may be underre-

ported by those for whom the disorder is either mild, transient, or simply unacknowledgeable for reasons of socialization or upbringing. It is not known what causes the disorder.

Some men with GID have reported awareness of their dysphoria as early as age 4, though most learn to suppress their difference as best they can since boys who want to play with girls and act like girls may be humiliated by others. Some boys will overcompensate, demonstrating overly aggressive "male" behavior. Only a very low number of effeminate boys later have GID as adolescents and adults.

What you can do Seek the help of a Gender Identity Program or one who is an expert in the treatment of gender dysphoria. Academic medical centers may assist in referrals. Support groups will tend to reinforce the cross-gender identity and behaviors.

When to call the doctor Living with gender dysphoria is not easy, and most individuals with this condition benefit from the help of a therapist. If you are depressed or have considered or attempted suicide, you should contact a doctor or mental health professional who specializes in such issues as soon as possible.

Treatment Psychiatric counseling is the best method of treatment, because it enables you to become more comfortable with your conflicting urges and provides you with ways of resolving your emotional conflicts. Sex change operations have been performed, but many experts do not regard this as an optimal way of helping people cope with GID.

FERTILITY AND INFERTILITY

The reproduction of human life is at once elegant in its simplicity and baffling in its complexity. The union of a prepared egg from the female with a single sperm from the male depends on the orchestration of interrelated mechanical, hormonal, and chemical forces.

Each month, a single egg is chosen from among the million or so contained in the ovary to awaken from a state of sus-

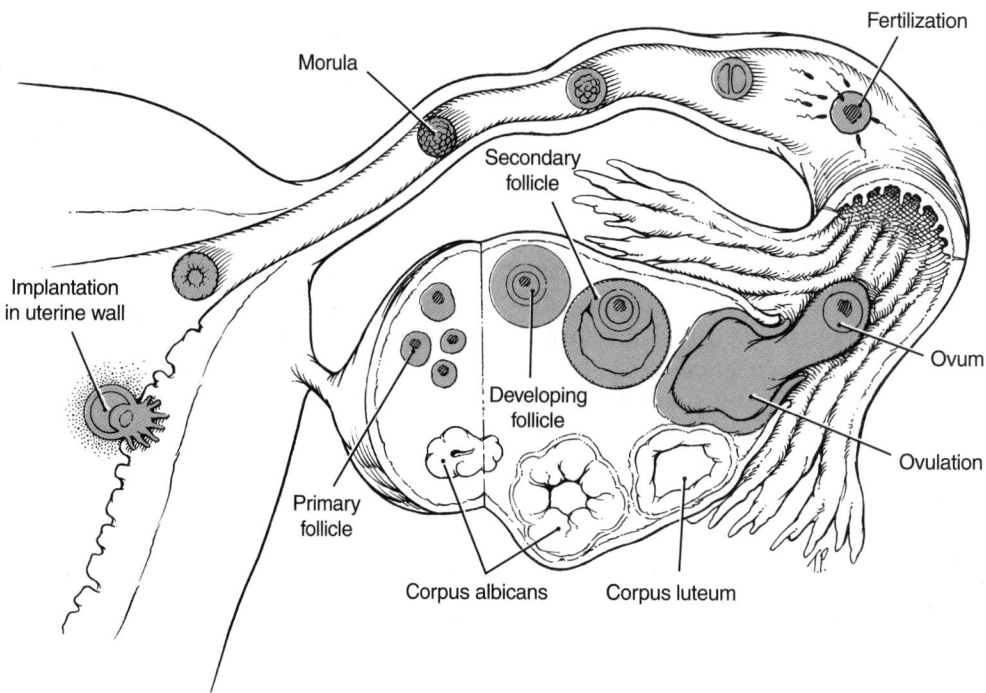

The egg develops inside the follicle, which passes through primary and secondary stages. The egg is released from the ovary (ovulation) about the 14th day of the menstrual cycle. A corpus luteum gland forms from the ruptured follicle. The egg travels down the fallopian tube, where fertilization with sperm may occur. Cleavage of the egg results in a ball of cells (morula), which enters the uterus and implants in the uterine wall. Unfertilized eggs degenerate after a few days. During pregnancy, the corpus luteum remains active for many weeks, but it eventually becomes an inactive corpus albicans.

pended animation and to mature. In some cases of multiple births, several eggs awaken. Under the influence of the correct hormonal signals, the egg ripens, bursts free from the ovary, and is gathered in by the waving fringed ends of one of the fallopian tubes. The muscular walls of the tube gently, over the next few days, propel the egg along its length in the direction of the womb. For fertilization of the egg to occur, it must encounter viable sperm within the few days after ovulation, a short window of opportunity.

With intercourse, ejaculation by the male propels millions of sperm (produced in the male testicle and mixed with secretions from the prostate gland to form semen) into the vaginal canal. The sperm must swim under their own power into the opening of the cervix, through the uterine cavity, and into the fallopian tube where they encounter the waiting egg. Usually fertilization occurs in the upper one-third of the tube and the now-fertilized egg continues its descent into the womb. The sperm surround the egg and must break through its protective "shell" to penetrate it. Millions may try, but only one sperm will succeed in reaching its ultimate goal.

For a human embryo to begin to grow and develop, it must have two copies of each of the 23 human chromosomes (structures containing the genetic material called DNA that directs all development and functions of life). The egg and sperm each contain one set of the 23 chromosomes; with the joining of sperm and egg, a new human embryo begins to grow. Barring any interruptions, if all proceeds according to plan, in approximately 9 months, a baby will be born.

Difficulties can arise at almost any point along the way, in either partner; often, a combination of factors, both male and female, may be at work when couples fail to conceive.

For example, a woman may experience difficulty ovulating, there may be scarring or other obstruction to the easy passage of the egg down the tube, structural problems in the uterus may impede normal implantation of the egg or make it difficult to carry a baby to term. Many of these disorders are covered here, but for more information about those related to pregnancy itself, once conception has occurred, see Chapter 7.

Men may experience problems in fertility ranging from impotence to difficulty in ejaculating to the production of weakly mobile or immotile sperm. About 30 to 40 percent of the time, a couple's inability to conceive a child results from problems of the male partner. In 10 to 20 percent of cases, infertility is due to both partners having problems. These disorders will be addressed in this section, but for more information, you may also refer to the discussion of the male reproductive system earlier in this chapter, page 1130.

Evaluation of Reproductive Difficulties

Human reproduction may seem all too simple in an age when teen pregnancy has soared to record highs, but as many as 25 percent of couples trying to conceive may experience infertility at some point in their reproductive lives. When this occurs, a variety of tests can help determine the cause and the most effective approach to treatment. Infertility, which simply means difficulty in conceiving, should not be confused with sterility, which means there is no possibility of conceiving under any circumstances, no matter what the intervention.

COMMON TESTS USED IN EVALUATING THE FEMALE PARTNER

Basal temperature records In this simple method, a woman will carefully chart her body temperature each morning. The measurement should be made immediately upon awakening, before arising, and with a minimum of muscle activity by the woman. The thermometer should be kept already shaken down (if applicable) and ready to use. There is a slight rise in the body's basal temperature at the time of ovulation, so that recording daily temperatures can help to pinpoint this critical time in the cycle.

Cervical mucus tests

- *Ferning test.* Cervical mucus collected near the time of ovulation will, when smeared onto a glass microscope slide, dry into a pattern that looks, under the microscope, like the fronds of a fern if estrogen levels are normal. This kind of mucus makes a more hospitable environment for sperm.

- *Postcoital test.* This test is used to evaluate whether viable sperm are arriving at the opening to the womb. The test must be performed just before ovulation. There should be an increased amount of thin, clear, elastic mucus at this time, conditions most favorable to the migration of sperm into the uterus. To be considered a satisfactory test, a drop of cervical mucus, collected and viewed under the microscope within 6 hours of intercourse, should show five or more active, swimming sperm. Sometimes this test will also detect an elevated number of white blood cells, a finding that could indicate infection of the female cervix or the male's prostate gland, or the presence of antisperm antibodies that clot and immobilize the sperm, rendering them ineffective. Either of these causes can contribute to difficulty conceiving a pregnancy.

Blood tests These tests may include determination of blood levels for estrogen, progesterone, prolactin, luteinizing hormone (LH), and follicle stimulating hormone (FSH) at various points of the menstrual cycle. Abnormalities in these hormones can explain lack of regular, predictable ovulation. Additionally, testing for specific immune system markers may be done, since couples that share certain of these markers have a greater tendency to be infertile; the reasons for this association are unclear.

X-ray studies In the hysterosalpingogram, an oil-based dye, visible on x-ray, is instilled into the uterus and fallopian tubes within 3 days after the menstrual period. The dye will fill the cavities and tubes, outlining the architecture of these structures. Polyps, partitions, benign tumors, and obstructions will all be visible on the x-ray. If a few days later repeat x-ray shows the dye dispersed widely within the abdominal cavity, the fallopian tubes can be said to be patent (open).

Laparoscopic surgery If infertility persists despite a normal initial evaluation, looking at the uterus, tubes, and ovaries with the laparoscope (a fiberoptic telescope inserted into the abdomen) may detect contributing causes to infertility in as many as one in four women; conditions commonly discovered include polycystic ovarian syndrome, scarring in and around the fallopian tubes, or pockets of stray uterine lining tissue (endometriosis).

COMMON TESTS USED IN EVALUATING THE MALE PARTNER

Semen analysis Examination of the semen should ideally be performed after a 72 hour abstinence from ejaculation, with the specimen analyzed within 1 hour of collection. The sperm should be evaluated for the number of sperm, which should exceed 20 million per mL; volume of ejaculate, which should range between 1.5 and 5 mL (about $^1/_4$ to 1 tsp); motility and morphology of sperm, 50 to 60 percent of which should be actively moving and 60 percent of which should be of normal shape and size.

DETERMINING IF THERE IS A PROBLEM WITH FERTILITY

Although many couples desirous of having children become concerned if conception fails to occur right away, most doctors will not recommend serious investigation of the problem until 6 months to 1 year of frequent unprotected intercourse has failed to result in pregnancy. For 75 percent of couples, giving nature adequate time is all that is necessary, and conception occurs within 1 year. If otherwise healthy couples have not made a concerted effort for this length of time, they should not become concerned about infertility.

About half the remaining 25 percent of couples will be able to conceive without medical intervention given slightly more time, but for 10 to 15 percent of couples evaluation will be necessary to determine the cause for the delay as well as the best course of action to alleviate the problem.

To increase chances of conception, a woman should track her menstrual cycle carefully (see Menstruation And Ovulation, page 1099) to determine as closely as possible when ovulation should occur; in most women, it should occur between days 12 and 14 of the menstrual cycle. Alterations in basal body temperature (a shift upward) can indicate approaching ovulation, as can the levels of luteinizing hormone (LH) in the urine. Over-the-counter kits are now available to detect these urine changes that herald ovulation. Sexual intercourse during this critical period will increase the likelihood that the prepared egg will meet viable sperm. ■

Blood tests In certain cases, the doctor may recommend measuring blood levels of testosterone, prolactin, LH, and FSH. These tests can help to determine if the problem lies in the testicle or in the pituitary gland that stimulates the testicle to produce sperm. Generally, these tests will only be performed if the sperm count is low or if there are other reasons to suspect a problem in the endocrine system (see Hypopituitarism, page 1203).

Ultrasound Rarely, the doctor may recommend a scrotal ultrasound to detect small, but potentially troublesome, varicose veins in the scrotum or within the spermatic cord. Usually, if this condition is detectable on physical examination, surgery to fix it does not improve infertility. For more information see Varicocele, page 1157.

Female Reproductive Abnormalities

UTERINE PROBLEMS

The disorders of the uterus that can hamper conception or successfully carrying a fetus to full-term primarily involve alterations in structure.

Septate or bicornuate uterus In these conditions, the uterine cavity develops partitioned into two chambers. The septate uterus may have a complete or partial interior wall, whereas in the bicornuate configuration, the uterus develops as two separate chambers, one for each fallopian tube. The two chambers usually join at the cervical end to form a single vaginal vault. Although these abnormal configurations may not prevent implantation of a fertilized egg, they may crowd the developing fetus and make it difficult to carry the baby for the full 9 months of growth. The disorders can be seen on ultrasound exam or with the use of a hysteroscope. These problems can often be corrected surgically.

Androgen insensitivity syndrome Regardless of genetic blueprint, for an infant to develop male characteristics, the cells must be able to respond to testosterone. In certain rare instances, a person is born with testosterone receptors that cannot respond to the male hormone. Consequently, this person will appear to be female in all respects, but will not menstruate and will not develop a uterus, without which, of course, conception is not possible. (For more information, see the discussion of this disorder in Congenital Abnormalities of the Reproductive Tract, page 1116.) This is a case of true sterility; there is no means available to make conception possible.

Implantation difficulties Under the influence of progesterone and LH, the uterine lining thickens into a soft, nourishing bed, rich in blood supply to receive the fertilized egg. If this development fails to occur, the egg cannot implant properly. This kind of problem can usually be corrected by administration of hormones.

FALLOPIAN TUBE PROBLEMS

Although the inside diameter of the fallopian tubes is quite small, no larger than a sewing needle, it is sufficiently roomy to accommodate the passage of the tiny egg. Difficulty arises, however, if infection, for example, from STIs or PID occurs; the inflammation and healing processes can result in scarring that blocks the tubes. Occasionally, the tubes are obstructed by a web or "kink." These obstructing abnormalities, whether the result of an infection or an anomaly of birth, can often be repaired by laser surgery performed with the laparoscope.

ANOVULATION

Conditions that suppress ovulation or make release of the mature egg erratic and unpredictable reduce fertility. A number of conditions can result in anovulation (lack of ovulation).

* *Polycystic ovarian syndrome.* The thickened outer covering of the ovary in this disorder may prevent the prepared egg from breaking free at ovulation. Without the release of a viable egg, conception cannot occur. A number of procedures have been developed to enhance the likelihood of regular ovulation in women with this condition. Weight loss (in obese women with this disorder) may help to normalize reproductive hormone levels. The administration of medications to stimulate ovulation (clomiphene or occasionally dexamethasone) or wedge resection of the ovary (surgically opening the thickened ovarian capsule to allow easier ovulation) may enhance the chance of conception. For more information, see Polycystic Ovarian Syndrome, page 1124.

  The tough, thick capsule may prevent the egg's release when it matures (see Polycystic Ovarian Syndrome, page 1124). Obesity often accompanies this syndrome, and sensible, healthy weight reduction can help to restore fertility by normalizing the amount of fatty tissue, where male hormone converts to estrogen compounds.

* *Premature menopause.* Normally, in the fifth or sixth decade of life, women experience anovulation and irregularities in menstrual cycling as ovarian hormonal function wanes. Sometimes this diminution of hormonal output begins earlier in life, a condition termed premature menopause. Simple blood tests demonstrate elevated levels of LH and FSH when premature menopause is the cause for anovulation. Consult a doctor to determine whether hormone therapy may be of benefit at this stage.

* *Discontinuation of oral contraceptive pills.* It is not uncommon for women to experience up to 6 months of continued suppression of ovulation after stopping the birth control pill. If conception fails to occur in the first 6 months after stopping the pill, you should not be unduly alarmed. If it fails to occur within the next 6 months, an evaluation is in order.

* *Thyroid imbalances,* of both the hyperactive and underactive variety, can disrupt menstrual cycling and ovulation and therefore be a cause of infertility. Correction of the imbalance will usually restore fertility promptly.

* *Extreme exercise.* Women who engage in excessive amounts of exercise, extensive daily training regimens, marathon and endurance running, and the like, can suppress ovulation both by disrupting the crucial timing of hormone flux

that prompts egg maturation and release and by excessive loss of body fat, a tissue necessary for conversion of androgens (male hormone) into certain estrogen compounds. Reduction of exercise frequency and intensity, coupled with a modest gain of weight and body fat (if deficient) will usually restore fertility.

- *Rapid weight loss* (particularly as seen with very low calorie dieting) can also disrupt the delicate hormonal balance necessary for regular, predictable ovulation. The condition is temporary, and fertility will usually return to normal within a few months after weight stabilizes or after returning to a balanced diet of sufficient calories to maintain the current weight. The exact mechanisms of this cause for infertility are unclear, but may relate to thyroid or reproductive hormone imbalances.

ENDOMETRIOSIS

Sometimes pockets of uterine lining tissue develop along the course of the fallopian tubes or scattered across the ovaries. Depending upon their location, they can occlude the tiny passageway inside the tube and hinder the egg's progress toward the uterus. Endometriosis on the ovary can inhibit ovulation. Surgically removing the pockets help to restore fertility. For more information, see Adenomyosis and Endometriosis, page 1117.

Male Reproductive Abnormalities

OLIGOSPERMIA (LOW SPERM COUNT)

Reduction in sperm production can account for difficulty conceiving. If a milliliter of collected semen contains fewer than 20 million sperm after 72 hours' abstinence from sex, the count is low. Causes for the reduced number can include previous injury (see Testicular Torsion, page 1142, Trauma to the Testes and Scrotum, page 1140, Cryptorchidism [undescended testicles] page 1143), testicular infection with mumps virus (see Mumps, page 880), excessive heat (fever, tight-fitting undergarments), radiation treatments, or medications (cimetidine, commonly used for ulcers; spironolactone used to treat blood pressure; anabolic steroids, commonly used by body builders and other athletes to build muscle bulk; phenytoin, a common seizure medication), and excessive alcohol or marijuana use. Many of these causes are reversible when the substance is stopped.

AZOOSPERMIA (ABSENT SPERM)

The sperm, produced in the testicles, travel through a duct system to the urethra where they are combined with prostatic and seminal vesicle secretions at the time of ejaculation. If something obstructs the ducts, the

SPONTANEOUS ABORTION

Miscarriage of a pregnancy can occur for a variety of reasons. The most common cause for a pregnancy to fail is a chromosomal (genetic) abnormality of the developing fetus, incompatible with life; these errors of development usually manifest early, with spontaneous termination of the pregnancy in the first trimester. Many women experience this kind of miscarriage once or twice in their reproductive years, sometimes so early as to be unaware of the pregnancy at all.

Sometimes, however, miscarriage occurs not because of abnormalities in the developing fetus, but from structural or hormonal abnormalities in the mother. In these cases, miscarriage can occur repeatedly and interfere with fertility. More than two or three pregnancies in a row ending in spontaneous abortion may require referral to a fertility specialist.

Structural abnormalities can usually be corrected surgically. These include the following:

- Congenital abnormalities of the uterus, such as septate or bicornuate uterus.

- Incompetent cervical os, in which the normally closed cervical opening is weak and unable to support the weight of the developing fetus.

- Endometriosis, in which deposits of uterine lining material may occlude the tubes, leading to tubal pregnancy

- Fibroid tumors in the uterine wall that could interfere with firm implantation of the fetus.

- Adhesions (scarring) from previous pelvic infection that can interfere with secure implantation or could limit fetal growth.

Hormonal imbalances, deficiency of luteinizing hormone, can leave the uterus inadequately prepared to receive the fertilized egg or to support the developing fetus in the early stages of growth. Such problems can usually be corrected with administration of hormones. ■

ejaculate will contain only the empty secretions from the prostate gland and seminal vesicles. These secretions contain no sperm. The obstruction could be scarring from previous infection (see Sexually Transmitted Infections, page 861) or be the intentional result of a vasectomy procedure.

In other cases, the ducts are not obstructed but the testes do not make sperm. The absence of sperm can result from deficiency of the brain hormones that stimulate sperm production. For more information see Hypopituitarism, page 1203.

IMMOTILE CILIA SYNDROME

In order to fertilize the female egg, sperm cells must be able to move under their own power. Once they are deposited upon ejaculation into the upper portion of the vaginal canal, the sperm must make their way through the cervical opening, up the length of the uterus, and into the fallopian tubes where they can encounter a mature egg (if intercourse occurs around the time of ovulation). Uterine contractions that occur with female orgasm help to create an upward flow to bring the semen in the correct direction, but from that point onward, the sperm cells rely on a vigorous whipping motion of their long tails to propel them forward. Once they encounter the egg, their beating tails help them as they try to penetrate the egg's protective outer layers.

In certain instances, although the testicles produce a sufficiently large number of sperm to ensure fertilization, they are immotile, that is, unable to "swim." Their immotility can stem from problems with their shape, from infection, or can, in some cases, be the consequence of antisperm antibodies produced by the female. Several medications including sulfasalazine, commonly used to treat ulcerative colitis and nitrofurantoin, used to treat urinary tract infections can also interfere with sperm motility.

In some cases, assisted reproductive technologies, such as in vitro fertilization, may enable a man with an unusually low percentage of active sperm to father a child because the sperm do not have to swim up the female reproductive tract. These technologies are expensive, however, and success rates with immotile sperm are not high.

VARICOCELE

A varicocele is a meshwork of varicose veins in and around the testicle that is associated with infertility. It is not known exactly how a varicocele interferes with fertility, but the most likely explanation is that it prevents the cooling needed for production of healthy, active sperm. Surgical repair of the varicocele can often restore fertility. See Scrotal Lumps, page 1139, for additional information.

OBSTRUCTION (VASECTOMY)

Although scarring from previous infections could obstruct the ducts that transport sperm to the ejaculate, the most common cause of obstruction is intentional via the vasectomy. For more information about vasectomy, refer to Vasectomy Reversal Procedures in this section, below. Obstructions can be surgically corrected and vasectomies surgically reversed should a man desire to father children; however, the reversal procedures can be costly and are not always successful.

IMPOTENCE

Inability to perform sexually, whether from loss of desire (libido), inability to achieve or

---

VASECTOMY REVERSAL PROCEDURES

In the vasectomy procedure, the urologic surgeon cuts the vas deferens (the sperm passageway from the testicles to the urethra) in two and usually seals the cut ends. By so doing, sperm can no longer enter the ejaculate. To reverse the procedure, the surgeon must reattach the cut ends, which sounds simple, but in fact is quite difficult, and must be performed using microsurgical techniques. Once the ends have sealed, the healing process causes formation of scar tissue that will further occlude the passageway. The scarred areas must be "pruned" back to allow healthy open ends to be sewn back together to recreate the tube; there may be insufficient slack in the tube, depending upon the length of the segment removed in the original vasectomy procedure, to allow the ends to realign properly. Even when the tissues cooperate, the healing of the new surgical violation may cause obstructive scarring to recur.

However, advances in microsurgical techniques have improved the rate of successful reversal. Even as long as 7 or 8 years after vasectomy, reversal can restore viable sperm to the ejaculate in as many as 80 to 90 percent of men. Rates of successful subsequent impregnation are slightly lower, about 50 to 60 percent. ■

REVERSIBLE CAUSES OF MALE INFERTILITY

A number of conditions can temporarily impair sperm production and motility and, therefore, fertility. In most cases, fertility will resume once the situation returns to normal. Many times, the cure is quite simple. In others cases, restoring fertility may take some time.

- Excessive heat to the testicles impairs production of live sperm. The heat could come from high fever or tight-fitting undergarments. *Remedy:* Bring fever down promptly with aspirin or acetaminophen. Wear loose-fitting undergarments such as boxer shorts to provide adequate room for proper cooling of the testicles. Avoid hot or whirlpool baths.

- Radiation or chemotherapy treatments for cancer can impair sperm production. In most cases, production of sperm resumes following cessation of treatment, but may take considerable time. *Remedy:* Discuss with a doctor whether it is advisable to bank sperm prior to treatments.

- Certain prescription medications, such as cimetidine (commonly used for ulcers), spironolactone (used to treat blood pressure), and phenytoin (a common seizure medication), can impair sperm production. *Remedy:* Request the doctor to prescribe alternate medications to treat these conditions where possible.

- Excessive alcohol or marijuana use or the use of anabolic steroids (commonly used by bodybuilders and other elite athletes to build muscle bulk) can impair sperm production. *Remedy:* Avoid these substances.

- Infection or injury to the testicles may cause impairment of sperm production that may only be temporary (although in some cases may be permanent). *Remedy:* Treat infection by taking all antibiotic medications to completion of the prescribed course. Try to limit swelling and bruising following injury. See The Bellevue Bridge for Testicular/Scrotal Swelling, page 1142 in this chapter. ■

maintain an erection, or inability to achieve orgasm, can impair fertility (see page 1153). These issues are also discussed in Chapter 11.

EJACULATORY PROBLEMS

If ejaculation fails to deposit an adequate volume of semen into the vaginal canal, the migration of sperm to the fallopian tube may not easily take place. Several conditions can result in insufficient ejaculation, including retrograde ejaculation (see page 1138), loss of emission due to obstruction, hypospadias (see page 1132), and premature ejaculation (see page 1137).

Optimizing Reproductive Ability

FERTILITY DRUGS

Fertility may often be restored by manipulation or normalization of hormone levels, not just of the reproductive hormones, but of other major metabolic hormones as well. For example, correction of thyroid imbalance (supplementing the hormone in hypothyroidism or reducing the levels in hyperthyroidism) will improve fertility.

But in many cases, the main thrust in fertility treatment is to stimulate ovula-

tion, and toward that end, most fertility specialists will recommend the use of clomiphene citrate, a medication that brings about the release of LH and a rise in estradiol. Shifting levels of these two hormones triggers ovulation. The treatment is successful in about 90 percent of cases of anovulation in the absence of other factors that impair fertility. Several eggs may release, leading to twin births in about 5 percent of cases and larger number multiple births in a few, rare (less than 0.5 percent) cases.

The medication can cause the development of painful ovarian cysts in about 1 in 12 women, with symptoms severe enough to warrant stopping therapy. Some studies suggest that prolonged use of clomiphene may increase the risk of ovarian cancer, although the connection is uncertain.

In women who exhibit elevated levels of male hormone, adding the corticosteroid dexamethasone to the regimen may improve response.

If there is no response to clomiphene, injections of gonadotropin-releasing hormone (GnRH) will reliably restore the menstrual cycle and improve response to ovulation stimulators, such as clomiphene.

Supplementation of the brain releasing hormones that stimulate egg or sperm production can also help to restore fertility. The medication Pergonal is a mixture of FSH and LH; it may be useful in correcting both anovulation in women and deficient sperm production in men.

SURGICAL REPAIR

Surgery can improve fertility in certain instances. It may be performed through the operating laparoscope (a lighted telescope equipped with a miniature camera and microscopic surgical instruments or a laser) or conventionally, opening the area and operating under direct vision. The situations best suited to surgical treatment include the following:

- Opening of blockages, such as those in the fallopian tubes or semen ducts, or removing the obstruction caused by misplaced pockets of uterine lining tissue in endometriosis.

- Correction of abnormalities of structure, such as the septate or bicornuate uterine cavity, the thick ovarian capsule in polycystic ovarian syndrome, or the varicocele in the male testicle or spermatic cord.

ARTIFICIAL INSEMINATION

Artificial insemination involves implanting sperm from an anonymous donor into the woman's uterine canal as close as possible to the time of ovulation. This technique is most commonly used in cases of absent sperm, but may also be recommended in other causes of male infertility unresponsive to medical or surgical remedies. When no female factors contribute to the couple's inability to conceive, success rates are quite high.

Although frozen and thawed sperm are less fertile than fresh sperm, the American Fertility Association recommends using frozen sperm to help prevent the spread of acquired immunodeficienc syndrome (AIDS). Freezing does not kill the AIDS virus, but it does allow time for donors to be tested properly for AIDS.

SPERM BANKING

Men can elect to "bank" specimens of their own sperm. Most commonly, this is done by men about to undergo vasectomy or those about to begin medical treatment that may affect fertility. The ejaculate is usually obtained manually, placed into specially prepared containers, and medically frozen.

ASSISTED REPRODUCTIVE TECHNOLOGIES (IN VITRO FERTILIZATION

Several procedures fall in this category, including in vitro fertilization (IVF), gamete intrafallopian transfer (GIFT), and zygote intrafallopian transfer (ZIFT). All of the procedures involve stimulating the female ovary to produce a number of prepared eggs, harvesting the eggs by using a needle guided by ultrasound, and bringing them outside the body.

In the case of IVF, the eggs will subsequently be fertilized with male sperm in a

(A) In gamete intrafallopian transfer (GIFT), an egg that has been harvested and removed from a woman is injected along with active sperm into the fallopian tube, where fertilization then occurs naturally. Although more invasive than in vitro fertilization (IVF), GIFT offers a better chance for success. (B) Intracytoplasmic sperm injection— an alternate method of promoting pregnancy—refers to the injection of sperm directly into an egg through a microscopic needle.

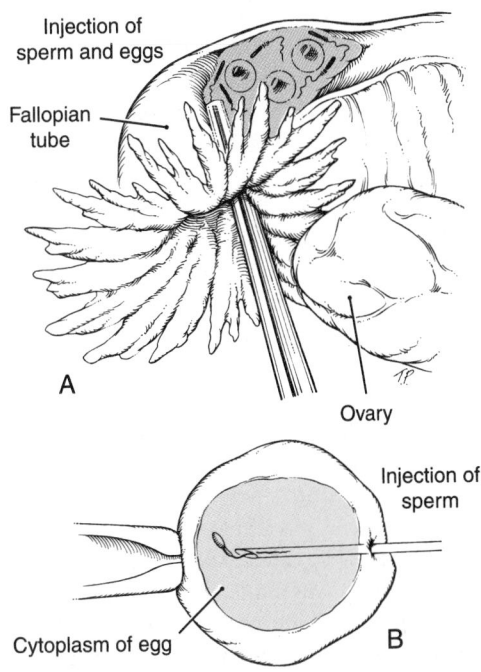

Injection of sperm and eggs

Fallopian tube

Ovary

A

Injection of sperm

Cytoplasm of egg

B

CAUSES OF AND TREATMENTS FOR INFERTILITY

CAUSE	EVALUATION	TREATMENT METHOD
Anovulation	Blood testing, endometrial biopsy	Hormonal therapy, fertility medication, lifestyle modification (decreased exercise and weight gain if indicated)
Fallopian tube blockage	Hysterosalpingogram	Surgery, assisted reproductive technologies
Polycystic ovarian syndrome	Ultrasound, laparoscopy, pelvic exam, blood testing	Surgery, hormone therapy, fertility medication, weight loss
Endometriosis	Laparoscopy	Surgery
Septate or bicornuate uterus	Hysterogram, hysteroscopy	Surgery
Absent sperm	Semen analysis, vasogram, blood testing	Life style modifications, sperm banking before vasectomy or medical treatment, artificial insemination
Low sperm count	Vasogram, blood testing	Life style modifications, assisted reproductive technologies, artificial insemination
Immotile cilia	Semen analysis	Artificial insemination
Varicocele	Ultrasound	Surgery
Duct obstruction	Vasogram	Surgery
Antisperm antibodies	Postcoital cervical mucus test	Condom use for 6 months to lower antibody levels

All the various factors affecting both the woman and man in concert need to be considered by the doctor when deciding what treatment to recommend.

"test tube" and the fertilized egg will be allowed to begin to divide. Depending on the number of duplications the fertilized egg goes through, it will be termed a zygote or embryo.

In IVF, several embryos will be returned to the mother's uterus to continue to grow and develop. Multiple births are possible following this procedure. Sometimes, extra embryos will be cryopreserved (medically frozen) to use in subsequent attempts if necessary.

The male sperm and female egg are also called gametes. In GIFT, the harvested egg and active sperm (the gametes) will be placed together into the woman's fallopian tube, where fertilization will occur in its natural setting. GIFT is a more invasive procedure than IVF, but offers a better chance for successful conception and delivery. In women with severe tubal disease, GIFT is not a safe option, since the risk for ectopic tubal pregnancy is much higher.

Success in all assisted reproductive technologies depends, among other factors, upon the age of the mother: Women under 40 (when the husband's fertility is not the problem) deliver 1 infant in 5 retrieval procedures (19.8 percent) with IVF and a little better than 1 in 4 with GIFT (26.3 percent). However, in women over 40, the success rate drops to around 1 in 10: slightly less (7.2 percent) with IVF and slightly better (11.9 percent) with GIFT.

In ZIFT, the sperm fertilizes the egg in the test tube, then after only a few divisions, the newly fertilized egg (a zygote) is implanted into the fallopian tube to complete its early development in a natural site and make its normal migration into the womb. Average delivery rates per retrieval are a little better than 1 in 5 (22.8 percent) in ZIFT procedures.

Intracytoplasmic sperm injection is one of the newest forms of IVF. In this procedure, a sperm is injected directly into the egg with a microscopic needle. Much higher success rates, up to 60 or 70 percent, have been reported for this procedure.

The chart above briefly summarizes the diagnoses and treatments of the various causes of infertility. Please note, however, that in many cases a couple may face several problems that inhibit fertility.

Contraception

A healthy sexual relationship is one of the most rewarding aspects of adulthood. We are one of the few animals that does not have a seasonal sex drive, that is, we are always prepared for sex, and it is one of the many mixed blessings we contend with. Although historically some have viewed it as solely for purposes of procreation, it is widely recognized that in human beings a sexual relationship plays a much more than utilitarian role. Indeed, according to many psychotherapy researchers, the ability to lose oneself in the act of love with another, loved human being is one of the hallmarks of adulthood.

A healthy sexual relationship requires taking mutual responsibility for staying healthy and avoiding pregnancy (when appropriate). Sexually Transmitted Infections (STIs) are a particular concern of sexually active adults, and this is another area where partners must be open with one another. Monogamy is the most sensible way to avoid contracting an infection; having multiple partners significantly increases your chances of becoming infected with chlamydia, gonorrhea, or even human immunodeficiency virus (HIV) (see Sexually Transmitted Infections, page 861 and Proper Use of a Condom, page 1162).

Abstinence, complete avoidance of sexual contact, is the only method of birth control that is 100 percent effective. Partners can also reduce the risk of pregnancy by avoiding coitus (penetration of the penis into the vagina). Using imagination and creativity, partners can engage in a range of alternative sexual activities such as oral stimulation. However, there is always a chance that sperm from the man's ejaculation can find their way into the vagina, even if penetration has not occurred. For this reason, people wishing to avoid pregnancy should take advantage of one or more of the many options for birth control.

There are many means of contraception available today. Deciding which method to use will be a matter of personal preference. A person's or couple's choice of contraception may also change several times over the course of adulthood. Discuss the choice with a doctor, who can give advice as to which method is the most appropriate. Doctors will recommend the method of contraception based upon a person's med-

ical history and lifestyle. Whatever method chosen, be sure to follow carefully the directions regarding their use; many contraceptives fail to prevent pregnancy because they are not used properly. (See Chart: Effectiveness of Contraceptives in Preventing Pregnancy and STIs, page 1167 for more information on the effectiveness of the various methods of contraception.

BARRIER METHODS

The term barrier refers to a method that physically prevents the sperm and the egg from coming into contact. The most com-

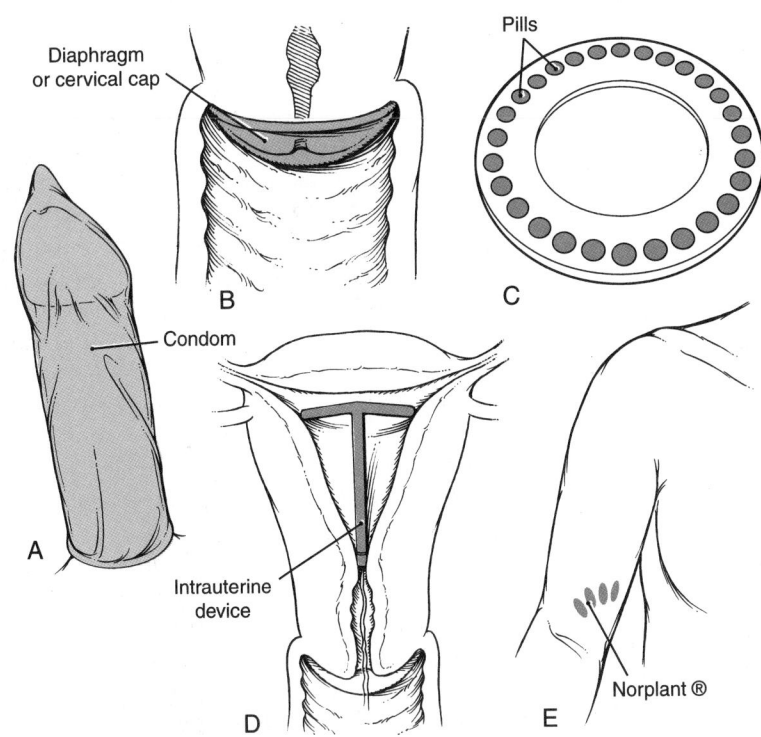

Several methods of preventing pregnancy are available. (A) The condom (see illustration, page 1164). (B) A diaphragm or cervical cap can be covered with spermicidal cream and positioned over the cervix to prevent entry of sperm, but it must remain in place for an extended period of time after intercourse. (C) Hormone-containing pills can be taken to prevent ovulation or fertilization of the egg. (D) An intrauterine device (IUD) can be inserted into and left inside the uterus, to prevent fertilization or implantation of a fertilized egg in the uterine wall. (E) Norplant is a hormonal capsule that is implanted under the skin of the arm, providing contraception for up to 5 years.

PROPER USE OF A CONDOM

Selecting a Condom

At this writing there are three kinds of condoms. Only one of them is adequate for preventing sexually transmitted infections (STIs) and pregnancy, and that is the men's latex condom. This is a latex sheath, often with a reservoir at the end. The condom, a barrier form of contraception, fits snugly over the penis and collects semen after ejaculation and protects the penis from vaginal secretions, both of which can carry STI viruses and bacteria. Also available are men's "natural" condoms, which are made of natural skins. These can be adequate protection against pregnancy but have pores large enough for the human immunodeficiency virus (HIV) to pass through and therefore are not adequate protection from STIs.

The third kind of condom is the female condom, approved in the mid1990s by the FDA. It is less effective than the male condom in preventing pregnancy, and may be similarly less effective in protecting against STIs.

Most experts on STIs recommend using a condom that is lubricated with a spermicide, such as nonoxynol-9, which has been shown to kill HIV as well as sperm. In some people, however, nonoxynol-9 causes burning and itching. It can also lead to higher incidence of urinary tract infection. There are condoms available with other spermicidal lubricants.

When choosing a condom, choose one with a reservoir end. The reservoir is an extension of the condom which is narrower than the penis and will collect semen after ejaculation, rather than forcing the ejaculate back along the length of the penis where it could leak.

There are different thicknesses of latex condoms available. The newest, thinnest condoms are as strong as thicker ones, but can be more difficult to handle properly than thicker ones. ▶

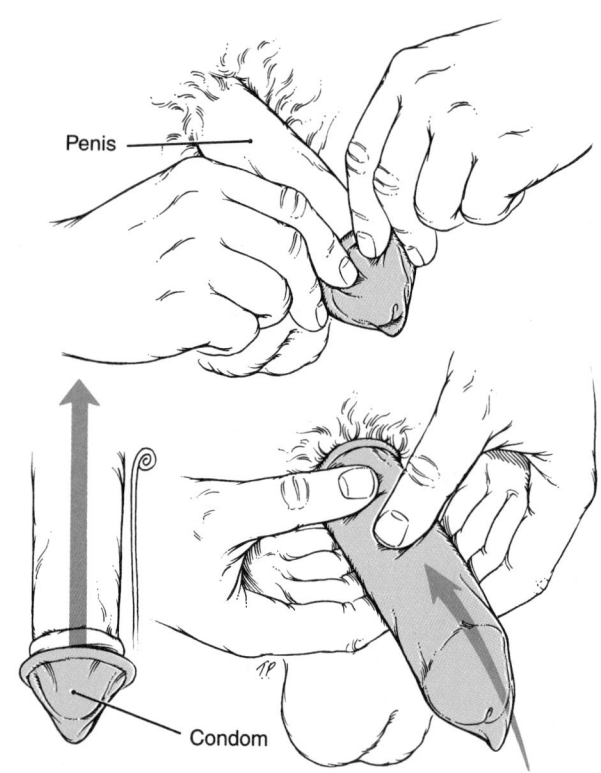

Penis

Condom

The most effective type of condom is the latex penile sheath with a reservoir at the tip. The condom is placed on the head (glans) of the erect penis and is unrolled toward the base of the penis. Avoid trapping air between the penis and condom. Never apply petroleum jelly, mineral oil, or body lotion to the condom, because these substances can weaken the latex. Once removed from the penis, a condom should never be reused.

mon method of barrier contraception is the condom, also called a prophylactic or a rubber. Condoms are rolled sheaths of latex, plastic, or natural animal tissue worn over the penis during intercourse. Since sperm can be released before ejaculation, condoms help prevent pregnancy and the spread of some STIs by collecting sperm before, during, and after ejaculation. Condoms can break, so if you feel the condom break or slip, withdraw immediately (see Proper Use of a Condom, above). The penis should be removed from the vagina immediately after ejaculation, before the penis softens and sperm has a chance to spill.

Female condoms (the vaginal pouch) are cylinders of polyurethane with heavier plastic rings attached at either end. One end is closed. This end is inserted into the vagina, with the other, open end left protruding about 1 in. from the opening of the vagina. Intercourse should be halted if the penis slips between the pouch and the wall of the vagina or if the outer ring is pushed inside the vagina. Some movement of the pouch is normal. Extra lubricant can be used, and then the pouch reinserted. All instructions explaining proper use of the female condom should be read carefully.

A diaphragm is a round, dome-shaped piece of rubber encircled with a thick, reinforced, flexible rubber rim. It is designed to cover the cervix and prevent sperm from entering. A cervical cap is also designed to cover the cervix and prevent the entry of sperm. It is hard plastic and thimble-shaped, and usually not the choice of younger women. Both must be used with a spermicidal cream or foam, and left in place for 6 hours after intercourse in the case of the diaphragm (to ensure that the spermicide has killed all the sperm), or for 48 hours in

All condoms are packed with an expiration date. Latex and urethane deteriorate over time, and a condom that has passed its expiration date should not be used.

Putting on a Condom Properly

Condom use can and should be a fundamental part of non-monogamous sex, and can be viewed as a part of foreplay, not as an unwanted interruption.

To put a condom on properly, first unwrap it. Do not unroll it yet. Examine it to determine in which direction it unrolls. Grasp the reservoir end with your thumb and forefinger and place the rolled-up condom on the head (glans) of the erect penis. If it has no reservoir end, grasp approximately a quarter inch of the tip of the condom between your thumb and forefinger, and place the unrolled condom on the head of the penis. Unroll the condom over the head of the penis, making sure there is no air in the condom. If there is, squeeze it out with your thumb and forefinger. When you are certain there is no more air in the condom, unroll it down the shaft of the penis until it will unroll no further. If for any reason you must take off the condom before ejaculation (having to urinate, losing your erection, cannot get in on properly), discard it and begin again with a new condom. Never reuse a condom.

How to Avoid Condom Breakage

Condoms break for two main reasons: air becomes trapped inside, causing the condom to burst, or lubricants are used improperly. If the vagina is not adequately lubricated during intercourse, friction can cause the condom to break. To avoid breakage, it is important for the vagina to be lubricated adequately and properly. Only use a lubricant designed for use with latex products. *Never* use petroleum jelly, mineral oil, or any sort of hand or body lotion. Many of these products contain petroleum-based ingredients and may contain other chemicals that should not be put in the vagina. Vegetable oil is also not recommended. Latex is made from petroleum-based materials and will dissolve or weaken in petroleum-based products.

Use a water-soluble lubricant such as K-Y jelly, which can be obtained at the drug store. For purposes of disease- and pregnancy-prevention, a spermicidal lubricant, such as nonoxynol-9, is better. If either person begins to experience discomfort during intercourse, check the condom and discard and replace it if it has become dislocated or stretched out of shape.

What To Do if the Condom Breaks

Women Wash thoroughly and use a spermicidal jelly or foam. You should follow washing by urinating. There is "morning-after" birth control available. If you are concerned that you might become pregnant, you should not wait, but contact Planned Parenthood and ask about the morning-after pill, which is actually a series of pills (see Contraception, page 1161).

Men and Women Although washing the genitals has not proven an effective method for preventing STIs, if a condom breaks, you should nonetheless wash thoroughly, and then urinate. If you suspect you might have contracted an STI, contact your doctor. If you would prefer to remain anonymous, you can call Planned Parenthood, which maintains clinics where medical services for family planning and treatment for STIs is available. You can obtain treatment for STIs without charge. ■

---

the case of the cervical cap. A woman must be fitted for a cervical cap or diaphragm by her doctor or a local family planning clinic; however, sexual intercourse must take place before a woman can be fitted with either of these contraceptive devices.

HORMONAL METHODS

In addition to their value in preventing pregnancy, birth control pills (the pill) can offer a number of substantial benefits. Women may experience milder premenstrual syndrome, have a reduced risk of PID, and have more regular periods. There are two types of birth control pills, combined and "mini." The former contains synthetic versions of the hormones progestin and estrogen that prevent ovulation. The latter, the minipill, contains only progestin, which thickens cervical mucus and prevents sperm from attaching to the egg. Both types of pill must be taken regularly and consistently. Missed pills can result in pregnancy.

Norplant consists of six timed-release capsules slightly smaller than matchbook matches, implanted just under the skin of the upper arm. The capsules contain levonorgestrel, a synthetic female hormone similar to those used in birth control pills. An advantage to Norplant is that the user does not need to remember to take pills. Undisturbed, the implants can provide protection against unwanted pregnancy for 5 years. If at any time the woman experiences unpleasant side effects (like any prescription medication, Norplant can cause side effects), or should she desire to become pregnant, the implants can be removed.

Depo-Provera is a synthetic hormone injected intramuscularly every 12 weeks. It works in a similar way to Norplant, but because people must return to their doctors several times over the course of a year to be injected, this method may be somewhat less effective than Norplant, which works continually for 5 years. When used consistently, however, Depo-Provera is still very effective. It causes fewer side effects than Norplant and also has a number of beneficial effects, such as the reduction of menstrual cramps and anemia, and protection against ovarian cysts. A woman's doctor can advise her if Depo-Provera is the right choice of contraception.

CONTRACEPTIVE FOAMS, GELS, CREAMS, AND SUPPOSITORIES

These preparations are spermicides and are most effective when used in conjunction with a barrier form of contraception, such as a condom or diaphragm. Less effectively, they can be used alone, and work by blocking entry of sperm into the uterus with foam or thick cream and creating an environment in which sperm cannot survive. Always read and follow directions carefully, some must be inserted into the vagina several minutes before intercourse and only remain effective for about 1 hour. Additional foam, cream, or jelly must be inserted every time you have intercourse.

INTRAUTERINE DEVICES

Intrauterine devices (IUDs) are devices placed inside the uterus to prevent pregnancy. A T-shaped device made of plastic and containing either copper or a natural hormone, the IUD works either to prevent sperm from fertilizing the egg, or to keep a fertilized egg from implanting itself in the uterine wall. The IUD is one the most popular birth control devices in the world, despite bad press in the United States. An IUD must be placed in the uterus by a doctor or a clinician.

Initial insertion of the IUD can be somewhat unpleasant, but any pain should abate after a few days. Antibiotics can be taken to head off any potential infection on insertion.

The IUD has a string that hangs down from the uterus into the vagina, and a user should check for the string on occasion to ensure that the device is in place. If not, she should see her doctor immediately. Some

IUDs can be left in place for 10 years; others must be replaced annually.

POSTINTERCOURSE OR EMERGENCY CONTRACEPTION

An egg that has been fertilized must embed itself in the lining of the uterus in order to begin pregnancy. Emergency contraception is an important adjunct to precautionary measures, and probably underused by women who do not know that it is available. It is very useful in people who may have had a condom break or who may have been forced into intercourse.

A hormonal method is available. One method involves a series of four pills that you can start taking up to 72 hours after intercourse. Similar to birth control pills, they prevent the fertilized egg from implanting in the lining of the uterus with a combination of synthetic hormones. This method is sometimes called the morning-after pill, but the name is misleading, because treatment can begin as late as 3 days after unprotected intercourse occurs.

A statistically more effective approach than the hormonal method is the IUD insertion method. It can be used up to 5 days following unprotected intercourse.

Either method will require a visit to the doctor or family planning clinic, an exam to rule out already-existing pregnancy, and careful instructions on how to use the methods, as well as their possible side effects.

RHYTHM METHOD (PERIODIC ABSTINENCE AND FERTILITY AWARENESS)

The rhythm method involves avoidance of sexual intercourse during those times of the month when conception is most likely to occur. Because this method is widely used in some cultures, it is discussed here. Keep in mind, however, that in most cases the rhythm method is not effective or appropriate as a means of preventing unwanted pregnancy.

Conception is only possible during certain days of the female reproductive cycle, 5 days prior to and 3 days following ovulation, or a total of approximately 9 days out of a typical 28 day cycle. These fertile days

ELECTIVE STERILITY (VASECTOMY AND TUBAL LIGATION)

Because no method of contraception is foolproof, at some point in their reproductive lives, some men and women may elect to undergo surgical sterilization. For men, the procedure is a vasectomy; for women, the procedure is a tubal ligation (having one's tubes tied).

Both procedures are relatively minor, but because they are intended to be permanent, they should not be undertaken unless you are completely certain that you do not now and will not in the future want to have any more children. Elective sterility in women can be reversed, but less than half of those who have had reversals have been subsequently successful in bearing a child. The risk for ectopic pregnancy (see page 150) increases following reversal. Reversing elective sterility in men is also possible, but difficult.

A vasectomy involves the severing of the vas deferens, the vessel that carries sperm from the testicles to the urethra in the penis. The man still produces semen, but this fluid contains no sperm. When couples seek surgical sterilization, the vasectomy is often the procedure of choice because it tends to be less serious with a quicker recovery time than the tubal ligation in women.

A vasectomy can be performed under local anesthesia in the doctor's office in about half an hour. After injecting an anesthetic in the scrotal area, the doctor will locate the patient's vas defer-ens (one at each testicle) and make a small incision in the skin of the scrotal sac. Through this opening, the doctor will withdraw a small segment of the vas deferens. The doctor will then surgically remove a short length of the tube and seal either end with stitches that will dissolve in several days. The severed ends are returned to the scrotum and the outer incision is stitched closed. The procedure is then repeated on the other side. When the surgery is complete, recovery will include a short observation and recovery period in the doctor's office. Strenuous activity (lifting, exercise, etc) should be avoided for the next couple of days. Following the procedure, it is normal to experience some pain and swelling in the area of the incision. As with any minor surgical procedure, however, if the pain persists for more than a few days or if a fever develops, call the doctor immediately. Returning to work as long as it does not involve strenuous activity is acceptable. ◗

Methods of surgical sterilization. (A) In a man, vasectomy involves cutting the ductus (vas) deferens that normally carries sperm from the testicles to the penile urethra. (B) In a woman, tubal ligation is 99 percent effective in preventing pregnancy. The fallopian tubes are cut and tied, preventing eggs from traveling from the ovaries to the uterus. Possible complications include infection, bleeding, and damage to internal organs. Compared to tubal ligation, vasectomy is usually a simpler operation with a faster recovery time.

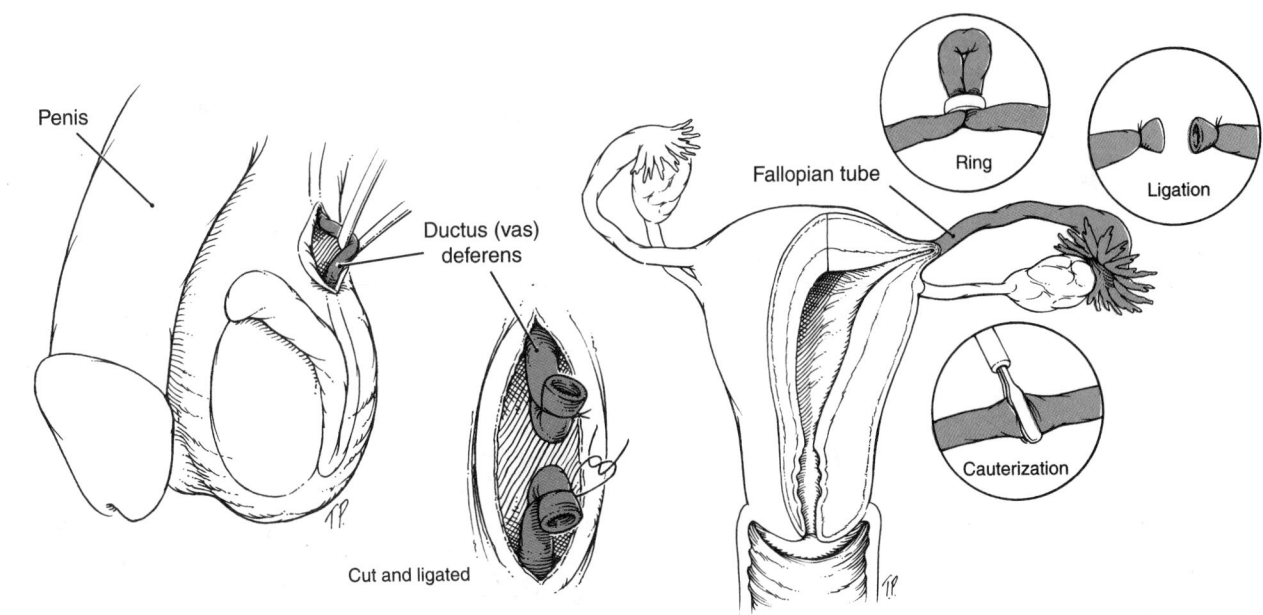

Penis

Ductus (vas) deferens

Cut and ligated

Fallopian tube

Ring

Ligation

Cauterization

require either abstinence from intercourse or the use of a barrier contraceptive (diaphragm or condom). Since it is difficult to know exactly when ovulation will occur, this method can be very unreliable and should be used only when no other, more reliable form of contraception is acceptable. Those who use this method most successfully are women whose cycles are predictable and regular, those who have had careful instruction, and those whose partners are as committed to the method as they.

◆ Approximately the first 10 to 15 ejaculations that follow surgery may still contain sperm, so it is important to use other forms of birth control for a short period of time. From that point on, vasectomy is quite effective as birth control, but it can have side effects. Sperm continue to be produced and though they are usually reabsorbed into the body, they can build up in the testes and create lumps or "granulomas" (see page 1139) that may require medical attention.

The tubal ligation procedure is 99 percent effective in preventing pregnancy. The tubes involve are the fallopian tubes, through which eggs travel after being released from the ovary. Tying the tube blocks eggs from making that journey and thereby prevents pregnancy.

In many cases, women choose to have the procedure performed immediately after giving birth. If the delivery was by cesarean section, the procedure can be performed directly and quickly, with no additional pain or anesthesia. If the delivery was vaginal, the tubal ligation procedure will require an incision, but the recovery period is simultaneous with recovering from childbirth.

When tubal ligation is not done postdelivery, it can be performed on an inpatient or outpatient basis, either under general anesthesia (you will be asleep), or under local anesthesia (which may also require the use of a tranquilizer to help you relax). The doctor will make a small incision through the wall of the woman's abdomen, near her navel. A harmless gas will be pumped slowly into the abdomen to separate the muscle wall from the organs. Using the laparoscope, a surgical tool equipped with fiber optics that enables the doctor to view the patient's internal organs without the large incisions that would once have been necessary, the doctor will identify the woman's reproductive organs. With another instrument, the doctor will clip, "tie," or seal each of the fallopian tubes by cauterization. Pregnancies are rare in women who have been tubally sterilized, but if they occur they may pose certain risks.

Following the procedure, the woman will experience some pain from the incisions and the ligation, but it should subside in a few days. Transient side effects from the procedure can include dizziness, nausea, and feeling bloated or tired, all of which should resolve in a few days. Because tubal ligation is a more major operation than vasectomy, there is more of a potential for complications. It is possible to become infected, have internal organs injured during the procedure, and to experience internal bleeding. These complications are rare, but a woman should discuss them with her doctor before she decides to undergo the procedure. The woman must know how to clearly tell if she is experiencing complications before she leave the doctor's office, clinic, or hospital. Fever should be immediately reported to the doctor. ■

There are several ways to approach predicting fertile days, but a combination of these methods is more effective than any of the first three alone.

- Body temperature changes during the menstrual cycle, rising approximately 0.4 to 0.8° F on the day of ovulation. It remains at that level until the next period. Take your temperature every morning before getting out of bed and record it on a calendar. You are fertile for 3 days after ovulation.

- Cervical mucus. Following your period, observe the consistency of your vaginal discharge. Immediately following the period, it should be cloudy and a little sticky. It will change consistency a few days before ovulation, becoming clear. This is your most fertile phase.

- The calendar or rhythm method works by charting your menstrual cycle on a calendar. This works effectively only if your periods are the same from month to month.

- The symptothermal method mixes the body temperature, cervical mucus, and calendar methods together.

- The postovulation method requires you to abstain from intercourse or use a barrier contraceptive from the beginning of your period until the morning of the fourth day after your predicted ovulation.

WITHDRAWAL

This method of contraception should only be seen as a stopgap, when nothing else (short of abstinence) is available. Withdrawal involves removing the penis from the vagina before ejaculation so that no sperm is released into the vagina. It has a significant failure rate because sperm can be released from the penis *before* ejaculation occurs. Proper implementation requires significant trust on the part of the female and self-control on the part of the male.

NEW METHODS OF BIRTH CONTROL ON THE HORIZON

While some methods of birth control have been around for years, researchers are con-

EFFECTIVENESS OF CONTRACEPTIVES IN PREVENTING PREGNANCY AND STIs

METHOD	TYPICAL USE[a]	PERFECT USE[b]	USEFULNESS IN PREVENTING STI
Latex condoms	12.0	2.0	After abstinence, the most effective (but by no means foolproof) method
Female condom (vaginal pouch)	24.8	5.2	Not as effective as the male condom, but more effective than using no protection
Diaphragm/cervical cap	18.0	6.0	Partly effective against HIV and some STIs (chlamydia, gonorrhea) when used with a spermicide such as nonoxynol-9, not as effective as latex male condoms
Birth control pills			No value
Combination pill (estrogen + progestin)	3.0	0.1	
Minipill (progestin only)	3.0	0.5	
Norplant	0.04 (first year of use)	0.04	No value
Depo-Provera	0.3	0.3	No value
Intrauterine Devices			No value[c]
ParaGard	0.8	0.6	
Progestasert	2.6	1.5	
Postintercourse or emergency contraception			No value
Hormonal (morning-after pill)	25.0	25.0	
IUD insertion	1.0	1.0	
Periodic abstinence and fertility awareness (rhythm methods)			No value
Postovulation	20.0	1.0	
Symptothermal	20.0	2.0	
Cervical mucus	20.0	3.0	
Calendar	20.0	9.0	
Withdrawal (coitus interruptus)	18.0	4.0 (estimated)	No proven value in preventing STIs
Elective sterilization			No value
Men	0.15	0.1	
Women	0.4	0.2	

[a]Percentage of failure among women whose use of the method is not consistent or always correct; 1.0 = 1 percent (1 woman in 100).

[b]Percentage of failure among women whose use is consistent and always correct.

[c]Some studies indicate a higher incidence of HIV infection among those using IUDs and having multiple partners, or having a single partner who has multiple partners.

stantly trying looking into different methods that could be more effective or relieve the woman of the primary responsibility for preventing pregnancy. Research is ongoing in many different spheres.

BufferGel has been around for years, but recently it has been given new life by Johns Hopkins researchers and may be on the market in the very near future. This contraceptive gel would be one of the first such products to be an effective preventive measure against many STIs. Laboratory research shows that, in addition to killing sperm,

BufferGel also destroys white blood cells in sperm and cervical mucus that can be infected with HIV. HIV, gonorrhea, syphilis, and genital herpes all would be destroyed in the environment created by this product. This new gel is an improvement over existing spermicides, such as nonoxynol-9, that are essentially detergents and can cause urinary tract infections. The researchers are also looking into the possibility that antibodies and vaccines could be added, and that the gel could be stabilized to provide protection that could last 24 hours.

Endocrine System

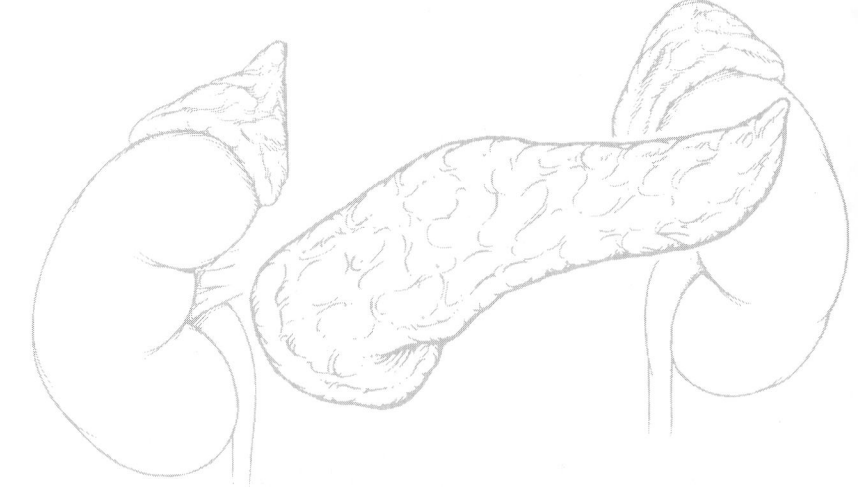

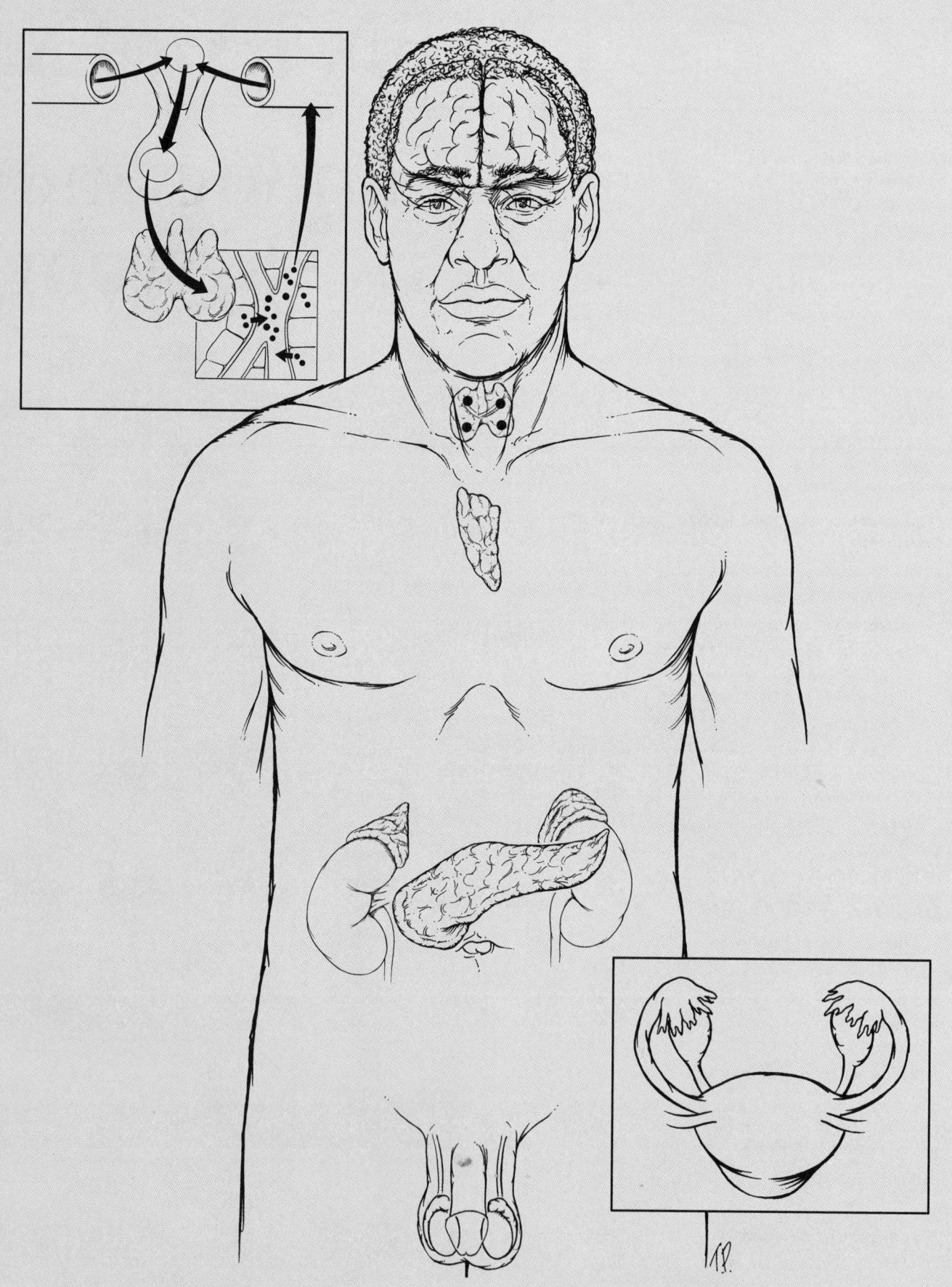

TWENTY-SIX

ENDOCRINE SYSTEM

How the Endocrine System Works

The endocrine system consists of various glands distributed throughout the body that serve as a main regulation, control, and signaling network for many body functions. The endocrine glands include the pituitary gland in the brain, the thyroid and parathyroid glands in the neck, the adrenal glands that lie atop each kidney, and the specialized cells within the pancreas in the midabdominal region. See the sections on disorders associated with specific endocrine glands for more information on those glands. The reproductive organs—ovaries in women and testicles in men—also have endocrine functions. See Chapter 25 for information on reproductive organs and their hormones.

The common feature shared by all endocrine glands is that, under the proper stimulation, they produce and secrete substances called hormones directly into the blood. A hormone is a chemical messenger; once released, it travels through the bloodstream to some distant part of the body in search of its target—an organ or tissue that bears specific and highly sensitive docking ports, called receptors, on its surface or inside its cells. Once the hormone locates its receptor, it locks into it in much the same way that a key fits into a lock and turns it. When a hormone joins with its receptor and, in effect, turns the lock, it transmits a message to that cell and causes the cell to respond with a specific action.

The actions of the major hormones influence body functions in four broad areas: regulation and distribution of nutrients in energy balance, growth and development, fluid and mineral balance, and reproduction. The major hormones (excluding those related to the reproductive organs) are discussed below.

INSULIN

Since its discovery in the 1920s, a wealth of information has been uncovered about this important metabolic hormone. Most people associate insulin with diabetes; however, its influence is much more far-reaching. The beta cells of the pancreas produce and release this hormone in response to the rise in blood glucose (sugar) that follows a meal. Insulin's primary purpose is one of building

and storage; it stimulates the packing away of nutrients into cells for later use in the following manner. When nutrients enter the bloodstream after a meal and the level of glucose in the blood rises, the pancreas releases insulin, which travels through the blood to its target tissues—primarily the cells of the liver, muscle, and fat, also called adipose, tissue. When insulin arrives at its target, it attaches to the insulin receptor on the cell's surface. Attachment of insulin to the receptor activates certain cellular functions that drive the nutrients—glucose, amino acids (protein subunits derived from dietary protein or muscle breakdown), and fatty acids (fats)—into the cell to nourish it, provide energy to it, or be stored within it. Regulating the flow of nutrients into the cells is insulin's primary job; however, it also has other functions. For example, insulin stimulates the kidney to retain salt and fluid, stimulates the production and storage of glycogen (the form in which carbohydrates are stored in the body) in liver cells, and stimulates the storage of fat in fat cells.

Disorders stemming from abnormalities in insulin regulation are type 1 diabetes mellitus (see page 1174), type 2 diabetes mellitus (see page 1179), syndrome X (see page 1178), insulinoma (see page 1183), and hypoglycemia (see page 1182).

GLUCAGON

The hormone glucagon—produced by the alpha cells of the pancreas—functions in direct opposition to insulin. Glucagon is involved in the burning and retrieval of stored fuels. Between meals, overnight, or during starvation (when the level of blood glucose falls too low) the pancreas releases glucagon to raise the blood glucose level. It does this by several methods: It stimulates the breakdown of glycogen in the liver; it stimulates the breakdown of stored body fat and burns it as a fuel source to provide energy to the tissues; and it stimulates a process in the liver called gluconeogenesis that creates new blood glucose from amino acids. In all respects, glucagon acts in an opposite fashion to that of insulin: It stimulates the kidney to waste excess salt and fluid and favors the burning of fuels instead of their storage.

Disorders resulting from abnormalities related to glucagon are diabetes mellitus

1171

and glucagonoma (see Islet Cell Tumors, page 1184).

THYROID HORMONE

Thyroid hormones exert some effect on virtually every tissue in the body, influencing such diverse areas as growth and development, basal metabolic rate (the minimal amount of energy expended to maintain vital bodily functions), temperature regulation, menstrual cycling in women, mood, and even mental and physical quickness or responsiveness as well as the metabolism (chemical conversion process that provides energy for vital bodily functions) of carbohydrates, protein, and cholesterol.

Manufacture of thyroid hormone depends on adequate dietary iodine. In fact, the thyroid hormones are the only substances in the body containing iodine. The availability of major dietary sources of iodine—such as iodized table salt, iodinated bread, seafood, and dairy products—has made deficiency of this crucial micronutrient rare in developed countries; however, prior to the routine addition of iodine to table salt, deficiency occurred commonly in the United States in areas having iodide-poor soils, resulting in abnormal, excessive growth of the thyroid gland—a condition known as a goiter.

Disorders of the thyroid gland can lead to hypothyroidism (see page 1188) or hyperthyroidism (see page 1185).

GROWTH HORMONE

Despite its name, growth hormone, produced in the anterior (forward) portion of the pituitary gland, does not actually stimulate growth itself. Instead, it causes the release from the liver of a substance called somatomedin-C, also called insulin-like growth factor 1, one of a number of growth factors the body produces. Children and adults produce about the same amount of growth hormone, but growing children are very sensitive to the various stimuli that release it from the pituitary and equally responsive to its effects. In adults, growth hormone's effects normally serve to maintain and repair the lean mass of the body.

The release of growth hormone is under the control of the brain through its production of a pair of substances from the hypothalamus (higher brain center that controls the pituitary). To stimulate release of growth hormone, the hypothalamus secretes a substance called growth hormone releasing hormone; to shut down the release, it secretes somatostatin, an inhibitor of growth hormone release. Factors that increase the release of growth hormone include a falling blood glucose level, stress, exercise, and sleep. Hyperglycemia (high blood glucose), the high adrenaline levels experienced with certain types of stress, and sleep deprivation all reduce the release of growth hormone.

Disorders associated with abnormal growth hormone effects include acromegaly (see page 1201), giantism (see page 1201), and dwarfism (see page 1202).

ANTIDIURETIC HORMONE

Antidiuretic hormone (ADH), also called vasopressin, is produced in the posterior (rearward) portion of the pituitary gland when the body needs to conserve water. If we are deprived of water, the brain senses the deficiency and stimulates the release of ADH, which in turn signals the kidneys to reabsorb water, resulting in a very concentrated urine. ADH also causes a strong constriction of certain blood vessels to provide more blood flow to vital organs in the event of a low blood pressure crisis.

Other factors that stimulate the release of ADH include significant blood loss, an abrupt fall of blood pressure such as might occur in prolonged periods of quiet standing, excessive sweating, and fever.

Disorders related to abnormalities in ADH secretion are diabetes insipidus (see page 1203) and the syndrome of inappropriate ADH secretion.

CORTISOL

Cortisol, made out of cholesterol in the middle zone of the adrenal cortex, is absolutely essential for life. It is chiefly responsible for maintaining vital processes during periods of sustained stress and for containing inflammation. It is termed a glucocorticoid because it increases the supply of glucose to the cells of the body during times of stress by stimulating the liver to manufacture new glucose from protein and from the breakdown of stored fat, and by increasing appetite. Cortisol's many other roles in the body include modulation of perception and emotion, maintenance of normal blood vessel integrity, preservation of normal kidney function, maturation of the fetal lungs and gastrointestinal (GI) tract, and possibly detoxification and containment of the chemical toxins released by the body's immune system during stress and in the case of major infections.

Disorders related to abnormal cortisol secretion include Addison's disease (see page 1197) and Cushing's syndrome (see page 1195).

ALDOSTERONE

Produced in the outer zone of the adrenal cortex, aldosterone acts to help regulate the fluid volume of the body and to conserve fluid by signaling the kidney to reabsorb salt. When the level of body fluid falls too low, specialized cells in the kidney sense the fall and call for aldosterone release. These cells produce renin, an enzyme that acts on a substance called angiotensin I, produced by the liver, to convert it to angiotensin II. It is angiotensin II that stimulates aldosterone release. One class of medications to lower blood pressure—called angiotensin converting enzyme (ACE) inhibitors—works to prevent the conversion of angiotensin I to angiotensin II and thus to stop the call for aldosterone. New medications for hypertension (high blood pressure), including losartan (Cozaar), block the receptor for angiotensin II. High levels of potassium in the blood and adrenocorticotrophic hormone (ACTH) also stimulate the release of aldosterone.

Aldosterone also causes sodium reabsorption from other body excretions such as saliva, sweat, and stool. These actions help the body adapt to a hot climate.

The disorder related to abnormal secretion of aldosterone is called hyperaldosteronism (see Adrenal Cortical Tumors, page 1199).

PARATHYROID HORMONE

Parathyroid hormone (PTH), the product of the two pairs of tiny glands located behind the thyroid gland, exerts its main effects in regulating the level of calcium in the blood. When calcium levels fall too low, PTH secretion rises—as much as 50 times over its normal rate—making more calcium available by prompting release of some of the mineral from bones, by increasing reabsorption of calcium by the kidney, and by enhancing absorption of calcium from the diet.

Disorders associated with abnormal release of this hormone include hyperparathyroidism (see page 1193), hypoparathyroidism (see page 1194), and pseudohypoparathyroidism (see Hypoparathyrodism, page 1194).

PROLACTIN

Most hormones produced in the pituitary gland do not act directly on target tissues in the body, but rather serve to prod specific glands to manufacture and release other hormones that actually do the work of stimulating the ultimate response. Prolactin, however, despite its pituitary origin, directly stimulates the mammary glands in the breast to produce milk. This stimulation normally occurs only during and following pregnancy in women; however, abnormal production sometimes occurs in both men and women as a consequence of a hormone-producing tumor (tissue mass) in the pituitary gland (see Prolactinoma, page 1200).

THE CATECHOLAMINES: EPINEPHRINE (ADRENALINE) AND NOREPINEPHRINE (NORADRENALINE)

These related hormones participate in the hormonal regulation and signaling functions of the body, but also serve as neurotransmitters (mediators in brain and nervous system signal transmission). As hormones, these substances are manufactured in the adrenal gland (hence their original names, adrenaline and noradrenaline) from the amino acid tyrosine and released into the bloodstream in response to fright, exercise, or exposure to cold temperatures or to low levels of blood glucose. Epinephrine and norepinephrine act primarily to elevate blood glucose, blood pressure, and heart rate and to ready the body for emergency action: to fight or flee. As neurotransmitters, they are produced and stored in nerve endings, where they carry signals across the gap between nerve cells.

Disorders can occur due to either an excessive production of epinephrine or norepinephine created by tumors of the adrenal gland (see Adrenal Tumors, page 1198) or due to a deficiency of these hormones.

Disorders of the Endocrine Pancreas

The pancreas is an elongated gland about the size of your hand that lies sideways deep in the abdomen behind the stomach. It is both an endocrine gland—that is, a gland that produces hormones for release into the blood—and a digestive gland, connected by a duct to the intestine into which it releases the other pancreatic products, digestive enzymes to aid in the breakdown of foods. See Chapter 23 for information about the digestive functions of what is termed the exocrine pancreas.

The endocrine functions of the pancreas are carried out by specialized clusters of cells called the islets of Langerhans that are scattered throughout the gland. The islets contain three types of cells—called

The pancreas secretes enzymes into the intestine to digest food into smaller nutrient molecules that are absorbed across the lining of the intestine. High blood glucose (sugar) levels signal the pancreas to secrete insulin, a hormone that aids in the removal of glucose from the blood. Low blood glucose levels stimulate the secretion of glucagon, a hormone that triggers the release of glucose from the liver.

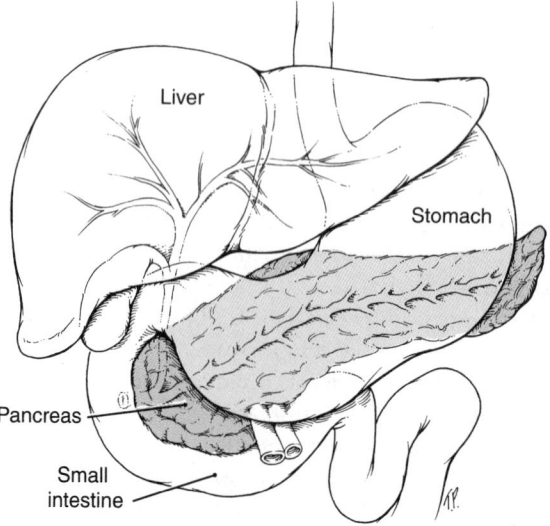

alpha, beta, and delta—each of which produces a specific hormone. The alpha cells produce glucagon; the beta cells, insulin; the delta cells, somatostatin. These hormones serve as the chief regulators of nutrient and energy utilization by the body.

❖ TYPE 1 DIABETES MELLITUS

Symptoms *(What you may experience)* Extreme thirst and hunger; unexplained loss of weight despite increased appetite; frequent urination of large volume; blurred vision; fatigue; decreased mental sharpness; nausea and vomiting (sometimes); frequent infections of skin, urinary tract, or vagina.

Emergency symptoms Shaking; confusion; loss of coordination; slurred speech; rapid breathing; fruity-smelling breath; abdominal pain; loss of consciousness.

Signs and laboratory findings *(What the doctor looks for)* Abnormalities in blood glucose (too high or, in the case of an insulin reaction, too low); glucose or ketone bodies (by-products of fat metabolism) in the urine, weight loss.

What is it? Also called juvenile-onset diabetes or insulin-dependent diabetes, this relatively uncommon disorder afflicts approximately 1 in 250 people in the United States and occurs more commonly among whites than among blacks or Asians. It occurs equally among males and females and is generally a disease of childhood, with most cases developing before age 20. The disorder clearly can be inherited, but the exact mechanism of its inheritance is not yet known, and environmental factors may play crucial roles in whether or not the disorder develops. Type 1 diabetes arises when something—usually a toxin or virus—prompts the body's own immune defense system to attack the pancreas. The resulting autoimmune destruction—termed an insulitis—damages the beta cells of the pancreas to such an extent that they can no longer produce sufficient insulin. Without insulin, the body cannot get nutrients such as blood glucose into the cells of the body's tissues, and the tissues, in effect, starve in the face of an abundance of incoming food.

The system of getting nourishment into cells normally works in the following manner: After a meal, food is digested and broken down into its most basic units for absorption into the body. Digestive enzymes transform protein into amino acids, starches and sugars into the simple single sugars that compose them, and fats (mainly triglycerides) into fatty acids. With absorption, blood glucose rises, and the rise signals the pancreas to release insulin. When the system functions as it should, the insulin acts to drive the nutrients into the cells of the tissues that need them and turn off the production of glucose by the liver as well as inhibit breakdown of fat stored in adipose tissue. Blood glucose then returns to the normal range. In people with type 1 diabetes, however, with no (or not enough) insulin, the level of glucose in the blood climbs higher and higher. When this happens, the glucose begins to escape through the kidneys into the urine, carrying with it large amounts of water, causing a significant increase in urine production that can lead to dehydration.

With no insulin to impede it, glucagon (insulin's opponent hormone) stimulates a massive breakdown of stored body fat, and this, together with the loss of glucose in urine, causes rapid and extreme weight loss. The fat pours out of the fat cells so rapidly that it exceeds the body's capacity to eliminate its breakdown products—called ketone bodies—and the dangerous condition of diabetic ketoacidosis (DKA) can develop. Although ketone bodies are natural by-products of normal fat metabolism and in a person without diabetes are readily used as fuels by the skeletal muscles and the heart, they can cause serious problems for the person with type 1 diabetes who has no ability to secrete insulin to shut down their production. Because ketone bodies are acids, their overwhelming, uncontrolled production can cause metabolic acidosis (excessive acidity of the blood). The body attempts to remove the excess of ketone bodies by sending them out in the breath—giving it a fruity smell—and through the urine, but after a time, production can outstrip removal capacity. DKA is a medical emergency that requires immediate treatment in a hospital. Untreated, DKA can be fatal, and is in as many as 10 percent of cases. Contrary to the warnings of some nonmedical nutritional information sources, people who are not diabetic need not fear ketone bodies, because anyone who can produce insulin can keep the rate of fat breakdown controlled and will not develop ketoacidosis.

Diabetes can predispose those who have the disease to two types of late complications: damage to small blood vessels and nerves due to hyperglycemia, and an increased risk of atherosclerosis (hardening) of large arteries, giving rise to myocardial infarction (heart attack), stroke, and insufficient blood flow to the legs.

The organs and tissues most susceptible to these late complications are the eyes—especially the retina (membrane that receives images formed by the lens)—the kidneys, the nerves supplying the extremities and GI tract, and the arteries supplying the heart, the brain, and the legs and feet. See Chapter 20 for information on how these complications can affect the heart and the blood vessels supplying the brain.

- *Retinopathy*. It occurs in 95 percent of people who have had diabetes for longer than 15 years, but fortunately only a minority of those people will develop significant visual problems because of it. The most common form of retinopathy develops because weak areas in the walls of the tiny arteries that nourish the retina balloon under pressure (the process of microaneurysm development) and may leak blood or rupture, causing microscopic hemorrhages of blood within the retina. Over time, obstruction of the tiny blood vessels impairs delivery of blood to the retina and tiny areas can die from lack of oxygen (termed microinfarctions). Hemorrhages can occur anywhere in the retina, but visual loss is most likely if they form near the macula—the area of sharpest vision. Left unabated, the ongoing rupture, the death of tiny areas of the retina, scarring, and formation of new blood vessels (neovascularization or proliferative retinopathy) can lead to detachment of the retina and blindness. Laser treatment to the retina has been demonstrated to preserve eyesight.

- *Kidney damage*. Although most people with diabetes of long duration develop some degree of retinopathy, only 35 to 45 percent of those with type 1 diabetes develop kidney damage, also called nephropathy. This complication, however, carries with it the highest mortality for this minority of people

BLOOD GLUCOSE SELF-TESTING

Blood glucose self-testing is crucial for all people with diabetes who are taking insulin, and valuable for most who are treated with oral medications. Typical times for self-testing might be upon waking in the morning, before meals, before or after exercise, and at bedtime. Your doctor will devise a schedule appropriate for your condition. Regular blood glucose self-testing will guide you and your doctor in determining how much insulin (or oral medication) you need and can help protect you from the many complications related to hyperglycemia. Equally important, it can protect you from the potentially dangerous consequences of extreme hypoglycemia (low blood glucose).

Many different blood glucose meters are on the market. They are small—often wallet-sized—electronic devices that analyze the level of blood glucose using one of two different methods. Each type of meter works by analyzing a sample of your blood placed onto a test strip. Some test strips change color, and the meter measures the change. Others are electrosensitive, and the meter measures the electric charge on the strip. They measure blood glucose in mg/dL, or milligrams of glucose per deciliter (one-tenth of a liter) of blood. Ask your doctor which ones are the most accurate and reliable before buying.

Before testing, rinse your hands with warm water—blood flows more freely from warm skin. Do not handle sweets, glucose tablets, or food immediately prior to testing. Do not use alcohol to clean the finger you plan to prick because it can dry your skin. Unless your hands are visibly dirty, you can do more harm than good by scrubbing them.

Using the finger-stick device supplied with the meter, prick your fingertip on the side. Some doctors recommend pricking the finger on the back, below the nail. Do not prick the pad of your finger. With your other hand, squeeze a drop of blood onto the test strip with a massaging action. Immediately but carefully insert the strip into the meter and start the timer. In a few moments, the device will give a reading of your blood glucose level. ■

with diabetes. The risk for kidney disease increases over time; however, if after 20 years the kidneys show no sign of allowing protein to escape into the urine, kidney damage is not likely to occur and will probably not develop at all. Aiming for control of blood glucose close to the normal range is the best hope for preserving kidney function, because hyperglycemia is the chief cause of damage to the kidneys. Control of hypertension and the administration of ACE inhibitors in people with diabetes who have kidney disease has been shown to aid in prevention of further progression of the disease.

- *Diminished sensation and poor circulation.* The damaging effect of hyperglycemia on the nerves and atherosclerosis of the large arteries creates a one-two punch of diminished sensation and poor circulation in the feet, making it easy for injury or infection to lead to serious problems. The lack of good sensation increases the risk of injury from blistering or pressure caused by tight or improperly fitted shoes, friction, or carelessly clipped nails; the decreased circulation impairs healing when the wounds occur. The risk of serious infection, leading possibly to gangrene, is real and significant for a person with diabetes. The risk of amputation of feet—or legs—is 40 times higher in people with diabetes than it is in people without the disease. (See also page 722.)

- *Neuropathy.* Damage to nerves due to hyperglycemia can also cause problems in the GI tract, especially in the stomach. Because nerves must adequately stimulate rhythmic contractions of the stomach in order to churn the food with stomach acid for proper digestion and then propel the food into the small intestine in a timely fashion, nerve damage can cause poor stomach function and a delay in emptying a meal. When the meal finally, through volume and pressure, forces open the outlet to the intestine, the entire meal may "dump" at once. Delay can cause blood sugar regulation problems in people taking insulin, because the insulin dose is already in the body, but the food is not—it is in the stomach waiting to pass into the small intestine from which it can be absorbed into the blood. Blood glucose falls too low during the lag, then rises too quickly for the insulin dose to control it during the dumping phase. Medications to help normalize stomach muscle contraction and speed up emptying, such as metoclopramide (Reglan), may help alleviate this problem.

Averting these serious complications means working diligently to keep blood glucose as close to normal as possible as much of the time as possible.

What you can do If any of the signs or symptoms of type 1 diabetes develop, do

HOW TO INJECT INSULIN PROPERLY

To administer a painless shot, speed is of the essence in piercing the skin. A quick, confident stick almost never hurts, whereas a tentative push through the skin can be quite uncomfortable. Insulin needles are short and very thin and designed for injection into the subcutaneous (beneath the skin) tissue. Any fleshy area with loose skin you can easily grasp will work—for example, the abdomen, thighs, or upper arm. You should bear in mind, however, that the absorption of the injected dose may vary from one site to another, so it is best to administer the shot in the same general area to keep absorption more predictable. To minimize trauma to the tissues once you have selected one region (the abdomen, for example), move your injection sites around within that area. It is helpful to devise a pattern of rotation. On the abdomen, you might select a snake-like pattern: Go up one side, down the middle, and up the other side.

To administer the dose, carefully withdraw the correct number of units of insulin into the syringe. (Note: You can mix regular insulin with the intermediate-acting forms, such as NPH and lente, in the same syringe. Mixing should be done immediately prior to injection. However, never mix regular and long-acting insulin in the same syringe. Mixing these two types alters the duration of action of both, makes timing of maximum effect unpredictable, and turns control of blood glucose into guesswork. If you must take both regular and long-acting, do so in two shots in two separate sites.) Hold the syringe in your dominant hand in much the same way you would hold a pencil or throw a dart. Grasp a good bit of the tissue of your abdomen (or other injection site) between the fingers and thumb of your other hand. Then using the kind of motion you would use to throw a dart (although you will not be letting go of the syringe as you would a dart), quickly and purposefully dart the needle into the skin at an angle of about 45°. Quick entry is nearly painless. (Do not place the needle on your skin and push; this method, while effective, can be painful). Once the needle is through the skin, gently push the plunger on the syringe to administer the dose. ■

not attempt to treat them yourself. See a doctor immediately. After diagnosis and treatment to stabilize blood glucose, you must learn how to recognize the symptoms of abnormal blood glucose levels, properly use a home glucose monitor (see Blood Glucose Self-Testing, page 1176), and treat blood glucose elevations and drops yourself. Always keep glucose tablets (or in an emergency, glucose containing candies such as Sweetarts) with you in your pocket or purse as protection against an insulin reaction—for example, following excessive exercise (see The Insulin Reaction—What to Do, this page). Wear a Diabetic Alert bracelet or dog tag to make medical personnel aware of your condition in case you should become unconscious.

After evaluation and stabilization by a doctor, the cornerstone of your therapy will be insulin administration, along with constancy in diet and exercise and a clear understanding of your disorder.

If you smoke, stop. Cigarette smoking compounds the tendency for cholesterol in the blood to imbed in the artery walls and vastly increases your risk for myocardial infarction and stroke. See page 795 for more information on the connection between smoking and cardiovascular disease.

Exercise helps to improve the control of blood glucose. The most recent evidence favors resistance exercise such as light weight training combined with aerobic endurance exercise (such as walking, jog-

THE INSULIN REACTION— WHAT TO DO

The most frequent complication of insulin therapy is the development of hypoglycemia due to too much insulin, too little food, too much exercise, or drinking alcohol. The hypoglycemia from excess injected insulin can be fatal if not recognized and treated. It is extremely important that people with diabetes, as well as their families and friends, recognize symptoms of hypoglycemia. Early signs to watch for include a racing pulse, headache, clamminess, hand tremors, hunger, strange tingling sensations, anxiety, and confused thinking or speech. Rapidly falling blood glucose can cause a person with diabetes to become irritable, hostile, combative, confused, and even to deny vehemently that there is a problem. Left untreated, the symptoms can progress to uncoordination, slurring of speech, sleepiness, unresponsiveness, loss of consciousness, convulsions, and coma. It may often fall to friends and family to notice the early warning signs of an insulin reaction and give help that may not be well received. During sleep, nightmares, unusual restlessness, excessive perspiration, or shouting may indicate hypoglycemia. Family members should keep in mind that in people who have had diabetes for many years, early warning signs may not appear, so that confusion leading quickly to coma may be the only manifestations.

Treatment involves rapidly raising blood glucose, usually by drinking juice or eating crackers or a sandwich. When food is not available, keep some source of glucose/dextrose, such as tablets, at hand. Remember: The larger the person is, the less effectively will a corrective glucose tablet raise that person's blood glucose. One dextrotab will raise blood glucose about 5 to 10 mg/dL in an average adult; one B-D glucose tablet will raise glucose about 20 to 30 mg/dL. One Sweetart candy will raise blood glucose 8 to 12 mg/dL on average. When possible, measure blood glucose with your home glucose monitor. If a person with diabetes has an insulin reaction that does not respond promptly to measures to raise blood glucose or the person loses consciousness, emergency medical care should be sought immediately. ■

GLYCOHEMOGLOBIN—A BETTER MEASURE OF BLOOD GLUCOSE CONTROL

Blood glucose levels change rapidly—rising and falling in response to food intake, stress, and exercise. Because the blood glucose level is so volatile, an isolated measurement of blood glucose only reflects what is happening at that precise moment, revealing little about how well or poorly the diabetes is responding to a particular regimen. Even if blood glucose is normal at the moment of the test, that does not guarantee good control on the whole.

To overcome the disadvantage of volatility in glucose levels, there is a blood test that takes advantage of a biochemical fact: the hemoglobin pigment in red blood cells interacts with glucose in the blood to form a product called glycohemoglobin or hemoglobin A$_{lc}$ that can be measured in the blood. The amount of the reaction increases as blood glucose levels increase, and red blood cells remain in the circulation for about 120 days. As a result, the glycohemoglobin measurement assesses not what the blood glucose is at one instant, but rather what the level has been on average for the past 90 days—a much more meaningful measurement of glucose control. This information can help the doctor better determine a person's adherence and response to diabetic therapy. ■

ging, swimming, or cycling) as the best means to improve insulin sensitivity. See Chapter 2 for more information about these and other forms of exercise.

Treatment Life long replacement therapy with insulin is essential, but the best therapy is the least therapy. Your doctor will prescribe the lowest possible insulin dosage regimen to deal with the specific eating and exercise plan that fits your state of health, age, and lifestyle (usually designed by a dietitian or nutritional consultant). It is imperative to stick as closely as possible to a prescribed routine: eat regularly spaced meals providing approximately the same amounts of carbohydrate and protein everyday and exercise at about the same intensity and for the same amount of time everyday.

People with type 1 diabetes should limit simple sugars such as sucrose (table sugar) or those found in corn syrup, honey, or fruit juices—except as emergency treatment for hypoglycemia associated with an insulin reaction (see page 1177). Try also to reduce the intake of quickly absorbable or refined starches such as those found in potatoes and white and processed flours and meals (including wheat flour and processed corn meals) and in foods made from these substances. The ideal diet for a person with type 1 diabetes would contain a variety of lean protein sources—lean meat, fish, poultry, egg whites, tofu, and low-fat dairy products—and also be rich in fresh, low-starch green and colorful vegetables and salad greens as well as in fresh fruits such as melons, berries, peaches, or apples. Starchier foods should be limited sharply in quantity and should come from beans and whole, unprocessed grains, especially oats and brown rice. Replacing some of the starch in the diet with low-fat protein and foods rich in monounsaturated fats—such as olives, nuts, seeds, avocado, and olive or canola oils—seems to offer better control of blood glucose than one weighted more heavily in favor of complex carbohydrates. The American Diabetes Association (ADA), which once recommended a diet very high in complex carbohydrates and lower in fat and protein, has recently reversed its stand in the face of the poor sugar control this regimen produces. In its stead, the ADA has adopted the policy that treatment should be tailored to the needs of the patient.

The more precisely you follow the nutritional regimen prescribed by your doctor, the less impact type 1 diabetes will have on your health.

Prognosis Good for a normal, productive life with early diagnosis and careful adherence to treatment. Poor if undiagnosed or carelessly treated.

❖ INSULIN RESISTANCE AND SYNDROME X

Symptoms *(What you may experience)* None.

Signs and laboratory findings *(What the doctor looks for)* Abdominal obesity; hypertension; abnormalities such as a low level of high density lipoprotein (HDL)—good cholesterol—and a high triglyceride (blood fat) level as detected by blood tests;

elevation of blood insulin; and glucose intolerance as demonstrated by increased fasting blood glucose or an abnormal glucose tolerance test.

What is it? Abdominal obesity has been linked with resistance to the action of insulin in tissues. The mechanism for this resistance remains unclear, but as a result, the pancreas produces and secretes more insulin.

The excess insulin in the circulation is not harmless—insulin is a powerful metabolic hormone. Its influence reaches a wide variety of organ systems, and for this reason people with excess insulin tend to develop the cluster of disorders referred to as Syndrome X. For example, an elevation of insulin signals the kidney to reabsorb sodium (salt) and fluid, leading to excess fluid retention. The hormone also stimulates thickening of and tension in the muscle layer of arteries. More volume in a tighter space equals elevated pressure—blood pressure rises. Insulin stimulates the liver to make more triglycerides, causing an increase in the release of triglyceride-rich lipoproteins into the blood and a rise in blood triglycerides. If insulin resistance and the necessity for higher and higher output of insulin continues, the pancreatic beta cells can suffer fatigue from overwork. When the pancreas can no longer produce enough insulin to overcome the resistance, type 2 diabetes mellitus (see below) will ensue. The disorders of hypertension, low levels of HDL cholesterol, elevated triglycerides, and diabetes and an increased risk of coronary artery disease are all related to each other through insulin resistance caused by obesity.

What you can do Weight loss is the most important goal, and careful adherence to diet and exercise is the cornerstone of your self-care. See Type 2 Diabetes Mellitus, below, for more information on controlling insulin resistance through diet.

If you smoke, stop. Cigarette smoking vastly increases your risk for myocardial infarction and stroke. See Chapter 20 for more information on the connection between smoking and cardiovascular disease.

Exercise helps to restore sensitivity of the insulin receptors. See Type 1 Diabetes Mellitus, page 1174, for more information on how exercise affects insulin receptors.

See Chapter 2 for information about forms of exercise.

When to call the doctor Insulin resistance develops gradually over many years, so there is no specific point at which to involve a doctor. The best time to take action is before you develop related problems and before any damage is done. If you have a strong family history of diabetes, hypertension, or cardiovascular disease but as yet do not suffer from any of them yourself, your best course of action is to begin now to reduce your risk of developing them by lifestyle modification. If you have begun to store excess fat—especially around the middle—have hypertension, HDL cholesterol or triglyceride problems, impaired glucose tolerance, or diabetes, you may already be under a doctor's care. If not, a visit to a doctor is overdue.

Treatment Your doctor will examine you thoroughly and probably will perform preliminary tests to determine your current status: checking blood glucose and your lipid profile (cholesterol, HDL cholesterol, and triglyceride levels) as well as assessing liver, kidney, and heart function. If diet and exercise do not achieve optimal results, the doctor may suggest treatment of one or more of these disorders using medication.

Prognosis Excellent with proper nutrition and regular exercise.

❖ TYPE 2 DIABETES MELLITUS

Symptoms *(What you may experience)* Fatigue, increased urination, and thirst; unexplained weight loss; frequent bladder and vaginal infections in women; chronic yeast infections occurring in areas between skin folds; poor wound healing; diminished sensation or numbness in the hands and feet; blurred vision; impotence.

Signs and laboratory findings *(What the doctor looks for)* Elevation of blood glucose and hemoglobin A_{1c}; increased blood triglyceride and low HDL cholesterol levels (often); and sugar or protein in the urine; microhemorrhages in the retina on eye examination; obesity; hypertension; decreased sensation in the feet.

What is it? Over 90 percent of the cases of diabetes in the United States fall into this category. Type 2 diabetes, also referred to as adult-onset diabetes or noninsulin dependent diabetes, and the related disorder termed type 1 diabetes share more than just a name. Although the two disorders arise from opposite causes, the late complications they both can lead to are the same. While in type 1 diabetes, people develop hyperglycemia because of a lack of insulin, those with type 2 diabetes develop hyperglycemia despite an initial abundance of insulin. The development of type 2 diabetes is the continued progression of the insulin resistance syndrome (see page 1178). As the disorder progresses, insulin resistance finally reaches a point at which the amount of insulin needed to effectively drive blood sugar and other nutrients into the tissues and to turn off production of glucose by the liver exceeds the amount the pancreas can produce. At that point, blood glucose rises and type 2 diabetes ensues.

The disease is quite common and becoming more so. The incidence of type 2 diabetes has tripled in the United States since 1960, bringing with it a rise in the host of medical disorders associated with the diabetic condition: hypertension, heart disease, stroke, and circulatory diseases of the feet and legs as well as disorders of the kidneys, eyes, and nerves. Unfortunately half of the approximately 16 million people in the United States with type 2 diabetes are undiagnosed and, therefore, not receiving proper treatment.

Although some people with type 2 diabetes are thin, the majority tend to store excess body fat, especially in the central abdominal area, both beneath the skin and in and around the organs in the abdominal cavity. Storage of fat within the liver (fatty liver) can lead to some disturbances in function that may elevate liver enzymes in the blood that can be detected by blood testing.

Hyperglycemia can lead to what is called glucose toxicity, which can further damage the overworked pancreas. When the production of insulin by the beta cells in the pancreas reaches maximum capacity, as further resistance to insulin's action develops and blood glucose escalates, the high level of glucose itself has a toxic effect on the beta cells. The one-two punch of overwork and toxicity finally overwhelms and damages the beta cells and their functional capacity declines. With the body now able to produce even less insulin in the face of escalating demand, blood glucose skyrockets and begins to damage other tissues such as the eyes, nerves, and kidneys. These changes mirror the complications faced by people with type 1 diabetes. See Type 1 Diabetes Mellitus, page 1174, for more information on damage to other organs. Patients with diabetes are at greatly increased risk for atherosclerosis, which can narrow blood vessels to the heart, brain, and legs.

Retinopathy is not the only eye problem that affects people with diabetes, both type 1 and type 2. Early development of cataracts (cloudiness of the lens of the eye) occurs quite frequently in people with diabetes. Their appearance seems to be a function of the length of time the diabetes has been present and the severity of the blood glucose elevations. Glaucoma (elevation of the pressure within the eyes) occurs in a minority (about 6 percent) of people with diabetics.

What you can do Educate yourself about this disorder and the exercise and dietary recommendations that apply. The cornerstone of successful therapy is weight control through a combination of appropriate diet and exercise. Eat well-balanced meals and snacks and exercise regularly, combining aerobic activities such as walking, swimming, or biking with resistance activities such as light weight training.

Treatment The mainstay of treatment for type 2 diabetes is nutritional. Restoring weight and blood glucose to the near-normal range is the single most important intervention. In some cases, medical therapy with oral blood-glucose-lowering medications or with insulin may be necessary; however, for many adults with type 2 diabetes, strict adherence to a proper nutritional and exercise regimen may be all that is needed to maintain control. People with type 2 diabetes should limit concentrated doses of simple sugars such as sucrose or those found in corn syrup, honey, or fruit juices—except as emergency treatment for hypoglycemia or insulin reaction (see The Insulin Reaction—What to Do, page 1177). Try also to eliminate or sharply reduce the intake of

ORAL MEDICATIONS THAT LOWER BLOOD GLUCOSE

Oral medications that lower blood glucose fall into four distinct categories: sulfonylurea derivatives, metformin (Glucophage), acarbose (Precose), and troglitazone (Rezulin). All can be used alone or in combination with each other or with insulin.

Sulfonylureas

The sulfonylurea family of medications includes tolbutamide (Orinase), chlorpropamide (Diabinese), tolazamide (Tolinase), and acetohexamide (Dymelor) and newer, second generation medications glyburide (DiaBeta, Micronase, and Glynase), glipizide (Glucotrol), glipizide GITS (Glucotrol XL), and glimepiride (Amaryl). These medications work by stimulating the pancreas to release more of its stored insulin. This family of drugs is the most widely prescribed group of oral medications to treat type 2 diabetes. They are used in nonobese or moderately obese people with this form of the disease. They are of no value in people with type 1 diabetes. The sulfonylurea medications all work in basically the same way; however, they vary widely in their potency and duration of action. Some act for only 6 to 8 hours while others act for 24 hours or more. The choice of a medication depends on the lifestyle and nutritional and exercise regimen of the person with diabetes. A common side effect is hypoglycemia.

Metformin

Metformin is the only currently available biguanide. Instead of stimulating the pancreas to release more insulin, the biguanides improve insulin sensitivity. By reducing the release of glucose from the liver and increasing its uptake by muscles, metformin decreases the amount of insulin needed to control blood glucose. For this reason, metformin is said to be insulin-sparing and may give the beta cells a much needed rest. Although metformin was approved in 1994 for use in the United States, its safety and effectiveness have been established over a period of more than 20 years in 70 countries around the world. People with diabetes who have liver or kidney disease cannot take metformin because of the risk of lactic acidosis (excessive amounts of lactic acid in the blood), a potentially fatal complication. Because it does not cause increased weight gain (it may lead to weight loss), this medication is especially useful in people with diabetes who are obese. The medication regimen usually consists of two tablets taken with meals two times daily. Used alone, metformin does not cause hypoglycemia, but that complication can occur when it is combined with a sulfonylurea or insulin.

Acarbose

Acarbose slows the breakdown of sucrose and starches by inhibiting the action of digestive enzymes—called alpha glucosidases—that convert these foods into the absorbable sugar, glucose. Acarbose should be considered an adjunct to proper diet and not a way to avoid dietary restraint. It is taken with meals and the dosage is increased gradually. The medication can be taken along with other oral diabetic medications such as the sulfonylureas; however, the additive effects of lowering blood glucose heighten the risk for hypoglycemia. Because the drug impairs the breakdown of table sucrose, episodes of hypoglycemia (if they occur) must be treated with glucose, not sucrose—in other words, the sugar in a soft drink or candy bar will not elevate the blood glucose. Instead people using acarbose will need to take glucose tablets or milk (which contains the sugar lactose that can be broken down while taking acarbose) to treat hypoglycemia. People are often troubled by the GI side effects that are common with acarbose, especially severe flatulence as well as diarrhea and abdominal cramping. These symptoms may diminish after 1 or 2 months on the medication.

Troglitazone

Like the biguanides, troglitazone also increases insulin sensitivity and has the theoretical advantage of resting the beta cells, decreasing insulin levels, and avoiding the harmful metabolic effects of high insulin levels (see Insulin Resistance and Syndrome X, page 1178). Troglitazone is the newest medication used to treat diabetes and the risk benefit ratio is still being studied. Concern has been raised about the possibility of harmful liver effects; people with liver disease should not take this medication. Liver enzymes must be measured every month for the first 6 months of treatment and then every 2 months for the next 6 months of treatment. ■

quickly absorbable starches such as those found in potatoes and white and processed flours (both wheat flour and processed corn meal) and in foods made from these substances. The ideal diet for a person with type 2 diabetes would contain a variety of lean protein sources—lean meat, fish, poultry, egg whites, tofu, and low-fat dairy products—and also be rich in fresh, low-starch green and colorful vegetables and salad greens as well as in fresh fruits such as melons, berries, peaches, and apples. Avoid foods high in saturated fats and cholesterol. Starchier foods should be limited in quantity per meal and should come from beans and whole, unprocessed grains, especially oats and brown rice. Replacing some of the starch in the diet with low-fat protein and monounsaturated fats—such as those found in olives, nuts, and seeds and in olive and canola oils—may offer better control of blood glucose than one weighted more heavily in favor of complex carbohydrates. The ADA, which once recommended a diet very high in complex carbohydrates and lower in fat and protein, has recently reversed its stand in the face of the poor sugar control this regimen achieved. In its

OBESITY

Obesity, the excess storage of body fat, is the most common chronic disorder in the United States and its incidence continues to rise. Approximately half of adult Americans are considered significantly overweight. The incidence of obesity has jumped sharply in the last few decades, increasing by 33 percent. The extent of obesity can be classified relative to ideal body weight—the weight expected for a person of a certain age, gender, and height. By that definition, obesity is considered to be mild in people weighing 20 to 40 percent above ideal body weight, moderate in those weighing 40 to 200 percent above ideal body weight, and severe or morbid in people weighing greater than 200 percent above ideal body weight.

While obesity usually results as a consequence of a sedentary lifestyle and chronic overeating, not everyone who pursues such a lifestyle develops significant obesity. The forces that drive the body to store excess calories as fat may be related to genetic inheritance and, in a few people, to metabolic imbalances that are a part of endocrine disorders such as hypothyroidism, Cushing's syndrome, and Turner's syndrome. Obesity is a serious, legitimate, and often frustrating metabolic problem deserving proper medical treatment.

The accumulation of excess body fat can occur all over the body, mainly in the hips and buttocks (called the female or gynoid fat pattern), or mainly in the abdomen (the male or android fat pattern). People suffering from significant obesity have an increased risk for medical problems as diverse as gout, gallbladder disease, degenerative arthritis, and sleep apnea (intermittent cessation of breathing during sleep). In addition, obese people more frequently experience other serious medical conditions such as hypertension, elevated blood triglycerides, low HDL cholesterol, atherosclerosis, coronary heart disease, stroke, and diabetes mellitus; these disorders occur more commonly in people with the android pattern of fat than in those with the gynoid variety.

Treatment of obesity is notoriously difficult and requires diligence and commitment for a long time on the part of both the obese person and the doctor. Although certain medications may help reduce weight in the short term, the cornerstone of therapy is lifestyle modification of diet and exercise. See Chapter 2 for more information on weight loss.

Medications useful in the treatment of obesity have begun to receive renewed medical interest in the last several years. Some of these medications are available over the counter (products containing phenylpropanolamine or ephedrine, both of which are mild stimulants and appetite suppressants) while others require a prescription (phentermine, mazindol, fenfluramine, dexfenfluramine, diethylpropion, phenmetrazine, and fluoxetine). These medications fall into two broad classes, the vasoactive amines and the serotonergic medications. The amines work to curb appetite in general and the serotonergics work to provide the brain with more of the feel-good brain chemical, serotonin. This chemical messenger quiets the brain centers controlling appetite, increasing the sense of satisfaction. Decreased production of or response to serotonin has been implicated in chronic overeating disorders, binge eating, and carbohydrate craving. (The medical community still debates whether carbohydrate craving or addiction even exists, with proponents on both sides of the issue.) The downside associated with use of medications to treat obesity are exemplified by the warning of the Food and Drug Administration (FDA) concerning the risk associated with ephedrine and by the withdrawal of fenfluramine (Pondimin) and dexfenfluramine (Redux) from the market. At present, cutting down on calories and increasing activity level are the primary, and safest, ways to accomplish weight loss. ■

stead, the ADA has adopted the policy that diet should be tailored to the needs of each patient.

The more precisely you follow the nutritional regimen prescribed by your doctor, the less impact type 2 diabetes will have on your health.

In people with diabetes who are troubled by delayed stomach emptying, medications such as metoclopramide may help to make absorption of food, and therefore blood glucose levels, more predictable.

Prognosis Good for a normal, productive life with early diagnosis and careful adherence to treatment. Poor if undiagnosed or carelessly treated.

❖ HYPOGLYCEMIA

Symptoms (*What you may experience*) Racing pulse; anxiety; headache; sweating; hand tremors; strange tingling sensations; hunger; confused thinking or speech; loss of consciousness.

Signs and laboratory findings (*What the doctor looks for*) Sweating; visible pallor; low blood glucose.

What is it? Hypoglycemia, which means low blood glucose, is a disorder of excess insulin action. There are two types of hypoglycemia: fasting hypoglycemia and postrandial hypoglycemia (the former is far more dangerous than the latter). Fasting hypoglycemia can occur for a variety of reasons including the following:

- *Excessive insulin administration.* Because people with type 1 diabetes have little or no ability to produce and release insulin on demand, they must estimate their insulin need to be able to administer set doses of insulin by injection. As a consequence, their chief means of keeping blood glucose within the normal range is constancy in meal content, meal timing, and daily exercise. If something disrupts their routine—for example, if they they administer their insulin doses as usual but fail to eat - sufficient amounts of food—they may experience hypoglycemia. The same phenomenon can occur if people with type 1 diabetes administer their usual doses of insulin or oral hypoglycemic medication and exceed their usual levels of exercise. (*Warning:* Rapid development of hypoglycemia can be life-threatening in people with diabetes taking insulin shots. See Type 1 Diabetes Mellitus, page 1174, for more information about this severe form of hypoglycemia.)

- *Insulinoma.* Since one of insulin's main roles is to regulate blood glucose in a controlled fashion, the secretion of insulin is governed by a variety of factors. The production of excessive amounts of insulin by insulin-producing tumors outside this carefully controlled system can result in unpredictable reductions of blood glucose with accompanying symptoms of hypoglycemia.

- *Liver disease.* Because of the central role played by the liver in supporting blood glucose levels (via its manufacture of new glucose from amino acids) during times of fasting, damage to the liver can impair this process. Hepatitis and liver tumors are the most common causes.

- *Adrenal insufficiency.* The corticosteroid hormone produced by the adrenal glands participates in regulation and support of blood glucose levels during periods of fasting. Inadequate amounts of cortisol can lead to impairment of glucose regulation and episodes of hypoglycemia. Replacement of corticosteroids, especially during stress periods, can relieve the problem.

Postprandial hypoglycemia occurs after meals. After we eat, we digest the meal, breaking down the foods into absorbable units. Upon absorption, among other things that happen, blood glucose rises. The rising glucose level in the blood signals the pancreas that it needs to release insulin, which will send the glucose into the cells of various tissues for immediate use or storage. When insulin does its job, blood glucose falls, returning the system to normal. Some people, however, exhibit an exaggerated release of insulin—or an exaggerated response to its action—and blood glucose falls too far and too fast, resulting in unpleasant symptoms. The symptoms of postprandial (meaning after a meal) hypoglycemia occur in response to the speed and degree of blood glucose drop, not necessarily to the blood glucose level itself. For example, a rapid drop in blood glucose from 180 to 100 mg/dL might cause symptoms of hypoglycemia, whereas a slow steady decline from 140 to 60 mg/dL might not even be noticed, even though 60 mg/dL is a much lower reading. For that reason, measurement of the blood glucose level may not always be a good indicator of the disorder. In addition, measuring blood glucose levels in the postprandial form of this disorder can be tricky because the very development of hypoglycemia causes the release of counter-regulatory hormones that rapidly raise blood glucose levels back to normal. Consequently, measuring glucose values must be done during the very short period before levels correct. The standard test for this disorder is the 5-hour glucose tolerance test.

What you can do In the postprandial variety of the disorder, preventing swings in blood glucose is important, and the best way to keep blood glucose stable is to reduce the dietary content of rapidly absorbed carbohydrates: simple sugars (such as sucrose or those found in corn syrup, fruit juices, and honey) and refined starches (such as those found in white or highly processed flours and meals and in foods made from these substances). Include some protein and a small amount of fat in each meal. Strive for constancy in nutrition and exercise to keep blood glucose stable. Never allow yourself to go for long periods without eating, and never eat too much at one meal. Smaller, more frequent meals will keep you in tighter blood glucose control.

Quickly restoring blood glucose to a normal level can be crucial if symptoms of hypoglycemia develop in people who have diabetes or other causes of fasting hypoglycemia. This is especially true for people with type 1 diabetes who develop hypoglycemia. Keep a supply of glucose tablets or small hard sugar candies that can be carried in a pill box with you at all times. Use only a few to bring blood glucose up a bit, then eat a well-balanced meal as quickly as possible. Avoid taking too much simple sugar to restore blood glucose, since you may drive your glucose up too high.

When to call the doctor If symptoms of hypoglycemia are frequent, severe, or do not respond to a stable, regimented diet and exercise schedule, other causes for your symptoms should be looked for. Unconsciousness or fainting demand immediate emergency treatment.

Treatment The swift restoration of blood glucose in response to fasting hypoglycemia will involve the administration of glucose solutions by vein if the symptoms have been severe enough to cause fainting or loss of consciousness. The cornerstone of treatment is nutrition and exercise. Careful adherence to dietary and exercise recommendations is all that should be required in postprandial hypoglycemia. A search for other causes—such as insulin-secreting tumors or other hormonal imbalances—may be necessary if the condition persists.

Prognosis Excellent in those people who commit themselves to following proper nutritional and exercise directions carefully.

❖ ISLET CELL TUMORS

Symptoms *(What you may experience)* Symptoms depend on which islet cell is involved: glucagonoma from alpha cells, insulinoma from beta cells, and gastrinoma from delta cells.

- Glucagonoma: weight loss; glossodynia (painful tongue); red rash, mild diabetes.

- Insulinoma: symptoms similar to those of insulin reaction (see page 1177)—sweating, mental confusion, rapid heart beat, seizures, coma, and more.

- Gastrinoma: gnawing, burning stomachache that progressively worsens despite eating food or taking antacid medications; watery diarrhea (sometimes).

Signs and laboratory findings *(What the doctor looks for)* Vary depending on the tumor. In insulinomas, markedly elevated blood insulin and low blood glucose. In glucagonomas, excessive blood glucagon and glucose along with a peculiar rash termed necrolytic migratory erythema. In gastrinomas, the stomach secretes excessive amounts of acid detectable by examination of the gastric juices.

What is it? The cells of the pancreatic islets of Langerhans can develop tumors, though this is a rare condition. These abnormal clusters of alpha, beta, or delta cells within the islets may produce and secrete exaggerated amounts of the hormonal product of that cell, sometimes giving rise to serious effects.

An insulinoma produces an unpredictable and exaggerated amount of insulin that acts to drive blood glucose too low in the same manner as does a shot of insulin. The reactions seem to occur more often with exercise or after an overnight fast (that is, before breakfast in the morning). More than 90 percent of insulinomas occur as benign, single, isolated tumors. Occasionally, they occur as a part of a syndrome—termed multiple endocrine neoplasias (MEN)—involving tumors of other hormone producing tissues, such as the pituitary or parathyroid glands. Less than 10 percent of insulinomas metastasize (spread) to other tissues.

A glucagonoma produces unpredictable and exaggerated amounts of glucagon. Since this hormone elevates blood glucose, the classic finding is hyperglycemia. The diagnosis often hinges on the appearance of a characteristic rash on the skin.

Because the hormone gastrin stimulates the stomach to secrete acid and juices of digestion, a gastrinoma—producing erratic release of abnormally high amounts of gastrin—causes severe ulcer disease. The ulcers may involve not only the stomach, but the duodenum (upper intestine) and small intestine as well. The standard therapies employed to treat ulcers usually do not work. Zollinger-Ellison is the name given to this disorder, in which excessive gastrin secretion causes ulcers, diarrhea, and stomach pain that are unresponsive to treatment. The excessive gastric acid in the intestine can lead to malabsorption of nutrients and watery diarrhea.

About 60 percent of both gastrinomas and glucagonomas are malignant and will spread to other organs.

What you can do For insulinoma and glucagonoma, small frequent meals may be helpful to stabilize blood glucose, but this should not replace a visit to a doctor. Gastrinoma usually does not respond to self-therapy.

When to call the doctor The appearance of the symptoms of islet cell tumors merits immediate investigation by a doctor, more specifically by an internal medicine specialist or an endocrinologist.

Treatment Definitive treatment involves locating and removing the offending tissue. Because insulinoma and glucagonoma tumors are richly supplied with blood vessels, they can probably best be identified by angiography. In these studies, dye (also known as contrast material) visible on x-ray is injected into arteries supplying an area near the suspected tumor. The rich blood vessel supply of the tumor will then show up on x-ray pictures, clearly outlining the extent of the tumor. Occasionally, they are too small to be visualized and the doctor will have to look directly by opening the abdominal cavity.

If removal of the tissue is not possible, chemotherapy (administration of a combination of powerful anticancer medications) can sometimes reduce tumor size and decrease hormone production.

Gastrinoma tumors may be small and difficult to locate, but angiography may occasionally find them as well. Computed tomography (CT) or magnetic resonance imaging (MRI) scans can locate more than 70 percent of tumors at least 1 cm in size and 90 percent of those at least 3 cm in size that have spread to the liver. Removal of the tumor should reduce gastrin production to normal; however, if surgery is not possible, or if surgical removal does not lower gastrin production sufficiently to improve symptoms, long-term treatment with the gastric acid inhibitor omeprazole may help. It may be necessary to remove the stomach surgically to prevent the formation of recurrent ulcers.

Prognosis Excellent in most cases if caught before significant metastases have occurred.

Disorders of the Thyroid Gland

The thyroid gland, shaped like a butterfly and lying across the base of the neck in front of the trachea (windpipe), produces thyroid hormone. This hormone affects nearly every tissue in the body, governing such diverse activities as protein building and breakdown, cholesterol production, the pace of cell activity, fat tissue breakdown, menstrual cycling, heart rhythms, and more.

In addition, specialized cells, called C cells produce a second hormone, calcitonin, which is involved in the maintenance of normal calcium balance and the preservation of bone density by preventing breakdown of bone.

A recent study at Johns Hopkins University suggests that screening people over age 35, especially women, for underactive thyroid hormone should become part of routine, periodic physical exams. Early detection and treatment of mild thyroid failure offer substantial health benefits, given the wide-ranging effect thyroid hormones have within the body.

❖ HYPERTHYROIDISM (GRAVES' DISEASE)

Symptoms *(What you may experience)* Sweating; heart palpitations; unusually rapid heart beat; muscle weakness; tremors; nervousness and irritability; difficulty sleeping; frequent stools; weight loss despite a hearty appetite; intolerance to warm temperatures; onycholysis or separation of nails from the nailbed (sometimes painful); bulging of the eyes. Sometimes: vision changes; reduced menstrual flow; impotence; gynecomastia (breast enlargement in men).

Signs and laboratory findings *(What the doctor looks for)* Prominent wide-eyed stare, also called exophthalmos; reddened palms; tremor; rapid pulse; changes in heart sounds (murmurs or scratches); onycholysis; plaques of thickened skin on the lower legs, also called pretibial myxedema; clubbed (misshapen) fingers; nontender goiter (swelling in the front of the neck due to enlargement of the thyroid gland); abnormal laboratory blood test results, specifically a low thyroid-stimulating hormone (TSH) level, elevated levels of thyroid hor-

BRAIN CONTROL OF HORMONES

Although the pituitary gland is located in the brain, its anterior portion is not true brain tissue, originating instead during fetal development from the structures that form the throat. This anterior part, which regulates the levels of many other hormones, is itself under the control of higher centers in the brain—located in the hypothalamus—which produces an array of hormones that either stimulate or inhibit the release of specific hormones by the pituitary. For example, if blood levels of thyroid hormone fall too low, this deficiency signals the hypothalamus to release thyrotropin-releasing hormone. Thyrotropin-releasing hormone stimulates the pituitary to release thyroid-stimulating hormone (TSH), which in turn stimulates the thyroid gland to manufacture and release more thyroid hormone. The higher levels of thyroid hormone in the blood will cause the hypothalamus to shut off its stimulation of the system.

Through this interplay of hormonal signals—called the hypothalamic-pituitary axis—the brain influences the production and release of thyroid and other hormones. For example, the pituitary produces luteinizing hormone (LH) to trigger the production of sex hormones and adrenocorticotrophic hormone (ACTH) to stimulate the release of cortisol from the adrenal gland. ■

The hypothalamus secretes thyroid-releasing hormone (TRH), which causes the anterior pituitary gland to release thyroid stimulating hormone (TSH). TSH triggers the thyroid's follicle cells to release thyroid hormone into the bloodstream. The amount of thyroid hormone in the blood is sensed by the hypothalamus and anterior pituitary gland. If there is too much thyroid hormone in the blood, the hypothalamus responds by reducing the production and release of TRH and the pituitary by reducing production and release of TSH. If there is too little thyroid hormone in the blood, the hypothalamus and pituitary respond by increasing the secretion of TRH and TSH, respectively. T3, triiodothyronine; T4, thyroxine.

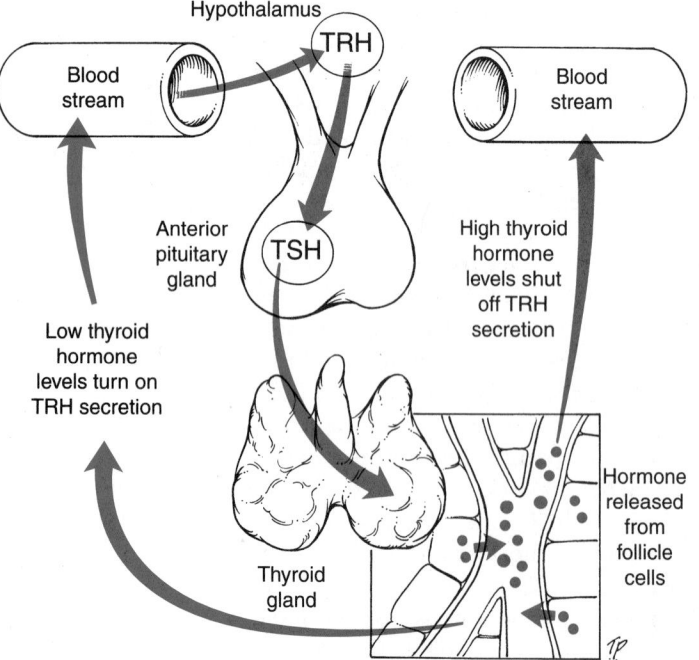

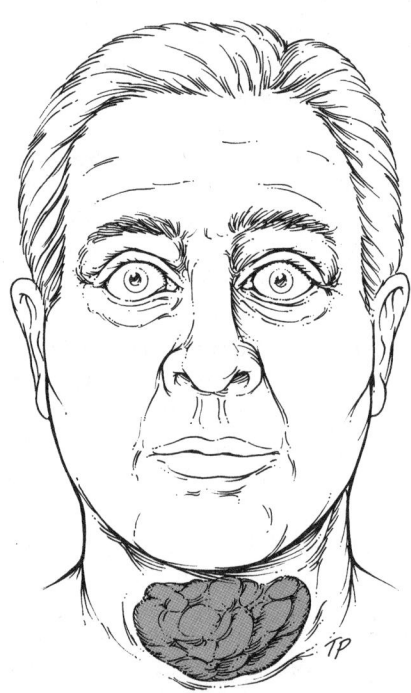

Graves' disease is caused by an overactive thyroid gland. People with Graves' disease have an enlarged thyroid gland and often bulging of the eyeballs (exophthalmos).

mones, and antibodies that mimic the function of TSH and cause inappropriate stimulation of thyroid hormone production (sometimes).

What is it? Graves' disease—also called diffuse toxic goiter—is the most common cause of hyperthyroidism (excess thyroid hormone production). Graves' disease is an autoimmune thyroid disorder (meaning that the body's immune defense system mistakenly attacks thyroid tissue) that occurs more often in women than in men. What causes the condition to develop is not yet clearly understood.

Often the most serious and difficult-to-manage problems associated with Graves' disease are those involving the eyes. For reasons that are poorly understood, the bulging of the eyes can in some instances be so severe as to cause paralysis of the muscles that move the eyeball in its socket. The conjunctivae (the filmy membranes covering the eye) and the eyelids can become inflamed and swollen and the cornea (the clear cover over the pupil and colored portion of the eye) can become ulcerated or infected, causing blurring and even loss of vision.

In elderly people, who may have some degree of heart disease, the diagnosis of hyperthyroidism may be missed because the increase in hormone production may not cause typical symptoms of hyperthyroidism, but might strain the heart. The added strain could cause or worsen angina (chest pain), stimulate abnormal heart rhythms (most commonly, the condition called atrial fibrillation, in which the upper small chambers of the heart contract in a disorganized, ineffective manner), or congestive heart failure. Heart-related symptoms in this group of people may be the first indication of thyroid hormone overproduction.

The use of beta-blocker medications—for example, propranolol (Inderal)—can mask some symptoms of excess thyroid hormone, such as rapid heartbeat, palpitations, and tremors, making the correct diagnosis a bit trickier. These medications do not alter thyroid blood test results, which can still be used to identify the condition.

What you can do There are no specific self-care remedies for Graves' disease; however, in the case of severe eye bulging, keeping the eyes well lubricated with artificial tears or saline solution can help to prevent drying and ulceration of the cornea.

When to call the doctor The symptoms of hyperthyroidism warrant a prompt visit to the doctor. Early identification and treatment may prevent the development of severe eye symptoms associated with Graves' disease. Treatment of the hyperthyroidism, however, may not change the course of eye disease once it is established.

Treatment Corrective measures for hyperthyroidism fall into three categories: administration of antithyroid medications, administration of radioactive iodine, and, least commonly, surgical removal of most of the gland (subtotal thyroidectomy). Each therapy has advantages and disadvantages.

Antithyroid medications, usually either methimazole (Tapazole) or propylthiouracil, act to block the formation of thyroid hormone. Because the treatment may need to continue for at least 12 to 18 months and thyroid hormone deficiency may occur, progress of therapy is followed by measuring blood thyroid hormone levels. Hypothyroidism caused by antithyroid medications usually is treated by reducing the dosage of the medication. A small minority of experts

THYROID STORM

Occasionally, in some people, hyperthyroidism escalates to a dangerous degree with a massive outpouring of thyroid hormone sufficient to produce a condition called thyroid storm. In this exaggerated form, people with stable or sometimes previously unrecognized hyperthyroidism develop severe symptoms consisting of extreme restlessness, high fever, very rapid heartrate, profuse sweating, and dehydration that could lead to circulatory collapse (shock) if not treated. The onset of thyroid storm may follow an infection, surgery, or trauma to the thyroid gland or may occur upon completion of courses of medication for hyperthyroid treatment. This condition demands emergency medical treatment, which usually corrects the condition promptly. ■

now use a combination of levothyroxine and antithyroid medications.

Since the 1940s several million people have been treated with radioactive iodine. Most cases of Graves' disease respond to this treatment, which relies on the fact that the thyroid gland uniquely gathers and concentrates iodine. This specificity allows the doctor to target only the thyroid gland with a dose of radiation, sparing the rest of the body. This method, like all therapies for hyperthyroidism, carries the risk of overshooting the mark and the subsequent development of thyroid deficiency. Treatment with radioactive iodine avoids the potential complications of any surgery (that is, the risk of bleeding or infection or risks associated with anesthesia) as well as the risks of accidental removal of the parathyroid glands and hoarseness. Radiation risk to the ovaries from radioactive iodine has never been proven, and although the risk exists for women of child-bearing age, administration of radioactive iodine is still a better option than surgery in this group. It should not be used, however, in pregnant women.

Surgical removal of most of the thyroid gland will halt the disorder. Although the procedure is not risky, the potential complications include the development of hypothyroidism, accidental removal of all four of the nearby parathyroid glands leading to hypoparathyroidism, or accidental damage to the nerve supply to the larynx (voice box), leading to vocal cord paralysis and hoarseness. In the hands of an experienced surgeon the operation rarely leads to these complications; however, surgery is now the last resort treatment, reserved primarily for people who cannot or will not take antithyroid medication or radioactive iodine.

Prognosis Excellent for alleviating all symptoms with the exception of the eye symptoms which often do not reverse upon normalizing thyroid function. Severe eye symptoms require the expert care of an ophthalmologist.

❖ HYPOTHYROIDISM

Symptoms *(What you may experience)* Intolerance to cold temperatures; fluid retention; changes in the texture of hair, skin, or nails; hoarseness; constipation; menstrual cycle changes (usually irregularly spaced, heavier periods), headache; pain in muscles and joints; abnormal nerve sensations such as the feeling of pins and needles, burning sensations, or numbness (sometimes). Fatigue, apathy, or depression may also occur.

Signs and laboratory findings *(What the doctor looks for)* Coarse hair; hair loss; dry skin; edema (swelling, especially in the legs and feet); gravelly hoarseness of the voice; slowed relaxation of reflexes; an enlarged, firm thyroid gland (often); decreased blood levels of thyroid hormones accompanied by an increase in the blood level of TSH.

What is it? Low levels of thyroid hormones result 95 percent of the time from inadequate production due to an abnormality in the thyroid gland, which can occur for a variety of reasons. Only 5 percent of cases of hypothyroidism occur because of deficiency of stimulating factors from the brain centers that regulate its release, the pituitary or hypothalamus. In these cases, the levels of TSH are not elevated.

Because thyroid hormone influences such a wide range of body functions, its deficiency can cause many seemingly disparate symptoms. The kind and severity of symptoms of hypothyroidism depend upon the degree of the deficiency as well as upon the age and gender of the person with the deficiency. In myxedema, the most severe degree of hypothyroidism, the affected person may exhibit not only the dry and thick skin, enlargement of facial features, constipation, cold intolerance, and menstrual changes that characterize the disorder, but also a significant degree of apathy. The depression and slowing of speech and reactions becomes so extreme in some cases—to the point of coma sometimes—that prior to the discovery of thyroid hormone and its effects, patients suffering from myxedema were often institutionalized in facilities for the hopelessly insane and left there while their disease became progressively worse.

In milder forms of the disorder—such as those that we usually see today—the symptoms arise gradually, and any one or group of the possible symptoms can predominate. Some people experience primarily hair, skin, and nail changes, while others complain of constipation or muscle and joint symptoms. Because the symptoms develop slowly and progressively, subtle changes in voice, facial features, hair, and skin may be apparent only to a person who has not seen the affected person for a long period of time.

Goiter does not always occur, but when present, may help clinch the diagnosis. The most common cause of hypothyroidism is autoimmune destruction of the thyroid gland, a condition termed Hashimoto's thyroiditis (see page 1189). Treatment of hyperthyroidism also can cause hypothyroidism, either temporarily, following therapy with medication to curb the excessive thyroid hormone output, or permanently, following radioactive iodine therapy or surgical removal of the gland as treatment for hyperthyroidism, thyroid nodules, or cancer.

Even though the problem is in the thyroid gland itself in most people with hypothyroidism, in some cases the disorder arises from lack of stimulation due to decreased secretion of TSH by the pituitary gland. This condition will cause low blood levels of both the thyroid hormones and TSH. Making this determination is critical, since hypothyroidism from this cause may represent the earliest evidence of a pituitary tumor.

When to call the doctor In the case of myxedema, immediate medical care is crucial. Otherwise, a doctor should be consulted promptly when symptoms suggestive of hypothyroidism appear.

Treatment After the diagnosis of hypothyroidism is made, treatment involves life-long replacement with thyroid hormone pills to restore the blood thyroid hormones to normal levels.

Prognosis Excellent with diagnosis and appropriate thyroid hormone replacement therapy.

❖ HASHIMOTO'S THYROIDITIS

Symptoms *(What you may experience)* Goiter with or without the symptoms characteristic of hypothyroidism (see Hypothyroidism, page 1188).

Signs and laboratory findings *(What the doctor looks for)* Diffuse swelling and firmness of the thyroid gland on physical examination; characteristic antithyroid antibodies in the blood; low levels of thyroid hormones (usually); elevation of TSH. Early in the course of the disease, thyroid hormone levels may be high.

What is it? Chronic thyroiditis, termed Hashimoto's thyroiditis, is responsible for virtually 100 percent of cases of primary hypothyroidism in adults. It occurs when the body's immune defense system mistakenly attacks the thyroid gland, setting off cycles of chronic inflammation, destruction, and scarring that limit the gland's ability to produce a sufficient amount of thyroid hormone to meet normal needs; any or all of the potential symptoms of hypothyroidism may follow. Hashimoto's thyroiditis may occur in conjunction with other autoimmune disorders such as Addison's disease (see page 1197), pernicious anemia, myasthenia gravis (neuromuscular disease causing progressive weakness), early ovarian failure, or diabetes mellitus.

When to call the doctor Any unusual swelling in the vicinity of the thyroid gland warrants a visit to the doctor; however, most cases of chronic thyroiditis are found incidentally on routine examination by a doctor. Development of the symptoms of hypothyroidism or of other associated autoimmune disorders warrants a prompt visit to the doctor.

Treatment The cornerstone of treatment

REPLACING THYROID HORMONES

Replacement of thyroid hormone is done with levothyroxine, a synthetic form of thyroid hormone. The dosage of levothyroxine depends largely on the body weight of the person being treated. The proper dosage is achieved by following the level of TSH until it returns to normal. Care must be taken not to over-replace the hormone—signaled by the TSH becoming too low—since excessive replacement can increase the risk of osteoporosis (weakening of bones due to loss of bone mass). Your doctor will follow your progress through periodic blood tests to measure thyroid hormone and TSH levels. In elderly people or those with known heart disease, replacement is started with a low dosage that is increased slowly to avoid the risk of over-stimulating the heart, which can cause rhythm disturbances, angina, or possibly a myocardial infarction. People taking medications that interfere with absorption of the hormone from the intestine or alter the metabolism of thyroid hormone may need higher dosages of thyroid hormone. The need to supplement with the hormone persists indefinitely. ■

is thyroid hormone replacement with levothyroxine (synthetic thyroid medication) in dosages sufficient to restore normal thyroid hormone levels. In many cases, the antithyroid antibodies disappear during thyroid hormone treatment, but once Hashimoto's produces hypothyroidism, thyroid hormone replacement must continue for life.

Occasionally, one area of the inflamed gland may seem firm enough to raise concerns of possible thyroid cancer. The doctor may recommend a fine needle biopsy (sampling of tissue for microscopic examination) to investigate this possibility. In fine needle biopsy, a slender needle is used to remove tissue.

Prognosis Excellent with timely diagnosis and proper medical treatment.

❖ GOITER

Symptoms *(What you may experience)* Swelling in the front of the neck on one or both sides of the trachea; difficulty swallowing or restriction in breathing (sometimes). Other symptoms that might occur depend on whether the enlarged gland produces an amount of thyroid hormone that is normal (causing no other symptoms), elevated (causing symptoms of hyperthyroidism), or reduced (causing symptoms of hypothyroidism).

Signs and laboratory findings *(What the doctor looks for)* Enlargement of the thyroid gland, lumps within the gland, and tenderness, firmness, or asymmetry of the gland; abnormal thyroid gland function or antibodies against thyroid tissue as detected by blood tests; signs of hypothyroidism (see page 1188) or hyperthyroidism (see page 1185).

What is it? Goiter is the term applied to enlargement of the thyroid gland. This condition once occurred commonly in many areas of the United States (called the goiter belt) in which the soil contained very little iodine. Because thyroid hormone production depends on iodine, a deficiency of iodine causes the gland to grow larger to compensate for the poor production of the hormone. The thyroid gland is usually able to compensate well such that blood levels of thyroid hormone are usually within the normal range and symptoms of hypothyrodism or hyperthyroidism are rare. Thanks to the routine iodizing of salt and the availability of seafood, goiter from iodine defi-

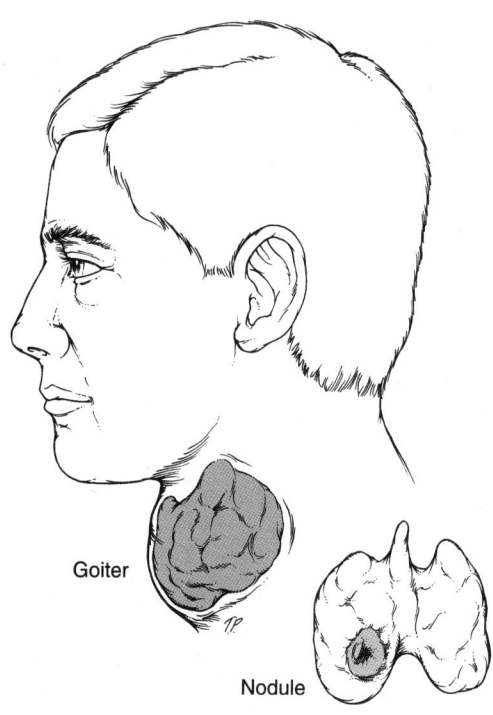

Goiter

Nodule

A goiter is any enlargement of the thyroid gland. One type of goiter, colloid goiter, can cause massive enlargement of the thyroid due to the presence of multiple nodules that give the gland a bumpy appearance. Thyroid nodules, however, are quite common and are generally not associated with noticeable enlargement of the thyroid.

ciency rarely occurs nowadays in developed countries.

When goiter does occur, sometimes the gland enlarges uniformly throughout both its lobes (simple goiter), but other times, only one lobe may enlarge (asymmetric goiter), or the swelling may be localized in one or more discrete lumps (nodular goiter). Depending on the degree of enlargement, because of the gland's location across the trachea the goiter may put pressure on the structures behind it and cause difficulty swallowing or restriction in breathing that may mimic asthma. Evaluation of the gland begins with the doctor feeling the gland to delineate its size and texture. Next, an ultrasound test—carried out by painlessly passing sound waves through the gland—can determine with 90 percent accuracy if the lumps are solid or fluid-filled cysts. Following these measures, the doctor may recommend scanning the gland (see What Does the Thyroid Scan Show?, this page).

What you can do Make certain your diet contains the recommended amount of

WHAT DOES THE THYROID SCAN SHOW?

The thyroid scan—called a radionuclide study—determines where the thyroid tissue takes up and concentrates radioactive iodine (^{123}I) or technetium (^{99}Tc). Where these radioactive substances concentrate and show up on the scan picture demonstrates the areas of functioning thyroid tissue. The scan is especially important when the physical examination detects lumps or nodules within the gland. If the thyroid scan shows that these nodules actively take up the tracer material, they are rarely cancerous. However, if the nodules show up cold on the scan, meaning the tissue took up none of the tracer and therefore does not produce thyroid hormone, the risk of thyroid cancer increases. As many as 10 percent of single, solid, cold nodules may prove cancerous. ∎

iodine, about 150 mcg per day. The easiest way to do this is to use iodized table salt (about 2 g of table salt provides the required minimum). Seafood is another excellent dietary source, especially important for people who must restrict salt consumption for other reasons.

When to call the doctor Although most goiters are benign, because the swelling of the gland may involve a thyroid cancer in a minority of cases, see your doctor if you discover a goiter.

Treatment Appropriate treatment depends on the nature and extent of the goiter. Minimally enlarged simple goiters usually demand no treatment. The presence of swallowing or breathing difficulty demands evaluation with x-rays (a regular x-ray and a barium swallow test) to determine how much the goiter compresses the trachea or esophagus. Significant compression usually requires surgery to remove part of the gland.

Lumps within the goiter present a different problem (see Benign Thyroid Nodules, below).

Prognosis Excellent with prompt diagnosis and appropriate surgical treatment when needed.

❖ BENIGN THYROID NODULES

Symptoms *(What you may experience)* None (usually).

Signs and laboratory findings *(What the doctor looks for)* One or more small, nontender lumps in the body of the thyroid gland and normal thyroid hormone levels (usually).

What is it? These usually harmless, small nodules in the thyroid gland may occur singly or in multiples (nodular goiter). Their cause remains unknown. Occasionally one nodule may become overactive and produce large enough amounts of thyroid hormone to suppress the release of TSH, resulting in reduced function in the rest of the thyroid gland. Small (less than 2.5 cm) nodules that still produce thyroid hormone (called hot nodules) can usually be watched safely without treatment. Larger hot nodules may cause severe hyperthyroidism and

require removal or destruction by radioactive iodine. Nodules that do not produce thyroid hormone (cold nodules) always require the consideration of surgical removal since they may represent thyroid cancer. The determination of whether a nodule is cold is made by performing a thyroid scan (see page 1190). The nodule is determined not to be cold if the radioactive tracer is concentrated in the area matching the location of the nodule.

When to call the doctor Any lump in the thyroid gland requires prompt investigation by a doctor.

Treatment Although most thyroid nodules are benign, thyroid cancer can be ruled out only by doing a fine needle biopsy of the nodules. Surgery is done to remove the whole lobe or whole thyroid if malignant cells are seen under the microscope. Benign nodules can be watched safely.

Prognosis Excellent with proper medical or surgical management.

❖ THYROID CANCER

Symptoms *(What you may experience)* A firm lump in the neck in the region of the trachea; painless swollen lymph glands in the neck; spinal or pelvic bone pain; fractures of the spine or pelvis with minimal trauma (rarely); hoarseness (occasionally); protracted diarrhea unresponsive to therapy (in some cases).

Signs and laboratory findings *(What the doctor looks for)* Firm to hard nodule on physical examination of the thyroid gland; firm, enlarged, nontender lymph nodes in the neck; pathologic fractures of the spine or pelvis as detected by x-rays (rarely); elevation of the hormone calcitonin in the blood (sometimes).

What is it? Thyroid cancers are uncommon, and most thyroid lumps prove to be benign nodules, but all lumps demand thorough evaluation to rule out cancer. Cancers of the thyroid gland come in four varieties: papillary or follicular cancers (or a mixture of the two), medullary cancers, and undifferentiated thyroid cancers. In the vast majority of cases, especially in people under age 40, thyroid cancers grow very slowly and remain close to their origin, rarely metastasizing beyond lymph nodes in the area close by. These cancers tend to be of the papillary or mixed papillary/follicular type and are so slow growing and mild that it is difficult to distinguish them from benign thyroid nodules. Follicular cancers occur less commonly and tend to spread via the bloodstream to the lungs and to the bone.

Medullary thyroid cancers arise from the thyroid C cells that produce calcitonin, and elevated levels of this hormone may be detectable on blood tests. This form of thyroid cancer may occur as a part of one of the inherited endocrine disorders called MEN 2 syndrome, also involving tumors of the parathyroid and adrenal medulla (pheochromocytomas). Medullary thyroid cancers often metastasize and are lethal unless removed early.

Only very rarely do cancers in the thyroid gland develop as the rapidly growing and invasive tumors called undifferentiated thyroid cancers. Progressively worsening hoarseness due to no other apparent cause and raspy, whistling breathing noises (also called stridor) may indicate compression of the trachea and larynx caused by this kind of cancer.

Although inheritance plays a role in thyroid cancer risk, especially in the case of medullary thyroid cancers, the most consistent risk factor for thyroid cancers is exposure to neck irradiation in childhood. In the past (30 or 40 years ago), doctors often used radiation to treat such problems as acne or enlargement of the tonsils or thymus gland. The long-term effect of what was then considered safe and effective treatment is an increased risk of thyroid cancer later in life. The risk increases directly with the amount of radiation used. The highest risk occurs in women who received irradiation in childhood.

What you can do Any persistent or growing, firm lump in the neck demands evaluation by a doctor. Do not attempt to treat yourself or to ignore such a finding.

When to call the doctor Contact a doctor as soon as possible after discovering a lump.

Treatment The direction therapy should take depends on the type of thyroid cancer involved. Your doctor may recommend a thyroid scan (see page 1190) to determine if the lump consists of functioning thyroid tissue or not; in many cases an ultrasound examination is conducted to determine if the lump is a fluid-filled cyst or solid mass. Fine needle biopsy is usually carried out. Many doctors initially do a fine needle biopsy, bypassing the thyroid scan or ultrasound, since the vast majority of nodules are cold. All cold nodules that can be felt, especially in people with a history of irradiation to the neck in childhood, demand medical evaluation and fine needle biopsy. The gland is removed surgically if cancer is detected.

Prognosis Very good for papillary and follicular thyroid cancers, especially in people under age 40 (cure rates are as high as 86 percent). The prognosis for these forms of thyroid cancer is not as good for people over age 60. Medullary cancers, if caught early and treated surgically also can be cured but do not have as good a prognosis as papillary tumors. Undifferentiated (primitive) cell cancers are more aggressive and survival rates are low.

Disorders of the Parathyroid Glands

The parathyroid glands, two pairs (occasionally more) of pea-sized collections of tissue, lie on either side of and behind the thyroid gland. They produce and release parathyroid hormone (PTH), the chief regulator of calcium balance through actions on the bone, the kidney, and the intestine. The level of calcium in the blood controls the release of PTH: a low level stimulates release and a high level shuts off release. PTH maintains the level of calcium in the blood by enhancing absorption of calcium from the diet by stimulating the kidneys to produce the active form of vitamin D. Once active, vitamin D prompts an increase in intestinal absorption of dietary calcium. PTH also increases calcium availability in the blood by slowing down the accumulation of calcium in bones as well as by speeding up its removal from them. In the kidney, in addition to its role of increasing production of active vitamin D, this hormone enhances the reabsorption of calcium from the urine. Abnormalities in the parathyroid gland can lead to a variety of problems relating to calcium metabolism.

❖ HYPERPARATHYROIDISM

Symptoms *(What you may experience)* Easy muscle fatigue and weakness; abdominal pain; constipation; loss of appetite; thirst; frequent urination; bone pain; spontaneous bone fractures; kidney stones; sleepiness; fatigue; depression; apathy; personality changes.

Signs and laboratory findings *(What the doctor looks for)* Elevated PTH and calcium levels in the blood along with low blood phosphate levels; calcium deposits in kidneys, pancreas, or conjunctival membranes covering the eyes; sluggish reflexes; excessive calcium in the urine; bone abnormalities on x-ray; hypertension; changes on the electrocardiogram; unexplained weight loss.

What is it? This disorder arises when the parathyroid glands produce an excessive amount of their hormone, PTH. The term primary hyperparathyroidism applies when the excessive production results from abnormal parathyroid tissue such as a benign or cancerous parathyroid tumor or from hyperplasia (overgrowth of normal glandular tissue). Both hyperplasia and benign tumors (also called adenomas) may have a genetic basis, meaning they are related to abnormalities in the chromosomes and either can occur alone or in conjunction with other endocrine abnormalities in MEN syndromes. Ninety-nine percent of tumors of the parathyroid glands are benign, but occasionally microscopic examination of the parathyroid glands (after they are surgically removed) discloses cancerous tissue. In primary hyperparathyroidism, blood tests always demonstrate an elevated level of calcium, because the hormone's main job is to increase calcium levels.

Secondary hyperparathyroidism denotes excessive PTH production by normal parathyroid tissue in response to increased stimulation to produce (for example, when there is too little calcium and too much phosphorous—calcium's counterbalancing mineral—in the blood). This form of the disease frequently occurs in people with severe kidney disease (see Kidney Failure, page 1078), disorders of the intestine that impair absorption of calcium and vitamin D, or certain bone disorders. The blood level of calcium in these cases could be low, normal, or high.

Hyperparathyroidism can cause acute pancreatitis. It also can cause kidney stones and calcium deposits to accumulate in the kidneys, leading to kidney stones and renal (kidney) failure.

What you can do If your blood has been tested and found to have increased calcium levels, you should stop taking supplements of calcium or vitamin D. You should also limit dietary sources high in calcium such as dairy products and soft bones in such fish as salmon, sardines, herring, and mackerel.

When to call the doctor Because blood tests done as part of routine physical exams generally measure calcium, most cases of primary hyperparathyroidism are discovered before problems arise. However, the appearance of any of the broad group of symptoms outlined above warrants a prompt visit to your doctor.

Treatment The only truly effective therapy for primary hyperparathyroidism involves surgical removal of one or more of the parathyroid glands. In overproduction caused by a benign parathyroid tumor—since these usually occur in only one of the four glands—the doctor can remove only the affected gland. In the case of hyperplasia, enlargement involves all four (or more) glands and adequate treatment may require removal of all but about one-half of one gland. This method of treatment must walk a fine line: remove too little, and hyperparathyroidism may recur; remove too much, and hypoparathyroidism may ensue. Extensive surgical removal of a cancerous gland and surrounding tissue offers the only successful control of parathyroid cancer.

Treatment for secondary hyperparathyroidism hinges decreasing the excess stimulation of the gland. In chronic kidney failure, for example, administration of vitamin D to improve intestinal absorption of dietary calcium or medications to decrease phosphorus absorption from the intestine may help normalize the release of PTH.

Elevations of the level of calcium in the blood exceeding 14 mg/dL require emergency measures to bring the calcium down.

HYPERCALCEMIA: ELEVATED BLOOD CALCIUM

The level of blood calcium reflects the balance between calcium absorption from the gastrointestinal tract, its reabsorption from or deposition in bones, and its loss in urine. Hypercalcemia—elevated calcium levels in the blood—occurs when the amount absorbed from food or reabsorbed from the bone exceeds the amount eliminated by the kidneys. The chief causes for this imbalance are hyperparathyroidism and various types of cancer. Other less common causes of elevated blood calcium include medications such as thiazide diuretics, excessive thyroid hormone replacement, vitamin D, and lithium; hyperthyroidism, sarcoidosis (see page 751), and prolonged immobilization.

Signs and symptoms of hypercalcemia, which depend not only on the degree of excess but on how rapidly it develops, can include mental and behavioral disturbances, muscle weakness, hypertension, excessive urination and thirst, nocturnal urination, dehydration, constipation, indigestion, loss of appetite, and nausea and vomiting.

Treatment is aimed at correcting the underlying cause, if possible. The administration of steroid hormone may be an effective treatment for the hypercalcemia resulting from a number of causes. When calcium levels exceed 14 mg/dL, urgent treatment is warranted to reduce the level. The first step is administration of fluids such as intravenous saline solutions accompanied by diuretics such as furosemide. A second step is the use of medications such as calcitonin, etidronate (Didronel), or pamidronate (Aredia) to slow the reabsorption of calcium from bone. ∎

This treatment usually involves the intravenous administration of fluid and potent diuretic medications (agents that increase sodium and water excretion in the urine) to increase the removal of calcium through the urine. Administration of calcitonin by injection twice daily helps in the short run, but its effects wane quickly. Long-term treatment may require the use of synthetic medications (such as etidronate, plicamycin, or pamidronate) that stop more calcium from coming out of the bones.

Prognosis Excellent if the cause is discovered and treated promptly. Benign parathyroid tumors are cured by surgical removal and the prognosis is excellent. For cancers of the parathyroid, early identification followed by aggressive initial surgery and appropriate medical therapy results in 85 percent survival at 5 years and about 60 percent at 10 years.

❖ HYPOPARATHYROIDISM

Symptoms (*What you may experience*) Fatigue; muscle aching and cramps; numbness and burning around the lips and fingers; restlessness; depression; emotional and intellectual changes.

Signs and laboratory findings (*What the doctor looks for*) Brisk, overly reactive reflexes; changes on the electrocardiogram; low levels of calcium and PTH in the blood.

What is it? Hypoparathyroidism can result from deficient production of PTH by the parathyroid glands, or it can be a consequence of resistance to the hormone's action in the body (pseudohypoparathyroidism). Deficient amounts of PTH occur most commonly following surgery on the thyroid gland with inadvertent removal of or damage to all the parathyroid glands. This form of the disorder develops quite rapidly following thyroid surgery. Deficiency of the mineral magnesium—a condition common in alcoholics and other malnourished people—can slow the release of PTH and blunt its effect in the body. Nutritional deficiencies usually develop slowly, and consequently the symptoms of hormonal deficiency develop slowly as well. In addition, hypoparathyroidism can occur in certain rare inherited conditions that exhibit either a decrease in production and secretion or a defect that renders the tissues unable to respond properly to the hormone.

When to call the doctor The appearance of symptoms suggestive of low parathyroid function warrant a prompt visit to the doctor for evaluation.

Treatment Unlike many endocrine deficiencies, administration of PTH is not a practical therapy. Because many of the calcium-elevating actions of the hormone occur through vitamin D activation, supplementation with this vitamin plus calcium will usually restore calcium balance. Some doctors may prefer to use synthetic vitamin D analogs of calcifediol, the forerunner of active vitamin D, or of calcitriol, which is active vitamin D. (An analog is a substance that mimics the action of another substance.) These synthetic medications work well to elevate calcium levels, but are much more expensive than standard vitamin D plus calcium, and seem to offer little advantage for the added cost. When the disorder occurs as a consequence of surgical removal of the majority of the parathyroid gland tissue, lifelong vitamin and calcium therapy is usually necessary.

Prognosis Excellent with prompt diagnosis and appropriate medical therapy.

Disorders of the Adrenal Glands

The adrenal glands, a pair of small glands 1 or 2 in. in length, sit like caps atop each kidney—the term *adrenal* is derived from the Latin *ad* (near to or next to) and *renal* kidney. Like the pancreas, they produce a variety of hormones in different parts of their structure. The glands are roughly divided into an outer portion, called the adrenal cortex, and an inner region, called the adrenal medulla. The cortex itself is further divided into three zones, each of which produces a specific hormone. The hormones of the cortex include aldosterone, important in regulation of blood pressure; cortisol, your body's natural steroid to help you withstand stress and infection; and dehydroepiandrosterone, the forerunner of the estrogens and testosterone produced outside the reproductive glands.

The adrenal medulla mainly produces epinephrine (also called adrenaline), important in the fight or flight response and involved in the regulation of blood pressure, heart rate, and numerous other functions. Epinephrine and the related hormone norepinephrine (also called noradrenaline), which is also produced in the adrenal medulla, have a wide range of other functions in the body. They regulate carbohydrate and fat metabolism and are involved in transmission of nerve impulses in the brain.

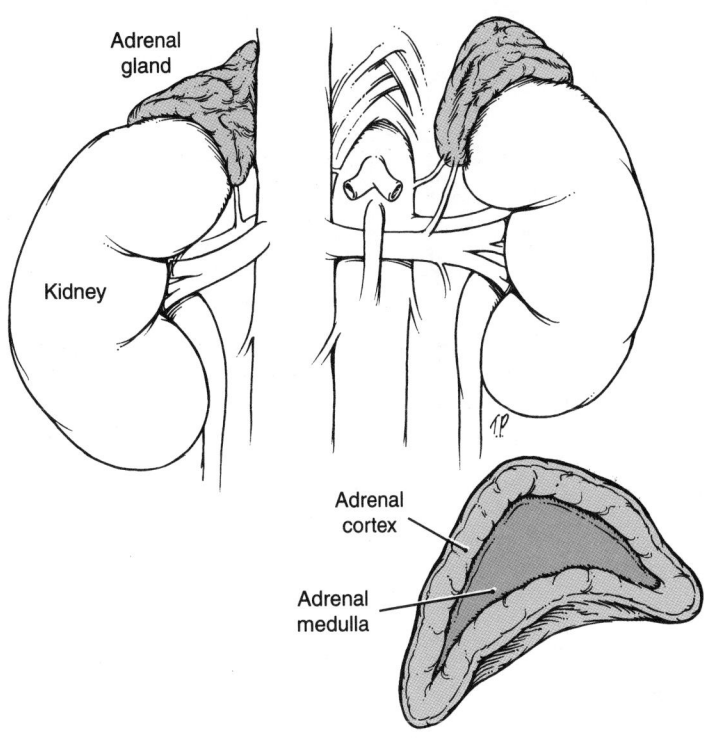

Seated atop each kidney, each adrenal gland consists of an outer layer (adrenal cortex) and inner layer (adrenal medulla). The cortex secretes steroid hormones that are involved in metabolism, sexual functioning, and the regulation of salts and water in the body. The medulla secretes hormones involved in sexual functioning and the body's response to stress.

❖ CUSHING'S SYNDROME

Symptoms (*What you may experience*) Obesity, with the fat gathering in the face, abdomen, and high on the back; hypertension; carbohydrate intolerance; fluid retention; purple stretch marks; poor healing of wounds; easy bruising; intestinal bleeding from peptic ulcer; blurred vision; bones fractures. Women may experience menstrual disturbances; excessive or unusual hair growth (facial); slight balding. Impotence may occur in men.

Signs and laboratory findings (*What the doctor looks for*) Striae (purple stretch marks on the abdomen, thighs, and elsewhere); characteristic development of fat in the face, the abdominal area, and below the neck between the shoulders (called the buffalo hump); cataracts; elevations of blood and urinary cortisol; unexplained low blood potassium level; pituitary tumor or enlarged adrenal glands as detected by imaging studies; characteristic response to

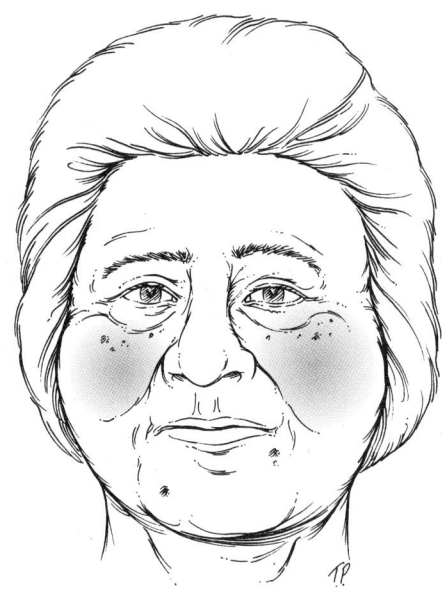

Cushing's syndrome is caused by an excess of corticosteriod hormones that are produced by the adrenal glands or taken in the form of medication. Excessive corticosteriods cause obesity, high blood pressure, and skin abnormalities in addition to other problems. The face often presents several clues to the disease, including puffy cheeks (moon face), red cheeks (plethora), and acne.

a dexamethasone (a corticosteroid) suppression test.

What is it? Cushing's syndrome—named for the Johns Hopkins-trained surgeon, Harvey Cushing, who first described the condition—results when the adrenal glands produce an excess amount of cortisol. Usually, the disease develops gradually, occurring most commonly in women of reproductive age. In two-thirds of cases, the overproduction results because the pituitary gland produces too much ACTH.

Because the pituitary itself bows to the higher influence of the hypothalamus, which produces corticotropin-releasing factor, Cushing's disease can develop from an increased release of corticotropin-releasing factor at this higher brain level. But the excess ACTH production also can occur from ectopic production (the production of ACTH by cancer cells) or it can result from a hyperplasia or a benign tumor of the pituitary gland. An ACTH-producing pituitary tumor is the most frequent cause for the disorder.

Hyperplasia or a benign tumor of the adrenal gland also can result in the production of excessive cortisol despite normal

amounts of pituitary or hypothalamic stimulation. Rarely, the syndrome is caused by adrenal cancer.

The syndrome also can occur as a consequence of prolonged use or excessive dosages of steroid medications, such as prednisone and other derivatives of cortisone, which might be used to treat asthma, rheumatoid or other inflammatory arthritic conditions, or severe skin conditions.

Diagnosis of Cushing's syndrome sometimes can be difficult because the disorder causes problems in so many different body systems—for example, osteoporosis, cataracts, and ulcers with gastrointestinal bleeding. Sometimes, people suffering from Cushing's syndrome may be treated by several doctors from different specialties before the correct diagnosis comes clearly into focus.

When to call the doctor Even though the syndrome usually develops gradually, early recognition and treatment can lead to full recovery and cure. Call the doctor if you develop more than one or two of the symptoms.

Treatment If x-ray studies—usually magnetic resonance imaging (MRI)—of the pituitary gland pinpoint a benign pituitary tumor of less than 1 cm as the cause of Cushing's syndrome, its removal (by a procedure called microadenomectomy) leads to cure in about 90 percent of cases. Larger tumors do not respond as well, making early diagnosis an important factor. Surgery to remove one or both adrenal glands (called adrenalectomy) is the most widely used option for the treatment of Cushing's syndrome resulting from benign adrenal tumors or hyperplasia of the adrenal glands (see Laparoscopic Adrenalectomy, page 1198). Although the adrenal glands produce many important hormones, after surgical treatment only long-term cortisol replacement therapy usually is necessary.

Several medications such as aminoglutethimide (Cytadren) and mitotane (Lysodren) have been developed to treat Cushing's syndrome; however, the development of toxic side effects of this therapy limits their use except in the most extreme cases, such as in adrenal cancer or when a person cannot withstand surgery.

Prognosis Good with early recognition and appropriate treatment. Complications of delayed treatment commonly include the development of diabetes, an increased tendency to develop spinal fractures from osteoporosis and atherosclerosis, which makes myocardial infarction or stroke more likely. Without treatment, Cushing's syndrome can be fatal.

❖ ADDISON'S DISEASE

Symptoms (What you may experience) Loss of appetite; weight loss; hypotension (low blood pressure); light-headedness or near fainting when rising from a lying or seated position; weakness; loss of libido; darkening of the skin of the palms, knees, elbows, and skin creases.

Emergency symptoms Vomiting or diarrhea leading to shock and loss of consciousness.

Signs and laboratory findings (What the doctor looks for) Orthostatic hypotension (sharp drop in blood pressure when rising after lying or sitting down); hyperpigmentation (darkening of the skin) of palms, soles, knees, elbows, and skin creases; elevated potassium in the blood (often). Blood tests may be entirely normal until symptoms reach critical severity, when blood tests will demonstrate low sodium, low blood glucose, high potassium, and elevated blood urea nitrogen (signs of body fluid depletion), and failure to respond to stimulation by ACTH.

What is it? Chronic insufficiency of the adrenal glands, called Addison's disease in tribute to English physician Thomas Addison who first described the condition, occurs due to an invasion or infiltration of the adrenal glands that disrupts their normal hormonal function. Usually the invasion limits itself to only the cortex of the gland, and the main hormonal deficiency is that of cortisol. In years gone by—in the 19th century during Addison's time, for example—tuberculosis of the adrenal glands caused most cases of insufficiency. Today tuberculous infections or fungal infections such as histoplasmosis cause a minority of cases of Addison's disease. More commonly, the invasion comes from the body's own white blood cell defenders in an autoimmune response. In these instances, the condition may occur in conjunction with an autoimmune disorder

of the thyroid gland called Hashimoto's thyroiditis (see page 1189). The invasion sometimes occurs in the course of acquired immunodeficiency syndrome (AIDS), when bacteria infect the adrenal glands or Kaposi's sarcoma (an unusual type of cancer seen frequently in AIDS) metastasizes to the glands. In people whose immune systems are not compromised by AIDS, infection in or metastasis of cancers to the adrenal glands occurs much less frequently. Adrenal insufficiency also occurs in persons who abruptly stop taking prednisone or other cortisone derivations after using them for a prolonged period of time. Rarely it occurs in people whose pituitary disease leads to inadequate release of ACTH.

Tests to uncover the disorder first involve measuring the blood and urinary cortisol levels, then stimulating the pituitary with ACTH and checking the blood for a rise in adrenal cortisol production to see if the deficiency is due to a pituitary or adrenal cause.

What you can do Once a doctor has established the diagnosis of adrenal insufficiency, self-care involves careful attention to the body's fluid and electrolyte balance. Replacing salts and body fluids lost due to exercise, fever, or minor diarrhea is of crucial importance. Even seemingly minor viral illnesses causing vomiting and diarrhea could lead to sufficient fluid loss in Addison's disease to bring on what is called Addisonian crisis—the rapid development of significant hypotension, low blood volume, and loss of consciousness; these symptoms may lead to death. It is important that every person with adrenal insufficiency wear a medical alert bracelet.

When to call the doctor The development of stable symptoms suggesting Addison's disease warrants a prompt visit to a doctor for testing. Any repeated episodes of vomiting or diarrhea demand hospitalization for intravenous fluid, salts, and hormone replacement. Severe symptoms suggesting Addisonian crisis demand immediate emergency treatment.

Treatment Although the cornerstone of therapy for Addison's disease involves replacing the deficient adrenal hormones, in those cases of Addison's disease caused by infection or tumor invasion, treatment must also include eradication of the infection or tumor. The usual method of long-term hormone replacement includes daily administration of cortisone and, in some cases, a small daily dosage of fludrocortisone to replace the salt-regulating action of aldosterone. In the case of infection or extra physical or emotional stress, dosage may be doubled.

Prognosis In most cases, the prognosis is good with prompt and adequate ongoing hormonal replacement therapy.

❖ ADRENAL HYPERPLASIA

Symptoms *(What you may experience)* Short stature (rapid growth early in childhood that ceases prematurely); excess body hair (facial hair in females); erratic or absent menstrual periods.

Signs and laboratory findings *(What the doctor looks for)* Hypertension (occasionally); low cortisol levels; high levels of male reproductive hormones in females.

What is it? Adrenal hyperplasia, usually congenital (present at birth), results from a genetic defect affecting the production of cortisol by the adrenal gland. The pituitary gland in the brain signals the adrenal gland to manufacture cortisol by producing ACTH. In adrenal hyperplasia, the problem lies in a reduced ability to produce the hormone, so no matter how great the signal from the brain, there is not enough cortisol to satisfy the body's need. The excess stimulation, however, leads to enlargement of the adrenal gland and overproduction of other adrenal hormones such as salt-retaining hormones (this can lead to hypertension) and androgens (male reproductive hormones). Both men and women produce androgens, but in normal circumstances women's adrenal glands produce only small amounts of male hormones. When adrenal hyperplasia affects females, the presence of excessive amounts of androgen can cause masculinizing effects such as excessive growth of body hair (also called hirsutism), absent mensturation or loss of normal menstrual function, and often polycystic ovary syndrome. (See Anovulation, page 1155, for information on polycystic ovary syndrome.) Milder forms of adrenal hyperplasia may not become evident until adolescence or adulthood. These signs and symptoms, so easily spotted in females, will not be evident in males.

When to call the doctor In young women, absent or erratic menstrual periods, in conjunction with any of the other symptoms of adrenal hyperplasia, should be investigated by a doctor. In mature women, the development of excessive body hair or loss of menstrual periods prior to menopause warrants a visit to the doctor right away to investigate the possibility of ovarian or adrenal tumors.

Treatment Hormonal replacement with cortisol corrects the deficiency and also stops the excessive production of ACTH from the pituitary that had overstimulated the adrenals. Once the excessive stimulation stops, the high levels of androgen and their masculinizing effects recede.

Prognosis Excellent if diagnosed and treated appropriately.

ADRENAL TUMORS

Adrenal tumors—all of which are rare—fall into four categories depending on which

---

LAPAROSCOPIC ADRENALECTOMY

Removal of the adrenal glands due to Cushing's syndrome or benign adrenal tumors once required a major surgical procedure. The procedure involved opening the abdomen and was followed by a lengthy hospital stay and a considerable recovery period. In the last few years, a new approach perfected at Johns Hopkins has allowed surgeons to operate with smaller incisions. The result is less postoperative pain and quicker recovery. In the new procedure, four tiny slits in the flank (the lower side of the back below the ribcage) allow the surgeon to insert a slender laparoscope (a flexible, lighted operating instrument) into the space in which the adrenal glands lie. The diseased gland is identified, freed from the surrounding tissues, and slipped into a pouch that is then gently pulled out through a slit. Recovery time is minimal—often the patient can go home the next day and may feel well enough to resume normal activities in 1 or 2 weeks. ■

part of the adrenal gland they arise from (either the adrenal medulla or the three zones of the adrenal cortex). Tumors arising in the three zones of the cortex can occur in the part that produces cortisol, causing Cushing's syndrome; aldosterone, causing Conn's syndrome (see Adrenal Cortical Tumors, below); or reproductive hormones, causing masculinization of women and very rarely the feminization of men.

❖ ADRENAL MEDULLARY TUMORS

Symptoms (*What you may experience*) Headache; rapid heart rate; profuse sweating; fainting; weight loss; constipation; changes in personality (sometimes).

Signs and laboratory findings (*What the doctor looks for*) Significant hypertension (which may be intermittent); elevation of epinephrine or norepinephrine in urine or blood or their breakdown products (metanephrine or vanillylmandelic acid) in urine collected over a 24-hour period.

What is it? Tumors arising in the adrenal medulla—called pheochromocytomas—produce epinephrine and norepinephrine. Because these substances increase heart rate and constrict arteries, pheochromocytomas uniformly cause hypertension that can be constant or may occur sporadically following seemingly minor emotional stress, mild exercise, or exposure to the cold. Tumors of the adrenal medulla tend to run in families and may occur as part of a multiple endocrine neoplasia (MEN) syndrome.

Treatment The only effective therapy for an adrenal medullary tumor is surgery. In most cases, removal of the tumor will eliminate the symptoms of the disorder. Hypertension may persist and continuing medication to control it may be necessary.

Prognosis Good with prompt diagnosis and surgery to remove benign tumors.

❖ ADRENAL CORTICAL TUMORS

Symptoms (*What you may experience*) Symptoms vary depending on the type of cortical tissue involved (see below).

MULTIPLE ENDOCRINE NEOPLASIA SYNDROMES

Some people inherit a tendency to develop tumors (also called neoplasias, which means new growths) of the endocrine glands. Two distinct types of inherited syndromes involving tumors of multiple endocrine organs have been termed MEN types 1 and 2.

In MEN type 1, symptoms usually do not appear before puberty, and some people who inherit the abnormal gene do not develop the disease. This syndrome involves tumors of the pituitary, parathyroid glands, and endocrine cells of the pancreas, more frequently of the delta type. The delta cells produce gastrin, which stimulates acid production by the stomach; serious gastric and intestinal ulcer disease often occurs in this syndrome.

MEN type 2 involves tumors of the thyroid (medullary carcinoma) and the medulla of the adrenal glands (see this page and page 1192). Benign tumors of the parathyroid glands, nerves, and skin can also occur in MEN type 2. ■

Signs and laboratory findings (*What the doctor looks for*) Computed tomography (CT) scan results.

What is it? Tumors of the adrenal cortex have been subdivided into those involving the aldosterone-producing cells and those involving the cells that produce sex hormones. In Cohn's syndrome, tumors arising in the aldosterone-producing zone of the cortex release excessive amounts of that hormone and cause such symptoms as hypertension, extreme thirst, excessive urination, or muscle cramping and weakness. Blood tests usually reveal elevated levels of sodium and reduced potassium levels as well as elevated levels of aldosterone.

Adrenal cortex tumors arising from cells that produce sex hormones are rare. When they do occur, the high levels of testosterone cause menstrual changes, excessive growth of body hair, and thickening of the vocal cords (deepening of the voice) in women. The increase in estrogen (female hormone) may cause gynecomastia, loss of body hair, and loss of muscle mass in men.

Treatment The only effective therapy for an adrenal tumor is surgery. In most cases, removal of the tumor will eliminate the symptoms of the disorder.

Prognosis Good with prompt diagnosis and surgery to remove benign tumors. Prognosis is poor with the rare malignant tumors of the adrenal cortex.

Disorders of the Pituitary Gland

The pituitary gland, sometimes called the master endocrine gland, produces hormones that exert their own effects as well as hormones that regulate the function of various endocrine glands. The pituitary gland is divided into two parts: the anterior pituitary, also called the adenohypophysis, which lies toward the front of the head, and the posterior pituitary, also called the neurohypophysis, which is oriented toward the back of the head. The two parts produce distinctly different products.

The anterior pituitary produces at least six hormones: growth hormone (necessary for normal growth and development), prolactin (necessary for mammary gland development and milk secretion), and the controlling hormones thyroid-stimulating hormone (TSH), ACTH, luteinizing hormone (LH), and follicle-stimulating hormone (FSH). TSH regulates the production and release of thyroid hormone by the thyroid gland; ACTH regulates the production and release of cortisol from the adrenal gland; LH and FSH regulate female reproductive cycling and have several important functions in men as well. See Chapter 25 for more information on LH and FSH.

The posterior pituitary produces two hormones, oxytocin and antidiuretic hormone (ADH). Oxytocin regulates and stimulates the expression of milk from the mammary glands and the rhythmic contractions of the uterus during labor in childbirth. During labor, doctors sometimes give this hormone as a medication (Pitocin) to enhance and sustain uterine contraction in childbirth. ADH stimulates the body to conserve water during periods of water deprivation or excessive loss of water.

The most common disorders of the pituitary gland are caused by tumors—almost always benign—which cause problems by secreting excess amounts of one of the hormones, by destroying normal pituitary tissue, or by creating pressure on the optic nerve or inside the skull.

❖ PROLACTINOMA

Symptoms (What you may experience) In women: disturbances of the menstrual cycle; unexplained breast milk production (occasionally). In men: reduced sex drive; erection difficulty; gynecomastia (less commonly); milk production (rarely).

Signs and laboratory findings (What the doctor looks for) High levels of prolactin in the blood; low levels of LH and FSH (sometimes); pituitary tumor as detected by CT or MRI scan.

What is it? Elevated levels of prolactin occur for many reasons, but often because of hormone-producing tumors in the pituitary. These small benign growths often can be detected by CT or MRI scans. Although a number of hormone-stimulating tests have been proposed to help distinguish between the tumors, also called prolactinomas, and other causes of prolactin elevation, none has proven to be a reliable indicator.

Because of the proximity of the pituitary to the optic nerves, enlargement from tumor growth can compromise vision.

Treatment Bromocriptine, pergolide, and recently approved cabergoline (Dostinex) effectively shrink the tumors and drop the blood level of the hormone. Side effects of these medications include fatigue, dizziness, nausea, and hypotension upon standing. (Side effects are less bothersome if the medication is taken at bedtime.) These effects may last for 7 to 10 days after stopping the medication. After 6 months of therapy as many as 50 percent of tumors have shrunk by half. If the tumor does not respond to medication or if the side effects are intolerable, the tumor should be removed. This procedure is called a transphenoidal hypophysectomy (removal of the pituitary tumor through the sinus cavity at the back of the nasal chamber).

Prognosis Good if the tumor is discovered promptly and treated appropriately.

❖ PITUITARY GIANTISM

Symptoms *(What you may experience)*
Excessive, rapid, and prolonged growth in children; headache; bone and joint pain; excessive sweating; visual disturbances.

Signs and laboratory findings *(What the doctor looks for)* Elevated levels of growth hormone as detected by blood tests.

What is it? Excessive production of growth hormone during childhood causes the condition referred to as giantism. If the growth plates of the bones have not yet closed, the excess growth hormone can stimulate rapid growth of bone and soft tissue, and the child grows exceptionally tall. The excess growth hormone comes in most cases from a small, benign tumor in the pituitary gland. As the tumor slowly grows it can put pressure on nearby areas of the brain and cause visual disturbances, runny nose, headache, and occasionally seizures. Rapid growth of long bones, especially in the legs, can result in bone pain.

When to call the doctor Seek medical attention right away for severe symptoms such as visual defects, loss of vision, or seizures. Other symptoms, including excessive height, warrant investigation as well.

Treatment Surgical removal of the pituitary tumor alleviates most of the symptoms and returns growth hormone levels to normal. In some cases, irradiation to the pituitary will suffice. This approach has the advantage of avoiding surgery but response to treatment may not occur for several years; when response does occur, it often leads to decreased pituitary function generally and the need for long-term hormone replacement therapy.

Prognosis Good with early diagnosis. Appropriate treatment can reverse many symptoms. The dramatic increase in height will remain.

❖ ACROMEGALY

Symptoms *(What you may experience)*
Swelling of the hands or feet; increasing shoe width; increasing ring or glove size; change in facial features to accomodate a prominent and jutting lower jaw; pro-

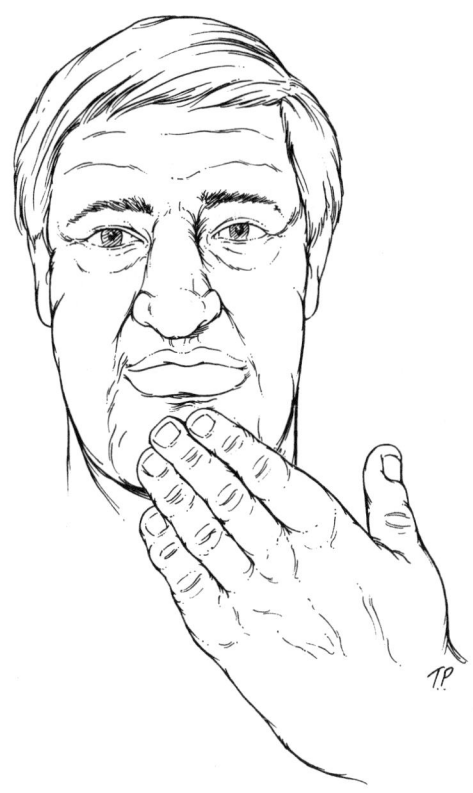

Acromegaly is caused by excessive production of growth hormone by a tumor in the pituitary gland. Common features include enlargement of the jaw, nose, brow, hands, and feet and a general coarsening of facial features.

nounced brow ridge; bone and joint pain (especially in the hips, knees, and spine); carpal tunnel syndrome (caused by compression of a nerve in the wrist and characterized by pain and numbness in the fingers or hand); thickening of the lips and tongue; spreading of the front teeth; excessive sweating; unpleasant body odor; thickening of the skin; oiliness of the skin; appearance of numerous skin tags (appendages); husky voice; restless or poor-quality sleep with snoring; headache; vision changes; seizures (possibly); loss of normal menstrual cycling; production of breast milk in women; impotence.

Signs and laboratory findings *(What the doctor looks for)* Alternations in facial features and voice; increasing hand and foot size; hypertension; enlargement of the heart; a swollen optic nerve as revealed by an eye examination; abnormally high levels of growth hormone and insulin-like growth factor 1 as detected by blood tests; diabetes mellitus or impaired glucose intolerance; a pituitary tumor as detected by an MRI.

What is it? Normal growth and repair of tissues depends on the release of growth hormone from the pituitary. This hormone does not itself increase growth but stimulates growth through the production of insulin-like growth factor 1 by the liver. When excess growth hormone output occurs in adults after the growth plates of the long bones have closed and sealed, increased growth can occur only in certain areas: the hands and feet, the facial bones, the internal organs, or the soft tissues. Overgrowth in these areas accounts for the alterations in appearance of people suffering from acromegaly.

Excess production of growth hormone occurs most commonly due to benign tumors of the pituitary gland; very rarely, excess production is caused by tumors of the lung or pancreas, which for unknown reasons produce growth hormone releasing hormone which stimulates the pituitary gland to produce excess growth hormone.

When to call the doctor The condition develops slowly and urgent medical care is not a concern; however, appearance of symptoms suggestive of acromegaly warrants a prompt visit to your doctor.

Treatment Microsurgical removal of the pituitary tumor usually results in rapid decline of growth hormone levels. Excessive sweating and carpal tunnel symptoms often respond promptly. Surgery brings about successful remission in 50 percent of cases. If surgery is not possible, a medication (bromocriptine or octreotide) injected 3 times a day may be of some help. A long-term medication (one injection of octreotide a month) may be available soon. Radiation to the pituitary gland also may reduce growth hormone production by the tumor, but may damage other hormone producing cells in the normal portion of the gland.

Prognosis Good with proper treatment. Untreated, the risks are high for early onset of heart disease and progression of symptoms. Patients with acromegaly have a higher risk of developing colon polyps.

❖ PITUITARY DWARFISM

Symptoms *(What you may experience)* Consistently short stature relative to age.

Signs and laboratory findings *(What the doctor looks for)* Persistently short stature without a family history of short stature; abnormal values on specific tests of pituitary hormones (such as growth hormone); abnormal bone age as detected by x-rays; low blood glucose.

What is it? Length and weight are measured at birth and periodically remeasured as a child grows. Children who consistently fall below the low end of the normal range for height and weight should be evaluated. In a small percentage of these cases, a child fails to attain normal stature because the pituitary gland produces insufficient amounts of growth hormone. The disorder can usually be detected in the first few years of life.

When to call the doctor In many instances, the doctor will note the lag in growth, as they record a child's height and weight during regular checkups. These values usually are plotted on a graph that outlines the normal ranges for children at each age. In other cases a parent may notice that a child appears small relative to peers or is not outgrowing clothes.

Many children, particularly boys, grow anxious about their heights when their peers experience growth spurts before they do. Usually these fears prove groundless, and their growth spurts begin later. Occasionally, growth lags behind persistently. If a child's growth is below normal relative to age and family history, investigation by a doctor is merited.

Treatment Children with growth hormone disorders can be treated with synthetic growth hormone. The hormone usually is prescribed as a daily injection.

Growth hormone injections are not appropriate for a child whose short stature is due to genetic inheritance. If a child's growth hormone levels are normal, growth hormone injections are not appropriate and are unlikely to increase height.

Prognosis Growth hormone replacement therapy usually results in growth of 3 to 4 in. in the first year of treatment and 2 to 3 in. in each successive year. Over time, the child's stature will gradually catch up to the normal range, unless treatment is started too late.

❖ HYPOPITUITARISM

Symptoms *(What you may experience)* Symptoms vary markedly depending on which pituitary hormone is deficient. Symptoms from loss of stimulation of reproductive hormones by LH and FSH: reduction of body hair; diminished beard growth (men); loss of menstrual cycling (women); erection difficulty (men); infertility. Symptoms from growth hormone deficiency: decreased muscle mass and increased body fat. Symptoms from deficient thyroid hormone stimulation: weakness; fatigue, weight gain. Symptoms from deficient ACTH: weakness; fatigue; weight loss; hypotension.

Signs and laboratory findings *(What the doctor looks for)* Signs of hypothyroidism (see page 1188) and adrenal insufficiency (see page 1197); note that adrenal insufficiency from hypopituitarism differs from primary adrenal insufficiency because the former condition is not associated with increased pigmentation. Signs also include low levels of blood sugar or sodium and low levels of specific hormones produced by the thyroid, adrenal, testes, or ovaries.

What is it? Many benign tumors of the pituitary gland do not produce excessive amounts of any hormone. Instead, these tumors take up space within the small area that confines the gland and crowd out normal pituitary tissue. Stimulating hormones normally produced in the pituitary become deficient and consequently the hormones under their control become deficient as well.

Deficient production of pituitary hormones also can occur in cases of starvation or if the blood supply to the pituitary is interrupted for some reason. Insufficient blood supply deprives the pituitary tissue of oxygen, and damage or death of certain areas can occur. Occasionally, Sheehan's syndrome (infarction of the pituitary gland) occurs in women after a complicated delivery. Whatever the initiating event, the disorder may cause a deficiency of one or more or all of the pituitary stimulating hormones, sometimes making the diagnosis a difficult one.

Treatment Surgical removal or radiation to the pituitary tumor offers the greatest success in the treatment of tumors. Replacement to correct hormonal deficiencies will usually be necessary before, during, and after surgery, and usually for the long term. The only exception is that of growth hormone deficiency, which is generally not replaced in adults because of its extreme cost and because there is no proven need for replacement in adults.

Prognosis Good. In cases of tumor, careful removal of the tumor may allow the remainder of the gland to recover and resume hormone production. In many cases (because of tumor size) functional recovery of the gland is not possible. In these cases, the disorder persists, but hormone replacement therapy allows for normal quality and length of life.

❖ DIABETES INSIPIDUS

Symptoms *(What you may experience)* Excessive urination, intense thirst (especially for ice water), and excessive fluid intake.

Signs and laboratory findings *(What the doctor looks for)* Inappropriately low specific gravity (very dilute) of the urine.

What is it? Diabetes insipidus occurs because of deficiency of ADH or a resistance to its action.

Deficiency, usually temporary, is quite common after surgery on the pituitary gland but can occur for a variety of other reasons: inherited lack of production or damage to the pituitary or hypothalamus.

Certain people have nephrogenic diabetes insipidus (inherited resistance to the effect of ADH in the kidney). These people produce plenty of ADH, but a defect in the kidney tubules interferes with the normal water reabsorption that the hormone should cause. Certain medications also can prevent normal water reabsorption, notably lithium (a medication used in manic depressive illness), methicillin and demeclocycline (antibiotic medications), and foscarnet (antiviral medication).

What you can do Always keep fluid available and monitor your intake. Intake should equal output in most instances. Failure to drink adequate fluid to replace the large volume of urine produced can lead rapidly to dehydration.

When to call the doctor Persistent symptoms suggestive of diabetes insipidus should prompt a visit to your doctor; the symptoms often are more inconvenient than actually dangerous.

Treatment Medications that mimic the action of ADH (desmopressin and lypressin) can be taken via nasal spray. Hydrochlorothiazide (normally thought of as a diuretic) may be helpful in patients with nephrogenic diabetes insipidus when taken with supplemental potassium. When some ADH secretion is still present, fine (partial) diabetes insipidus can be treated with chlorpropamide (Diabinese).

Prognosis Excellent with appropriate medical treatment.

Mental Health

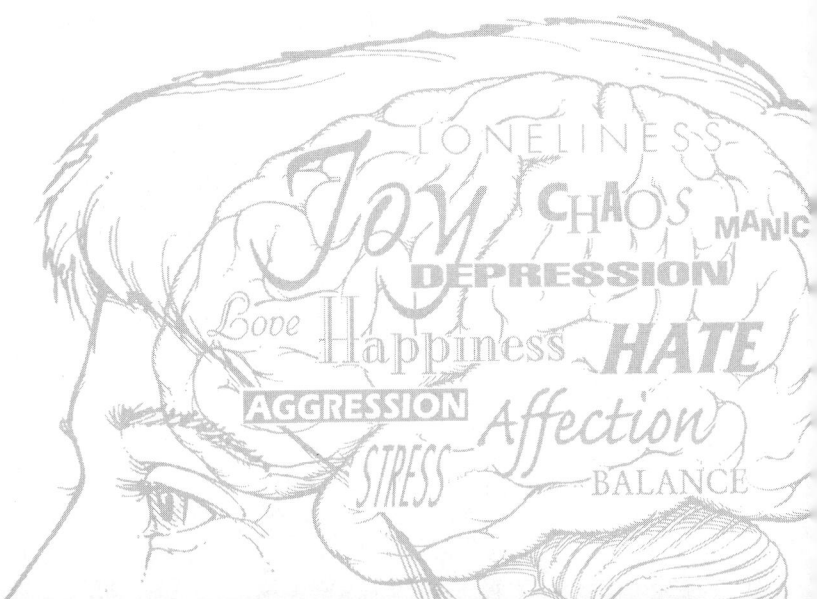

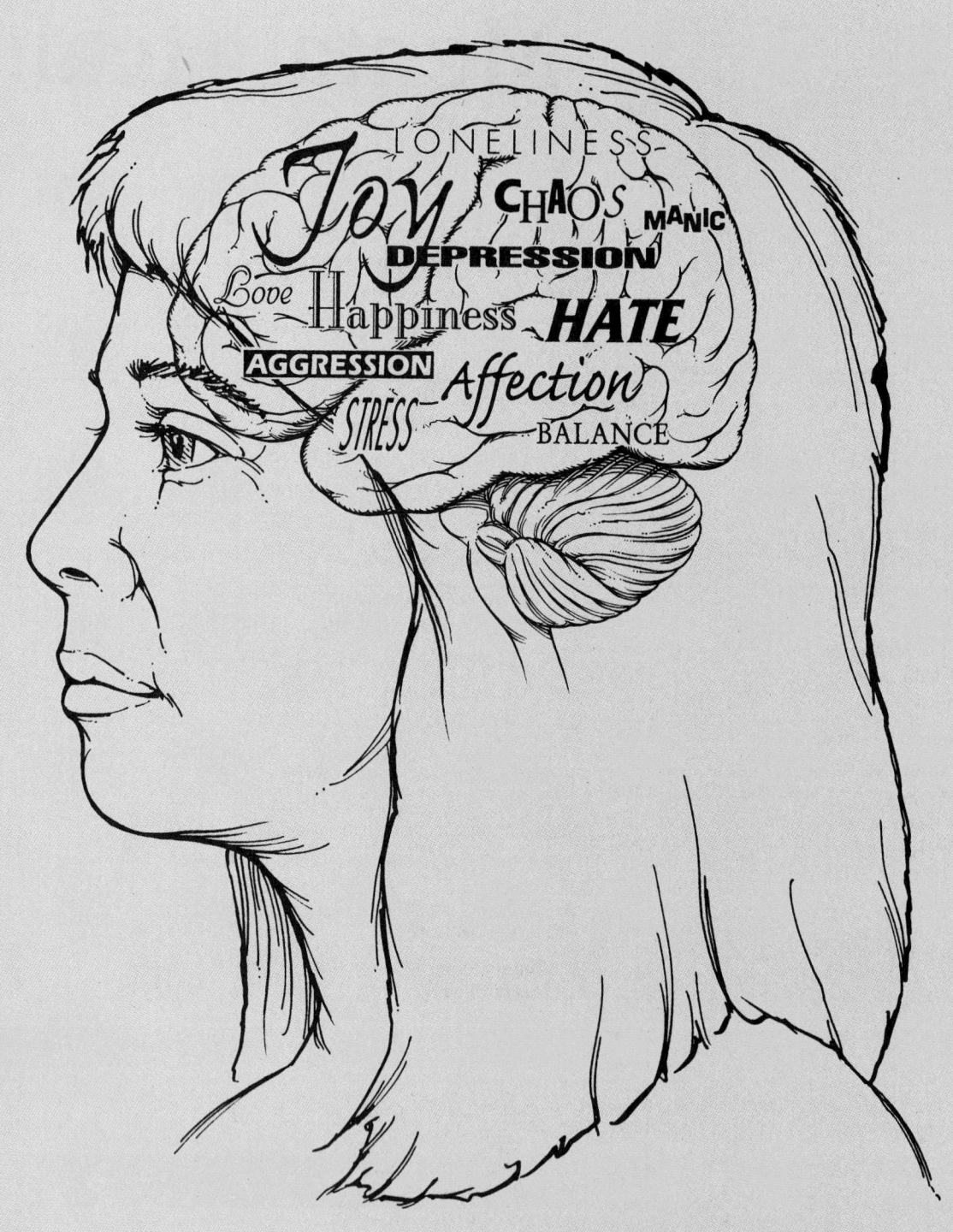

MENTAL HEALTH

What is Mental Health?

When a patient comes into a doctor's office with a medical complaint, there are usually specific, identifiable symptoms and signs that he is suffering: a fever, localized pain, a lump, or swelling. In most cases, the symptom can be isolated and gauged. Health and illness can be measured within a relatively narrow range by quantifiable measures—a blood pressure reading, for example. However, when someone seeks professional help in the field of mental health, the symptoms are often vague: a feeling, a sensation, or a behavior that is slightly exaggerated. Even the most severe psychiatric disorders must be evaluated and understood within the broad context of the person's life: his interpersonal relationships, work role, and family life.

Moreover, the diagnosis of emotional and psychiatric conditions—which can range from problems of everyday living to severe mental illness—relies heavily on the person's descriptions of internal states and subjective experiences that are, often, hard to describe. There are no quantifiable gauges or data to confirm or deny with absolute certainty the existence of a mental or emotional disorder. Instead, mental illness and psychological problems are described in terms of emotions, thoughts, behavior, and physical signs, and they are measured in terms of excess or deficits, duration, intensity, timing, and rigidity.

Trying to define mental and emotional health is made even more complex and ambiguous when you consider the fact that the scope of individual differences is enormous. We are each born with a distinct disposition—a characteristic emotional repertoire and range—that colors our attitudes about and responses to our world. What, then, exactly is a healthy mood? Even when the symptom involves behavior, the extent of what is normal is so sweeping that labeling a behavior disorder is seldom unequivocal. An emotion, response, or attitude that seems completely in keeping with one person's temperament may be an indication that something is wrong for another.

Add to individual variations in emotions and behavior the variations that arise in regard to context and culture. Certain subjective experiences, emotions, and behavior that may be defined as disordered in one context or one culture may be perfectly acceptable and within normal boundaries in another. For example, it is considered normal to giggle at a party but not at a funeral. At the same time, it may be normal to enjoy yourself at a wake.

Thus, given the wide range of normal emotional states and responses, as well as the capriciousness of life circumstances, it is seldom easy to define with great precision just what constitutes mental and emotional health. Almost always, mental health or mental illness is determined on an individual basis. As with physical illness, some mental disorders are diseases, arising from biologic imbalance and disruption. Often, however, mental health and emotional well-being are the products of the struggle between a person's vulnerabilities and strengths as they surface in his interactions with his world.

In this chapter, we examine those feelings, behaviors, thought patterns, and physical signs that, because they linger over a long stretch of time, because they are excessive or exaggerated, or because they interfere with a person's day-to-day functioning, may well signal the existence of an emotional disturbance or psychiatric disorder.

Most of the chapter is devoted to mental health issues that affect adults. However, there is no question that children and adolescents frequently experience and manifest emotional problems differently than adults. For youngsters, intense or persistent emotional upset may interfere not only with their day-to-day functioning but with their psychological, intellectual, and social development as well. Furthermore, in one way or another, a child's inner disturbance affects those around him, and, as a result, it is usually necessary that parents and sometimes siblings involve themselves in a child's psychiatric treatment. Given the singular and complicated nature of childhood mental health, those disturbances that commonly affect children and teenagers—depressive, anxiety, and behavioral disorders—are covered in their own section within the chapter. Eating disorders—affecting older children, teens, and adults—are covered in a separate section.

Other subjects that naturally arise when discussing mental health—choosing a clinician, the difficulties posed in establishing a psychiatric diagnosis, the various types of treatment, the use and overuse of medications, substance abuse, suicide, the stigma surrounding mental illness, and the like—are also considered in some detail.

It is important to mention that the purpose of this chapter is not to enable you to diagnose mental illness within yourself or in those around you. Rather, the information provided here can help you make an informed decision as to whether you or a loved one could benefit from professional mental health intervention. Should you decide to seek help, this chapter can guide you in finding the right kind of help for you and your family, in asking the right questions along the way, and in establishing a productive working relationship with your mental health clinician.

Seeking Help

Even when you are reasonably clear that you (or someone you love) are having problems managing the demands and details of day-to-day living or experiencing significant internal upset, it is not always clear if the problems require professional treatment or if they will resolve themselves on their own. Sometimes, just talking to your doctor will help. Other times, a brief consultation with a mental health clinician will clarify things sufficiently to put you back on track or start you on the track of long-term, intensive treatment.

Many people seek professional treatment in response to a feeling: They feel bad for no obvious reason; they feel anxious or disheartened beyond what seems reasonable; they feel out of control. Often, a person is prompted to seek help by a significant change or crisis in his world. Work presents daunting challenges, or job security seems tenuous; a love relationship ends; a loved one dies. A person may come into treatment to address apparent problems—a strained marriage, a child who is acting out, various physical complaints—only to find that what he has been struggling with is actually a depression, anxiety disorder, or post-traumatic stress disorder. And sometimes, a person contacts a mental health clinician to deal with troublesome habits or behaviors: alcohol or drug use, obsessive gambling, and the like.

Most of the time, it is the combination of internal distress and the observations or reactions of others—spouse, parents, friends, work colleagues, or supervisors—and sometimes, a life crisis, that brings someone into the world of mental health

professionals. Nevertheless, there are a few general symptoms and signs that, when present over an extended period of time, point to the need for psychiatric treatment. These include

- Marked decline in work or school performance

- Poor performance at work or grades in school despite diligent work

- Excessive worry or anxiety, especially when it manifests in regular refusal to go to work or school, regular sleep difficulties, inability to enjoy and engage in normal activities, or problems in establishing or maintaining friendships and love relationships

- Constant fidgeting, uneasiness, worry, or dread

- Alcohol or drug abuse

- Inability to cope with problems and demands of daily life

- Irrational fears

- Dramatic weight loss or weight fluctuation that is not related to medical condition

- Obsessive preoccupation with food and fear of becoming obese with no relationship to actual body weight

- Significant change in sleeping or eating habits

- Persistent physical ailments and complaints

- Aggressive or nonaggressive violation of other people's rights, opposition to authority, truancy, thefts, fire setting, or vandalism

- Suicidal thoughts, the urge to hurt oneself or others

- Self-mutilation, self-destructive, or dangerous behavior

- Sustained, prolonged sadness, withdrawn mood and attitude, often accompanied by poor appetite, difficulty sleeping, or thoughts of death

- Frequent outbursts of anger and frustration that seem way out of proportion to one's circumstances

- Hallucinations and abnormal perceptions

Having decided to seek help, you may find the mental health system confusing. Chances are that finding your way through

CHOOSING A CLINICIAN

Many times, people seek treatment during a time of crisis around, for example, an intense period of marital conflict, divorce, grief, substance abuse, or an active episode of a psychiatric illness. At those times, few feel that they have the internal stability to make sober determinations about where to go to find the best treatment. Even if you are not in crisis, selecting the right mental health clinician can be a daunting task.

If you are unsure where to look for a mental health clinician, start by asking your doctor. Then ask friends or family members; you may be surprised to learn how many people you know are currently involved in psychiatric or psychological treatment or have sought help in the past.

If you are looking for someone to treat your child, check with his pediatrician and school counselor. If there is an employee assistance program through your work, speak to its representative. If you belong to a health maintenance organization, you can ask for their list of mental health providers. Many insurance providers include certain mental health benefits within their coverage. Often, they will supply you with a phone number so that you can discuss your needs and complaints with a mental health professional who will then provide a referral. In addition, local hospitals, teaching hospitals, and medical centers frequently extend mental health services and/or referrals.

Chances are you will be referred to a hospital outpatient clinic, a free-standing mental health clinic, or private practitioners. If you receive names of psychotherapists, psychiatrists, psychologists, and social workers, you may wonder what the difference is and which is most suitable to your situation. The term *psychotherapist* does not denote any specific professional degree or training; anyone with any kind of background can call himself a psychotherapist. Most states, though, regulate and certify psychiatrists, psychologists, and social workers.

While the fact that a therapist possesses a certain degree and/or specific credentials does not ensure that he is a skilled and effective clinician, it is more likely that those who hold state-licensed degrees will have a more extensive professional background and skills.

There are a range of different training and educational programs within the mental health field: counseling, pastoral counseling, and psychiatric nursing, among others. In actual practice, the differences among a psychiatrist, psychologist, social worker, or other types of mental health clinicians may not be immediately discernible. However, there can be very real and important differences in terms of education, training, and orientation. Briefly, some of the distinctions follow:

Psychiatrist A psychiatrist is a medical doctor whose training and education include medical school and at least 4 additional years of study, research, and clinical training in adult and possibly child and adolescent psychiatry. Because of their medical training, psychiatrists bring into their practice a thorough understanding of medical as well as mental issues. In addition, psychiatrists generally possess an in-depth knowledge of medication and its effects and limitations as a treatment modality. Among mental health professionals, only psychiatrists can prescribe drugs. If you are struggling with a serious mental illness or with a severe emotional disorder, you may want to see a psychiatrist for a thorough diagnostic workup to evaluate your need for medication.

Psychologist The majority of psychologists who practice psychotherapy hold a PhD in clinical, educational, or experimental psychology. A doctorate in psychology usually entails detailed study of research and psychological testing procedures. Many who practice clinically have also engaged in some postgraduate training.

Social Worker Social workers usually hold a master's degree. Their education typically focuses on the individual within the context of his social environment—his family, relationships, and community. Social workers often provide what is referred to as concrete services; that is, they help people negotiate such social systems as the community, its institutions, and local and governmental social service agencies. Psychiatric or clinical social workers typically work as psychotherapists, either in agencies, hospitals, or in private practice.

Psychotherapist The term *psychotherapist* refers only to the fact that one is engaged in the professional practice of psychotherapy (see page 1213). It does not refer to any particular educational discipline or training. However, in many cases, a person who practices psychotherapy holds a professional degree and has postgraduate training in one or more methods of therapy.

As important as professional credentials and degrees may be, finding a comfortable and productive match between you and the clinician is equally important in choosing a clinician. And often, these days, finding the right clinician includes considering whom your insurance plan will cover. ■

the system to the right kind of professional help will be clouded by abundant and often conflicting feelings, not least of which are distress, vulnerability, guilt, and shame—on top of the feelings produced by the disorder. If the problem concerns your child or other members of your family, you may feel that somehow you are to blame, and you may worry that others, including medical and mental health professionals, will blame you as well.

If you seek help for yourself, you may be nagged by the feeling that you should be able to resolve the problems on your own, that mental illness or an emotional disorder is a sign of weakness. On the contrary, seeking help is a sign of strength, demonstrating your awareness that something is wrong and change is necessary. Furthermore, many mental disorders are illnesses just like diabetes and asthma. No one expects people suffering from asthma to control their

MEDICATION

Psychopharmacology, the treatment of psychiatric disorders and emotional distress with medication, has developed over the last 50 years, as our understanding of the workings of the brain has increased in sophistication. When medication is prescribed for mental and emotional illness, the most frequent goal is to restore the chemical balance within the brain, thereby restoring equilibrium to the entire system. Certain drugs function to address certain symptoms, such as when sedatives are prescribed for insomnia. Medications can work to slow disease processes, such as when antioxidants are used to treat Alzheimer's disease. Still other medications control cravings and curb other problematic behaviors, such as when naltrexone (Revia) is taken to control alcoholism.

In many instances, medication is essential. If you suffer from mania, a major depression, or a paranoid disorder, medication may actually be able to restore you to your normal self. For other conditions, such as schizophrenia, medication controls and modifies symptoms to the degree that a person can stay in his community. Medications also ease the more distressing symptoms, allowing a person to engage in a therapeutic relationship and reengage in the activities of daily life. Sometimes a medication is a useful additional measure during particularly stressful times, perhaps in the initial stage of treatment or at a time of crisis. People with thought disorders or hallucinatory experiences can be maintained only with appropriate antipsychotic medications.

It is not entirely clear why psychotropic medications work; yet, they appear to reestablish balance within the chemistry of the brain. Behavior is determined through messages transmitted within the brain from one nerve cell to another through various chemicals.

These chemicals are called neurotransmitters. Through the millions of nerve cells within the brain, chemicals trigger memories, sleep patterns, perceptions, feelings, moods, and thoughts. The electric current that carries the messages is received by nerve ends, called synapses, which then release the neurotransmitter. These chemicals, in turn, propagate the message by stimulating the next nerves in line to send on the electrical message. Once used, the neurotransmitter chemical is returned and stored in the nerve end. This recycling process is called reuptake. When this signaling process goes askew, the effects are seen in a person's behavior and experienced in his emotions, perceptions, sensations, and ideas.

Although numerous chemicals perform vital functions within the brain, three basic chemicals, or neurotransmitters, seem most critical in regulating this process and maintaining balance: serotonin, which is related to anxiety, depression, and aggression; dopamine, which affects reality perception and pleasurable experiences; and norepinephrine, which affects attention, concentration, and mood.

Medication is most helpful when there is a clear disorder or, sometimes, a specific target symptom for a particular drug. Usually, a pattern of symptoms points to a specific chemical imbalance. Whenever an imbalance appears evident through a person's disordered behavior and emotional state, medication centers on modifying the strength of the signal or readjusting the balance among them. In psychopharmacology, the relationship between drug and chemical action is as follows:

- A group of drugs called selective serotonin reuptake inhibitors (SSRIs) addresses serotonin; the most widely known are fluoxetine (Prozac), sertraline (Zoloft), and paroxetine (Paxil).

- Neuroleptics affect dopamine; the most commonly ▶

breathing difficulties or to get over the condition on their own. People who suffer from emotional disorders, likewise, need the expertise, experience, and guidance of well-trained, well-educated professionals to help them manage their condition sufficiently so that they can get on with the business of their lives.

THE CONTINUUM OF CARE

As a rule, professional treatment for a psychiatric illness or emotional disorder starts with a comprehensive psychiatric evaluation. Whether you come to a private therapist, a mental health clinic, or hospital emergency room, the problem must be understood before treatment begins. Typically performed by a psychiatrist, psychologist, clinical social worker, or a team of mental health professionals, the psychiatric evaluation will establish a working diagnosis, which then directs treatment.

During a series of interviews, which usually takes several hours over one or more office visits, the clinician, individual, and, frequently, the family work together to gather information and formulate a diagnostic picture. Based on the information, a broad hypothesis is formulated concerning the nature of the presenting problem, likely causes, circumstances that may exacerbate the problem, and any related problems that may coexist. In addition to assessing the current problem, the clinician will ask about such areas as the patient's current functioning, his individual and family history, his health (both mental and physical), any past experience with mental health treatment, and drug or alcohol use. Whenever necessary, the therapist may refer the patient out for other tests such as special psychiatric, psychological, educational, speech or language assessments, blood tests, x-rays, or neurologic tests.

Once the clinician has evolved a reasonably full diagnostic picture of the person

▶ prescribed are fluphenazine (Prolixin), haloperidol (Haldol), chlorpromazine (Thorazine), and thioridazine (Mellaril).

- There are many tricyclic antidepressants (TCAs), which are typically prescribed to address both norepinephrine and serotonin; among the best known are imipramine, amitriptyline, desipramine, and nortriptyline.

- Atypical antipsychotics affect serotonin and dopamine; the most commonly prescribed are risperidone, clozapine, and olanzapine.

- Monamine oxidase inhibitors (MAOIs) are prescribed to affect all three basic neurotransmitters; the most commonly prescribed MAOIs are phenelzine (Nardil) and tranylcypromine (Parnate).

- Lithium carbonate is a naturally occurring salt that controls mood disorders by directly affecting internal nerve cell processes in all the neurotransmitter systems.

- Anticonvulsants, such as divalproex sodium (Depakote) and carbamazepine (Tegretol), are also used for mood and aggressive disorders. Just how they work on neurotransmitters is not known, however.

- Benzodiazepines affect another neurotransmitter system, gamma-aminobutyric acid, which is involved in anxiety, alertness, and sleep. These include alprazolam, clonazepam, and diazepam.

Usually, these medications either increase the availability of these chemicals and strengthen their messages or decrease the availability of the chemicals and weaken the signal.

The treatment of mental illness with medication can be complicated because the brain is a complex organ. Mental illness or emotional disorders are likewise complicated; often more than one condition exists simultaneously. Add to this the fact that each individual is unique and complex in his own way. As a result, finding the right medication and the right dosage often is a painstaking process.

Usually, the process begins with a medical consultation. It is best if psychotropic medications are prescribed by a psychiatrist or psychopharmacologist, although many times a general practitioner will write the prescription.

During the consultation, the doctor will specify what disorder and which symptoms are to be addressed by the medication, and what the person can expect in terms of benefits and side effects. In addition, the doctor will discuss how long treatment should last, what sort of follow-up will be given, and at what point or under what conditions medication will be adjusted or discontinued.

Before prescribing a specific medication, the doctor will take a careful history, including information about previous physical illnesses or allergies and any previous drug experience. The person's physical health will be reviewed, and a baseline mental status examination will be performed, against which progress will be measured. After the course of medication therapy has begun, the prescriber will review reaction and progress on a regular basis, making adjustments whenever necessary.

Of course, not all disorders should be treated with medication. For some people, psychotherapy alone is sufficient to address their distress. For many, though, medication is the mainstay of treatment. Frequently, the combination of therapy and medication, at least initially, can mean the difference between living in this world or living trapped inside a psychiatric disorder. ■

and his problem, he will likely recommend a course of treatment. Treatment usually involves a specific treatment modality: individual psychotherapy, for example, or day treatment. Frequently, psychotropic medication is suggested, either as the primary therapy or as an adjunct to other treatment methods. In many cases, treatment entails more than one modality, so that an individual may be referred to a residential treatment facility while the family is advised to engage in family therapy.

While not every community has every type of treatment program and service, most offer a range of options for treating mental illnesses. A complete range of programs and services is called the continuum of care. The more common services are described below.

Outpatient treatment The term outpatient treatment describes treatment conducted in a private office, a mental health clinic, or an outpatient clinic within a hospital. A clinician may meet with individuals, children, couples, families, and groups, conducting psychotherapy in sessions that typically last somewhere around an hour (see Psychotherapy—What Is It?, page 1213). The number of visits per week depends on the needs of the patient. Some psychiatrists provide psychopharmacologic treatment in conjunction with counseling, support, and guidance (see Medication, page 1210). Other clinicians perform psychological testing or address specific behavioral problems in an outpatient setting.

Hospitalization Hospital treatment is usually recommended in response to an acute crisis when issues of safety become paramount: a suicide attempt, an uncontrollable manic or psychotic episode, or a serious incident of aggression or violence. Psychiatric emergencies often result when resources in the person's family and community break down or become overwhelmed. Once a person is hospitalized, he will receive a comprehensive psychi-

WHEN SOMEONE IS NOT WILLING TO SEEK TREATMENT

Someone you love is clearly troubled. You can see that he needs help. He cannot. With a child, you have the authority and responsibility to find the appropriate help. With adolescent children and adult family members—your spouse, sibling, elderly parent—the issue becomes trickier.

If the trouble involves problems in everyday living—he is constantly frustrated and discontented at work or at school, or he feels unaccountably anxious much of the time—you can gently suggest that talking with a mental health professional might help. Sometimes you can enlist other family members, your minister or rabbi, or your doctor to encourage him to see a therapist. But then again, you may have to stand on the sideline and hope that he finds his way through it. Ultimately, the difficulty is his, and he will have to find his own motivation and his own solution. Even when the problem is more severe, causing you concern about the effect on the quality of his life, as with alcohol or substance abuse or depression, you may still have to wait it out until he rouses himself sufficiently to do something. In some cases, a person needs to hit bottom before he can reach out for help. In the meantime, you may want to seek help and support for yourself, either finding your own psychotherapist or joining a self-help group such as Al-Anon.

But there are times when the problem holds the potential for danger, in which case you may think about having the person committed. The protocol and procedures for involuntary hospitalization vary from state to state. When children appear to be seriously suicidal or threaten violent endangerment, they can be hospitalized at the request of a parent or guardian. As a rule, adults are admitted to psychiatric hospitals or wards only as voluntary patients or pending a full judicial hearing.

In many states, there are procedures by which you can make a request of a judge to have a loved one taken by the police to a psychiatric hospital or emergency room for an emergency psychiatric evaluation. At that point, involuntary hospitalization may be considered.

Ordinarily, the legal system will mandate hospitalization only in cases of a clear and immediate danger to the person or someone else. However, it is not always clear that these dangers exist. In many instances, a person exhibits questionable judgment that invites trouble: An elderly woman, for example, walks in the park alone late at night, her handbag dangling from her arm; during a manic episode, a man goes about muttering wildly to himself, cursing and angrily provoking others. When someone constantly puts himself in harm's way, does that constitute a clear and immediate danger?

Most often, the request for involuntary hospitalization comes from police following a violent incident or from family members who worry about the safety of their loved one. Although procedures differ in each state, psychiatric commitment can follow a common course. Generally, when a person in a psychiatric crisis is brought into a hospital emergency room, any request for involuntary admission begins a complicated process of evaluation. The psychiatrist will assess whether the person meets the legal criteria for involuntary hospitalization. During the process, the psychiatrist may try to negotiate with the person for a less restrictive situation. However, if the person refuses and continues to appear agitated, violent, or dangerous, the doctor can require hospitalization and a period of further evaluation before the judicial hearing.

Again, the length of stay for involuntary evaluation varies according to state guidelines, but it is usually quite short, perhaps 3 days or less. If after that time the person still seems suicidal or homicidal and continues to refuse treatment, the family or hospital must turn to the judicial system to detain him. The court decides if it is in the best interest of the person with mental illness to remain in the hospital, weighing the individual's freedoms and rights against his need for care.

At the same time, hospital mental health staff will work with the family to take greater control of the situation, consider their options, and make appropriate decisions. If the court rules against the request for involuntary hospitalization, the hospital will help provide services—visiting nurses, meals on wheels, day hospital treatment, for example—that the family may need until the person is willing to seek treatment. Nevertheless, the person will have the right to refuse any and all services. ■

---

atric evaluation. The length of treatment varies.

Residential treatment facility Occasionally, when an individual is too disturbed to live at home or his family is too chaotic or overtaxed to provide him with the support and structure he needs, he may live in a residential treatment facility. In these campus-like settings, patients receive intensive and comprehensive treatment that typically includes psychotherapy, both individual and group, occupational therapy, medication, and education, over a long period of time.

Intensive case management This type of comprehensive treatment approach is usually offered by a hospital, community mental health center, or, increasingly, a private or public insurance carrier and managed care organization. Through intensive case management, specially trained individuals coordinate and provide psychiatric, financial, legal, and medical services to help the patient stay at home and in the community. Often, such services are provided as part of follow-up services when a patient is discharged from a hospital or residential treatment facility.

Day treatment programs Developed to serve people with substance abuse problems, psychiatric disorders, and other conditions that require a range of intensive services, day treatment programs provide psychiatric treatment coupled with special education, vocational rehabilitation, and socialization groups. The patient usually attends 5 days a week but returns home in the evening and on weekends. Many times, these types of programs are offered as part of partial hospitalization or day hospital programs.

Therapeutic group home or community residences These special residences generally accommodate small groups of children and adults whose home life is chaotic, whose families are overtaxed, or whose illness is severe to the degree that they are unable to receive the type of support, structure, and nurturance that would allow them to stay in their own home. For many, community residences and group homes provide the only opportunity they have to live independently. The scope of psychiatric and medical services provided varies from site to site. However, these homes are commonly connected to a day treatment, special educational, or vocational rehabilitation program.

PSYCHOTHERAPY— WHAT IS IT?

To many, psychiatric treatment is synonymous with psychotherapy. While that is not the case—the array of effective psychiatric treatments has become, in recent years, impressively broad—"the talking cure," or psychotherapy, is a valuable, widely used method of treating psychiatric disorders, emotional distress, and the problems of everyday living.

Simply put, psychotherapy is a process in which a caring, mutually trusting relationship develops between a person who is suffering and a psychotherapist who possesses the training, skill, and motivation to ease that suffering. Within a very special and specialized human relationship, the person is heard, understood, and comforted. His choices, decisions, and feelings are considered and discussed, and he is offered insight and, at times, guidance. Usually, in time, he discovers that he actually feels better and is able to proceed with the business of life—work and relationships—with greater vigor, efficacy, and satisfaction.

A psychotherapist usually has advanced degrees in one of the mental health professions—psychiatry, psychology, social work, nursing—as well as specialized training in performing therapy and possibly in other related areas. The psychotherapist brings to the therapeutic relationship an in-depth understanding of human development, mental disorders, and psychological processes. He also brings a nonjudgmental attitude, an honest curiosity, and, perhaps most importantly, a vision that the person can be helped to get better.

Yet, it is not the therapist alone who advances change and healing; psychotherapy works on the assumption that the capacity for cure lies within each person. To some degree, the goal of all psychotherapy is to foster, within the person, a full and complex understanding of his abilities, worries, difficulties, relationships—of himself. As the person gains greater curiosity and insight, many of his thoughts, feelings, and behaviors naturally become modified. Many of the internal (intrapsychic) struggles that pose obstacles to normal psychological growth and functioning diminish. As he develops greater insight into himself and greater understanding of the way he operates in the world, he will likely be able to manage the demands of everyday living more effectively. Consequently, over time, a person develops a sense of mastery over his feelings, thoughts, behavior, and troubles.

Individual psychotherapy Depending on the person's age and diagnosis as well as the therapist's custom, individual psychotherapy is typically divided into periods of 30 to 50 minutes. These meetings can be held anywhere from one to four times a week, although once a week is customary. Usually, therapy sessions take place in a suitable office setting. During these sessions, the person is encouraged to explore his thoughts, choices, intimate experiences, and feelings while the therapist listens without moral judgment or criticism. From time to time, the therapist may ask for clarification, offer interpretations of internal conflicts, make connections between current problems and past experiences, and suggest different ways of coping.

Although the goal of individual therapy varies, therapy usually works to reduce anxiety, improve self-esteem, increase one's ability to tolerate frustration, modify symptoms, encourage better coping strategies and appropriate independence, and foster better relationships and more satisfactory and satisfying work. In short, when psychotherapy is successful, it enhances feelings of pleasure, joy, and competence. Child and adolescent therapy usually aim at freeing youngsters from internal and external conflicts to the degree that they can reengage in the normal process of development.

While there are many approaches to psychotherapy, psychoanalysis, analytically oriented psychodynamic psychotherapy, and behavioral and cognitive therapies are the most widely used. Individual intensive or psychodynamic psychotherapy is based on psychoanalysis, which emphasizes insight and understanding. More specifically, psychoanalysis and psychoanalytically oriented psychotherapy place great importance on interpretation—making the unconscious, that which exists outside of the person's awareness, conscious. In many cases, it entails understanding the person's unconscious as it is communicated through his feelings about the therapist, that is, interpreting the transference. Transference is the unconscious mechanism whereby a person assigns to his therapist the qualities, attitudes, and feelings of an individual (or individuals) significant in his earlier emotional development.

Cognitive and behavioral perspectives also inform most psychotherapies. These techniques focus on modifying the symptoms by correcting distorted thinking or dysfunctional behavior. In practice, most psychotherapists draw on a variety of theories, styles, approaches, and interventions, depending on the person's problem, personality, capacities, and needs. Most therapies encourage self-exploration while offering support and direction.

Psychodynamic psychotherapy The essence of psychodynamic psychotherapy—also called psychoanalytically oriented psychotherapy—is the communication and exploration of the person's inner state and beliefs even when they are dimly perceived by the person or reside almost completely within his unconscious.

As a process, psychodynamic psychotherapy typically unfolds in three phases. During the initial phase, a therapeutic alliance, or working relationship between the patient and clinician, is fostered. This is usually achieved when the patient experiences the therapist's nonjudgmental, understanding response to his behavior, responses, and feelings.

Ordinarily, the middle phase includes the interpretation of the transference and working through. By this time, the patient understands the fundamental intent of psychotherapy: to understand the way he feels and behaves. This includes the way he feels and behaves toward the therapist. *Working through* refers to the repeated examination of the patient's conflicts as they manifest in his day-to-day life, as well as in the patient-therapist relationship. What is more, many theories suggest that the relationship between the patient and therapist provides a corrective experience and thereby fosters psychological growth and healing.

The final phase of therapy centers on termination, which is usually marked by some actual achievement of the goals of therapy. There is no such thing as a perfect or complete therapy. However, all therapy ends at some point—with many things accomplished during the process and many other things left to be done outside of therapy. The termination phase provides an invaluable opportunity to explore issues of dependency and independence separation, and reactions to loss. Quite often, people temporarily fall back during this phase, and symptoms reappear. Others are able to recall the beginning of their treatment rather than reenact it through regressive behavior. Usually, a reasonable period of time is required to deal with termination so that the gains achieved during therapy can be consolidated.

Variations of psychodynamic psychotherapy arise from other theories, such as those that work toward self-mastery as well as insight. Although the method and the specific stages of treatment may differ slightly, these, too, rely heavily on the experience shared between the therapist and patient as they work together to help the patient.

Cognitive therapy Cognitive therapy addresses the thoughts and beliefs that a person develops early in life that color the ways he feels and behaves. For various, complicated reasons, some people develop negative core beliefs about themselves and their world that distort their interpretations of events and their expectations. Cognitive theories suggest that when people are helped to examine and correct their thinking—how they interpret events, what they expect from the world, and how they talk to themselves—their moods and behavior naturally improve.

In most cases, cognitive therapy is short term. Typically, a course of cognitive therapy runs once a week for 3 to 6 months. It focuses on the present and tends to be problem or symptom specific. The therapist takes an active role, guiding the person toward more accurate and realistic thinking, questioning the person's explanations, and teaching more effective coping strategies.

During therapy sessions, the therapist directs the person's attention to those automatic thoughts that seem to produce feelings of anxiety or depression. Facing a new task, a person may automatically think, "Why try? I'll only mess up." After a disappointment, he might think, as always, "I'm nothing but a loser."

The person is helped to recognize how he exaggerates the sense of threat, for example, anticipates disaster, overgeneralizes from negative experiences, and ignores when things go well. He is then encouraged to examine how realistic these thoughts are and to consider alternative interpretations and outcomes. So, for instance, someone who has panic attacks would be encouraged to see that the physical symptoms—the palpitations, hyperventilation, and dizziness—are not actually an overture to a heart attack.

Unlike a psychodynamic psychotherapist, who may help a demoralized person understand the origins of the feelings and defeatist thoughts that underlie his demoralization, cognitive therapists teach him to identify and label his negative thoughts, recognize their erroneous nature, and devise a plan to assess things more positively and deal with them more realistically.

In essence, cognitive therapy is a self-help approach that provides tools—specific ways of thinking—that a person can apply on his own whenever he finds himself slipping into old patterns of thought and behavior.

Behavioral therapy Rooted in learning theory, behavior therapy rests on the assumption that problematic behavior has been learned; it can therefore be unlearned, or replaced with new, more adaptive behavior. Once behavior is changed or modified, the thinking goes, a person will function more effectively in his world and therefore feel better.

Like cognitive therapy, behavior therapy tends to be active and directive. Unlike psychodynamic therapy, which assumes that insight and choice are the primary mechanisms for change, behavior therapy assumes that action motivates change. Direct symptom change is the focus of treatment. Therefore, behavior therapists frequently assign homework to complete between sessions, regularly discuss and review specific treatment strategies and goals, and negotiate behavioral contracts and expectations in the sessions. A person is encouraged to practice what he learns in therapy, interpretation is rarely used, and most of the therapist's interventions aim at helping the person accomplish behaviorally based treatment objectives.

Behavior therapy uses a number of specific techniques to advance behavioral change. Many times, the therapist relies on the person's environment—specifically, his family—to collaborate with and strengthen the process. Techniques include reinforcement, whether positive or negative, in which behavior is modified by imposing consequences; contingency contracting, which uses verbal or written contracts to identify, clarify, and reinforce desired behaviors; modeling, in which the person observes a model engaged in relevant behaviors; skills training techniques, which teaches social skills, cognitive skills, parenting skills, self-control, problem solving; and punishment and response cost, in which a person loses privileges, which aims at reducing or eliminating problem behaviors. These techniques work especially well with children or when an adult problem is expressed through disordered, destructive, or addictive behaviors.

Desensitization refers to a broad spectrum of exposure training behavior techniques that are based on conditioning principles. These techniques are often used to treat anxiety disorders. Ordinarily, these techniques use a detailed list of the person's fears, typically developed in hierarchical form by the person and therapist. In systematic desensitization, the therapist encourages the person to imagine a scene or object from the list, beginning with the least distressing. This is repeated until the person no longer responds to the imaginary exposure with distress.

In vitro desensitization uses exposure to actual scenes or circumstances to help lessen the person's anxiety. Flooding involves having the person come into contact with the most frightening object or situation on the list, either directly or imaginatively, until the fear is extinguished.

Play therapy Children naturally have trouble identifying and expressing their feelings. Play therapy—the use of simple toys, drawing, and play acting as symbolic, meaning-laden language—provides an indispensable venue for children to communicate their distress. Play can allow children to explore and communicate their inner state with their therapist, even when their feelings and conflicts remain largely unconscious.

Through play therapy, traumatized children might feel safe enough to reenact the event, for example, or depressed children, to act out their feelings of loss, powerlessness, aggression, and danger. Eventually, most children move from play to verbal expression. When children are having difficulty dealing with painful life circumstances, play therapy gives them the chance to resolve some of the feelings and accept even an unhappy reality.

While we commonly conceive of psychotherapy as a one-on-one process, it is very often conducted in family and group configurations as well. Indeed, rarely does a single form of psychiatric treatment suffice. In many instances of mental and emotional disorders, various combinations of treatment modalities are necessary, including individual psychotherapy, psychopharmacology (see Medication, page 1210), cognitive-behavioral therapy, family therapy, and group therapy.

Family therapy Family therapy, which aims at understanding individual problems within the context of the family, has proved helpful in treating a wide range of emotional disorders, including psychotic disorders, depression and manic-depressive disorder, anxiety disorders, substance abuse, eating disorders, and conduct disorders. Family treatment considers those aspects of family life that cause or maintain the problems, as well as family strengths and resources available to help resolve the problem.

In many cases, family therapy provides support and education as each member tries to live with another's emotional distress. Concurrently, issues within the family—problems in the marriage, unresolved grief, or a family secret—actually cause or worsen an individual member's emotional symptoms. Family therapy routinely speaks to certain problems that unwittingly perpetuate or promote symptoms in individual members, including a lack of generation boundaries, severe marital conflict, rigid or chaotic rules, projection of parental feelings onto a child, or neglectful or overly involved relationships.

In general, therapy offers families the opportunity to learn more productive ways of communicating with each other. It fosters mutual support, positive reinforcement, direct communication, and more effective problem solving within the family. It may offer instruction on conflict resolution as well.

Group therapy Group therapy uses the power of group dynamics and peer interaction to further understanding and hope. In addition, group process can have a very real influence on symptom reduction and internal change within the individual. It is an invaluable treatment modality for various types of people who come together around a wide range of emotional, behavioral, and life problems. Group therapy can be long term or time limited (usually 10 to 20 sessions). Each session typically meets for 1 to 2 hours each week. While self-help groups may not have a leader, psychotherapeutic groups most often are led by a trained group therapist. Frequently, a group will center on a specific issue or theme or on a particular population, such as rape victims, parents of manic-depressive children, or living with agoraphobia. Moreover, groups are particularly effective in addressing specific problematic behaviors, such as eating disorders and substance abuse.

Group therapy—whether it is a support or insight-oriented group—can help people develop social and coping skills, greater insight, and self-esteem. Many people find it easier to express feelings in a supportive group of their peers than in individual therapy. Often, an individual will feel supported and understood and will gain helpful insight and practical skills. For most people, hearing others talk about their problems and the ways they are trying to resolve them can have powerful therapeutic effects.

Anxiety Disorders

Everyone experiences anxiety from time to time. In fact, anxiety is an extremely useful emotion; feelings of uneasiness and distress work to signal us whenever an unfamiliar, challenging, or threatening situation is at hand.

There are times, however, when feelings of anxiety are so intense or long-lasting that they interfere with day-to-day functioning. And there are people for whom feelings of anxiety consistently intrude on their lives, making enjoyment and accomplishment nearly impossible. In these cases, anxiety is more than a normal emotion and is a serious emotional problem.

❖ GENERALIZED ANXIETY DISORDERS

Symptoms and signs Inexplicable feelings of impending doom; unfounded or excessive worry; trembling, twitching, shaky sensations; clammy hands, dry mouth, trouble swallowing; heart palpitations, sweating, tightness and pain in the chest, frequent urination, gas pains, nausea, muscle spasm, headaches, neck pain; difficulty paying attention, remembering, and learning; fatigue and difficulty sleeping; irritability.

What is it? A generalized anxiety disorder manifests in a vague, uncontrollable hum of worry, distress, uneasiness, and apprehension. You may feel restless, on edge, or all keyed up. You may harbor inexplicable feelings of approaching doom or menace. Even when there is little actual cause, you may constantly fret about the success of your business, your health, your child's safety, or the fate of your marriage.

When faced with particularly stressful circumstances or events, feelings of anxiety flair up. A person who is naturally timid, anxious, or wary may suddenly experience an irrational acute fear of a situation, such as

attending a party; an activity, such as driving; or an object, such as an animal.

The anxiety ripples out, affecting an individual's thinking, perception, memory, and learning. People suffering from anxiety disorders may find themselves forgetful or confused about time or place. They may interpret people's intentions or the meaning of events in more negative, menacing terms, and therefore feel unsafe in the world.

Approximately 5 percent of all Americans suffer from severe anxiety at some point in their lives. Most report that they were nervous as children and have been overly anxious throughout their lives. Although over half of those who seek treatment for anxiety disorders claim that they first felt anxious in childhood or adolescence, it is not all that uncommon for onset to occur after the age of 20. Slightly more women than men suffer from anxiety disorders.

Anxiety disorders seem to have a genetic component: The tendency toward anxiety seems to run in families. Also, studies show a connection to the brain chemicals norepinephrine, the neurotransmitter that governs concentration and attention, and serotonin, which is related to feelings of anxiety, depression, and aggression. It is not uncommon for depressive symptoms to exist side by side with anxiety. For information on anxiety disorders in children, see page 1231.

When to seek treatment Anxiety and fear are normal emotions, but if the following conditions apply, you should consult your doctor: Your worry outlasts or seems out of proportion to your circumstances; your anxieties interfere with your work and relationships; profound fear, restlessness, fatigue, or anxiety is present most of the time over a period of at least 6 months; you experience feelings of apprehensive expectation that cannot be soothed or controlled; physical symptoms, disturbed sleep, and difficulty concentrating seem to be getting out of hand.

Treatment Once it is clear that anxiety symptoms are not due to drug abuse, medication, or such general medical conditions as thyroid disorders and hypoglycemia, generalized anxiety disorders can be treated through individual psychotherapy or medication. In many cases, treatment that combines the two works best.

THE DANGERS OF TRANQUILIZER OVERUSE

In the last 50 years, as our understanding of the brain and the way it works has become more sophisticated and detailed, numerous new drugs have been developed to treat mental illness and emotional problems. In many instances, the effects of these psychotropic medications have been quite dramatic; in most instances, the benefits are unquestionable.

One such group consists of the antianxiety medications benzodiazepines. Popularly referred to as tranquilizers, this family of drugs includes diazepam (Valium), triazolam (Halcion), alprazolam (Xanax), chlordiazepoxide (Librium), and lorazepam (Ativan). These are typically prescribed to treat anxiety disorders and post-traumatic stress disorders.

Occasionally, these medications are prescribed in smaller dosages to ease the nervousness and stress related to everyday living. Using antianxiety drugs to manage lesser states of unease is a questionable practice. When a person does so, it is best if he takes them only for a short period of time. These medications are highly addictive. If the dosage is sufficiently high, they can, within short order, become physically and psychologically addictive. If taken over a long period of time, even a low dosage can lead to addiction. Indeed, even a patient who follows the prescribed dosage closely over a few months can develop withdrawal symptoms when he attempts to discontinue the medication.

During withdrawal, symptoms of addiction include nausea, anxiety, loss of appetite, restlessness, difficulty sleeping, blurred vision, tremors, twitching, and muscle pain. In extreme instances, withdrawal can prompt convulsions, delirium, seizures, paranoia, hallucinations, and psychotic-like breaks with reality.

In addition, problems arise when a patient takes other medications or drinks alcohol while taking antianxiety medication. If you have or have had a problem with alcohol dependency, be sure to alert your doctor. Before you take any other medication in combination with tranquilizers, consult your doctor. Avoid alcohol altogether. Drinking while you are taking any psychotropic medication is always risky. The combination of tranquilizers and alcohol can interfere with memory, make you drowsy, and speed up intoxication. Sometimes, the mixture can be deadly.

Every year, thousands of people go to emergency rooms or enter drug rehabilitation centers because their use of tranquilizers has gotten out of hand and become dangerous. Therefore, if you are currently taking antianxiety medications, do so only according to your doctor's instructions. And do not discontinue or alter your dosage without checking with your doctor first. ■

Antianxiety drugs, called benzodiazepines—clonazepam (Klonopin), lorazepam (Ativan), diazepam (Valium), and alprazolam (Xanax)—often bring relief. These medications work quickly to even out a person's mood. When side effects appear—agitation, giddiness, and impulsiveness—the dosage may need to be lowered. These drugs must be slowly discontinued and only under the direction of the prescribing physician or psychiatrist (see The Dangers of Tranquilizer Overuse, above). A group of drugs called selective serotonin reuptake inhibitors (SSRIs)—fluoxetine (Prozac), sertraline (Zoloft), paroxetine (Paxil)—and another called tricyclic antidepressants (TCAs)—clomipramine (Anafranil), amitriptyline (Elavil), desipramine (Norpramin), imipramine (Tofranil)—are also used to lower basic anxiety. SSRIs and TCAs have the added benefit of being nonaddictive.

Psychotherapy can help you understand what experiences, conflicts, and beliefs are at the root of your anxiety. Cognitive techniques that can help you examine the nature and reasonableness of your fears, and behavioral techniques that can guide you to confront, test, and tolerate those fears, have proven to be particularly effective in dealing with generalized anxiety disorders. Relaxation techniques such as square breathing, meditation, and visualization can relieve some of the more disconcerting physical symptoms; once these subside, you may be able to focus more clearly on what is causing the upset (see Techniques for Managing Stress, page 308).

Prognosis Good. Generalized anxiety disorders respond well to treatment. Many people with the disorder continue to experience higher than usual anxiety throughout their lives, which will likely intensify during times of stress. Yet, with treatment, anxiety becomes less debilitating.

❖ PANIC DISORDERS

Symptoms and signs Sudden, unexpected rush of anxiety; sweating, heart palpitations, trembling or shaking; shortness of breath; sensations of choking, chest pain, nausea, dizziness, light-headedness, or numbness; feelings of unreality or being detached from oneself; fear of dying, losing control, or going crazy; chills, hot flushes, or tingling sensations.

What is it? Panic attacks are discrete, recurrent periods of profound fear or discomfort in which sudden rushes of fearfulness are accompanied by such physical symptoms as hyperventilation (labored breathing), palpitations (rapid heartbeat), and dizziness. A person who suffers from panic attacks may experience feelings of unreality and fear of dying. These intense, sudden surges of anxiety typically reach intensity within seconds and subside between 5 and 20 minutes later, although less intense, vague feelings of panic may linger for an hour or so.

The symptoms that accompany a panic attack are responses that the body normally experiences in dire situations. But because no real threat has caused the response, the person may worry that she is having a heart attack or is suffering from some other life-threatening illness that has gone undiagnosed by her doctors. She may worry that she is going crazy.

For many people, panic attacks occur spontaneously without the presence of an identifiable trigger. In fact, a person may awaken from sleep in the throes of a panic attack.

For others, panic attacks may have a recognizable trigger. They may occur, for example, immediately upon exposure to or in anticipation of specific objects, such as snakes or dogs. In other instances, panic may be associated with certain situations, particularly those in which fleeing may be impeded or help is not immediately available, such as when one is riding on public transportation, driving across a bridge, standing in a crowd, or waiting in line. Sometimes, a person begins to avoid particular objects or situations in order to avoid panic attacks. When fearful anticipation begins to encircle her life, she may begin to manifest phobic behavior (see Phobia, page 1220). Because the occurrence of panic attacks is not always predictable, a person who is prone to them may become preoccupied with worry that they will return without warning.

Between 1.5 and 3.5 percent of the general population experiences panic disorders within their lifetime. Women are twice as likely as men to suffer from panic disorders, and when the disorder includes agoraphobic tendencies (see page 1220), women are three times as likely to be affected.

On the average, people begin to first experience severe panic symptoms between late adolescence and their mid-30s. In rare instances, though, panic disorders begin in childhood or after age 45.

There is considerable evidence that panic disorders are rooted in genetic disposition. In addition, risk for such disorders increases not only when there is a family history of anxiety disorders but when family members suffer from other mood disorders, alcoholism, or somatization disorder. At the same time, the biologic symptoms—hyperventilation, palpitations, and dizziness that bring on the panic—can be precipitated, exacerbated, and modified by external and internal events and influences.

The course and severity of panic disorders vary from person to person. In rare instances, people have continuous symptoms. In most instances, though, there is a waxing and waning rhythm to the disorder. Some people have moderately frequent attacks, once a week regularly for a month, for example. Others report short bursts of more frequent attacks, daily or many times a day for a week separated by weeks or months with no or fewer attacks. Some people have episodic outbreaks with periods of remission in between.

When to seek treatment People often are referred for psychiatric treatment by their general physician after a medical consultation fails to uncover a physical explanation for the sensations.

Treatment The combination of medication and cognitive-behavioral therapy has been found to be successful in treating panic attacks. Benzodiazepines, or antianxiety medications such as clonazepam, diazepam, and alprazolam, can take some of the edge off the feelings of panic. Also, low dosages of the antidepressants fluoxetine or sertraline or of the TCAs—clomipramine, amitriptyline, desipramine, imipramine—seem to be able to modify some of the more debilitating symptoms. Frequently, the right dosage of the right medication can eliminate symptoms altogether.

Therapy generally includes a strong educational component. The nature of panic attacks is described. Together with the therapist, the person looks at how realistic her fears are. Reassurances that there is no real physical or mental danger and that the symptoms are invariably time limited may make the attacks seem more manageable. Therapy may also help the person learn to read bodily sensations more accurately, rather than interpreting them all as anxiety responses.

Other behavioral techniques can also be effective in dealing with feelings of panic, particularly when panic attacks have specific triggers. Exposure techniques introduce the feared object or situation in a controlled and measured way. The therapist may then gently encourage confrontation.

In systematic desensitization, the person is encouraged to visualize whatever causes anxiety with the help of tranquilizers, hypnosis, and muscle relaxation techniques. Flooding, or exposing the person to the feared object or situation as long as she can tolerate it, is another approach.

Prognosis Good.

❖ PHOBIA

Symptoms and signs Continuous, excessive, or unaccountable fear triggered by the presence or anticipation of a particular object, activity, or situation; feelings of panic; avoidance, crying, freezing.

What is it? Phobias—intense, unreasonable fears of a specific activities, objects, or situations—are actually quite common in our society. In many cases, phobias do not pose any significant restrictions or disruptions to a person's life. However, when phobic anxiety begins to interfere considerably and consistently with a person's functioning, it becomes a serious disorder. If, for example, a person cannot step on an elevator, he will have to limit where he lives and works. A person who fears crowded or closed-in places may find his social activities severely restricted.

A person may develop a phobia following a traumatic event or after observing someone undergoing an intensely upsetting or horrific experience. It is not uncommon for a person to respond with phobic anxiety, for example, after being trapped in a closet, being attacked by an animal, or watching someone fall from a great height. Phobias may arise after a person experiences an unexpected panic attack. Milder phobias may result from repeated parental warnings about danger or after hearing media coverage of some disastrous event.

Commonly, phobias center on fear of animals, storms, heights, water, and blood. Some people have phobic reactions to medical objects and settings—hospitals, needles, testing equipment, and procedures. Other phobias involve such situations as flying, driving, riding in tunnels or over bridges, being on public transportation, elevators, and other enclosed places. For some individuals, circumstances that require them to perform or interact socially fill them with phobic dread. Still others have great anxiety around the possibility of choking, vomiting, or contracting an illness, and they limit their activities accordingly.

People who fear going out in public are said to suffer from agoraphobia. Agoraphobia often arises out of a dread of being in places or situations from which escape might be difficult or embarrassing, or in which help might not be available should a panic attack occur.

Another relatively common phobic disorder is called social phobia. People who suffer from this type of phobia experience a constant dread of the possibility that they might have to interact with unfamiliar people, be subject to the scrutiny of others, or be humiliated or embarrassed. For example, people with a social phobia may avoid eating in restaurants because they believe that others will comment negatively on their eating habits or manners. Social phobia may preclude people from writing in front of others or using a public bathroom.

When to seek treatment Seek treatment when you find yourself avoiding particular situations, activities, or objects to the point that your life is seriously circumscribed.

Treatment Phobias—like other anxiety disorders—can be treated in a variety of ways, although combined use of medication and cognitive-behavioral therapy has been found to be widely successful. Antipanic medications—diazepam, lorazepam, and alprazolam—are often prescribed to modify some of the more debilitating panic symptoms. In some cases, antidepressant medications—fluoxetine or sertraline—are given in dosages generally lower than for depression.

Therapy may include insight and examination of feelings, especially when a phobia has arisen in response to a specific event or situation. When a phobia reflects other problems—depression, for example, or post-traumatic stress disorder—those will be addressed in therapy as well. Certain behavioral techniques have proved particularly effective in treating phobias: exposure, which encourages controlled and measured confrontation with the object of the phobia; systematic desensitization, which uses tranquilizers, hypnosis, and muscle relaxation techniques and then encourages visualization and confrontation; and flooding, in which a person is brought into contact with the feared object or situation for as long as he can tolerate it. Once the phobia is controlled through behavioral techniques, frequent practice or reexposure to the phobic stimuli is usually needed to maintain the benefits of treatment.

Prognosis Fairly good. However, phobias that persist into adulthood tend to be tenacious.

❖ OBSESSIVE-COMPULSIVE DISORDER

Symptoms and signs Persistent unwanted thoughts, images, impulses, doubts, or ideas that intrude repeatedly and involuntarily on a person's consciousness (obsession), often concerning cleanliness, contamination, safety, and sexuality; irresistible, repetitive performance of irrational actions (compulsions based on underlying obsessions), such as hand washing, hair pulling, ordering, and checking, or such mental acts as counting, praying, and repeating words silently.

What is it? People who suffer from obsessive-compulsive disorder get caught up in uncontrollable rituals and rumination. Many times, the rituals and ruminations—which can be relatively benign or quite bizarre—began as a way of imposing order on intense internal feelings of chaos. These repetitive thoughts and actions constitute a disorder when they become a source of considerable anxiety and distress and when they interfere dramatically with normal functioning. Although individuals with obsessive-compulsive disorder may recognize that their thoughts, impulses, and urges make no sense, and may well resist them, they nevertheless feel that they have no control over them.

The most common obsessions involve repeated thoughts about contamination and germs (worries that shaking hands will cause disease); constant doubts (anxiety that the gas stove was not turned off in the house); order and organization (distress when papers are not stacked just so); aggression (fear that one will inflict pain on a child); sex (a recurrent pornographic image).

Frequently, attempts to ignore, neutralize, or suppress such thoughts develop into compulsive habits. A woman who worries about contamination may begin to wash her hands countless times during the day, until they are red and raw. A man who worries that he will yell out obscenities at work may count backward from 100, countless times a day. Usually, people with obsessive-compulsive disorder will be able to delineate elaborate rules for chronology, rate, order, duration, and number of repetitions involved in their compulsive behavior.

Until recently, the prevalence of obsessive-compulsive disorder was thought to be relatively rare; however, it now appears that within the general population, 2.5 percent suffer from this disorder within their lifetime. It usually begins in early adolescence or adulthood, although it may appear in childhood. For men, the average age of onset is between age 6 and 15; for women, it is between age 20 and 29. Usually, onset is gradual, and in most instances, there is a fluctuating pattern to the illness. Symptoms tend to worsen during stressful times.

Current studies suggest that a vulnerability to obsessive-compulsive disorder is transmitted genetically. In addition, there seems to be a strong link between the disorder and the neurochemical serotinin and perhaps norepinephrine and dopamine as well.

When to seek treatment Obsessive-compulsive disorder seldom disappears on its own. In the vast majority of cases, professional treatment is necessary to alleviate the symptoms, address the anxiety or depression underlying the behavior, and minimize the disruption it causes in a person's social, intimate, and occupational functioning.

Treatment Treating obsessive-compulsive disorder usually combines a number of elements over an extended period of time, including medication, family, and individual therapy.

Often, antidepressant medications—specifically, those that influence serotonin, the nerve cell chemical that acts as a brain messenger—can reduce the frequency and intensity of the more problematic symptoms and may be prescribed, at least initially, in conjunction with therapy. The medications most often prescribed for obsessive-compulsive disorder are SSRIs, such as fluoxetine, sertraline, paroxetine, and fluvoxamine (Luvox). TCAs, particularly clomipramine, also are effective in treating obsessive-compulsive disorder.

Because this disorder can be so very disruptive to family life, family therapy is frequently recommended. Therapy can support family members as they learn about the disorder. In addition, therapy can identify ways in which family members unwittingly perpetuate symptoms as well as identify other problems that could be promoting symptoms.

Individual therapy is an important, though demanding, aspect of treatment. Behavioral and cognitive techniques have proven quite useful in treating people with obsessive-compulsive disorder. These people may be brought into contact, through either gradual direct confrontation or imaginary exposure, with the feared object or event; then their attempts to engage in obsessive-compulsive behavior are gently thwarted. At the same time, they can begin to examine and evaluate their distorted, fearful thinking and to consider alternate ways of dealing with their anxiety.

Prognosis Fairly good. However, because obsessive-compulsive disease can be a chronic condition, treatment may be necessary for years.

❖ POST-TRAUMATIC STRESS DISORDER

Symptoms and signs Different people develop different symptoms in response to trauma, depending on their age when the traumatic event occurred, the nature of the event, and the way in which the trauma was handled by others at the time. Related symptoms include intense feelings of fear, horror, and helplessness; flashbacks; persistent avoidance of reminders of the trauma; psychic and physical numbness; intensified distress, especially on anniversaries of the event; distressing dreams and nightmares; hypervigilance; tendency to startle easily; irritability and outbursts of anger; preoccupation with randomness, ruminating why the event occurred, its purpose, and ways it could have been averted; an ominous sense of life's destiny. Symptoms tend to change and evolve over time.

What is it? First identified as "shell shock" in World War I, and brought to prominent attention in veterans of the Vietnam War, post-traumatic stress disorder has since been recognized in the larger population. The term is used to describe a broad pattern of emotional and behavioral symptoms that arise as a result of direct exposure to or participation in intensely frightening, often violent events or circumstances. Psychic trauma occurs when people are involved in horrible external events over which they have no control and which render them temporarily helpless.

There are three basic types of psychic trauma: single-blow trauma, which arises from a single, sudden, and unexpected blow such as a rape, a car accident that kills someone else, or a destructive flood; repeated trauma, which arises from long-standing, anticipated blows, such as political torture, sexual or physical abuse; and long-term trauma, in which a single, sudden shock results in homelessness, disability, disfigurement, prolonged hospitalization or pain, or serious injury or death of a loved one.

Post-traumatic stress symptoms appear and evolve over time. At the moment of the event, a person usually retains full physical and emotional control. In retrospect, it may be noted that he remained remarkably calm. Yet, within days, the full impact of the experience may hit. He might begin to wonder why it happened, whether he was chosen in particular for the experience, and what he could have done to prevent it. In time, this may evolve into a belief that his future is limited, and his destiny grim.

With a single-blow trauma, a person is likely to remember the event with dazzling clarity. Yet the details may become distorted; time becomes protracted or condensed.

For people who are subjected to repeated trauma, there is a greater tendency to become numb. Take, for example, the experience of sexual or physical abuse; once a child comes to understand that the abuse will happen again, and that she has no control over it, her dread may eventually translate into physical and emotional numbing. Or, as she comes to accept the terrible inevitability, she may begin to dissociate, cutting that part of her life, and herself, off, and forcing herself not to feel. As an adult, she will likely experience a reduced ability to feel emotions, especially those associated with tenderness, intimacy, vulnerability, and sexuality.

Even so, trauma may lead a person to experience vivid and unwelcome imagery from the event, especially during leisure times, when he is bored at work or school, falling asleep, listening to the radio, or watching television. Some people experience flashbacks years after the traumatizing event.

It is not at all unusual for people with post-traumatic stress disorder to be preoccupied with the event or experience for years. Feelings of fearfulness, panic, and menace tend to pervade most areas of their life. Traumatic episodes tend to drain the enjoyment from activities that used to interest them. They may feel estranged from other people, even those who are dearest to them. In addition, they may experience unremitting sadness and generalized rage. Occasionally, a traumatized person expresses that rage in self-mutilating and self-endangering behavior or physically damaging suicidal gestures.

When to seek treatment Depending on the severity of the event or circumstances, and the persistence of your reaction, it is usually wise to consult a mental health clinician following a disastrous experience.

If traumatizing episodes are not dealt with immediately, it may be discovered, years later, that trauma lies at the root of other conditions, including depression, behavioral disorders, and anxiety or panic disorders. During subsequent psychiatric treatment, the existence and impact of earlier trauma will be uncovered.

Treatment Often, when a single-blow episode, such as a hurricane, flood, tornado, a violent act at the local school, or the suicide of a classmate, affects large groups of people, the community will step forward and provide emergency interventions. After such disastrous events, early responses from mental health professionals, community assemblies, and school-centered groups allow for immediate exploration of the impact. By providing the forum for sharing experiences, feelings, and reactions, these interventions may well act to circumvent later problems and symptoms.

When symptoms in response to a traumatic episode or experience take root, other treatment may be necessary. Occasionally, medication is recommended in the early course of post-traumatic or acute stress disorder, particularly to treat trauma-related depressions, anxiety, or compulsive behaviors. Also, therapy that, over time,

allows the person to talk about the trauma can be instrumental in allowing him to get on with his life.

Prognosis Good. Although few people get over traumatic events completely, with the support and love of family members, and appropriate psychosocial interventions, most are able to gain greater perspective and understand the experience within the larger context of their past and go on to engage in productive and healthy lives.

Depressive Disorders and Mania

Each and every one of us manifests, within our basic temperamental makeup, an emotional baseline of sorts. Made up of characteristic moods and responses, a distinct disposition is, in most instances, discernible within the first few months of a child's life. And unless something dramatic intervenes, a child brings his emotional and behavioral endowment into adulthood.

At the same time, disposition accounts only partially for a person's mood patterns and attitudes toward life. Environmental factors—both the family circumstances into which each one of us is born and the events that meet us along the way—play a crucial role in the development and expression of emotions.

Periods of sadness are inevitable throughout life. There are times when everyone feels blue, even when life circumstances seem uneventful or reasonably happy. All this is as it should be.

However, some people feel a profound and constant sense of hopelessness and despair. For those who suffer from a depressive illness, feelings of black, impenetrable despair and often unaccountable irritation color every experience, perception, thought, activity, and reaction. Most times, when such people are depressed, their mood has little relation to the life around them. When there is a connection, the emotional response seems completely out of proportion to the circumstances. Yet, they may well blame themselves for their troubles. Indeed, depression actually makes circumstances seem worse, because all experiences are filtered through feelings of hopelessness, self-blame, and negative implications.

For some people, feelings of despair are occasionally interrupted by episodes of euphoria. When this is the pattern, the disorder is called bipolar disorder, or manic-depressive disorder.

Studies indicate as many as 25 percent of all women and 12 percent of men will at some time suffer from some sort of depressive illness. Regardless of ethnicity, education, income, or marital status, serious mood disorders affect millions of people in the United States each year.

Mood disorders—whether depression or bipolar disorder—can range from a mild, persistent condition to a profound and dramatic emotional state. Some people with chronic depression and bipolar disorder function reasonably well most of the time. Others find that their functioning and social relationships are severely circumscribed by their illness, either consistently or periodically.

Both depression and bipolar disorder have roots in the physiology and chemistry of the brain. In people who suffer from mood disorders, the mechanism that maintains an even chemical level in the brain goes askew, and the imbalance results in a dulling or frenzy of mood. The vulnerability to depressive and manic illness is clearly inherited. It is not uncommon to find that depression and bipolar disorder run in families.

In addition, life circumstances, especially early in a child's development, may pave the way for depression. Some studies draw a link between depression and the early loss of or unsuccessful attachment to a nurturing figure. Other theories point to a connection between depression and a habitual pattern of negative thinking. Most researchers and practitioners, however, assume that a combination of factors contributes to a vulnerability to depressive or bipolar disorder.

❖ REACTIVE AND GRIEF-RELATED DEPRESSION

Symptoms and signs Feelings of despair, helplessness, and fatigue following a significant event, change, or loss; uncharacteristic feelings of worthlessness, guilt, irritability, and uneasiness; withdrawal from relationships and depressed sex drive; lack of concentration and reduced motivation; change in eating and/or sleeping patterns; when related to grief, vague and acute feelings of sorrow, shock, disbelief, anger, protest, and despair that persist long after the actual loss.

What is it? Reactive depression describes a condition of gloom, sadness, and other depressive symptoms that exceeds—in terms of intensity and duration of the feeling—what would be expected in response to a given disappointment, loss, or significant change.

When a loved one dies, a person naturally goes through a complicated process of grieving. (For more information on grief, see The Five Stages of Grief, on page 1488.) In addition, feelings of shock, despair, and anger may follow many other experiences involving loss, such as the end of a relationship, the loss of a job, a divorce, or serious illness or accident. Even when events seem generally happy, when a child begins kindergarten or leaves home for college, for example, or during a move to another community or another job, you may find yourself feeling bereaved. Everyone has characteristic ways of responding to the expectable and unexpectable events in one's life, and a common reaction to disappointment, change, and loss is to feel blue.

Such feelings are normal; they indicate a serious problem only when they persist for a long period of time, seem extraordinarily intense given the nature of the circumstances, or when there is a continued pattern of responding to most every kind of stress with depressive reactions.

What you can do Frequently, feelings of depression are exacerbated when you are taken off guard. Being able to anticipate which experiences regularly evoke depressive reactions for you—the beginning of the school year, for example, or after you have completed a complicated job assignment—may offer some protection from the full impact of the feelings. Also, knowing that the depression will diminish when the stress fades may also soften the edge. For some people, exercise and relaxation techniques may also help.

When to seek treatment If you tend to react to situational problems with mild symptoms of depression, you may want to seek the emotional support and guidance of a therapist. Through psychotherapy, you can

ADDICTION, DEPENDENCY, AND SUBSTANCE ABUSE

The relationship between mental illness and substance use and abuse is a complicated one. Alcohol and psychoactive drugs alter a person's perceptions, feelings, and behavior, and some people use these substances for just that reason. Many people who suffer from emotional disorders or mental illness turn to drugs and alcohol to self-medicate, as a way of tolerating feelings that are intolerable. Yet, ironically, this method of self-treating seldom works in the long run and frequently makes matters worse.

A person may take a drink or two, or smoke marijuana when he is having a tough time in response to trouble at the office, a divorce, the death of a loved one, or the diagnosis of an illness. Problem drinking or drug use often starts out as a relatively moderate way of soothing upset, perhaps as a way of falling asleep. Yet, because drinking or using drugs only masks the problem, dulls the senses, and compromises judgment, this is a self-defeating, futile solution. The difficulty that led to the drink or the joint lingers, after the glass is empty or the ashes are cold.

For others, drinking or drug use may be a way of breaking out of a chronic, mild depressive or anxious state. Methylphenidate (Ritalin) or the designer drug "ecstasy," a psychostimulant, may give a person just the right "high" he needs to enjoy his evenings, or it might be that reward at the end of a tedious day. In the same way, a person finds that a few beers at lunch and then a few more at night take the edge off anxiety or angry feelings. However, usually when the drug wears off, or the alcohol-induced mellow haze fades, the blues, irritability, and agitation return, often with a vengeance. In more severe cases of self-medicating, opiates, specifically, heroin, are used to temper psychotic symptoms. Frequently, psychotic episodes occur during and after detoxification.

Using drugs and drink to self-medicate is only one side of the equation. During a psychiatric evaluation, it is always necessary to rule out drug or alcohol use, because they can produce symptoms that mimic those of mental illness. Hallucinogens, for example, can cause hallucinations, dissociative states, and bizarre, manic-like behavior. Depressive symptoms can arise as a result of cocaine withdrawal. Alcohol usually exacerbates anxiety or depression. With people who use recreational depressants—such as diazepam, lorazepam, alprazolam, and triazolam—barbiturates—such as pentobarbital (Nembutal) and secobarbital (Seconal)—and other hypnotics—such as glutethimide (Doriden), methaqualone (Quaalude), and ethchlorvynol (Placidyl)—there can be increased aggressiveness and violent behavior because these medications lower inhibitions. Stimulants can produce a cycle of rush-high-crash-anxiety-depression that imitates a manic-depressive cycle. They can also prompt suicidal or violent behavior. Cocaine can cause manic-like symptoms, panic attacks, hallucinations, paranoia, and, in withdrawal, depression and suicidal behavior. Opiates frequently cause depression, and withdrawal can result in criminal acts or suicidal behavior.

In short, alcohol and drugs—no matter how tempting—do not provide any real, enduring relief from emotional problems. And in almost all instances, they make things worse. For more information on the dangers of substance abuse and on ways to break addiction, see Chapter 5. ■

learn to manage such episodes in a more even-handed way and to cope with the day-to-day stresses in your life. Also, if the signs and symptoms become more acute or persistent, contact a therapist.

When sharp feelings of grief do not subside with time or seem to be expressing themselves in physical or emotional symptoms, call your doctor.

Treatment The best treatment for depressive disorders combines antidepressant medication and psychotherapy. Generally, your doctor will prescribe SSRIs such as fluoxetine, sertraline, paroxetine, and fluvoxamine. Another type of medication, TCAs, is also commonly prescribed. These include imipramine, nortriptyline (Pamelor), amitriptyline (Elavil), and desipramine (Norpramin) (see Antidepressant Medication, page 1227).

Once symptoms are relieved, psychotherapy can work to help you understand what precipitated the depression and what resources are available to relieve some of the stresses within your life (see Recognizing Stress, page 305, and Managing Stress, page 307).

Prognosis Good. Reactive depression responds well to both medication and psychotherapy. During the course of treatment, an underlying predisposition toward depression may be uncovered, in which case, longer-term therapy may be recommended to address the deeper mood disorder (see Major Depression, below).

❖ MAJOR DEPRESSION

Symptoms (*What you may experience*) An acute or lasting sense of despair, hopelessness, and guilt that seems to have little or exaggerated relation to life circumstances; a lack of interest or pleasure in most activities; deep feelings of sluggishness, fatigue, or agitation; certainty that everything is worthless and hopeless; preoccupation with thoughts of suicide or death; a precipitous change in appetite and/or weight; difficulties in sleeping or a tendency to oversleep; diminished ability to concentrate and make decisions; dramatic changes in working and social patterns.

Signs and laboratory findings *(What the doctor looks for)* A sustained and pervasive change in mood. Loss of interest in normal pleasures of life: food, sex, friends, work, family, sports, hobbies; a family or personal history of depression or suicide attempts, alcohol or drug use; a change in the way one thinks about oneself; a pattern of negative, pessimistic, self-blaming, or self-critical thinking; suicidal thoughts and behavior.

What is it? There is a tendency today to use the word *depression* to describe the inevitable periods of sadness that each of us experience from time to time. And indeed, for many, during these periods, it is not always easy to discern where normal sorrow ends and clinical depression begins. Yet, anyone who has ever experienced a major depression knows—at least after the depression has lifted—that what they feel is more than just persistent sadness.

Clinical depression is an illness characterized by a cluster of feelings, thoughts, and behaviors that are strikingly distinct from a person's normal range of feelings and functioning. Caused by a complex interaction of biologic, social, and psychological factors, a major depressive disorder can make a person exquisitely sensitive to life circumstances, the least of which can throw him into total black despair.

During a major depression, a person becomes enveloped by feelings of sadness, emptiness, and worthlessness. Like an impenetrable curtain descending, these feelings distort every thought and experience, rendering life meaningless and hopeless. Feelings of being deeply, continually deprived, insignificant, inadequate, and guilt-ridden build on feelings of sadness. At the same time, a depressed person may feel chronically irritated, occasionally erupting in frustration and anger.

While a major depression may be triggered by some life circumstance or event, the mood reaction seems greatly exaggerated. In all likelihood, depression has less to do with events than with a person's inherent vulnerability to the condition.

In rare cases, a person may experience a major depression as a single episode.

However, in most instances, clinical depression tends to recur periodically, reactively, or cyclically. A major depression may last up to 2 years.

Milder depressive states are called dysthymic disorders. It is likely that these low-grade, intermittent, or chronic depressive states form in some people the temperamental basis from which major depressions arise. For those with dysthymic disorder, certain life circumstances—the end of a relationship, the loss of a job, going away to college, for example—might provoke a deeper depression.

For some people, there is a seasonal aspect to their depression. Seasonal affective disorder (SAD) is a form of reactive depression that is more prevalent in northern parts of the country where the climatic extremes are greater. Typically affecting people in the fall or winter, seasonal affective disorder is characterized by fatigue, sugar craving, overeating, and oversleeping. While the exact cause of the disorder is not certain, it may be related to the way in which the light-responsive pineal gland in the brain functions.

For information on depression in children, see page 1235.

What you can do During the time that you feel despondent, seek the emotional support of family and friends. For milder depressions of short duration, the support of loved ones may help you through. But in most cases, you will not be able to fight depression on your own, and you should not try to. Like asthma or hypertension, depression is an illness and requires medical attention so that it can be managed effectively. If you are suffering from a depression, it is important that you seek professional help.

If you suffer from SAD, you may respond to spending at least an hour a day outdoors, even in winter. Increase the amount of natural light in your house. Whenever possible, take trips in winter to warmer and sunnier climates.

When to seek treatment If you are in the throes of depression, you may well believe that you are beyond help. Yet depression can be effectively treated and managed. If your state of gloom persists more than 2 weeks, you find that you cannot get out of bed, you are increasingly isolated from fam-

ANTIDEPRESSANT MEDICATION

Regardless of life circumstances—which can indeed be depressing from time to time—it is the chemistry of the brain that determines whether a person will respond to those circumstances with depression or develop depressive symptoms quite apart from his circumstances. Consequently, depression is quite responsive to antidepressant medications.

Children inherit their basic chemistry from their parents; thus, depression runs in families. Any imbalance in that chemistry—specifically, among the neurotransmitters dopamine, serotonin, and norepinephrine—might trigger depression. However, it is thought that underactivity of serotonin or norepinephrine is the true culprit. When a person inherits such a chemical vulnerability, any internal or external stress can alter the balance and produce depressive symptoms.

In the past 50 years, it has become increasingly clear that the best treatment for almost any kind of depression is the combined use of antidepressants and psychotherapy. The most effective and widely prescribed medications for depression are selective serotonin reuptake inhibitors (SSRIs)—fluoxetine, sertraline, and paroxetine. These medications work fast; symptoms may disappear as soon as 3 weeks after treatment begins. Side effects tend to be mild and infrequent: nausea, diarrhea, sexual dysfunction, and insomnia. (See Medication, page 1210, for more information on how these and the other antidepressant medications work.)

Another group of antidepressants consists of the tricyclic antidepressants (TCAs)—imipramine (Tofranil), nortriptyline (Pamelor), amitriptyline (Elavil), and desipramine. These medications usually take up to 4 to 6 weeks before their effects are felt. Mild but frequent side effects include dry mouth, drowsiness, and constipation. However, these medications can, in rare cases, affect the cardiovascular system, so they require careful monitoring.

When patients do not respond well to either TCAs or SSRIs, atypical antidepressants such as bupropion (Wellbutrin), trazodone, nefazodone (Serzone), and venlafaxine (Effexor) may be prescribed. Side effects for bupropion—irritability, agitation, and restlessness—are usually mild and transient. There is, however, a small risk of seizures associated with this medication. Side effects with trazodone and nefazodone are also mild and short lived; these include sleepiness, increased blood pressure, nausea, and dizziness. However, in rare cases, trazodone can cause priapism in men, a prolonged erection without sexual stimulation. Possible side effects for venlafaxine are similar to those seen with SSRIs (see Medication, page 1210), plus a significant increase in blood pressure.

Sometimes monoamine oxidase inhibitors (MAOIs), such as phenelzine or tranylcypromine, will be prescribed. These require some restrictions in terms of diet: Foods rich in tyramine—red wine, beer, smoked fish, aged meats and cheeses—can produce serious hypertensive reactions, including sweating, palpitations, headaches, and nausea.

Some people worry that they will become addicted to antidepressant medications. Unlike benzodiazepines (see The Dangers of Tranquilizer Overuse, page 1218) or drugs of abuse, antidepressants are not addictive. Rather, like antihypertensive medications, antibiotics, or insulin, antidepressants are needed by the body to treat and prevent certain conditions or illness. As such, you may need to take them for long periods to manage the illness and prevent relapse.

A more serious problem occurs when people simply take themselves off the medications, even when the benefits have been apparent for some time. If the drug is abruptly discontinued, symptoms can return and stronger than ever.

Finally, the fact that these medications work quickly to modify depressive symptoms, often without serious side effects, is certainly a blessing for those who suffer from severe depression. However, it also poses a rather troublesome quandary. Fluoxetine, especially, has become widely used to medicate even the mildest depressive symptoms, raising concern that it is inadvisable to provide medication as an antidote for life's ups and downs without helping an individual learn to deal with life's vicissitudes in other ways. Fluoxetine is best used in well-defined circumstances, for example, when a specific diagnosis, such as clinical depression, has been made. Although medication may be a treatment in and of itself, it is often an important component of a more comprehensive treatment plan. And no matter how effective and compelling a medication is in treating a disorder, it simply cannot smooth out the distresses and disorders of the human condition. ■

---

ily and friends, and you have lost any sense of enjoyment or interest in your usual activities, call your doctor. Also, if you find yourself ruminating about death and the meaningless of life, and you are considering suicide, seek help immediately. (see Spotting the Warning Signs of Suicide, page 1228, for more information.)

Treatment Mild depression can be effectively treated through psychotherapy. Even short-term therapy can help you understand your natural inclination toward more negative and somber moods. In addition, you can learn to cope better with life's upset and triumphs. When depression is triggered by seasonal change, light therapy, which extends exposure to bright light for measurable periods of time, may work to relieve symptoms.

In cases of more severe depression, medication will provide the main avenue for treatment. At the same time, psychotherapy is usually an important complement to medication. By restoring chemical balances within the brain, psychotropic medication will lift the veil of sorrow. The most commonly prescribed antidepressant medications are SSRIs (fluoxetine, sertraline, paroxetine,

SPOTTING THE WARNING SIGNS OF SUICIDE

Caught in feelings of desperation and hopelessness, thousands of people—some estimates put the number as high as 30,000—commit suicide each year in the United States. The number of people who attempt suicides may be eight to ten times higher.

Suicide is the eighth leading cause of death in this country. Men commit suicide more than three times as often as women, perhaps because they tend to choose more violent, efficient methods, such as jumping from high places or hanging or shooting themselves. Women are four times more likely to make attempts, typically using poison or drug overdose. The greatest number of male suicides happens after age 45. Women tend to be most vulnerable to suicidal behavior after age 55.

People who live alone with few social connections are at high risk. A person is more likely to attempt to kill himself during a period of unemployment. Overall, suicides go up during recessions, depressions, and periods of high unemployment.

For many, suicide seems the only solution to intractable problems and feelings of emptiness, inertia, and helplessness. Often, people who are profoundly depressed lack the energy to kill themselves. As they begin to respond to treatment and feel better, they stand at higher risk for suicide, because they regain sufficient direction and energy to act.

Individuals in the following circumstances may be at greater risk for attempting suicide:

- Someone who has experienced a recent and significant loss

- Someone who suffers from a serious depression, schizophrenia, or other mental illnesses

- Someone with a personal or family history of suicidal behavior and depression

- Someone with an alcohol or drug problem and depression

- Someone who suffers from serious physical illness and has depression

- Someone who has a chronic illness or has been in a serious accident that has resulted in unremitting pain, diminished mobility, or disfigurement

- Someone who abruptly withdraws from his normal activities and involvements

- Someone who exhibits a sudden and profound change of personality

- Someone with an impulsive or aggressive disposition and depression

You need to be particularly alert for the possibility of suicide if someone in the above circumstances appears to lack a vision or plans for the future and sees nothing to live for, starts giving away cherished possessions and makes a will, or talks with great specificity of killing himself.

If you suspect that someone close to you is at risk for suicide, talk frankly with him. You may worry that a candid discussion about thoughts and intentions will encourage action. However, this is seldom the case. When someone threatens to kill himself, take such threats seriously. People who succeed at suicide almost always talk about it and give a warning first.

Suicide prevention centers, telephone hot lines, and, of course, emergency rooms are available in most communities, and they can move a person beyond the immediate crisis. However, over time, drug therapy and long-term psychotherapy may be necessary to address the underlying depression and life circumstances that lead someone to contemplate such a drastic and absolute step as suicide. ■

ABOUT ELECTROCONVULSIVE (SHOCK) THERAPY

Despite the bad press, electroconvulsive (shock) therapy is one of the safest and most effective treatments for symptoms of depression and mania, especially when those symptoms have not yielded to other forms of treatment, such as medications and psychotherapy.

Simply put, electroconvulsive therapy (ECT) uses electrical current, passed through the brain, to induce generalized seizures. These seizures, usually lasting between 25 and 150 seconds, seem to restore balance within the chemical makeup of the brain and decrease symptoms of serious mental illness.

Before ECT can be used, the person must give informed consent. He must understand his illness, the exact nature and procedure of the treatment, the reasons for recommending ECT, alternative treatments, and what will likely happen if he refuses ECT.

Then, a comprehensive evaluation is conducted, including psychiatric, medical, and neurologic assessments. Generally, the person will undergo an electrocardiogram and complete blood analysis.

During the procedure, the person receives a short-acting general anesthetic to prevent discomfort, a drug called muscarinic anticholinergic, to dry secretions, and a skeletal muscle relaxant to block abrupt muscular convulsions and induce deep relaxation. Then two electrodes are placed, either bilaterally, one on each side of the head around the temples, or unilaterally, both on the right side of the head, near the language center of the brain.

A patient receives treatment usually two to three times a week until symptoms are gone. ■

and fluvoxamine) and TCAs (imipramine, nortriptyline, amitriptyline, and desipramine hydrochloride) (see Antidepressant Medication, page 1227). Despite the fact that general practitioners can prescribe these medications, it is probably wisest to consult a psychiatrist or psychopharmacologist who is specially trained to evaluate and monitor the need for and use of antidepressant medication.

For many different reasons, treatment with antidepressants takes time to work. Because every person and his depression differ, finding the most effective medication is often a process of trial and error. While the process may be frustrating, you and your doctor will eventually find the right treatment.

During a severe episode, there may be severe paranoid persecutory delusions or even hallucinations. There may be suicidal behavior (see Spotting the Warning Signs of Suicide, page 1228). When these occur, hospitalization, antipsychotic medication, or electroconvulsive therapy (see About Electroconvulsive (Shock) Therapy, page 1228) may be necessary. After the acute phase has subsided, psychopharmacologic treatment should be continued to decrease the likelihood of relapse or future recurrence.

Unlike medications for physical illness, psychotropic medications do not work to cure the depressive illness; rather, they work to relieve acute episodes and prevent recurrences. For many people, medications work most effectively in conjunction with psychotherapy. Insight-oriented therapy can allow you to consider how such contributing factors as early experiences of loss and cumulative negative life circumstances and disappointments have colored your disposition. Cognitive techniques can also provide significant relief insofar as they address the negative and distorted thinking that typically characterizes depression.

Prognosis Good. Recent progress in the development of new medications that act directly on specific parts of the brain make the treatment of depression even more promising. SAD responds well to light therapy.

In some instances, one course of treatment is sufficient to manage or remedy major depressive illness. However, for many others, depression is a chronic, lifelong condition that requires continued or episodic intervention. Even after a successful round of treatment, it is important that you remain sensitive to stresses that are likely to trigger a depression. If you are able to recognize early signs, you will be able to contact your clinician before you find yourself deep into another depressive episode. Learning to manage depression through therapy, medication, and lifestyle will lessen the likelihood that it will overshadow your life.

❖ BIPOLAR DISORDER (MANIC-DEPRESSIVE DISORDER)

Symptoms *(What you may experience)* In bipolar disorder, or manic-depressive disorder, a person usually experiences severe depressive symptoms along with alternating or intermittent manic symptoms. The manic phase of this illness includes euphoric or expansive mood; unrealistic or inflated self-esteem; feelings or irritability, anger, agitation, and impatience; decreased need for sleep; increased distractibility and talkativeness; rapid and pressured speech; hyperactivity and agitation; frenetic, frantic activity.

Signs and laboratory findings *(What the doctor looks for)* Pattern of depressive symptoms alternating with periods of manic symptoms: loud, racing speech that is hard to follow and interpret; attention that shifts from one focus to another; inability to complete tasks before going on to others; a tendency to pace and to hold more than one conversation at a time; poor judgment and unwarranted optimism; grandiosity; tendency toward anger outbursts.

What is it? According to some estimates, as many as 2.5 million Americans suffer from bipolar disorder. This psychiatric illness involves manic episodes of euphoric or elated moods, pressured and racing thoughts and speech, and often uncontrolled, reckless behavior. While a few people experience only manic episodes, most often mania is experienced along with depressive episodes. Two-thirds of those who suffer from bipolar illness have numerous recurrences of alternating or cyclic phases; others experience mixed states of simultaneous depressive and manic symptoms. Some people experience only small, occasional manic blips interrupting a more constant hum of depression. For others, it is a constant up-and-down churning.

The milder, chronic form of bipolar disorder is called cyclothymic disorder. It appears that cyclothymic disorder, in which numerous brief periods of mania alternate with numerous brief periods of depression, provides, for some people, the temperamental foundation from which major manic-depressive episodes spring.

When people are in the grips of a euphoric episode, their behavior may seem a bit odd, or, in some instances, completely bizarre. They may become increasingly involved in such goal-oriented activities as sex, work, school, or social relations. However, this behavior may have problematic consequences; they may become involved in gambling, unprotected or indiscreet sex, reckless spending, or irresponsible business or financial ventures. Typically, during a manic phase, a person's appearance changes abruptly: The style of dress may become more sexually provocative or flamboyant, or disheveled and slovenly.

Some people enjoy the sensations and energy that accompany manic episodes and maintain that their success or particular genius derives from it. While it is true that milder forms of manic disorders can contribute to success in business or the arts, recurrence of even the mildest mania can be disruptive. An elated mood, for example, can lead to impulsiveness and overoptimism concerning one's abilities, which can lead to such unfortunate consequences as a bad business venture or financial investment, sexual indiscretions, or imprudent expenditures.

Regardless of the different symptomatic picture, mania is closely linked to depression. Some of the symptoms—irritability, anger, insomnia, agitation, and tendency toward outbursts—occur in both.

Like other mood disorders, bipolar disorder has a genetic component and runs in families. And like diabetes, hypertension, and cancer, bipolar disorder is a complex disease with many causes and variations. It is theorized that the presence of a predisposing genetic foundation, coupled with something in the environment—a virus, a brain injury, a chaotic family circumstance—triggers the symptoms.

When to seek treatment Just like asthma or diabetes, bipolar disorder is an illness and as such requires medical attention. Unless your condition is extremely mild, you should consult a mental health practitioner—probably a psychiatrist who can prescribe medication—to diagnose, treat, and monitor your bipolar disorder.

Treatment Most psychiatrists treat bipolar disorder as a chronic illness that needs to be managed and controlled. At this time, it is not possible to eradicate or cure the disease. However, treatment that combines the drug lithium with psychotherapy can be relatively effective in bringing bipolar disorder under control or into remission.

Lithium, a natural salt, evens out the highs and lows of the mood disorder. When it is prescribed, lithium addresses current manic and depressive symptoms and, in the vast majority of individuals, reduces the frequency and severity of subsequent manic episodes.

Lithium requires regular monitoring. Right after it is initially prescribed, your psychiatrist will want to watch your response. If it seems that the medication is not working optimally, he may want to add another medication or adjust the dosage.

Monitoring entails assessing levels of lithium within the blood. Lithium can suppress thyroid functioning. In addition, dehydration can cause lithium to concentrate dangerously within the blood. During the summer months or if you are involved in strenuous activity, you may experience unpleasant side effects. Both of these conditions can be checked with blood tests. Thyroid problems can be addressed with a synthetic hormone.

Other potential side effects include hand tremors, increased thirst, the need to urinate frequently, acne, or weight gain. In most cases, these represent only slight nuisances. Almost always, the benefits of the medication outweigh the problems. With some individuals, lithium is not effective. Carbamazepine (Tegretol) or divalproex sodium (Depakote), both anticonvulsants, can be used to stabilize a person's mood. Your psychiatrist will work with you to find the right medication and the lowest dose that maximizes the benefits and minimizes side effects.

There may be the temptation, once you begin to feel better, to discontinue the medication. However, almost 90 percent of the time, symptoms recur within a year and a half of stopping the drug.

Occasionally, before the illness has been correctly diagnosed, or if medications are abruptly discontinued, a person with bipolar disorder may experience severe persecutory delusions or suicidal behavior (see Spotting the Warning Signs of Suicide, page 1228). In those instances, hospitalization, antipsychotic medication, or electroconvulsive therapy (see About Electroconvulsive (Shock) Therapy, page 1228) may be necessary. After the acute episode has passed, psychopharmacologic treatment may need to be monitored closely for a while to decrease the likelihood of relapse.

Supportive psychotherapy provides the opportunity to monitor your medication as well as to learn ways of managing and coping with your illness. Living with a chronic illness will always stir up strong feelings, and therapy is the place to deal with them. Therapy can also furnish practical information to help you cope. You can learn to detect the early signs of a relapse and to identify stresses that might trigger an episode.

In addition, because bipolar disorder can be hard for others to live with, family or couples' therapy may be recommended. When someone in the family has bipolar disorder, it is advisable to remain vigilant, on the lookout for possible signs of mania. Manic episodes can be embarrassing, disruptive, and sometimes dangerous. Family therapy can provide some very practical information on living with the illness and can offer the opportunity to consider ways in which family patterns exacerbate symptoms.

Although treatment for bipolar disorder may seem complicated and cumbersome, complying with treatment is crucial if you have this illness. Hospitalization may be necessary from time to time, specifically, when manic symptoms become extreme or dangerous. When the disorder is not treated or when treatment recommendations are not followed, it can lead to alcohol and drug abuse and even suicide. Fifteen percent of all individuals with bipolar disorder commit suicide.

Prognosis Fairly good. However, bipolar disorder is a chronic illness that needs to be managed and monitored throughout life. If drug regimens are not closely followed, relapse is likely. Even when one phase has been successfully treated and it looks like the illness is in remission, it is important that you resume treatment at the first signs that symptoms may be breaking through.

Psychiatric Disorders in Children and Teens

Like the adults they will become, young children and teens feel anxious, sad, angry, and frustrated at different times, and in different measures. In most instances, these and other emotions are passing, healthy responses to life. Occasionally, when internal and external circumstances exert unusual stress upon the child, these emotions may feel overwhelming and menacing to the child and seem disconcerting to the parents. Yet, in most instances, when circumstances smooth out, the upset will dissipate.

Some children and teens, however, are particularly vulnerable to extreme or persistent feelings of anger, depression, and anxiety. And because youngsters have difficulty identifying and describing exactly what is bothering them, many communicate their distress in their behavior.

Of course, all children misbehave on occasion. Usually, their misbehavior is normal misbehavior. However, in some instances, disordered behavior is a very eloquent expression of an emotional disorder.

Whether a youngster internalizes her upset and feels depressed or externalizes it, flinging it out into her world through troublesome behavior, it is not always easy for parents to discern when their child is suffering from an emotional or psychiatric disorder. In this section, we look at some of the more common disorders that affect children and the indications that professional help is needed. Eating disorders, which usually first appear during the teen years, are covered in their own section (see also Chapter 10).

❖ ANXIETY DISORDERS

Symptoms *(What your child may experience)* Unrelenting and overwhelming worry, fearfulness, wariness, and agitation in the absence of an actual danger or threat; the need to cling or withdraw, especially in social situations; phobias; panic attacks; ritualistic behavior and obsessive thinking; vigilance and suspicion; trouble falling asleep or staying asleep; nightmares; stomachaches, headaches, muscle tension and cramps; frequent urination.

Signs and laboratory findings *(What the doctor looks for)* Behavior that is clingy, needy, dependent, withdrawn, uneasy, and overly vigilant, beyond what would be expected at the child's developmental age. Excessive tantrums, thumb sucking, hair twirling, and other self-soothing behaviors; desperate attachment to a blanket, stuffed animal, hat, or other soothing objects; the tendency to sweat, blotch, and startle easily; regressive or anxious behavior that interferes with the ability to make and keep friends, to operate and cooperate within the family, and to manage the challenges of school; alcohol or drug use in older children and adolescents.

What is it? Anxiety is a natural and important emotion during childhood. With each stage of development—infancy, the toddler years, young childhood, and adolescence—a youngster experiences new fears and anxieties. Because growth and development depend on and necessitate that a child interact with an ever-expanding environment, feelings of apprehension and fearfulness arise naturally.

Anxiety helps guides a child on his journey toward adulthood. The degree to which a child is able to move successfully through his environment and master his anxiety largely determines his sense of competence and self-esteem. In addition, without fear or worry, a child would never learn to watch both ways before crossing the street or feel motivated to get that book report done on time.

However, there are children who do not come through periods of natural anxiety. For them, anxiety looms out of proportion to their circumstances. These children literally become sick with fear. Sometimes their anxiety manifests itself in an overall feeling of unease. At other times, it surfaces in panic disorders, panic attacks, and phobias.

Depending on the child's age, anxiety will express itself in different behaviors and concerns. Insofar as these manifestations of fearfulness become persistent or seriously interfere with the child's development or ability to engage in the normal activities of childhood, they indicate the existence of a generalized anxiety disorder.

At around 8 months, babies experience fear of separation from parent figures and fear of strangers; unless the child experiences intense and persistent separation disorder, tangible comforts such as blankets and stuffed animals will effectively soothe this anxiety.

Preschool children may regress when they feel anxious. A child who has mastered toilet training, for example, may begin to wet his bed at night or soil his pants (see Enuresis and Encopresis, page 1234). At this age, when separating from parents is a daily challenge and accomplishment, a child may suddenly worry that he will hurt himself or something bad will happen to his parents while they are apart.

Once they are in school, youngsters tend to worry that peers and important adults such as teachers will disapprove of them. They express their anxiety in trembling voices, biting their nails, chewing on clothes, or licking their lips raw. They may have headaches or stomachaches. They may become perfectionists, unable to complete their schoolwork for fear that it will not be good enough. Some children act aggressively and argue continually with other children.

Teenagers may turn to drug and alcohol to dull their feelings of uneasiness (see Addiction, Dependency, and Substance Abuse, page 1225). Many times, a child or teenager who seems overly anxious or suffers from a generalized anxiety disorder goes on to develop a panic disorder or phobia.

Although panic disorders most commonly appear in early adulthood, the disorder is not rare in adolescence. In addition, symptoms that precede panic attacks in adulthood may appear in children who suffer from depression or severe separation anxiety. A panic attack is a discrete episode of anxiety combining emotional and physical symptoms. Children may feel an intense fear or discomfort when an attack suddenly seizes them, along with a sense of impending doom, fear of going crazy, or sensations of unreality. Physical symptoms include shortness of breath, palpitations, sweating, choking, chest pains, nausea, dizziness, and numbness or tingling in the extremities. Following a panic attack, children may feel apprehensive that they will have other attacks. Sometimes children develop phobias in response.

An exaggerated and usually inexplicable fear that focuses on a specific object or situation, a phobia typically limits a child's activities. Children may focus their phobic anxiety on strangers, blood, fire, germs, insects, snakes, spiders, dirt, heights, small or closed spaces, darkness, or thunder.

Older children become phobic about social and school situations, which can pose significant complications to their day-to-day life. School phobias center on apprehension about performance or social pressures and result in refusal to attend school. Usually, a cycle of anxiety, physical complaints, and school avoidance escalates until it becomes almost impossible for these children to overcome their fear. The longer they stay out of school, the more likely they are to feel different from other kids and left out of normal activities.

Social phobia grips some youngsters as they approach new social situations in which they anticipate other people's judgment or expectations. As a result, they may cry, throw tantrums, freeze, or cling to a familiar person. Although restless, they tend to shrink from contact with others, refuse to participate in group play, and stay on the periphery of social activities. They may also complain of pain, fatigue, and stomachaches and seem preoccupied with worries about their health or appearance.

Approximately 1 million children have obsessive-compulsive disorder, an anxiety disorder characterized by obsessions (unwanted, repeated thoughts and urges) and compulsions (repetitive, purposeless behaviors). This disorder can appear in children as young as age 3, although it more commonly appears around age 10. Many children become obsessed with germs, contamination, lucky or unlucky numbers, superstitions, religion, and bodily functions. The most common compulsions involve hand washing, touching, counting, and hoarding. Obsessive-compulsive disorder causes considerable upheaval in the child's family, social, and academic life.

Over half of all children who have anxiety disorders also have major depressive disorders (see page 1223). In older children, persistent anxiety may be accompanied by suicidal feelings or other self-destructive behaviors. Often, children experiment with drugs or alcohol in an attempt to soothe or mask anxious feelings.

When to seek treatment If you suspect that your child is engaged in self-destructive or self-mutilating behaviors, that he is preoccupied with thoughts of suicide, or that he is involved in alcohol or drug use, call your doctor immediately. If it seems that your child is involved in obsessive-compulsive behavior, call your doctor; this condition requires professional intervention. In the absence of these behaviors, the need for professional help will be indicated by the degree of distress and disorder that the feelings of anxiety generate.

When your child's fear or fearfulness begins to invade his life and limit his activities, or when it persists for more than 6 months, call your child's doctor or talk to his school counselor. They will be able to recommend a mental health professional specializing in childhood anxiety disorders.

Treatment When a child is brought to a mental health clinician for an anxiety disorder, any suicidal or self-destructive behavior or any attempt to self-medicate through alcohol or drugs will be assessed and addressed at once. If it seems that a child is at risk for harming himself, hospitalization may be recommended.

In most cases, though, treatment for childhood or adolescent anxiety disorders involves individual psychotherapy, family therapy, and, in many instances, medication. Treatment will attempt to reduce the symptoms of anxiety, relieve distress, prevent complications associated with the disorder, and minimize the effects on the child's social, school, and developmental progress.

Childhood anxiety disorders commonly are treated with a group of antianxiety medications called benzodiazepines: clonazepam, diazepam, and alprazolam. These medications work quickly to even out a child's mood. Occasionally, they cause agitation, giddiness, and impulsiveness; when these side effects appear, the dosage may need to be lowered. If these drugs are to be discontinued, it must be done gradually and only under the direction of the doctor who wrote the prescription.

Psychotherapy that focuses on behavior seems to be best suited to children with this disorder. It tends to be active, helping these children think about and confront their fears. Children may also learn relaxation techniques such as breathing exercises and visual imagery.

Treatment for obsessive-compulsive disorder may be slightly different. The drugs most often prescribed for obsessive-compulsive disorder are SSRIs, such as fluoxetine, sertraline, paroxetine, and fluvoxamine.

TCAs, such as clomipramine, are also effective in treating obsessive-compulsive disorder. Effects are usually seen within 2 to 6 weeks. Therapy for obsessive-compulsive disorder usually includes specific behavioral techniques, including exposure and response prevention, in which a child is exposed to situations, activities, or objects that provoke anxiety; the child's automatic obsessive or compulsive reactions are then thwarted.

Parents and siblings may also engage in family therapy in which they will learn to help the child manage anxiety in more effective and less disruptive ways. Parents may also learn ways in which they unwittingly perpetuate the symptoms.

Prognosis Good, although there may be occasional relapse, especially at stressful times.

❖ ENURESIS AND ENCOPRESIS

Symptoms and signs Wetting or soiling the bed at night or clothing during the day well past the age when a child has gained control over his bowels and bladder.

What is it? More common in boys than girls, enuresis describes the condition when a child age 5 or over wets himself at least twice a month. If he has never been totally dry for a year, the condition is called primary enuresis. Secondary enuresis refers to the condition when a child seems to regress from complete bladder control.

Encopresis is also seen more often in boys than in girls. This diagnosis is made only after age 4 to describe the condition in which a child defecates in his underwear or on the floor. Typically, because the child has withheld his bowel movements for extended periods of time, stools are hard and painful.

In the vast majority of instances, primary enuresis and encopresis are symptoms of gastrointestinal problems or delayed physical development, and they do not require the attention of a mental health professional. Secondary enuresis can arise temporarily in relation to a stressful circumstance such as the birth of a sibling, entering preschool, or an extended separation from parents. In rare instances, encopresis can be an indication of anxiety or an expression of oppositional behavior (see Behavior Disorders, page 1238).

Twenty-five percent of all children diagnosed with one condition also have the other.

What you can do Even after your child has become completely toilet trained, accidents will happen. It is important that you remain calm and casual as you change the bed sheets or your child's underpants. Never shame, scold, or punish your child when he loses control over his bladder or bowels. And try not to show disgust or disappointment.

If from the time he begins to show curiosity about the toilet, you gently encourage but resist pushing or prodding, you may avoid power struggles that can center on toilet training. Ultimately, it is his body and his body's rhythm; if left to his own devices, he will likely learn to go to the bathroom when he needs as often as he needs.

Provide your child with a high-fiber diet. Limit the amount of liquids he consumes before bedtime. If your child is wetting the bed consistently, it might help to wake him in the middle of the night so that he can urinate in the toilet. Some children respond to token and reward systems. Keep track with gold stars on a colorful chart whenever he stays dry during the night. When the chart is filled, let him select a modest reward.

When to seek treatment If you suspect that secondary enuresis has a physical root, call your doctor so that he can rule out such conditions as diabetes or infection. If stresses in your child's life—a divorce, for example, or a loss—are playing a role, consider calling your doctor for a referral to a child or family therapist.

Treatment If your child has encopresis, your doctor may recommend a stool softener or suppository to ease impaction and irritation around the rectum.

If it looks as those these conditions are not rooted in physical problems, but reflect oppositional behavior, family therapy may help you look at the ways in which your family communicates and handles discipline.

Also, therapy that focuses on the behavior and coaches the child and his family in systematically altering the behavior can be helpful. In some cases, a nasal spray, Desmopressin, which is a synthetic antidiuretic hormone, can decrease the number of times a child wets his bed at night. The medication can cause mild nasal irritation and headaches. In very rare instance, it may also cause seizures in children who already have a seizure disorder. However, most children respond well to the medication, and though it does nothing to alter behavior in the long run, it can help in the early stages of therapy.

Prognosis Good. Prognosis depends very much on your energy and willingness to work consistently and sympathetically with your child.

❖ DEPRESSIVE DISORDERS

Symptoms *(What your child may experience)* Lasting sense of despair and, in some cases, intermittent episodes of elevated, expansive, or irritable mood, that has no discernible roots in a life event, is an exaggerated response to circumstances, or arises out of a traumatic event; consistent fatigue or lack of energy; loss of appetite or overeating; difficulty concentrating or making decisions; feelings of worthlessness, silent anger, or guilt; suicidal thoughts or ruminations about death; marked drop in school, athletic, or other performance; lack of interest in social activities; headaches, muscle pains, heaviness in arms or legs. When the depressive illness has a manic component, periodic feelings of inflated self-esteem, grandiosity, pressured speech, racing thoughts, and impulsive behavior may be present.

Signs *(What the doctor looks for)* Persistent lethargy and loss of interest in normal pleasurable experiences: food, friends, pets, sports, hobbies; a family or personal history of depression or suicide, self-mutilating or self-destructive behavior, alcohol or other drug use; uncharacteristically tearful, withdrawn, listless, dull, or agitated appearance; failure to achieve the expected weight gain for a child his age or a sudden drop in weight; change in personal habits; slow movements, monotonous voice; negative self-references: "I'm stupid," or "No one loves me," or "I'm bad."

What is it? All children feel sad or needy from time to time. Usually, these feelings are perfectly normal reactions to the inevitable bumps and bruises that life dishes up. However, there are some youngsters who seem perpetually wrapped up in sorrow and frustration. Seriously depressed youngsters exist in a state beyond sadness; their symptoms tend to interfere with their emotional development and interrupt the normal business of childhood: family interaction and academic and social performance in school. In addition, they may express their feelings in disturbing symptoms, including suicidal gestures, self-mutilation, substance abuse, obsessive-compulsive rituals, or delinquent behavior.

Some children suffer from major depressions, periods of depression that last for at least 2 weeks and that seem to have very little connection to actual events. Other youngsters have what is called a dysthymic disorder, in which a depressed mood seems to underlie their general mood. In dysthymia, symptoms tend to be milder but constant.

During depressions, signs and symptoms—despairing, irritable, and volatile mood; appetite and sleep changes; diminished energy; low self-esteem; feelings of hopelessness; poor concentration and indecisiveness—color every experience, impression, and response. These children look out onto their life and see only a grim, barren, and pointless future.

Sometimes, the emotional disturbance combines both depressed and euphoric moods. This type of depression is known as bipolar disorder, or manic-depressive disorder. Bipolar disorder is characterized by episodes of mania, or exuberant highs. In some children, their mood may swing from one extreme to the other; in other children, there is a simultaneous jumble of both highs and lows. Mania is also characterized by irritable mood.

During manic states, a child may have an inflated self-esteem. His speech becomes constant and rapid, and he may have difficulty focusing on one idea or subject at a time. A manic child becomes easily distracted, appears agitated and restless, and sleeps very little. Most alarming, he may engage in activities that have a high potential for painful consequences.

When the disorder is milder and chronic, the mood disturbance is called cyclothymic disorder. In cyclothymic disorder, numerous manic and depressive episodes occur over a period of time without marked social or academic impairment. In children under age 9, their sadness, mania, and agitation are often intermixed; they may appear extremely moody and irritable. Older children show distinct signs of euphoria, elation, paranoia, and grandiose delusions, and as puberty begins, extremes of depression and manic excitement become more pronounced.

Children with bipolar disorder may be extremely hard to tolerate. Hyperactive, silly, and aggressive in their verbal communications, their speech may be littered with profanities and sexual innuendo. Delusions of grandeur—believing one is Superman, for example—can lead to dangerous behaviors, like running in front of cars or jumping off roofs. A manic child paces. He refuses to eat and sleep. One moment, he is ridiculing others, and the next, he is accusing others of making fun of him or conspiring against him.

It is likely that depression and bipolar disorder arise out of a complex combination of factors. Almost certainly, there is a biochemical predisposition toward mood disorders. In addition, mood disturbances tend to run in families, suggesting a genetic component.

The family environment may build on these biologic vulnerabilities. When parents, for example, suffer from emotional disturbances, which are left untreated, their ability to be consistently responsive and nurturing may be compromised. Because bipolar disorder, for example, is episodic, an adult's ability to parent may be erratic and unpredictable. When a parent is depressed, she may be less responsive to her child, which in turn can precipitate depressive symptoms in the child.

In many cases, depression reflects elements of unresolved grief, possibly in response to early real or imagined losses of nurturing figures. Depression may also indicate that children have learned to embrace feelings of helplessness rather than to seek solutions for life's problems. Depressed thinking tends to be negative, hopeless, and self-defeating, which in itself reenforces feelings of depression.

In some cases of childhood or adolescent depression, a youngster has experienced early life trauma (see Post-Traumatic Stress Disorder, page 1222) or loss. Many depressed children have family lives that are consistently bleak, chaotic, neglectful or abusive.

Depression and bipolar illness generally interfere with a child's social or academic functioning. When a child is depressed, school performance deteriorates. He loses interest in extracurricular activities and drops out. He may complain of headaches or stomachaches, especially before entering a new situation. Phobias may develop (see page 1220).

What you can do   It is not always easy to determine just when a child's behavior and mood are sufficiently troubled to seek professional help, but the place to start is to talk with your child. Acknowledge his sadness, and let him know that feelings of loss, loneliness, inadequacy, or silent anger are normal. Reassure him that no matter how deeply isolated, worthless, or despondent he feels, these feelings will pass. Your interest and concern will go a great length in soothing your child.

Gently encourage him to engage in activities he enjoys and at which he excels. Whenever you recognize his accomplishments and admire his abilities, you help build up his self-esteem, which will counteract feelings of depression. If possible, help him stay connected with friends. Encourage him to exercise and play sports. Keeping a journal and talking to friends are other ways of sorting out feelings that can threaten to envelop him. In all things, be encouraging but be careful not to push.

When to seek treatment   If you suspect that your child may be ruminating about the meaning of life and considering suicide, seek professional help immediately. Depressive symptoms, particularly when they persist or seriously interfere with social and academic functioning, are hard for a child and his family to manage on their own. Ask your child's doctor for names of clinicians who could conduct a psychiatric evaluation if your child's depression continues.

Treatment   Treatment for a child's mood disturbance will begin with a full evaluation, which usually includes the whole family. An assessment will be made to rule out simple bereavement, substance abuse, or any medical conditions that could produce depressive or manic symptoms. The clinician will look at the family context and his-

TEEN SUICIDE

More and more, teenagers seem to be turning to suicide as a desperate solution to seemingly insoluble problems and feelings. Suicide is the sixth leading cause of death for 5- to 14-year-olds, and the third leading cause of death for 15- to 24-year-olds. Alarmingly, the numbers are growing.

Whether a teenager actually wants to die or not, suicidal behavior speaks of deep feelings of impotence and helplessness. Given the changes and challenges that adolescence poses—including physical, hormonal changes, social and academic demands, and a shifting role in the family—youngsters may well feel overwhelmed and alone. In addition, today's society offers up a series of environmental stresses—divorce, single-parent homes, blended families, poverty, overtaxed school systems, negative peer pressure, as well as increased exposure to violence and illicit drugs—that even the most resourceful youngster can have difficulty managing.

Most young people feel depressed from time to time. And most will wonder what it would be like if they killed themselves. In adolescence, the notion of suicide may even take on a romantic quality. But most teenagers do not kill themselves or even attempt it.

Suicidal attempts are not uncommon with children and adolescents who have drug problems or conduct disorders or whose behavior seems aggressive rather than despondent. Though it may be tempting to dismiss such attempts as manipulative, they must be taken seriously, not only in terms of their immediate danger, but as possible expressions of extreme frustration, pain, anger, and impulsiveness. Youngsters with conduct disorders are notoriously inarticulate and may illustrate their pain with self-destructive acts.

At the same time, teenage behavior may seem perplexing to parents. You may wonder if what you observe is indeed a cause for concern. From time to time, you will likely notice a number of problematic behaviors in your teenager that could be warning signs. These include

- An abrupt change of personality, dress, style, interests, and friends

- Withdrawal or isolation, especially if your child has always been gregarious and outgoing

- Alcohol or other drug use

- Signs of self-mutilation

- Violent behavior—punching holes in walls, getting into fights, or self-destructive violence

- A consistent pattern of running away from home

- Significant change in sleeping patterns: suddenly sleeps all the time or does not sleep at all

- Neglect of personal appearance (most adolescents always want to look their best, even if their idea of looking good is completely at odds with yours)

- Lingering lethargy, a drop-off in schoolwork, loss of interest

- Loss of interest in recreational activities

- Lack of interest in praise or rewards

- Weepiness; abrupt or constant crying

- Expressions of low self-esteem; feelings of worthlessness: "I'm simply no good."

- References to the fact that he will not be around much longer to be a burden to everyone

- Indications that he is completely overwhelmed: *"What difference does anything make?"* or *"Life makes no sense."*

- Actions that reflect sudden interest in giving important or favorite possessions away, putting his affairs in order, making amends, and saying good-bye

- Sudden and unaccountable cheerfulness, sense of relief, or resoluteness after an extended period of depression

If you suspect your teenager is depressed, ask him. Be tentative and respectful, but do not worry that if you ask about suicidal thoughts you will put it in his mind or encourage the act. Your child may feel comforted by your concern. He may want more than anything to talk about what he is feeling. Just listening may counteract some of his feelings of worthlessness. And your interest and willingness to help may counteract his feelings of hopelessness.

Other adolescents may be so depressed that they may not talk about it directly. They may not be able to identify or put into words just what is making them feel so despondent.

If you have any doubts, contact your doctor or your child's doctor. Therapy may be prudent, not only for your child but also for you and the rest of the family. Learning to recognize and live with depression can head off a suicide attempt and other related problems down the road.

For more information on teen suicide and hotline numbers, see page 286. ∎

tory as well as the specific manifestations of the illness.

When the depression seems mild, psychotherapy with a therapist who specializes in treating children or adolescents may be all that is called for. However, the more serious the disorder, the more comprehensive the treatment will be.

A seriously depressed child will be assessed for the risk of suicidal or self-endangering behavior. If a child is obsessed with suicide or has a well-thought-out plan, hospitalization may be suggested. Occasionally, manic-depressive episodes can be so dramatic and, in rare cases, self-destructive, that hospitalization may be necessary. Otherwise, as long as the child is able to function and his family can provide sufficient support, intensive therapy can proceed on an outpatient basis.

Treatment for a major depressive disorder frequently combines psychotherapy and antidepressant medications. If medications are needed, a doctor, either your pediatrician or a psychiatrist, will prescribe them. While psychotropic medications do not cure the illness, they can relieve an episode and lift the veil of sorrow so that the child can engage in a therapeutic relationship and reengage in the social and academic business of life.

Your child's doctor or psychiatrist will monitor the effects of antidepressant medication. Because this medication takes time to work, and because it works differently with each child, there will be a period of trial and error until the right dosage is determined.

When there are manic as well as depressive symptoms, treatment will probably combine the drug lithium with psychotherapy. Lithium works to stabilize mood and manage more troublesome symptoms. The most common side effects are stomach upset or nausea, increased appetite, weight gain, bed-wetting, tremors, and acne. As with all psychiatric medications, it is important to work together with your doctor to arrive, over time, at the right dosage so that side effects are minimal.

When the child is stabilized or when the symptoms are milder, psychotherapy is an important source of continued care, support, and education. Therapy offers support and empathy while encouraging exploration of feelings.

For younger children or children who have trouble expressing themselves in speech, play therapy can provide an opportunity to communicate feelings and perceptions. Through play, for example, depressed children can act out feelings of loss, powerlessness, aggression, or danger—and eventually deal with them.

In cases when a specific circumstance or event has precipitated the depression—divorce or some disastrous event, for example—therapy gives children a chance to resolve some of their feelings and accept even an unhappy reality.

Frequently, psychotherapy also provides a forum in which depressed youngsters can examine negative beliefs and distorted thoughts that generally inform their view of themselves, their environment, and their future.

Group therapy is an important modality for children and adolescents. In a supportive group of their peers, youngsters can develop social skills that in turn can lead to a greater sense of mastery and self-esteem.

Families who live with depressed or manic-depressed children might find help through family therapy. Many times, families learn to modify certain behaviors that commonly exacerbate depression in children—lack of generational boundaries, severe marital conflict, rigid or chaotic rules, projection of parental feelings onto a child, or neglectful or overly involved relationships—as well as ways of dealing with the problems wrought by an emotionally disturbed child. In addition, other depressed family members can be identified in family sessions.

Prognosis Good. As long as parents are involved and supportive, early and comprehensive child-oriented therapy, coupled often with medication, will address a child's mood disorder sufficiently to free him up to reengage in the business of childhood.

❖ BEHAVIOR DISORDERS

Symptoms and signs Behavior that is consistently impulsive, antisocial, defiant, argumentative, or dangerous; poor school and/or social functioning; low self-esteem; inability or unwillingness to comply with rules and limits; difficulty in concentrating, completing tasks, and achieving up to potential; depressive or anxious symptoms; disruptive or intolerable conduct; restlessness; intense, unrelenting excitability, distractibility, and impetuosity. In very young children, hard to soothe or cuddle; use of such self-soothing behaviors as excessive thumb sucking, head rolling, head banging, or rocking; accident prone; intense tantrums. In school-aged children, trouble cooperating with others in play or on tasks; delayed or impaired fine motor coordination and language development; sleep problems; little awareness of or concern about the pain they inflict or the damage they cause.

What is it? Behavior disorders are a group of often intertwined disruptive disorders in which a child's distress is expressed primarily in the way he acts. These include attention-deficit/hyperactivity disorder, conduct disorder, and oppositional defiant disorder.

Attention-deficit/hyperactivity disorder Once called hyperkinesis or minimal brain dysfunction, attention-deficit/hyperactivity disorder (ADHD) affects between 3 to 5 percent of all children—perhaps as many as 2 million children. Two to three times more boys than girls seem to manifest the disorder, though it is increasingly being identified in girls. On the average, at least one child in every classroom in the United States needs help for the disorder.

Characteristic behaviors are inattention, hyperactivity, and impulsiveness. Children with ADHD have a hard time keeping their mind focused on any one thing and become easily bored or distracted. They seem to be in continual motion. They are unable to curb their automatic reactions; it appears as if they fail to think before they act.

However, because all children display occasional hyperactivity, short attention spans, and impulsive thinking and behavior, especially during times of stress, it is often difficult to diagnose ADHD with great certainty. ADHD symptoms can be milder or more severe, depending on the individual child and circumstances. Even a child with severe symptoms may be able to focus and contain himself when he enjoys the activity or the supervising adults.

ADHD appears to arise out of a neurologic or genetic vulnerability; if the child's environment is consistently chaotic or troubled, the genetic vulnerability is particularly likely to be triggered. When ADHD goes unrecognized and untreated, a child can experience a lifetime of emotional pain, frustration, academic failure, and social isolation.

Conduct disorders This category of behavioral disorders describes those children who engage in antisocial or delinquent behavior. Far more common, at any age, in boys than in girls, conduct disorders are one of the most frequently diagnosed conditions in outpatient and inpatient mental health facilities for children. It is estimated that 6 percent of all children have some form of conduct disorder.

In normal circumstances, children misbehave for a number of reasons: because they do not comprehend what is expected of them; because they wish to assert their independence and individuality; or because they want to test the rules and limits imposed on them. Sometimes their behavior is simply an expression of the anger or frustration they feel.

However, when a child's behavior is consistently disturbing, destructive, and aggressive, it leaves little doubt that the child is disturbed. Whether it is a chaotic or abusive life circumstance or internal deficits and disabilities that produce distress, the child's disturbed behavior ripples out, causing disturbance all around.

The degree of severity of objectionable behaviors will vary from child to child. In general, these antisocial behaviors—excessive disobedience, truancy, repeated physical aggression, stealing, running away, fire setting, cruelty to animals, lying, stealing, inappropriate sexual behavior, and substance abuse—are tenacious enough to draw attention to themselves.

Usually, in children who engage in such problematic behavior, a predisposition or genetic vulnerability interacts with environmental forces and individual characteristics to produce the disorder. Behavioral problems may also reflect brain damage, brain dysfunction, or neurologic problems that express themselves early on in poor fine motor coordination, impaired short-term memory, poor judgment, and difficulty regulating feelings and controlling actions.

There seems to be a link between conduct disorders and mild intellectual deficits, especially in the area of verbal skills. Learning disabilities and intellectual difficulties that go unrecognized and untreated seem to contribute to problem behavior.

More and more, mental health and education professionals are beginning to recognize that physical, sexual, and emotional abuse often play a role in the genesis of certain kinds of aggressive and inappropriate sexual behaviors. In addition, when parents are antisocial or suffer from psychosis, severe depression, or manic-depressive disorders, their own conduct, which may include addiction and antisocial behaviors, will likely have a grave impact on a child.

Oppositional defiant disorders When children express their aggression and noncompliance indirectly, their behavior is commonly referred to as passive-aggressive. The psychiatric diagnosis is oppositional defiant disorders.

All children are oppositional, forgetful, and inattentive from time to time, particularly at certain times in their development such as around the ages of 2 and 3 and in early adolescence. However, a child's disrespectful and hostile behavior may be a serious concern if it is so incessant and fierce that it stands out when compared with his peers or interferes with his social and academic performance.

Symptoms of an oppositional defiant disorder are common child-rearing struggles gone awry. If a child suffers from this disorder, he exhibits a pattern of uncooperative, defiant, and hostile behavior toward authority figures that seriously interferes with his daily interactions. He may lose his temper, argue with adults, actively defy adult rules, or refuse adult requests. Deliberately acting in ways to annoy others, he will blame others for his difficulties. He may seem touchy or easily annoyed, angry, resentful, spiteful, or vindictive. And although children with oppositional defiant disorder tend to express their aggression passively rather than actively, they may regularly use obscene language and mild physical aggression.

In its most extreme, a child may refuse to speak, develop an eating (see Eating Disorders, page 1242) or sleeping disorder, wet his bed, or soil his pants (see Enuresis and Encopresis, page 1234). Certain types of learning difficulties and academic underachievement can also be expressions of oppositional tendencies.

Before puberty, the rate of this disorder is higher in boys than in girls. In adolescence, the disorder is equally shared between boys and girls. It appears that for both, the disorder arises out of a circular family dynamic. Typically, a child is temperamentally fussy, colicky, and harder to soothe. Anticipating noncompliance, parents may try to assert control in such areas as eating, toilet training, sleeping, speaking, and separating. The child then increases his resistance by withholding or withdrawing.

The more a child reacts in defiant, provocative ways, the more he elicits negative reinforcement from his parents: nagging, lectures, reprimands, and physical punishment. But far from diminishing oppositional behavior, these tend to increase the intensity of the child's noncompliance.

At school, this pattern of passive-aggressive, oppositional behavior may provoke teachers and other children as well. At school as at home, a child is met with anger, punitive reactions, and criticism. The child then argues back, blames others, and loses his temper.

These children tend to have difficulty adapting at school. They disrupt the classroom, and their conduct runs contrary to their social and academic interests. As a result, oppositional children often experience school failure and social isolation. This, coupled with chronic criticism, can lead to low self-esteem.

For more information on learning disabilities and conduct disorders, see also Chapter 9.

What you can do Providing support, stability, educational stimulation, and hope can compensate over time for whatever physical vulnerabilities your child has. Children who seem to have a temperamental oppositional predisposition to defiant disorder do better when their parents develop an effective, flexible disciplinary style. In addition, it helps to find a school or classroom setting that can provide structure, organization, and appropriate expectations for your child.

When to seek treatment Because behavior disorders can be so hard to live with, and so often mask other emotional illnesses, professional intervention is frequently needed to modify the symptoms.

However, because it is often difficult for parents to judge exactly what level of activity and misbehavior is considered normal in young children, treatment is usually not sought before a child enters school. Most children with behavior disorders are referred to mental health professionals between the ages of 6 and 9. Once a child enters elementary school, he is expected to sit still and stick with a task for increasingly longer periods of time. If a child is unusually disruptive, antisocial, fidgety, and impulsive, there is a very good chance that he will be noticed. At that point, you may be called into your child's school, and a referral for treatment will be made.

Nevertheless, if your baby is extremely hard to soothe, seems particularly accident prone, needs constant close supervision, or if your school-aged child's behavior has you frankly concerned, speak to your child's doctor.

Treatment Treatment for behavior disorders usually requires a comprehensive approach that may combine medication, individual therapy, social skills training, family support and therapy, and in some instances, remedial education.

Based on a comprehensive evaluation, treatment usually addresses the condition underlying the behavior. If, for example, intellectual and learning problems are uncovered, those will be addressed. When a child is found to be suffering from an anxiety or depressive disorder, a psychosis, or ADHD, those conditions will be addressed, most likely, through medication and psychotherapy. In addition, when oppositional defiant disorder manifests in eating disorders, enuresis or encopresis, or selective mutism (inability to speak), those conditions will be addressed.

Psychopharmacology Since the 1930s, stimulants have been used to treat ADHD. More recently, there has been considerable success in treating oppositional defient disorders with stimulants as well. Methylphenidate (Ritalin) has had dramatic results in children with these types of disorders. This medication helps a child focus by stimulating the production of dopamine and norepinephrine within the brain and nervous system. Children who take methylphenidate are able to perform and complete tasks with fewer errors. They are less impulsive and more attentive, both in the classroom and with their peers. They can control themselves and act in ways that earn them praise and lessen criticism.

When methylphenidate does not produce the desired effects, dextroamphetamine (Dexedrine) and pemoline (Cylert) may be prescribed. In general, stimulants are less reliable in children under age 6. When

they fail to modify the symptoms or cause problematic side effects, many clinicians consider antidepressants, such as TCAs—nortriptyline and imipramine. Clonidine (Catapres) and guanfacine (Tenex) are also commonly prescribed for ADHD, particularly when a child is prone to tics.

Despite the striking effects of medication, considerable controversy surrounds diagnosing and medicating ADHD. Many believe that the diagnosis of ADHD is used too loosely and medication given too readily in order to control children who are too active or difficult for the adults around them.

If your doctor or mental health clinician is recommending medications for your child, take the time to evaluate the necessity, benefits, and possible side effects. Ask your doctor to describe how he decides when and how to prescribe medication and the kind of follow-up he will conduct.

Psychotherapy While medication may be an important component of treating behavior disorders, especially early in treatment, they work best as an adjunct to psychotherapy. Individual therapy can help children gain greater self-control and insight into their social conduct and develop more thoughtful and efficient problem-solving strategies. But perhaps most important, it gives them the opportunity to understand and express their feelings with words instead of through their behavior.

Frequently, treatment will include behavioral modification techniques, such as social skills training through which children can learn to evaluate social situations and adjust their behavior accordingly. In addition, children with serious behavior problems often need to have some kind of remedial education or special tutoring to compensate for their learning difficulties or to address any reading disorders, learning disabilities, or language delays they may have.

Many times, treatment for behavior disorders is family focused. Family therapy or behavioral therapies, such as parent training programs, address the family stress normally generated by living with a disturbed child. Such treatment modalities provide strategies for managing a child's behavior, often helping parents encourage appropriate behaviors in their children and discipline them in more effective ways. By involving the entire family, treatment fosters mutual support, positive reinforcement, direct communication, and more effective problem solving within the family.

Prognosis Fairly good, especially when the condition is recognized and treated early. ADHD can be a lifelong disorder; yet it can be effectively managed, and a child's life can be full and accomplished.

If your child is diagnosed with a conduct disorder, it is important to remember that, despite the rather dramatic and disturbing quality of some of the symptoms, the majority of behaviorally disturbed children do not go on to become antisocial or criminal adults. Many of the underlying causes, including family violence and abuse, can be prevented and addressed with relative success. It is important, therefore, to look beyond the hodgepodge of superficial behaviors to the more subtle indications of potentially treatable biologic, emotional, or social vulnerabilities underneath.

With more severely disturbed children, ongoing, adequate medical, emotional, educational, and social supports are often required for many years.

Eating Disorders

In a way, eating disorders are the perfect psychiatric illness for our times. In the past generation or two, we Americans have become almost fanatic in our interest in food and dieting. At the same time, as a society, we are deeply intolerant of obesity while we glorify thinness. Add to this our dependency on the opinions of others for our sense of who we are, and our insistence on being in control in most all areas of our lives, and you have fertile ground for anorexia nervosa and bulimia nervosa, illnesses characterized by pathologic preoccupation with food, weight, shape, thinness, and control.

Eating disorders as a whole display varying progressions, ranging from a single, mild illness in adolescence to a lifelong disorder, which is either persistent or fluctuates, with remissions and exacerbations.

Besides the clear impact of cultural factors, as mentioned above, eating disorders seem to spring from a multitude of sources.

There has been considerable debate about the role of faulty parenting and dysfunctional family dynamics in eating disorders. Specifically, studies have looked at the power struggles that tend to be established early in childhood around food. However, genetic and hormonal factors may in fact be much more significant factors. People who suffer from eating disorders very likely have a genetic predisposition to the illness: Where there is a family history of depression, alcoholism, obesity, or eating disorders, individuals are at higher risk. In addition, there is a neurologic relationship between eating patterns—specifically, dieting and starvation—and the neurologic and hormonal systems, because craving (hunger) and its satisfaction through eating are regulated drives in certain areas of the brain.

❖ ANOREXIA NERVOSA

Symptoms *(What you may experience)* Preoccupation with one's body, weight, and eating; profound dread of obesity; distorted body image; malnutrition; cessation of monthly periods (menses); irritability, depression, and inability to concentrate; dehydration; faintness; slow heart beat.

Signs and laboratory findings *(What the doctor looks for)* Weight of at least 15 percent less than minimal normal weight for age and height; continual loss of weight; low blood pressure and pulse; dizziness; abnormal estrogen, progesterone, and cortisol levels; symptoms of malnutrition.

What is it? Anorexia nervosa is deliberate, self-imposed starvation. In relentless pursuit of thinness and fear of obesity, anorexia invariably leads to varying degrees of emaciation, malnutrition, and related health problems.

More than 90 percent of all those diagnosed with anorexia are female. In a distorted way, the illness reflects our society's obsession with thinness and personal control as well as the tendency to rely on the opinion of others for self-affirmation and self-esteem. It is a disorder of dieting.

There has been considerable discussion both in the medical and mental health professions and in the popular press pointing to the link between anorexia and faulty family communications and power struggles.

Yet the illness is just as likely rooted in the chemistry of the brain and a genetic predisposition.

Recent studies suggest that people with anorexia respond to dieting differently from other people. While most people feel uncomfortable when their calories are restricted, people prone to anorexia are not sensitive to the discomfort. As they begin to starve, they experience a sense of euphoria, as the brain releases opioids. Much like a long-distance runner whose brain releases the chemical, producing "runner's high," individuals with anorexia feel disciplined and successful. As they become emaciated, they feel genuine, palpable pleasure.

Individuals with shaky self-images and a family history of depression, weight problems, and substance abuse seem to be at higher risk for the disorder. Those who participate in activities that require thinness or weight control—such as ballet, gymnastics, or modeling in girls and wrestling in boys—are most vulnerable.

While the disorder can manifest itself in children as young as age 7 and as late as age 25, the average age of onset is 14. At that age, a child is moving into adolescence, a girl's body is changing, and her breasts and hips are developing. The disorder often starts when a young girl, who may be a bit overweight, attempts to diet, but keeps on dieting after she achieves a sensible weight range. If the onset of anorexia nervosa is before puberty, a girl's sexual development will stop and menstruation will not begin. If it appears after a girl has begun to menstruate, her monthly cycles may stop. (They should resume once the she has achieved adequate weight.)

Even when she is emaciated, someone who suffers from anorexia maintains with absolute certainty that she is fat. She may diet all the time and often will abuse over-the-counter weight-control drugs, diuretics, and laxatives in her determination to lose weight. Even as she refuses to eat, she may obsess about food, perhaps collecting recipes and cooking lavishly for others. She may hide food around the house, carry candy in her purse, and constantly scoot food around on her plate.

In some instances, when a person does not sufficiently control her food intake, she may binge. From 30 to 50 percent of people with anorexia also suffer from bulimia nervosa (see page 1224). Often rigid and perfectionistic, those with anorexia may obsess about exercise as well as diet. Severe anorexia leads to chronic malnourishment, which takes its toll throughout the body, particularly in the thyroid, heart, and digestive and reproductive systems. Untreated anorexia can prove fatal. For more information on anorexia, specifically, anorexia in teens, see page 287.

When to seek treatment People with anorexia rarely acknowledge that they have a problem other than weight. Unless they are seen for another illness, anorexia may not be assessed until family members and friends notice a significant weight loss or until a number of consecutive menstrual periods have been missed.

In addition, people with the disorder seldom want treatment. It is therefore often up to family members and friends to recognize the disorder and urge them to get help. In very few cases, anorexia subsides on its own. You need help to conquer and manage this condition.

Call your doctor if you have any of the symptoms of anorexia. Abuse of laxatives or diuretics and the like can pose a threat to your life and health.

Treatment The largest obstacle to treating anorexia is that those who suffer from the disorder do not want to be treated. Yet it is essential that they get treatment quickly. Anorexia nervosa can be fatal.

In all cases, the immediate goal of treatment will be to get the person to eat and gain weight. Because in general the anorectic does not consider her behavior abnormal, convincing her to eat may not be easily accomplished. When the condition has progressed to the point of emaciation or when outpatient treatment is not effective, hospitalization may be necessary. In the hospital, the patient is weighed daily and monitored until her weight reaches normal levels.

Once the immediate medical crisis subsides, and in more moderate cases of the illness, individual and often family therapy are recommended to address the underlying psychosocial contributors to the disorder. Drug therapy has proved successful only occasionally with anorexia and only in the most acute cases. Yet medication is crucial when, as is often the case, the person also has a depressive or obsessive-compulsive disorder.

In general, a person with an eating disorder is distrustful of health care practitioners, suspecting them of wanting to feed her, break her will, and make her fat. Therapy that is educationally or behaviorally based—offering information about body weight regulation, normal eating habits, nutrition, and the effects of starvation, vomiting, and laxatives on the system—is usually a good place to start. Behavioral-cognitive therapy that includes weekly weigh-ins and ongoing assessments of the person's distorted perceptions about self-image, food, and thinness has proven to be extremely successful.

Depressive disorders exist in almost one-half of all individuals with anorexia, and when this is the case, the depression will also be addressed in therapy. Antidepressants—fluoxetine or sertraline—may be prescribed as well.

Prognosis Good. Although anywhere from 5 to 18 percent of all people who suffer from anorexia will die within 10 years (mostly from suicide or related health complications), about 70 percent of all those who receive treatment in a timely manner make a full medical, social, and psychiatric recovery. At the same time, anorexia can be a lifelong pull, even when it is not an active condition; as such, it often requires long-term treatment and management. Even when the disorder is managed effectively, some people continue to manifest peculiar habits or ideas concerning food for many years.

❖ BULIMIA NERVOSA

Symptoms *(What you may experience)* Episodic patterns of binge or compulsive eating that lead people to feel they have lost control, frequently followed by efforts to control body weight through self-induced vomiting, use of laxatives and diuretics, periods of fasting and excessive exercise; obsessive fear of obesity; feelings of shame, self-reproach, and guilt.

Signs *(What the doctor looks for)* Dehydration and depletion of electrolytes and other significant nutrients as a result of diuretics and laxatives, which are apparent on blood tests; tooth decay and erosion caused by regurgitated stomach acid; low blood pressure, constipation, swollen cheek glands, and hormonal changes.

What is it? Ninety percent of all people who suffer from bulimia nervosa—an eating disorder that involves compulsive binge eating—are women. Most often, the condition involves purging through self-induced vomiting and abuse of laxatives, enemas, suppositories, or diuretics. Some people with bulimia do not purge but compensate for episodes of bingeing with other behaviors such as fasting or overexercising. Most male bulimics are the nonpurging type.

Although people with bulimia are afraid of becoming fat, unlike those with anorexia nervosa, they can look perfectly normal; most are of normal weight, and some may be a bit heavy. Women with bulimia tend to be high achievers. Unlike people with anorexia, who may wish to deny or reverse their sexual development, many individuals with bulimia obsess about their sexual attractiveness.

While they fear food, they consume huge quantities of it—sometimes up to 20,000 calories at a time. The foods on which they binge tend to be "comfort foods": sweet foods, high in calories, or smooth, soft foods like ice cream, cake, and pastry. An individual may binge anywhere from twice a day to several times daily.

In many instances, after the binge comes the purge. A bulimic may use as many as 20 or more laxatives a day. Others compensate by fasting, dieting too strictly, or exercising obsessively. And like anorexia, bulimia wreaks havoc on the body. At its most destructive, purging can cause permanent heart damage.

Commonly, bulimia appears in the latter part of adolescence, between age 18 and 20, but it can develop at an earlier or later age. Unlike those who suffer from anorexia, people with bulimia are aware of their difficulties with food. Yet, they do not feel in control of the problem. People with bulimia are often impulsive and more likely to be involved in other addictive behaviors than people with anorexia.

There is almost certainly a genetic predisposition to the disorder as well as a neurochemical component. Studies show that people with bulimia produce less serotonin and respond strongly to changes in serotonin levels.

Many people with bulimia also have a history of anorexia or obesity. They may have a concomitant major depressive disorder, anxiety disorder, social phobia, or panic disorder. Other addictive behavior—specifically, drug or alcohol abuse—may also be present. For more information on bulimia, specifically, bulimia in teens, see page 288.

When to seek treatment As with anorexia, the vast majority of people who suffer from bulimia need professional help to fight the disorder. Many individuals with bulimia experience depression or post-binge anguish, and subsequent remorse. They may have the awareness that what they are doing is not normal. And while they may try to keep their behavior a secret, once found out, many experience great relief. The ability to experience direct feelings in relation to their acting out may make them more willing to seek and respond to help.

Treatment As a rule, people with bulimia can be treated as outpatients, usually with a combination of cognitive-behavioral therapy and medication. Antidepressants, such as fluoxetine, imipramine, and trazodone (Desyrel), can help to cut down on food cravings and on the frequency of bingeing and purging. Psychotherapy can be used to monitor and increase awareness of eating habits. In addition, it may address distorted thinking and attitudes about calories, weight, and body image. This kind of treatment will also alleviate any underlying depression.

Group therapy can provide the opportunity to discuss the eating disorder candidly and to feel less isolated. Family therapy can also help with the inevitable conflicts that arise at the dinner table as well as the general feelings of helplessness and anger that may ripple throughout the household.

Because many binge eaters appear only to have a weight problem, it is not unusual for them to be present at diet centers rather than mental health settings. Many times, their eating problem will be addressed by their doctor as a general health issue. Still others find help in such self-help organizations as Overeaters Anonymous.

Prognosis Good. Seventy percent of all people with bulimia recover with treatment and suffer no long-term ill effects.

Somatoform Disorders

There are very few purely physical or purely psychological conditions. More often than not, where there is a medical condition, there will be psychological components, and where there are psychological conditions, there will be physical aspects. Although a rather daunting term, somatoform disorder describes those conditions in which physical symptoms or complaints are not fully explained by a medical or physical condition. In somatoform disorders, the ever-present interplay between mind and body manifests in a complex, dramatic fashion.

A person is said to have a somatoform disorder when his physical complaints or his problematic bodily sensations and functions are influenced primarily by the mind. Unlike the popular and demeaning notion of hypochondria, in which a person is thought to be faking illness in order to get attention, people with somatoform disorders are sincerely convinced that they have serious physical problems. Within this category, the more prominent diagnoses are conversion disorder, hypochondriasis, and somatization.

❖ CONVERSION DISORDER

Symptoms *(What you may experience)* Episodic, often dramatic physical symptoms or deficits that seem real but in fact have no relation to an actual medical condition. Symptoms arise from psychological conflicts or stress. Symptoms include difficulties and deficits that mimic sensory, motor, or neurologic disorders. People who suffer from conversion disorder think that their symptoms are real; symptoms are experienced as real. Not only are people with conversion disorder unaware that they are producing their symptoms; they also do not recognize that they are reacting or adopting this behavior as a coping mechanism.

Signs and laboratory findings *(What the doctor looks for)* No actual physical cause is found for the symptoms, despite adequate medical attention; inconsistencies in the presentation of symptoms.

What is it? Once referred to by the term hysteria, conversion disorder describes those not uncommon conditions in which extreme emotional or psychological stress is dissociated from conscious awareness and converted to physical symptoms in both men and women.

When someone has a conversion disorder, it may indeed appear as though he has a medical condition. However, a careful medical examination will likely reveal little connection to an actual physical illness or problem. In fact, the symptoms typically fail to conform to physical mechanisms or disease processes. Rather, they are shaped more often by the individual's understanding, however faulty, of anatomy and physiology. Yet, this is not to say that the symptoms are consciously constructed or intentionally faked. The intent and construction of symptoms are unconscious to the individual who suffers from conversion disorder.

The actual manifestation of conversion disorder is varied. In some cases, the disorder mimics neurologic problems with symptoms such as poor coordination or balance, paralysis, and the inability to speak. Some people who suffer from this type of somatoform disorder experience weakness in their limbs, difficulty swallowing, or the feeling that there is a constant lump in their throat. Sometimes conversion disorder appears in tics or tremors. The inability to walk or stand is an especially dramatic symptom. In other cases, there may be sensory symptoms or deficits such as double vision, tunnel vision, blindness, deafness, hallucinations, or the absence of touch or pain sensation.

Many times, unexplained pain can signal a conversion disorder. Headaches especially can occur alongside motor, sensory, or neurologic symptoms, or they can occur alone. Constant coughing, sneezing, or hiccuping, as well as stomachaches or recurrent vomiting are often attributed to conversion disorder, but some of these conditions may also depend on a gastrointestinal physiologic mechanism; they are not the sole creation of the unconscious mind. Conversion symptoms are restricted to ones that mimic neurologic disorders. Hysterical seizures, which may mimic petit

mal, grand mal, or psychomotor seizures (see Chapter 14), are common conversion symptoms.

Generally, conversion disorder arises as a time-limited episode, characterized by one or a few symptoms. It is often the case, although not always, that this disorder develops as a result of or concurrently with a general medical condition; frequently, a mild illness or injury prompts or precedes a conversion disorder.

Many times, conversion symptoms come on with little warning. On the other hand, they can begin as vague sensations or difficulties and progress gradually or haltingly. Sometimes there is one dramatic symptom. At other times, the symptoms are many or changing. When there are many conversion episodes over time, it is likely that the person has somatization disorder.

Conversion symptoms may arise in relation to specific emotional triggers: a move to a new community, family conflict, unresolved grief, sexual or physical abuse. They can also arise as a response to a natural disaster or other fear-inducing situations. In many instances the physical symptoms work to deflect from the actual trouble and to reduce anxiety. There may also be a secondary gain associated with the symptoms; a person may derive concrete benefits from the appearance of the condition or may be excused from troubling duties and responsibilities. Despite the fact that a person derives benefits from appearing ill, it is not necessarily the case that the symptoms are conscious.

Conversion disorders seem to be more common in women than men. Although this type of disorder can occur in people with any type of personality, those with histrionic personality (see Histrionic Personality Disorder, page 1259) and antisocial personality traits (see Antisocial Personality Disorder, page 1269) are thought to be more likely to develop conversion symptoms. In fact, conversion symptoms frequently occur as part of a variety of psychiatric conditions, ranging from anxiety disorders to depression, from psychosis to dissociative disorder.

If certain conversion symptoms last over time, there is some risk of actual physical harm. So if you have conversion paralysis, for example, the fact that you do not use your muscles can lead to muscle atrophy or damage as well as demineralization of the bones. In addition, you may engage in unnecessary diagnostic tests, therapeutic trials of various medications, and surgery, all of which carry a real risk of harmful side effects.

When to seek treatment Most people who are eventually diagnosed with conversion disorder find their way to a mental health clinician after a series of physical examinations, medical tests and procedures, and treatments fail to yield fully satisfactory results. Between 1 and 3 percent of all referrals to outpatient treatment have conversion disorder as their focus.

Treatment If it seems that your physical symptoms are related to emotional illness, treatment will begin with a thorough evaluation that includes taking an in-depth medical and psychosocial history and mental status examination. Any recent stressors or history of early losses and crises will be especially noted.

You may find that once the diagnosis of conversion disorder is made, you begin to feel better and symptoms abate a bit. Since the condition involves both physical and emotional realms, any type of treatment usually includes both medical and mental health professionals.

Treatment can often encompass a full range of psychotherapeutic approaches: Individual, family, and behavioral group therapy can work together to modify symptoms and address emotional conflicts or stresses. Cognitive-behavioral therapy can help you identify the ways that your physical symptoms function as well as any secondary gains involved. During therapy, you will probably work on developing more adaptive ways of coping. Physical therapy and prescribed exercises are often used if your symptoms involve restricted movement, paralysis, or weakness.

Whenever psychiatric illness, such as psychosis, depression, or anxiety, underlie or exist alongside conversion disorders, appropriate medications will be prescribed.

Prognosis For a single conversion episode, excellent. For multiple episodes, fairly good.

Whenever the conversion symptoms are transient, the prognosis tends to be quite good. Many symptoms abate on their own within a few days or weeks. If you require psychiatric treatment for the disorder, you may respond immediately to the knowledge that your physical symptoms are actually rooted in emotional or psychological trouble.

In most cases, the success of treatment depends on the person's acceptance that the symptoms are a direct manifestation of a psychological problem. For those who do not respond to treatment, the course of the condition can be chronic and fluctuating. In rare cases, conversion disorder can evolve into chronic somatization disorder (see page 1249), which can be quite disabling.

Treatment that combines psychotherapy and medication works best when there is another condition such as anxiety disorder or reactive depression or when the disorder has an identifiable stressor.

❖ HYPOCHONDRIASIS

Symptoms (*What you may experience*) Obsessive convictions and fear that one has developed a serious disease, which interferes with the ability to function at work and in relationships.

Signs and laboratory findings (*What the doctor looks for*) No physical cause is found for the symptoms, despite adequate medical attention.

What is it? A person may be diagnosed with hypochondriasis when he is preoccupied with the fear that he has developed a serious disease. Usually, the person notices an ache, pain, lump, or other bodily signs and assumes, with great certainty and considerable anxiety, that he is truly ill. As a result, he then frets about the illness, to the point that his normal activities, work, relationships, and the like, are dramatically disrupted.

When people suffer from hypochondriasis, they focus on body functions, heartbeat or respiration; on minor physical problems, a small sore, an occasional cough; or on vague or minor physical sensations, a pang around the ovaries, a "tired heart." They then become extremely concerned about just what these signs mean and what causes them. In addition, they fixate on certain parts of the body, their heart, for example.

As a rule, hypochondriasis is a chronic condition, with a waxing and waning rhythm. Symptoms tend to flair up during times of stress. Almost uniformly, the concern is not about some transient minor disease but, rather, a serious, life-threatening condition. The object of concern, however, can change from time to time.

If you suffer from hypochondriasis, you may suspect that you are overreacting or exaggerating. Yet, no amount of reassurance from your doctor or negative readings on various tests and examinations will assuage your anxiety. Every article you read or story you hear only fuels your anxiety and the certainty that you suffer from an actual illness. Sometimes, when you learn of someone else's illness, you may become additionally alarmed that you suffer from the same condition.

Frequently, the conversations, self-image, and daily involvements of people with hypochondriasis will center on their health. They may join special self-help and support groups, buy books about the conditions, and shape their lifestyle as if they actually suffer from the disease.

People who suffer from hypochondriasis shop around for doctors. As frustration and anger builds on both sides, their relationship with their doctors deteriorates, and they move on to the next one. They may insist that they are not getting proper care and attention. In addition, they subject themselves to unnecessary medical procedures and tests, even when these carry considerable risks and offer little actual benefit. After time, because they have had so many complaints, they may not be taken seriously should an actual medical condition arise.

Social relationships frequently become strained as a result of this disorder. People with hypochondriasis are preoccupied with their own physical condition and may expect special treatment and consideration. Family life becomes troubled as it centers more and more on one member's physical well-being. In addition, in their pursuit of medical attention, they may miss work frequently and become less productive.

People who have been seriously ill as children or who have been involved in another's illness are more likely to become concerned about their own health. In some cases, the death of a loved one may also prompt hypochondriasis (see Reactive and Grief-Related Depression, page 1224). In general, the disorder seems to first appear in early adulthood.

Within general medical practice, between 4 and 9 percent of all patients actually suffer from hypochondriasis. In popular usage, the term *hypochondria* is adopted to dismiss someone's illness as being all in his head, but hypochondriasis may veil a serious depressive or anxiety disorder.

When to seek treatment Most people with hypochondriasis consult their doctors for medical concerns. As a rule, the doctor will first rule out possible physical conditions that could explain the symptoms: early stages of such neurologic conditions as myasthenia gravis or multiple sclerosis; such endocrine conditions as thyroid or parathyroid disease; and other conditions such as lupus or occult malignancies. When test after test fails to uncover a medical condition, or after a series of such complaints, the doctor may refer the patient to a mental health clinician.

If your worries about your health begin to interfere with your work and social relationships and the doctor cannot reassure you, ask her to recommend a therapist.

Treatment When hypochondriasis masks depressive or anxiety symptoms, medication will be prescribed. Antianxiety medications—such as lorazepam, clonazepam, and alprazolam—and antidepressant medications—such as fluoxetine, sertraline, paroxetine, fluvoxamine, imipramine, nortriptyline, amitriptyline, and desipramine—seem particularly effective in curbing some of the more distressing symptoms so that the person can engage in therapy.

Psychotherapy is usually recommended, with or without medication. Insight-oriented therapy can help the person understand his feelings underlying the symptoms. Behavioral techniques can help the person examine his preoccupations and worries; eventually, he may be able to make judgments about how realistic they are.

Education about the nature and development of hypochondriacal symptoms can have significant therapeutic effects. Once the person with hypochondriasis understands that worrying and focusing on his symptoms actually exacerbates them, he may begin to reduce his anxiety and the tendency to self-monitor.

Marriage and family therapy may be necessary to deal with the strain of the disorder. Also, group therapy can provide the support and education for an individual with hypochondriasis.

Prognosis Fair. Too often, the condition is not recognized and diagnosed, and care remains within the domain of the primary care doctor. The success of treatment depends on the person's acceptance that the symptoms are a direct manifestation of a psychological problem. Approximately half of all people with the diagnosis of hypochondriasis improve in response to treatment. The rest show a chronic, fluctuating course. When another, treatable condition, such as anxiety disorder, major depression, or reactive depression, is the cause, or when the condition has an identifiable stressor, therapy is better able to address the disorder.

❖ SOMATIZATION DISORDER

Symptoms *(What you may experience)* Various recurring physical complaints—headaches; stomachaches; nausea or abdominal bloating; backaches; achiness in the joints, arms, or legs; or problems in menstruation, sexual functioning, or urination—that cannot be traced to any specific medical condition or to substance use and that cause serious problems in day-to-day functioning.

Signs and laboratory findings *(What the doctor looks for)* No physical cause revealed on tests, x-rays, and diagnostic procedures; a pattern of complaining of many symptoms in many parts of the body; also a pattern of hospitalizations coupled with anxiety or depressive symptoms.

What is it? Somatization disorder is a chronic or recurrent condition characterized by many unexplained somatic, or physical, complaints. Most commonly diagnosed in women, it often appears comingled with substance abuse, depression, suicidal behavior, and histrionic or antisocial personality disorders (see Histrionic Personality Disor-

der, page 1259, and Antisocial Personality Disorders, page 1260). Many times, people with this disorder also tend to be impulsive, dependent, and perfectionistic.

The majority of people who are diagnosed with this disorder report four basic symptoms usually in many manifestations: pain, gastrointestinal discomfort, sexual or reproductive trouble, and neurologic impairment. Nausea and abdominal bloating, vomiting, diarrhea, and food intolerance are frequent complaints. Women with somatization disorder often have a history of irregular menstruation, menorrhagia, or vomiting throughout pregnancy. Men typically recount difficulties in achieving an erection or ejaculating. Both men and women with this disorder report little interest in sexual relations.

People who suffer from somatization disorder may complain of symptoms that suggest some type of neurologic problem: impaired coordination or balance; paralysis or localized weakness; difficulty swallowing or a lump in the throat; loss of touch or pain sensation; aphonia (loss of speech); bladder problems; double vision; blindness; deafness; seizures; amnesia; loss of consciousness.

Untreated, this disorder tends to have a chronic course, with relapses occurring during times of stress. Typically, a new physical symptom will appear with each emotional distress. Episodes generally last from 6 to 9 months. It is unlikely that people with somatization disorder will go an entire year without developing a new symptom and seeking medical attention.

People with this disorder may submit to numerous medical examinations, diagnostic procedures, surgeries, and hospitalizations—many of which are unnecessary and may increase the possibility of developing a serious medical problem. Their frequent use of medication may lead to significant side effects.

The lives of people with somatization disorder tend to be chaotic. Too self-involved to maintain a mutual relationship, they may divorce a number of times. Too disabled to hold gainful employment, they may have trouble holding down jobs.

When to seek treatment Because the symptoms tend to be physical, people with somatization disorder almost always consult doctors first. They may then be referred for psychiatric treatment by the hospital or doctor as test after test yields little conclusive results. Occasionally, people with somatization disorder will contact a mental health professional because they feel depressed or anxious.

Treatment Psychotherapy for somatization disorders usually involves identifying and addressing the precipitating stress. Therapy that is supportive and fosters a trusting relationship can help the person begin to trust his doctor as well. He may then begin to accept medical reassurances and understand the psychological implications of his illness. A psychodynamic approach that fosters understanding of how internal conflicts and psychological factors influence the development and maintenance of

symptoms can be quite beneficial. Cognitive and behavioral principles can also help the individual understand the secondary gain, or unspoken benefits, derived from the symptoms and the behavior. Time-limited group therapy provides opportunity for people with somatization disorder to feel supported and share methods of coping.

When there are significant depressive or anxiety symptoms, antidepressant and antianxiety medications, such as lorazepam, fluoxetine, sertraline, paroxetine, fluvoxamine, imipramine, nortriptyline, amitriptyline, and desipramine, will be prescribed.

Prognosis Fairly good. Just as with hypochondriasis, a person with somatization disorder must be able to accept that his physical symptoms reflect a psychological

WHERE TO FIND HELP

While mental health services may be appropriate and quite helpful after the crisis of abuse has passed, or as support as a person tries to extricate herself from an abusive situation, the problem of abuse requires a complex intermeshing of various community services. Depending on what is needed, most communities offer social, legal, financial, housing, educational, and preventive services for abuse victims, and, often, the abusers.

In the case of sexual or physical child abuse, it must be reported immediately to Child Protective Services. If you have any questions or concerns, you can call the National Child Abuse Hotline number, (800) 4-A-CHILD.

With other types of abuse, the primary and most effective way to initiate help is by calling the appropriate hotline. Most communities have confidential hotlines for sexual abuse and domestic violence, and most of these hotlines are linked to free-standing centers. If you call the national hotline, they will refer you to or connect you directly with your local hotline.

- Child Abuse: (800) 4-A-CHILD

- Domestic Violence: (800) 799-7233

- Sexual Assault: (800) 656-HOPE

Once a person calls the hotline, the hotline volunteer will immediately ask about her safety, current health, and circumstances. During the aftermath of a rape or episode of domestic violence, the hotline may offer options—to call the police, to go to the hospital—and advise the victim what she can expect if she chooses to do so. If a person has already called the police or gone to the hospital, chances are that people there will report the abuse or rape to the hotline; if the victim chooses, a volunteer will

come to support, advocate, and calm her during the height of the crisis.

After the crisis passes, and the victim is stabilized, hotline volunteers, who are often linked to free-standing service centers, will likely make appropriate referrals. Even if someone calls the hotline because his current crisis is rooted in a childhood experience of sexual abuse or incest, the volunteer will help stabilize him and make appropriate referrals. Depending on the circumstances, these may include

- Legal services and advocacy

- Individual counseling and support groups

- Testing for acquired immunodeficiency syndrome (AIDS) and sexually transmitted diseases, as well as providing other medical services

- Divorce workshops and counseling around custody issues

- Women in transition programs that help women leave abusive home situations

- Emergency shelter and transitional housing

- Employment and financial counseling

- Counseling and other help for the offender or batterer

The National Coalition Against Sexual Assault and The National Coalition Against Domestic Violence sponsor the national hotlines. They also lobby for legislation and funding, organize and fund local free-standing centers, disseminate information, and coordinate much of the local services around these issues. ■

condition. Those who are able to accept treatment generally do well.

Physical, Sexual, and Emotional Abuse

People who are subjected to continuous abuse—whether emotional abuse, domestic abuse or battering, or sexual assault, incest, or rape—often develop clusters of symptoms that, depending on the nature and duration of the event, resemble symptoms of other psychiatric disorders. These include anxiety disorders, depressive disorders, and post-traumatic stress disorder. Despite the fact that the implications and manifestations of abuse may be psychological, abuse is actually a complex social and legal issue. Dealing with abuse involves preventive, active policy, and often legal intervention as well as psychological treatment.

❖ BATTERED SPOUSE SYNDROME

Symptoms and signs Feelings of depression, anxiety, hypervigilance, extreme timidity, and hopelessness in response to abuse and battering by one's spouse; lack of self-confidence and poor self-esteem; actual signs of beatings, including black eyes, cuts, swollen face, welts, broken bones.

What is it? People suffer from battered spouse syndrome after being continually subjected to domestic violence, that is, abuse between married or unmarried partners. Coercive by nature, domestic abuse, whether physical, emotional, sexual, or economic, aims at controlling or dominating the other. Ninety-five percent of victims of domestic abuse are women. Each year, 2 million women are battered or abused by their partners. One-third of all female murder victims are killed by their partners.

Typically, abuse escalates in relationships. An abusive event—a slap, forcing unwanted sex, taunting, throwing objects at another—is rarely isolated. Violence may be one aspect of a batterer's abuse: He may be possessive and jealous, withhold money or control assets and access to family finances, or force his partner to dress in an uncomfortable sexually provocative way.

Many times, women stay in abusive relationships because they fear retaliation or death if they leave. Some wish to preserve the family and their roles as wife, mother, and homemaker. Many lack the financial resources or the confidence in their ability to earn a living (especially if they have small children) to live on their own. And many face the very real possibility that they will lose custody of their children if they leave. In addition, many women lack the self-assurance to leave. Years of abuse have made them feel helpless and fearful. Many women who are abused as adults were abused as children; they have come to believe that they deserve the abuse.

But women are not the only victims of domestic abuse. Today, a staggering number of young children witness violence. Believing that they can protect their children from domestic violence, many parents may wait until the children are asleep or fight in other parts of the house. Yet, children know what goes on in their homes. They hear the screaming, threats, broken glass; they see the holes in the wall, the broken furniture, their mother's bruises and cuts. When arguments become violent, when father batters mother, children are traumatized (see Post-Traumatic Stress Disorder, page 1222).

Perhaps most troubling, though, is the fact that when a child watches his father use violence to assert dominance and power over his mother, he is at heightened risk for developing aggressive and violent behavior, not only as an expression of his rage, but also as a hedge against his own feelings of helplessness. He then is at high risk for aggressive behavior that becomes increasingly more dangerous as he gets older (see Behavior Disorders, page 1238).

When to seek help The first time your partner strikes you or inflicts some other form of violence, leave if at all possible. If he hurts you once, chances are he will hurt you again. Let him know that you will return when he gets proper help. If it is not possible for you to leave at present, contact the Domestic Violence Hotline—(800) 799-7233—so that you can get the information you need to give careful thought to your situation and your options. You may want to begin to make preparations to leave in the event that the abuse repeats itself.

Regardless of the action you choose to take, do not dismiss an abusive incident as unimportant. Whenever a person uses physical force or violence to assert himself, it is a warning that he is troubled.

Whenever your home life leaves you feeling helpless, powerless, depressed, anxious, or actually unsafe, speak to your doctor or call the Domestic Violence Hotline, (800) 799-7233.

Treatment The first step for getting help for battered spouse syndrome is to call the Domestic Violence Hotline, if you are still in an abusive relationship and in crisis as well as after the crisis has passed. The hotline volunteers can advise you on the appropriate steps to take to resolve the crisis and to stabilize yourself and your children once the crisis has abated.

Dealing with domestic abuse involves a complex interweaving of services to address housing, financial, legal, and other matters (see Where to Find Help, page 1250). Once the practical matters are taken care of—or during the process—counseling is usually necessary to help you manage the complicated feelings that inevitably arise. Long-term therapy may be called for to examine the way past experiences or abuse may predispose you to current violent situations.

Medication may be prescribed to relieve some of the depressive or anxiety symptoms that develop as a result of the abuse.

Finally, if you are a batterer, or fear that you may become one, call the hotline. There is help—perhaps in the form of group or individual counseling—for you, too.

❖ CHILD ABUSE

Symptoms and signs Although it is hard to judge whether a child is being abused solely on appearances, abused children generally appear excessively aggressive or sexually provocative and may lag behind in academic achievement. Other symptoms and signs of abuse include extreme anger, impulsiveness, fearfulness, or depression; sleep problems; exaggerated startle response; panic; irritability; immature or regressed behavior; and hypervigilance.

What is it? Child abuse is a pattern of mistreatment, abusive behavior, sexual abuse, or extreme neglect by a parent or another adult in authority. Adults inflict physical abuse by deliberately hitting, kicking, and beating the child. Sexual abuse includes both sexual assault and sexual exploitation. Emotional abuse includes acts of emotional cruelty that harm the child. Neglect is considered abuse when it results in harm or the threat of harm to the child's welfare and health, including actual abandonment, inadequate supervision, and denying medical care.

Children who withstand multiple or long-standing abuse develop a kind of survivor's syndrome. Because their trauma is repeated or prolonged, shock following the first blow evolves into sickening anticipation or expectation. After being repeatedly brutalized, children may withdraw or become numb. They may try to look normal but seem zombie-like. Indeed, many abused children forget what it is to feel alive. They frequently become indifferent to pain, lack empathy, and fail to read or acknowledge their own feelings.

Long-standing or repeated abuse can produce extreme, often muted rage in children. Anger festers, occasionally exploding in tantrums and violent behavior. A child may turn the rage against herself, engaging in self-mutilating and self-endangering behavior or making physically damaging suicidal gestures. She may enact her anger through habitually aggressive or delinquent behavior, or she may identify with the aggressor, so that she victimizes and humiliates other children. This kind of behavior may fluctuate with extreme passivity, because the child experiences any kind of aggression as dangerous.

Abuse shatters a child's natural sense of invincibility and basic trust. When the abuse persists over a long period, children tend to limit their expectations: They do not anticipate a career, a marriage, children, or a normal life span. Abuse may affect their attitudes about people. After years of abuse, children may come to believe, with good reason, that they cannot trust anyone. Children who are sexually abused may shrink from men or approach them with overly friendly advances. These children tend to recognize the profound vulnerability in all people, especially themselves (see Post-Traumatic Stress Disorder, page 1222).

Many extremely abused children continue to foster one or two trauma-related fears well into adulthood. For example, sexually abused children may grow up to fear sex. Abuse can set in motion internal changes that last throughout life. If childhood abuse is not treated, it can account for a number of adult character problems including psychotic thinking, violent behavior, extremes of passivity and victimization (people who were raped or incestuously abused as children are often raped again and again as adults), self-mutilation, suicidal or self-endangering behavior, and a variety of anxiety disturbances.

What you can do If you suspect that a child you know is being abused, either sexually or physically, or neglected, you must contact your local child protective services agency. It is crucial that the child's safety be secured directly and immediately before any of the other issues are considered.

It may not be clear to an outsider if a child is being subjected to extreme corporal punishment or physical abuse. Bruises, black eyes, bloody noses, lacerations, and marks that stay red for a long time may be signs that a child is being abused. If you think that you are abusing your child or that someone else in the family is abusing your child, call one of the emergency hotlines and get help (see Where to Find Help, page 1250).

Treatment More often than not, children who have been abused need treatment to be able to talk about their pain, anger, and concerns about safety. Play therapy allows young children to reenact the traumatic events in a safe environment. Being able to build a trusting relationship with an adult during therapy in which the child will not be betrayed, exploited, or hurt is immensely valuable.

Involving abusive parents in the treatment of children and adolescents is also necessary to reduce the possibility that the abuse will continue and to establish a sense of safety for the child. In therapy, parents may learn more effective and appropriate parenting skills. In addition, they can receive the support, understanding, and encouragement they need to be better parents.

Occasionally, medication is recommended in the early course of treatment, particularly to treat abuse-related depressions or compulsive behaviors.

Prognosis When people who have experienced childhood abuse are able to feel safe again, and when their issues are addressed effectively, they are generally responsive to treatment.

❖ ABUSE OF THE ELDERLY

Signs and laboratory findings *(What a doctor looks for)* In an older person: increased depression and unresponsiveness, anxiety, withdrawal, or timidity; uncharacteristic confusion and hostility toward others; new poverty or unexplained loss of resources; longing for death or an end to it all; vague health complaints, insomnia, or psychosomatic symptoms. In caregivers: mounting resentment against the older person or the situation; aggressive and/or defensive behavior toward others; preoccupation and/or depression; shifting blame and excusing their own failure.

What is it? Elder abuse is the maltreatment or neglect of dependent older people. It can be passive neglect, psychological abuse, financial abuse, active neglect, or physical abuse. Except in the instance of passive abuse, which is not intentionally caused and arises when a caregiver is overworked or underinformed, elder abuse is a deliberate act of a hostile perpetrator.

Unlike children, the elderly are responsible for themselves unless they are declared incompetent. Yet many are frail, dependent, and vulnerable, and as such, subject to abuse. Elder abuse cuts across gender, class, race, and age lines. In 60 percent of elder abuse cases, the abusers are spouses; 20 percent are adult children; and 20 percent are siblings, grandchildren, boarders, and caregivers.

Often, in cases of passive neglect, tensions from complicated, conflicted, or unresolved family relationships result in neglect. Occasionally, caregivers and family members find themselves stressed by the responsibility and thus become neglectful.

In more active forms of abuse, there is actual intent to inflict harm or deprivation on the older person. In many cases, the caregiver is motivated to abuse by his own greed or wish to exploit his charge. Or he may become increasingly resentful of his situation and his responsibility.

Treatment Intervening in cases of elder abuse means locating the resources that provide protection and health care for the older segment of our population in a timely and ongoing manner. Many times, finding such resources begins with a call to your state or local protective services agency to find out what social, legal, and criminal recourse is available.

In some communities, local hospitals, medical schools, universities, and mental health centers provide resources specially tailored to the needs of seniors. Also, if possible, finding a geriatric physician or a psychiatrist who is trained in recognizing disturbances and susceptibilities particular to seniors is often helpful. Geriatric physicians will likely be able to distinguish between fear arising from actual life circumstances and those arising from anxiety disorders, clinical depression, and dementia. They will be able to review any medication the person is taking and consider any undue side effects. Because they have a better understanding of the factors that are specific to old age, geriatric specialists are more likely to understand the nature and severity of abuse.

Schizophrenia and Delusional Disorders

Schizophrenia and delusional disorders fall under the diagnostic umbrella of psychosis. A psychotic illness is a brain disorder, characterized by an impaired perception of reality, often coupled with mood disturbances. Psychosis can be either progressive or episodic. Although this is a serious illness, the prognosis varies according to severity and type.

❖ SCHIZOPHRENIA

Symptoms *(What you may experience)* Delusions (false beliefs), hallucinations (per-ceptions without external stimuli), incoherence, bizarre ideas and behavior; dramatic moodiness and mood swings as well as flat emotional tone; inability to socialize and work normally; agitation; occasionally violent eruptions; profound withdrawal; loss of interest in hygiene or personal appearance.

Signs and laboratory findings *(What your doctor looks for)* Disorganized speech and behavior; a flat emotional quality; expressions of profoundly paranoid or grandiose thinking; deteriorating social and vocational functioning; grossly chaotic appearance. For a clinician to arrive at a diagnosis of schizophrenia, a combination of symptoms and signs must be present for a significant portion of time during at least a 1-month period with some aspects of the disorder persisting for over 6 months.

What is it? Schizophrenia is a brain disorder that affects approximately 1 percent of the population. The National Institute of Mental Health puts the number of people currently being treated as outpatients for this psychotic disorder at around 1 million. Thought to be a disturbance in the brain's chemistry, schizophrenia is a mental illness characterized by prominent and persistent disturbances in the way a person thinks, sees, and hears. These cognitive and perceptual disturbances are often coupled with disturbances in mood. Psychosis can be either progressive or episodic. Although this is a serious illness, the prognosis varies.

On the average, men experience their first psychotic episode in their early to mid-20s, and women in their late 20s; however, it may strike in late adolescence when, it seems, the pressures exerted during the transition into adulthood overtax the system. Schizophrenia can emerge during middle age, particularly in women. As a rule, when the disorder appears early, the course tends to be more severe.

Schizophrenia may initially appear as a gradual decline in behavior or a dramatic break with reality. When the latter is the case, the psychotic break can seem profoundly abrupt and alarming: A person can seem perfectly normal one day, then, for all intents and purposes, lost the next. In other cases, there is a sense that the person, even in childhood, has never been quite normal.

Schizophrenia involves disordered thinking (reflected in a disturbance in the logical and coherent structure and form of speech), delusions or fixed beliefs that are odd or highly unusual, and hallucinations (hearing sounds or voices and seeing things that do not exist for others). Usually, a person with schizophrenia has trouble distinguishing what is real from what is in his head.

Referential delusions—the belief that everyday things within one's environment (advertisements, newscasts, passages from books, song lyrics, and the like) are directly addressed to him—are common. Persecutory delusions are also typical of the illness. An individual with schizophrenia may truly believe that others are spying on him, tormenting him, following him, making fun of him or trying to trick him. Schizophrenic thinking may also include delusions of influence, the belief that outside forces are directly affecting or controlling one's thoughts, actions, or sensations. This delusional thinking goes beyond strongly held beliefs; rather, it involves complete and utter convictions in the face of all contradictory evidence.

Feelings are also affected. A person suffering from schizophrenia may be extremely moody or his feelings profoundly flat. Almost always, his feelings are not appropriate to his situation. He may laugh or be silly at somber or serious occasions and appear to have no reaction to clearly upsetting circumstances.

The behavior of an individual with schizophrenia may also be grossly disturbed: His actions will appear strange, bizarre, or disorganized. He will likely withdraw from all social interactions. In many cases, a person with schizophrenia is unable to perform even the simplest of daily tasks. He may dress in an unsuitable or disheveled fashion and have trouble maintaining basic hygiene. He may exhibit inappropriate sexual behaviors. Consequently, people suffering from schizophrenia tend to live in a world circumscribed by disordered perceptions, emotions, and behavior, most of which are beyond their control.

Although there is little doubt that schizophrenia is a brain disorder, it is not clear just what causes the brain to malfunction. Studies indicate that genetic and environmental factors play a role. Other studies point to such biologic components as gestational and birth complications (a viral condition present during pregnancy, for example), genetic mutation, or a delay in a child's neurologic development that combine to cause brain distortions that manifest usually during young adulthood. Recently, research into the brain's chemical balance, specifically, the levels of dopamine in the brain, has yielded some promising results.

When to seek treatment Once you begin to experience psychotic symptoms, you may not be able to judge that they are unusual; it may therefore be up to friends and family members to recognize the problem and seek help. If you begin to experience, or notice in someone close to you, any of the symptoms listed above, call your doctor immediately.

Treatment The first and most effective form of treatment for schizophrenia is medication. Neuroleptics that affect dopamine neurotransmitter systems are effective in managing and reducing psychotic symptoms. This group of drugs includes haloperidol (Haldol), fluphenazine (Prolixin), chlorpromazine (Thorazine), and thioridazine (Mellaril). At the same time, these drugs can produce problematic side effects including low blood pressure, drowsiness, dry mouth, blurred vision, lethargy, constipation, and weight gain. The high-potency medications like haliperidol and fluphenazine may produce restlessness, muscle spasms, and tremors as well but tend to cause fewer problems with blood pressure, blurred vision, dry mouth, and drowsiness. The most disturbing side effect, tardive dyskinesia, an involuntary series of tics in the tongue, facial muscles, arms, and legs, can occur after years of taking the drugs.

The novel neuroleptics, including risperidone (Risperdal), olanzapine (Zypnexa), and clozapine (Clozaril) work particularly well on the more tenacious forms of schizophrenia. And because they work more selectively among the brain's dopamine neurotransmitter systems, they tend to have fewer side effects. They may not cause tardive dyskinesia at all. However, because clozapine can cause a dangerous drop in the blood's white cells, which can interfere with the body's ability to fight infection, it must be monitored closely with weekly blood counts. In fact, the use of all

LIVING SITUATIONS FOR THE MENTALLY ILL

Only four decades ago, people who suffered from serious mental illnesses lived in state hospitals or institutions. For better or for worse, today, most have been relocated to the community. Even when they are involved in community-based rehabilitation programs, finding supportive and affordable housing has become a real issue for many.

When residential treatment and housing programs are available and adequate, they can increase the level of a person's functioning and reduce the social handicap of limited access to appropriate housing that arises from disabilities and the social stigma connected to being mentally ill.

Linear Continuum One type of residential program is called linear continuum, in which a person progresses toward higher functioning and less restrictive settings. The basic types of residential care settings are transitional half-way houses, long-term group residences, nursing homes, foster care, board and care homes, and total rural environments. Each setting differs in terms of the length of time a person is allowed to stay, the intensity of on-site staff supervision, and the degree to which it emphasizes clinical and rehabilitation services as opposed to simple housing.

Supportive Housing A second type of residential housing is referred to as supportive housing. These mainstream housing programs, set within a populated neighborhood, offer support services as needed but not on site. The housing is conceived as a normal living environment rather than a treatment or service setting, and the focus is on individual choice and normalization of the person's living environment.

For many, these alternative, supervised living situations offer the only opportunities they have to lead independent lives. ■

such antipsychotic medication requires close monitoring.

Once the more troubling symptoms recede, individuals may be tempted to discontinue the medications. Yet, once the medications are stopped, the voices will return, and the disorder will reemerge full force, sometimes immediately, sometimes after a delay of a few months, but always, sooner or later.

For this and other reasons, drug treatment is almost always one aspect of a more elaborate plan for treating schizophrenia. Because the illness is severe and chronic, and invariably interferes with normal functioning, treatment usually includes day or partial hospitalization, rehabilitative therapy, training in social skills, and vocational training. In many cases, assisted or supervised living situations make it possible for adults with schizophrenia to lead relatively independent lives. In addition to psychiatric

management, individual supportive therapy, family support, and education are regularly part of the treatment plan.

During an acute psychotic episode—during the first psychotic break, when medications have been discontinued, or when an attack forces its way through the preventive effects of the medication, for example—full hospitalization may be required. Also, a doctor may decide to hospitalize the patient in order to work out the right medication protocol. If the diagnosis follows an attempt at suicide, the individual may also be hospitalized until it is established that he no longer presents a danger to himself.

As with any chronic disease, relapses may occur, often following stressful events. Schizophrenia is a serious illness that requires long-term intensive treatment.

Prognosis Fair. The later the onset, the better the prognosis. Many patients experience a full or almost full recovery from schizophrenia, although this might take many years. However, for others, the cumulative effect of schizophrenia is severe and long lasting. Some schizophrenics continue to decline, and few return quickly to the level of functioning they had achieved before their first psychotic episode. Many people with schizophrenia find it hard if not impossible to hold a significant job or sustain a long-term relationship. Between 25 and 50 percent of all individuals with schizophrenia abuse drugs or alcohol, and there is a high rate of suicide associated with the disorder.

Yet, this does not mean that the diagnosis of schizophrenia automatically assigns a person to a lifetime of institutions or homelessness. Most people who suffer from schizophrenia can be treated, and the condition can be managed with reasonable success. Many recover in time, and others are helped substantially with medications, family support, and special living arrangements (see Living Situations for the Mentally Ill above) to lead fully satisfying lives.

❖ PARANOIA AND OTHER PSYCHOSES

Symptoms (*What you may experience*) Delusional thinking that centers on a specific theme but does not otherwise interfere significantly with a person's ability to function; hallucinations that have to do with such sensations as touch or smell; irritable or depressed mood; anger and violent behavior; litigious behavior (tendency to sue in court).

Signs and laboratory findings *(What the doctor may look for)* Delusions that involve profound preoccupations with beliefs about things that could be happening but are not; such beliefs may have some connections to a person's ordinary experiences; poor social relationships.

What is it? Delusional disorders may well account for 2 percent of all admissions to mental health facilities. Usually appearing in middle or late adult life, these disorders involve distorted thinking that, while not particularly bizarre, becomes so obsessive and consuming that it has significant impact on a person's relationships and, at times, his work. Focusing on specific themes and concerns, the delusional thoughts tend to have some connection to the person's real life.

These disorders tend to be chronic, although there may be an intermittent quality to them. Delusions may become especially apparent during times of stress.

Predominant delusional themes are described below.

Paranoid delusions Also called persecutory delusions, a person with this type of delusional thinking holds the conviction that other people are out to get him. He feels persecuted, pathologically certain that others are conspiring against him, trying to trick or cheat him, spying on him, following him, poisoning or drugging him, harassing, slandering, or preventing him from achieving his goals. Small slights are exaggerated. As a result, a person may react with litigious behavior. He may consistently seek restitution and protection from imagined persecutors through the court system or other governmental agencies. In addition, people who are preoccupied with paranoid or persecutory thoughts often are resentful and angry; they are prone to violent outbursts and behavior when they believe that others are attacking them.

Somatic delusions These delusions center around physical preoccupations and sensa-

tions. A person who suffers from this form of psychosis is sure that he is infested with insects or emitting a foul odor from certain areas of her body: her mouth, skin, rectum, or vagina. Or a person may be convinced that insects are crawling around his skin, he has an internal parasite, or that, contrary to all evidence, certain parts of his body are misshapen, ugly, or not functioning.

Grandiose delusions People who harbor grandiose delusions are convinced that they have some great, but as yet unrecognized, talent or insight. Some people who suffer from this form of delusional disorder believe that they have made a significant discovery without receiving the recognition and reward they deserve. Some assert with all certainty that they occupy a position of privilege or enjoy a special relationship with a prominent public figure; a person may claim to be a special advisor to the president or the mistress of the Dali Lama, for example. Some maintain the conviction that they, themselves, are prominent. Occasionally, there is a religious component to these delusions, so that a person, for example, may believe that he is the sole chosen messenger from God.

Delusions of jealousy These appear when someone is preoccupied with the certainty that his partner is unfaithful. Even in the face of reasonable evidence to the contrary, a person with jealous delusions will sustain and support the belief with incorrect inference and slim evidence. He may spend inordinate amounts of time collecting such evidence and justifying the delusion. In all likelihood, he will confront his partner, and then attempt to control her behavior, attacking her, restricting her autonomy, stalking her, and investigating the imagined lover.

When to seek treatment People who suffer from delusional disorders may not recognize that they have a disorder that can be treated, although they may seek treatment for other conditions—marital conflict, a medical problem, and the like—which may lead to treatment for delusional disorder. Or, because such delusions can cause problems in personal relationships, people with these disorders may be urged to seek treatment by friends and family members.

Treatment Hospitalization is occasionally required during the acute phase of these disorders, especially when a person poses a danger to himself or to others. Medication treatment typically includes antipsychotics to reduce or eliminate the delusion and to address agitation and possible violent behavior. When there is a manic quality to the grandiose or jealous delusions, the diagnosis may be bipolar disorder and lithium is often prescribed. When there is a depressed quality to the paranoid or somatic delusions, major depression may be the primary disorder and an antidepressant might be used.

Family therapy can help spouses and families deal with the unpredictability of the disorder. Individual behavioral therapy can help a person examine and evaluate his distorted thinking, as well as identify and anticipate factors that could possibly trigger more acute episodes.

Personality Disorders

People seek therapeutic help for a number of reasons. Some contact a mental health professional following a crisis or traumatic experience: a death in the family, a divorce, a rape, an illness, the loss of a job. Others seek therapy to help them deal with specific issues: finding a more satisfying career; raising a difficult child; dealing with teenagers at home; making the transition from adolescence to adulthood, from childless adult to parent. Still others begin therapy to help them manage a persistent psychiatric disorder: depression, eating disorder, panic attacks, and the like.

Yet there are many other people whose reason to seek therapy is less conspicuous. These people seem to have crisis after crisis, their intimate relationships and friendships seem consistently stormy or ungratifying, or their work patterns tend to be frustrating and self-defeating. They come to therapy because their lives never seem to go the way they want. They feel essentially unhappy. Many of these patients suffer from personality disorders.

The term *personality* refers to the individual, ingrained, pervasive, enduring, and habitual ways a person operates. Made up of attitudes, perceptions, habits, emotions, and behaviors, one's personality is one's style. More than a collection of traits and dispositions, personality is characterized by the way in which a person perceives, relates to, and thinks about himself and his environment.

In contrast to the term *character*, which refers to a person's distinct nature, an individual's personality traits are both based on his inherent character and shaped by his unique developmental process and life experience. In other words, personality is a product of both nature and nurture, of constitutional attributes, early developmental experiences, and ongoing life circumstances.

Personality traits transform themselves into personality disorders when they become so rigid that a person cannot respond spontaneously or appropriately to his environment and life circumstances. Personality disorders can be detected in the ways an individual acts, feels, thinks, and relates. Generally, a disordered personality is evident when a person has persistent problems in maintaining intimate relationships, holding jobs, or advancing in a career. Usually apparent since late adolescence or early adulthood, the pattern of difficulties and distress caused by a personality disorder is consistent and long lasting.

There is considerable debate as to what actually accounts for personality disorders, but recent theories suggest that in addition to inherited and constitutional qualities, these more or less distorted personality styles are also products of a child's early relationships with his parents or primary caregivers. Simply put, because the fit between a child's inborn temperament and the parents' child-rearing practices is an important determinant of how a personality develops, a disordered personality may in fact originate in less than adequate parenting or troubling childhood experiences.

Because many of the signs and symptoms of personality disorders are exaggerations or slight distortions of normal personality traits, they are not always easily diagnosed. What is more, personality disorders can complicate other psychiatric and emotional disorders, making diagnosis more difficult and rendering the difficulties more tenacious (see page 1263). Between 70 and 85 percent of all criminals have personality disorders; between 60 and 70 percent of people with alcohol-related problems and between 70 and 80 percent of those who abuse drugs have personality disorders. People with personality disorders are more likely to commit violent crimes, attempt and commit suicide, have accidents, and receive hospital emergency room treatment.

The most common types of personality disorder—histrionic, antisocial, borderline, dependent, obsessive-compulsive, passive-aggressive, and schizotypal—are described in greater detail below. Information on treatment for the various personality disorders begins on page 1258.

It is the nature of a personality disorder that those who have one are unlikely to recognize it. Instead, if you have one, you are more likely to see yourself as a victim of circumstances. You may find yourself feeling unjustly picked on, criticized, and rejected, and, most importantly, you may feel unaccountably dissatisfied and malcontent. At the same time, chances are that because you are functioning reasonably well, it may not occur to you, or to those in your life, that you could benefit from professional help.

The following descriptions of symptoms may help you identify some aspects of your own distress and functioning and perhaps even help you acknowledge that you, in fact, suffer from an emotional disorder. While it may be unsettling to see yourself in the descriptions below, you may at the same time feel relieved to realize that what you feel and experience has a name and a cause, and that, in most cases it can be effectively dealt with through psychiatric treatment.

❖ HISTRIONIC PERSONALITY DISORDERS

Symptoms and signs Essential feeling of emptiness and helplessness; an automatic, compelling need to use physical appearance or seductive and provocative behavior to secure attention and approval; constant craving for the center of attention; rapid-shifting and somewhat shallow expression of emotions; tendency toward self-dramatization, theatricality, and flamboyance; excessive reliance on outside influences and measures of self-worth.

What is it? The flamboyant, dramatic, attention-seeking, and self-centered quality of a histrionic personality disorder is popularly associated with women. And, indeed, more women seek treatment as a result of the disorder. However, community studies show that histrionic personality

disorders in fact exist equally in men and women in our society. Individuals with histrionic personality disorders generally have tempestuous and unsatisfying personal relationships.

Many of those who have this type of disordered personality developed as children a style of relating that is indirect, seductive, and often manipulative. Current psychodynamic theories suggest that the histrionic personality may have arisen over time out of a pattern of interactions with parents who were extremely competitive or seductive. For these children, receiving the attention, care, nurturing, approval, and acknowledgment that they needed seemed both uncertain and dangerous. Now as adults, they still feel unable to negotiate directly with their world and incapable of remedying their deep sense of emotional deprivation.

If you suffer from a histrionic personality disorder, chances are that you have a seductive, sociable, and extravagant style that attracts others to you. Your general presentation may be lively and flirtatious, and you may have the tendency to express ordinary emotions with extra flair and color: Warmth becomes passion, anger becomes rage, sadness becomes heartbreak, and disappointment becomes tragedy.

Even though many of the qualities characteristic of histrionic personality are quite appealing to others, the person may nevertheless feel like a fraud, and the dramatic displays can come across as insincere or embarrassing. Underneath the flamboyance, there usually lies a deep emotional emptiness and hunger. Failure to achieve constant attention and approval compounds feelings of distress and depletion. And ultimately, nothing received from the outside works for long to address a profound internal need.

Frequently, people with histrionic personality disorders feel trapped within their compulsion to be at the center of attention, to be constantly complimented and flattered, to maintain a veneer of sexual or physical attractiveness. An inordinate amount of time may be spent dressing and grooming. At the same time, the individual may worry about being found out, believing himself to be an impostor.

People with histrionic personality disorder are easily frustrated and find it hard to delay gratification. They look to others, particularly strong authority figures, to solve their problems and relieve their sense of inner emptiness.

❖ ANTISOCIAL PERSONALITY DISORDERS

Symptoms and signs Impulsiveness and a seeming lack of concern for consequences; a pattern of unlawful behavior, lying, and deceit for personal profit or pleasure; lack of empathic feelings; irritability, aggressiveness, and violent behavior; disregard for safety or responsibility; lack of remorse.

What is it? Three to four times more common in men than in women, antisocial personality disorders are marked by a consistent disregard for the rights and rules of others and behavior that reflects that disregard. Antisocial personality disorders exist in 2 to 3 percent of the general population. The popular term used to describe an individual with antisocial personality disorder is sociopath.

Research suggests that there is a genetic factor underlying antisocial personality disorders. At the same time, regular exposure to substance abuse and criminal behavior as well as a childhood characterized by chaotic, neglectful, harsh, or abusive parenting seem to increase a person's risk for developing the disorder. Attention-deficit/hyperactivity disorder (ADHD) and conduct disorders in childhood can presage adult antisocial personality disorders.

If you have an antisocial personality disorder, others may view you as emotionally cold and insensitive. Or you may come across as charming, but conning and insincere. You, in turn, may value others primarily for what they can provide. It may seem perfectly evident to you that if you are to survive, you need to manipulate, deceive, and do whatever else is necessary; otherwise, you will go without. Consequently, people with antisocial personality disorders engage in questionable, perhaps even unlawful, activities, believing that the laws and customs do not or should not apply to them.

Individuals with antisocial personality tend to push others around, for fear others will get the better of them. As a result, they may bristle at any kind of coercion and authority—the boss, the police, the legal profession—and may be vexed by financial obligations such as debts and taxes. They

are often cruel and have little remorse or conscience about the harm they do to others. This lack of concern marks most of their interactions, not only with strangers, but also with those they say they care about.

If you have an antisocial personality, you may worry about being weak or victimized. To guard against someone victimizing, exploiting, or simply getting the better of you, you may become malicious or cruel. You may have trouble being faithful, empathic, responsible, and honest in your relationships.

People with antisocial personality disorders are impulsive and often careless—engaging in promiscuous sex, for example, or reckless driving. This disregard for safety may reflect a need for excitement and sensation to counteract their flat and empty feelings.

❖ BORDERLINE PERSONALITY DISORDERS

Symptoms and signs Pattern of unstable relationships that alternates between idealizing and devaluing the other; precarious sense of self; wide mood swings; intense anger; angry and violent outbursts; panic around separation or loss; chronic feelings of emptiness.

What is it? Borderline personality disorder is thought to originate in early childhood experiences: significant loss; profoundly unstable attachment to parental figures; or trauma, abuse, or deprivation. Over half of all individuals who receive the diagnosis of borderline personality disorder were physically or sexually abused as children. Estimated to occur in 2 to 3 percent of the population, it is by far the most common personality disorder in mental health settings.

If you have a borderline personality disorder, you are constantly trying to ward off panic around real or imagined abandonment. As a result, your behavior may be impulsive and erratic, your moods volatile, and your relationships extremely stormy and intense.

You are likely to alternate between frantic efforts to hold onto the people you care for, and, in an attempt to avoid feelings of loss, discounting these same loved ones. To avert feelings of loneliness, you might surround yourself with people, despite the fact that you may not get along with them.

Stressful circumstances, especially within relationships, usually worsen symptoms.

Because people with borderline personality disorders have extremely fragile identities and self-esteem, they tend to be highly sensitive to social rejection or acceptance. If you have this disorder, you will feel, even when you are in a relationship, essentially isolated and lonely. Whenever you are threatened by impending loss, separation, or abandonment, you may react with sudden rage, devaluation, or paranoid accusations.

It is not uncommon for people with borderline personality disorders to use alcohol, drugs, binge eating, self-mutilation, or suicidal actions to ward off feelings of isolation and abandonment.

❖ DEPENDENT PERSONALITY DISORDER

Symptoms and signs A compelling and enduring need to be taken care of; submissive and clinging behavior; intense anxiety around separations; indecisiveness; excessive reliance on others' advice and reassurance; reluctance to express disagreement or assert differences.

What is it? More often diagnosed in women than men, dependent personality disorder is thought to be rooted in early experiences of parental deprivation, or in inconsistent parental responses that alternated between intrusiveness and criticism at the child's natural assertions of autonomy.

If you have a dependent personality disorder, you lack confidence in your ability to care for yourself and rely on others to look after you. Threatened with separation or solitude, you may panic with feelings of profound helplessness. Regardless of evidence to the contrary, you tend to be convinced that you are incapable of functioning on your own. You seek direction from others, no matter how insignificant the issue. As a way of securing the care and support you seek, you likely subordinate your own wishes and needs to those of others. You avoid disagreeing with others, and as a result, you may appear to be self-effacing, obsequious, and ingratiating.

The relationships of individuals with dependent disorder are usually unbalanced, as they seek all-powerful helpers, people they believe can protect them from deep feelings of loneliness. They may hop from relationship to relationship, and when one ends, may latch on to another quickly and perhaps indiscriminately. All the while, they may be experiencing acute anxiety, depression, and somatic concerns.

❖ OBSESSIVE-COMPULSIVE PERSONALITY DISORDER

Symptoms and signs Preoccupation with orderliness, perfection, and control that becomes rigid and inefficient; obsession with details, rules, lists, order, organization, and schedules; perfectionism; excessive and inflexible moral scrupulousness; inability to delegate tasks or to discard worn-out or worthless items; excessive hoarding or penny-pinching.

What is it? Twice as common in women as in men, obsessive-compulsive personality disorder represents a maladaptive extreme of normal traits. Perseverance, methodical attention to detail, and focus on facts and figures are all qualities that can serve a person well, especially in our culture, which values hard work, punctuality, and orderliness. However, when these personality traits become so rigid or extreme that work and productivity overshadow all other activities and interactions, or when they become ends in themselves, obsessive-compulsive personality disorder may be diagnosed.

Many people rely on lists and schedules to maintain a sense of control. However, if you have an obsessive-compulsive personality disorder, it is likely that the details, rules, organizations, and lists overshadow the larger projects. Even when you engage in hobbies and recreational activities, you have trouble relaxing; instead you approach leisure time seriously and laboriously. Frequently, in your drive toward perfection, you may fear that you can never live up to your own standards; therefore, you put off or leave projects and tasks uncompleted. Your perfectionism also surfaces in indecisiveness and procrastination.

Many people with obsessive-compulsive personality disorders are workaholics. Delegating tasks does not come easily to them; they may try to maintain control by giving highly detailed instructions.

People with obsessive-compulsive personality disorder find it difficult to give time, money, or gifts, and they may be viewed by others as ungenerous. They tend to be loyal and attentive in their relationships, yet may be seen by others as controlling. They may have difficulty expressing affection. Although they frequently feel angry, especially when others fail to live up to their standards, they have trouble expressing it. When they do express anger, it is usually in a self-righteous outburst.

This disorder seems most prevalent in oldest children and in those individuals who have chosen professions that require perseverance, methodical attention to detail, or involvement with facts and figures. Psychodynamic theories suggest that obsessive-compulsive personality disorders arise out of early, intense power struggles between a child and her overambitious, demanding, and impatient parents. When a child's expression of her drives, emotions, and autonomy are met by excessive parental control and disapproval, the child may stifle these expressions. In addition, the child may become preoccupied with the details of her tasks and try to perform perfectly as a way of winning approval. As adults, these people tend to feel that their lives offer little pleasure and fulfillment.

Unlike the psychiatric condition called obsessive-compulsive disorder (see page 1221), obsessive-compulsive personality disorder does not entail significant repeated, unwanted ruminations (obsessions) and ritualized behavior (compulsion).

❖ PASSIVE-AGGRESSIVE PERSONALITY DISORDER

Symptoms and signs Negative attitudes and passive resistance to the demands for adequate performance in routine social and occupational tasks; feelings of being misunderstood and unappreciated; sullen and argumentative; tendency to criticize and scorn authority; inclination to express envy and persistent complaints of personal misfortune and to appear alternately hostile and defiant on the one hand and contrite on the other.

What is it? Also known as negative personality disorder, a passive-aggressive personality disorder is apparent when a person consistently expresses the word "no" in passively defiant ways. This may be because as a child, he was unable to express his anger, autonomy, and negative feelings directly. There is also some evidence that people with this type of personality disorder were responded to, throughout their childhood, with extreme inconsistency, ambivalence, and perhaps neglect. Because parental authority was unpredictable, erratic, and maddening, the child felt captured by his anger and resentment, able neither to let it go nor express it.

If you have a passive-aggressive personality disorder, you likely feel deeply burdened by even the most moderate demands of those around you. You generally resent and envy the authority of others, even when that authority is benign. Most of the time, you feel beleaguered, harassed, and overwhelmed. Both in your work and in your personal relationships, you feel misunderstood, unappreciated, and overextended. Many times, you feel angry and resentful, and you reflexively react negatively.

The natural mood of people with passive-aggressive personality disorder is pessimistic, cynical, and skeptical. They generally anticipate difficulties and disappointments, and feel cheated, unappreciated, victimized, and hapless. When things do not go as they wish, they become more sullen, defeatist, antagonistic, and irritable.

People with passive-aggressive disorder have difficulty confronting others, and they are likely to express differences, disappointment, or resentment indirectly. Procrastination, stubbornness, or inefficiency are typical behaviors that are likely to enrage those around them.

At work, individuals with passive-aggressive disorder may have difficulty advancing, since they tend to undermine their own success. Often, they alienate those who could help.

People with passive-aggressive personalities tend to be moody—easily nettled, offended, or provoked. And often, their behavior alternates between hostile self-assertion and guilty contrition; they find fault, remain uncooperative and resentful, yet are excessively dependent.

Deep down, individuals with passive-aggressive personality disorder feel powerless, at the mercy of others, aggrieved, misunderstood, and anguished. It is not uncommon for someone with this type of personality disorder to assume the role of the martyr.

❖ SCHIZOTYPAL PERSONALITY DISORDER

Symptoms and signs Acute discomfort and reduced capacity for relationships; distorted thinking and perceptions about other people; personal habits, mannerism, and appearance that are off-putting; inappropriate or constricted expressions of emotions; suspicious or paranoid thinking; extreme social anxiety; lack of close friends.

What is it? If you have a schizotypal personality disorder, you feel extremely uncomfortable with intimacy. In most situations, but especially those involving unfamiliar people, you experience profound anxiety that tends to be associated with fear that others will judge you or impose their expectations on you. As a result, you have considerable trouble establishing and maintaining close relationships.

For individuals with schizotypal personality disorder, the profound social discomfort and anxiety they experience may translate into distorted thinking and perceptions. For example, such an individual may get the eerie feeling that someone else is present in the room or may believe that others are talking about him.

Individuals with schizotypal personality disorder may present themselves in ways that attest to their social anxiety. Their speech may be vague, for instance, their language full of exaggeration, metaphors, or clichés, and their mannerisms and appearance may in some ways be odd and uninviting. They may find it difficult to engage in either casual or meaningful conversations; instead, they tend to relate in a stiff, awkward, or constricted manner.

There is evidence that schizotypal personality disorder has a strong genetic component; in fact, there seems to be a genetic link between this personality disorder and schizophrenia (see page 1254). An estimated 10 to 20 percent eventually develop schizophrenia. However, about the same percentage show considerable improve-

ment in their general ability to function over time, especially in response to psychiatric treatment. At the same time, as many as half of those with schizotypal personality disorder also have a depressive or anxiety disorder.

TREATMENT OF PERSONALITY DISORDERS

The fact that personality disorders develop early and are, in fact, the natural way people operate and define themselves complicates the treatment picture. For treatment to be effective, it must address a person's basic, ingrained behavioral patterns, attitudes, relationship styles, and functional capacities. Although, in most cases, personality disorders are responsive over time to psychotherapy, changing these durable habits of thought, feeling, and behavior requires extensive and repetitive examination, evaluation, and relearning.

For example, long-term individual psychotherapy can be extremely helpful for those with borderline personality disorders. However, given their difficulties with relationships, the course of therapy is often volatile and uneven. Therapy typically must weather the intense feelings, demands for care, and repeated crises that the individual brings to the process. Even then, the individual with borderline personality disorder is likely to discount the therapy and therapist and, many times, to abruptly and angrily end treatment. In these cases, therapy may take at least 5 years.

Nevertheless, even with the most tenacious difficulties, classic psychoanalytically oriented, psychodynamic psychotherapy and, in some cases, psychoanalysis, can be impressively effective. Other types of talk therapies that take a more here-and-now approach are also quite effective with personality disorders.

Cognitive-behavioral techniques and family and group therapy have proved useful. For example, when a person has a dependent personality disorder, assertiveness training and group therapy may help increase social self-confidence, encourage autonomy, and provide the forum in which self-denigrating thoughts and behavior can be examined. With schizotypal disorders, psychoeducational methods—along with supportive psychotherapy—can help the individual develop more appropriate social skills.

The use of medication in treating personality-disordered patients varies, but is, in many instances, quite effective, especially when used in conjunction with psychotherapy. Furthermore, a person with a personality disorder often comes into therapy reporting vague feelings of depression, anxiety, or certain physical complaints. In those instances, such psychiatric disorders will also be addressed with the appropriate medications. Sometimes, selective serotonin reuptake inhibitors (SSRIs)—paroxetine, fluoxetine (Prozac), sertraline, and fluvoxamine—may diminish impulsiveness, the tendency to worry, and depressed mood in people with personality disorders who do not have another diagnosable psychiatric disorder.

In some instances, especially at times of crisis, suicidal threats, or acting out, a person with a personality disorder may need to be hospitalized for a short period. Furthermore, when severe personality disorders persist or when a person's home life cannot provide the support and structure he needs, a specialized therapeutic community can furnish firm structure, close supervision, immediate confrontation around the consequences of behavior, group meetings with peers, and a structured work program to foster vocational skills. This is often necessary when a person has an antisocial personality disorder.

Prognosis Fairly good. Studies show that, because personality traits are enduring characteristics, personality disorders tend to persist over the years. However, some seem to burn out. It is likely that through life experience, a person learns to modify the

COPING WITH THE STIGMA OF MENTAL ILLNESS

The more severe the psychiatric illness, the more disruptive it is to a person's everyday life and relationships. When treatment is continuous or extensive, such as with hospitalization, day treatment, or residential treatment, it is inevitable that a person will receive a diagnosis. Upon learning his diagnosis, a person may feel great relief; at least now he knows why he has been feeling the way he has. However, in many cases, diagnosis becomes a label, and as such, it becomes a double-edged sword.

Frequently, a person's label will follow him throughout life: His school, work, and medical records may document it, his school or work may learn of it, or perhaps his housing and credit applications may inquire about it. Even when the circumstances are not particularly dramatic, such as when a child who receives the diagnosis of learning disability or attention-deficit/hyperactivity disorder, the label can have powerful effects, influencing the way people come to view him and the way he comes to think of and value himself.

A person may be tempted to use the label to demean himself or magnify his sense of social isolation. When the person is a child, the sense of stigmatization can be extreme. Children are more likely to accept a simplified explanation—he is just plain crazy—and his peer group is less likely to tolerate differences. Parents of children who have serious emotional or psychiatric disorders may also usually feel left out of the mainstream; many of the considerations that occupy other parents—sports, academics, arts activities, college applications—may seem tangential or indulgent. Instead, they feel lonely, isolated, or odd.

Typically, stigmatization results in shame, guilt, and low self-esteem, and it may lead to self-destructive or suicidal acts. Unfortunately, unlike physical illness, which is usually met with true sympathy and compassion, with mental illness, there is a tendency in our society to blame the victim, to point to flaws in his character or weakness in his makeup. Even with victims of sexual or physical abuse, there is a tendency to consider them as responsible or even culpable: "She asked to be raped in the way she dressed." Or, "If he was beating her, why didn't she just leave?"

The most effective way of coping with stigmatization is by learning all you can about the specific illness or disorder you are dealing with or by seeking out a local support group. You can contact the appropriate national organization that will be able to provide you with information and support. If you feel completely weighed down by feelings of isolation and shame, contact a mental health professional.

Following are organizations that offer support and information:

- American Academy of Child and Adolescent Psychiatry
  3615 Wisconsin Ave. NW
  Washington, DC 20016–3007
  Phone: (800) 333–7636

- American Anorexia/Bulimia Association, Inc.
  293 Central Park West, Suite 1R
  New York, NY 10024
  Phone: (212) 501–8351

- Anorexia Nervosa and Related Eating Disorders, Inc.
  P.O. Box 5102 ▶

▶ Eugene, OR 97405
Phone: (503) 344–1144

- Anxiety Disorders Association of America
  6000 Executive Blvd. #513
  Rockville, MD 20852
  Phone: (301) 231–9350

- Center for Mental Health Services
  5600 Fishers Lane
  Rockville, MD 20857
  Phone: (301) 443–1333

- Children and Adults with Attention Deficit Disorders
  499 Northwest 70th Ave., Suite 109
  Plantation, FL 33317
  Phone: (305) 587–3700

- Council on Anxiety Disorders
  P.O. Box 17011
  Winston-Salem, NC 27116
  Phone: (910) 722–7760

- Depression and Related Affective Disorders Association
  Meyer 3-181
  600 North Wolfe St.
  Baltimore, MD 21287–7381

- Federation of Families for Children's Mental Health
  1021 Prince St.
  Alexandria, VA 22314–2971
  Phone: (703) 684–7710

- National Alliance for Research on Schizophrenia and Depression
  60 Cutter Mill Rd.
  Great Neck, NY 11201
  Phone: (516) 829–0091

- National Alliance for the Mentally Ill
  200 North Glebe Rd., Suite 1015
  Arlington, VA 22203–3754
  Phone: (800) 950-NAMI

- National Association of Anorexia Nervosa and Associated Disorders
  Box 7
  Highland Park, IL 60035
  Phone: (708) 831–3438

- National Depressive and Manic-Depressive Association
  730 Franklin St., Suite 501
  Chicago, IL 60610–0049
  Phone: (800) 826–3632

- National Foundation for Depressive Illness
  P.O. Box 2257
  New York, NY 10116
  Phone: (212) 268–4260

- National Institute of Mental Health
  5600 Fishers Lane, Room 7C-02
  Rockville, MD 20857
  Phone: (301) 443–4536

- National Mental Health Association
  1021 Prince St.
  Alexandria, VA 22314–2971
  Phone: (703) 684–7722

- OCD Foundation Inc.
  P.O. Box 70
  Milford, CT 06460–0070
  Phone: (203) 878–5669

basic aspects of his personality and avoid relationships that do not work. For example, a person with an antisocial or borderline personality disorder can learn to curb his more impulsive and socially unacceptable behaviors over time. This may be due to the consistently negative legal, social, and economic consequences that a person with these disorders experiences.

With treatment, the prognosis improves, especially when the person seeks treatment on his own, cooperates with the treatment, and takes responsibility for his problems. People can learn to modify the expression of these traits through effort; the change in their actual behavior that results can reduce their vulnerability to circumstance. On the other hand, when a person projects his difficulties out into his environment, denies responsibility, and claims that he is powerless to correct his own problems, treatment tends to be less effective.

Family Issues and Mental Illness

The relationship between mental illness and family is a complicated and interconnected one. On the one hand, when one member of a family is troubled, the upset usually ripples throughout, causing distress in the entire family system. On the other hand, when the family system is disturbed, individual members may develop their own symptoms, or their own vulnerabilities are triggered.

Many times, problems in and between the adult members of a family cause or exacerbate individual problems. When, for example, the relationship between parents is highly conflictual, consistently angry, or deeply frustrated, children are inevitably affected. By the same token, when one parent suffers from psychiatric disorders or severe personality disorders—depression, panic disorders, antisocial personality disorders, for example—or when they engage in addictive behaviors, other members feel the impact.

No matter how much the parents may try to protect their children from their conflicts and disturbances, children are by their very nature sensitive to their parents' internal and actual experiences. In many cases, it is not so easy to disguise the fact that one is deeply angry, disappointed, or distressed. Some parents communicate their troubles directly, in what they say. But many more communicate indirectly, through their parenting. Frequently, the result is parenting that is abusive, neglectful, flagrantly inconsistent, and unpredictable.

All this can, and does, cause children pain. And when the trouble and pain are incessant, children may develop emotional or behavior problems in response. Or, whatever internal difficulties or biologic vulnerabilities children carry become exacerbated.

When children develop symptoms, parents often feel that they are to blame. In addition to feelings of guilt, if they must seek outside help, they frequently feel shame. They worry that others will blame them as well. In fact, most parents want their children to be happy and well adjusted. When they see their child in pain, they are themselves in pain. This adds to the upset that a child's troubles cause within the family.

Living with someone who has a mental disorder—someone who is sick—is never easy. No matter what the illness, there is always guilt, anger, and confusion. Sometimes, there are feelings of desperation. And from time to time, mental illness escalates into crisis: Someone makes a suicide attempt and must be hospitalized; someone is arrested for speeding and drunk driving during a manic episode. A behaviorally disordered child sets a fire.

Moreover, each psychiatric and personality disorder carries its own characteristic strain that can be felt throughout the family. Living with someone who has an eating disorder necessarily means that there are power struggles that often erupt into tantrums or angry outbursts around the dinner table. While a depressed person may seem lost and dismally unhappy, his disorder exerts profound strain on the others around him. He cannot go out because he feels so bad. He cannot help with chores in the house because he has no energy. In addition, other people's feelings, their anger, distress, joy, and pain, are often squeezed out by the overbearing weight of another person's depression.

Although all mental disorders bring with them their own stresses, perhaps the most perplexing and heartbreaking is schizophrenia. It often happens that, once a person develops schizophrenia, no matter at what age, he reverts back to the care of his parents. Even if he has been out of the family home and living on his own, after his first psychotic break, chances are that he will return home.

Beyond the practical matter of caring for an adult with severe mental illness, parents usually also contend with deep feelings of guilt. Even though we now know that schizophrenia is an illness of the brain just as hypertension (high blood pressure) is an illness of the cardiovascular system, it was not too long ago that people commonly referred to the "schizophrenogenic mother," the mother who literally drove her child crazy. Still, today, many parents look on the disease, and wonder mournfully what they could have done differently to prevent their child's breakdown.

It is not hard to understand that parents would want to make sense of a disease that can be so catastrophic, especially because there are no clear explanations. Yet, schizophrenia is no one's fault; no stress is so extreme as to bring on a psychotic episode on its own.

Many parents' dreams, hopes, and visions for their child dissolve with his first psychotic break with reality. A child with schizophrenia will probably never be independent, capable of having a mature enduring love relationship, or holding a good job. A large part of living with a mentally ill child involves coming to terms with the reality of the illness.

Many families faced with the challenge of managing and living with mentally ill family members find guidance and solace through family therapy or support groups.

Yet, it must be noted that when all is said and done, most psychiatric disorders are very responsive to treatment. Getting better with the help of the right treatment is more often the rule than the exception—both for the person with the disorder and his family. But good results cannot happen if care is not sought.

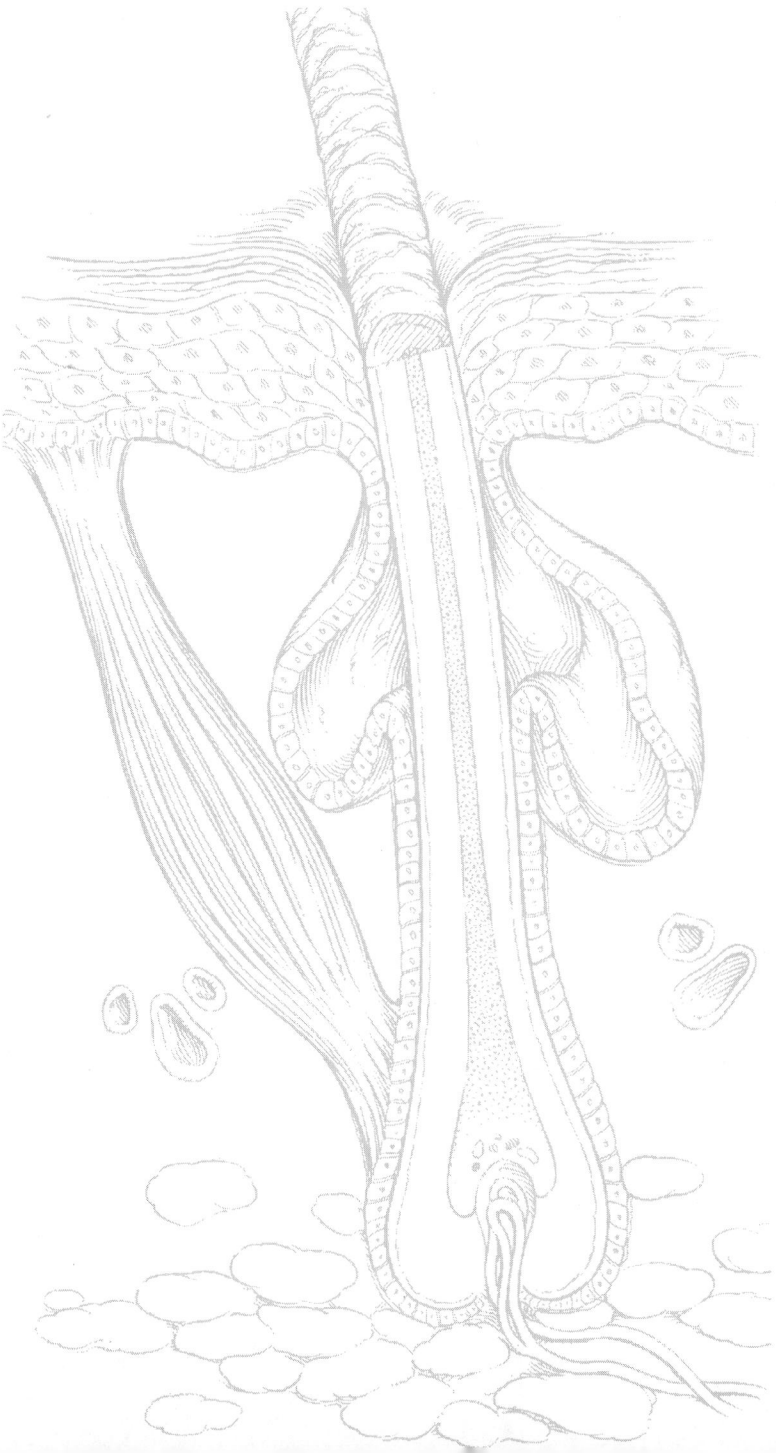

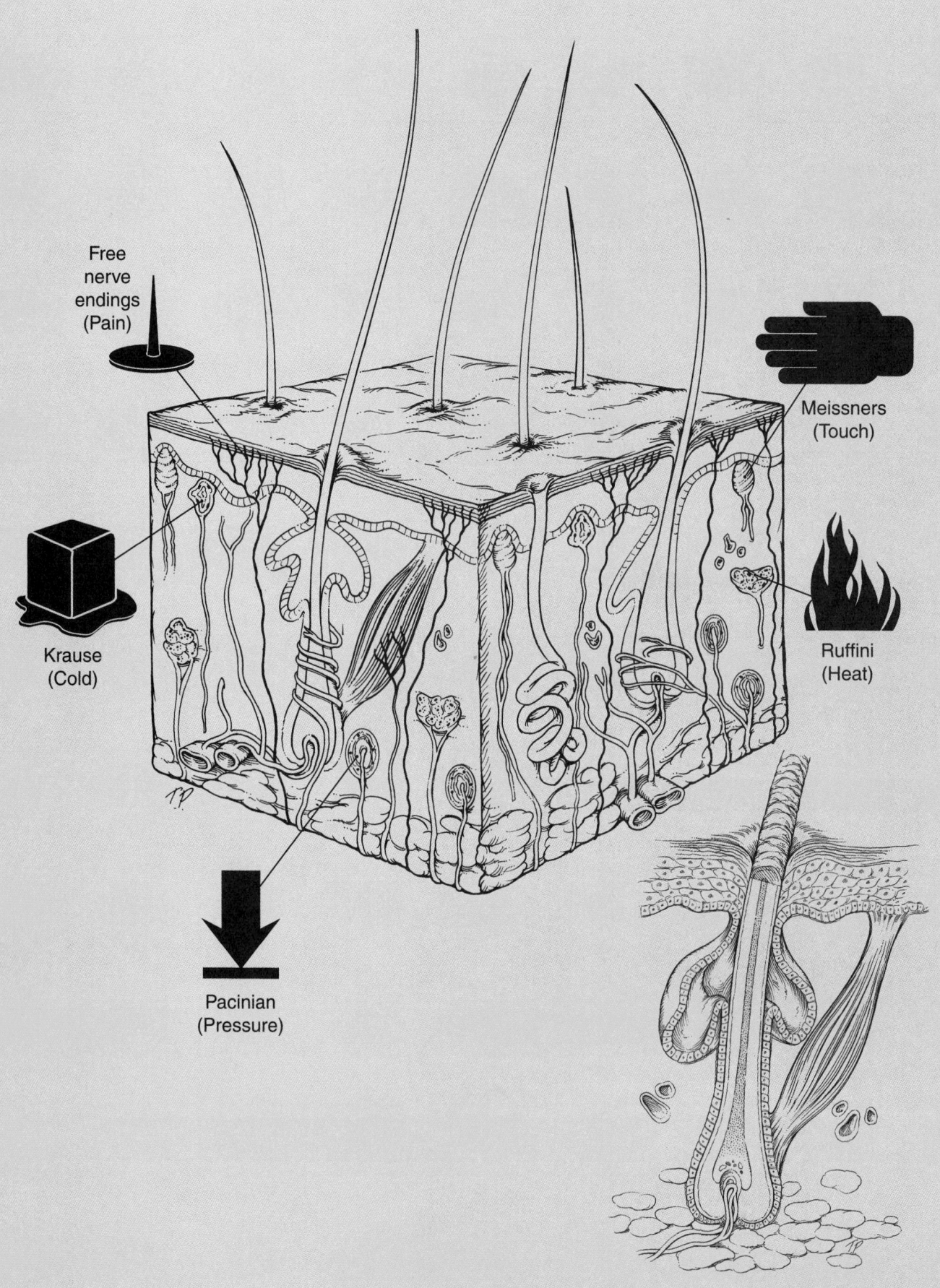

Free
nerve
endings
(Pain)

Meissners
(Touch)

Krause
(Cold)

Ruffini
(Heat)

Pacinian
(Pressure)

SKIN, HAIR, AND NAILS

The skin is the largest organ of the human body, and it is called upon to play many roles. It serves on the front line as the body's buffer against infectious invaders, such as bacteria and viruses. It assists in preventing dehydration, and it produces vitamin D when exposed to the sun. Because it contains millions of tiny nerve endings, the skin plays an important part in sensing (and sending messages to the brain about) pain, pressure, and touch.

There are about 2 square yards of skin on the typical adult. The skin is amazingly resilient, particularly in light of what we put it through. It is subjected to the freezing weather of winter and the heat waves of summer. It is exposed to wind gusts, rain torrents, hail storms, and snow flurries. We poke, puncture, shave, and scrub it. Yet it almost always bounces back, seemingly oblivious to the punishment it takes.

The thickness of the skin varies from one part of the body to another. For example, the soles of the feet and the palms of the hands have the thickest skin; the eyelids are the site of the thinnest skin.

To some extent, your body temperature is dependent on your skin. As the body senses the need to raise or lower its temperature, the skin's blood vessels and capillaries widen or constrict. For example, in very cold weather, blood vessels constrict, causing less blood to travel through the skin, which reduces the loss of body heat. When the weather is hot, blood vessels dilate, which increases heat loss, and the sweat (or eccrine) glands secrete perspiration, which cools the body as it evaporates.

The Anatomy and Structure of the Skin

The skin has two layers. They are the epidermis and the dermis. A layer of subcutaneous fat lies under the skin.

The epidermis is the outermost layer of the skin. Though very thin, it contains several layers of different types of cells. It is a dynamic structure that is constantly active. It is the place where skin cells are manufactured, all in a very orderly way. In this process, cells at the base of the epidermis, called the basal cell layer, divide and create new skin cells. As that occurs, the new cells push older ones upward toward the skin's surface, where they flatten and become squamous cells. When cells eventually reach the top layer (the stratum corneum), they are sloughed off or shed. The average life expectancy of a skin cell is about 1 month; thus, your skin is constantly turning over and renewing.

Cells called melanocytes are individually scattered throughout the basal layer of the epidermis, and provide the skin with melanin, the darkly pigmented substance that gives skin its tan or brown coloring. The more melanin in your skin, the darker your skin will be, and the greater your protection from natural sunlight and artificial ultraviolet (UV) light (such as suntan parlor lights).

The dermis, the next layer of skin, is mostly composed of collagen that serves as supportive, connective tissue. The dermis is filled with blood vessels, nerve cells, muscle cells, lymph vessels, hair follicles, and sweat and sebaceous (oil-secreting) glands. The sebaceous glands are found on every part of the body except the palms and the soles, and keep the skin soft and moist; as their output decreases with aging, the skin is more prone to drying.

The other secretory glands in the dermis are of two types: Eccrine glands are found throughout the body, but primarily on the palms, soles, and forehead; they help regulate the body temperature; apocrine glands are located in the underarms and in the genital region; they are responsible for body odor. Blood vessels carry whole blood through the dermis while lymph vessels carry fluid containing disease-fighting white blood cells.

The bulk of the dermis is made of fairly rigid fibers (collagen), along with scattered elastic or flexible fibers called elastin, which together keep the skin strong yet supple; as we age and are exposed to the sun, these fibers decrease in number and become damaged, which causes the skin to gradually lose firmness and elasticity.

The subcutaneous tissue lies just below the skin. This layer is composed primarily of fat, which serves as an insulator and shock absorber. Certain structures of the skin may extend into the fat, such as the sebaceous and sweat glands. Also, nerves and blood vessels traverse through the subcutaneous tissue. The anatomy and growth of the hair and nails is also related to the skin (see page 1316 and page 1320 for more information on hair and nails).

Skin Conditions

Unlike conditions affecting other organs of the body, skin problems are visible to the eye; thus, we may think that we know a lot more about them than we really do. In fact, there are so many skin conditions with overlapping symptoms that it is often easy to mistake one for another.

Myths surrounding many skin conditions have created additional confusion. For example, although regular cleansing is important, poor hygiene is infrequently the cause of skin disease. Once a proper diagnosis is made, treatment—some of it self-care—is usually available to cure or control the condition.

❖ ACNE

Symptoms and signs Whiteheads; blackheads; inflamed red bumps (pimples); and/or large cysts or nodules; most often on the face, chest, and back; with or without pain or tenderness. (See page C-26.)

What is it? Acne (also called acne vulgaris) is the most common skin disease among Americans. It is a condition that usually starts during puberty, affecting at least 85 percent of individuals in their teen and young adult years. In some individuals, acne may persist well into adulthood.

Acne occurs when rising hormone levels during adolescence trigger an overproduction of oil (sebum) that combines with surface skin cells to clog pores or hair follicles. When the follicle is completely blocked, a whitehead is created. When the follicle remains open, the sebum that is clogging it is visibly dark; hence the common name blackhead. Pimples, or red bumps, can form from the whiteheads and blackheads when bacteria that normally live on the skin increase in number in the clogged follicles.

Small acne lesions can sometimes progress to large, deep nodules or cysts (sacs filled with sebum, bacteria, and reactive immune cells). The diameter of these cysts can be as great as an inch. They can be painful and may last for many weeks. They are also the lesions most likely to leave scars or pits after they heal.

Acne most frequently occurs on parts of the body where the sebaceous glands are most dense—that is, the face, back, and chest.

Acne is not contagious, nor is it caused by chocolate or greasy or fatty foods, such as potato chips or pizza. However, it can be provoked or worsened by factors such as stress; use of oil-based cosmetics; hormonal fluctuations that stimulate the sebaceous glands, such as those that accompany menstruation;

PROPER SKIN CARE

Like many other parts of the body, the skin requires care and attention. The most important thing you can do to keep your skin healthy and attractive is to protect it from excessive exposure to the sun. Like the safety precautions regarding seat belts, warnings about sun exposure are well known and too often ignored. It is difficult, particularly for younger people, to give proper weight to health threats that lie far in the future. Nonetheless, skin cancer is far and away the most commonly diagnosed cancer in this country. The ability of skin cancer to disfigure your looks or even kill you greatly exceeds the temporary ability of a suntan to enhance your looks.

The *best* single strategy for preventing skin damage, premature aging, and skin cancer is to reduce your direct exposure to sunlight, particularly between 10 AM and 3 PM (the time period when radiation is most intense). Wear a sunscreen with a sun protection factor (SPF) of 15 or greater, applying it generously and reapplying it as necessary, and cover exposed parts of the body with clothing whenever possible. (See The Risks of Sun Burn and Sun Damage, page 1300, for more information.)

Skin also needs to be well cleansed. Regular use of soap and water removes bacteria, dirt, and body oils. Washing your face once in the morning and once at night is fine for most people, although those with oily skin may wash up to three times a day. Use lukewarm rather than hot water on your face, washing gently rather than scrubbing. Bathing or showering more than once a day can lead to excessive dryness; for some adults, even once a day may cause enough drying to require the use of a moisturizing soap and an after-bath moisturizing lotion.

Any soap will clean the skin. For people with normal skin, a mild, preferably antibacterial soap is all you need. It need not contain fancy-sounding or expensive lotions, perfumes, or deodorizers. If you purchase a "special" soap with "extra" ingredients, evaluate its effects on your skin. For example, certain soaps may produce dry skin and rashes in some people. Fragrances in soaps are sometimes responsible for skin irritation, so avoid them if your skin is particularly sensitive. If your skin tends to be dry and is easily irritated, consider using a superfatted (moisturizing) soap or applying a light moisturizer to the skin while it is still damp after washing, thus trapping the water in the skin; moisturizers help replace the oils that are lost by the skin. Although drinking eight glasses of water in the course of the day will also help keep your body well hydrated, it will not effectively treat dry skin; dry skin requires topically applied moisturizing skin-care products.

Other suggestions for keeping the skin healthy: Eat a well-balanced diet; get plenty of rest and regular exercise; do not smoke cigarettes; and do not abuse alcohol. ■

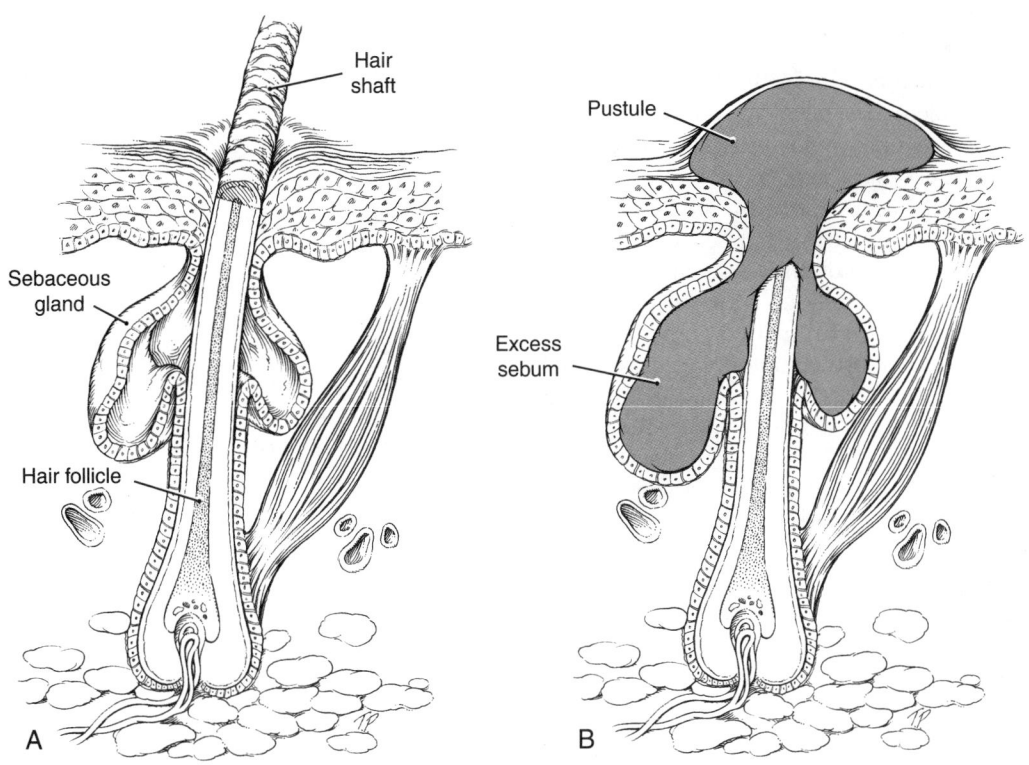

(A) The surface of the skin has thousands of tiny pits called hair follicles that support the growth of individual hairs. Hair grows within the hair bulb at the bottom of each follicle. In a normal hair follicle, sebaceous glands secrete oil (sebum) into the follicle, and the smooth arrector pili muscle causes "goosebumps" or erection of hair. (B) Acne is the most common skin disease in the United States, affecting at least 85 percent of people during adolescence. Hormones trigger overproduction of sebum, which combines with shedding skin cells to clog follicles and create a whitehead. A blackhead forms when sebum resides in but does not completely block the follicle. Pimples form when skin bacteria multiply in the whiteheads. Acne sometimes creates deep nodules or large cysts. Do not squeeze or scratch acne lesions. Remember that tanning the skin does not unblock the follicles and that acne is not caused by eating chocolate or other fatty foods.

and hereditary factors. Certain medications (corticosteroids, phenytoin, lithium) can aggravate acne; so can high doses of vitamins B_2, B_6, and B_{12}.

What you can do Gently wash the affected area two to three times a day, using a mild antibacterial soap (such as Dial, Almay, Lever 2000); washing will reduce the surface oil and bacteria. When washing, do not scrub or you may irritate the skin, which can make the acne even worse. Do not squeeze or scratch acne lesions, because this usually makes them both redder and larger, and may even cause scarring.

Choose cosmetics that are labeled non-acnegenic or noncomedogenic, which should not contribute to the development of acne.

People with acne often believe that tanning can improve it; however, tanning only camouflages acne—and ultraviolet rays increase the risk of skin cancer and should be avoided.

Over-the-counter acne creams, lotions, and gels, such as those containing benzoyl peroxide, accelerate healing in many people.

When to call the doctor If self-help measures are ineffective, see a doctor for prescription medications and other strategies.

Treatment Tretinoin (Retin-A) cream or gel—with or without a topical (applied to the skin) antibacterial medication such as benzoyl peroxide, erythromycin, or clindamycin—is effective for many people. Tretinoin can cause side effects such as redness and peeling, but these can usually be remedied by less frequent application. Oral antibiotics such as tetracycline and erythromycin are often added when topicals alone don't work; they reduce the density of bacteria and associated inflammation or redness. One brand of birth control pill (Ortho Tri-Cyclen) has been approved for use in acne; it works by lowering levels of active hormones that can provoke acne outbreaks.

For severe acne with nodules or cysts, aggressive treatment is needed to prevent scarring. Isotretinoin (Accutane) is effective in about fully clearing 70 percent of people who are treated; however, side effects are more common and close monitoring is needed. While taking isotretinoin, pregnancy *must* be avoided—the simultaneous use of two contraceptives is required—because the medication causes major birth defects.

Prognosis Although most people outgrow acne in early adulthood, some people may continue to experience acne for years or have the initial onset of acne in their 20s or 30s. If acne is severe, it can leave behind permanent scarring; therefore, treatment is important whenever the disorder is present.

❖ ROSACEA

Symptoms and signs Ruddy or flushed complexion, most often on the nose and cheeks, and occasionally involving the chin and forehead; red bumps and pimples (papules and pustules); tiny, thread-like blood vessels visible on the skin surface (telangiectasias); a red, sometimes swollen nose, with or without burning and stinging of the eyelid margins and eyes. (See page C-26.)

What is it? Rosacea is a progressive disorder that occurs most often in fair-skinned, young and middle-age adults. Women experience rosacea more often than men, but it is frequently more severe in men.

The redness on the face is caused by telangiectasias or dilated small thread-like blood vessels. In the early stages, this red, flushed appearance may come and go. Occasionally, the sebaceous glands of the nose can become enlarged, giving the nose a red, bumpy appearance (a condition called rhinophyma). The eyelids can become inflamed, causing the margins to redden and feel "gritty." (See also Ocular Rosacea, page 513.)

The underlying cause of rosacea is unclear. Rosacea is also called acne rosacea or adult acne because of the resemblance to acne. But unlike acne, rosacea is neither related to excess sebum production, nor is it associated with comedones (blackheads and whiteheads).

What you can do Lifestyle adjustments help reduce redness and flushing of the skin. These include avoiding exposures and situations that make you flush: spicy foods, very hot beverages, alcohol, sunny or very hot or cold environments, scrubbing or rubbing the face, and stressful circumstances.

Some people with rosacea can benefit from keeping a diary, helping them to identify and subsequently avoid those environmental factors that cause their condition to worsen.

When to call the doctor Rosacea rarely goes away on its own. Early therapy is helpful, so see your doctor for care, which can keep the condition from progressing. Self-treatment is not advisable, since many non-prescription "acne" products can irritate and worsen rosacea.

Treatment Doctors individualize therapy for each patient, depending on the severity of symptoms. Treatment may involve a combination of approaches, aimed at stabilizing the disorder and reducing the symptoms.

Oral antibiotics such as tetracycline or erythromycin are often prescribed. The dosage can be decreased gradually in patients who show a good response; some patients can stop taking the antibiotic after several months. Alternatively, prescription metronidazole gel or cream applied to the face may provide effective control.

The tiny blood vessels (telangiectasias) can be eliminated with a laser or electrocautery; the latter is an electric current that, like the laser, destroys the telangiectasias.

Prognosis Rosacea can usually be controlled effectively with medication, and the long-range outlook is good. However, if rosacea is left untreated, it can continually worsen, gradually thickening and distorting the skin surface.

❖ PITYRIASIS ROSEA

Symptoms and signs Multiple oval, flaky, pink or salmon-colored patches ($1/2$ to 2 in. in size), primarily on the chest and back; occasionally, associated itching.

What is it? Pityriasis rosea is a common rash that most often starts with an oval, pink patch on the back or chest. Similar but smaller patches then develop elsewhere on the body, typically confined to the back, chest, and abdomen. The spots often follow a "Christmas tree" pattern, with oval spots scattered over the back in a distribution similar to branches reaching outward and angling downward.

Pityriasis rosea is thought to be caused by a virus; however, it is not contagious. It occurs most often in young adults, although it can develop in anyone.

The rash is typically mild. Itching may occur, increasing in intensity when the skin is warmed by exercise or a hot shower. The rash usually disappears in 4 to 8 weeks; occasionally, it may persist for months.

When to call the doctor Pityriasis rosea usually does not require treatment, but because it can mimic other skin conditions, you should generally see your doctor. He can differentiate the rash from similar-appearing conditions, including ringworm, guttate (waterdrop-shaped) psoriasis, nummular (coin-shaped) eczema, and secondary syphilis. Also, some people may develop similar-appearing skin eruptions when taking antibiotics, diuretics (water pills), and gold salts (used for treating arthritis). At times, the doctor may need to perform a biopsy to make a conclusive diagnosis.

Treatment While mild cases of pityriasis rosea may not require treatment, topical (applied to the skin) corticosteroid creams can be prescribed to relieve itching. If itching is interfering with sleep, sedating antihistamines may be prescribed. In some instances, a dermatologist (skin doctor) may recommend in-office ultraviolet light treatments or a short course of oral corticosteroids.

Prognosis Although the rash usually resolves uneventfully in several weeks, people with darker skin may notice residual dark spots; these may take many months to vanish.

❖ PSORIASIS

Symptoms and signs Raised skin patches (plaques) less than $1/4$ in. to several inches in diameter, deep pink to dark red in color, with a silvery-white scaly surface; most often on the scalp, elbows, knees, navel, lower back, and buttock fold; itching, burning or stinging lesions; ice pick–like pits in the fingernails or heavy white scaling and thickening under the nails. (See page C-26.)

What is it? Psoriasis (pronounced sor-EYE-a-sus) is a chronic, noncontagious skin condition. In the most common form, called plaque psoriasis, skin lesions are sharply defined, inflamed (pink to red), and covered with silvery-white scales. In most people, the plaques are few in number, being present on the elbows and/or knees; however, some individuals develop generalized plaques, affecting almost all body regions. Very rarely, the disorder can be even more severe, with total body redness and pustules (pimple-like lesions) covering the body. Psoriasis is often associated with arthritis, which usually is fairly mild but may be as severe and deforming as rheumatoid arthritis.

An estimated 6.4 million people in the United States have psoriasis. It can develop at any age, although it most often develops in adolescence or young adulthood. The condition is sometimes inherited; if a parent has psoriasis, the children have a 10 to 25 percent chance of developing the disorder.

Although the underlying cause of psoriasis is unclear, it is known that in this condition the skin cells reproduce and mature many times faster than they should, resulting in thickening and scaling of the skin. In most cases, the condition cycles, with flares, defined as enlarging or thickening of plaques or new plaques of psoriasis, lasting several weeks to months, followed by improvement and subsequent flares. Flares of disease can sometimes be triggered by infections, dry or injured skin, stress, excessive alcohol intake, changes in climate, or sunlight deprivation. Some medications can also cause flares—including lithium and antimalarials (for example, hydroxychloroquine, chloroquine).

What you can do? To soothe the skin, remove scales, and ease itching, soak in a warm bath containing an over-the-counter, coal-tar preparation made for psoriasis. Mild psoriasis also often responds to moisturizing ointments and creams.

Avoid trauma to the skin (for example, cuts, scratches, scrubbing the floor on your knees, resting on your elbows, knocking the backs of your hands on surfaces), which can trigger localized psoriasis plaques (called the Koebner phenomenon). Also, because infections (such as strep throat) are believed to trigger psoriasis in some people, treatment of infections should be started as soon as possible. Although sunlight can help psoriasis, sunbathe only in moderation; apply sunscreen to areas of the skin not affected by psoriasis.

When to call the doctor Because treatments are available to ease psoriasis, a doctor should be contacted when this skin condition is suspected. Urgent medical care is needed if the entire skin surface is affected, because this degree of involvement places extreme stress on the entire body.

Treatment Various therapies are available for psoriasis; the treatment regimen should be tailored for each individual. Medications applied to the skin are often the first-line therapy. These include topical corticosteroids and newer topicals including a vitamin D derivative (calcipotriene [Dovonex]) and a vitamin A derivative (tazarotene [Tazorac]).

Light treatment (phototherapy) is frequently given in combination with a medication called psoralen, which sensitizes the skin to ultraviolet A (UVA) light and slows down the accelerated growth of skin cells. Treatments (called PUVA; the P is for psoralen) are typically given three times a week, and are administered only in a dermatologist's office or a hospital. Oral medications for psoriasis include methotrexate, which retards cell multiplication and inflammation, and etretinate, which is derived from vitamin A and, like vitamin A, helps normalize cell developments. Either of the medications is an option when psoriasis is very extensive, and methotrexate is usually indicated when psoriatic arthritis is severe. People who are taking these medications need to be monitored closely because of the risk of serious side effects, particularly liver toxicity with methotrexate. Also, alcohol ingestion is prohibited with methotrexate, because it increases the risk of liver damage.

Prognosis There is no cure for psoriasis, but treatment can often minimize itching, inflammation, and scaling. In some cases, treatment can eradicate skin lesions, which dramatically enhances the quality of life in people with this frequently quite visible and potentially embarrassing disorder. Some people with psoriasis experience spontaneous remission (clearing up without any treatment).

❖ SCLERODERMA

Symptoms and signs Uncomfortable tightening, thickening, and hardening of the skin; puffiness in the hands and feet; swelling and redness of the nail folds around the cuticles (caused by dilated blood vessels); itching; pain, numbness, or color changes in the hands when exposed to cold or stress; stiffness in the joints; difficulty swallowing; high blood pressure. (See page C-27.)

Signs and laboratory findings Usually a biopsy is performed, in which a small plug of skin (usually a sample about the size of the eraser on a pencil) is removed for microscopic examination; blood tests and other tests (such as a kidney function test) may be recommended if internal organ involvement is suspected.

What is it? Scleroderma is a disease that occurs when the body produces excess amounts of collagen (the protein that normally makes up over 75 percent of the skin thickness), giving large areas of skin the appearance of a scar, similar to healed areas in a burn victim. The tissue feels hardened, stiff, and "bound down." Scleroderma generally begins and may even remain localized to the fingers. Along with swelling of the fingers and the "bound down" feeling of the overlying skin, affected people also experience Raynaud's phenomenon when their hands are exposed to cold; see Raynaud's Disease/Raynaud's Phenomenon, page 1277, for more information.

About 300,000 people in the United States have scleroderma. While it occurs in individuals of all ages, it develops most often in middle-aged women.

In serious forms of the disease, organs such as the lungs, kidneys, and esophagus may also be affected. (For more information about scleroderma, see page 643.)

What you can do Because bathing can dry the skin, use moisturizing soap, avoid very hot water, and always apply a moisturizer immediately after bathing to trap moisture in the skin. Apply a heavy hand cream or petroleum jelly after each handwashing.

In cold weather, wear warm clothing and gloves to avoid numbness or color

COLOR ATLAS
Anatomy, Disorders & Diseases

Frontal View of the Skeleton

The adult skeleton is composed of more than 200 bones, connected to one another at joints. The bones impart strength and structure, supporting the soft tissues of the body and giving them shape.

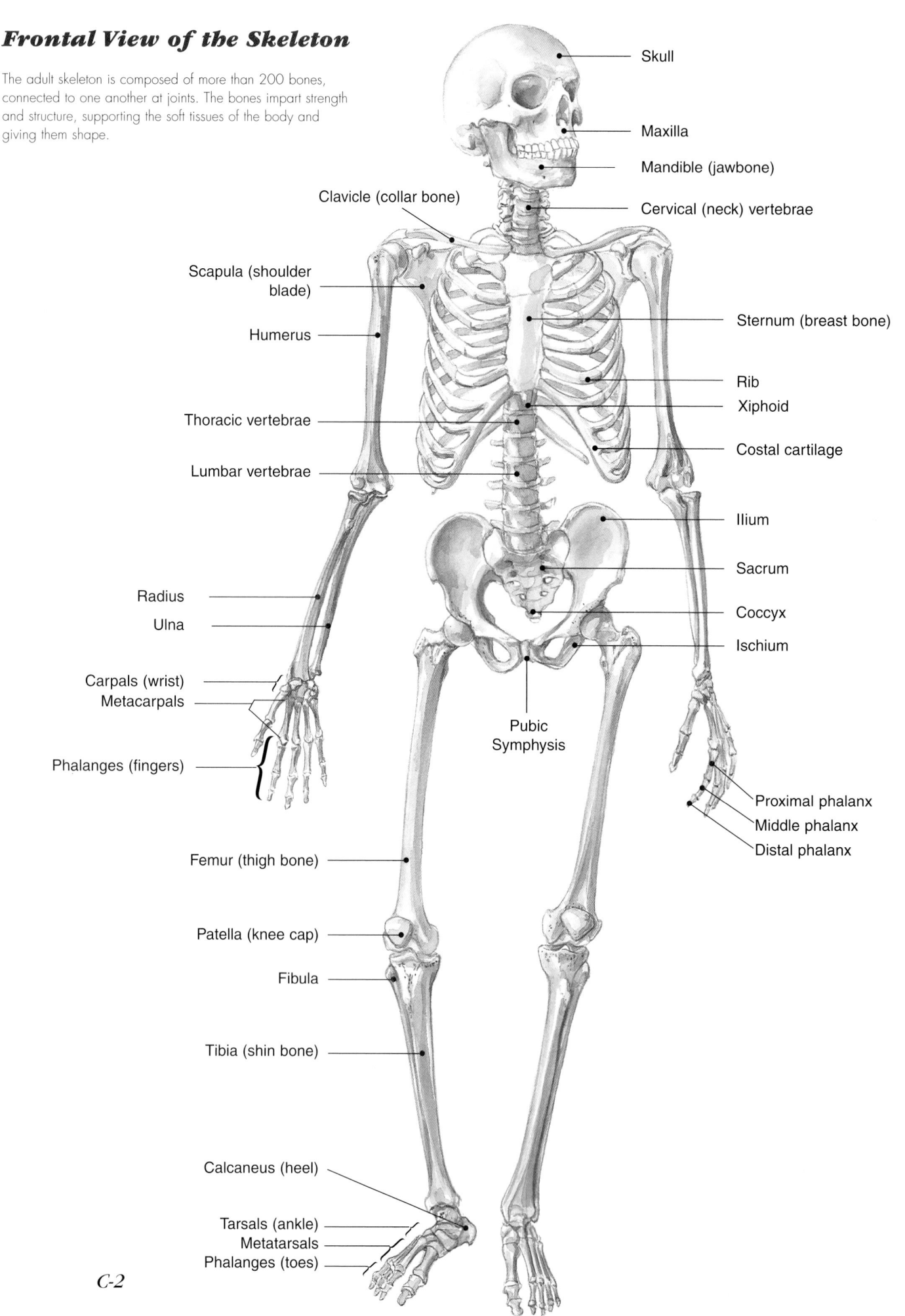

Skull

Maxilla

Mandible (jawbone)

Cervical (neck) vertebrae

Clavicle (collar bone)

Scapula (shoulder blade)

Sternum (breast bone)

Humerus

Rib

Xiphoid

Thoracic vertebrae

Costal cartilage

Lumbar vertebrae

Ilium

Sacrum

Coccyx

Radius

Ischium

Ulna

Carpals (wrist)

Metacarpals

Pubic Symphysis

Phalanges (fingers)

Proximal phalanx

Middle phalanx

Distal phalanx

Femur (thigh bone)

Patella (knee cap)

Fibula

Tibia (shin bone)

Calcaneus (heel)

Tarsals (ankle)

Metatarsals

Phalanges (toes)

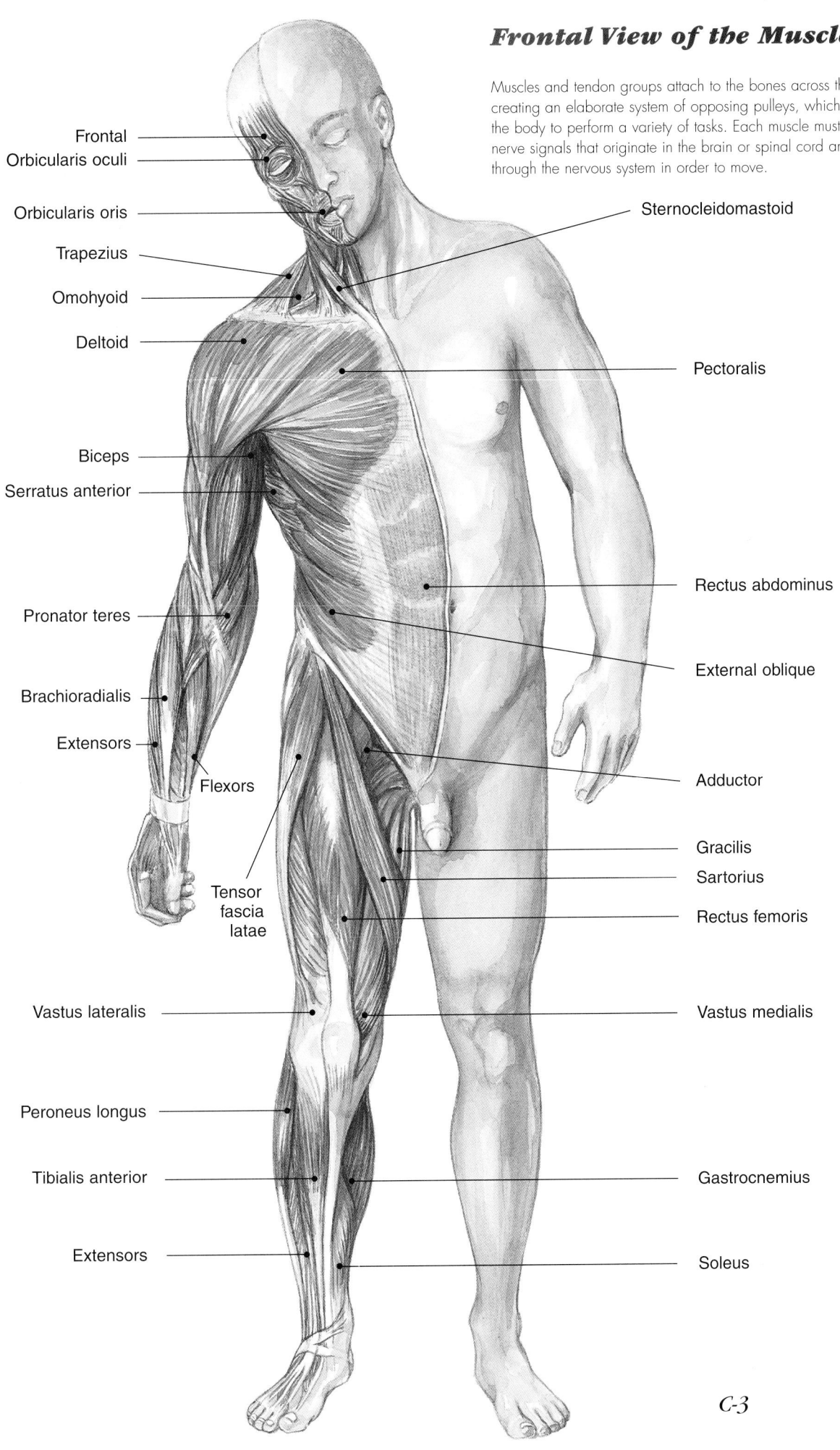

Frontal View of the Muscles

Muscles and tendon groups attach to the bones across the joints, creating an elaborate system of opposing pulleys, which enables the body to perform a variety of tasks. Each muscle must receive nerve signals that originate in the brain or spinal cord and travel through the nervous system in order to move.

Frontal
Orbicularis oculi
Orbicularis oris
Trapezius
Omohyoid
Deltoid
Biceps
Serratus anterior
Pronator teres
Brachioradialis
Extensors
Flexors
Tensor fascia latae
Vastus lateralis
Peroneus longus
Tibialis anterior
Extensors

Sternocleidomastoid
Pectoralis
Rectus abdominus
External oblique
Adductor
Gracilis
Sartorius
Rectus femoris
Vastus medialis
Gastrocnemius
Soleus

C-3

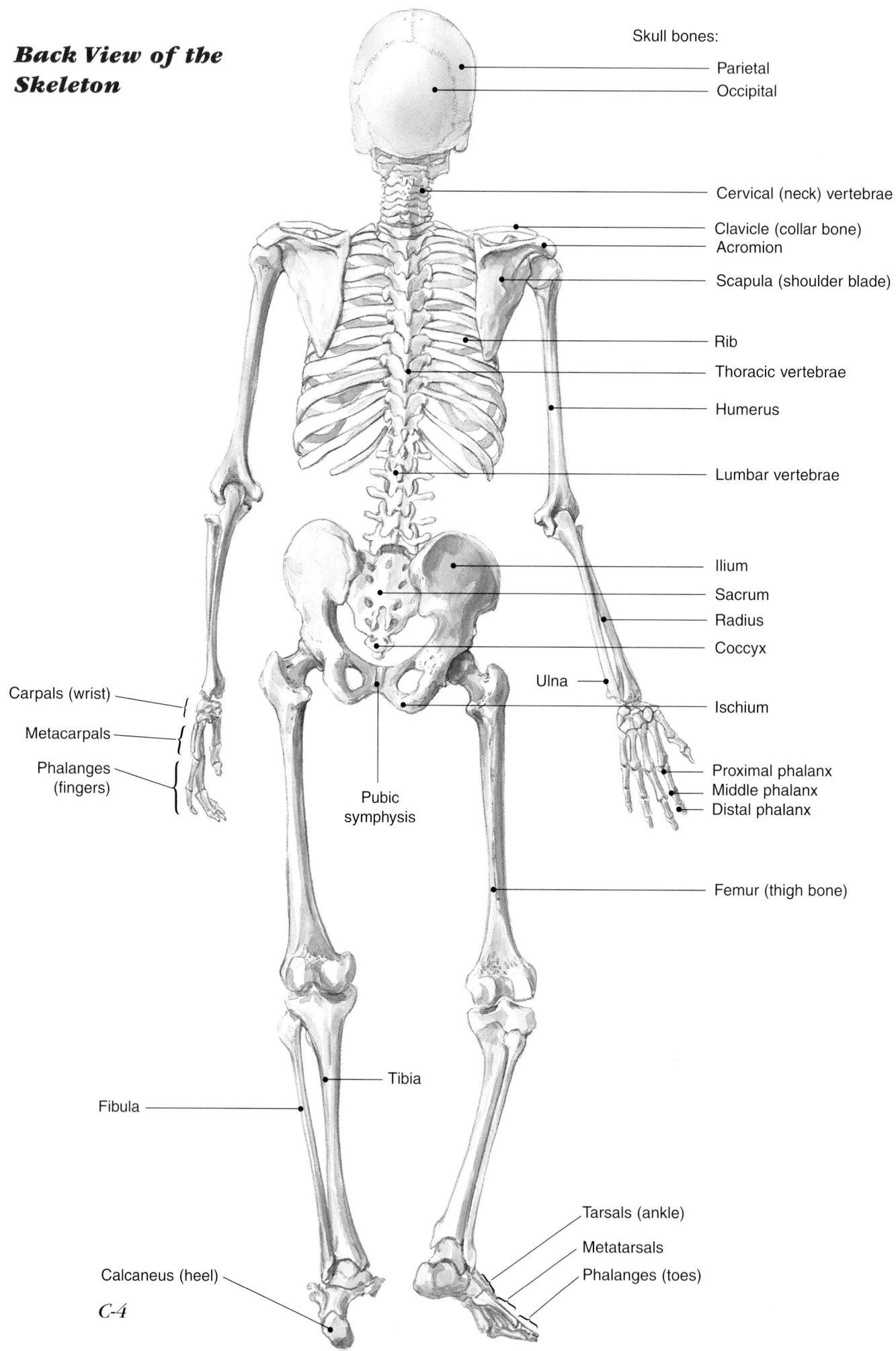

Back View of the Skeleton

Skull bones:

Parietal

Occipital

Cervical (neck) vertebrae

Clavicle (collar bone)

Acromion

Scapula (shoulder blade)

Rib

Thoracic vertebrae

Humerus

Lumbar vertebrae

Ilium

Sacrum

Radius

Coccyx

Ulna

Ischium

Carpals (wrist)

Metacarpals

Phalanges (fingers)

Proximal phalanx

Middle phalanx

Distal phalanx

Pubic symphysis

Femur (thigh bone)

Tibia

Fibula

Tarsals (ankle)

Metatarsals

Phalanges (toes)

Calcaneus (heel)

C-4

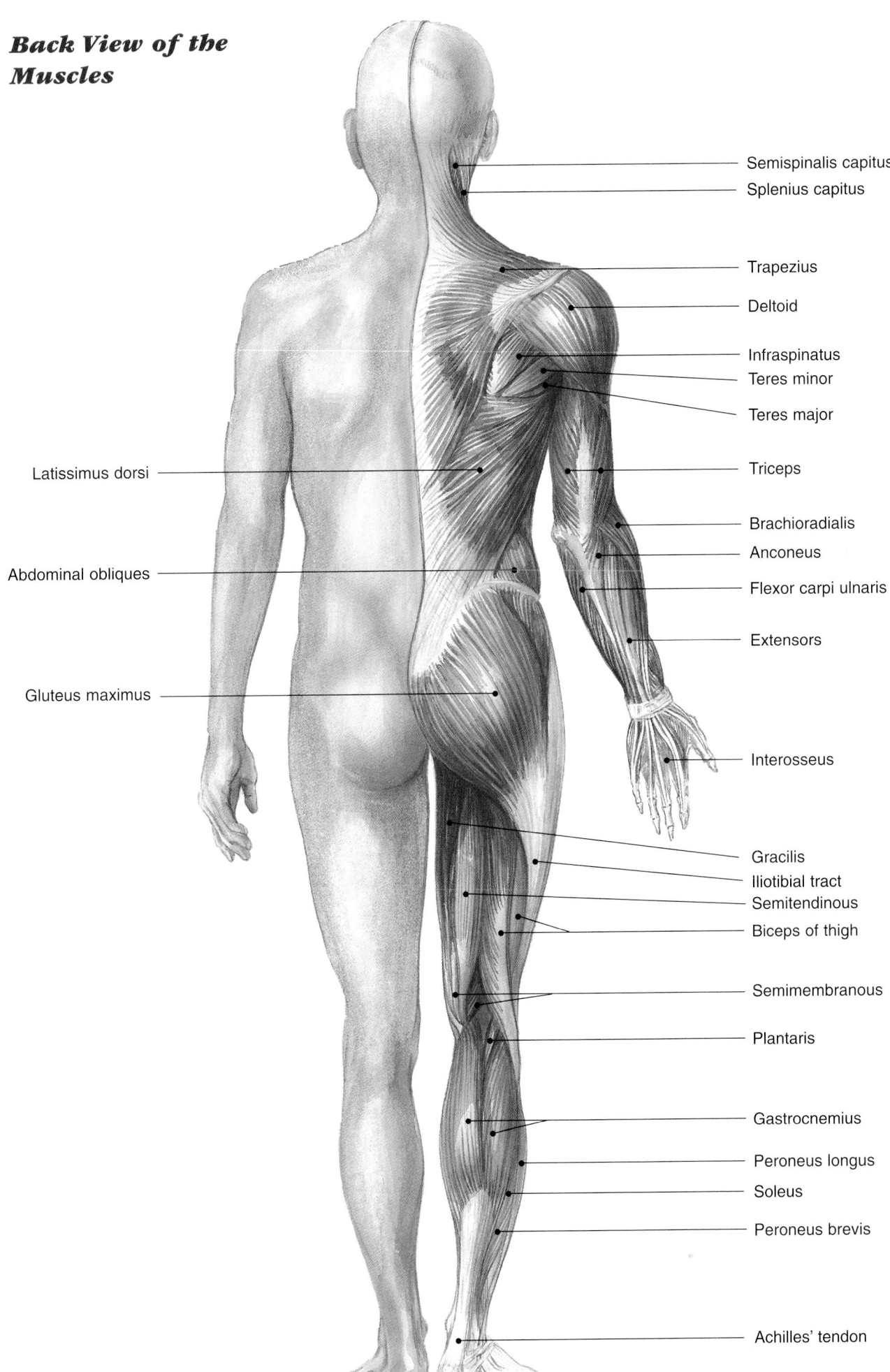

Back View of the Muscles

Semispinalis capitus

Splenius capitus

Trapezius

Deltoid

Infraspinatus

Teres minor

Teres major

Latissimus dorsi

Triceps

Brachioradialis

Anconeus

Flexor carpi ulnaris

Abdominal obliques

Extensors

Gluteus maximus

Interosseus

Gracilis

Iliotibial tract

Semitendinous

Biceps of thigh

Semimembranous

Plantaris

Gastrocnemius

Peroneus longus

Soleus

Peroneus brevis

Achilles' tendon

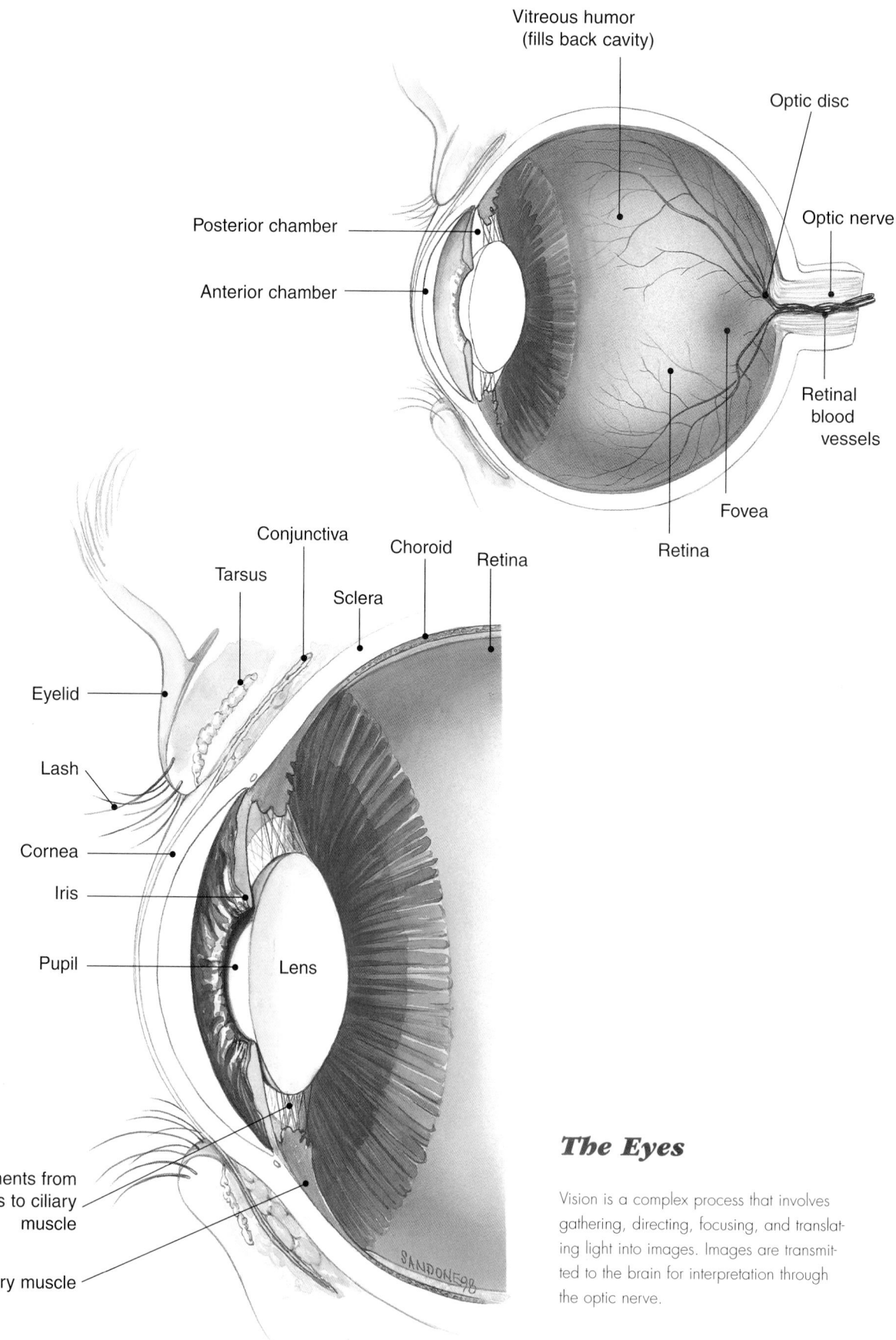

Vitreous humor
(fills back cavity)

Optic disc

Optic nerve

Posterior chamber

Anterior chamber

Retinal
blood
vessels

Fovea

Retina

Conjunctiva

Choroid

Retina

Tarsus

Sclera

Eyelid

Lash

Cornea

Iris

Pupil

Lens

Ligaments from
lens to ciliary
muscle

Ciliary muscle

SANDONE98

The Eyes

Vision is a complex process that involves gathering, directing, focusing, and translating light into images. Images are transmitted to the brain for interpretation through the optic nerve.

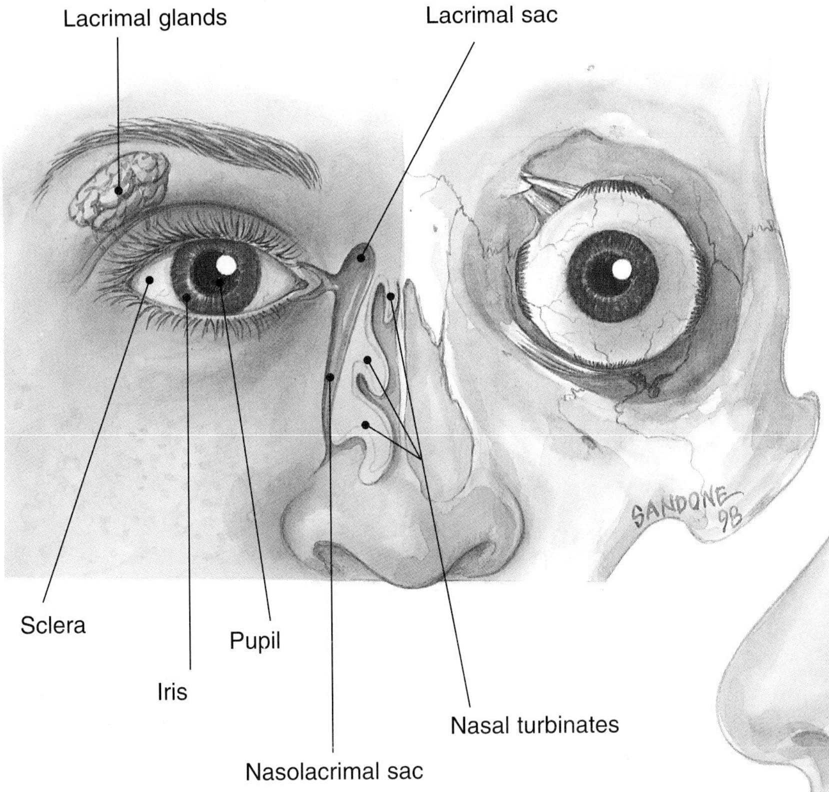

Lacrimal glands

Lacrimal sac

Muscles of the eye

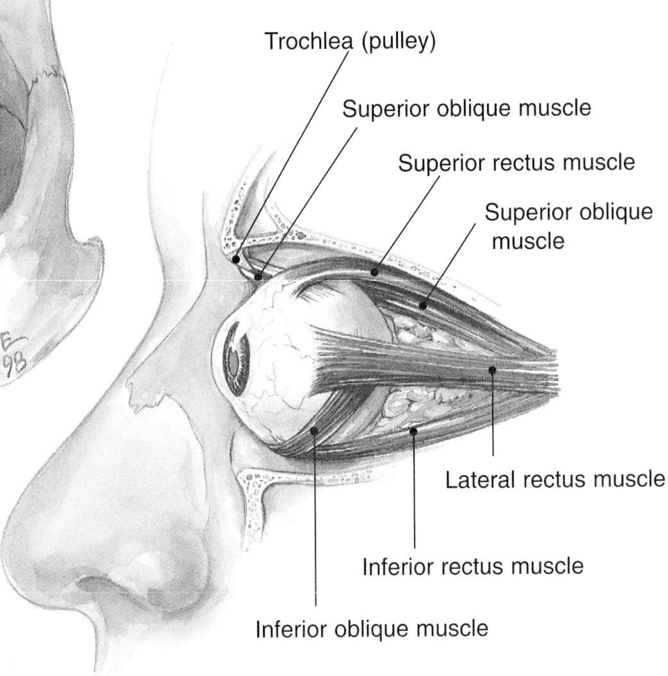

Trochlea (pulley)

Superior oblique muscle

Superior rectus muscle

Superior oblique muscle

Lateral rectus muscle

Inferior rectus muscle

Inferior oblique muscle

Sclera

Pupil

Iris

Nasal turbinates

Nasolacrimal sac

**Fundus
(back of the eye)**

Optic disk

Fovea

Retinal blood vessels

Retina

C-7

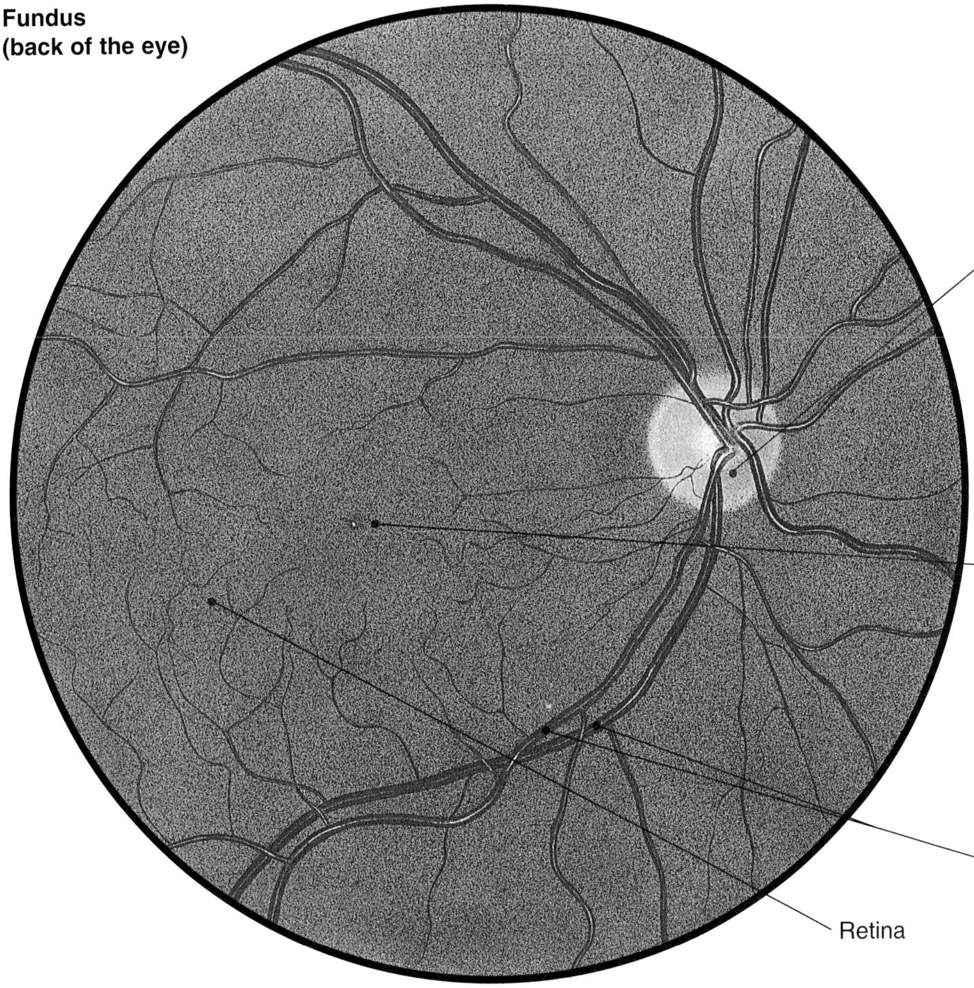

Ears, Nose, and Throat

The ears, nose, and throat are closely related in structure and function. For example, the ear chamber is connected to the throat through the eustachian tube, and the nose and sinuses drain into the throat. Infections and tumors in one area may spread to others because of these connections. The ears are responsible for hearing as well as our sense of balance. The nose provides our sense of smell and is the opening to the respiratory tree. The throat functions as the common pathway for the respiratory and digestive systems.

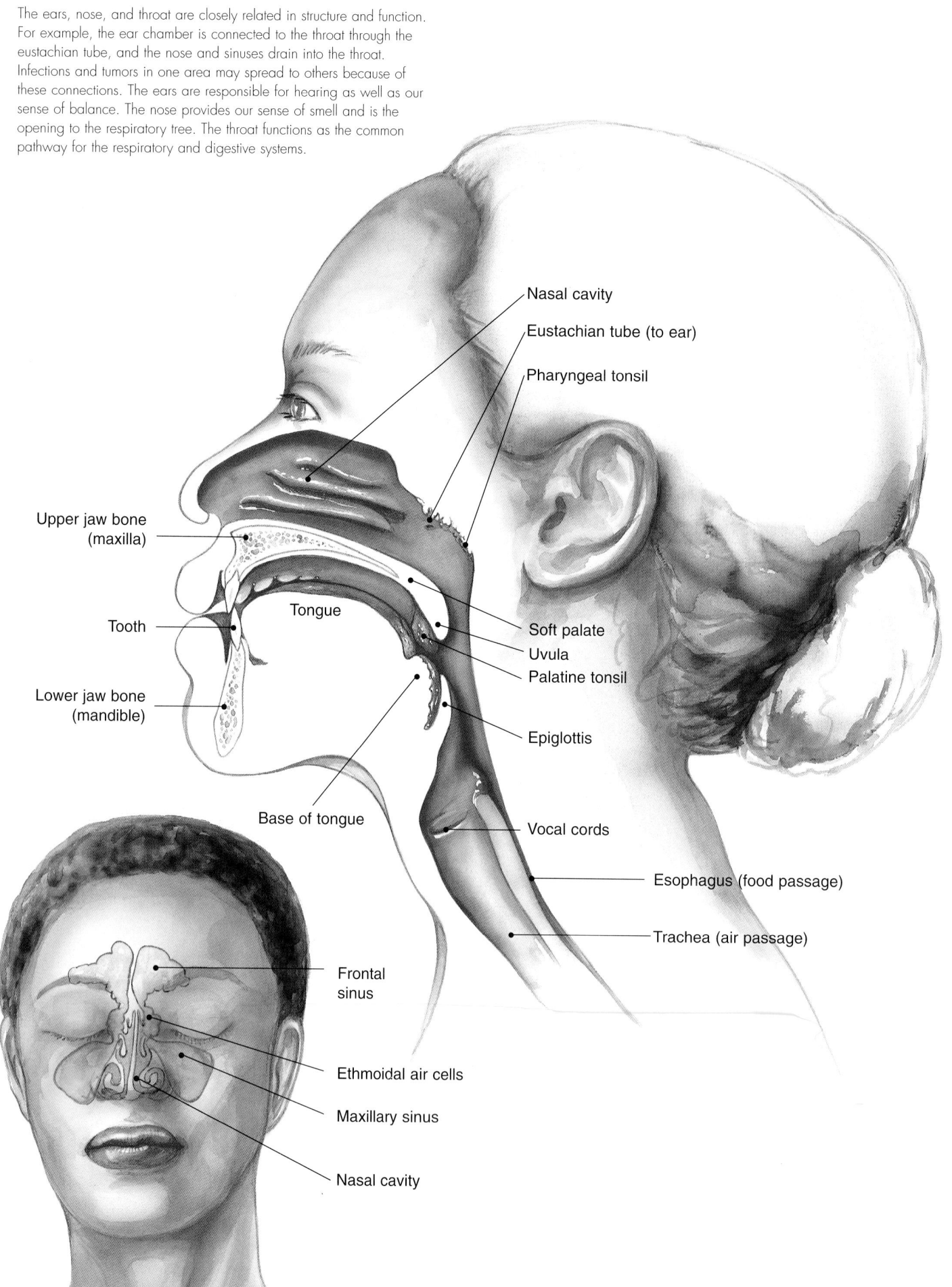

Nasal cavity

Eustachian tube (to ear)

Pharyngeal tonsil

Upper jaw bone (maxilla)

Tooth

Tongue

Lower jaw bone (mandible)

Soft palate

Uvula

Palatine tonsil

Epiglottis

Base of tongue

Vocal cords

Esophagus (food passage)

Trachea (air passage)

Frontal sinus

Ethmoidal air cells

Maxillary sinus

Nasal cavity

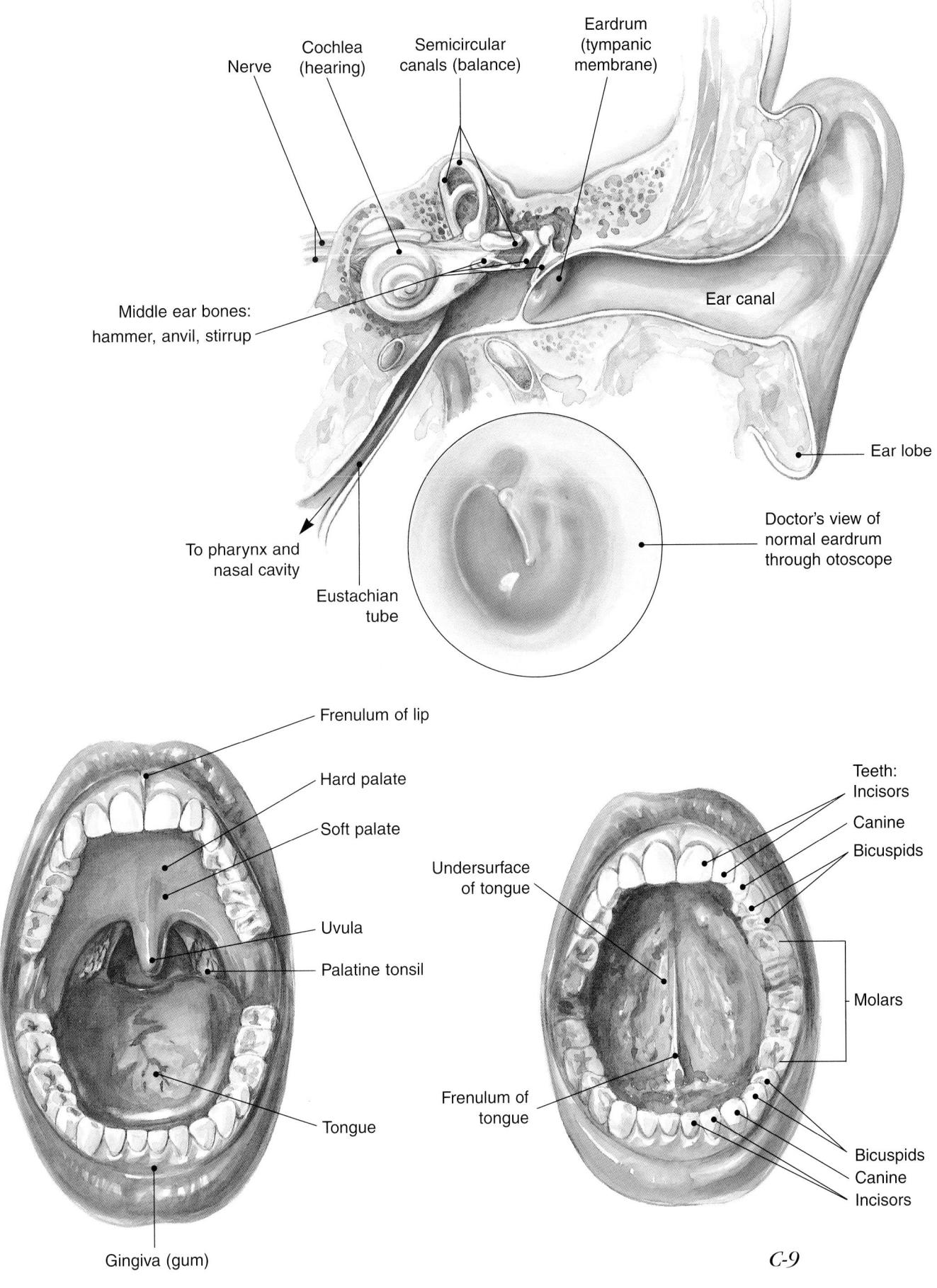

Nerve

Cochlea (hearing)

Semicircular canals (balance)

Eardrum (tympanic membrane)

Middle ear bones: hammer, anvil, stirrup

Ear canal

Ear lobe

To pharynx and nasal cavity

Eustachian tube

Doctor's view of normal eardrum through otoscope

Frenulum of lip

Hard palate

Soft palate

Uvula

Palatine tonsil

Tongue

Gingiva (gum)

Teeth: Incisors

Canine

Bicuspids

Undersurface of tongue

Molars

Frenulum of tongue

Bicuspids

Canine

Incisors

Cardiovascular System

The heart and its blood vessels, a 60,000–mile network of arteries, veins, and capillaries, make up the cardiovascular system. Arteries (red) deliver blood, with oxygen and nutrients, to the tissues of the body and veins (blue) carry away carbon dioxide and other metabolic wastes. The heart pumps about 2,000 gallons of blood through the body every day.

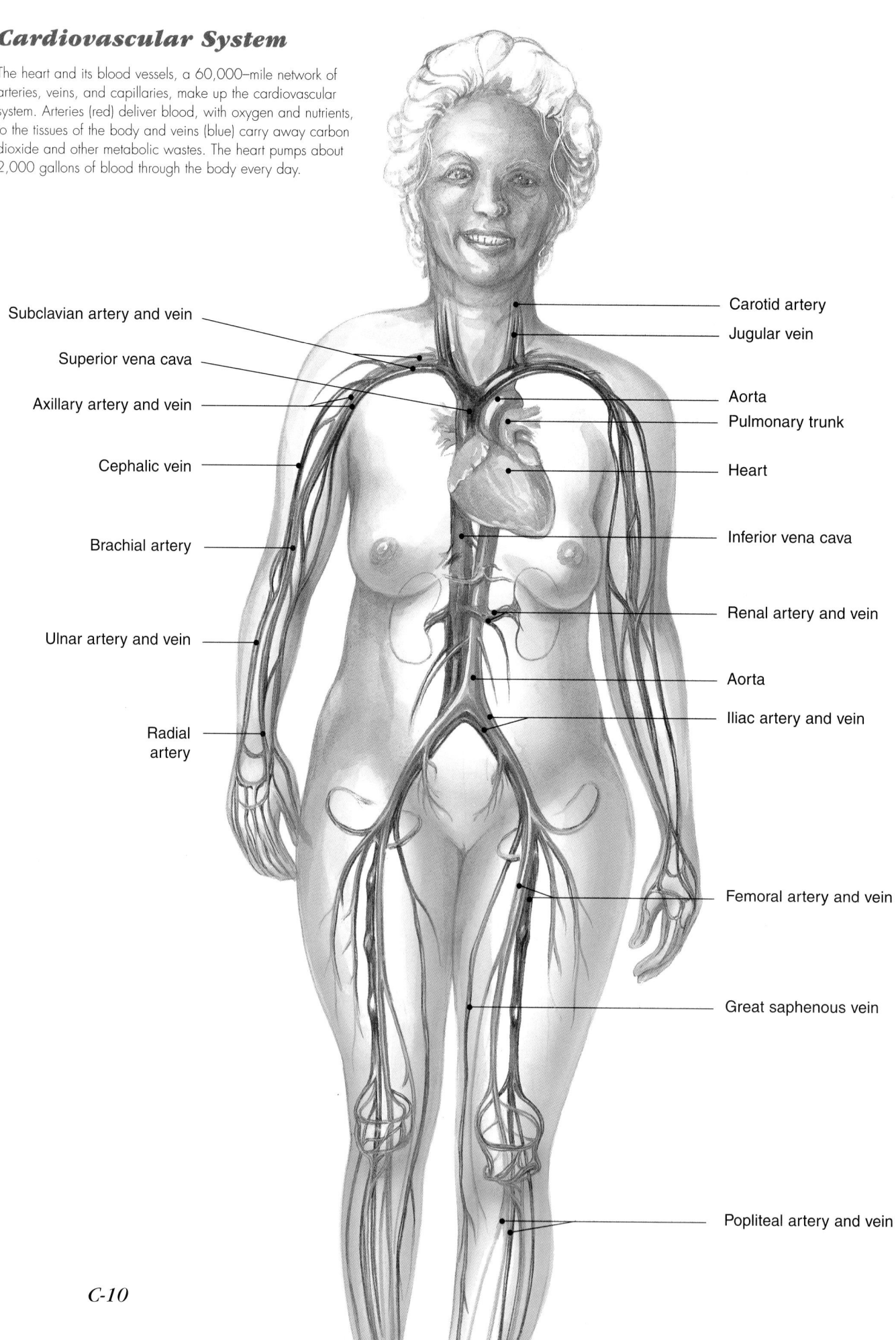

Subclavian artery and vein

Superior vena cava

Axillary artery and vein

Cephalic vein

Brachial artery

Ulnar artery and vein

Radial artery

Carotid artery

Jugular vein

Aorta

Pulmonary trunk

Heart

Inferior vena cava

Renal artery and vein

Aorta

Iliac artery and vein

Femoral artery and vein

Great saphenous vein

Popliteal artery and vein

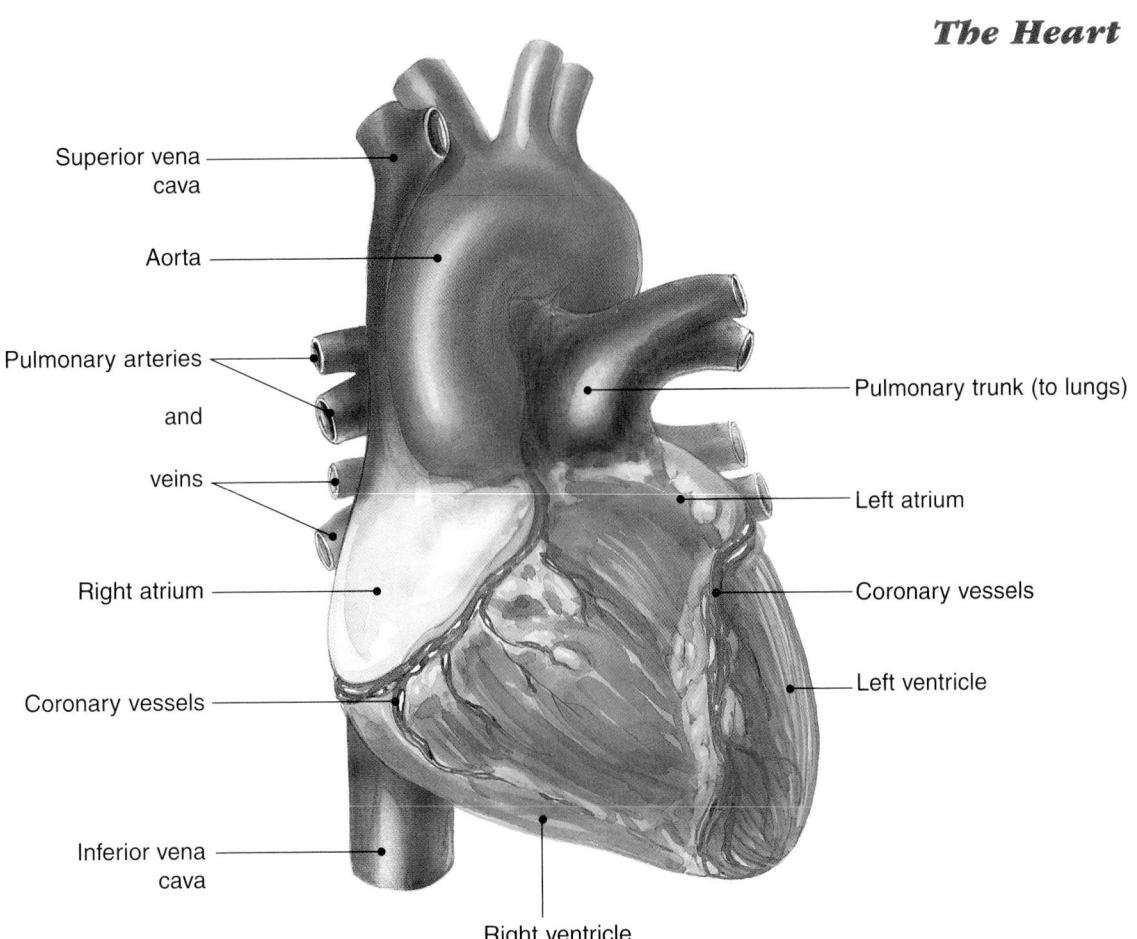

Superior vena cava

Aorta

Pulmonary arteries

and

veins

Right atrium

Coronary vessels

Inferior vena cava

Pulmonary trunk (to lungs)

Left atrium

Coronary vessels

Left ventricle

Right ventricle

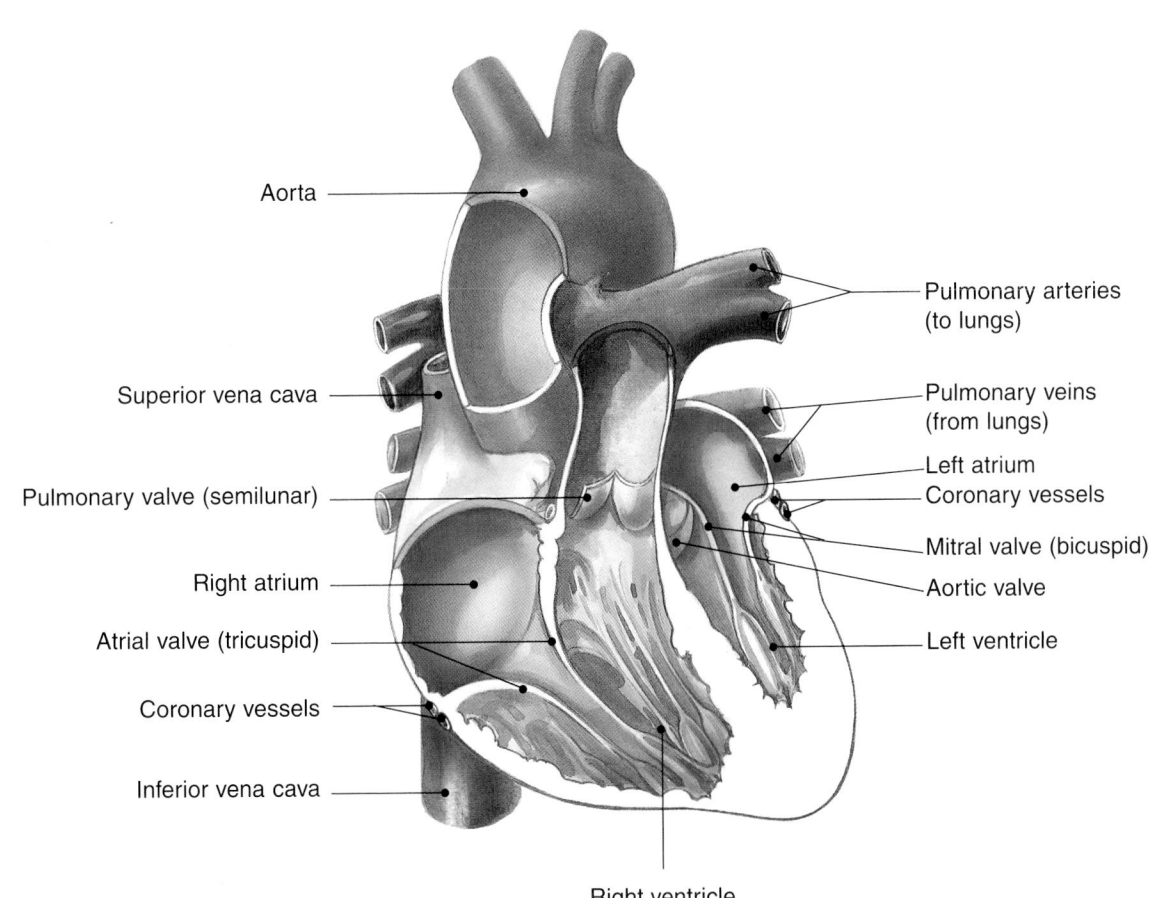

Aorta

Superior vena cava

Pulmonary valve (semilunar)

Right atrium

Atrial valve (tricuspid)

Coronary vessels

Inferior vena cava

Pulmonary arteries (to lungs)

Pulmonary veins (from lungs)

Left atrium

Coronary vessels

Mitral valve (bicuspid)

Aortic valve

Left ventricle

Right ventricle

Lymphatic (Immune) System

The lymphatic system is made up of lymphatic vessels and capillaries that lie close to the veins and arteries in most tissues. Just as blood circulates through the blood vessels, lymphatic fluid, or lymph, circulates between the cells that make up the different tissues carrying oxygen, nutrients, and water from the bloodstream to them. Cell waste products such as carbon dioxide and water are picked up by the lymph and transported back to the bloodstream. Along the vessels lie lymphatic nodes or glands. They function primarily to filter out bacteria and other toxic substances flushed out from the tissues by the fluid.

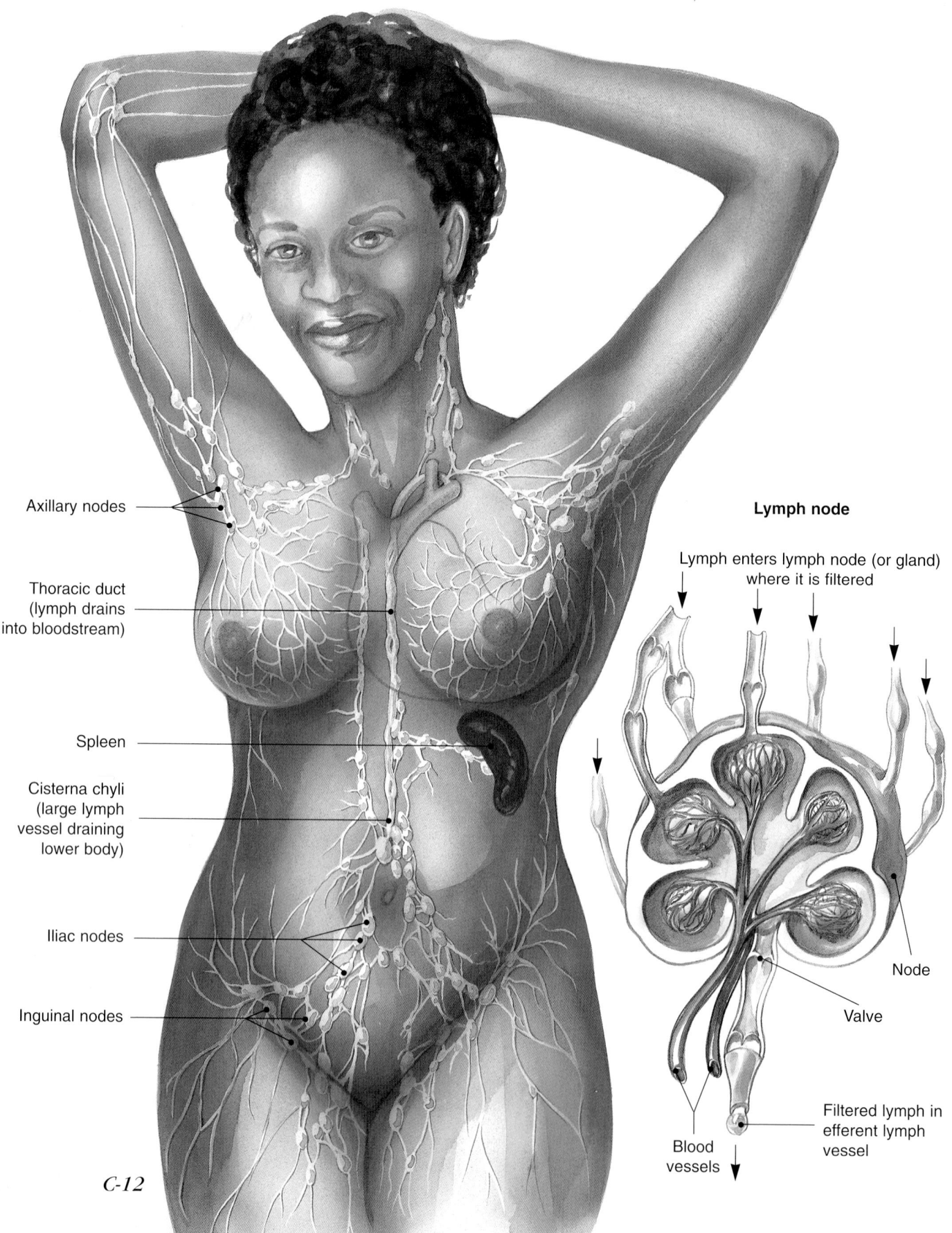

Axillary nodes

Thoracic duct
(lymph drains
into bloodstream)

Spleen

Cisterna chyli
(large lymph
vessel draining
lower body)

Iliac nodes

Inguinal nodes

Lymph node

Lymph enters lymph node (or gland)
where it is filtered

Node

Valve

Filtered lymph in
efferent lymph
vessel

Blood
vessels

C-12

Respiratory System

Air enters the respiratory system through the act of inhalation. During inhalation, the diaphragm contracts causing the lungs to expand and air to rush in. During exhalation, the diaphragm relaxes and the expanded lungs deflate pushing carbon-dioxide-filled air out. Oxygen is exchanged for carbon dioxide in the alveoli.

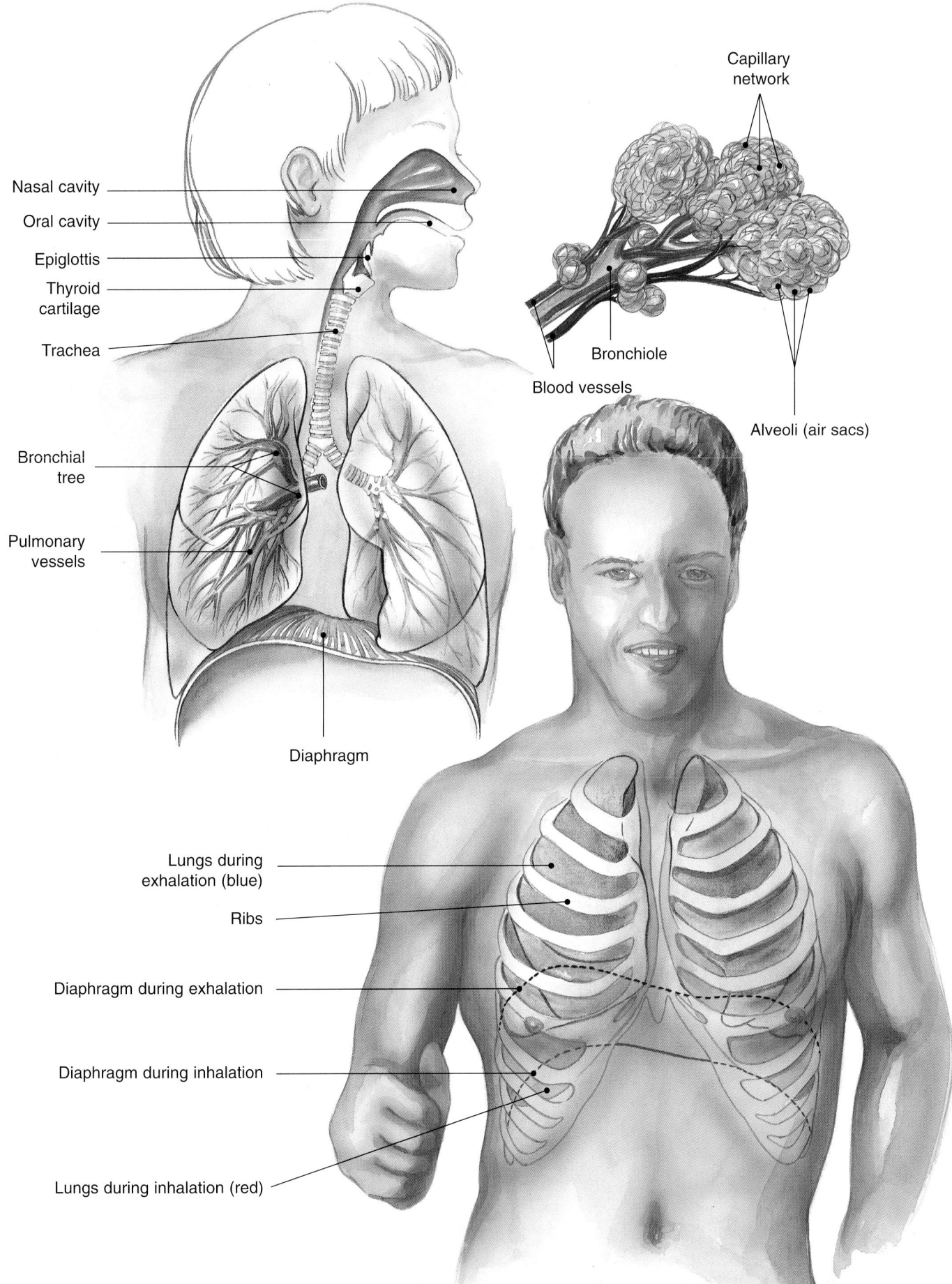

Capillary network

Nasal cavity

Oral cavity

Epiglottis

Thyroid cartilage

Trachea

Bronchiole

Blood vessels

Alveoli (air sacs)

Bronchial tree

Pulmonary vessels

Diaphragm

Lungs during exhalation (blue)

Ribs

Diaphragm during exhalation

Diaphragm during inhalation

Lungs during inhalation (red)

Digestive System

Digestion begins when food is chewed in the mouth and swallowed. The chemical breakdown of the food, which began in the mouth, continues in the stomach. Gastric juices in the stomach activate an enzyme called pepsin, which digests protein. The food, by now in small particles, is released by the stomach into the small intestine, where digestion continues and nutrients are absorbed. Food is pushed into the colon, or large intestine, which is responsible for removing salt and water from what is left of the food. The digested mass becomes more solid and, in its final form, travels through the rectum where it is expelled.

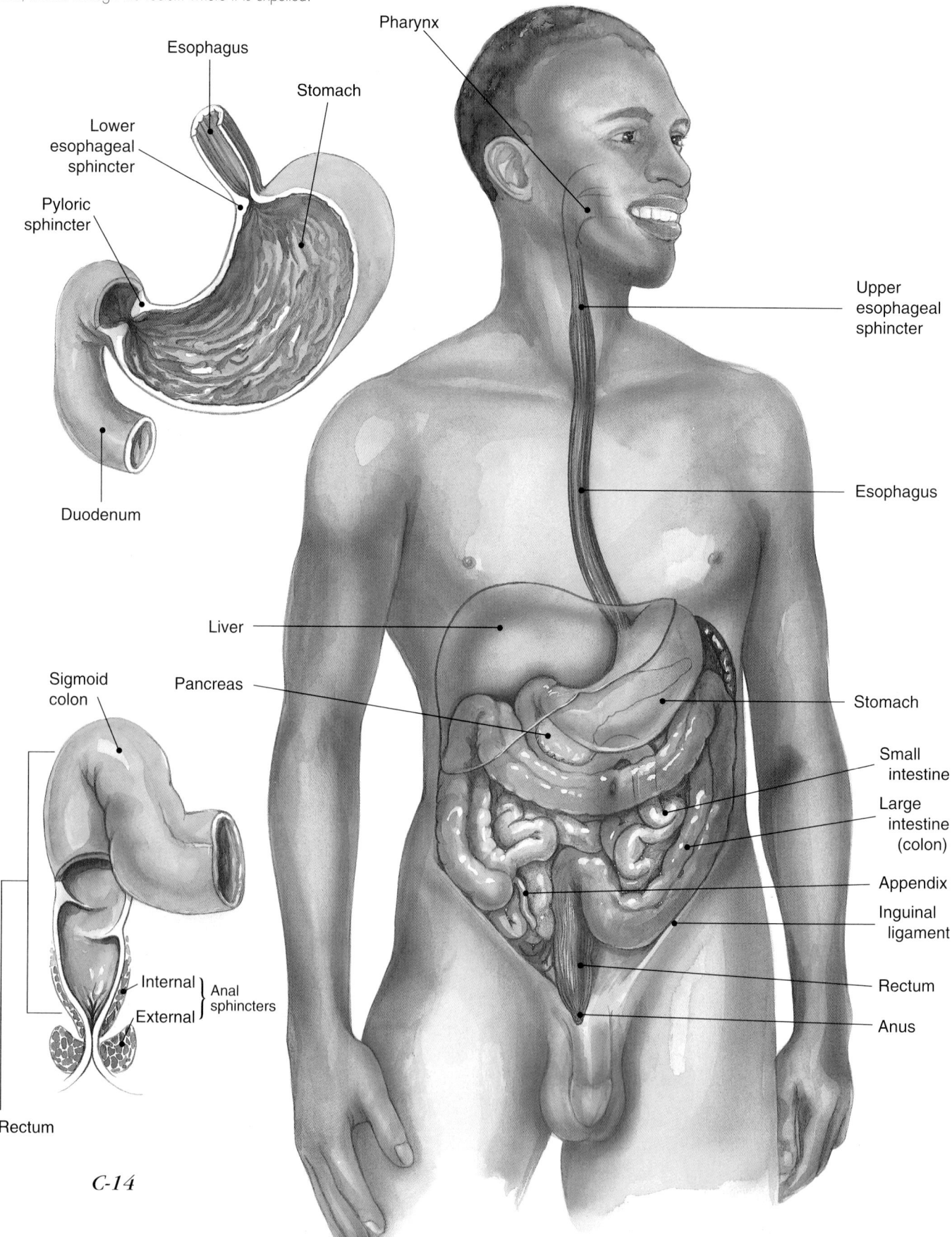

Pharynx

Esophagus

Stomach

Lower esophageal sphincter

Pyloric sphincter

Duodenum

Upper esophageal sphincter

Esophagus

Sigmoid colon

Liver

Pancreas

Stomach

Small intestine

Large intestine (colon)

Appendix

Inguinal ligament

Rectum

Anus

Internal
External } Anal sphincters

Rectum

Abdominal Organs

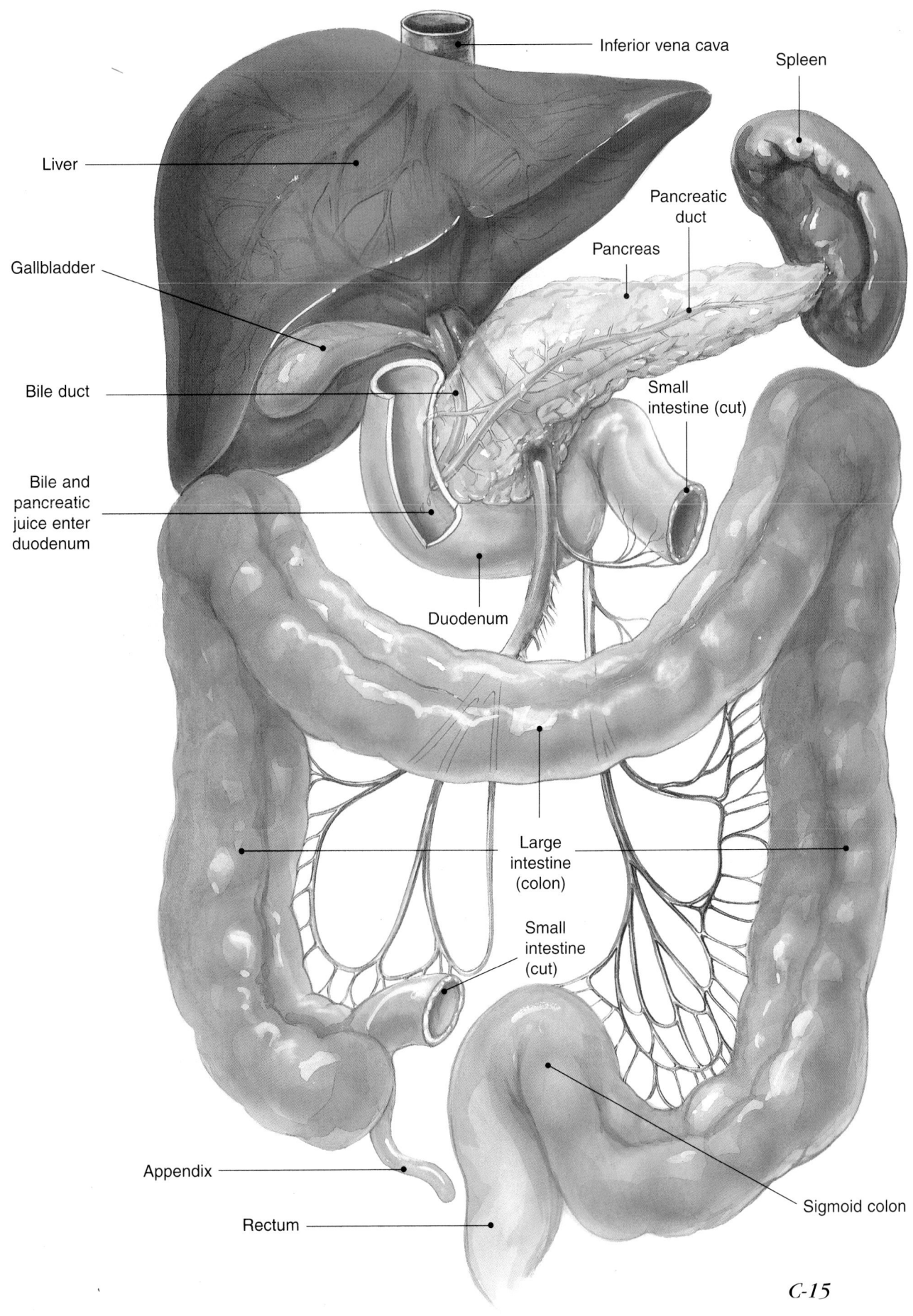

Inferior vena cava

Spleen

Liver

Pancreatic duct

Pancreas

Gallbladder

Bile duct

Small intestine (cut)

Bile and pancreatic juice enter duodenum

Duodenum

Large intestine (colon)

Small intestine (cut)

Appendix

Sigmoid colon

Rectum

C-15

Male Reproductive and Urinary Systems

The male reproductive and urinary systems are more closely related than the female systems because the penis serves as a sexual organ and a urinary tract organ (due to the urethra running through its center). The urethra carries urine or sperm through the penis. The kidneys are composed of millions of filtering units called nephrons. Each nephron has two parts. The glomerulus filters waste and fluid from the blood to create urine, and the tubule concentrates and excretes the waste products into the urine, while allowing water and essential salts, minerals, and nutrients to be reabsorbed back into the bloodstream.

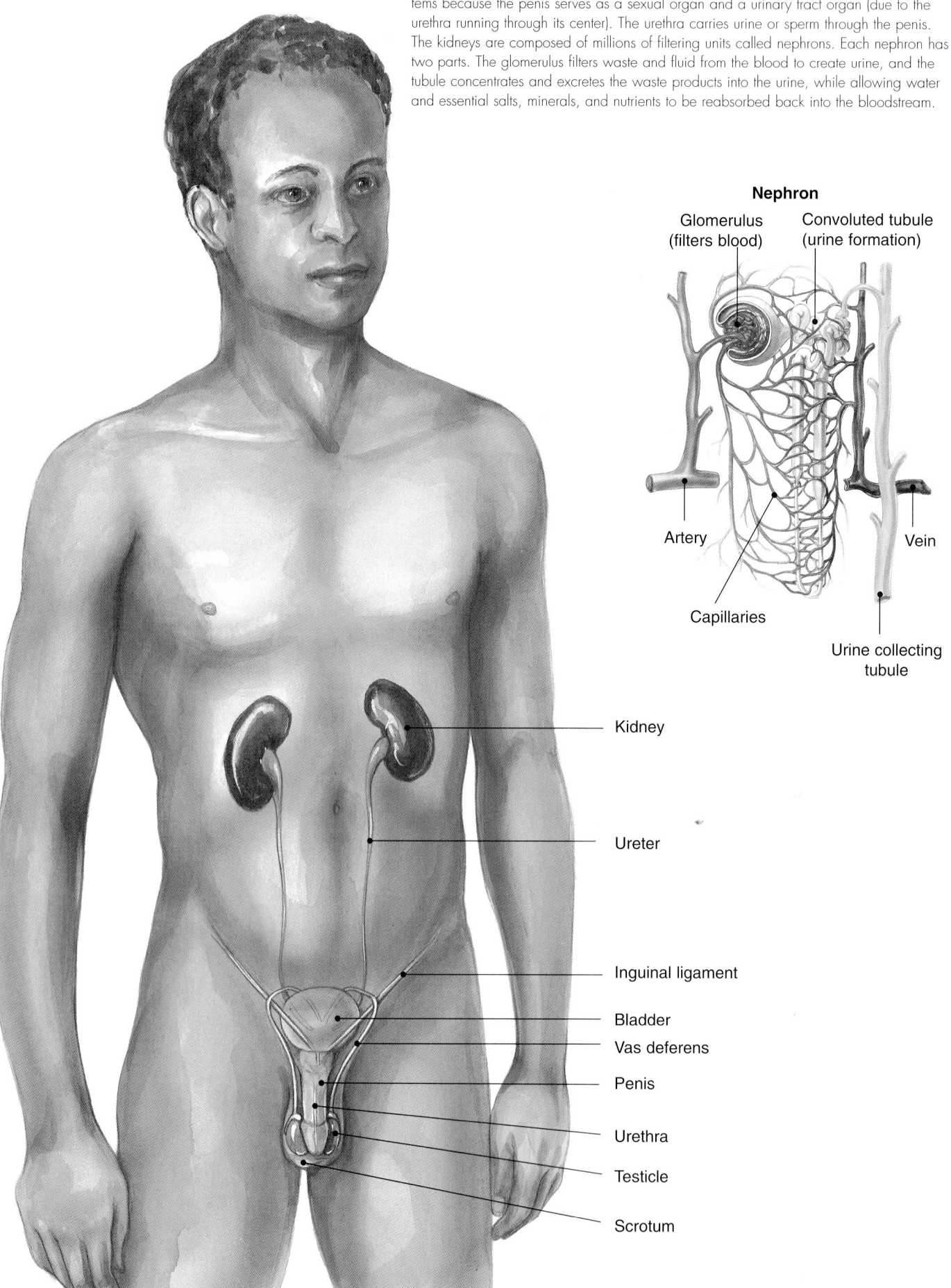

Nephron

Glomerulus (filters blood)

Convoluted tubule (urine formation)

Artery

Vein

Capillaries

Urine collecting tubule

Kidney

Ureter

Inguinal ligament

Bladder

Vas deferens

Penis

Urethra

Testicle

Scrotum

Male Reproductive System

Male Urinary System

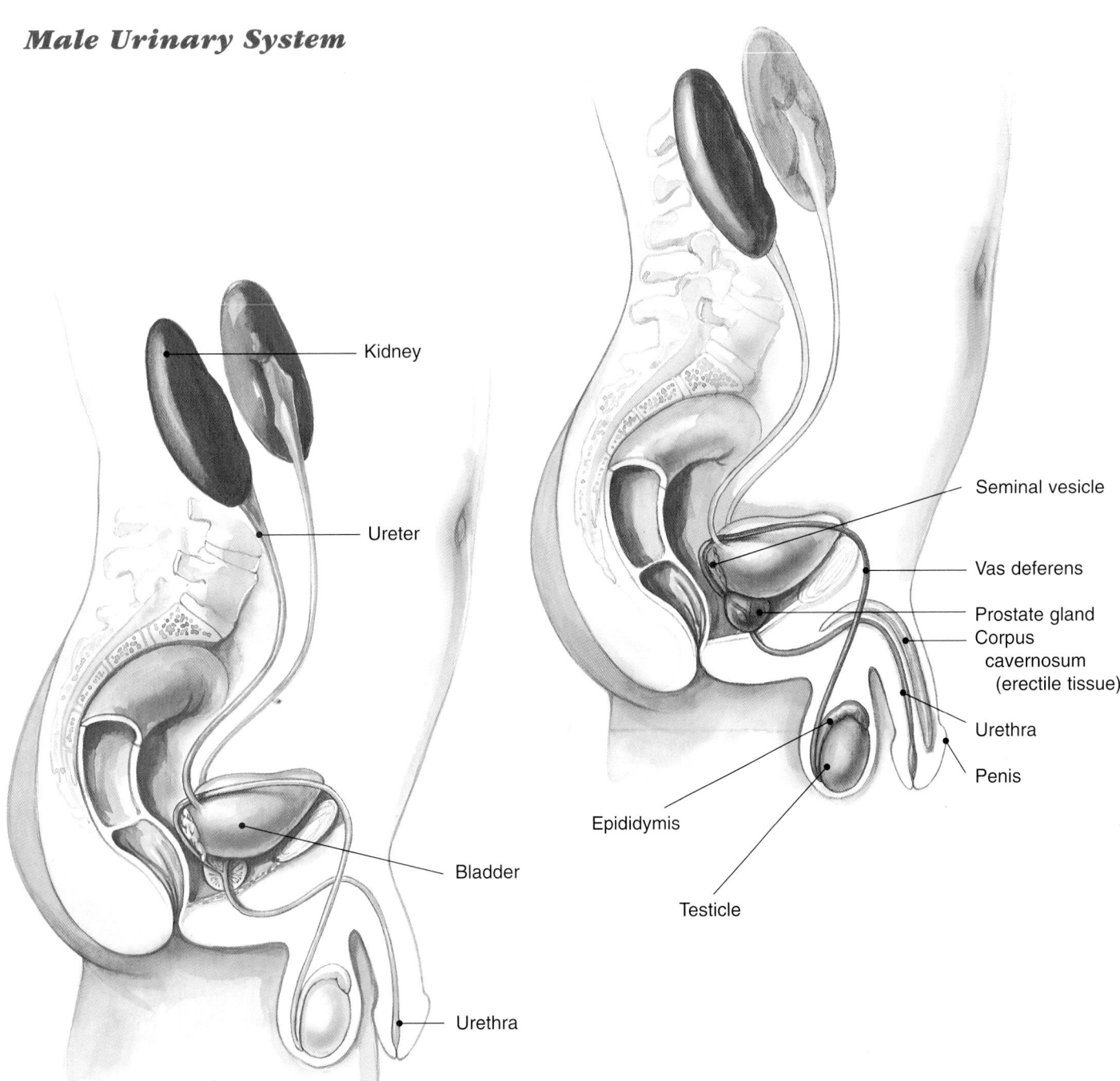

Kidney

Ureter

Seminal vesicle

Vas deferens

Prostate gland

Corpus cavernosum (erectile tissue)

Urethra

Penis

Epididymis

Bladder

Testicle

Urethra

C-17

Female Reproductive and Urinary Systems

The female reproductive system consists of the ovaries, fallopian tubes, uterus, and external genitalia. Usually, a single egg is released by the ovaries for fertilization during a monthly cycle. The urinary tract in both genders consists of a pair of kidneys each attached by its ureter to the bladder, which empties to the outside through the urethra. The urinary tract serves to eliminate waste from the body.

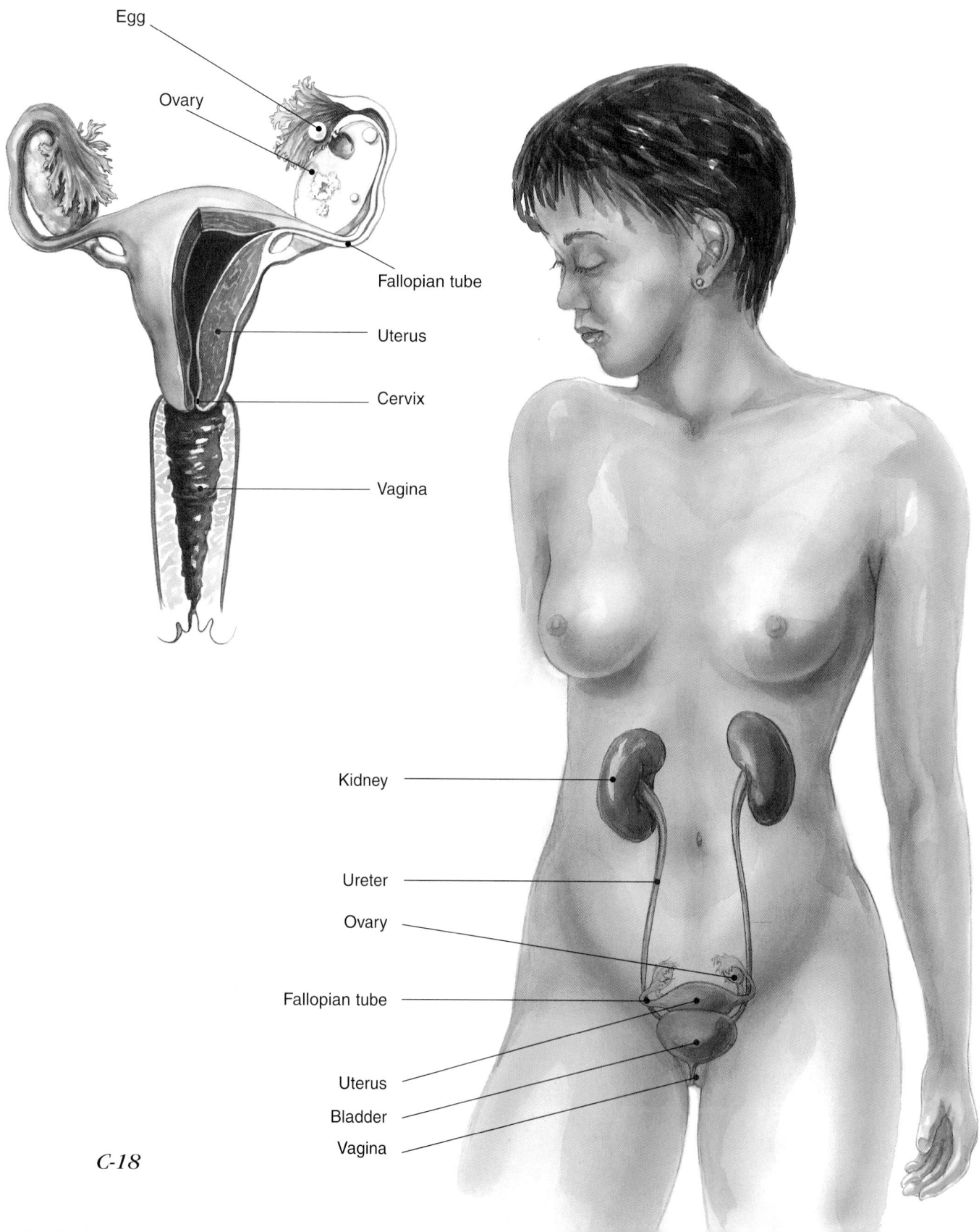

Egg

Ovary

Fallopian tube

Uterus

Cervix

Vagina

Kidney

Ureter

Ovary

Fallopian tube

Uterus

Bladder

Vagina

Female Reproductive System

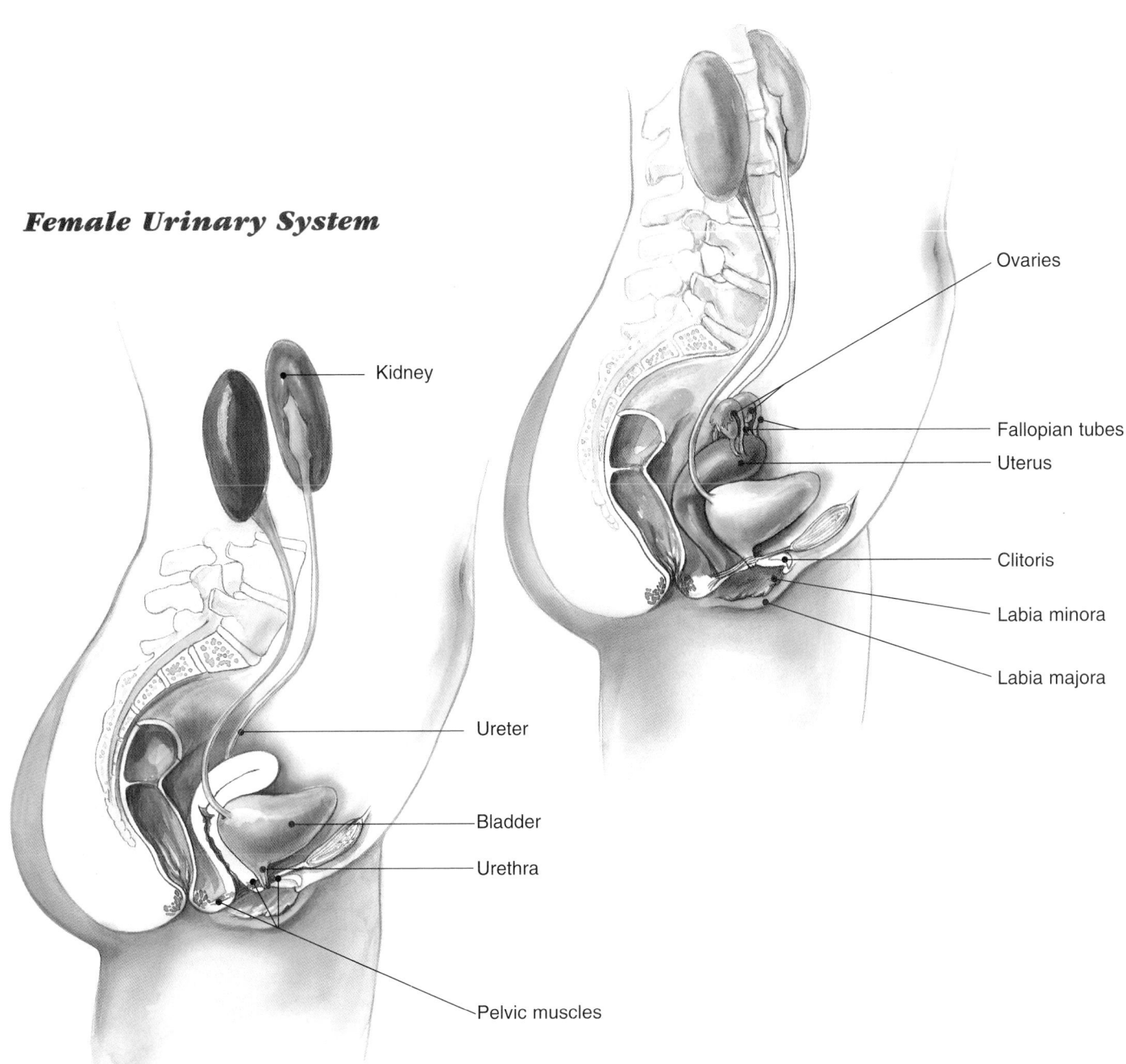

Female Urinary System

Kidney

Ovaries

Fallopian tubes

Uterus

Clitoris

Labia minora

Labia majora

Ureter

Bladder

Urethra

Pelvic muscles

Pregnancy

During the first trimester of pregnancy a woman's body goes through many changes. She may experience morning sickness and exhaustion. By the end of the first trimester, the critical structures of the baby are formed. During the second trimester the mother will feel her baby's first movements as it continues to grow. The nausea and fatigue have usually disappeared by this time. Throughout pregnancy, a woman's breasts will increase in preparation for breast-feeding. Toward the end of the third trimester the baby has shifted position and "dropped" into the pelvic area to prepare for labor.

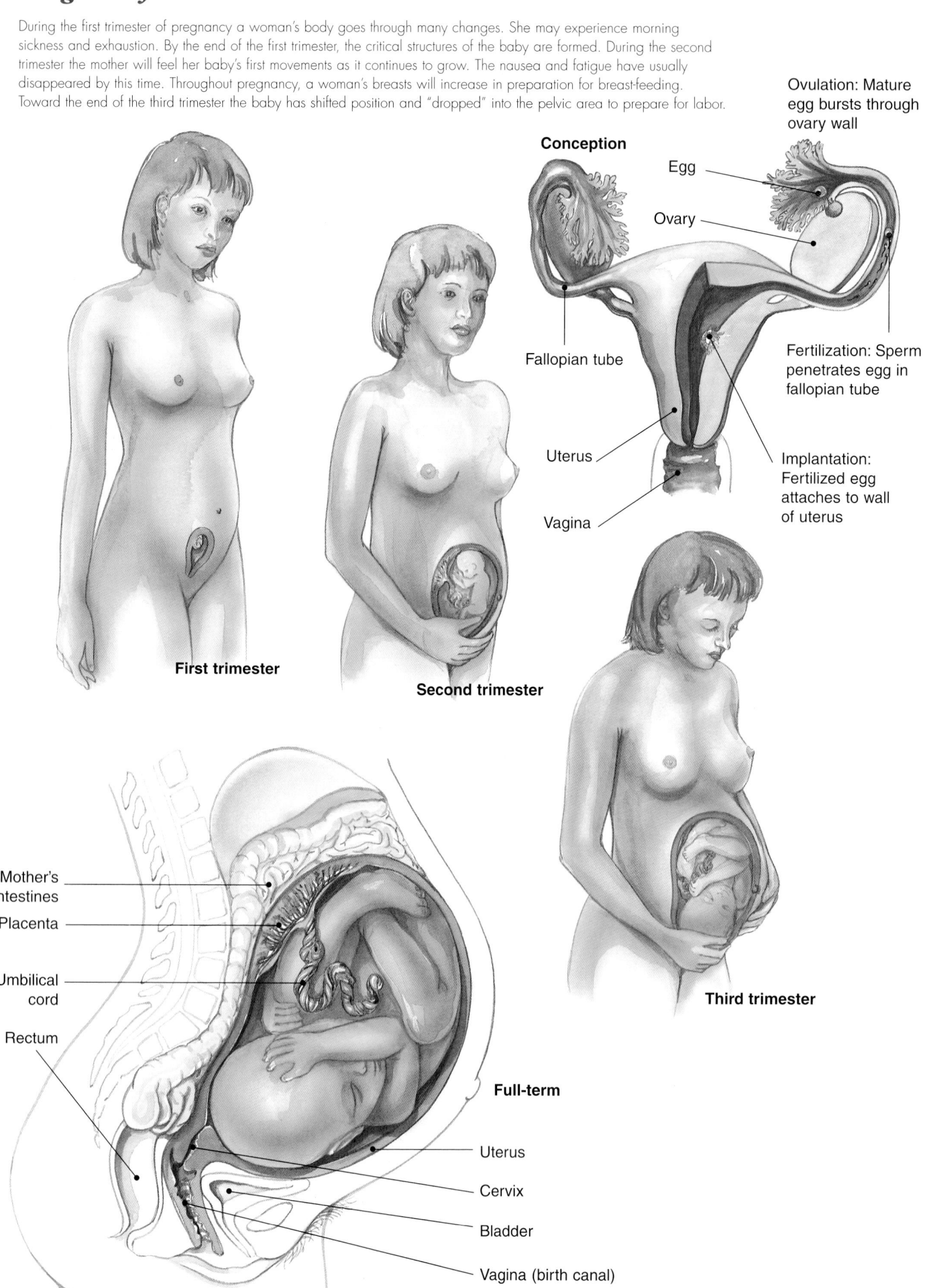

Ovulation: Mature egg bursts through ovary wall

Conception

Egg

Ovary

Fallopian tube

Fertilization: Sperm penetrates egg in fallopian tube

Uterus

Implantation: Fertilized egg attaches to wall of uterus

Vagina

First trimester

Second trimester

Third trimester

Mother's intestines

Placenta

Umbilical cord

Rectum

Full-term

Uterus

Cervix

Bladder

Vagina (birth canal)

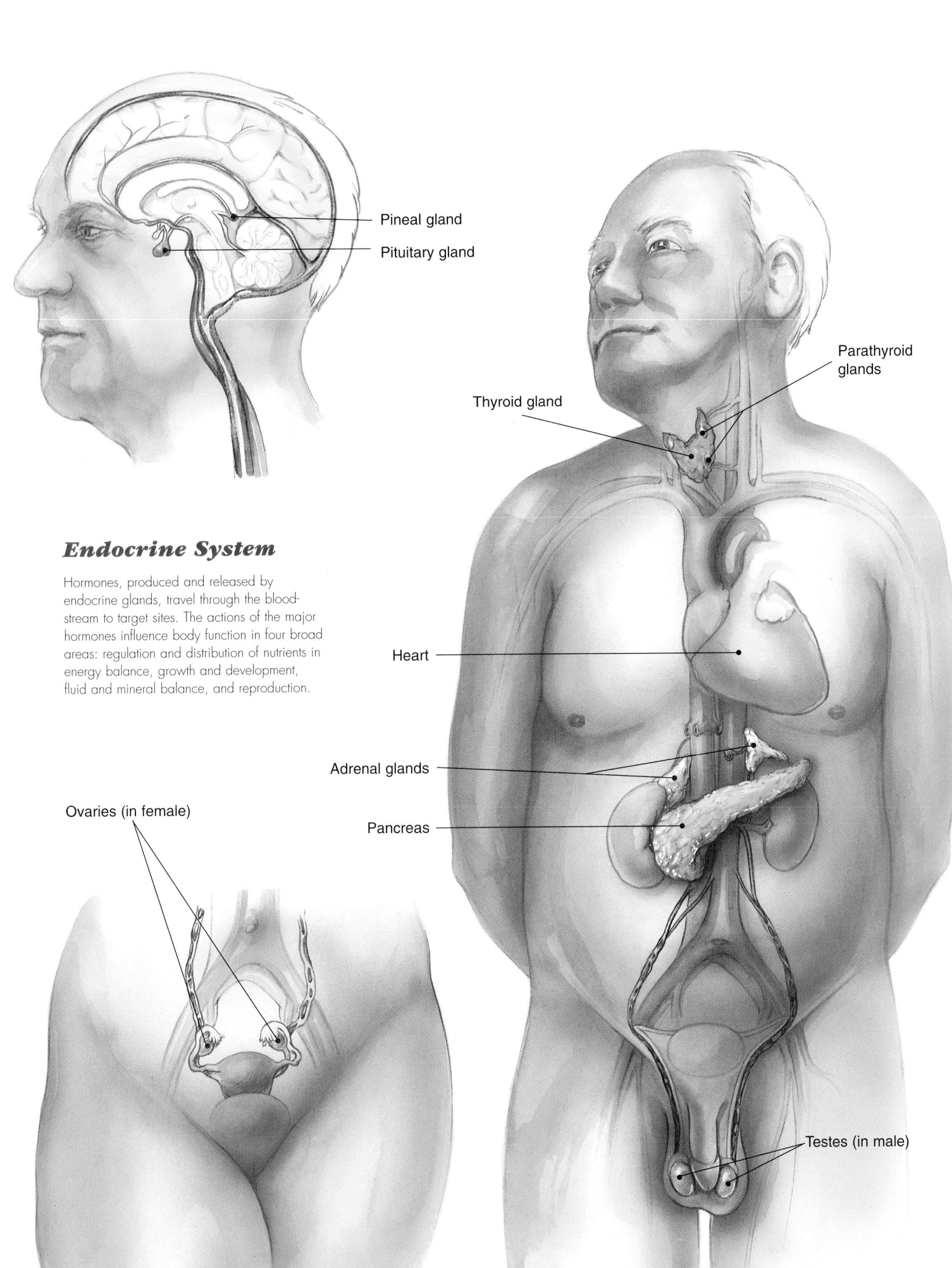

Pineal gland

Pituitary gland

Parathyroid glands

Thyroid gland

Endocrine System

Hormones, produced and released by endocrine glands, travel through the bloodstream to target sites. The actions of the major hormones influence body function in four broad areas: regulation and distribution of nutrients in energy balance, growth and development, fluid and mineral balance, and reproduction.

Heart

Adrenal glands

Pancreas

Ovaries (in female)

Testes (in male)

Brain and Nervous System

The brain and spinal cord make up the central nervous system, which communicates with the rest of the body through the spinal nerves, or peripheral nervous system. Spinal nerves enter and exit the spinal cord through gaps in the vertebrae. The 31 pairs of spinal nerves are divided into five sections: 8 cervical, 12 thoracic, 5 lumbar, 5 sacral, and 1 coccygeal.

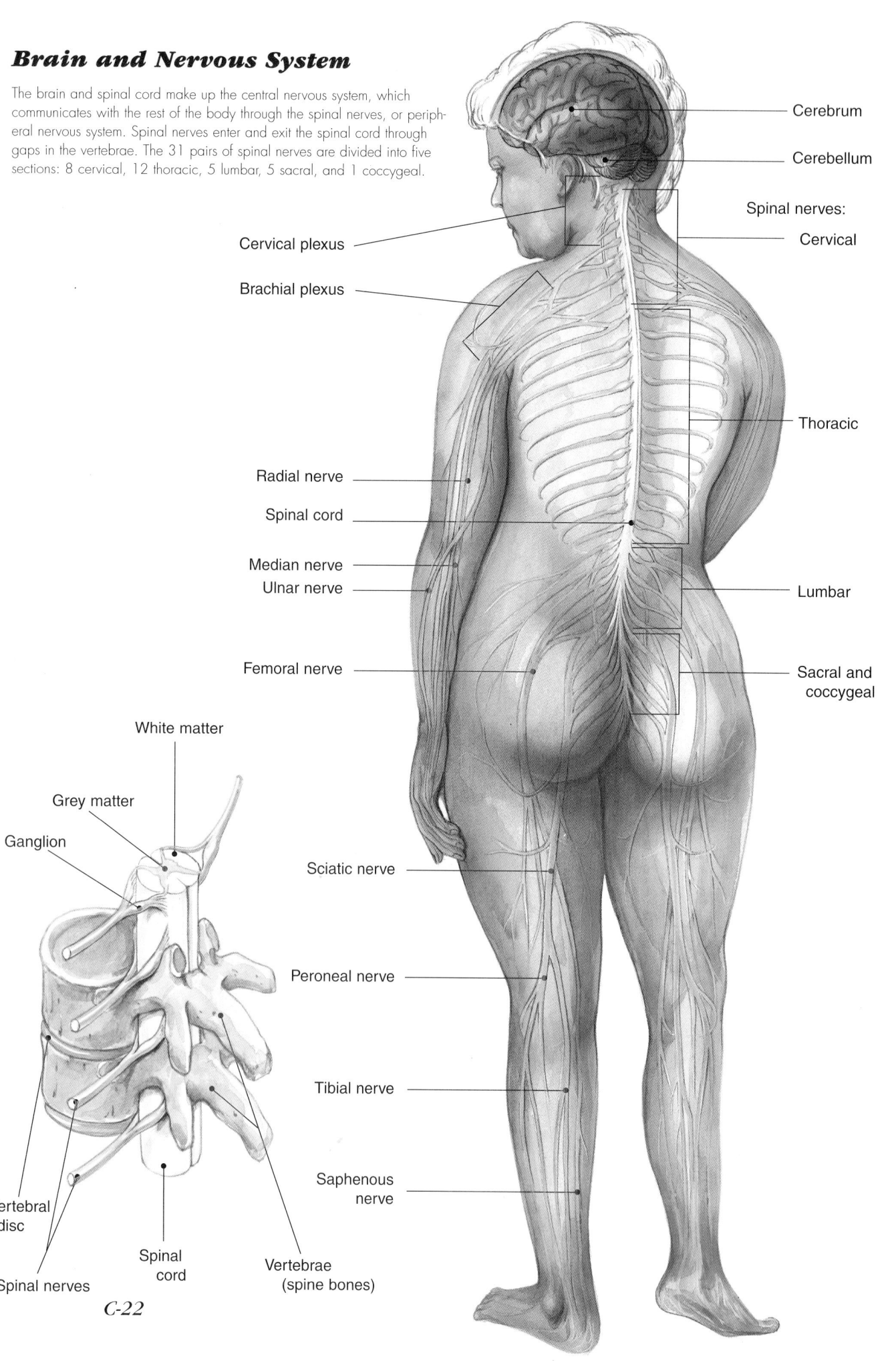

Cerebrum

Cerebellum

Spinal nerves:

Cervical

Cervical plexus

Brachial plexus

Thoracic

Radial nerve

Spinal cord

Median nerve

Ulnar nerve

Lumbar

Femoral nerve

Sacral and coccygeal

White matter

Grey matter

Ganglion

Sciatic nerve

Peroneal nerve

Tibial nerve

Saphenous nerve

Vertebral disc

Spinal nerves

Spinal cord

Vertebrae (spine bones)

C-22

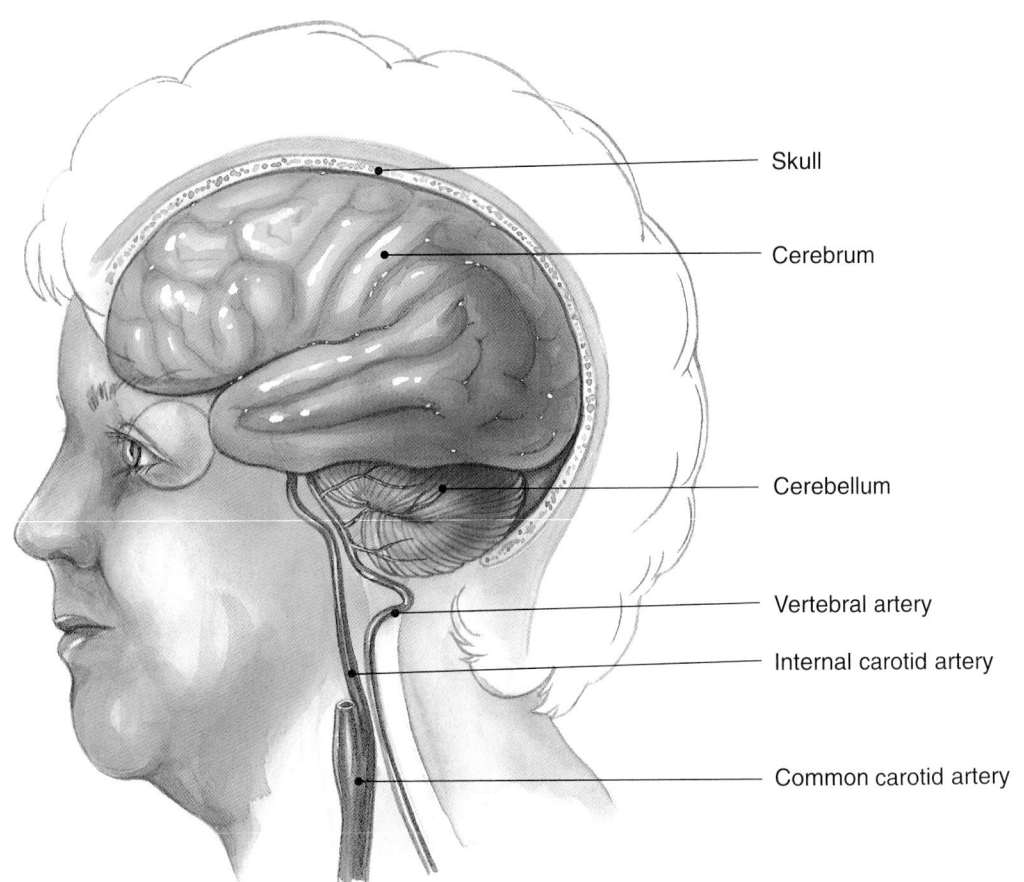

Skull

Cerebrum

Cerebellum

Vertebral artery

Internal carotid artery

Common carotid artery

Brain and Nervous System

The brain is the most complex organ in the body. It is divided into three main sections: the cerebrum, the cerebellum, and the brain stem. The four lobes of the cerebrum coordinate such functions as speech, vision, thought, and memory. The cerebellum controls coordination and balance, and the brain stem maintains the body's vital functions, such as breathing, digestion, heartbeat, and sleep.

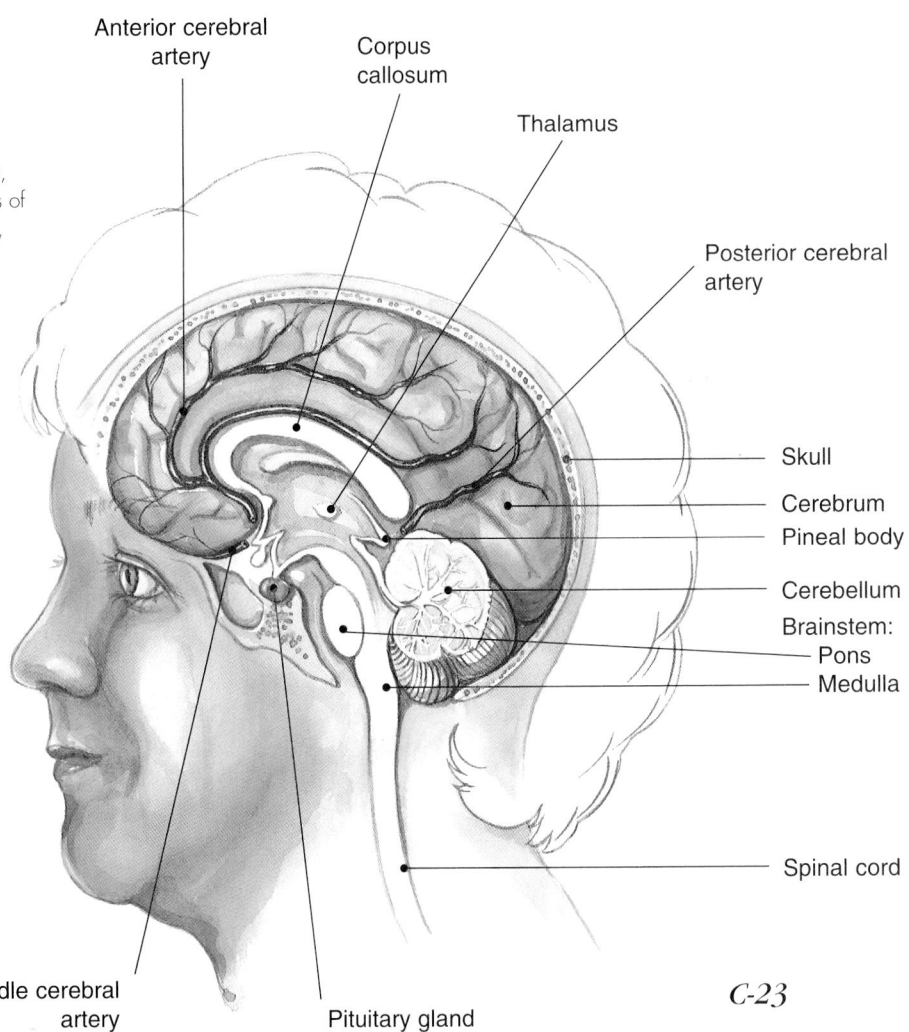

Anterior cerebral artery

Corpus callosum

Thalamus

Posterior cerebral artery

Skull

Cerebrum

Pineal body

Cerebellum

Brainstem:
Pons
Medulla

Spinal cord

Middle cerebral artery

Pituitary gland

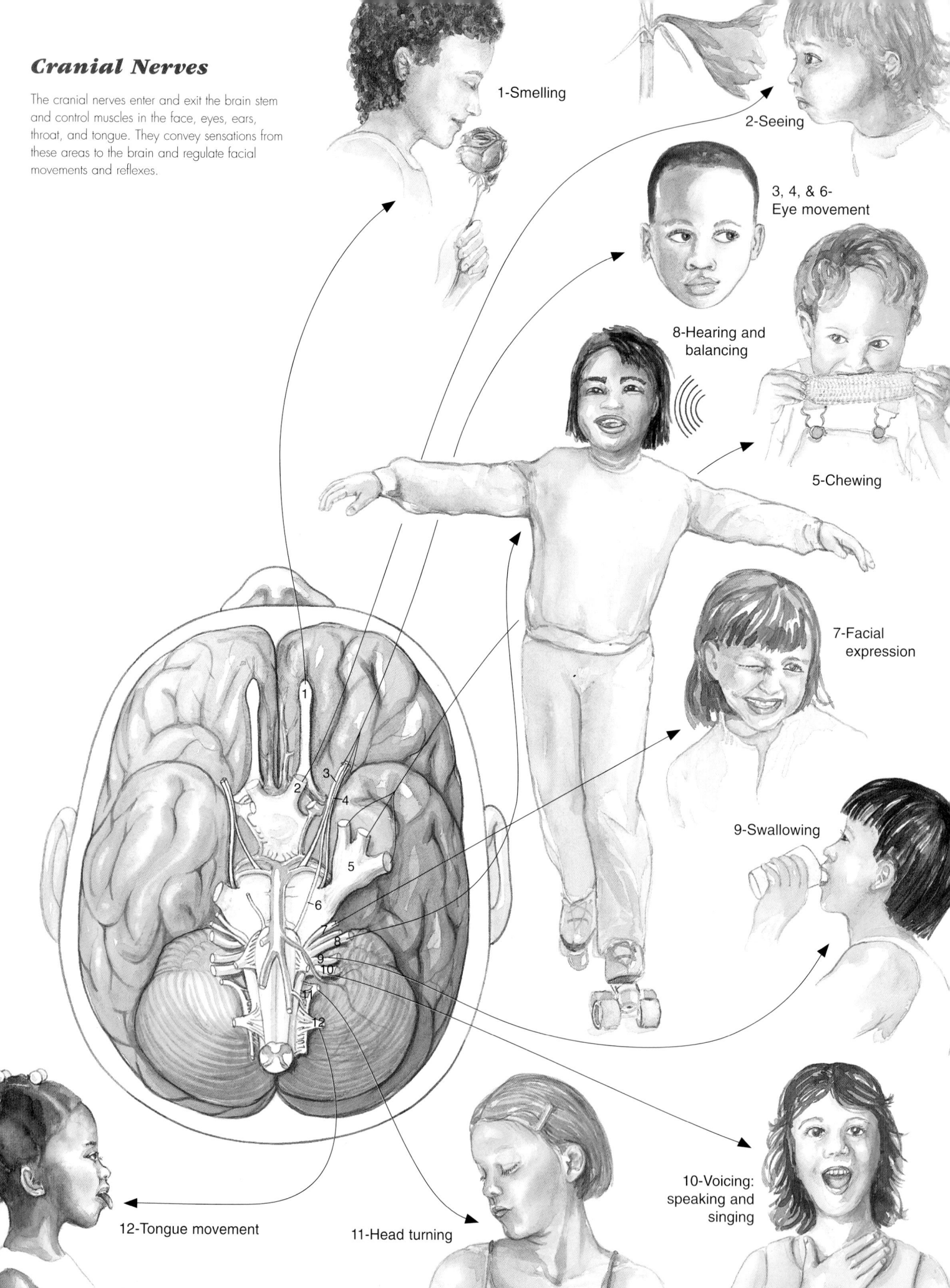

Cranial Nerves

The cranial nerves enter and exit the brain stem and control muscles in the face, eyes, ears, throat, and tongue. They convey sensations from these areas to the brain and regulate facial movements and reflexes.

1-Smelling

2-Seeing

3, 4, & 6- Eye movement

8-Hearing and balancing

5-Chewing

7-Facial expression

9-Swallowing

10-Voicing: speaking and singing

11-Head turning

12-Tongue movement

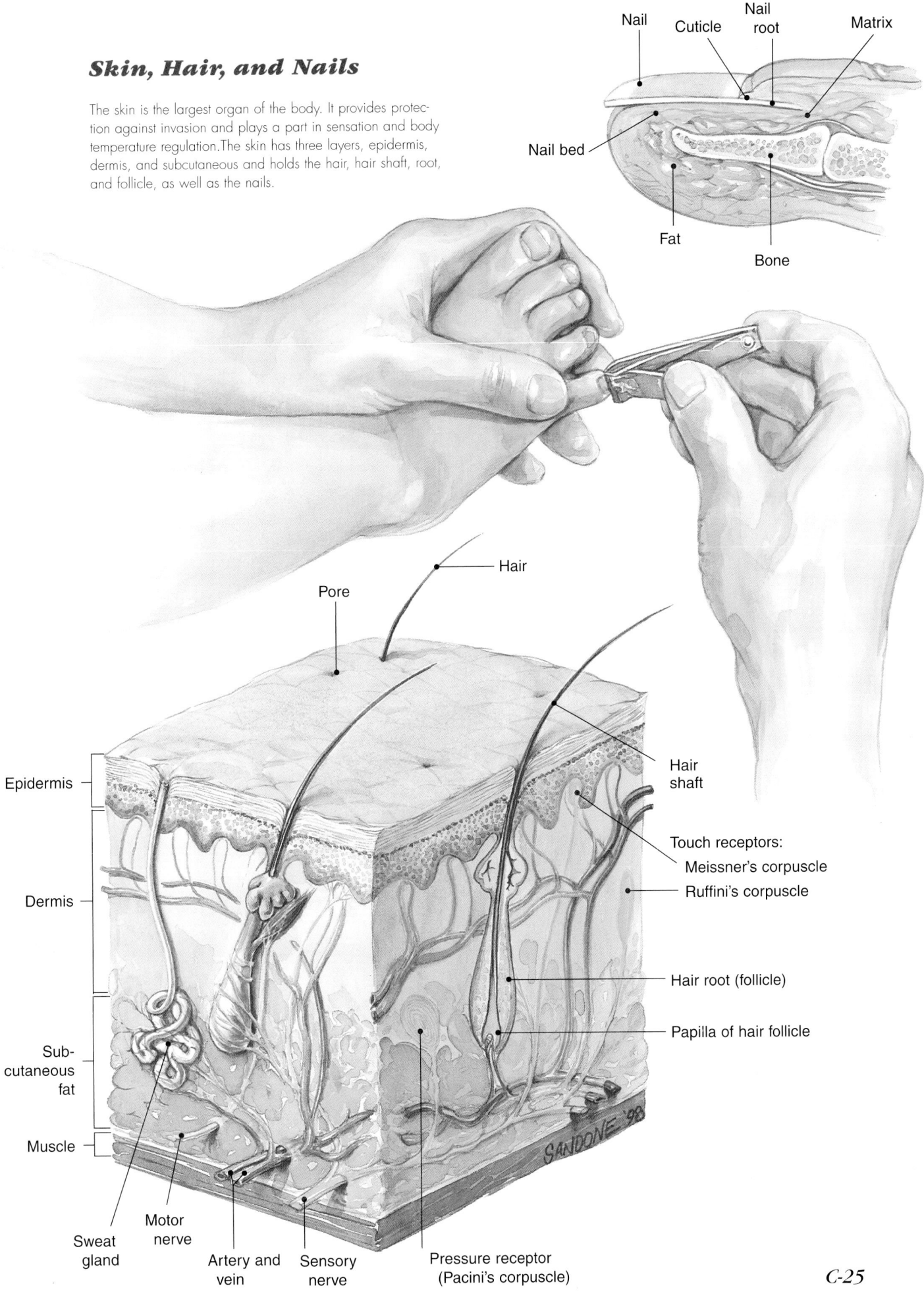

Skin, Hair, and Nails

The skin is the largest organ of the body. It provides protection against invasion and plays a part in sensation and body temperature regulation. The skin has three layers, epidermis, dermis, and subcutaneous and holds the hair, hair shaft, root, and follicle, as well as the nails.

Nail

Cuticle

Nail root

Matrix

Nail bed

Fat

Bone

Hair

Pore

Epidermis

Dermis

Sub-cutaneous fat

Muscle

Hair shaft

Touch receptors:

Meissner's corpuscle

Ruffini's corpuscle

Hair root (follicle)

Papilla of hair follicle

Sweat gland

Motor nerve

Artery and vein

Sensory nerve

Pressure receptor (Pacini's corpuscle)

SANDONE '98

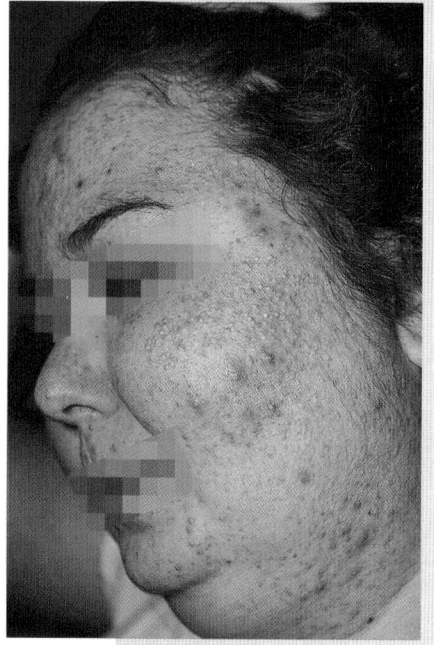

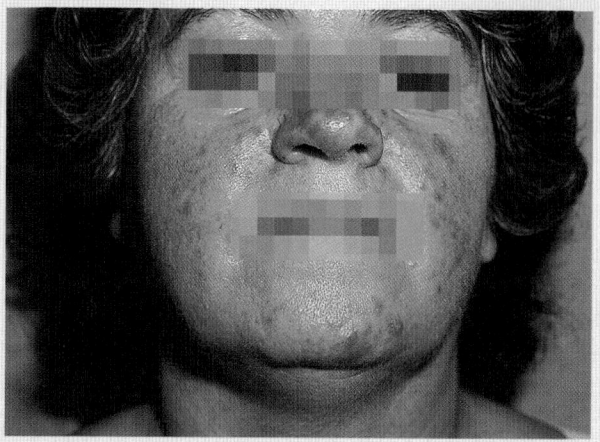

Rosacea is a skin disorder characterized by a ruddy complexion and pimples on the cheeks and nose and occasionally the chin and forehead. It occurs most often in fair-skinned, middle-age adults and is more common in women. (See page 1274.)

Acne, a common skin disease, develops when rising hormone levels during adolescence trigger an overproduction of oil which clogs pores and hair follicles. Pimples (red, inflamed bumps) can form when bacteria living in the skin increase in number in clogged follicles. (See pages 290 and 1272.)

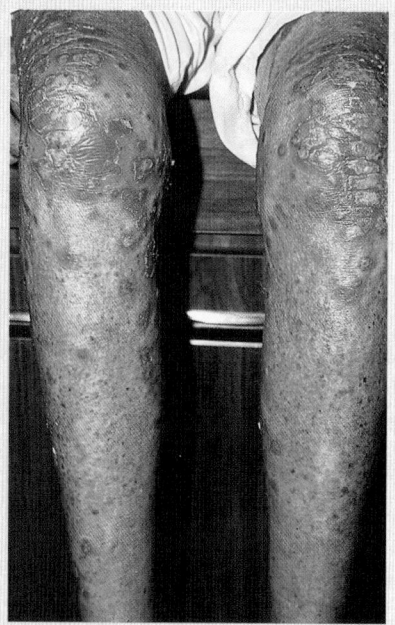

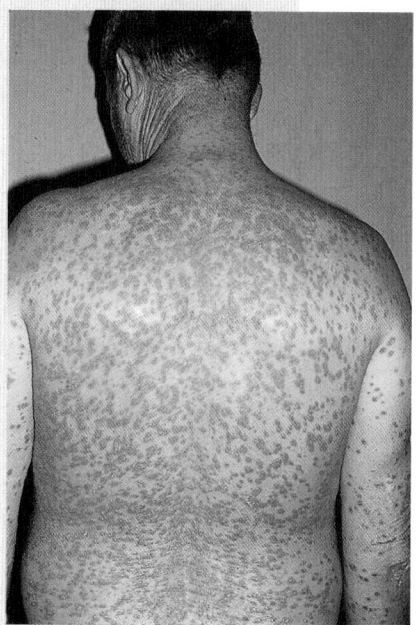

Psoriasis in its most common form is a chronic skin condition marked by inflamed, sharply defined lesions covered with silvery-white scales. In most people, psoriasis appears on the elbows and knees, but it can be more severe, covering the body. (See page 1275.)

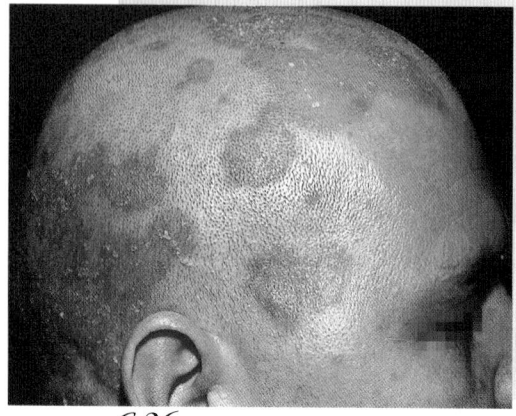

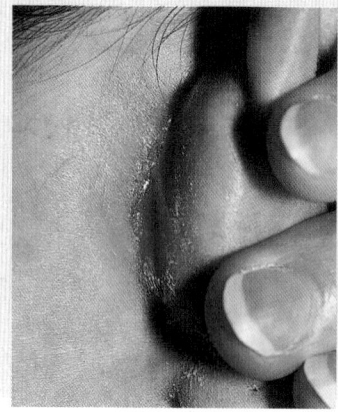

Seborrheic dermatitis is a rash that occurs most frequently on the parts of the body with the largest concentrations of sebaceous (oil) glands including the scalp, the sides of the nose, between the eyebrows, and behind the ears. The rash is characterized by red and flaky skin and a greasy appearance. (See page 1279.)

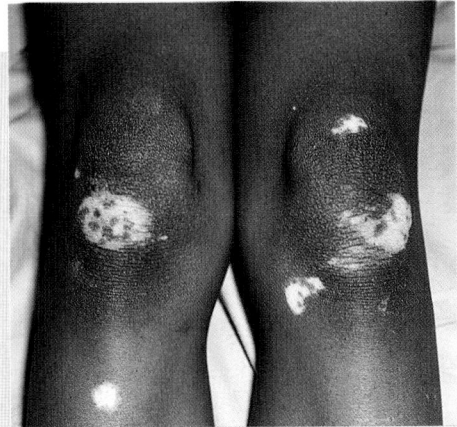

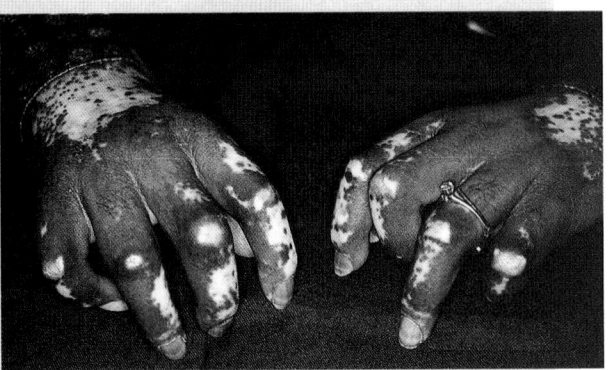

Vitiligo is caused by the loss of pigment-producing cells in the affected areas. It may occur as one or two small patches or large areas of pigment loss. Vitiligo often runs in families, although the exact cause is unknown. (See page 1309.)

Scleroderma is a disease that occurs when the body produces too much collagen, giving large areas of skin a scar-like appearance. The affected skin feels tight, thick, and hardened. (See page 1276).

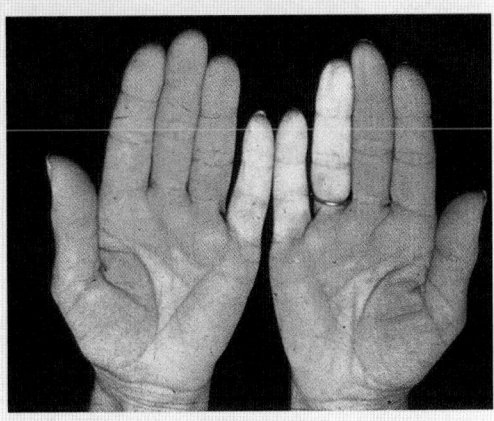

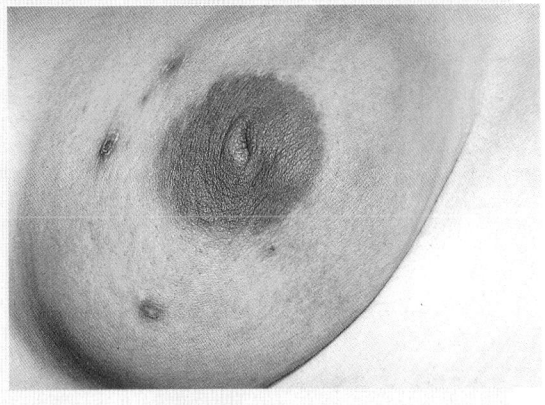

Mastitis is an inflammation of the mammary gland caused by bacterial infection in the milk ducts. Mastitis is most commonly found in breast-feeding mothers and causes the skin of the breast to become red, warm, and tender or painful. The redness and warmth of the breast help to differentiate mastitis from other causes of breast pain. (See page 772.)

Raynaud's phenomenon is not a disease of the skin but rather a circulatory disorder causing the fingers and sometimes toes to become white when exposed to cold temperatures. As the affected extremities warm, they turn a bluish purple and then return to normal color. In primary Raynaud's phenomenon, all of the fingers or toes are affected. This photograph depicts secondary Raynaud's in which just a few fingers change color. (See pages 842 and 1277.)

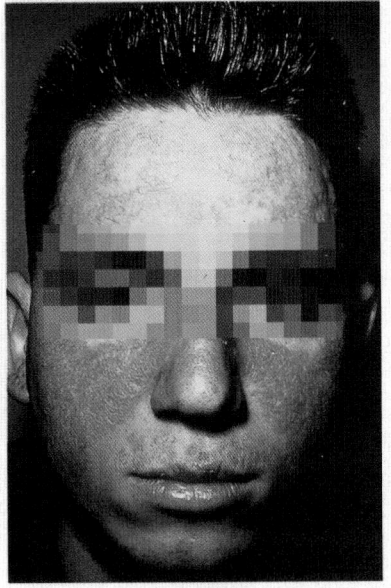

Butterfly rash of lupus. Systemic lupus erythematosus is an autoimmune rheumatic disorder of unknown cause. Lupus involves multiple body systems (systemic), but its effects on the joints and skin are most apparent. The classic red rash of lupus, called a malar or butterfly rash, erupts across the bridge of the nose and cheeks. (See page 642.)

Contact dermatitis is an inflammatory reaction to direct contact with a substance.

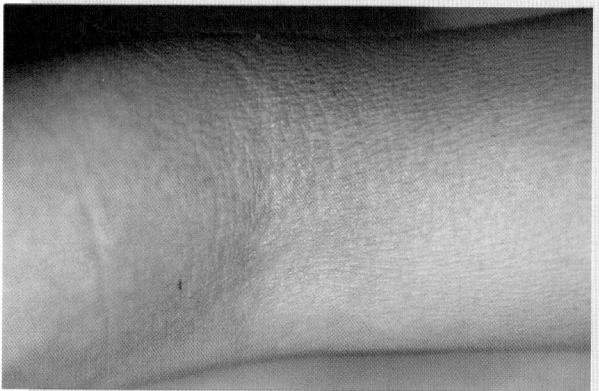

Irritant contact dermatitis. This common type of contact dermatitis occurs when an external substance such as the chemicals found in dishwashing liquids or other cleaning agents irritates the skin. (See page 1290.)

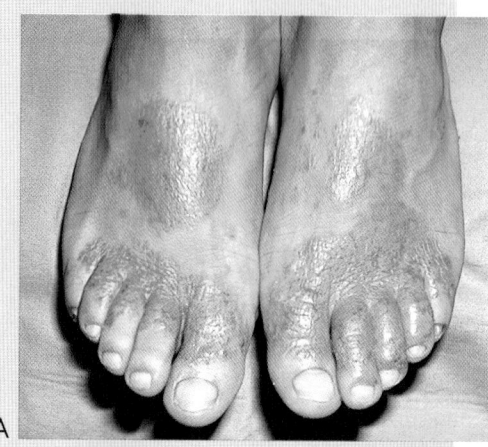

A

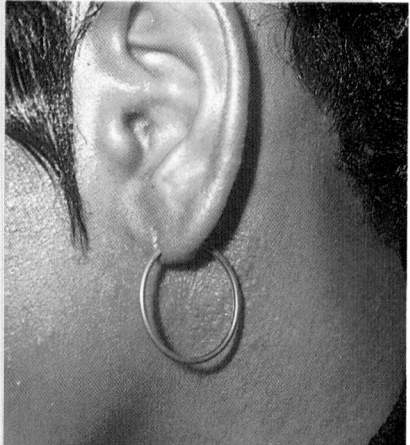

B

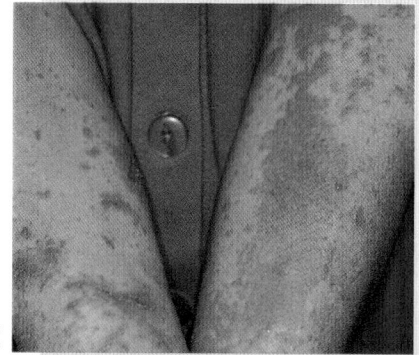

C

Allergic contact dermatitis (A & B) occurs when the body produces an allergic reaction after exposure to a particular substance, such as the nickel found in some jewelry. Allergic contact dermatitis causes itching and dryness. (See page 1290.)

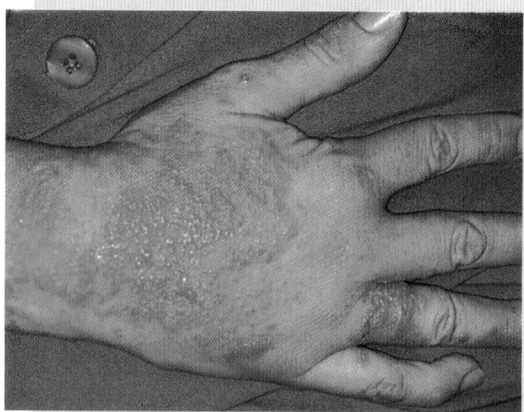

D

Allergic contact dermatitis—poison ivy rash (C & D). A common form of allergic contact dermatitis occurs after exposure to the poison ivy plant. A poison ivy reaction includes swelling, redness, itching, and blistering. (See pages 407, 1290, and 1335.)

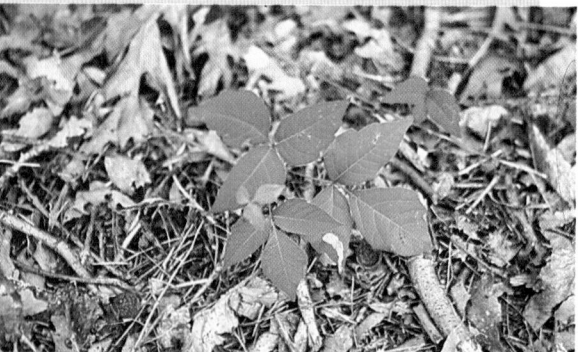

Poison ivy plant

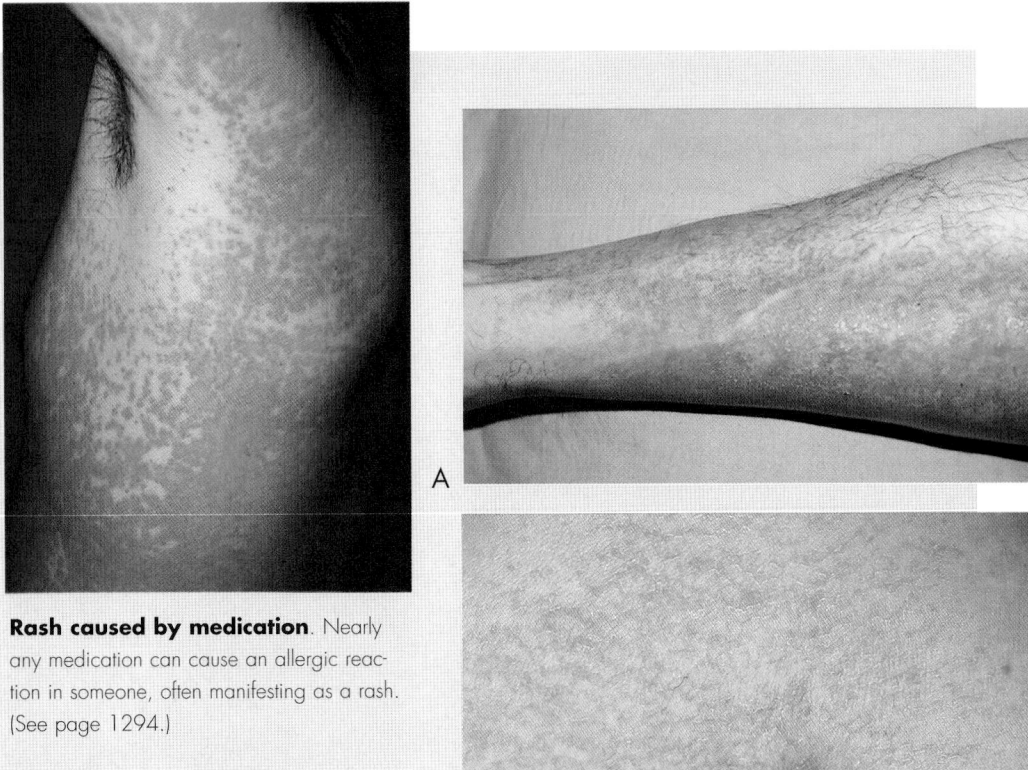

Rash caused by medication. Nearly any medication can cause an allergic reaction in someone, often manifesting as a rash. (See page 1294.)

Atopic dermatitis (allergic eczema) (A & B) is a skin condition characterized by a hereditary tendency to develop allergic reactions that cause dry, itchy, inflamed skin. (See pages 1292 and 1334.)

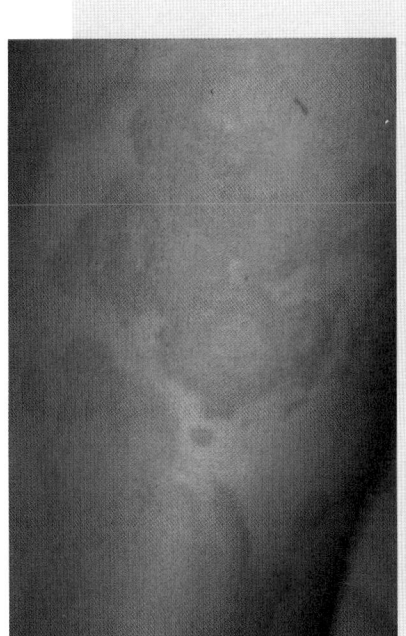
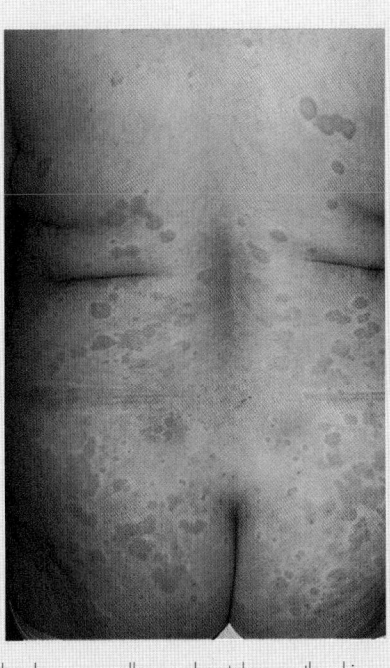
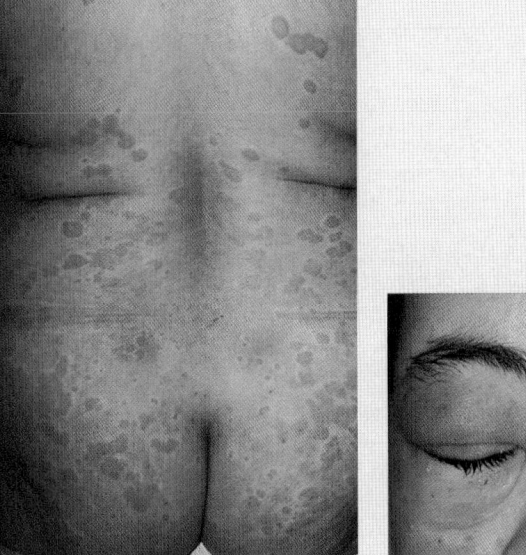
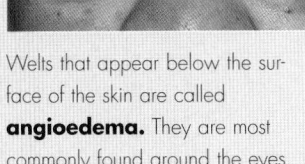

Hives, also known as uticaria or wheals, are swollen, red patches on the skin causing itching and occasionally burning. An individual spot usually lasts less than an hour and never over a day. Hives occur often as the body's allergic reaction to certain medications, infections, insect bites, or foods. (See page 1293.)

Welts that appear below the surface of the skin are called **angioedema.** They are most commonly found around the eyes.

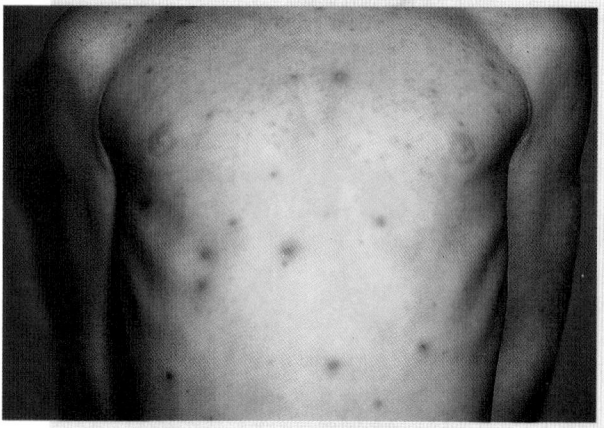 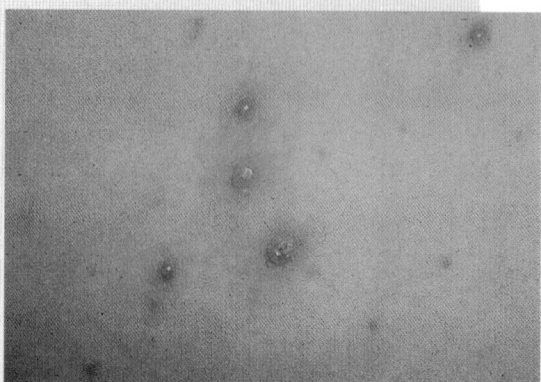

Chickenpox, also known as varicella, is a highly contagious viral illness with a rash of itchy, red bumps. The bumps develop into blisters and then rupture to become crusty sores. (See pages 238 and 883.)

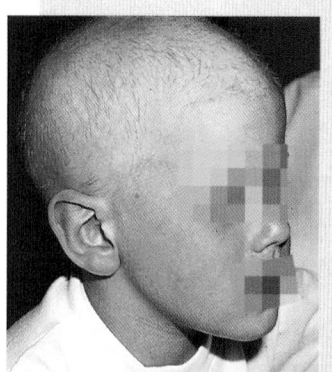 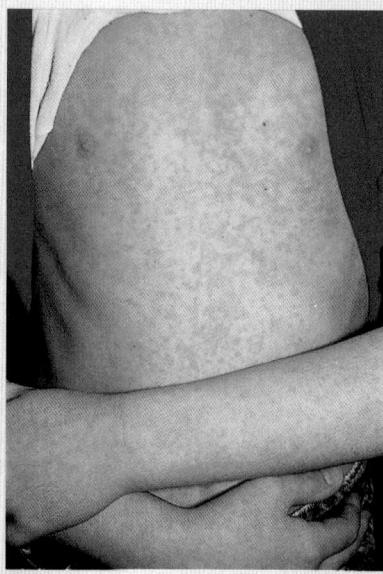 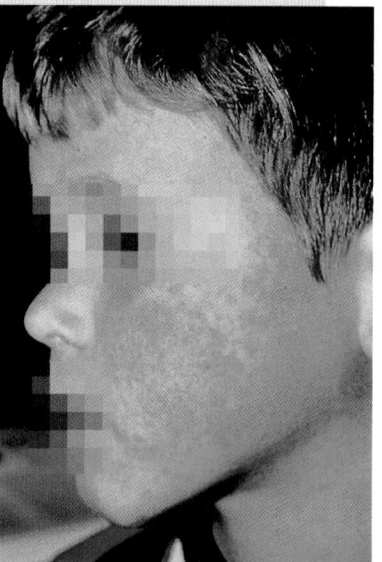

Erythema infectiosum (fifth disease). The onset of this viral disease is characterized in children by fiery red cheeks. A few days later a red rash that comes and goes develops on the body. (See pages 239 and 882.)

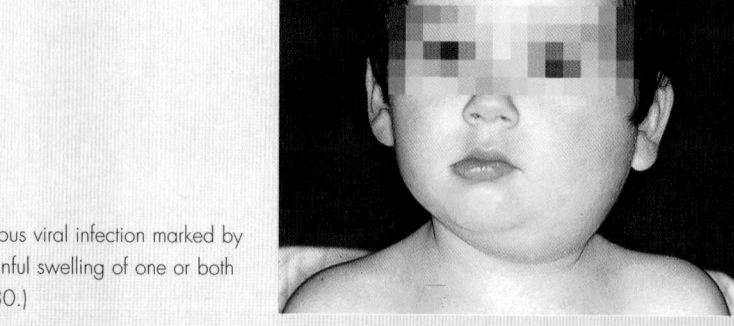

Mumps is a contagious viral infection marked by fever, fatigue, and painful swelling of one or both cheeks. (See page 880.)

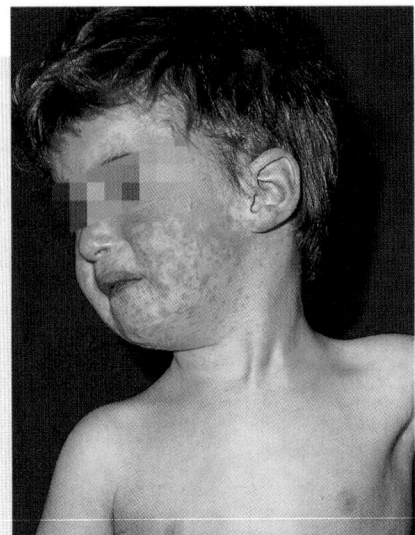

Rubella (German measles), unlike rubeola, often has no accompanying rash. When a rash does appear, it is usually a fine, pink rash showing first on the face, then on the trunk, and finally on the arms and legs. Other symptoms include mild fever, sore throat, and tender lymph glands at the back of the neck or behind the ears. (See page 881.)

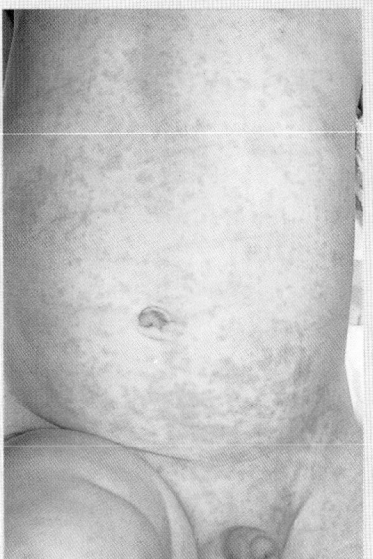

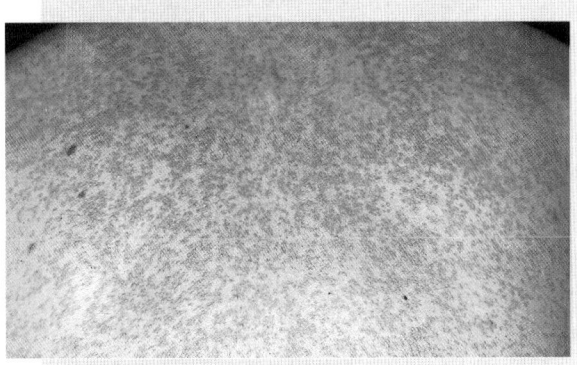

Rubeola (red measles) is a viral infection causing cold-like symptoms, with malaise and fever. About 4 days after the initial onset of symptoms, a blotchy red, slightly raised rash begins on the face, moves down to the trunk, and then to the arms, legs, and palms and soles of the feet. (See page 879.)

Roseola infantum is caused by a virus and occurs most frequently in the first year of life. It has symptoms of unexplained fever and a fleeting, pinkish, spotty rash that occurs in 10 to 20 percent of affected babies. (See pages 212 and 883.)

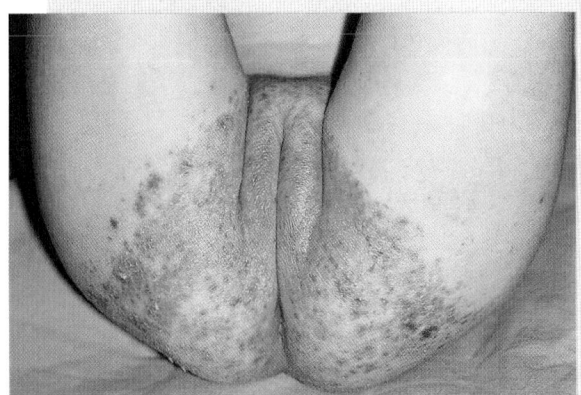

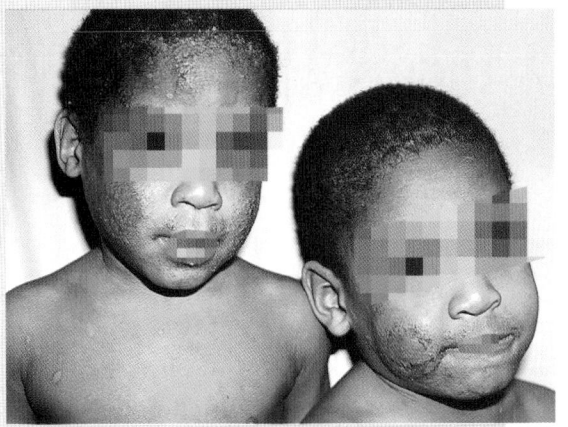

Diaper rash. Nearly all babies will develop diaper dermatitis (diaper rash) at some time during infancy. Many causes contribute to this rough, red, skin irritation including the chronic moisture in the diaper area and the presence of urine and stool. (See page 204.)

Infantile eczema. The first signs of infantile eczema generally appear as a rash on the face, arms, legs, and trunk. Dry, scaly, red patches appear that are intensely itchy. Scratching may lead to oozing and crusting. (See page 212.)

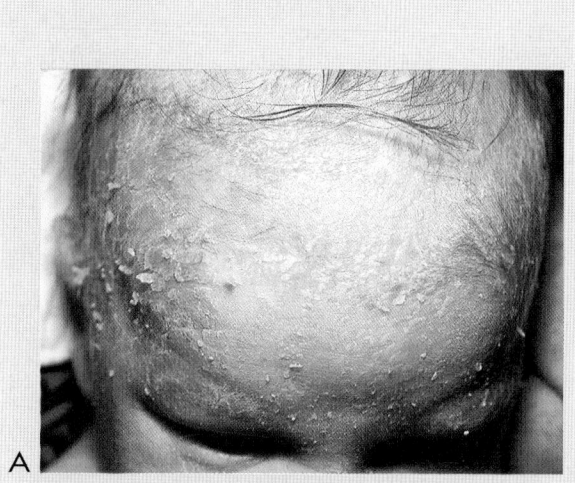
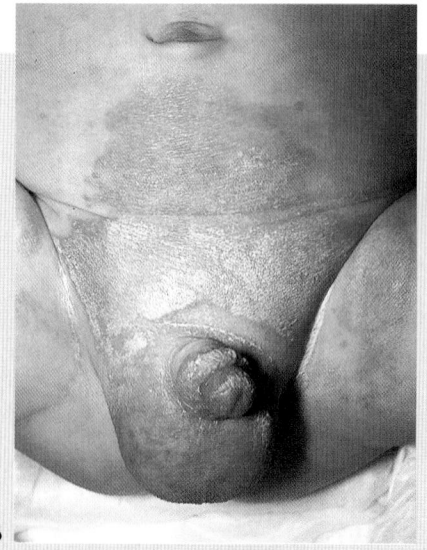

A   B

Cradle cap, or seborrheic dermatitis, is a skin condition common in newborns that is characterized by dry, scaly or crusty skin that may occur in patches or all over the scalp (A). It may extend down the forehead to the eyebrows and ears. Seborrheic dermatitis may also be found in creases under the arms or neck and in the diaper area (B). (See page 182.)

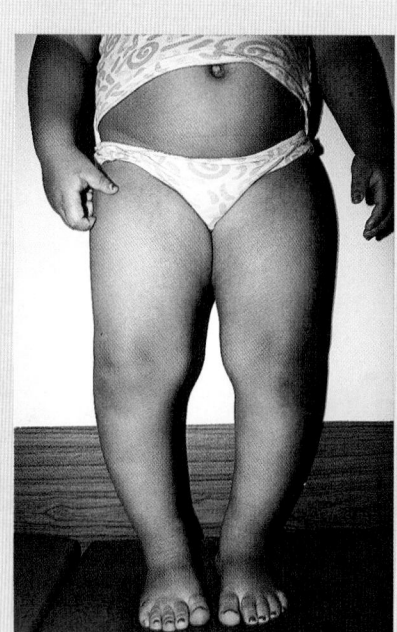

A

Bowed legs (A) and knock knees (B). These conditions present at birth are normal phases of development that correct themselves and are rarely a problem in otherwise healthy children. (See page 216.)

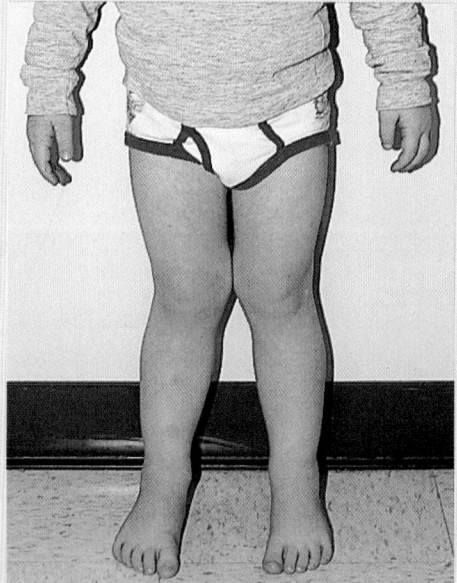

B

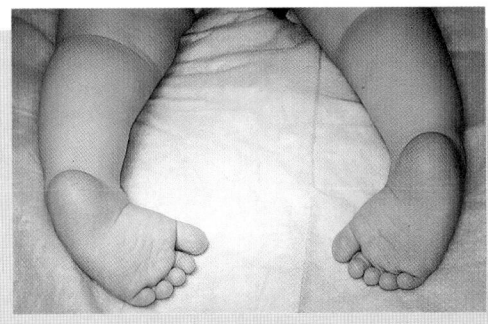
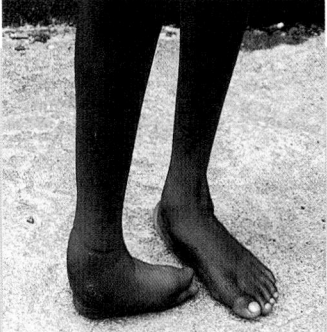

A   B

Clubfoot is one of the most common birth abnormalities of the feet and with early, skilled care usually results in normal walking and running ability. (A) With clubfoot, the foot turns inward toward the other leg and the side of the foot faces down. (B) If uncorrected the child would eventually walk on the side of the foot. (See page 215.)

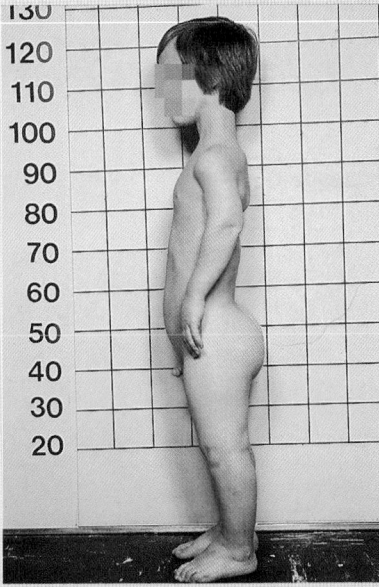

Dwarfism. The most common form of dwarfism, or skeletal dysplasia, is achondroplasia. The trunk is short and the limbs are disproportionally shorter. (See pages 217 and 659.)

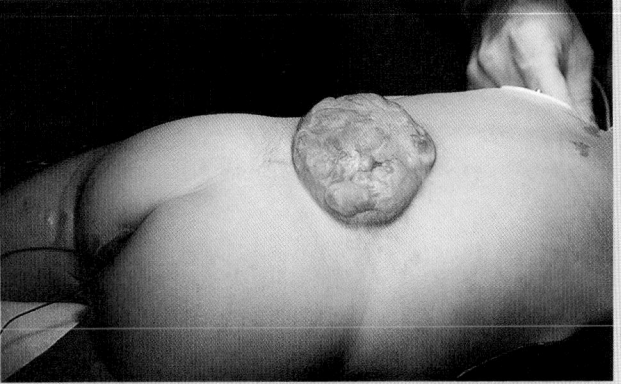

Spina bifida. At birth the spinal cord is normally enclosed beneath the skin within soft covering tissue layers (meninges) and the bones of the spine. Spina bifida occurs when the closure is incomplete. The opening can be very tiny or large enough so that part of the spinal cord and its coverings protrude (myelomeningocele). (See pages 223 and 472.)

Birthmarks

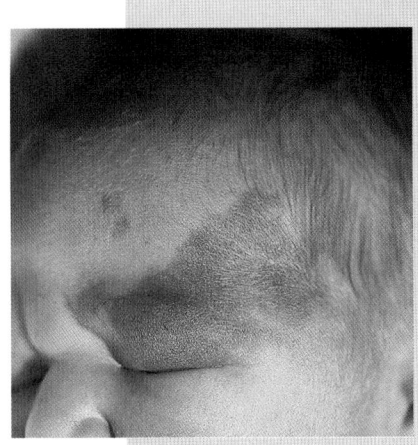

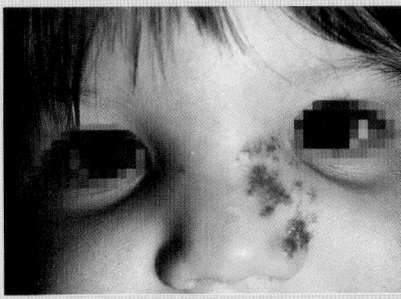

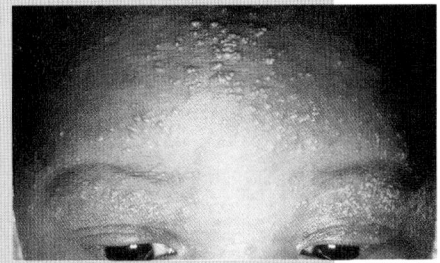

Strawberry hemangioma is a red, slightly raised lesion, which increases in size in infancy but gradually shrinks and disappears by age 7 to 9 years. (See pages 181 and 1297.)

Milia are miniature cysts present on a baby's face at birth or within the first few month of life. They disappear without treatment. (See page 182.)

Port-wine stain is a flat patch of pink, red or purplish skin most commonly found on the face, side of the neck, or an arm or leg. (See pages 181 and 1297.)

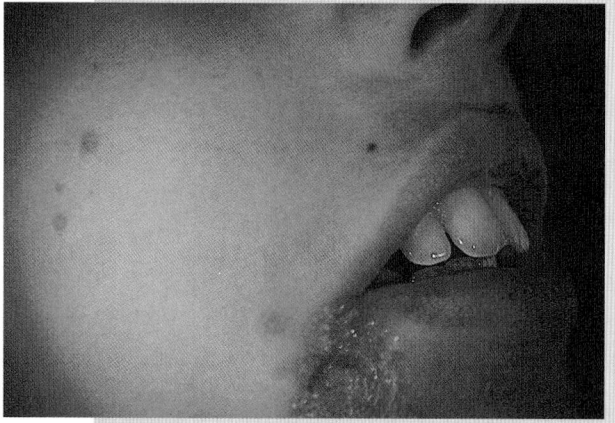
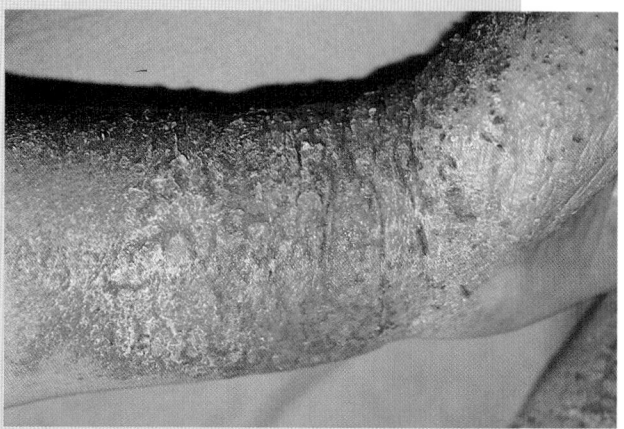

Impetigo typically begins as small blisters that rupture easily forming a sticky yellow crusting. Impetigo is most common in young children and appears most frequently on the face, scalp, arms, legs, and sometimes at the site of a cut, scratch, or insect bite. (See pages 239 and 1281.)

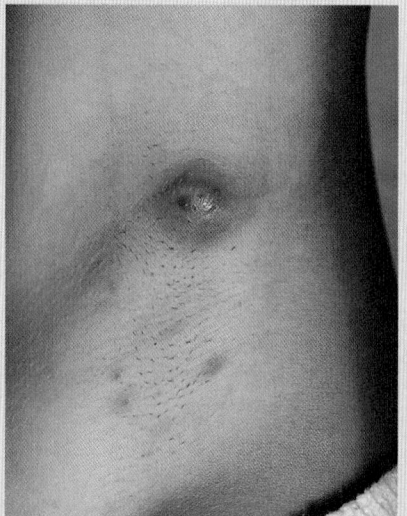
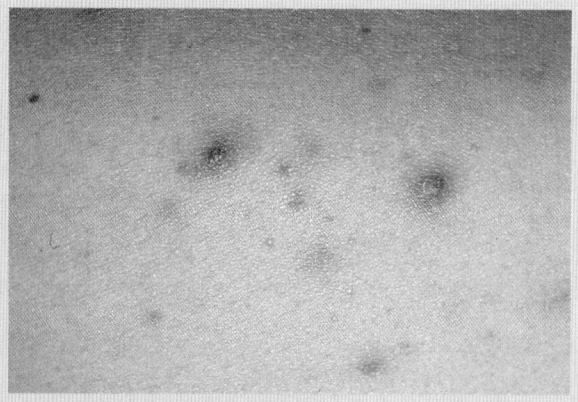

A **boil** is a bacterial skin abscess that starts in a hair follicle. It begins as a small, firm, tender nodule and turns shiny and bright red as it enlarges. Eventually the boil ruptures, draining pus, and subsides. (See page 1281.)

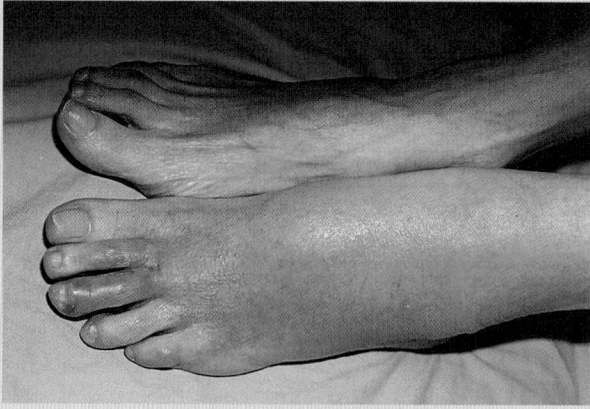

Cellulitis occurs when bacteria enters the skin through an opening such as a cut, scrape, or bite causing a skin infection. The affected skin is red, swollen, warm, and tender or painful. (See page 1282.)

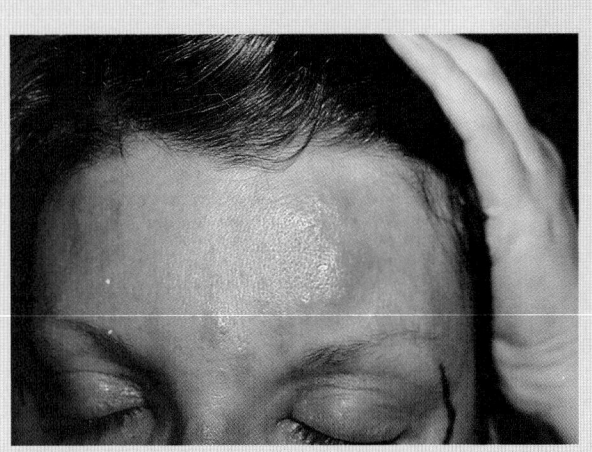
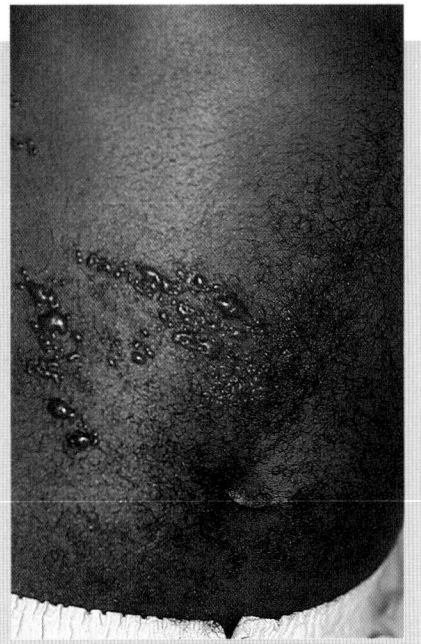

Shingles, also known as herpes zoster, is caused by the same virus that causes chickenpox. The virus causes a red rash that evolves into multiple clustered blisters accompanied by a tingling sensation that may turn to burning or severe pain. (See page 1284.)

A **wart** is a small flesh-colored, pink, white, or tan bump on the skin, usually found on the hands or feet. Warts are caused by the human papillomavirus (HPV) which is transmitted through direct or indirect contact. Warts are usually painless unless they occur on weight-bearing portions of the feet. (See page 1286.)

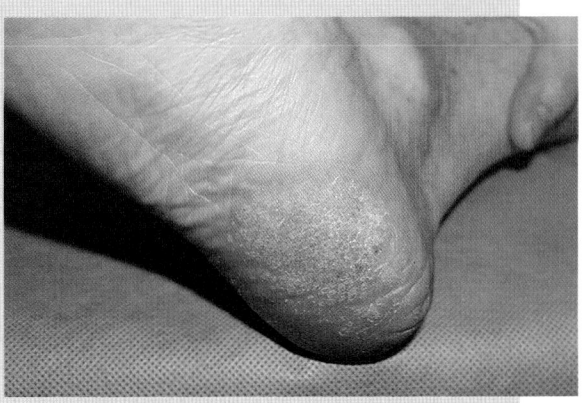

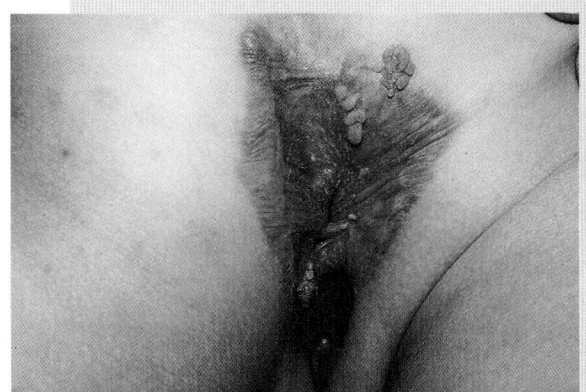

Genital warts are caused by a different strain of the same virus that causes common warts. They are small, flesh-colored or pink bumps that occur on the genitals or anus. Genital warts are sexually transmitted. (See pages 865 and 1286.)

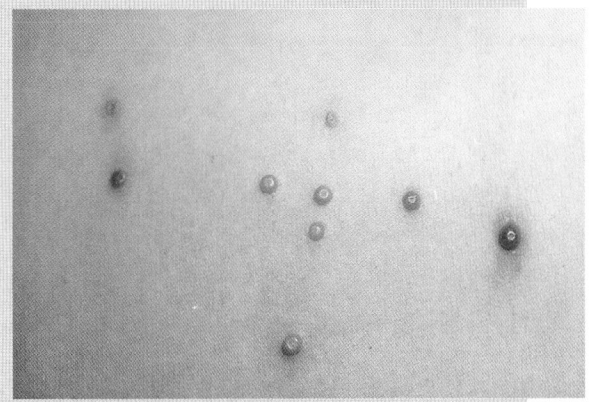

Molluscum contagiosum is a contagious viral infection characterized by pea-sized, flesh-colored or seemingly translucent growths, often mistaken for warts. There are usually multiple lesions. (See page 1285.)

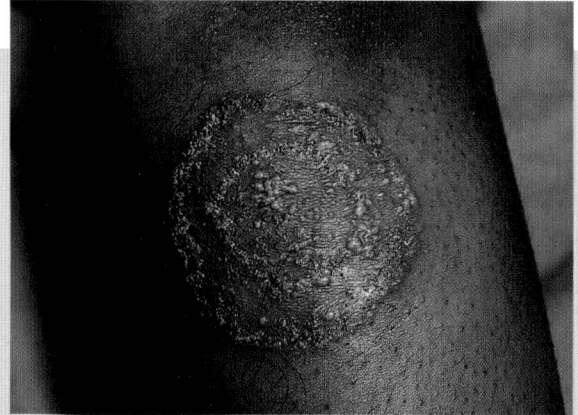

Ringworm, also known as tinea corporis, is a fungal skin infection that has nothing to do with worms. It causes a red, ring-shaped, itchy patch that can expand to several inches in diameter with a slightly elevated scaly border. (See page 1288.)

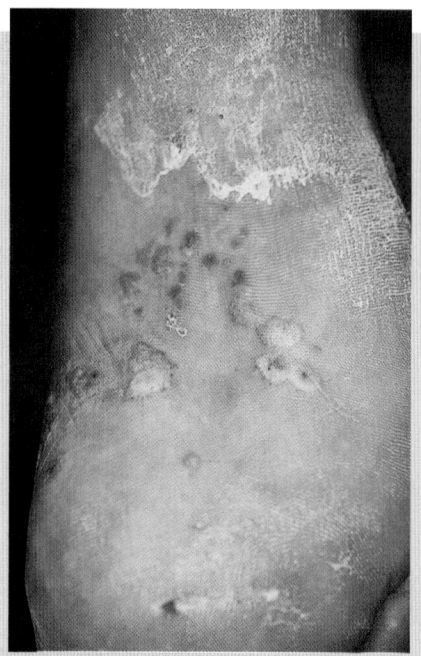

A

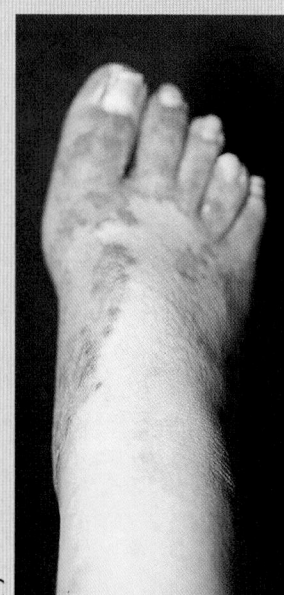

B

C

Athlete's foot (A–C), also known as tinea pedis, is a fungal infection involving the toe web spaces and/or the soles of the feet. It causes scaling, cracking, and flaking of the skin between the toes, scaling and redness on the soles and sides of the feet, itching, and occasionally burning. (See page 1287.)

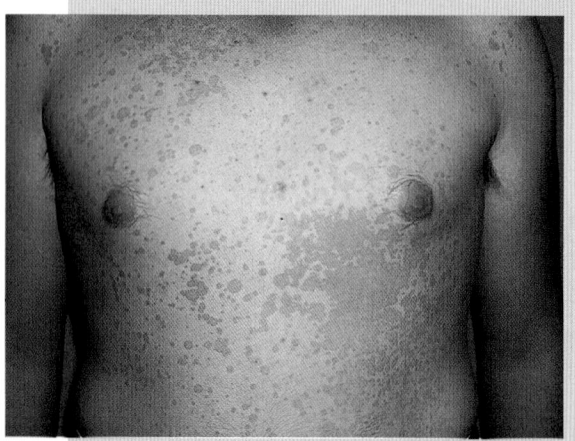

Tinea versicolor is a mild skin infection caused by a slow-growing yeast. This yeast can multiply in areas of the body that have many oil or sebaceous glands, such as the upper chest, back, and neck. It is characterized by multiple pink or tan, oval, scaly spots causing mild itching. (See page 1289.)

A **nevus**, or mole, is a spot on the skin, usually round and symmetrical with a sharply defined border and uniform color. It can be flat or raised like a dome or bead of water. (See page 1296.)

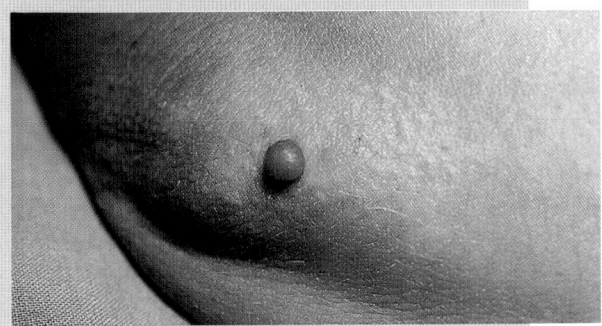

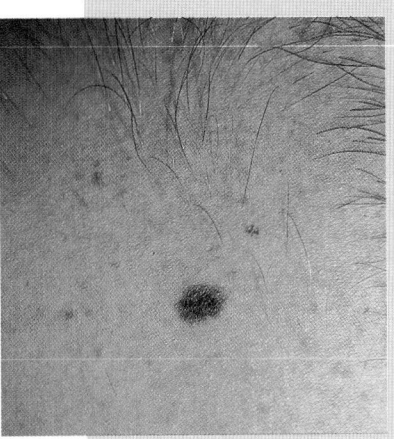

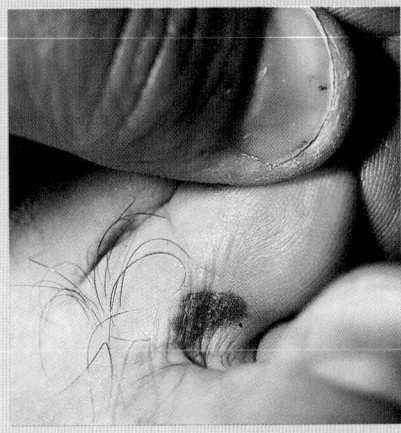

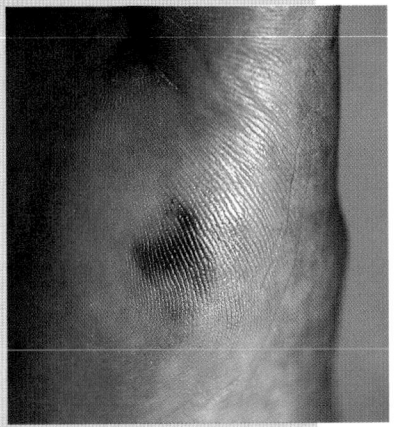

Dysplastic nevus. Moles with an increased chance of developing into cancer are called dysplastic. These moles are more irregular in shape with less defined borders and less even color. These moles should be inspected monthly for changes. (See page 1296.)

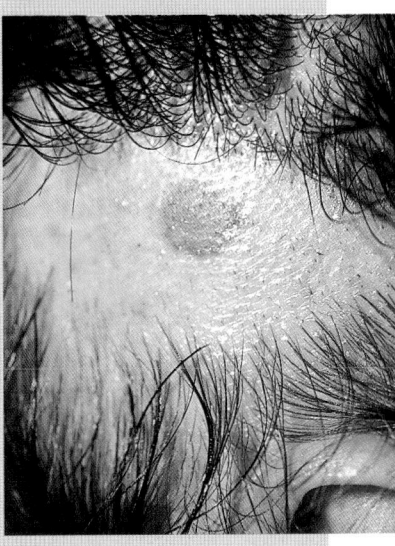

Cherry angiomas are clusters of small, dilated, red blood vessels visible beneath the skin. They may be as small as a pinhead or as large as an eraser on a pencil. (See page 1296.)

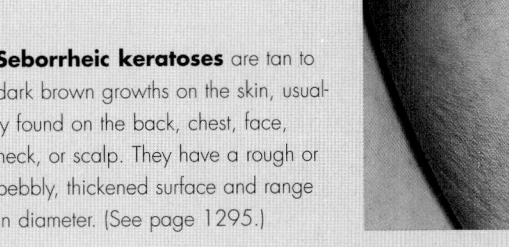

Seborrheic keratoses are tan to dark brown growths on the skin, usually found on the back, chest, face, neck, or scalp. They have a rough or pebbly, thickened surface and range in diameter. (See page 1295.)

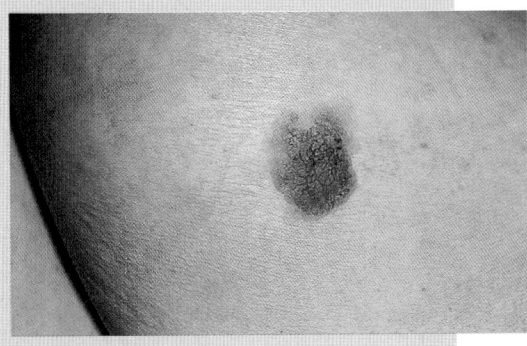

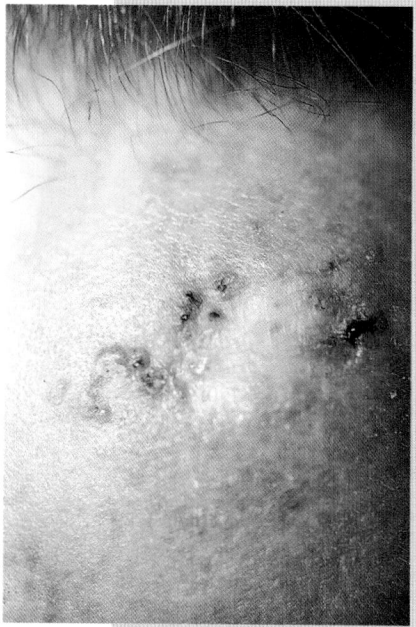
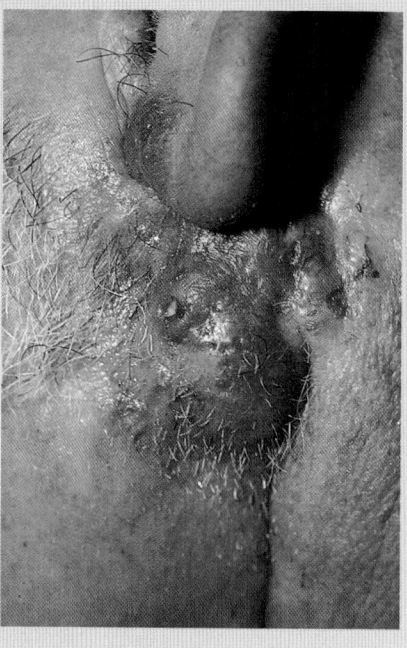
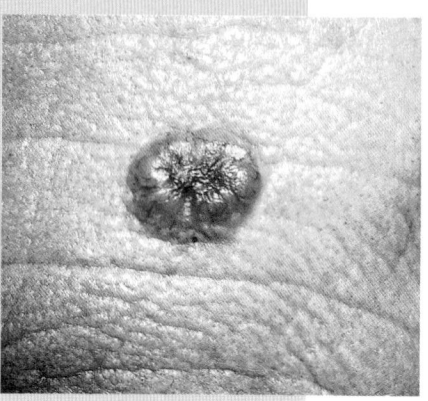

Basal cell carcinoma can appear as a small, smooth or waxy-appearing bump that grows slowly. It can be whitish to pink in color and may become an ulcer or sore. (See pages 1300 and 1358.)

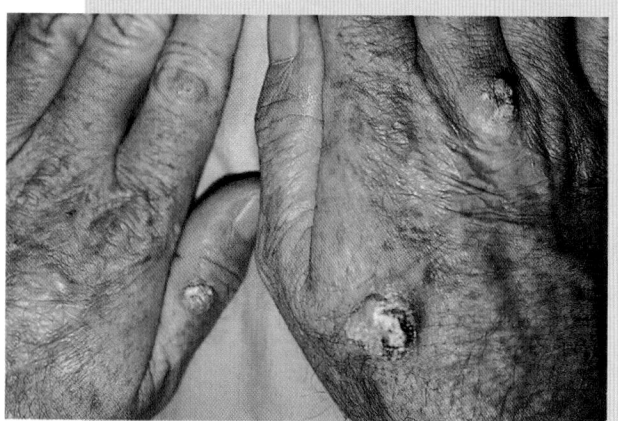
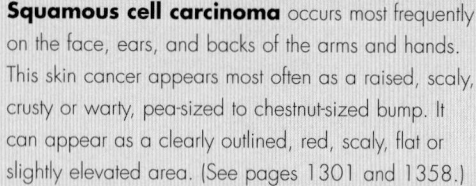
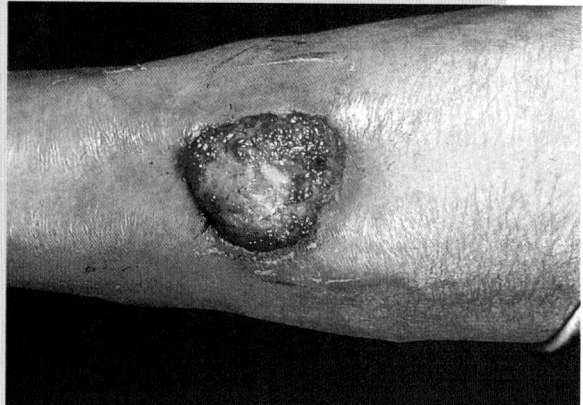

Squamous cell carcinoma occurs most frequently on the face, ears, and backs of the arms and hands. This skin cancer appears most often as a raised, scaly, crusty or warty, pea-sized to chestnut-sized bump. It can appear as a clearly outlined, red, scaly, flat or slightly elevated area. (See pages 1301 and 1358.)

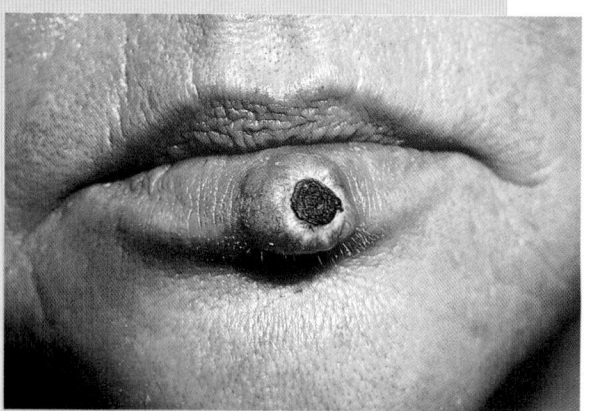

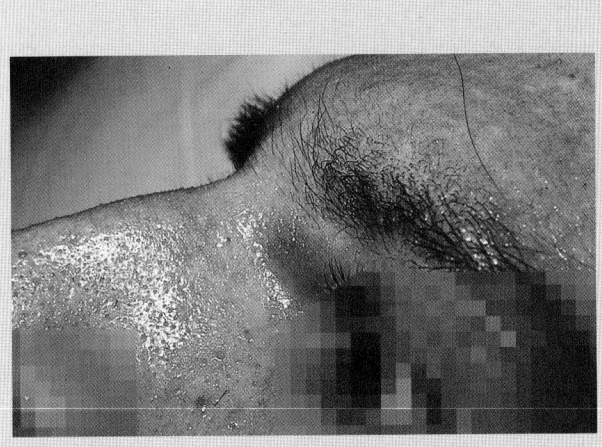
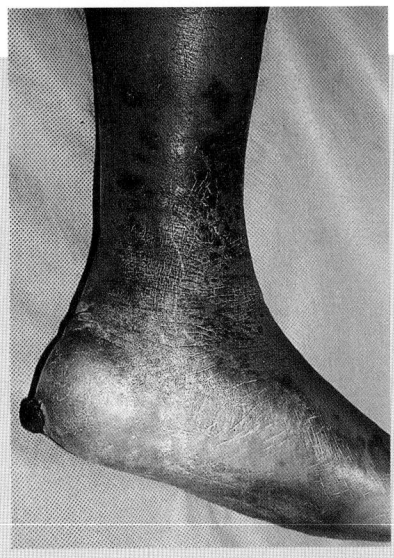

Kaposi's sarcoma is a cancer of the skin appearing most frequently in AIDS patients. It appears as a flat patch or pea-sized or larger bump with a bruise-like coloring. (See page 1303.)

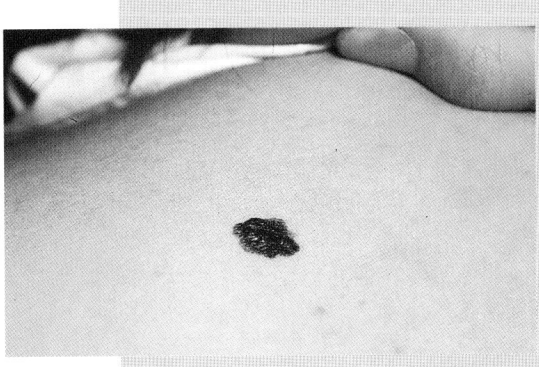
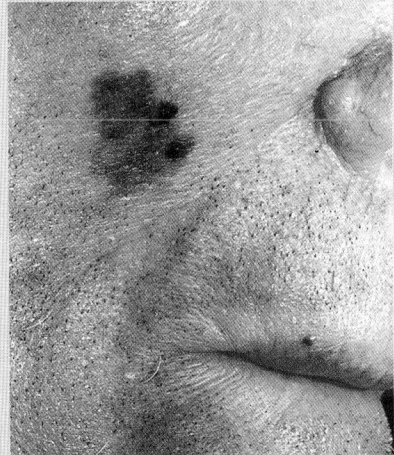
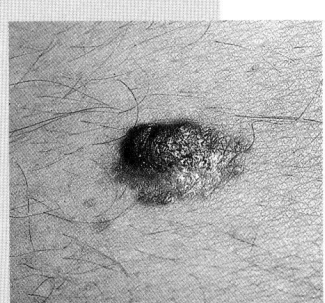
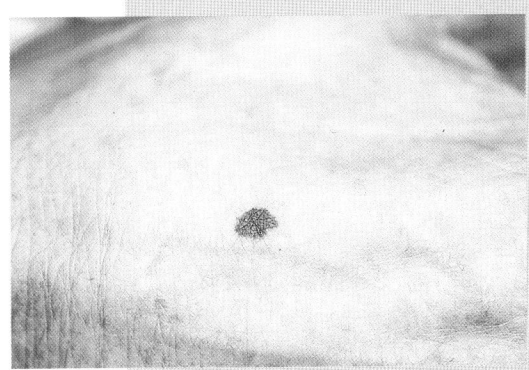
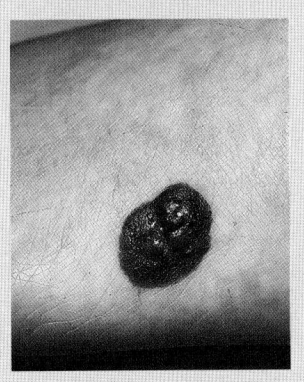
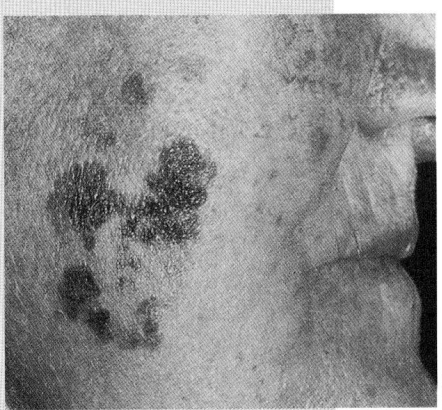

Melanoma is the least common but most dangerous of the skin cancers. Melanoma develops from melanocytes, the cells that produce pigment in the skin. Although melanomas may appear within normal skin, nearly one-third develop in a pre-existing mole or other dark spot. Moles should be checked periodically for changes in Asymmetry, Border, Color, or Diameter (ABCD's). (See pages 1302 and 1358.) If a mole has an irregular shape or hazy edges, varies in color, or changes in size, it should be examined for melanoma.

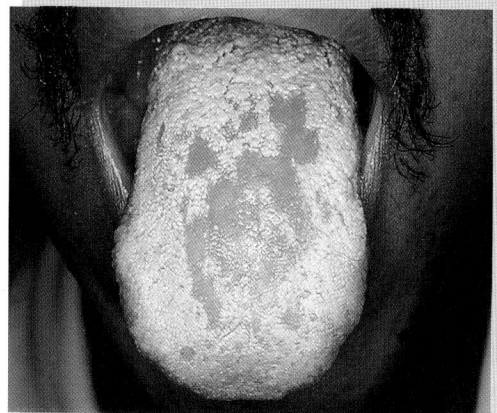 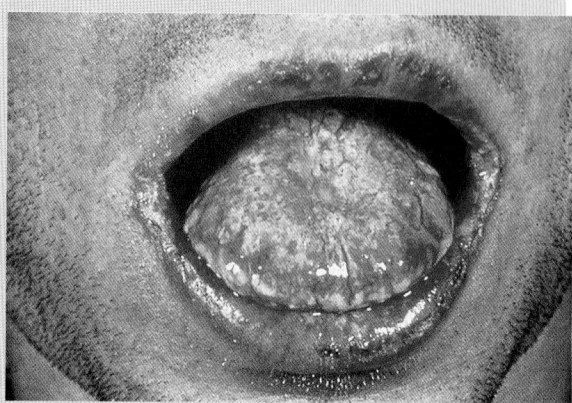

Oral candidiasis (thrush) is a fungal infection of the mouth caused by the yeast fungus *Candida albicans*. Many people carry this yeast in the gastrointestinal tract normally but under certain conditions it can overgrow and cause disease. Thrush appears as painful, white, elevated patches on the tongue and lining of the mouth that can be wiped away easily. (See pages 184 and 605.)

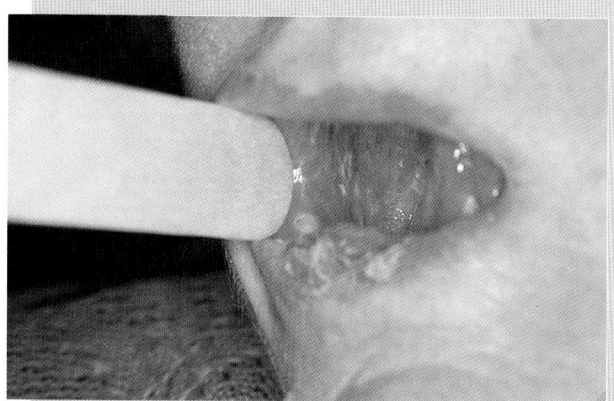

Oral lichen planus is characterized by pale bumps, a lacy white network, and shiny, raised, red patches on the inner cheeks and tongue. It may be triggered by emotional stress, reaction to medication, or in association with cigarette smoking. (See page 608.)

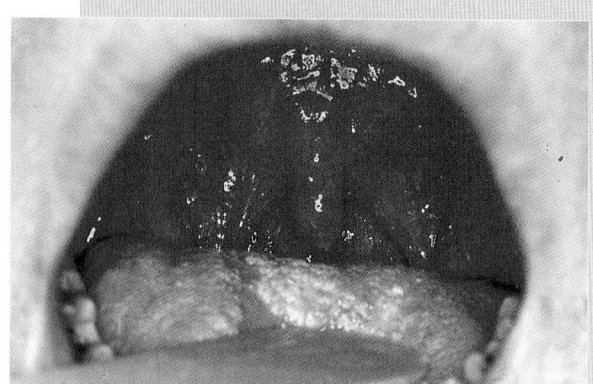 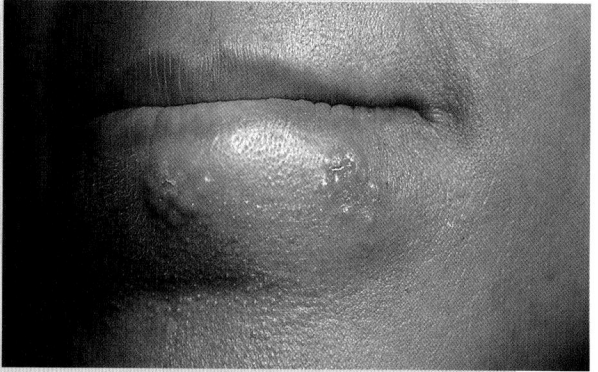

Strep throat. The most common cause of pharyngitis (sore throat) is a bacterial infection commonly known as strep throat. The throat is red; tonsils are swollen and often white patches are present. (See pages 240 and 592.)

Cold sores. Herpes simplex virus is a member of the herpes virus family, which causes chickenpox and shingles. Under certain conditions, such as ultraviolet light, fever, or impairment of the immune system, the virus can erupt into what are commonly called cold sores or fever blisters. A tingling sensation may precede this outbreak of clusters of small, painful blisters on the lip. (See pages 603 and 1283.)

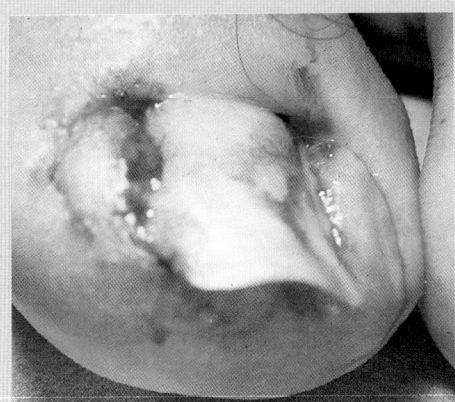

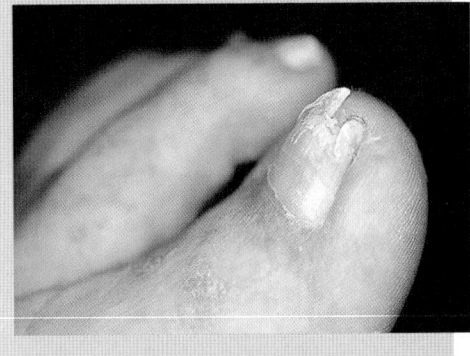

Ingrown toenail occurs when a corner of the toenail (often of the big toe) grows into the surrounding skin, piercing the skin and causing redness, swelling, pain, and occasionally a pus discharge. This case of ingrown toenail has become infected. (See page 1324.)

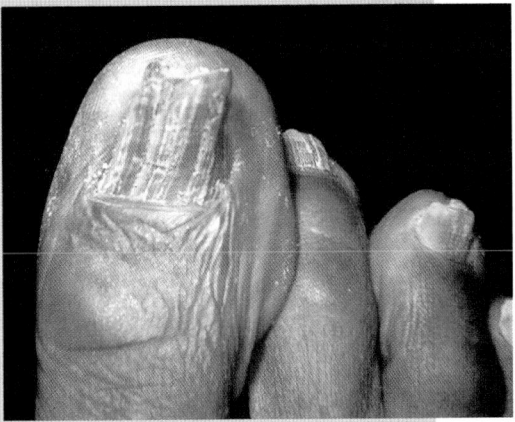

Onychomycosis is a fungal infection of the nail causing discoloration and thickening of the nail, separation of the nail from the nail bed, and itching and flaking of nearby skin. (See page 1320.)

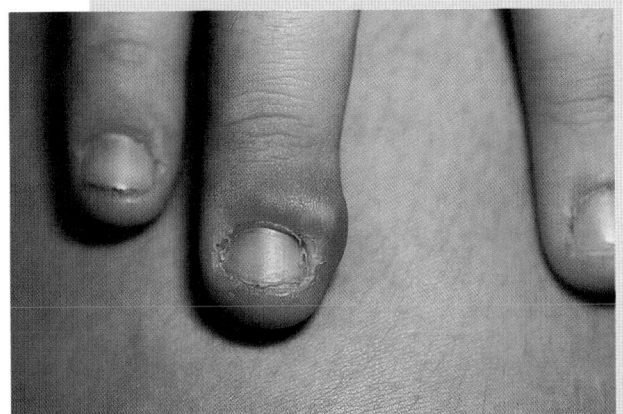

Paronychia is a bacterial infection of the skin adjacent to the nail causing tenderness and pain, redness, and bulging. (See page 1322.)

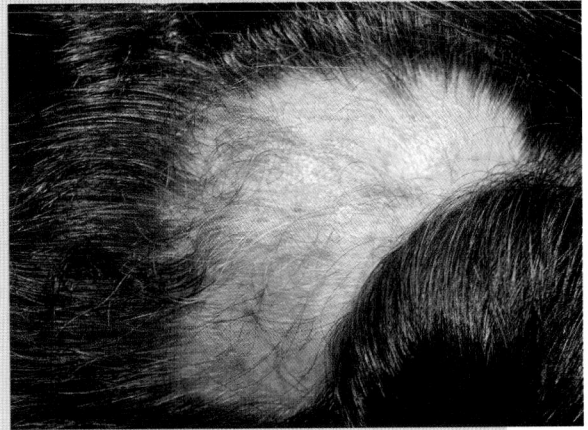

Alopecia areata is most commonly one or more patches of hair loss on the scalp or elsewhere on the body. In rare cases, it can cause a total loss of body hair. (See page 1318.)

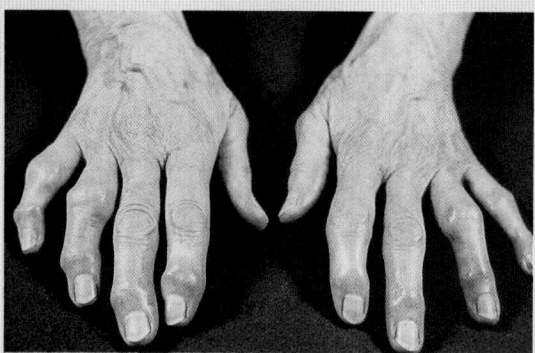

In **osteoarthritis**, the most common form of arthritis, the wearing away of the slick cartilage surface that coats the bone ends occurs in conjunction with the new growth of bone spurs (also called osteophytes). Although the bony spurs may deform the external appearance of the hands and make the joints stiff and painful, this type of arthritis rarely causes significant crippling. (See page 651).

Gout is an inflammatory disease of joints caused by the deposition of needle-like crystals of uric acid in the joints. Gout occurs most often in the first joint of the big toe, where it joins the foot, but it can affect other large joints, such as the ankles and knees. Gout can cause intense pain and redness and swelling of the affected joints. (See page 652.)

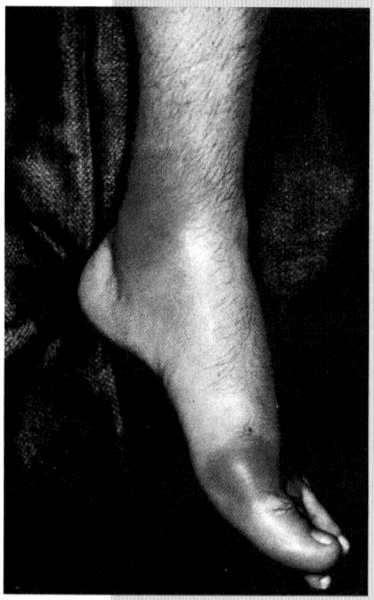

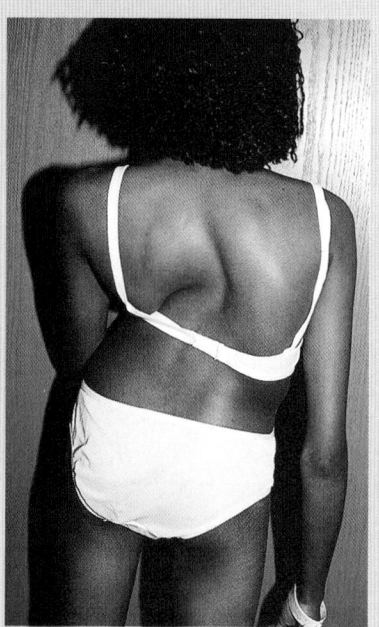

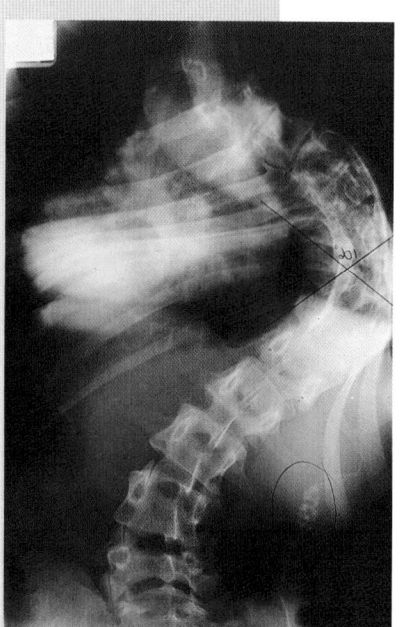

Scoliosis. A normal spine curves gently in several places when viewed from the side but should run straight when viewed from the back. Sometimes, more commonly in adolescent girls than in boys, the spine develops a curve causing an uneven bulge of the shoulder blades. X-rays confirm the diagnosis. This case of scoliosis is severe enough to be visible externally. (See pages 292 and 685).

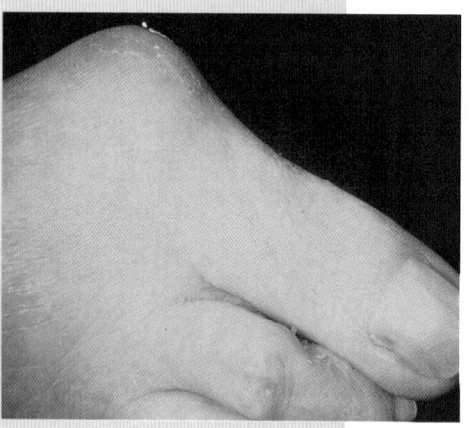

Bunions. When the big toe turns inward toward the other toes, it pushes the base outward, creating a bony hump called a bunion. Because the bunion sticks out beyond the normal curve of the foot, it is vulnerable to excess pressure and friction from shoes, causing tenderness and pain. (See page 714).

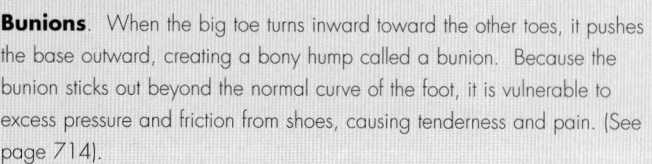

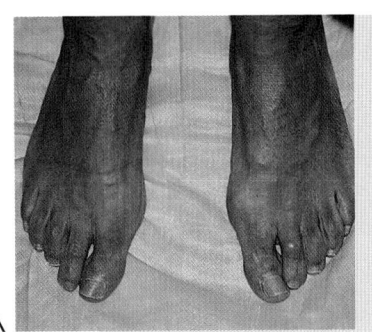

A

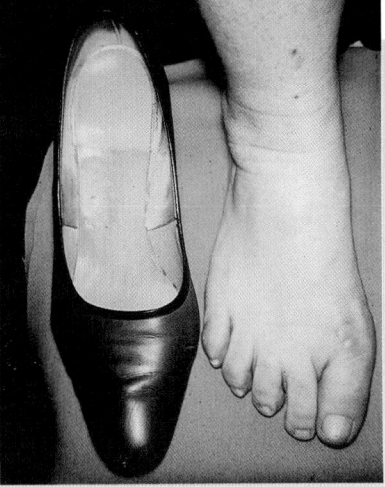

B

Corns occur as a result of external pressure, such as tight-fitting or pointed shoes, on bony projections in the toes. The layer of skin over the projections thickens, creating the corn. Corns can occur on the outer surface or between the toes. In (A), the corn is on the second toe of the foot on the right. In (B) the corn is on the little toe. (See page 722).

Disorders and Injuries of the Eye

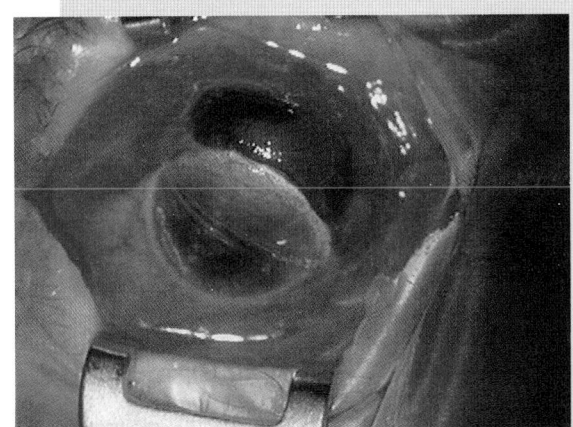

Direct trauma. Traumatic injury to the eye occurs as a result of a direct blow. In this case a cataract wound was ruptured during injury. (See page 392.)

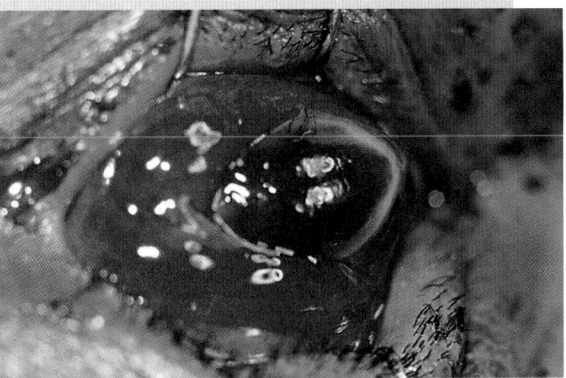

Open globe. The globe of the eye can rupture or break open from blunt trauma such as the impact of a baseball, or from penetrating injury such as piercing. (See page 548.)

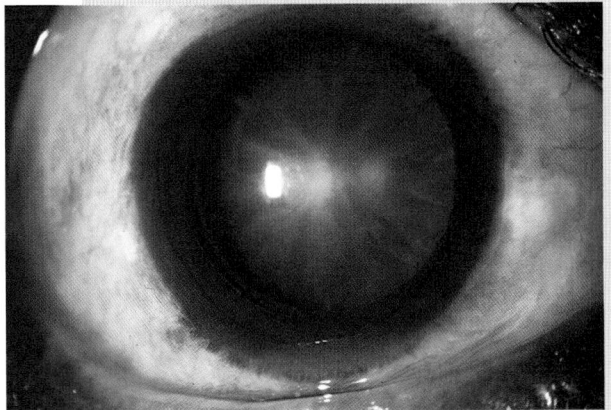

Cataract is the progressive clouding of the eye's normally clear lens causing blurring or dimming vision. Cataracts vary in size and in the loss of vision they cause. (See page 524.)

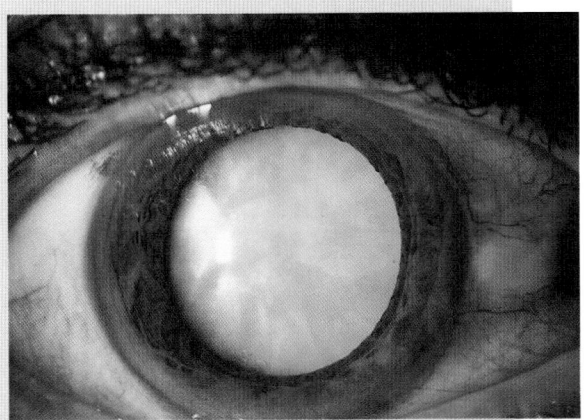

Mature cataract.

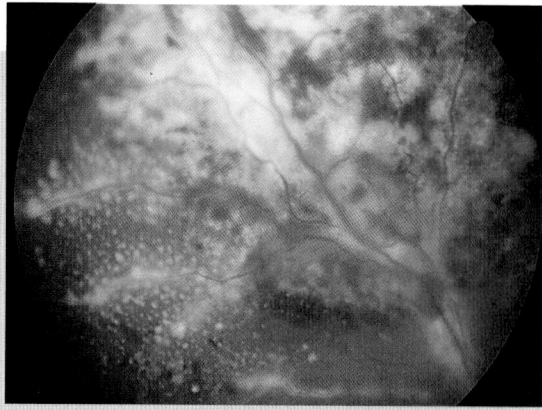

Cytomegalovirus (CMV) retinitis. CMV is a form of herpes virus, which is present but dormant in most healthy people. Under certain conditions, such as a weakened immune system, the virus can be reactivated and cause disease of the eye and other organs. A person with CMV retinitis may experience blurred or decreased vision and pain behind the eye. Large yellow-white lesions develop on the retina. (See page 541.)

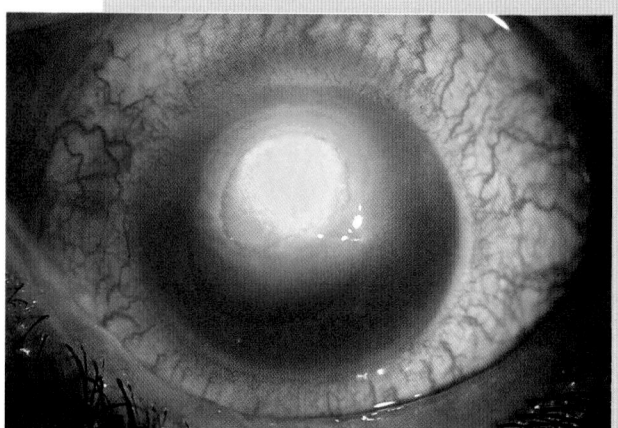

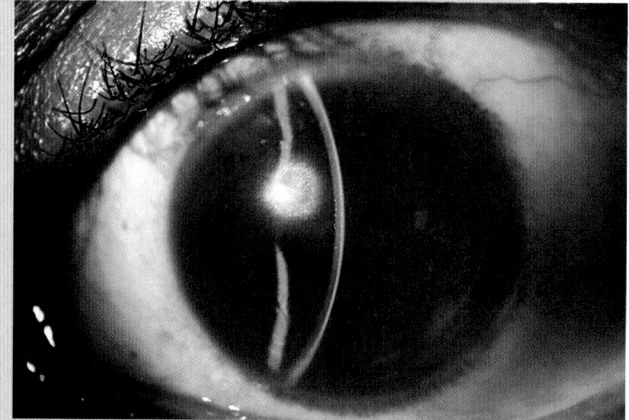

A **corneal ulcer** is an open sore on the cornea. A corneal ulcer looks like an opaque, white spot on the cornea and causes pain, sensitivity to light, and decreased vision. (See page 521.)

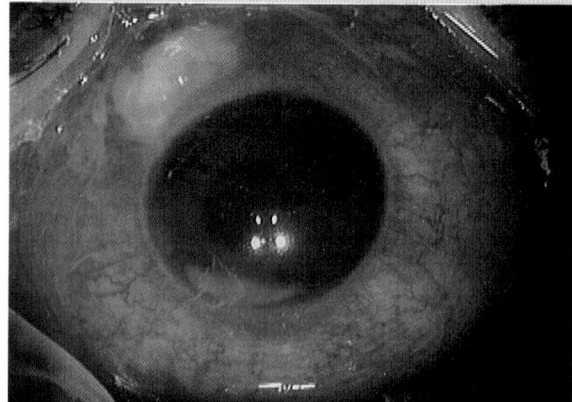

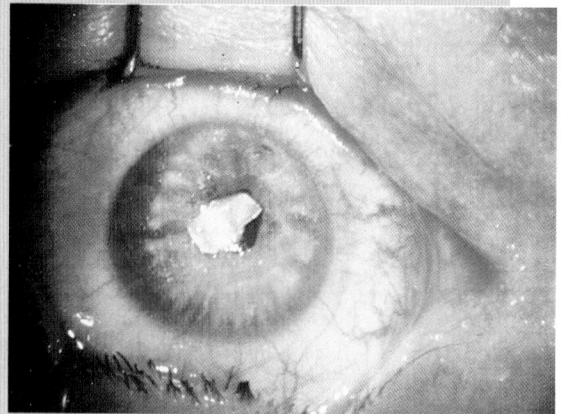

Endophthalmitis is an inflammation inside the eyeball usually caused by a bacterial or fungal infection. The symptoms of endophthalmitis are redness, sensitivity to light, and decreased vision. (See page 536.)

Foreign body in the eye. This eye has a metallic foreign body in the pupil causing tearing, redness, and irritation. (See pages 392 and 551.)

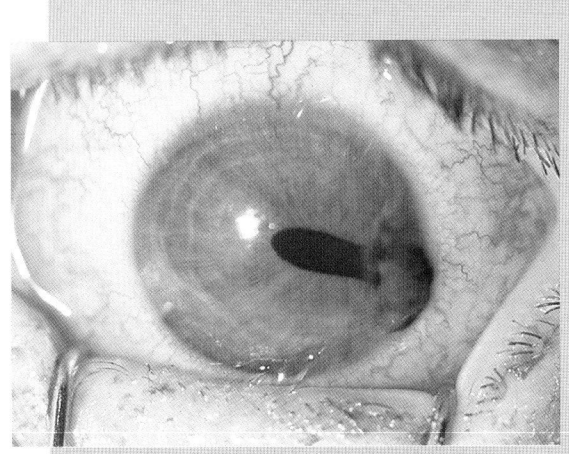

Penetrating trauma to the eye refers to an injury in which an object has become imbedded in the eye. (See page 393.)

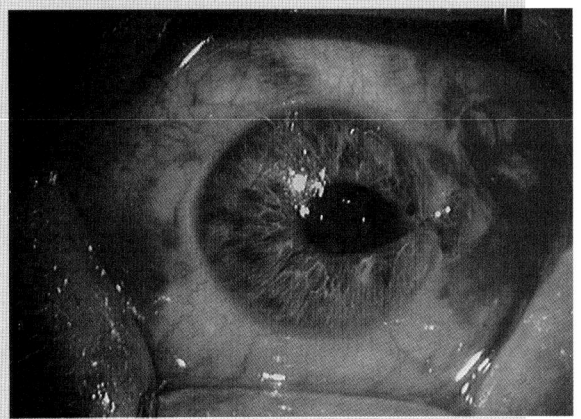

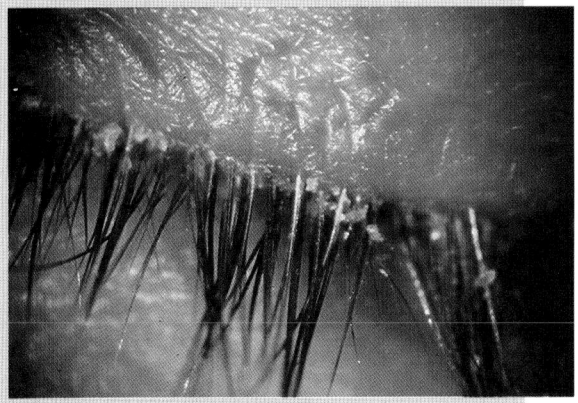

Blepharitis is an inflammation of the edges of the eyelids. Symptoms of blepharitis include swollen, red, and irritated eyes with itching, tearing, and burning. The eyelid margins have a crusty, red, thickened appearance with mild mucous discharge and dandruff-like flakes. (See page 513.)

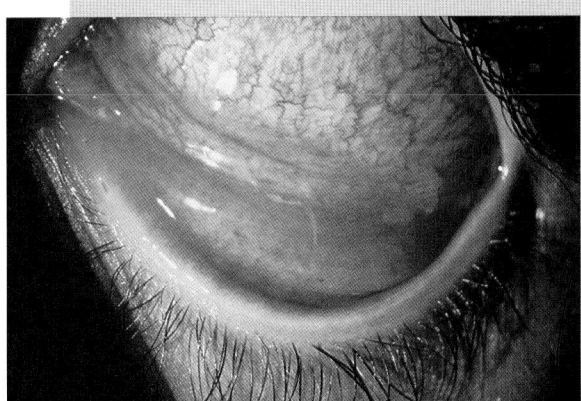

Conjunctivitis is an inflammation of the conjunctiva, the thin transparent tissue that lines the inner surface of both eyelids and the sclera until it meets the cornea. Conjunctivitis, or pink-eye as it is commonly called, causes symptoms of redness, pain, tearing, blurred vision, and sticky discharge upon awakening. (See pages 238 and 519.)

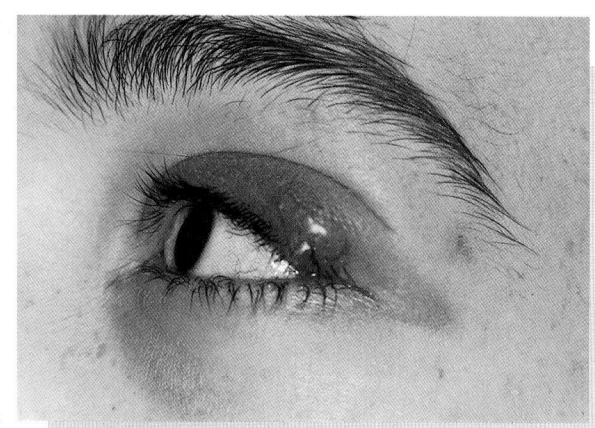

A

Stye and **chalazion** are two common conditions that can cause lumps on the eyelid. A stye (A) occurs when the eyelid glands and their ducts become infected or clogged. Styes are most commonly seen on the upper eyelid but can occur on the lower eyelid as well. A chalazion (B) is caused by the blockage of one of more of the meibomian glands in the eyelid. The accumulated secretions harden and form a bump. A chalazion is generally painless but a stye can be tender and sensitive. (See page 514.)

B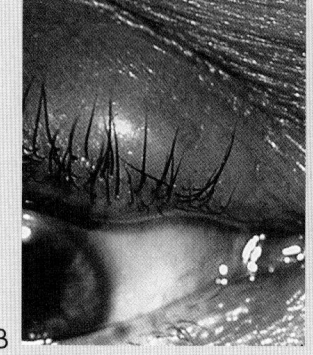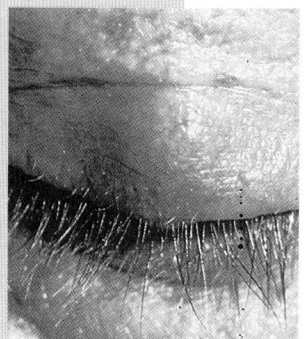

Color blind test. These figures are used as part of a series to test for color deficiency. In Figure A, an average person will see the number 3 embedded in the dots. A person with red-green weakness will see a 5, and a red-green blind person will see no number. In Figure B, an average response is 15, a red-green weak response will be 17, and a red-green blind response will be nothing. (See page 502.)

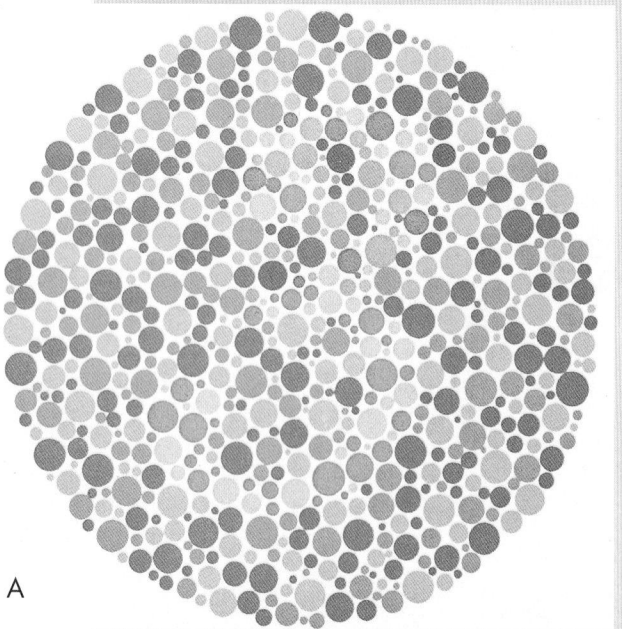

A

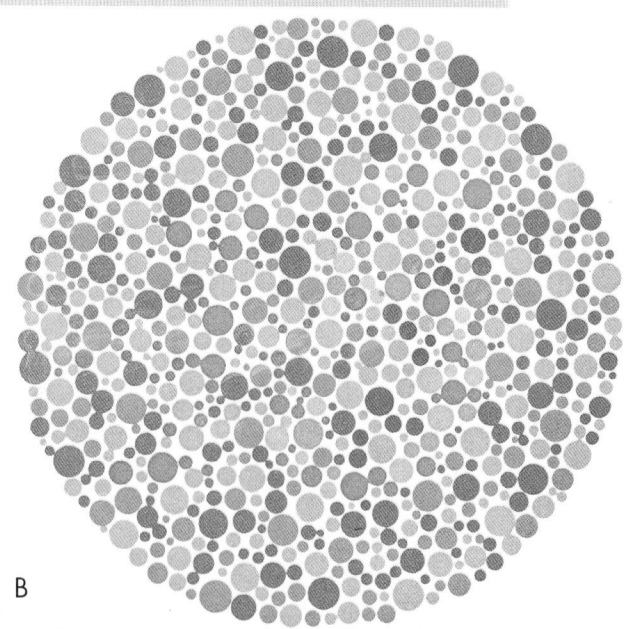

B

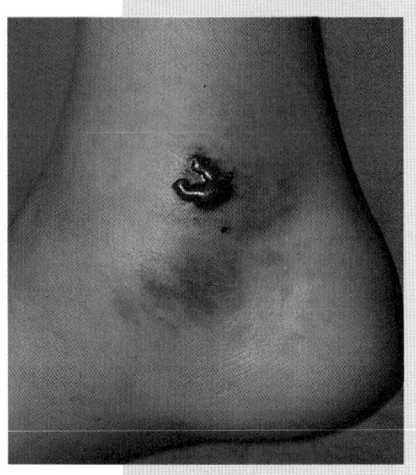

Copperhead bite. Of the hundreds of types of snakes found in the United States, only four types are poisonous: copperheads, coral snakes, rattlesnakes, and water moccasins. A snake bite causes discoloration, pain, and swelling of the area of the bite. (See page 401).

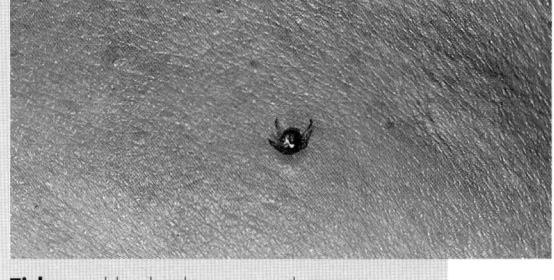

Ticks are blood-sucking insects that can carry serious diseases such as Lyme disease and Rocky Mountain spotted fever. Ticks imbed themselves in the skin and feed on blood. (See pages 400 and 1306.)

Lyme disease. After a tick is removed, the area should be watched for signs of the rash that accompanies Lyme disease. The rash is usually an expanding red circle with central clearing, resembling a bull's eye. (See page 886 and 1306.)

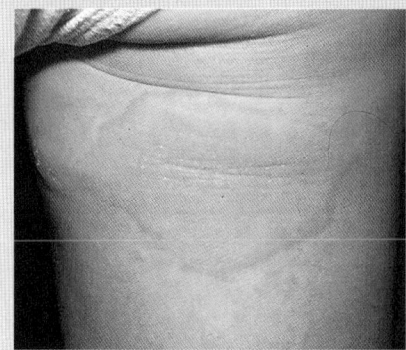

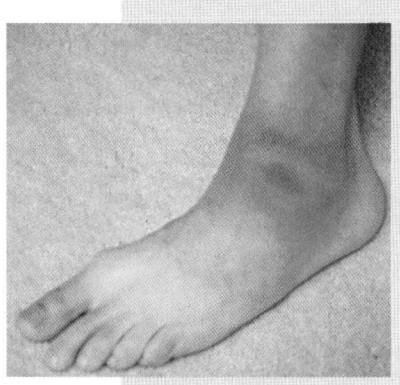

Brown recluse spider bite. Certain spiders, including the brown recluse, carry a venom that is poisonous when injected through a bite. A bite from the brown recluse spider causes swelling, redness, and pain. A blister forms at the site and then ruptures to leave a growing sore. (See page 398.)

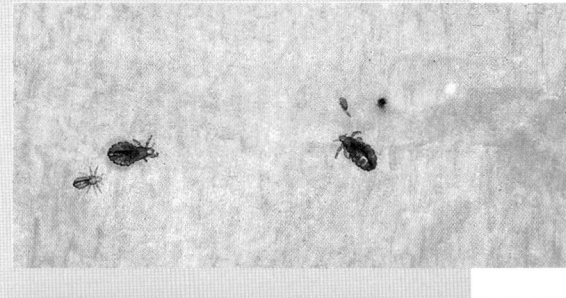

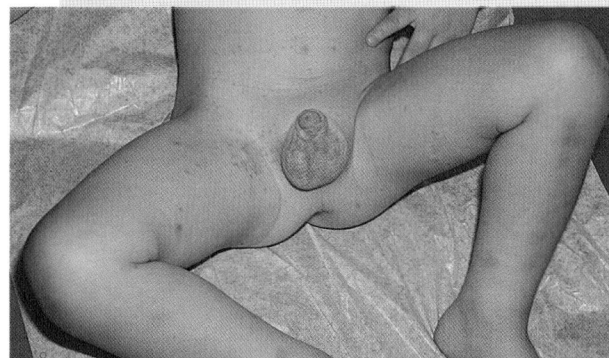

Scabies is an infestation caused by a microscopic mite that burrows in the skin, prompting an allergic response. Severe itching and a rash develop. The rash may progress from small, red bumps to scattered scaly or crusty lesions. Commonly affected areas of the body include crevices such as underarms, buttocks, and the genital area, particularly the scrotum and penis in males. (See page 1304.)

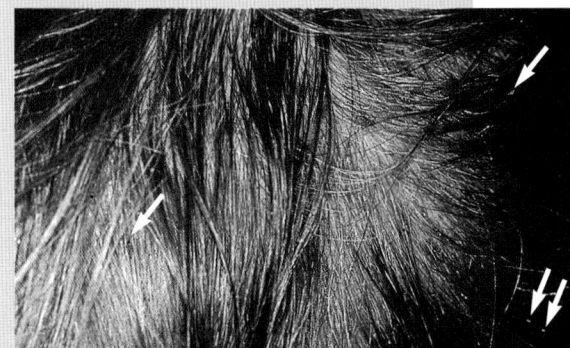

Lice are tiny, blood-sucking, wingless insects that can live in the hair, on the body, or in the pubic area. Head lice may resemble dandruff but are firmly attached to the hair shaft. (See page 1305.)

Many common home or garden plants can be poisonous when ingested (see page 410). Some poisonous plants include the following.

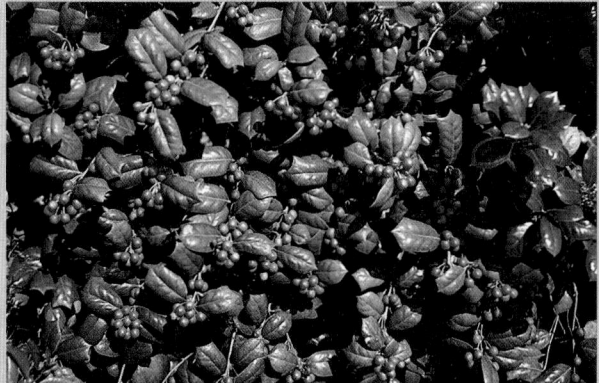

Holly berries

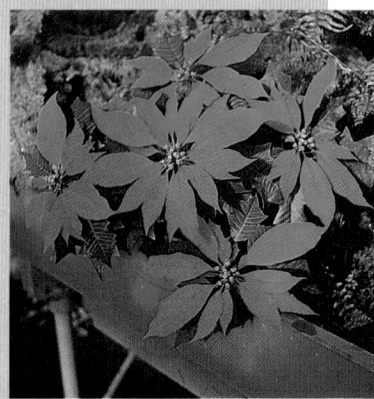

Poinsettia

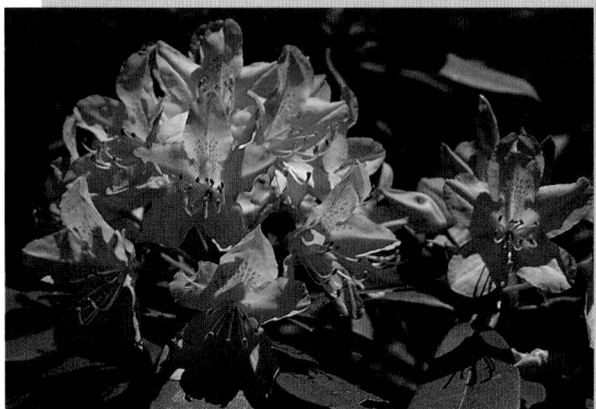

Rhododendron

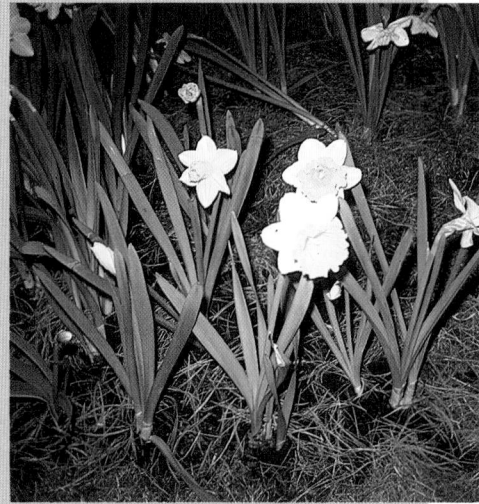

Daffodil buds

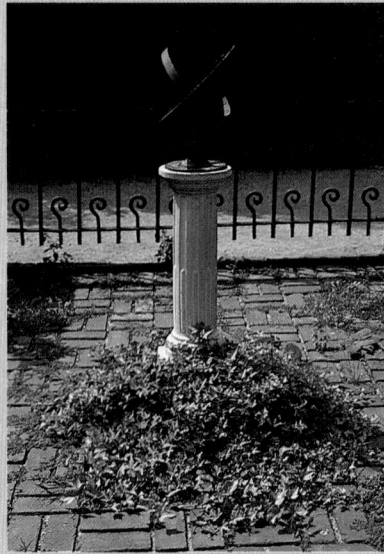

Common English ivy

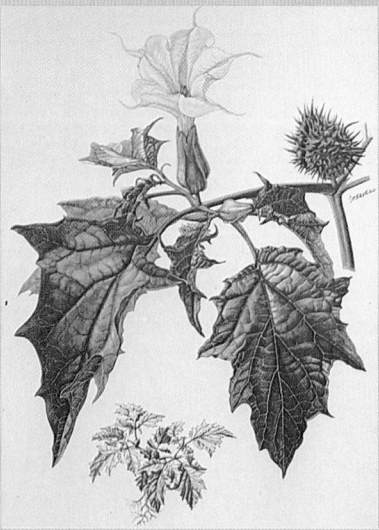

Jimson weed

changes in the hands (Raynaud's phenomenon). Stretching exercises help to gently stretch the tightened skin and to sustain maximal skin and musculoskeletal flexibility. Smoking should be avoided because it worsens the Raynaud's and other symptoms of scleroderma. (See Chapter 4 for help with quitting smoking.)

When to call the doctor Anyone with scleroderma should see their doctor regularly. Initial and ongoing checkups for internal organ involvement are mandatory.

Treatment The doctor may recommend corticosteroid ointments, which can minimize itching. (For treatment of internal organ involvement, see Scleroderma, page 643.)

Prognosis Although no cure exists for scleroderma, symptoms can often be effectively managed. The condition, however, may be very serious and life-threatening, due to internal organ involvement.

❖ RAYNAUD'S DISEASE/PHENOMENON

Symptoms and signs White or pale color changes in the tips of the fingers or toes upon exposure to cold; extremities turn white, then bluish or red when warmed, gradually returning to their normal color; infrequently, similar discoloration of the nose or earlobes may also occur; tingling or pins-and-needles sensation during episodes. (See page C-27.)

What is it? Raynaud's disease is not a disease of the skin, but rather a circulatory disorder that manifests as color changes of the skin of the fingers and sometimes toes (see Primary Raynaud's Phenomenon, page 842, for more information). It occurs when emotional stress or cold temperatures produce constriction and temporary spasms of the blood vessels of the digits (fingers or toes) reducing or totally shutting off blood flow. The cold exposure may take place in cold weather outdoors, while holding a glass of ice water, or when reaching into the freezer. The extremities become very sensitive to cold, and quickly turn pale or white; then, in the presence of warmer temperatures, a bluish purple followed by normal coloring as the blood vessels relax.

Raynaud's disease is an isolated (not associated with other disorders) circulatory disorder of unknown cause that occurs most commonly in young women. At times, the symptoms that are characteristic of Raynaud's disease may accompany other disorders—for example, connective tissue disease such as scleroderma and lupus erythematosus (see pages 643 and 642)—in which case it is called Raynaud's phenomenon.

What you can do Keep warm; minimize time outdoors during extremely cold weather. When exposed to cold, layer clothing and take steps to ensure that your hands and feet stay warm. Wear silk-lined gloves, and warm socks or stockings on cold days. Avoid touching very cold objects (for example, use a hot pad or glove when handling frozen items).

Stop smoking cigarettes; smoking causes blood vessel constriction or narrowing. (See Chapter 4 for help with quitting smoking.)

When to call the doctor You should see a doctor to confirm that you have only Raynaud's disease—not Raynaud's phenomenon, which can be an early manifestation of a connective tissue disease. The latter can be very serious and is important to diagnose, treat, and follow closely.

Treatment At times, drugs that dilate the blood vessels may be prescribed to treat Raynaud's disease. These include calcium channel blockers (nifedipine, diltiazem). Positive results have also been seen with biofeedback techniques that can help prevent the abnormal constriction of the blood vessels. It is generally recommended that people with Raynaud's disease avoid medications that can make their symptoms worse, such as decongestants or diet pills that contain phenylpropanolamine.

Prognosis Raynaud's disease, although often quite bothersome, is not a severe disorder. In most cases, preventive measures (such as avoidance of cold) can reduce the frequency and severity of symptoms.

❖ DRY SKIN

Symptoms and signs Dry, itchy skin; cracking; flaking.

What is it? Even though the skin is always being coated by its own oil (sebum), ambient humidity is an important source of moisture. While high humidity during parts of the year provides moisture the skin can absorb, low humidity usually becomes a problem in the winter months when people spend most of the day inside where dry, forced heat is used. This can cause skin dehydration and symptoms that include cracking, flaking, and itching. As the skin develops microscopic or visible openings from cracking or scratching, it is prone to further damage due to soap, clothing irritation, or bacterial infection. Dry skin can then become complicated by irritant dermatitis (a red, itchy, stinging rash) or even cellulitis (a serious bacterial skin infection requiring immediate antibiotic therapy).

Dry skin is more common in seniors, because aging is associated with a decrease in production of skin sebum. Dryness also occurs more frequently in people who wash their hands many times each day (for example, health care professionals, restaurant employees, hairdressers), because washing can rinse away the natural oils. In some parts of the country where the humidity is always low, such as the Southwest, dry skin is a year-round concern.

What you can do Use warm instead of hot water for bathing; cut down on the number and length of showers and baths; and use superfatted soaps that include moisturizers and that do not wash away the body's own oils.

After washing, dry all skin folds well (that is, underarms, groin, under the breasts, between the toes). But everywhere else just pat yourself dry, leaving some moisture on your skin. Then, apply heavier lotions (for example, Eucerin) to trap this moisture in your skin. Petroleum jelly is an extremely effective moisturizer; to eliminate the sticky feeling after it is applied, gently remove any excess with a damp washcloth. Also, alpha-hydroxy acid lotions are helpful to soften the skin and remove the surface scale (for example, Aqua Glycolic, Am-Lactin, Lac-Hydrin V, Eucerin Plus).

Wear gloves or mittens outdoors during the winter to retain moisture and avoid strong winds. If other health problems do not require avoiding a humidifier, use it during the cold-weather months to increase the relative humidity in your home to 40 percent or more.

When to call the doctor If your own efforts do not prevent the skin from becoming cracked and irritated, see a doctor, who may recommend prescription ointments. If you suspect that a secondary infection has developed—characterized by redness, warmth, tenderness or pain—see your doctor immediately; this infection is serious and requires antibiotic therapy and sometimes hospitalization.

Treatment If you have dry skin only, a prescription-strength alpha hydroxy acid moisturizer, such as Lac-Hydrin 12 percent lotion or cream, may be prescribed. If you have developed an irritated dry skin rash, a corticosteroid ointment will probably be needed.

Prognosis Most cases of dry skin will heal with self-help or doctor-prescribed measures. Also, prevention is the key; if dry, winter weather has caused your dry skin, anticipate and prevent the problem in the future by using moisturizers in the early fall.

❖ ICHTHYOSIS

Symptoms and signs Extremely dry, "fish-scale" skin; in some cases, the skin becomes tight and may crack, burn, and sting.

What is it? Ichthyosis from the Greek word *ichthys* (fish)—is a genetic skin disorder that begins in infancy or early childhood and often worsens with age. Ichthyosis that begins early in life is called ichthyosis vulgaris. It occurs when too many skin cells build up on the outermost skin layer due to inadequate shedding. This results in thickened, dry skin and the appearance of being covered with white "fish scales." Although abnormal scaling is present everywhere on the body, it is heaviest on the legs and arms. Symptoms tend to become worse in the dry, low humidity of winter. When ichthyosis is severe, the skin feels inelastic and may crack, making the person susceptible to irritant rashes and infections.

What you can do Heavy lubricants (for example, petroleum jelly, or lubricants that contain petrolatum or mineral oil) and urea-containing lotions (Carmol-10, Carmol-20) can be used to trap moisture in the skin. Alpha hydroxy acid lotions or creams, such as Aqua Glycolic, Am-Lactin, Lac-Hydrin V (5 percent), and Eucerin Plus, help shed the scales. All lubricants should be applied after soaking in a bath; this not only hydrates the skin but also allows the scales to soften and shed. Superfatted or moisturizing soaps are helpful in preventing the removal of natural skin oil when bathing.

When to call the doctor If you were diagnosed with ichthyosis in infancy or early childhood, you probably have already been informed about this condition and general skin care measures. However, if you developed dry, "fish-scale" skin after your early childhood years, you may have another condition, such as "acquired" ichthyosis. This may be due to a medication (for example, cholesterol-lowering agents). It may be associated with an internal disease (for example, kidney failure, cancer, acquired immunodeficiency syndrome [AIDS]). You should consult a doctor regarding the diagnosis.

Also, people with ichthyosis vulgaris beginning in childhood should be counseled regarding the autosomal-dominant inheritance of this condition; each of their children carries a 50 percent chance of having this disorder.

Treatment Prescription alpha hydroxy acid moisturizers (for example Lac-Hydrin 12 percent) are usually recommended, since they are more effective than lower concentration over-the-counter products.

Prognosis Ichthyosis cannot be cured; however, proper treatment can ease symptoms and make the condition more tolerable.

❖ SEBORRHEIC DERMATITIS

Symptoms and signs Reddened and scaly (flaky) skin; dry or greasy appearance; dandruff; itching. (See page C-26.)

What is it? Seborrheic dermatitis is a common rash that occurs most frequently on the parts of the body with the largest concentrations of sebaceous (oil) glands. These include the scalp, portions of the face (nose, eyebrows, eyelids), behind and inside the outer ears, the breast bone area (sternum), the navel (umbilicus), and in the buttock fold. The condition can occur in cycles, waxing and waning over time.

Seborrheic dermatitis is thought to be associated in part with increased growth of a yeast (*Pityrosporum ovale*) normally

DESCRIBING A SKIN PROBLEM TO YOUR DOCTOR

When a rash or other skin problem develops, a phone call to a doctor is often the first step in getting the treatment process under way. To help the doctor decide what the problem may be and whether a doctor's attention is necessary, describe the affected area clearly and in detail. Jot down some notes before contacting your doctor to be sure you can answer the following questions:

- Where is the rash or other skin change located? On the face? Neck? Arms or legs? Chest or back? Other bodily area?

- What are the characteristics of the affected skin? What color is it? Is it bumpy, scaly, or smooth? Does it have a blisters? Is the skin thickened? Is it painful? Does it itch? Has it caused numbing or tingling? How large is the affected area?

- How long has the lesion been present? Have you ever had this skin disorder before? If so, has it always occurred during the same time of year or on the same part of the body?

- Has the appearance of the rash changed since it first surfaced? Has it gotten larger or smaller? Has its texture, coloring, or degree of itchiness or discomfort changed?

- Did the rash seem to develop after exposure to a particular chemical, cosmetic, clothing material, or other substance?

- Have other members of your family had the same skin disorder?

- Did you self-treat the lesion in any way in the days before calling the doctor? ■

found on the skin; this organism thrives in oily and warm areas.

What you can do Seborrheic dermatitis cannot be cured, but it can be effectively controlled with treatment. For the scalp, over-the-counter shampoos can help; look for ingredients such as selenium sulfide, zinc pyrithione (found in Head & Shoulders, for example), tar (found in Neutrogena T/Gel, for example), or sulfur (found in Sebulex, for example). Avoid scratching the affected area, which can make symptoms

SKIN CLUES TO HEALTH PROBLEMS

Glowing skin may be the ideal—but when illness strikes, it can manifest itself in your skin, even when the actual underlying problem is not a primary skin disorder. If you have developed a rash, itchy skin, or changes in your skin color, this may be a sign or symptom of another health condition.

Here are the skin manifestations of some common medical problems, which help doctors in diagnosing these conditions

- *A butterfly-shaped rash across the nose and cheekbones,* sometimes accompanied by red, raised rashes on other parts of the body, may be signs of lupus erythematosus, which is an autoimmune disease in which the disease-fighting immune system attacks the body's own healthy cells. Other skin symptoms of lupus include photosensitivity, or sun sensitivity, which causes the development of skin rashes after sun exposure. (See page 642 for more information on systemic lupus erythematosus.)

- *Dry skin and hair* may be symptoms of an underactive thyroid (hypothyroidism), in which the metabolic rate slows down in response to a shortage of thyroid hormone. The disorder may also cause a thickened and dry, rough skin, brittle nails, and an intolerance to cold temperatures. Ironically, the opposite condition—an overactive thyroid, or hyperthyroidism, in which the metabolic rate accelerates—can cause skin symptoms as well, including flushed skin, excessive sweating (particularly of the palms), and an increased sensitivity to warm environments. (For information on hypothyroidism and hyperthyroidism, see pages 1185 and 1188.)

- *Tiny, firm, painful blisters or red spots* on the palms of the hands, the soles of the feet, and inside the mouth are signs of hand-foot-mouth disease, which most often affects children. It is caused by a virus called Coxsackie. Signs and symptoms include a mild fever and a sore throat. (See page 212 for more information on hand-foot-mouth disease.)

- *Bluish coloring, and tenderness, numbness, or burning in the toes and fingers* may be caused by Buerger's disease (also called thromboangiitis obliterans), which is a disease of the blood vessels, leading to an inflammation and thickening and, in some cases, the gradual blocking of these vessels. Though the precise cause is not known, the disease can cause ulcers on the skin and even the loss of fingers if it progresses; it occurs primarily in young men who smoke cigarettes. (See page 841 for more information on Buerger's Disease.)

- *Skin thickening* may develop in people with diabetes. This velvety thickening of the skin, usually around the sides and back of the neck and over the backs of the hands, is called acanthosis nigricans. Persons with diabetes also may have tremendous difficulty with their feet, leading to loss of sensation, nonhealing ulcers, and underlying bone infections. Anyone with diabetes, no matter how mild, should be educated about meticulous foot care and inspection, both of which should be performed once or twice daily. (See Chapter 26 for more information on diabetes.)

- *Yellow coloring of the skin* may be an indication of a liver disorder called hepatitis. The yellowish skin color (which also affects the whites of the eyes) occurs when the liver and kidneys cannot efficiently remove bilirubin (a breakdown product of red blood cells) from the blood. Caused by a virus, hepatitis also produces achiness and fever. (See page 1035 for more information on hepatitis.) ■

worse. Over-the-counter hydrocortisone clear lotion may relieve itching: after shampooing, while the hair is still damp, a few drops may be rubbed into each quarter-sized affected area of the scalp.

When to call the doctor If seborrheic dermatitis does not improve with these measures, see a dermatologist to make sure the diagnosis is correct or for additional treatment.

Treatment Prescription-strength, topically applied corticosteroid creams and shampoos as well as antifungal preparations (ketoconazole) may be needed to control your condition.

Prognosis Even after seborrheic dermatitis is treated successfully, it often recurs when treatment is stopped; therefore, prevention with ongoing use of a therapeutic shampoo is frequently necessary.

Skin Infections

The skin is an important line of defense, protecting the body against attacks by organisms such as bacteria, viruses, and fungi. However, sometimes the skin itself can become infected with these germs.

While the infections described next can be cared for with medications, they need to be properly diagnosed. Although some of these skin disorders are more of a nuisance than a serious health threat, certain infections that go undiagnosed or that are inappropriately treated may progress to more serious and even life-threatening conditions.

BACTERIAL INFECTIONS

Bacterial infections of the skin include impetigo, furuncles, boils, carbuncles, cellulites, and erysipelas.

❖ IMPETIGO

Symptoms and signs Tiny blisters, usually already ruptured when first noticed; honey colored, crusty scabs; itching or burning. (See page C-34.)

Signs and laboratory findings Although usually not necessary, a culture may be taken to determine the specific bacteria causing the infection.

What is it? Impetigo is a contagious bacterial skin infection most common in young children. It may also occur in adults, but usually only as a complication of another skin disorder, such as eczema. Impetigo typically begins as tiny blisters that rupture easily; the clear, yellow fluid discharge dries and forms sticky, honey-colored crusts. It appears most frequently on exposed sites, such as the face, scalp, arms, and legs, and sometimes at the site of a cut, scratch, or insect bite.

What you can do Do not scratch the impetigo lesions; they are loaded with bacteria. The infection can easily be spread to another part of the body or to another person through direct contact or shared items (such as clothing, washcloths, or towels). Frequent handwashing and avoidance of sharing towels and clothing are essential in preventing the transmission of impetigo to others. The lesions should be gently washed a few times a day with an antibacterial soap.

When to call the doctor If impetigo is suspected, contact a doctor. Untreated impetigo can spread quickly. In rare cases, the infection can cause a severe autoimmune kidney disease called poststreptococcal glomerulonephritis.

Treatment. Impetigo is usually treated with a 10-day course of antibiotics—most commonly, dicloxacillin (a form of penicillin), cephalexin, or erythromycin. Alternatively, the infection may be treated with a topical ointment, mupirocin.

Prognosis Impetigo should heal without scarring as long as the lesions are not scratched or picked. Routine handwashing with an antibacterial soap, if not already being used, should be started.

❖ BOILS AND FURUNCULOSIS

Symptoms and signs Red, shiny, swollen, pus-filled, warm or hot, tender lumps or cyst-like lesions; when ready to rupture, white or yellow central area "points." (See page C-34.)

What is it? A boil, or furuncle, is a bacterial skin abscess that starts in a hair follicle. It begins as a small, firm, tender nodule that becomes inflamed (red, warm); as it enlarges, the skin turns shiny and bright red, and the tenderness may progress to "throbbing pain." Within several days, the nodule becomes distinctly outlined and a point forms on the surface; often it spontaneously ruptures and drains pus, leading to the gradual subsiding of the boil.

Boils can occur on any part of the body where hair is present, but are found most commonly on the scalp, back, underarms, and buttocks. The term furunculosis is applied to the condition when a person has recurrent and multiple boils or furuncles, developing one after another over several weeks or months.

Boils are common, and no one is immune to them. Some people are more prone to the infections, including people with diabetes or with compromised immune systems due to certain diseases (such as AIDS) or conditions requiring drugs which suppress the immune system (including autoimmune diseases and organ failure requiring an organ transplant).

What you can do Do not squeeze or pick at the lesions; this can cause spreading of the infection. Apply warm, moist compresses to the affected area several times a day. Self-care measures frequently lead to healing within 1 to 2 weeks.

When to call the doctor Contact a doctor if you have a boil that does not heal within 2 weeks, is very painful, does not spontaneously drain on its own, or develops redness extending outward into the surrounding skin or if you develop a fever or are immunocompromised for some reason.

Treatment A doctor may nick or lance the lesions with a small blade to facilitate drainage and healing. A topical or oral antibiotic will be prescribed. To prevent frequently recurring boils, a daily dose of antibiotics may be prescribed, often for a period of 3 months or more. Also, vitamin C seems to help reduce the number and frequency of furuncles, which develop in some persons with furunculosis.

Prognosis Although boils typically heal without complications, regular cleansing with antibacterial soap is advisable to help prevent recurrences.

❖ CARBUNCLES

Symptoms and signs Adjacent boils (see Boils, page 1281) forming connections deep in the skin and raised from the skin's surface; clusters of boils that are red, shiny, tender, and very painful; fever; fatigue.

What is it? Carbuncles are clusters of interconnected, deep boils. They are highly inflamed and pus-filled, and occur most commonly on the back of the neck, underarms, shoulders, and buttocks.

Carbuncles begin as tender, red lumps that enlarge and develop pus-filled centers. They can be extremely painful, and can be accompanied by a fever. The pain subsides when the lesions break open and release pus, typically through multiple openings.

Some research shows that carbuncles may occur later in life than boils and affect men more often than women. The incidence is much greater in persons with diabetes than in healthy people.

What you can do Apply warm, moist compresses to the affected areas several times a day; this can promote natural drainage of the pus, which stimulates healing and relieves pain. Gently wash the area with antiseptic soap. Do not squeeze or pick at the lesions.

When to call the doctor Contact a doctor if you develop a carbuncle, especially if you have diabetes or a condition causing you to be immunocompromised. Carbuncles require medical attention.

Treatment To promote drainage of the pus, a doctor may lance or surgically open the lesion. Oral antibiotics may also be needed.

Prognosis Although very painful, carbuncles generally heal within 2 weeks. However, they can recur due to bacteria that may linger on the skin. To reduce this risk, good hygiene is important, including washing with an antibacterial soap.

❖ CELLULITIS

Symptoms and signs A red, swollen, warm or hot area of skin; pain; tenderness; fever and chills as the infection progresses; headache, sometimes. (See page C-34.)

What is it? Cellulitis is a very serious, rapidly progressive, bacterial skin infection that primarily involves the underlying fat. It usually occurs with some other skin disorder, such as venous stasis dermatitis (eczema of the legs associated with varicose veins and swelling) or chickenpox, or after a skin injury, such as a cut, a bite, or a healing surgical wound. Cellulitis causes warmth, pain, redness, and swelling of the skin. The texture of cellulitis has been compared to that of an orange peel.

This infection occurs most often on an extremity, although it can develop anywhere. It starts when bacteria enter the skin through an opening (such as an erosion in an area of dermatitis) or a cut, scrape, or bite, which may not even be apparent.

What you can do To prevent cellulitis from occurring, thoroughly wash all cuts, scrapes, puncture wounds, and bites, using antibacterial soap and water.

When to call the doctor If cellulitis develops, see your doctor immediately for treatment.

Treatment Your doctor will prescribe immediate antibiotic therapy. If cellulitis is caught very early and involves only a small area of skin, your doctor may put you on oral antibiotics, cautioning you to call immediately if, despite therapy, the redness continues to spread outward or does not improve. Very often, however, cellulitis requires hospitalization for intravenous antibiotic therapy. If not appropriately treated, the infection can spread into the bloodstream (septicemia) and cause a severe, life-threatening infection.

Rarely, another type of infection may mimic or develop from cellulitis (a condition called fasciitis). Also known as the "flesh-eating bacteria," this infection spreads very rapidly, dissecting through the connective tissue underlying the fat, destroying wide areas of tissue. This condition is a surgical emergency, as the infected tissue must be excised (cut out) to prevent continued extension, tissue destruction, and, ultimately, death. Intravenous antibiotics are concurrently administered with the surgery.

Prognosis Cellulitis is clearly a serious infection that must be recognized and treated as soon as possible. The prognosis depends on the type of bacteria causing the infection, the general health and immune system of the person, and timing of the initiation of therapy.

Some people who have had one episode of cellulitis may begin having recurrent episodes; this is particularly true in persons with varicose veins and resultant leg ulcers causing the initial episode of cellulitis. These people should be followed very closely in an effort to prevent recurrent cellulitis and recognize recurrences early.

❖ ERYSIPELAS

Symptoms and signs A warm or hot, sharply defined area of skin; shiny; red; tender; a visible red streak extending to the lymph nodes draining the area (sometimes).

What is it? Erysipelas is a bacterial skin infection that is sometimes called superficial cellulitis. Although similar to cellulitis, it involves primarily the skin instead of the underlying fat. Erysipelas has a vivid red color; the affected area is hot and painful, and slightly elevated from the surrounding skin.

The infection occurs most often on the face and extremities. It tends to develop primarily in infants, young children, seniors, and people who have had lymph nodes removed from the groin or underarm area (for example, women who have had lymph nodes removed as part of their treatment for breast or uterine cancer).

What you can do Be alert for possible signs of erysipelas. Hospitalization is required in serious cases, such as when the face is involved, and when the affected individual has an impaired immune system or other medical problems. Fever, chills, and vomiting are signs that could indicate a serious

infection and the immediate need for a doctor's attention and hospital care.

When to call the doctor Erysipelas can spread rapidly. If you suspect the presence of this skin infection, contact your doctor for prompt treatment. As with cellulitis, erysipelas can progress to, or be mistaken for, fasciitis (the "flesh-eating" bacterial infection of the skin; see the preceding discussion of cellulitis).

Treatment Antibiotics, given orally to an outpatient or intravenously to a hospitalized inpatient, will be prescribed. Improvement should begin within 24 to 48 hours; this therapy is generally continued for 2 weeks.

Prognosis If untreated, erysipelas is a potentially fatal infection, while prompt treatment is usually fully successful. However, persons having conditions predisposing them to this skin infection (such as prior lymph node removal during breast cancer surgery) often have recurrent episodes of erysipelas; these persons may require ongoing antibiotic therapy or the daily use of antibacterial soap to reduce these recurrences.

VIRAL INFECTIONS

Viral infections of the skin include cold sores, shingles, molluscum contagiosum, warts, and genital warts.

❖ COLD SORES (FEVER BLISTERS)

Symptoms and signs Small, clustered blisters on the lips or elsewhere on the face (nose, chin, cheeks), and occasionally elsewhere on the body; tingling sensations; pain; itching. (See page C-40.)

What is it? Cold sores, sometimes called fever blisters, are painful sores that usually form on or at the edge of the lips. They are caused by the herpes simplex virus. While the sores will disappear in 7 to 14 days, the virus stays in the body, living within nerve root cells, thereby allowing recurrences to develop. These recurrences are often triggered by stress, fatigue, exposure to sunlight, menstruation, or an infection such as the common cold. The virus is contagious and can be transmitted most easily by kissing or other direct contact with an infected individual.

What you can do Most cold sore outbreaks are mild and heal fairly quickly without specific treatment. Make efforts to avoid spreading the virus to other people or to other places on your own body. Most importantly, do not touch the sore and then your eye, since that could lead to a serious corneal (eye) infection which, if left untreated, could produce permanent vision loss.

For symptomatic relief, try placing ice on the lip sores. If the surface becomes crusty, gently apply warm water compresses (for 5 to 10 minutes, several times a day). As the area is drying and healing, apply over-the-counter antibiotic ointment to prevent splitting and secondary bacterial infection.

To help minimize sunlight-associated recurrences at the beach and on ski slopes, frequently apply sunscreen-containing lip balm to the lips and sunscreen lotion to the rest of the face.

When to call the doctor Cold sores pose no serious dangers to your overall health. However, if they persist or recur quite frequently, consult your doctor.

Most doctors are so familiar with the appearance of the sores that no testing is required to properly diagnose the condition. Laboratory tests are available, however, that can identify the presence of the herpes simplex virus.

Treatment Antiviral medications such as acyclovir can slow down the replication of herpes simplex virus. These medications, both topically applied and orally administered, are available by prescription. They are used in the early stages of a cold sore outbreak—such as when a person feels the tingling and itching that are often present just before an outbreak.

Prognosis No medication is available to wipe out the herpes simplex virus. Thus, if you are prone to recurrences, you may have to learn to live with this, knowing that it is annoying but not serious.

❖ SHINGLES (HERPES ZOSTER)

Symptoms and signs Burning, tingling, or painful sensation wrapping around one side of the body or face, or down an arm or leg; associated with a similarly distributed red rash that evolves into multiple clustered blisters (from half-dollar to palm-sized); hypersensitivity to touch; possibly associated headaches and mild fever (sometimes preceding development of other symptoms). (See page C-35.)

What is it? Anyone who has ever had chickenpox is a candidate for developing shingles (also known as herpes zoster). Both conditions are caused by the varicella-zoster virus.

After a person has chickenpox, typically in childhood, the virus lies dormant or "hibernates" within a nerve root in the spine. Many years later it can become active again, inflaming the nerve and traveling from the nerve root into the skin that the root serves.

Doctors do not know why the virus reactivates, but a transient and otherwise inconsequential weakening of the immune system probably plays a role in the majority of affected persons. Shingles is also more likely to occur in people receiving treatment for certain types of cancer, those receiving immunosuppressive medications, and persons infected with the AIDS virus.

Although shingles may be painless, it frequently is extremely painful and occasionally itchy. It usually begins with a sensation of tingling that may become a burning or stabbing pain as the reactivated virus spreads along the nerve. As the virus reaches the nerve endings in the skin, redness and blisters develop. Because these fluid-filled, clustered blisters follow a nerve, they may begin on one side of the body and wrap around to the front of the body on the same side; alternatively, they may originate on the buttocks and travel down the leg, or cover the forehead and cheek on one side of the face. These blisters can also be itchy. They may linger for 2 to 3 weeks before they crust, scab, and finally disappear.

Unfortunately, the pain from herpes zoster may persist after the blisters are gone. In fact, in about 10 percent of people who have had shingles, constant pain—called postherpetic neuralgia—can continue for months and even years after the rash and blistering are gone, sometimes causing not only debilitating discomfort but also depression.

Prevention For people who have never had chickenpox, a relatively new varicella vaccine may provide protection not only from the chickenpox but also from shingles. Although not yet tested, it is possible that if this vaccination is given to a person who has had the chickenpox earlier in life, it may prevent the development of shingles.

The varicella virus that causes both chickenpox (the initial viral infection) and shingles (the reactivation of the virus) is not contagious to someone who already had chickenpox, but those who have never had chickenpox can develop it if exposed to a person with either active shingles or chickenpox infection.

What you can do Cool, tap water compresses can be placed on the blisters for 15 minutes several times a day to promote drying. Over-the-counter analgesics, such as ibuprofen, may be useful, too.

When to call the doctor If shingles is diagnosed within the first 72 hours of its appearance, antiviral medication may be used with the intent of bringing a quicker resolution of symptoms and reducing the chance of consequent long-term pain or postherpetic neuralgia. The sooner the medicaiton is started, the better the outcome. If shingles occurs on your face, it may affect your eyes and cause permanent vision impairment. Therefore, it is important to consult your doctor promptly. A doctor should also be contacted immediately if you are immunocompromised due to an illness or a medication; in such circumstances, you are at risk for becoming seriously ill from shingles and need antiviral medication intravenously or by mouth.

Treatment Treatment is most effective if begun within days of the onset of the first symptoms of shingles. Antiviral medications such as acyclovir and famciclovir may be given if they are started within 72 hours of the appearance of the rash. Cool compresses for blisters, followed later by topical antibacterial ointment for scabs, may also be applied to help stimulate healing and prevent secondary bacterial infections.

For people who develop persistent pain (postherpetic neuralgia) after the skin lesions have healed, both analgesics and low-dose antidepressants may be prescribed with variable success. Some people are helped by over-the-counter capsaicin, a topical cream with pain-relieving properties; and transcutaneous electrical stimulation (TENS), in which low-intensity electric currents are used to ease discomfort.

Prognosis The rash and blisters associated with shingles usually run their course in 2 to 4 weeks; however, postherpetic neuralgia may last for months to years, and it can be extremely painful.

❖ MOLLUSCUM CONTAGIOSUM

Symptoms and signs Bumps that are flesh-colored, pink or seemingly translucent, pea-sized or smaller, and dome-shaped, with a central dimple. (See page C-35.)

What is it? Molluscum contagiosum is a contagious viral infection, causing tiny skin-colored growths that are often mistaken for warts (they are sometimes called water warts). However, the smooth, shiny surface and the centrally located depression set it apart from the common wart. There are usually multiple lesions, most often distributed on the chest, abdomen, or chin, although a single molluscum lesion can exist on the body.

This infection is common in young children, transmitted by person-to-person contact, or through shared towels or clothing. When it occurs in adults, it is often transmitted through intimate sexual contact, and the growths concentrate on the genital area and inner thighs.

What you can do In children, molluscum contagiosum frequently resolves on its own within several months; when it does not or when lesions are increasing in number, treatment can eliminate the growths. Over-the-counter wart preparations are frequently effective against this viral infection. Adults with sexually transmitted molluscum should see their doctors for evaluation for other sexually transmitted diseases.

When to call the doctor If initial treatments do not work or lesions are multiplying, see a doctor. If the diagnosis is questionable, the presence of the infection can be confirmed by the doctor through microscopic evaluation of a scraping from the lesion. Adults with genital lesions should be evaluated for other coexisting sexually transmitted diseases. Adults with numerous lesions on the face or body should be evaluated for immune suppression, as occurs with AIDS and some cancers.

Treatment Cryosurgery with liquid nitrogen can be used to freeze and destroy the growths. They can also be scraped away with an instrument called a curette. Although both approaches may be successful after an initial treatment, the lesions may frequently require multiple freezing or scraping sessions. However, neither treatment is painless or guaranteed to be successful.

Prognosis Molluscum eventually disappears without treatment in persons with normal immune systems. Before the decision is made to remove molluscum with liquid nitrogen, it must be recognized that this procedure can leave behind a permanent depigmentation or whitening of the skin. People with darker skin in particular may find this cosmetically unappealing.

❖ WARTS

Symptoms and signs Rough or "warty" bumps that are skin-colored, white, tan, or pink; typically pea-sized or smaller; usually on the hands and feet; pain in warts that occur on weight-bearing portions of the feet. (See page C-35.)

What is it? A wart, or verruca, is a small bump on the skin (most often on the hands and feet) caused by a virus that infects the top layer of skin cells. Warts are believed to be transmitted through direct or indirect contact (via a gym or shower floor) with a person carrying the virus. This virus, called human papillomavirus (HPV), is easier to "catch" if there is a cut or an abrasion on the skin.

Two of the most prevalent types of warts are common warts and plantar warts.

Common warts These warts most often occur on the fingers (near the fingernails) or on the backs of the hands. Although they are more prevalent in children and young adults, they can develop at any age. They tend to be free of pain.

Foot (or plantar) warts These warts occur on the bottoms of the feet. They frequently are studded with pinpoint dark spots, which are tiny, clotted blood vessels. When they occur on portions of the feet that bear weight, they are flattened by the weight placed on them, and can be quite painful. They can be confused with corns; however, corns lack surface pinpoint dark spots.

What you can do Over-the-counter liquids and patches containing salicylic acid are widely available.

When to call the doctor Warts do not necessarily require treatment. They are neither cancerous nor precancerous. About one-half to two-thirds of all warts disappear spontaneously within 1 to 2 years without any therapy. However, warts can be treated by a doctor to alleviate pain and to prevent them from spreading to other areas of the body and to other individuals.

Treatment A doctor can remove a common wart by freezing it with liquid nitrogen, by using laser vaporization, or by surgically removing it in a procedure called curettage and electrodesiccation.

Your doctor should explain that no single treatment is guaranteed to work, and a given form of treatment may need to be repeated several times. Unfortunately, the wart virus can be very resistant to therapy. Even after an apparent complete cure, it may pop up again in the same spot years later.

Plantar warts are even more difficult to successfully treat; treatment options are the same as those used for common warts.

Prognosis Because existing warts shed virus, new warts can surface nearby, even as others are vanishing. Unfortunately, warts can be a recurring, chronic problem for some people.

❖ GENITAL WARTS

Symptoms and signs Small, flesh-colored or pink bumps on the genitals or anus; asymptomatic. (See page C-35.)

What is it? Genital warts are a common sexually transmitted infection. Like common warts, they are caused by the human papillomavirus (HPV), although it is a different subtype or strain that infects the genital area. HPV is transmitted by direct contact with the skin of an infected person, usually during sexual activity (see Sexually Transmitted Infections, page 861). As the virus multiplies in the skin cells, it forms one or more small, painless, wart-like bumps on the penis, labia, within the vagina, cervix, or anal region. These sores tend to be softer and smoother than other types of warts, particularly when they are on moist areas.

The greatest risk associated with genital warts is that of cervical cancer. Some strains of HPV are associated with the development of cervical cancer, and, much less commonly, rare anal-rectal cancer and penile cancer.

What you can do Use condoms to help prevent sexual transmission of HPV; condoms are not foolproof, however, since they may not cover all areas to and from which HPV may be transmitted.

When to call the doctor If you suspect you have genital warts, consult your doctor. Do not try to self-treat this problem. Your doctor will confirm the diagnosis, screen for other sexually transmitted diseases, and in women, perform a Papanicolau (Pap) smear and examine the cervix and vagina to screen for any precancerous or cancerous changes. Your sexual partner should also be checked by a doctor.

Treatment Genital warts can typically be identified by their appearance, although a biopsy may be performed to confirm the diagnosis. Prescription home therapies, such as topically applied podofilox (Condylox) or imiquimod (Aldara) may be successful in some cases. Physician administered topical podophyllin, liquid nitrogen, and laser vaporization are alternative approaches.

Prognosis Recurrences of genital warts are common. Very importantly, women with this infection should have yearly or more frequent Pap smears to detect precancerous or cancerous lesions of the cervix. Notably, most women with HPV never develop cervical cancer, but given the known increased risk and the tremendous advantage of the early diagnosis of cancer, women with HPV

should have Pap smears performed every 6 to 12 months, or as recommended by their doctors.

FUNGAL INFECTIONS

❖ ATHLETE'S FOOT (TINEA PEDIS)

Symptoms and signs Scaling, cracking, and flaking of the skin between the toes (toe webs); scaling and redness on the soles and the sides of the feet; itching and occasional burning. (See page C-36.)

What is it? Athlete's foot, (also called tinea pedis) is a fungal infection involving the toe web spaces and/or the soles of the feet (see Onychomycosis, page 1320, for a discussion of fungal nail infections). The fungus grows in moist, warm environments, and is usually acquired initially in public or private showers/bathing areas (such as home and hotel bathrooms, gym floors, and locker rooms in sports clubs). The condition typically occurs between the toes, most frequently between the fourth and fifth toes; however, it also may cover the soles and sides of the feet and is frequently mistaken for dry skin. It is most common among males, both adolescents and adults. As many as 80 percent of males develop athlete's foot at some time.

Prevention To reduce the risk, feet should be washed with an antibacterial soap and dried thoroughly, especially between the toes, once or twice a day. Also, shower stalls and bathtubs should be disinfected regularly (every 1 to 2 weeks). An inexpensive cleanser, made of a mix of one part bleach to 10 parts water, can be used to wipe down the shower, and is very effective. Make sure to wear gloves and ventilate the bathroom adequately when using this mixture. Also, change your socks if they become wet. Athlete's foot is contagious, so avoid sharing towels and wear rubber thongs in public showers. Also, dry your feet carefully after showering or swimming.

What you can do If athlete's foot develops, a number of over-the-counter, antifungal foot powders, creams, and sprays containing clotrimazole or miconazole are available to treat the problem. These treatments should be continued for 2 weeks after the infection has cleared up, to minimize the chance of recurrence.

When to call the doctor Because other skin conditions affecting the feet (such as eczema or psoriasis) can sometimes be confused with athlete's foot, see a doctor if the rash does not clear up after 2 to 4 weeks of self-care. On occasion, an untreated or mistreated case of athlete's foot can be complicated by a secondary bacterial infection.

Treatment In most instances, athlete's foot responds well to treatment. Over-the-counter and prescription antifungal creams usually work well. If the problem persists, antifungal medications, taken orally, may be prescribed.

Prognosis Although annoying, athlete's foot is rarely a serious condition. Most cases can be treated successfully, without requiring a doctor's attention.

❖ JOCK ITCH (TINEA CRURIS)

Symptoms and signs Semicircular, scaly rash in the groin region, including the upper, inner thighs; itching; burning.

What is it? Jock itch, also called tinea cruris, is a common fungal infection that causes an itchy, red rash in the groin area and upper, inner thighs. Although it occurs primarily in men, it occasionally affects women.

The condition develops when moisture and heat trapped by tight underwear or athletic garments set up an environment favorable for fungal growth. Fungi multiply and flourish in this environment. Not surprisingly, this condition is most likely to occur in warm weather.

Prevention To prevent jock itch, cleanse the groin region with antibacterial soap and dry well. During warm weather, wear loose clothing. Change underwear and athletic garments frequently. Wash body towels after each use and do not share towels, as they may carry the fungus.

What you can do If jock itch develops, apply an over-the-counter antifungal powder or cream. Continue using it for 2 weeks after the rash has cleared.

When to call the doctor If jock itch persists despite the self-treatment described above, call a doctor, because it is possible to confuse this rash with other skin conditions, such as contact dermatitis and psoriasis. A doctor can confirm the diagnosis by taking a skin scraping and examining it under a microscope.

Treatment If tinea cruris has been diagnosed, the doctor may recommend a prescription antifungal cream or lotion, which in some instances may be more effective than the over-the-counter antifungal product that you may have been using.

Prognosis Although jock itch can be treated successfully, it often recurs—particularly if the predisposing environmental factors (in other words, wearing tight underwear or athletic garments, sharing or reusing towels) have not been modified.

❖ RINGWORM (TINEA CORPORIS)

Symptoms and signs Red, ring-shaped lesion, with a slightly elevated, scaly border; itchy. (See page C-36.)

What is it? Ringworm, or tinea corporis, is a contagious fungal skin infection. Despite its name, it has nothing to do with worms. Although it may develop in anyone, it most often affects children.

Ringworm can appear on any part of the body, but it is seen most frequently on the scalp (tinea capitis), arms, legs, chest, and back. When it occurs on the scalp, it produces hair loss, redness, and flaking on the infected area. The ringworm patches usually expand to several inches in diameter, and several may cluster in one area of the body.

The fungus responsible for ringworm is usually transmitted by person-to-person contact and by sharing combs, brushes, hats, towels, and clothing. Even pets can carry the fungus and infect family members.

What you can do Ringworm on the skin, other than the scalp, can be treated with over-the-counter antifungal creams (such as clotrimazole or miconazole). However, self-diagnosis can be difficult, because ringworm may look very similar to other skin eruptions, including eczema and psoriasis.

When to call the doctor To confirm the diagnosis, see your doctor. He will likely take a scraping to confirm that fungus is present, and recommend an over-the-counter or prescription antifungal cream. If you have a scalp infection, see your doctor as soon as possible, because permanent scarring and hair loss may occur if the infection progresses. Also, scalp infections cannot be treated with topical creams alone.

Treatment Over-the-counter antifungal creams (for example, clotrimazole) are usually effective for these skin infections. However, sometimes fungi can be resistant to this treatment and require a different chemical class of prescription antifungal cream. Occasionally, oral antifungal medication is needed for extensive and widespread lesions. Unlike skin infections, a scalp infection (tinea capitis) must always be treated with an oral antifungal medication. A selenium sulfide shampoo is usually also recommended to reduce shedding of the fungus and the spread of the infection to others.

Prognosis Ringworm is cosmetically unattractive—but in most cases it is not a serious condition, and it can be treated successfully with antifungal medications.

❖ TINEA VERSICOLOR

Symptoms and signs Multiple, $1/4$- to-1-in. oval, scaly spots; pink or tan in color; when fully merged or coalesced, may cover the entire upper chest, upper back, neck, or upper arms, and occasionally the face; mild itching, which may be aggravated by perspiration. (See page C-36.)

What is it? Tinea versicolor is a common, mild skin infection caused by a slow-growing yeast, called *Pityrosporum orbiculare*. Although this yeast normally exists on everyone's skin, it can multiply in regions of the body that have a dense population of oil or sebaceous glands—such as the upper chest, back, and neck—and produce oval, scaly spots or patches on the skin, usually pale, pink, or tan in color. These spots become more noticeable after suntanning due to the lack of tanning in the involved areas, which contrasts with the normal surrounding suntanned skin. Affected people often find tinea versicolor unattractive due to the color variation, or are bothered by mild itching that tends to worsen when heavy perspiring takes place.

Most people with tinea versicolor are adolescents or young adults. The condition often wanes on its own during the colder seasons of the year, only to reappear when warm, humid weather returns.

What you can do Apply selenium sulfide 1 percent shampoos (such as Head & Shoulders Intensive Treatment, Selsun Blue) from the neck down to the waistline and wrists, rinsing after 10 to 15 minutes. Performing this daily regimen for 2 weeks may be effective. If it is successful, then a single application once a week during the summer months should be continued to prevent recurrences.

When to call the doctor If the shampoo treatments mentioned above do not work, see your doctor so that he can confirm the diagnosis.

Treatment Prescription topical antifungal lotions and shampoos (such as selenium sulfide 2.5 percent and ketoconazole 2 percent) may be used to treat tinea versicolor. They are typically applied for 10 to 15 minutes and rinsed each day for 2 weeks, and repeated less frequently, as described above, to prevent recurrences. In resistant cases, oral antifungal medications—such as ketoconazole or fluconazole—are prescribed for this condition. In most people, a 5- to 7-day course of these oral medications clears the infection; however, recurrences are still common, because some people seem to have an increased susceptibility to this infection.

Prognosis Tinea versicolor is usually a mild infection. Although it can be treated successfully with lotions or medications, the condition may be a chronic recurring problem.

Allergic Skin Conditions

An allergy is the response of the body's immune system to a foreign, yet otherwise harmless, substance—perhaps a cosmetic, a food, or ragweed pollen—often manifesting as an itch, skin rash, or swelling. In the first type of reaction, the immediate allergic reaction, which includes hay fever and skin swelling or hives, reactions are triggered by specific antibodies (immunoglobulin E; IgE) to an allergy-producing protein; the antibodies activate the body's mast cells, which release histamine in the eyes, nose airway, and/or the skin—a process that repeats itself each time you come in contact with the allergenic substance. In the other type of reaction—the delayed allergic reaction or allergic contact dermatitis (see below)—the itchy, bumpy, and often blistering rash is caused by immune cells in the skin called Langerhans' cells.

The skin manifestations (hives) of "immediate" skin allergies begin within minutes of the allergen exposure and last for just a few hours or even less; notably, however, new hives may occur in adjacent or distant skin for days or even years if exposure continues. In contrast, the skin changes of "delayed" allergic reactions (such as poison ivy) initially begin about 8 to 72 hours after the exposure and may take 1 to 2 weeks to go away. (See Chapter 29 for more information on allergic reactions.)

Poison ivy can be identified by its three distinct leaves. After repeated exposures on different occasions, plants such as poison ivy may suddenly cause allergic contact dermatitis, with severe itching, inflammation, or blistering of the skin. The reaction is triggered by an oily resin in the sap of the plant. If you develop contact dermatitis, flush the affected area with warm water before using soap, which could spread the allergen. Affected clothing should also be washed thoroughly. Over-the-counter creams are available for relief of itching and inflammation. Although the fluid inside blisters will not spread the dermatitis, scratching the skin excessively can cause damage that allows infections to develop.

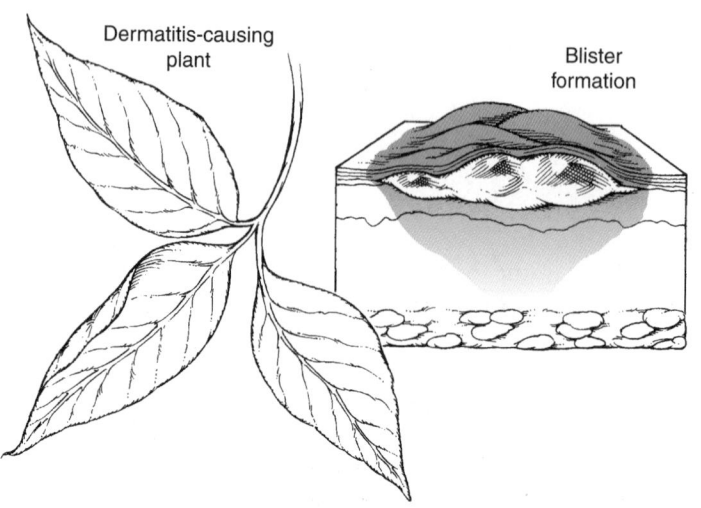

Dermatitis-causing plant

Blister formation

❖ CONTACT DERMATITIS

Symptoms Redness; blisters; weeping; oozing; flaky; intense itching. (See page C-28.)

Signs and laboratory findings If a delayed allergic reaction is causing the symptoms, "patch testing" may be performed to determine the specific cause or causes.

What is it? Contact dermatitis is an inflammatory reaction to a substance. There are two types of contact dermatitis: irritant contact dermatitis and allergic contact dermatitis.

Irritant contact dermatitis This type of contact dermatitis is the more common type, occurring when an external (often chemical) irritant touches the skin. A common example of contact dermatitis is "hand eczema," in which the skin develops a red, rough, thickened rash in response to harsh chemicals in soaps, dishwashing liquids, solvents, and other cleaning agents.

Allergic contact dermatitis This type of contact dermatitis occurs when an allergic reaction takes place after exposure to a particular substance. Allergic reactions never occur on the first-ever exposure to a substance. Any exposure may sensitize an individual (sensitization may occur following the first, the tenth, the hundredth, or any exposure, depending upon the individual), and then an allergic reaction will occur upon subsequent exposures. Common allergens or substances that cause allergic contact dermatitis include plants (for example, poison ivy, oak, and sumac) and nickel (found in jewelry and wrist watches). Less common allergens include fragrances, preservatives and other additives found in personal-care products, and many chemicals used in various manufacturing processes.

The allergic reaction occurs when the body recognizes and reacts to a substance by turning on immune cells that release very potent chemical mediators in the skin at the area of contact, producing itching, and an oozing, often blistering, red rash, typically within 8 to 72 hours after exposure to the substance, and continuing to develop on subsequent days.

The best-known forms of allergic contact dermatitis are reactions to poison ivy (see page C-28) sumac, and oak. The sap of

REDUCING OUTBREAKS OF POISON IVY/OAK

If you work outdoors or enjoy a recreational outdoor life, and you react to poison ivy or oak, your summer can become an endless round of itchy ivy rashes and trips to the doctor or drugstore. Here are a few tips that may help to reduce your outbreaks.

- Protect yourself from direct contact with plant oils. Wear protective clothing covering as much of your skin as temperature and humidity allow. Apply available barrier lotions or creams to all exposed skin. Currently available products that work by forming a barrier to prevent the ivy/oak oils from making direct contact with your skin include Ivy Block and Stokogard. You can obtain these or similar products at most drugstores.

- Quickly flush plant oils from your skin. After outdoor activity where you have or may have come into contact with poison ivy or oak, remove all clothing and immediately run the cloth-

ing through a warm-water washing machine cycle. Shower thoroughly in warm water to remove the allergic oil resin, and then you may wash with soap as well. Any boots, gloves, other durable clothing, tools, or equipment you used should also be rinsed thoroughly, preferably by someone else who is not sensitive to ivy. Oils can remain active on these objects forever, creating a potential hidden ivy/oak exposure in the future.

- Remember that if pets accompany you into the outdoors, they can pick up the ivy/oak plant oils on their fur, creating another possible source of exposure for you. Bathe them or allow them to swim after the outing to remove the oils.

- Poison ivy or oak clinging to dry firewood can also pose a hazard to allergic people. Burning the vines with the wood produces smoke that may contain the allergen and could provoke a reaction in those people exposed to it. ■

these plants contains an oily resin called urushiol, which triggers the allergic reaction. The result of exposure is swelling, redness, itching, and blistering of the skin.

The same type of allergic reaction occurs with other allergens; however, it tends to be much less intense, lacking the oozing blisters. For example, women allergic to nickel who wear costume jewelry earrings tend to experience itching, drying, and thickening of the earlobe skin instead of explosive blistering.

See Plant Dermatoses in Chapter 29 for more detailed information on reactions to poison ivy, sumac, and oak.

What you can do The most effective remedy for contact dermatitis is avoiding substances that trigger it. Stay away from poison ivy, sumac, and oak. Follow the motto, "Leaves of three, let them be." These plants tend to grow in wooded areas and adjacent lakes and streams. If you do come into contact with one of them, immediately flush the affected area thoroughly with warm water—then, use soap and water. If you lather with soap before flushing the skin, you may spread the allergen to previously unexposed areas of the skin. Minimize touching exposed clothing which has come into contact with the poison ivy until it can be thoroughly washed. Rinse all washable tools with a garden hose. If a rash does appear, take cool showers or apply cool compresses to dry the blisters and to relieve the itching, and apply Sarna lotion or calamine lotion for further relief

of the itch. Refrain from scratching, as this may lead to a secondary bacterial infection. (See Reducing Outbreaks of Poison Ivy/Oak, above, for more detailed information.)

When to call the doctor If there is extensive poison ivy with blistering, contact a doctor. Prescription corticosteroids are generally very helpful.

With other allergic skin reactions, such as those due to fragrances, additives, or preservatives in cosmetics, patch testing must be conducted to determine the responsible chemical. In this process, small amounts of about 30 to 50 different chemical allergens are placed on the skin of the back for 2 days to determine the exact chemical causing the allergy.

Treatment For cases of blistering poison ivy, the doctor will usually recommend compresses to dry the blisters and a potent topical corticosteroid cream or oral corticosteroid tablets.

The most important measure to prevent future contact dermatitis is avoidance of the substance or substances that cause the reaction. This is why the previously mentioned patch testing is so important if you do not know what triggered your allergic contact dermatitis. Patch testing, performed with chemicals by dermatologists in search of skin allergies, differs from the "scratch" or "prick" testing performed with dust or pollen, done by allergists trying to identify breathing allergies. (See Chapter 29 for more information on the diagnosis and treatment of breathing allergies such as hay fever and asthma.)

Prognosis Outbreaks of contact dermatitis can be prevented if triggering substances—such as poison ivy or cosmetics containing specific allergenic chemicals—can be identified and avoided.

❖ ATOPIC ECZEMA (ATOPIC DERMATITIS)

Symptoms and signs Persistent red, dry, flaky, irritated skin, particularly in the folds (inside the elbows, backs of the knees, back of the neck); oozing and crusting (occasionally). (See page C-29.)

What is it? Atopic eczema (or atopic dermatitis) is a common condition that causes dry, itchy, inflamed skin. It has been called "the itch that rashes." Atopic refers to a hereditary tendency to develop allergic reactions because of the presence of a circulating antibody (atopic reagin) in the blood. Although the cause of the condition is not known, it tends to run in families, particularly in those in which allergy-related conditions such as asthma or hay fever are also present. People with atopic eczema typically develop the condition in infancy or early childhood.

Atopic eczema can affect any area of the body. However, in children and adults, atopic eczema most often affects the folds of the elbows, the back folds of the knees, the face, the scalp, the neck, and the front of the ankles. In contrast, infants generally experience changes on the cheeks, the top surfaces of the forearms, and the front of the thighs; notably, these are the areas that babies can most easily rub (that is consistent with the idea that rubbing itchy areas aggravates the rash). The extreme itchiness can lead to scratching of the skin, causing the affected area to bleed, crust, and sometimes become infected.

Atopic eczema tends to improve as people progress through childhood and into adulthood; it often shows improvement by age 4 years, but symptoms can recur throughout one's lifetime. Recurrent secondary infections caused by bacteria invading the affected skin are not uncommon and should be treated promptly.

What you can do Do not wear tight or large-fiber, rough-textured clothing (wool) that can irritate the skin. Cotton fabrics worn in layers are among the best choices of clothing; layers may then be removed if you feel too warm, because excessive warming often triggers itching.

Bathe in warm (not very hot) water, using one of the new moisturizing, antibacterial soaps. Apply a good moisturizer immediately after patting dry; try to leave a little moisture on the skin so that the moisturizing lotion or cream can seal this moisture in the skin.

If you find that you tend to itch and then scratch in stressful situations, find alternative or subsequent activities that help you wind down and refocus. Strategies such as biofeedback, meditation, yoga, or taking a brisk walk may be helpful diversions. (See page 305 for information on the relief of stress.)

When to call the doctor See a doctor if you suspect that you have atopic eczema. He will make the diagnosis by taking a history and examining your skin. Occasionally, a skin biopsy may be necessary for diagnosis.

Treatment Corticosteroid creams and ointments, which reduce the inflammation causing the itch and rash, may be prescribed to normalize the skin changes of atopic eczema. Nighttime itching can be relieved by taking oral, sedating antihistamines before bed. Sedating antihistamines help induce sleep (although histamine is not thought to play a role in atopic eczema). Notably, nonsedating antihistamines are not effective, except in rare individuals.

In cases in which these treatments are not effective, ultraviolet light therapy, administered by a dermatologist in his office, might be needed to control the condition. (See Atopic Dermatitis (Allergic Eczema), page 1334, in Chapter 29 for more information.)

If a secondary bacterial infection such as impetigo, cellulitis, or erysipelas develops, see a doctor immediately for prompt treatment with oral or intravenous antibiotics.

Prognosis If appropriately treated, the symptoms of atopic eczema can be effectively controlled.

❖ HIVES (URTICARIA)

Symptoms and signs One or many pink, red or white raised circles, semicircles, or rings on the skin; less than one inch to several inches in diameter; intense itching, occasional burning or stinging; occasional associated flushing or wheezing. (See page C-29.)

What is it? Hives, also called wheals, are swollen red patches in the skin. They can occur on any portion of the body, may be smaller than a penny or as large as a plate, and their centers are often paler than their outer portions (central clearing). An individual spot is typically present for an hour or less, and always disappears in less than 1 day. New spots may continue to come and go for hours, weeks, or, in unfortunate persons, years. Hives are common, affecting 15 to 20 percent of people at some time in their lives.

Hives occur when a chemical called histamine is released by the body, often in reaction to the presence of certain medications, infections, insect bites, or foods. Chocolate, shellfish, nuts, cheese, tomatoes, and fresh berries commonly cause hives. Less often, hives are due to physical factors such as stress, exercise, or exposure to sunlight or cold. (For more information on causes of allergic reactions, see Chapter 29.)

An individual wheal will go away, after a few hours (or sometimes as short a time as under 1 hour), but new ones usually continue to erupt elsewhere. Several are usually present at the same time. The entire outbreak may last for a few days or as long as several weeks or even years. In the latter instance of "chronic hives," a person may continue to have daily hives for years without a known trigger.

What you can do Whenever possible, pinpoint the suspected substances triggering the hives and avoid them. Because hives are a histamine reaction, antihistamines are the treatment of choice. Prescription antihistamines, which come in nonsedating varieties, are the best form of treatment during the daytime. Over-the-counter antihistamines such as diphenhydramine (Benadryl) and chlorpheniramine (Chlor-Trimeton) are sedating, and thus are excellent before bedtime; unfortunately, they should not be taken when you are required to be alert— for example, while driving, operating heavy equipment, or test-taking. Cool compresses applied to the affected area, for periods of about 10 minutes, may temporarily relieve symptoms but are usually not practical.

When to call the doctor Difficulty in breathing is a potentially life-threatening reaction that may develop in people with hives or histamine reactions. If you have trouble catching your breath or are wheezing, it is due to the swelling of your airway, similar to the hive swelling in your skin. If this swelling blocks the airway completely, you will die. Therefore, if you experience wheezing or swelling of your lips or tongue, you need to receive immediate medical care.

Even if you have an episode of hives, that does not involve swelling of your airway, the next time you are exposed to your "trigger"—for example, shellfish—you may indeed develop breathing difficulties. This risk in itself makes it important to try to identify the trigger so that you can prevent future episodes. If you are unable to pinpoint the trigger, it is best to see your doctor for help; however, you must realize that triggers cannot always be identified. It is important to be prepared for the possibility of a severe allergic (anaphylactic) reaction. (See Anaphylaxis: A Life-Threatening Reaction, page 1341.)

Also, if your hives persist, see your doctor for nonsedating prescription antihistamines for daytime use. And if you have had hives for weeks, months, or even years, but have never contacted a doctor about them, you should be evaluated. Sometimes, chronic hives may be caused by autoimmune diseases or chronic, low-grade infections, which are important to diagnose.

Treatment Prescription nonsedating antihistamines—for example, cetirizine (Zyrtec), loratadine (Claritin)—are usually recommended for people with hives.

Individuals with difficulty breathing requiring immediate medical attention will usually be treated with an epinephrine (adrenaline) injection, an intravenous antihistamine, and often a short course of a corticosteroid medication.

Prognosis For most people, hives are transient and cause no serious or lasting health problems. However, emergency treatment is needed if the hives are accompanied by potentially life-threatening difficulties in

RASHES CAUSED BY MEDICATIONS

Nearly every prescription and nonprescription medication can cause an allergic reaction in some people, often manifesting itself as a rash. (See page C-29.) Problematic over-the-counter medications include laxatives and analgesics (painkillers), while problematic prescription medications include many antibiotics (such as penicillin), seizure medications, diuretics (water pills), and other blood pressure medications and analgesics. Penicillin, for instance, can cause a skin rash, itching, or wheezing in some people. In the worst cases, some people may experience a potentially life-threatening anaphylactic reaction: hives on their skin, swelling of their tongue or throat, serious breathing problems, choking, and/or loss of consciousness; these people require immediate medical attention. (See Anaphylaxis: A Life Threatening Reaction, page 1341.)

If you experience a rash or other allergic response that appears to be related to a medication you are taking, notify your doctor. Often a reaction to a medication may be a side effect of that medication rather than a true allergic reaction. (See Telling a Medication Allergy from a Side Effect, on page 1343.) Your doctor may suggest an alternative medication that you can take in place of the one that may be causing the problem. Your doctor can also advise you whether you should take antihistamine or steroid medication to resolve the symptoms of an allergic reaction, such as a skin rash or itching. Anaphylaxis or other reactions associated with difficulty breathing or a faint feeling are potentially life-threatening and require immediate medical care. ■

breathing or swallowing. See Anaphylaxis: A Life-Threatening Reaction, page 1341, for more information.

❖ PHOTOSENSITIVITY

Symptoms and signs Red blotches, bumpy rash, and itching on sun-exposed skin.

What is it? When the skin is exposed to sunlight, suntan parlor bulbs, or sometimes even overhead fluorescent light, a number of abnormal reactions, all categorized under "photosensitivity," may occur. A common type of photosensitivity involves a medication taken by mouth that causes rapid sunburning. Specifically, this is called a phototoxic medication reaction, and occurs when an individual taking, for example, the medication doxycycline (a tetracycline derivative) is exposed to the sun or suntan parlor bulbs. This same reaction happens with a number of quinolone medications—such as ciprofloxacin (Cipro) and ofloxacin (Floxin). In a similar way, chemicals in limes, celery, and figs can cause localized phototoxicity or sunburn on areas of the skin on which they have been rubbed or spilled.

Less commonly, photoallergic medication reactions may occur; they affect only certain allergic people, who develop a red, bumpy, itchy rash on sun-exposed areas after sun exposure, but only during times when they are also taking the medication to which they have developed a photoallergy. Medications that may cause these reactions include thiazide diuretics (water pills), piroxicam (a nonsteroidal anti-inflammatory agent; NSAID), and sulfa medications. Also, ingredients in cosmetics, perfumes, soaps and even suntan lotion can cause photoallergic reactions in some people, producing this same type of itchy, bumpy rash, limited to the body areas in which the products are applied and exposed to the sun.

Another type of photosensitivity is called polymorphous light eruption. Independent of the use of any medication or topically applied chemical, an itchy, bumpy, red rash develops with the first few intense sun exposures of the summer. With subsequent exposures, the skin tans, and seems to become resistant or desensitized, no longer breaking out after sun exposure. This sensitivity tends to develop for the first time in persons in their 20s to 40s, and generally recurs at the beginning of each summer. Polymorphous light eruption needs to be distinguished from lupus erythematosus, a serious autoimmune condition that may be associated with internal organ disease. Persons with lupus frequently develop photosensitivity; however, unlike polymorphous light eruption, their skin sensitivity continues throughout the entire summer if sun exposure is continued.

Rare photosensitive disorders include sun-induced hives (solar urticaria) and several of the inherited porphyrias, in which affected persons have elevations of certain chemicals in their blood, which cause photosensitivity, and burning and stinging or blistering of the skin.

Most photosensitivities are at least in part triggered by long-wavelength ultraviolet light, which is most intense in suntan parlor lamps and also passes through the window glass of cars and buildings.

What you can do Many medications, including some blood pressure medications, analgesics, antibiotics, antidepressants, and oral contraceptives, may cause photosensitivity. When your doctor prescribes medications, ask whether there is any problem with sun exposure while taking the medication. If there is a possible problem and you anticipate sun exposure, ask your doctor if you can take the medication later in the day, after your sun exposure. Also, read the patient information sheet that the pharmacy provides with your prescription medication.

If you are taking a potentially photosensitizing medication, avoid sunlight as much as possible. When outdoors, wear protective clothing as well as a sunscreen with a broad spectrum and a high sun protection factor (SPF).

When a photosensitive skin reaction occurs, wet compresses or lukewarm baths can soothe the rash or blistering. An over-the-counter oral antihistamine can relieve the itching through its sedating effects.

When to call the doctor If you have a severe reaction with intense redness and discomfort or with blisters, contact your doctor immediately. Also, if you suspect that you have developed photosensitivity in association with a medication, inform the doctor who prescribed it. He may want to change your medication or work out ways to avoid future reactions.

Treatment If the skin reaction is severe, medications (such as topical or oral corticosteroids) may be prescribed to minimize symptoms.

Prognosis The prognosis depends on the specific type of photosensitivity you have. Your doctor should discuss your particular prognosis with you once a diagnosis is made.

Noncancerous Growths and Tumors

As people pass through their 20s and 30s, they may begin to notice small new growths on their bodies. Most of these skin manifestations, such as skin tags and liver spots, are not worrisome; however, they may be considered unattractive, or cause irritation, anxiety, and concern. For these reasons, people frequently bring them to the attention of a doctor, asking about treatment and removal.

If you have a new or undiagnosed growth on your body, have it evaluated by a doctor. Do not rely on your own diagnostic efforts for determining whether a particular skin condition is cancerous or not. Remember, undiagnosed melanomas are potentially fatal.

❖ SEBORRHEIC KERATOSIS

Symptoms and signs Tan to dark brown growths; rough, or fine-pebbly, thickened surface; commonly dime-sized or smaller. (See page C-37.)

What is it? Seborrheic keratoses are growths on the skin, most frequently on the back or chest, face, neck, or scalp. Their diameter can range from just a fraction of an inch to more than an inch, and they may slowly enlarge. There may be a single lesion present or, less often, literally hundreds of lesions over the back or chest. They often have the appearance of sitting atop or being "stuck on" the skin. Seborrheic keratoses become more common in middle and old age. In fact, nearly everyone eventually develops at least some of these growths.

Many people mistake their seborrheic keratoses for warts; indeed, they are sometimes called senile warts. Others think they have skin cancer or a precancerous condition. But seborrheic keratoses are neither warts nor cancer. They are not caused by viruses or exposure to sun. The cause of seborrheic keratoses is unknown.

What you can do Seborrheic keratoses do not require medical treatment.

When to call the doctor Seborrheic keratoses can sometimes be hard to distinguish from moles and even melanomas. If you have any doubts about what you have, see a doctor to make sure that you do not have a cancerous growth. This examination may be lifesaving.

Treatment If seborrheic keratoses become irritated (by rubbing against clothing, for example), or if you find them itchy or unsightly, a doctor may advise removing them. Because they are not deep in the skin, removal is usually easily performed. They can be frozen using liquid nitrogen, scraped with a currette, or vaporized with an electric current or laser.

Prognosis These growths are harmless and generally painless. Persons who develop them tend to develop additional seborrheic keratoses as they age.

❖ CHERRY ANGIOMAS

Symptoms and signs Cherry-red dots on the skin. (See page C-37.)

What is it? Cherry angiomas are clusters of minute, dilated, red blood vessels visible beneath the skin. Although many are the size of a pinhead, they can also be as large as the eraser on a pencil. The trunk is the most common site for these angiomas, although they are often seen on the arms, legs, and other parts of the body.

Cherry angiomas tend to appear for the first time in adulthood and increase in number with age.

What you can do There is no self-treatment for cherry angiomas. Do not scratch them, or they may bleed.

When to call the doctor There is no medical reason to undergo therapy for cherry angiomas, although treatment is available if you find them cosmetically unattractive.

Treatment Cherry angiomas can be easily removed using a laser or an electrical needle. Lesions sometimes recur or need to be treated more than once.

Prognosis Cherry angiomas are benign (noncancerous) and do not turn into cancer.

❖ MOLES (NEVI)

Symptoms and signs Roundish, skin-colored to deep brown spots on the skin, sometimes raised above the skin's surface, smaller in diameter than a pencil head eraser. (See page C-37.)

What is it? Moles are spots on the skin, most of which are present by age 20. They can be found on any part of the body; they are usually round and therefore symmetrical, with a sharply defined border. They have a uniform color, ranging from flesh tones to deep brown/black. They may be flat, or raised like a miniature dome or a bead of water. They may slowly increase in size over time, such that flat moles may become raised; however, they should always maintain their symmetrical character and their even coloring.

Most moles never become problematic; however, all moles should be inspected on a regular basis for abnormal changes (see below). Those with an increased likelihood of becoming malignant are called dysplastic nevi. (See page C-37.) They are usually larger in size, and have irregular shapes, mottled coloring, and hazy borders; unlike normal moles, they may continue to increase in number well into adulthood. Also, moles that you are born with (congenital nevi) have a greater tendency to develop into cancer, so these must be vigilantly inspected on a monthly basis, looking for any changes.

What you can do Conduct regular self-exams of your skin, looking for any suspicious changes in moles. Get someone else to inspect your scalp and any other areas you cannot see. To help determine whether a mole is abnormal, or may be a potentially life-threatening melanoma, refer to the ABCDs listed below. These are the early warning signs of a mole cancer.

Also, never sunbathe or visit a suntan parlor for the sake of tanning. Enjoy the outdoors, but use high-SPF sunscreen, wear protective clothing, and avoid being outdoors during the peak sun intensity hours from 11 AM to 3 PM.

When to call the doctor Too often, people ignore the warning signs and delay having a suspicious mole checked by a doctor. Melanoma is the deadliest form of skin cancer and early diagnosis can save your life. If a mole is Asymmetrical, has an irregular Border or Color, or has a Diameter bigger than a pencil eraser (the ABCDs), have it checked by a doctor. He will decide to perform a biopsy if the mole appears abnormal. Always remember, just because a doctor has told you that a mole looks normal does not mean that it cannot later go on to be a mole cancer; so if you notice any new changes, have the mole reexamined. Also, if you have dysplastic nevi or a history of melanoma in your family, have a doctor check all of your moles at regular intervals.

Treatment If a mole appears to be abnormal, it should be removed surgically for microscopic pathologic examination. If it is found to be cancerous, additional surrounding skin will also need to be removed (see Melanoma, page 1302). Moles can also be removed for cosmetic reasons, often with a procedure called shave excision.

Prognosis Although moles may become cancerous, most remain benign throughout a person's lifetime, and pose no health problem.

❖ HYPERTROPHIC SCARS AND KELOIDS

Symptoms and signs A firm, raised scar, often lighter than the surrounding skin; occasional itching.

What is it? A hypertrophic scar is a scar that is raised instead of being flat. A keloid is like a hypertrophic scar but is larger, extending outward beyond the original scar line. Also, a keloid may develop spontaneously, without any prior injury or cut in the skin. Both are more of a cosmetic concern than a genuine health problem. For individuals prone to keloids, any kind of skin injury—a relatively minor cut or a vaccination, a surgical incision site—can result in a hypertrophic scar or keloid upon healing. This thick scar tissue reaction is seen more frequently in people with dark skin than in those with light skin.

What you can do Sometimes, a hypertrophic scar or keloid will become smaller or even disappear without any treatment. However, this is more often the exception than the rule. So before undergoing any surgery, particularly elective procedures, discuss the possibility of keloid formation with your surgeon.

When to call the doctor If you find a keloid or hypertrophic scar unsightly, contact a dermatologist or cosmetic surgeon to see if any of the therapies described below might be worthwhile.

Treatment No treatments are guaranteed to be successful. Injections of corticosteroids (such as triamcinolone) or topically applied silicon patches (such as CicaCare) may be used to aid in the flattening of keloids; laser and routine surgeries may also be used, often in combination with corticosteroid injections.

Prognosis Although laser and routine surgeries are effective in many cases, new

keloids may form in the aftermath of these procedures. Again, no treatment is guaranteed to be successful.

❖ SKIN TAGS (CUTANEOUS TAGS)

Symptoms and signs Soft, often floppy outpouchings of skin; minute to pea-sized; flesh-colored to dark brown.

What is it? Skin tags are tiny protrusions of skin that occur most often on the neck, underarms, groin, and under the breasts. They often develop during pregnancy, and are more common in individuals over age 50.

Although skin tags generally cause no pain of their own, they can become irritated by clothing, necklaces, and underarm shaving.

What you can do Do not try to snip off skin tags yourself; complications such as bleeding and infection can develop.

When to call the doctor If your skin tags often become irritated by clothing or shaving, see a doctor to discuss possible removal. If you feel that they are merely cosmetically unsightly, they may also be removed for cosmetic (nonmedical) purposes; this would be considered a cosmetic procedure by most insurance companies.

Treatment Skin tags can be removed by excision with a scissors or scalpel, destruction with heat from an electrical needle (electrodesiccation), or freezing with liquid nitrogen applications.

Prognosis Skin tags are a benign condition. If they are taken off, they generally do not regrow, but new ones usually develop over the years.

❖ VASCULAR BIRTHMARKS

Symptoms and signs Port-wine stain (nevus flammeus): Flat, pink, red, or purplish patch of skin; occasional elevation with tiny bumps, or thickening with time; variable fading of discoloration.

Strawberry hemangioma: Red, slightly raised lesions; rapid increase in size; nonmalignant.

What is it? Vascular birthmarks are discolorations of the skin. They are present at or shortly after the time of birth, and are composed of clusters of blood vessels in the skin (see Chapter 8). Two of the most common are port-wine stains and strawberry hemangiomas.

Port-wine stain A port-wine stain is a flat patch of pink, red, or purplish skin. It typically occurs on the face, side of the neck, or an arm or leg, and may cover a large area of skin. (Mikhail Gorbachev has a port-wine stain on his forehead.) Some may fade almost completely with time (particularly pink or light-red spots between the eyebrows (Angel's Kiss) or at the nape of the neck (Stork Bite); others thicken and may develop tiny bumps. (See page C-33.)

Strawberry hemangioma A strawberry hemangioma (or strawberry mark) is a bright red spot. It occurs most commonly on the face, chest, or back. In early infancy, it increases in size, sometimes rapidly. Although disconcerting, its growth eventually stops; even without treatment, a hemangioma shrinks in size and has usually disappeared by age 7 to 9 years. (See page C-33.)

What you can do Self-care options are limited with birthmarks. If desired, you can use opaque cosmetic cover-up creams to help camouflage flat birthmarks.

When to call the doctor Doctors should evaluate birthmarks soon after they appear, and on a regular basis thereafter, so they can be properly diagnosed and their development followed.

If a port-wine stain is present around the eyes and/or over one-half of the forehead, a doctor should examine the baby very carefully; the port-wine stain could be associated with the development of the eye disease glaucoma, or even with underlying blood vessel growth within the brain, resulting in an increased chance of an associated seizure disorder.

Treatment Laser surgery can be used to remove both port-wine stains that persist and hemangiomas. However, because hemangiomas tend to disappear spontaneously, they are usually treated only when they interfere with a vital function. Treatment is indicated if a hemangioma is over an eye and is affecting vision, around the mouth and nose and is interfering with breathing, or within the ear and is affecting hearing.

Doctors may recommend treatment with oral prednisone (a steroid medication), alone or in combination with surgery.

Prognosis Strawberry hemangiomas typically disappear on their own, often vanishing completely by mid-childhood. Although port-wine stains may almost totally fade away, some may worsen over time. Fortunately, laser surgery is usually very helpful in the latter cases.

❖ SEBACEOUS CYSTS

Symptoms and signs A whitish-yellow or skin-colored lump underneath the skin; slow-growing; painless.

What is it? A sebaceous cyst or epidermal inclusion cyst is a common growth. It forms when the skin turns underneath itself, creating a small sac or cyst. The cell layer that is normally produced and shed from the top of the skin (stratum corneum) is trapped within this sac and, because of this occlusion, forms a thick, soft cheese-like yellow substance, which is quite odoriferous. Though many of these cysts are small, they can enlarge to the size of a golf ball over a period of years.

Sebaceous cysts develop most frequently on the scalp, the back of the neck, and the upper back. They do not cause pain unless they spontaneously rupture underneath the skin or become infected. Both of these events result in sudden redness, swelling, and tenderness of the cyst.

When to call the doctor If a sebaceous cyst ruptures or becomes infected, see a doctor. Talk to a doctor about removing a cyst if it becomes irritated or tender, frequently because of friction against clothing, or if you consider it cosmetically unattractive.

Treatment For an inflamed and infected sebaceous cyst, a doctor may recommend any combination of surgical drainage (performed in-office), antibiotics, and warm compresses applied several times a day. Once the cyst is no longer painful or red, it can be surgically excised after it has been numbed with a local anesthesia injection.

Prognosis Sebaceous cysts generally do not pose any health risks, although they should be treated if they become inflamed or infected.

❖ DERMATOFIBROMA

Symptoms and signs A firm, pea-sized, slightly elevated growth; from flesh-toned to purplish or dusty brown in color; usually painless or only slightly painful when direct surface pressure is applied.

What is it? A dermatofibroma is a pea-sized growth that appears most often on the lower legs and, less frequently, on the arms or trunk. While common in adults, they occur only rarely in children. The cause is not known.

To confirm whether a lesion really is a dermatofibroma, a doctor may pinch the growth; if it dimples into the skin, it probably is a dermatofibroma.

What you can do Most dermatologists believe that the best approach for the majority of dermatofibromas is to do nothing. They are benign growths and do not require treatment.

When to call the doctor If you find a dermatofibroma to be cosmetically unacceptable, talk to your dermatologist about the feasibility of removing it, as well as the expected resultant scarring (This scarring is sometimes more noticeable than the dermatofibroma itself.)

Treatment Dermatofibromas can be removed completely (surgically excised), or only the elevated portion can be removed, leaving the base remaining in the skin; the former requires stitches, while the latter does not. Cryosurgery with liquid nitrogen is another option that only partially removes the dermatofibroma. None of these steps is medically necessary unless the diagnosis is in question because the lesion does not have the characteristic appearance or if it is growing suddenly. In these cases, it should be biopsied to exclude the possibility that it is actually another type of growth that may be malignant or cancerous.

Prognosis Typical-appearing dermatofibromas are benign growths and are not a cause for concern.

Skin Cancer

Skin cancer is the most commonly diagnosed form of cancer in the United States. Possible signs and symptoms of skin cancer should never be ignored. Specifically, in the case of melanoma, early diagnosis may be lifesaving.

Even better, prevention is the key. As you will read, minimizing your exposure to the sun is the most powerful step you can take to minimize your risk of skin cancer.

❖ ACTINIC KERATOSIS

Symptoms (What you may experience) Rough, reddish spots or patches, frequently on sun-exposed areas of the skin; usually half-dime to nickel-size; fine to coarse sandpaper-like surface texture; asymptomatic.

What is it? An actinic keratosis is a precancerous lesion or spot that can in a small percentage of lesions progress to a skin cancer (see Squamous Cell Carcinoma, page 1301). The most susceptible people are those who are fair-skinned with a history of frequent sun exposure and who have other visible evidence of sun damage (such as freckles, liver spots, uneven pigmentation, and wrinkles). Although actinic keratoses usually begin to develop in people after the age of 30, they are occasionally seen in teenagers.

What you can do Avoid the sun. Conduct regular inspections of your body for changes on the skin to detect lesions early in their development.

When to call the doctor If you have spots or patches that you suspect could be actinic keratoses, see a doctor. These spots are best detected by feeling for fine sandpaper-like areas, or by closely inspecting the skin after putting on a light facial powder or watery (thin) foundation; these spots stand out, because they tend to take up the powder or liquid makeup differently than the surrounding skin, creating difficult cosmetic coverage.

Treatment The lesions can be removed with cryotherapy, in which liquid nitrogen is used to freeze and destroy the lesion; heal-

THE RISKS OF SUNBURN AND SUN DAMAGE

Many people think that a suntan gives them a healthy look. If they could see what lies in the future, they'd head to the beach with not only a beach towel, but a full bottle of sunscreen and a wide-brimmed hat—or they wouldn't go at all. That's because sun exposure cannot only cause minor skin changes (such as freckles), but it is responsible for cosmetically unattractive ones (wrinkles) and even life-threatening conditions (skin cancer).

When you overdo it in the sun (the length of time is different for each person), you will develop a sunburn, with the skin reddening in the hours that follow; this sunburn is often accompanied by pain and swelling. A severe sunburn can cause blistering, chills, and fever, and a doctor's attention is necessary. Too much sun also makes you more susceptible to the most common types of skin cancer (see Basal Cell Carcinoma, page 1300, Squamous Cell Carcinoma, page 1301, and Melanoma, page 1302), which may not develop for decades until after the sun exposure itself.

Due in large part to our society's devotion to the sun, the average American's risk of developing malignant melanoma will be 1 in 75 by the year 2000; that is twice what the risk was during the mid-1980s.

Among regular sun worshipers (including construction workers and others who are in the sun for hours every day), the skin is likely to show signs of early aging, including premature wrinkling, a leathery appearance, and "liver spots." The sun can alter the skin's texture, and lead to sagging skin at an earlier age (see Wrinkles and Liver (Age) Spots (Solar Lentigo), pages 1312).

When choosing a sunscreen, select one with not only a high sun protection factor (SPF) of 15 or more, but also with a broad spectrum (meaning that it can guard against both ultraviolet A and B sun radiation). Be sure you apply it liberally to every exposed area of your body, including earlobes and lips.

Plan your time outdoors by paying attention to the new Ultraviolet (UV) Index, which was created by the National Weather Service and the Environmental Protection Agency and is published each day in many newspapers. You need to be particularly careful if the UV Index (which is a 0 to 10+ scale) is in the moderate to very high range (5 and over). This means that UV radiation can be particularly problematic to your skin. ■

ing should be complete in 1 to 2 weeks. Cryotherapy can sometimes cause loss of pigment (depigmentation) or leave a white patch of skin at the site.

Other treatment options include a topical cream called 5-fluorouracil (Fluoroplex, Efudex) applied at home twice daily for about 4 weeks, and various in-office chemical and laser peel procedures.

Prognosis Actinic keratoses are not cancers; however, they are an indication of previous sun damage and are associated with a greatly increased risk of skin cancer on sun-exposed areas. For this reason, people who have had these lesions treated should usually be reexamined yearly and should perform self-examinations every 1 to 2 months, looking for the development of more actinic keratoses and new skin cancers.

❖ BASAL CELL SKIN CANCER (BASAL CELL CARCINOMA)

Symptoms and signs Most commonly, a small bump that appears smooth or waxy; whitish to pink in color; slowly growing; may open to become an ulcer or sore as it grows. Less commonly, (a) a small, red, flat spot with a fine, thread-like border; (b) a sore that persists, heals, then recurs repeatedly; or (c) a "spontaneous" scar with no history of a preceding injury. Usually asymptomatic. (See page C-38.)

What is it? More than 1 million skin cancers are diagnosed yearly in the United States, making them by far the most prevalent cancers in humans. Of the various types of skin cancer, basal cell cancer or carcinoma is the most common, eventually developing in one of every six persons in this country. It occurs most often in people with light skin, hair, and eyes. It only rarely develops in black people.

Although this form of cancer is painless and slow growing, it can bleed, ulcerate (become an open sore), and crust or scab.

What you can do To try to prevent this and other skin cancers, limit your exposure to sunlight to avoid sunburning and suntanning.

When outdoors, generously apply a sunscreen with a sun protection factor (SPF) of 15 or greater. Most people use less than half the amount of lotion needed to get the sunscreen's claimed SPF. Wear a wide-brimmed hat and sunglasses.

Every 1 to 2 months, conduct a full-body-skin self-exam with another person's assistance or by using mirrors so that you do not miss areas that are difficult to see. Examine every region of your body, including the scalp, the soles of the feet, and the toe webs. Look closely at moles, freckles, and other spots to check for changes from one month to the next.

When to call the doctor If you suspect that you may have a skin cancer, see your primary care doctor or dermatologist.

MOHS' SURGERY FOR REMOVAL OF CANCEROUS SKIN

When doctors surgically remove skin cancers, they can now use a technique called Mohs' surgery. Named after its creator, Dr. Frederic Mohs, it is usually performed under local anesthesia in an outpatient surgical suite. Mohs' surgery demands great precision on the part of the surgeon; it involves shaving away slices of cancerous skin, one layer at a time. As each layer is removed, it is checked under the microscope, examining all the surgical margins. This process is continued until no abnormal cells are seen.

Mohs' surgery attempts to guarantee that all of the cancer is removed, while conserving as much healthy tissue as possible, thereby reducing the amount of scarring that is left behind after surgery. This technique is used most often for poorly defined cancerous lesions. It is also used to remove lesions on parts of the body—such as the nose, lips, ears, or eyelids—where it is important to remove the least amount of healthy skin possible. Mohs' surgery is being used primarily for squamous and basal cell cancers and, more recently, for some melanomas. Studies have shown that Mohs' surgery has produced 5-year cure rates of 99 percent for primary basal cell carcinoma, and 96 percent for recurrent basal cell cancers.

Depending on the amount of tumor removed, Mohs' surgery may be followed by reconstructive surgery to improve the postoperative cosmetic appearance. ■

Treatment Treatment of basal cell skin cancer involves removal of the lesions. One of the most common surgical techniques is called curettage and electrodesiccation, in which a very small, spoon-shaped blade (a curette) scrapes away the cancer, and then a probe with a high-frequency electric current destroys the remaining cancer cells. Alternatively, the cancer may be removed with a scalpel blade and then closed with sutures (stitches). Mohs' surgery (see above) is also used to remove skin cancer, particularly in areas such as the face; this is where the smallest possible scar is desired and where it is also most difficult to ensure complete removal of the cancer because the skin surface curves, making the exact extent of the cancer more difficult for the surgeon to appreciate.

Prognosis The cure rate of basal cell cancer is 95 percent with early and proper treatment. Although basal cell skin cancer does not spread internally, if it is not fully removed it may recur, typically within 5 years of initial removal. Recurrent cancers should be removed, and this is usually performed with Mohs' surgery. If you have had basal cell cancer, you should protect yourself scrupulously from further sun damage by using high SPF sunscreens, clothing coverage, and avoidance of sun exposure during the midday hours (11 AM to 3 PM) of late spring, summer, and early fall.

❖ SQUAMOUS CELL SKIN CANCER (SQUAMOUS CELL CARCINOMA)

Symptoms and signs Most often, a raised, scaly, crusty or warty pea-sized to chestnut-sized bump; less often, a clearly outlined, red, scaly, flat or slightly elevated $1/4$-in. to 1-in. sized area; asymptomatic. (See page C-38.)

What is it? Squamous cell cancer is second only to basal cell cancer as the most common skin cancer. In the United States, there is one squamous cell skin cancer for every four basal cell skin cancers. Squamous cell skin cancer appears most frequently on the ears, face (including the lips and inside the mouth), and the backs of the arms and hands. In women, squamous cell cancers are frequently found on the legs.

Unlike basal cell skin cancer, squamous cell cancers can spread internally. Usually this occurs only if the cancer is neglected and is allowed to grow for a long period of time.

What you can do As with other forms of skin cancer, the risk of squamous cell carcinoma can be decreased significantly by reducing sun exposure and applying a sunscreen (SPF 15 or greater) when outdoors. Regular self-examinations of the skin are important, because early diagnosis and treatment offer a cure rate of 95 percent. This self-examination in an effort to provide early diagnosis is even more important for cancer of the lips and the inside of the mouth, as these cancers have a much greater chance of spreading internally or to another part of the body (metastasizing).

When to call the doctor At the first signs of lesions that may be squamous cell cancer, see your doctor for a checkup. Although squamous cell cancers grow slowly, the sooner the cancer is diagnosed, the less extensive the surgery to excise it may be; also, suspected cancers inside the mouth should be examined as soon as possible.

New molecular screening techniques are being developed that may allow for earlier detection of cancer recurrences and greater precision in the initial excision of the cancer. A molecular probe can seek out individual cancer cells that have not yet developed the visible microscopic cell changes used to identify cancer cells, but that have developed the gene mutations that precede these visible changes.

Treatment Treatment depends on the size and location of the cancer. Surgical excision of the tumor and a small margin of surrounding skin is most often used to remove squamous cell skin cancer. Mohs' surgery (see page 1301) is another option; it is often used for cancers of the lips, nose, and ears, as well as recurrent cancers in any location. If a large lesion is removed, a skin graft (skin transplanted from another part of the body) may be performed to cover the area where the cancer had been. In unusual cases where the cancer has spread internally or metastasized, referral to a medical or surgical oncologist is usually necessary. (See Chapter 30 for more information on the diagnosis and treatment of cancer.)

Prognosis When treated in a reasonable amount of time after its initial development, squamous cell skin cancer has cure rates as high as those of basal cell cancers. However, in the unusual cases where it has metastasized, it is usually eventually fatal.

❖ MELANOMA (MOLE CANCER)

Symptoms and signs Changes in the appearance of an existing common mole or birthmark; or a new, developing mole, which shows the ABCDs: Asymmetry, Border irregularity, Color variation, and/or a Diameter greater than that of a pencil eraser. (*Note:* There are two melanoma variants *not* detectable based on the ABCDs: Nodular melanoma may show none of these features; it usually is a "new mole" with very sharp and even borders, and a dome shape; it is symmetrical, and it has an even brown or dark coloring. Amelanotic melanoma is not brown; instead, it is white, red, purple, or various shades in-between.) (See page C-39.)

Signs and laboratory findings A biopsy and pathological exam showing cancerous cells.

What is it? Melanoma (sometimes called malignant melanoma, even though *all* melanomas are malignant) is the rarest but most worrisome of all the skin cancers. It strikes about 38,000 Americans each year, eventually killing more than 20 percent of these people. The incidence of melanoma has steadily increased over the years. Although melanoma strikes men and women in nearly equal numbers, men have a higher mortality rate.

Melanoma can occur on any part of the body. It develops from melanocytes, which are the cells that produce melanin, the pigment in the skin. Melanoma occurs most often in fair-skinned, blue-eyed redheads or blonds who sunburn easily. However, no one is immune. In fact, black people may develop this skin cancer, most often on the palms, soles, or under the nails.

Although melanomas may appear within normal skin, almost one-third of them develop in a preexisting mole or other dark spot. For this reason, watch your moles for any changes suggestive of melanoma (especially, the ABCD changes; see page 1303).

What you can do Like other forms of skin cancer, melanoma is associated with sun exposure. More specifically, it occurs in people with a history of severe and blistering sunburns that have occurred prior to the age of 20. For these reasons, generously apply sunscreen (with an SPF of 15 or greater) when outdoors, wear protective sunglasses, hats, and clothing, and avoid the peak sun intensity hours of the day (11 AM to 3 PM). Also, avoid tanning parlors.

Fortunately, unlike internal cancers, which are difficult to detect early on, melanoma is visible on your skin, just waiting to be noticed—and early detection saves lives! Therefore, examine your entire skin surface once a month, using both a full-length mirror and a hand mirror. Have someone else examine your scalp. Keep an eye on any moles you might have, and on any brown birthmarks, as the latter are at greater risk for developing cancers within them. Look for changes in the shape, border outline, color, and size of moles (the ABCDs), and for any new moles or unusual marks on your body. Think of the ABCDs when examining *each* mole (one or more of which is usually present in a melanoma).

- **A**symmetry (one half of the lesion does not match the other)

- **B**order irregularity (ragged, notched edges)

- **C**olor (multicolored lesions, with various shades of tan, brown, blue, or black)

- **D**iameter (greater than the size of a pencil eraser, although an early melanoma will often be smaller than this)

Because melanoma can arise from normal skin as well as from existing moles, closely inspect any new growths or spots on your body. Call them to the attention of your doctor, particularly if you notice any of the ABCD characteristics, such as multiple colors or an asymmetrical shape.

When to call the doctor Early treatment of melanoma is crucial. If you detect any of the ABCD signs described above, or any other suspicious changes in the skin, contact a doctor *soon* (not next month or when you "get around to it"). Suspected melanoma should never be ignored for weeks or months. If untreated, melanoma can and generally does kill.

If there is a history of melanoma in your family, be especially vigilant about having skin changes checked; heredity may play a role in melanoma development in your family.

A biopsy and pathology examination will indicate whether the suspected lesion is cancerous. If melanoma is diagnosed, other evaluations are generally performed, including a thorough physical examination, liver function tests, and a chest x-ray. If the doctor suspects that the cancer may have spread to other areas of your body, additional studies may be needed, including tracer dye studies, lymph node biopsy, and computed tomography (CT) scans.

Treatment If melanoma is present, the lesion will be excised using conventional surgery, usually performed under local anesthesia.

When there is a suspicion that the cancer may have spread, removal of nearby lymph nodes may be necessary. Depending upon where the disease has spread, chemotherapy and immunotherapy may be recommended. (See Chapter 30 for more information on the treatment of cancer.)

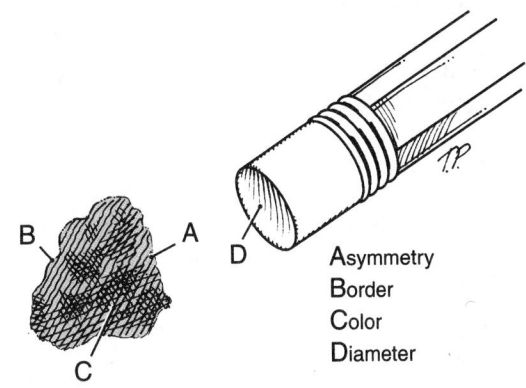

Asymmetry
Border
Color
Diameter

Skin marks, or lesions, may indicate the presence of skin cancer. Melanoma cancer can often be identified by looking for four main lesion characteristics: asymmetry, border irregularity, color variation, and diameter greater than that of a pencil eraser (remembered by the letters A, B, C, and D). Any skin lesion with one of these features should be examined by your doctor. Melanoma occurs most often in fair-skinned, blue-eyed, red-haired, or blond-haired people who sunburn easily. Although rare, melanoma kills more than 20 percent of affected people.

Prognosis Melanoma is usually curable if treated early. If treatment begins in the very earliest stages of melanoma, the survival rate is 95 percent. However, that positive prognosis declines as the lesion grows and spreads, with a poor 5-year survival rate if the cancer has spread to distant regions of the body.

❖ KAPOSI'S SARCOMA

Symptoms and signs Flat patches with a bruise-like appearance; or reddish-purple to brownish-blue, pea-sized or larger bumps, which eventually may grow to cover larger areas. (See page C-39.)

What is it Kaposi's sarcoma is a cancer of the skin that is seen most commonly in the United States in people with acquired immunodeficiency syndrome (AIDS), (see page 858). AIDS (as well as other diseases involving deficiencies in the immune system) allows this cancer to appear and grow. Kaposi's sarcoma develops in about one-fourth of people with AIDS who have acquired the infection through sexual exposure; it is rarely seen in persons infected with AIDS through blood transfusions or intravenous drug abuse. Kaposi's sarcoma can occur anywhere on the body, although in AIDS patients, lesions tend to favor the upper trunk.

Another form of this cancer, referred to as classic Kaposi's sarcoma, was the most common form of this disease prior to the AIDS epidemic. In the United States, this form of Kaposi's is found primarily in otherwise healthy older males of Italian or Jewish descent; in classic Kaposi's sarcoma, lesions tend to appear on the legs.

When to call the doctor If you have skin changes that fit the description of Kaposi's sarcoma, see a doctor. He may perform a skin biopsy for microscopic pathologic examination to confirm the diagnosis. The doctor will likely ask you about risk factors for, or symptoms of, AIDS (such as, swollen lymph nodes, night sweats, fatigue, fever, and weight loss). A blood test for the AIDS virus (called human immunodeficiency virus, or HIV) will also be performed.

Treatment For smaller lesions, local injection into the lesion of chemotherapeutic agents or topically applied liquid nitrogen cryotherapy may be used. If larger lesions are present or if there is involvement of the lymph nodes or internal organs, chemotherapy or radiation therapy may be recommended. (See Chapter 30 for more information on the treatment of cancer.)

Prognosis If Kaposi's sarcoma has developed within lymph nodes, it may lead to swelling of the extremity that normally drains into this lymph node region; if Kaposi's invades internal organs, it may interfere with normal functioning and ultimately be life-threatening.

Infestations, Bugs, and Ticks

When tiny, living creatures attach themselves to the body or the hair, they can cause conditions that may lead to very aggravating or, on occasion, very serious medical disorders. You can take steps to avoid or resolve these problems in their earliest stages, thus keeping serious risks to a minimum.

❖ SCABIES

Symptoms and signs Small, red bumps; intense itching and secondary changes (scaling, crusting, redness) from scratching. Burrows, or slightly raised, thread-like lines less than $1/8$ in. in length, sometimes with a minute black speck visible at one end; the burrows occur most commonly in the finger web spaces and the inner wrists. (See page C-47.)

What is it? Scabies, from the Latin word for to scratch, is an infestation caused by a microscopic mite that burrows in the skin, prompting an allergic response. *Sarcoptes scabiei*, the mite, lays eggs just under the top surface of the skin. Seven to 10 days later, the allergic response to the mites and their waste products occurs, and severe itching and a rash develop. Itching can become almost intolerable, and tends to intensify at night. The rash may progress from small, red bumps to scattered scaly or crusty lesions. The favored parts of the body are crevices such as the finger web spaces, wrists, underarms, elbows, breasts, buttocks, and genital area, particularly the scrotum and penis in males.

Scabies is highly contagious. It is usually contracted by physical contact with another person, but it can also be transmitted by sharing towels or clothing. Pets with scabies infestations can transmit animal scabies to humans; however, these mites, unlike the human scabies mite, do not persist on humans after the initial bite.

A secondary bacterial infection sometimes occurs in people with scabies, especially when breaks have occurred in the skin due to scratching.

What you can do Even if your personal hygiene is excellent, you may still develop scabies if you are in contact with someone with this infestation. Nevertheless, maintain good hygiene.

When to call the doctor If the symptoms of scabies develop, see a doctor as soon as possible. When scabies infestation is diagnosed, treatment should be started that night.

Treatment Scabies can be treated effectively with products your doctor can prescribe, such as permethrin cream (Elimite) or lindane lotion (Kwell). These preparations should be used on all household members; the doctor will make special considerations for infants, persons with a history of seizures, and women who are pregnant or breast-feeding. The treatment cream or lotion should be applied to the body from the neck down, in the evening at bedtime, and then washed off in the shower the following morning. Also, prior to showering in the morning, all family members' bedsheets and recently worn clothing should be put into the washer. The "laundry person" may then shower, after which he should place the newly washed clothing in a hot dryer (it is this heated drying that kills the mite). Alternatively, clothing or garments which you prefer not to wash and dry may be sealed in plastic trash bags for 10 days; this will also kill the mites.

All family members and others who have direct contact with the affected person are also candidates for treatment. They may be unaware of the infestation, because the allergic response, with the rash and itching, may not occur for 1 to 3 weeks after the initial exposure.

To relieve itching, oral sedating antihistamines may be prescribed for their sedating effects. If a secondary infection has developed, antibiotics will also be prescribed.

Prognosis As miserable as the itchiness and aggravation of scabies can be, it is an otherwise benign, curable condition.

❖ LICE

Symptoms and signs Visible, black mites (lice) and white flakes (eggs or nits) on the hair shaft which, unlike dandruff, are firmly attached to the hair. (See page C-47.)

What is it? Lice are tiny, wingless insects that make themselves at home on the head, body, or genital area. While head lice may attach themselves to the hair shafts of the scalp, body lice usually live on the skin and hide in the seams of underclothing, while pubic lice live in the pubic area.

These small parasites thrive on blood from their hosts. They are about the size of the head of a pin, and their nits or eggs are often mistaken for dandruff on the scalp. Lice occasionally may be found in the eyebrows and eyelashes. These nits are affixed to hair shafts, thereby allowing the eggs to hatch on the host.

Pubic lice, also known as crab lice or crabs, exist in pubic hair. They are spread most often through intimate sexual contact.

Head lice are common in children, occurring most often in the young, school-age group. Every year, up to 12 million youngsters develop head lice. They are usually spread from child to child in school settings when children have direct contact with one another, or share a baseball cap, hooded coat, comb, or brush. While many people believe that a child with head lice simply has poor hygiene habits, this is not the case. In contrast, body lice are rare in people with good hygiene who bathe regularly.

What you can do To prevent lice infestations, encourage your family members to avoid sharing hairbrushes, hats, bicycle helmets, scarfs, towels, clothing, and bedding.

When one member of the family has developed lice, all members are at risk and should be examined. In addition, the school or day care facility which the child attends should be notified so other children may be checked for lice.

Nonprescription antilice shampoos, lotions, and creams (such as permethrin or pyrethrins) will kill the live lice; follow the product's label instructions carefully. Call the product manufacturer's 800 number if you have any questions about methods of application or special considerations in persons with different hair types. The nits (eggs) must be physically removed. These nits are oval, pinhead-sized or smaller, and white or gray. While the antilice medication is still in the hair, use a comb with closely spaced teeth to comb them out; or instead, pick them out by hand or with a tweezers, or use safety scissors to cut away individual hair strands that have nits.

The shampoo treatment is usually repeated in 7 to 10 days. Reinspection and removal of nits is done again at this time. To control the itching, an over-the-counter clear hydrocortisone lotion can be used.

Lice infestation can persist due to inadequate or unsuccessful treatment, or it can recur. This risk can be reduced by washing clothing, bedspreads, blankets, and linens, and then putting them through a hot dryer cycle. Thoroughly vacuum couches and chairs. Wash hairbrushes and combs with a disinfectant.

Warning: Do not use lice sprays that are designed to be applied to bedding, furniture, rugs, and clothing on the human body.

When to call the doctor If a case of lice persists, or a secondary bacterial infection develops because of "scratching and digging," see a doctor. Also, in people who are pregnant, breastfeeding, or have epilepsy or a history of seizures, a doctor's advice should be sought before self-treating.

Treatment If you believe that the over-the-counter antilice products have been unsuccessful, your doctor will be able to determine if the infestation is still present; if it is, he may advise you on variations in treatment regimens. Also, if a secondary infection has developed, oral antibiotics will be prescribed.

Prognosis The presence of lice is not a serious condition; although it may be very frustrating, it is treatable.

❖ TICK BITES

Symptoms and signs Lyme disease: A red, expanding circle with central clearing, resembling a bull's eye.

Rocky Mountain spotted fever: A rash starting on the palms and soles, and then spreading to other parts of the body.

What is it? Ticks are tiny insects that live on animals, in bushes, grass, or forests; they can imbed themselves into the human skin, where they feed on blood. They may be as small as poppy seeds or as large as a nickel (see page C-47). Although the bite of a tick may not hurt and frequently is not even noticed, it can carry bacteria, viruses, or toxins that cause infections and illnesses, such as Lyme disease and Rocky Mountain spotted fever.

The rash associated with Lyme disease is usually an expanding red circle with a central clearing that resembles a target or bull's-eye. The rash of Rocky Mountain spotted fever begins with pinpoint-sized red dots on the hands and feet, which later spread over the body. Neither rash itches or causes pain.

What you can do Protect yourself from tick bites by wearing a long-sleeved shirt and long pants (tucked into socks or boots) when in grassy fields, wooded areas, or other places where ticks may live. Apply an insect repellent containing DEET to exposed skin. Stay on cleared paths whenever possible. When you return home, inspect skin and hair thoroughly, particularly areas where detection may be difficult,

HOW TO REMOVE A TICK

When you discover a tick, you should remove it promptly. Grasp the tick with fine-tipped tweezers firmly, as near to its attachment to the skin as possible (to try to grab its mouthparts and not just its body). If you squeeze too tightly, you may inject tick saliva into the body. Pull slowly, gently but firmly until the tick releases its hold. Put the tick into a bottle of alcohol for later identification if needed. If not, destroy the tick with an object—do not crush the tick with your fingers or pinch it apart with your fingernails. Cleanse the bite area with soap and water, dry

Petroleum jelly can be used to smother a tick and make it fall away from the skin. If this method is unsuccessful after 30 minutes, tweezers can be used gently to lift off the tick. Using the tweezers, grasp the tick firmly as close to its attachment to the skin as possible, without squeezing too tightly. Pull slowly but firmly, and then put the tick into a bottle of alcohol for later identification if needed. Do not use your fingers, a lit match, a cigarette, or a cigarette lighter to remove a tick. Clean the bite area with soap and water and apply a small film of antibiotic ointment to the skin at the affected site. Follow similar procedures when removing ticks from animals.

well, and apply a small film of topical antibiotic ointment to the bite site.

To avoid the risk of infection from ticks carrying organisms that cause Lyme disease or Rocky Mountain spotted fever, do not use your bare hands when removing ticks from yourself, others, and your pets. ■

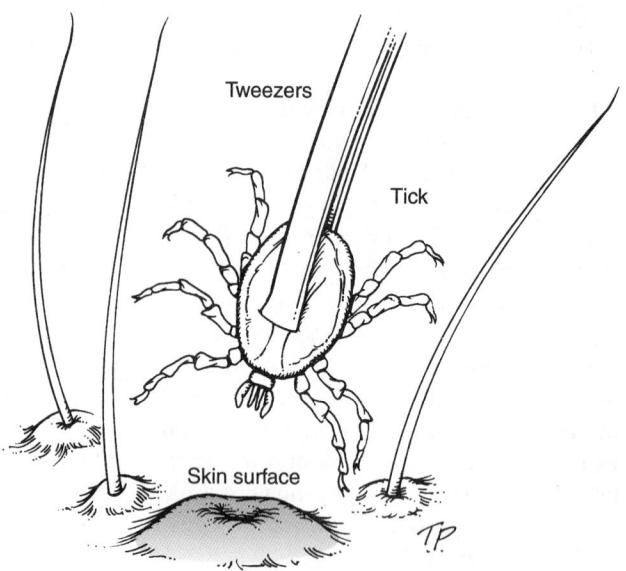

Tweezers

Tick

Skin surface

such as the groin and underarms. If a tick is found, remove it immediately (see How to Remove a Tick, page 1306) to minimize the chance of transmission of Lyme disease or Rocky Mountain spotted fever.

When to call the doctor When the rashes of either Lyme disease or Rocky Mountain spotted fever develop, you *must* see a doctor; with Rocky Mountain spotted fever, seek a doctor's (or emergency room) care immediately; time can literally mean the difference between life and death in this rapidly progressive and potentially fatal infection.

Treatment For information about treating Lyme disease or Rocky Mountain spotted fever, see pages 886 and 888.

Pressure, Friction, and Heat

Through the wear and tear of day-to-day life, the skin can develop a number of conditions, which may be bothersome or painful, and trivial to quite serious. Blisters, for example, can be painful, but are usually more of a nuisance than a potentially serious problem. In contrast, bed sores, which may develop in bedridden people, may be very serious and require prompt intervention and treatment. Prevention is important to keep at bay skin conditions related to pressure, friction, and heat.

❖ FRICTION BLISTERS

Symptoms and signs A thin-walled "bubble" of skin filled with clear fluid; pain when pressure is applied.

What is it? Friction blisters are caused by shearing friction forces or pressure. When they occur on the feet, the culprit is often poorly fitting shoes or wearing shoes without socks. As blisters form, clear fluid accumulates in a pocket formed between the separated layers of skin. If a small blood vessel is broken as the blister is forming, the fluid will contain blood instead of clear fluid (a blood blister).

What you can do No treatment is necessary for most blisters. It is usually best not to "pop" the blister to drain it, nor try to remove the damaged skin by cutting it away; the intact blister roof provides a sterile, protective, natural bandage.

If left alone, the fluid will gradually be absorbed by the body and the blistered skin will fall off, and be replaced by new skin forming below it. Until healing happens, keep the area clean. If a blister is located in a place on the body where it may be subjected to continued friction, cover it with a bandage to protect it from further injury. Whenever a blister accidentally breaks, gently wash the area with an antibacterial soap, place a bandage over it, and allow it to heal.

On occasion, you may need to drain a blister if it is very large and interferes with walking or the use of your hands. First, disinfect the blister and surrounding skin by cleansing with an antibacterial soap, followed by a 30-second gentle rubdown with rubbing alcohol. Then, use a sterile needle to pierce the blister at its edge and allow complete drainage of the fluid. Apply an antibiotic ointment to the puncture site, and cover with a bandage. The fluid will frequently reaccumulate and need to be drained again in the same fashion.

To prevent blisters on the feet, choose shoes and socks that fit properly. If you have sandals with straps that rub, wear socks with them or use mole skin or adhesive bandages to cover areas that are rubbed.

If you have diabetes or any other condition predisposing to or causing neurologic or vascular problems of the feet, you should inspect your feet daily for blisters, redness, and sores, because these changes are often painless and therefore go unnoticed. Ask your doctor to recommend a daily foot-care regimen and what to do if blisters or other foot problems develop. If your doctor is not familiar with foot care, contact the American Diabetes Association for literature.

When to call the doctor If a blister is very painful or develops redness extending outward from it, contact a doctor; these factors may be signs of a secondary infection requiring therapy. Also, keep an eye on any blister that has accidentally broken; continue to watch for indications that an infection has developed (surrounding redness, crusting, red streaks). If you suspect an infection, consult your doctor promptly.

Treatment A doctor may decide to drain a blister that is very large and painful. After the procedure, an antibiotic cream may be recommended to minimize the chance of an infection. Oral antibiotics will be given if a secondary infection has developed.

Prognosis Most blisters will heal on their own. Efforts should be made to ensure that a secondary infection does not occur, or is treated promptly.

❖ CANKER SORES (APHTHOUS ULCERS)

Symptoms (What you may experience) Painful sores inside the mouth; grayish white or milky colored, with white halos.

What is it? A canker sore (aphthous ulcer) occurs inside the mouth. It can make eating or speaking painful and difficult. This is particularly true when several are present at the same time. Although doctors do not know what causes canker sores, some people appear more susceptible to them than others. Infrequently, certain nutritional deficiencies (of vitamin B_{12}, folic acid, and iron) may play a role in their development; they may also occur after trauma has occurred inside the mouth (accidentally biting down on the skin, dental work or prosthesis placement, orthodontic work). Ulcers often develop in association with stress, fatigue, or the onset of menstruation. They are neither infections nor contagious.

What you can do Rinsing with antiseptic mouthwashes or warm salt water may ease the discomfort of sores in the mouth. Eating bland food can cut down on the pain and irritation from canker sores.

When to call the doctor Canker sores are not a serious problem. However, for people who have frequently recurring or large ulcers, doctors can conduct screening tests for nutritional deficiencies and other, more serious disorders in which mouth ulcers may occur. For example, some persons may have mouth sores in association with noncancerous bowel disease (ulcerative colitis), as part of a disorder involving the eyes and genitalia (Behçet's disease), or as part of an autoimmune blistering skin disease (bullous pemphigoid, pemphigus vulgaris, and paraneoplastic pemphigus). All of these diseases are significant medical conditions requiring timely diagnosis.

Treatment Although the most painful phase usually ends after 3 to 4 days, canker sores may take up to 2 weeks to completely disappear. For recurrent canker sores, doctors may recommend the use of topical corticosteroids or other medications to ease the ulcer severity and speed healing.

Prognosis Canker sores will go away on their own. However, there is no way to prevent them from recurring.

❖ PRICKLY HEAT

Symptoms and signs Small, itchy, red bumps on the back and sometimes on the chest and abdomen.

What is it? Prickly heat (or miliaria rubra) is a condition related to overheating. It tends to occur most often in active people when the sweat ducts become inflamed and obstructed or plugged; this causes perspiration to be retained within the skin rather than being excreted onto the surface. The ensuing irritation produces small red bumps, usually on the chest or back.

Another condition, miliaria crystalina, is very similar, although the sweat is trapped within the sweat ducts right at its exit point from the skin, just below the most superficial layer of skin. This produces tiny, delicate blisters that look like beads of sweat, which remain after trying to "blot" them off.

Both types of miliaria occur most frequently in hot, humid conditions, although they can develop in cool weather in individuals who are overdressed and therefore perspire more heavily.

What you can do Wear lighter-weight clothing. Take cool baths or showers, and dry the skin thoroughly. Avoid hot environments and physical activities that cause heavy sweating. Spend time in air-conditioned rooms. For itching, apply an over-the-counter anti-itch lotion, such as Sarnol HC or Aveeno Anti-Itch.

When to call the doctor The symptoms of prickly heat generally last for no more than a few days, resolving on their own. However, if the rash does not go away, see a doctor to make sure you have made the correct diagnosis.

Prognosis Prickly heat is a benign, self-limiting condition; the prognosis depends on measures taken to prevent recurrences.

❖ BED SORES

Symptoms and signs Ulceration or sore formation on pressure-bearing sites of the skin in bedridden patients; surrounding warmth, tenderness, and swelling; drainage of yellow or green fluid from the ulcer base indicating secondary bacterial growth; pain in the area.

What is it? When people are confined to a bed or a chair, perhaps because of weakness or paralysis, their inability to turn can cause unrelieved pressure on certain parts of the body. As blood flow in the tiny blood vessels nourishing the skin is reduced by this pressure, skin and tissue damage occurs at these pressure points—most commonly on the buttocks, hips, heels, lower spine, shoulder blades, elbows, and ankles.

Also called pressure sores or decubitus ulcers, bed sores begin with mild redness or duskiness of the site; this is the first and often only warning of imminent tissue breakdown, sometimes leading to very deep ulcers that may extend into the underlying fat, muscle, and bone. Healing is usually very difficult, because many elderly, bedridden individuals have low physical reserves and poor or delayed healing ability.

What you can do A person who is confined to a bed or a chair should change position at least every 2 hours to relieve pressure upon particular body areas. When lying on the back, pressure can often be eased by placing a pillow under the lower legs. "Egg-crate" pads, air mattresses, and other specially designed cushions can be used to redistribute weight to prevent sores from developing. Also, make sure that the bed sheets are smooth and not wrinkled.

Poor nourishment and anemia may contribute to the development of bed sores and slow their healing—so it is important to eat a nutritious, balanced diet. Exercise can help maintain blood flow; if the bedridden person is not capable of exercising, others can administer passive movement or exercise. (See page 1482 for more information on prevention of bed sores.)

When to call the doctor If a part of the body becomes red or purple, this could be the initial sign of a developing bed sore. Call the doctor immediately to begin treatment. Also, if an existent ulcer becomes infected (characterized by redness moving outward into the surrounding skin, pus, and foul odor), see a doctor immediately.

Treatment Bed sores typically require a long healing period. Care must be taken to avoid putting pressure on the sore. Antibiotics (oral or topical) may be prescribed. Bed sores must be cleaned frequently, rinsing away dead tissue, and then bandaged. Recommended bandages range from Telfa pads to newer self-adhering occlusive dressings, such as DuoDerm and Opsite.

Surgery is sometimes necessary to repair injured tissue.

Prognosis Proper care can prevent and stimulate the healing of most bed sores. However, healing is often a long process.

Pigmentation Problems

The differences in skin color among humans are determined by the activity of melanocytes, which are pigment-forming cells. At times, problems with pigmentation can arise, most often due to trauma or insult to the skin, and less commonly due to an abnormal immune response.

Fortunately, people with abnormal pigmentation conditions usually enjoy good overall health. While resolution of pigmentary problems can be challenging, approaches can be used to make these conditions more cosmetically acceptable.

❖ VITILIGO

Symptoms and signs Irregularly shaped, stark white patches of skin; these patches tend to occur on particular areas (face, lips, neck, arms, underarms, hands, feet, genitalia), although any part of the body can be affected; body hair in affected areas usually turns white; absence of other symptoms. (See page C-27.)

What is it? Vitiligo is caused by the loss of the pigment-producing cells (the melanocytes) in the affected areas. Some people have one or two small patches, while others have many and/or large areas of pigment loss. It is more noticeable in people with dark skin, due to the greater contrast involved.

Although the precise cause of vitiligo is not known, one theory is that the immune system of people with this condition produces cells or antibodies that destroy the body's own pigment-producing cells, mistaking them for a foreign invader. There may be a genetic predisposition to vitiligo, because it often runs in families.

While most people with vitiligo have no associated health problems, the incidence of autoimmune disorders—such as thyroid disease, pernicious anemia, and diabetes—is greater than that of the general population. For this reason, it is a good idea to see your doctor, who will take a medical history and conduct a physical examination to screen you for these disorders.

Vitiligo is sometimes mistaken for so-called chemical leukoderma, in which phenol-containing substances, commonly found in industrial cleansers, may cause depigmentation in areas of skin contact. Although unusual, this occurs most often in persons working for professional cleaning services who use the cleansers without wearing gloves. Similar to vitiligo, the melanocytes in the skin are absent in these areas of contact.

What you can do Most people with very light-colored skin find that their vitiligo can be best camouflaged by simply keeping their unaffected, normal-colored skin from becoming suntanned. Over-the-counter cosmetic products, manufactured in various skin tones and in waterproof formulations, are available to camouflage vitiligo patches. Skin dyes and self-tanning products are also available.

One very important point to remember is that the patches of vitiligo have no "pigment protection" to prevent sunburn and possible skin cancer. Thus, you need to protect these patches with a high-SPF (30) sunscreen.

When to call the doctor As mentioned above, see a doctor for a history-taking and physical examination. Also, consult a dermatologist if you are interested in attempts at possible repigmentation, or if the diagnosis itself is in question.

Treatment Medical therapies include psoralen photochemotherapy—an ultraviolet A (UVA) light therapy combined with use of a drug called psoralen, which sensitizes the skin to UVA light. This therapy, done under a doctor's care, requires several in-office treatments three times a week for a period of many months. It may repigment and darken vitiligo patches; however, results are variable.

If begun early in the course of the disorder, use of steroid creams may occasionally bring color back to the depigmented regions. Results are seen after about 4 to 6 months of treatment.

In individuals who have lost pigment almost everywhere, another approach may be taken that involves depigmenting the skin that has still remained normally pigmented. A substance called monobenzyl ether of hydroquinone may be used in this process. Extensive consultation with your doctor and much personal consideration must go into the decision to use this treatment, because once it is done, it is irreversible.

Prognosis Pigmentation of the skin generally does not return without therapy. In fact, the disorder is often progressive, with patches gradually spreading to other parts of the body.

❖ MELASMA/CHLOASMA

Symptoms and signs Irregular, dark browns patches that occur on the face, most often on the upper cheeks and forehead.

What is it? Melasma, or chloasma, is a facial discoloration that occurs most frequently in association with pregnancy—hence, its alternate name, the mask of pregnancy. The skin on the upper cheeks and, often, on the forehead and upper lip, experience a localized tan to light brown color change. In melasma, color pigment is deposited in excess in the skin's upper layer. Female hormones are believed to be largely responsible for this condition. In fact, the hormonal changes that occur when taking oral contraceptives (birth control pills) or estrogen replacement therapy (ERT) may produce these skin changes. Notably, however, some women who develop melasma are neither pregnant nor taking birth control pills or ERT.

The skin coloring may gradually return to normal when hormone levels return to normal, either after childbirth and once a

WHAT IS A FRECKLE?

Freckles are common tan or brown spots on the skin.

They are small areas of increased skin pigment or melanin, and are a sign of sun damage to the skin.

Because there is a genetic tendency to freckle, you are more likely to have them if other family members do, too. They appear for the first time during early childhood, mostly on the face, arms, and other areas of the body that are sun-exposed. They fade in the winter and darken in the sun-drenched summer months. Although freckles themselves pose *no* health risks, they are a marker of increased risk for all types of skin cancer. ■

woman goes off birth control pills or ERT. (However, melasma is not a good reason to give up either therapy.) The return of normal coloring can be a painfully slow process. In fact, melasma can persist for many months after the baby is born or after a woman stops taking oral contraceptives or estrogen supplements.

What you can do Bleaching creams containing hydroquinone 2 percent may be helpful in lightening the skin discoloration. However, they are fairly weak and often produce less than acceptable lightening.

Because melasma can become worse due to exposure to sunlight, always wear high SPF sunscreen whenever you are outdoors.

When to call the doctor If you would like more aggressive therapy, see a doctor, who can prescribe various topical agents or recommend cosmetic procedures.

Treatment Doctors may prescribe a hydroquinone 4 percent bleaching cream (twice the strength of the over-the-counter cream) and/or tretinoin (Retin-A). These two agents are often used in combination to produce maximal improvement. Chemical peels and laser treatments can also lighten melasma.

Prognosis Melasma discoloration may eventually fade, although it may take months or sometimes even years to do so. Sunscreen should always be used to prevent recurrences.

Skin Changes With Aging

As we grow older, changes in the skin are common. Although most of them may not qualify as medical conditions, and do not require treatment, people often find them disturbing, particularly the development of wrinkles. As with other skin conditions, many of those associated with aging can be minimized by cutting down your exposure to the sun. In fact, despite the claims of many cosmetic companies, your best bet to retard the aging process is to avoid sunlight.

❖ WRINKLES

Symptoms and signs Creases on the face that increase in number with age, often concentrated on the forehead and around the eyes and mouth.

What is it? Wrinkles are a part of aging. They appear when connective tissues—collagen and elastin—in the skin are weakened or decline in number. As this occurs, the thickness of the skin declines; its fat content decreases; it loses some of its elasticity, resiliency, and smoothness; and it starts to sag. Also, underlying fat in the face is usually lost during the aging process, making facial skin wrinkling most pronounced.

The decrease in skin elasticity can be accelerated by damage caused by ultraviolet (UV) light—related not only to recent sun exposure, but also to the amount of sun exposure over a lifetime. A person's tendency to develop wrinkles is also influenced by heredity.

What you can do To decrease your risk of developing wrinkles, cut down your sun exposure, particularly during the peak sun intensity hours of 11 AM to 3 PM. When outdoors, apply a sunscreen with an SPF of 15 or greater.

Research suggests that smokers are more susceptible to collagen damage and skin wrinkling—yet another reason to quit smoking.

Many over-the-counter "wrinkle creams" are available. The alpha-hydroxy acids have been shown to improve the quality of the epidermis, thereby potentially improving very tiny, fine wrinkles. They also cause the outermost cells to shed more quickly, causing fine peeling and mild irritation of the skin. Some, but not all, individuals have found the peeling "refreshing" and "renewing," and have responded positively to the added pinkness that is associated with the mild irritation. Alpha-hydroxy acid, however, has not been proven in well-executed studies to increase skin collagen (which makes up the bulk of the skin content); it is the loss of collagen that plays the major role in wrinkling.

When to call the doctor Consult a doctor if you are interested in a prescription anti-wrinkle cream or the cosmetic surgical procedures described below.

Treatment Research has shown that tretinoin cream, an acne therapy, and more recently, a moisturizing retinoic acid cream formulation (Renova cream), can reduce fine wrinkles, thicken the epidermis, and add substance to the dermis, albeit by a very small amount. Renova and Retin-A must be used under a doctor's supervision, because they have side effects (including increased sensitivity to the sun, peeling, and redness).

Collagen, injected directly into wrinkles, may be used to fill out facial lines. The procedure is done in a dermatologist's office. The benefits are only temporary, however, because the body absorbs the injected collagen over a period of months. Reinjection is required every 6 to 12 months to maintain the desired effect.

Dermabrasion and laser resurfacing may also be used for treatment of wrinkles (see Plastic and Reconstructive Surgery, page 1313).

Prognosis Although wrinkles are a natural part of the aging process, you need only compare your facial skin to your buttock skin to appreciate the marked difference between sun-induced damage (photoaging) of the skin on the sun-exposed face in contrast to the inherent, natural physiologic aging of skin on the sun-protected buttocks. The "take-home message" is "Use sunscreen daily!"

❖ LIVER (AGE) SPOT (SOLAR LENTIGO)

Symptoms and signs A tan to dark brown, evenly colored, often dime-sized flat spot on sun-exposed sites; asymptomatic.

What is it? Despite the common name liver spot, these spots have nothing in common with the liver, except their color. They are caused by ultraviolet sun exposure. The spots occur most often on the face and the back of the hands of people over age 40.

What you can do Over-the-counter "fade" creams, such as Porcelana (hydroquinone 2 percent cream), will help lighten these spots, but it is unlikely that they will actually vanish. Opaque cosmetic coverup creams may camouflage these spots.

You can reduce the chances of developing new liver spots—or of experiencing a darkening of existing spots—by wearing sunscreen (SPF 15 or greater) when outdoors.

When to call the doctor Liver spots may be considered cosmetically unattractive by some people, but they pose no health risks. Nevertheless, if you have a spot that changes, has variable coloration in it, or just appears different from your other liver spots, you should have it examined by a doctor to ensure that it is not an early melanoma, a potentially fatal skin cancer.

Treatment A dermatologist may offer you various treatment options, including: prescription fading agents (hydroquinone 4 percent creams), which are stronger than those available over the counter; cryosurgery (destroying the lesions by freezing with liquid nitrogen); chemical peeling; or laser surgery.

Prognosis Liver spots are harmless, and treatment is not required.

❖ SPIDER VEINS

Symptoms and signs Fine, red to bluish-purple blood vessels, usually on the legs or thighs; burning, pain (occasionally).

What is it? Spider veins are small, visible, superficial blood vessels, typically on the legs or thighs. Although patterns can vary considerably, they get their name from the spider web–like patterns in which they are often distributed. When they cover wide areas of skin, many people find them unsightly, even though they are harmless.

Doctors do not know what causes spider veins, although hormones may be involved. They are more common in women than men, and often become more pronounced during pregnancy or while taking oral contraceptives or hormone replacement therapy. Exposure to the sun commonly produces similar, but finer, thread-like spider telangiectasias on the nose and cheeks, especially in people with fair skin.

Burning or pain of the legs, particularly after long periods of standing, may be associated with spider veins.

What you can do Spider veins are difficult to prevent; however, wearing support hose and low-heeled shoes, avoiding motionless standing, losing excess pounds if needed, and increasing physical activity may all be helpful. To reduce the likelihood of sun-induced facial telangiectasias, wear sunscreen when outdoors.

When to call the doctor Spider veins are not needed to transport blood in the body. They are mostly a cosmetic problem. However, if they cause pain or if you find them unattractive, talk with a dermatologist or cosmetic surgeon about methods available to eradicate them.

Treatment In a technique called sclerotherapy, a sclerosing solution (hypertonic saline) is injected directly into each spider vein, which eliminates it or makes it less apparent. Some vessels may need a number of injections over several weeks. Compression leg bandages (such as Ace Bandage wraps) are often worn following the injections. An alternative to sclerotherapy is laser surgery; lasers are now available that can destroy these vessels.

Prognosis People whose spider veins are treated with sclerotherapy can anticipate a 50 to 90 percent improvement; a series of injections over weeks or months is often required. Ask your doctor how many treatment sessions should be anticipated and approximately how much the total cost will be. Also, ask for his personal "success rate" in eradicating these vessels.

Plastic and Reconstructive Surgery

Plastic (cosmetic) and reconstructive surgery is performed for a variety of reasons, but all of them relate to enhancing the appearance of the skin or the underlying bone structures. An individual may want to make wrinkles less obvious, change the shape of her nose, or remove sagging skin. The surgery may be done to make minor or even major scars less noticeable, or to remove tattoos.

ARE YOU A GOOD CANDIDATE?

Ideal candidates for cosmetic surgery should have resilient skin and good overall health. They also must have realistic expectations regarding what surgery can accomplish. Although some degree of pain can be expected after these procedures, this discomfort can usually be managed with oral analgesics (pain killers), which may have to be taken for at least several days.

Before meeting with a doctor and agreeing to the surgery, collect as much information as possible about the operation. Make sure you understand what the surgery can and cannot accomplish. For more information about these operations, you can contact the following organizations:

- American Academy of Facial Plastic and Reconstructive Surgery
  1110 Vermont Ave., N.W.
  Suite 220
  Washington, DC 20005
  Phone: (202) 842-4500

- American Society of Plastic and Reconstructive Surgeons
  444 E. Algonquin Rd.
  Arlington Heights, IL 60005
  Phone: (847) 228-9900

- American Academy of Otolaryngology—Head and Neck Surgery
  1 Prince St.
  Alexandria, VA 22314
  Phone: (703) 836-4444

- American Society for Dermatologic Surgery
  P.O. Box 4014
  Schaumburg, IL 60173
  Phone: (708) 330-0230

SELECTING A SURGEON

Dermatologic surgeons, plastic surgeons, and ear, nose, and throat surgeons perform procedures on the face and/or other parts of the body. Do not choose a surgeon by impulsively contacting one who advertises in local newspaper or television ads. Ask a family doctor for a referral to a surgeon who specializes in these types of operations. Also ask family members and friends about their experiences with these surgeons, and whether they were pleased with the results.

In your first meeting with the surgeon, inquire about his training, board certification, and experience. You can find much of this information in the public library in the reference book, *The Official American Board of Medical Specialties Directory of Board Certified Medical Specialists*. Look for a surgeon who is board-certified in dermatology, ear, nose, and throat, or plastic and reconstructive surgery—meaning that he has completed a residency involving training in this particular area and has passed an examination demonstrating competency in the field. Ask about the surgeon's hospital affiliations, which indicate that he has met the criteria to receive hospital privileges. (For more information about selecting a surgeon, see Chapter 32.)

In the initial or subsequent consultations with the surgeon, get all your questions answered about the operation you are considering. Schedule a date for the surgery only after your feel comfortable that you have all the information you need about the operation and the doctor.

Ask the surgeon questions such as, "How many of these operations have you done?" "Do I make a good candidate for this particular operation?" "Do you recommend that the surgery be done on an inpatient or outpatient basis?" "What kind of anesthesia will be used?" "How long will the surgery take?" "After the surgery, how much pain will I feel, and how will it be managed?" "When will I feel normal again?" "When will I be able to return to work?"

Be sure to let the surgeon know about any special circumstances in your medical history, such as allergies to medications, bleeding problems, and abnormal healing or scarring.

Also ask about the risks associated with surgery. *No* operation is risk-free. Although complications are uncommon, they can include excessive bleeding, blood clots, unusual swelling, infections, nerve injury, and anesthesia-related problems. Ask the surgeon about how these risks can be minimized.

SURGICAL TECHNIQUES

The most frequently performed plastic and reconstructive surgical procedures include:

Rhytidectomy This facelift surgery is performed to minimize sagging skin and creases on the face and neck. Incisions are made on the face's perimeter, above the hairline at the temple, and are extended behind the ear; then the skin is raised, and the muscle and tissue underneath are tightened and repositioned. Excess skin and fat are excised (cut off), and the incisions are closed. The average facelift takes between 2 and 4 hours. About 2 weeks are needed for recovery (including the resolution from bruising, swelling, and puffiness). Activity levels should be reduced for several weeks after the operation, and a high-SPF sunscreen should always be used to prevent future wrinkling.

Blepharoplasty This eyelid surgery involves the removal of fat, muscle, and excess skin from around the eyes. It can get rid of bags under the eyes and drooping layers of skin on the upper eyelids. The incisions are made along the natural folds and lines of the eyes. The operation takes 1 to 3 hours. Although the stitches are usually removed within 5 days, the recovery takes 2 to 4 weeks.

Rhinoplasty In this surgery of the nose, some bone and cartilage are removed, thus allowing the nose to be reshaped and reconstructed to create a smaller or narrower nose. During the operation, the skin of the nose is lifted while the underlying structures are being worked on. Although most often done for cosmetic reasons, this procedure is sometimes performed to improve breathing or to repair a nose injury. It is a common operation in adolescents, although a teenager should reach complete growth before the procedure is considered. After the operation, a splint is usually worn on the nose to hold the new shape in place during the healing process.

About a week is needed for recovery. (See Chapter 16 for more information on rhinoplasty.)

Chemical peel Also called chemabrasion, this procedure uses chemicals to produce a "controlled (chemical) burn" of the skin. It is designed to peel away the top layer of skin, which leaves behind skin with new, growing cells that provide a smoother, more evenly colored skin surface and a more even tone. It is often used for sun-damaged, wrinkled, or blemished skin. The chemicals typically sting when they are applied, and the procedure takes as long as 2 hours. Swelling will occur afterward, and the normal recovery time is 7 to 14 days.

Laser resurfacing Laser (high-intensity light) resurfacing is used to remove wrinkle lines, precancerous spots (actinic keratoses), superficial acne or chickenpox scars, and some pigmented birthmarks. It is a noninvasive procedure (requiring no incisions), in which unwanted skin is vaporized without injuring the remaining skin structures.

The technique typically takes 30 to 60 minutes. The recovery requires about a week, and most doctors recommend avoiding direct sunlight during that time.

Another procedure, called laser destruction (rather than resurfacing), uses other types of lasers to remove unwanted blood vessels or vascular birthmarks, warts, tattoos, and even unwanted hair.

Dermabrasion This procedure involves using a power-driven wire brush to gently abrade or "sand" away the outer layer of skin. It is performed to eliminate or reduce acne scars, fine wrinkles, and some tattoos. Recovery time averages 7 to 10 days.

Liposuction (or suction-assisted lipectomy) In this body-contouring procedure, one or more small incisions are made, through which a tube (called a cannula) is inserted; the tube is attached to a vacuum-like machine. As the surgeon moves this tube back and forth, it breaks up the fat and sucks it out from under the skin. The most common sites for this surgery are the buttocks, thighs, abdomen, face, neck, back, and arms. Local anesthesia is usually used,

unless fat is being removed from large areas of the body. The procedure can take an hour or more, depending on how extensive the surgery is. Patients are typically attached to an intravenous drip to replenish the body with fluids that may be lost during the procedure. Some bruising and swelling occurs afterwards. Individuals are often advised to wear a snug, elastic garment around the treated area during the recovery period of 1 to 2 weeks.

Other procedures Other plastic and reconstructive surgical procedures include submental lipectomy (fat removal, and tightening of the skin and muscles to eliminate a double chin); otoplasty (pinning back protruding ears); and abdominoplasty (a tummy tuck involving the tightening of abdominal muscles).

SCAR REVISION SURGERY

An increasingly important application of plastic surgery involves scar revision, which is designed to improve the appearance of scars. Although scars are part of the normal healing of the skin—occurring in the aftermath of an operation, injury, or burn—they are often considered unsightly, depending on their texture, color, depth, and location.

Scar revision surgery may involve surgical removal of the scar itself, and then rejoining the skin with very fine stitches in a way that produces a narrower, less noticeable scar. Or it can involve changing a scar by creating irregular incision lines that give the scar a broken, less noticeable appearance. Other scar revision techniques include surgical excision of the scar and, in its place, grafting healthy skin from elsewhere on the body. Sometimes, a flap of skin next to the scar can be lifted and stretched over the site where the scar had been.

As with other types of plastic surgery, scar revision procedures can frequently be done in the surgeon's office or an outpatient surgical center, using a local anesthetic.

In the hands of a skilled surgeon, scar revision surgery produces good results in most cases.

HAIR

The skin is the site of many thousands of hair follicles; there are about 100,000 on the head alone. They are present everywhere except the lips, palms, and soles. The hair bulb at the base of each follicle is the site where new hair is made. The coarse terminal hair on the scalp, beard area of the face, underarms, and pubic area is of a greater caliber or diameter than the fine vellus hair found on other areas of the body.

Every hair strand has two layers: the outer cuticle and the inner cortex. Oil (sebum) secretion from the sebaceous glands gives the hair its glossy appearance. The capillaries leading to the follicles supply the hair with nutrients, including vitamins and minerals. Just as melanin determines skin color, it also is responsible for the color of hair.

Hair grows in cycles. While some strands are growing, others are dormant. The average scalp hair grows about one-third to one-half inch per month, although hair growth cycles may be affected by seasonal temperature changes and illness. While scalp hair will typically grow to about 20 in. in length if it is not cut, hair on the arms has a much shorter growth cycle and a much longer resting cycle, so that its maximal length is about 1/2 in. Scalp hair is normally lost each day, with 50 to 100 strands shed.

The hair on our heads and bodies has only limited functions—for example, it provides sun protection for the scalp. However, most of us value hair primarily for cosmetic reasons. When something goes awry with our hair, it can deflate our self-esteem and even our outlook on life. For some people, "bad hair days" are predictive of "bad days." For this reason, many people are willing to expend both their time and money to address concerns regarding too much or too little hair.

❖ HEREDITARY PATTERNED BALDNESS

Symptoms and signs Overall thinning of hair; receding hairline; bald spot on the crown.

What is it? Although various factors can interfere with normal hair growth—such as diet, weight loss, illness, and the use of certain medications—the vast majority of people with hair loss have what doctors call male- or female-pattern baldness. As we age, all of us experience some hair loss; however, some people show much greater or much earlier hair loss than others.

Researchers do not know the complete cause of pattern baldness, but heredity and hormonal factors play major roles, as does the maturing process. Contrary to one popularly held belief, the genes of both parents, not just the mother's genes alone, help determine patterned hair loss. When patterned baldness occurs in men, it most often starts with thinning on the temples, and a bald spot at the top of the head. Women experience a more gradual and subtle hair thinning over the entire top part of the scalp, notably sparing the frontal margin and temples.

What you can do Although many "hair restoration" treatments are aggressively advertised, only minoxidil (Rogaine and

The surface of the skin has thousands of tiny pits called hair follicles that support the growth of individual hairs. Hair grows within the hair bulb at the bottom of each follicle. In a normal hair follicle, sebaceous glands secrete oil (sebum) into the follicle, and the smooth arrector pili muscle causes "goosebumps" or erection of hair.

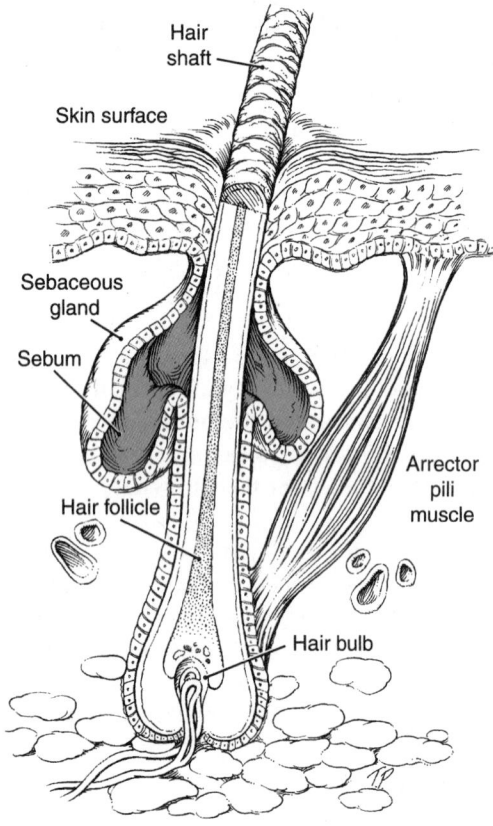

Hair shaft

Skin surface

Sebaceous gland

Sebum

Hair follicle

Arrector pili muscle

Hair bulb

Rogaine Extra Strength) and finasteride (Propecia) have been proven effective in controlled studies. Both Rogaine Extra Strength and Propecia produce improvement in hair growth or preservation of hair in most persons. Rogaine must be applied twice daily for about 6 months before it can be determined whether it is helpful in a given individual; to maintain any new hair growth that is achieved, its use must be continued indefinitely.

When to call the doctor Women who have signs of possible androgen (male hormone) excess—such as facial hair growth, deepening of the voice, irregular menses, or infertility—should be medically evaluated with hormone blood level testing. Both men and women who have undiagnosed signs or symptoms of possible internal illness should be evaluated, with the doctor keeping hair loss in mind as a possible indication of such internal disease or problems (for example, thyroid disease; malnutrition with protein deficiency due to uncontrolled inflammatory bowel disease; an "incomplete" or protein-deficient vegetarian diet; anorexia nervosa; and AIDS).

Also, consult a dermatologist or cosmetic surgeon if you are interested in any surgical treatments for baldness.

Treatment Surgical hair replacement has become a popular way of treating pattern baldness, most often involving a procedure called "pinch grafting." In this technique, round plugs of skin are surgically removed from a part of the scalp that is hair-bearing, and these are transplanted into bald or thinning areas. The latest refinements of this grafting treatment use micrografting techniques, which can provide a restored hairline that appears finer and more natural than was possible through surgery in the past.

The prescription medication finasteride is also available for the treatment of male-pattern baldness. It is a lower dosage of the same drug already in use in this country for the treatment of benign prostate disease (under the trade name Proscar). Finasteride blocks the conversion of the male hormone testosterone to its most active form in the prostate and on the scalp.

Prognosis When baldness is due to male- or female-pattern baldness, the hair loss is permanent, although treatments, including surgical transplants, may be able to restore variable amounts of hair growth.

❖ HIRSUTISM

Symptoms and signs Applies only to women: excessive body hair growth, in areas dependent on male hormone stimulation for growth (moustache, sideburns, beard areas, upper chest, upper trunk).

What is it? Hirsutism is the medical term used to describe abnormal hair growth stimulated by (a) an increased sensitivity of the hair follicles to normal blood levels of androgens (male hormones), or (b) elevated blood levels of androgens. By definition, it occurs only in women, because men normally have hair in these body areas.

The amount and distribution of normal hair growth is dependent on hereditary and hormonal factors. It varies significantly, particularly among different ethnic groups. Individuals of Mediterranean descent tend to have more hair in androgen-dependent areas, while Asians tend to have less hair. Also, even within particular ethnic groups, some families tend to have more hair than "average," while others have less. Hormonal factors, including the balance of estrogen and testosterone, also contribute to the amount of body hair. Hirsutism, therefore, is defined by whether hair is excessive for a particular woman compared to her sisters and/or other women of the same ethnicity.

Many women also experience slight increases in hair growth after menopause in the beard and moustache regions. At the time of menopause, estrogen levels plummet, while testosterone levels remain stable or slowly decline over the postmenopausal years. This new balance—with a relative excess of the male hormone testosterone—may stimulate facial hair growth. Some women are also given a postmenopausal hormone replacement containing a small amount of testosterone, which may produce hair growth in some cases. Topical testosterone cream, sometimes used to treat genital disorders, may be absorbed into the blood well enough to cause facial hair growth. Danazol, a drug used to treat endometriosis, occasionally may cause hirsutism.

In women who lack one of the above possible causes of hirsutism, a thorough examination for clinical and laboratory evidence of excess androgen hormones must be conducted to exclude the presence of disorders such as polycystic ovary disease, adrenal disorders, and adrenal and ovarian tumors. Most women whose hirsutism is due to one of these disorders have other evidence of androgen excess—for example, patterned scalp hair loss, acne, irregular menses, or infertility.

What you can do This is a condition that can be treated cosmetically. Unwanted hair can be shaved, waxed, plucked, chemically dissolved (using depilatories), or bleached; however, all of these are temporary solutions. Electrolysis is a permanent treatment that destroys individual hair follicles. Even when performed by an experienced electrologist, it can in some cases lead to infections and scarring, so proceed with caution. Lasers have recently become available for removing hair; these likely will be improved and perfected over the next few years.

When to call the doctor Because hirsutism is sometimes related to hormonal abnormalities and, albeit very rarely, to tumors, you should see a doctor for evaluation and laboratory tests to rule out any abnormalities that require therapy.

Treatment Birth control pills alone or in combination with a diuretic drug called spironolactone, which has an effect on hormones, may be prescribed to help control hirsutism. If the doctor concludes that excessive hair growth is associated with medications being taken for other medical conditions, alternative medications may be available instead.

Prognosis Some persons treated successfully with birth control pills and spironolactone who stop this therapy may experience a recurrence of hirsutism; more prolonged therapy may be necessary in these individuals.

❖ TELOGEN EFFLUVIUM

Symptoms and signs Shedding of greater than normal amounts of hair diffusely over the scalp; occasional scalp soreness.

What is it? Telogen effluvium is a common disorder involving the loss of hair. The strands involved are the telogen hairs, which are those in the resting phase of the normal hair-growth cycle. People may be most aware of this hair loss when they see loose strands entangled in their brush, comb, or the shower drain.

Telogen effluvium tends to develop during or after a variety of health-related events. For example, it often occurs 2 to 4 months after childbirth, and excessive hair loss can continue for 1 to 6 months. Thyroid hormone abnormalities and surgical procedures, which can place tremendous stress on the body, can produce this hair loss. So can a high fever lasting many days, a severe infection, rapid weight loss, a protein- and iron-deficient diets, or the use of particular medications (anticoagulants, isotretinoin, etretinate, lithium, birth control pills).

What you can do Once the causative factor of telogen effluvium is resolved, the hair loss should cease within two to three months. Thus, if a crash diet is identified as contributing to the hair loss, nutritional changes may end the problem.

When to call the doctor For help in pinpointing the cause of telogen effluvium, contact a doctor for a history-taking and physical examination. Expect blood tests to exclude the possibility of thyroid disease and anemia.

Treatment The hair loss associated with telogen effluvium should stop spontaneously about 2 to 3 months after its cause is resolved—such as the healing of an infection, or recovery from surgery. If the use of a particular medication is responsible for this condition, your doctor may be able to recommend a substitute drug.

Prognosis Telogen effluvium will tend to cease when both patient and doctor deal with causative factors such as illnesses, diet, or medications.

❖ ALOPECIA AREATA

Symptoms and signs One or several coin-sized patches of hair loss on the scalp or elsewhere on the body (see page C-41).

What is it? Alopecia areata is most commonly a localized, limited type of hair loss; however, in unusual cases, it can cause a total loss of all body hair. In this condition, the hair follicles that normally produce hair become dormant.

The first sign of alopecia areata is often one or two coin-sized patches in which the hair is totally absent. It is frequently first noted by a hair stylist in a client. The condition may progress no further, or unusually, it may eventually involve the entire scalp—and in some cases, the entire body, including the loss of eyebrows, eyelashes, moustache, and hair in the underarms and the pubic area. Alopecia areata may be associated with nail changes, too, including pinpoint pits, ridging, and roughening with a loss of shine.

Alopecia areata can affect both adults and children. The cause is not known, but research suggests that the immune system may inappropriately attack and interfere with the normal activity of hair follicles. Heredity appears to play a role as well.

The incidence of autoimmune thyroiditis and pernicious anemia is greater in people with alopecia areata than in the general population; therefore, screening for these two disorders is appropriate.

What you can do Wigs and hairpieces are available to camouflage alopecia areata that affects the scalp. In most people, however, only one or a few patches of hair loss develop, and these are easily covered with the remaining hair.

When to call the doctor People with alopecia areata should have their condition evaluated, and screenings should be performed for thyroid disease and anemia by a doctor. Also, because this condition understandably can be emotionally devastating to individuals who suddenly find themselves with little or no hair, a referral to a mental health professional for counseling should be requested if desired.

Treatment Most often, alopecia areata is short-lived; hair growth may begin on its own without any therapy, often within months after the first symptoms appear. A number of treatments are also available, aimed at stimulating hair follicles to grow hair in a normal manner, but none are guaranteed to work. For people whose hair loss is modest, small amounts of cortisone can be applied or injected directly into the hairless areas. The regrowth of hair typically begins within weeks after the treatment, although new

hairless patches can arise. These injections are usually repeated about every 4 weeks.

Another treatment option is the application of anthralin cream, which is a medication used to treat psoriasis. When placed on bare areas of the scalp each day (and rinsed off within an hour), new hair growth frequently occurs in 2 to 3 months.

For hair loss ranging from most of the scalp to large portions of the entire body, there are no proven effective therapies. However, research is ongoing in the areas of both cause and treatment of this disorder. The National Alopecia Areata Foundation, 710 C Street, Suite 11, San Rafael, CA 94901 (415-456-4664) is an excellent resource for additional information.

Prognosis The primary health risks associated with extensive alopecia areata tend to be psychological in nature, causing depression, embarrassment, and social withdrawal. Thus, when appropriate, it is important to obtain psychological care, and perhaps invest in a natural-appearing wig that can boost self-confidence and self-esteem.

With the more common forms of alopecia areata involving just a few patches of hair loss, hair regrowth is usually complete in less than 1 year from the initial hair loss.

❖ DANDRUFF

Symptoms and signs Flakes of dead skin, itching, scaling on the scalp.

What is it? Dandruff is a condition in which dead skin cells are shed by the scalp in sufficient quantity to be noticeable. When cells stick together, often due to surface debris and oil in the hair, they are noticeable as unsightly flakes in the scalp and on one's clothing.

Dandruff is a mild form of seborrheic dermatitis (see page 1279) of unknown cause. It is more of a nuisance and a cosmetic problem than a medical one.

What you can do Frequent shampooing can not only remove the flakes, but can help control dandruff outbreaks by slowing the production and subsequent shedding of skin cells on the scalp. When selecting an over-the-counter shampoo, look for antidandruff ingredients such as salicylic acid (Neutrogena T/Sal) and zinc pyrithione (Head & Shoulders).

When to call the doctor If dandruff symptoms persist or worsen—with severe flaking, itching, scaling or redness—see a doctor for more intensive therapy.

Treatment Your doctor may prescribe an alternative shampoo (ketoconazole, Nizoral) or a corticosteroid lotion to control the redness and itching.

Prognosis Once dandruff has been eradicated, there is a good chance that it will recur. For this reason, some doctors recommend frequent shampooing and at least weekly use of an antidandruff shampoo as a preventive measure.

NAILS

Nails are composed of skin cells that are made hard by a tough protein called keratin. Nails protect the tissue underneath them and improve manual dexterity.

Each nail consists of several parts:

- The nail plate is the visible nail itself.
- The nail bed is the skin underneath the nail. The nail gets its pink appearance from the capillaries coursing through the nail bed.
- The cuticle is the fold of the skin at the base of the nail plate. It serves as a seal, keeping bacteria, yeast, and debris in the environment from entering the adjacent skin.
- The matrix is located under the cuticle; it is composed of cells that produce the nail plate.
- The lunula is the portion of the nail matrix that looks like a whitish crescent; it is often referred to as the half moon.

Nails grow slowly but steadily. Fingernails grow about one-eight of an inch or less per month, while toenails grow at only one-third this rate. As we age, the nails tend to become more brittle and the growth rate slows.

Because we use our hands primarily to interact with the environment, the fingernails are subjected to frequent trauma. Nails can be nicked, torn, or bruised during normal activities. Fortunately, most of these are little more than cosmetic insults.

Even so, a number of conditions can affect the structure of the nails, such as nail splitting related to exposure to chemicals. Nail infections can develop from fungal or bacterial invasion. Thus, you need to pay attention to the appearance of your nails and intervene if you suspect that an infection or other problem is present.

❖ ONYCHOMYCOSIS (TINEA UNGUIUM)

Symptoms and signs Whitish nail discoloration with thickening, due to accumulation of scales under the nails; separation of the nail from the nail bed; often, itching and flaking of nearby skin between the toes or around the nails; pain when footwear presses on the nails. (See page C-41.)

What is it? Onychomycosis (or tinea unguium) is a fungal infection of the nail; it most often affects toenails, although it can occur on the fingernails as well.

The fungus thrives in moist, warm areas, such as sweaty feet. It digests the nail keratin, which is the protein that makes up the nail. The color of the infected nail ranges from white to yellow, and less often from green to black. The surrounding skin may also be infected with the fungus, as demonstrated by itchy dry white scaling or flaking on the toes, between the toes, and sometimes on the entire sole of the foot. People usually mistake their flaking, dry feet for "dry skin." In some cases, the nearby skin of the foot or hand can develop a secondary bacterial infection, becoming warm, red, swollen, and itchy. The infection may even cause cellulitis in the leg, which needs immediate attention from a doctor. (See Cellulitis, page 1282.)

What you can do Try to prevent fungal infections by minimizing exposure to infection-promoting dampness. Following a bath

BASICS OF NAIL CARE

Nails require very little attention. If you trim them regularly and keep them clean, you can significantly reduce your risk of nail problems.

Nails should be trimmed at least once every 2 to 3 weeks. Trim the toenails straight across, rather than curving them at the edges; this reduces the risk of an ingrown toenail (see page 1324). If your nails tend to be thick or brittle, they will be easier to trim after bathing or showering.

Do not trim the cuticles. They are there for a reason: to prevent organisms from invading the adjacent skin and nail. Also, if they are cut or pushed back, the cuticles and perhaps the underlying matrix can be injured. If you have poor vision or problems with hand dexterity, see a podiatrist for nail care.

Avoid biting your nails. Nail biting can lead to infections and hangnails (as well as unsightly nails). Although having manicured nails help some people to stop biting them, the manicure itself can sometimes make the nails vulnerable to other problems. For example, the acetone in nail polish remover can worsen nail brittleness. So, if you are prone to weakened, brittle, and cracked nails, limit the use of nail polish removers to once a week or even less or use one of the new acetone-free nail polish removers. If you use artificial nails, be sure that there is no gap or opening between the artificial nail and your own nail; bacteria or fungi can find their way in and cause an infection. Make certain that sterile or brand-new filing tools are used, to further guard against infections.

Hardening substances in nail polish often contain chemicals, such as formaldehyde, which can cause an allergic reaction (redness, itching and swelling around the cuticle, or even on other parts of the body); if this problem develops, switch to a hypoallergenic polish that is free of formaldehyde and fragrances. Glues used for artificial nails can provoke similar allergic responses.

Avoid direct contact with harsh chemicals; these can injure or weaken the nails, leaving them susceptible to infections. Wear rubber or latex gloves when using household detergents and cleansers. Also, after washing your hands, use lotions (such as those with alpha-hydroxy acids), which can minimize the risk of split nails.

Hangnails are tears in the edge of the nail near the skin, or projections or splits of the skin that surround the nail. Hangnails can be painful, and they can cause an inflammation and infection if bacteria enter small openings in the skin. To resolve the problem, use nail clippers or nail scissors to cut away the hangnail as close to the skin surface as you can. Then, to speed healing, use an antibiotic ointment for several days.

Eat a healthy diet. If you have a nutritional deficiency, it may be reflected in your nails—perhaps slowing their growth, or causing splitting or ridges. ■

---

or shower, dry the feet completely, including between the toes. Use a foot powder or spray designed to kill fungi. Change socks a few times a day if needed, and use an "extra-strength" antiperspirant on your feet. Do not walk barefoot in locker rooms, public bathrooms, or at public swimming pools.

To cut down the likelihood of fingernail infections, wear latex or vinyl gloves if your hands are frequently immersed in water. The use of artificial nails increases the likelihood of a fungal infection. If you see any discoloration, be sure to have the artificial nails removed. (See The Risks of Artificial Nails, page 1322, for more information.)

Any time you have a manicure or pedicure, be sure to choose a nail salon that is scrupulous in its observance of sterilization procedures—or, better yet, bring along your own nail implements for the manicurist to use.

When to call the doctor Fungal infections are difficult to treat. Even oral medication does not guarantee eradication of the infection, although newer drugs are usually successful and well tolerated (see below). If a fungal infection is accompanied by pain and swelling, suspect that a secondary bacterial infection has developed and see your doctor immediately.

Treatment A relatively new oral drug—itraconazole (Sporanox)—is winning favor among many doctors for treating fungal infections. Itraconazole clears about 50 to 70 percent of treated patients after 3 to 4 months of therapy. Another more recently released drug, terbinafine (Lamisil), has similar cure rates and requires the same length of therapy. Due to the unlikely possibility of liver toxicity and other rare abnormalities, blood tests are usually done before the medication is administered and then repeated monthly for monitoring purposes throughout the course of treatment. (See page 850 and Chapter 22 for more information on the difficulty of treating fungal infections.) Because toenails grow so slowly, it can take many months or even a year to judge the effectiveness of treatment. Notably, even after you stop these medications, they continue to be active in the nail for about 9 months.

To prevent future infections doctors also sometimes recommend applying an

THE RISKS OF ACRYLIC NAILS

Artificial nails made of acrylic are often used for cosmetic reasons, to enhance the nails or to camouflage chipped, damaged, or injured nails. However, these artificial nails can cause damage to the nails and surrounding tissues.

A common problem is the tendency of artificial nails to trap moisture in the underlying natural nail. This can create a breeding area for secondary infections, particularly those caused by fungi.

Some people have allergic responses to acrylics. This reaction may irritate and cause swelling, soreness, and itching in the surrounding skin. In persons who develop this allergy, the artificial nails must be removed; otherwise, the condition will only worsen. A dermatologist can evaluate the changes and test for an allergy. ■

antifungal cream or polish to the nail itself, either instead of the medication or once treatment with the oral medication is completed. Use of the cream alone may occasionally eradicate the infection.

Prognosis Onychomycosis is difficult to treat. It may take many months—sometimes a year or more—for the infection to completely clear.

❖ PARONYCHIA

Symptoms and signs Pain, tenderness, redness, occasional trapped pus and swelling of the skin adjacent to the nail. (See page C-41.)

What is it? Acute (sudden-onset) paronychia is a bacterial infection of the skin adjacent to the nail. This infection tends to occur following a minor break in the skin near the nail. This may be caused by the pulling or biting off of a hangnail or the trimming of cuticles, or it may be due to a cut or abrasion, a splinter, or a prick from a thorn. The skin on the sides of the nail, or sometimes near the cuticle, will become red and bulging. Pus may be visible at the infection site. The pain can become severe.

Chronic paronychia differs from the acute form by its long-term course and lack of intense pain, swelling, and pus. It appears as redness and flaking of the skin surrounding the nail. It may be caused by a yeast

(*Candida*) infection, or a primary skin disease such as eczema, psoriasis, and lupus erythematosus.

What you can do In acute paronychia, if pus can be released by gently pressing on the nail, the infection may heal on its own in a few days. In the meantime, soak the affected nail in warm salt water ($^1/_4$ tsp of salt per 8 oz of water).

When to call the doctor Contact a doctor when pain, bulging, and redness are present, and when the above measure does not lead to immediate relief of pain and subsequent healing.

Treatment If drainage of the pus has not occurred and redness and swelling persist, the doctor may lance the sac containing the pus. The subsequent drainage will ease the pain and speed up the healing process.

For an acute bacterial paronychial infection, oral antibiotics such as dicloxacillin, cephalexin, or erythromycin are typically prescribed. For chronic paronychia caused by *Candida*, an antifungal cream will be used.

Prognosis Paronychia usually heals promptly with proper therapy.

❖ FELON

Symptoms and signs Severe finger pain; accumulation and/or discharge of pus in the finger pad; warmth and swelling in the region.

What is it? Felon is an infection of the finger pad. It usually occurs after a relatively minor injury to the finger, such as a splinter, pinprick, or thorn prick. The area of inflammation tends to enlarge if the infection is not treated promptly.

What you can do Over-the-counter analgesics (painkillers) and warm compresses may help relieve the discomfort of felon until a doctor can be seen.

When to call the doctor If symptoms are present that suggest the presence of felon, see a doctor as soon as possible.

Treatment Doctors can perform a minor surgical procedure, which involves making

CHANGES IN NAIL SHAPE AND COLOR

When nails change their appearance—for example, with the development of ridges or pits, or an alteration of their color—an underlying disease or an inadequate diet is often to blame. Thus, these nail abnormalities may be symptoms of medical conditions, many of which are described in detail elsewhere in this book. Here are some of the more common nail changes:

- A person with anemia may notice vertical ridges in her nails, along with brittleness and a concave or spoon-shaped surface. Anemia can also cause the nail bed to become pale. (See page 920 for more information on anemia).

- A concave shape to the nails, when accompanied by thickened nails, could be a sign of an overactive thyroid (see Chapter 22 for more information on hyperthyroidism).

- If the nails assume a club-like appearance (turning downward at the tips), this could indicate a variety of medical problems, from chronic infections to emphysema to lung cancer (see page 756 and 762 for more information on emphysema and lung cancer).

- Small pits on the nail—accompanied by thickening or splitting of the nail, or its partial detachment from the skin underneath it—may be a symptom of psoriasis. A yellowish nail color may also indicate the presence of psoriasis (see Psoriasis, page 1275).

- When the nails become bluish or bluish-gray (a condition called cyanosis), this might be a sign of chronic lung or heart problems. (See Chapters 18 and 20.)

- White nails can be produced by chronic diseases affecting the kidneys or liver. If the whiteness is limited to small spots on the nails, it might be caused by a vitamin deficiency or trauma.

For other causes of discoloration, see descriptions of bacterial and fungal infections of the nails, Onychomycosis, page 1320 and Paronychia, page 1322.

Doctors do not know why some of these nail abnormalities develop in conjunction with various diseases—but because most of the underlying disorders require treatment, see a doctor for proper diagnosis and therapy. In fact, the presence of these nail changes often helps doctors make the correct diagnoses. With several of these diseases or disorders, successful treatment may lead to a resolution of the related nail abnormalities. For example, if you are found to have iron-deficiency anemia, dietary iron replacement will lead to a normalization of your nails as they grow. ■

an incision at the site of the infection to allow for proper drainage. Antibiotics are also usually prescribed.

Prognosis Early treatment can resolve the infection quickly and prevent very serious complications such as an infection ascending up the finger and into the hand or the underlying bone (osteomyelitis).

❖ FOREIGN BODIES UNDER THE NAIL

Symptoms and signs Object imbedded under the nail; redness, swelling, and pain with progression of condition.

What is it? A foreign body (for example, a splinter of wood) can accidentally make its way between the nail and the skin underneath it. If not cared for properly, an infection can develop at the site of the injury.

What you can do If the foreign body is protruding from beneath the nail and can be grasped with a tweezers, gently remove it.

After the object has been extracted, soak the nail in warm water and an antibacterial soap, cleansing it thoroughly. In addition, update your tetanus vaccination, if needed.

When to call the doctor If you are unable to easily remove the foreign body, do not continue to try. See a doctor for proper extraction of the object.

Treatment After the doctor removes the object from under the nail, a topical antiseptic may be recommended. Antibiotics may be prescribed if an infection has developed in the area.

Prognosis Most of these injuries heal rapidly once the foreign object has been removed. However, continue to watch the nail for several months for possible development of a fungal infection.

❖ SUBUNGUAL HEMATOMA (BLOOD UNDER THE NAIL)

Symptoms and signs Bleeding and accumulation of blood under the nail; red discoloration, ultimately turning dark blue and black; swelling; pain; tenderness; pressure.

What is it? When a nail becomes injured—for example, when a finger becomes caught in a closing door—bleeding can occur, and blood can collect underneath the nail. That often leads to pain, tenderness, and a dark red color under the nail. The pressure from the trapped blood can be extremely uncomfortable.

It is possible for an injury to a nail to occur without your being aware of it at the time; for example, a toenail might be injured during sports activities if poorly fitting shoes are worn.

Research studies suggest that hematomas are more common in people who take aspirin or other nonsteroidal anti-inflammatory drugs (such as ibuprofen); these medications slow the normal blood coagulation process.

What you can do With time, the pain and tenderness associated with subungual hematomas will subside. Until then, apply ice to the nail to help ease discomfort and swelling. The redness under the nail will eventually turn dark blue.

When to call the doctor If your nail is still painful, see a doctor for treatment and also to exclude the possibility that you have a more serious problem—such as a fracture of the finger.

Also, if you "just happen" to notice what looks like a healing hematoma—deep blue, black, or brown in color—but you cannot recall an event in which the injury has occurred, a doctor should evaluate the nail to make sure that the problem is really a hematoma rather than a mole or melanoma (mole cancer) under the nail.

Treatment A doctor can relieve pressure and pain associated with a subungual hematoma by piercing the nail with a needle and allowing drainage of the trapped blood. If an infection has developed, antibiotics may be prescribed.

If the doctor suspects a broken bone in the finger, an x-ray will be ordered; if a fracture is detected, a referral to an orthopedist may be appropriate.

Prognosis With time, subungual hematomas will heal with little or no medical intervention.

❖ ONYCHOLYSIS

Symptoms and signs Partial separation of the nail from the underlying or nail bed; asymptomatic.

What is it? Onycholysis is a painless condition in which the nail loosens or separates from the underlying nail bed. It can have a number of causes. For instance, it can develop when the nails are exposed to household and occupational chemicals or other substances, including nail polish, nail acrylics, detergents, soapy water, or moisture. Runners sometimes suffer from onycholysis, when their toenails are struck repeatedly by the interior of their shoes.

Also, onycholysis may be a sign of a primary skin disease, most commonly psoriasis. In people with psoriasis, tiny nail pits are also often present. Less commonly, onycholysis is a presenting sign of thyroid disease. (See Psoriasis, page 1275.)

In people with onycholysis, organisms can invade the separated nail region, leading to the development of fungal or bacterial infections.

What you can do Wear gloves when working with household cleaners and other chemical irritants that may cause this disorder. Do not use your nails as "tools" for opening things. If you work at a computer keyboard or use your hands for other activities in which you repeatedly strike your fingernails, you may need to cut your nails shorter.

Wear properly fitting shoes, particularly for sports activities. Avoid shoes that press on or "knock" your toenails.

When to call the doctor If you have onycholysis and are not able to pinpoint a chemical exposure or some kind of trauma causing it, contact a doctor. You will likely be screened for thyroid disease or primary skin disorders that may have caused this nail change.

Treatment Doctors can advise patients on how best to avoid irritants in the future. If secondary infections have developed, the responsible fungi or bacteria need to be readicated with appropriate medications.

Prognosis Onycholysis typically resolves once the cause is identified and avoided—as with irritants or trauma—or treated—as with hyperthyroidism (over-active thyroid).

❖ INGROWN TOENAIL

Symptoms and signs Edge of the toenail growing inward into the surrounding skin (nail fold) with redness, swelling, and occasionally visible pus; severe pain (frequently). (See page C-41.)

What is it? An ingrown toenail occurs when a corner of the toenail (often the big toe) pierces the nail fold skin that surrounds the nail. As the toenail jabs into the tissue, it causes intense pain and tenderness (particularly when walking or wearing shoes), redness, and swelling.

A common cause of ingrown toenails is improper trimming of the nails—specifically, cutting them too short.

What you can do To prevent ingrown toenails, cut the nails straight across the top. Do not wear tight or poorly fitting shoes that squeeze the toes and promote ingrown nails.

To treat this problem, soak the affected toe in warm water and antibacterial soap; this will help reduce the discomfort and soften the nail. Next, raise the edge of the nail tip slightly by placing a tiny wisp of cotton between the nail and the skin. Apply an antibiotic ointment to the affected skin. Wear open-toed shoes—or a loose, comfortable pair of regular shoes—until the inflammation is gone and healing is complete. Soak the toe and replace the cotton at least twice a day.

Persons with diabetes, or with vascular or neurologic deficits in their feet, should undergo intense training on proper foot care by a doctor or nurse if they have not in the past, or if they need a "refresher course."

When to call the doctor If the above measures do not solve the problem, or if pus is present, see a doctor. You probably have a secondary bacterial infection. Also, if you have diabetes, or vascular or neurological deficits in your feet, see your doctor whenever an ingrown toenail develops.

Treatment If pus is present, the doctor will drain it by lancing the skin. An oral or topical antibiotic may be prescribed for an infection at the site of the ingrown nail.

If a tiny portion of the nail has embedded itself under the skin, this will also need to be removed. Later, after the inflammation and pain have subsided, a surgical procedure can be used to permanently remove the lateral-most portion of the nail to prevent recurrences.

Prognosis Ingrown nails due to physical factors are usually easily prevented once these factors are identified and avoided (such as tight shoes) or corrected (such as abnormal lateral nail growth requiring minor surgical correction).

TWENTY-NINE

Allergies

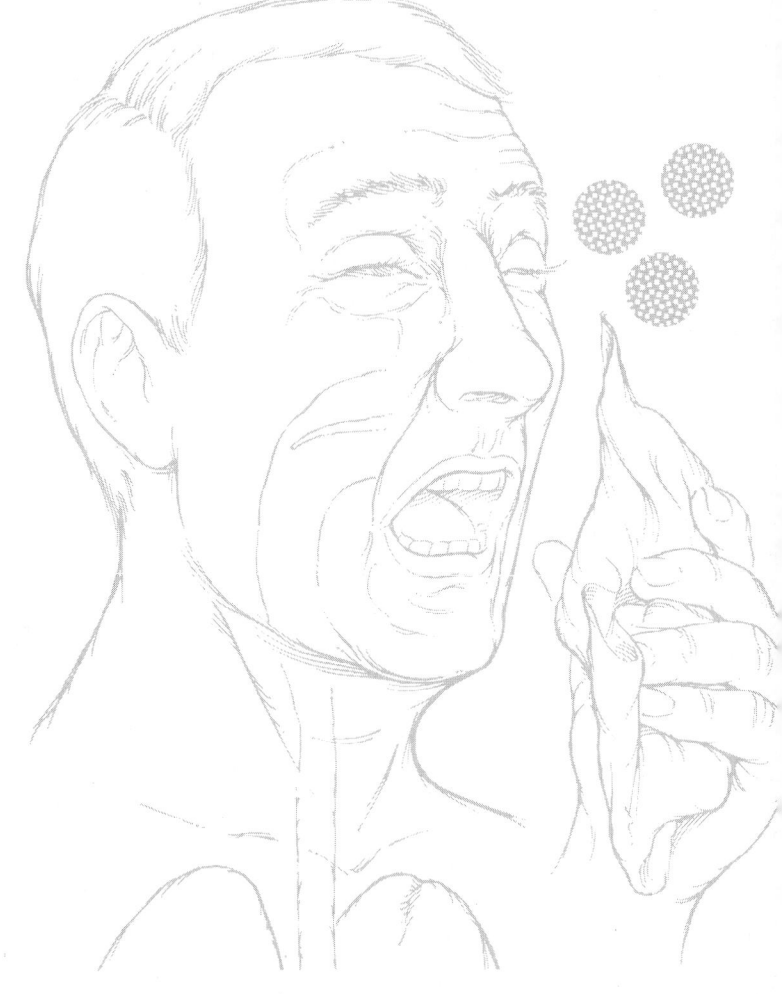

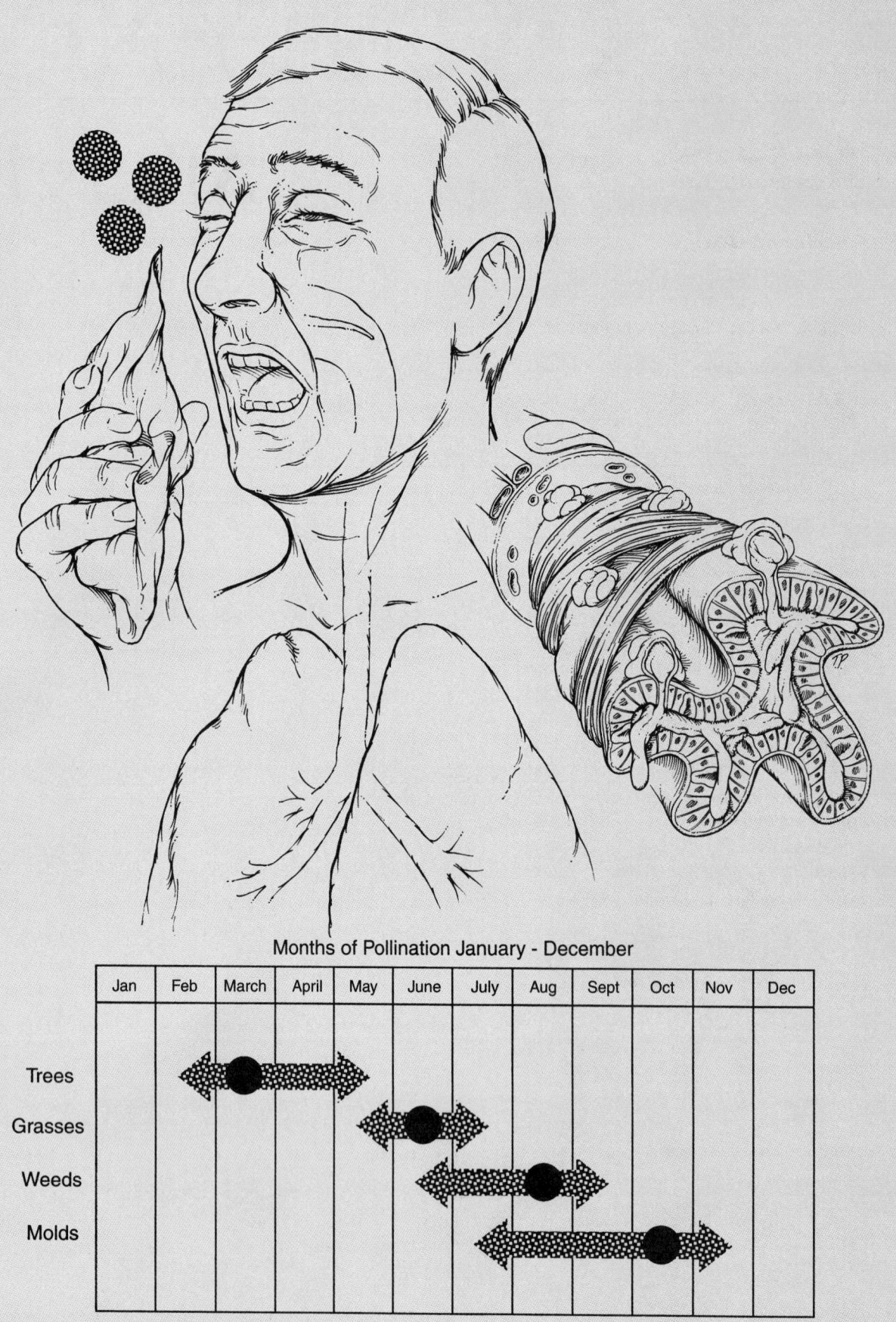

Months of Pollination January - December

Jan	Feb	March	April	May	June	July	Aug	Sept	Oct	Nov	Dec

Trees

Grasses

Weeds

Molds

ALLERGIES

What Is Allergy?

Allergy—the most common disorder of the immune system—afflicts at least 2 in 10 Americans. The allergic reaction is the result of an overzealous response on the part of the immune system in reaction to substances from the external environment known as allergens.

The most common causes of allergic response are pollen grains, mold, dust mites, animal danders, foods, medication, insect venom, and plant oils (see page 1335). Since the allergens usually come from the environment around us or from something we consume, the body systems most vulnerable to allergic responses include the eyes, the respiratory system, the skin, and the intestinal tract—areas directly exposed to the external environment.

The symptoms of allergy vary depending on the site. The eyes may become weepy, red, and itchy; the eyelids and sometimes even the conjunctivae (the filmy clear covering over the eyes) may become swollen. In the nose, the symptoms typical of allergy include watery clear discharge, sneezing, itching, and often swelling in the nasal passages sufficient to obstruct free breathing. The nasal symptoms can promote drainage down the back of the throat, or postnasal drip, leaving it itchy or irritated and occasionally even irritating the vocal cords and causing hoarseness. In the breathing passages of the lung, allergy can cause constriction and tightness of the chest, production of phlegm (clear or white mucous secretions discharged through the mouth) with coughing and wheezing. Although some cases of asthma (a condition characterized by breathlessness and wheezing) do not arise as a consequence of allergies, they can be a major contributing cause, especially in children (see Chapter 18).

Allergic skin reactions can include itching, redness, dry scaly rashes, blistering rashes, and hives, which are irregularly shaped patches on the skin that are swollen and itchy, much like a large mosquito bite. In the intestinal tract, allergic reactions to foods can cause abdominal cramping, vomiting, diarrhea, or bloating.

UNDERSTANDING THE ALLERGIC RESPONSE

It is sometimes difficult to understand why some people suffer mightily from the environment around them and other people are undisturbed. In part, the answer lies in our genes; some of us inherit a tendency to react in an allergic way to substances—pollen grains, mold, dust, foods, medication, insect venom, plant oils, and the dander (shed skin debris) of furred animals—that surround us, and others do not. We call these substances allergens because for susceptible people they are capable of stimulating an allergic response after sensitization has occurred. It is an interesting phenomenon of allergy that you cannot be allergic to something to which you have never been previously exposed. Allergy requires an initial exposure to the substance, which sensitizes the immune system. Subsequent reexposure can then activate immune mechanisms to bring about allergic symptoms.

Allergic reactions are dependent on several factors, the most important of which are the individual's sensitivity level and the environmental exposure level. Both of these factors may wax and wane over time. For example, a person may be stung once a year by a honeybee and never react, perhaps because sensitivity declines and disappears between stings. But then one month the person gets stung twice 2 weeks apart and suffers a severe allergic reaction for the first time ever after the second sting.

Within a similar group of allergens, some substances cause more trouble than others. In the case of animal dander, for example, cats induce allergic symptoms far more frequently than other animals. The dander itself—just like human dander or dandruff as we usually call it—is nothing more than flakes of shed skin that may shake loose from the animal's coat or remain loosely attached to the fur. Because cats groom themselves by licking, their dander has the added element of saliva, which is very rich in allergens. In contrast, dogs are less of a problem than cats, in part because they preen less and in part because dogs do not usually invade the space of their masters as much as cats do.

When allergens come in contact with the lining of the nose or eyes of a previously sensitized person, tissue mast cells are activated. These mast cells carry specialized immune molecules, called IgE antibodies (allergy-triggering proteins made by the body in response to a specific allergen), on their surfaces. These antibodies

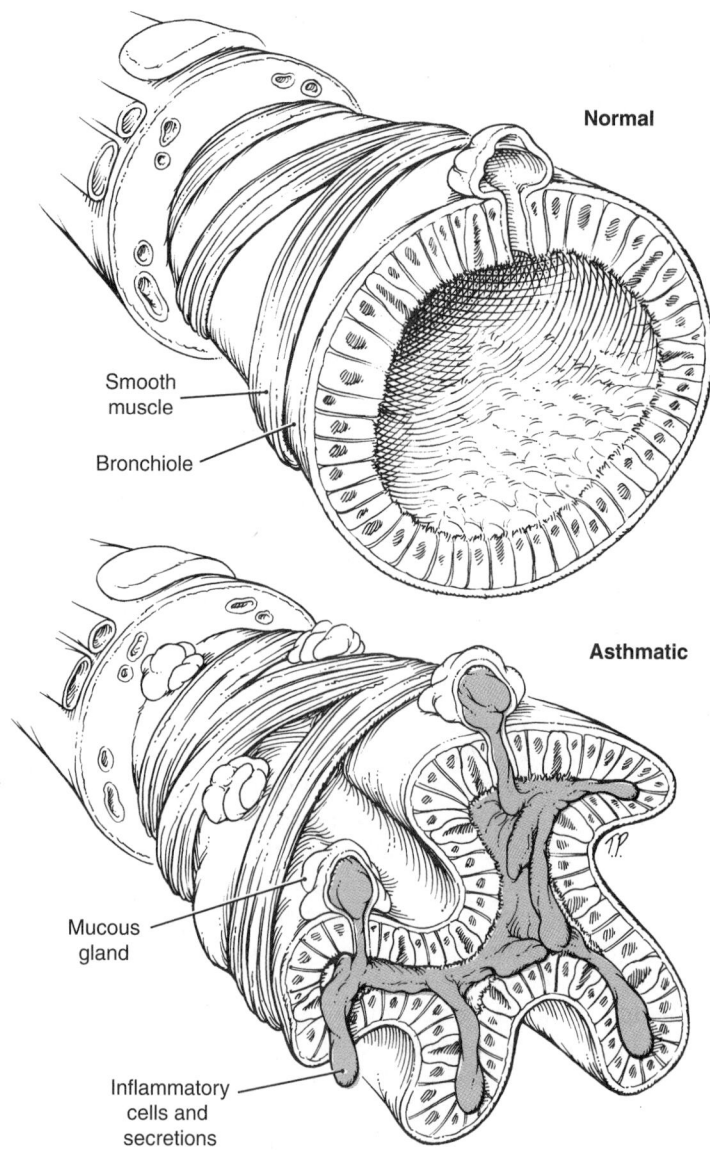

Normal

Smooth
muscle

Bronchiole

Asthmatic

Mucous
gland

Inflammatory
cells and
secretions

Asthma commonly causes recurrent attacks of breathlessness. Exposure to allergens and other environmental
agents leads to inflammation, increased mucus production, and constriction of the bronchioles. Your doctor
can prescribe inhaled medications to reduce inflammation and relieve bronchial constriction (See page 1333
for more information.)

bind to the allergens which then bridge
multiple antibodies. This bridging activates
biochemical reactions that culminate in
the release of histamine and other mast
cell-derived chemicals. These chemicals
cause the tissues lining the nose or eyes to
swell, increase the production of mucus,
cause itching, sneezing, and irritation, and
even stimulate constriction of the breathing passages in the lungs.

Because histamine is one of the major
causes of the allergic inflammation, an early
focus of treatment for allergies has for many
years been antihistamine medications,
which block histamine's action and thereby
reduce symptoms. But blocking histamine is
not the only option for allergy treatment,
and depending on the symptoms, antihistamines may not be the most appropriate
medication (see page 1333). In some cases,
allergen injection treatments can be used to
mitigate the symptoms of respiratory
allergy (see page 1332). Some allergies
respond better than others to injection
treatments. Allergies to dust mites and pollens often respond favorably to shots; allergies to molds and animal danders, less
favorably; and allergies to food, most medications, and chemicals are not treated with
injections since avoidance of the offending
food or medication is usually possible. Your
allergist can help to determine if your allergies will respond to allergen injections.

Treatment of Allergies

Allergies are managed, not cured. Fortunately, the treatments used to manage allergies can provide considerable relief. The
effective management of allergies frequently requires that the doctor, the person
with allergies, and the person's family work
together to control allergic reactions.

The first step is to find out what is causing your allergic symptoms, particularly if
they are severe. Because there are many
allergy-provoking agents in the environment, trying to sort out the cause on your
own can be difficult. It is best to seek the
help of a qualified allergist (a doctor who
specializes in the diagnosis and treatment of
allergic conditions) who can both determine the cause of your allergy and devise a
comprehensive treatment plan to minimize
the symptoms. The allergist will take a careful history, perform a relevant physical
exam, and recommend appropriate allergy
testing as indicated by the individual case
(see page 1331).

Knowing what is causing your allergic
reactions is essential, because it enables you
to take steps to avoid the offending sub-
stance(s) as much as possible. Your doctor
will advise you on ways to begin to eliminate allergens from your environment and
on lifestyle changes that can bring relief, but

it is up to the allergy sufferer and his family to be vigilant, particularly in the case of life-threatening food or bee sting allergies. Avoiding the offending allergen is the treatment of choice whenever possible.

There are many situations, however, where allergens cannot be avoided. In these cases, your doctor may recommend either immunotherapy (see page 1332) or long-term drug therapy (see page 1333). The newer antihistamine medications and nasal steroid sprays have been a tremendous boon to allergy sufferers because they do not cause one of the most frequent side effects of the older antihistamines—drowsiness.

Each case of allergy is different, and your doctor will customize a treatment plan for your needs and lifestyle. A well thought out strategy incorporating one or more of the mainstays of allergy management—avoidance, immunotherapy, and medication—can make an enormous difference in quality of life. In the sections that follow, you will learn in detail how allergic disorders can be diagnosed and treated.

DIAGNOSIS OF ALLERGIES

When you suffer from allergies, discovering what substances cause your symptoms can make the difference in being able to live with your problem or being made miserable by it. The search for causes, however, is not always easy, even if you have an idea about the allergens that are troubling you. The wisest and most direct approach may be to enlist the aid of a qualified allergist who can perform a variety of appropriate tests to help determine the precise cause of your allergic symptoms. Once your allergist determines what is causing your allergic symptoms, he can formulate an effective treatment plan to prevent or reduce your allergic symptoms. There are several types of tests an allergist can perform to determine the cause of allergic symptoms. The following are examples of some commonly used allergy testing methods.

Skin testing The mainstay of the allergist's testing armory involves skin testing using a standard panel of common pollens, animal danders, dust mites, and molds found in the region of the country where the allergy sufferer lives. The allergist first places a drop of

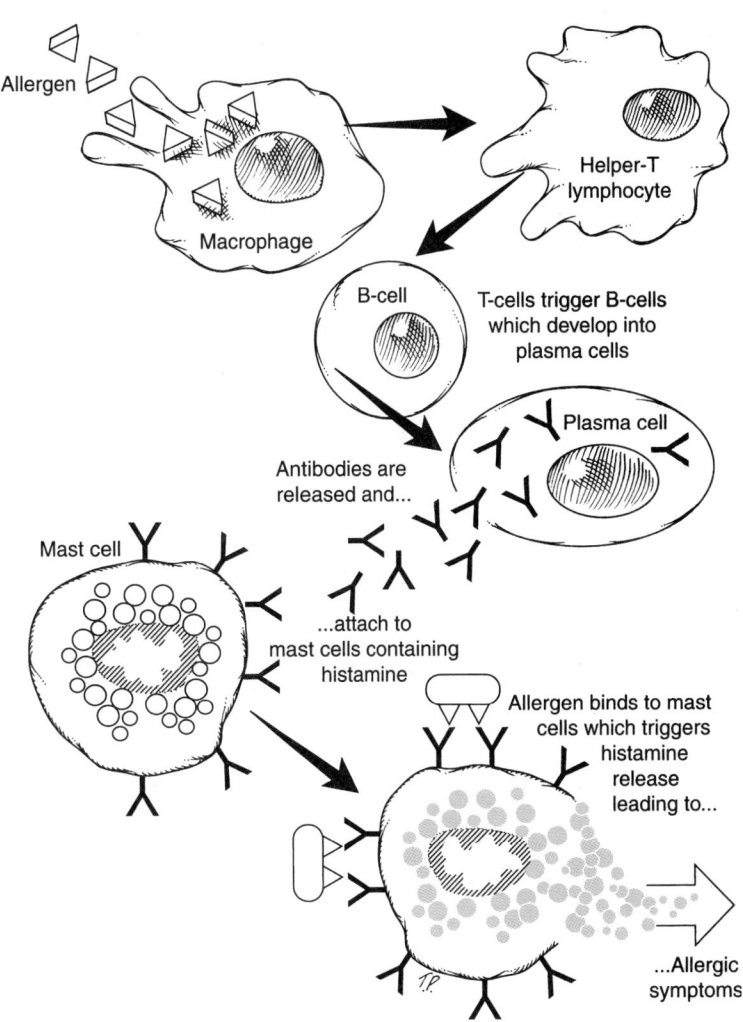

An allergic reaction results from recognition of a foreign substance (allergen) by the body's immune system.

fluid containing an allergen onto the skin and makes a small puncture or prick through the drop that allows a minute amount of the allergen to penetrate into the skin. If positive, the puncture test causes redness (or a flare), and a hivelike swelling of the skin (or a wheal) similar to a mosquito bite reaction, within 15 to 20 minutes. The size of the flare and wheal correlate with the degree of sensitivity to the allergen. If there is no reaction to the superficial prick/puncture test and yet the allergist still has reason to suspect that particular allergen, an injection of a small amount of the allergen under the skin is also commonly done to provide a more sensitive test for allergic sensitivity.

Skin tests are most commonly used for respiratory allergies, which may produce symptoms including nasal congestion and drainage, sneezing, itchy eyes, and wheezing, but they can also help to detect those food and drug allergies that arise within 2 hours after eating a food or taking an allergic medication (for example, penicillin). Skin tests are also used to determine allergy to insect stings.

To be sure of the accuracy of the results the allergist will recommend discontinuing antihistamine medication prior to testing because the development of a positive skin test result depends on the release of histamine into the skin. A positive skin test result causes some discomfort (primarily itching) and, very rarely, can precipitate a more severe bodywide allergic reaction, which is why it is important to have a qualified doctor present during testing to handle any untoward reactions. Despite these minor inconveniences, this method of allergy testing is relatively inexpensive, safe if properly performed, readily available, and gives immediate results.

Blood testing Recent advances in medical technology have given doctors several new tools to test for allergies: the radioallergosorbent test (RAST) and the enzyme-linked immunosorbent assay (ELISA). Both of these tests are designed to detect the IgE antibodies. These tests mix blood from the allergy sufferer in a testing chamber containing an insoluble form of the suspected allergen. If the blood contains antibodies to that allergen, the antibody will recognize and bind with the allergen; in a second step, a tracer tag glows to demonstrate the allergen-antibody binding and a positive result. Although it is not necessary to discontinue the use of antihistamines to verify the accuracy of these tests, they are not quite as sensitive as skin testing. Lack of sensitivity is generally not a concern for airborne and food allergens, but is a reason to prefer skin tests for serious medication or insect sting allergies.

The radioallergosorbent test and the enzyme-linked immunosorbent assay usually cost substantially more than skin testing, but since both tests are lab tests, they are totally safe, with no uncomfortable wheals and no chance of inducing allergic reaction.

Patch testing This kind of allergy testing involves the application of small amounts of individual allergens beneath adhesive patches applied to the skin of the back. The allergen patches, which are left in place and gener-

ally checked after 48 hours and again after 72 hours, will cause redness and sometimes swelling of the skin in positive tests. This method of testing works best for metals (notably nickel) and allergy-provoking chemicals such as formaldehyde and some cosmetic additives.

Provocative testing This method of allergy testing, also called challenge testing, may sometimes prove necessary to implicate a substance as the definite cause of symptoms. Provocative testing involves physically administering the suspected substance to an individual in a controlled setting (usually the doctor's office) to see if it provokes the allergic symptoms. Examples of provocative testing might be the administration of an inhaled aerosol containing an airborne substance to attempt to provoke nasal, bronchial, or lung allergy symptoms, or giving the person a certain food or medication to see if it provokes the allergic symptoms. Provoking symptoms in a person with anaphylactic reaction to a food or medication should rarely be done because it can be dangerous (see page 1341). A positive challenge test brings with it the discomfort of unpleasant and potentially severe symptoms. For this reason, very small doses of the substance are used initially, and increases in amount are gradual in order to minimize the risks.

ALLERGY DESENSITIZATION INJECTIONS

Allergy desensitization injections (allergy shots), or immunotherapy, consist of a series of injections that can serve to desensitize you to an allergen by slowly increasing your immune defenses to this foreign matter in a controlled setting (usually the doctor's office). Immunotherapy is most effective in the treatment of allergies caused by airborne allergens or insect stings.

The allergist will compound a mixture in solution containing the allergens to which you react most strongly. Your desensitization will begin with weekly injections of a very dilute solution of these allergens. The injection treatments progress slowly, with incremental increases in volume and concentration. This process is repeated until the allergist feels you have reached the optimal dose or until treatment cannot advance

MEDICATIONS USED TO COMBAT ALLERGIES

Medications that are commonly employed to treat allergies fall into three basic categories: those that block or counteract the action of histamine, those that block the release of histamine and other medications, and corticosteroids that block the inflammation associated with allergy. The medications may be administered as pills, capsules, or liquids taken by mouth, as sprays inhaled into the nose or lungs, as injections, and, in some cases, as creams or lotions applied to the skin.

Following are descriptions of the three basic categories of allergy medications, the symptoms they treat, and the various forms in which they may be administered.

Antihistamines

Antihistamines act to block the action of histamine, the body chemical released in allergic reactions that is responsible for allergic symptoms such as itching, sneezing, and production of secretions in the nose, throat, and larynx and constriction of the bronchial tree; cramping and bloating in the upper gastrointestinal tract; or itching and hives in the skin. Common antihistamines that are available over-the-counter include diphenhydramine, clemastine, and chlorpheniramine (found in Dristan and a wide variety of cold/sinus/allergy medications). Some of these antihistamines, such as clemastine, are lower-dose formulations of prescription-strength antihistamines. Although they are slightly different in chemical structure, all of these products work to counteract histamine and all can cause some degree of drowsiness and dry mouth in about 20 percent of people. These medications are available as pills or liquids.

Among the antihistamines available only by prescription, several medications block the action of histamine but do not cause drowsiness. These include loratadine (Claritin), fexofenadine hydrochloride (Allegra), astemizole (Hismanal), and cetirizine (Zyrtec).

Be aware that Hismanal can cause potentially life-threatening interactions with such medications as erythromycin (and clar-ithromycin) and with antifungal medications such as Nizoral and Sporanox. These reactions can include irregular heart beat, fainting, dizziness, and cardiac arrest and death. You should always advise your doctor of other medication you may be taking to prevent dangerous interactions. Terfenadine (Seldane), another antihistamine with potentially life-threatening reactions with certain medications, was taken off the market because of potential side effects. Terfenadine has been replaced by fexofenadine hydrochloride, which does not appear to have these interactions. Loratadine and cetirizine also appear safer.

Nasal Inhalers (Nasal Sprays)

Nasal inhalers containing corticosteroid medication such as beclomethasone (Vancenase, Vancenase AQ, Beconase), fluticasone (Flonase), triamcinolone (Nasacort), and others work by delivering a fine mist of steroid to the lining of the nose. The steroid acts both to reduce inflammation and swelling of the nasal chamber and also to reduce histamine release by stabilizing the mast cells and reducing their number. Two other medications commonly used in inhaled nasal sprays, cromolyn sodium and nedocromil, also block the release of histamine from the mast cells and may have other anti-inflammatory properties. Cromolyn sodium can also be taken orally to combat food allergies or inhaled into the lungs to relieve the asthmatic wheezing that sometimes accompanies allergy.

Injectable Medication

Corticosteroids, antihistamines, and epinephrine can also be administered by injection to combat allergy. Epinephrine, which is produced in the adrenal glands, is also called adrenaline; in the event of serious allergic reaction, a synthetic form of this body chemical is commonly used as an injectable medication. Its actions are many, but its chief roles in allergy treatment are to open constricted breathing passages in severe asthma, to constrict the dilated blood vessels and elevate lowered blood pressure, and to stop the angioedema (skin swelling) and wheal formation that are characteristic of hives. ■

---

further because of allergic reaction to the injection.

Along the way, as the pollen seasons peak or the allergen loads in your environment increase, you may have a few setbacks. You may not tolerate the progression in volume or strength of the injections for a few weeks because of local swelling, redness, tenderness, and heat at the site of your injection, or you may experience more serious systemic reactions such as hives, asthma, or shock.

Although the mechanisms by which allergen injections treat allergies are complex, one way this stepwise administration of progressively larger amounts of the offending allergen acts is to gently prompt the immune system to produce a blocking antibody of a different type—an IgG antibody—that competes with the allergy antibodies (IgE) for the allergen, sops it up, and prevents the activation of mast cells and histamine release.

Allergen injection treatments do not offer a cure for allergies, but they can be a tremendous benefit to some people, particularly for those with pollen allergies whose allergic symptoms may be reduced to an occasional inconvenience rather than an ongoing daily misery. The process of desensitization may require several years of regular shots with the continuing risk, albeit low, of acute allergic reactions. This is why injection treatments must always be given in a supervised medical environment. Injection therapy has no place at all, however, in the treatment of many other types of allergy, most notably those to food, medication, and chemical sensitivities.

How long must the injections go on? It is not always clear when to stop the shots, but most allergists agree that after 5 years of treatment, a trial off the injection schedule may be reasonable. Your allergist can advise you whether this kind of therapy might benefit you and, if so, how long it should be given.

Allergic Disorders

❖ ATOPIC DERMATITIS (ALLERGIC ECZEMA)

Symptoms *(What you may experience)* Red, itchy, weeping, or leathery rash on the face, neck, behind the ears, hands, the bend of the elbows, or behind the knees. (See page C-29.)

Signs and laboratory findings *(What the doctor looks for)* History of hay fever or childhood-onset asthma; family history of the same allergies; allergic sensitivity to foods, dust, or other allergens demonstrated by allergen tests.

What is it? Atopic dermatitis is a common inflammatory skin disorder that is characterized by a red, itchy, scaly rash that can cause considerable discomfort. Atopic refers to a hereditary tendency to develop allergic reactions due to IgE (allergic) antibodies. In the case of atopic dermatitis, the allergic reaction takes place in the skin. Atopic dermatitis may first begin in infancy or early childhood and often remits during adolescence, only to recur in a milder form after age 20. The rash develops because of an inflammation of the top layer of the skin that appears as rough red patches. In children the patches may appear in what has been described as a monk's cowl distribution that involves the face, neck, upper chest, and shoulders. Other areas typically involved include the bends of the elbows and knees, behind the ears, and on the wrists and the hands. Repeated eruptions over time leave the skin thickened, dry, and leathery. In blacks, the chronic rashes may cause patchy loss of skin pigment in these areas.

Allergy to foods may be a cause of atopic dermatitis in as many as 30 percent of cases. In children in particular, identifying and avoiding foods that cause atopic dermatitis may bring major relief. Milk, eggs, and wheat—including both flour and other products made from wheat—are common offenders. And since animal danders can be a possible cause of atopic dermatitis, if you have a furred pet at home you may need to ask the allergist to check for allergy to pet dander.

What you can do The most effective way for you to deal with atopic dermatitis is to scrupulously avoid known triggers. You can relieve itching with over-the-counter antihistamines, such as diphenhydramine (Benadryl) or clemastine (Tavist). Topical application of over-the-counter corticosteroid creams may help, although adequate therapy may require higher potency prescription-strength formulations. To relieve itching and stop weeping of rashes, apply astringent soak solutions such as Domeboro tablets dissolved in 2 cups of water, or bathe in a colloidal oatmeal soap such as Aveeno.

When the rash is dry and scaly, bathe in warm (not hot) water, use a moisturizing soap such as Dove, Aveeno, Basis, Alpha Keri, or Purpose, and avoid irritating the skin with washcloths, loofah pads, or brushes. Gently pat the skin dry with a soft cotton towel and immediately apply an emollient lotion such as Alpha Keri, Nivea, Vaseline, Aquaphor, Eucerin, or Derma-Sil. For the most effective relief of your symptoms, apply emollient lotions or over-the-counter corticosteroid ointments, such as hydrocortisone 0.5 percent, after bathing at bedtime. Cover the affected areas (excluding the face or neck) overnight by wrapping them with plastic wrap and then securing the wrap with tape. This method both prevents the medication from being rubbed off and allows it to penetrate the thickened, scaly areas. Do not wrap so tightly that you cut off circulation.

Avoid wearing scratchy fabrics such as wool and acrylic, and when possible use natural fibers, such as 100 percent cotton or silk, next to the skin.

When to call the doctor Seek medical help for skin infections that are painful, with evidence of pus and fever, or if a rash is persistent or worsening.

Treatment Moderate to high potency prescription corticosteroid, or steroid lotions, creams, or ointments are the most effective method of dermatitis control when skin care and topical emollients fail; the more severe the dermatitis, the stronger the steroid cream required. Lower to moderate strength preparations should be used to treat children. These treatments should not be used continuously because they can cause abnormal skin thinning and pigment changes with long-term use. The frequency of application of higher potency formulations should be tapered over several weeks to avoid rebound recurrence of the rash and itching.

In hard-to-treat, thick, scaly patches that do not respond to potent steroid creams, preparations containing coal tar (5 percent in Aquaphor or Fototar cream) may help. Occasionally, none of these therapies applied to the skin will be sufficient to alleviate the chronic itchy rashes. In these instances, relief of symptoms may require taking systemic steroid medication orally.

Prognosis Atopic dermatitis waxes and wanes. It is at its worst in infancy (less than 2 years old), often remits in adolescence, and can recur in adulthood. Lasting remission occurs in about one-half the cases.

❖ PLANT DERMATOSES (POISON IVY, OAK, AND SUMAC)

Symptoms *(What you may experience)* Red, intensely itchy, slightly swollen rash (in patches or often lines) that develops into blisters that weep and finally crust and peel. (See page C-28.)

Signs and laborating findings *(What the doctor looks for)* A rash in a distribution that is consistent with plant contact; known sensitivity to ivy or oak; a history of physical contact with these plants.

What is it? Exposure to the oils of certain plants—such as poison ivy, oak, or sumac—causes an intensely itchy type of contact dermatitis in people who are sensitive to these plant oils. These plants belong to the family Toxicodendron and account for the vast majority of plant-related rashes in the

United States. They share a toxic sap resin called urushiol, which is a strong allergen that will sensitize 70 percent of people who are exposed to it. The plants contain the resin from one end to the other—in the leaves, stems, seeds, flowers, berries, and roots—so that no part of the plant is safe to touch for a sensitive person. The rash spreads only by contact with the plant oils; contrary to popular myths, the fluid from skin blisters cannot spread the rash.

Sensitization can occur from contact with bruised stems or leaves of the plant, from the smoke of the dried vines when they are burned, or from subsequent contact with clothing, pet fur, tools, or other equipment that may have the plant resin on it.

The ivy, oak, or sumac rash begins as red, itchy, slightly swollen patches or lines on areas of skin that came in direct contact with the plant oils by some means. The severity of the outbreak depends on both the degree of

Direct skin contact with a wide variety of plants, medications, chemicals, cosmetics, or metals can cause an allergic skin reaction known as contact dermatitis. Poisonous plants such as ivy, oak, and sumac are common causes. The itching, burning, blistering, and redness are caused by an allergic response to oil in the leaves.

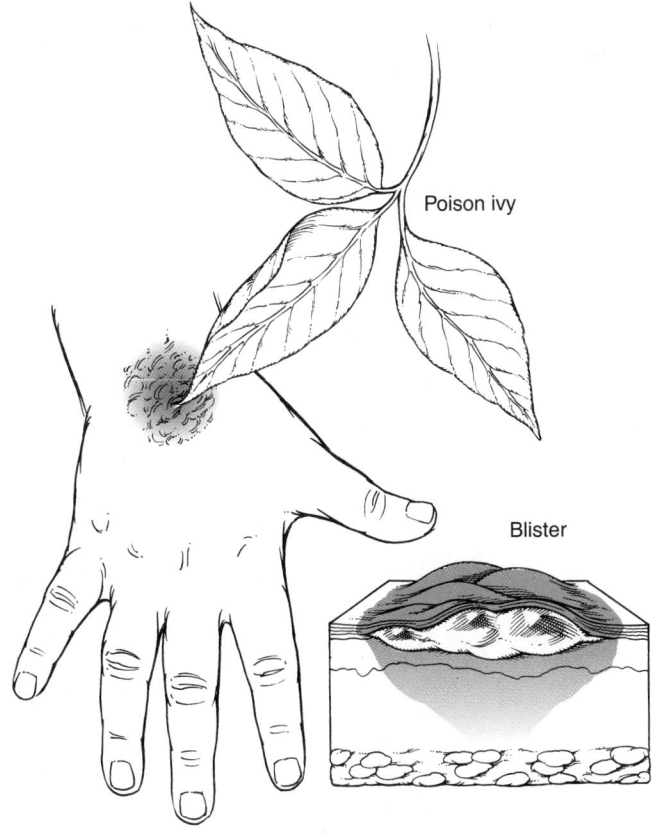

Poison ivy

Blister

OTHER CAUSES OF ALLERGIC CONTACT DERMATITIS

Although most people are aware of poison ivy and oak as causes of blistering rashes, many other substances can have the same effect. Typical among them are metals (nickel, in particular), cosmetics, chemicals, dyes, the tanning agent in leather (which may cause allergies to shoes, for example), the sizing chemicals in fabrics, perfumes, and the ingredients in topical creams and ointments.

Although a contact rash looks the same no matter what triggered it—red, itchy, swollen areas that blister, weep, and crust—the location of the rash gives clues to what may have caused it. A pattern behind the ears, on the sides of the neck, the pulse points on the wrist and bend of the elbow suggests an allergy to perfume. An outbreak encircling the neck or wrist suggest allergy to metals in jewelry. Rashes on the hands suggests allergy to cleaning solutions or food substances. With common sense and a little detective work, it is possible in most instances to track down probable causes of the problem. Once a list of reasonable suspects is made, an allergist or dermatologist can use patch testing to further narrow the field. In a patch test, the allergist or dermatologist tapes small cotton pads containing test amounts of suspected allergens onto the skin of the back. After 48 hours the pads are removed and the degree of reaction to each allergen is noted. Identifying an allergen allows you to avoid it and prevent the contact rash from recurring. Following is a list of some substances that commonly cause sensitivities.

- Adhesives
- Cleansers
- Clothing (rabbit hair, elastic waistbands)
- Cosmetics
- Detergents
- Dyes (hair, leather, cloth)
- Fragrances
- Leather (tanning agents)
- Ointments or creams containing medication such as neomycin or bacitracin
- Metal jewelry
- Paints or varnishes
- Preservatives such as formaldehyde that are used in sunscreens, antifungals, over-the-counter steroids, and other lotions
- Rubber products (latex, elastic bands in clothing, shoes, gloves)
- Shampoo
- Shoes (containing leather tanning agents or rubber chemicals)
- Soaps
- Sunscreen
- Toothpaste

What is a Photosensitive Reaction?

In some cases of contact or allergic dermatitis, the offending substance alone is not sufficient to cause the skin reaction but instead it acts as a photosensitizer—a substance that causes a rash only after subsequent exposure to sunlight. The pattern of the rash gives the strongest clue to its photosensitive origin—it will appear only in areas of skin exposed to the sun, typically the face, neck, backs of the hands, and lower arms. Areas that are covered by clothing will not be affected. Common topical photosensitizers include perfumes, colognes, or aftershave lotions containing oil of bergamot or synthetic fragrances such as musk ambrette; many soaps, cosmetics, detergents, and sunscreens containing derivatives of warfarin sodium (a blood-thinning medication); certain fruits and vegetables, particularly limes, celery, parsley, figs, and parsnips that contain a component of certain plants collectively known as psoralens. A number of oral medications can also act as photosensitizers including tetracycline, doxycycline, and trimethoprim-sulfamethoxazole, all of which are commonly prescribed antibiotics. ∎

sensitivity of the person exposed and the amount of plant oil that touched them. The rash develops into blisters usually within 2 days of plant exposure, although this reaction may occur as quickly as 6 hours or as long as 2 weeks afterward. The rash may appear sooner in some areas than others and may appear different depending on location; areas where skin is thin—the eyelids, for example—may swell dramatically.

These weepy rashes can easily become infected with bacteria if scratching breaks the skin, but severe complications from this type of allergic rash seldom occur unless a critical organ, such as the eye, becomes involved.

What you can do Avoid these plants! You can learn to spot the plants in the wild, and you can become very familiar with their appearance in all seasons, (see illustrations on pages 1335 and C-28).

For mild plant dermatitis, topical application of over-the-counter corticosteroid creams may help, but adequate therapy for more severe cases may require higher potency prescription-strength formulations or even oral steroids. To relieve itching and stop weeping of rashes, apply astringent soak solutions such as Domeboro tablets dissolved in 2 cups of water or bathe in a colloidal oatmeal soap, such as Aveeno.

When to call the doctor If the methods of self-care given on page 1336 fail to relieve the itching and weeping from the rash, if the rash involves the eyes or extensive body surface, if the rash begins to weep cloudy or discolored fluid, if you develop fever, or if you feel generally ill from the rash, contact your doctor as soon as possible.

Avoid topical creams or ointments that contain anesthetic agents such as lidocaine or benzocaine to relieve itching. These topical formulations, when applied to open skin, can themselves cause allergic sensitization and worsen the rash.

Treatment If over-the-counter creams containing cortisone products and drying solutions (such as Domeboro's Soak Solution) have not relieved the symptoms, the doctor may prescribe a short, tapering course of high-potency prescription topical steroid cream or ointment or administer these potent antiallergy medications by mouth. Studies have also shown reduction of sensitivity by the administration of ivy or oak resin in progressively stronger doses by mouth over a period of 4 months, although this treatment has not gained general acceptance. Side effects from this treatment limit its use.

Prognosis Although the allergic reaction will repeatedly recur with exposure to the plant, it responds well to treatment and rarely causes severe complications.

❖ ALLERGIC RHINITIS (THE ALLERGIC NOSE)

Symptoms *(What you may experience)* Sneezing; clear, thin nasal secretions; itching of the nose; red, watery or itchy eyes.

Signs and laboratory findings *(What the doctor looks for)* Swollen pale mucous membranes in the nose; clear, watery nasal secretions; dark circles under the eyes; mouth breathing; retraction of the ear drum; or demonstration of specific allergic response to common airborne allergens on skin or blood testing.

What is it? When an allergen—most commonly pollen but also dander, mold, dust mites, and a host of other offending airborne substances—land on the moist lining of the nose or the eyes, a chain reaction begins in sensitive people (see page 1329). The reaction culminates in the release of histamine and other substances that cause the tissue lining the nose or eyes to swell, promotes secretion of mucus, causes itching and irritation that results in sneezing, and even stimulates constriction of the breathing passages in the lung, which can lead to wheezing and chest tightness.

Discovering the cause of allergic rhinitis may require enlisting the aid of an allergist who can perform and interpret specific tests for a wide range of airborne allergens. Collecting a few clues can help the search. For example, do the symptoms occur seasonally—that is, for 2 or 3 weeks in the spring or the fall? Do the symptoms occur only when you mow the yard or garden? These patterns would suggest pollen allergies or hay fever (seasonal allergic rhinitis). Do the symptoms occur only for a week or two at the change of seasons? That might indicate airborne allergens from the cooling or heating system. Do the symptoms always seem to occur with exposure to a pet or only in homes where pets live? This pattern suggests a cat or dog allergy. Are the nose and eye symptoms worse in the morning than later in the day? That pattern may suggest bedroom allergens such as dust mites as the culprits. Finding the causes will be of great help in alleviating the symptoms, because avoidance of allergen triggers offers the most effective therapy.

What you can do If possible, you should avoid known or suspected triggering substances. If you suspect dust or dust mites as triggers, dust proof the bedroom (see page 1339). If you have pollen and dust allergies, wear a filtration mask and safety goggles (available at most large home improvement or hardware stores) when you mow, weed, or clean to reduce the level of allergens entering the nose or eyes.

Over-the-counter antihistamines such as diphenhydramine or clemastine can offer some relief of the sneezing, drippy nose, postnasal drip, and itchy or watery eyes. Nasal stuffiness that makes nose breathing difficult may respond better to medications that combine antihistamines with decongestants. Most over-the-counter forms contain the decongestant pseudoephedrine in combination with the antihistamines chlorpheniramine, diphenhydramine, or clemastine.

Warm salt water gargles (1 to 2 tsp table salt dissolved in 8 oz warm water) may relieve a mild sore throat from postnasal drip.

When to call the doctor If the symptoms of allergic rhinitis fail to respond to over-the-counter remedies and avoidance measures, it is time to contact your doctor. The development of more than a low-grade fever, a nasal discharge that becomes discolored, thick, or bloody, a persistent sore throat, or a throbbing earache could indicate that a bacterial infection has begun in the sinuses, throat, or middle ear. If you experience any of these symptoms you should call your doctor right away.

Treatment Identification and elimination of the suspected allergen offers the most benefit to allergy sufferers. Sometimes, however, elimination is not possible—a beloved pet, for example, is not likely to be eliminated from the household, and no one can totally avoid pollen and still live a reasonably normal life. In these instances, there are two treatment options. The first order of business after allergy testing to determine specific triggers will be to attempt to relieve symptoms by interrupting the chain of events that leads to the release of the histamine in the first place. Several medications may help: steroid nasal sprays such as Beconase, Vancenase, Nasacort, or Flonase, a cromolyn sodium spray such as Intal, or the newer nedocromil spray called Tilade. The steroid sprays may take a few days of regular use to control the symptoms, but once the sprays reach an effective level they work quite well and offer the advantage of not causing drowsiness (like many antihistamines) or overstimulation (as do many decongestants) (see page 1333). Cromolyn sodium and nedocromil sprays offer the same benefits. In addition, these preparations can even be used as preventive sprays if you can anticipate your exposure to the trigger.

THE DANGER OF DECONGESTANT NASAL SPRAY ABUSE AND HOW TO KICK THE HABIT

Although many more serious allergic symptoms exist, none is more aggravating than the allergic nose—the chronically plugged up, swollen nasal passages that leave many allergy sufferers longing for just a few clear, deep, unobstructed breaths through their noses. That longing leads many people with chronically stuffy noses to use decongestant nasal sprays for the immediate relief they can provide. That relief is not without consequence, however.

Decongestant nasal sprays constrict the blood vessels in the swollen tissues inside the nose, and they quickly—but temporarily—open a larger passage for the free flow of air. Unfortunately when the blood-vessel-constricting effect of a decongestant spray wears off, a rebound blood vessel dilation follows that swells the passages to their previous state, and sometimes they may swell to an even greater degree. The natural inclination is to spray again to reopen the passages, but, again, a rebound swelling will follow. Too frequent application of these decongestant sprays can lead to rebound swelling that produces nearly constant congestion. The abuse of decongestant sprays can become so extreme that some people may stash bottles of nasal spray in their pockets or purses, glove compartments, desk drawers, kitchen cabinets, bathroom shelves, bedside tables—in short, anywhere they might be in order to always have one nearby.

The consequence of this degree of nasal spray abuse can be far greater than rebound nasal congestion because overuse of decongestant medication can increase the heart rate and elevate the blood pressure. The sprays, which are designed for topical application to the nasal lining, can be absorbed into the body through the many blood vessels that fill the nose. With frequent use, the level of decongestant in the blood climbs, sometimes to dangerous levels.

Because the rebound nasal congestion that attends spray abuse causes such misery, a nasal spray habit can be difficult—but not impossible—to break. Although you may need to enlist the aid of your doctor here are some tips that may help.

How to Kick the Nasal Spray Habit

1. Discard all stashed bottles of decongestant nasal spray.

2. Substitute a nonmedicated salt water nose spray to moisturize and soothe the nasal lining. Since it contains no medication, you cannot overuse this kind of spray.

3. Purchase an over-the-counter decongestant medication such as pseudoephedrine, preferably long-acting (8 to 12 hours) in tablet or capsule form, and take it by mouth according to manufacturer's directions for a week, then taper off to discontinue it over the second week.

4. If significant congestion is intolerable during the first days of your effort to kick the nasal spray habit, enlist the aid of your doctor, who may prescribe a short course of oral steroids or a nasal steriod spray.

5. In the future, select nonmedicated nasal sprays and decongestant medication that can be taken by mouth. If a decongestant spray is needed, use the spray in only one nostril at a time, no more than manufacturer's suggested frequency, and for no longer than 2 or 3 days. ■

CREATING A DUST-FREE ROOM

Because of the number of hours we sleep, we spend more time in the bedroom than any other room in the house; children and teenagers tend to spend even more time there. For children and adults who suffer from dust and dust mite allergies, creating a relatively dust-free environment in the bedroom will help to relieve symptoms.

House dust is not dirt that comes in from the outdoors; rather it is produced indoors in the breakdown of plant and animal materials in the home. These include fibers from furniture, carpets, and pillows as well as animal dander, molds, and dust mites. It is possible to be allergic to one or many of the components of house dust although for many people, it is the waste products of dust mites—microscopic creatures that live chiefly in pillows, mattresses, carpets, and upholstery and feed off shed scales from human skin—that are most problematic. Here are several tips to help reduce dust and dust mites to the lowest possible level.

1. Keep the bedroom uncluttered; smooth, easily-cleaned surfaces can help in the control of dust. Objects on which dust can gather—including all clothing, small appliances, children's stuffed toys, and knickknacks—should be kept in closed drawers or closets.

2. Encase pillows, mattresses and box springs in airtight, allergen-impermeable covers. Your allergist can recommend sources for commercial products such as mattress covers that help with allergy control.

3. Wash all bedding weekly in hot (130°F) water. If the water is not hot, the dust mites will not be killed. Avoid using down or wool blankets, which are great reservoirs for dust.

4. Use hardwood, vinyl, or tile floor covering instead of carpeting, where feasible. Carpeting laid over concrete may have particularly high levels of dust mites.

5. Avoid heavy curtains; use pull-down shades or wooden shutters instead. If curtains are used, wash them frequently. Avoid fabric wall-hangings or other dust-collectors. For children, select toys for sleeping that are the least fuzzy possible, or wash stuffed animals weekly.

6. Cleaning and vacuuming is essential, but it is preferable that the individual with allergies does not do the cleaning. If you must do the cleaning yourself, wear a well-fitting face mask. Vacuums with high-efficiency particulate-arresting (HEPA) filters are very effective in preventing dust from becoming airborne during cleaning. Be sure to vacuum all upholstered furniture.

7. Dust mites and molds thrive in high humidity. Keep your indoor humidity levels below 50 percent but above 30 percent, if possible. Air-conditioning will help in summer. Avoid window fans that pull outside allergens, such as pollen, into the house. ■

For example, if you are allergic to cat dander and will be visiting a relative with a cat, pretreatment an hour or two before the visit, during it, and for a day or two afterward may prevent your symptoms. For prolonged seasons or moderate to severe symptoms, your doctor may recommend a course of allergen injections to reduce your sensitivity to the triggering substances (see page 1332).

Prognosis Although allergic rhinitis is a chronic condition, it is usually more a nuisance than a serious risk to well-being. And with the identification of allergens, avoidance or elimination of them, modern antiallergy medication, or allergen injection treatments, the prognosis for good control of this condition is excellent.

❖ INSECT STING ALLERGIC REACTIONS

Symptoms *(What you may experience)* Swelling of the lips, face, or hands; the development of hives; difficulty swallowing or breathing; fainting, usually occurring within minutes of the sting.

Signs and laboratory findings *(What the doctor looks for)* Prior sting history is relevant as it may reveal the likely insect; demonstration of sensitivity to insect venom on allergy testing.

What is it? The venom of a number of insect species contains protein components called allergens that stimulate allergic sensitization. When these allergens enter the skin through the stinger of the insect, they bind to specialized immune molecules, or IgE antibodies, on tissue mast cells. The binding of antibodies by allergen sets off a chain reaction of events that culminates in the release of histamine and other substances that cause swelling of the tissues, dilation of the blood vessels, and the development of hives. In cases of severe allergy the chain reaction becomes widespread and causes the development of symptoms throughout the body that are far removed from the site of the sting—the serious condition called anaphylaxis (see page 1341).

Nonfatal bee sting reactions occur in 8 of every 1,000 bee stings, with 40 deaths

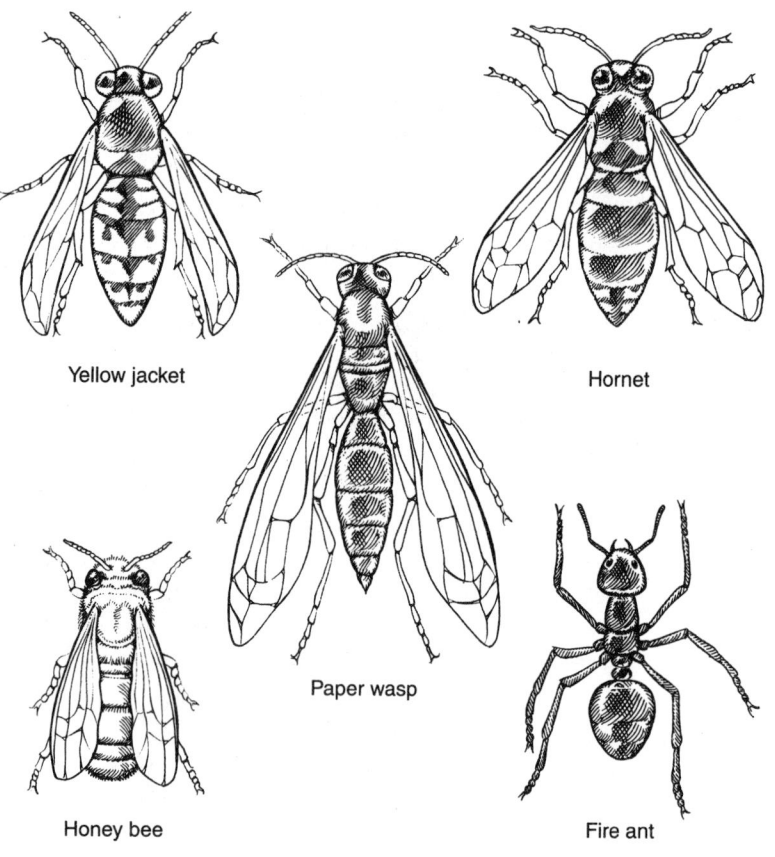

Yellow jacket

Hornet

Paper wasp

Honey bee

Fire ant

Stinging insects such as bees, wasps, hornets, yellow jackets, and fire ants can cause a severe allergic reaction in a person who has been sensitized by a previous sting.

occurring annually in the United States each year.

Common offending insects include: honeybees, wasps, yellow jackets, hornets, and fire ants.

What you can do A person known to be allergic to insect stings should wear no perfume or perfumed cosmetics, soaps, hair sprays, or toiletries that might attract insects and should wear neutral-colored clothing to avoid mimicking the bright colors of flowers. People who are known to be allergic to insect stings should never walk barefoot outdoors because bees love clover, and yellow jackets and hornets may build their nests in the ground. Always look before you sit and lean back in outdoor settings.

After an insect sting you should remove the stinger as quickly as possible. Studies have shown that the more quickly the stinger is removed, the less severe the reaction. Apply cold compresses to the area and take antihistamines such as diphenhydramine or clemastine. Every person who is allergic to insects should have a bee sting kit available (see below).

When to call the doctor Any exaggerated response to a sting should prompt a visit to the doctor right away. Severe reactions demand immediate (within minutes) treatment to prevent a possible fatal reaction and immediate transport to the closest hospital.

Treatment The mainstays of treatment for severe insect sting reactions include epinephrine and antihistamines and sometimes the administration of intravenous fluids (see below). Some reactions may require a short course of oral or injected steroid medication. For adults, the allergist will usually recommend allergen injection treatments to prevent severe reactions to insect stings that may occur in the future.

INJECTABLE EPINEPHRINE— A LIFESAVER

Although bee sting allergy is perhaps the most common reason to carry injectable epinephrine for emergency use, anyone with severe allergic reactions to foods or idiopathic anaphylaxis should also have one. Your doctor or allergist will need to write a prescription for injectable epinephrine for you. One such device is sold under the name EpiPen (or Epi-Pen Jr. for children); it provides a premeasured dose of the proper dilution of epinephrine in a spring-loaded single use syringe that requires no measuring of doses, handling of needles, or special expertise. Simply remove the cap, hold the pen in your fist, and hit it against your thigh with a quick firm blow, even through light clothing if necessary. The spring mechanism injects the dose of medication for you. This means that even the allergy victim can administer the dose to himself. Some injectable epinephrine kits also contain a capsule of diphenhydramine (or some other antihistamine), which can be taken to quell hives and itching. The dose of epinephrine should last about 15 minutes, which will give you time to call 911 for help or to proceed with assistance to an emergency facility.

Keep a fresh device at home, at work, and with you in the car or on vacation. If your travel distance is greater than 15 to 20 minutes from civilization (if you are camping or backpacking, for example), you should probably take several doses of epinephrine along. The medication will expire and you must replace it regularly to keep it fresh, but having it ready may one day mean the difference between life and death. ■

ANAPHYLAXIS—A LIFE-THREATENING REACTION

The most serious of all allergic reactions—anaphylaxis—can begin within seconds of exposure to an allergen and if not immediately and appropriately treated can prove fatal in a matter of minutes. Although the symptoms may vary, they may include widespread red flushing and itching of the skin, the eruption of hives, swelling of the lips and eyelids, tightening of the throat, sudden hoarseness, nausea, vomiting, and abdominal pain. The disorder may progress to constriction of the breathing passages with wheezing and extreme dilation of blood vessels throughout the body that causes the blood pressure to drop dangerously low. Death can occur from extreme swelling of the throat that blocks the breathing passages, from severe bronchospasm, or from loss of blood pressure, also called anaphylactic shock.

Allergens that have been identified as common causes of anaphylaxis include such diverse substances as extracts of inhalant allergens administered in allergen injection treatments, insect venom, latex from surgical gloves and other rubber products, many foods (especially peanuts, eggs, seafood, nuts, and seeds), cottonseed oil, certain hormones and vaccines, some antibiotics (especially penicillin and the related cephalosporins), and other medications such as protamine insulin and anesthetic medications.

Symptoms may appear very suddenly upon exposure to the triggering allergen and survival may depend on the immediate administration of an injection of epinephrine (for adults and children over 12 years old) that is repeated every 15 to 20 minutes.

Because there may not even be enough time for emergency help to arrive, all people who are highly allergic to unavoidable allergens, such as insect stings or some foods, or people who have spontaneous anaphylaxis of unknown cause—a condition called idiopathic anaphylaxis—should have a preloaded syringe

Anaphylaxis is a severe allergic response that can be deadly. An anaphylaxis kit is important to have if you have suffered a severe allergic reaction to an insect sting or ingested food or medication that may be difficult to avoid. This kit contains instructions, epinephrine, alcohol pads, antihistamine pills, and a tourniquet. Instructions should be read at the time of buying the kit. Kits should be replaced after the expiration date.

of epinephrine available for self-administration in the event of a severe allergic response (see page 1340). Administer the epinephrine dose immediately and go to an emergency medical facility right away; the injection may mean the difference between life and death and it will give you enough time to get help. ■

Prognosis Most large topical reactions are not followed by more severe systemic reactions. Severe reactions, treated promptly and appropriately, also carry an excellent prognosis for full recovery; however, delay of treatment of anaphylaxis can be fatal in a few minutes. Allergen injection treatment are 99 percent effective in preventing reactions to single stings.

❖ MEDICATION ALLERGIES

Symptoms *(What you may experience)* Variable (one or all may develop): rash, hives, itching, tissue swelling, joint aches or swelling, tender lymph glands, and fever.

Emergency symptoms Swelling of the lips, eyelids, tongue, throat; sudden hoarseness; difficulty breathing; fainting (see Anaphylaxis: A Life-Threatening Reaction, above).

Signs and laboratory findings *(What the doctor looks for)* Skin rashes, low blood pressure, rapid heart beat, swelling of the larynx (visible only with a laryngoscope); skin or blood tests demonstrating specific antibodies against the suspected medication.

What is it? Although unpleasant reactions to medication occur quite commonly, true allergic reactions account for fewer than 10 percent of them (see page 1343). By their very nature, medications of all types are substances foreign to the body and therefore could induce an allergic antibody, or IgE, response, which sensitizes the individual for a subsequent allergic reaction (see page 1329). In most instances, however, the allergic antibodies stimulate no response because, in general, the small size of the drugs allows them to escape detection by the immune system. Some allergenic medications may attach to larger protein molecules (the body's own proteins) in the bloodstream, creating a protein-medication complex large enough to attract the attention of the immune system. Once the immune system has been sensitized to the medication, an allergic reaction may occur. Therein lies the root of one of the basic truths of allergic reactions—you cannot be allergic to something to which you have never been exposed. True allergy requires an initial exposure, sensitization, and subsequent re-exposure for a reaction to occur.

Of all the many medications currently on the market, the antibiotic penicillin not only accounts for more allergic reactions than any other (occurring in 1 to 5 out of every 100 people who receive it), but penicillins also account for a majority of the 300 fatal allergic reactions to medication that occur annually in the United States.

Sometimes medication allergy develops within a few minutes of taking a trigger medication, often as hives, but occasionally as the more severe form of immediate allergic reaction, anaphylaxis (see page 1341). But in most cases, the reaction develops more insidiously, occurring between 6 days and 2 weeks after beginning a medication. These late-appearing allergic medication reactions may make their appearance in a variety of ways: as itching or a rash, painful or swollen joints, swollen or tender lymph glands, fever, or vague flu-like symptoms. The symptoms can be mild or severe, but in either event they usually disappear within several days to a week after discontinuing the medication.

What you can do Know the specifics of your medication allergy history—know the names of the medication you cannot take as well as the names of medication in the same family that might also cause a reaction. Keep this information written down and in your wallet at all times.

If you react to a medication and it is a mild reaction, it may require only symptomatic treatment such as an antihistamine to stop itching, cool baths for a rash, or mild pain medication such as ibuprofen or acetaminophen for joint or body aches.

If you have responded with anaphylaxis to one type of medication, it is possible to do so to others in the same chemical family. If you have had a life-threatening response

to a medication, you should wear a medical identification bracelet that names the medication and reaction.

Medications commonly found to trigger allergic reactions include the following types:

- Antibiotics (penicillins, cephalosporins, sulfonamides)
- Antituberculous medications
- Diuretics (thiazides, diazoxide)
- Diabetic medications (sulfonylureas, insulin)
- Medications for ulcerative colitis (sulfasalazine)
- Hormones and organ extracts (adrenocorticotropic hormone, whole thyroid, insulin)
- Seizure medications
- Barbiturate general anesthetic agents (thiopental)
- Muscle relaxants (those used for general anesthesia, for example, curare)
- Heart rhythm medication (quinidine)
- Enzymes (chymopapain, asparaginase)
- Vaccines and foreign antitoxins (horse serum)
- Anticancer medications (cisplatin)

Although these are the common offenders, remember that any medication can cause an allergic reaction in a sensitized person.

When to call the doctor A reaction that causes any of the emergency symptoms listed on page 1341 should prompt you to seek immediate emergency medical care. A less severe reaction at least warrants a call to the doctor to discuss the reaction, to see if other treatment is needed, and to be certain it gets recorded in your medical record.

Treatment The first principle of therapy is to stop the suspected offending medication. Antihistamines may reduce the itching from a rash or other mild allergic symptoms. Occasionally steroid medications such as prednisone may be necessary to control the allergic response. Although in most cases it is possible to avoid the medication that is causing your allergic reaction, occasionally no other medication will work to treat a particular condition. In

TELLING A MEDICATION ALLERGY FROM A SIDE EFFECT

Medications can sometimes cause unpleasant, unwanted effects above and beyond their intended ones. Although people may describe themselves as being allergic to the medication they are taking, most of the problems people experience with medications are not true allergies. In fact, allergy to medication accounts for less than 10 percent of the adverse reactions. The remainder of the problems fall into the category of side effects or idiosyncratic reactions (an unusual response that is peculiar to that person) to a medication.

For example, hives are a common side effect some people may suffer when taking narcotic pain relievers like codeine, but it is not an allergy. Certainly hives are unpleasant, and perhaps sufficiently so that you would not wish to take the medication again, but codeine does not stimulate the immune defense system to produce antibodies against codeine, so the hives and itching are not due to true allergy. On the other hand, hives that are the result of taking penicillin, which may be equally unpleasant, are not just a side effect; they are a true allergic reaction complete with specific antipenicillin antibodies that are detectable in the bloodstream or on a skin test. And because an allergy to penicillin is a true acute allergy, it carries the risk of developing a life-threatening reaction (see page 1341).

Some idiosyncratic medication reactions, such as developing hives after codeine or other narcotics, are called pseudoallergic reactions because they produce symptoms that mimic allergic reactions. Unlike true allergic responses, pseudoallergic responses can occur the first time you are exposed to a medications. For example, some people who take aspirin or other nonsteroidal anti-inflammatory drugs experience hives or worsening of asthma that resemble allergic reactions. It is unclear what causes these reactions, but those who experience them should not only avoid the offending medications but sometimes related medications as well. Your doctor can advise you about which medications can be effective and safe substitutes.

Although it may be difficult to tell the difference between an allergic reaction, a side effect, and an idiosynaratic reaction, here are some tips.

• An allergic reaction to a medication never occurs on the first exposure to it, but it can occur even with small amounts of the medication at any subsequent exposure. The reaction to a particular medication will usually be of the same type in every instance be it a rash, itching, abdominal complaint, or respiratory symptom, however, the severity of the symptoms may vary.

• A side effect is an undesirable but known action of a medication that is most often uncovered during clinical testing of the drug. Whether or not the side effect occurs often depends on the strength of the dose; the larger the dose, the more likely it will be to cause a side effect. That means that—unlike allergy—you may not experience the unpleasant effect at a lower dose.

• An idiosyncratic reaction, unlike allergy, can occur on first exposure to the medication, and unlike a side effect, the reaction occurs only in susceptible individuals, presumably due to a genetic or metabolic abnormality. ■

---

these instances, a qualified allergist can devise a regimen to desensitize you to the triggering medication, thus making its use possible again. For the safety of the individual, this is usually done in a hospital inpatient unit.

Treatment of anaphylaxis requires immediate treatment with epinephrine; antihistamines and steroids may be used as well. In most cases hospitalization, intravenous fluids, oxygen, and steroids and supportive care will be necessary until the reaction subsides.

Prognosis Until proven otherwise, once allergic, always allergic. However, 80 percent of people with penicillin allergy will lose their allergy over 2 to 4 years and can take the medication safely thereafter. A pair of skin tests can usefully evaluate penicillin allergy. For most episodes of medication allergy, although the symptoms may be uncomfortable, the reaction usually lasts only a short time and resolves completely without consequence.

❖ FOOD ALLERGIES

Symptoms (*What you may experience*) Swelling or itching of the lips or mouth lining; nausea; cramping stomach pain; bloating; vomiting; diarrhea; gas; red, itchy skin rash or hives; drippy nose; wheezing.

Emergency symptoms Major swelling of the lips or throat; difficulty breathing; hives within minutes of eating the food (see page 1341).

Sign and laboratory findings (*What the doctor looks for*) Physical signs; a history of past exposures and reactions to similar foods; demonstration of specific antibodies to the suspected food on allergy blood or skin tests.

What is it? When food enters the intestinal tract, its foreign nature can sometimes attract the attention of the immune system, which mounts a response that culminates in

PEANUT ALLERGY IN CHILDREN

Peanuts are one of the leading causes of food-allergic reactions in the United States, and, more significantly, they are one of the leading causes of fatal and near-fatal food-induced anaphylactic reactions (see page 1341).

Although children commonly outgrow milk, egg, and soy allergies, they rarely outgrow peanut allergies. And unlike shellfish, the source of another lifelong and serious food allergy, peanuts can be difficult to avoid in the United States. The average American consumes 11 lbs of peanut products each year, and peanut products are often added to soups and desserts in a way that is hard to detect. Indeed, researchers believe that it is the ubiquity of peanut products and the fact that peanuts are introduced into children's diets so early (in the form of peanut butter, peanut butter crackers, and the like) that has contributed to the surprising upsurge in peanut allergies. For this reason doctors advise the exclusion of peanuts from the diets of children less than 3 years old who have a family history of food allergies or asthma or eczema.

In a country where peanut-butter-and-jelly sandwiches are a lunchroom staple, parents of a child with a severe peanut allergy face the difficult but essential task of preventing their child from eating, and in some cases, even coming in contact with, peanuts or peanut products. Affected individuals must avoid ground nuts, mixed nuts, artificial nuts, peanut butter, and peanut flour. Because peanuts can be a hidden ingredient in many prepared and packaged foods, you must check package labels carefully or ask chefs how food was prepared. Here is a list of some foods and food products that may contain this legume.

- African, Chinese, and Thai foods, notably egg rolls

- Baked pastries and cookies

- Ice cream, desserts, and garnishes

- Candy, particularly chocolate products, marzipan, and nougat; enriched cocoa

- Chili, brown gravies

- Hydrolyzed plant protein and hydrolyzed vegetable protein

Simply removing peanuts from a prepared dish will not remove the contaminating protein that causes the allergic reaction. Foods prepared using utensils that were used to make a food containing peanuts must be avoided. Many affected individuals can safely eat foods containing peanut oil but must avoid cold-pressed peanut oil.

Children and adults who have experienced severe allergic reactions should carry an injectable form of epinephrine (see page 1340). ■

the release of histamine and other chemicals that cause the symptoms of food allergy described on page 1329.

As is often the case with other allergies, determining which food causes the symptoms can sometimes prove difficult. We seldom eat one specific food; rather, we eat combinations of food, with additives, preservatives, or coloring agents that may confound the search for the offender. And to further confuse the issue, other factors may make the allergic response variable; for example, the amount of the food eaten, other foods eaten at the same time, how the food was prepared (cooked, dried, or raw), what parts of the food (skin, seeds) were eaten, the degree of freshness of the food, and whether eating the food was followed by rest or exercise.

What you can do The prevention of symptoms hinges on identifying the offending foods and avoiding them. The best first step in this determination involves keeping a detailed food and symptom diary in which you note the components of each meal and the timing of any symptoms that occur. This kind of record will also help the allergist if consultation becomes necessary. Even if you think you have discovered a trigger food, it can be both uncomfortable and dangerous to test your theory by attempting to provoke an allergic response with food on your own. ***Warning: You should never attempt to provoke allergy if your symptoms suggest anaphylaxis or are severe in nature.***

When to call the doctor The development or persistence of symptoms suggesting food allergy should prompt a visit to the doctor if you cannot determine the likely cause on your own or if the symptoms are severe enough to interfere with your daily activities. Symptoms suggesting anaphylaxis demand immediate emergency attention. If you discover a pattern tying a certain food to symptoms, you should next undertake an elimination trial under the guidance of an allergist. For a period of at least 3 weeks the allergist will require strict avoidance of the suspected food and anything that contains even small amounts of it. Then, under supervision, you will be given a meal or a capsule containing the food to see if symptoms recur.

Treatment Unlike respiratory allergies, food allergies are not treated with immunotherapy. Elimination of the offending food

IS IT FOOD INTOLERANCE OR ALLERGY?

Foods themselves and the additives, preservatives, or coloring agents used in them can sometimes cause unpleasant symptoms, but only 6 percent of the time are those symptoms the result of a true allergic response. Much more often the symptoms come about because of chemical intolerance to the food—that is, the body (chiefly the intestinal tract) reacts abnormally or simply is not able to handle the food or some component in it.

Two familiar examples of such an intolerance occur to wheat (actually the gluten of wheat, a gluelike component that holds pasta or dough together) and to dairy products (see Chapter 23). These two food-related disorders occur fairly commonly and cause considerable discomfort (such as bloating, diarrhea, abdominal cramping) to those who suffer them.

An intolerance to food can develop because of an unusually strong response to a druglike component in foods such as caffeine, alcohol, or other chemicals; from an inborn lack of the helper enzymes needed to process the food properly such as the lactose (milk sugar) in dairy products for lactose deficient people;

or in conjunction with other medical conditions such as gastritis, colitis, gallbladder disease, or peptic ulcers.

Symptoms of intolerance to caffeine or alcohol sometimes include gastrointestinal irritation but, particularly in the case of caffeine, these substances may cause disturbances in the heart rate or rhythm or a sense of nervousness or agitation.

A less common and more curious example of heightened sensitivity to a naturally occurring plant chemical involves solanine, which is found in members of the nightshade vegetable family that includes white potatoes, tomatoes, and peppers (except black pepper). In people sensitive to solanine, eating these foods can produce the symptoms of arthritis—joint tenderness, swelling, and even warmth to the touch that may mimic true inflammatory arthritis (see Chapter 17).

You and your doctor should identify foods that cause you problems because avoiding them offers the best hope of alleviating symptoms or preventing them in the first place. Eliminating the food for a substantial period (usually at least 3 weeks) and then reintroducing it in a controlled setting under the guidance of your doctor can help verify allergic or adverse responses to particular foods (see page 1330). ■

from the diet and medication to alleviate symptoms in the event of inadvertent consumption of the food are the cornerstone of therapy for food allergies.

Treatment for food allergy falls into two basic groups. Medication (the chief one being cromolyn sodium) can be used to blunt your allergic response to a food if it is taken before eating. Otherwise the appropriate treatment depends on the symptoms the food causes. For mild itching or rash, minor swelling of the lips or tongue, nasal drainage, or headache, antihistamines such as Benadryl, Tavist, Claritin, or Hismanal often provide relief. For abdominal cramping and bloating, nausea, or diarrhea, antispasmodic products such as hycosamine (Levsin, Anaspaz) will usually help.

The other course of treatment for food allergy is for people with known anaphylaxis to foods that are difficult to avoid such as peanuts and by-products. The doctor will usually recommend that you take a kit containing emergency epinephrine with you when you eat in restaurants or outside the home (see page 1340).

Prognosis Once you have developed an allergy to a certain food, you may or may not react to that food in the future. But if you work to identify the culprit and avoid it, and if you are prepared to deal with an accidental consumption of the food, the prognosis for remaining symptom free is excellent.

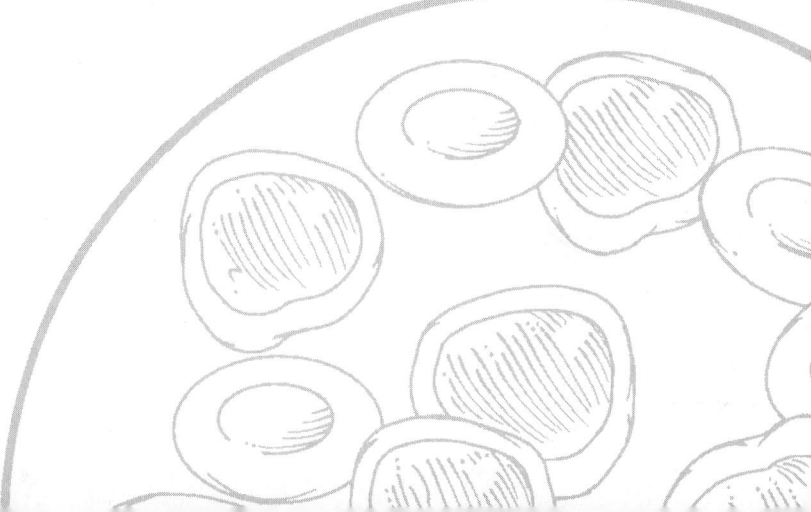

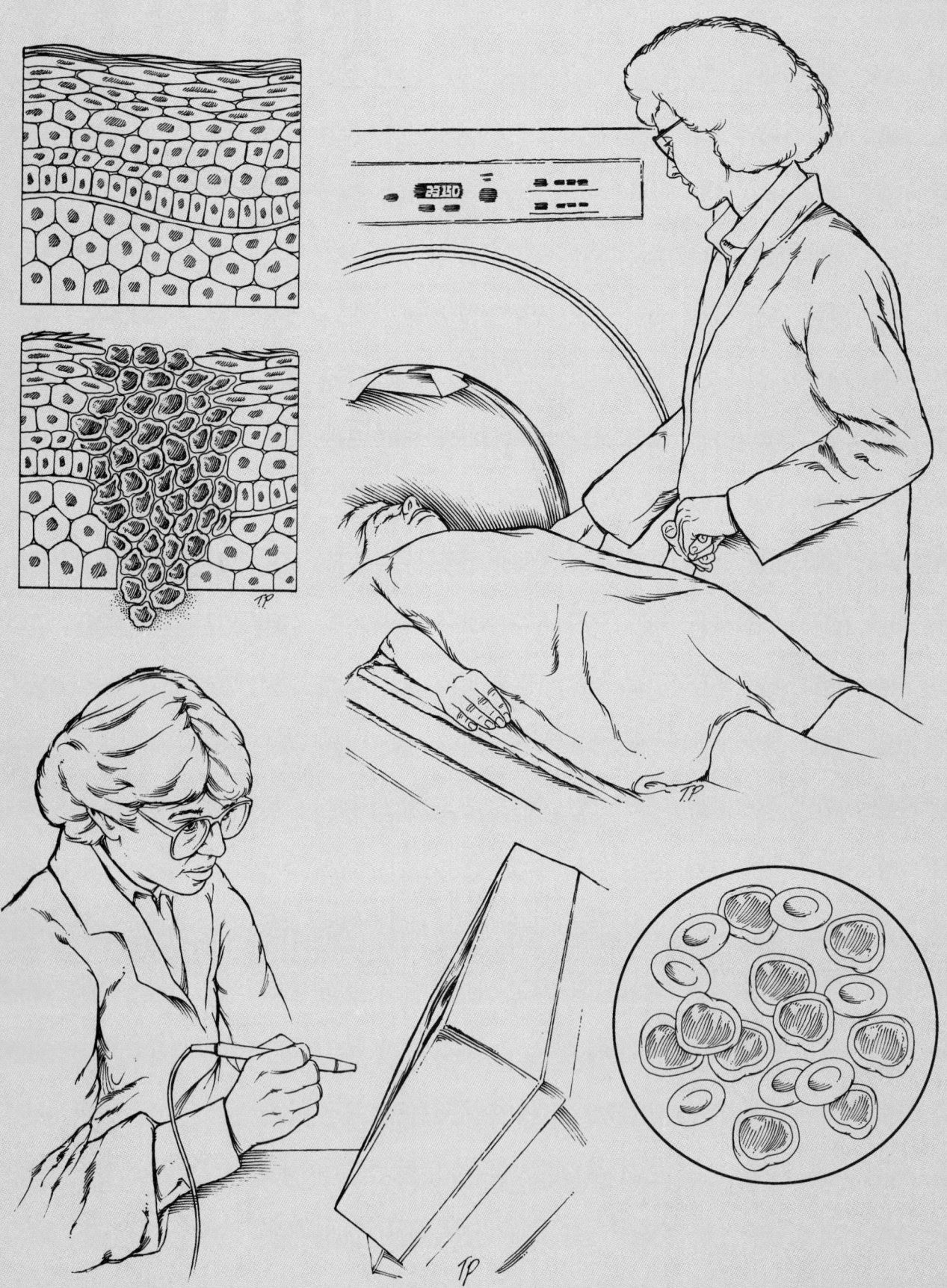

CANCER

Understanding Cancer

When we talk about cancer, we use a single word to refer to a number of diseases and stages of disease. In fact, there are over 100 different types of cancer. Information on a particular cancer can be found in the chapters in Part IV: Body Systems and Disorders; this chapter offers more general, yet vital, information on what cancer is and how and where it is treated, on the importance of regular screenings and early diagnosis, and on how to cope with the treatment of cancer. The aim of the chapter is to give you the information you need to get the right care and to manage your treatment effectively.

CARCINOGENESIS: THE BIOLOGY OF CANCER

The human body is composed of billions of cells. The following are the three main kinds of cells:

- Undifferentiated (or expanding) cells, also called committed cells. These include the cells of the liver, the kidney, and the glands (hormone-producing organs). These cells have a limited capacity to reproduce. If the tissue is damaged or a portion of an organ is removed, the cells "turn on" and begin to replicate, regenerating the organ to partial or, sometimes, full capacity.

- Differentiated (or static) cells, also called specialized cells. These include the cells of the muscles and the nerves. Once these cells reach their adult size they cannot be replaced if damaged or lost because they cannot reproduce themselves.

- Renewing cells, also called stem cells. These include the cells of your skin and hair, the cells that line your intestinal tract, and the cells that make up your blood. Stem cells reproduce continually throughout a person's lifetime.

The process of orderly replication through division is called mitosis. Cells that undergo mitosis are called somatic cells (from *soma*, the Greek word for "body"). During its lifetime, a normal somatic cell acts in ways that are strictly governed by genetic information contained within the cell. The cells in our body know when to divide and when to stop dividing. For exam-ple, the heart grows only to a certain size and then stops growing. The cells also know what their function is: eye cells develop into eyes, liver cells into the liver. These cells cannot continue to divide and multiply indefinitely. Part of their genetic instruction tells them when their lifespan has ended. At that point the cell dies a natural death and its functions are taken over by fresh young cells. The process of programmed cell death is called apoptosis.

The orderly process of human growth and development depends on the increase in the number of cells (cell reproduction), and the specialization of cells into the different types of human tissue (cell differentiation). Normal human growth is a balance of cell reproduction and cell death. These processes are orchestrated by instructions contained in the genetic material called DNA (deoxyribonucleic acid). Once physical development is complete, only the stem cells and the undifferentiated cells continue to reproduce, and they do so only in a regulated fashion.

But sometimes something happens to disrupt the cell's normal life cycle. The instructions governing the cell's activity become garbled, resulting in a loss of balance between cell reproduction and cell death. This imbalance causes the cell to multiply out of control and to produce the growth known as a tumor. Some tumors are benign; others are cancerous. Benign tumors do not invade surrounding tissues or spread to distant sites. Cancerous tumors have the ability to migrate to other parts of the body. Cancer cells have lost the ability to respond to signals to specialize, stop dividing, or die.

Carcinogenesis—the process by which a normal cell becomes cancerous—alters life at the genetic level. Carcinogenesis results from mutations (alterations) in the DNA of individual cells. Normal cells of any type in any organ may mutate into altered, cancerous cells. These mutated cells will then reproduce with the altered DNA. Cells are exposed constantly to substances, produced both within our bodies and in the external environment, that have the potential to alter genetic material. Usually the cell is able to fend off attacks from harmful substances or repair itself and prevent long-term damage, such as cancer. But if the damage does not get fixed, then each time the cell reproduces it copies the same altered DNA.

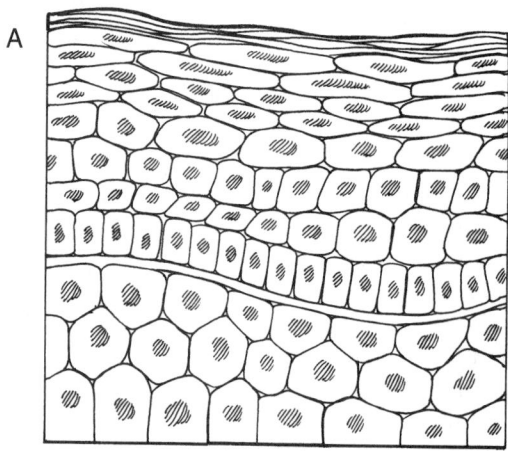

Normal cells

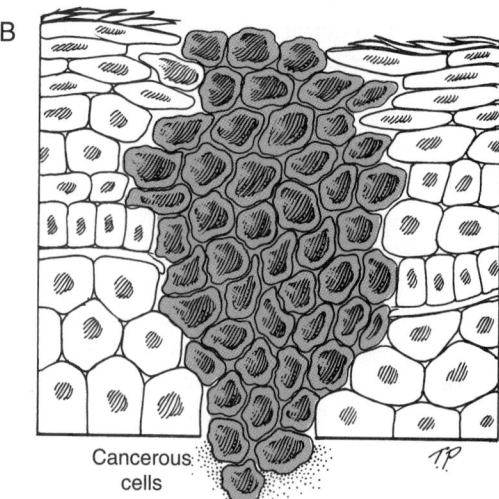

Cancerous cells

(A) In normal human tissue, cells develop specialized functions, and their reproduction typically leads to organized structure. (B) Cancerous tissue contains cells whose reproduction and function are improperly regulated, leading to disease and often to spread of the tumor.

DNA resides in the nuclei of all cells in the body except red blood cells, which lack a nucleus. DNA possesses two unique characteristics: it makes an exact copy of itself, and it tells the cell when and how to make the proteins necessary to carry out all of the functions of a living organism. DNA is shaped like a double helix, which resembles a twisted ladder. The complete set of genetic information, called the human genome, is contained in approximately 100,000 distinct segments of DNA, called genes. These genes are assembled into 23 matched pairs called chromosomes. Each normal human cell thus contains two copies of every gene; one of each pair was inherited from one of the parents (see Chapter 6).

Different genes are responsible for different functions within the cell. One important type is a growth-promoting gene, or proto-oncogene. There are between 300 and 400 proto-oncogenes within the human genome. Normally, proto-oncogenes assist in regulating cell division and differentiation and are strictly controlled. But proto-oncogenes are delicate structures. If they become damaged, they can transform into oncogenes (*onc-* is the root of the Greek word for "tumor").

A proto-oncogene can become an oncogene in one of three ways: point mutation, translocation, or amplification. Point mutation refers to a specific alteration at some point along the strand of the DNA. Mutations can occur spontaneously as a result of some accident or disruption in the process of cell division, or they can arise due to the presence of a cell-damaging substance known as a carcinogen. Approximately 20 percent of all human cancers (including colon, lung, and pancreatic cancers) are associated, along with other changes, with mutations in a certain gene known as *ras*. The *ras* gene produces a protein whose function is to maintain the cell's ability to send signals between its various parts.

In translocation, a segment of a chromosome, which may contain more than one gene, breaks off and becomes joined to another chromosome. Amplification refers to an increase of 10 to 100 times the normal rate at which proto-oncogenes are copied. Translocation and amplification are associated with cancers involving white blood cells, such as leukemias and lymphomas.

Carcinogenesis is a complex process. It takes time for the series of spontaneous mutations that eventually produce a malignant cell to occur, which is why the risk of developing most kinds of cancers increases with age. The conversion of a proto-oncogene to an oncogene is just one of many steps in the process. Normally, after this conversion occurs, the cell's built-in protection mechanism goes to work to repair or minimize the DNA damage. In carcinogenesis, however, there may also be changes in tumor suppressor genes. The normal function of these genes is to repair DNA and to control cell growth; they can be thought of as the brakes of a car. Each cell has two copies of a tumor suppressor gene, one

CANCER MYTHS/CANCER FACTS

One in four Americans will receive a diagnosis of cancer at some point in his or her lifetime. After heart disease, cancer is the second leading cause of death in the United States, and each year more than 1.6 million Americans develop cancer. However, among women under age 65, cancer is the leading cause of death, a fact that is due mainly to the rising rate of lung cancer in women. In children, only accidents surpass cancer as the leading cause of death. By the year 2010, it is predicted that cancer will be the leading cause of death in the population. The myth is that cancer is on the rise because of environmental pollution. In fact, cancer is on the rise chiefly because the risk for most cancers increases with age, and Americans are living longer.

The second reason for the rise in cancer can be expressed in one word: smoking. The lung cancer mortality rate continues to rise, and approximately 85 percent of all lung cancers are caused by smoking.

Smoking is the largest preventable cause of premature death and disability in the United States. Because of the extraordinary impact of the incidence of lung cancer on the cancer statistics, the strides being made in curing cancer are often overshadowed. It is important to remember that these numbers would be markedly diminished but for tobacco use and that real progress has been made in detecting and curing cancer.

At the beginning of this century, a diagnosis of cancer meant almost certain death. By as early as the 1930s, however, one out of five people diagnosed with cancer survived for 5 years or more. Today fully half of those diagnosed with cancer survive for 5 years or more and are considered to be cured. And those who have been cured of cancer will have the same life expectancy as a same sex person in their age group who has not had cancer. Yet the myth that a diagnosis of cancer is equivalent to a death sentence persists. This ongoing dread of cancer and cancer treatment inhibits many cancer patients from seeking medical attention early enough so that their cancer may be diagnosed at a treatable stage. And at present, early detection is the best weapon in combating cancer successfully. ■

---

from each parent. Cancer may result if both copies are damaged.

Proto-oncogenes and tumor suppressor genes can be damaged by continual environmental insults, including chemical carcinogens (such as cigarette smoke) and physical carcinogens (such as x-rays and certain other forms of radiation). There are also naturally occurring carcinogens, such as toxins made from some molds. Infections by viruses, including papillomaviruses, hepatitis, and retroviruses, may also trigger oncogene activity.

Normal cells grow and stay in one place in the body. When cells divide uncontrollably, they can grow to form tumors. What makes cancerous tumors different from benign tumors is that cancer cells have the ability to spread into neighboring tissues and migrate (metastasize) to other places in the body if the cancer is not detected early. Once cancerous cells lodge in tissue, they can produce new tumors. Tumors that spread and metastasize are known as malignant tumors. Tumors that do not spread are considered noninvasive or benign.

Cancer cells divide more frequently and live longer than normal cells, and thus accumulate. They compete with the surrounding healthy tissue for oxygen and nutrients in the blood. Eventually they also begin to vie for territory, crowding out healthy cells, inhibiting normal function, and causing further complications.

CANCER AND TUMOR TYPES

The following are the four major groups of cancers:

- Carcinomas. Carcinomas are tumors that begin in the exterior or interior linings (epithelial tissue) of the internal organs and also on the exterior surface of the body, also called the epithelial tissue.

- Leukemias. Leukemias are cancers of the blood-forming tissues.

- Lymphomas. Lymphomas are tumors that originate in the lymphatic system.

- Sarcomas. Sarcomas are tumors that originate in the connective tissues, in particular, muscles, bones, and cartilage.

While these cancers may spread from the organ where they originate to other organs, they will retain their initial cellular distinction. In other words, a breast cancer that spreads to the lungs does not become lung cancer; rather, it remains characteristic of breast cancer, although in another location.

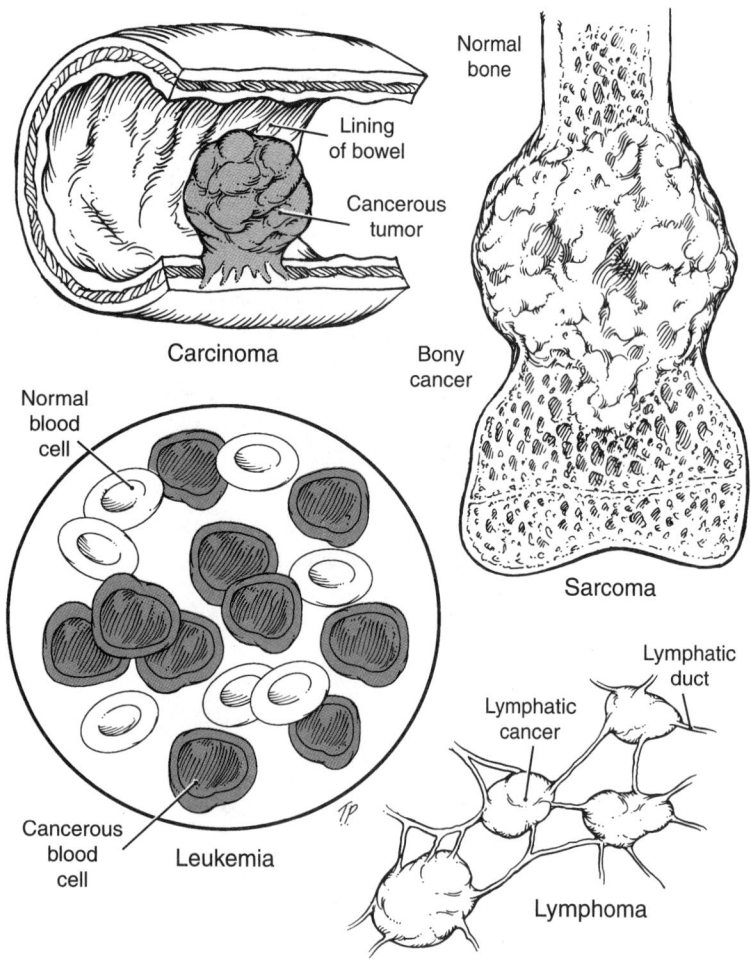

Cancers are grouped according to the types of cells from which they develop. Carcinoma begins in the skin or linings of internal organs. Leukemia begins in blood. Sarcoma begins in connective tissue such as muscle or bone. Lymphoma begins in the lymphatic system of special ducts and nodes.

HEREDITY AND CANCER

In a way, each chromosome is like one volume in your body's vast biologic encyclopedia. The pages of the volume are your genes. These genes, alone or in concert with other genes, are responsible for every trait you possess: body size and shape, hair color, even your emotional responses to the world. Certain traits such as eye color are passed from generation to generation.

Only a small proportion of all cancer types—perhaps less than 10 percent—are due to an inherited predisposition. Far more common are the carcinogenic mutations of somatic cells, which are mutations that occur within the individual's life and that arise as a result of environmental factors such as cigarette smoke or radiation.

However, some people are born with genes that are already damaged. Like a misprint in a book, these faulty genes contain erroneous information. Ideally, any defective gene inherited from one parent will be canceled out by a normal, healthy gene passed along from the other parent, which, in fact, is the biologic advantage of sexual reproduction. Ideally, by mixing up the genes over generations, certain problem genes will eventually be replaced by healthy ones. This does not always happen, however. Most hereditary cancers occur when a defective copy of a tumor suppressive gene is inherited from a parent; later in life a mutation occurs in the single remaining normal gene. The normal function of the gene to act as a brake on cell growth or to repair DNA is then lost and cancer occurs.

That is what is meant when it is said that a disease "runs in the family." Depending on how the genes were inherited, some members of a family are more or less likely to experience the same type of health problems. Keep in mind that cancers themselves—that is, the actual defective cells that form the tumor—are not passed from the mother to the fetus in the way that viruses or bacteria can be transmitted. Cancer is not contagious. Instead, what is inherited is the risk that a person will develop the certain kind of cancer later in life.

The task of genetic research is to identify specific genes that cause cancer. Often, the research into the inherited mutations of familial cancers results in knowledge that helps in the battle against noninherited forms of the cancer as well.

A person who inherits certain damaged genes is more likely to develop cancer than a person who does not inherit these genes. However, having a predisposition does not necessarily mean that a person will definitely develop cancer. It simply means that fewer mutations must occur before cancer arises. The inherited predisposition to cancer explains less than 10 percent of cancer cases. At present, the following cancers are known to be linked to heredity.

Breast and ovarian cancer About 5 percent of all breast cancer cases are associated with an inherited predisposition. Two mutated genes known as BRCA1 and BRCA2 have been discovered to be associated with

ADVANCES IN GENETIC RESEARCH

A massive research effort known as the Human Genome Project is underway in laboratories around the world. The goal is to decode the entire genetic library contained in human DNA. By translating the vast amounts of information contained within each cell, scientists are learning more about how our bodies function and how problems such as cancer can arise.

In addition to uncovering information on inherited cancers, researchers are discovering more about how mutations occur. Mutations are abnormalities that develop in DNA at some point during the cell's life cycle. Some mutations are inherited, but others arise due to damage over the course of time. For example, some cells can lose part of their DNA. If that happens, each subsequent cell that results from division will lack that same DNA particle. Sometimes a piece of DNA breaks off but becomes reattached at the wrong place in the DNA strand. Over time, as the mutated cell continues to reproduce, it may become cancerous.

In 1995, scientists at Johns Hopkins used a special technique to speed up the search for gene mutations. The technique is known as representational difference analysis. Using representational difference analysis, researchers can quickly compare two pieces of DNA to see if either or both of the pieces are missing a segment. In one experiment, scientists found that some people who are prone to pancreatic cancer are missing a certain piece of DNA from both of the genes in a pair. Consequently, their cells lack the ability to produce an important tumor-suppressor protein whose job is to prevent tumors from developing.

Knowing what "words" in the genetic code are missing or "misspelled" is the first step in developing a gene therapy—a treatment designed to replace the defective segment with a new, fully functioning part—or it may lead to treatment in which patients take doses of the missing tumor-suppressing protein.

Genetic research is still in its infancy. The discovery of a gene involved in a disease does not necessarily mean we know how to treat the disease more effectively. As time goes on, we are finding that genes do not necessarily act alone; many genes, even genes on separate chromosomes, may interact with each other in complex ways that could not have been predicted. Parts of genes we originally thought were meaningless are turning out to play key roles in cell function.

It may take many years, even decades, before we can translate our growing knowledge of the genetic code into practical strategies for diagnosing and curing cancer—or better yet, preventing cancer altogether. But progress is being made every day. ∎

---

an increased risk of breast and ovarian cancer (BRCA simply stands for "*breast cancer*"). These two genes explain about 50 percent of the inherited form of breast cancer. Women who have strong family histories of breast or ovarian cancer in close relatives may possess a BRCA1 mutation. Those that do have about a 50 to 80 percent risk of being diagnosed with breast cancer in their lifetime; they are also at a substantially higher risk for ovarian cancer than the general public. Normally, the BRCA1 is a tumor-suppressor gene; it produces a protein that protects against uncontrolled cell division. If both copies of the BRCA1 gene are mutated or inactive, the cell no longer produces the protective protein and thus is susceptible to uncontrolled growth, which leads to breast or ovarian cancer. Loss of both copies of the BRCA1 gene usually occurs when a mutated, abnormal copy is inherited and the second normal copy becomes damaged. A related gene, BRCA2, is also a tumor-suppressor gene. People who inherit the mutant form of this gene are more likely to develop breast cancer and are also at increased risk of developing other cancers.

Colon cancer Colon cancer is sometimes an inherited disease, particularly in association with familial adenomatous polyposis, a rare hereditary condition characterized by the occurrence of hundreds of polyps in the colon. Johns Hopkins researchers, led by Dr. Bert Vogelstein and Dr. Kenneth Kinzler, have shown that mutations in the APC tumor suppressor gene switch on the powerful c-MYC oncogene, leading to colon cancer.

Retinoblastoma The deletion or damage of a tumor-suppressor gene known as Rb has been linked to retinoblastoma, a rare cancer that affects the eye and that occurs most often in infants and children under the age of 5. Both copies of the Rb gene must be affected for the disease to develop, as is true for other cancers due to genetic mutations.

Inherited genetic linkages in other cancers are being discovered with increasing frequency, including linkages for certain lung cancers and a form of malignant skin cancer called melanoma. While research into inherited forms of cancer is promising, its findings directly pertain to only a small fraction of cancers. If you have concerns about your family history, you should discuss them with your doctor and see a genetics counselor. In the meantime, scientific advances leading to earlier detection and more effective treatment of cancer are likely to benefit more people with the disease.

HEREDITARY NONPOLYPOSIS COLORECTAL CANCER

HNPCC is a condition that involves an inherited tendency to develop cancer of the colon or rectum. Affected women are also at increased risk of endometrial cancer. Other names for HNPCC are Lynch syndrome and cancer family syndrome. In the mid-1990s, researchers at Johns Hopkins identified three defective genes that cause at least 60 percent of all cases of HNPCC.

Most types of colon cancer arise from polyps, which are abnormal mushroom-shaped growths in the lining of the large intestine. While most polyps are harmless, some can progress to become cancerous. Cancer in persons with HNPCC also starts from a polyp. The term nonpolyposis is used to distinguish HNPCC from familial polyposis where dozens, or even hundreds, of polyps are present.

People with HNCPP inherit defective genes that produce abnormal cells in the intestine. People who have the HNPCC gene have a 50–50 chance of passing the gene along to each of their children. The gene can be passed on even if the parent has had surgery to remove the colon, because the instructions for producing the disease are contained within each cell.

The majority of people who have the HNPCC gene will develop cancer in the colon or rectum, usually by age 45. Women with the HNPCC gene are at high risk of developing endometrial cancer. Early diagnosis is especially important in these individuals because the sooner the cancer is detected, the more effective the treatment will be.

People from families that are prone to HNPCC should have a colonoscopy (an exam using a viewing scope inserted through the rectum) every 1 to 3 years starting by age 25 or 5 to 10 years before the age of the earliest case of colorectal cancer diagnosed in the family. People who start having colonoscopies should also have annual tests for hidden blood in the stool (feces). People with HNPCC are also more likely to develop other types of cancer. For that reason, women with the HNPCC gene should have a biopsy of the lining of the uterus (the endometrium) every year to check for signs of uterine cancer.

People who have undergone genetic testing and in whom the HNPCC gene has been identified need to take special precautions. In addition to the tests just described, some people with a known HNPCC risk may need to undergo surgery to remove part or all of the colon as a way to prevent cancer from developing.

CANCER ON THE INTERNET

The Internet offers a great deal of information on cancer, from material provided by the National Cancer Institute a wide range of online support groups. Here are just some of the resources you can find on the Internet.

Cansearch (http://www.access.digex.net mkragn/cansearch. html) If you are looking for information on cancer, this is the place to start. Cansearch is organized to show you where to go first to research your disease, how to use each resource, and where to go for more information. Cansearch is the home page for the National Coalition for Cancer Survivorship, and it will help you find the resources to understand your disease medically and cope with it emotionally.

Cancer-L (e-mail: listserve@wnvm.bitnet) CANCER-L offers an online way to discuss cancer with fellow patients and survivors. CANCER-L offers emotional support and information and can form the basis of your online support group. New members are welcome, and members follow each other's progress, sharing good news and bad, clinical information, and practical tips.

Cancernet Data (e-mail: cancernet@icicb.nci.nih.gov; Internet: http://www.nih.gov) Using e-mail through CANCER-NET, you can request various types of information from the National Cancer Institute including material from the Physician Data Query (PDQ) database, fact sheets from their Office of Cancer Communications, and abstracts on various topics from the CANCERLIT database. Much of the information is also available in Spanish.

OncoLink (http://cancer.med.upenn.edu) OncoLink is offered by the University of Pennsylvania Medical School and is an excellent reference for information on every aspect of cancer including medical, emotional, spiritual, and financial issues.

American Cancer Society (http://www.cancer.org) The American Cancer Society's Web Site offers a variety of topics including general information on specific cancers, updates on research progress, and listings of programs and events, as well as information on local American Cancer Society offices.

CANCERGUIDE (http://bcn.coulder.co.us/health/cancer/canguide.htm) CANCERGUIDE is devoted to helping you research the treatment options for your particular cancer.

There are many more options for finding the information you need on cancer on the Internet, and you can find most of them through Cansearch. ■

Genetic tests are not yet perfect; they may not identify everyone who actually has the HNPCC gene. For that reason, people at risk—that is, those who have a family history of colon cancer—should discuss their genetic susceptibility and the advisability of genetic testing with their doctor and a genetic counselor. They also need to work closely with their doctors to watch for early signs of colorectal cancer.

EXPOSURES THAT CAN CAUSE CANCER

Tobacco Smoking is the leading cause of preventable death in the United States. Smoking is responsible for approximately 85 percent of the deaths caused by lung cancer. It is also associated with an increased risk for cancers of the mouth, larynx, esophagus, pancreas, bladder, and cervix. There are many hazards to our health over which we may have no control, but smoking is not one of them. People who continue to smoke are choosing to jeopardize their own health and the health of their families on a daily basis. While quitting smoking is difficult, there are many excellent programs designed to help smokers quit smoking (see Chapter 4).

Chemicals Environmental pollutants pose a persistent health risk, particularly for those workers who are continually exposed to high levels of carcinogens. The link between cancer and exposure to asbestos, industrial dyes, nickel, chromate, vinyl chloride, and especially a chemical called benzene has been well established. Protective clothing is essential for those who work with asbestos or other dangerous substances.

Ionizing radiation The term ionizing means that energy levels are high enough to knock tiny particles called electrons out of their orbits around the nucleus of an atom. Ionized particles are highly active and can damage other molecules, including molecules of DNA. In fact, ionizing radiation is often used in the treatment of cancer for this reason. Research has shown that there is a small but significant risk that second tumors can develop in patients who have been treated with ionizing radiation. Diagnostic x-rays contain ionizing radiation but

at about one-thousandth of the dose used in cancer treatment. The connection between ionizing radiation and cancer has been documented, but the amount of radiation exposure that significantly increases the risk of cancer is still unknown and is a matter of much public debate.

Viruses Human immunodeficiency virus (HIV), the virus that causes acquired immunodeficiency syndrome (AIDS), is associated with increased risk of hepatoma (liver cancer) and of lymphomas and sarcomas (cancer of connective tissue). Hepatitis B viral infection, common in those who suffer from AIDS, is associated with an increased risk of hepatoma. It may be that other sexually transmitted diseases cause an increase in certain cancers. Venereal warts, which result from infection with certain kinds of human papilloma virus, are associated with an increased risk for cancer of the cervix. And the virus that causes genital herpes—herpes simplex virus 2, or HSV-2—may be a cofactor in the risk for cervical cancer.

Sunlight Sunlight contains ultraviolet (nonionizing) radiation, and prolonged exposure causes damage to the skin that may result in skin cancer. Artificial sources of ultraviolet radiation, such as tanning lamps, also cause damage. While most skin cancers, such as basal cell and squamous cell cancers, are benign, they can cause local damage and can be disfiguring. They do not usually cause death. A melanoma (a malignant skin tumor), however, can be deadly. To minimize risk, experts urge people to limit their exposure to the sun, wear hats and long sleeves when the sun is strongest, and always use adequate sunscreens, at least SPF 15.

Diagnosing Cancer

Cancer is not a diagnosis anyone wants to hear. But if you do have cancer, the sooner you find out about it, the better your chances for a full recovery and a normal life. The tools that we now have to fight cancer are most effective when the cancer is diagnosed early. To maximize your chances of full recovery, you need to be constantly vigilant—watching for warning signs of cancer, undergoing all recommended screening tests, and seeing a doctor as soon as possible if a cough persists, a sore does not heal, a bowel habit changes, or any other physical concern arises.

Often, however, cancers in the early stages have no symptoms, so your yearly checkup is vitally important in detecting cancer early. As you age, certain screening tests will become routine parts of your physical exam. Everyone should be screened at certain ages for particular cancers, such as breast and colon cancers, and people with a very strong family history of cancer may be urged to have screening tests at an earlier age than the general population. Too often, regular screening tests are neglected because a person feels fine, but that is precisely the point of regular screening—to catch cancer early before it has grown sufficiently to cause warning signs. Regular screening saves lives.

WARNING SIGNS FOR THE MOST COMMON CANCERS

The American Cancer Society lists seven classic warning signs for the most common cancers. The warning signs may occur in people who do not have cancer, and they may also be absent in those who are diagnosed with cancer. Despite this variability, it is important to take these warning signs seriously and contact your doctor immediately should you develop one or more of them.

1. Any change in bowel or bladder habits
2. Any sore that does not heal
3. Unexplained bleeding or discharge
4. Any lump or thickening in the breast or prostate or elsewhere on the body
5. Difficulty in swallowing, or unexplained or chronic indigestion
6. Any changes in a wart or mole
7. A chronic cough or persistent hoarseness

The seven classic signs are the most common; the following are other possible signs of cancer, though they may be signs of many other disorders as well:

- Unexplained appetite loss or weight loss
- Unexplained and persistent headaches that may be accompanied by changes in vision or behavior
- Excessive bruising
- Unusual pallor
- Unusual tiredness
- Pain in the bones or elsewhere that cannot be easily explained

THE STAGES OF CANCER

When a tumor is found to be malignant, your doctors need to determine how far and to what parts of the body the tumor has spread. This process is called staging, and it involves classifying the cancer by the size of the primary tumor, the involvement of malignant cells in adjacent lymph nodes, and the spread to other organs. Because there are so many different types of cancer, there are several types of staging systems in use, and the systems are constantly being revised. The following are some of the terms your doctor may use in describing a cancer:

- *In situ.* The Latin term means "in its original place" or "at the place of origin." Carcinoma in situ is a cancer that has not spread into surrounding tissue or to other parts of the body. If this term is used in your diagnosis, it is good news. The chances of complete recovery are good.

- *Metastasis.* The spread of a tumor from the site of origin to other organs or tissues.

- *Necrosis.* Cell death.

- *Occult.* Occult means undetectable without magnification. The term often applies to the situation in which cancer cells are found in the sputum although there is no visible tumor in the lung.

- *Stage 0.* Stage 0 may also be referred to as precancer. Cancer cells have been found, but no cancerous invasion or spread is present.

- *Stage 1.* A stage 1 tumor has not spread beyond the organ where it originated.

- *Stage 2.* For most cancers, a stage 2 cancer has reached a certain size or spread to adjacent lymph nodes or to other tissue within the organ of origin.

- *Stage 3.* Stage 3 often refers to a cancer that has spread to multiple lymph nodes or to adjacent tissue.

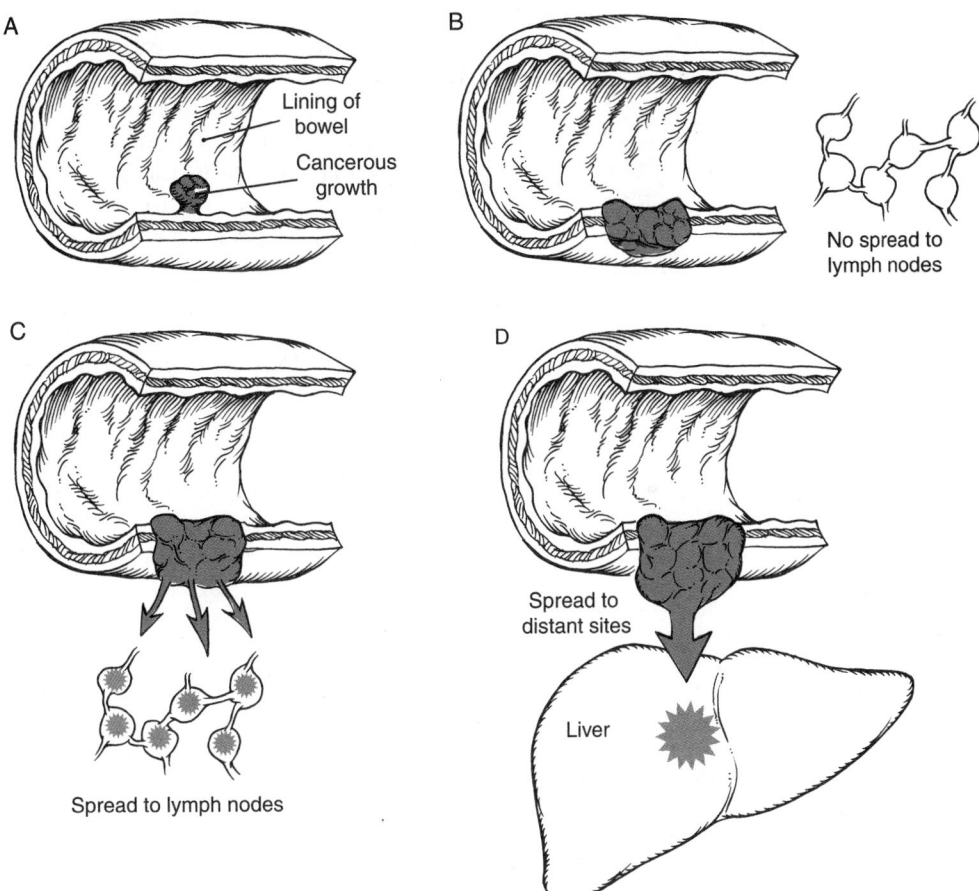

(A) Cancer *in situ* (stage 0) has not spread into nearby or distant sites. (B) In Stage 1, cancer invades local tissue but has not spread elsewhere. (C) Cancer in stage 2 or 3 has spread to lymph nodes or other regions within the original organ. (D) In stage 4, distant spread has occurred.

- *Stage 4.* For most cancers, a stage 4 cancer has spread to other organs.

THE MOST COMMON CANCERS

The most common form of cancer in the United States is skin cancer. However, the vast majority of skin cancers are benign—that is, they are not likely to spread and are easily cured. The exception is melanoma, a malignant and often fatal form of skin cancer.

Confusing the statistical picture is the fact that some cancers occur only in one sex or the other. Virtually all cases of breast cancer occur among women, although in rare cases men can also develop breast can-

1998 ESTIMATES OF THE MOST COMMON TYPES OF CANCER

SITE OF CANCER	NUMBER OF NEW CASES PER YEAR
Prostate	184,500
Breast	180,300
Lung	171,500
Colon and rectum	131,600
Lymphoma	62,500
Bladder	54,400
Melanoma of the skin	41,600
Uterus	36,100
Oral	30,300
Kidney	29,900
Pancreas	29,000
Leukemia	28,700
Ovary	25,400
Stomach	22,600
Liver	13,900
Cervix	13,700

The above table was compiled from the 1998 estimates from the American Cancer Society of the most common types of cancer (other than benign skin cancer) in terms of the approximate number of new cases per year.

THE MOST FREQUENT CAUSES OF CANCER-RELATED DEATH

SITE OF CANCER	NUMBER OF DEATHS PER YEAR
Lung	160,100
Colon and rectum	56,500
Breast	43,900
Prostate	39,200
Pancreas	28,900
Lymphoma	26,300
Leukemia	21,600
Brain	17,400
Stomach	13,700
Liver	13,000
Esophagus	11,900
Bladder	12,500
Kidney	11,600
Multiple myeloma	11,300

cer. Prostate cancer occurs only in men, while cancers of the ovaries, uterus, and cervix affect only women. Apart from skin cancer, prostate cancer is the most common cancer; for every 10 men with prostate cancer there are approximately 6 women with breast cancer.

Some types of cancer are more dangerous and are harder to treat than others, and thus are more likely to be fatal. Lung cancer is by far the most deadly form of the disease. Although prostate cancer is the most frequent type of cancer in terms of number of cases, it is less often the cause of death than some other forms of cancer; for example, women are more likely to die of breast cancer than men are to die of prostate cancer.

The last few years have seen significant improvements in survival times—that is, the length of time people live after their disease is diagnosed. In 1930, for example, only about 20 percent of people with cancer—one out of five—lived 5 years or more after their disease was detected. Today, more than 50 percent of people with cancer survive 5 years or longer, an improvement that is due largely to earlier detection and improved treatment.

Despite these advances, however, the overall death rate from cancer is on the increase. This is due primarily to the rapid increase in the number of lung cancer deaths, which rose from approximately 5,000 per year in 1930 to nearly 50,000 per year by 1990. There has also been an increase, although less dramatic, in the rate of deaths from leukemia and from cancer of the pancreas and prostate in the same period. Death rates from cancer of the uterus, stomach, and liver have declined significantly.

Each of the specific types of cancer is covered in detail elsewhere in the chapters in Part 4: Body Systems and Disorders. Whether you have a family history that might lead you to suspect that you are at risk for a particular cancer or not, we are all at greater risk for cancer as we age. Following is a brief introduction to symptoms and screening procedures that might help you detect a cancer early or avoid cancer altogether. The cancers are discussed in the order of their frequency.

❖ SKIN CANCER

While skin cancer is common, it need not be fatal. The key to detecting all skin cancers before they become a problem is observation. Of the three types of skin cancers, basal cell, squamous cell, and melanoma, melanoma is the most dangerous. Men have a higher mortality rate from melanoma than women, perhaps because more men work outdoors, where they are more likely to be exposed to sunlight.

Symptoms Any change in the shape, size, or color of a mole or any bleeding from a mole may be a sign of skin cancer. (See pages C-38 and C-39.)

What you can do Wear sunscreen and cover exposed skin. Do not stay in the sun for long periods of time and avoid being in the sun altogether in the middle of the day. When checking moles, remember your ABCDs: A stands for asymmetry (irregular shape); B stands for borders that are notched; C stands for color variation within the mole, and D stands for diameter greater than 6 mm. If any of these conditions exist, see your doctor immediately.

Screening If you have any suspicious moles, your dermatologist will probably want to check them every 6 months for any visible changes. If there are visible changes, the doctor will probably remove the suspicious mole before it becomes a problem.

US PREVENTIVE SERVICES TASK FORCE SCREENING GUIDELINES

CANCER TYPE	TEST	AGE AND RECOMMENDED FREQUENCY
Breast	Breast self-exam	No recommendation (C)
	Doctor's exam	50 to 69, once every 1–2 years (C)
	Mammography	50 to 69, once every 1–2 years (A)
Cervical	Physical exam	No recommendation
	Pap smear	Onset of sexual activity, (A)
		At least every three years, until age 65
Colorectal (bowel)	Digital rectal exam	No recommendation (C)
	Fecal occult blood test	50 and above, yearly (B)
	Proctosigmoidoscopy*	50 and above, instead of fetal occult blood test or in conjunction with fetal occult blood test (B), frequency unspecified
Uterine (endometrial)	None	
Head and neck	Physical exam	No recommendation (C)
Lung	None for nonsmokers	
	Chest x-ray	Not recommended (D)
Melanoma**	Skin self-exam	No recommendation (C)
	Physical exam	No recommendation (C)
Prostate	Digital rectal exam	Not recommended (D)
	Prostate specific antigen (PSA) blood test	Not recommended (D)
Testicular	Testicular self-exam	No recommendation (C)
	Physical exam	No recommendation (C)

These guidelines are based on evidentiary findings; in other words, they are made only after there is clinical evidence of the effectiveness of each screening procedure for the recommended age group. For example, the Task Force is not recommending against a mammogram under age 50 but rather is merely clarifying that there is not sufficient data to support the actual effectiveness of mammography as a screening technique for women under age 50. The Task Force uses an A to E rating system, which is defined below. Based on your family or personal health history, your personal doctor may recommend screening at an earlier age or may use screening techniques that do not currently receive a recommendation by the Task Force. These screening procedures may be effective although there is not yet enough clinical evidence to support a recommendation by the US Task Force standards.

*Recommendations for the periodicity of this test may vary.

**It is recommended that high-risk persons wear protective clothing and avoid the sun.

A indicates there is good evidence to support routine screening with this technique in this age group.

B indicates there is fair evidence to support routine screening with this technique in this age group.

C indicates there is no evidence for or against the inclusion of the screening technique in routine health exams.

D indicates there is fair evidence to recommend against including the screening technique in routine health exams.

E indicates there is good evidence to recommend against including the screening technique in routine health examinations.

Screening People at increased risk may be referred to a skin specialist for evaluation and surveillance.

❖ PROSTATE CANCER

As men age, the risk of prostate cancer increases. Men with a family history of prostate cancer need to be particularly vigilant. Blacks are also at higher risk.

Symptoms Most prostate cancers cause no symptoms, especially in the early stages. Difficulty in urination, back pain, and blood in the urine may be symptoms of more advanced prostate cancer. Such symptoms are reported by approximately one out of four men in whom prostate cancer is diagnosed.

What you can do Prostate cancer is most common in men over age 70 but it is recommended that men over age 50 discuss screening options with their doctors.

Screening tests Many doctors recommend that men over age 40 undergo an annual digital rectal examination, which can detect changes in the prostate gland. A blood test is also available to measure the levels of a substance called prostate specific antigen, or PSA, which is produced by cells in the prostate. Benign enlargement of the prostate and prostate cancer may both cause an increase in PSA levels. If the PSA level is elevated, other tests will be done to find out the cause. Although PSA testing is widespread, its use as a screening test is controversial (see below and page 1149).

❖ BREAST CANCER

Breast cancer is the fourth most common cancer in the United States, and it ranks behind only heart disease and lung cancer as a cause of death among women each year. Yet it is the first disease on most women's minds. The oft-repeated statement that one in nine women will get breast cancer in their lifetime is partly responsible for this increased awareness. This is a lifetime average risk. A particular woman may be at more or less risk based on her personal risk factors. The greatest risk factor is age, hence the recommendation that all women age 50 and older should have a mammogram.

Symptoms A lump in the breast; any thickening in the breast; discharge or bleeding from the nipple.

PROSTATE SPECIFIC ANTIGEN TESTING: PRO AND CON

The prostate specific antigen (PSA) test is a blood test that measures the level of a protein produced by the prostate cells. The PSA test has been available since the 1980s. It was developed as a screening test for prostate cancer. Hundreds of thousands of men have this test annually. Benign prostate hypertrophy and prostate cancer both increase PSA levels. A PSA level under 4 suggests that prostate cancer is unlikely, although it can occur; when the PSA level is over 10 the probability of cancer is high. The probability of cancer increases as the PSA level increases. But again, this is a test that indicates the possibility of cancer. If the level is elevated, further tests will need to be done to determine the cause.

The American Cancer Society recommends yearly PSA testing combined with a rectal exam. For men at high risk for prostate cancer, such as black men or men with a strong family history of prostate cancer, the American Cancer Society recommends that screening should begin at age 40.

While PSA testing increases the possibilities of early diagnosis, what happens after prostate cancer is diagnosed early is what makes PSA testing controversial. There has been some concern that PSA test results would lead to aggressive treatment in men with insignificant cancers, that is, cancers that would not spread or cause problems in a man's lifetime. Overtreatment may include a prostatectomy (the complete removal of the prostate), the side effects of which may include impotence or incontinence. While technological improvements in the procedure continue to reduce the chances of these complications, the risk of such complications may be greater than the risk involved in simply watching the cancer to see if it progresses. A slow-growing prostatic tumor in an older man is often not worth the quality of life changes that may occur with the surgical procedure. In addition, there have been no studies to determine whether early detection and early treatment actually improves outcomes, as measured by mortality from prostate cancer.

Experts disagree on whether the PSA test should be a recommended routine laboratory evaluation for every adult male over age 50. The test is not perfect, a low reading does not always mean a clean bill of prostate health and elevations do not always means cancer. Questions persist about how to interpret the results of the test and how to proceed based on that interpretation.

Still, the PSA test is a worthwhile screening test for prostate cancer when used in conjunction with diagnostic techniques such as surgical biopsy, and when all treatment options, including watchful waiting, are considered before surgery is recommended. You should discuss the value of this test in your specific case with your doctor (see Prostate Cancer, page 1147). ◼

What you can do Have a yearly gynecologic exam that includes a physical exam of your breasts for lumps or changes by your doctor or nurse practitioner. Practice breast self-exam. To make self-exams worthwhile in detecting changes in your breasts, you should examine your breasts once monthly at the same time each month, about 3 days after the end of your period. Although clinical trials have yet to offer conclusive evidence that breast self-exam improves the chances of early diagnosis, detecting an irregularity during such an exam may be the motivation to have the mammogram that detects a cancer early on.

Screening tests Women between the ages of 50 and 69 should have a mammogram every 1 to 2 years. Some groups, such as the American Cancer Society, recommend mammography beginning at age 40. Women between the ages of 40 and 50 and those with a strong family history of breast cancer should discuss when to start mammography with their doctor.

❖ LUNG CANCER

Symptoms and signs The most common symptom of lung cancer is a chronic cough often referred to as smoker's cough. Frequently, such a cough persists for months or years before the cancer can actually be diagnosed. If you cannot quit smoking or if you are a former long-time smoker, you should see your doctor every year for checkups, and if you have a persistent cough you should see your doctor immediately. An ache in the chest and increased sputum or blood in the sputum are also warning signs of lung cancer. Unfortunately, it is often the case that by the time lung cancer patients have symptoms, the cancer is inoperable or has metastasized.

What you can do If you have never smoked, do not start. If you smoke, stop. If you have quit smoking and started again, you should try to quit again. Studies show that those who have quit smoking before have a greater chance of quitting for good (see Chapter 4 for help on quitting smoking).

Screening tests No effective screening tests for lung cancer exist. Periodic chest x-rays of smokers' lungs have not proven to be an effective measure in early detection because they rarely detect a cancer in its early stages. Similarly, sputum examination to check for cancer cells in the sputum has not been found effective in early detection.

❖ COLON AND RECTAL CANCER

Symptoms and signs The most common sign of colon or rectal cancer is a change in bowel habits, such as blood in the stool or constipation. Other gastrointestinal symptoms include abdominal cramping, loss of appetite, alternating constipation and diarrhea, and weight loss. Rectal bleeding is the most serious symptom, and while rectal bleeding is usually the result of hemorrhoids, you should contact your doctor if bleeding lasts for more than a day or two.

What you can do If you experience a change in bowel habits, you should tell your doctor immediately. Eating a low-fat diet that is high in dietary fiber and includes lots of fresh fruits and vegetables is an effective strategy for lowering the risk of colon and rectal cancer.

Screening tests If you are age 50 or older, your doctor may recommend a digital rectal examination as part of your annual checkup. After age 50, you should have an annual fecal occult blood test, which is a stool sample test that can detect occult blood (blood that is invisible to the human eye). A sigmoidoscopy should also be done and if the results are normal, these tests should be repeated every 3 years. These endoscopic tests are not usually recommended on a yearly basis unless you have already had an occurrence of colon or rectal cancer. If you have a family history of colon cancer or familial adenomatous polyposis, you should discuss a screening strategy including colonoscopy that may start before age 50.

❖ NON-HODGKIN'S LYMPHOMA

Non-Hodgkin's lymphoma is the most common of the lymphomas (cancer of the lymph glands) and is slightly more common in men than in women and in whites than in blacks. Non-Hodgkin's lymphoma may start almost anywhere in the body because the lymph system is so far-reaching, and it may spread to almost any organ. While the risk for non-Hodgkin's lymphoma increases with age, it also strikes people in the prime of life (about age 40). Lymphomas are becoming more common in the United States. The reason for the increase is unknown, though it is suspected that exposure to chemicals and certain viruses including Epstein-Barr virus, human T-cell leukemia virus (HTLV), and HIV may play a role.

Symptoms Pain or swelling of the lymph nodes in the neck, underarm, or groin is a common symptom. Other symptoms include fever; fatigue; skin rashes; weight loss; lumps in the skin; bone pain; swelling of the abdomen.

What you can do If you have been exposed to industrial or farm chemicals over a long period of time or if you have had a virus such as Epstein-Barr virus or HTLV or are HIV-positive, you should have a regular physical exam that focuses on your increased risk for lymphoma.

Screening tests There are no screening tests available at present for non-Hodgkin's lymphoma, although many tests exist that may be used in diagnosing lymphomas if symptoms and physical findings warrant their use.

❖ BLADDER CANCER

Smokers are at increased risk for bladder cancer. Bladder cancer is more common in men over age 50 and in people with a history of recurrent or chronic bladder infections.

Symptoms Blood in the urine is the most common symptom of bladder or urinary tract cancer and should always be evaluated by a doctor.

What you can do If you smoke, stop. The residue of tar present in the urine of smokers has been linked to an increased risk for bladder cancer. Since the dawn of the 20th century, bladder cancer has been linked to exposure to certain industrial chemicals and dyes. If you work with chemicals or other carcinogenic material, you should discuss with your doctor whether diagnostic tests for bladder cancer are advisable.

Screening tests There are no established screening tests for bladder cancer. Diagnostic tests, such as urinary cytology, cystoscopy, and intravenous pyelogram (see Chapter 24) should be performed in people with blood in their urine.

❖ UTERINE OR ENDOMETRIAL CANCER

Symptoms Early symptoms of uterine cancer include abnormal vaginal bleeding. The blood may be red or brown in premenopausal women and a watery, bloody discharge in postmenopausal women. Bleeding after intercourse may also be a symptom.

What you can do Women with few or no children are at higher risk for endometrial cancer. If you are in this category you should be particularly aware of symptoms and have a yearly pelvic exam.

Screening tests There is no screening test for endometrial cancer that has proven to be effective. Because endometrial cancer occurs in the uterus, the Papanicolaou (Pap) smear will not detect it. If endometrial cancer is suspected, at present the best test is an endometrial biopsy, which can detect the cancer in its earliest stages. The use of ultrasound exam and endometrial biopsy as screening tests in high-risk women are under study.

❖ CANCER OF THE ORAL CAVITY

Most cancers of the tongue, mouth, throat, or vocal cords are preventable because most of these cancers are related to the use of tobacco. Tobacco products of all kinds, including snuff, chewing tobacco, cigars, and pipes, increase the risk for cancers of the oral cavity.

Symptoms Often cancer of the tongue or mouth presents itself as a small sore that will not heal. Cancer of the vocal cords may be preceded by persistent hoarseness and changes in voice quality.

What you can do The best way to lower your risk for all of these cancers is to stop using all tobacco products. You should have frequent checkups and see your doctor immediately if you notice any symptoms.

Screening tests If cancer of the oral cavity is suspected, the area will need to be biopsied.

❖ LEUKEMIA

Leukemias are cancers of the blood, characterized by the production of abnormal white blood cells. While leukemias are less common in children than in adults, they are the most common cancers among children (see page 1376).

Symptoms The symptoms for leukemia are often similar to those for more minor conditions and are often not distinctive enough to call attention to themselves. Bruising and nosebleeds may become more frequent. Pallor and tiredness may also be symptoms that are caused by the anemia associated with leukemia. Joint pain, skin lesions, fever, and chronic infections, such as a sore throat, are also symptoms of leukemia. In acute leukemias, symptoms may develop in days; in chronic leukemia, symptoms may take months or years to develop.

What you can do Avoid exposure to radiation and chemicals, particularly benzene, which is a byproduct of coal and a known carcinogen. If you have been exposed to certain medication used in the treatment of other cancers or to the HTLV virus, you also have an increased risk of leukemia. Prompt treatment of acute leukemia is essential. Leukemia may be diagnosed by screening tests that show an abnormal amount of a particular type of blood cell or by observing abnormal blood cells on a blood smear under a microscope. However, in both cases only minor abnormalities may be apparent and further testing may be necessary.

❖ OVARIAN CANCER

Women with a family history of breast cancer are at a higher risk for ovarian cancer. When caught early, ovarian cancer has one of the highest cure rates of any of the cancers that affect women. Seventy percent of women diagnosed with ovarian cancer are diagnosed with advanced disease, however, and there is approximately a 70 percent

mortality rate within the first 5 years of the disease.

Symptoms Detecting ovarian cancer early is difficult because there are no consistent early symptoms. Some women do complain of early satiety (feeling full soon after they start eating) and bloating, but the disease is usually advanced by this time.

What you can do Have a yearly pelvic exam with bimanual palpation. This means that one of the doctor's fingers is in your vagina and another is in your rectum while the other hand is pressing down on your abdomen.

Screening tests There are no consistently reliable screening tests for ovarian cancer at present, although work is being done on a procedure that involves measuring levels of CA-125, a compound found in the blood serum. Because CA-125 is not specific to ovarian cancer and may be elevated for a number of other reasons, including pregnancy and endometriosis, it will probably never achieve the degree of reliability as a screening technique as the Pap smear has for cervical cancer. In addition, CA-125 screening has not proven effective in detecting ovarian cancer in its earliest stages. A vaginal sonogram is another possible way to detect early ovarian cancer. The efficacy of either CA-125 or vaginal sonogram as screening techniques for ovarian cancer have yet to be supported by controlled trials, but trials are underway. However, if you have a family history of ovarian or breast cancer, your doctor may recommend making a vaginal sonogram and the monitoring of CA-125 levels as part of your yearly gynecologic exam.

❖ PANCREATIC CANCER

While the causes of pancreatic cancer have not been established, smoking is a factor that is known to increase your risk for pancreatic cancer.

Symptoms Dull upper-abdominal pain that often radiates to the back is a common symptom of pancreatic cancer. Other common symptoms are weight loss, jaundice (yellowing of the skin), and constant itching. Recent onset of diabetes may also be a clue to the presence of pancreatic cancer.

What you can do If you smoke, quit. If you have trouble quitting, see your doctor for regular checkups.

Screening tests There are no reliable routine screening tests for pancreatic cancer. Once the disease is suspected, a computed tomography (CT) scan and endoscopic retrograde cholangiopancreatography are reliable tests for diagnosis.

❖ CERVICAL CANCER

Cervical cancer is a cancer of the uterine cervix, and the highest incidence is between the ages of 35 and 55. The cancer is slow-growing, and when caught at the precancerous stage (called cervical dysplasia), it is almost always curable.

Symptoms Cervical cancer is almost entirely without symptoms. However, bleeding between periods or unusual discharge may be symptoms. In advanced stages, a dull backache may occur.

What you can do Multiple sex partners may put a woman at increased risk for cervical cancer. For this and many other reasons, you should practice safe sex (see STI Prevention and Condom Use, page 860). You should also have a yearly Pap smear accompanied by a vaginal exam.

Screening tests The Pap smear is one of the best screening tests available and is recommended for all sexually active women. The test is not specifically recommended for women over age 65 unless a woman has not had regular Pap smears before age 65.

Treating Cancer

There are two basic goals of cancer treatment. The first is to control the primary tumor which may include surgery or radiation. The second goal is to destroy cancerous cells that may have spread from the primary tumor. Treatment involving drugs that kill or control the spread of tumor cells is called drug therapy. Drug therapy generally refers to chemotherapy, although biologicals are also used. Biologicals include hormones, interferons, interleukins, growth factors, and vaccines.

The cancer patient has many options in terms of how and where this treatment proceeds today. In fact, there are as many options in how to manage cancer treatment surgically, medically, psychologically, and financially as there are cancers. When a person is first diagnosed with cancer, the difficult and important decisions that must be made may seem overwhelming. Therefore the person should be accompanied by one or two close family members or friends at every consultation with a doctor or caregiver. Questions regarding treatment should be written down beforehand and notes should be taken during the meeting to ensure that the person has all the necessary information to make an informed and accurate decision.

One important component in obtaining all the information a person needs to make an appropriate treatment decision is a second opinion. Many insurance carriers even require a confirming second opinion before they will cover cancer treatment.

WHERE CANCER IS TREATED

When you are considering treatment for cancer, one of the most important early decisions to make is where to go for treatment. Often a family doctor is the first doctor to detect a cancer, but often such doctors do not have all the medical expertise needed to treat the cancer. When it comes to treating cancer, all hospitals are not equal in the options and expertise they offer, and the hospital in the immediate vicinity is not always the right choice for cancer treatment.

The National Cancer Institute supports 58 Cancer Centers nationwide based on their excellence in scientific research. These include 10 basic science centers, 13 clinical centers that couple basic research with clinical (patient-oriented) research, and 35 comprehensive centers that integrate basic and clinical research with population-based cancer prevention programs. For contact information, visit the NCI Web

NATIONAL CANCER INSTITUTE-SUPPORTED CANCER CENTERS

- Alabama
  Comprehensive Cancer Center
    University of Alabama

- Arizona
  Comprehensive Cancer Center
    Arizona Cancer Center

- California
  Comprehensive Cancer Centers
    Jonsson Comprehensive Cancer Center at UCLA
    USC/Norris Comprehensive Cancer Center
  Clinical Cancer Centers
    City of Hope National Medical Center/Beckman
      Research Institute
    University of California-Irvine Cancer Center
    University of California-San Diego Cancer Center
  Basic Cancer Centers
    The Burnham Institute
    The Salk Institute for Biological Studies
  Consortium Center
    Drew-Meharry-Morehouse Consortium Cancer Center

- Colorado
  Clinical Cancer Center
    University of Colorado Cancer Center

- Connecticut
  Comprehensive Cancer Center
    Yale Cancer Center

- District of Columbia
  Comprehensive Cancer Center
    Lombardi Cancer Center/Georgetown University
      Medical Center

- Florida
  Comprehensive Cancer Center
    University of Miami Sylvester Comprehensive
      Cancer Center

- Illinois
  Clinical Cancer Centers
    University of Chicago Cancer Research Center
    Lurie Cancer Center/Northwestern University

- Indiana
  Basic Cancer Center
    Purdue Cancer Center

- Maine
  Basic Cancer Center
    The Jackson Laboratory

- Maryland
  Comprehensive Cancer Center
    Johns Hopkins Oncology Center

- Massachusetts
  Comprehensive Cancer Center
    Dana-Farber Cancer Institute
  Basic Cancer Center
    Center for Cancer Research/MIT

- Michigan
  Comprehensive Cancer Centers
    Karmanos Cancer Institute
    University of Michigan Cancer Center

- Minnesota
  Clinical Cancer Center
    Mayo Cancer Center

- Nebraska
  Basic Cancer Center
    Eppley Institute for Cancer Research/UNMC

- New Hampshire
  Comprehensive Cancer Center
    Norris Cotton Cancer Center/Dartmouth-Hitchcock
      Medical Center

- New York
  Comprehensive Cancer Centers
    Memorial Sloan-Kettering Cancer Center
    Kaplan Cancer Center/New York University
    Roswell Park Cancer Institute
    Columbia-Presbyterian Cancer Center
  Clinical Cancer Centers
    Albert Einstein College of Medicine
    University of Rochester Cancer Center
  Basic Cancer Centers
    American Health Foundation
    Cold Spring Harbor Laboratory

- North Carolina
  Comprehensive Cancer Centers
    Duke Comprehensive Cancer Center
    UNC Lineberger Comprehensive Cancer Center
    Comprehensive Cancer Center of Wake Forest
      University at the Bowman Gray School of Medicine

- Ohio
  Comprehensive Cancer Center
    The Arthur G. James Cancer Hospital and Research
      Institute/Ohio State
    University Comprehensive Cancer Center
  Clinical Cancer Center
    University Hospitals Ireland Cancer Center/Case
      Western Reserve University

- Pennsylvania
  Comprehensive Cancer Centers
    Fox Chase Cancer Center
    University of Pennsylvania Cancer Center
    University of Pittsburgh Cancer Institute ▶

▶ Clinical Cancer Center
Kimmel Cancer Center/Thomas Jefferson University
Hospital
Basic Cancer Center
The Wistar Institute

- Tennessee
Clinical Cancer Centers
St. Jude Children's Research Hospital
Vanderbilt Cancer Center

- Texas
Comprehensive Cancer Centers
The University of Texas M.D. Anderson Cancer Center
San Antonio Cancer Institute

- Utah
Clinical Cancer Center
Huntsman Cancer Institute/Utah Regional Cancer
Center/University of
Utah Health Science Center

- Vermont
Comprehensive Cancer Center
Vermont Cancer Center/University of Vermont

- Virginia
Clinical Cancer Centers
Massey Cancer Center/Medical College of
Virginia/Virginia Commonwealth University
University of Virginia Health Sciences Center

- Washington State
Comprehensive Cancer Center
Fred Hutchinson Cancer Research Center

- Wisconsin
Comprehensive Cancer Center
University of Wisconsin Comprehensive Cancer Center
Basic Cancer Center
McArdle Laboratory for Cancer Research ■

site at http://www.nci.nih.gov. See the list on page 1365 for a breakdown of centers by state.

If your cancer is not a complicated case and does not require extensive or experimental treatment, most large local hospitals or medical centers will be able to provide you with appropriate treatment. If this is not the case, your cancer team will recommend the nearest center equipped to manage your cancer treatment.

YOUR CANCER TEAM

When you are diagnosed with cancer, the best antidote to feeling helpless is to begin to play an active role in your treatment. The more informed you and those closest to you are about how and where cancer is treated, the better your chances of receiving the best treatment possible.

Generally, it is your family doctor or internist who will diagnose the cancer. Your doctor will then consult with you regarding the best oncologist to treat your particular condition. Your primary oncologist will be your cancer team leader and is responsible for coordinating the various aspects of your treatment. For example, if surgery is necessary, a specialist will perform the surgery in consultation with your oncologist who will then oversee any additional (adjuvant) treatment. Because there are often many members to a cancer team and many stages of treatment to coordinate, you will want to pay particular attention when choosing your oncologist as she will be responsible for assuring that your treatment proceeds smoothly and effectively. Other members of your team may include a surgical oncologist, a pathologist, a radiation oncologist, nurses, rehabilitation therapists, a nutritionist, a psychologist or psychiatrist, and a clergy member. ■

SURGICAL TREATMENT

Surgery was the first and is still the most common treatment for many cancers. Cancer treatment may involve surgery at one or more points during the treatment of the disease. A surgical biopsy is often performed to determine the type of cancer and whether a cancer has spread or not. Surgery is also used to remove a tumor that has not spread to other organs. In some advanced cancers, such as ovarian or colon cancer, surgery is used to remove as much of the cancer as possible; any remaining cancer is then treated with chemotherapy or radiation therapy. Surgery may also be used in cancer emergencies, such as in relieving an obstruction in the intestine.

Surgery is more likely to be successful if the tumor has not spread. When the complete removal of the tumor is possible, no further cancer treatment may be necessary. If, however, the cancer is likely to metastasize, then adjuvant therapy (surgery in conjunction with chemotherapy or sometimes radiation therapy) may be recommended. If the cancer has metastasized, then chemotherapy may be recommended. If a cancer is widespread, surgery is unlikely to cure the cancer or prolong life and may not be recommended.

RADIATION THERAPY

At present, some form of radiation treatment is used to treat approximately half of all cancer patients. Radiation refers to high-energy beams of invisible particles that penetrate body tissues and destroy cells. In some cases, radiation therapy alone can eradicate a cancer. In other cases, it may be used along with surgery or chemotherapy (or both) to enhance the effectiveness of treatment. For example, radiation can shrink a tumor and make it easier to remove during surgery. Radiation may also be used to relieve pain and discomfort in some advanced cases of cancer.

There are two main approaches of radiation therapy used in cancer treatment. External beam radiotherapy (sometimes called teletherapy) involves use of a machine that is positioned outside the body and that directs radiation to the affected tissue. Internal radiation therapy, or brachytherapy, is the term used when a radioactive source is surgically implanted directly into or near the tumor.

The intensity of the dose of radiation used in treatment depends on the location and extent of the cancer. Low-energy or electron (superficial) external beam radiation does not penetrate very far into the body, and is often used for the treatment of cancers on or near the surface, such as skin cancer. High-energy (or megavoltage) radiation penetrates more deeply and is used to treat most other forms of cancer. The rays can be narrowly focused to a site deep inside the body, which helps minimize side effects that may develop on the surface of the skin. In preparation for bone marrow transplantation, whole-body radiation may be used to eradicate cancer cells that have spread throughout the body.

The treatment regimen depends on the type and extent of cancer. In some cases, the entire dose of external radiation is administered at one time, but more often treatment involves a cycle. Doses are given 5 days a week and then followed by a weekend of rest; the pattern may be repeated for up to 8 weeks. Patients who receive radioactive implants or other forms of internal radiation therapy receive radiation 24 hours a day until the desired dose is given.

Although radiation is aimed at the tumor, it can also affect healthy cells near the tumor, as well as any cells through which it must penetrate to reach its target. Damage to healthy cells is responsible for the troublesome side effects of radiation treatment. While side effects are a possibility, many cancer patients experience none at all. The type and severity of side effects can range from mild to severe. A common reaction to external-beam radiation is weariness and lethargy. Other side effects the patient experiences depend on where the radiation is given. Some patients having treatments to their head or neck experience hair loss. The skin may darken or become dry, red, or itchy. Nausea and vomiting may develop; such problems often can be controlled with antinausea medication. If you are losing weight because radiation therapy is causing a lack of appetite and nausea, a nutritionist will become an important member of your cancer team (see page 1366).

Much progress has been made in protecting normal cells from the effects of radiation during radiation treatment; however, radiation still may cause some late effects or aftereffects. These effects may occur days, months, and sometimes years after your treatment is completed and usually affect the radiated regions of your body. The frequency of these problems varies depending on the dose and type of radiation. Examples of such effects include changes in circulation that may cause scarring or malfunctioning of an organ, scarring of the lungs or bowel, changes in the function of the thyroid, loss of normal cells from an organ, and changes in the skin including rashes. Extreme side effects include chronic disruption of bone marrow activity (bone marrow suppression) and, in rare cases, secondary cancers. Discuss the possibility of late effects with your doctor and contact your doctor if you notice any symptoms.

CHEMOTHERAPY

Chemotherapy involves the treatment of tumors with anticancer drugs. In a larger sense, any form of medicine involving chemicals is chemotherapy, but the term usually refers specifically to cancer treatment. Surgery, and in many cases, radiation, are local therapies—that is, they are designed to address cancer in a specific part of the body. In contrast, chemotherapy is referred to as systemic treatment, because it can affect the body's entire system, not just the target tissue where the cancer originally arose. The anticancer chemicals in a drug circulate in the bloodstream to reach tissues and cells that other forms of treatment may be unable to reach. For this reason, chemotherapy is often given to people whose tumors cannot be removed fully through surgery or radiation. It is also given to people whose cancer has metastasized. In other cases, chemotherapy is given as a strategy to prevent metastasis from occurring (referred to as adjuvant therapy), especially if there is a chance that a few cancer cells may have spilled into the bloodstream during an operation.

Chemotherapy generally refers to the use of cytotoxic chemicals, or chemicals that kill cells. Because cells go through various stages as they mature, the following different classes of chemotherapy agents may be prescribed depending on the type of tumor and what stage of growth its cells have reached.

- Alkylating agents prevent cells from dividing at any stage. Examples include cyclophosphamide (Cytoxan) and cisplatin (Platinol).

- Antimetabolites work by taking the place of nutrients a cell normally needs to survive, thus starving the cell to death. Examples include fluorouracil and methotrexate.

- Alkaloids interfere with division at specific stages of growth. Examples include vincristine (Oncovin), vinblastine (Velban), and taxol.

- Antitumor antibiotics destroy the DNA inside the cell's nucleus, thus blocking the cell's ability to make viable copies of itself. Examples include doxorubicin (Adriamycin) and bleomycin (Blenoxane).

Hormonal therapy—treatment that alters the activity of the body's chemical messengers—is another type of chemotherapy. Certain types of cancerous tumors, such as those that develop in the breast or the prostate, often depend on having a supply of hormones to grow. Blocking the activ-

ity of hormones can disrupt the growth or spread of the tumor. For example, tamoxifen is often prescribed for women whose breast cancer tumors contain large numbers of estrogen receptors. Tamoxifen attaches to the receptors and prevents the body's estrogen hormones from reaching the tumor and stimulating their growth.

Cytotoxic drugs are indiscriminate—that is, they kill healthy cells along with cancer cells. This is why chemotherapy can affect the entire body, not just the cancer it is meant to destroy. The systemic effect of chemotherapy is a double-edged sword; it is responsible both for the effectiveness of treatment and its often troublesome side effects.

The side effects of chemotherapy vary according to the treatment chosen and to the individual. While side effects are a distinct possibility in chemotherapy, many cancer patients encounter none at all, and very effective medication is available to minimize side effects such as nausea and vomiting. Common side effects of chemotherapy are hair loss, nausea, vomiting, and loss of appetite. Mouth sores, conjunctivitis (pinkage), runny nose and eyes, diarrhea, and constipation are also possible side effects. Severe side effects include chronic bone marrow suppression and, in rare cases, secondary cancers.

Fortunately, modern advances in chemotherapy have reduced the incidence and severity of side effects compared to the early days of anticancer drug treatment. Furthermore, there are several effective strategies available that can alleviate many of the discomforts associated with chemotherapy.

COPING WITH THE SIDE EFFECTS AND AFTEREFFECTS OF CHEMOTHERAPY

With the many advances in chemotherapy itself and in coping with the treatment's side effects, facing chemotherapy need not be the ordeal it once was. Having the right expectations and planning ahead are key to allaying your anxiety. To do this you will need to learn all you can about the drugs you will be taking.

Different drugs are responsible for different side effects. For example, the drug cyclophosphamide almost always causes nausea while tamoxifen does not. However, tamoxifen is often responsible for hot flashes. Doxorubicin generally causes hair loss while some other drugs may not. Discuss the drug you are taking with your doctor and research the drug further if you can. Knowing what to expect usually makes your symptoms easier to manage.

If your research indicates that the drug you are taking causes nausea, plan your meals around your treatment. It is a good idea to eat a very small meal just prior to your treatment and small but frequent meals after your treatment. You can also take medication to reduce nausea. Ondansetron (Zofran), for example, can be given by pill or intravenously before you start your chemotherapy regimen and continued afterwards. Also ask your doctor for a prescription for antinausea medication that you can use at home. Make sure to take the medication at the first sign of discomfort. Do not wait until you feel like you are going to be sick; then it is already too late for the medication to help. Prochlorperazine (Compazine) has been proven effective when taken at the earliest sign of discomfort.

Hair loss is still a common side effect of many chemotherapy drugs; the best way to cope with hair loss is to plan for it before it occurs. If you think that you will be uncomfortable wearing hats or scarves or simply being bald, shop for a wig before your treatment begins.

Try to make the actual treatment experience as tolerable as possible. If there is no music in the chemotherapy room at your hospital, bring your own and your headphones, too. Music, books-on-tape, or relaxation tapes may help to alleviate your anxiety and also to distract you from the unpleasant side effects you may anticipate.

IMMUNOTHERAPY

Immunotherapy involves enhancing the body's natural immune reaction toward cancer cells. The immune system is the body's policing system; it guards the body's health by recognizing and eliminating foreign substances that might pose a threat to the body. Lymphokines, normally produced by the white blood cells, are the biologic agents that form the basis for immunotherapy.

Interferon (a glycoprotein that exerts antiviral activity) is the best studied of these agents and is produced by the body in response to a viral infection. Interferon has proven remarkably effective in treating a rare form of leukemia called hairy cell leukemia. It has also provided some benefit in fighting certain types of lymph tissue cancer.

❖ ALTERNATIVE TREATMENTS

Surgery, chemotherapy, and radiation are all forms of what is often called traditional, mainstream, conventional, or standard medicine. Treatments that are currently being studied in controlled trials but whose benefits are not yet known are called experimental or investigational therapies (see page 1370). Other methods of treatment that have not been subjected to rigorous scientific study are often referred to as alternative or complementary treatments.

At this time, no alternative treatment has been proved to be an effective means of curing an existing cancer. For some people, alternative therapies may be helpful in relieving the stress and side effects of cancer treatment. As a rule, however, people who decide against pursuing their doctors' recommended, traditional treatments in favor of alternative treatments offered outside mainstream medicine are likely putting themselves at risk and making the cancer harder to treat later on. Unlike investigational therapies, which are carefully regulated and supervised, the techniques and medicines used in alternative medicine have not been approved for use on cancer patients.

Despite the lack of evidence that alternative treatments are effective in the fight against cancer, alternative cancer therapy is a multibillion dollar business. Those who champion alternative treatments tend to be well-meaning people who genuinely believe that their treatments will be helpful. Cancer patients who are emotionally distraught and who feel helpless are often susceptible to such claims. Even people who are knowledgable about the proven benefits of traditional treatments may spend thousands of dollars on useless therapies and remedies when they are diagnosed with cancer. Such desperation keeps the business of alternative treatment thriving, even though none of the therapies offered have any proven success. The vulnerability of the cancer patient is yet another reason why the support and guidance of the cancer team is invaluable during the course of cancer treatment.

Many practitioners of alternative medicine claim that their treatments have failed to receive the endorsement of the mainstream medical community because doctors fear the possible loss of revenue. In reality, the medical community as a whole is interested in arresting and curing cancer. Most practitioners will endorse any treatment methods that can be shown to offer measurable efficacy. The National Cancer Institute currently sponsors research on alternative treatments, including the use of natural herbal remedies. The National Institutes of Health maintains an Office of Alternative Medicine devoted to rigorous research into those practices that appear to be the most promising. Mainstream medicine is dedicated to exploring all avenues that may lead to a cure for cancer, but until results show that alternative methods work, doctors will be reluctant to endorse them.

When alternative treatments are used in conjunction with traditional radiation therapy or chemotherapy, positive results may be achieved in controlling nausea and boosting nutrition and in achieving a greater sense of personal well-being. In addition, many people report that techniques such as acupuncture, hypnosis, meditation, visualization, or yoga can help in coping with discomfort and pain. Hypnosis, for example, has been found to be effective in managing both the anxiety associated with chemotherapy and the nausea that accompanies treatments. Such therapies have also been found to be effective in relieving anxiety and depression and in helping the patient psychologically—all of which can help the patient in her battle with cancer.

Alternative treatment should be undertaken only in conjunction with traditional methods of treatment, including routine evaluation to measure the size of the cancer and whether it has spread. Discuss the risks and possible benefits of the alternative treatment with your oncologist. If your oncologist adamantly opposes the combination of an alternative therapy with your ongoing cancer treatment, you should consider giving up your plans for alternative therapy. If you are committed to doing both, the safest way to proceed is to find another reputable oncologist who will continue your treat-ment and monitor your alternative therapy to make sure it is not interfering with your conventional therapy.

When considering any alternative treatment, patients and their families should not be afraid to ask questions and should consult with their personal doctors. The following are important questions to ask if you are considering an alternative treatment:

- Is there any documented proof that this treatment has been effective for other cancer patients?
- What is the background and what are the credentials of the person who will be giving the treatment?
- Are there any risks or side effects from this treatment?

You should also be wary of any self-published reports that advertise the value of the treatment. Try instead to find out if the treatment has been described in qualified medical journals that subject their articles to review by experts (peer review) prior to publication. Also find out if the treatment is monitored by any regulatory agencies. As a general rule, alternative medicine clinics located outside the United States tend to offer forms of treatment that are ineffective or, worse, dangerous.

People with cancer have sought cures from alternative treatments for centuries. It is only in the past few decades, however, that large numbers of people with cancer have enjoyed full remission and long survival rates, and this recent success is due to advances in modern medicine.

DRUG TRIALS AND EXPERIMENTAL TREATMENTS

Cancer treatment centers and university hospitals are involved on a daily basis not only in treating people with cancer but also in exploring experimental treatments in the laboratory and in clinical trials of new treatments. The opportunity to be involved in clinical trials of new treatments (also called investigative therapies) is first offered to people who have not been helped by any conventional treatment. The decision to participate in a clinical trial is a personal one that you should make with the help of your cancer team. If you are healthy except for the diagnosed cancer, and your prognosis with standard therapy is considered poor, participating in a clinical trial may be the right choice for you. Since clinical trials are often small, not all people who wish to participate may have the opportunity to do so.

The following are the four phases of clinical trials.

Phase 1 trials involve new drugs and other remedies and are offered to people who have not benefitted from traditional treatment. Such trials may be risky as they can involve chemicals whose toxicity level in humans has yet to be determined. The trials are small, usually including between 10 to 20 patients, and are used to determine the appropriate drug dosage and schedule and to observe possible side effects. These are the riskiest trials and are only appropriate where traditional therapy has failed.

Phase 2 trials determine the responsiveness of a tumor to a new therapy. These trials are also small (including between 20 to 40 patients) and involve people with a single kind of advanced cancer.

Phase 3 trials become necessary when a preliminary trial indicates that a new therapy may be more promising in treating patients than the therapy currently used. This type of trial compares the standard treatment to the experimental treatment to see which is more effective.

Phase 4 trials are important in readying a new treatment for general use once it has already been found to be more effective than the traditional treatment.

Among the experimental therapies currently being investigated are the use of biologicals and monoclonal antibodies. Biologicals are natural products obtained from living organisms. These substances are first isolated and then cloned for administration in large doses to patients. The purpose of biologicals is to stimulate or manipulate the immune system to mobilize its efforts to fight cancer. At present the studies of biologicals are purely investigative, but the hope is that biologicals will prove to be instrumental new weapons in controlling and curing cancer. Monoclonal antibodies are genetically engineered substances that have the ability to find and attach themselves to cancer cells. Monoclonal antibodies can be helpful in determining whether a cancer has spread to other sites in the body. Researchers hope that in the future these antibodies can be attached to anticancer

drugs to facilitate carrying the drugs directly to the cells they are targeted to destroy, thereby reducing systemic side effects that occur because of the destruction of healthy cells.

For information about current clinical trials call (800) 4-CANCER.

RELIEF OF CANCER-RELATED PAIN

Some cancers are silent cancers that give almost no warning of their presence prior to diagnosis, some cancers may cause little or no pain, and other cancers and many cancer treatments cause at least temporary and sometimes chronic pain. About a third of the patients who undergo ongoing treatment will experience severe pain.

What kind of pain you experience depends on you as an individual, the type of cancer that you have, and the stage of the cancer. Your pain may be constant or intermittent, dull or aching, mild or severe. The severity of pain can change over time.

As with all aspects of your cancer treatment, it is important to take an active role in how your pain is treated. If and when you begin to suffer pain, keep a record of the type of pain you are feeling and what time of day and night you are suffering pain. Share this information with your cancer team on a continuing basis. Never suffer cancer pain in silence or assume that there is no way to alleviate it. Not only will your personal analysis of your pain help you get the appropriate pain relief, it will also help doctors to identify if your pain is from pressure from the tumor on a nerve or a blocked internal organ. This information can help avoid unwanted cancer complications.

Many treatments are available to relieve pain. Mild discomfort may be relieved by acetaminophen and other non-narcotic painkillers. NSAIDs (nonsteroidal anti-inflammatory drugs, such as aspirin or ibuprofen) are also excellent pain relievers. People who find aspirin alone inadequate to relieve pain may be prescribed aspirin or acetaminophen with codeine, which can be extremely effective in relieving most mild to moderate cancer pain. If your pain is more severe, stronger narcotics such as morphine may be prescribed, but they will be administered carefully. Some patients are afraid that if they take narcotics they will become addicted or tolerant to the medication and that it will not be effective when they need it. These fears are unfounded because the chance of addiction has been shown to be very low and the medication remains effective. The importance of pain relief should outweigh any concerns about addiction. Antidepressants in combination with narcotics may also be effective in controlling severe pain without significantly impairing mental ability. In some cases of severe pain tranquilizers may also be used. Tranquilizers do not relieve pain, but they improve a person's ability to tolerate the pain. Nerve blockers may also be used to relieve severe pain arising from specific nerves. In advanced cases of pain, it is important for family members, as well as the patient, to insist that morphine, methadone, or other opiates be prescribed in sufficient doses to relieve the pain. If you are not getting the relief you need, make your situation known.

WEIGHT LOSS IN CANCER

Many cancer patients suffer from extreme weight loss, which is known as wasting or cachexia. Researchers have recently identified a chemical released by tumors that seems to cause the wasting by breaking down muscle and fatty tissue. Wasting is a serious illness itself; in some cases, it is the wasting rather than the cancer that causes the death of a patient. In addition, cancer treatment often interferes with a person's appetite and ability to swallow foods and liquids. Treatment can also disrupt the ability to digest food and absorb nutrients. As a result, a nutritionist is almost always a part of the cancer team.

The lack of interest in eating and drinking is something that should be addressed by the medical staff and members of the cancer team, particularly when a patient is undergoing intense therapy. If you suffer from loss of appetite or nausea, it is important that you get help from nutritional supplements to stem your weight loss and to make sure you are getting the vitamins and nutrients you need to help restore your body to health.

In many cases dehydration is a more acute problem than weight loss. Both you and your cancer team must be vigilant in monitoring your intake of liquids during chemotherapy or other treatment. If you are

home from the hospital after a treatment and you find that you cannot manage to drink the necessary amount of liquid, a family member should notify your doctor who will probably give you intravenous fluids to hydrate you until you are able to hold liquids down.

When you have an appetite, a diet rich in fresh fruits and vegetables, high in protein, and low in saturated fats and that includes complex carbohydrates (legumes and grains as well as fresh vegetables) while minimizing simple carbohydrates (sugars and starchy foods) is the most healthful. During your chemotherapy cycles, however, you'll probably find most of these foods unpalatable and you will be advised to maintain your weight with foods you can tolerate, such as ice cream and other soft foods, particularly if you have trouble chewing or swallowing. Frequent, small meals during the day will also be recommended. With recent nutritional advances, including the ready availability of protein powders and liquid supplements, the problem of weight loss during cancer treatment has become manageable in most cases. Once again, what is most important is that you, the patient, are vigilant about your nutritional needs and problems. Keep a record of what you are able to eat and drink during the day and keep track of your bowel habits and share the information with your doctor and family. If you have trouble swallowing or your mouth is sore or if you have chronic indigestion, be sure to discuss it with your cancer team (see Chapter 1).

DEALING WITH THE COMPLICATIONS OF CANCER

Cancer is often an aggressive disease, and cancer treatment is frequently aggressive as well. This takes its toll on the patient's body and as a result, cancer emergencies and complications may occur. Cancer emergencies require immediate treatment, and this treatment takes precedence over the treatment for the cancer itself. Common emergencies that may occur in cases of advanced cancer include intestinal obstruction, which is a frequent complication of colon cancer, pressure of the tumor on other organs, and spinal cord compression. Metabolic imbalances, such as a dangerously high calcium level, can develop. In advanced cases of cancer, internal bleeding may also occur.

When you are diagnosed with cancer, you should discuss possible emergency symptoms with your doctor and keep a list of what to watch for during cancer treatment. Being able to identify a symptom early will help save precious time in an emergency.

MANAGING THE FINANCIAL COSTS OF CANCER

Treating cancer is expensive, and in many cases your insurance carrier will not cover certain risky or experimental treatments. The first step in assuring that your cancer costs do not get out of hand is to check with your insurance company regarding your policy as soon as you are diagnosed. If facing the tedious task of tracking down a person to talk to in a resistant bureaucracy seems overwhelming to you, assign a family member or a member of your cancer team to help out. When you are interviewing doctors, one of your questions should always be how insurance coverage will be handled.

One way of keeping track of the cost of your treatment is to make discussing treatment costs part of the agenda for you and your cancer team on a monthly basis. Any changes in therapy that may affect your insurance coverage and other issues should be discussed at this meeting. Though your cancer treatment is and should be your priority, the issue of financial costs will only become more difficult to handle if the subject is postponed or avoided.

If you are part of a managed care plan you will probably need to obtain a second opinion before beginning your treatment. Many plans will also require that you receive treatment from an in network doctor (a doctor who accepts your insurance plan). If you see a doctor who is out of network, you may have to obtain a referral by an in network doctor. Many managed care plans cover all costs of chemotherapy and other cancer treatment except for your copayment. However, it is a good idea to review your policy and discuss it with a representative of your plan before you choose a doctor or begin treatment.

Sometimes during the course of treatment an insurance company may revise the list of doctors and hospitals it covers, thus leaving you in a situation where your oncologist is no longer covered. Most cancer patients find the proposition of funding such expensive treatment daunting, if not impossible, but before you change doctors you should find out the following information:

- Is there a particular expertise your doctor provides that would qualify for out-of-network coverage by your insurance company?

- Will your insurance company pay a portion of your medical fees if you continue to see your doctor?

- Can you influence your doctor to stay in the plan or your company to continue coverage until the end of your treatment?

If you find that you must change doctors, ask your current doctor for recommendations and discuss recommendations with other cancer patients who use the same insurance company. See below for more information on insurance and health plan issues.

If at any time during your treatment a claim has been unfairly rejected by your insurance company, you should resubmit the claim. If it is rejected again, you can request an explanation from your insurance company for the rejection. You may also ask your doctor to write a letter to the insurance company describing your medical condition and the treatment you have been receiving.

MANAGING INSURANCE ISSUES

If you are having trouble with your insurance company or if you have been dropped by your carrier and are having trouble getting insurance, the following is a listing of organizations that can assist you:

- The National Coalition for Cancer Survivorship. Staff members are devoted to helping members cope with insurance problems. Phone (301) 650–8868

- The Cancer Information Service's toll-free hotline will provide information and further sources. Phone: (800) 4CANCER

- The local division of the American Cancer Society will provide information regarding state and local laws and regulations and inform you of your rights as a patient.

- Your local insurance agent can advise you.

- "What You Should Know about Health Insurance" is a pamphlet published by The Health Insurance Association of America. You can obtain the pamphlet by writing to The Health Insurance Association of America, 1850 K St. NW, Washington, DC 20006.

Living With Cancer

Studies show that patients who take charge of their therapy by seeking proper treatment, asking questions, and participating in the decision-making process cope best over the long term. Managing cancer is a long-term proposition, and your emotional and physical endurance are of the utmost importance. Work in tandem with your cancer team, including your nutritionist, to establish short-term and long-term goals and to devise a modest exercise plan you can follow, even if in only limited fashion at first. For example, lightweight free weights may be used to strengthen muscle tone even if your mobility is impaired (see Chapter 2).

To maintain as positive an outlook as possible you will need the help of family and friends. While many cancer sufferers choose not to share their fears and discomfort with others for fear of upsetting them, such a strategy may have the opposite effect. Your friends and family want to know how you are feeling and what they can do to help. Sharing your condition with them will help them feel less helpless, and it will help you get the support you need. Just as taking an interest in your treatment will help garner the most positive results, remaining interested in life will help you maintain the most positive attitude possible. If you are bedridden for a time, you may want to consider reading the books or magazines you never managed to find time for. Maintaining a favorite hobby or taking up a new one, returning to work as soon as you are able, or simply taking a walk outside every day are all helpful strategies in remaining interested in and enjoying life. Relaxation and meditation techniques may also be helpful in stabilizing your mood (see page 1369). Maintaining a sense of well-being will be invaluable in facilitating your long-term cancer treatment.

LONG-TERM REHABILITATION AND RECOVERY

In many cases, life after cancer is different from the life one lived before cancer. For some people life is different because they must learn new ways of talking or walking or even of eliminating bodily waste. But rehabilitation after cancer must be psychological as well as physical. The body has undergone a harrowing experience and so has the mind, and lingering fears about the recurrence of cancer are inevitable. Many of the cancer patients who survive 5 years or more and are considered cured are haunted by such reminders and need help adjusting to the changes in their lives that cancer has caused. The purpose of rehabilitation is to help those who survive cancer achieve the best quality of life possible.

In 1952 the first cancer rehabilitation program, the International Association of Laryngectomies, was founded. This organization was dedicated to teaching new ways of speaking to people who had had their larynxes removed. Reach to Recovery was also founded in the 1950s and was dedicated to helping women cope with mastectomy. Now there are programs for amputees, colostomy and ileostomy patients, and those who are terminally ill. Many of these programs are staffed by volunteers who are cancer survivors themselves. They have first-hand experience that can be extremely helpful in coping with the disease.

The goal of every rehabilitation program is to help the cancer survivor function as well as possible. While most cancer survivors return to work, some lose their jobs because certain employers are reluctant to hire cancer survivors because they fear that the disease might return or that a person's productivity will be affected. One of the goals of rehabilitation centers is to change this misperception by sharing the results of recent studies that show that cancer survivors often have better work records than those who have never suffered from cancer. Legislation has recently been passed that supports this goal by pre-

SUPPORT GROUPS FOR CANCER SURVIVORS

Anyone can create a support group simply by talking with others who are suffering from the same disease. Sharing your big fears and little problems can offer not only tremendous relief but also vital information. While many people are initially reluctant to talk with strangers about what they are going through, joining a cancer support group usually becomes invaluable to cancer patients and cancer survivors. Sharing your feelings about what you are going through will help to alleviate your sense of isolation and help you cope. Your support group can also be a valuable resource for tips on managing your cancer therapy and guidance in choosing specialists as well as advice on coping with the side effects of your treatment.

The American Cancer Society sponsors many support groups nationwide; information may be obtained through your local American Cancer Society chapter or by calling (800) ACS-2345. You can also start your own support group (see page 1354). Sharing your experience can be invaluable in helping you manage your recovery. ■

venting job discrimination against former cancer patients.

In the past 2 decades cancer rehabilitation has made tremendous strides so that now rehabilitation services are available in most communities and included as part of cancer treatment itself. As cancer treatments become more sophisticated and effective, so does our knowledge of the need for physical and psychological rehabilitation after treatment. Now rehabilitation is considered essential to a patient's full recovery.

WHEN CANCER RECURS

The fear of recurrence often haunts cancer survivors. Like the sword of Damocles, it hovers permanently and sometimes it curtails the ability to appreciate the daily pleasures of life. That you have a history of cancer is a fact that cannot be changed; what can be changed is how you choose to live with it.

To help manage your fear it is important to remind yourself that just as a diagnosis of cancer is not a death sentence, neither is a recurrence of cancer. It is also important to face the fact that you are afraid. To be afraid is natural; to cope with your fear by facing it is to take control. Once you have learned to manage your fear of recurrence, that fear can actually work to your advantage by motivating you to be vigilant in pursuing follow-up care.

Vigilant care can minimize the risk of recurrence and the seriousness of a recurrence, particularly in certain cancers such as colon cancer and breast cancer. In the case of colon cancer, for example, a yearly colonoscopy to check for precancerous polyps lowers the risk of recurrence significantly.

While the desire to put off an unpleasant, though necessary, screening procedure is a natural one, delaying such a test will not delay the recurrence of the disease. If cancer cells are multiplying in your body once again, they do so whether or not you see your doctor. Hiding from this reality wastes precious time and only worsens the problem, which should be tackled sooner rather than later to ensure the best outcome. Obtaining a clean bill of health after a screening procedure may help to remind you that not every bruise or cough is a sign of cancer.

Sometimes medication may be used to help prevent the occurrence of a second cancer that is different from a person's first cancer. Treatment involving use of chemotherapy as a primary preventive measure is called chemoprophylaxis. Prevention of both primary and secondary cancers through the use of drugs is an exciting new area of cancer research, and trials are now underway to confirm which medications offer the best protection. Adjuvant tamoxifen, for example, has been shown to prevent the recurrence of breast cancer as well as the development of a new (primary) breast cancer in the unaffected breast.

HOSPICE CARE

Nearly half of all cases of cancer do end in death. Many people are reluctant to discuss death openly: the person who is terminally ill may want to spare family members, and family members wish to protect the person who is dying from further concern. The hospice movement was designed both to help families face death and the questions and conflicts it involves and to give the patient the maximum degree of comfort possible. A hospice is defined as a facility that provides physical, emotional, social, and spiritual care for the dying and for their families. Hospice support may be offered in a separate area of a hospital, a separate facility altogether, or at home. In other words, what a hospice offers can be provided anywhere there is a need and there are sensitive, well-trained people who can supply the required support (see Chapter 35).

Cancer in Children

Fortunately, cancer is rare in children, but when it does occur the impact on everyone involved is profound. What is heartening, however, is that the greatest progress in curing cancer has been made in curing those cancers that affect children. As recently as 2 decades ago, most children diagnosed with cancer died from it within a year. While cancer is still responsible for more deaths in preschool and school-age children than any other disease, today at least half of all American children diagnosed with cancer survive it, and in the case of acute lymphoblastic leukemia, the most common leukemia in children, the cure rate is approximately 80 percent.

Leukemia is the most common childhood cancer, followed by cancer of the brain or brain tumors. Other cancers in children include kidney cancer, bone cancer, soft tissue sarcomas, and lymphomas. The causes for these cancers are still not known, although certain chemicals (such as benzene), viruses (such as HTLV), and medication are suspected of altering the genetic material of healthy cells and putting children at greater risk for cancer. Retinoblastoma, a rare cancer of the retina, also occurs in children, particularly under the age of 3. When diagnosed and treated early, retinoblastoma is curable approximately 80 percent of the time. About half of all cases of retinoblastoma are hereditary.

DIAGNOSIS AND TREATMENT

Usually the family doctor or pediatrician first discovers cancer in a child. The doctor—who may often suspect anemia—does a blood test and identifies the cancer. Your child's doctor will then help you choose a cancer center for your child's treatment. It is generally recommended that the child be treated at a specialized cancer center because all cancers in children are special and often complicated situations. A child with cancer has the best chance of receiving the most effective, state-of-the-art treatment at a cancer center, a children's hospital, or a large, university affiliated hospital (see page 1365).

If your child has been diagnosed with cancer and you live far away from an appropriate cancer center, you will still be able to get the help you need by initiating the treatment at a cancer center and then continuing treatment with a local doctor. The cancer treatment will be planned, initiated, and then supervised by the staff of the cancer center in conjunction with your local doctor, with periodic visits to the cancer center when necessary. In addition, if your child's treatment necessitates ongoing chemotherapy, your local doctor can learn to administer the chemotherapy and do the necessary bloodwork so that your child's life will be disrupted as little as possible.

A pediatric oncology team usually consists of a primary oncologist, other doctors, nurses, social workers, and clergy, when appropriate, all of whom are skilled in coping with serious illness in children. Members of this team will help you with the emotional issues surrounding the disease and treatment. Children need to be assured both by their parents and the doctors they see most frequently that everything possible is being done to make them well and that the pain of treatment is temporary and necessary to help them get better. While children need to be told the truth, they also need such statements to be simple and comforting and to have them repeated often for reassurance and to maintain their sense of security.

You, as a parent, can help your child immeasurably during treatment by being both informed and vigilant. As excellent as any pediatric oncology team may be, it is important to remember that you are the only continuous source of care for your child. Shifts may change, residents may go off rotation, but you or your spouse or other family member will always be there. You will know better than anyone whether or not your child had the medication she was supposed to have had 2 hours ago. The more constant your involvement, the more confident you will feel about your child's treatment.

PSYCHOLOGICAL EFFECTS ON THE CHILD AND THE FAMILY

It is never easy when a child is seriously ill, but it is particularly devastating when a child gets cancer. If you or someone you know is facing the diagnosis of cancer in a child, the most important thing to realize is that cancer affects the child not only physically but emotionally as well and that the entire family will be in crisis. This happens to all families when a child gets cancer, and all families need at least some help in coping.

When a child is diagnosed with cancer and a treatment plan is initiated, a psychiatric social worker is usually part of the cancer team. The social worker works with the child and the child's family during the initial treatment in the hospital and throughout the course of treatment. Many parents are particularly grateful for help in structuring how they will talk about the disease with their child. In many cases, more personal and intensive help may be necessary for a child or the child's family, and the social worker can help in finding the appropriate therapist or counselor for the family.

The child with cancer needs ongoing help in sharing her feelings and fears and in coping with the physical discomforts of treatment. If there are other children in the family, they too will need support in managing the new situation. In addition to coping with feelings of fear and concern for their sister or brother, your other children often feel some resentment toward their sibling who is getting all the attention and they may become withdrawn and isolated if attention is not paid to their needs. This is a tall order for parents who are struggling with the early stages of their child's cancer treatment. For these reasons, the ongoing involvement of the social worker or a therapist is recommended. Family counseling can prove instrumental in making the transition from the hospital back home a smooth one and in facilitating the child's return to school and reentry into normal activities.

WARNING SIGNS IN CHILDREN

As with cancer in adults, often there are no warning signs when a child gets cancer, particularly for leukemia, the most common childhood cancer. However, there may be symptoms that can be indicative of certain cancers that parents should be aware of and that may necessitate further investigation by a doctor.

Leukemia In some cases, anemia may be diagnosed prior to the diagnosis of leukemia. A child may complain of bone or joint pain or back pain in the early stages of leukemia. Often complaints such as lethargy and a general, aching, rundown feeling, like that prior to a flu, may be the symptoms that cause parents to take a child to the doctor. If a general blood test indicates anemia, the doctor may suspect leukemia and may do further bloodwork. Excessive bruising and chronic nosebleeds and fevers and infections, such as a sore throat that lingers, may also be symptoms of leukemia. In children, enlarged lymph nodes, spleen, or liver are indications of leukemia, as are skin lesions and swollen or bleeding gums.

Retinoblastoma Symptoms of retinoblastoma include a yellow or white spot in the pupil or crossed eyes (strabismus). Approximately 50 percent of all cases of retinoblastoma affect both eyes.

Brain Tumors A brain tumor or tumors can cause extremely diverse symptoms. If the tumor is increasing the pressure on the brain, headaches, blurred vision, vomiting, and a lack of mental acuity may be indicative of a tumor, although sometimes there are almost no symptoms. If a tumor has begun to destroy parts of the brain that regulate certain functions such as motor control or language, signs of dysfunction in these areas will probably occur. While these symptoms in adults may indicate other conditions, such as stroke, such symptoms in children are more likely to indicate a tumor, although sometimes they may be caused by an infection or a subdural hematoma (hemorrhage) caused by head trauma. ∎

HELPING CHILDREN THROUGH SURGERY AND CHEMOTHERAPY

Chemotherapy for childhood leukemia is a long-term proposition that often lasts as much as 2 years or more. During this time numerous side effects may occur and adjustments in the therapy regimen may have to be made. The side effect that causes the most concern for many children is hair loss. While the quality of wigs keeps improving, many children feel uncomfortable wearing a wig and would rather wear a cap, which often makes them feel more at ease with their friends and classmates at school.

Other side effects that may occur and recur during the course of treatment include nausea, vomiting, weight loss, stomach pains, constipation, muscular aches, and severe nosebleeds. Pain is also a common side effect of chemotherapy. Fortunately, successful relief of pain is a major focus of cancer treatment in children. Usually, morphine drips are administered during the chemotherapy treatment. The steroids used in some treatment courses may cause extreme mood swings in the child, a side effect for which many parents are not adequately prepared.

A child who is undergoing an intensive, long-term course of chemotherapy is at increased risk for any and all infections. When the child returns to school, the school should be made aware of this increased risk. A child with cancer should not be exposed to children who may have a fever, a cold, or any possible virus. Exposure to chickenpox is extremely dangerous for a child with cancer.

Parents can help their child endure the rigors of cancer care by offering comfort and reassurance and by being vigilant in monitoring the child's treatment. Parents can be instrumental in managing side effects such as constipation, chronic nose bleeds, and muscle soreness before they become serious problems. It is also the parents who will have the most insight into how much pain or discomfort their child is suffering, as well as how to seek relief for the child.

As with adults, rehabilitation forms an important part of a child's treatment. Since children are often on chemotherapy for 2 years, rehabilitation efforts begin during treatment to help the child cope with reentering school and making the transition back into her normal activities with the limitations her therapy may necessitate. Children often encounter difficulties returning to school and other activities, particularly when they are not allowed to swim or join in other physical activities because of either a surgically inserted line for chemotherapy treatments or overall weakness and muscle soreness. Rehabilitation efforts for children include offering counseling to the teachers and to parents of other children in the school the child attends and coming up with a daily game plan that includes school activities that will be substituted for gym class or other classes in which the child may not be able to participate. Paying attention to the feelings and questions of the child's schoolmates and teachers can make a child's reentry into school positive not only for the child, but for all of those in the school system who want to know what they may be able to do to help.

LONG-TERM EFFECTS ON GROWTH AND DEVELOPMENT

Growth Cancer therapy in children may affect growth in two different ways: either by damaging hormone producing glands or by affecting the lengthening of the bones themselves. Both kinds of damage can be caused by deep x-ray treatment to the brain or spinal cord. The higher the dose, the greater the chance for damage. In children surviving leukemia, growth hormone deficiency occurs in approximately 10 to 20 percent of those receiving deep x-ray treatment. Children who have had brain tumors have a much higher incidence of effects on growth and development.

Development Cancer therapy may also cause other hormone producing glands to malfunction including the pituitary, the thyroid, and the reproductive organs. Damage to the sex organs may cause either early puberty or delayed puberty. Children whose development has been affected are treated with hormone therapy, which is highly effective.

Fertility Male fertility may be affected by cancer therapy while female fertility, depending on the age of the child, usually is not. Boys who have undergone testicular radiation therapy become sterile. Many boys who have undergone a full course of treatment for leukemia are often subfertile and will have difficulty fathering children later in life.

Intellectual damage X-ray treatment of the brain in very young children may impair intellectual development depending on the dose of radiation and other factors. Research has shown that these children remain mildly to moderately mentally handicapped, although basic bodily functions are not impaired. Older children are usually not affected by x-ray treatment, although in rare cases they do suffer intellectual damage to a lesser degree. Sometimes older children also develop seizures.

Other organ damage In some treatments involving anthracyclines, damage to the heart muscle may occur. Anthracyclines are powerful antileukemic agents that kill many types of cells and, at higher doses, damage the heart muscle. This side effect is usually observed years later in severe breathlessness and swollen ankles when strain is put on the circulatory system. Other organs that may be damaged by chemotherapy or radiation therapy are the kidneys, lungs, liver, and bowels. However, none of these problems are common.

Second cancers When children survive one cancer they are often put at increased risk for developing another form of cancer later in life. This predisposition occurs because of the paradox inherent in both chemotherapy and radiation therapy: That which cures cancer can also cause cancer. A genetic factor may also be involved. While the role of heredity in causing second cancers is still speculative, that of chemotherapy and radiation therapy is very real.

5

PART FIVE

Becoming *a* Partner *in* Your Health Care

THIRTY-ONE

Taking Charge of Your Health Care

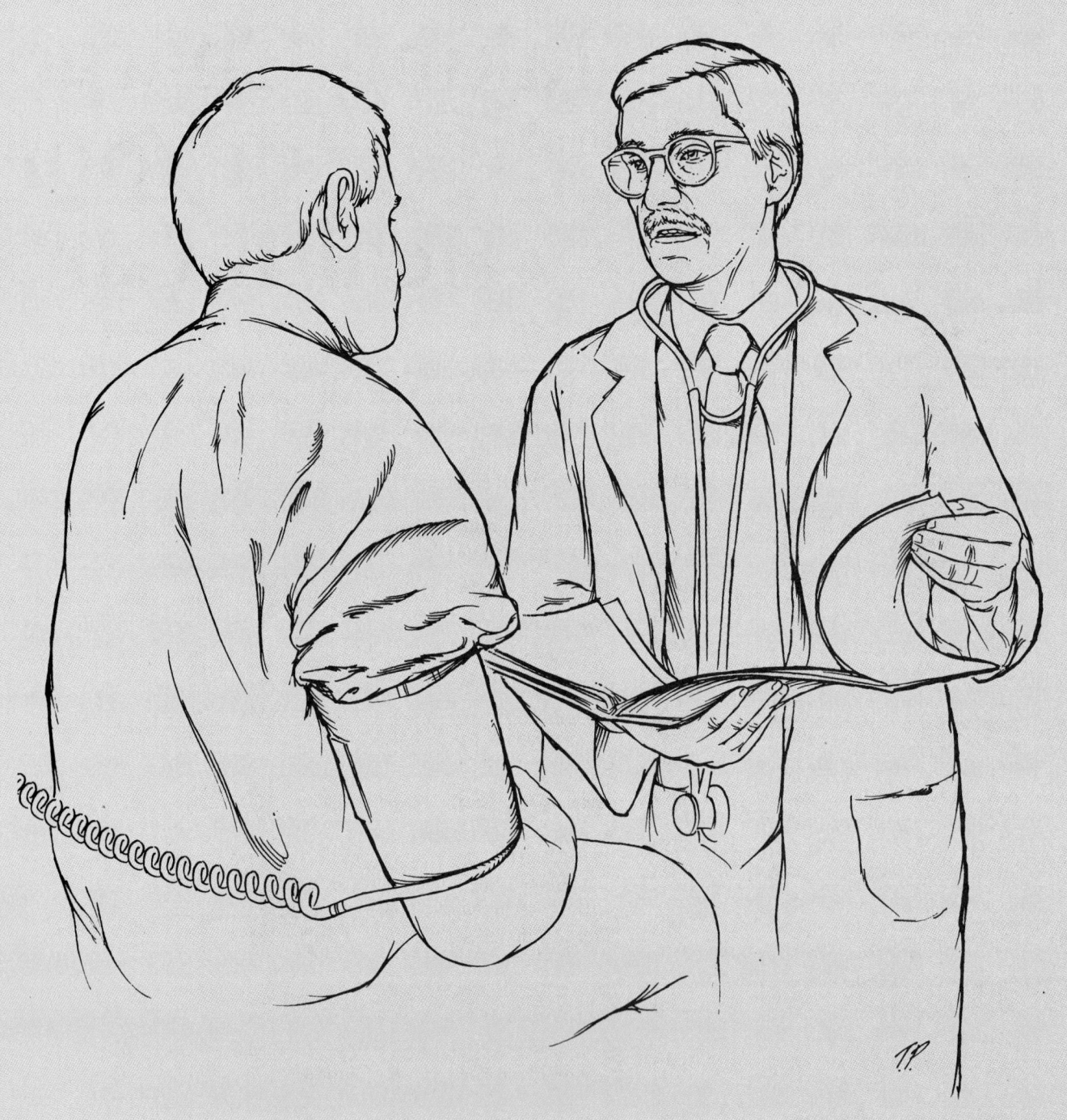

TAKING CHARGE OF YOUR HEALTH CARE

The Changing Health Care Scene

Advances in medical science and public health have transformed disease prevention and treatment in this country and as a result, most people lead longer and healthier lives. Someone born in the United States in 1920 had a life expectancy of 54.1 years; today Americans are born expecting a life 2 full decades longer, with reduced risk of illness from many diseases that once threatened quality of life.

These advances have translated into a technologically sophisticated system of medical care that would not be recognizable to even the most far-seeing of our grandparents and great-grandparents. It is sometimes a little harder to understand that not only has the science of medicine changed but so, too, have the organization and delivery of medical care.

Several interrelated factors, including economics and the aging of our population, have played a large part in fueling the changes in the health care system. With people living on average two decades longer, increased demands are made of medical resources. State-of-the-art technology is expensive, and the skyrocketing costs of medical care demand a hard look at how medical dollars are spent. This scrutiny has resulted in an upheaval that has been difficult both for the public—the health care consumers—and the medical practitioners who provide the care.

Sometimes these changes can seem confusing and even disturbing. No longer can we count on the comfortable notion of the family doctor who knows us personally, who treated our families, and who is familiar with our medical histories and life circumstances. The Marcus Welby type of doctor who makes house calls has become a rarity today. This is no longer an efficient way to practice modern medicine, which often relies on documentation, supervision, and access to equipment and technology. Today doctors are more likely to be members of large groups and organizations than the independent private doctors who were once the bedrock of primary health care. The health insurance plan that your employer offers may necessitate that you switch doctors, change from one group to another, or become a member of a health maintenance organization (HMO).

HMOs and the concepts of managed care they are based on are gradually changing the way medical care is delivered in this country. In 1997, three-quarters of working Americans with health coverage and more than 5 million Medicare recipients received their health care from some sort of managed care organization, and the number continues to grow.

This chapter explains what is meant by managed care and shows the different faces it can assume. It is necessary to understand the changes that are taking place and what they mean for you in order to take charge of your health care, learn the options that are available, and make the best decisions for you and your family.

UNDERSTANDING PREVENTIVE CARE

Prevention of illness and disease—including early detection to prevent disease progression—is one of the key principles in our evolving health care system.

But health care—always imbued with the goals of saving and improving lives—has adopted the companion goal of being cost-effective. Managed care is based on the premise that the most economical health care is that which prevents disease. There is no doubt that prevention saves money. Studies have found, for example, that for every dollar spent on school-based tobacco, drug, alcohol, and sexuality education programs, $14 is saved in avoided health care costs. Other examples abound. Immunizations against common childhood diseases save the expense of treating those diseases. Diabetes education programs save the costs of treatment of the many potential serious complications of diabetes.

According to the National Health Information Center, half of all deaths in the United States result from preventable or controllable risk factors. These include smoking, poor nutrition, sedentary lifestyle, alcohol or other drug misuse, unprotected sexual intercourse, and inadequate health care services. As the growing body of medical research has pinpointed these factors and linked their effects, a large focus of primary care medicine has shifted to preventive care.

Never before has medicine had so many techniques, strategies, and interventions to offer people who want to take an active role in the promotion of their own health. The idea of prevention has permeated our health institutions. Preventive medicine has now become a specific medical specialty, like surgery or cardiology. The US Public Health Service sponsors an Office of Disease Prevention and Health Promotion. The Centers for Disease Control recently changed its name to the Centers for Disease Control and Prevention.

At the start of this book, we looked at ways people can lay the foundation for disease prevention and a healthy life with good nutrition and physical activity (see Chapters 1 and 2). Nothing is more important in taking charge of your health than these two components of daily life. We also looked at safety measures everyone can take to lower the risk of illness or injury (see Chapter 3) as well as at substances to avoid that can substantially increase your risk for diseases (see Chapters 4 and 5). But there is also a multitude of resources for prevention that are delivered through the health care system, and this chapter will provide you with tips and strategies for negotiating the system in a manner that will best take advantage of these resources.

There are many areas where prevention is still neglected, both by individuals and medical professionals. One of the most important strategies for disease prevention is education—simply talking with your doctor about personal health habits such as smoking, diet, exercise, drinking, injury prevention, and sexual practices. As we explain throughout this chapter how to optimize your health care, we will also give you specific tips for communicating with your doctor to help her assess as accurately as possible what your risks are and how to minimize them.

Prevention is classified in three categories: primary, secondary, and tertiary. Primary prevention gets in on the ground floor by preventing a disease or disability from ever occurring. One example of primary prevention is immunization against the diseases of childhood (see page 194). Another is stopping cigarette smoking—or never starting—to prevent the development of cardiovascular or lung diseases (see Chapter 4). Another widely publicized means of primary disease prevention is the use of condoms to prevent the spread of sexually transmitted diseases (see page 860).

Secondary prevention is an intervention that occurs in the early stages of a disease, before any symptoms are apparent. Screening tests are one example of secondary prevention; mammograms and Pap smears are tests that can detect breast and cervical cancer before a woman can feel a lump in her breast or has any symptoms of gynecologic abnormalities. Another example of secondary prevention is weight reduction for an overweight person with impaired glucose tolerance. In this case, the intervention could prevent diabetes.

Tertiary prevention means preventing a disease from progressing, or preventing complications from a chronic disease. For example, careful monitoring and tight control of blood glucose levels by the person with diabetes will prevent the blindness, kidney failure, amputations, and cardiovascular problems that can be associated with poorly controlled diabetes. Physical and occupational therapy for stroke victims can prevent further muscular deterioration.

Screening tests, such as the mammogram and Pap smear mentioned above, are an important component of preventive care. These tests are discussed in detail throughout this book in the context of the various diseases they screen for. In the section of this chapter about the physical exam, we will give you a list of screening tests and recommendations for when they should be used. And the physical exam itself, which will be described in detail, is one of the most important elements of preventive health care.

Before we discuss the exam, however, we will look at who will be providing your health and medical care.

Who Are the Caregivers?

As you proceed through the health care system, you will interact with a variety of personnel who will each have a certain role to fulfill in the delivery of care. Your initial contacts will probably be with a primary care doctor. Primary care is the point of entry and the foundation of managed care systems, so it might be helpful to understand just what this phrase means.

The Institute of Medicine defines primary care as "the provision of integrated, accessible health care services by clinicians who are accountable for addressing a large majority of personal health care needs, developing a sustained partnership with patients, and practicing in the context of family and community."

The American Academy of Family Doctors emphasizes that primary care is an inclusive discipline that covers health promotion and maintenance, disease prevention, counseling, patient education, and treatment of acute and chronic illnesses in a variety of settings (see page 1413). Mental health as well as physical health is in the domain of the primary care doctor. Another important role of the primary care doctor is patient advocacy. Ideally, the philosophy of primary care is to encourage open doctor-patient communication and to consider the individual as a partner in health care.

PRIMARY CARE DOCTORS

We use the phrase "primary care doctor" to refer to the person who has traditionally been known as a family doctor. While the primary care doctor is a generalist who is trained to provide care for a broad variety of needs, she is no longer the general practitioner of years past. A primary care doctor has specialty training in one of the following disciplines.

Family practice Family practice is the contemporary version of general practice, and the family practitioner is a generalist who provides comprehensive care for all members of a family without limitations due to age, gender, organ system, or type of health problem. But family practice is now a specialty in its own right, with specific training in a three-year residency program, accreditation, and certification. The family practice doctor is trained to treat each family member in the context of the family and the community. With this comprehensive role, family doctors will usually perform the basic functions of the internist, the pediatrician, the gynecologist, and the psychiatrist. They will not delve too deeply into these specialties, however, as referral for specialty care is an important function for the family doctor or any other primary care doctor.

Pediatrics Pediatricians are doctors who care for children and teenagers in every stage of development, from infancy to adulthood. Like family doctors, pediatricians evaluate children and adolescents in the context of their families and are often involved with behavioral and social as well as strictly medical issues. Just as in adult medicine, there are many pediatric subspecialities for diseases and organ systems and for surgery and psychiatry. A residency in general pediatrics lasts 3 years.

Internal medicine Internists or internal medicine specialists treat the wide range of nonsurgical medical problems of adults. Internists are trained to look at the whole person; their training puts a special emphasis on clinical skills, problem-solving, and diagnostic abilities. Internists are board-certified by the American Board of Internal Medicine following completion of a 3-year residency and passing an examination. While many internists pursue subspecialties in fields such as cardiology, endocrinology, hematology, infectious diseases, or oncology (to name just a few), many training programs also have a primary care track for internists who wish to keep their approach more general and comprehensive.

Obstetrics/gynecology Many women will go to an obstetrician/gynecologist (OB/GYN) for their reproductive health care needs but will not seek any other medical or preventive care. Because of this, many OB/GYNs have stepped into the gap and have broadened their services to provide more inclusive care. A recent study by the American College of Obstetrics and Gynecology found that 54 percent of women who see a gynecologist used these doctors for their primary care. The OB/GYN in this role has been somewhat controversial. Many OB/GYNs do not wish to fill the role of primary care doctor, and other professionals may question their ability to perform these services. But there are also many OB/GYNs who enjoy a more general approach to the people they treat and can competently provide care for more than the reproductive system.

MDs and DOs There are two types of doctors you are likely to use for primary care: medical doctors or MDs, or doctors of osteopathy or DOs. While MDs are far more common, osteopathic doctors are fully accredited and licensed to provide care and write prescriptions in all 50 states and the District of Columbia.

Medical doctors receive an intensive medical education that begins with an undergraduate college degree, usually in a subject that lays some groundwork for medicine. This is followed by 4 years of medical education at a university-based medical school. Medical school provides a scientific and clinical orientation to health care. Doctors are taught to prevent, diagnose, and treat diseases, and to promote overall health for their patients. Medical education in the United States emphasizes the interrelation between teaching, research, and health care. Each year over 15,000 medical students are awarded the MD degree from one of 125 medical schools.

For most MDs, graduation from medical school marks just the halfway point of their professional education. MDs continue their education in residency programs, usually in hospitals, where they get hands-on training in the specialty they have chosen. Residency programs generally last from 3 to 7 years, depending on the specialty. Subspecialties may demand even more years of training. Fellowship programs are another type of postresidency training. In the United States, approximately 80,000 doctors are in residency or fellowship training programs at any given time.

Every state has licensing requirements for medical doctors. Certification by specialty boards assures you that a doctor is competent in a specialty. Most doctors pursue their medical education throughout their careers by taking advantage of continuing education programs.

Osteopaths represent about 5.5 percent of all doctors in the United States and account for about 100 million patient visits a year. "Osteo" refers to bones, and osteopathic medicine has focused historically on the musculoskeletal system—your bones and muscles—and the interconnectedness of this system throughout the body. Osteopathic doctors have 4 years of medical school and clinical training as interns and residents and use traditional medical methods such as medications, various diagnostic techniques, and surgery, just like other doctors. Some also use osteopathic manipulative techniques for diagnosis and treatment. These are hands-on techniques that move joints and extremities through their range of mobility.

Because prevention is such an important part of primary care medicine, you should think of your primary care doctor as someone who will see you in sickness and in health. The primary care doctor will treat you as a whole person. She should know your medical history, your family history, and, ideally, be able to recognize changes over time in your health. That means continuity in care—but even if you change your primary care doctor, your new doctor should be able to study your history and talk with you so that there is minimal interruption in continuity of care. An important thing to remember about primary care doctors is that in most managed care systems they serve as the gatekeeper to specialty services in the system. Usually your plan will only pay for care from a specialist if you have been referred by your primary care doctor.

NURSES, NURSE PRACTITIONERS, AND NURSE-MIDWIVES

Nurses are playing an important and growing role in the delivery of primary care. The evolution of advanced practice nursing has gone hand in hand with this role. Advanced practice nurses have a graduate degree in nursing, specialized education that emphasizes primary care, and are certified by taking nationally recognized examinations specific to their area of specialization, similar to board certifications for doctors.

Many primary care facilities use nurse practitioners, and nurse practitioners have taken on many of the duties traditionally performed by doctors. While these nurses work primarily in communities that are medically underserved, they also apply their comprehensive education and training in a range of medical settings including hospitals, private practices, and managed care organizations. Nurse practitioners have master's or postmaster's degrees and many have further specialty training in fields such as adult medicine, pediatrics, family medicine, gerontology, emergency medicine, or OB/GYN.

Nurse practitioners work closely with doctors, but also often have an independent role to play in the delivery of care. Nurse practitioners are taught to diagnose health problems and to prescribe medications or other therapies. They are licensed to write prescriptions for most medications in most states, although some states require a collaborative association with a doctor. Often the nurse practitioner's role is to manage your total care. This includes taking health histories, performing physical exams, ordering or performing diagnostic tests, determining and evaluating care, and collaborating with other health care professionals in meeting your needs.

Nurse-midwifery is a more specialized form of advanced practice nursing that focuses on pregnancy, childbirth, postpartum care, care of the newborn, and the family planning and gynecologic needs of women. Certified nurse-midwives practice in freestanding birth centers, in hospitals in collaboration with OB/GYNs, in health departments or community clinics, or in their own private or group practices. Like OB/GYN doctors, nurse-midwives today are prepared to provide primary care to women.

PHYSICIAN ASSISTANTS

Physician assistants, or PAs, work under the supervision of doctors to provide a range of direct services. This is a relatively new discipline that was begun in the mid-1960s in response to the shortage and uneven distribution of primary care doctors.

Many physician assistants are specifically trained to work with family practice doctors. In many practices, physician assistants, like nurse practitioners, will often perform most of the tasks of a physical exam. Physician assistants, who are trained in special accredited programs, are usually qualified to take a medical history, monitor patient care and patient management plans, and use routine diagnostic procedures to determine deviations from the norm. They also perform routine procedures such as administering immunizations and other injections, simple wound care, and managing uncomplicated illnesses. Physician assistants are also frequently involved in counseling and referral when necessary.

Physician assistants are allowed to prescribe medications in 42 states and the District of Columbia. In some states, they are restricted to certain classes of medications (for example, noncontrolled substances).

OTHER HEALTH CARE WORKERS

Many other people with special training in various aspects of health care will have a role in provision of health services. The list below profiles some of these health care workers.

Physical therapists help people recovering from an injury or illness to regain their physical function through a program of therapeutic exercise, massage, and other physical activity. A physical therapist considers a person's joint motion, muscle strength and endurance, muscle tone and reflexes, heart and lung function, and functional ability in preparing a rehabilitation program. Modern physical therapy takes advantage of the latest technological advances in medicine and may use traction, ultrasound, diathermy (heat treatment), electrotherapy (treatment using electricity), cryotherapy (cold treatment), hydrotherapy (the application of water in the treatment of disease), and laser therapy.

Occupational therapists work with people who have physical, developmental, mental health, or aging problems that result in obstacles to the successful completion of self-care, work, or recreational activities. Occupational therapists usually focus on the activities of daily living such as dressing, grooming, bathing, and eating and may use assistive devices when necessary.

Dentists take care of your teeth and gums. In some ways dental care is a model for preventive health care in general, since many people make regular visits to their dentist for teeth cleaning and evaluation even though they do not give the same type of preventive attention to the rest of their bodies (see Chapter 16).

Dietitians help you achieve and maintain a healthy diet. Nutritional therapy may be essential for people with particular health conditions such as hypertension, cardiovascular disease, diabetes, or kidney disease.

Podiatrists diagnose and treat diseases, injuries, and malformations of the foot. Doctors of podiatry must be certified by the state they practice in after finishing a 4-year postgraduate education and training program.

Chiropractors: Chiropractic has become an increasingly popular form of adjunct therapy for people with back problems. Some studies have shown that this discipline, which emphasizes realignment of the spine by physical manipulation, can be effective for lower back pain. Many chiropractors also use massage, nutritional therapy, and alternative therapies. Because alternative therapies may be harmful, it is a good idea to check with your doctor before seeing a chiropractor (see page 1404).

Optometrists diagnose and treat vision problems that are not related to disease. Optometrists measure your vision and prescribe glasses or contact lenses, and they often work closely with ophthalmologists, who are doctors who treat eye disease.

Home health aides assist in a variety of capacities for people who need assistance and care in their homes.

Mental health workers include psychiatrists, psychologists, and clinical social workers who provide therapy and counseling. These practitioners may employ a variety of therapeutic techniques, but the psychiatrist is the only one who can prescribe medication (see Chapter 27).

Medical technologists and other technicians usually work behind the scenes in laboratories analyzing material and data to provide you with the test results that will help determine the health care you receive.

Choosing a Primary Care Doctor

The primary care doctor is your lifeline to health care. The changes that managed care is bringing emphasize the importance of choosing a primary care doctor. Your health plan or managed care organization may have a great deal to say about the person you choose for your primary care doctor, but that does not mean that you do not have important input into the decision-making process.

As you weigh the factors involved in this decision, it might help to give some thought to what your role will be. In the traditional doctor-patient relationship the role of the patient has generally been to do what the doctor says without much input into determining the care that is delivered. The popular phrase "You're the doctor" amounts to an abdication of responsibility for many individuals for their own health care.

The notion of preventive care is changing all that. The patient is no longer necessarily a sick person, and the passive role is no longer appropriate. As you make the decisions involved in choosing a doctor and obtaining the best health care possible, it

might be helpful to think of yourself as a health care consumer or customer, with control over the course of your treatment. You can also think of yourself as a partner with your doctor, an active participant in establishing your health goals and determining courses of treatment.

Making decisions about your care means judicious use of health care resources. As your health care system changes, you will be assuming new responsibility for your own care. Some people tend to neglect signs and symptoms, while others may pay too much attention. Unfortunately, some studies have found that in some managed care arrangements, where a set fee pays for most services, some people may be inclined to unnecessarily overuse services. In this chapter, and throughout this book, you can find guidelines that will help you determine when to seek medical care.

HOW TO FIND THE RIGHT DOCTOR FOR YOU

If you are looking for a doctor, you may have moved or changed your health plan or you may be dissatisfied with the care you are receiving. There are several different ways to find a doctor, and many resources are available to help you.

As you begin your search, be clear in your own mind what you are looking for. Surveys about people's satisfaction with their medical care often find that satisfaction is related more to interpersonal skills than to quality of care. While it is important that you trust and feel comfortable with your doctor, it is also important to know enough about her background, training, and reputation to be able to judge the quality of care you will be receiving. The following is a list of possible resources for finding a doctor.

- If you are moving, your current doctor may be able to provide a referral. Most doctors are in contact with colleagues in various areas through their professional societies or through associations made in medical school or residency programs. Make sure, however, that your doctor knows something about the colleague's present practice.

- The time-honored custom of word-of-mouth referral can be a very effective method. Ask your friends, relatives, or business associates if they have a primary care doctor that they can recommend. Remember, though, that a relationship with one's doctor is individualized and what works for someone else may not work for you.

- Another possible means of finding a doctor is through a hospital doctor referral service. Most hospitals offer a service that will furnish you with the names of staff doctors who meet your requirements, such as specialty, geographic location, and gender. However, these services will probably not tell you anything about the doctor's credentials or qualifications.

- Your health plan or managed care organization will also have a provider list, and you may be restricted to the doctors on your plan's list. In most cases, the organization will also provide information about the doctor's credentials and what services are offered.

- Medical society directories, usually published by local societies, include all members of the society and will give you information about specialties and location, but no details on qualifications. In addition, you can find a directory of certified medical specialists in your public library. This book lists doctors by training. Or call the alumni office of a medical school in your area for a list of doctors.

- Finally, as you search for both general and specific information, one of the most comprehensive resources is one of the newest—the Internet. This massive—and ever-growing—aggregation of information can be a powerful tool to aid you in seeking health care. You do not even need your own computer; most public libraries now have computers connected to the Internet that are available for the public to do research. The abundance of different sources makes it impossible for us to recommend specific Internet sites to visit for your information. Most major health institutions now have home pages, from government agencies (for example, the National Institutes of Health, the Centers for Disease Control and Prevention) to managed care organizations and advocacy groups such as the Ameri-

can Heart Association and the Juvenile Diabetes Foundation. Private medical facilities such as the Johns Hopkins Medical Institutions also have an online presence and often offer lists of doctors, which can be a valuable aid if you are looking for a doctor. Be sure, however, that the source you consult is an authoritative one and that the information provided is documented by information published in scientific journals. Anyone can create a Web page and give it an impressive name; just because information appears on the screen does not ensure its validity.

QUALIFICATIONS TO LOOK FOR

Having a list of names is only the first step in choosing your doctor. It is important that you check the qualifications and professional credentials of any doctor you consider as the quality of doctors varies widely.

Your doctor should have a medical degree from an accredited medical school. The best qualified doctors have usually completed residencies in academic medical centers and are board certified.

Board certification is one of the best ways to evaluate doctors in practice. When a doctor is board certified in a specialty (and remember, family practice is a specialty), she will have completed a prescribed term of residency in the specialty, passed oral and written examinations, and handled a minimum number of cases. Doctors who are board certified have surpassed the requirements necessary to get a medical license. The American Board of Medical Specialties oversees the board certification process and will provide information to the public about whether a doctor is board certified. To learn if a doctor is board certified, you can call the American Board of Medical Specialties at (800) 776-2378.

Other considerations that you should weigh in selecting a doctor are likely to be more personal and subjective. Among the factors you may want to consider are:

- Is the office conveniently located, with nearby parking?

- What are the office hours? Does the doctor respond to weekend or night calls?

WHEN IT'S TIME TO CHANGE DOCTORS

You want your needs to be met, and so does your doctor. She should be willing to listen to your questions, and she should be able to explain to you what is happening in your body in a way that is understandable. If you do not feel that this is happening, say so. If you continue to feel dissatisfied with your care, it is time to consider finding another doctor.

There are many reasons you may want to switch doctors. You may feel uncomfortable talking to your doctor, or may want to find someone with a philosophy that is more compatible with your own. You may feel that your doctor is not keeping up with the latest developments in medicine. Or you may think that your doctor is too willing to try something new before it is proved to be safe and effective. You may want to find a doctor who has a more nutritional approach to health, or who is more open to alternative treatments.

Other reasons that are often cited for changing doctors include lack of empathy or an evasive approach to your questions. If your doctor is evading your questions, she is not including you as a partner in health care. You also have the right to expect that your doctor will respect your confidentiality in all medical issues.

Sometimes more practical concerns will be the reason you decide to change your doctor. While medical emergencies can sometimes wreak havoc with a doctor's appointment schedule, if you consistently have to wait for long periods of time to see your doctor, it may be a sign that she does not respect your time.

Changing doctors can be a sensitive issue. Many people feel somewhat intimidated in the doctor-patient relationship and are uncomfortable questioning the doctor. Many people are not aware of the rights they have in this context (see page 1424). You have the right to switch doctors if this is your wish, and the right to ask your current doctor to transfer all your files to your new doctor. Ultimately, you are the person who is in control of all aspects of your health care and everything related to it. ∎

- Is coverage available from the doctor's partners or colleagues when she is not available?

- What health insurance plans does the doctor accept?

- What is the doctor's hospital affiliation? Does she have admitting privileges?

- Have there been any complaints or actions taken against the doctor? If a doctor has been disciplined for unprofessional conduct or found liable for malpractice, these actions will be on file with the National Practitioner Data Bank. This information is not available to the public, but if a doctor has a file, you can find out from your state medical board. For information about how to contact your state medical board, call the Federation of State Medical Boards, (817) 868-4000.

When you are considering using someone as your doctor, call her office and ask for information about office policies, billing procedures, and the doctor's education and training. Finally, you will want to meet the doctor. It is important that you feel comfortable with your doctor and that you trust her and feel that the the two of you will be able to work together as partners in health care. A face-to-face meeting is important before making a final decision. Many doctors will charge for such a visit.

Checkups

Regular medical checkups are a key component of preventive health care. The physical exam, which includes taking your medical history and doing laboratory tests is a fundamental part of primary medicine. As you might expect, though, with the changes that are causing a reshaping of the system of health care delivery in this country, even this consistent feature of medical practice is undergoing some changes.

WHO NEEDS A CHECKUP, AND WHEN?

The physical exam serves two main purposes—to diagnose health problems and assess risks, and to provide a structured forum for the doctor (or nurse practitioner or physician assistant) to present information about good preventive care. Annual comprehensive physical exams were once recommended for everyone. In reality, it is doubtful that more than a small proportion of the population ever followed that guideline. It is also true that many of the standard procedures of the routine physical—listening to chest sounds, probing the abdomen, tapping the knees—are unlikely to turn up a previously unsuspected illness.

Current recommendations are evolving more toward targeted screenings for people at high risk for certain conditions rather than periodic comprehensive physical exams for everyone. In 1995, the US Preventive Services Task Force, a panel convened by the US Public Health Service, published clinical guidelines about preventive services, including routine physical exams. The Task Force found that a standardized annual physical exam is not a very effective tool for

COMMUNICATING WITH YOUR DOCTOR TO STAY HEALTHY

Effective communication between you and your doctor is not just a matter of pleasant social graces. Productive communication, researchers have found, translates to appropriate follow-through on the doctor's recommendations regarding medication and lifestyle modifications. That, in turn, translates to better control of disorders and chronic diseases and more effective prevention. So listen to what your doctor is telling you, and make sure that she is listening to you.

Unfortunately, noncompliance with medical recommendations is more common than you might think. From 30 to 60 percent or more of people do not take the medication that has been prescribed for them. In the management of chronic diseases, researchers have found that 40 to 50 percent of people with diabetes, 40 percent of people with hypertension, and as many as 70 percent of people with arthritis do not follow their recommended medication regimens. A study of noncompliance conducted by the National Pharmaceutical Council's Task Force for Compliance blamed this problem on poor communication between doctors and patients.

Developing a good rapport is a significant component of the doctor-patient relationship. While you are working to make good communication with your doctor your priority, it may be encouraging to know that your doctor is doing the same. The importance of open communication and the issue of patient autonomy—patients being able to make their own decisions based on medical advice—are principles of medical ethics that are taught in medical schools.

It is important that you feel comfortable talking about personal and intimate issues with your doctor. Sexual function and changes in bowel and urinary habits, for example, might be important clues about things going on with your health. So, too, are emotional problems. Emotional and physical health are usually closely intertwined. If you cannot feel comfortable with these discussions, you may want to consider a new doctor (see page 1392). Think about whether it might be easier for you to talk about these sensitive topics with someone who is close to you in age, or the same gender.

As you strive for good communication, focus on your medical visit and what you hope to accomplish. According to Debra L. Roter, a Johns Hopkins faculty member who studies doctor-patient communication, people should be very clear about the purpose of their visits and let the doctor know what they expect so that their needs will not go unmet.

Roter points out that it helps to know a little about the doctor's perspective, particularly the fact that medical exams usually follow a routine. Most doctors follow a "script" that includes taking a medical history, discussing your specific complaints, the actual physical exam, then the consultation after the exam. If you do not get your concerns on the table and your problems remain unmentioned, it is likely that they will not be addressed at all.

Keep in mind a list of details about each problem you want to talk to the doctor about.

- When the problem began
- What the symptoms are, and what they feel like
- When the symptoms occur (for example, at what specific times of the day)
- How long the symptoms last
- Severity of symptoms. Do they affect your daily functioning?
- Anything that seems to trigger or is associated with the symptoms
- Whether you have ever experienced a similar problem
- What you think (or fear) is the problem

As a patient, then, you must take an active role in directing the communication with your doctor. You know your body better than anyone, and it is up to you to figure out your agenda. Begin before your visit to make a list of specific questions you want to ask the doctor (see page 1399). From the time you start thinking about making an appointment, keep a pad handy so you can jot down things that occur to you.

Ask yourself, for example, "Am I seeing the doctor just for this persistent cough, or are there other things I want to talk about?" Make note of any health problems that are secondary to the major reason for your visit. Tell the doctor at the beginning of the visit that you have other areas of concern that may or may not be relevant to the central reason for your visit. If you have heard of a specific medication or treatment that you think may be helpful for you, make a note of it and ask the doctor about it. Ask every question that comes to your mind. Remember—the only stupid question is an unasked question. ■

improving people's health. As an alternative, they recommended that the content and frequency of physicals be adapted to the age, health risks, and individual needs of each person. They emphasized that counseling people about personal health practices and risk behaviors is one of the most important parts of the health visit, although it is often overlooked by many doctors.

Everyone needs periodic examinations of some sort, from the well-baby checks for infants to the frequent exams that are often needed by seniors to monitor chronic or acute health problems. Physical exams are often required by health insurers, employers, or for participation in organized sporting activities. It is usually a good idea to get a comprehensive physical exam when you begin a relationship with a new primary care doctor, so she can have a baseline against which to judge your subsequent health.

After your initial exam, talk to your doctor about how often physical exams are necessary and how they can be targeted to your individual health needs. For preventive health care to be effective, productive communication between you and your doctor is essential (see page 1393).

MEDICAL HISTORY

A doctor takes your medical history by asking you questions about your current health, your health history, and your family history. The purpose of a medical history is to allow the doctor to develop an individualized risk profile for you and gain an understanding of what should be looked for in the physical exam. The medical history should be comprehensive and include your medical, family, social, and occupational background. While some of these factors may not seem directly relevant to your health, there may be an active interplay between these aspects of your life and your physical and mental health.

The history may be taken by a doctor, a nurse practitioner, or a physician assistant. A sensitive doctor will take your history in a quiet, private, comfortable place. The interview will consist of two types of questions. Direct questions will require an answer of only a couple words, often just yes or no. Open-ended questions will require more input on your part. An example of an open-ended question is, "Describe the symptoms that have brought you here today."

Different health care organizations and practitioners use a variety of questionnaires or formats for taking your medical history. Some may have you fill in the answers on a preprinted form or on a computer, although there will usually be a personal question and answer period for at least part of the medical history.

The person taking your health history will begin by asking you for simple biographical information: name, address, birth date, gender, marital status, race, occupational history, and current job. The history-taker will then focus on the current reason you are seeking care. Even if this is a routine physical, it is likely that there are symptoms or concerns that you want to bring to the doctor's attention. Doctors are trained to look for the following nine characteristics to describe the symptoms:

- Location. Where, specifically, are the symptoms occurring?
- Exact nature. What is the quality and character of the symptoms?
- Quantity and severity. How often do the symptoms occur, and how serious are they?
- Timing. This includes when the symptoms began, how long an episode occurs (or if it is continuous), and the frequency of episodes. Also, have the symptoms changed over time?
- Setting. Where do the symptoms occur?
- Things that make the symptoms better or worse, including medication.
- Other factors that you think may be associated with the symptoms.
- What you think the symptoms mean.
- Functioning. How are the symptoms affecting your daily functioning?

After you have reviewed the details of your current concerns with the doctor, she will move on to your past medical history. Of particular interest will be anything in your past that may be related to the current problem. In addition, you should be prepared to talk about the following subjects:

- Childhood illnesses
- Previous accidents or injuries
- Serious or chronic illnesses
- Any previous hospitalizations or surgeries
- Obstetric history (for women)
- Immunization record, including recent flu or tetanus shots
- Allergies
- Medications you are currently taking
- Your family's history of illnesses, including the age of onset and treatments given
- The last time you had a physical exam, and what tests were done. Also, the dates of your most recent dental and vision exams

In this part of the interview the doctor will also talk to you about lifestyle issues that affect your health. These include smoking, diet, alcohol consumption, other substance use, exercise habits, sleeping patterns, work, potentially harmful occupational or hobby exposures, and stress and other emotional issues in your life. Thinking about these issues before your exam will help you compile your own risk profile, which can be helpful for the doctor. Remember that all this information is confidential and that providing truthful answers is essential for proper medical care. If you hide embarrassing information from your doctor, you will be harming yourself.

Your sexual history also has potential implications for physical and mental health. Some people may find their sexual history embarrassing to talk about, but the doctor should be able to handle this topic sensitively. Your sexual history includes whether you are sexually active or not, your sexual orientation, number of partners, types of sexual activity you engage in, contraceptive and disease-prevention methods you use, whether you have had any sexually trans-

mitted diseases, and whether you have any concerns about your sexual function.

As part of your family history the doctor will want to know the age and health of your spouse and children as well as the age and health or cause of death of blood relatives: your parents, grandparents, and siblings. Specifically, she will ask if any of these family members have or have had any health problems that may have a genetic component. These include cardiovascular disease, hypertension (high blood pressure), diabetes, cancer, blood disorders, arthritis, allergies, obesity, mental illness, seizure disorder, or kidney disease (see Chapter 6). The illustration below shows you how the doctor may illustrate your answers by sketching a family tree, or genogram, depicting this information.

The next part of a comprehensive medical history is a review of systems. The doctor will ask you specific questions about problems or concerns with each of your organ systems. After your doctor asks you about your general overall health status, she

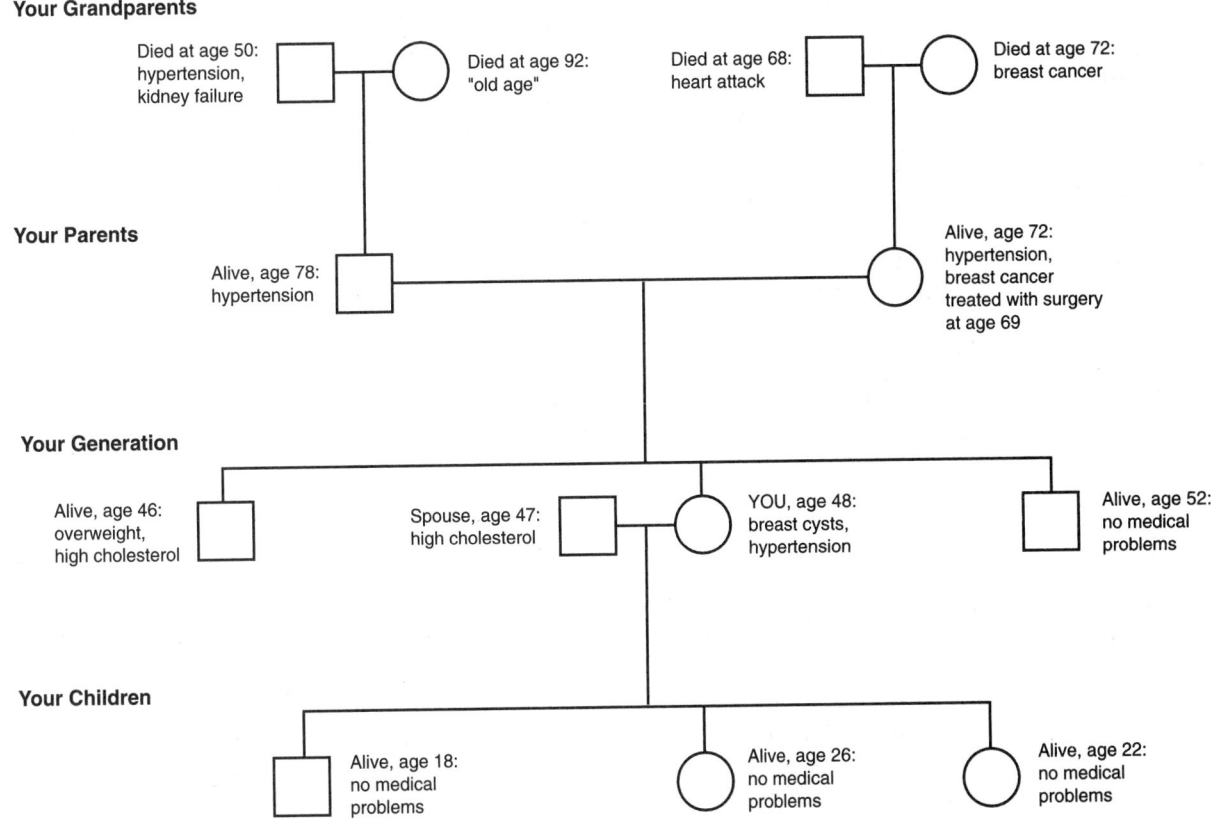

Example of a family tree, or genogram.

Your Grandparents

Died at age 50: hypertension, kidney failure

Died at age 92: "old age"

Died at age 68: heart attack

Died at age 72: breast cancer

Your Parents

Alive, age 78: hypertension

Alive, age 72: hypertension, breast cancer treated with surgery at age 69

Your Generation

Alive, age 46: overweight, high cholesterol

Spouse, age 47: high cholesterol

YOU, age 48: breast cysts, hypertension

Alive, age 52: no medical problems

Your Children

Alive, age 18: no medical problems

Alive, age 26: no medical problems

Alive, age 22: no medical problems

may then ask, for example, questions about fatigue, weight gain or loss, weakness, or malaise.

Finally, the medical history part of your checkup will include a functional assessment, which is done to gauge how well you take care of yourself in the routine activities of daily living such as eating, sleeping, grooming, and interpersonal activities. This part of the history may also include questions about stress in your life and your performance on the job.

MENTAL STATUS

Your doctor will also assess your mental status during your medical history and subsequent physical exam. Your mental status is how well you are functioning emotionally and cognitively—your perception, memory, judgment, and knowledge of the world around you. While it cannot be measured like pulse or blood pressure, the perceptive doctor can evaluate mental status with cues from several different areas. These include

- Appearance: your posture, body movements, dress, grooming, and hygiene
- Behavior: awareness and alertness, facial expression, and mood affect
- Cognitive functions: memory, orientation (for example, do you know the date, do you know where you are?), ability to concentrate, and judgment

Sometimes a distinct mental status evaluation will be done, but usually the doctor can gather the necessary data for this from the other components of the exam.

THE PHYSICAL EXAM

The physical exam is the part of the checkup when the doctor (or other clinician) examines your body to ascertain information about your health. The following are four different assessment techniques used to gather this information—inspection, palpation, percussion, and auscultation.

Inspection Inspection is observant, careful visual examination, first of you as a whole and then of each of your body systems. It begins the moment you and your doctor meet each other. In the general survey, the doctor will closely observe your physical appearance, body structure, mobility, and behavior. She will then apply these observations to each of the viewable body systems including skin, hair, and nails; head and neck; eyes, ears, nose, and throat; breasts and underarms; chest, back, and abdomen; genitalia; and extremities.

Palpation When the doctor palpates, or examines by touching, she is following up on points noted during the inspection and applying the sense of touch for a more detailed assessment. The doctor will use different parts of her hands for different kinds of palpation.

- Fingertips, to feel detailed features such as skin texture, swelling, pulsation, or lumps
- Grasping with the fingers will ascertain the position, shape, and consistency of an organ or mass
- The back of the hands and fingers are often applied to determine temperature, because the skin on the back of the hand is thinner and more sensitive than that on the palm.
- The base of the fingers (from the end of the hand to the first finger joints) is applied to detect vibration.

Percussion When the doctor taps your skin with short, sharp strokes she is using percussion to get a feel for underlying structures. The sharp tap will produce a vibration that gives the experienced examiner information about the location, size, and density of the underlying organ.

Auscultation Auscultation, from the Latin word for listening, means listening to body sounds through a stethoscope. The doctor can hear activity in your heart, blood vessels, lungs, and abdomen in this manner.

Conducting the exam For a comprehensive physical exam, the doctor will usually ask you to remove your clothing and change into an examining gown to make the examination easier. The doctor will begin the exam by taking several measurements: weight, height, and, in some cases, skinfold thickness (to estimate body fat). For infants and children younger than 6 years old, head and chest circumference will also be measured.

If there has been a notable change in your weight—either loss or gain—your doctor will want to talk to you about the reasons for it. Weight change can be an important indicator of a number of diseases, and preventive counseling may be needed.

Your doctor will also take your vital signs. These are your temperature, pulse, respiration, and blood pressure. Irregularities in any of these measurements may be indicators of health problems, although there is a fairly wide range of normal levels for pulse and blood pressure, and many transitory conditions (for example, emotions or stress) can affect these measurements.

Another part of the physical exam will test your neurologic or nervous system. This includes assessing the sensory system for reaction to superficial pain and sensation of vibrations (using a tuning fork); testing the ability to recognize objects by feeling their form, size, and weight (stereognosis); and testing reflexes.

Depending on how comprehensive it is, the physical exam will take from a few minutes to a half hour or more. A directed exam focusing on particular symptoms and complaints will be briefer than a full physical. As a partner in your health care, you should feel comfortable asking the doctor what she is doing and why at any point in the exam.

LABORATORY TESTS

Laboratory tests serve a number of purposes. They may screen for a disease or potential health problem. They may confirm a tentative diagnosis or, conversely, rule out a possible diagnosis. They can be used to monitor treatment progress. They can provide reassurance about health status or evaluate the functioning of any of your body's systems.

As cost considerations continue to play a bigger part than ever before in the delivery of health care services, diagnostic laboratory testing has become the object of increased scrutiny. Anyone who has ever had a series of tests knows that the costs can mount quickly, from the more moderate expense of lab tests examining blood and urine to the hundreds and even thousands of dollars for today's technologically sophisticated imaging procedures.

In decades past, with malpractice suits a looming threat, many doctors chose to err on the side of overprescribing diagnostic and screening tests rather than underprescribing in order to reduce the possibility of liability. There does not appear to be a relation between amount of testing and better medical outcomes. In the 1990s, as the medical profession has taken a good hard look at bottom lines, attitudes and recommendations about testing have shifted. Some procedures have been found to have limited diagnostic value, such as routine electrocardiograms for healthy adults, or ultrasound scans in low-risk pregnancies. Some procedures are associated with potential health risks for the individual, as well as expense.

Changes are slow in coming, and many critics still feel that some tests are overprescribed. There is a wide geographic variation in the way diagnostic tests are used. What you encounter in common medical practice may not, in fact, coincide with what major medical authorities recommend. Part of this variation is in response to pressure from the consumer—you—who may feel reassured by negative test results, even if there was no indication that you had any problem in that area. But it is true that many doctors are becoming more discriminating about offering tests. You should have the same attitude. Whenever a test is recommended, you should make sure you understand why the test has been suggested, what it will tell you, and whether the results will affect treatment decisions.

In its 1995 *Guide to Clinical Preventive Services*, the US Preventive Services Task Force recommended for and against the routine administration of a number of medical procedures. Their report emphasizes the preventive value of counseling and education; for example, informing people about the health risks of smoking is a much more effective means of preventing lung cancer than routine chest x-rays for healthy adults.

The Task Force recommended in favor of certain screening procedures:

- Hypertension should be screened for at least every 2 years for everyone. Blood pressure should be measured at every visit to the doctor.

- Periodic screening (every 5 years) for high blood cholesterol is recommended

RECOMMENDATIONS FOR PREVENTIVE MEDICAL CARE

Screening

- Blood pressure
- Height and weight
- Pap smear
- Fecal occult blood test and/or sigmoidoscopy[a]
- Mammography with or without breast exam[b]
- Assess for problem drinking
- Total blood cholesterol (men aged 35 to 64, women aged 45 to 64)
- Vision screening[c]
- Assess for hearing impairment[c]

Counseling

- Tobacco cessation
- Avoidance of alcohol and drugs when driving, swimming, boating
- Limitation of fat, cholesterol
- Maintenance of caloric balance
- Emphasis on grains, fruits, vegetables in diet
- Adequate calcium
- Physical activity
- Lap/shoulder belts
- Motorcycle and bicycle helmets
- Smoke detectors
- Storage or removal of firearms
- Sexually transmitted infection prevention
- Dental visits, fluoride, flossing
- Contraception
- Fall prevention[c]
- Cardiopulmonary resuscitation (CPR) training for household[c]
- Hot water heater less than 120°F[c]

Immunization

- Tetanus-diphtheria
- Pneumococcal vaccine[c]
- Influenza vaccine[c]

Chemoprophylaxis

- Discussion of hormone replacement therapy with perimenopausal women ∎

[a]After age 49.

[b]After age 49; before 70.

[c]Ages 65+.

Source: Adapted from the US Preventive Services Task Force Guide to Clinical Preventive Services. Consult full report for details and recommendations for high-risk individuals. From Harrison's Principles of Internal Medicine. McGraw-Hill, New York, 1998; used with permission.

for men ages 35 to 65 and women ages 45 to 65. Seniors, young adults, and adolescents should only be screened if there are major coronary risk factors such as hypertension, diabetes, or smoking. The Task Force noted that elevated blood cholesterol is one of the major modifiable risk factors for coronary heart disease, which is the leading cause of death in this country (see Chapter 20).

- Mammograms to screen for breast cancer are recommended every 1 or 2 years for all women ages 50 to 69. There has been controversy about the benefits of routine mammography for women under the age of 50 (see page 778), and this is something every woman should discuss with her doctor while taking into account family history and the existence of other risk factors.

- Women should have a Pap smear to screen for cervical cancer every 1 to 3 years, beginning at the age of 18 or at the beginning of sexual activity.

- Colorectal cancer is the second most common form of cancer in the United States, and the Task Force recommended screening for this cancer for everyone over age 50 using either sigmoidoscopy, annual fecal occult blood testing, or both. Unless there are other indications, a sigmoidoscopy every 10 years is usually sufficient.

The Task Force also recommended against the following screening tests that many doctors have been performing routinely:

- Little benefit was found from routine blood tests of asymptomatic adults without risk factors for diabetes, thyroid diseases, or anemia.

- Chest x-rays are not recommended for routine screening for lung cancer. By the time a malignancy shows up on an x-ray, it is often too late for treatment.

- Electrocardiograms are not recommended for routine screening for heart disease.

- The Task Force also recommended against routine screening for prostate cancer by measurement of prostate-specific antigen or the use of digital rectal examination (DRE). The prostate-specific antigen (PSA) test produces a high incidence of false-positive results (see Chapter 25).

- Routine electronic fetal monitoring is not recommended for low-risk women in labor as long as adequate clinical monitoring by trained personnel is available.

- Routine urine tests for early detection of bladder cancer or asymptomatic urinary tract infections are not recommended.

See the list showing recommendations for preventive medical care on page 1398.

Making Treatment Decisions

In the rapidly changing world of medical care, there is probably only one thing we can be sure of—that the systems will continue to change. With the pattern of evolving health plans and switching doctors that has become the norm in modern health care, the only constant in your medical history might be yourself. It has never been more important to be informed and knowledgeable about your medical care.

This can be a daunting prospect. After all, your doctor had years of technical education and clinical training to learn about the human body, what can go wrong with it, and how to fix it. It is up to you to work together with your doctor to apply her knowledge to your specific needs. No one knows your body the way you do. This knowledge gives you the tool to be an equal partner in your medical care. You can move from this starting point to educate yourself so that you are competent to participate in treatment decisions for yourself and your family—from your first decision to seek medical treatment through the continuing health care process.

HOW TO BE AN INFORMED PATIENT

Individual autonomy and self-determination have become increasingly important in American medicine. This concept is in direct contrast with many other cultures, where decision making is almost totally relinquished to the doctor. Even in the United States, this attitude of autonomy is relatively new; as recently as the 1960s, 90 percent of doctors did not tell patients of a cancer diagnosis. Today, nearly 100 percent of doctors do tell people when they have cancer. This policy is institutionalized in the Ethics Manual of the American College of Physicians, which explicitly states that all people have the right to be informed of their medical condition, their prognosis, and the various treatment alternatives.

The most knowledgeable health care consumers make the healthiest lifestyle choices and take best advantage of available medical services. The Joint Commission on Accreditation of Healthcare Organizations describes the goals of patient education as the following: "To improve patient health outcomes by promoting recovery, speeding return to function, promoting healthy behavior, and appropriately involving the patient in his or her care decisions." In fact, education is directly linked to improved outcomes. People who are knowledgeable about their health care have shorter hospital stays, experience fewer complications, feel less

CHECKLIST: QUESTIONS TO ASK YOUR DOCTOR

- What caused my health problem?
- How can it be treated? What are the treatment alternatives?
- Is medication necessary?
- How long is it likely to continue?
- When can I expect improvement?
- How will this problem affect my general health?
- Is the problem likely to recur?
- Can it be prevented in the future?
- Is further testing needed?
- What are the tests for, and what are they expected to show?
- What do my test results mean?
- Is referral to a specialist necessary?
- Are there lifestyle changes (for example, diet, exercise, smoking, drinking) that you can suggest to promote better health for me? ■

anxious, and are generally more satisfied with the health care they receive.

The first step toward being informed about your health care is to use the communication skills we have discussed in this chapter. The importance of asking questions cannot be overemphasized. If you do not feel comfortable asking your doctor questions, you should think about finding another doctor. In this important interaction, do not be satisfied with a relationship you are not comfortable in. Getting accurate and understandable answers to your questions is critical. Knowing what to expect will be a tremendous help in whatever health care situation you find yourself.

Many people find that it is helpful to take notes in conversations with their doctors. Jotting down words and phrases can help you focus on what the doctor is telling you and give you a tool for further investigation on your own. Do not be afraid to request correct spellings of words you do not understand.

Unfortunately, studies have shown that many people feel intimidated in the doctor's office. Some people may feel that they do not have the right to ask questions, or they may fear that they will not understand the doctor's answers. It is necessary to overcome these feelings. You have the right to ask questions, you need to ask questions, and you have the right to explanations that make sense to you.

You might be hesitant to raise issues because you think your doctor does not have time to answer your questions. Often, you may find that a nurse in the office can answer many of your questions and can also serve as a go-between between you and the doctor.

You might also find that your doctor does not know the answers to all your questions. This is an era of rapidly proliferating knowledge, fragmentation of information because of specialization, and an ever-increasing array of diagnostic and treatment options. It is impossible for every doctor to keep up with every new development. Your doctor might need to do research on her own to come up with answers to your questions.

There is a wealth of printed material available today to help you learn about the health issues that concern you. Books like this one can give you information about almost any medical condition you might encounter. You can find many books about specific diseases in libraries and bookstores. Many doctor's offices have pamphlets about prevalent health problems such as diabetes, hypertension, coronary artery disease, and obesity. If you want material about something that you do not see, ask for it. Your doctor will be happy to help you. It is much easier to formulate your questions if you have read background literature about the subject, and it helps the doctor to know that you have some basic information.

Another resource is the Internet. You can find information about almost any health problem you can think of on the Internet at sites maintained by federal agencies, state governments, researchers, consumer organizations, doctors with private practices, and others. A master list of health information from federal government agencies can be found at www.healthfinder.gov. Consumer health news and information from Johns Hopkins is posted at www.intelihealth.com. You can also exchange information with others who have the same health problem you do and learn about treatment options they may have tried or heard about. You will notice that many of the Web sites include disclaimers warning that the information provided should not be used instead of professional medical consultation. Use written information for background and explanation but never as a substitute for professional diagnosis and treatment recommendations.

DOCTRINE OF INFORMED CONSENT

The doctrine of informed consent is an integral part of the concept of being well informed about your medical care. The fundamental principle of informed consent is that a person has the right to an understanding of the risks, benefits, and alternatives of any medical therapy before making a treatment decision. For surgical procedures and research protocols the doctrine is presented in the form of a legal document to be signed that stipulates that this information has been offered.

True informed consent implies a doctor and patient working together to share information and communicate about the person's health problem, treatment possibilities, and realistic expectations. At its worst, the process of informed consent may be a perfunctory form-signing with the person not really understanding what is being presented and the doctor going through the formalities primarily to protect against litigation.

Do not sign anything without reading and understanding what you are signing. Remember that your consent is given voluntarily and it may be withdrawn if you change your mind. Unless the case is an emergency, take time to think about the treatment you are consenting to. Do not rush into treatment unless there is a real medical reason for urgency.

Informed consent forms relating to specific procedures should present a comprehensive list of risks associated with the procedure. Reviewing the form with your doctor is often a good way to address your concerns about these risks. Ask about the severity of the potential harm of each risk. Any risk of death or disability should be discussed. This is also the time to talk about the risk of alternative treatments or the risk of no treatment.

You are entitled to this information about any procedure or therapeutic approach. The process of getting your informed consent is not likely to be overlooked for surgery, for example, or for participation in an experimental drug trial. However, simpler procedures that are carried out in a doctor's office may be handled more casually. Even when a doctor prescribes medication, you should be fully informed about any possible side effects or contraindications before you consent to take them.

Informed consent has a somewhat different context when children are involved. For younger children, a parent or other surrogate must make the treatment decisions. But children too, should be partners in health care decisions. Even elementary school-aged children should be informed about issues with their health and involved in decision making about medical treatment. Adults may have the protective instinct to shield children from harsh medical realities. In fact, most children sense when information is being withheld. Not knowing can be more stressful than knowing, for children as well as adults.

In a policy statement about informed consent, the American Academy of Pediatrics emphasized the importance of respecting children's own wishes about medical treatment and obtaining the assent of the child for treatment whenever possible. Once children are 14 and older, the statement notes, they often have decisional skills that are as well developed as those of adults for medical decision making.

WHEN DO YOU NEED A SECOND OPINION?

There is as much art as science to medicine. For many problems there is no single correct answer. Decisions are based on objective findings, but many subjective elements are also involved in the process. Only with hindsight is it possible to know for sure. Many medical conditions offer choices for treatment. Surgery or medication or lifestyle changes may all be viable treatment options for the same problem, each with its own risks and benefits.

Seeking a second opinion does not mean you do not trust your doctor, nor does it mean you are changing your doctor. Different doctors offer different approaches. Some are more conservative, some more aggressive. They may come to a problem from differing perspectives. Doctors see things from the point of view of their own specialty. A cardiologist is more likely to think of a heart problem when making a diagnosis, for example, while a pulmonologist will focus on the lungs.

Research shows that when a person seeks a second opinion, it lowers the likelihood of surgery. In one study, when a Chicago hospital began requiring a second opinion before performing a cesarean section, the cesarean section rate dropped from 18 to 11 percent.

People most frequently seek a second opinion when surgery is recommended. In the past, insurance companies usually required a second opinion validating the necessity of an operation before they would pay for it. Many HMOs (Health Maintenance Organizations) and health insurers will pay for a second opinion regarding surgery and other treatments. If a surgeon has recommended surgery, it is often a good idea to get a second opinion from someone who is not a surgeon. If back surgery has been advised, for example, a neurologist may offer another perspective. If a hip replacement has been suggested, consider seeing a rheumatologist.

LIST OF MEDICAL SPECIALTIES

Most of the time when you need the services of a medical specialist, your primary care doctor will refer you to someone. If your medical coverage is through a managed care organization, the referral to a specialist by the primary care gatekeeper will probably be required if you want the visit paid for. However, there are many cases when people call a specialist on their own, particularly if they are not covered by managed care.

The basic rule for this sort of self-referral is to use common sense. In nearly every case, it is not a bad idea to check first with your primary care doctor. While you may feel positive that you know exactly what body system is in need of treatment and which specialist to turn to, you may not possess the professional diagnostic skills needed for this type of decision. However, if you are certain of the type of care you need, and especially if you already know a specialist—maybe you were treated previously by an orthopedic surgeon for a broken bone, for example, or a dermatologist for skin rashes—you may feel comfortable making an appointment with the doctor on your own volition. If you have a chronic disease, something that requires continuing treatment, you will probably have an ongoing relationship with a specialist. If you are seeking a specialist on your own, be sure to check for board certification in the specialty.

There are many specialties in medicine. The following list identifies specialties along with the different body systems and populations that they treat.

Anesthesiology The administration of anesthesia, as for surgery

Cardiology The study of the heart and diseases related to the heart

Dermatology The diagnosis and treatment of diseases of the skin

Emergency Medicine Care in the emergency room

Endocrinology The study of the endocrine system and diseases related to the hormones secreted by the endocrine glands, such as diabetes or thyroid disorders

Gastroenterology The study and treatment of conditions associated with the digestive system (stomach and intestines); doctors specializing in this field are called gastroenterologists or GI specialists

Geriatrics The study and treatment of problems related to aging

Genetics The study of hereditary diseases that are passed from parent to child through the genes

Gynecology/Obstetrics The study and treatment of conditions of the female reproductive system (gynecology) and those of pregnancy and childbirth (obstetrics)

Hematology The study and treatment of blood diseases and disorders

Infectious Diseases The study and treatment of diseases that are spread by infectious agents such as viruses or bacteria

Internal Medicine A broad specialty that covers the nonsurgical diagnosis and treatment of disease in adults; these doctors are called internists, and many of the specialties listed here are subspecialties of internal medicine

Immunology The study and treatment of diseases of the immune system

Neurology The study and treatment of conditions associated with diseases of the nervous system (the brain and spinal cord)

Nephrology The study and treatment of conditions associated with the kidneys

Oncology The study and treatment of cancer in its many different forms

Ophthalmology The study and treatment of the eye and diseases of the eye

Orthopedics The study and treatment of diseases and injuries involving bones

Otorhinolaryngology The study and treatment of the ear, nose, and throat and their related conditions; these doctors are sometimes referred to as ear, nose, and throat, or ENT, specialists

Pathology Laboratory study of tissues to determine what causes diseases

Pediatrics Treatment of babies, children, and adolescents for diseases and disorders as well as monitoring normal growth and development; there are also many pediatric subspecialties, such as pediatric oncology or pediatric surgery

Pharmacology/Toxicology The study of drugs, medications, and poisons and their antidotes

Public Health The science of applying medical solutions to broad populations, not just individuals

Pulmonology The study and treatment of the lungs and lung diseases

Rheumatology The study and treatment of diseases of the joints and muscles

Psychiatry The study and treatment of mental and emotional disorders

Radiology The use of x-rays to diagnose and treat diseases

Sports Medicine The study and treatment of injuries and health conditions related to sports and physical training

Surgery The treatment of disease or injury with an operation; there are many surgical subspecialties—for example, cardiothoracic surgery (heart and chest), neurosurgery (brain and spine), and pediatric surgery (for the treatment of injury or disease in babies, children, or adolescents)

Urology The study and treatment of the urinary system and the male reproductive system ■

You should get a second opinion not just when surgery is recommended but any time you are not certain where a treatment course is leading. You should seek a second opinion if the problem you are seeing the doctor about is not getting better, or if your doctor cannot figure out what is wrong with you. You should seek a second opinion any time you do not feel comfortable with your doctor's recommendations. If a laboratory finding is equivocal, it is a good idea for a second pathologist to look at the slides. If you have been given no hope about your condition, you will probably want to get another opinion. If your condition is borderline—for example, a tumor that the doctor says is "almost operable"—you should get a second opinion.

Getting a second opinion not only gives you another professional perspective but also keeps you better informed about your treatment options. Most doctors will be very open to your desire to get another opinion, particularly if they can refer you to someone who has more experience with the problem.

There are arguments for and against using someone your doctor knows for a second opinion. The two doctors' relationship could facilitate record-sharing and consultation and continuity of care. However, it is also possible that your doctor will refer you to someone who has the same treatment philosophy (that is, conservative or aggressive) that she does, as well as a similar background. In order for you to know that you will be receiving independent advice, it is usually a good idea to at least go to someone in a different practice or group than your own doctor.

The second doctor will examine you and go over your records and then talk to you about her findings. She may feel that more diagnostic tests are necessary. If she agrees with the first doctor, you will probably feel comfortable about proceeding with the treatment that has been recommended. Differing opinions do not mean that one doctor is right and one is wrong. The practice of medicine is not that clear-cut. If there is a disagreement, you will want to carefully consider your own preferences and let that be your guide. You may want a third opinion to reconcile the conflicting ideas you are hearing. Some health plans will pay for a third opinion if the first two differ.

CHOOSING AMONG TREATMENT OPTIONS

In health and medicine, as in anything else in life, decision making is a process of weighing the odds. When you make decisions about medical treatment you need to assess the risks, benefits, and costs of the various options. One thing to keep in mind is that the choices you make do not necessarily limit you to a single treatment option. You may want to begin with a more conservative form of treatment, and then move on to others if the first approach does not work.

Consider, for example, the person with lower back pain, one of the most common complaints that brings someone to the doctor's office. The first—and most conservative—course of treatment might be simple bed rest and nonsteroidal anti-inflammatory drugs. The severity of the pain, whether it changes, and other related factors about your health will determine how long you will try this conservative approach. If this course of treatment does not seem to be working, the next step would probably be to get a clearer picture of what is going on with diagnostic imaging such as magnetic resonance imaging, or an MRI. That would probably be followed by an orthopedic or neurosurgical consultation and perhaps physical therapy. If that is not helping, you may decide that surgery is necessary.

Some medical decisions will be more urgent than others. For emergency treatment, you will not have time to weigh the options or wait out a conservative approach. The same might be true for treatment of some cancers or any other rapidly progressing disease.

Of course, your doctor's recommendation will have a great deal to do with the choices that you make. It is helpful to understand what these recommendations are based on. Doctors make decisions based on complicated formulas, but they also put an issue in the context of their personal experience. If they have seen a number of people with the same condition who have responded well to a particular treatment, they will most likely lean toward that treatment for another person with a similar problem.

Recommendations are often based on statistical odds, but statistics are not always as clear-cut as they might seem. The impli-

ALTERNATIVE MEDICINE

Alternative medicine, also known as complementary or non-traditional medicine, continues to have an increasingly significant impact on the American health care system. A recent study found that one-third of Americans who seek medical care turn to alternative practitioners, at a cost of $13.7 billion.

Alternative medicines encompass a variety of philosophies and therapies. The National Institutes of Health's Office of Alternative Medicine broadly defines alternatives as "those treatments and health care practices not taught widely in medical schools, not generally used in hospitals, and not usually reimbursed by medical insurance companies." Usually their medical effectiveness has not been proven scientifically.

Some alternative therapies are well known, and their value in particular situations is accepted by some medical doctors. These include chiropractic, acupuncture, and biofeedback. Others are of more questionable value, and some alternative care may be outright quackery with the potential to do considerable harm.

Are alternative therapies useful? The problem is, there is very little direct scientific evidence showing this. Alternative medicines have simply not been studied and tested in the rigorous ways that are standard for conventional therapies. Some treatments once considered alternative have been shown variously to be effective, to have no effect, or to cause harm. Until evidence from such studies is available, most traditional doctors are likely to be dubious of alternative therapies.

However, in recent years the scientific method has been applied to some alternative medicines. The Office of Alternative Medicine funds a range of studies of alternative treatments. Examples of just a few of the treatments being studied include acupuncture, Chinese herbal medicine, hypnosis, massage therapy, macrobiotic diets, and antioxidant vitamins.

As this brief list illustrates, alternative medicine spans a wide range of approaches. Other examples of alternative medicine include aromatherapy, in which you inhale or massage into your skin the aromatic oils distilled from certain plants and herbs; homeopathy, the use of tiny amounts of substances to combat various conditions; naturopathy, which emphasizes the body's ability to heal itself when free of toxins and uses natural medicine; yogic breathing; therapeutic massage; and even prayer intervention.

The Office of Alternative Medicine recommends the following steps when considering alternative therapy:

- Assess what is known about the safety and effectiveness of the treatment.

- Investigate the credentials of the practitioner.

- Consider how the treatment will be administered and if it conforms to recognized standards of medical safety.

- Consider the costs. Your health plan probably will not cover alternative treatments, although some alternatives are now reimbursable by some companies.

- Talk about the alternative treatments with your doctor.

Some alternative treatments may have serious negative side effects. "Natural" is not synonymous with "harmless." Many of medicine's most powerful drugs are naturally occurring substances that have the potential for great benefit or harm. And just as you should inform your doctor of any medication other doctors may have prescribed, you should also inform her of any alternative therapies or remedies you may be taking to be sure they are safe and do not conflict with more conventional treatments you may be receiving. One of the greatest dangers of using alternative therapies is that you may ignore conventional therapies that have been proved useful.

There are many sources for information about alternative medicine. The Office of Alternative Medicine has a toll-free number for consumers: (888) 644-6226. Many of the disciplines have their own professional associations. Although the Internet is teeming with information and discussions about alternative treatments, much of it is opinion rather than fact, so use your judgment when you review material that you find on Web sites. ■

cations of diagnostic testing, for example, can be less than definitive. A good example is the treadmill test for heart problems for young women. This test turns up a large number of false-positives—positive results when there really is no disease present. A premenopausal woman who tests positive for heart disease on a treadmill test should be aware that there is a greater likelihood that the test is wrong than there is that she actually has heart disease. This is an important factor to keep in mind when making treatment decisions.

You may decide to forgo medical treatment. In some instances, this is a valid choice. You may feel that treatment is futile, or that the risks are not worth the possible benefits, or that the potential benefits of the treatment are dubious. Again, this is a decision you should discuss with your doctor to be sure that you understand the consequences of your decision.

Sometimes there will be disagreements among family members about treatment decisions. This can be a difficult and stressful time for you and your loved ones. If family members disagree about a proposed course of treatment, it is often a good idea to meet together in a group with the doctors and nurses who are involved with treatment and discuss the conflicts. Medical social workers can also offer helpful input. Sometimes, if there is a family member who is a medical professional, she can be helpful in providing insight and understanding about the situation.

Making decisions about medical care is not always easy. End-of-life decisions can be particularly difficult. Consider, for example, the person who remains unconscious following a stroke and requires life support to stay alive. The family may want to cling to the chance that some form of recovery is possible while the doctor may advise that there is no hope for recovery or meaningful life and it is time for life support to be withdrawn. In extreme situations such as this one, the hospital ethics committee can often offer compassionate guidance and counsel. For more information on these committees, which are composed of doctors, nurses, social workers, and lawyers, see below.

In today's world of rapid technological advances, many of us have come to take for granted the effective treatments and cures that medicine offers. The fact is, though, that not everyone will be cured of everything. We all die eventually. There are limits to what medical science can accomplish, and all of us need to be aware of these limits even as we take advantage of the marvelous opportunities that the scientific discoveries of this century have made possible.

ETHICAL CONSIDERATIONS

Ethics are the shared values of a group of people that govern decision making. Ethics provide the basis of laws. Ethical considerations have always been an underpinning of the medical and nursing professions, dating back to the Hippocratic Oath directing doctors to first do no harm, and then to heal whenever possible—the basic ethical philosophies of medicine.

These basic philosophies have developed to encompass several specific principles of medical ethics:

- Beneficence—working for the benefit of others

- Justice—the right of all people to be treated equally

- Prognostic uncertainty—the fact that it is impossible to predict exactly how a person will respond to a treatment

- Autonomy—the right of the individual to determine her own medical care

- Quality of life—the complicated issue of the worth of life in the context of the extraordinary measures that are now available to prolong life at a relatively low level of functioning

- Honesty—the right of people to expect the truth from doctors

- Respect—treating people with respect, including the confidentiality of medical information

- Futility—the knowledge that all conditions will not respond to treatment

While medical treatment can be clear-cut and unequivocal, that is not always the case. Many different medical situations arise in which difficult questions must be resolved by the application of ethical principles. There are a number of areas of medical practice and research where ethical considerations play a critical role, including abortion, determination of death, organ transplantation, withdrawal or withholding of life supports, treatment of disabled newborns, new reproductive technologies, euthanasia (assisted suicide), genetic counseling, animal research, treatment of incapacitated people, and cloning. The advances of technology in medicine, in fact, have spawned a whole new area of ethical studies—bioethics.

ETHICS COMMITTEES

The American Medical Association and the American Nurses Association have written Codes of Ethics that govern the practitioners in these professions. However, because ethical considerations involve subjective decision making, there are many gray areas. Ethical conflicts often arise. For that reason, most health care facilities now have ethics committees or people designated as consultants in ethics to consider these thorny questions when they come up.

A hospital ethics committee includes doctors, nurses, social workers, clergy, administrators, and other representatives. Members of the committee have expertise in dealing with the technological issues that often raise ethical questions associated with hospital care. The committee provides a forum for rational discussion of ethical issues. Its role, in part, is to clarify the debate and facilitate communication between the involved parties. Usually hospital ethical committees meet regularly, but they can call a special meeting when necessary to handle specific acute circumstances. If you are involved with an issue that you feel requires guidance or intervention from an ethics committee, you should talk with whatever hospital personnel you feel most comfortable with—a doctor, nurse, social worker, or chaplain, for example—to find out how to enlist the aid of the committee.

ETHICS, RELIGION, AND MEDICINE

Ethics are often linked to religion and for many people their ethics are reflected in their religious beliefs. Health care today is a largely nonsectarian enterprise and has little connection with organized religion. However, many hospitals were founded by religious groups, and for many people any ethical decisions they must make are deeply rooted in their religious beliefs.

Religion and spirituality can play a role in medical treatment in a number of different ways. More and more doctors are beginning to see that there is a very strong link between a person's spiritual life and her ability to heal or recover from illness. Hope can be a potent medicine, and for many people their religious beliefs or spirituality play a major role in fostering hope. Often people become increasingly spiritual with advancing age or health problems.

Religion can become an issue of another sort in health care when people refuse treatment because of their religious beliefs. Although this does not occur frequently, it gets considerable attention when it does, sometimes ending up in courts of law. This is particularly true in the case of minors whose parents make medical decisions for them.

Generally, the religious beliefs of a person and her family should be taken into account, and if there is any way to avoid an objectionable treatment, the alternative should be attempted. It is vitally important that people and their families understand the risks and benefits of a proposed treatment and that they understand the consequences of withholding treatment.

EXPERIMENTATION ON HUMANS

Ethical questions frequently come up in the context of experimentation on humans. In the abstract, no one wants to be a guinea pig—to try out something that may have unknown effects. In reality, though, the medical profession experiments on humans all the time. Most of the treatments that are available today have had a period in their development when they were tested on humans. Advances in medicine and science come from new ideas that are developed and refined and applied to the solution of problems through research. There is no way for sure to know how a product or a method of treatment will affect humans until it is used on humans.

Drug trials are the most widespread form of human experimentation. This process is tightly regulated by the federal Food and Drug Administration. Most drugs are extensively tested in test tubes in a laboratory and on animals before they are ever given to a human. Clinical trials—actually giving the drugs to people—have three phases (see below).

While history is full of unfortunate stories of people who have unwillingly or

---

THREE PHASES OF CLINICAL DRUG TRIALS

In a process closely regulated by the Food and Drug Administration, new medications are tested in clinical trials on humans to find out if they are safe and if they are effective. Each phase of testing builds upon information learned from the previous phases. Testing is conducted in the following three phases.

Phase I Drugs are tested for their toxicity, that is, for what harm they may cause. These tests are done on a small number of people and help determine the best way to give a new drug and how much is safe to use. Often when a new drug is tested, the trial will begin with very small doses, which are slowly increased. People in Phase I trials are closely monitored for side effects.

Phase II In the second phase of testing, drugs are given to a larger number of people to see if they work. People in this phase of a trial have often not responded to more conventional treatments—for example, people with cancer whose tumors have not been reduced, or have continued to grow, despite chemotherapy, might be placed in a Phase II trial. People are closely monitored for response to the drug as well as side effects.

Phase III If a treatment is judged successful in Phase II trials, the drug will be given to a larger group of people to continue to study how well it works and what side effects it causes. In Phase III trials, standard treatments are often compared with the product under investigation. Sometimes Phase III trials will continue for many years in order to look for long-term effects of the drug. ■

unknowingly become the subjects of medical testing, this is not likely to happen to anyone in the modern system of American medicine. Drug trials are conducted by voluntary enrollment. You will not be given an untested drug or subjected to an unproved procedure without being fully informed about the status of this intervention.

If a technology or drug is new, your doctor should also inform you of that and clearly review the risks and benefits with you. Again, as we have emphasized throughout this chapter, the issue for you as a health care consumer is to be as well informed as possible so that you can make the best decisions for yourself about your care.

Ethical considerations are considered in the context of patients' rights later in this chapter.

Choosing a Health Plan

In the not too distant past, a relatively small number of large health insurance companies provided coverage for most people, usually through a plan with their employer. In recent years that system has changed dramatically, and the changes continue at a rapid pace. Never before have Americans been faced with such a dizzying—and shifting—array of options for health care. The health care system in the United States is in such a fluid state that any detailed description given here would be out of date by the time you read this book. Even the language is changing, and you may feel you need a glossary to understand the vocabulary of modern health care (see below).

INDEMNITY INSURANCE

The traditional system of medical care is called indemnity insurance—also called fee-for-service—and it means just that: you go to your doctor, or to the hospital or clinic, and you pay a set fee for the service that you receive. If you have indemnity insurance, your insurance company covers all or part of your medical costs.

While more and more people are moving into managed care organizations, a substantial number are still covered by the indemnity insurance systems that finance fee-for-service medicine. In general, traditional indemnity insurance offers an unlimited selection of doctors and hospitals. However, the cost is usually higher than managed care, and the services covered may not be as comprehensive. Health insurance plans were originally established to cover hospital charges, and while most have expanded considerably, you may find that some companies do not cover visits to the

---

THE ALPHABET SOUP OF HEALTH CARE: A GUIDE TO ACRONYMS

The following is a list of abbreviations that you may encounter as you learn more about the health care system.

DRG Diagnosis-related group. A system used by many insurers, including Medicare, to classify illness according to diagnosis and treatment and thus allocate reimbursement.

EPO Exclusive provider organization. A network type of managed care organization in which people may only use network doctors and will not get reimbursement for services outside the network.

FFS Fee for service. The traditional payment method in health care.

HEDIS Health Plan Employer Data and Information Set. A measure of health plan performance.

HMO Health maintenance organization. Health plans that use staff providers or contract with medical groups to provide comprehensive services for their members for a prepaid fee.

IPA Independent practice association. An HMO that contracts with network of independent doctors to provide care.

NCQA National Committee for Quality Assurance. Independent nonprofit organization that evaluates and accredits managed care organizations.

PCP Primary care physician

PHO Physician hospital organization. An organization that integrates the services of private doctors and a hospital.

PPO Preferred provider organization. A system where members get discounted rates from the organization's network of affiliated doctors.

POS Point of service. An option that some HMOs provide that allows members to seek care from non-HMO doctors, but at a higher premium.

UR Utilization review. The process by which health plans measure the amount and appropriateness of services used by members. ∎

BUYING YOUR OWN HEALTH COVERAGE

The majority of Americans get health insurance paid for at least in part by their employer. This limits their options and their financial obligation. However, there are many people who are self-employed, who work part-time jobs, or who work for small businesses or in positions where health coverage is not offered. Millions of Americans must shop for and buy their own health insurance, or go without.

It is wise to spend time researching the alternatives that are available in your area and to compare the costs and components of each plan. If you or someone in your family develops a chronic illness, it can be difficult to change coverage, so it is important to make your selection with care. Managed care plans and indemnity insurance companies do most of their business contracting with groups, and their cost for individual premiums may be high. Speak with friends who have had to buy their own coverage to see if they can recommend their plan or an insurance agent. Meet with insurance agents and see what they have to offer. You might also investigate whether a group you are a member of or can join offers health coverage. Many self-employed people buy their health insurance in a group plan by affiliating with an organization such as the National Association for the Self-Employed, or professional or trade groups.

Be sure to read the fine print of a coverage plan you are considering to see what conditions are covered and what is excluded (see page 1412). All insurance plans are different, and you will want to consider your individual health care needs as you shop for insurance. If you are thinking of having children, for example, obstetric coverage will be important, but if you are past childbearing age it will not be a consideration. If you have a family history of mental health problems, you will want to look closely at what the insurer covers, since this is an area where coverage can vary considerably. Often, you will not see all the details of the contract until you have agreed to buy a particular coverage. In most states there are laws that protect you and that give you a certain amount of time (usually 30 days) to review a contract and to change your mind if you wish. In general, premiums for managed care plans will be lower, but indemnity insurance plans offer more freedom in your choice of doctors and care settings. In the case of indemnity insurance, always make sure that the lifetime cap—the total dollar amount of coverage that the company will pay—is sufficient. A lifetime cap of $100,000 may seem like a lot of money, but it can be used up very quickly should a family member develop a serious disorder or if several members of a family are in a car accident.

If you are healthy and seeking health insurance as an individual, you will not have any problem finding coverage, though it may be expensive. If you have been sick or are disabled, your task will be more difficult, although the 1996 Health Insurance Portability and Accountability Act prohibits denying coverage for preexisting conditions for longer than one year. Many insurance companies now offer open enrollment periods when anyone may be insured.

Your state insurance commission and local insurance agents can give you specific information about what options are available in your area for individuals buying health insurance. ■

doctor's office or prescriptions or some diagnostic tests.

Indemnity means protection from loss. These policies reimburse either the doctor or the individual for a portion of the costs they incur according to the terms of the insurance contract. Usually, the insured person is solely responsible for paying a predetermined deductible—a certain dollar amount of costs each year. Depending on the type of coverage, the deductible may be minimal—$25 to $150—or as high as $5,000. Once the deductible has been earned, the insurer will begin paying a percentage of the costs. The most common arrangements are 80/20—with the insurer paying 80 percent of the cost and the individual 20 percent—or 50/50. Usually there is a limit—called a stop-loss clause—on the amount that you must copay, and once that limit is reached the insurance company pays 100 percent of the cost. However, most policies also have a lifetime cap that puts a top limit on how much the company will pay for you in your lifetime.

While it may seem to a healthy person that she could never run up $1 million in medical expenses, for example, the costs of catastrophic illnesses or injuries can be astronomical.

There are a number of other points to be aware of if you have or are thinking of getting indemnity health insurance. Apart from the 80/20 or 50/50 copayment, your insurer may pay only what it considers "reasonable and customary" charges, which are the common charges for services in your geographic area. Some doctors will agree in advance to accept what the insurer pays, but some may not. If your doctor is recommending a particular treatment that may be costly, it may be wise to check with your insurer in advance about the extent of coverage you can expect. Insurers may also specify limits for hospital care for each illness. In addition, deductibles may have certain qualifications—for example, you may have a separate deductible for each hospitalization you experience. You will also have a separate deductible to pay for each family member, although there may be a cap on that payment.

You or your employer will pay a monthly premium for your insurance coverage. The provisions of your coverage will, to some extent, determine the amount you pay each month. For example, a 50/50 copay plan will cost less each month than an 80/20 copay plan, though your costs on the 50/50 company plan for each medical visit will, of course, be higher. If you have the opportunity to make certain choices (50/50 versus 80/20 or high deductible versus low, for example), the insurance math can be complicated because you may need to consider not only your present medical expenses but also future ones, which no one can know for certain (see Buying Your Own Health Coverage, page 1408).

THE INS AND OUTS OF MANAGED CARE

Managed care is the general term used to describe an organizational approach to health care and the delivery of medical services that seeks to control the costs and quality of health care and to coordinate and integrate medical and other health-related services. When we talk about managed care, we are not talking about a single system or type of system but a large array of methods and strategies for organizing the delivery of health care. No two health plans work the same way or offer the same services.

The most common feature of managed care organizations is their emphasis on cost controls. Ideally, costs are controlled by highlighting preventive care, eliminating unnecessary services whenever possible, and monitoring outcomes of treatment to determine what works and what does not. However, the common complaint about managed care organizations is that they save money by limiting care and cutting corners in a way that compromises the quality of care. This is a complaint that must be confronted because for all the different forms that managed care takes, there is little disagreement that it is here to stay and will continue to be the framework of health care delivery in this country in the years and decades to come.

Managed care organizations actually began as long ago as the 1930s, with the first HMOs. These companies represented only a small portion of the health care marketplace until the 1980s, when the numbers started to grow rapidly. In the 1970s, just over 3 million Americans belonged to HMOs. By 1980, that number had risen to 9 million. In 1995, as many as 115 million Americans received their health coverage from some type of managed care plan. As millions of Americans who are covered by Medicare and Medicaid move into managed care, the numbers will continue to grow substantially. Even in rural America, where indemnity insurance has continued to predominate, managed care is making its presence felt.

As managed care evolves, it is experiencing the growing pains of any system that has faced a skyrocketing increase in participants—both individuals and doctors. The people who pay for much of managed care—usually our employers—are called the purchasers. In many areas, purchasers are banding together in order to improve their bargaining position for financial negotiation with the health care companies.

While costs are important, most purchasers are also interested in providing their clientele with care that meets their needs. Ultimately, American health care consumers will not accept a system that does not emphasize quality and access to care. In these transitional times, the challenge is to discover which systems work best to provide the best possible care for the most people at the least cost.

Purchasers are not the only ones who have banded together in order to better negotiate the complexities of managed care. Doctors are forming groups at an ever-increasing rate, with some doctors' groups joining together to form supergroups, to enhance their bargaining position with the managed care organizations. Large academic medical centers are linking together with community hospitals in their region and home health care companies in another grouping. In yet another form of organization, physician-hospital organizations integrate the resources of private practice doctors (both primary care and specialists) and a hospital and work with a variety of insurers to provide services.

Your choice of plans will be limited by the options your employer offers you. Even with limited options, this can be confusing. Health care is a fiercely competitive marketplace, and companies will vie for your attention with television commercials, glossy pullouts in national magazines, and giant billboards along the highway. Every individual and family has different health care needs, and it is up to you to read the literature offered by the various plans, weigh the services that are offered against each other, think about what you need, and consider the cost.

In order to make informed choices it is helpful to know a little about the different types of managed care organizations and how they work.

TYPES OF MANAGED CARE

There are three major types of managed care organizations: HMOs, preferred provider organizations, and point of service plans.

HMOs HMOs are health plans that contract with groups of doctors to provide comprehensive medical services for their enrolled members. Members are required to use participating providers for all health services. You will pay a fixed fee for your care, no matter how extensive or limited your use of services actually is. In other words, a person in good health who just requires routine preventive and screening services pays the same fee as someone with serious health problems who requires considerable treatment. This is the principle of capitation, explained more fully below. Members may have additional financial obligations in the form of deductibles or copayments, also explained below (see The Principle of Capitation, page 1411).

There are three different types, or models, of HMOs:

- Staff model HMOs employ doctors, nurses, physician assistants, and other health care providers in salaried positions. These professionals work full-time for the HMO.
- Group model HMOs contract with multispecialty medical groups for care for their members. Members are required to see a doctor in a contracting group unless an outside referral is made.
- Independent practice association model HMOs contract with groups of independent doctors who provide care in their own offices. Independent prac-

tice associations will often contract with more than one HMO and their doctors may also do fee-for-service work as well.

Preferred provider organization A preferred provider organization has an arrangement in which participants receive care from a network of doctors who furnish medical services for members at discounted rates. If members want to use "non-preferred" doctors they may, but the rate is considerably higher. An exclusive provider organization is a variation in which participants may only use network doctors and will not get reimbursement for services outside the network.

Point of service Point of service plans allow HMO members to seek care from non-HMO doctors, but members who choose this option will pay higher premiums than members who stick to the HMO's more limited selection of doctors. This arrangement, also known as an open-ended HMO, encourages members to choose a primary care doctor, but may not require it.

Whatever the model, the primary care doctor is the heart of managed care. The primary care doctor serves as your initial contact with the system and your conduit through it. Usually her authorization is needed for consultations with other doctors. This gatekeeping function, ideally, helps streamline the process, coordinate your care, and avoid unnecessary duplication of services or inappropriate referrals. The primary care doctor may be assisted in this role by a case manager, usually a nurse or social worker, who has the responsibility of coordinating services and ensuring continuity.

JUDGING QUALITY

With all the information provided here, the advice and guidance you get from your friends, and the material you read, you may still find yourself wondering: How can I be sure that I am getting quality health care?

Quality of health care is a subjective thing, but there are some guidelines that have been established to help you become more knowledgeable about the quality of care you are receiving. Many large health care companies have research branches that study treatments and their outcomes and analyze such factors as cost effectiveness and patient satisfaction.

The plans themselves are accredited by a number of different independent organizations including the National Committee for Quality Assurance (NCQA), the Joint Commission on the Accreditation of Health Care Organizations, the Utilization Review Accreditation Commission, or the Accreditation Association for Ambulatory Health Care.

The NCQA is the largest accreditation organization for managed care companies and confers full, 1-year, or provisional accreditation. Since 1996, the NCQA has made the results of its accreditation reports available for purchasers and consumers. It rates performance in the following six categories:

- Quality of care
- Relationship with members
- Doctor qualifications and evaluation
- Preventive health services
- Decision making on services
- Medical records

The NCQA provides graphs that compare the scores of individual health plans with the national average.

The NCQA also sponsors an information-gathering program called HEDIS, the Health Plan Employer Data and Information Set. The Health Plan Employer Data and Information Set is a defined set of measures that evaluate areas such as quality and access to care, patient satisfaction, membership stability, and internal management, and the plan also includes a number of measures designed to assess the quality of preventive care.

State and federal regulation through licensure requirements can also provide a measure of quality assurance. The federal government is becoming increasingly involved with this process as more and more Medicare and Medicaid clients move into managed care.

HOW TO GET MANAGED CARE TO WORK FOR YOU

The best way to get the most you can from a managed care system is to become well-informed about what is happening in the health care arena. Know what managed care is, and explore the options that you have. Read the fine print in the literature and contracts. Talk to others and learn from their experiences. Ask questions. Most large employers have personnel who answer these questions every day and will be able to help you. Or call a company directly with your specific questions.

Weigh what the various plans offer against your needs. One plan might be better for covering regular checkups but it may not cover more extensive procedures. If you are a woman thinking of having chil-

THE PRINCIPLE OF CAPITATION

Another shared characteristic of most managed care organizations is the principle of capitation. Capitation is the process whereby insurance plans or managed care companies pay doctors a set amount per month per enrolled person, regardless of how often or how rarely the doctor sees that person and what services are provided. Capitation rates are determined by defining the population that the doctor treats and estimating what the average health care costs are for this group.

Ideally, this system allows doctors to be more efficient and encourages preventive care. In recent years capitation has played a key role in holding down health insurance rates. However, the concern among individuals, consumer groups, and many doctors is that capitation rewards doctors for restricting care and may create a financial incentive to undertreat. Compounding this concern are the bonus plans that many health plans offer their doctors. Bonus plans, while sometimes associated with quality of care and patient satisfaction, are often added reimbursements for doctors who keep expenses down.

For doctors, the other side of the capitation coin is the financial risk they take. In general, the cost of caring for a person with complex and expensive medical needs is offset by the lesser costs associated with healthier people. However, if a practice has a predominance of less healthy people, the doctor who is reimbursed through a capitated system may end up bearing some of the costs herself.

Different managed care organizations apply the principles of capitation in slightly differing forms. Sometimes capitation applies only to primary care services. With a more comprehensive approach called global capitation, other services such as referrals to specialists and hospitalization are covered, and the reimbursement to these providers is "subcapitated" or "carved out." It will help you understand how your health care dollars are being spent—and what the limits are on your coverage—if you know how capitation works in your health plan. ■

TWENTY QUESTIONS TO ASK BEFORE YOU ENROLL IN A MANAGED CARE PLAN

1. What does the plan cover?

2. Does the plan cover adjunct services such as dental, optometry, mental health counseling, prescription medication, and substance abuse treatment programs?

3. What is my monthly premium?

4. Is there a deductible or copayment for services? What is the maximum out-of-pocket cost?

5. Are there annual or lifetime maximums?

6. Is there a limit to the number of visits for specific services that will be covered—for example, mental health, home health care, or transplantation?

7. Does the plan exclude any preexisting conditions? Which ones, and for how long?

8. Can I choose my primary care doctor in the plan? If I am not satisfied, will I be able to switch doctors?

9. What percentage of plan doctors are board-certified?

10. If I already have a doctor, is she one of the participating providers in the plan?

11. Is the primary care doctor's office convenient to my home or office, and are the hours convenient for me and my family?

12. How long is the typical waiting time for a new appointment with my primary care doctor?

13. Does the plan allow me to access doctors outside the network? What is the added cost of this for me?

14. Are the hospitals I might use part of the managed care plan's network?

15. What are the procedures for reimbursement for emergency care?

16. Does the plan have a grievance procedure, to challenge claims that are not allowed?

17. Is the plan certified by the NCQA (National Committee for Quality Assurance)?

18. How long will it take to get an appointment with a primary care doctor?

19. Where would I be referred for specialty care?

20. How much of its budget does the plan allot for administrative costs and profit, and how much for patient care? ■

INSURANCE MATH

With the traditional form of indemnity insurance in a fee-for-service medical marketplace, you were reimbursed for all or part of your medical expenses by your insurance company. With managed care and capitation that system is becoming less common, but a number of the concepts and methods are also incorporated in managed care payment arrangements.

Deductible This is the amount of money that you must pay out of pocket for medical expenses before your company picks up on reimbursement. The amount of the deductible can vary greatly and is specific to each insurance plan; in fact, to each policy. A higher deductible will usually mean a lower premium, which is the cost that you pay for your insurance.

Copayment Many insurers will require you to cover a portion of your medical expenses after the deductible is paid. Sometimes the copayment is a percentage of the cost, or it may be a flat fee, such as $5 or $10 for every prescription or office visit. A common arrangement is for the insurer to cover 80 percent of costs after the deductible and the individual to pay 20 percent.

Out-of-Pocket Limits Most companies will set a maximum of what you must pay for your health care. This means that once your deductible and copayments add up to a certain amount, the insurer will pick up full coverage. Usually the out-of-pocket maximum will be per person per calendar year. ■

dren, obstetric benefits will be an important consideration. If you are a senior, you may be interested in at-home care or long-term care.

How the company covers preexisting medical conditions is very important if you or a member of your family already has a diagnosed health problem. In the past, some companies would not accept someone with a preexisting condition, or would accept the applicant, but not cover the preexisting condition for a certain period of time. This depends on the contract your employer has negotiated with the insurer. You will pay less for a contract that allows the health plan to exclude coverage of preexisting conditions.

In many cases this exclusion has caused considerable hardship for people with medical problems who switched jobs, or if their employer switched the insurance options that were available to them. While this practice still continues, it has attracted a great deal of attention, and legislators have attempted to address the problems it creates. The Health Insurance Portability and Accountability Act, passed by the US Congress in 1996, says that insurers cannot deny coverage for preexisting conditions for longer than 1 year.

WHEN YOUR HEALTH PLAN SAYS NO

Up until recently health insurers covered nearly every medical treatment and procedure that was offered and people could be fairly certain that whatever their doctor prescribed for them would be paid for. With the advent of increasingly expensive medical technology, services are scrutinized more closely. It is not unusual for an insurer or managed care company to deny reimbursement for care in some instances.

If you are denied reimbursement, sometimes there is no choice but to pay the medical expenses out of pocket. But often there are alternatives. Most organizations have an appeals or grievance procedure. There are a number of principles to keep in mind and steps you can take when your health plan says no.

- Make sure you have followed the proper procedure. Most plans will not cover services unless they are derived from referrals by your primary care doctor.

- Document all of your diagnoses and treatment suggestions and the reasons for them.

- Read your contract and follow the steps that are outlined for filing grievances.

- If there is no specified grievance procedure, write the company and explain your complaint. Include copies of all relevant documentation.

- Send copies of your complaint to your state's department of insurance and your employer. If you feel the rejection is particularly outrageous, you might write to your congressman or the health reporter at your local newspaper as well.

The Care Settings

Seeking medical care, whether it is for a routine exam, a suspected problem, or a health crisis can be an anxiety-provoking experience for many people. It helps if you know what to expect. There are several different settings in which you are likely to receive medical care. In this section we will look at three: the doctor's office, the outpatient center, and the emergency room.

DOCTORS' OFFICES

Most of us are familiar with doctors' offices, but you may encounter a variety of arrangements depending on the type of practice your doctor is in and what kind of doctor you are seeing. The solo office, with one doctor and her supporting staff, is an expense that few doctors can bear alone in this era of expensive medical equipment. It is rapidly being replaced by the clusters of offices that are necessary to serve the needs of group and multispecialty practices.

Most doctors' offices will include a reception area and waiting room, a business office, a referral desk, several exam rooms, and a consultation room. There may be a procedure room and an x-ray room.

You should expect to fill out a number of forms in the doctor's office, particularly if this is your first visit. You will probably be moved from room to room during the course of your visit, depending on the reason for your visit and the complexity of your medical needs. The procedures that are performed in the doctor's office depend on what the doctor feels comfortable doing in this setting, and the type of practice. Many subspecialty surgeons perform minor procedures in their offices. Examples include minor skin procedures such as biopsies or removal of lesions, x-rays and other diagnostic imaging procedures, or colposcopy or biopsy at the gynecologist's office. A neurologist may do a spinal tap at the office; an orthopedist may set a broken bone.

If your doctor is in a staff model HMO, the office is likely to be more like a clinic than a traditional private practice office. From your perspective, this can mean convenience for referrals and other auxiliary services.

Another version of doctors' offices can be seen in community health centers, which are often located in urban areas. These storefront one-stop centers can be particularly useful for people who do not have a primary care doctor. Community health centers offer more continuity of care than a hospital emergency room, which many people also use for primary care (see page 1414).

OUTPATIENT CENTERS

Outpatient centers have sprung up in recent years to provide an alternative for people who do not want to deal with the daunting labyrinth of a big city hospital, and as entrepreneurial enterprises aimed at providing more cost-effective care. Outpatient centers are designed to be accessible, streamlined, efficient, and user-friendly. Because they are new, they usually offer the latest technology.

Outpatient centers, also called ambulatory care facilities, may be freestanding or associated with hospitals. Generally they require accreditation but are not subject to the same regulations applied to hospitals. They usually offer the convenience of many specialists and subspecialists grouped together, making for ease of referral and document-sharing. X-rays and other lab tests can be done quickly, and the results are reported back while the person is still receiving care. Outpatient centers are not intended to replace primary care doctors, but some primary care doctors may have their offices in outpatient centers.

The growth of these centers in the past decade has a great deal to do with the technological advances that have led to less invasive surgery for many conditions. The tiny incisions needed for laparascopic procedures heal much more quickly than the large open incisions that were once necessary for an operation. Laparascopes and other fiberoptic equipment mean that gallbladder surgery, biopsy, cataract removal, or any of dozens of other procedures that once required days of hospitalization can now be done on an outpatient basis.

Not all procedures can be done in outpatient centers, and they are not appropriate for everyone. People with complicating conditions or risk factors may need the more comprehensive care a hospital can provide. If you are uneasy about whether the care at an outpatient center will meet your needs, discuss your concerns in detail with your doctor.

Outpatient centers go hand in hand with the notion of people assuming a role in their own care. For example, at one time, preoperative care involved checking into the hospital the night before surgery and letting the staff take care of you. If your surgery is being done in an outpatient center, you will arrive in the morning and leave that same day. The responsibility for your care the night before will be in the hands of you and your family, based on your doctor's orders and recommendations, and the same is true of your postoperative care.

EMERGENCY ROOMS

Emergency rooms—also referred to as ERs or EDs (emergency departments)—exist to deal with medical emergencies. Unfortunately, many people also use emergency rooms for their primary health care needs. Chapter 13 of this book discusses emergency first aid care, how to handle emergencies, and when you should take yourself or someone else to the emergency room.

It is not a good idea to use the emergency room for primary care. Unfortunately, this is too frequently the case. A 1992 study of hospital emergency departments found that 55 percent of emergency room visits were for non-urgent situations, and that people came to the emergency room almost as frequently for coughs and sore throats as they did for chest pain.

Disadvantages of using the emergency room for your primary health care services include:

- *Expense* Hospital charges for this type of care are typically two to three times higher than what the same service would cost in a doctor's office.

- *Lack of continuity* Emergency room records will not include your complete medical history. Unless you are an emergency room regular, it is unlikely you will be treated by someone who knows you.

- *Convenience* While an emergency room offers 24-hour service, if your problem is minor you may have to wait for hours while more serious cases get treated first.

Some HMOs have implemented strategies to discourage the use of emergency rooms for anything but a genuine emergency. These strategies include both positive measures—for example, extending doctors' office hours so that coverage is available on evenings and weekends—and negative measures, such as making it difficult to get reimbursed for emergency room care.

In some areas, a new type of service called urgent care is available through HMOs or clinics. Often this service is offered during evening and weekend hours when your doctor is not available. You may need urgent care for something like a sprained ankle or an ear infection—a condition that requires prompt attention, but is not a serious or immediate threat to your health.

WHAT TO EXPECT IN THE EMERGENCY ROOM

Unless your situation is urgent, when you enter the emergency room you will be asked to fill out registration and insurance forms. You will also be asked to sign a form consenting to treatment.

Most emergency rooms are set up in a very organized way, with a triage system to determine the order in which people are seen and treated. It is not a first-come, first-serve system, but a need-based system. If you have a serious or life-threatening condition, you will be seen very quickly. But if your problem is not that acute, you may have to wait a while. Usually the triage—the order in which people are seen—is determined by a nurse.

Most emergency room patients are treated and released, but if your condition requires, you will be admitted to the hospital. If you have a primary care doctor, she may meet you at the emergency room, particularly if you are going to be admitted.

Managing Your Hospital Stay

No one wants to stay in a hospital, but there are times when hospitalization is necessary in order for you to receive the best care. While it may be frightening to have a condition serious enough to warrant hospitalization, it can also be reassuring to know that you are in a place where expertise and advanced technology come together to serve you. The medical team, nursing staff, and support personnel will be working together and on call to take care of your needs.

Many of the same points that we discussed in this chapter about communicating with your doctor and making informed decisions are applicable to your hospital stay. Ask questions. You have the right to know about every procedure that is performed, every medication that is given, and every test that is done. You have the right to know not only what is happening, but also why. Be persistent if necessary. Sometimes—especially if you are in a big teaching hospital—it might seem that most of the people you see are medical students and nursing aides who do not have the answers you need. However, often they can answer many of your questions, and if they cannot, they can relay them to your doctor or nurse.

It is usually helpful, especially in the case of a child or a senior who is hospitalized, to have an advocate who stays with the person during as much of the hospital stay as possible. This includes staying overnight, particularly in the case of children. Pediatric units will nearly always provide some sort of sleeping arrangement for parents, either in the child's room, or in a nearby guest room. An advocate can pursue questions for you, make phone calls, talk to personnel at the nursing station, run errands, and help make your stay smoother and more comfortable.

You do not need to take many personal items to the hospital, but there are some things that may make your stay easier. You will probably want to bring along some basic toiletries, slippers, a bathrobe, and clothes for your return home. The hospital will provide a gown, but you may feel more comfortable in your own pajamas, and this is often permitted. Boredom can be a problem for many people and it is helpful to bring along reading material, music, or games to pass the time. Your meals will be provided, but you may be able to have some of your favorite foods brought in if your diet is not restricted by your medical condition.

Hospitals can be busy, noisy places, and there are steps you can take if this bothers you. Asking that your door be kept shut can make a big difference. Check what the additional charge is for a private room; you might be willing to pay for one even if your insurance company does not cover it.

WHEN DO YOU NEED TO GO TO THE HOSPITAL?

There is no definitive rule to determine when a person must be hospitalized, but there are a number of guidelines that can

SYMPTOMS INDICATING
THE NEED FOR
HOSPITALIZATION

- Severe pain
- Bleeding
- Loss of consciousness
- Difficulty breathing
- Loss of vision
- Inability to urinate or move bowels
- Choking
- Extreme frailty, especially in seniors
- Debilitating chronic diseases
- High fever or convulsions, especially in babies and young children
- Persistent diarrhea, especially in babies and children who can quickly become dehydrated
- Sudden severe headache, weakness, or numbness of face, arm, or leg on one side of the body, which may indicate stroke. ■

help you make this important decision. Often hospitalizations, particularly those for surgery, are planned ahead of time and you will have plenty of time to get ready. The opposite of that is the emergency admission, which comes through the emergency room and is usually the result of an accident or injury or a sudden health crisis such as a heart attack.

The decision to admit a person to the hospital is in the hands of the professionals—your primary care doctor, the specialist you have been referred to, or the emergency room staff. However, it is helpful to know some symptoms that indicate hospitalization should be considered (see above).

TYPES OF HOSPITALS

There are more than 6,500 hospitals in the United States, with more than 1 million beds. Like everything else in modern medicine, America's hospital system is in a state of change. Many of these hospitals are in the process of merging, downsizing, affiliating, integrating services, or diversifying and generally trying to move into a future where

the roles of medical institutions are being redefined.

The majority of hospitals are nonprofit institutions that are often community-owned and run by a board of trustees. However, a growing trend is toward for-profit hospitals, which may be owned by managed care or other corporations.

Until the twentieth century, hospitals were usually medical centers for the poor; wealthier people usually got their health care at home. Hospitals were often thought of as places where diseases were spread. Throughout this century, with the advent of sophisticated and expensive technological equipment, the specialization of doctors, and the concentration of specialty care at the hospital, hospitals have come to be the focal point of the health care system.

Now the movement is going the other way. With their intensive services, specialized staff, and high-tech equipment, hospitals are very expensive to manage and maintain. The shift to managed care and its emphasis on cost control means that hospital expenses are being scrutinized more closely than ever before. Well-equipped outpatient centers and refined surgical techniques mean that fewer and fewer people require overnight hospitalization. Home health care is also filling the needs of many people who were once treated in the hospital. Usually only the more serious medical conditions and surgical procedures require hospitalization today, and the hospital of the future will probably resemble today's intensive care unit.

Your choice of a hospital may be controlled by your health plan. However, you will probably have some choice, and there are some factors to consider. One of the most important things to think about is the experience that the facility offers in the procedure or medical condition being treated. For example, if you need coronary bypass surgery, the American Heart Association and American College of Cardiology recommend that you select a hospital where at least 200 open heart surgeries a year are performed.

It may be difficult to choose among a number of hospitals, especially in an urban area. One resource that might help you is "America's Best Hospitals," a ranking of over 1,000 hospitals nationwide that is compiled annually by the newsmagazine *US News & World Report.* This survey—which has consistently conferred its highest rating on

Johns Hopkins Hospital—rates hospitals overall and according to specialties and provides information about size, staffing, certification of staff, and mortality rates.

The largest hospitals are generally academic medical centers like Johns Hopkins. Academic medical centers, or teaching hospitals, not only offer care, but also serve as research and teaching centers, thus offering people the advantages of the most up-to-date procedures, techniques, and medications. Academic medical centers, even as they are training doctors and nurses, also place an emphasis on patient education with nursing and medical students both providing education for patients.

Usually there are more levels of nursing care in an academic medical center than in other hospitals. These centers also tend to attract a high level of nursing and medical personnel. However, the high costs of specialized treatment and state-of-the-art equipment are forcing many academic medical centers to streamline their services and pay closer attention to budget considerations than was necessary in the past.

Another form of hospital is a large medical center that is not an academic center. Often these hospitals also have a teaching component and are also associated with medical schools, but you will find less structure in relation to education and teaching, and less cutting-edge research.

Community hospitals vary in size; they usually have between 300 and 500 beds. Community hospitals may seem friendlier than large medical centers, with more personalized attention. A good hospital will be accredited by the Joint Commission on the Accreditation of Health Care Organizations, and you do not need a big-name teaching hospital for most routine surgeries and treatment of illnesses. If your case becomes more complicated, you might be transferred to a medical center that can provide a higher level of care. In some areas, the distinction between community hospitals and academic centers is becoming blurred as the smaller facilities become affiliated with academic centers and staff members have multiple associations.

The following are examples of specialized hospitals that provide care for people with special needs.

Rehabilitation (or rehab) hospitals and centers These are facilities that help peo-

ple regain function that has been lost due to disease or injury. They also help people adjust to and compensate for permanent physical changes, and help to make people become as independent as possible. Rehab is applied to a variety of medical conditions, from sports injuries to strokes to degenerative disease. Large hospitals often have rehab departments, but many rehab centers are freestanding facilities.

People with intensive rehab needs, such as those with serious head injuries, may be hospitalized for lengthy stays at rehab hospitals. However, much rehab therapy is also accomplished on an outpatient basis. Rehab work is done by a team that includes a physiatrist (rehabilitation medicine specialist), physical therapist, occupational therapist, speech therapist, nurse, social worker, and psychological counselor, depending on the person's individual needs. Many assistive devices are available, such as feeding implements and writing implements, to help people with disabilities master the routine activities of daily living.

People in rehab are reviewed frequently and their programs reassessed and adapted to their improvement and changing needs. Advancing technology is having a large impact on rehab medicine, and if you or a family member needs rehab, you should look for a well-equipped facility with the latest equipment and experienced personnel.

Psychiatric hospitals Psychiatric hospitals provide for mental health needs. Large hospitals have psychiatric units, but longer-term care is often provided by freestanding hospitals. The increasingly widespread use of psychiatric medications, along with changing attitudes and financial considerations, has drastically decreased the number and length of psychiatric hospitalizations in the past couple decades. Conditions that once required months of psychiatric hospitalization are now treated in weeks or days.

Psychiatric hospitals vary in quality, and it is a good idea to visit in advance before an admission, if possible. Some psychiatric units are locked for security reasons and to protect the patients.

Psychiatric treatment is provided by psychiatrists, nurses, psychologists, and other therapists. Freestanding psychiatric hospitals usually do not have extensive physical medicine resources, and people with medical needs will need to be transferred to a general hospital.

Private psychiatric hospitals may have waiting lists for admission. These hospitals can also be very expensive, and most health insurers limit psychiatric coverage. Check with your health plan about what your coverage allows. Unfortunately, insurers and psychiatric treatment teams may have differences of opinion about how many days of hospitalization are required for treatment, and the insurer will have the last word about what is covered.

Nursing homes With the aging of America's population, nursing homes and other extended care facilities are facing growing demand for their services. Nursing homes are residential care facilities for seniors or the infirm. They offer a range of services to fill social, psychological, and medical needs. Usually nursing homes are classified as intermediate care facilities, which assist with activities of daily living and routine medical and nursing services, or as skilled care facilities, which provide more intensive nursing and medical care.

Nursing homes are part of an increasingly complex system of care for seniors that includes home health care, assisted living, senior housing, and other arrangements that work to allow seniors as full a life as possible.

Hospices Hospices are programs and facilities that help people and their families through terminal illnesses. Hospice care emphasizes compassionate pain control and death with dignity. Many hospice services are provided in the person's home, which enables them to stay at home through the terminal phases of an illness and to die at home if desired and possible. Families are closely involved with hospice care (see Chapter 35).

ADMISSION PROCEDURES

Often much preadmission paperwork and diagnostic testing is done prior to your actual hospitalization. You may go to the hospital itself or an affiliated outpatient facility for this. It is usually during this period that you will be told what to bring with you to the hospital and what instructions you should follow, such as fasting

before surgery. You will also be consulted about what type of room you want (private or semi-private), auxiliary services such as telephone and television, and dietary needs and options. This is the time to find out about visiting policies; for example, what the visiting hours are and if children are allowed.

Admission forms will ask you for basic information such as name, address, employer, and health insurer. You will also be asked to name a person to contact in case of emergency. When you sign the admission form you are agreeing to be treated at the hospital, pay the charges, and authorize the release of medical and billing information to your insurance company. Admission forms should also include the American Hospital Association's Patient's Bill of Rights (see page 1424).

When you arrive at the hospital for admission, your first stop will be the admissions desk, where a clerk will process your paperwork, answer questions about hospital policies and procedures, and direct you to your next destination. Do not bring cash or valuables to the hospital. It is not a good idea not to wear jewelry, except perhaps a watch and wedding ring. All of your belongings will be listed, and a plastic identification bracelet will be put on your wrist.

At the admissions desk you may also be asked to sign an advance directive form. Advance directives specify your wishes about choices in your medical care and are discussed more fully in the next section of this chapter.

An orderly or volunteer will probably take you to your room. You may have stops to make on the way for x-rays or other lab testing. You probably will not see your doctor when you are first admitted. Most of your contact will be with the nursing staff, and a nurse will be assigned to you as your primary nurse.

WHO WILL BE TREATING YOU?

During a single day of hospitalization you are likely to see dozens of people, and it may be difficult to know who is who and to keep their roles straight. The next day, many of the faces may have changed. Expect to see a changing array of personnel throughout your hospital stay. Your world will be populated not only by doctors and nurses but also by x-ray technicians, phlebotomists (technicians who take blood), dietary aides, physical therapists, social workers, and others, according to your needs and the size of the hospital. In an academic medical center, your case will probably be discussed daily by a team of doctors, nurses, and students who move from room to room on their rounds.

Since most of your contact will be with the nursing staff, there is a nursing hierarchy that is useful to understand. This varies somewhat from hospital to hospital, and we will use the Johns Hopkins Hospital model as an example. As far as clinical care is concerned, the top of the hierarchy is the nurse manager. The nurse manager may supervise one or several units, depending on the size of the unit. If the nurse manager supervises more than one unit, there will often be a charge nurse for the individual unit. Working under the supervision of the charge nurse are staff level nurses, who are registered nurses, or RNs, but may have a range of training and experience. Registered nurses have different levels—Nurse Clinician I, II, or III—based on their experience and expertise, and have different roles to play. There may also be nurse practitioners on the unit. Generally, sicker people are cared for by the more senior nurses.

Nursing assistive personnel help people with grooming and feeding.

The backbone of medical care in a hospital, particularly an academic medical center, is provided by the resident staff. Residents are medical school graduates who are completing their training in the hospital in a medical or surgical specialty. Residents are on duty round-the-clock in the hospital and are usually the first to respond to a call for services needing a doctor. Residents are differentiated by their specialty, and by their experience (usually first, second, or third year), and they assume increasing responsibility as they go through the years of their residency. A chief resident oversees all the residents in each specialty area.

Attending doctors are more senior doctors who are on the faculty or staff of the hospital or in private practice in the community with hospital privileges. Their role in the hospital is to make regular visits to their own patients and serve as consultants to the residents. If you have a specialized problem—for example, you need eye surgery, or you need chemotherapy for cancer—your attending doctor will be the specialist in that area.

Generally you will see your primary care doctor when you are in the hospital, but if you have a specialist attending doctor, your own doctor will take a background role. Your primary care doctor may confer and consult with the specialist, answer your questions, and serve as an advocate for you.

The nursing staff also often fills a consulting or advocacy role for people. Often nurses will serve as go-betweens by facilitating contact between you and the doctor. You may ask your nurse about a change in medication, for example, and she will relay your request to the doctor and come back with the necessary adjustments. Nurses will be on duty throughout an assigned shift, whereas the attending doctors come and go and can be much harder to track down. Residents are also on duty for an assigned shift, but they may have responsibilities that take them around the hospital, while the nurse will usually be assigned to a specific unit.

HOW LONG WILL YOU STAY?

Hospital lengths of stay are quite variable, but no matter what your condition, the current trend in medicine emphasizes a shorter hospital stay. There has been considerable debate over this trend in some areas, and what some view as unreasonably brief hospitalizations has even prompted legislation in some states, particularly regarding childbirth.

While the trend is clear toward shorter hospital stays, shorter stays do not lead to adverse outcomes such as increases in readmission rates or increased mortality.

To be sure, most of us would prefer a shorter hospital stay. For many conditions, the length of stay is predetermined by a treatment plan called a critical pathway. The critical pathway is a day-by-day plan that plots the course of treatment based on previously proven treatment strategies. It is individualized for the seriousness of each case and complications for each person. Critical pathways help predict the course of treatment. These blueprints for care are designed for use by hospital staff so that doctors and nurses can anticipate an expected length of stay and what services will be needed. However, if you ask to see your critical pathway, most staff will comply with your wishes, and you may find that this document helps you know what to expect in the hospital. Some hospitals will also prepare critical pathways for you and your family so you will know exactly what to expect in the course of your hospitalization (see below and pages 1421 to 1423).

GOING HOME FROM THE HOSPITAL

Shorter hospital stays mean longer recovery time at home. Your doctor will determine when you will be released, but this determination may have a great deal to do with the coverage allowed by your insurer.

Your discharge plan will help you know what to expect at home, what your limitations will be, and the schedule for resuming normal activities. Be sure to talk with your doctors about the various details that you will have to be aware of, including the following:

- Mobility. How well will you be able to move around? Can you walk up stairs?

- Bed rest. How much time must be spent in bed?

- Diet. Can you eat a normal diet?

- Driving. When will you be able to resume driving?

- Medications. What should you take and when?

Also talk to your doctor about when she wants to see you next. Follow-up visits are a crucial part of aftercare to monitor the course of your recovery.

Many people can benefit from home health care after a hospitalization (see Chapter 34).

Patient's Rights

One of the hardest parts about being a patient and requiring medical care is the feeling of helplessness that can go with it. Throughout this chapter we have tried to give you tips on how to take control of your care and become a partner in treatment decisions.

It can be all too easy, in the complex health care system we must deal with, to lose the focus on the needs and rights of the patient. But a number of reassuring protections are in place. On the individual level, the Joint Commission on the Accreditation of Health Care Organizations requires that every hospital have a committee to represent patients. More globally, the American Hospital Association issued "A Patient's Bill of Rights" in 1973 that is supported by US hospitals. These rights include your access to care, your right to privacy, your right to accurate and complete information, and your right to make decisions for yourself. These rights are posted in most hospitals, and whenever you are admitted to a hospital you will receive a copy as part of the admission process.

To conclude this chapter about taking charge of your health care, we will discuss

---

PATHWAY TO RECOVERY: MYOCARDIAL INFARCTION (HEART ATTACK)

A Guide for Patients and Families

Welcome to the cardiology service. This pathway was developed to let you know what to expect during your hospital stay and recovery period. Upon admission a collaborative team of doctors, nurses, case managers, physical therapists, nutritionists, pharmacists, and social workers will develop a plan of care or "Pathway to Recovery" which is unique to you. If you have any questions about this plan or your progress, please talk to any member of your team.

Your cardiologist is _____   Your nutritionist is _____

Your case manager is _____   Your pharmacist is _____

Your social worker is _____   Your physical therapist is _____

Television services can be activated using the handset at your bedside or by calling 5-5409. Education channels are 30 and 31.

Telephone service is available by purchasing a phone in the admitting office. A phone jack is located in each patient room. If you need assistance obtaining the phone, please contact your nurse.

Visiting hours are 12 to 8 PM. Children under age 12 are not permitted. Some restrictions may apply due to your need for rest and medical treatment. ▶

◗ Patient/Family Pathway Myocardial Infarction (Heart Attack)

	CRITICAL CARE UNIT (FOR STABILIZATION)	INTERMEDIATE CARE	READY FOR DISCHARGE
Monitoring	Your heart will be monitored continuously. Your blood pressure and heart rate will be checked every 1 to 2 hours or more. You will have a pulse oximetry probe on your finger that measures oxygen in your tissues. You may need a urinary catheter.	Your heart will be monitored continuously. Your blood pressure and heart rate will be checked every 4 to 8 hours, or more, if needed.	Your blood pressure and heart rate will be checked every 8 hours.
Activity	You may be on bedrest. You may be out of bed to chair for meals.	You may be out of bed with assistance. Physical therapy or cardiac rehab may assist you to walk in the hall and prescribe an individualized exercise program.	You may perform warm-up exercises and walk in the hall. Physical therapy/cardiac rehab may assist you with stairs.
Diet	You may not be allowed to eat or you will be on a low cholesterol, low saturated fat, no added salt diet.	Your diet may advance. You will be on a low cholesterol, low saturated fat, no added salt diet.	You will be on a low cholesterol, low saturated fat, no added salt diet.
Medication	You will be receiving medications intravenously (IV) and/or by mouth. You may be taking aspirin, blood thinners, stool softeners, and other medications. You may have oxygen through a mask or nasal cannula.	You may be on at least one IV. You will be taking medications by mouth.	Be sure to learn about your medications. Your nurse and pharmacist will provide you with important information.
Test and Procedures	You will receive electrocardiograms (ECGs) daily and as needed. A blood test may be taken every 4 to 8 hours. Additional tests or procedures may include an echocardiogram, temporary pacemaker, cardiac catheterization, balloon procedure, or stents.	You will receive ECGs daily and as needed. A blood test may be taken 1 to 2 times each day or more often as needed.	You may have further tests to evaluate your heart function such as a stress test or a Holter monitor.
Important Issues	Report any chest pain, radiating (spreading) pain, or shortness of breath. Report any bleeding or strange bruising, which may result from blood thinning medications.	Report any chest pain, radiating (spreading) pain, or shortness of breath. Report any bleeding or strange bruising, which may result from blood thinning medications. A social worker may visit you to see if you have any concerns about discharge such as financial issues/insurance, family issues, or home care needs. A nutritionist may visit you to review your diet. A pharmacist will visit you to review your medications.	Be sure that you understand all discharge instructions, including your medication usage, activity level, diet, return to driving/work, and follow-up appointment. Notify the person planning to pick you up the night before you are scheduled to go home.

Source: The Johns Hopkins Hospital, Department of Medicine, Baltimore, Maryland.

	DAY BEFORE SURGERY	DAY OF SURGERY	1ST DAY AFTER SURGERY	2ND DAY AFTER SURGERY	3RD DAY AFTER SURGERY
ACTIVITY	As usual	Bed rest	Out of bed to chair	Walk in room	Walk in hall
		Begin to wake 6 to 8 hours after arrival to intensive care unit	Breathing exercises every 2 hours	Breathing exercises every 2 hours	Breathing exercises as needed
DIET	Regular diet/Nothing to eat or drink after midnight (starting day before surgery)	Nothing to eat or drink	Fluids (broth, tea) started in limited amounts (beginning first day after surgery)	Progress to a no added salt diet with limited fluids (beginning second day after surgery)	
			Stomach tube removed		
		Stomach tube to drain stomach contents			
			(May experience some nausea from medications given during surgery)		
MEDICATIONS	Bring a list of medications you are currently taking	Intravenous (IV) medications for blood pressure to assist heart to pump better	Oral medication for blood pressure as needed (beginning first day after surgery)	Oral medication for blood pressure as needed	Oral medication for blood pressure as needed
	Sleeping pill	IV furosemide (Lasix, "water pill") and potassium	Furosemide and potassium pills two times a day	Furosemide and potassium pills two times a day	Furosemide and potassium pills two times a day
		Pain medication as needed	Pain medication: Tylox as needed	Tylox	Tylox
			Warfarin (coumadin) to prevent blood clots around the new valves	Warfarin	Warfarin
				Docusate sodium (Colace, stool softener) two times a day (beginning second day after surgery)	Docusate sodium
TESTS	Blood tests	Blood tests (from IV)	Blood tests	Blood tests	Blood tests
	Electrocardiogram (ECG)	ECG	ECG		
	Chest x-ray	Chest x-ray	Chest x-ray		
	Weight	Weight (bed-scale)	Weight (standing)	Weight	Weight
MISCELLANEOUS	Shower with medicated soap to chest/arms/legs three times to decrease germs	Heart monitor to watch heart rate	Heart monitor to watch heart rate	Heart monitor to watch heart rate	Heart monitor to watch heart rate
			Dressing changes on incisions	No dressing on incisions	
		Breathing tube connected to breathing machine (respirator)	Breathing tube removed		
			Oxygen by face mask or nasal prongs	Oxygen by face mask or nasal prongs	Oxygen by face mask or nasal prongs
			Removal of various tubes put in during surgery		

4TH DAY AFTER SURGERY	5TH DAY AFTER SURGERY	6TH DAY AFTER SURGERY	7TH DAY AFTER SURGERY	
Walk in hall	Walk independently	Walk independently	Walk independently	
	Physical therapist will review exercise program			
Breathing exercises as needed	Breathing exercises as needed	Breathing exercises as needed	Breathing exercises as needed	
No added salt diet with limited fluids	No added salt diet with limited fluids	No added salt diet with limited fluids	No added salt diet with limited fluids	
	Nutritionist will review diet and will assist with meal/food selections			
			Discharge medications: Tylox, docusate sodium (Colace stool softener)	
Until you are at pre-surgery weight and have no swelling				
Tylox	Tylox	Tylox	Tylox	
Warfarin	Warfarin	Warfarin	Warfarin	
Docusate sodium	Docusate sodium	Docusate sodium	Docusate sodium	
Blood tests	Blood tests	Blood tests	Blood tests	Blood tests
ECG				
Chest x-ray				
Weight	Weight	Weight	Weight	
Pacemaker wires removed	Staples removed			
Oxygen stopped				
IV catheter in hand/arm removed				

*The above table is an adapted example of an educational tool for patients and families that explains critical pathways. Every procedure will have its own critical pathway. This example is for coronary artery bypass. Source: The Johns Hopkins Hospital, Baltimore, Maryland.

Tylox is a brand name for acetaminophen and oxycodone hydrochloride.

A PATIENT'S BILL OF RIGHTS

1. The patient has the right to considerate and respectful care.

2. The patient has the right to obtain from her doctor complete current information concerning her diagnosis, treatment, and prognosis in terms the patient can be reasonably expected to understand. When it is not medically advisable to give such information to the patient, the information should be made available to an appropriate person on her behalf. She has the right to know by name the doctor responsible for coordinating her care.

3. The patient has the right to receive from her doctor information necessary to give informed consent prior to the start of any procedure or treatment. Except in emergencies, such information for informed consent should include but not necessarily be limited to the specific procedure or treatment, the medically significant risks involved, and the probable duration of incapacitation. Where medically significant alternatives for care or treatment exist, or when the patient requests information concerning medical alternatives, the patient has the right to such information. The patient also has the right to know the name of the person responsible for the procedures or treatment.

4. The patient has the right to refuse treatment to the extent permitted by law, and to be informed of the medical consequences of her action.

5. The patient has the right to every consideration of her privacy concerning her own medical care program. Case discussion, consultation, examination, and treatment are confidential and should be conducted discreetly. Those not directly involved in the patient's care must have the permission of the patient to be present.

6. The patient has the right to expect that all communications and records pertaining to her care should be treated as confidential.

7. The patient has the right to expect that within its capacity a hospital must make a reasonable response to the request of a patient for services. The hospital must provide evaluation, service, or referral as indicated by the urgency of the case. When medically permissible a patient may be transferred to another facility only after she has received complete information and an explanation concerning the needs for and alternatives to such a transfer. The institution to which the patient is to be transferred must first have accepted the patient for transfer.

8. The patient has the right to obtain information as to any relationship of her hospital to other health care and educational institutions insofar as her care is concerned. The patient has the right to obtain information as to the existence of any professional relationships among individuals, by name, who are treating her.

9. The patient has the right to be advised if the hospital proposes to engage in or perform human experimentation affecting her care or treatment. The patient has the right to refuse to participate in such research projects.

10. The patient has the right to expect reasonable continuity of care. She has the right to know in advance what appointment times and doctors are available and where. The patient has the right to expect that the hospital will provide a mechanism whereby she is informed by her doctor or a delegate of her doctor of her continuing health care requirements following discharge.

11. The patient has the right to examine and receive an explanation of her bill regardless of source of payment.

12. The patient has the right to know what hospital rules and regulations apply to her conduct as a patient. ∎

some of the concepts covered in the Patient's Bill of Rights, including the rights of people who are no longer competent to make their own decisions. These rights are not just well-meaning promises—in many cases patients' rights are backed up by laws. Laws vary from state to state and you may have to do some research to find out exactly what the provisions are in your jurisdiction, but many of the principles are shared nationwide.

THE RIGHT TO PRIVACY

The right to privacy and the confidentiality of your medical records are among the most basic ethical tenets of medicine and nursing. There are provisions in the codes of ethics for all of the various medical professions recognizing the patient's right to privacy and the need to preserve the confidentiality of information about patients and their medical condition.

The right to privacy is motivated by respect for the individual, but there is another more practical reason for this right. Health care providers need to know personal, intimate details of your life in order to treat you. You cannot be expected to talk openly and provide the information they need without the assurance that this information will remain confidential.

This means that you can expect that conversations between you and your doctor, information in your record, and results of your tests will remain private between you and your doctor and any other medical professionals who need to know to be involved in your care. It is unethical for doctors to even talk about your condition or care in an elevator or corridors where conversations might be overheard.

You may sometimes be asked to waive confidentiality rights so that others with an interest in your care can consult or participate in your medical treatment. This includes your health insurer, to whom all medical records must be released in order for you to receive reimbursement. You may also be asked to waive confidentiality for your employer, for schools, or for other agencies.

There are other exceptions to the right to privacy. A doctor has the duty to report a medical condition if the welfare of others is concerned. For example, when a doctor in the emergency room treats a child with injuries that appear to be the result of child abuse, most jurisdictions require that this be reported to law enforcement officials. Another example is sexually transmitted diseases—reporting to sexual partners is often required. In a well-known legal case (*Tarasoff* v. *Regents of University of California et al*, 1976), when a psychiatric patient threatened to kill his girlfriend—and then did exactly that—the mental health counselor was held liable for not disclosing information that could have saved the woman's life. "Privilege ends where public peril begins," the court ruled.

MAKING YOUR OWN MEDICAL CHOICES

There are a number of mechanisms in place in the American health care and legal systems to ensure that you are able to make your own medical choices.

Consenting or refusing treatment As a patient, you have the right to know the risks and benefits involved for any treatment or procedure that is suggested, and the right to consent to the treatment or refuse it. Consent forms are generally very straightforward and written at a level that most people can understand.

The concept of informed consent gives people control of their care. It is explained in detail, in the section of this chapter about being an informed patient (see page 1399).

When a person is not capable of informed consent, they can give the power of attorney to someone, usually a spouse or other relative or close friend. This person is designated as your proxy to make medical decisions for you if you should become incapacitated. If no family member is available, hospital lawyers or ethics committees may become involved.

Obviously, you will want to designate the power of attorney before your capabilities are so compromised that such a decision is impossible. Known as durable power of attorney, this decision making power is granted to someone—known as an agent or proxy or surrogate—and continues (is durable) after you become incompetent. The person to whom you assign power of attorney should be someone who understands your feelings about health care, particularly terminal care, supports your feelings, and would probably make the same decisions you would make.

Advance directives Advance directives are orders made in the present, while you still have all your mental capabilities, to apply to the future, when you may not have the capability to make decisions regarding your medical care (see Chapter 35 and page 1589). Advance directives are legal arrangements that either consent to or refuse certain treatments. They should be very specific about what you want or do not want for a period in your life when you may be unable to make decisions for yourself. In practice, most advance directives refuse treatment, and many advance directives amount to do not resuscitate orders. Do not resuscitate orders are discussed in greater detail in Chapter 35.

Advance directives have developed as a means for people to spare themselves unwanted care, particularly at the end of life. Advance directives are usually in the form of durable powers of attorney or living wills (see Chapter 35 and page 1589). Each state has its own laws regarding advance directives and these laws are new and evolving. All states now have laws on the books requiring that living wills or durable power of attorney for health care be honored.

Patient Self-Determination Act The authority of advance directives was strengthened in 1990 when the federal government passed the Patient Self-Determination Act. This legislation says that any health care facility that receives federal funds (usually Medicare money) is required to inform people of their rights to accept or refuse medical or surgical treatment and of their right to have—or not have—advance directives.

Some people are troubled by the movement to advance directives and living wills because they believe that this trend is prompted by economic rather than humanitarian concerns and will sometimes unnecessarily hasten death. Another concern is that people at one stage of life may not be able to predict how they will feel about critical life and death issues when they are at another stage of life.

It is also true that in practice, living wills are sometimes not followed. For example, if a living will specifies not to prolong life with a feeding tube, but a person's family wants the feeding tube used, often the doctor will honor the family's wishes rather than the living will. It is important for you to discuss the specific provisions of your living will with your family so that when the time comes for the provisions to be invoked, there will be no confusion about intent.

WHEN A PATIENT IS NOT COMPETENT

More and more people, especially seniors, are using advance directives to control medical decisions that will be made when they are no longer competent to be full participants in the decision-making process. There are cases, however, when a person becomes incapacitated or is not competent to make decisions and has not named a medical proxy to assume the responsibility.

When this happens, someone—usually a close relative—must petition a court to be named as guardian. In order for the guardianship to be granted, the court will determine whether the person is truly incapacitated. Usually a guardianship is for an unlimited period of time, but the court may limit it.

Critically ill babies and young children also need a guardian to make medical decisions for them. In most cases it is the parents, although often grandparents are involved. Children have the same rights as everyone else, and the same issues are involved that we have been discussing throughout this chapter. When they are old enough and able to participate, children should be included in the decision-making processes about their treatment.

Preparing for Surgery

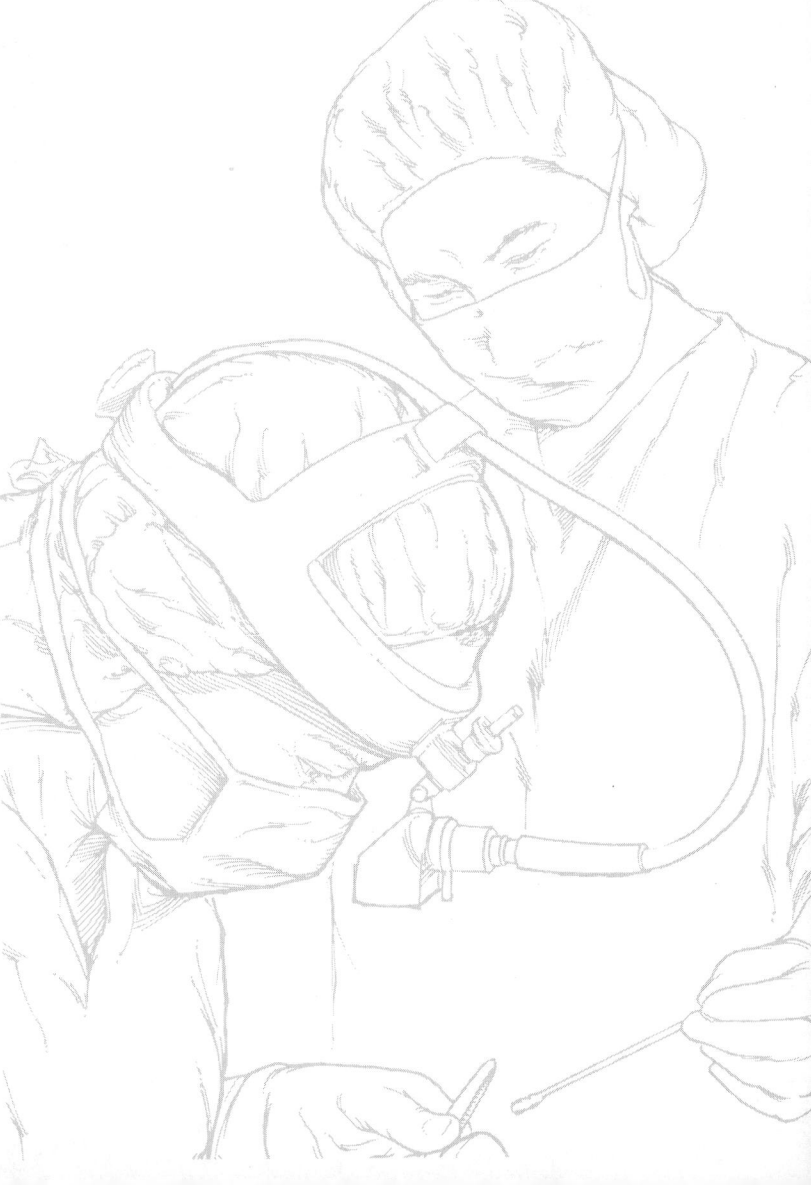

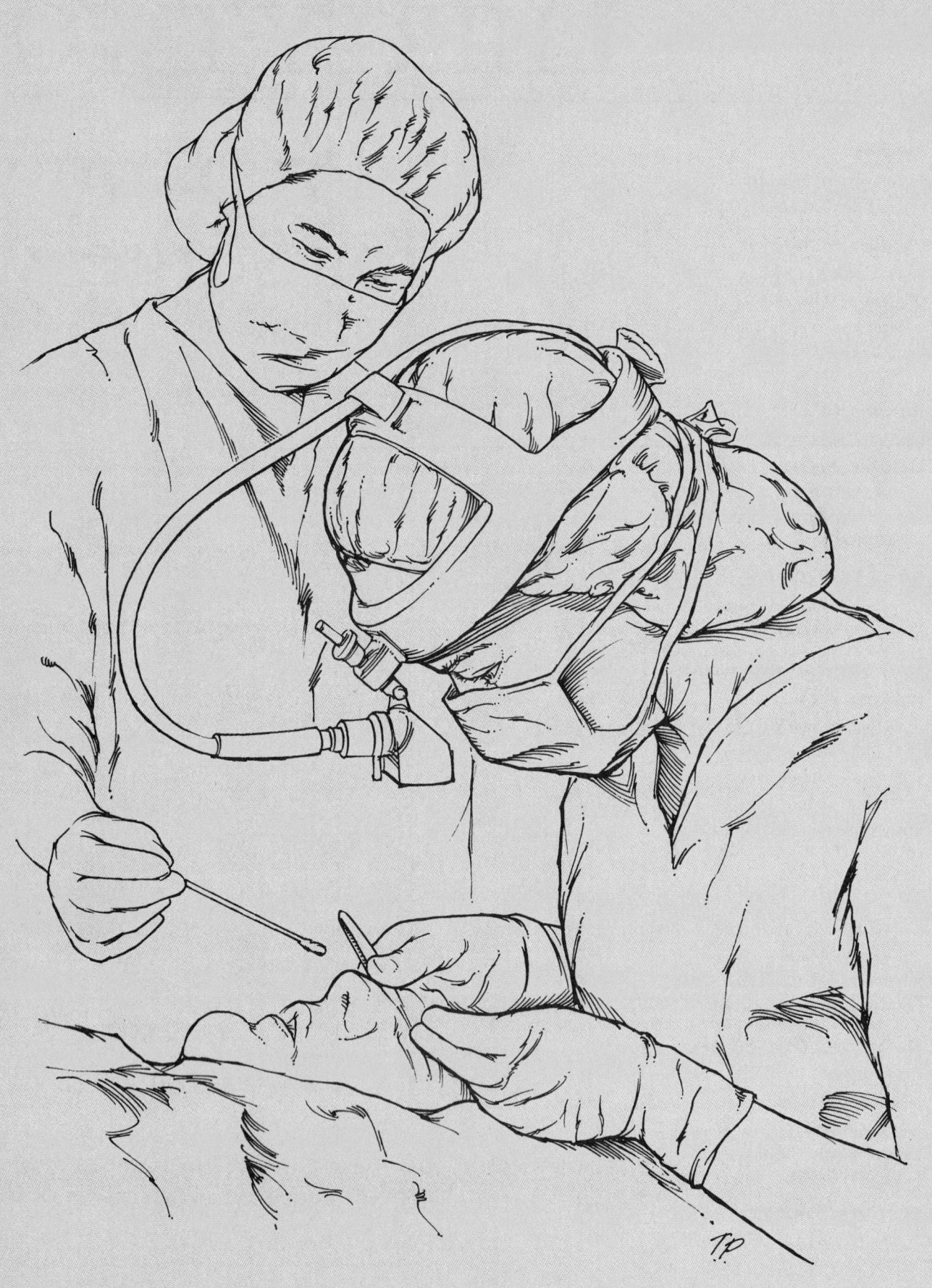

PREPARING FOR SURGERY

Surgery

More than 30 million major surgical operations are performed in hospitals in the United States every year. An even greater number of surgeries, both major and minor, are performed in outpatient clinics and doctors' offices. Tremendous technical strides have been made, making more and more complicated procedures possible and safer. This chapter offers detailed information to help you make decisions regarding surgery, prepare for your surgery, and speed your recovery. By taking an active role in your surgical care, you will be taking the first step towards a positive outcome.

IS YOUR SURGERY NECESSARY?

The decision to have surgery should only be made after careful consideration of your options. Make certain that the particular surgery you are contemplating is the best treatment for you.

The first step is to explore the alternatives with your doctor. There are several questions you should review with your doctor, as well as with the surgeon:

- Why is the surgery being recommended?

- Are there alternative forms of treatment that might be tried first?

- What risks are involved in the surgery?

- What sort of complications may develop?

- What is the risk of death from the surgery?

- How will the surgery improve your health and quality of life?

- How often are second or third revision surgeries necessary?

In many cases it may be worthwhile to get a second opinion, and in some cases, your insurance company will insist on a second opinion before approving coverage of the surgery. A consultation with another surgeon allows you to explore your options more fully and to learn whether there is agreement or disagreement regarding the recommended treatment. The best opinion is the one that most fully considers the range of options and their likely outcome.

COMMON SURGICAL PROCEDURES

The most commonly performed surgical procedures in all age groups are circumcision, tube placement for middle-ear fluid drainage, and cataract surgery. The frequency of other common surgical procedures varies by sex and age group.

In women of all ages, the most frequently performed operations include:

- Procedures to assist delivery such as forceps delivery or episiotomy

- Hysterectomy (although the frequency of this procedure has undergone a dramatic decline)

- Cesarean section

- Breast biopsy

- Cholecystectomy (gallbladder removal)

In women over age 65, the most frequently performed operations include:

- Arthroplasty (joint surgery) and hip replacement

- Pacemaker insertion or replacement

In men of all ages, the most frequently performed operations include:

- Prostatectomy (surgical removal of all or part of the prostate gland)

- Fracture reduction (repair)

- Disk excision and spinal fusion

- Coronary bypass

- Hernia repair

- Cholecystectomy

In men over age 65, the most frequently performed operations include:

- Prostatectomy

- Pacemaker insertion or replacement

- Hernia repair

- Cholecystectomy ■

Choosing a Surgeon

A surgeon is a qualified medical practitioner who specializes in surgery, the branch of medicine concerned with disorders that require operative treatment. Choosing a surgeon carefully is the best way of ensuring that your experience with surgery will be positive. While surgery is never risk free, the more experienced your surgeon, the lower the risk involved in surgery. The level of your surgeon's skills will greatly influence how you fare—regarding both postoperative complications and survival rates—and the effect on your quality of life will be felt for many years after the operation.

If your primary care doctor or the specialist who has been treating you suspects you may need surgery, he will recommend a surgeon to you and a hospital or clinic where the necessary diagnostic tests can be performed.

A qualified surgeon must be board certified. This means the surgeon has been certified by a surgical board that has been approved by The American Board of Medical Specialties (ABMS)—each surgical specialty has its own national board—and has successfully completed years of residency training in surgery and an examination approved by the ABMS. You will also want to check on the surgeon's specific board certification to ascertain that his expertise coincides with your needs. To find out if your surgeon is board certified, you may call the ABMS at (800) 776-2378 or check the Directory of Medical Specialists, which is available at your local library. You may also be able to find basic directory information from a credible source on the Internet, such as the American Medical Association (www.ama-assn.org).

You will also want to find out whether the surgeon you are considering is a fellow of the American College of Surgeons. If the letters FACS appear after the surgeon's name, you can be assured that the surgeon has passed a thorough examination designed to test professional competence and ethical standards. You may also want to inquire whether the surgeon is a member of any other medical societies, many of which require the continuing education of their members in new procedures and techniques and utilize peer review procedures to ensure ongoing quality of service. These safeguards can assure that your surgeon is up to date on the most advanced medical techniques and is maintaining the highest standards in his practice. It is equally important to find out whether the surgeon you are considering has been subject to discipline, has had his license suspended, or has been the subject of a professional peer review. To discover if there is a medical society for specialists who perform the procedure you are contemplating, check the Encyclopedia of Associations at your local library.

While being board certified and a fellow of the American College of Surgeons indicate general competence, being experienced in performing a certain procedure increases a surgeon's proficiency. Before deciding on a surgeon, you should find out how many times the surgeon has performed the particular surgery and for how long. In addition, you may want to ask how the surgeon's other patients have fared, though you should be aware that a person's preexisting health status affects the success of a surgical procedure.

Another way to find a surgeon is to ask your friends and other people you trust for referrals. Keep in mind, however, that your symptoms are individual to you and a surgeon who treated your friend may not be the most appropriate person to treat you. Find the doctor most appropriate to treat your condition.

Most importantly, when you choose a surgeon you are also choosing the hospital with which that surgeon is affiliated. Make sure your surgeon is affiliated with an accredited health care facility, and then obtain information regarding the hospital's record on the surgery you are contemplating. You will want to ask how often the procedure is performed there and how frequently complications occur. People undergoing high-risk, complex operations experience significantly better results when the surgery is performed at major medical centers where the surgery is performed frequently. If your surgery is to take place in an office or surgical clinic, you should make sure the doctor you choose has privileges at the local hospital in case an emergency admission is necessary. Ask how emergencies are handled in an outpatient clinic setting.

When you feel you are deciding between two equally competent surgeons and institutions, consider the rapport you feel you have with the surgeon. Feeling positively about your surgeon can add to your sense of confidence, which can have a positive impact on your surgical outcome.

THE FINANCIAL COST OF SURGERY

Modern surgical therapy requires the use of advanced techniques and technology as well as the safeguards that Americans consider standard. No surgery is inexpensive, and certain major surgeries can cost a substantial amount of money. For this reason you should go over the cost of surgery and its attendant procedures with your doctor or his office staff prior to surgery. Ask your surgeon's billing personnel what the fee will be and precisely what it covers. For example, the fee may cover only the surgery, or it may include postoperative visits to the surgeon as well. The anesthesiologist and other care providers will bill you separately; determine whether members of your surgeon's team will accept your medical benefits plan.

Health insurance reimbursement for surgery varies widely depending on the kind of coverage you have. It is therefore extremely important to speak to a representative of your medical benefits company before your surgery and find out what costs are covered and what costs you will have to pay yourself. You will be billed separately for your hospital stay, so you should inquire how many nights of hospitalization your benefits plan will cover for the planned procedure. Some medical plans require a second opinion before approving surgery; others will not pay for nonemergency surgery that they have not approved in advance. Read your benefits plan carefully and speak to a representative to be certain you have met all the requirements. Many health insurance plans have a recommended cost for individual surgical procedures. If your surgeon's fee exceeds this figure you will have to pay a portion of the bill yourself. If your medical plan will not pay all of the costs and you cannot afford to pay the difference, discuss the problem with your surgeon to see if a solution can be worked out. The more you know regarding your insurance coverage, billing procedures, and reimbursement before surgery, the fewer frustrations and annoyances you will face after surgery.

Throughout this whole process, keep in mind that you should always pursue the best possible medical care, which may well be outside of your plan, particularly if the procedure required is complex and fraught with serious complications. It is important to remember that such a procedure may save the medical plan money in the long run if a better outcome is achieved.

SURGERY IN SENIORS

Any surgical procedure involves risk, and as we age the risks we face when confronting surgery and anesthesia increase. Seniors are more likely to have preexisting conditions such as diabetes or hypertension that may increase the risks associated with surgery. It should be noted, however, that for seniors who are in good health, the increase in risk is not great. For example, hip replacement surgery, which is often performed on seniors, is one of the most successful surgeries.

Seniors do have a greater risk of contracting pneumonia after surgery. To minimize this risk, the nurse in the recovery room will ask you to begin breathing exer-

LASER SURGERY

One recent surgical development has been the introduction of laser surgery. A laser is a concentrated beam of light that produces a tremendous amount of heat and can therefore be used in place of a scalpel to cut or otherwise destroy tissue. Using a laser, a skilled surgeon may be more precise in making incisions, causing less blood loss for the patient. In some cases, laser surgery can be performed using scopes, which are illuminated optical instruments that allow the surgeon to make smaller incisions that speed recovery and minimize pain (see page 1432). While laser surgery may be less invasive than surgery performed with a scalpel, all surgeries are invasive. Also, as with any surgery, laser surgery is not risk free and complications can occur. Conventional surgery is often preferable to the use of a laser, particularly when laser heat may be damaging to nerves or blood vessels or the use of a laser excessively prolongs the procedure.

If you are contemplating surgery, you should consult your doctor regarding the possibility of laser surgery. Be as careful in choosing a surgeon to perform laser surgery as you would be in choosing any surgeon. The American College of Surgeons recommends that all surgeons performing laser surgery have credentials in both the appropriate surgical specialty and in the use of lasers. Also make sure that your surgeon has successfully performed the surgery you are contemplating many times and that the hospital with which he is affiliated has a similarly high success rate for the particular surgical procedure. Be wary of any doctor who represents laser surgery as a perfectly safe, 100 percent successful alternative to traditional surgery. All surgery involves risk, and situations do exist in which traditional surgery is safer and can achieve better results than laser surgery. ■

MINIMALLY INVASIVE SURGICAL TECHNIQUES

New surgical techniques allow doctors to perform major surgeries in ways that are far less grueling for patients. These techniques reduce pain and trauma to the body as well as recovery time, and they are helping to increase the possibilities of what can be accomplished with surgery.

Most new surgical techniques are first applied and made available at teaching hospitals and are not immediately available to the general public. If you are contemplating major surgery, you should investigate whether new, less invasive techniques are available for the procedure and whether there are any hospitals in your area where these techniques are in use. The following are examples of minimally invasive surgical techniques.

Laparoscopic Procedures

Laparoscopic procedures have been instrumental in making major internal repairs possible with minimally invasive surgical procedures. The endoscope is a long, flexible tube with a miniature camera and light source at the end that allows the surgeon an internal view of the patient's organs and body cavities on a television monitor in the operating room. The endoscope may be inserted through a natural opening in the body or through an incision. A laparoscope is a type of endoscope used for several surgical procedures including cholecystectomy, small bowel resection, colon resection, and tubal ligation, and for examination of the colon and ovaries. It is inserted through a small incision in the abdominal wall. The thoracoscope, which is inserted through a small chest incision, is useful for cardiac and lung procedures. Both scopes eliminate the necessity for huge incisions and the resultant trauma to the body, thus making many major surgeries far less invasive. Endoscopy and laparoscopy have revolutionized the operating room by reducing the risk and trauma of certain surgeries and increasing the accuracy of many complicated procedures including gallbladder surgery, adrenalectomy (surgical excision of one or both of the adrenal glands), back surgery, and heart bypass surgery.

Coronary Artery Bypass Grafting and Minimally Invasive Direct Coronary Artery Bypass

In traditional bypass surgery, the surgeon makes a foot-long incision in the chest to cleave the patient's breastbone, spreading it open to expose the heart. Both coronary artery bypass grafting (CABG) and minimally invasive direct coronary artery bypass (MIDCAB) eliminate the need to completely expose the heart, although the status of the MIDCAB procedure is still experimental.

In CABG, which is used for single bypass surgery, a catheter to the heart carries both a medication to stop the heartbeat and a balloon that expands in the aorta to block the flow of blood. Then a heart-lung machine is attached at the femoral artery in the leg rather than at the heart itself. The endoscope is used to free a healthy artery to replace the damaged one. Finger sized ports (tiny cuts into the body) in the chest allow entry of the endoscope

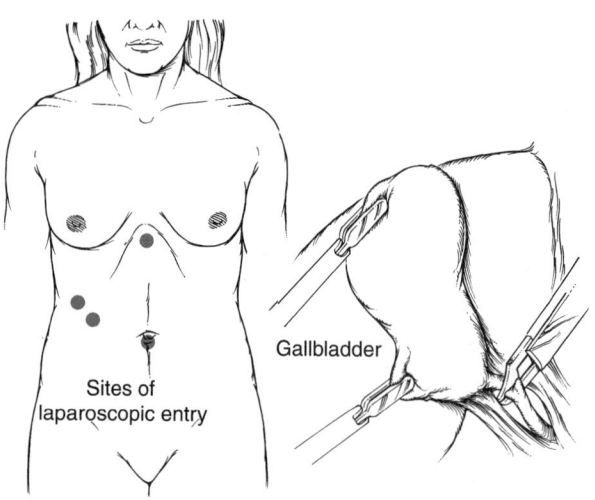

Laparoscopic removal of gallbladder. (A) Four small incisions allow tubes containing a video camera and surgical instruments to be passed into the abdomen. (B) Instruments hold the gallbladder while the cystic duct is cut and stapled closed.

and of the customized long tools that are used to perform the surgery itself.

MIDCAB surgery is restricted to those patients who only have one or two diseased arteries. During the procedure a small opening in the chest is made and a small piece of rib is removed so that the heart can be seen and touched. The heart is slowed with beta blockers but unlike traditional bypass surgery, where the heart is stopped, the heart continues to beat during MIDCAB surgery. Sutures, soft snares, and clamps are used to almost completely immobilize the heart so that the surgeon can operate. After CABG and MIDCAB most people go home in a matter of days and complete recovery takes approximately 3 weeks instead of the 3 months recuperation that follows traditional bypass surgery.

Neurosurgery

Many of the most high-tech advances in minimally invasive surgical techniques have been made in the field of neurosurgery, including stereotactic devices, which are finely tuned head frames attached to patients' skulls, and the sterile wand, which allows a neurosurgeon to work within brain tissue and view the exact location on a television monitor in the operating room. This procedure can limit injury to surrounding brain tissue.

Telesurgery

Telesurgery allows two surgeons in different locations to advise each other, and it also allows a surgeon to supervise an operation taking place in another location. Robotics, the use of robots to hold endoscopes and other equipment steady, are under development. ■

cises immediately and to use a breathing machine, called an incentive spirometer, to encourage you to breathe more deeply. Many people who have had major surgery use an incentive spirometer following surgery, but it is particularly important for seniors to heed the advice of the nurses and the doctors and to practice deep breathing exercises. Doing so will help to ensure your safe recovery and avoid those common complications involving the lungs.

If you are a senior contemplating an operation, it is important to weigh the risks you face if you undergo a surgical procedure against the quality of life you may face if you do not. Be sure to give consideration to how your life will be changed if you have the surgery and your recovery does not go as smoothly as you may wish. Whatever the procedure you are contemplating, it is important to have a frank discussion with your doctor regarding its risks, the possible outcomes, and the changes in your quality of life that you might expect. Ask your doctor or surgeon for an honest appraisal. Also see if you can speak to people who have had the procedure and attend a support group meeting if possible. Your doctor's recommendation that you have the surgery is a good indication that a favorable outcome can be expected.

Anesthesia

When you select a surgeon, you are also choosing the team that will assist with your surgery. One of the most vital members of this team is the anesthesiologist, whose skilled administration and monitoring of the anesthesia can support a positive surgical outcome and speed recovery. Your anesthesiologist will not only administer the medications that will keep you from feeling pain and sensation but will also be responsible for making informed judgements in regulating critical life functions during surgery. The anesthesiologist is also responsible for diagnosing and treating any medical problems that may arise during surgery. At the conclusion of the surgery, it is the anesthesiologist who reverses the effects of the anesthesia and helps to restore consciousness. Your anesthesiologist is also trained in pain management and will oversee initial pain control after surgery.

After your surgery you will receive a separate bill for professional anesthesia services, which will include the cost for pain management after surgery. The anesthesiologist's bill covers only professional services. You will receive a separate bill from the hospital for equipment and medications used during surgery.

Anesthesia has multiple definitions depending on the goals of surgery and type of anesthesia. Most importantly, it refers to the lack of normal sensation, especially the sensitivity to pain. It also may include a lack of movement in response to the surgery, and amnesia if general anesthesia is administered. Anesthesia is induced by a medication that prevents pain or brings about unconsciousness for the duration of a surgical or diagnostic procedure. There are three broad categories of anesthesia: general, regional, and local. Advances in anesthesia and its administration, such as improved equipment and techniques and new or faster-acting, predictable drugs, have simplified many common surgeries and allowed faster discharge to home without the aftereffects commonly associated with general anesthesia.

Advances in anesthesia have also led to better pain management. Patient-controlled analgesia (PCA) is a novel approach to controlling pain after surgery—that is, pain levels that are inadequately treated with conventional approaches to analgesia (pain relief without a loss of consciousness). If PCA is prescribed by your doctor, a pump loaded with pain-relieving medication is attached to your intravenous line, which allows you to administer your own pain medication as needed. The PCA pump also protects you from overdosage. Epidural analgesia, for example, is used to relieve pain after major surgery. A fine plastic catheter is inserted in your back, which allows for the continuous delivery of anesthetic around the nerves in your spine.

Most major surgical operations, particularly those involving the abdomen, chest, and brain, will require general anesthesia. Regional or local anesthesia may be used for minor surgical procedures, particularly those involving the extremities or superficial parts of the body. Regional anesthesia, particularly spinal or epidural techniques, may also be used for selected major operations such as cesarean section; pregnant patients frequently prefer to be awake to see and bond immediately to their newborn child. Additionally, many patients prefer to be conscious during surgery and therefore more in control. In certain procedures, such as prostate or hip surgery, a regional anesthetic may also offer advantages in reducing blood loss and risk related to surgical outcomes and may facilitate earlier recovery. Local or regional anesthesia may also be combined with general anesthesia to reduce the amount of general anesthesia needed and provide pain relief after surgery. It is best to discuss the potential advantages of any one anesthesia technique with the anesthesiologist, who can provide you with the potential benefits and risks associated with each technique for a particular surgical procedure.

Local, regional, and general anesthesia are all safe procedures, and the risk due to complication from an anesthetic is extremely low. It has been estimated that deaths related directly and totally to the anesthetic used during a surgical procedure occur in only about 1 in 185,000 cases. This rate may even be lower in the outpatient setting, where the surgery is less intense. The primary determinant of risk related to surgery and anesthesia is the patient's coexisting disease. Even in patients with heart disease, there appears to be no one best anesthetic technique. Therefore it is best to discuss your history and preferences with the anesthesiologist and an informed decision can be made regarding what technique will provide you with the best outcome for any given surgical procedure.

Anesthesia is administered by an anesthesiologist or by a certified registered nurse anesthetist. The American Society of Anesthesiologists recommends that an anesthesiologist be present throughout the administration of either general or regional anesthesia and that during the administration of any anesthesia the level of blood oxygen, the temperature, and the circulation of the patient be continually monitored. Local anesthesia used for in-office procedures may be administered by the doctor without the presence of an anesthesiologist. Increasingly, anesthesiologists are available to provide anesthesia in an office-based setting for complex cases; this can frequently be arranged by the doctor or dentist performing the procedure.

Most people are not admitted to the hospital until the day of surgery, especially with today's tendency toward shorter hospital stays. You may be evaluated in a preoperative evaluation clinic by members of the department of anesthesiology or your primary care doctor may complete a questionnaire, which is sent to the anesthesiologist and surgeon. If you are undergoing surgery in an outpatient facility, personnel from the facility may call you several days prior to surgery to discuss your history and provide you with information regarding your anesthetic. On the day of surgery, the anesthesiologist will meet you prior to undergoing surgery and further discuss your history, medications, and how the anesthesia will be administered. Medication to help relieve anxiety can be given prior to entry into the operating room if you desire. If you are admitted to the hospital the day prior to surgery, a member of the anesthesia team will visit you there, and medication can be given to you prior to coming to the operating room.

GENERAL ANESTHESIA

General anesthesia induces a reversible loss of awareness to enable major surgical procedures. When the patient is unconscious, the brain does not receive pain signals from the nervous system, so there is neither pain nor any other conscious sensations. General anesthesia also inhibits the body's response to stimulation, which can be helpful in limiting reactions such as sweating and muscle movement during surgery. General anesthesia is achieved by the administration of intravenous sedatives, narcotics, and other medications, and/or by inhaling vaporlike agents that produce a deep sleep.

While undergoing general anesthesia, you may or may not require the insertion of a breathing tube. The breathing tube is used to assist in the delivery of the vaporlike agents as well as in ventilation of the lungs. The decision regarding a need for a breathing tube depends on both the patient and surgery-specific factors. Placement of a breathing tube may cause chipping of a tooth during insertion or removal and a sore throat.

General anesthesia will be administered while you are lying down in the operating room. You will be hooked up to an oxygen monitor and electrocardiograph (ECG) monitor, and a blood pressure cuff will be placed on your arm before the anesthesia is administered intravenously. The time of recovery from general anesthesia varies. Immediately after surgery you will remain in the recovery room, where your vital signs will be monitored.

REGIONAL ANESTHESIA

Regional anesthesia is used to eliminate pain in a large segment of the body by blocking the transmission of nerve impulses in groups of nerves or in the spinal cord. Regional anesthesia may be administered by injection or continuously through a catheter (a small plastic tube). The following are the most common forms of regional anesthesia.

Nerve block Regional nerve blocks are used for surgery on the extremities and in some cases of gynecologic surgery and anorectal surgery. A regional nerve block may be used in conjunction with an inhalation anesthetic or heavy sedation. Either a surgeon or an anesthesiologist will administer the nerve block (see illustration below). Nerve blocks may also be used to relieve pain during labor.

Spinal and epidural anesthesia There are two types of anesthesia that act by blocking the nerves of the spinal cord: epidural, also called extradural, and spinal, also known as intrathecal and commonly called a spinal block. Both forms of anesthesia may be used for surgeries that involve the lower half of the body including cesarean section, hip and knee surgery, surgery on the foot or leg, hernia repair, and some prostate surgery. Spinal and epidural anesthesia have been combined in cesarean section surgery to reduce sensation during surgery and also to reduce recovery time.

An epidural involves the injection of local anesthetic agents into the epidural

space around the casing of the spinal cord. An epidural can be administered at any level of the spinal column and is usually administered continuously throughout surgery and may be continued after surgery. A catheter is inserted at the site where the original injection was given to administer the anesthesia during the operation. You can assist the anesthesiologist by remaining as still as possible while the tube is being inserted.

A spinal block is similar to an epidural, but it usually involves a single injection. Spinal anesthesia is performed through a lumbar puncture—a needle inserted between the vertebrae in the lower back. The needle is removed after injection of the medication. A spinal anesthetic takes effect more quickly than epidural anesthesia. For this reason spinal anesthesia may cause a rapid drop in blood pressure because of the temporary blockage of the nerves that regulate blood flow in the legs. Once again the patient can assist the anesthesiologist by staying as still as possible while the needle

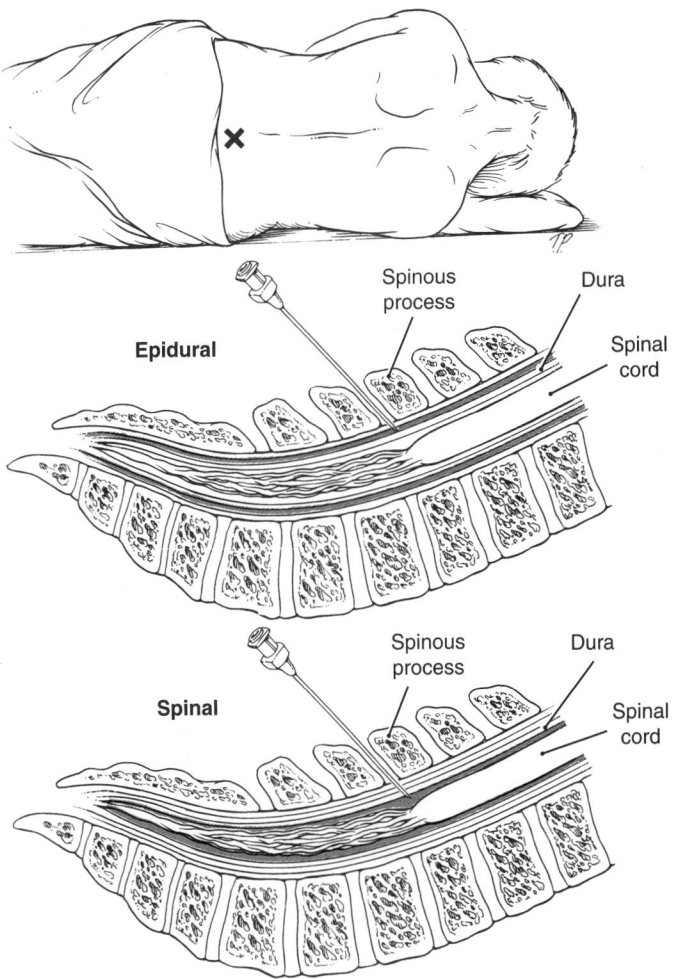

Epidural and spinal anesthesia. Both techniques allow for temporary pain blockage below the level of the chest. The techniques differ by the depth of the needle when the pain medication is infused, although both are performed below where the spinal cord ends to reduce the risk of damaging the cord. These blocks are commonly used in childbirth and procedures performed within the pelvis and on the lower extremities.

is being inserted. After a spinal block, numbness in the lower body may last up to 6 hours. Until recently, painful headaches were a common aftereffect of spinal anesthesia, but the use of new, small specially designed needles has almost eliminated this aftereffect. Epidural analgesia may also be used to relive pain after major surgery (see page 1435).

LOCAL ANESTHESIA

A local anesthetic blocks transmission of impulses along the nerve fibers. Local anesthesia allows an operation to be carried out painlessly within a localized region by blocking the sensory nerves. Local anesthesia is usually used for dental or brief surgical procedures on the skin surface. It is administered as a surface preparation or by using a syringe or needle to inject the drug in the correct location. The injection may sting initially, but the discomfort passes as soon as the anesthetic takes effect. During surgery, you may still be able to feel pressure or tugging, but you should not experience pain. Local anesthesia may also be used to relieve postoperative pain. The following are the most common forms of local anesthesia.

Topical anesthesia Topical anesthesia involves the application of an anesthetic agent to the surface of the surgical site. The anesthetic may be administered as a spray, gargle, cotton soak, gel ointment, or eye drop. Topical anesthetic is often used in surgery of the mouth, pharynx, larynx, and eyes. It may also be used in conjunction with other local or general anesthesia. The anesthesia takes effect rapidly and lasts for 30 to 60 minutes.

Local infiltration Local infiltration (injection of an anesthetic with a very small needle) may be used to deliver local or regional anesthesia and is often used for many plastic surgeries, anorectal procedures, ear and eye procedures, and for stitching small cuts and the removal of small skin lesions.

Additional sedation can be given during the surgical procedure if an anesthesiologist is present. Many of the new, short-acting medications available to the anesthesiologist allow you to undergo procedures using local anesthesia that would previously have required general anesthesia. The level of sedation is quite deep and the effects may mimic those of a general anesthetic, including amnesia of the operation, but you may not require placement of a breathing tube.

In general, no particular type of anesthesia is safer than another. However, there are particular individuals in whom there are distinct advantages to regional, as described previously. Additionally, in people who have bad lung disease, or for whom there is concern regarding placement of a breathing tube for administration of general anesthesia, a regional anesthesia may offer distinct advantages. The risks associated with local anesthesia specifically include administration of the medication directly into a vein or inadequate blockade of the pain of surgery. In either case, the complications can be treated but general anesthesia may be required.

COPING WITH THE AFTEREFFECTS OF ANESTHESIA

Recent advances in the administration of anesthetic drugs have minimized the aftereffects of general anesthesia, but these drugs may still exacerbate your discomfort after surgery. At first you will be unable to drink even water. You will probably feel nauseous and may even need to vomit. Your voice may be hoarse. Your mouth and throat will feel dry and sore, and your desire to sip something to relieve your thirst and dryness will be at war with your inability to hold anything down. When you are able to, you may be given ice chips to suck on. In a few hours, you may be able to sip a clear liquid. As soon as you are able to drink liquids, you should keep increasing your intake steadily.

The most common aftereffect of local anesthesia is a temporary weakness or paralysis of the area. Spinal anesthesia, such as a spinal block, may leave the extremities without feeling for a number of hours. After general and spinal anesthesia, many people complain of a headache and sometimes an ache in the shoulder area. You may be able to reduce some postoperative pain by asking your surgeon to add pillows under your knees or otherwise adjust your positioning on the operating table. If you have pain, request medication for pain relief. The headache and achiness should pass quickly as you begin to get up and move around.

Before your surgery, you should discuss with your anesthesiologist how the anesthesia will affect you and whether you can choose one drug versus another. Anesthesiologists are also pain relief experts, and your anesthesiologist will work with you to minimize the pain of surgery and the aftereffects of anesthesia.

Blood Transfusion

Blood is a living tissue that is pumped through the heart and circulates throughout the body via the arteries, veins, and capillaries. Blood transports essential substances—including electrolytes, hormones, vitamins, antibodies, and oxygen—between organs and tissues to meet the body's metabolic needs. Blood also removes carbon dioxide, the waste product generated by the body's metabolic activity, from the body's tissues. The carbon dioxide passes through the veins to the lungs, where it is expelled into the exhaled air. Any operation entails a certain amount of blood loss, but in most cases this does not necessitate a blood transfusion. However, about 14 percent of all people who undergo surgery require blood transfusions, and many surgeries could not be performed without transfusion support.

Emergency transfusions in people who suffer major trauma, such as car accidents, account for far more transfusions during surgery than planned transfusions. While blood units are still kept in reserve during major surgery, transfusions are less frequently performed because of the advances in surgical techniques that have reduced blood loss and made less invasive procedures possible.

Blood transfusion is safe only when the donor's blood and the blood of the recipient are compatible. There are four main blood groups—A, B, AB, and O—and each is divided into two Rh types, Rh negative and Rh positive. The surface of each red blood cell is coated with proteins known as antigens that differ for each blood type. Because each of us forms antibodies (molecules that attack foreign substances—antigens—in the body) against antigens our body lacks, transfused and native blood should match. Before any transfusion, small amounts of the donor blood and the recipient's blood are mixed in a lab to ensure compatibility. Blood may be transfused as whole blood, or one or more of its components may be transfused (see page 1438).

Blood transfusions can be lifesaving but as with any treatment, there are risks involved. These risks include hemolytic reaction (a breakdown of red blood cells that usually results in anemia) because of incompatibility, the transmission of disease, fever, and allergic reactions. The most common infection transmitted by blood transfusion is hepatitis C, but the risk of this transmission is less than 1 in 3,000 per unit of blood or blood product. The risk of transmission of the human immunodeficiency virus (HIV) is between 1 in 40,000 and 1 in 225,000 per unit of blood or blood product.

Overall, the risk of contracting any infection from a blood transfusion is extremely low. All donated blood is screened for possible infectious diseases. Before 1985 blood was tested only for hepatitis B and syphilis, but now each unit of donated blood undergoes eight tests for infectious diseases, including HIV and hepatitis C. In addition, a new test for HIV, the monoclonal HIV-1p24 antigen test, can detect the virus more quickly, this further assuring the safety of the blood supply. The safest blood of all, however, is still your own (see page 1438).

The most common immunologic complication that occurs because of a blood transfusion is fever and chills. Almost all deaths that occur because of blood transfusion are due to blood type incompatibility, which can occur because of an error in patient identification. If you are preparing to have surgery, make sure you know your blood type and that your patient identification bracelet identifies you correctly. Double check with your doctor if you have any doubts.

The most common reason for a blood transfusion is to replace blood volume. In a healthy person the body will naturally replace blood volume, even when moderate blood losses occur during surgery, but in people with preexisting conditions or who experience significant blood loss during surgery, transfusion may prove necessary.

In discussing your upcoming surgery, review the possible need for blood transfusion with your doctor. You will want to discuss why a transfusion might be necessary

BLOOD COMPONENT THERAPY

The process of transfusing only that portion of the blood needed by the patient is called blood component therapy; it allows a single unit (1 pint) of donated blood to benefit more than one patient. The blood components that are transfused most frequently are red blood cells and platelets. Blood products used in blood transfusions include the following.

Whole Blood Whole blood consists of red blood cells, white blood cells, and platelets, all of which float in a colorless, watery fluid called plasma. Transfusions of whole blood are rarely required. However, if a person has undergone certain types of major surgery or has suffered major trauma such as a car accident or gunshot wound prior to surgery, a transfusion of whole blood may be necessary. Whole blood can be stored for 5 weeks.

Packed Red Cells and Frozen Red Cells Red blood cells contain hemoglobin, the protein that carries oxygen throughout the body. Packed red cells have about 40 percent of the volume of whole blood. Using frozen red cells reduces the risk of infusing antigens, or foreign bodies, that the body might regard as potentially dangerous. Recent advances have made it possible to store red blood cells for up to 42 days. A transfusion of red blood cells may be necessary for people who have suffered acute trauma prior to surgery or for people who are anemic who are having surgery.

Platelet Concentrates Platelets are small-scale cellular components that help in the clotting process. A platelet transfusion is used if there is a platelet disorder or when massive blood loss has occurred. Platelets are stored for up to 5 days at room temperature. A platelet transfusion may be necessary after prolonged surgery.

Cryoprecipitated Antihemophilic Factor Cryoprecipitated antihemophilic factor, an antihemophilic concentrate, is prepared from plasma and is rich in clotting factors. It is used in people with hemophilia or von Willebrand's disease and other major coagulation abnormalities to prevent or control bleeding. ∎

and how it might be avoided. You should also discuss the blood bank capabilities at the hospital where you are having your surgery and whether or not it is advisable to bank your own blood. At present, the only source of blood and blood products continues to be blood donors or the patient, but research in developing synthetic blood substitutes is underway.

BANKING YOUR OWN BLOOD

Autologous blood donation and transfusion, or using your own blood for your transfusion needs, is appropriate for many medically stable people and may even be appropriate for children. Between 4 and 5 percent of all blood donated is autologous blood. Approximately half of all the autologous blood donated is not used by the person who donated it and then discarded because it may not be suitable for transfusion to another person.

If you and your doctor have decided that preoperative autologous donation is appropriate, you can begin to donate your own blood up to 6 weeks before surgery. For example, you might give 1 unit of blood every week for 6 weeks prior to your surgery because blood can be stored in its liquid form for 42 days. The donation procedure is painless, safe, and takes approximately 10 to 20 minutes each time. Frequency of donation is highly individualized but usually no more than once each week after the first 2 units are donated. Since you may feel tired after donating blood, you should have someone drive you home. Your blood will then be stored until the time of your surgery. Since the process of donating blood stimulates the bone marrow to produce new red blood cells, your bone marrow will easily replace the blood you have donated.

Your red blood cell count (hematocrit) must be at least 33 percent at each appointment or you will not be allowed to donate blood. If you have been taking antibiotics, you cannot donate blood until 3 days after the last dose was taken. It is also important that you do not donate blood if you have a cold, flu, or other infection. If you have been sick, you should be free of symptoms for at least 3 days before donating blood. If you are donating your own blood, an iron supplement may be prescribed to aid your body in replacing the red blood cells it has lost. You should take this supplement up until the day of your surgery. While it will take your body 3 to 6 weeks to replace the red blood cells it has lost, it will take only a few hours for your body to replace the fluid it has lost.

Blood dilution, or hemodilution, is another method of autologous transfusion. One or more units of blood are removed from the patient in the operating room, prior to surgery, and reserved for transfusions during or at the end of surgery. Intravenous fluids are given to replace the volume of blood that has been removed. Because the number of red blood cells has been diluted, fewer red blood cells are lost when bleeding occurs during the operation. If a transfusion is not necessary during surgery, the patient's blood is transfused at the end of surgery.

Intraoperative blood collection is another method that minimizes the risk of blood transfusion. In this procedure the blood that is lost during the surgery is recovered and recycled when necessary throughout the operation. The red blood cells are then concentrated and washed prior to transfusion. This procedure is often used when the anticipated blood loss is at least 20 percent of the patient's blood volume such as in cardiac, gynecologic, vascular, orthopedic, urologic, and transplant surgery.

Your Surgical Experience

The need for surgery places you in the same position as a passenger boarding an airplane. In fact, one of the hardest aspects of the surgical experience is accepting that you are not in control. You are, literally, in someone else's hands. The more you can do to ensure you have chosen the right surgeon and the right pair of hands, the better prepared you will be to accept the prospect of surgery calmly (see page 1429). If you have considered your options carefully, you will know that surgery is the best decision to maintain your health, and you will be better able to approach the experience with a positive outlook.

GETTING IN SHAPE FOR SURGERY

Whether you are in the best of health or sick before your surgery, there are always steps you can take to improve your general health as well as your chances for a successful surgical outcome. The following is a list that will help you to get in shape for surgery:

- If you smoke, try to quit as far in advance of your surgery as possible. If you cannot quit, at least cut down on your smoking before your surgery to give your lungs an opportunity to increase their capacity to take in oxygen.

- Tell your doctor if you take birth control pills. You will probably be asked to stop.

- Tell your doctor if you take aspirin or ibuprofen. Your doctor may request you stop taking these medications a week or two before surgery as they can inhibit the blood's ability to clot.

- Eat a healthy diet rich in fruits and vegetables and drink plenty of water.

- Consult your doctor about an appropriate exercise regimen for your age and condition and exercise regularly. Aerobic exercise, such as a regular, long walk, will increase your lung capacity.

- Consult your doctor about the vitamins you take; ask whether the dosage of any of your vitamins should be increased. When you go to the hospital, bring items from home that will help make you more comfortable and your stay more pleasant, including a toothbrush, toothpaste, hairbrush, and slippers. Both women and men who suffer from dry skin may want to bring a moisturizer or moisturizing spray because hospital air tends to be dry. Encourage friends and family to bring fresh fruit and other healthy snacks if you are going to be hospitalized for a while. ■

Whatever your condition, there are things you can do to prepare your body and mind for surgery (see above).

PREPARING FOR SURGERY

Before your operation (if it is outpatient, or ambulatory), your doctor will schedule an

THE DAY BEFORE SURGERY

If you are going to be admitted to the hospital the day of your surgery, you will be given a list of presurgical instructions by your doctor. It is essential that you follow these instructions exactly. Usually, you will be forbidden to eat or drink anything, even water, from midnight on. In some cases you will be requested to make other preparations, such as giving yourself an enema. All of these preoperative preparations are important and help to lower the risk of complications during surgery and to facilitate a problem-free recovery. If you have any questions about what you are supposed to do or not do the day before your surgery or if you feel you may be unable to follow your doctor's instructions, you should discuss this with your doctor. In many cases, your surgery will have to be postponed if you have not followed your doctor's presurgical instructions. ■

SURGICAL EMERGENCIES

Trauma, including burns, wounds, and multiple injuries, often necessitates emergency surgery. While it is impossible to prepare in advance for emergency surgery, it is wise to keep vital information with you at all times. You should carry the address and phone numbers of your next of kin and other family members in your wallet. You should also carry a list of any allergies or ailments. Make sure that you know your blood type and have it written down on the list. If you have diabetics or any chronic condition, wear a Medic Alert bracelet for your own protection. ■

outpatient visit to assess whether you are fit for surgery. Your presurgical physical exam will include an assessment of your general health, including taking a history that includes whether you have had any bleeding disorders or have taken any medication that might affect coagulation (the clotting of your blood). Your respiratory and cardiovascular system will be evaluated. A urine sample will also be taken to check for the presence of sugar and metabolic waste products, which may indicate underlying problems.

During this exam you will be asked questions regarding previous surgeries and experiences with anesthesia as well as any previous allergic reactions to medication or anesthetic agents. Women of childbearing age will be asked if they use oral contraceptives, which should not be taken for at least 4 weeks prior to any major surgery and any operations on the legs to reduce the risk of thromboembolism (blood clot). In cases of emergency surgery, when such advance discontinuation of oral contraceptive use is impossible, low dose heparin may be given to minimize the risk of thromboembolism. You will be interviewed regarding your use of alcohol, psychotropic drugs, and tobacco. Be sure to answer these questions accurately; your answers will be confidential and holding back information may put your health at risk. Any use of medication will be reviewed. In addition to revealing valuable information regarding your med-

OUTPATIENT SURGERY

Outpatient surgery refers to any surgery in which a person spends less than 24 hours in the hospital or in the facility where the surgery is performed. The term same-day surgery is used when someone is operated on and admitted on the same day. The terms ambulatory and outpatient surgery are used interchangeably: you are in and out of the hospital the same day. Local, spinal, and even general anesthesia are usually used when outpatient surgery is performed; all are feasible.

In 1985, inpatient surgeries outnumbered outpatient surgeries almost two to one. By 1993, however, these numbers had changed radically, with outpatient surgery having surpassed inpatient surgery in numbers of surgeries performed. This trend is due to advances in surgical and anesthesia procedures that make recovery time shorter but also to changes in insurance coverage, including the advent of managed care plans. Many surgeries that only a few years ago were covered by insurance plans for a 2 to 3 day hospital stay, are no longer covered. Depending on your age and the nature of your surgery, you

should discuss with your doctor whether or not outpatient surgery is the right choice for you. In some cases it is advantageous for a person to return home directly following surgery. In other cases the risk of accident and complications may be increased because the person is not closely monitored after surgery.

If you are going to undergo surgery on an outpatient basis make sure a friend or family member is available to take you home after the procedure and to assist you afterwards at home if necessary. Check with your doctor about when you will be able to drive again and about whether there will be any restrictions on your daily activities, and make plans accordingly.

When a person has no one to take him home and lives alone, most hospitals help make arrangements for a visiting nurse or home care assistant to make home visits. Such arrangements may be made by a nurse, via a home care agency, or through the social services department of the hospital. Before your surgery, ask your doctor or the nurse who is managing preoperative instructions how such arrangements can be made. ■

ical history and your health, the preoperative interview gives your doctor a chance to detect any undiagnosed conditions, such as hypertension (high blood pressure) or diabetes mellitus, that may increase your risk of complications during and after surgery.

ADMISSIONS PROCEDURES AND PREOPERATIVE PROCEDURES

If you are not already in the hospital, you will be admitted to the hospital the day of the surgery or the night before, depending on the need for preparations for surgery. Ambulatory surgery typically means that you are admitted and released from the hospital on the same day; same-day surgery typically means that you are admitted after surgery. You should inform friends and family members that delays are common and your time in the recovery room may be lengthy so that they do not worry unnecessarily.

Often admissions procedures take time, and you might find yourself waiting. To avoid becoming more nervous while you wait, bring books and magazines to read or a personal cassette player and tapes so that you can listen to music. Ask a friend or family member to come along with you so you do not have to wait alone.

Once you have filled out all the forms and have been admitted to the hospital, a staff doctor, physician's assistant, or nurse practitioner will examine you and take a brief medical history. You will be asked if you are taking any medications. If you have the medications with you, you will be asked to send them home with a family member unless your doctor has written a specific order allowing you to continue to take them while in the hospital. The staff doctor or your own doctor will then explain the surgery you are about to undergo and ask you to sign a form, called an operative permit, giving your consent to the surgery. This is a good time to ask any questions you might have about your surgery. Your anesthesiologist will also meet with you before the surgery to ask you some of the same questions you may have already answered and to answer any questions you may have about the anesthesia. If you begin to feel that you are repeating the same information

SURGICAL ONCOLOGY

Surgical treatment is the most successful and most commonly used method of cancer therapy available today. More radical and extensive surgical therapies for cancer are now more available than ever before due to improved surgical techniques, advances in anesthesiology, and additional supportive care. In many cases adjuvant therapy, such as chemotherapy or radiation therapy, is used to supplement surgical treatment.

Surgery for cancer usually involves a more extensive treatment team than other surgeries. Your oncologist will work with your surgeon to determine the most advantageous treatment for you. Surgery for cancer also differs from other surgeries because it may be used in conjunction with other treatments that may make you sicker before they make you well and will certainly prolong your recovery period (see Chapter 30). ■

over and over, remember that your doctors and the rest of the medical staff are trying to ensure that no mistakes are made.

Before you are taken to a preanesthetic care unit where you will wait to be taken to the operating room, or OR, you will have to remove all of your clothing and wear only a hospital gown. You will also be asked to remove all your personal belongings including your watch, rings, earrings, and other jewelry as well as dentures, hearing aids, glasses or contact lenses, hairpieces, and hairpins. If you wear nail polish you should

AMPUTATION

Amputating a limb or part of a limb is an extreme measure, but in some cases it is the only way to save a person's life. Amputation is used as a last resort when more conservative treatment has failed. It may become necessary as a result of traumatic injury, in cases of malignant tumors that are unresponsive to other treatment, extensive infection, necrosis, or advanced peripheral vascular disease.

All amputations are major surgical procedures involving a hospital stay and sometimes a protracted recovery period. The recovery period may be lengthy because your physical recovery is accompanied by a period of adjustment to a new way of life and rehabilitation therapy that may involve learning to use a prosthetic limb. In addition the loss of any extremity, whether it be part of a limb or only a toe or finger, takes an emotional toll.

If you are facing the possibility of amputation make sure this surgery is the only option open to you before you proceed. Knowing that this radical step is the only measure that can save your life will make your adjustment to a life-altering surgery easier. Make sure, too, that you arrange for emotional as well as physical support after the surgery. The more help you accept in learning to manage your new life, the more successful your recovery will be. Great strides have been made recently in the development of highly functional artificial limbs that allow many people who undergo amputation to lead full and normal lives. ■

TRANSPLANTATION SURGERY

Organ transplantation makes possible the replacement of damaged or nonfunctioning organs and is one of the greatest advances in medicine in the last 3 decades. Conditions that only a short time ago had mortality rates of 100 percent now have survival rates of 80 percent or more because of organ transplantation, and people usually enjoy a normal or nearly normal life after transplantation surgery. The biggest obstacle to successful transplant surgery is the lack of donor organs (see Chapter 35).

Ever since organ transplantation became a possibility in the 1960s the number of transplantable organs has increased progressively. At present transplantable organs include kidney, liver, heart, heart and lung together, and single or double lung. Pancreatic transplantation is also possible but is not as well established as other organ transplantation surgeries. Some minor success has also been achieved with intestinal transplantation, but the surgery is not used routinely. Kidney transplantation is the most common transplantation surgery. Advances in transplantation surgery also extend to children, although adults have benefited more in terms of numbers. Technologic developments in liver transplantation have made this surgery more successful in the past decade, and kidney transplantation is highly successful in children. Cardiac transplantation in children has also become more common.

The greatest risk involved in transplantation surgery is rejection. The general rule is that the greater the genetic difference between the recipient and the graft—the organ or living tissue—the greater the possibility of rejection. Grafts between identical twins or from an individual to himself (such as a skin graft) survive indefinitely. To maximize the chances that an allograft (transplantation of tissue between two genetically different individuals of the same species) will be successful, a person undergoing transplant surgery will be treated with medication that suppresses the body's automatic rejection response to the foreign tissue. Advances in the development of immunosupressive agents have revolutionized transplantation surgery.

After rejection, the most common complication of transplant surgery is infection. The use of immunosuppressive agents increases the risk of viral, fungal, and bacterial infections. Viral infections are particularly common in kidney transplants. However, improved antibiotics and immunosuppressive agents have lowered the risk and severity of infections.

In recent years bone marrow transplantation has become a particularly successful procedure in cases of aplastic anemia, irradiation exposure, leukemia, and disseminated breast cancer that has spread. Autologous bone marrow transplantation (from self to self) has also proven highly successful in allowing cancer patients to receive high doses of radiation to irradiate the cancer when needed. ■

remove it to enable the anesthesiologist to readily check your circulation by examining your nail beds. Your money and other valuables can be given to a family member to take home for safekeeping, or they may be locked in the security office of the hospital.

While you are waiting to be taken to the operating room you will probably receive a medication to relax you and keep you calm. Be aware that delays are common and that surgery schedules cannot always be strictly met. Depending on the type of surgery you are having, an operating room escort will take you to the operating room in a wheelchair, on a stretcher, or in your bed. You may want to request a blanket since the operating room may be cool. In addition, the combination of anesthesia, intravenous fluids, and an open incision can lower body temperature as much as 4°F. Recent research has shown that keeping the surgical patient warm can help improve outcome.

The anesthesiologist will discuss the steps in undergoing anesthesia, and a nurse will help you to the operating table and place a safety strap across your legs. The anesthesiologist or anesthetist will remain present during the operation to monitor your condition.

THE RECOVERY ROOM

After your surgery is completed you will be taken to the recovery room, also known as the postanesthesia care unit, or PACU. There may be other patients in the recovery room with you. Beds will be separated by curtains to provide each patient with some privacy. Generally, you are not allowed to have visitors in the recovery room. However, some hospitals will allow a family member to visit someone in the recovery room if the surgery has taken longer than expected or if the move from the recovery room to a hospital room has been delayed and the person is alert. Prior to surgery, inquire into the hospital's visitation policy so that those who accompany you to surgery will know what to expect.

Your stay in the recovery room will last a minimum of 2 hours and will vary in length depending on the type of anesthesia you received and the procedure you have undergone. During this time your vital signs will be monitored continually. If you had a breathing tube inserted in the operating room it will now be removed. You may find your throat is sore for a day or two after the tube is removed. You may find that your mouth is dry from the anesthesia. You may also have nausea or vomiting. Drinking or eating will exacerbate your nausea, but you can request ice chips to relieve your dry mouth. Later, you may feel that you can hold down liquids. If you are being sent home

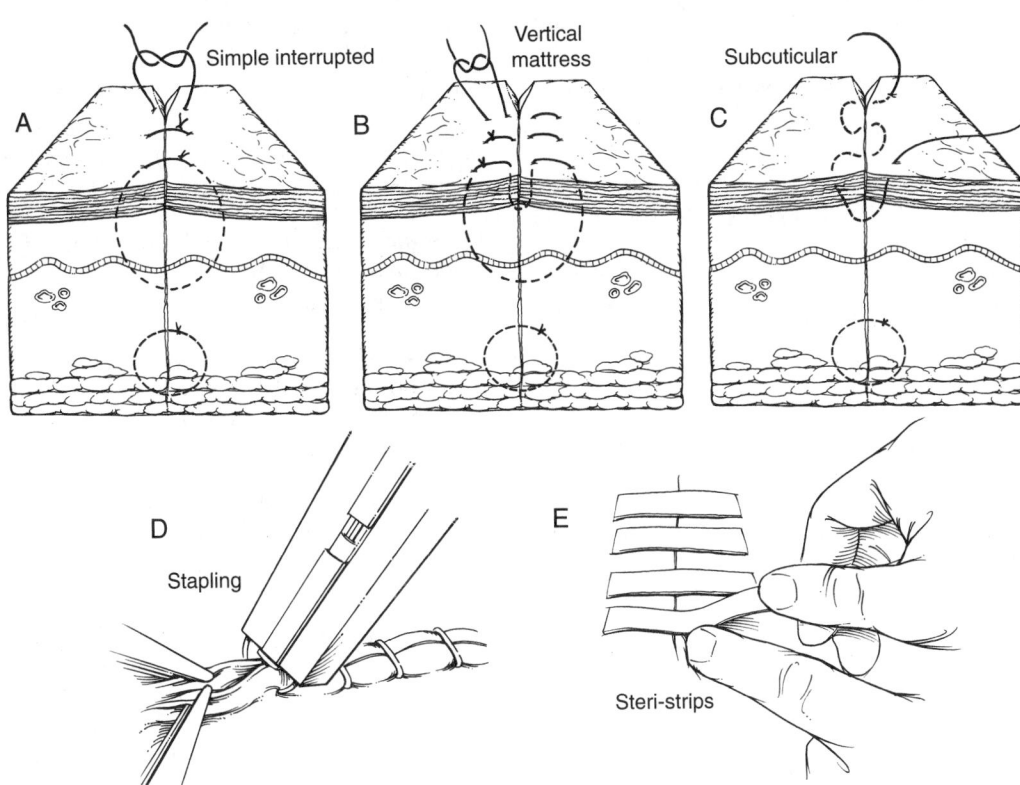

A — Simple interrupted

B — Vertical mattress

C — Subcuticular

D — Stapling

E — Steri-strips

Methods of surgical wound closure. (A–C) Stitches (sutures) are placed by different techniques depending on skin tension and the location and depth of the wound. (D&E) Removable staples and adhesive strips are alternatives to sutures.

directly after recovery, be sure to attempt to drink liquids. You will not be allowed to leave the hospital until it is clear that your urinary tract is functioning. This can be difficult to ascertain without drinking liquids. A good rule is to resume eating only after hunger returns.

If you feel pain or discomfort, you will be given medication. Do not hesitate to ask for pain relief. After surgery, you may receive PCA if the procedure is commonly associated with pain. If your doctor has ordered PCA, a PCA pump will be prescribed and the anesthesia pain service will teach you how to use it (see page 1433). Epidural analgesia is also used to control pain after major surgery (see page 1435).

If you were given a spinal or epidural anesthetic you will be unable to move your legs at first, and you will remain in the recovery room until sensation and movement return to them. If you had a spinal anesthetic it will take longer for the sensation to return to your legs. The anesthesia usually wears off from the toes up.

After major surgical procedures that require close monitoring of neurologic status, vital signs, and fluid balance, you may be required to stay overnight in the recovery room. If you are required to stay overnight, you will probably be allowed to have visitors for a short period of time. In addition, some major surgeries require that you spend the first part of the recovery in the intensive care unit, so that your vital signs can be monitored more closely. Intensive care units have special visiting hours.

POSTOPERATIVE HOSPITALIZATION

The length of your hospital stay will vary depending on the type of surgery you underwent and how well your immediate recovery period goes. In most cases, when you return to your room you will still have an intravenous (IV) line in one arm. It will remain there until you are able to drink fluids and take medication orally. The nurse will check your IV line to make sure it does not dislodge from the vein and infiltrate surrounding tissues with fluid. Your vital signs will be checked periodically, as will the dressing covering the incision. This dressing will probably be changed within 24 to 48 hours after your surgery, at which point the doctor will inspect your incision. Unless your hospital stay lasts longer than a week, the stitches or staples used to close the wound will probably be removed in your doctor's office after you have been discharged. However, practice patterns among surgeons have moved away from using external stitches to using those that are placed deep in the skin and are absorbable. This type of stitch is also called "the melting kind of stitch."

After your surgery you may feel sore and uncomfortable. The site of your surgery may ache or burn. If you are in pain, be sure to ask for pain medication before the pain begins to feel unbearable. Making sure you receive medication for pain when you need it is an important part of participating in your own recovery. The more comfortable you are, the sooner you will feel able to get out of bed and move about. The sooner you begin walking, the sooner your digestive system will begin to return to normal and the sooner you will be able to leave the hospital. After you leave the hospital there are exercises that you can do—whether you are bedridden or ambulatory—to aid in your recovery (see page 1446).

Try to make your time in the hospital as pleasant as possible. If you can afford it, order phone service and television service. Many hospitals now provide a patient education channel that is offered free of charge and covers health issues, patient information, patients' rights issues, and nutrition and fitness, all of which may provide you with useful information to aid in your recovery. If your recovery will necessitate physical or occupational therapy, many hospitals include a rehabilitation unit where you will be transferred to pursue a comprehensive treatment program that will meet your medical, physical, cognitive, and communication needs and that will also help you cope with emotional and social issues surrounding your rehabilitation and any disability you may have.

Before you are discharged from the hospital, you should ask your doctor or nurse about your diet, any limitations in your daily routine, what medication you will be given, and what medication you may take to control pain. You should also discuss care of the incision, warning signs of infection, precautions regarding bathing and showering, and follow-up care. You should also inquire about any limitations regarding your exercise routine.

POSTOPERATIVE COMPLICATIONS

In all surgical procedures, there is some risk of both minor and major postoperative complications, including the following:

Pulmonary Pulmonary complications include atelectasis, which is a collapse of a portion of the lung, and pneumonia.

Wound infection Symptoms of wound infection may include swelling or discoloration of the surrounding tissue and elevated temperature.

Fever Low grade fever is a very common postoperative complication. Low grade fever is usually not indicative of infection; rather, it usually indicates inadequate aeration of the lungs. A postoperative fever unrelated to the lungs or to wound infection usually occurs either because of a pre-existing infection or it may be caused by the operation itself. A medication reaction or a reaction to a blood transfusion may also cause a fever.

Urinary retention Urinary retention and other complications are more common in older men, especially men who have a history of prostate problems. A catheter may be used to prevent bladder distension. Postoperative urinary retention may signal the need for urologic evaluation.

Cardiac complications Cardiac complications may also arise after surgery. The most common cause of death in surgical patients is myocardial infarction, or heart attack. The most common cardiac complication is a cardiac arrhythmia or abnormal heartbeat. If an arrhythmia persists, medication will be prescribed based on the rate and nature of the palpitations. There is a greater risk of cardiac problems if the patient has suffered a previous heart attack.

Psychiatric complications Psychiatric complications may occur after surgery. The most common of these are confusion and depression. Depression is common in the first 2 to 4 weeks after surgery. Senior patients may get confused at night, particularly if they are staying in a hospital. When delirium occurs, withdrawal from alcohol or drug addiction may be suspected. Medication combinations used in the postoperative period may also be responsible. People who begin the recovery period in the intensive care unit, or ICU, may experience "ICU psychosis," a disorder based on anxiety and disorientation. Treatment involves managing anxiety, occasionally with a tranquilizer, such as haloperidol, and diagnosis and treatment of other precipitating causes.

Recovering from Surgery

Depending on your surgical procedure, you may feel well in a matter of days, or your recovery period could last a month or more. People who make the most rapid and complete recovery are those who actively participate in the recovery process. If your "old self" was not really doing all that well, you can use your surgical experience as a source of motivation to change your lifestyle and to improve other aspects of your life. If you were a smoker and gave up smoking temporarily in preparation for surgery, use this opportunity to quit for good. If you had bypass surgery and are overweight, use this opportunity to change your diet and permanently lower your blood pressure and cholesterol level. In all cases, when you have undergone major surgery because of a life-threatening disease or condition, this is the time to reevaluate your life and habits so that you can lower your level of stress and get more enjoyment out of life.

GOING HOME

The length of your hospital stay will vary depending on the procedure and the presence of any complications. The average length of stay for a woman who has had a cesarean section or a hysterectomy is between 3 and 4 days. The average length of stay for a man who has had a prostatectomy is between 5 and 6 days. If you have had a traditional coronary bypass, you may be hospitalized for 4 to 7 days.

Once your doctor says you are ready to go home, you will begin the next stage of your recovery. If you will be bedridden at home, or if your activities will be limited, try to work with family members, friends, and your physical therapist or nurse so that your home is adapted to your special needs before you get there. If you will need nursing care at home, make arrangements for it before you leave the hospital. When you return home have your nurse or home care practitioner visit as soon as possible to assess the setting and help you determine whether there are any home aids or devices that might ease your recuperation. See Chapter 34 for detailed information on making changes at home that can speed your recovery.

In most cases, when you are discharged from the hospital you will travel from your room to the lobby of the hospital in a wheelchair, for your safety. Even if you are feeling fine, you should have someone accompany you home from the hospital. Your level of activity will increase immediately on discharge and you will probably need assistance.

When you do return home, you should begin to establish a daily routine as soon as possible. If you will be bedridden for a while or cannot manage your old routine, set up a new routine and establish goals for yourself, whether they are as simple as walking from the bedroom to the kitchen or as challenging as returning to work in a week. If you need assistance shopping for food and other necessities and preparing meals, call upon friends and make doing errands a social event. If you have help with your home care and convalescence, you should still make every effort to do more for yourself every day. Use your doctor's instructions as a guide. The more you do to participate in your own recovery, the more you will be able to do.

A RECUPERATIVE DIET

Good nutrition is always important, but it is particularly important when you are recovering from surgery. A healthy diet can help you feel better and help you recuperate more quickly. Above all you should drink plenty of fluids, including plenty of water. Drinking water is always necessary for good health, but it is particularly important during a recovery period. You should also try drinking herbal teas or vegetable or chicken broth. If you avoid drinking in order to save yourself an arduous trip to the toilet, you will be impeding your recovery. Fluids are essential to the healing process.

Depending on your medical condition, your doctor will give you a recommended diet. As soon as possible, you should begin to eat solid foods, concentrating on a diet rich in fresh fruits, vegetables, and grains. Concentrate on fruits and vegetables rich in vitamins A and C. Good sources of vitamin A include dark green or deep yellow fruits and vegetables such as spinach, carrots, peaches, and apricots. Good sources of vitamin C include green and red peppers, oranges, and strawberries. If you are recovering from heart surgery, you will want to follow a recommended diet for heart patients to lose weight and maintain a lower cholesterol level (see Chapter 1).

EXERCISING AGAIN

Adding exercise to your routine as soon as possible is one of the best ways to facilitate recovery. In fact, except for the period immediately following your surgery, you should continue to exercise, even if this means merely rotating your feet and ankles while you are bedridden. Your body needs to be used. If you do not exercise, your muscles may atrophy and your recovery will simply take longer.

As soon as you are ambulatory, the best and easiest exercise to incorporate into your routine is walking. Begin with short walks and work up to a half hour daily. Once you are comfortable walking for 30 minutes a day, consult your doctor about returning to your exercise regime and any sports in which you participate. If you were not in the habit of exercising before surgery, now is the time to make exercise a part of your life (see Chapter 2).

EXERCISES FOR THE PARTIALLY DISABLED PERSON

As soon as you are able to move after your surgery, you should begin to do so as much as possible without wearing yourself out. As soon as you are able to get out of bed, do so often, even if it is only to walk across the room and back. Exercise will help your digestive system to function properly again, it will increase your circulation, and it will help you to heal and to regain your strength.

If you must remain in bed you can practice deep breathing: breathe deeply and slowly 10 times in a row as often as possible. If you are able to move your feet, bend your ankles up and down. Bend each ankle up and down 10 times and repeat this exercise every hour. Bending your ankles will help maintain flexibility. If you are able to move your legs, tighten your thighs and buttocks by pressing the backs of your knees into the bed. Then bend your legs at the knees. Bend each leg 10 times to increase circulation and avoid bedsores on your heels. To increase the flexibility of your hands and wrists, place your fingertips together, press hard, hold for a count of 10, and then repeat 10 times. Then hold your hands out in front of you with your wrists limp. Rotate your wrists away from each other, and then towards each other, 10 times. If you can use your legs, leg lifts will also improve circulation and keep your muscles from atrophying. If you are lying in bed, raise each leg as high as you can, keeping the leg straight, then lower it and repeat 10 times. If you can sit up in bed, sit on the edge of the bed with your legs dangling, lift each leg to knee height, or as high as you can, and then lower it. Do this 10 times with each leg, if possible. If you can, add shoulder rolls to your routine to help keep your upper body limber. While either lying in bed or sitting on the edge of your bed, roll each shoulder forward 10 times and then back 10 times. Try to repeat these exercises at least twice a day and once every hour if you feel able to. It is important to move your body as much as you can to keep muscles from atrophying and to increase mobility and circulation.

If you will be hospitalized for a while, you may also want to ask a friend or family member to bring you some lightweight free weights. While you are bedridden, if you are able to, begin to do gentle arm lifts with your free weights. Begin with a few and work up to repetitions of 10 (see Chapter 2).

If you are wheelchair bound, your physical or occupational therapist will work with you to develop an exercise program that will help you maximize your muscle strength and improve your ability to carry on with activities of daily living.

Pediatric Surgery

Pediatric surgery may be necessary to correct congenital abnormalities or it may become necessary following an injury. Children who suffer from cancer may require surgery as a part of their treatment. The saying that a pediatric patient is not a "small adult" holds true not only because the equipment necessary for pediatric surgery and pre- and postoperative procedures may vary from standard adult procedure, but also because the emotional needs of the infant and young child differ from those of an adult.

The surgical experience for children has improved dramatically in the past 2 decades. Years ago children who were in the hospital for something as routine as a tonsillectomy had to stay in the hospital overnight by themselves. Now, in many cases, a parent may stay overnight with the child for the duration of the hospitalization to offer reassurance and care.

If your child is facing surgery, you will be counted on for stability just when you may be confronting your own fears about the upcoming procedure. If you feel you need more support, ask your doctor to recommend a family or child therapist.

All children worry about what is going to happen when they go to the hospital to undergo surgery. They share common fears centering on why they have to have the surgery, whether the procedure will hurt and how much it will hurt, where their parents will be, whether or not they will look different after the surgery, and when they will be able to come home again. It is important that you reassure your child that you understand that he is afraid and that you will always be there to listen and offer comfort. Show understanding and encourage your child to share feelings and ask questions.

Very young children are most fearful about being separated from their parents. Make every effort to stay overnight with your child to avoid separation at a traumatic time. School-aged children tend to be most concerned about what is happening to their bodies and whether or not they will be like other kids. They have difficulty accepting that a procedure that hurts will actually make them well. Some children also feel that going to the hospital is a punishment for having done something wrong. Teenagers

WHAT TO TELL YOUR CHILD

When a child must be hospitalized for surgery, he should be encouraged to bring his favorite things to the hospital, to ask questions whenever he does not understand something, and to let someone know when he is scared or when something hurts. He should also be informed that there are people who will help when more help is needed. If there is a playroom on the children's ward you may want to let your child know that there will be a place for him to play and to meet new friends as soon he is ready. After the surgery it is important to encourage your child to talk about his surgical experience at home, with friends, and at school. Writing a book or drawing a picture about the experience may also be helpful for school-aged children.

You can help your child cope with the hospital stay by sharing the following information:

- If there is something your child doesn't understand, he can ask a nurse or a doctor; if he is scared or if something hurts, he should tell an adult.

- If the hospital allows you to stay overnight, reassure your child that you will be there overnight. Remember to pack your own overnight bag and bring snacks for yourself. Hospitals provide meals only for patients.

- Explain that the doctors and nurses are there to provide the extra care children need when they aren't feeling well.

- Remind your child periodically that he will be coming home soon. When you have a specific discharge date, plan a coming home party with your child that includes writing a book or organizing a scrapbook about his hospital experience. ∎

have somewhat different concerns; often they want some sense of control in a situation that is beyond their control. They may want their privacy, and they may also want to be with their friends. Teenagers do best when they are allowed to participate in their care and treatment. They should be encouraged to share their questions about their illness and surgery with the doctors and nurses and to investigate the process for themselves.

For parents, the news that a child requires surgery can be overwhelming. Finding out all that you can about what to expect from the procedure and your child's hospitalization will help you feel more in control and allow you to convey this feeling of control to your child. The calmer and more informed you are, the calmer your child will be.

Admission to the hospital may occur because of an emergency illness or injury, which leaves you no time to prepare your child or yourself. When the situation is an emergency, staying calm and being with your child as much as possible are the best ways you can help your child. Ask as many questions as possible about the procedure and what will happen next. If your child needs an IV, tell your child about the IV ahead of time and be there when it is inserted. If your child needs stitches, explain that numbing medicine will be given before the stitches so that the stitches will not hurt. In most situations, you will be able to stay with your child while he receives the stitches. In some cases you may be requested to help hold your child still during the procedure. If you feel you cannot do this well, tell the doctor so that other arrangements can be made to ensure your child's safety. In some cases restraints—such as a mummylike wrap for newborns, infants, and small children—may be necessary when a procedure is performed under local anesthetic.

How to Use Medications

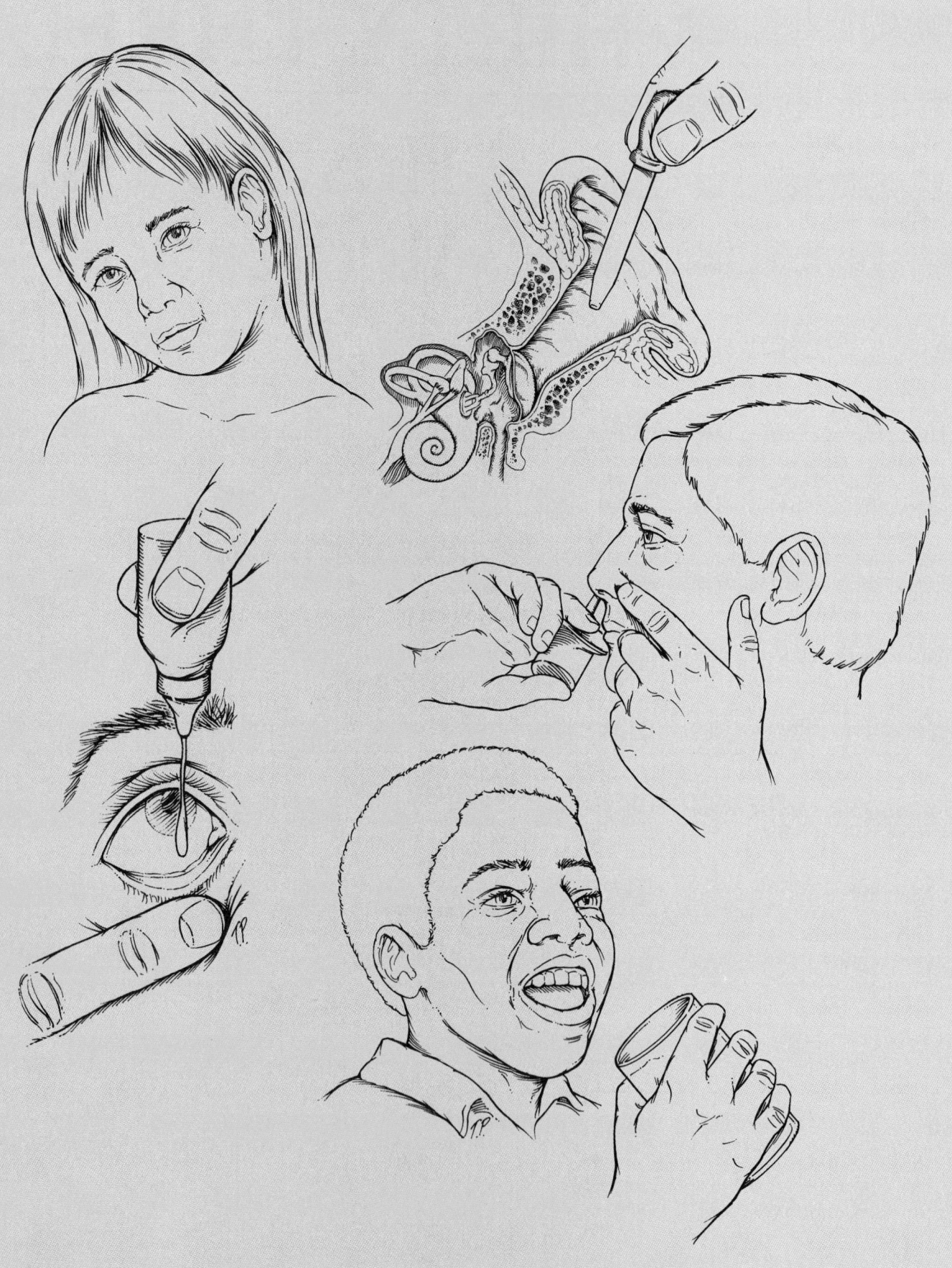

HOW TO USE MEDICATIONS

Modern medications represent a wondrous tool in modern health care. When used properly they can alleviate pain, slow the progression of illness, and in some cases even cure disease and save lives. But their power must be respected. Medications are not magic; all medications can cause side effects, and all too often medications are taken improperly, sometimes to disastrous effect.

This chapter will help you understand the diverse ways medications work, while advising you on ways to use them wisely. Modern medications can help you and your family stay healthy, fight off disease, and ease many aches and pains over the years if you use them properly.

What Is a Medication?

Medications (or medicines) are substances—commonly referred to as drugs—that a person swallows, smoothes onto the skin, has injected into a vein, or takes in a myriad of other different ways for the purposes of healing. In common vernacular the word drugs also refer to substances that influence behavior and mood and that pose the risk of dependence. Caffeine is a widely used drug in this sense, as are illegal substances such as marijuana and cocaine. Unless otherwise noted, the word *drugs* in this text refers to medications that are used to heal the body.

While some medications actually cure disease, most simply enable the body's natural recuperative powers to take over. Many antibiotics work this way; for instance, by interfering with the growth or multiplication of bacteria, antibiotics make it easier for the body's natural defense system to eliminate the invader. Some antibiotics, however, kill germs. There are drugs that are designed to kill abnormal cells, such as cancer cells, directly, while other medications are used to replace substances that need replenishing, such as insulin for people with diabetes and thyroid hormone for people with hypothyroidism. Some drugs actually alter the way cells work by intensifying or increasing their activity; others, by reducing their activity. Often scientists are not yet sure exactly how a drug works.

Medications are available either by prescription or over-the-counter. The US Food and Drug Administration (FDA) decides which medications can be obtained only with a prescription—through a licensed pharmacy with a doctor's written order—and which medications can be sold over-the-counter—without a doctor's written order and at various retail stores including, but not limited to, pharmacies.

THE DRUG APPROVAL PROCESS

Before a drug enters the US marketplace it must undergo a rigorous approval process overseen by the FDA. The drug developer must not only prove that the drug is effective in humans—meaning it produces the intended effect—but also that it is acceptably safe. To prove safety, the developer first tests the drug in small animals such as mice, rats, dogs, and monkeys. Promising results lead to studies in which carefully controlled doses are given to small numbers of healthy human volunteers. Observers carefully monitor reactions to the drug.

If the drug passes these and other safety tests, double-blind trials in large groups of both healthy and sick people are initiated to measure its effectiveness. In a double-blind trial, neither the participant nor the doctors running the trial know whether the participant is taking the test drug or a placebo (or in some cases, a particular concentration of a drug); this is done to minimize bias.

A company that has developed a drug that manages to fulfill all of these safety and efficacy qualifications—a lengthy process costing many millions of dollars—will then petition the FDA for the right to market the drug. FDA approval endows the manufacturer with the right to market the drug exclusively under a brand (or trademark) name of their choosing. This right to exclusive manufacture and sale, called a patent on a drug, lasts for a period of time; when the patent expires other manufacturers may produce the same drug under a different brand name or in a generic form.

Occasionally, authorities will recall a drug released onto the market because a severe, unintended reaction develops in some of the thousands of consumers taking the drug which had not shown up in smaller test groups. In order to recall a drug, the adverse reaction must be deemed excessive in comparison with the drug's benefits, or unnecessarily risky given the existence of other drugs that can be used for the same problem.

GENERIC AND BRAND NAME MEDICATIONS

You may know the medication you take by two names: its generic name and its brand name. The generic name reflects the medication's active substance and fits into a classification scheme that holds meaning for doctors and pharmacists. The generic name is designated during development of a drug. An organization called the US Adopted Name Council decides on this name. The US Adopted Name Council consists of representatives of the American Medical Association (doctors), the American Pharmaceutical Association (pharmacists), and the US Pharmacopoeia (doctors and pharmacists). A medication's brand name represents its registered trade name; the manufacturer chooses (or creates) this name for marketing purposes, usually selecting a name that they hope will be easy for the public to recognize and remember. Zantac is the brand name for ranitidine, for example. Drugs also have chemical names, but these are usually too technical for consumers to understand or retain—ranitidine's chemical name, for example, is extremely long and complex.

MANAGING MEDICATION EXPENSES

Some insurance plans cover nearly the whole cost of a prescription medication and require the subscriber to pay only a small portion called a copay. But insurance plans—and the cost of medications—vary widely. Keep in mind that generic medications tend to be much less expensive than their brand name equivalents. Government assistance programs such as Medicaid cover or significantly contribute to the reimbursement for, or payment of, prescription medications. Some manufacturers have programs to help defray the cost of their products for people with limited funds. Seniors may want to consider getting their medications through the American Association of Retired Persons, an organization that offers deep discounts on many medications. ∎

Chemical names are generally only used by scientists and developers.

A patent on a drug lasts 20 years from the date of filing. Once it has expired, other companies may start to competitively manufacture and market the substance under their own brand name. The differences among these brand name medications are often negligible, although manufacturers often try to distinguish their product by giving it a memorable name, packaging it in a particularly appealing way, or offering it in a convenient or easy-to-digest form. Competition among manufacturers often results in lower prices for the consumer.

Generic medications tend to be less expensive than their brand-name equivalents. The price gap does not reflect a difference in quality as much as a difference in marketing and advertising costs. Your doctor and pharmacist may be able to help you select a generic version of a medication that is cheaper than the brand-name product you might be using. Be aware, however, that prices for the same generic medications as well as for brand-name medications can vary widely from one pharmacy or drug outlet to the next.

Most pharmacists will dispense the generic version of a drug unless your doctor specifies that you should be given a particular brand-name product by noting on the prescription itself to "dispense as written." However, the pharmacist is required to pass some savings along to the consumer if a generic is substituted for a brand. Laws regarding the pharmacist's ability to substitute generics or another brand-name version vary from state to state.

THE PROBLEM OF NONCOMPLIANCE

As many as one-third to one-half of Americans reportedly fail to comply with their medication regimen in one way or another. They may measure out an incorrect dose, take it at the wrong time, or even forget to take the medication altogether. The reasons for such behavior varies, from forgetfulness to a fear of adverse reactions (real or imagined), concerns about addiction, frustration over being dependent on a medication, avoidance of an unpleasant taste or smell, or a desire to cut costs. Some people stop tak-

THE PLACEBO EFFECT

A placebo is a chemically inert substance made to look like an active drug. Placebo means "I will please" in Latin. The placebo effect or placebo response refers to a physical or emotional change a person may experience after being administered a placebo. Approximately 30 percent of people who receive a placebo will derive benefits from it simply because they anticipate that the "drug" will help them in some way. A certain proportion of placebo-takers report side effects as well, ranging from nausea to dizziness, insomnia, depression, itching, hives, diarrhea, and headache. If these people had not received a placebo they might have gone on to experience these symptoms anyway, but because they received a placebo they attribute them to the placebo.

A placebo-controlled clinical trial aims to determine the true efficacy and safety of a proposed drug by giving a portion of trial subjects a placebo, such as a sugar pill, instead of the presumably active drug. Placebo-controlled trials are intended to discern the true effects—wanted and unwanted—of the test drug itself, as distinct from the placebo effect.

There is a lot we do not understand about how the body heals itself, including the beneficial response many people experience when given a placebo. The placebo effect is sometimes referred to when describing the power of positive thinking in speeding recovery. ■

ing their medication once symptoms are relieved even though the prescription calls for the medication to be taken until used up. Other people may avoid taking their medication because it reminds them that they are ill while still others may feel the medication causes more annoying symptoms than their condition does. This common reaction often occurs with so-called silent diseases that cause few if any symptoms, such as high blood pressure, and with certain chronic diseases that tend to flare in cycles, such as systemic lupus erythematosus.

Whatever the reason, the results of noncompliance can be extremely serious. Failing to take blood pressure medication, for example, can lead to potentially fatal consequences. Even something as mundane as failing to take a medication with food when the prescription recommends it can cause serious problems.

Talk to your doctor if you find yourself altering your medication regimen for any reason. Discuss your concerns about expected or unexpected reactions before stopping a medication, changing the dosage, or adding another medication on your own. There may be solutions that surprise you, such as an alternative medication with fewer side effects, or ways to consolidate or simplify your medication regimen. See page 1465 for tips on following your medication regimen properly.

ALTERNATIVE MEDICINES

The popularity of alternative medicines has mushroomed over the past few years, as increasing numbers of Americans turn to herbs, homeopathic medicines, and other natural remedies for minor as well as occasionally for serious ailments. In fact, although the majority of medications available in industrialized countries today consist of chemical compounds synthesized in the laboratory, it was only a few decades ago that pharmacy shelves were stocked with formulations of roots, leaves, and other plant parts, not to mention animal extracts. Pharmaceutical companies continue to search for new drugs in the natural world as well as in the laboratory.

There is no question that many natural substances can be medicinally effective. As many as a quarter of all prescription medications are, in fact, derived from natural substances. Aspirin, for example, consists of a purified form of salicin (acetylsalicylic acid), originally isolated from the bark and leaves of certain willows and poplars. Some herbalists recommend taking willow bark as an aspirin substitute to break a fever, treat headache pain, control inflammation, and allay various other symptoms. This and other herbs contain active ingredients, and a few, such as saw palmetto for prostate enlargement and St. John's wort for mild to moderate depression, have proved somewhat effective in human trials.

Most herbs and other natural remedies, however, have yet to be carefully examined in humans to assess the safety and efficacy of these herbs. This situation is unlikely to change any time soon because herbs cannot be patented and their sale cannot be controlled. Thus manufacturers are unwilling to devote the time and money necessary to officially prove that an herb is medically safe and efficacious.

In America today, herbs and other natural remedies are officially categorized as dietary supplements, which means the packager or manufacturer is barred from making claims regarding their medicinal effect in humans. More importantly, it means that the careful review that the FDA provides for drugs is not extended to dietary supplements. At the same time, the packager is free to sell the substance without proving its safety or effectiveness to health authorities. As a result, the quality of dietary supplements varies widely. Random testing has shown that some herbal products on the market contain little if any of the designated herb.

If you are considering taking a dietary supplement, it is important to keep in mind not only general risks but risks that your particular condition may pose. Are you taking prescription medications, or are you pregnant, nursing, suffering from kidney or liver disease (organs involved in metabolizing and eliminating medications), or very old or very young? While everyone should talk to a doctor before taking a dietary supplement—just as you would if you were going to take any medication—it is particularly important to do so if any of these conditions apply to you. Potential risks almost always outweigh potential benefits in such cases unless the safety of the substance has been carefully studied. Remember that natural does not equal harmless. Consider the poppy flower: natural, no doubt, but also the source for the highly potent and potentially destructive substance we know as opium. The long-term effects of such popular hormones as melatonin and dehydroepiandosterone, or DHEA, have yet to be determined. Even certain common foods can be harmful if taken in high doses and under certain circumstances.

Wise Medication Use

Medications can offer everyday relief and can even be lifesaving, if used properly. If medications are used improperly, however, they can pose significant risks to your health. Review the following tips to ensure that you are taking the proper precautions.

WHAT YOU SHOULD TELL YOUR DOCTOR

Your doctor can prescribe medication most effectively if she is thoroughly familiar with your medical history. While your doctor will doubtless ask you about your medical history initially, make it a practice of keeping her updated on new developments. It is vital to mention other medications you are taking whether they are prescription, over-the-counter, or alternative. Do not hesitate to mention medications you are taking that another doctor has prescribed. If you use recreational drugs or alcohol, be sure to tell your doctor; hiding this information can put your health at risk. Even over-the-counter medications such as aspirin and vitamin supplements should be mentioned because some over-the-counter medications can interact in unwanted ways with prescription medications. Acetaminophen, for example, can interfere with the prescription medication warfarin, which is an anticoagulant (a substance that prevents blood clotting). You should also report any new symptoms or problems and any unusual or unexpected reactions to medications, including allergic reactions that may have occurred in the past. It is important to also inform your doctor when you stop taking medication, which is as important for your doctor to know as when you start to take a medication. This information should be provided to anyone who may be prescribing medications for you including primary care doctors, specialists, and dentists.

SIDE EFFECTS AND ADVERSE REACTIONS

It is not surprising that any effective medication that can treat an illness or relieve a symptom may have an impact on other parts of the body as well. Extensive testing in thousands of people before the release of a drug onto the market usually reveals common side effects. Take a look at the product insert to a medication and you will find a list of potential side effects—often an extensive list—that may give you pause. Most people find side effects bothersome but tolerable given the benefits the medication offers them. There are three things to keep in mind

ALLERGIC REACTIONS: HOW TO IDENTIFY THEM AND WHAT TO DO

Virtually any medication has the potential to cause an allergic reaction in a susceptible individual. There is almost no way to predict whether you will develop an allergic reaction to a medication. In general, however, people who are allergy-prone are more likely to develop medication allergies. Be sure to tell your doctor about allergies you have as well as any unusual reactions you develop with a medication.

An allergic reaction can occur regardless of how much medication is taken or what the medication is designed to treat. The reaction may include an unexpected rash—mild redness and itching ranks as the most common type of reaction—or it may include swelling, hives, fever, blood changes such as anemia, or a host of other symptoms and signs. These reactions may appear suddenly or become apparent gradually, over time. Your doctor can help you determine whether your side effect is, in fact, an allergic reaction.

Anaphylaxis is the most severe and dangerous type of allergic reaction, and penicillin is the drug most often implicated in anaphylaxis. Anaphylaxis can be fatal in some cases if not treated promptly and properly. An anaphylactic reaction causes the victim's breathing passages to rapidly swell and spasm, which can make it difficult or even impossible to breathe. Life-threatening shock can also develop, with a precipitous drop in blood pressure and associated pallor, fast pulse, confusion, and nausea, with a potential loss of consciousness and cardiovascular collapse. People who know they are at risk for this type of severe allergic reaction should wear a bracelet (or necklace or card) that indicates that they have this allergy and they should also carry a solution of epinephrine (adrenaline) to inject immediately should they be exposed to the offending substance, known as the allergen. Epinephrine opens tightened airways, making it easier for the person to breathe, and constricts blood vessels to normalize blood pressure. Emergency medical help should be sought immediately.

Most allergic reactions to medication, however, are not life threatening. Consult your doctor regarding whether you should stop taking the medication. Antihistamines or steroids may be recommended. The most effective way to manage a medication allergy is to prevent yourself from becoming exposed to the allergen. Familiarize yourself with the genetic and brand names of the medications. Always examine over-the-counter medication labels to see if the allergen is among the ingredients.

Medications that bear a chemical relation to the one you are allergic to may cause problems as well. If you are allergic to a cephalosporin antibiotic such as cephalexin, for example, you may well react to another drug in the same chemical class. Unfortunately, people are seldom aware of chemical relations between drugs. Furthermore, the chemical similarity between drugs does not necessarily mean that there will be cross-reactivity. Before receiving medication remind your doctors, from your primary care doctor to your dentist, of any history of allergies or allergic reactions. ■

when weighing the benefits and risks of a medication: how likely each side effect is to occur, if the side effect is reversible once it occurs, and what is the overall chance and magnitude of harm, pain, or discomfort that may accompany taking the medication. For example, hay fever sufferers put up with the drowsiness that many antihistamines tend to generate if they effectively relieve nasal stuffiness and other symptoms. The actions of certain medications are considered so valuable—such as controlling seizures—that even significant side effects like drowsiness and loss of balance are considered acceptable given the benefits of the medication. Most medications, however, pose little risk of serious side effects. An adjustment to the dose may reduce or clear up the reaction altogether. Sometimes the body simply needs time to adjust to the medication and the side effect wanes or disappears altogether. If you develop a side effect with a medication, ask your doctor about whether you should change the dose or even switch your medications.

The exhaustive drug approval process in the United States tends to weed out drugs that cause side effects that are more serious or hazardous than the symptoms or condition they are designed to treat. For instance, side effects noted during initial testing of a headache medication may be deemed unacceptable given that most headaches are transient and not life threatening. But the same side effects may be considered acceptable in a cancer drug, for example, given the seriousness of the disease.

Adverse reactions differ from idiosyncratic reactions in several important respects. Idiosyncratic reactions are unexpected, unpredictable reactions that can actually be quite serious. Abuse or misuse of a medication, such as intentional or accidental overdose, can cause adverse reactions, as can the presence of another disorder. Allergic reactions are a risk as well. Call your doctor right away if you develop an unusual, unexpected reaction to a medication. Groups at particular risk for side effects and adverse reactions include the very young, the very old, and

MEDICATIONS: DO'S AND DON'TS

Do

- Follow prescription instructions exactly

- Read all warning labels

- Familiarize yourself with the medication's generic and brand names

- Confirm a refill is identical to the medication you received before

- Get all prescriptions filled at the same place; this may help prevent your being given medications that interact with another medication

- Make sure you have and understand instructions that come with the medication; the pharmacist may be able to supply you with a printed information sheet

- Take the medication your doctor has prescribed for as long as recommended, even if your symptoms have disappeared; be patient—some medications take some time to work

- Tell your doctor if you become pregnant while taking a medication of any type whether it is prescription, over-the-counter, or alternative; also inform your doctor of any alcohol or recreational drug use

- Confirm that it is safe to drive a car, operate heavy machinery, or participate in other potentially hazardous activities while taking your medication

- Place all medications out of the reach of children

- Ask your pharmacist for another type of packaging if you have trouble opening the one you have

- Keep medications in a cool, dry place unless otherwise directed

- Discard all outdated medications (many deteriorate with time); look for an expiration date; dispose of outdated medication properly (see page 1467); consult your pharmacist if you have any questions

- Discuss potential side effects with your doctor when you start taking a medication for the first time

Don't

- Share prescription medications

- Mix different medications in one container

- Take more of a medication than the prescribed dose

- Change the amount or timing of a prescription medication without the doctor's approval

- Demand overtreatment

- Be unduly influenced by advertisements; bear in mind the advertiser's motivation

- Keep a medication on your bedside table, unless you are supposed to use it in urgent situations, such as nitroglycerin for chest pain; this avoids the risk of taking the wrong medication while still groggy

- Take medications in the dark; always turn on the light first and make sure you are alert enough to take the correct medications at the proper dosage

- Assume that over-the-counter medications can do no harm; many can cause serious complications if misused

- Take any medication—prescription or over-the-counter—if you are pregnant or trying to conceive, unless your doctor confirms that it poses little risk to you or your unborn child ■

---

people with kidney or liver dysfunction, because both of these organs are vital to proper processing and excretion of many medications.

If you take two or more medications at the same time they may interact with one another in unwanted ways such as cancelling out the effect of one or both, for example, or altering the intended effect in some other way. Not all such drug interactions are necessarily negative; sometimes two medications are prescribed to take at once because one enhances the impact of another or in some other way produces a favorable reaction. Medication and food interactions can frequently be anticipated by your doctor or pharmacist, so consult with one of them before adding a new medication to your regimen.

WHAT YOU SHOULD ASK YOUR DOCTOR

Much of the responsibility for taking the proper medication—and taking it in the right way—rests with you. It is also important to establish with your primary care doctor that she will know about all of the medications that you are taking. Before using any new medications, whether prescription or over-the-counter, be sure you can answer the following questions. If you cannot, ask your doctor or pharmacist for guidance.

- Why have I been prescribed (or recommended) this medication?

- What is the medication treating? A symptom or the ailment itself?

- What can I expect in terms of my condition? How quickly will the medication take effect?

- When should I take the medication? How often? At what times of the day? Along with other medications, or alone?

- How should I take the medication? With food or milk, or on an empty stomach?

- Does the medication interact with any other medications, foods, or drinks, including alcohol?

- Are there any side effects commonly associated with the medication?

NAVIGATING THE PHARMACY

The modern pharmacy can be a dizzying—and daunting—place to shop for medications. There are ways to simplify the task, however.

Establish a relationship with the pharmacist Fill all your prescriptions at the same pharmacy (or pharmacy network); as the pharmacist gets to know you, they can alert you to the potential interactions that your prescription(s) may have with other medications and can help ensure that you consistently get the same brand of medication. You should also familiarize yourself with the generic name (and brand name, if applicable) of the prescription and over-the-counter medications you take. It is important to have one doctor who coordinates your medical care and who is aware of all the medications that you take.

Select over-the-counter medications wisely Many over-the-counter medications treat symptoms but will not actually cure you of an ailment. Cold medications address symptoms such as congestion and cough, for example, but do nothing to actually rid the body of the cold-causing virus. Many over-the-counter medications contain substances that certain groups of people should avoid. Alcohol and aspirin (and other salicylates) are prime examples of ingredients that are in many medications that should not be given to children in many cases. The pharmacist should be able to offer you guidance on over-the-counter medications.

KEY QUESTIONS FOR YOUR PHARMACIST

Take advantage of your pharmacist's knowledge about medication. Be sure to ask the following questions if you are not sure of the answers yourself:

- Will this over-the-counter medication interact negatively with any prescription medications I take?

- Is this medication available in a cheaper, generic form that would be appropriate for me?

- Does this medication come in a container that is easier to open? This question is appropriate only if no children live at home or visit regularly.

If any aspect of taking your medication confuses you, ask the pharmacist for guidance. In most cases she will know, for example, what time of day to take it, whether or not to take it with food, and what side effects to anticipate. If you notice that a prescription refill differs from what you have been receiving, be sure to ask your pharmacist why. ■

Respect the power of over-the-counter medications You may not need a prescription to buy them, but many over-the-counter medications pose their own risks of side effects or more serious reactions if not properly used. Never send your child to pick up a medication from a pharmacy; too many mishaps can occur in the hands of a curious child.

ORDERING MEDICATIONS BY MAIL

Ordering medications by mail offers two important benefits: convenience and a potentially lower bill. Ask your doctor or health coverage company if they can refer you to mail-order outlets or special plans. The American Association of Retired Persons Pharmacy Service, for example, is widely used by members of the association to order medications.

If you order by mail, make sure that you have enough medication to tide you over until the order arrives, which can take several weeks. To avoid a gap, your doctor may be willing to write you two prescriptions: a smaller one to get filled at a local pharmacy first, and a larger one to order from a mail-order outlet. When you receive your order, check that the correct prescription has been sent to you. Confirm your name, the name of the medication, and the dosage. Only order by mail if your delivery is secure. ■

USING OVER-THE-COUNTER MEDICATIONS SAFELY

Walk into any drugstore or supermarket and you can buy dozens of drugs without a doctor's prescription, from cold medications to pain relievers. These over-the-counter, or OTC, medications generally boast a wider safety margin than medications that require a prescription; they tend to cause fewer or less severe side effects and they are much less likely to pose the risk of addiction. Most over-the-counter medications are intended for minor ailments and complaints that do not demand professional medical care.

Just because an over-the-counter medication can be bought without a prescription does not mean it is necessarily free of side effects or potential hazards. Read the package label carefully and follow dosage instructions as written. All too often people who fail to get complete relief from an over-the-counter medication will take more than the recommended dose or will take the medication more frequently than is recommended on the package. Dosage restrictions on over-the-counter medications exist to protect your health—exceeding them can put your health at risk. Most labels will warn you of conditions under which the medication should not be taken, individuals for whom it is not appropriate (such as children or pregnant women), and circumstances under which it is advisable to see a doctor. Do not treat an apparently serious illness with an over-the-counter medication unless a doctor has reviewed your condition and recommended one. Your pharmacist may be able to advise you on an appropriate over-the-counter medication and also on when to see a doctor if symptoms persist or your condition worsens. Some over-the-counter medications can interfere with other medications you take, so be sure to check with your pharmacist or doctor if you already take a prescription or over-the-counter medication.

TAKING AN EXTRA STEP

It has never been easier to get information about illnesses, both common and obscure, and the medications used to treat them. There are national and international foundations for a host of diseases, such as diabetes, arthritis, and lupus. Many of these foundations publish fact sheets and newsletters that cover recent drug developments and some run hotlines that can field basic informational calls. Community health services may offer medication information as well, and some major university hospitals run health information libraries for their patients and the public. Bookstores now sell various consumer medication information guides. The Internet can also be mined for drug information, although much of what can be found there is wrong or promotional; always consider the source. Remain wary, particularly of sources that promote "quick fixes." The Food and Drug Administration (FDA), National Institutes of Health, universities, and sources that have undergone FDA review, such as pharmaceutical companies, are the most reliable sources.

As part of the development process of new drugs or treatment protocols, drug studies are conducted to examine safety and efficacy. Sometimes individuals are presented with the opportunity to participate in drug trials. Taking part in a drug study offers you a chance to help advance medical care and knowledge.

There are several places you can look for information on becoming part of a drug study. First, ask your doctor if she knows of one. Local hospitals, senior centers, and other community-based organizations may have listings to recruit volunteers. The public information office at the National Institutes of Health in Bethesda, Maryland, will have information on the trials they are conducting around the country. Information may also be available through your nearest university or teaching hospital. Lastly, directions of ongoing clinical trials are available on the Internet. See the Web site at http://www.centerwatch.com for more information.

ABUSE OF PRESCRIPTION AND OVER-THE-COUNTER MEDICATIONS

Recognizing and doing something about drug abuse in yourself or someone you care about can be frightening and challenging. Drug dependence usually implies an inability to moderate or alter one's intake of a substance. One can be dependent on an apparently innocuous substance such as caffeine or a dangerous substance such as heroin. Americans have long struggled with problems of dependence on sleeping medications, tranquilizers, and pain killers (see Chapter 5).

There are several types of drug dependence. Physical dependence implies a physiologic reliance and adaptation to a drug; the body has actually adjusted to a new chemical environment. Sometimes violent and even potentially fatal physical symptoms known as withdrawal symptoms, can develop upon stopping the drug. Withdrawal from a physical dependence on a drug demands expert medical supervision. Many of the drugs that tend to cause physical dependence are mood- or behavior-altering substances, such as antianxiety drugs and central nervous system stimulants like nicotine and cocaine, but chronic pain medications can also cause physical dependence. Psychological dependence often accompanies physical dependence. Psychological dependence is a deep emotional craving for a drug. Scientists commonly refer to addiction as a condition that encompasses these various types of dependence. The addicted person compulsively uses a substance even though it incurs physical, social, or psychological harm.

Some people taking prescription medications worry that they will become dependent on them. Dependence occurs infrequently when the medication is taken properly as prescribed. If you are worried that you will become dependent on a medication, discuss your concerns with your doctor. The fear of becoming addicted is often unfounded and can lead to a serious underdosing of pain medication, which can have deleterious consequences.

RISKS OF MIXING MEDICATIONS WITH ALCOHOL OR RECREATIONAL DRUGS

Alcohol is a potent drug that depresses the central nervous system and can damage the liver. Mixing alcohol with a prescription or over-the-counter medication poses several risks; in some cases even small amounts of alcohol can increase the drowsiness experienced with sedatives, pain relievers, and antihistamines, for example. These types of reactions can even occur from the alcohol actually present in many over-the-counter

medications. With some medications having even a few drinks can cause serious harm, including liver damage and central nervous system depression, beyond just drowsiness. Serious cases of liver toxicity have resulted from combining alcohol and acetaminophen, and barbiturates and alcohol can form a deadly combination.

Alcohol is a common ingredient in many types of medications, although often the consumer may be unaware of the alcohol content. Over-the-counter cough syrups and decongestants are good examples of this. The manufacturer may add the alcohol for various reasons, such as to dissolve the contained active ingredient or to add a sedative component. Check all medication labels for alcohol if you wish to avoid it. Be sure that you take alcohol-containing medication at the proper dose, especially if you are taking multiple alcohol-containing medications. This is especially true for children, seniors, and people with serious stomach or liver problems or people whose systems may be more sensitive to alcohol.

Taking Your Medication: General Guidelines

ORAL MEDICATIONS

Most medications you take by mouth are absorbed into your bloodstream through the walls of your intestine. The medication has to get to this area intact to work properly. You can help ensure this by taking the medication with plenty of water (at least half a glass) while standing or sitting

---

MEASURING THE DOSE PROPERLY

When you measure a liquid medication, use only a standardized measuring device. If a medication comes with a special measuring cup or other unit, always use that. If 1 tsp is the prescribed dose, use a spoon specially designed for measuring medication or a standard teaspoon used for cooking measurements. Under no circumstances rely on household teaspoons for measurement; they vary widely in size.

When measuring out medication from a dropper, do not take extra to compensate for the small amount that typically remains inside the dropper; this has been accounted for in setting the dosage.

Shake all liquid medications well before measuring out the dose; this helps ensure that the active elements are fully distributed. ■

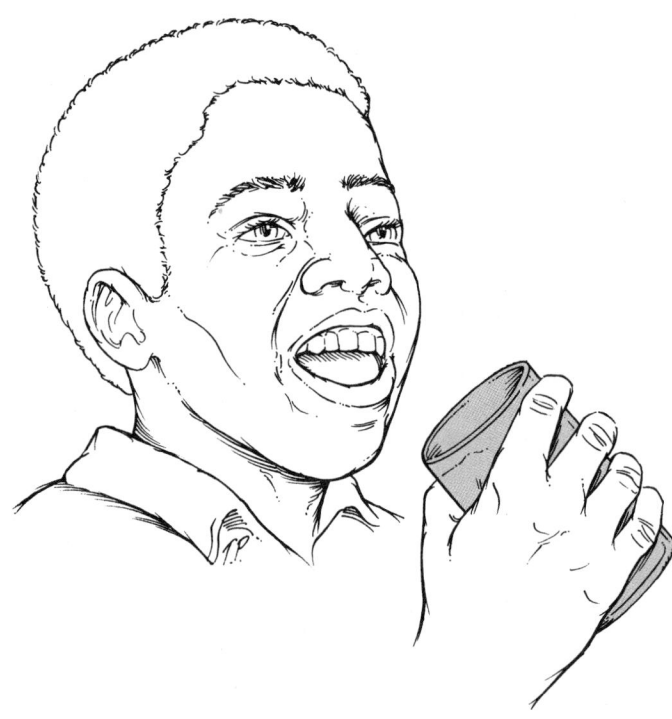

Use plenty of water when taking tablets or capsules by mouth, and be sure to follow instructions about whether to take oral medications with food or on an empty stomach (1 hour before or 2 to 3 hours after eating). To make sure you swallow the medication properly, stay in an upright position for a minute or two after taking it (note that some medications require an even longer period). If medication becomes stuck in the esophagus, eat a soft, bulky food such as a banana or a slice of bread, and drink some additional water. Do not crush, cut, chew, or open a tablet or capsule without consulting your doctor. Do not take medications at nonprescribed times, and if you miss a dose, do not take additional doses later unless your doctor advises you to do so. Pharmacists are excellent sources of information about medications—especially side effects and interactions—but they may be unaware of your specific medical conditions.

upright. Stay in this upright position for a minute or two after taking the medication; this reduces the risk of a tablet, capsule, or other hard medication from getting stuck in the esophagus, the tube that connects your throat to your stomach. If a medication gets stuck it could damage the esophagus or the medication's actions could be delayed. Drinking plenty of water also aids absorption. If a pill does get stuck in your esophagus, eat a soft, bulky food such as a banana or a slice of bread and drink some water to help wash it down.

Always check with your primary care doctor, pharmacist, or a reliable reference book before manipulating—crushing, opening, cutting, or chewing—a medication in any way. Some tablets and capsules that seem too large to swallow may be crushed or mixed with a soft food such as applesauce. The same is true for liquids whose taste you dislike. If you mix a liquid medication with food, take the mixture immediately so that no one else takes it by accident. A number of medications are also available in a variety of forms, including easy-to-swallow liquids.

Long-acting or extended-release tablets or capsules should always be swallowed whole. Chewing or breaking open these types of pills will cause the medication to be released into your system rapidly, rather than gradually as intended. As a result, the medication may not work properly and may even cause harm.

Timing is often critical to the effectiveness of oral medications, yet the instructions that accompany many medications may seem unclear. A prescription that calls for you to take three doses a day, for example, may mean three doses during waking hours, or three doses spread out over a 24-hour period—that is, every 8 hours. Ask your doctor or the pharmacist for more specific guidance if you are not clear on what you should do. In general, medications that you are taking regularly should be taken at the same time every day. A schedule that is consistent from day to day will not only help you remember to take the medication but will also ensure that your body is exposed to relatively constant levels of the active substance in the medication.

Food can alter the effectiveness of a medication, so carefully follow the medication's instructions as to whether or not the medication should be taken with food. Most medication works more quickly when taken on an empty stomach. Sometimes the presence of food reduces the amount of medication free to be absorbed into the body or it affects the speed at which the medication is absorbed into the body. However, in certain cases, some medication is better absorbed when taken with food. The type of food you eat makes a difference with medication. Certain medications, for example, bind to milk or milk products, thus hindering their absorption into the bloodstream. Some medications should be taken with food to minimize stomach irritation. As a general rule, avoid taking medications with hot drinks such as coffee or tea, because they can reduce or even erase the effectiveness of many medications.

If a prescription insert (or label in the case of over-the-counter medications) instructs you to take the medication on an empty stomach and offers no specifics on how to do this, take it at least 1 hour before or 2 to 3 hours after eating.

THE MANY FORMS OF TABLETS, CAPSULES, AND LIQUIDS

Tablets, typically round in shape, contain the medication compressed into a solid form along with substances that bind the tablet together. Tablets come in many forms. Enteric-coated tablets are designed to dissolve in the small intestine rather than the stomach, which they pass through first. Chewable tablets, often tailored to appeal to children, should always be chewed thoroughly to avoid stomach irritation. Effervescent tablets are fashioned to dissolve completely in a liquid. Be sure to drink all the liquid. Sublingual tablets are placed under the tongue, and buccal tablets are tucked between the cheek and teeth. As these last two types of tablets dissolve, the medication quickly enters the bloodstream through the dense network of blood vessels lining the mouth. These types of tablets can prove quite valuable when fast action is needed; many people with angina (chest pain), for example, rely on sublingual nitroglycerin tablets when their condition flares. Never swallow a sublingual or buccal tablet. Caplets are tablets shaped into capsule form for easier swallowing. A lozenge is a tablet in which the medication has been incorporated into a sugar- or fruit-based paste; most lozenges are designed to be sucked on until they dissolve, much like a hard candy.

Capsules, typically cylindrical in shape, come in either soft gelatin form, with a liquid inside, or in hard gelatin form, with timed-release beads or powder inside. Sustained-release, slow-release, or timed-release pills (tablets or capsules) are designed to release medication slowly over time as they dissolve in the gastrointestinal tract.

Liquid medications come in several forms. Some are made into the following forms from granules, powders, effervescent tablets, or other dry substances:

- A syrup consists of the active medicinal ingredients dissolved in a sugary flavored solution. Syrups are usually quite thick.

- An elixir consists of the active medicinal ingredients mixed in a flavored and sugary alcohol base.

- A suspension contains powdered or otherwise solid medication that has been suspended rather than dissolved in a liquid. Because the medication often settles down to the bottom, it is particularly important to shake a suspension well before measuring out a dose. Some formulations require that you mix the medication with a liquid (called a diluent) yourself.

- A solution consists of a clear liquid in which the medication has been dissolved.

- A mixture contains one or more medications, dissolved to form a solution or suspension.

- An emulsion is a medication contained in an oil-and-water base.

TOPICAL MEDICATIONS

Medications that are applied to the skin and surface tissues of the body—also called topical medications—come in a wide array of forms, from creams and ointments to solutions, dusting powders, nasal drops, suppositories (rectal and vaginal), and ear and eye drops. Because topical medications deliver the medication directly to the problem site, topical medications generally do not cause the complications that systemic medications can. It is also much easier to control the impact of topical medications. Many infections and irritations of the skin, ears, and eyes are treated with topical medications.

As with other forms of medications, the belief that, with topical medications, more is better is not only misguided but potentially hazardous. Sometimes the risks of applying more medication than necessary can add up to more than mere skin irritation; topical steroids, for example, can cause body-wide side effects if taken in higher than recommended doses or repeatedly placed on large or damaged areas of skin. Avoid leaving any topical medication on for longer than is recommended.

Always wash your hands before and after applying a skin medication. Dab the prescribed amount onto the center of the affected area and spread the medication out from there in an even and thin layer. Unless otherwise directed, a spray should be held at least 6 in. from the skin. Shake the container well before spraying.

EYE MEDICATIONS

Always wash your hands before applying eye medication and lie or sit down before applying the medication to make sure that you do not lose your balance and can focus on what you are doing. Eye medications typically come in ointment or drop form.

Ointment If the ointment tube is cool, warm it up by rolling it between your hands. With a gauze, wipe away any crusting or secretions that have built up on the eye. Tilting your head back, gently pull down your lower eyelid by drawing down the skin below it, or pinching the skin directly under the lower eyelid to form a pocket between the eye and the lower eyelid. Look upward toward your forehead and squeeze a small amount (about a $\frac{1}{2}$ in.) of ointment onto the inside margin of the eyelid. Close the eye for 1 to 2 minutes to help the medication absorb into the eye. Try to avoid blinking because that will flush the medication out of the eye. Gently wipe away any excess medication on the eyelashes or cheeks with a clean tissue. Your vision may be blurry for a few moments after applying an ointment. To avoid contamination, never actually touch your eye, eyelid, cheek, or fingers with the medication tube opening. To help prevent contamination, end by squeezing a small amount of ointment onto a tissue and throw the tissue away.

Drops Bring drops that are cool to room temperature by rolling the bottle between your hands. Shake the bottle. With a gauze, wipe away any crusting or secretions that have built up on the eye. Tilting your head back, gently pull down your lower eyelid by drawing down the skin below it, or pinching the skin directly under the lower eyelid to form a pocket between the eye and the lower eyelid. Squeeze the drops behind

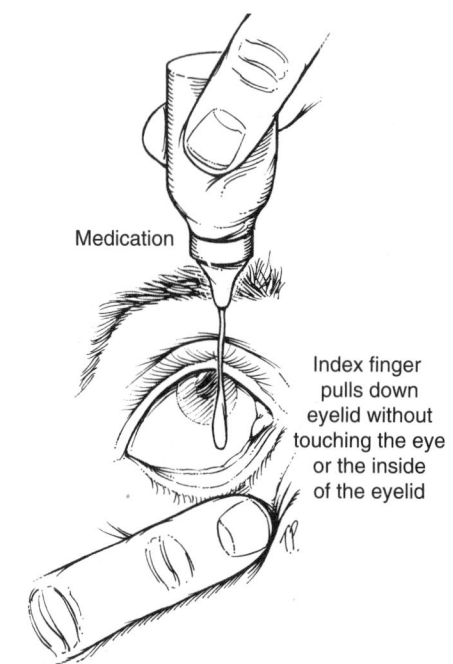

Medication

Index finger pulls down eyelid without touching the eye or the inside of the eyelid

Eye medications typically come in drops or ointments. Always wash your hands before applying medication to an eye, whether it is your eye or someone else's. If you are using eyedrops, shake the bottle to mix the medication. Roll the bottle or tube of medication between your hands to warm it. Steady yourself by lying or sitting down. Next, use a gauze pad to wipe away any secretions from the eye. Tilt your head back, and gently pull down your lower eyelid by pinching or drawing down the skin below the eyelid. Squeeze the drops into the area behind the lid without touching your fingers or the dropper to any part of the eye. Close your eye for 1 or 2 minutes to allow the medication to spread. Gently wipe away any extra medication with a clean tissue. Use a similar procedure for applying ointments. For medications that are absorbed into the bloodstream, such as beta blockers, press your finger in the corner of the eye near your nose for 1 minute. This pressure prevents side effects due to the medication being absorbed rapidly.

your lower eyelid. To help prevent contamination, carefully avoid touching the dropper to any part of the eye, including the eyelashes, skin around the eye, or fingers. Close your eye for 1 to 2 minutes to keep the medication in and to allow it to be absorbed. Gently wipe away any extra medication on the eyelashes or cheeks with a clean tissue.

EAR MEDICATIONS

Be gentle when administering ear medications; rough handling can damage the eardrum and ear canal. Never actually insert

Always wash your hands before and after applying medication to an ear, whether it is your ear or someone else's. Shake the bottle to mix the medication and then roll the bottle between your hands to warm it. Use a gauze pad to wipe away any crusting or drainage from the outer ear. Tilt your head sideways so that your ear points upward. Pull the side of the outer ear up and back. Without touching the ear canal with the dropper, instill the prescribed number of drops and hold your head steady for several minutes. When you are finished, place the dropper back into the bottle without rinsing it. Never insert anything past the outer ear, and remember not to share ear medications.

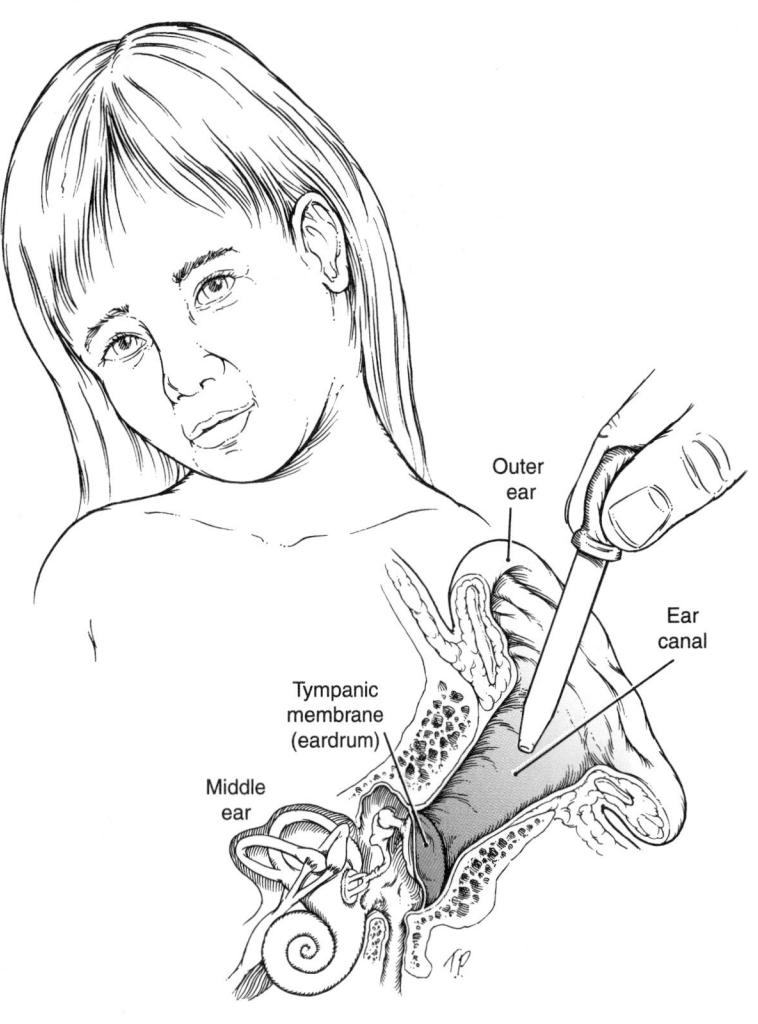

anything—especially not a cotton swab—past the outer ear. Avoid touching the ear canal with the dropper. To prevent spreading an infection, do not share ear medications. Most ear medications come in liquid form contained within a dropper.

Drops Always wash your hands before and after administering an ear medication. Cool medication may make you feel dizzy or even nauseous, so warm it up, if needed, by rolling the bottle between your palms or running it under warm water for a few minutes. Also make sure the tip of the dropper is not cracked or chipped. Shake the bottle. Use gauze to gently clean away any ear drainage or crusting on the outer ear. Tilt your head sideways so that your ear faces the ceiling. To straighten the ear canal so that the medication can penetrate it well, draw your earlobe down and toward the back of your head. However, if you are administering drops to a child more than 3 years old, pull the side of the outer ear or the ear lobe up and back. Instill the prescribed number of drops. Hold your head in the same position for several minutes to allow the medication to absorb into the ear. Repeat these steps for the other ear if needed. Do not rinse the ear dropper; simply place it back into the bottle.

NASAL MEDICATIONS

Nasal medications are available in several forms including drops, sprays, ointments, and aerosols. Gently blow your nose before administering a nasal medication and always wash your hands before and after applying it.

To avoid passing infection from one person to another, never share nasal medications.

Nasal drops If the drops are cool, bring them to room temperature by rolling the container between your hands. Shake the container. Lie or sit down, and tilt your head back. Breathing through your mouth, slowly instill the prescribed number of drops into a nostril, carefully avoiding touching the sides of the nostrils with the dropper. After instilling the drops, keep your head tilted back for several seconds to allow the medication to absorb into the nasal cavity. Repeat this procedure for the other nostril if necessary. When finished, wash the dropper in hot, soapy water and dry it.

Nasal spray Sit or stand with your head tilted back. Close off the opposite nostril by pressing against it with one finger, and with your other hand insert the tip of the sprayer (or pump bottle) about $1/2$ in. into the nos-

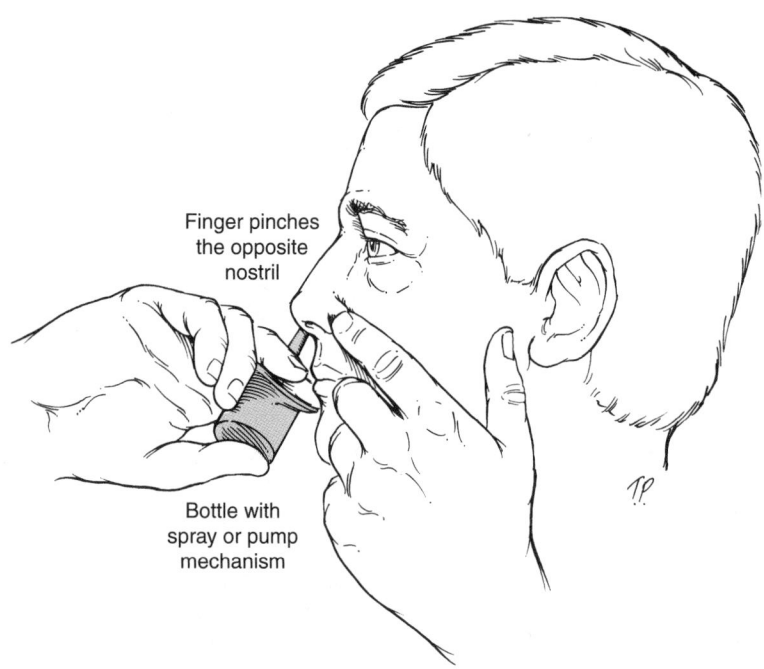

Finger pinches
the opposite
nostril

Bottle with
spray or pump
mechanism

To use nasal spray, sit or stand with your head tilted back. Close the opposite nostril with one finger and insert the tip of the bottle about ½ in. into both nostrils, with the tip pointing straight back. Keeping your mouth closed, spray or squeeze the bottle while inhaling through the nostril. Avoid blowing your nose for 2 minutes. Clean the tip of the bottle with warm water, dry it with a clean cloth, and replace the cap.

tril, with the tip of the container pointed toward the inner corner of the eye. Simultaneously squeeze the container and sniff in. Treat the other nostril the same way if needed. Avoid blowing your nose for 2 minutes or so if possible to allow the medication to do its work. Clean the sprayer tip with warm water and dry it well with a clean tissue. Always replace the cap.

RECTAL MEDICATIONS

There are several reasons for taking a medication rectally. Nausea or other complications may make it impractical to take the medication by mouth, for example. The stomach's digestive juices can destroy certain medications, or the rectum or anal area may need to be treated directly.

A few rectal medications—mostly those for constipation or inflammatory bowel diseases—are prescribed in enema form. Ene-

mas are liquid medications inserted into the rectum with an applicator. But most medications designed for rectal administration come in the form of a suppository. These solid, bullet-shaped suppositories dissolve gradually, releasing the active ingredients that go on to affect the body as a whole. Some suppositories are solid when cold—for example, when kept in the refrigerator—but melt quickly at room temperature. These suppositories must be inserted quickly and efficiently.

Wash your hands before and after inserting a rectal suppository. Wear latex gloves or a finger cot, which covers one finger. The suppository should not be too soft; run the package under cool water for a few minutes to firm it up if necessary. Lie on your side, separate the cheeks of the buttocks, and gently insert the suppository high into the rectum, with the pointed end entering first. If the suppository slips out, simply reinsert it higher in the rectum. If you sense you need to lubricate the suppository, smear it with a small amount of water to make it slide in more easily. Holding the cheeks of the buttocks together for a few minutes may also encourage the suppository to stay in and will also give it time to dissolve.

VAGINAL MEDICATIONS

Most vaginal medications are designed to treat conditions affecting the vagina alone, such as local yeast infections. Gels, foams, and creams are just a few of the forms of vaginal medications available.

Clean your hands before and after administering a vaginal medication. Empty your bladder. Spread the lips of the vagina and insert the medicine—typically an applicator or suppository—a few inches (or as directed) into the vagina. Do not use a tampon directly afterwards as it is likely to absorb the medicine. Wash reusable applicators with warm, soapy water and dry them well. A panty liner will protect underwear from medication that may leak out.

INHALATION MEDICATIONS (ORAL AND NASAL)

Inhalation medications may affect the respiratory tract directly—a benefit widely valued in asthma and emphysema medications—or produce a general effect by entering the bloodstream through the lungs. Inhalation medications come in several forms, from metered dose inhalers, or MDIs, which often come with an attachment device called a spacer that makes them easier to use, to capsules delivered through an inhaler. Administering these types of medications correctly can prove challenging. Errors are common. So, in addition to getting a handout from your doctor that describes how to administer the medication—these also can be found in virtually all inhalation medication packages—you should periodically demonstrate your technique to your doctor or pharmacist. See page 747 for more detailed information on the use of inhalers.

INJECTION MEDICATIONS

There may be several reasons why you have been prescribed an injection medication. Speed is one of the most common; a medication that is injected into your body will circulate quickly through your system. Minutes and even seconds can be critical when attempting to treat a severe allergic reaction, for example. Sometimes an injection medication is prescribed because the stomach destroys the active substance when taken orally (insulin is an example of this) or the medication may fail to pass into the bloodstream because it cannot penetrate the walls of the intestine. Nausea or other adverse reactions to an oral medication may also justify the use of an injection medication.

Depending on the type of medication and the condition it is being used to treat, an injection will be administered one of three ways. Intramuscular injections are administered into a muscle, characteristically the buttock, thigh, or upper arm. Subcutaneous injections are delivered under the surface of the skin. Intravenous injections are administered directly into a vein.

Unless you have been carefully instructed on how to administer an injection medication a doctor or nurse should perform the procedure. If you have been shown how to administer an injection medication and have been prescribed needles to do so, make sure to dispose of them properly. This is important to avoid spreading infection as well as misuse of needles for illegal drug injection. Never use another person's needles because it can lead to the spread of hepatitis, bacterial infections, or infection with the human immunodeficiency virus (HIV), which causes acquired immunodeficiency syndrome (AIDS). Place used needles (and extra, unused needles) in a "sharps" container (sold in drugstores) and return them to your pharmacist.

TRANSDERMAL PATCH MEDICATIONS

One of the newest methods for administering medications is by transdermal patch, a medication-impregnated pad you place on the skin. These patches can offer steady and constant delivery of medication; the adhesive material releases a premeasured supply of medication gradually over a designated period of time. The patch also liberates the user from having to remember to take a medication every day. Medications that are commonly available in this form include estrogen, nitroglycerin (for angina), and nicotine (for smoking cessation), although there are many others. The packaging (or your prescription) should provide instructions on where to place the patch. To avoid excessive skin irritation, apply it to a relatively hair-free area of skin and remember to rotate the patch to a different spot every once in a while. Let your doctor know if the transdermal patch is irritating your skin; she may have strategies for relieving this reaction.

TIMING: WHEN TO TAKE YOUR MEDICATION

Prescription medications are most effective when taken at the same time every day. In addition to jogging your memory, a consistent medication schedule will encourage a steady level of the medication's active ingredient in your system. A weekly pill box or medication calendar can serve as a valuable memory aid. Weekly pill boxes, available at most drugstores, feature medication storage compartments for each day of the week. Checking the compartment for a given day will let you know if you have already taken a certain medication. A medication calendar can also help. If, for example, you take several separate medications—a diuretic every day for high blood pressure, sumatriptan as

MISSED DOSES

To err is human, and while it is best never to miss doses of a medication most people do at one point or another. In most cases, a missed dose will cause no major problems. If you are taking medication on a regular basis, it is a good idea to consult your doctor regarding what to expect in terms of a potential change in symptoms following a missed dose, and what to do next. In general, if you miss one dose of a medication you take regularly, take the missed dose as soon as possible and then resume your regular schedule. If you only remember that you missed a dose when preparing to take the next scheduled dose, skip the dose you missed. Do not take two doses at once. If you miss more than one dose, ask your doctor for guidance.

Some medications do not last long in your system and must be taken very regularly to ensure adequate concentrations in your body. These types of medications are particularly important not to miss. Insulin is just one example. Find a strategy for remembering to take your medication if you find that you are frequently missing doses. ■

MEDICATION PRECAUTIONS WHEN TRAVELING

When preparing for a trip, make sure you have extra medication with you in case your return home is delayed. Keep important prescription medications with you at all times and a few doses in your luggage to avoid the risk of having none should you be separated from your luggage or get robbed. These precautions are particularly important to take if you are traveling abroad. Whenever you travel, carry a card with your doctor's name and number on it, your medical condition, and the medications you take for it. Medical alert bracelets can be useful as well. Ask your doctor or call the consulate for the country you will be visiting or a reputable travel clinic for information on immunizations you should get (for more detailed information, see page 74).

Exercise care in obtaining medications overseas, particularly in underdeveloped countries where standardization of medications and expiration dates are not always honored. Consulates can offer referral to doctors who speak your language. Make sure you know the generic name of your medication should you absolutely need to get more medication abroad; the generic name is more globally recognized than a brand name. ■

needed for migraines, and a benzodiazepine for insomnia—you can faithfully note each dose and the time you took it on your medication calendar. Not only do you have a ready memory aid, but you also provide your doctor with a useful tool. By looking at the patterns of medication use that appear on a weekly calendar, your doctor may find ways to combine, alter, or even eliminate certain medications.

You and your primary care doctor can draw up a medication calendar together. This will encourage her to take a close look at all the medications you take and possibly eliminate unneeded ones or find ways to simplify your medication regimen, such as consolidating certain medications you take to a particular time of day.

A MEDICATION'S JOURNEY THROUGH THE BODY

Most oral medications follow a specific route through the body: After being swallowed, it travels to your stomach and intestines, where it is absorbed and transported to the liver by blood vessels. Some medications are simply released from the liver into the general circulation; others must first be broken down by the liver into their active form. Typically, however, the liver converts the medication into a more soluble form that can be eliminated in the urine. Some medications are designed to remain within the stomach and intestines and to only affect these organs. Ideally, medications would only have an impact on the organs they are intended to treat. But since oral medications are delivered by the blood, which circulates throughout the body, tissues and organs everywhere may be affected. This helps explain why toxic reactions to certain medications occur; a chemotherapy drug taken to kill cancer cells, for example, will also destroy normal, healthy tissue that turns over quickly, such as blood-producing cells.

Unlike medications that are swallowed, orally inhaled, or injected, those applied to the body—such as skin creams and eye, ear, and nose drops — primarily affect the specific tissue to which they are applied. There is little absorption and distribution around the body, although small amounts may enter the circulation. When you apply eyedrops, for example, some of the medication will be absorbed by the blood vessels of the eye and some will drain through the tear ducts down into your nose, where additional absorption occurs. The amount of medication absorbed into the circulation is usually not enough to exert any notable or widespread effects on the body.

Medications and their by-products eventually leave the body through the urine, feces, sweat, or tears. Some medications can stain sweat and tears—such as rifampicin, which stains red—but the staining is unimportant. In some unusual cases, medications leave the body through other body tissues such as the lungs. Many of the instructions given along with a medication, such as what time of day to take it and whether or not to take it with food, reflect various characteristics of the particular medication including the length of time it takes to be absorbed, exert its intended effect, and exit the body.

STARTING AND STOPPING A MEDICATION

Call your doctor right away if you develop worrisome, persistent, or apparently significant reactions to a medication. Do not abruptly stop a regular prescription medication on your own, however, unless you believe you are having a serious adverse reaction or an allergic reaction. Stopping a course of medication treatment before the time recommended is fraught with hazards. Depending on the medication, your ailment may recur, complications may develop, or withdrawal symptoms may set in. Many people fail to complete a course of antibiotics because they feel better after just a few doses; the risk in such cases is that the infection will linger quietly in your body and the disorder will in time reemerge and will probably require another round of antibiotics. Long-term oral corticosteroids, on the other hand, are important to withdraw from gradually under the careful guidance of a doctor, because the medication has probably shut down the adrenal glands and they must be slowly coaxed back into action. Fight the temptation to stop taking a medication because of an unpleasant side effect; talk to your doctor about your concerns. Often the side effect will dissipate with time or your doctor may prescribe another medication that suits you better.

THERAPEUTIC MEDICATION MONITORING

People vary in the way they respond to medications and in many cases your doctor may work with you to fine-tune your dosage to maximize effectiveness and minimize side effects. Some medications, however, need to be monitored more closely. These medications have narrow safety margins, meaning the level at which they are toxic closely straddles the level at which they are effective. These medications also may need to be monitored closely because they can cause toxic reactions that could elude easy detection because they resemble symptoms of the disorder the medication aims to treat. One of the tools at the doctor's disposal in such murky circumstances is therapeutic medication monitoring; by measuring blood levels of certain medications, your response to medication can be predicted more precisely, the risk of toxicity reduced, and the dosage adjusted accordingly. Blood tests are typically done when the medication either drops to its lowest point in your body—the trough level—or its highest point—the peak level. Therapeutic medication monitoring is commonly conducted on people taking medications such as theophylline and various cardiac antiarrhythmia and antiseizure medication. For medication monitoring it is important to accurately time the blood test and the exact time the last dose or few doses were given.

YOUR MEDICINE CABINET

Your medicine cabinet should be stocked with the supplies necessary for treating minor aches and pains and handling minor home emergencies. It is a good idea to store some first aid items in your car as well (see Chapter 13).

Despite popular thinking, the bathroom is one of the worst places to store medications because heat and humidity are often damaging to many medications. If you have children (or frequent young visitors) it may also give them unwanted access to your medications. Find another place in the house; a locked closet in the bedroom is the best selection in homes with children. Store all your medications in this place including iron tablets, oral contraceptives, and commonly used over-the-counter medications. Put away all medications immediately after using them. Securely replace caps, lids, and other container tops to prevent leaks and premature deterioration.

The area you choose for storage should be cool, dry, and away from direct sunlight. Only refrigerate a medication if you are specifically advised to do so. Keep medications in their original container along with any accompanying instructions to avoid confusion.

Periodically review and clean out your medicine cabinet and discard expired medications or those that show signs of breaking down. Medications deteriorate over time: Aspirin and acetaminophen tablets may smell of vinegar; liquids may become discolored or take on a different consis-

KEEPING MEDICATIONS AWAY FROM CHILDREN

The safest place for medications in a home with children is a locked medicine cabinet in the bedroom. To be useful, the cabinet must actually be locked all the time, even when you are in the room. Medications that require refrigeration should be kept in the refrigerator on a high shelf behind other items, well out of reach. Make sure to discard the medication properly once you have taken the prescribed amount. Older children may take a medication that they need to administer to themselves, such as a bronchodilator during an asthma attack. This should be kept where only they—and no other children—will have easy access to it.

Too often in households the medicine cabinet is kept locked, but medications in daily use are left out. Do not leave the container out to remind you to take the medication; find another way to jog your memory, or leave an empty bottle. Never characterize medications as candy when trying to coax your child to take them.

Ask for childproof tops for all your medications if the pharmacist does not give them to you automatically. Keep in mind that these tops do not make it impossible for a child to get into them; it simply makes it more challenging. Do not forget to properly secure childproof tops after taking medication—if you leave the little arrows aligned, for example, you have defeated the safety feature. ■

tency, taste, or smell; tablets may crack or soften; and ointments and creams may discolor or harden. If you have any doubts about the contents of a container, discard it immediately. Flush unused prescription medications and any deteriorated or outdated medications down the toilet, or give them back to your pharmacist. Never put them in the garbage. Always discard syringes in a special sharps container and arrange to return them to your pharmacist.

Key items to store in your medicine cabinet include the following:

- *Pain relievers and fever reducers.* Acetaminophen, ibuprofen, and aspirin are a few of the standard medications effective for these purposes. Do not give aspirin to a child or teenager under age 18 unless you are specifically instructed to do so by your doctor. Chewable acetaminophen tablets are a good choice for households with children past infancy but less than 12 years old.

- *Antiseptics and bandages* for minor wounds. Antiseptics include hydrogen peroxide solution to help clean a wound and a disinfectant cream or ointment. Keep adhesive tape and scissors handy. Elastic bandages are valuable for stabilizing a sprained or otherwise traumatized joint.

- *Thermometer.* If you have children, consider getting a rectal, oral digital, or tympanic (ear) thermometer. Rectal thermometers give very accurate readings (see Chapter 8). Oral digital and tympanic thermometers enable you to take a temperature quickly, which can be particularly valuable if you have an uncooperative child.

- *Tweezers* come in handy for removing splinters and small objects from a wound. Disinfect the tweezers in boiling water first. Never probe or dig into a wound.

- *Syrup of ipecac* to induce vomiting in the case of an accidental poisoning. Syrup of ipecac is particularly important for families with children less than 12 years old. Use syrup of ipecac only under the instruction from a doctor, a pharmacist, or a poison control center because some poisons can cause even more damage by being vomited.

A simple first aid book that fits into your medicine cabinet may come in handy. Depending on your family's medical conditions, you may also want to stock the following items:

- Rubbing alcohol and absorbent cotton for disinfecting minor wounds
- Cold and cough medications
- Antihistamines and nasal preparations for allergy symptoms
- Bulk laxatives such as psyllium for constipation
- Antacid for stomach upset
- Sodium fluoride to help prevent dental problems in regions where the local water supply contains no fluoride
- Eye drops and artificial tears for eye irritations
- Diarrhea medications
- Antifungal preparations for fungal infections
- Hemorrhoid preparations
- Bee or wasp sting kit (these are available by prescription only)
- Sunscreens

IN AN EMERGENCY

Drug overdose is the leading cause of fatal poisoning in the United States. Some of these cases are accidental, others intentional. You are unlikely to suffer complications if you mistakenly take an extra dose of a medication. However, if you cannot remember whether or not you took a dose of your medication, call the pharmacist or your doctor for guidance. To avoid an accidental overdose, never attempt to speed up or reinforce a medication's effect by taking more than the stated dose; not only will this strategy fail, but it may cause harm. Measure out medication doses carefully and in full light and check the label for the dosage every time you take the medication; never take a guess. Seniors are particularly prone to forgetfulness and are therefore at risk for taking extra doses. Dangerous medication buildups can also occur if the liver or kidneys are not functioning properly and processing the medication as needed. Poisoning symptoms may develop as medication levels in the bloodstream rise; these

symptoms may become apparent right away or they may appear within days or even weeks.

If you suspect an overdose, be it unintentional or deliberate

- Do not panic.
- If the suspected overdose has occurred in a child, check her mouth for any pills or other medication and quickly remove what is there.
- Check to make sure the victim is breathing; a lack of oxygen may cause her to turn blue.
- *If the victim is unconscious and not breathing,* remove any obstacles to breathing, lay the victim on her back, open her collar, place a hand on her forehead and gingerly push her head back at the same time that you lift, push, or pull her jaw so that it juts outward. This will open the airway as far as possible. Only proceed with mouth-to-mouth resuscitation if the victim is still not breathing. Shout for help. Call a rescue squad (for more information on CPR, see page 361).
- *If the victim is conscious and breathing,* give her an 8 oz glass of water to dilute the poison.
- *If the victim is breathing but having convulsions,* lay her onto her stomach

GETTING MEDICATIONS IN THE HOSPITAL

If you are admitted to a hospital, tell the doctor about all the medications you take as soon as possible. Depending on why you are admitted, the doctor may allow you to take your regular medications form home rather than pay for them through the hospital, which can be quite costly. For instance, if you are admitted for an infection and you take medications for your headaches and asthma, taking your own medications will likely prove much cheaper than acquiring them through the hospital pharmacy. Check first with your doctor or pharmacist to verify any medications you might bring in. When you are discharged from the hospital, the doctor or nurse will explain how to take your new medications and discuss possible side effects or interactions with other medications you take. ■

and turn her head to one side so that any vomit is not inhaled. Do not give anything by mouth. Keep her warm until help arrives.

- Take the medication container to the phone with you and try to keep the victim in sight. If the victim is a child, take her with you. Watch for reactions to the medication including sleeping, vomiting, and convulsing.

- Call a poison control center, your doctor, or an emergency department. You will get instructions on what to do.

- You may be asked what type of medication and how much the victim took, her approximate age and weight, and what medications she takes regularly (if any).

- Only give the victim ipecac syrup (to induce vomiting) or any other substance by mouth if specifically instructed to do so. Likewise, do not induce vomiting unless directed to do so; some substances may cause as much harm coming back up as they did going down. Ipecac syrup is the ideal way to induce vomiting. Follow instructions from the health care professional you talk to for inducing vomiting in other ways.

See Chapter 13 for more information on what to do in emergency situations. Always bring an apparent deliberate overdose to the attention of the victim's primary care doctor; many such cases represent calls for help.

Special Groups

Certain people should exercise extreme care in taking medications because their bodies are likely to process them differently. These include infants and children, seniors, pregnant or nursing women, immunocompromised individuals such as those suffering from HIV infection or AIDS, and people with liver or kidney disease.

MEDICATIONS IN INFANTS AND CHILDREN

When it comes to medications infants and children are not just small adults. They cannot simply be given smaller dosages of a medication, for example. Much more complex calculations must be done that take into account such factors as weight and relative maturation of organs that are critical to metabolizing and excreting medications (that is, the liver and kidneys). The capacity to digest, store, and eliminate medications evolves quickly in the newborn period. Many medications have not been tested or widely used in children, although this situation may be changing due to governmental pressure to initiate such investigations. Sometimes a medication will actually affect a child in a completely different way than it will an adult. Methylphenidate (Ritalin), for example, functions as a stimulant in adults but calms hyperactive children.

Talk to your doctor before giving a child less than 2 years old any over-the-counter medication. Consider carefully whether a child of any age really needs the medication you are considering giving them. Do not give aspirin to a child or teenager under age 18. This is particularly important if she is suffering from a fever of unknown cause, a cough, sore throat, cold, a viral infection, or chickenpox symptoms. Giving aspirin to a child with any of these conditions poses the risk of a rare but potentially fatal disease called Reye's syndrome. Carefully examine the ingredients listed on an over-the-counter medication as some unexpected ones contain aspirin. Look for the presence of alcohol in medications and carefully avoid giving these to small children. Acetaminophen is a good choice for children under age 18 suffering from pain or a fever. Whenever you give your child a medication, check the label twice to confirm the dosage for your child's age. Do not give her more than one over-the-counter medication; many contain identical ingredients that can result in hazardous accumulations.

Select liquid medications for children less than 5 years old whenever possible because they may have difficulty swallowing a pill. Only give chewable tablets to children more than 2 years old who have enough teeth to chew a tablet well. If your child spits out medication that you have just given her, consider it a partial dose and call the doctor or pharmacist for directions. Do not automatically give a second dose to make up for the lost medication.

MEDICATIONS IN THE PERSON OVER AGE 65

As we get older, the way our bodies metabolize and respond to medications changes. There are several reasons for these changes. The capacity of the liver to break down medications and the capacity of the kidneys to excrete them is often compromised, which poses the risk of medications accumulating to dangerous levels and causing adverse reactions. Dosages for seniors must often be lowered for this reason. As the body ages, its ability to maintain constant, even levels of a medication also deteriorates. Certain parts of the body, such as the nervous system and brain, become more sensitive to a medication's actions. Immune system changes may cause unexpected reactions in some cases. The digestive system may also become less efficient, which interferes with the absorption of medications. Medication dosages may ultimately need to be readjusted more frequently to avoid or minimize adverse reactions.

Failure to take a medication correctly or on schedule is another major problem with seniors. Sometimes this problem is attributed to everyday forgetfulness—was a dose already taken?—and other times to senility, drowsiness, or other problems. Seniors also tend to have prescriptions for multiple medications, which increases the risk for adverse reactions among medications as well as errors in taking them all properly. For seniors taking several medications each day, the prospect of coordinating them can be daunting indeed. Work with your doctor to make your dosage schedule as uncomplicated as possible; opt for single daily doses of a medication whenever possible and for taking as many of the medications as possible at a designated time so that you are less likely to forget any one in particular. Your doctor and pharmacist should be able to help you make these consolidations when possible. Your doctor should be encouraged, when necessary, to review the various medications you are taking and confirm that they are all still relevant and necessary.

There are a number of other important measures you can take. Make sure all of your medication containers are clearly labelled with the medication name and directions in oversized, easily legible type. Informational leaflets should come with the medication; keep these together. The pharmacist may be able to dispense medication in easy-to-open containers. Use of weekly pillboxes should help prevent confusion about what medications have already been taken for the day, thus preventing double dosing.

MEDICATIONS IN THE PREGNANT OR NURSING WOMAN

Most women today recognize that pregnancy and nursing are important times to avoid unnecessary medications—including basic over-the-counter medications such as aspirin—given the risks that many medications pose to unborn children or nursing infants. Almost all medication crosses the critical filter between mother and child—the placenta—and enters the fetal bloodstream. The rapidly growing and developing fetus can occasionally be very vulnerable to the effects of a medication the mother takes. Reactions can range from birth defects or mild developmental deformities to slowed growth or death. Sometimes medication affects the pregnant woman adversely or interferes with the normal progression of labor. The potential for harm to the developing fetus has shown to be greatest at exactly the time that many women are not even aware that they are pregnant—the first 3 months of gestation. Medications that pose a risk to the normal development of the fetus are called teratogens. Although investigators have assessed the safety of some medications for use during pregnancy, there is scant evidence for safe use during pregnancy for the majority of medications. Limiting your intake of all medications is wise for this reason. Alcohol, nicotine, caffeine, and recreational drugs should be avoided.

If you become pregnant do not suddenly stop taking prescription medications you regularly take for a chronic or serious condition such as epilepsy; talk over your pregnancy plans with your doctor and together you may be able to find a safe solution for modifying your medication regimen. Similarly, consult your doctor before starting any medication (prescription or over-the-counter) during the time you are trying to conceive. Some medication is considered safe to the mother or fetus during one of the three trimesters of pregnancy but potentially damaging in another.

Most medications can pass to a baby through breast milk as well; the medication finds its way into the milk through the fine blood vessels that surround the breast's milk-producing glands. However, only occasionally does the infant get enough of a medication in breast milk to produce any effect. If you plan to nurse, talk to your doctor about the medications you take.

MEDICATIONS IN THE TEENAGER

When it comes to good medical care, teenagers constitute one of the most neglected age groups. They no longer seem to belong in the pediatrician's office and they are too young to be accepted into an adult practice. Many teenagers remain on medications that were appropriate for them when they were younger—asthma medications are a good example of this—although they may have outgrown the condition or need a different amount of medication now that their bodies are larger and more mature. As with every other age group, a doctor should review the medications an adolescent takes. It is also wise to ask your doctor to review with your adolescent the health risks involved in the use of illegal drugs and alcohol.

MEDICATIONS IN THE PERSON WITH HIV INFECTION

One of the challenges that HIV-infected people face is taking a cocktail of medications on time, several times a day, in some cases with certain foods only. You may have trouble complying with what will likely be a dizzying regimen, and you may struggle with side effects produced by many of the medications. If you still feel well, you may especially resent or resist taking medications.

Standard care for people infected with HIV now involves medications designed to prevent opportunistic infections (infections caused by a virus, bacterium, or other pathogen that is not usually harmful to a person with normal immune function) as well as medications designed to block the virus from replicating. Complying with the regimen may be one of your most challenging tasks—and also one of the most important measures that you can take to ensure con-

tinued health. Missing doses can have serious consequences because the virus can take advantage of even minimal drops in the level of medications designed to prevent it from replicating.

Given the difficulty in discerning which medication should be blamed for a side effect or a negative interaction with another medication, medications should be added one at a time when possible. Scientists continue to search for ways to simplify the HIV medication regimen by looking into strategies for consolidating various medications into single pills.

For more information on HIV and AIDS, and how to take part in a drug trial, see pages 855 and 1370.

MEDICATIONS IN THE PERSON WITH LIVER OR KIDNEY DISEASE

The liver and kidneys are critical to the normal processing of medications. One of the primary responsibilities of the liver is to break down certain medications into forms that the body can then eliminate. When the liver fails to function normally, as in the case of severe cirrhosis, for example, the liver's ability to metabolize medication is impeded and dangerously high levels of certain medications may accumulate, which can cause potentially adverse reactions.

Similarly, people with poor kidney function are at increased risk for side effects. When kidneys fail to function properly and process medications as needed for elimination through the urine, dangerous accumulations in the body can occur. The protein loss caused by some types of kidney disease can also complicate the situation, because a number of medications rely on protein to bind to in the bloodstream. With less protein to bind to, the medication is free to circulate through the body and may cause unwanted side effects or damage.

People with liver or kidney disease should check with a doctor before taking any medication including those that are over-the-counter. The doctor will attempt to avoid prescribing medications that may actually strain or damage these organs further, she may prescribe adjusted doses to avoid unwanted medication accumulations.

For a guide to specific medications, see page 1503.

THIRTY-FOUR

Home Care and Long-Term Care

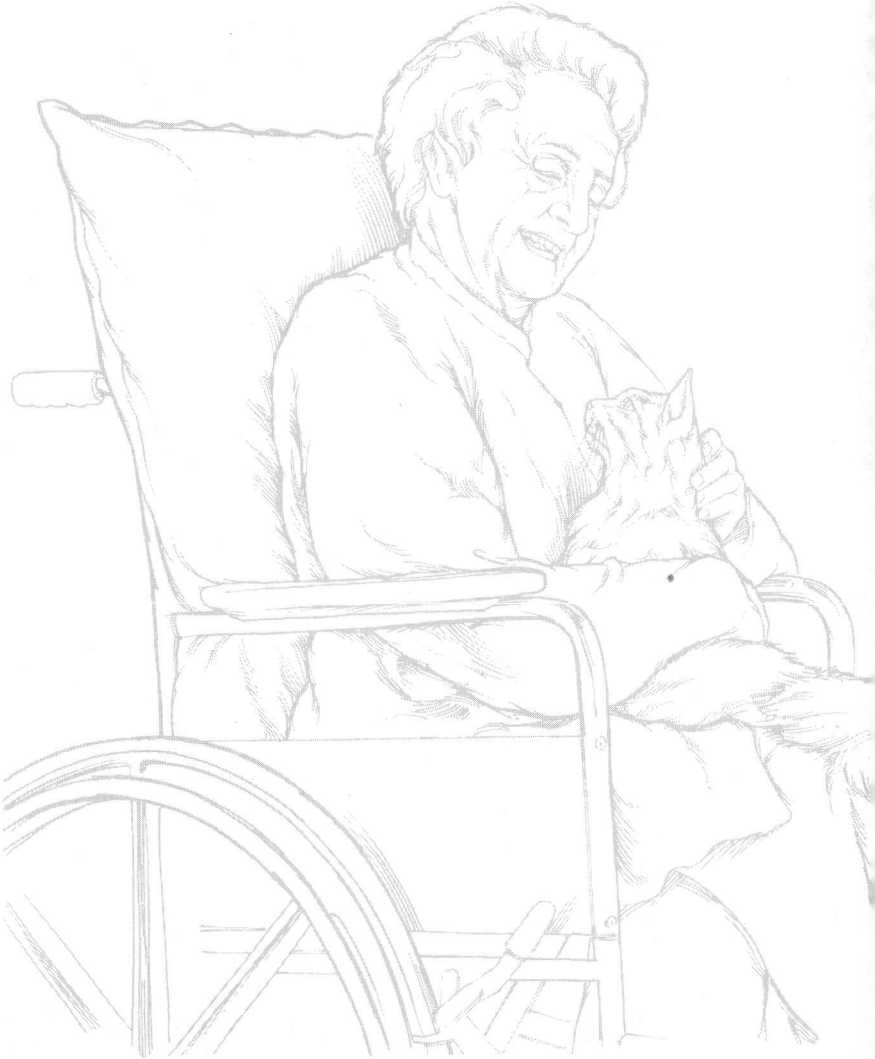

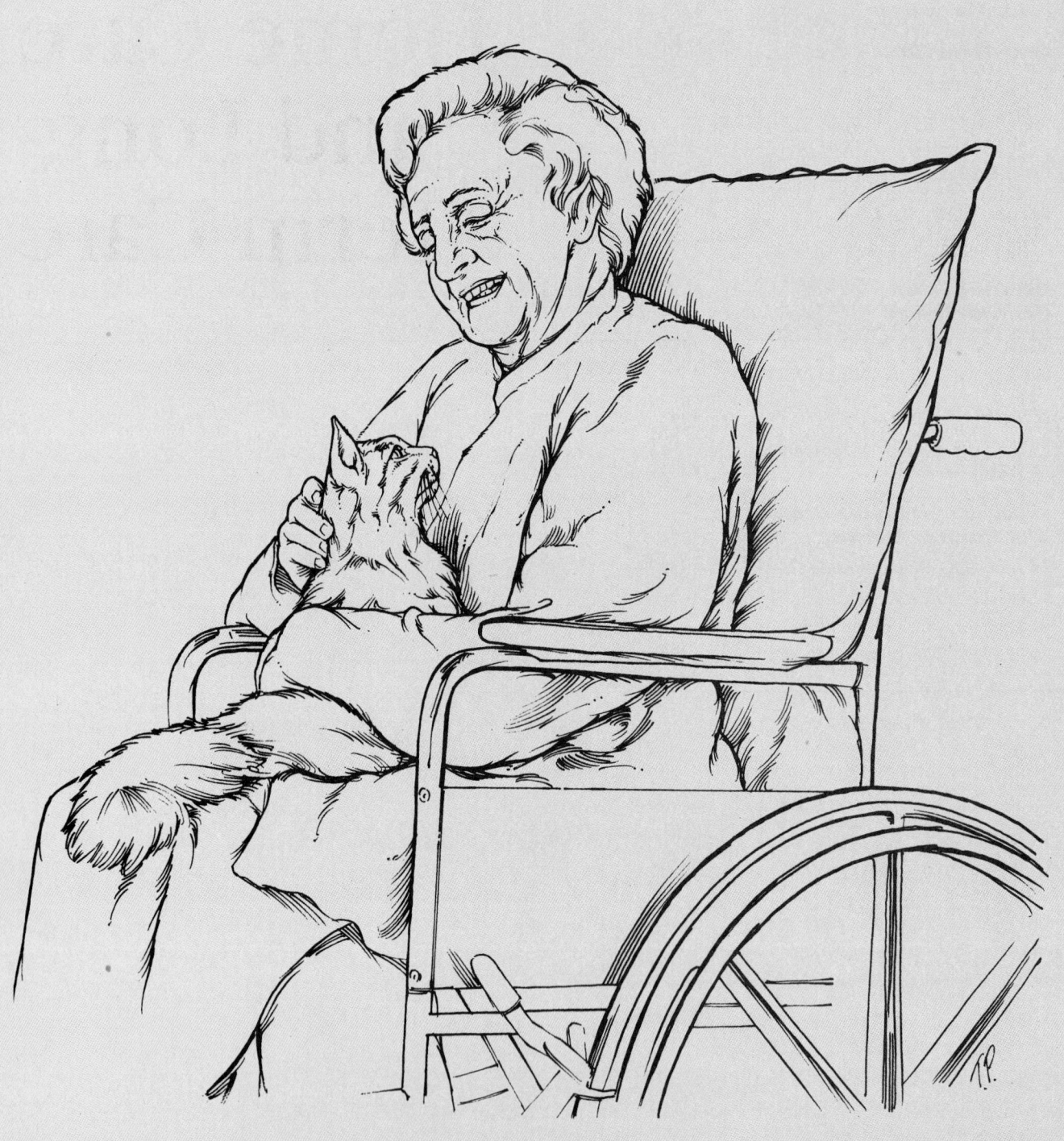

HOME CARE AND LONG-TERM CARE

Given the choice, almost everyone would opt to be cared for at home if they became ill or incapacitated. But for the adage "There's no place like home" to hold true, accommodations must be made so that both the care and the home itself can be kept running smoothly for all involved.

Whether a person is old or young, moderately or severely disabled, terminally ill or on the road to recovery, a variety of services are available to treat him and assist the caregiver. They include nursing care (both full- and part-time), rehabilitative services, custodial care, personal care, and social services. Some or all of these resources are often covered by insurance, depending on the insurance company's assessment of the person's condition and eligibility for coverage. Before embarking on any home care or long-term care plan, be sure to examine your insurance coverage and query your insurance carrier regarding reimbursement; this can be a complex issue (see Insurance and Reimbursement, page 1478).

There are two types of care given at home: acute and long term.

Acute Home Care

Acute home care is a finite period of caring for someone who has just had an operation, a serious disease, an acute exacerbation of a chronic condition, or a trauma of some kind. The person has been discharged from the hospital but is not yet able to take care of himself or has an unstable condition that does not require hospitalization. The type of continuing care needed is delivered by health care professionals and is taught to family members or friends.

Third-party payers (both public, such as Medicaid and Medicare, and private) usually provide coverage for professional home care, although the amount of coverage and the time such coverage is available are often limited. The health care professional not only cares for the person but also teaches family members how to provide specialized care once professional care ceases. If you are responsible for someone's home care, be sure to contact the person's insurance company to clarify exactly what is covered and what isn't; these "allowables" vary greatly, and you must educate yourself about what sort of financial help is available to you.

It is critical that caregivers be given as much support as possible to help them successfully balance the demands placed on them by the person they are caring for, their families, and often their outside jobs. Caregivers should educate themselves about counseling opportunities and various ways to obtain relief. See The Caregiver, below.

The home in which the home care is given may have to be adapted, at least temporarily, to make care easier and to ensure the ill or disabled person's safety (see Setting up a Room for Home Care, page 1477, and Home Safety, page 1477).

Long-Term Home Care

Long-term home care is rendered to people who need supervision and personal care because of some chronic condition or illness such as Alzheimer's disease or Parkinson's disease, a stroke, or other such disability. The care they need may be required for months or years. They may become increasingly disabled, requiring more and more intense and complex supervision and care, in some cases ultimately relying on intravenous (IV) therapy and other devices more characteristic of acute care.

Fully two-thirds of those individuals receiving long-term care are cared for at home either by family or by community services, while only one-third live in an institutional setting, such as a nursing home. Of those living at home, the majority are elderly. Approximately 7 million Americans received some form of long-term care in 1990, and it is estimated that as the population ages, by 2040 as many as eighteen million people will require some form of long-term care.

THE CAREGIVER

Approximately 75 percent of home caregivers are women. Often wives, mothers, daughters, or daughters-in-law forgo employment to attend to the responsibilities of caregiving, though 25 percent of this group also work outside the home.

Caring for someone who is ill is a hard job, and it can take a heavy toll on both caregivers and their families. In all home care situations, the welfare of the primary

MEDICATIONS

Most people who receive acute or long-term care take one or more medications, which often causes problems. Many studies have shown that seniors in particular are likely to take medications improperly. Common problems for people who are taking one or more medications are:

- *Missed doses*—If a person misses a dose, he should not double the next one. If only one dose a day is prescribed, giving it a few hours late usually will not cause problems. In all other cases, the doctor should be consulted.

- *Wrong dose or wrong medication*—If a person takes the wrong dose or medication, the doctor should be notified immediately.

- *Polypharmacy*—This word describes the situation of a person who is taking many medications, often prescribed by more than one doctor. In such instances, medications may interact with each other to cause severe side effects; establishing a reasonable schedule can be a problem, and there is a greater risk of side effects. To prevent polypharmacy, a list of all the person's medications (both prescribed and over-the-counter) should be presented to each of his doctors. Many home care agencies have a pharmacist who can provide consultation.

- *Compliance*—Often, particularly among the elderly, medications either are not taken or are taken in excess because of increasing forgetfulness or addiction. Addiction is most likely to occur when a person is being treated by more than one doctor; if addiction is suspected, all doctors must be contacted and an alternative medication plan should be instituted. Sometimes, compliance wavers because the person becomes incapable of administering the medication properly. In such situations, the caregiver should offer to help the person. If assistance is refused, the caregiver will have to insist and may want to ask the doctor to make it clear to the person that help is necessary. If training in administering the medication is required, one or two visits from a nurse may help. Another reason a person may stop taking a medication may be that it is inconvenient. Diuretics, for example, cause frequent urination, so some people will resist taking them. (Alternatively, some people may restrict their fluid intake, which can also be dangerous.)

Certain types of prescription medications cause particular difficulty for the elderly. When an elderly person is taking one or more of the following types of medications, the doctor should be consulted regarding the types of problems to look for, such as side effects, signs of intolerance, and any other indications that the medication may not be appropriate: analgesics, antidepressants, antihypertensives, dementia treatments, muscle relaxants and antispasmodic agents, nonsteroidal anti-inflammatory drugs, and sedative or sleeping agents.

The best way to prevent medication problems is to keep a detailed daily record of the medications being taken, the time of day they should be taken, and the number of daily doses that are prescribed. The medications should be checked off as they are taken. When a person is being cared for at home, this schedule should be kept by the bedside. Keeping track of medications that have been given should be a part of the daily routine for all caregivers.

Also, since a big problem for people on multiple medications is trying to remember if they took a particular dose, it can be very helpful to use a mediplanner, which is a special container that holds a week's worth of daily doses of all the various medications. The individual or his family can tell by a glance at the mediplanner if the morning medications, for example, were taken.

Some medications are absorbed better on an empty stomach or when taken with food. This adds another level of complexity to the situation.

Medications should be stored in their original containers (except the doses in the mediplanner), kept out of the reach of children, and taken only when the lights are on and what and how much is being taken can be clearly seen. If there are no children in the house, request that the pharmacy dispense the medications in easy-to-open non-childproof containers.

Side effects are a common problem when a person is receiving one or more medications. In fact, the literature accompanying some prescription medications may list up to 50 possible side effects. In managing the side effects of any medication, observing and questioning the person taking them is the best way to monitor and control any problems. Many side effects may be mild and will disappear over time on their own. Mild stomach or gastrointestinal discomfort may be resolved by giving the medication with a meal, or it may resolve itself. Certain medications may cause mental changes. If this occurs, consult the doctor immediately.

For free publications on medications and the elderly, contact the National Institute on Aging at (800) 222–2225. ■

---

caregiver must be considered to be as important as that of the person who is receiving care. Caregivers must be regularly encouraged by other family members to take care of their own needs and other responsibilities.

Caregivers may find it helpful to get counseling on how to manage the burdens of home care; without the necessary support, caregivers may find that they are not able to successfully fulfill their various roles. In such cases, families are often taxed beyond their physical and emotional capacities.

Also, caregivers must be relieved of their healthcare responsibilities periodically. Respite care, in which a substitute paid caregiver comes into the home for a few days or more, can be very helpful. In addition, the person who requires care may perhaps be admitted into a hospital or nursing home for a short stay to provide relief.

Stay alert for signs of alcohol abuse, physical and emotional abuse, neglect, or other such problems, as these may be indications that caregivers are overburdened or unable to cope with their responsibilities and may be placing the person they are caring for in danger.

SETTING UP A ROOM FOR HOME CARE

The room should be located on the ground floor and as close to a bathroom as is feasible to make things as easy as possible for both caregiver and the person receiving care. Still, as many essentials as possible of the person's old life should be maintained. Try to strike a balance between the person's new needs and his identity and sense of independence. For example, use the person's old bed and keep other favorite objects in the room, including photographs of family members.

There are many aids now available to ensure safe and comfortable care in the home, including air mattresses, bed rails, grab bars for the shower and toilet, elevated toilet seats, and room monitors. You may also need to acquire a bedpan, bedside commode, urinal, and special pillows. If the person can use the telephone alone, make sure it's accessible; if he can't handle a regular phone, consider acquiring an adaptive telephone system. Such aids will make your job as caregiver easier and ensure the person's comfort and safety.

Equipment may be rented or purchased through a home medical equipment company or at a surgical supply store. Such stores are usually found near hospitals, or the local drug store staff will be able to tell you where the nearest one is located. If the person you are caring for needs nursing or rehabilitative services, the home care agency you are using will help arrange for the equipment. In addition, there are now a number of mail-order catalogs that sell an astonishing variety of home health care merchandise at reasonable cost.

HOME SAFETY

When a person is receiving care at home, safety precautions should be taken not only in the person's room, but also throughout the areas of the house that are accessible to him. These precautions include functioning smoke detectors, bright lights in the hallways, night lights, nonskid rugs and low-pile carpeting, a rubber bath mat and grab bars for the shower or tub, and railings approaching the house. Whenever possible, glass tabletops, scatter rugs, and highly waxed floors should be avoided. Ramps for easy wheelchair access may be necessary if certain areas of the house are not easily accessible.

If the person feels capable of driving but should not get behind the wheel, car keys should be kept out of reach.

When the person receiving home care is elderly and lives alone or may sometimes be left alone at home, it is advisable to install an emergency alerting system that will automatically dial the police or an ambulance when the device is triggered. Neighbors may serve as an informal warning system for elderly or incapacitated people living alone. Neighbors can check that mail is picked up and that lights are turned off and on and can contact family members if anything seems amiss.

Issues of Daily Life

Caring for a loved one who is not independent enough to care for himself, whether temporarily or permanently, must be incorporated into the structure and routine of the family's life. Life does go on, and other family members, especially children, have needs that must be tended to. The person who needs care must not dominate life at home. Striking this balance is difficult for almost all families coping with home care issues.

Daily tasks will have to be integrated into the family routine. They include the following categories.

Feeding Most people want to eat with the family and feed themselves if at all possible. Utensils geared to accommodate special needs are available. If the person is confined to bed, try to keep him company during meals; an adjustable bedside tray table may be useful. If he does not eat or seems to be losing weight, be sure to inform the doctor.

Bathing For adults, bathing is an intensely personal experience. Caregivers who are

BATHING THE BEDRIDDEN PERSON

To ensure comfort, it is important to gather what you need before the bath so that you never leave the person being bathed damp or exposed while you retrieve necessary equipment. You will need a basin filled with warm water, mild soap, washcloth, dry towels, and a basin of warm water for rinsing. You should wear gloves while bathing the person if there is any chance of contact with their body fluids.

After each area of the body has been washed, it should be dried immediately to avoid chills and discomfort. Areas not being washed should be kept covered. When possible, the face, genitals, and underarms should be washed daily, as should the hands and feet. In some cases, the person may need to be bathed more frequently, for example, if vomiting, diarrhea, incontinence, or a fever occurs. The skin should be carefully inspected for bruises, rash, areas of discoloration, blisters, or open wounds. If noted, these conditions should be treated per the doctor's advice. A medicated soap may be recommended, and cornstarch can be applied very sparingly in skin folds to keep them dry if necessary. If dry skin or pressure ulcers are an issue, a moisturizer may be added to the bathwater and should be applied after the bath. Massage of the skin over bony prominences should be avoided. Perfumed lotions, bath oils, and bubble bath should be avoided. If the person is incontinent, a protective cream or ointment and absorbent pads or briefs that keep moisture away from the skin should be used. ■

family members often have the greatest degree of difficulty dealing with this aspect of personal care. Bathing a parent can be especially awkward, while bathing a spouse or older child is not necessarily as difficult. Bathing a small child can actually be one of the most pleasurable parts of home care. If this routine is difficult for you or the person you are caring for, consider having a home care or personal care aide take on this responsibility. When this is not possible and the person is ambulatory, bathing aids in the bathroom, such as a seat in the shower stall, water-temperature regulating devices, and an intercom in the bathroom can help the person maintain privacy and avoid accidents, including burns, which often occur when an elderly or partially disabled person is unable to regulate the hot and cold water.

Making the bed In all cases, cotton sheets are preferable. If the person cannot get out of bed, the sheets should be changed every day and arranged twice a day to ensure comfort. If the person is immobile, special devices are available to prevent skin irritation and sores from developing.

Toilet needs When a person cannot leave the bed, or the bathroom is located at some distance, a bedpan or urinal may be neces-

sary or a bedside commode might prove convenient, especially at night. The bedpan should be placed under the buttocks, and the person should then be given privacy. Keep comfort in mind—don't offer an ice-cold bedpan, for example. A bedpan should be cleaned directly following use. Once again, if part-time nursing care is possible, the person may prefer to handle this activity with the nurse or aide, and not a family member. Nights and evenings are often when such help is needed.

Vomiting When necessary, the person should have a basin for vomiting within easy reach. Afterwards, the person should be made as comfortable as possible; give him water to clear his mouth and a washcloth to wipe his face. Tea, broth, or other clear liquids should be offered. If vomiting is a new symptom, the doctor should be contacted.

Transportation Families that do not have a car can find transporting an ill or incapacitated person particularly challenging. Some disabled people may require a specially equipped van or bus.

Recreational and emotional needs Be sure the person has physical exercise whenever possible, as well as recreational activities such as games or hobbies, reading material (including talking books), radio, television, and social activities. Phone visits with family and friends may break up the monotony of a long afternoon, and helping with meal preparation or easy household chores when possible can help make the person feel useful and included. Comfort, conversation, and a sense of community should always be part of daily life in the home care situation.

Insurance and Reimbursement

While both acute and long-term home care can be very expensive, long-term care is especially costly whether it is provided at home or in an institutional setting. In most cases, insurance covers part, but not all, of the costs, and often families find their own finances jeopardized in the process. If you or a family member are facing the possibility of long-term care—at home or in an institution—learning everything you can about the ins and outs of insurance coverage will save you time, money, and a good deal of frustration.

MEDICARE AND MEDICAID

Unfortunately, there is quite a bit of confusion about the differences between the Medicare and Medicaid programs. Medicare, which is not based on financial need, is the largest insurance program serving the elderly. Its financing of health care for the elderly is unique: fully 65 percent of the funding for health care for the elderly comes from public sources, as opposed to only 30 percent for those under age 65. Medicare covers medical, but not custodial, needs. People who are eligible for Medicare include those over age 65 and those who are disabled and have been receiving Social Security disability payments for 24 months or more. Enrollment is not automatic for people eligible for Medicare; they must enroll. Those who are covered by Medicare may receive coverage for home care when the following conditions are met:

- A doctor has certified that there is a need for home health services and has set up a treatment plan. The need for treatment must be periodically recertified.

- The person is homebound. This does not mean bedbound; nor does it mean that the person never leaves the home. If the person goes out, it must be infrequently and with considerable effort.

- The care falls into the following categories: intermittent nursing care, physical therapy, and speech therapy. If the person qualifies for one or more of these services, he may also receive occupational therapy, medical social services, and/or personal care.

- The home health services agency is certified by Medicare.

When these conditions are met, Medicare covers "reasonable cost" for these visits as long as the person requires intermittent and skilled services and the condition is improving.

Many elderly Americans assume that Medicare will cover their health expenses, both in and out of the hospital, and are often dismayed and overwhelmed to find out how complicated and limited the coverage is in most cases. Therefore, it is important to understand Medicare's limits and consider other coverage alternatives before a family member turns 65 in order to avoid the loss of a lifetime's savings in covering medical care costs.

Medicare coverage is divided into two types. "Intermediaries" (Part A) will pay for the cost of hospitalization (after the deductible, which was $760.00 in 1997) and covers home care services as well. "Carriers" (Part B) provides standard medical insurance and pays for 80 percent of all approved doctors' fees (after the deductible, which was $100 a year in 1997) as well as outpatient hospital services, diagnostic tests, ambulance transportation, and also medical equipment, such as wheelchairs.

While Medicare may cover a large portion of medical expenses, it will not cover all of them. The following is a list of services *not* covered by Medicare.

- Ongoing institutional nursing home services

- Prolonged home care services when the condition has stabilized

- Prescription medications except for those administered in the hospital and, in special circumstances, in a doctor's office or a nursing facility. Some medications requiring IV administration may be covered.

- Immunizations, except hepatitis and pneumococcal vaccines

- Routine physical, eye, and dental exams

Almost anyone over age 65 can enroll in Medicare. If the necessary amount of Social Security has not been paid, however, a small monthly payment must be made in order to obtain coverage. Publications on Medicare are available free by calling (800) 638-6833 or on the World Wide Web at http://www.medicare.gov/publications.html.

Unlike Medicare, Medicaid is need-based and does pay for custodial care and long-term custodial care. Medicaid was created solely to serve those below the poverty line. Seniors who begin a program of long-term care often are covered by Medicare initially and then, eventually, by

Medicaid. Understanding the Medicaid program may be challenging, as the administration varies from state to state. Therefore what is and what is not provided by Medicaid may differ from state to state. Medicaid is available to all Americans regardless of age. For those over age 65, it is provided under a provision made for the "blind, disabled or aged" if their income, including Social Security benefits, is below a specific level set by the federal government. To qualify for Medicaid, a person cannot have more than a limited amount of cash or other available assets in his possession. If he does, he is required to use those monies to pay for care before the state will pay. Often, people admitted to nursing homes "spend down" their incomes until they are poor enough to be eligible for Medicaid coverage. Anyone considering long-term care should exhaust all other options before depleting a life's savings simply to be eligible for Medicaid coverage.

PRIVATE LONG-TERM CARE COVERAGE

Because long-term care is extremely costly and few insurance carriers cover it for more than a limited amount of time, the interest in long-term care coverage is growing. Over 40 percent of all individuals will spend some time in a nursing home during their lifetime; the average stay is 2.8 years. The current average annual cost of care in a nursing home is $34,500. Nine percent of individuals stay in a nursing home for more than 5 years. The costs of care escalate as the person deteriorates, but the overall average is more than $122,000 per person annually.

The impact of private insurance coverage on nursing home costs is still small, but it is growing. In 1986, fewer than 100,000 people held private long-term insurance policies. In 1990, more than 2 million people held policies, and 5 percent of all people over age 65 now hold some kind of long-term care policy. Many long-term care policies sold by private companies are called Medigap. A person deciding to buy such a policy should buy only one—more than this is generally a waste of money. Most such policies still will not cover private duty nursing care, rest homes, or routine health care not covered by Medicare. Such policies should be carefully considered, with family, friends, and other policy holders consulted before a plan is purchased. The plan should clearly cover aspects of care that are not already covered by existing coverage; for example, medication, nursing services, or additional rehabilitative equipment. All checks should be made payable to the insurance company and not an insurance agent, and records of all payments should be kept easily accessible.

Rehabilitation

Although the elderly comprise the majority of those who receive home care, long-term care and nursing home care, there are many people young and old who suffer acute illnesses, incapacitating accidents, or traumas that require rehabilitation. In addition, 49 million Americans are disabled and require some form of ongoing home care.

Hospital outpatient services offer specialized rehabilitation programs for many acute illnesses and conditions, including stroke, paralysis, and amputation. Many hospitals are also affiliated with rehabilitation centers to which people may be referred. In inpatient, outpatient, or home-based rehabilitation programs, a physical therapist works to reestablish normal physical functioning or help the person learn to cope with the disability by developing other physical skills to compensate.

Most programs also include occupational therapy, which is geared to helping

---

THE ROLE OF THE OCCUPATIONAL THERAPIST

The occupational therapist is an integral part of the home care team. The occupational therapist evaluates the person who is being cared for at home and focuses on deficits in self-care, home management, cognition, and physical functioning. A collaborative treatment plan is developed that includes the goals of the person receiving care and those of the caregiver. The occupational therapy intervention plan includes strategies and skilled techniques that facilitate independent functioning in the home.

Occupational therapists have special skills and training in the area of corrective and preventive splinting, home modification, and durable medical equipment recommendations for the home. The occupational therapist also assists individuals in learning coping strategies and compensatory techniques after an illness or injury. A qualified certified occupational therapy assistant (COTA) may also implement a treatment plan under the guidance and supervision of the registered therapist. ■

the person begin to cope with everyday tasks. Many occupational therapists will visit the home, establish a regimen, and will even help to rearrange household furniture to minimize the number of obstacles that might prevent a return to normal functioning. The occupational therapist will also offer suggestions on managing daily hygiene and on minimizing the complications that may arise.

If a person is newly disabled, job or vocational training will also be made available through the rehabilitation program. Usually these services will also help with job placement.

Speech and language pathologists assist with swallowing problems, speech difficulties, cognitive patterning to improve memory, reasoning, and communicating abilities.

Independent Living Centers and Nursing Homes

When a person needs some assistance but is not incapacitated, an independent living center may allow the individual to maintain a sense of personal independence while still receiving the care that is needed. The autonomy of the living arrangements varies from center to center, but for the most part separate quarters are available for all individuals or couples. The center makes certain services available to all residents, including everything from emergency medical care and treatment of symptoms of existing conditions to meal preparation, though each residence usually has a kitchen so that meals can be prepared at home. Ongoing daily nursing care is not provided by independent living centers, but home health service agencies and other sources can arrange for nursing care to be made available.

The most common type of independent living center is the retirement community, but other options include nonmedical residential institutions, which offer help with personal care, housekeeping, and shopping. Nonmedical residential institutions are sometimes referred to as board-and-care homes. Nursing care can be made available in board-and-care homes.

When individuals can no longer manage independently, it may be necessary to

A NURSING HOME CHECKLIST

There are many questions to ask and concerns to be addressed when selecting a nursing home. This list will help get you started.

- Is the home licensed by the state?

- Is the home certified by Medicaid?

- Is the home clean and odor-free?

- Are there grab bars, railings, and other appropriate safety features?

- Is the room that will be provided adequate?

- Do the residents seem well cared for?

- How much does it cost? What services are provided? What costs are covered by insurance?

- Is the home within reasonable traveling distance for family members?

- What is the food like? What meal choices are provided?

- Are there recreational spaces for residents?

- Are there special areas for people with Alzheimer's disease that allow free movement yet prevent wandering away from the home?

- Are there private spaces for residents?

- Are restraints used? Under what circumstances?

- Can family members visit at any time?

- What is the ratio of nurses to residents? The higher the ratio, the better the care you can expect.

- Does the staff have special training in geriatrics and long-term care?

- Are medical professionals full-time or part-time staff members? If part-time, inquire into how many hours a week they are on the premises. The fewer the hours, the less attention they may provide.

- What happens if funds run out?

- Does the facility have hospice capability?

- Does the hospital or home care social worker recommend this home? ∎

PRESSURE ULCERS

The best way to cope with pressure ulcers, also called bed sores or pressure sores, is to prevent them from happening, although this is not always possible.

Pressure ulcers are a form of skin damage that can range from small, slightly reddened areas to severe, deep wounds. They occur in areas where bony parts of the body press against other body parts, a mattress, or a chair. They most often occur on the tailbone, hips, and heels, but can also form on the elbows, ankles, or shoulders. Pressure ulcers cost more than $5 billion a year in health care expenditures and result in more than 17,000 lawsuits.

Pressure ulcers may be prevented by meticulous skin care, relief of pressure over bony prominences, and good nutrition. Good skin care includes daily inspection (especially over bony prominences) and bathing, keeping the bedding clean, dry, and wrinkle-free, and protecting the skin from urinary or fecal incontinence. When repositioning, it is important to lift the person with a sheet, rather than dragging them in the bed. Relief of pressure is achieved by shifting or turning the person who is bedridden once every hour during the day and every 2 to 3 hours at night. The use of pressure-reducing mattresses that are filled with air, gels, or foam help to reduce the pressure on bony surfaces. Soft foam pillows, foot protectors, and wheelchair cushions may also be helpful. Good nutrition helps to prevent skin breakdown. A balanced diet with adequate protein and calories is very important. Weight loss may indicate the need for a special diet and vitamin supplements.

Proper care of a pressure sore includes frequent repositioning, pressure reduction, good nutrition, and keeping the sore clean and properly bandaged. Cleaning usually involves rinsing or irrigating the ulcer. Loose material may also be gently wiped away with a gauze pad. Use only cleaning solutions recommended by health care professionals. If the ulcer is not kept clean, healing can be slowed, and infection can result. Choosing the right dressing is important to pressure sore care. The choice of dressing is based on the type of material that will best aid healing, how often dressings will need to be changed, and whether the ulcer is infected. The doctor or nurse will consider the location and condition of the pressure ulcer when recommending dressings. ■

SIGNS OF ABUSE OF THE ELDERLY AND INCAPACITATED

The elderly or incapacitated person may be abused in nursing homes or other long-term care facilities or even when being cared for in a home environment. Some neglect and abuse may be deliberate, but in many cases, particularly in the case of home care, it may be unconscious and due mainly to family members' feeling overworked and overwhelmed by the responsibilities of full-time care.

Family members must be responsible for monitoring the long-term care of a loved one and for notifying the doctor if they feel that neglect or abuse is a possibility. Signs of abuse or neglect include the following:

- Bruises, cuts, or burns
- Poor hygiene
- Dehydration
- Untreated or poorly treated bedsores; bedsores that do not heal
- Fractures
- Malnutrition
- Painful constipation or impaction
- Urine burns or excoriation (abrasions)
- Withdrawal, depression

If any of these conditions occur and persist, the doctor should be contacted and measures should be taken to find an alternative long-term care arrangement. ■

place them in a nursing home. Approximately 5 percent of older adults live in nursing homes. However, the numbers increase dramatically with age. Only 1 percent of people aged 65 to 74 live in nursing homes, whereas 6 percent of people aged 75 to 84 and 22 percent of people over age 85 live in nursing homes.

Often the hardest part of choosing a nursing home for a loved one is deciding that a nursing home is necessary in the first place. This process necessitates the admission of a certain loss of independence on the part of the individual and also an acknowledgment of the need for help on the part of the rest of the family.

Choosing the right nursing home or other long-term care facility is a very important decision (see page 1481). While no nursing home or residential center is perfect, some are a great deal better than others. If long-term care has been recommended, the family doctor will probably provide a list of nursing homes to choose from, but further recommendations may be obtained from other health care professionals. It is a good idea to obtain as many suggestions as possible and to compose a list of needed medical services and of other important requirements such as transportation needs, safety features, assistance with shopping and other parts of daily life, recreational facilities, and social activities. The time and consideration invested in making this choice may save a great deal of concern, aggravation, and unhappiness later on.

While Medicare does not pay for nursing home costs per se, the Medicare Catastrophic Coverage Act (MECCA), passed in 1988, does allow Medicare to pay for up to 100 days of nursing home treatment for rehabilitative purposes.

For further information on long-term care alternatives contact Elder Care Locator at (800) 677-1116.

To ensure that the person in a long-term care facility receives safe and appropriate care, family members need to visit on a regular basis. Any signs of abuse or neglect should immediately be reported to the doctor (see page 1482). If the problem is not quickly resolved, the family should consider transferring their relative to another facility.

THIRTY-FIVE

Death and Dying

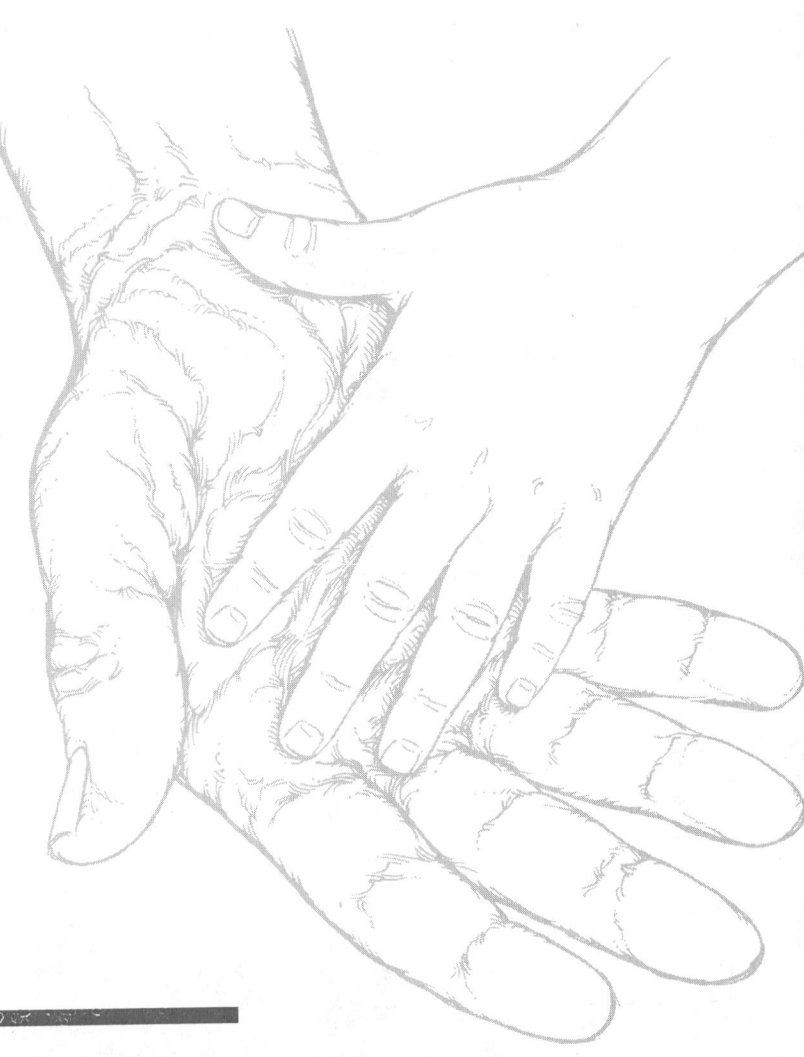

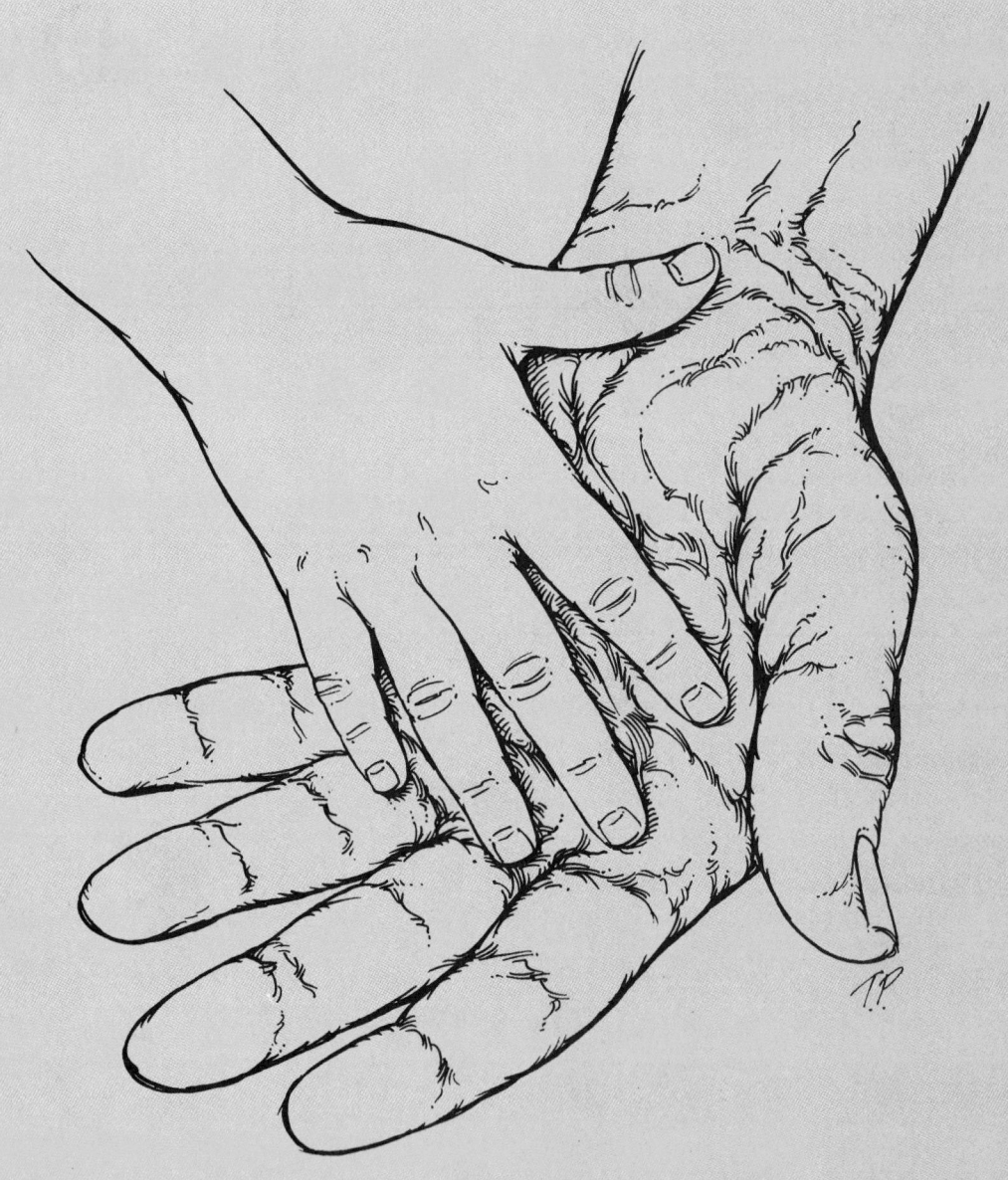

DEATH AND DYING

Coping with Death

The knowledge that death is inevitable does not lessen the tragedy of losing a loved one, though it may help us come to terms with our loss. Most of us have little contact with death in our modern, technological world. Few of us have nursed a dying person and fewer still have experienced a loved one's dying and death at home. This cultural alienation from death makes the dying process all the more difficult for many of us to cope with. In the antiseptic atmosphere of a hospital where a loved one may lie connected to myriad tubes and seem unrecognizable, the meaning of death and dying can elude us. We may agonize over how best to offer love and support and wonder what behavior or conversation is appropriate because we have had little experience dealing with this important passage.

Facing our fears and insecurities is a difficult challenge, but it is essential if we are to help our loved ones face overwhelming fears of their own. Above all, those who are sick and dying fear pain and abandonment. Loved ones can ease the difficult process of dying by trying to relieve these anxieties. Education, understanding, and planning ahead can make a tremendous difference in how friends, family, and the dying person manage this final stage of life.

Offering Comfort to the Dying Person

The period before death, which we call dying, is a stage of life that can be managed with varying degrees of success.

Because of modern medicine's capacity to diagnose terminal illnesses and also to sustain life, the dying process often lasts longer than ever before. For this reason it is all the more important to treat the dying process as one of the stages of life and to continue to treat the dying person as a living person with wishes and desires and a right to control this part of his life.

We tend to view the dying differently, not so much out of prejudice as out of fear. We hide from death and we hide death away. While we have at our disposal the medications and technology to allay pain and unnecessary physical suffering, too frequently we let the dying person suffer emo-

DEALING WITH SUDDEN OR UNEXPECTED DEATH

The unexpected loss a sudden death brings can be overwhelming to the bereaved. Being denied both the chance to say good-bye and the opportunity to show how much they cared can be a crushing burden. In addition the survivors may be faced with new and immediate worries such as arranging for burial and managing the deceased's affairs.

In some situations the griever may have an unrealistic perception of the death's preventability and may experience ongoing feelings of blame and guilt. Shock may also accompany grief, further limiting the griever's capacity to cope. A feeling of apprehension that something terrible may happen at any time may also linger.

When sudden death occurs, there is a greater likelihood that grievers will not completely recover from the loss. For example, widows who did not have the opportunity to experience anticipatory grief are less likely to remarry than those who do. Those mourning a sudden death should be encouraged to accept the reality of the enormous loss gradually. The bereaved should be encouraged to seek therapeutic help to avoid the bereavement complications that often arise when sudden death occurs. The consequences of sudden death on survivors can be long-lasting, and those around them should be alert for signs of depression, which may occur or recur months or years following the death of a loved one. ∎

tionally by leaving him alone with his fears and contemplation of death.

The following is a list of several ways in which you can offer comfort and support to someone who is dying.

Make the dying person as comfortable as possible The dying person will need to have help in establishing the personal control that was once assumed. Things that were once easy to do—bathing, trimming finger and toenails, and going to the bathroom—may become difficult or impossible to do alone. Ensuring that cleanliness, ventilation, and room temperature are maintained can offer simple relief. The family can assist the person in these areas and inform health care professionals when assistance is necessary. Family members can also ensure that pain is managed imme-

THE FIVE STAGES OF GRIEF

According to Elisabeth Kübler-Ross, MD, author of the classic work *On Death and Dying*, the dying person comes to terms with death in five stages: denial and isolation, anger, bargaining, depression, and acceptance. These stages need not be experienced in this order; indeed a dying person may move on and then return to a previous stage of grief during the dying process.

When confronted with the news that they are dying, most people react by saying or thinking "No, not me." Death seems impossible; a mistake must have been made. The person then progresses to feeling anger at this gross injustice. "Why me? How could this be happening? I object," becomes his bitter lament. Eventually the person begins to try to reason with death by bargaining for both more time and less pain, and by bargaining event by event to extend his life. "Please, let me see my child graduate," or "Please let me reach my next wedding anniversary," become common bargaining chips at this imaginary negotiating table. When it becomes clear that the bargaining is not working, the person finally becomes depressed. Life is ending. The realization of this certainty is bleak and can leave the person despondent and sometimes inconsolable. If the person has enough time and has been able to discuss his feelings with family members, a therapist, or clergy member, a certain sense of acceptance can be reached. This acceptance may be more accurately described as facing the inevitable.

Few people are willing to let go of life or to reflect on their own passing with peaceful equanimity, and this should not be expected of the dying person. Rather, how the dying person feels about death should be accepted for what it is—his personal feelings. As family members continue to maintain their relationships with the dying person and to offer him support and understanding, it may become easier for the dying person to accept what is happening to him. ■

diately and as well as possible. The person's thirst should always be quenched, and if he has an appetite, small portions of favorite foods should be provided. Family and friends can and will make a great difference in determining the quality of life for the person who is dying. Perhaps there is no other time in which maintaining quality of life is more important than in this final stage of life.

Continue to communicate with the dying person One of the most common mistakes that even the best-intentioned of us may make is to assume that the dying person does not need or want to be included in the ongoing decision-making process. Even if a dying person is unable to speak he usually can hear what is being said. Family members should continue to speak to the dying person whether or not he appears to understand. Family members should take care to discuss difficult issues involving the person's death out of his earshot. If the dying person can no longer speak, there are many other ways to communicate with him. Holding someone's hand lets them know you are there. Body massage is also a way to soothe and show you care, if you and the dying person are comfortable with this type of physical contact. Often, simply being near the person can be a great comfort to someone who fears being abandoned at the end of life.

Be aware of the dying person's fears The fear of being left alone is almost always

A CHECKLIST FOR EVERY ADULT

Many of us avoid decisions that affect where we die, how we die, and how we are buried in a futile effort to avoid the inevitable. To better serve our own needs and the best interests of our loved ones, it is best to pay attention to these matters before a crisis intervenes and takes the power of choice from us.

The following is a checklist of issues that each and every adult should address while they are healthy. If you or a loved one is ill, these issues must be addressed immediately.

- Maintain a current last will and testament. Notify your lawyer and update your will as life changes occur.

- File a living will. Living wills are available through many organizations including Choice in Dying (see page 1495).

- Designate a durable power of attorney or a health care proxy who can act on your behalf if you are physically or mentally

incapacitated. Make sure your proxy is intimately familiar with the choices you wish to have made and that he has a copy of your living will and any other end-of-life directives. Your doctor can help you obtain these forms.

- Consider whether or not you wish to participate in an organ donation program.

- Decide whether or not you wish to be buried or cremated. If you wish to be buried, choose a cemetery or graveyard for the burial. If you wish to be cremated, decide also in what way you wish your ashes to be disbursed or commemorated.

- Make clear to family members, your clergyperson, or your proxy what type of funeral or memorial service you prefer, and if you are in a position to do so, allocate funds for this service.

- Notify family members or a legal consultant where important documents are located. ■

TALKING ABOUT DYING

Most people who are dying need to be told the truth about their condition. In general, this includes informing the dying person that he is dying. Rather than upsetting the person, the information often gives him the opportunity to prepare for death and to formulate how he will say good-bye to family and friends.

Knowing that he is going to die also gives the dying person the chance to discuss death with those closest to him. At this time it is important for family members to reassure the dying person that he will not be abandoned or left alone at the time of death. The dying person should also be encouraged to share his fears about death and not to feel the need to be stoic in the face of impending death. Many people who are dying feel more comfortable discussing their fears and concerns with someone outside their family, which may enable them to be frank without worrying that they are burdening family members with their own fear and emotional pain. Hospitals usually provide psychiatric social workers and an appropriate clergyperson who is available to talk with the dying person. The dying person's own clergyperson may also become his confidante.

Some people who are sick may request family members not to tell them if they are dying. You may choose to respect their wishes, but you should not blame yourself if they discover the truth. In all cases open awareness is preferable to secretiveness and offers the dying person opportunities to gain strength from those around him and to make his peace with the help of others.

Family members and the attending doctor can discuss how best to inform the person who is dying. When the person is given the news, he will invariably suffer an acute crisis. This stage usually involves a period in which the recognition of nonexistence becomes clear, after which extreme anxiety occurs. The person should not be left alone during this time. Of all the periods in the dying process, the time of diagnosis is considered to be the hardest for both the dying person and his family. Denial, confusion, shock, and anxiety all characterize the moment and period directly following the diagnosis, and all of those reactions inhibit the task of assimilating the knowledge of one's own dying. Family members close to the dying person need to understand that the intensity of this reaction is normal and that they should support the dying person through this time rather than to react to his responses. As the initial moment passes family members may begin to focus on reducing the person's anxiety by turning to practical issues while continuing to offer their consistent emotional support. ■

present for the dying person, and assuaging this fear is one of the greatest services family members can provide. If one family member must leave the bedside, it is important to let the dying person know that another family member will take their place.

Prepare for signs of approaching death

While we often feel helpless when faced with a loved one's impending death, our mere presence can make the difference between a person's terror of death and his calm acceptance. You should be aware that often a person who is facing immediate death is more agitated than usual. At this time the dying person is still able to hear those around him though he may be unable to respond. Thus, your soothing words are never wasted, and the comfort of touch continues to be important.

Being there when your loved one dies

The presence of family members at the moment of death brings comfort to the dying person. Often death occurs in the intensive care unit or in a hospital room. These are difficult settings for such an emotional moment, but what is most important is that the dying person is not alone and that loved ones are present at the time of death. Often the dying person will struggle against giving up life, and it is appropriate for close family members to tell the dying person that it is okay to let go.

What to do if your loved one dies alone

Some people may take months to die, and as much as family members may strive to be there 24 hours a day, this may be impossible. In such circumstances there is always the chance that the person may die alone, and family members need to accept this possibility. Family members should try not to feel guilty when this happens. It may even be inevitable, and many hospice nurses report that the dying person often refuses to die until family members leave the room because he is holding on to life for the loved ones' sake. Family members should find consolation in the fact that they provided care and comfort during this period and that they expressed their love and said their good-byes before the actual moment of death.

WHEN A CHILD DIES

The death of any loved one calls into question the meaning of life and how fleeting it can be, but the death of a child is particularly difficult to accept. Children are not supposed to die and yet they do, and we must find ways to cope.

In recent years tremendous strides have been made in how we care for and communicate with the dying child. Only 20 years ago the ego of the young child was considered too fragile to process information regarding his illness and impending death. But current research and literature show that children's passivity or silence regarding their own illness is often cued by adult behavior. When children are encouraged to communicate regarding their illness they do, and when they are given clear, straightforward information, they are comforted. All findings show that the family that deals openly with the anxieties surrounding a child's illness and suffering copes with the illness more successfully. Open communication also helps the family through the grieving process after the child's death. More and more doctors, psychotherapists, and medical professionals who treat and work with terminally ill children have begun to accept that the cues should come from the children rather than the adults. Research has also shown that it is important to make the child part of the treatment team. The more involved the child is, the greater his sense of control.

In general, information about death should be offered in an age-appropriate manner. The medical professionals caring for the child can advise parents on what level of information is appropriate for the child's age. Infants are solely aware of the physical distress of dying and, therefore, offering maximum comfort and relief should be the major goal of treatment. Toddlers will respond according the reactions of those around them and should be offered reassurance. Because hospitalization will involve feelings of separation, a continual parental presence or parental substitute can offer a sense of security and constancy.

The very young school-aged child has begun to experience punishment and reward. The child may believe that an unpleasant experience, such as hospitalization, is a consequence for some wrongdoing. As the child's illness progresses and the bodily functions that have provided him with a sense of mastery begin to deteriorate, he may begin to blame his parents for what is happening to him. These reactions should be accepted as natural and even nec-

essary. The school-aged child is able to understand what is happening, and parents should be truthful with the child while avoiding unnecessarily lengthy explanations. Parents should offer concrete details about the illness along with reassurances that while what the child is experiencing is painful it is not a punishment for anything he has done. Above all, parents should be willing to listen.

When an adolescent is dying, accurate communication about the prognosis and expectations of quality of life is essential to maintain the mutual trust and respect the adolescent demands. The adolescent should be allowed to maintain as much control over his life as possible. Parents can help by respecting the need for privacy and reinforcing the adolescent's individuality by accepting his choice of friends and activities. Parents should also encourage the expression of angry feelings, and they also should offer comfort and reassurance. The dying adolescent's needs and fears are much like those of the dying adult's. Above all he fears being alone and in pain, and although newfound autonomy needs to be respected, love and comfort should always be offered, particularly by the parents.

The following information is important to share with the dying child when he is ready.

- Death is a part of life.

- When you want to talk, we will always want to listen.

- If you do not know what to say, we understand. Adults do not always know what to say either. Sometimes, we can communicate without words just by being together or holding hands.

- To cry and feel sad is okay and appropriate.

- To be angry about the situation is natural.

- You will not be alone when you die. We (your parents) will be with you then and always. The child needs the assurance of parental presence even after death, and it is important that he be given that assurance, even if you simply tell him "We will always love you."

- Your life has been important. You have made a difference in the lives of your friends and family, at school and at home. You will always matter. To have made the most of one's life, whatever the duration, is a universal human concern. Children, as well as adults, need the assurance that they have lived life as best they could and to the fullest.

- You will always be with us in some way. How this information will be conveyed depends on the religious beliefs of the family. This assurance may take the form of the parents' reassurance that the child will always be part of their lives in terms of memories and contributions to the family or it may be conveyed by assuring the child that he will live on in body and soul for eternity. However this is conveyed, it is important that the child know he will be remembered and included.

When a child is very close to death it is also important to assure the child that death will not hurt. The dying process may be painful, even when the doctors are doing all they can to eliminate the pain, but the child should know that his pain will cease. Children, just as adults, fear abandonment and pain when they are dying as much as they fear death. They should be assured at all times that they will not be alone, that they will always be a part of their parents' lives and the life of the family, and that the pain they are suffering will never return.

TELLING CHILDREN ABOUT THE DEATH OF A LOVED ONE

Even if children are not informed that someone they love is dying, they will understand something is wrong simply because of the way the adults in the house are behaving. There are more phone calls. The adults they trust whisper and become upset, though they may insist nothing is wrong. Because children will inevitably understand that they are not being told important information, they may begin to imagine the worst. For this reason, it is advisable to inform them about what is going on without giving them more information than they can process. Keep the facts simple and listen to their questions. Too much explanation is difficult for younger children and will begin to confuse and frighten them unnecessarily. The child should always be assured that the

dying friend or relative will be made comfortable, that he will not be left alone, that he will have what he needs, and that he will not be left to suffer.

The grieving process varies greatly depending on the age, maturity, and support system of the child. If the mother of a newborn or very young infant dies, the infant may cry and become distressed because his basic needs, such as nursing and being held, are not being met. Surrogate mothering may ease the infant's suffering. Infants from 4 months to $2\frac{1}{2}$ years may express ongoing, nonspecific distress when the mother dies. These are the earliest manifestations of grief.

When another family member dies, the infant will react according to the mother's reactions. Children from the age of $2\frac{1}{2}$ years on experience similar grief responses to those of adults, though they may be unable to verbalize their feelings and memories of the deceased. Children between the ages of 2 and 5 may have grief responses that are variable and intermittent. A lack of any noticeable reaction does not mean the child is not grieving.

If a parent dies, a young child will worry about the survival of the other parent. A child experiences the loss of a parent as abandonment or desertion, so it is important to reassure a child that the deceased parent loved them. Avoid using euphemisms when referring to death, and always speak truthfully. The child may react to grief by clinging, misbehaving, or withdrawing. Offer comfort and support and be open to questions about death and loss.

Between the ages of 5 and 8, a child will have a clearer understanding of death but will not know how to cope with his feelings of grief. Children in this age group often behave as if nothing has happened to protect themselves from their feelings. Talking to a favorite teacher or a counselor may help the child express grief. The child should also be reassured that nothing he did or thought caused the parent's death.

Children between the ages of about 8 to 12 may be shocked by death or may react by being anxious and distressed or by denying the death occurred. Children in this age group are still unable to accept the finality of death and loss; they may yearn for the dead parent and at the same time they may repress this yearning because they consider it childish. A child may also feel anger and express it through difficult behavior. Difficult behavior should not be punished but instead should be seen as a plea for help. Children need to share their complex and often conflicting feelings and should be encouraged to do so.

Adolescents often feel helpless and frightened when they experience the death of a parent and may retreat back into childhood in search of protection from the consequences of death and loss. Such feelings may result in ongoing depression. Adolescents are threatened by mortality and also are fearful of losing control of their intense emotions. The adolescent may respond to grief by acting out, for example, performing poorly in school or engaging in indiscriminate sexual activity. Adolescents may also be conflicted about expressing their feelings because they feel alienated from the adults around them. An adolescent should be encouraged to share feelings with friends, teachers, a favorite coach, or a mentor.

Children also need to share their own grief and have their grief acknowledged. They need to talk about death, to share their ideas about death, and to be reassured that the death of a loved one does not mean that other family members will soon die as well. Teaching children about the ritual and ceremony surrounding death is also important, although younger children and some older children may not feel comfortable attending funeral services or participating in extended periods of mourning. As much as possible, children should be allowed to decide how they wish to mourn the loved one and commemorate the death. Writing a poem, drawing a picture, or visiting a grave site with flowers can often be more helpful to a grieving child than attending a funeral service.

By not informing your children about illness, dying, and death you are potentially leaving these very important aspects of living to become part of your child's fertile imagination, where they may become terrifying and distorted if they are left unexplained. When we do not share information about death or inform children of the death of a loved one, we begin to teach them that the best way to cope with pain and suffering is to ignore or avoid it, which does not prepare a child to manage the inevitable challenges of life. Pain and loss are unavoidable, and learning how to face them openly and constructively can be an important aspect in the growth and development of a child.

DYING AT HOME

Years ago people died at home as a matter of course unless an accidental death occurred far from home. Now if a person is terminally ill to die at home is the exception, not the rule, and may even be considered something of a privilege. In certain cases, such as those of acute infection, dying at home may be impossible. But in other cases the option of dying at home is one that may be considered by the terminally ill person, the family, and the doctor.

More and more people who are able to are choosing to die at home in an effort to ensure a compassionate death in a warm and familiar place. The support of the family is the pivotal factor in making such a death possible. Caring for the very ill at home, however, can be arduous and stressful and should not be undertaken without first considering the physical, emotional, and financial tolls that are always involved.

Even when a family decides that death at home is the right choice for them, family members will have to be prepared for the possibility that despite all of their efforts, death at home may still not be feasible. A person may be well cared for at home for weeks or months only to have a medical complication force him return to the hospital. In caring for the dying in general, it is always important to remember that despite the best preparations and the best intentions death, just like life, often takes its own course.

After a death at home, a death certificate will have to be obtained, usually from the attending doctor, and in most cases the funeral director is notified and the body will be taken to the funeral home.

HOSPICE CARE

If home care is not feasible and the hospital seems like an impersonal place to die, hospice care is an option that is being chosen by more and more people and their families.

The hospice movement has gained popularity at the same time that modern technology has made it possible to prolong life.

Hospice care addresses the needs of the dying person and his family by helping families make the important and difficult decisions necessary to ease the passage into death. This all-inclusive approach is aimed at relieving the two greatest fears associated with dying beside the fear of death itself: the fear of isolation and the fear of pain.

Hospice care emphasizes control of pain and management of other symptoms. Usually the dying person chooses to remain at home as long as possible, and many people choose to die at home, if possible. Much of the home care is managed by the family, with assistance from the hospice team when necessary. If a person needs to be admitted to the hospice facility the same team will oversee treatment. The support team consists of a doctor, nurses, home health care aides, counselors, and other team members, such as physical therapists or nutritionists, when necessary. Bereavement counseling and group therapy are also among the services offered, but these options are rarely covered by insurance carriers.

A person is accepted into a hospice program at his own request, along with a referral from the doctor. A stipulation of hospice care is that the person's prognosis be no more than 6 months of life. This can be a problem for those people who are terminal but whose illnesses are highly unpredictable, though hospices try to be as flexible as possible to meet people's needs. To find a hospice program in your area, contact the National Hospice Organization, 1901 N. Ft. Myer Dr., Arlington, VA 22209.

Ensuring a Death with Dignity in a Technological World

The best way for any person to ensure that his wishes are followed at the end of life is to communicate his wishes clearly and in detail, both verbally and in writing, with their closest family members, their doctor, their lawyer, or their clergyperson.

Approximately 2 million Americans die every year. Of this number, 80 percent die in hospitals, nursing homes, or hospices. Two out of every three of these deaths are caused by a chronic illness such as cancer, acquired immunodeficiency syndrome (AIDS), heart disease, and advanced diabetes. These are conditions that often involve extensive end-of-life care. Of those who die yearly in the United States, it is now estimated that about 70 percent decide to refuse life-sustaining treatment at the end of life. In 1990 the US Supreme Court recognized that the refusal of unwanted medical care is an issue of personal liberty and is therefore constitutionally protected.

We now have the capacity to maintain the body even after the mind that animates life has ceased to exist, and it is estimated that each year 5,000 people are kept alive in a permanent vegetative state. The prolongation of dying or the maintenance of a person in a vegetative state when there is no true chance of recovery is a dilemma that the medical community and society have only now begun to address fully.

The person who enters the hospital with pneumonia may find himself in an intensive care unit being faced with immediate intubation before discussion of such matters is even possible. Family members are often pressured to make decisions that they may have to live with for the rest of their lives. At such times confusion often prevails and there is sometimes a blurring of the lines that separate a doctor's responsibility to treat from the patient's right to make choices in his own best interest. The doctor's creed, "First do no harm," becomes obscured by the dominance of technology. It is therefore the obligation of every person to consider in advance the choices that may have to be made regarding end-of-life care and empower a spokesperson or surrogate to speak for him should the person be unable to do so.

Death with dignity is the term used to describe a compassionate or appropriate death in which the person who is dying does not suffer needlessly or in solitude and has his wishes regarding care respected. Life-support technology is utilized only when there is some chance of partial recovery and not simply to sustain bodily functions after natural respiration has ceased and is irreversible or after the person has been declared brain dead.

Continued communication between the dying person and his family and doctor regarding his wishes while he is still conscious is essential. If you or your family have questions regarding what issues to expect and what decisions might need to be made, ask your doctor. A simple question such as

MAKING YOUR LIVING WILL WORK

Almost all 50 states have enacted laws that respect living wills, but these laws vary widely from state to state. A living will that is valid in your state may not be valid in another state. Most states that do not authorize living wills per se allow similar rights through other legal channels. It is in your best interest to familiarize yourself with the laws in your state to ensure that your living will is respected.

At best, a living will is the commencement of a dialogue between you and those who are important to you regarding your wishes for medical care should you become terminally ill. At worst, the living will is a document that is signed and filed away and disregarded when the time comes for it to be of use. One way to make your living will an active declaration of your wishes is to give copies of the document to family members and to your doctor and other health care providers. Take the time to discuss your choices and decisions for care with your doctor and those closest to you. A living will is most effective when it is a catalyst for discussion rather than only a contract.

When you are discussing your living will with your doctor you may also want to discuss organ donation and whether or not you want to donate your body to science (see page 1498). It is essential to review your living will periodically with your primary doctor, and to discuss your living will and choices for the end of life with your new doctor should you change doctors or see more than one, such as a specialist. Your doctor may have to advocate on your behalf in medical situations when you may be unable to make your wishes known, so it is imperative that you make your choices clear. In many instances the hospital or nursing home staff may have trouble accepting a directive of "comfort measures only," and your doctor's support will help ensure that your wishes are respected.

Living wills apply only to terminal illness. They may or may not apply when dealing with a person who has had a severe stroke or who is in a form of coma referred to as a persistent vegetative state. To ensure that your wishes are respected in all medical situations, you should also designate a durable power of attorney for health care decisions. Having a person who can speak on your behalf affords you greater control over situations that may arise at the end of life (see page 1589).

When you are appointing a surrogate to make these decisions for you it is important to have a thorough conference with that person in which you specify all of your medical choices and desires regarding treatment for terminal illness and the dying process. If you address medical situations now that may arise in the future, you are not only ensuring that your wishes will be respected, but you are also ensuring that your surrogate is more secure in doing what is a very difficult and stressful job.

You can obtain a state-specific living will from Choice in Dying, a national not-for-profit organization that pioneered the living will over 25 years ago. Forms for appointing a health care proxy are also available from Choice in Dying, 1035 30th St. NW, Washington, DC 20007; phone (202) 338-9790; fax (202) 338-0242. You may also obtain a living will by dialing (800)-989-WILL. ■

"How will treatment decisions be made if I am too ill to let you know my thoughts?" will help you get the information you need to make informed choices. It is a good idea to be as specific as possible regarding choices at the end of life. Using general terms such as "heroic" or "extraordinary" measures is far less instructive, for example, than specifying that you do or do not wish to be given antibiotics for pneumonia should pneumonia arise during chemotherapy for cancer. A do not resuscitate (DNR) order, for example, is a request that is exact and can be followed to the letter, unlike a general directive to avoid heroic measures (see below).

The issues of treatment at the end of life may involve highly technical procedures, such as mechanical ventilation, which may be considered a heroic measure, or "ordinary" care, which may include the use of intravenous fluids, but at the end of life these distinctions blur. If your goal is to avoid unnecessary suffering and make possible a death that is in accord with your dying wishes, planning ahead for your compassionate death is the best insurance that it will come to pass.

UNDERSTANDING DNR ORDERS AND OTHER END-OF-LIFE CARE REQUESTS

DNR refers to the request that cardiopulmonary resuscitation (CPR) not be used on a person when his heart action or breathing ceases. CPR is an aggressive treatment that includes the insertion of many tubes, the vigorous massage of the chest, and the repeated administration of electrical shocks to the heart. Hospitals routinely perform CPR on all heart attack and heart failure cases unless a DNR order has been written, even though CPR is not successful in a majority of cases. CPR can be an effective treatment in the event of sudden illness, but it is generally not effective for people whose death is expected, and the outcome is particularly poor for older people. Less than 10 percent of those over age 70 who have CPR leave the hospital alive. When requesting that a DNR order be written, you should be sure to discuss with your doctor why CPR may not be indicated in your case.

A DNR order must be written and signed by a doctor to be valid. Some states now recognize nonhospital DNR orders, which apply when emergency medical technicians respond to a 911 call. Emergency medical technicians are legally required to perform CPR in all circumstances. If you are planning for a death at home, you may want to discuss a nonhospital DNR order with your doctor as well.

When you are requesting that a DNR order be written, you may also want to discuss your overall treatment plan to decide what supportive care and treatment you would accept once your DNR order becomes effective. Whether or not artificial feeding methods should be used at the end of life is a decision that is best made by individuals and their families via a living will or proxy agreement prior to the time that the person becomes terminally ill. Hospitals readily insert feeding tubes, and family members may find it difficult to order their removal without feeling that they are making a decision to kill the person. Family members may also worry that they are causing their loved one additional suffering if the tubes are removed.

Clearly, tube feeding is advisable if it helps to provide the time needed to treat successfully the underlying condition or if the person requests such feedings. But if invasive life support measures merely prolong the dying process they can do more harm than good. Few people realize that the dying usually do not suffer hunger or thirst, and a feeding tube may cause rather than relieve suffering by reviving a sense of hunger in the dying person. The refusal of food and drink is a natural part of the dying process, and in fact artificial nutrition and hydration are not forms of comfort care for the dying.

In all cases of end-of-life orders your wishes are best served by appointing a health care proxy or by designating a durable power of attorney for your health care needs. If someone has been appointed to act on your behalf should you lose consciousness or be unable for any reason to make your own wishes known, it is best to

ASSISTED SUICIDE

Assisted suicide is defined as providing someone with the means to commit suicide with the understanding that he is going to use the means provided to take his own life.

Doctor-assisted suicide refers to a situation in which a medical doctor knowingly provides medication that will cause death to a person who wishes to die. The legalization of assisted suicide is an issue of ongoing debate in the United States. Polls show that the number of Americans who support the legalization of assisted suicide for those who are ill with incurable, painful, or terminal diseases is increasing steadily. At present, over 60 percent of Americans support doctor-assisted suicide legislation. The debate over the issue focuses primarily on whether or not the "right to die" will indeed begin to be perceived as a "duty to die," particularly among seniors, and on whether doctor-assisted suicide is compatible with the life-saving role that is the doctor's first responsibility.

Despite increasing popular support, assisted suicide is still an explicitly criminal act in 33 states. The District of Columbia and 10 other states criminalize assisted suicide through the common law of the state. Recently, Oregon passed a law permitting doctor-assisted suicide in limited circumstances. That law was struck down in a higher court and later upheld, which made Oregon the first jurisdiction in the world to pass legislation legalizing assisted suicide. Recently, New York State declared it illegal to criminalize assisted suicide. The US Supreme Court is expected to rule on the matter soon, but legislative and social debate should continue in the years ahead. ■

have someone in charge who is intimately familiar with the choices you would want to make at such a time (see page 1589). Using an advance directive, with specific instructions provided by you to your proxy, protects you better than all the best intentions.

Further information on DNR orders is available from Choice in Dying, 1035 30th St. NW, Washington, DC 20007; phone (202) 338-9790; fax (202) 338-0242.

The Aftermath of Dying: Survivor's Grief

Just as death is inevitable, grief is a universal experience in life, a necessary and natural aftermath of loss. Grief is the actual psychological, social, and somatic reaction that we experience when we undergo tremendous loss.

In trying to offer comfort to the bereaved, friends too often feel they must avoid mentioning the deceased for fear of upsetting those in mourning. On the contrary, remembrances of the deceased brings comfort to those who miss him most.

SURVIVOR'S DEPRESSION

It is common for a grieving person to feel a sense of guilt that he is still alive when a loved one is dead, but there are certain cases where guilt occurs more frequently and can lead to depression. This type of depression frequently occurs in accidental death cases where the trauma is shared and the survivors often suffer from what is termed survival guilt. This reaction is also common when a child dies and his parents or other family members experience guilt for having violated the natural expectation that children should outlive their parents and other elders.

Parents who must endure the death of a child are most prone to feelings of guilt. No parents wish to survive their own child. For many parents such a reversal of the natural order of things is unimaginable and, when it happens, almost unendurable. The guilt that parents of a deceased child feel is multifold. Their survivor guilt may have a moral component to it, as the parents may see the child's death as a form of terrible retribution for a past moral transgression of their own. The parents may also feel responsible for not having lived up to their parental role in a general sense and in particular, regarding the child's illness and death. If the child's death was accidental the parents may also feel responsible for the death by having permitted the child to go swimming or by having purchased the bicycle the child was riding, for example. A range of guilt and self-recrimination often overwhelms the parent who is already having a difficult time coming to terms with a child's death. Many parents require assistance with the grieving process and should understand that counseling or other therapeutic assistance is healthy and natural and can help them to better process their feelings of grief and guilt. Parents should be encouraged to seek help for their own sakes, for the sake of the other children in the family, and for the sake of their marriage. ∎

Everyone experiences grief when they experience loss, though grief, like pain, is a subjective experience, varying from person to person. However, the same five stages that are applied to the ways a person copes with imminent death are also used to map the grieving process (see page 1488). Denial or isolation refers to the period of shock that directly follows death and serves to protect us from the overwhelming significance of the loss for a time. Anger follows, as does a bargaining process, either with God or with oneself, to avoid the grieving process: "If I do this, the loss will hurt less." Eventually, the actuality of the loss begins to sink in and depression occurs before the final acceptance of the loss.

Often, religious, cultural, or spiritual rituals, such as the funeral, offer emotional and social support to those who are grieving. The temporary idealization of the deceased may be a facet of the grieving process. A successful grieving or mourning process, in which the survivor is able to remember the loved one both comfortably and realistically, may take a year or more.

Common responses to grief include the following:

- Crying
- Inability to sleep
- Physical exhaustion
- Shortness of breath
- Tendency to sigh
- Lack of energy
- Lack of strength
- Anxiety
- Weight loss or weight gain
- Gastrointestinal disturbances
- Lack of sexual desire or hypersexuality
- Feelings of emptiness

Sometimes there are problems encountered in the grieving process that lead to unresolved grief. The most common of these is absent grief reaction, in which the grieving process appears to be totally absent, either because the grieving person has totally denied the loss or remains in a

SUPPORT GROUPS

Support groups for widows, widowers, and others who have lost a loved one exist throughout the country and on the Internet. To find a bereavement group in your area consult your clergyperson, doctor, or hospital social service worker. There are many widow/widower support groups such as Widow-to-Widow, Parents without Partners, and They Help Each Other Spiritually (THEOS), which have local chapters in most areas. Most churches and synagogues also offer such support groups, as do many social service organizations. The Candlelighters Foundation is a national organization that offers support to parents who have lost children. Hospitals also offer support groups for parents whose children are terminally ill.

There are also several sites on the Internet that offer support for mourners.

Grief, Death, and Dying GriefNet (at http://www.rivendell.org) is an online resource for information on grief and bereavement, including resource listings, topical articles, and more.

Emotional Support and Grief Discussion Growth House Inc. (at http://www.growthhouse.org) points to Internet resources concerning hospice and home care, grief, pain management, and bereavement. Growth House also has a chat room for grief discussion. ∎

perpetual state of shock. In our society we tend to admire those who are serene in the face of difficulty. Such respect may impede a person suffering from absent grief reaction from getting help.

There are other common forms of unresolved grief. Inhibited grief occurs when the grieving person may be able to mourn only some of the aspects of the deceased, such as the positive ones, without incorporating the negative ones into the grieving process. Delayed grief occurs when a mourner feels unable to grieve because of the burden of pressing obligations and responsibilities at the time of the death. In cases of delayed grief a relatively minor incident that may occur as long as a year or more later, such as watching a sad movie or losing a wallet, may trigger the latent grieving response. Conflicted grief is similar to inhibited grief. If a person is experiencing conflicted grief the grieving process is suppressed either because of extreme anger at the deceased or extreme guilt about the deceased. A mourner suffering chronic grief continues to express the kind of intense grief appropriate when a loved one is newly deceased long after the loss has occurred. The grieving process fails to reach a natural conclusion, and the loss is perceived as always new. Such a reaction often occurs when a relationship has been particularly dependent. It is as if the mourner is trying to keep the loved one alive with their grief.

A person who is experiencing grief may also withdraw socially, which may make the grieving process longer and more difficult since isolating oneself offers little opportunity for the creation of new relationships or relief from the stress of the grieving process. When a person is having trouble resolving their grief, they should consider seeking help. Otherwise, their unresolved grief may begin to manifest itself in physical complaints or in depression, which may strike months or even years following the death. Grief is natural and to grieve well and fully is a healthy response to loss.

The Bureaucracy of Death

Death is often made more difficult for the grieving family because of all the business that must be handled just as the grieving process commences. The life insurance company must be notified if the deceased had such a policy, medical insurance issues must be dealt with, bank accounts must be closed, and business associates and personal friends must be notified. All of this takes time and may seem overwhelming at first, so it is best if tasks can be delegated among family members and close friends.

If your loved one dies in a hospital the practical necessities of death begin when the heart stops and the doctor requests that all machines be disconnected. At this time the clothing and possessions of the deceased will be returned to the family if the family wishes to have them.

The first order of business is to obtain a medical death certificate. Such a certificate formally registers the death and must also state the cause of death. If the cause of death is potentially a homicide or a suicide or if the death is accidental or otherwise unexplained, an autopsy may have to be performed before such a certificate may be granted. Usually the doctor who was in attendance at the time of death completes the death certificate. If an autopsy is necessary the coroner or medical examiner will sign the certificate in most cases.

Once the death certificate has been obtained the business issues regarding death are basically twofold: to prepare for and manage the funeral service or memorial service and burial (see page 1499) and to arrange for the reading of the deceased's last will and testament and the appropriate management of his personal business matters and personal effects.

As soon after the death as possible a funeral director should be appointed (see page 1499). Once the family has chosen a funeral director and funeral home with which they are comfortable, the director can assist them in all aspects of planning the funeral and the burial or cremation. This process may be started prior to death if a long, terminal illness is involved, but many families prefer to wait until the actual death has occurred (see page 1499).

Generally, the funeral director who is chosen will come to the hospital or home where the person died to collect the body, which is then brought to the funeral home. In the following days, family members will meet with the director to go over the details of the funeral arrangements. During these meetings it is up to the members of the fam-

ORGAN DONATION

Organ transplantation surgery offers the possibility of survival to people with terminal illnesses. At present the transplantation of hearts, kidneys, livers, corneas, and many other organs is possible, but healthy human organs are the rarest medical resource. For this reason, many programs have been initiated to encourage all of us to become organ donors and to make it easy for us to do so. Indeed, many families find solace at a time of loss in giving the gift of health to someone else in need.

In 1995, despite a record number of transplants, the shortage of donor organs was also greater than ever before because of the rise in the number of people seeking transplants. More than eight people died each day waiting for an organ to be donated. The number of people waiting for an organ transplant continues to increase much more rapidly than the number of organ donors as the clinical results on organ transplantation continue to improve. Today there are more than 50,000 people on the national waiting list for organ transplantation. The total of organ donations at this time is approximately 19,000. Clearly, organ donation can save lives and is becoming more and more necessary. Making the choice to become an organ donor is a generous and lifesaving act.

The following is a list compiled by the United Network of Organ Sharing in January 1997 of the number of people waiting for the most common transplant surgeries:

- 34,604 registrations for kidney transplants
- 7,511 registrations for liver transplants
- 3,683 registrations for heart transplants
- 2,317 registrations for lung transplants
- 1,458 registrations for kidney-pancreas transplants
- 328 registrations for pancreas transplants
- 233 registrations for heart-lung transplants
- 87 registrations for intestine transplants
- 69 registrations for pancreas islet cell transplants

For many people the knowledge that they may be responsible for saving another person's life often makes the thought of their own death or the death of a loved one easier to bear. If you wish to become an organ donor, you can discuss the registration procedure with your doctor. Many states provide a place for you to note your organ donor status on the back of your driver's license, though the state may also require the signature of the next of kin at the time of death. Donor cards may also be obtained from certain medical organizations. Your doctor or a hospital administrator can provide you with further information on who to contact to obtain a donor card or you may call the branch of the United Network for Organ Sharing in your area. ■

AUTOPSIES

An autopsy is defined as the examination of a body after death to determine the cause of death. A pathologist performs the autopsy and reports his findings to the attending doctor. The doctor will then discuss the findings with the family if the family requests this information.

Generally autopsies are required by state law when a suicide or homicide is suspected, when a death is either sudden or unexplained, or if the cause of death is considered to be the result of an accident. In any other case an autopsy cannot be performed without the consent of the next of kin. Consent forms offer a choice between a limited autopsy, in which only specific parts of the body are examined, or a complete autopsy, in which the entire body is examined. The choice between these two types of autopsies should be considered carefully by family members. If you choose a limited autopsy, for example, you may be left with the same unanswered questions that you had before the autopsy. These same consent forms will also permit the removal of tissue and organs from the body if the deceased or his family elected to donate organs.

Since the 1940s there has been a major decline in the numbers of autopsies performed in all hospital deaths. Autopsies were once performed about 50 percent of the time; currently they are performed about 10 to 15 percent of the time. This decline has occurred chiefly because many doctors believe that diagnostic techniques performed while the person was alive define the cause of death clearly enough.

However, there are many situations in which autopsy is still a useful procedure. An autopsy can reveal hereditary disorders that may affect siblings, children, or other relatives of the deceased, and autopsies have also been useful in identifying newly emerging illnesses such as acquired immunodeficiency syndrome (AIDS). Autopsies are also useful to medical science because they can confirm and expand on what is known about diseases. An autopsy may also be useful to the family in settling any insurance disputes that may arise regarding the death and to give family members the assurance that there was nothing further they could have done to save the loved one.

A properly conducted autopsy will not result in the body becoming disfigured. Embalming may be handled after the autopsy and an open-casket funeral service will still be possible. Alternatively families may choose to will the body for science in hopes that the knowledge gained may benefit others. ■

ily to make clear the type of funeral they would like and how elaborate and expensive a ceremony they envision. The family members will also want to consider the requests of the deceased, if any. At all times, the funeral director should take directions from the family. It is particularly important to be aware of the cost of the funeral and burial—something the newly bereaved may not want to cope with. If these decisions seem overwhelming to the family of the deceased, it may be helpful to ask for the help of a family friend or their clergyperson to facilitate this decision-making process.

Once funeral and memorial services are completed a probate judge—a judge who determines the validity of a will—is appointed. This judge then designates the executor of the will or the representative of the estate. Usually the executor is a family member, the deceased's personal attorney, or a very close friend. The executor will also be responsible for the personal affairs of the deceased, which may or may not include funeral expenses. If the deceased's personal possessions are not designated in the will, the executor and family members will also need to manage these effects in an appropriate manner.

Burial or Cremation

The traditional method of disposing of the deceased is burial, but cremation can be chosen as an alternative means of dealing with the body and honoring the dead. If the choice of burial or cremation is not made by the deceased before death, the burden of this difficult choice is placed on the family. Therefore, it is important to consider this choice at the same time that you make out a living will, appoint a health care proxy, or decide on a DNR order to make sure your wishes are honored and to save your family the anguish of trying to make that choice for you. In all cases, the more specific the deceased is about his wishes before dying, the less difficult the mourning process will be for the survivors.

When cremation occurs immediately after death with no funeral service, it is referred to as disposition. Usually cremation occurs in conjunction with the funeral or memorial service or directly following such a service. In the first case, the funeral director cremates the body prior to the service. In the second case, after the funeral the family can accompany the body to the crematory where it is cremated.

After the body has been cremated there are several choices regarding how the ashes of the decreased will be commemorated. They may be placed in a small stone or metal urn or other container in a procedure called an inurnment. The urn is then buried in a plot, as a body would be, or placed in a mausoleum called a columbarium. Many families forgo these choices in favor of scattering the deceased's ashes in a favorite location usually of the deceased's own choosing, such as a favorite beach or lake or woods. In this case a tree may be planted in memory of the deceased or a plaque inscribed at the site in lieu of a final resting place. Some families also choose to keep the remains with them in the family home.

Funeral and Memorial Services

Almost every culture uses a funerary ritual of some kind to commemorate death. The association of ritual commemoration with death appears to have developed very early in human history. Even the Neanderthals, more than 60,000 years ago, buried their dead in a ceremonial ritual. While such ritualistic partings with the deceased vary immensely, there are also many similarities among these rituals. Such similarities include the provision of support for the grievers; a ritual or ceremony marking the passing from life to death; a viewing of the body or a similar, ritualistic action; a gathering of the family; and a sanitary, ritualistic disposal of the body.

A funeral or some other form of ceremony is a rite of passage and a formal goodbye to the deceased. Modern funerals are often criticized for being overembellished. Family members should remember that what is most important about a funeral is that it is meaningful to those who are grieving. Mortuaries and funeral homes may try to encourage grieving members of the family to buy the most expensive coffin, as if this were a symbol of the importance of the dead person. Family members should understand that a memorial service will be meaningful and memorable based on how the deceased was honored, not by the cost of the event.

Funerals and other similar ceremonies benefit mourners psychologically and spiritually. A funeral confirms the reality of death, eradicating the option of denial. Mourning in such a public and controlled manner also allows those who are grieving to express their feelings and to acknowledge the depth of their grief. The funeral also gives mourners a structure in which to remember the deceased and to recreate their relationship with the deceased as one based on memory and the recollection of past experiences rather than one based on physical presence and interaction. Spiritually, funerals allow mourners to place their loss within the context of their faith and in so doing to give it meaning and purpose.

If a family is religious, their clergyperson will aid in planning the service and will also officiate. If there is no church or synagogue affiliation, funeral homes and other locations are prepared to accommodate funerals and memorial services.

Funeral services pertain to the burial or cremation of the dead. Memorial services are held after the body has been buried or cremated. Memorial services may be held in the week following the funeral service or they may be held at a later time. One advantage of a memorial service is that it focuses on the life of the deceased rather than the death of the deceased, which allows mourners to begin to create an enduring picture of the person who has died.

An average funeral, including burial, costs approximately $5,000, and the cost is rising. The financial differences between burial and cremation may become substantial. Burial plots are costly, as are caskets and coffins. The cost of a burial plot may range between $1,000 and $2,000. Caskets may range in cost anywhere from $500 to $2000 or more. Cremation in a wooden casket costs between $100 and $200, approximately. Costs vary from location to location, but burial is always more costly than cremation. Many funeral homes ask for payment up front to avoid situations in which family members spend more than they have in an effort to give their loved one the very best. It should be noted that after death, family members often feel obligated to give their loved one the best funeral they can. If you personally would prefer to be cremated, this is another reason to make your wishes known before you are unable to do so.

As with other issues at the end of life, planning ahead may help to avoid having funeral or memorial services take an added toll on the already strained finances of a family who has just experienced the financial and emotional drain of a terminal illness. Many funeral homes offer prearrangement plans or general preplans.

Prearrangement planning is done when a loved one does not have long to live and planning the event beforehand may save the additional emotional strain of making funeral arrangements directly following a death. Preplans offer people the opportunity to plan ahead for funeral expenses including offering the option of a funeral account, which is in trust with the funeral home. Money deposited in such an account earns interest at a higher rate than an ordinary savings account. This trust is not tied to the funeral home, however, and with presentation of a death certificate the money may be used for services at any other location. Planning ahead absolves survivors from feeling they must do more than they can afford to do.

In addition, to counteract the rising cost of funerals, memorial societies have been founded in most areas of the United States. Such societies endeavor to promote more economic funeral services. They recommend foregoing embalming, which is not required by law, and choosing cremation. For more information contact the Funeral and Memorial Societies of America, Inc., 6900 Lost Lake Road, Egg Harbor, WI 54209-9231.

PART SIX
Appendices

Medication Directory

Generic name Acyclovir

Brand name Zovirax

Principal uses

Acyclovir is prescribed for herpes virus infections affecting the skin, eye, brain, genitals, and other parts of the body. Some people with recurrent genital herpes outbreaks take acyclovir regularly to prevent new episodes and reduce the severity of outbreaks. Acyclovir is also taken to reduce the severity and duration of chickenpox. The topical form of acyclovir is used to treat herpes virus infections of the genitals and mucous membranes, such as oral herpes and fever blisters; however, when studied in most people with normal immune systems, this ointment did not show any benefit.

How does it work?

Acyclovir fights such illnesses as genital herpes and chickenpox by preventing the virus responsible for these ailments—the herpes virus—from multiplying. This reduces pain and discomfort and accelerates the healing of any sores that might be present. Acyclovir is also given by injection, but this form of administration is not discussed here.

Administration

Follow prescribing information from the doctor and pharmacist. Also:

- Acyclovir may be taken without regard to food.

- When applying acyclovir ointment to a herpes sore on the mouth or the genitals, cover the lesion completely with a thin layer of the medication. To prevent spreading infection, use a finger cot or rubber glove when applying the ointment.

- Check the expiration date. Once it has passed, the medication is not likely to work as well.

- It is particularly important to avoid missing doses of acyclovir.

If you miss a dose of the oral form: Take the missed dose right away, unless it is almost time for the next dose, in which case you should skip the missed dose. Do not take two doses at once.

If you miss a dose of the ointment: Simply apply some as soon as possible and resume the regular schedule.

How quickly will it take effect?

Acyclovir will shorten the duration of a first-time case of genital herpes by as many as 3 to 5 days if you start to take it within 3 days of the outbreak. It can also shorten the duration of recurrent cases and help control pain when it is taken at the first symptoms of an outbreak. In the case of chickenpox, acyclovir will encourage the sores and other manifestations of the infection to clear up more quickly and cause less pain, although it may still take 3 to 5 days for you to notice any benefits. Although the topical ointment helps speed up healing in primary infections, it is not nearly as effective as the oral form for recurrent ones.

Side effects and severe reactions

Side effects that are generally of no concern unless they are persistent or severe include:

- For the oral form: headache, light-headedness, nausea, vomiting, diarrhea, constipation

- For the topical form: transient mild pain, stinging, or burning. In unusual cases, itching or a skin rash may develop.

Contact the doctor if any unusual, worrisome, or severe reactions occur.

Seek emergency care if you develop:
- Seizures, coma

Warnings

- Acyclovir will not cure your condition. *It does not prevent your being able to spread it to others.* Discuss with your doctor the risks of sexual contact during a genital herpes outbreak.

- Even if your condition appears to be improving, take the full regimen prescribed. Also take care not to exceed the dosage because this increases the risk that the virus will find a way to resist the medication.

- Contact the doctor if your condition fails to improve—or if it worsens—within 1 week.

- Avoid getting the ointment around the eyes. Never insert it inside the vagina.

Tips and other important things to know

- Acyclovir is a powerful medication, but it will fight only certain viruses. It will not work for a common cold, for example.

- Acyclovir is most effective when taken at the first sign of symptoms, such as tingling, pain, and burning. For chickenpox, acyclovir is most effective when taken right after the chickenpox rash appears, ideally within 24 hours.

- Try to keep the affected area clean and dry. Wear loose clothing to avoid irritating the lesions.

- Acyclovir is not used to prevent chickenpox in otherwise healthy children. It is typically reserved for children who have an underlying chronic illness, who have a weakened immune system that would make it harder for them to fight off the infection, or who have been taking aspirin for long periods. Adults who acquire chickenpox usually have more severe illness than children, so acyclovir is commonly prescribed in adults.

Special precautions

- If you are pregnant or breast-feeding, discuss with your doctor the use of this medication *before* you start taking it.

Generic name Albuterol

Brand names include Proventil, Ventolin, Vomax

Principal uses

Albuterol is prescribed to prevent and treat asthma and bronchospasm (narrowing of the airways). It relieves wheezing, cough, breathing difficulty, and shortness of breath. Albuterol is commonly prescribed for exercise-induced asthma.

How does it work?

Albuterol is a beta agonist. In an action known as bronchodilation, it opens up the airways, helping to prevent an asthma attack as well as making it easier to breathe during one. It promotes bronchodilation by acting on certain receptors in the muscles of the airways. *Salmeterol*, another commonly used beta agonist, is very similar to albuterol except that it is long-acting rather than short-acting (fast-acting). For this reason, it is used to prevent asthma attacks rather than treat those that have already begun.

Administration

Follow prescribing information from the doctor and pharmacist. Also:

- Take albuterol exactly as prescribed; resist the temptation to take it more frequently or use more of it than recommended if your condition is acting up. Overuse could cause an actual worsening of symptoms, called "paradoxical bronchospasm."

- Albuterol is administered by metered-dose inhaler, by nebulization, or by means of a special brand-name oral inhaler. See page 1464 for guidance on how to administer inhalation medications. Also carefully read the package insert.

- Albuterol tablets are most effective when taken on an empty stomach (1 hour before or 2 hours after eating). Take them with food or milk if stomach upset develops.

- Swallow extended-release tablets whole. Never chew or crush them.

If you miss a dose and take this medication regularly by mouth or by inhalation: Take the missed dose as soon as possible, then take the day's remaining doses at evenly spaced intervals. Do not take two doses at once.

How quickly will it take effect?

When using the inhalation form of this medication, you should start to feel some relief from asthma symptoms within 15 minutes. The medication will continue to exert its effect for about 3 to 4 hours. Regular albuterol tablets will start to relieve symptoms within 30 minutes, with a peak effect in 2 to 3 hours. The tablets will work for 8 hours overall. The long-acting tablets continue working for up to 12 hours.

Side effects and severe reactions

Side effects that are generally of no concern unless they are persistent or severe include:

- Unusual or unpleasant taste, nervousness, restlessness, trembling, trouble sleeping, weakness, coughing or other bronchial irritation, dryness or irritation in the mouth or throat

Contact the doctor if any unusual, worrisome, or severe reactions occur or if you develop:

- Numbness in the hands or feet, unusual bruising, rapid heartbeat, hallucinations, chest pain, irregular heartbeat, severe dizziness or feeling faint, bluish discoloration of skin; skin rash, hives, or itching; swelling of face, lips, or eyelids; persistent flushing or redness of skin

- Persistent or worsening trouble breathing

Warnings

- Consult your doctor without delay if you find that albuterol fails to work as effectively as it used to or if you find yourself needing increasing numbers of doses to control your symptoms.

- Use albuterol only if it has been prescribed specifically for you.

- Do not expose the inhalation canister to extreme temperatures: avoid placing it in direct sunlight or other hot and potentially humid places such as a car glove compartment.

Tips and other important things to know

- Proper technique will make all the difference in making this medication effective for you. Ask your doc-

tor for guidance if you have any questions.

- Inhaled albuterol is most effective when taken at the first symptoms of bronchospasm: coughing, wheezing, tightness in the chest, shortness of breath.

- If you are bothered by dryness of the mouth or throat with the inhaled medication, try rinsing your mouth with water, sucking on ice chips or hard candies, or chewing sugarless gum.

- If you are having trouble sleeping, try taking the day's last dose several hours before going to bed.

- Albuterol appears to affect the heart less than do other bronchodilators. This makes it a good choice, in many cases, for people with heart conditions.

- Certain side effects are more likely to occur in children between the ages of 2 and 12 years than in older children or adults. Ask the doctor what to expect if you have a young child taking albuterol.

Special precautions

- If you are pregnant or breast-feeding, discuss the use of this medication with your doctor *before* you start taking it.

Generic name Alprazolam

Brand names include Alprazolam Intensol, Xanax

Principal uses

Alprazolam is prescribed for short periods of time to reduce symptoms of anxiety and tension, anxiety associated with depression, panic disorder, and insomnia.

How does it work?

Benzodiazepines, such as alprazolam, depress (slow down) certain parts of the central nervous system. This produces relaxation and feelings of tranquility and sleepiness. Some benzodiazepines— although not alprazolam—also suppress the release of chemicals that enable a seizure to spread through the brain. Common benzodiazepines, in addition to alprazolam, include *clonazepam* and *lorazepam*.

Administration

Follow prescribing information from the doctor and pharmacist. Also:

- Alprazolam may be taken without regard to food.

- Alprazolam will work best if you follow the dosing schedule exactly. Most prescriptions advise taking it at evenly spaced intervals throughout the day.

- Avoid taking antacids unless the doctor prescribes them, as they may delay the absorption of benzodiazepine.

If you miss a dose: Take the missed dose right away if you remember within 1 hour or so of the scheduled time. If you remember the missed dose later than that, skip the missed dose and resume the regular schedule. Do not take two doses at once.

How quickly will it take effect?

You will likely start to feel alprazolam's effects within 15 to 30 minutes, with a peak effect in 1 to 2 hours.

Side effects and severe reactions

Side effects that are generally of no concern unless they are persistent or severe include:

- Drowsiness, dizziness or lightheadedness (especially caused by sudden changes in position), impaired motor function, unsteadiness or clumsiness, slurred speech. These effects are of special concern when first starting these medications and whenever operating machinery or a motor vehicle.

Contact the doctor if any unusual, worrisome, or severe reactions occur or if you develop:

- Such uncommon or even rare symptoms as confusion or mental depression, problems concentrating, outbursts of anger, muscle weakness, skin rash or itching, uncontrolled body movements

- Agitation, stimulation, sleep problems, hallucinations, and other unwanted reactions. These rare "paradoxical reactions" are the opposite of what you would expect from the medication.

- Withdrawal symptoms upon abruptly stopping the medication include increased anxiety, insomnia, vomiting, sweating, mental depression, fast or pounding heartbeat, unusual irritability, and seizures. These symptoms appear around the time you decrease or stop taking the medication, as opposed to symptoms of your actual illness that may have been present for some time.

Seek emergency care if you develop:

- Symptoms of benzodiazepine overdose, including continuing confusion or slurred speech, staggering, and severe drowsiness or weakness

Warnings

- A benzodiazepine, such as alprazolam, may be habit-forming. Withdrawal symptoms may develop when you stop taking it.

- The potential benefits of a benzodiazepine must be carefully weighed against the risks associated with taking it for long periods. Concerns include dependence on the medication, withdrawal symptoms, and reappearance of the underlying condition.

- The risk of emotional or physical dependence is present even at recommended doses and after taking the medication for a relatively short period of time. It is greatest, however, in people treated with relatively high doses (more than 4 mg a day) for long periods (longer than 8 to 12 weeks).

- Never alter your benzodiazepine dose in any way without consulting your doctor. The dosage has been carefully tailored for you. Doses must be changed only under professional supervision: increased gradually so that dependence can be monitored and decreased gradually so that withdrawal symptoms can be monitored.

- Ask your doctor about the risks of taking other central nervous system depressants, such as antihistamines, painkillers, and antidepressants, when you are taking alprazolam. There are also serious risks associated with drinking alcohol at the same time as taking the medication. You must not drink alcohol while taking this drug.

- Contact the doctor if you feel the medication is not working as well as it did the first few weeks.

Tips and other important things to know

- Benzodiazepines are not appropriate for managing anxiety associated with the everyday stresses and tensions of life.

- Keep all appointments for follow-up visits so that your doctor can monitor your condition and reaction to the medication.

- Withdrawal reactions are more likely to occur when you abruptly stop or rapidly reduce a relatively high dose that has been taken over a long period of time.

- To minimize lightheadedness or dizziness when rising from a sitting or lying down position, get up slowly.

- Seniors tend to be more sensitive than others are to the central nervous system effects of benzodiazepines.

- Smoking cigarettes may reduce the effectiveness of benzodiazepines; it speeds up the rate at which the body breaks down the medication. Talk to your doctor about the risks.

Special precautions

- Until your reaction to this medication has been established, avoid activity that requires mental or physical alertness.

- If you are pregnant or breast-feeding, discuss with your doctor the use of this medication *before* you start taking it.

- Ask your doctor about risks of taking this medication at the same time as alcohol or other central nervous system depressants (these slow down the nervous system).

Generic name
Amitriptyline

Brand names include
Amitriptylene, Elavil, Endep, Enovil

Principal uses

Amitriptyline is prescribed for depression. It has also been used to treat anxiety conditions such as panic disorder and obsessive-compulsive disorder, post-herpetic neuralgia (a type of severe nerve pain), anorexia or bulimia (eating disorders) associated with depression, and intractable hiccups and to prevent migraine and cluster headaches.

How does it work?

Amitriptyline belongs to a class of medications known as tricyclic antidepressants. It is believed to help relieve the symptoms of depression by blocking the reuptake of certain chemicals (serotonin and norepinephrine) in the brain, leading to a greater concentration of these stimulant chemicals. Much remains to be learned about how tricyclic antidepressants work, however. Amitriptyline is taken orally as well as given by injection. The injection form of administration is not discussed here.

How quickly will it take effect?

In the case of depression, you will likely start to feel an improvement in 2 to 4 weeks.

Administration

Follow prescribing information from the doctor and pharmacist. Also:

- Take amitriptyline with food or milk to reduce the risk of stomach upset.
- Your doctor may advise you to take the full dose at bedtime to help decrease sedation the next day or to take it in the early evening to avoid a "hangover" feeling the next morning.

If you miss a dose: Skip the missed dose and take the next prescribed dose at the usual time. Do not take two doses at once. If you miss your once-a-day bedtime dose and do not remember until the next day, skip it. Amitriptyline may cause side effects if taken during the day.

Side effects and severe reactions

Side effects that are generally of no concern unless they are persistent or severe include:

- Drowsiness, weakness, dizziness when standing, dryness of the mouth and mucous membranes, headache, increased appetite, weight gain, nausea, unpleasant taste

- Temporary (and harmless) blue-green tint to urine

Contact the doctor if any unusual, worrisome, or severe reactions occur or if you develop:

- Confusion, fast heartbeat, fainting, difficulty urinating, disorientation, stuffy nose, constipation, sweating, muscle spasms or tremors, blurred vision

Seek emergency care if you develop:

- Seizures

Warnings

- Your dosage has been carefully tailored to you and your condition. Do not change it in any way without consulting your doctor.
- Abruptly stopping this medication increases the risk of withdrawal symptoms (anxiety, malaise, chills, vomiting, headache, dizziness), especially if you have been taking the medication for a long time or at high doses.
- Amitriptyline should be discontinued a minimum of 48 hours before elective surgery; your doctor should oversee this withdrawal.

Tips and other important things to know

- To minimize side effects, this medication is started at low doses and gradually increased to higher doses. Levels of the medication in your blood are monitored to maximize the effectiveness of the medication. After the first few doses of this medication—until you know if you will get dizzy or experience other reactions to it—lie down for 30 minutes. Always get up slowly to prevent dizziness or fainting.
- If dryness in the mouth becomes bothersome, try chewing sugarless gum or sucking on ice chips or hard candy. Take good care of your teeth to reduce the increased risk of cavities associated with mouth dryness.
- As with any antidepressant medication, amitriptyline should constitute part of a broader regimen that includes psychotherapy, if necessary.

Special precautions

- Until your reaction to this medication has been established, avoid activity that requires mental or physical alertness.
- If you are pregnant or breast-feeding, discuss with your doctor the use of this medication *before* you start taking it.
- Ask your doctor about risks of taking this medication at the same time as alcohol or other central nervous system depressants (these slow down the nervous system).
- This medication may increase sensitivity to the sun; discuss appropriate precautions with your doctor.
- If you have a cardiac condition, discuss the risks of contraindications with your doctor.

Generic name Amlodipine

Brand names include Lotrel, Norvasc

Principal uses

Amlodipine is prescribed to manage hypertension (high blood pressure) and certain types of angina pectoris (chest pain).

How does it work?

Amlodipine belongs to a class of medications known as calcium channel blockers, a class that also includes such medications as *diltiazem* and *nifedipine*. Calcium channel blockers promote relaxation of smooth muscle in the walls of certain arteries and the heart muscle by blocking the effect of calcium on these tissues. This reduces the contraction of these muscles. The arteries dilate (or "open up"), become less likely to spasm and blood pressure is lowered. The heart requires less oxygen because it is not working as hard and more blood and oxygen make their way to the heart muscle as well. These effects help reduce and prevent chest pain.

Administration

Follow prescribing information from the doctor and pharmacist. Also:

- Amlodipine may be taken without regard to food.

- Never abruptly stop taking this medication if you have been taking it regularly for some time. If the dosage is not reduced gradually, your condition may worsen. Your doctor should give you guidance on tapering the dose.

If you miss a dose: Take the missed dose immediately unless it is within 8 hours of the next one, in which case you should skip the missed dose and resume the regular schedule. Do not take two doses at once.

How quickly will it take effect?

Amlodipine reaches peak concentrations in your system in 6 to 12 hours, but it varies widely in the amount of time it takes to lower blood pressure.

Side effects and severe reactions

Side effects that are generally of no concern unless they are persistent or severe include:

- Headache, nausea, flushing, weakness, notable tiredness

Contact the doctor if any unusual, worrisome, or severe reactions occur or if you develop:

- Fluid retention leading to swelling of the ankles or feet (relatively common), dizziness, lightheadedness, sensation of a pounding heartbeat
- Unexpected chest pain or difficulty breathing, unexplained bruising or black and blue marks, unusual bleeding

Warnings

- Take this medication as prescribed even if you feel well; hypertension is a largely symptom-free disease until organs become damaged.
- Rarely, people with severe heart disease may experience more severe and frequent chest pain (and heart attack in some cases) when starting calcium channel blockers or undergoing a dosage increase. The doctor should be fully informed of any heart conditions you have before you start taking this medication.
- If you are taking amlodipine for chest pain, take care not to overexert yourself. This can be tempting to

do if your symptoms subside. Discuss with your doctor safe levels of exercise.

Tips and other important things to know

- Calcium channel blockers may help control your high blood pressure, but they will not cure it.
- Your doctor should give you guidance on lifestyle measures you can take to control high blood pressure, such as weight control, moderate exercise, and following a healthy diet.
- Keep all appointments for follow-up visits so that your doctor can monitor your condition and examine your reaction to this medication.
- There is considerable variation in the amount of time that calcium channel blockers take to start working and how long they continue working.
- If you are taking amlodipine for chest pain, your doctor may advise you to keep taking sublingual nitroglycerin (taken as a tablet placed under the tongue) for symptoms when they develop. Make sure you clearly understand when and if you should continue to take these tablets.
- In some people, amlodipine causes gums to swell, bleed, or become tender. Discuss these reactions with your doctor or dentist if they occur. Careful flossing and brushing may help prevent them, as may regular cleanings done by your dentist.

Special precautions

- If you are pregnant or breast-feeding, discuss with your doctor the use of this medication *before* you start taking it.

Generic name Amoxicillin

Brand names include
Amoxil, Polymox, Trimox, Wymox

Principal uses

Amoxicillin is prescribed to treat bacterial infections that affect the lower respiratory tract (bronchitis, for example),

throat (such as "strep throat"), skin, sinuses, middle ear, genitals, urinary tract, and other parts of the body. It is also used to prevent a bacterial infection of the heart lining called endocarditis.

How does it work?

This penicillin antibiotic fights infection-causing bacteria by preventing them from forming cell walls. Only certain types of bacteria are susceptible to amoxicillin.

Administration

Follow prescribing information from the doctor and pharmacist. Also:

- Amoxicillin may be taken without regard to food.
- To help ensure effectiveness, take amoxicillin at evenly spaced intervals around the clock, or as otherwise prescribed.
- It is preferable but not necessary to refrigerate the oral suspension and pediatric drops. Discard any unused portion 14 days after opening the bottle.
- The pediatric drops should be placed directly onto the tongue (aim toward the side of the mouth to avoid gagging) or may be mixed in with milk, formula, fruit juice, soft drink, or another cold drink. Your child should ingest the entire mixture right away.
- Thoroughly chew chewable tablets before swallowing, and drink them with a liquid to encourage absorption. These tablets may also be crushed and mixed with a small amount of soft food, such as apple sauce; consume this entire mixture immediately after mixing.

If you miss a dose: Take the missed dose unless it is almost time for the next one. If you are scheduled to take two doses a day, take the missed dose immediately and the next dose 5 to 6 hours later, then resume the regular schedule. If you are scheduled to take 3 or more doses a day, take the missed one immediately and the next dose 2 to 4 hours later, and then resume the regular schedule. Do not take two doses at once.

How quickly will it take effect?

Although it will depend partly on the type and severity of your infection, your condition will likely improve notably within 24 to 48 hours of the first dose.

Side effects and severe reactions

Side effects that are generally of no concern unless they are persistent or severe include:

- Diarrhea (mild). Consult your doctor before taking an antidiarrheal medication.
- Nausea, vomiting, mouth or tongue irritation

Contact the doctor if any unusual, worrisome, or severe reactions occur or if you develop:

- Muscle aches, diarrhea (severe), mild skin rash, itching, or hives
- Symptoms of a new infection

Seek emergency care if you develop:

- Lightheadedness, peeling skin, seizures
- Symptoms of a severe allergic reaction, such as increasing itching, hives, skin rash, breathing difficulty or wheezing, peeling skin, swollen or painful joints, sore throat, abnormal bleeding or bruising. These symptoms may develop several days after you stop taking the medication.

Warnings

- Take all the prescribed medication even if symptoms of the infection have cleared; otherwise, the infection may linger and reappear later.
- Failure to take the full course of prescribed medication for "strep" infections in particular increases the risk of such serious conditions as rheumatic fever, an ailment that can cause permanent heart damage.
- As with any medication, it is important to mention all your allergies to your doctor before taking it for the first time. In the case of amoxicillin, it is particularly critical that you make note of a history of allergies (hay fever, asthma) or an allergic reaction to any medication (prescription or over-the-counter), amoxicillin, or especially another penicillin antibiotic.
- Contact the doctor if your condition does not improve—or if it worsens—within a few days.

- Amoxicillin may decrease the effectiveness of estrogen-containing oral contraceptives; discuss with your doctor whether you should temporarily supplement your birth control method. It may interact with other medications in notable ways as well; make sure to tell your doctor about all the other medications you take.

Tips and other important things to know

- Amoxicillin is a powerful antibiotic, but it can fight only certain susceptible bacteria. It will have no impact on an infection caused by other organisms, such as viruses (as in the common cold), fungi, or parasites.
- If you have diabetes, be aware that the medication may cause false positive results with some tests for urine sugar.

Special precautions

- If you are pregnant or breast-feeding, discuss with your doctor the use of this medication *before* you start taking it.

Generic name Amoxicillin Clavulanate

Brand name Augmentin

Principal uses

This medication is used to treat bacterial infections affecting the sinuses, skin, middle ear, lower respiratory tract (including pneumonia), urinary tract, and other parts of the body. It is commonly given to children.

How does it work?

Amoxicillin and clavulanate are combined to create a more powerful antibiotic than amoxicillin alone. Like many penicillin antibiotics, amoxicillin destroys susceptible bacteria by inhibiting them from creating new cell walls and being able to reproduce. Clavulanate contributes by inactivating enzymes created by certain bacteria to break down amoxicillin. With these two medications at work, amoxicillin clavulanate successfully treats infections that amoxicillin alone might not cure.

Administration

Follow prescribing information from the doctor and pharmacist. Also:

- Take this medication at evenly spaced intervals throughout the day. This helps ensure a constant level of medication in your system.
- This medication may be taken without regard to food. Taking it with food or milk will reduce the risk of stomach upset, however.
- The suspension may be mixed with formula, milk, or juice. This may make it easier to give to a child. Make sure the child consumes the entire mixture right away.
- The suspension can be kept at room temperature for 7 days and in the refrigerator for 14 days. Discard any unused portion of either after this amount of time.
- Drink a glass of cold water (8 oz) after taking the tablet.

If you miss a dose: Take the missed dose right away, unless it is almost time for the next dose. If you have been prescribed two doses a day, take the missed dose right away and the next one 5 to 6 hours later. If you have been prescribed three or more doses a day, take the missed one right away and take the next dose 2 to 4 hours later, and resume the regular schedule. Do not take two doses at once.

How quickly will it take effect?

You will likely have to take this medication regularly for a day or two before your condition improves, although a severe infection may take longer. Ask your doctor what to expect.

Side effects and severe reactions

Side effects that are generally of no concern unless they are persistent or severe include:

- Diarrhea (mild). Consult your doctor *before* taking an antidiarrheal medication.
- Stomach upset, nausea, vomiting, gas, indigestion, loss of appetite, mouth or tongue irritation

Contact the doctor if any unusual, worrisome, or severe reactions occur or if you develop:

- Diarrhea (severe or bloody), fever, muscle aches, mild skin rash, itching, or hives
- Symptoms of a new infection

Seek emergency care if you develop:

- Lightheadedness, peeling skin, seizures
- Symptoms of a severe allergic reaction, such as increasing itching, hives, skin rash, breathing difficulty or wheezing, peeling skin, swollen or painful joints, sore throat, abnormal bleeding, or bruising. These symptoms may develop several days after you stop taking the medication.

Warnings

- Take all the prescribed medication even if symptoms of the infection have cleared; otherwise, the infection may reappear.
- Failure to take the full course of prescribed medication for "strep" infections in particular increases the risk of such serious conditions as rheumatic fever, an ailment that can cause permanent heart damage.
- As with any medication, it is important to mention all your allergies to your doctor. In the case of amoxicillin and clavulanate, it is particularly critical that you make note of a history of allergies (hay fever, asthma) or an allergic reaction to amoxicillin, other penicillin antibiotics, or any other medication, prescription or over-the-counter.
- Contact the doctor if your condition does not improve—or if it worsens—within a few days.
- The amoxicillin in this medication may decrease the effectiveness of estrogen-containing oral contraceptives; discuss with your doctor whether you should temporarily supplement your birth control method.

Tips and other important things to know

- This is a powerful medication, but it can fight only certain susceptible bacteria. It will have no impact on an infection caused by other organisms, such as viruses (as in the common cold), fungi, or parasites.

- This medication may alter the results of certain diagnostic tests. Make sure the tester knows that you are taking it.
- If you have diabetes, be aware that the medication may cause false positive results with some tests for urine sugar.

Special precautions

- If you are pregnant or breast-feeding, discuss with your doctor the use of this medication *before* you start taking it.

Generic name Atenolol

Brand name Tenormin

Principal uses

Atenolol is prescribed to manage hypertension (high blood pressure) and chronic, stable angina pectoris (chest pain). It is also given to reduce the risk of future heart attacks in heart attack victims. Some doctors have prescribed it to help manage alcohol withdrawal and prevent migraines.

How does it work?

Atenolol is a beta adrenergic blocker (a "beta blocker"). Beta blockers work by blocking a certain class of nerve receptors in the body, helping to control high blood pressure and angina by decreasing the work that the heart needs to do.

Atenolol is taken orally as well as given by injection. The injection form of administration is not discussed here.

Administration

Follow prescribing information from the doctor and pharmacist. Also:

- Atenolol may be taken without regard to food.
- Take this medication at the same time every day; this will help you remember to take it.

If you miss a dose: Take the missed dose as soon as possible. If you normally take two doses a day and it is within 4 hours of the next scheduled dose, skip the missed dose and take the next dose at the regular time. If you take one dose a day and it is already within 8 hours of the next scheduled dose, however, skip the missed dose and take the next dose at

the regular time. Do not take two doses at once.

How quickly will it take effect?

Atenolol will start to alter the heart rate within 60 minutes or so, with a peak effect in 2 to 4 hours. Its antihypertensive action lasts for approximately 24 hours.

Side effects and severe reactions

Side effects that are generally of no concern unless they are persistent or severe include:

- Dizziness, lightheadedness, slight drowsiness, notable fatigue or weakness, trouble sleeping, decreased sexual ability

Contact the doctor if any unusual, worrisome, or severe reactions occur or if you develop:

- Cold hands and feet; swelling of ankles, feet, or lower legs; slow heartbeat (particularly fewer than 50 beats per minute); breathing difficulty (that develops gradually)
- Unexpected chest pain, sudden shortness of breath, general feeling of discomfort or weakness, trembling, sweating, fast or irregular heartbeat

Warnings

- Take this medication as prescribed even if you feel well; hypertension is a largely symptom-free disease until organs become damaged.
- Never suddenly stop taking this or any other beta blocker, regardless of the reason for taking it. Doing this could not only cause discomfort but also severely worsen angina or even instigate irregular heart rhythms or a heart attack, especially in people with coronary artery disease.
- When you are stopping the medication, the dosage must be reduced gradually over a period of about 2 weeks. Follow your doctor's instructions carefully.
- If you are taking a beta blocker for chest pain, take care not to overexert yourself. This can be tempting to do if your symptoms subside. Dis-

cuss with your doctor safe amounts of exercise.

- Do not take over-the-counter cold preparations, nasal decongestants, or other medications without checking with your doctor first. As with any medication, it is important to tell your doctor about all the medications you take.

- Beta blockers can worsen asthma and must be used carefully, if at all, in persons with this condition. Let your doctor know if you have ever had asthma or wheezing.

Tips and other important things to know

- Beta blockers do not cure high blood pressure, but they may help control it. Discuss with your doctor lifestyle measures that you can take to control your high blood pressure such as losing weight, exercising moderately, and following a healthy diet.

- Withdrawal of atenolol should be monitored with particular care in people with hyperthyroidism.

- If you experience dizziness when getting up from a sitting or lying position, try to avoid sudden changes in position, rise slowly, and talk to your doctor about taking the medication at bedtime.

- Inform any doctor about to perform major surgery on you that you take a beta blocker, as he or she may want to stop the medication before the surgery. This practice is controversial, however.

- Ask your doctor for guidance on monitoring your own pulse rate while taking a beta blocker.

- If you have diabetes, be aware that a beta blocker may alter blood sugar levels or mask symptoms of low blood sugar. Ask your doctor for guidance.

Special precautions

- If you are pregnant or breast-feeding, discuss with your doctor the use of this medication *before* you start taking it.

- When first starting this medication, avoid activity that requires mental or physical alertness until reaction to medication has been established.

Generic name Atorvastatin
Brand name Lipitor

Principal uses

Atorvastatin is prescribed to lower high levels of cholesterol in the blood. This is done in an attempt to prevent heart complications of coronary artery disease with cholesterol-clogged blood vessels.

Administration

Follow prescribing information from the doctor and pharmacist. Also:

- Take this medicine exactly as prescribed. The dosage has been carefully tailored to your body's requirements and response. Do not take it in larger or smaller doses, more often, or for longer than recommended.

- Atorvastatin may be taken without regard to food. Taking it in the evening enhances its effectiveness.

If you miss a dose on one day: Skip the missed dose and resume the regular schedule the next day. Do not take two doses at once.

Tips and other important things to know:

- Atorvastatin belongs to a class of medicines called HMG-CoA reductase inhibitors (statins). Medicines in this class may vary slightly as to when they are best taken, the side effects they produce, the research they have been used in, and the amount of experience doctors have with them.

See the *simvastatin* entry for more information on how statins work, what to expect in terms of speed and side effects, and when to call the doctor if problems develop. (Unless otherwise noted, the information in *simvastatin* is common to all statins.)

Generic name
Azithromycin

Brand name Zithromax

Principal uses

Azithromycin is prescribed for bacterial infections that affect the skin, middle ear, and upper and lower respiratory tracts, such as "strep throat," pneumonia, and

---

tonsillitis. It is also used for, among other things, acute exacerbations of chronic obstructive pulmonary disease (COPD) caused by bacterial infection, venereal ulcers, and sexually transmitted chlamydial infections.

How does it work?

Azithromycin belongs to a class of antibiotics known as macrolides. Macrolide antibiotics fight infection by directly killing susceptible bacteria or by slowing them down so that your body's natural defenses can eliminate them. Other important macrolide antibiotics include clarithromycin and erythromycin. Azithromycin is actually a derivative of erythromycin.

Administration

Follow prescribing information from the doctor and pharmacist. Also:

- For the medication to work properly, prescription instructions must be followed carefully in regard to the spacing of doses and the number of days the medication should be taken.

- Take azithromycin on an empty stomach (1 hour before or 2 hours after a meal); food reduces its absorption. Single-dose packets for oral suspension that you mix with water are an exception, however. They may be taken without regard to food.

- Drink the oral suspension you make with a single-dose packet immediately after mixing the medication with a glass of water (8 oz). Drink the entire mixture. Then add water to the same glass, mix it around to catch any residual medication, and drink all of this liquid.

- If you are taking an aluminum- or magnesium-containing antacid, take it at least 2 hours before or after the azithromycin.

If you miss a dose: Take the missed dose right away unless it is already the next day, in which case you should skip the missed doses and resume the regular schedule. Do not take two doses at once.

How quickly will it take effect?

Macrolide antibiotics, such as azithromycin, will reach peak concentrations in your bloodstream within 2 to 3 hours, although you will likely have to take the medication regularly for 3 to 5 days before noticing an improvement in your condition.

Side effects and severe reactions

Contact the doctor if any unusual, worrisome, or severe reactions occur or if you develop:

- Severe nausea, vomiting, loose stools or diarrhea, indigestion, abdominal pain and stomach gas, abnormal taste, skin rash, headache, fainting, drowsiness, tiredness, vaginal irritation, unusual sensitivity to the sun

- Symptoms of a new infection

- Heart palpitations, chest pain, yellowish skin or eyes

- Severe diarrhea or diarrhea that persists for more than 24 hours; diarrhea such as this may indicate a rare but serious form of bowel inflammation: pseudomembranous colitis.

Seek emergency care if you develop:

- Symptoms of a serious allergic reaction, possibly including swelling of the face, lips, tongue, and neck; or difficulty talking, swallowing, or breathing

Warnings

- Take all the prescribed medication even if you feel better; otherwise, the bacteria may linger in your system and cause an infection later. In the case of "strep throat" especially, there is an increased risk of rheumatic fever (a heart condition) and glomerulonephritis (a kidney disease) if you do not take the medication regularly for at least 5 days.

- Contact the doctor if your condition fails to improve—or if it worsens—within approximately 5 days.

- As with any medication, it is important to mention all medication allergies to your doctor. In the case of macrolide antibiotics, it is particularly important to mention reactions to any medications in this class, such as erythromycin.

Tips and other important things to know

- Macrolide antibiotics are powerful and often very effective medications. They work against only certain susceptible bacteria, however. They will not help fight infections caused by viruses (such as the common cold and flu), fungi, or parasites, for example.

Special precautions

- This medication may increase sensitivity to the sun; discuss with your doctor what precautions are appropriate.

- If you are pregnant or breast-feeding, discuss with your doctor the use of this medication *before* you start taking it.

Generic name
Beclomethasone

Brand names include
Beclovent, Beconase, Vancenase, Vanceril

Principal uses

Beclomethasone is used in the form of an oral inhalant to treat severe, chronic bronchial asthma. It is used in the form of a nasal spray and aerosol to treat hay fever symptoms and nasal stuffiness and irritation, and to prevent the recurrence of nasal polyps.

How does it work?

This adrenal corticosteroid ("steroid") helps open up the lungs and nasal passages by reducing inflammation in these areas. It accomplishes this by suppressing many of the chemical and cellular reactions responsible for inflammation. *Triamcinolone*, another corticosteroid medication, is used similarly as an oral and nasal inhalant.

Administration

Follow prescribing information from the doctor and pharmacist. Also:

- To function as intended, the oral and nasal forms of this medication must be used every day and at evenly spaced intervals, as directed by your doctor.

- Carefully read the package insert. For extra guidance on administering oral inhalation steroids, see page

1464. For extra guidance on nasal steroids, see page 1464.

- To reduce the risk of harmful reactions, do not use the oral inhalation medication more frequently, in larger doses, or for longer than recommended. Likewise, do not suddenly stop taking it; withdrawal should be gradual, as directed by your doctor.

- After using the oral inhaler, rinse out your mouth or drink a glass of water.

- Clean the inhaler regularly in warm water. Dry it thoroughly.

If you miss a dose of the oral inhalant: Take the missed dose as soon as possible unless it is almost time for the next dose, in which case you should skip the missed dose and resume the regular schedule.

If you miss a dose of the nasal medication: Take the missed dose right away if it is within 1 hour of when you should have taken it. Otherwise, skip the missed dose and resume the regular schedule. Do not take two doses at once.

How quickly will it take effect?

The full benefits of oral inhaled beclomethasone are usually felt within a few days of regular use, although it may take up to 4 weeks of regular treatment in some cases. Benefits of the nasal medication may take 1 to 3 weeks to become evident.

Side effects and severe reactions

Side effects that are generally of no concern unless they are persistent or severe include:

- *For the oral inhalation:* irritation or dryness of the nose, mouth, tongue, or throat; cough, headache, nosebleeds

- *For the nasal spray or aerosol:* mild and transient sensations of burning or irritation in the nose, headache, cough, hoarseness, sneezing attacks, transient and mild nosebleeds, nausea, runny or stuffy nose, mild throat irritation, tearing of the eyes

Contact the doctor if any unusual, worrisome, or severe reactions occur or if you develop:

- A nasal condition other than the one for which the medication is prescribed, as many types of nasal infections should not be exposed to a steroid.

Oral inhalation:

- Fast or pounding heartbeat, skin rash, fever, increased susceptibility to infection, creamy white patches in the mouth or other symptoms of a mouth, lung, or throat infection, persistent hoarse voice

- An asthma attack that fails to improve with the use of a bronchodilator

Nasal spray or aerosol:

- Hives; itching; rash; dryness or bad taste in the mouth; sore throat; symptoms of a nose, sinus, or throat infection; fever; notable fatigue or weakness; swelling of the face, eyelids, or lips

Seek emergency care if you develop:

- Difficulty breathing, increased shortness of breath, wheezing, tightness in the chest, swelling of the tongue or lips

Warnings

- Contact the doctor if you are taking an orally inhaled steroid and your condition fails to improve—or if it worsens—within 4 weeks. Do not increase the dosage on your own. Also contact the doctor if you undergo a period of great physical stress.

- Contact the doctor if you are using a nasal steroid and your condition fails to improve within 3 weeks.

- Many people with severe asthma are prescribed a tablet or other oral form of steroid, such as prednisone, to take along with an orally inhaled steroid. Even if your asthma seems to have improved, do not stop taking either medication without consulting your doctor.

- If your doctor has advised you to transfer from an oral steroid to an inhaled one, contact him or her for guidance if you experience a severe asthma attack or anticipate undergoing a period of physical stress, such as surgery. You may need supplementary steroids during this time.

- It is important to act on symptoms that your system is not handling a switch from oral to inhaled steroids, because the situation can become very dangerous. Look for muscle or joint pain, fever, abdominal or back pain, dizziness or fainting, shortness of breath, unexpected weight loss, and other unusual or worrisome developments.

- Children should be very carefully monitored while taking a steroid in any form, as the medication can slow growth in some cases. Discuss with your doctor any concerns you have.

Tips and other important things to know

- Proper technique in administering this medication will make a big difference in how effective it is for your condition.

- Orally inhaled steroids will not relieve an asthma attack that is underway. They are used only to help *prevent* asthma attacks.

- Because steroids suppress the immune system, you may be more susceptible to infections than if you were not taking them. Such infections as chickenpox and measles can cause more serious complications, for example. Avoid exposure to these illnesses and contact your doctor immediately if you are exposed.

- The benefit of an inhaled steroid is that much less gets absorbed into the body as a whole than would be the case with a steroid pill, reducing the likelihood that unwanted side effects will occur.

Special precautions

- If you are pregnant or breast-feeding, discuss with your doctor the use of this medication *before* you start taking it.

Generic name Benazepril

Brand name Lotensin

Principal uses

Benazepril is prescribed to treat mild to severe high blood pressure (hyperten-

sion). It belongs to a class of medications called angiotensin converting enzyme (ACE) inhibitors.

Administration

Follow prescribing information from the doctor and pharmacist. Also:

- Benazepril may be taken without regard to food.

- Take benazepril at the same time every day; this will help you remember to take it.

- Do not alter the dosage on your own; your doctor has tailored it carefully to meet your body's needs and its response to the medication.

See the *enalapril* entry on page 1522 for more information on how ACE inhibitors work, what to expect in terms of time of onset and side effects, and when to contact the doctor if problems develop. Unless otherwise noted, the information for *enalapril* applies to all ACE inhibitors.

Generic name Buspirone

Brand name BuSpar

Principal uses

Buspirone is used short term to treat nervousness and anxiety and to manage anxiety disorders.

How does it work?

It is not clear exactly how this antianxiety agent works. It appears to affect various chemical transmitters in the central nervous system.

Administration

Follow prescribing information from the doctor and pharmacist. Also:

- To avoid unwanted reactions, take this medication exactly as prescribed: do not take more of it, take it for longer, or take it more often than recommended.

- Buspirone may be taken without regard to food.

- Store buspirone in a cool, dark place.

- Take buspirone at the same time every day; this will keep a constant level in your system and help you remember to take it.

If you miss a dose: Take the missed dose as soon as possible, unless it is almost time for the next dose, in which case you should skip the missed dose and resume the regular schedule. Do not take two doses at once.

How quickly will it take effect?

You may notice an improvement in your condition within 7 to 10 days, although many people do not feel the medication's full benefits until 3 or more weeks of regular use.

Side effects and severe reactions

Side effects that are generally of no concern unless they are persistent or severe include:

- Drowsiness, dizziness, headache, lightheadedness, restlessness, unusual excitement, nervousness, dry mouth

Contact the doctor if any unusual, worrisome, or severe reactions occur or if you develop:

- Muscle spasms; uncontrolled tongue or jaw movements; uncontrolled twitching in the face or body; chest pain; blurred vision; nausea; stomach upset; diarrhea; confusion or mental depression; or numbness, tingling, weakness, or pain in the hands or feet

Warnings

- Ask your doctor about the risks of drinking alcohol or taking other central nervous system depressants, such as antihistamines, while taking this medication. Buspirone may increase the drowsiness and sedation that these substances can produce.

Tips and other important things to know

- It is not appropriate to use buspirone for anxiety associated with everyday stresses and tensions.
- Discuss with your doctor what to expect from this medication.
- Do not expect the same reactions to buspirone that you may have had with benzodiazepines or other standard sedative and antianxiety medications; buspirone is not chemically

or pharmacologically related to these. It produces little of the sedation, sluggishness, or other slowed movement that a number of these medications do. It does not relax muscles or have anticonvulsant actions.

- Research indicates that buspirone is not habit forming.
- If you are taking buspirone regularly, be sure to keep all appointments for follow-up visits so that your doctor can monitor your condition and check for unwanted reactions to the medication.

Special precautions

- Until your reaction to this medication has been established, avoid activity that requires mental or physical alertness.
- Ask your doctor about risks of taking this medication at the same time as alcohol or other central nervous system depressants (these slow down the nervous system).
- If you are pregnant or breast-feeding, discuss with your doctor the use of this medication *before* you start taking it.

Generic name
Carbamazepine

Brand name Tegretol

Principal uses

Carbamazepine is used to control certain types of epileptic seizures. It has also been prescribed for pain associated with trigeminal neuralgia (tic douloureux), a type of facial pain, as well as pain from peripheral nerve disorders, such as diabetic neuropathy. Less common uses include the treatment of bipolar disorder, acute mania, schizophrenia, certain types of diabetes insipidus, and pain caused by ailments ranging from multiple sclerosis to diabetes.

How does it work?

Carbamazepine controls seizures in several ways. It not only reduces the likelihood that a seizure will occur but it also limits the ability of a seizure to spread through the brain. Seizures are therefore less severe. Carbamazepine helps relieve

the pain of trigeminal neuralgia and various other ailments by interfering with critical nerve impulses that transmit pain signals.

Administration

Follow prescribing information from the doctor and pharmacist. Also:

- Follow prescription instructions carefully; your doctor will slowly adjust the dosage on the basis of your particular condition.
- Take carbamazepine with food to reduce the risk of stomach upset.
- To reduce the risk that carbamazepine tablets will harden and lose potency, store them in a tightly closed container in a cool, dry place. Avoid storing them in humid environments, such as bathrooms.
- Store the oral suspension in a light-resistant container. Do not expose it to high heat or freezing temperatures.

If you miss a dose: Take the missed dose right away, unless it is almost time for the next dose, in which case you should skip the missed dose and resume the regular schedule. Do not take two doses at once. Consult your doctor if you miss more than one dose in a day.

How quickly will it take effect?

Carbamazepine is typically taken for 3 months or more, with frequent adjustments, before its capacity to control seizures and severe pain can be determined.

Side effects and severe reactions

Side effects that are generally of no concern unless they are persistent or severe include:

- Mild drowsiness, dizziness, lightheadedness, unsteadiness or clumsiness, nausea, or vomiting

Contact the doctor if any unusual, worrisome, or severe reactions occur or if you develop:

- Blurred or double vision, odd eye movements, agitation or confusion, behavioral changes (watch for these in children in particular), unexpected hostility, severe diarrhea, persistent headache, notable drowsiness, severe nausea and vomiting

- Darkening or obvious appearance of blood in the urine; painful or difficult urination; unusual bleeding or bruising (including unexpected nosebleeds); stools that are pale, black, tarry, or bloody; shortness of breath; pinpoint red spots on the skin; swollen or painful glands; abdominal pain; chest tightness; yellowing of the eyes or skin; bone or joint pain; cough or hoarseness; fever; mouth sores

Seek emergency care if you develop:

- Bleeding problems, excessive bruising
- Unexplained, persistent fever

Warnings

- Never suddenly stop taking this medication, particularly when it has been prescribed for epileptic seizures. The medication is withdrawn slowly to reduce the risk of severe seizures or severe, continuing seizures (status epilepticus).
- Because carbamazepine can cause potentially severe or even fatal blood reactions, regular blood checks are usually necessary.
- Make sure the doctor in charge of a surgical or dental procedure is aware that you are taking this medication.

Tips and other important things to know

- Carbamazepine will affect only certain types of seizures: grand mal, partial, and mixed seizures.
- Keep all appointments for follow-up visits so your doctor can properly monitor your condition and check for unwanted reactions to the medication.
- Carbamazepine is appropriate to take for true trigeminal neuralgia pain but not for simple aches and pains.

Special precautions

- If you are pregnant or breast-feeding, discuss with your doctor the use of this medication *before* you start taking it. If you are at risk of

pregnancy or on birth control pills, discuss with your doctor the use of this medication. Carbamazepine can increase metabolism of birth control pills and make them ineffective.

- Ask your doctor about risks of taking this medication at the same time as alcohol or other central nervous system depressants (these slow down the nervous system).
- This medication may increase sensitivity to the sun; discuss with your doctor what precautions are appropriate.
- Until your reaction to this medication has been established, avoid activity that requires mental or physical alertness.
- Wearing a medical alert bracelet or necklace is advised.

Generic name Cefprozil
Brand name Cefzil

Principal uses

Cefprozil is prescribed for bacterial infections that affect the middle ear, skin, tonsils, throat (such as "strep throat"), lower respiratory tract, and other parts of the body.

How does it work?

Cefprozil is a second-generation cephalosporin antibiotic distantly related to penicillin. It destroys susceptible bacteria by interfering with their ability to synthesize new, protective cell walls. Cefuroxime is another commonly used second-generation cephalosporin antibiotic. Some medications in this class immobilize bacteria so that the body's natural immunity can destroy it.

Administration

Follow prescribing information from the doctor and pharmacist. Also:

- Cefprozil may be taken without regard to food. Take it with food if it causes stomach upset, however.
- Store the suspension in the refrigerator. Shake it well before measuring out the dose. Discard any unused medication after 14 days.

If you miss a dose: Take the missed dose right away, unless it is almost time for the next dose, in which case you should skip

the missed dose and resume the regular schedule. Do not take two doses at once.

How quickly will it take effect?

Your condition will probably start to improve within a few days, although this will depend in part on the type and severity of the infection.

Side effects and severe reactions

Side effects that are generally of no concern unless they are persistent or severe include:

- Mild diarrhea, sore mouth or tongue, mild stomach cramps, nausea, vomiting

Contact the doctor if any unusual, worrisome, or severe reactions occur or if you develop:

- Symptoms of a new infection
- Diarrhea that is severe, watery, and possibly bloody; severe abdominal pain or stomach cramps and pain; fever. These reactions may develop several weeks after you stop taking the medication.
- Persistent or severe diarrhea; in some uncommon cases, this could indicate the development of a serious bowel inflammation. Do not take an antidiarrheal medication unless the doctor recommends it.
- Dizziness or lightheadedness, joint pain, loss of appetite, seizures
- Symptoms of an allergic reaction, such as shortness of breath, skin rash, itching, or redness

Seek emergency care if you develop:

- Symptoms of a severe allergic reaction, such as increasing swelling of face, lips, or tongue or difficulty breathing

Warnings

- Take this medication only for the infection for which it has been prescribed. Do not share it with family members or friends.
- Take all the prescribed medication even if symptoms of the infection have cleared; otherwise, the infection may linger and reappear later.
- Contact your doctor if your con-

dition fails to improve—or if it worsens—over several days of treatment.

- As with all medications, it is important to mention medication allergies to your doctor. In the case of cephalosporin antibiotics, it is particularly critical to mention past allergic reactions to other cephalosporin or penicillin antibiotics.

- If you suffer from phenylketonuria (PKU), check with your doctor before taking the oral suspension form of cefprozil; it contains phenylalanine.

- Although alcohol does not cause a problem with cefprozil, other cephalosporin antibiotics should not be taken with (or within several days of taking) alcohol or alcohol-containing products. Ask your doctor or pharmacist for guidance.

- Use of this medication in patients with renal failure or those receiving diuretics may require close monitoring by a physician.

Tips and other important things to know

- Cephalosporin antibiotics are powerful medications, but they can fight only certain susceptible bacteria. They will have no impact on an infection caused by other organisms, such as viruses (as in the common cold), fungi, or parasites.

- If you have diabetes, be aware that the medication may cause false positive results with some tests for urine sugar.

Special precautions

- If you are pregnant or breast-feeding, discuss with your doctor the use of this medication *before* you start taking it.

Generic name Cefuroxime

Brand names include
Ceftin, Kefurox, Zinacef

Principal uses

Cefuroxime is prescribed for bacterial infections that affect the throat (such as bronchitis, tonsillitis, and pharyngitis), middle ear, skin, lungs, urinary tract, and other parts of the body. It is a second-generation cephalosporin antibiotic related to penicillin.

Administration

Follow prescribing information from the doctor and pharmacist. Also:

- Take cefuroxime with food to increase its absorption.

- If the tablet proves distasteful (it has a strong, bitter taste) or difficult to swallow, you may crush it and mix it with a small amount of soft food, such as pudding. Swallow—do not chew—this entire mixture right away. You may also mix it with a beverage, such as orange juice or chocolate milk.

- Store the suspension in the refrigerator. Shake it well before measuring out the dose. Discard any unused medication after 14 days.

- Cefuroxime is used in injection form for very serious infections. This form of administration is not discussed here.

If you miss a dose: Take the missed dose right away, unless it is almost time for the next dose, in which case you should skip the missed dose and resume the regular schedule. Do not take two doses at once.

Tips and other important things to know

- Certain types of cefuroxime contain sodium, an important consideration for people who are following sodium-restricted diets.

- Cefuroxime may alter the results of certain diagnostic tests. Make sure that all doctors treating you are aware that you take this medication.

See the *cefprozil* entry on page 1514 for more information on how second-generation cephalosporin medications work, what to expect in terms of speed and side effects, and when to contact the doctor if problems develop. (Unless otherwise noted, the information for *cefprozil* applies to all second-generation cephalosporin.)

Generic name Cephalexin
Brand names include
Keflex, Keftab

Principal uses

Cephalexin is prescribed for bacterial infections that affect the respiratory and urinary tracts, skin, joints, middle ear, and other body parts.

How does it work?

Cephalexin is a first-generation cephalosporin antibiotic related to penicillin. It stops susceptible bacteria from growing and reproducing by interfering with their ability to create new, protective cell walls.

Administration

Follow prescribing information from the doctor and pharmacist. Also:

- Take cephalexin on an empty stomach (1 hour before or 2 hours after eating) unless it upsets your stomach, in which case you should try taking it with food.

- Store the suspension in a tightly closed container in the refrigerator after mixing it. Discard any unused medication after 14 days.

If you miss a dose: Take the missed dose as soon as possible, unless it is almost time for the next dose, in which case you should skip the missed dose and resume the regular schedule. Do not take two doses at once.

How quickly will it take effect?

Cephalexin will reach peak concentrations in your system within 1 hour, but you will probably have to take it regularly for 3 to 5 days before noticing an improvement in your condition. This timing will also depend, in part, on the type and severity of your infection.

Side effects and severe reactions

Side effects that are generally of no concern unless they are persistent or severe include:

- Mild diarrhea or stomach cramps, nausea and vomiting, loss of appetite

Contact the doctor if any unusual, worrisome, or severe reactions occur or if you develop:

- Genital or anal itching, unusual vaginal discharge, headache, fatigue, agitation, confusion

- Symptoms of a mild allergic reaction, such as a skin rash, itching, redness, or hives

- Diarrhea that is severe, watery, or possibly bloody; severe abdominal pain; stomach cramps or pain; fever. These reactions may occur weeks after stopping the medication.

- Persistent or severe diarrhea, because in some uncommon cases it could indicate the development of serious colitis (bowel inflammation). Do not take an antidiarrheal medication unless the doctor recommends it.

- Symptoms of a new infection, possibly including creamy white patches in the mouth or vagina

- Seizures; decreased urine output; unusual bleeding; arthritis; joint pain; dizziness; loss of appetite; skin that is peeling, loose, or blistering

Seek emergency care if you develop:

- Symptoms of a severe allergic reaction, including possible swelling, trouble breathing, or severe skin rash, itching, hives, or redness

Warnings

- Take all the prescribed medication, even if symptoms of the infection have cleared; otherwise, the infection may linger and reappear later.

- Contact the doctor if your infection fails to improve—or if it worsens—within 3 to 5 days of starting this medication.

- Take this medication only for the infection for which it has been prescribed. Do not share it with family members or friends.

- As with all medications, it is important to tell your doctor about medication allergies. In the case of cephalosporin antibiotics, it is particularly important to mention past allergic reactions to other cephalosporin or penicillin antibiotics.

Tips and other important things to know

- Cephalosporin antibiotics are powerful medications, but they can fight only certain susceptible bacteria. They will have no impact on an infection caused by other organisms, such as viruses (as in the common cold), fungi, or parasites.

- If you have diabetes, be aware that cephalexin may cause false positive results with some tests for urine sugar.

Special precautions

- If you are pregnant or breast-feeding, discuss with your doctor the use of this medication *before* you start taking it.

Generic name Cerivastatin

Brand name Baycol

Principal uses

Cerivastatin is prescribed to lower high levels of cholesterol in the blood. This is done in an attempt to prevent heart complications of coronary artery disease associated with cholesterol-clogged blood vessels.

Administration

Follow prescribing information from the doctor and pharmacist. Also:

- Take this medicine exactly as prescribed. The dosage has been carefully tailored to you, based on your body's requirements and response. Do not take it in larger or smaller doses, more often, or for longer than recommended.

- Cerivastatin should be taken with food. Taking it in the evening enhances its effectiveness.

If you miss a dose on one day: Skip the missed dose and resume the regular schedule the next day. Do not take two doses at once.

Warnings

- Patients with moderate or severe kidney failure will need a lower dosage.

Tips and other important things to know

- Cerivastatin belongs to a class of medicines called statins. Medicines in this class may vary slightly in price, when they are best taken, the research they have been used in, the side effects they produce, and the amount of experience doctors have with them.

See the *simvastatin* entry for more information on how statins such as cerivastatin work, what to expect in terms of speed and side effects, and when to call the doctor if problems develop. (Unless otherwise noted, the information under *simvastatin* is common to all statins.)

Generic name Cimetidine

Brand names include Tagamet, Tagamet HB

Principal uses

Cimetidine is prescribed as a short-term treatment for active duodenal (intestinal) and gastric (stomach) ulcers and as a maintenance therapy to help prevent the recurrence of duodenal ulcers. Cimetidine is also prescribed to treat conditions involving excess stomach acid, to control gastroesophageal reflux disease (GERD; backflow of stomach contents), and to treat heartburn, sour stomach, and various other disorders.

Administration

Follow prescribing information from the doctor and pharmacist. Also:

- Cimetidine may be taken without regard to food.

- If you are taking an antacid, avoid canceling out cimetidine's effects by taking the antacid 2 to 3 hours before or after the cimetidine, unless your doctor recommends otherwise.

- Cimetidine is taken orally as well as given by injection. The injection form of administration is not discussed here.

Side effects and severe reactions

Contact the doctor if any unusual, worrisome, or severe reactions occur or if you develop:

- Mild transient diarrhea, dizziness, mild skin rash, headache, drowsiness

- Symptoms of blood complications: unusual bleeding or bruising, weakness, notable tiredness

Warnings

- Side effects with this medication are uncommon; however, there are rare but potentially life-threatening blood complications associated with the use of cimetidine. Discuss with your doctor any concerns you have.

- Do not take enteric-coated tablets with cimetidine, because the altered stomach acidity caused by cimetidine may make the tablet disintegrate before it is supposed to.

Tips and other important things to know

- Cimetidine was the first H_2 (gastric histamine) blocker on the American market. It is the least potent of the medications in this class.
- Cimetidine is available without a prescription.

See the *ranitidine* entry on page 1556 for more information on how H_2 blockers work, what to expect in terms of speed and side effects, and when to contact the doctor if problems develop. (Unless otherwise noted, the information for *ranitidine* applies to all H_2 blockers.)

Generic name
Ciprofloxacin

Brand name Cipro

Principal uses

Ciprofloxacin is prescribed for bacterial infections affecting the urinary tract, lower respiratory tract (including pneumonia and bronchitis), bone and joints, prostate, skin, and other parts of the body. It has been used to treat infectious diarrhea, gonorrhea, and typhoid fever. Ciprofloxacin is also available in injection form and as an eye solution, but neither of these is discussed here.

How does it work?

Ciprofloxacin is a fluoroquinolone antibiotic. It is believed to fight infection by interfering with bacteria's ability to replicate and multiply. Only certain bacteria are susceptible to it.

Administration

Follow prescribing information from the doctor and pharmacist. Also:

- Take this medication exactly as prescribed. Do not take more or less of it or take it for longer or less time than recommended. This is impor-

tant for avoiding unwanted reactions or a resurgence of the infection.

- Ciprofloxacin may be taken without regard to food.
- Take ciprofloxacin with a full glass (8 oz) of water and drink lots of fluids between doses.
- Do not drink milk or consume any other dairy products within 2 hours of taking this medication.
- Take ciprofloxacin at evenly spaced intervals throughout the day and try not to miss any doses so that the level of infection-fighting medication in your system remains constant.
- Avoid taking ciprofloxacin with antacids, calcium, or multivitamin or mineral supplements. Separate the doses of these substances from ciprofloxacin by at least 2 hours.

If you miss a dose: Take the missed dose as soon as possible, unless it is almost time for the next dose, in which case you should skip the missed dose and resume the regular schedule. Do not take two doses at once.

How quickly will it take effect?

Although this medication starts to fight infection quickly, it may take 1 to 2 weeks of regular use to bring the infection under good control, and possibly longer—4 weeks or more—in the case of joint or bone infections.

Side effects and severe reactions

Side effects that are generally of no concern unless they are persistent or severe include:

- Abdominal or stomach discomfort or pain, nausea or vomiting, mild diarrhea, dizziness, headache, lightheadedness, drowsiness, trouble sleeping

Contact the doctor if any unusual, worrisome, or severe reactions occur or if you develop:

- Severe sun reaction, blurred vision or other vision problems
- Symptoms of a new infection
- Seizures, hallucinations, agitation or confusion, shakiness or tremors, peeling skin, tendon rupture

Seek emergency care if you develop:

- Shortness of breath; skin rash, itching, or redness; swelling of the face, neck, lips, or tongue, unusual bleeding

Warnings

- Take all the prescribed medication, even if you feel better; otherwise, the bacteria may linger in your system and cause an infection later.
- Contact the doctor if your condition fails to improve—or if it worsens—after several days.
- Fluoroquinolone antibiotics are not recommended for use in pregnant or breast-feeding women and in infants, because studies indicate that they cause joint disease in immature animals. This antibiotic is also rarely prescribed in children and adolescents; however, as joint disease due to ciprofloxacin has not been observed in humans, more pediatricians are prescribing this drug.
- As with any medication, it is important to mention all your allergies to your doctor. In the case of fluoroquinolone antibiotics, this is particularly critical because of the risk of very severe allergic reactions.
- Take this medication only for the infection for which it has been prescribed. Do not share it with family members or friends.

Tips and other important things to know

- Fluoroquinolone antibiotics are powerful and often very effective medications. They work against only certain susceptible bacteria, however. They will not help fight infections caused by viruses (such as the common cold and flu), fungi, or parasites, for example.

Special precautions

- Until your reaction to this medication has been established, avoid activity that requires mental or physical alertness.
- If you are pregnant or breast-feeding, discuss with your doctor the use of this medication *before* you start taking it.

- This medication may increase sensitivity to the sun; discuss with your doctor what precautions are appropriate.

Generic name Cisapride

Brand name Propulsid

Principal uses

Cisapride is prescribed to treat nighttime heartburn caused by the backward flow of gastric acid into the esophagus, a condition known as gastroesophageal reflux disease (GERD). It is also a treatment for patients with gastroporesis (difficulty with stomach motility).

How does it work?

Cisapride increases the tone of the sphincter at the bottom of the esophagus, which normally prevents acid from leaking back up out of the stomach. Also, both liquids and solids are encouraged to move through the stomach more quickly.

Administration

Follow prescribing information from the doctor and pharmacist. Also:

- To help ensure a relatively constant rate of absorption of the medication into the gastrointestinal tract, take cisapride with a beverage at least 15 minutes before meals or at bedtime, unless directed otherwise by your doctor.

If you miss a dose: Take the missed dose as soon as possible, unless it is almost time for the next dose, in which case you should skip the missed dose and resume the regular schedule. Do not take two doses at once.

How quickly will it take effect?

Cisapride starts to work in approximately 30 to 60 minutes.

Side effects and severe reactions

Side effects that are generally of no concern unless they are persistent or severe include:

- Diarrhea, constipation, nausea, gas, abdominal cramping or pain, headache, unusual tiredness or weakness,

insomnia, runny nose, sinusitis, upper respiratory tract infection

Contact the doctor if any unusual, worrisome, or severe reactions occur or if you develop:

- Fever, symptoms of a urinary tract infection (increased urination, burning or stinging sensation when urinating)

Seek emergency care if you develop:

- Convulsions

Warnings

- Because of potentially serious interactions, it is particularly critical that you tell your doctor about all the medications you take, including over-the-counter ones.
- When you are taking this medication, alcohol may be absorbed more quickly than it normally would be; ask your doctor about the risks.

Tips and other important things to know

- A medication for nighttime heartburn should be considered only when other measures have failed. Your doctor should discuss poor diet, overeating, and other lifestyle habits that may be contributing to your condition.

Special precautions

- If you are pregnant or breast-feeding, discuss with your doctor the use of this medication *before* you start taking it.
- Ask your doctor about risks of taking this medication at the same time as alcohol or other central nervous system depressants (these slow down the nervous system).
- This medication has a number of potentially hazardous interactions. Discuss with your doctor all the medications you take—including over-the-counter ones—before taking this one.
- Until your reaction to this medication has been established, avoid activity that requires mental or physical alertness.

Generic name Clarithromycin

Brand name Biaxin

Principal uses

Clarithromycin is prescribed for bacterial infections that affect throat and tonsils (as in "strep throat" and tonsillitis), sinuses, skin, upper respiratory tract (as in bronchitis and pneumonia), skin, middle ear, and other body parts. It has also been used to help treat ulcers caused by the bacteria *Helicobacter pylori*. Clarithromycin belongs to a class of medications called macrolide antibiotics.

Administration

Follow prescribing information from the doctor and pharmacist. Also:

- For this medication to work properly, you must carefully follow prescription instructions regarding the spacing of doses and the number of days to take it.
- Clarithromycin may be taken without regard to food.
- Do not refrigerate the suspension made with granules. Shake it well before use. Discard any unused portion after 14 days.
- Take clarithromycin at the same time every day; this will help you remember to take it.

If you miss a dose: Take the missed dose right away unless it is within 4 hours of the next regularly scheduled dose. If this is the case, skip the missed dose and resume the regular schedule. Do not take two doses at once.

Warnings

- Clarithromycin should not be taken during pregnancy unless absolutely necessary, because of the risk of pregnancy complications and harm to the fetus.

See the *azithromycin* entry on page 1510 for more information on how macrolide antibiotics work, what to expect in terms of speed and side effects, and when to contact the doctor if problems develop. (Unless otherwise noted, the information for *azithromycin* applies to all macrolide antibiotics.)

Generic name Clonazepam

Brand name Klonopin

Principal uses

Clonazepam is used to prevent certain types of seizures, including petit mal seizures, and to suppress attacks of unwanted leg movements during sleep. It is also used for anxiety, panic attacks, and treatment of chronic pain. It has been prescribed for a variety of other disorders—mania, nerve pain, schizophrenia—although its value for these remains to be fully examined. Clonazepam belongs to a class of medications known as benzodiazepines.

Administration

Follow prescribing information from the doctor and pharmacist. Also:

- Take this medication exactly as prescribed. Do not stop taking it abruptly or in any way alter the dosage without specific instructions from your doctor. The dosage must be slowly and carefully adjusted.

- To help keep a constant level of this medication in your system and to prevent seizures (when this medication is taken for a seizure disorder), take clonazepam at the same time every day.

- Take clonazepam on an empty stomach (1 hour before or 2 hours after eating), unless it causes stomach upset, in which case you should try taking it with food.

- If you take antacids, separate the antacid dose from clonazepam by at least 1 hour to avoid problems with absorption of clonazepam.

- Clonazepam is also used in injection form, but this form of administration is not discussed here.

- Clonazepam will start to work within 20 to 60 minutes, with its effects lasting 6 to 8 hours in infants and young children and up to 12 hours in adults; thus, it is a long-acting benzodiazepine. Its usefulness in controlling a seizure disorder may take 2 to 3 weeks to determine, however.

If you miss a dose: Take the missed dose right away, unless it is already more than 1 hour past the time that you should have taken it, in which case you should skip the missed dose and resume the regular schedule. Do not take two doses at once.

Warnings

- Contact the doctor promptly if side effects develop.

- Follow the doctor's instructions carefully when you stop taking this medication. Stopping abruptly after long-term use increases the risk of withdrawal symptoms, such as tremors and vomiting, as well as status epilepticus, a condition of severe repeated seizures.

- Clonazepam may cause behavioral disturbances, particularly in children. These may include aggressiveness, agitation, irritability, and excessive movement. Contact the doctor if these types of reactions appear to be developing.

Tips and other important things to know

- The doctor should tell you exactly why he or she has prescribed this medication for you and discuss its associated risks and benefits.

- Clonazepam is usually prescribed for seizure disorders that have not responded to other anticonvulsants. It is commonly combined with other anticonvulsants. Make sure you know what to expect from all the medications you take.

- The doctor may recommend periodic dosage increases. This is to ensure that the medication continues to work for you in the same way.

- Talk to your doctor about wearing a medical alert bracelet or necklace that indicates that you take clonazepam to treat a seizure disorder.

- Check the prescription you get from the pharmacist to make sure you have been given the proper medication. Clonazepam's brand name *Klonopin*—sounds similar to the unrelated generic name medication, clonidine.

See the *alprazolam* entry on page 1504 for more information on how benzodiazepines work, what to expect in terms of speed and side effects, and when to contact the doctor if problems develop. (Unless otherwise noted, the information for *alprazolam* applies to all benzodiazepines.)

Generic name
Clotrimazole and Betamethasone

Brand name Lotrisone

Principal uses

This medication is prescribed to treat athlete's foot, jock itch, and other fungal skin infections.

How does it work?

This medication combines clotrimazole, an antifungal agent, with betamethasone, a corticosteroid ("steroid"). Clotrimazole damages or kills susceptible fungal cells by causing essential elements within the cells to leak out. Meanwhile, the betamethasone suppresses chemical and cellular reactions that cause inflammation, itching, redness, and other characteristic symptoms of fungal or inflammatory skin conditions.

Administration

Follow prescribing information from the doctor and pharmacist. Also:

- Gently massage the cream into the affected area.

- Particularly when treating an infection in the groin area, take care to apply the medication sparingly.

- This medication is for external use only. Never apply it to raw, broken, or otherwise damaged skin unless the doctor specifically advises you to do so.

- Never apply this medication in or around the eyes.

If you miss a dose: Apply the missed dose right away, unless it is almost time for the next dose, in which case you should skip the missed dose and resume the regular schedule.

How quickly will it take effect?

Redness and itching typically lessen within 3 to 5 days, although this depends in part on the body part being treated. For jock itch or general fungal skin infection, symptoms should lessen within 7 days; for athlete's foot, symptoms should lessen within 2 weeks.

Side effects and severe reactions

Contact the doctor if any unusual, worrisome, or severe reactions occur or if you develop:

- Abnormal sensations in the treated area, such as persistent burning, tickling, tingling, or prickling

- Evidence of a new rash, swelling, stinging, redness, blistering, intensive itching, cracking, fine reddish lines, irritation, dryness, or acnelike eruptions
- Symptoms of a new infection

Warnings

- Take the full course of this medication, even if your condition appears to be improving; otherwise, the infection may linger and resurface later.
- Take this medication exactly as prescribed to avoid unwanted reactions. Do not place it over larger amounts of your body than recommended or continue using it for longer than advised. Do not use occlusive dressing or cover the treated area with a tight bandage, tight-fitting diapers, plastic pants, or other wrapping that does not let oxygen circulate. Do not apply other steroids to the area unless specifically advised to do so. Doing these things could dangerously increase the steroid's potency and increase the risk that the medication will absorb into your system and cause complications.
- It is not appropriate to use this medication for more than 4 weeks.
- Take this medication only for the condition for which it has been prescribed.
- Take particular care in applying the exact dosage to children because they are more susceptible to toxic reactions due to systemic absorption of the medication.
- Never use this medication to treat diaper rash.

Tips and other important things to know

- This medication will not work for an infection caused by a bacteria or virus.
- Avoid reinfection by refraining from scratching itchy areas.
- Keep the affected area as cool and dry as possible. Shower frequently and wear fresh socks, underwear, or other undergarment in the affected area daily. Change quickly out of damp gym clothes.

- If you are treating the groin area, wear loose-fitting clothing so that the area can "breathe." Wear cotton underwear. Fight athlete's foot with well-ventilated shoes and socks made of cotton or another porous material.

Generic name Codeine with Acetaminophen

Brand name Tylenol with Codeine (Tylenol No. 3)

Principal uses

Codeine with acetaminophen is prescribed to treat moderate to moderately severe pain.

Administration

Follow prescribing information from the doctor and pharmacist. Also:

- Take this medication exactly as prescribed. Do not take it in larger doses, more frequently, or for longer periods of time than recommended. There is a risk of dependence (physically and psychologically habit forming), overdose, and liver damage in such cases.

If you miss a dose and normally take this medication regularly: Take the missed dose as soon as possible, unless it is almost time for the next dose, in which case you should skip the missed dose and resume the regular schedule. Do not take two doses at once.

Warnings

- People who have had allergic reactions to sulfites should not take the tablets, as they contain sodium metabisulfite.

See the *hydrocodone and acetaminophen* entry on page 1535 for more information on how narcotic (opioid) analgesic and acetaminophen combination medications work, what to expect in terms of speed and side effects, and when to contact the doctor if problems develop. (Unless otherwise noted, the information for *hydrocodone and acetaminophen* applies to all narcotic [opioid] analgesic and acetaminophen combinations.)

Generic name Digoxin

Brand names include
Lanoxicaps, Lanoxin

Principal uses

Digoxin is prescribed for congestive heart failure and to help prevent and control certain heart rhythm disorders.

How does it work?

Digoxin strengthens the heart and enables it to work more efficiently. It encourages the weakened heart to pump more forcefully and helps regulate the heartbeat by changing the way in which electrical signals are carried through the heart muscle. As a result, heart function improves in people with some kinds of heart problems. Digoxin is also used in injection form, but this form of administration is not discussed here.

Administration

Follow prescribing information from the doctor and pharmacist. Also:

- Take digoxin at the same time every day; this will help you remember to take it.
- Digoxin may be taken without regard to food.

If you miss a dose: Take the missed dose right away if you remember within 12 hours of when you should have taken it. If it is later than 12 hours after the missed dose, skip that dose and resume the regular schedule. Do not take two doses at once. Contact your doctor if you miss 2 days or more of digoxin treatment.

How quickly will it take effect?

You will likely have to take digoxin for 7 to 10 days before the doctor can determine how effectively it is controlling your heart failure or heart rhythm disorder.

Side effects and severe reactions

Contact the doctor if any unusual, worrisome, or severe reactions occur or if you develop:

- Skin rash, hives
- Possible symptoms of overdose, in the order they may develop: loss of appetite, nausea or vomiting, pain in the lower stomach, diarrhea,

unusual tiredness or extreme weakness, notably uneven or slow heartbeat (below 60 beats per minute; may actually be rapid in children), blurred vision or yellow-green halos around visual images, drowsiness, confusion, mental depression, headache, fainting

Warnings

- Keep taking this medication exactly as prescribed, even if you are feeling well.

- Do not change the dose you take—increase it, decrease it, or in any other way alter it—without specific instructions from your doctor.

- Do not switch brands unless the doctor specifically recommends it; brands may differ in important ways.

- The dose at which this medication is toxic is very close to the dose at which it is beneficial. Stay alert for symptoms of an overdose (see above under *Contact the doctor ...*).

- Changes in pulse rate, rhythm, or force may signal the development of side effects. Ask your doctor for guidance on checking your own pulse daily and contacting him or her if needed.

- As with many medications, it is important not to mix this one with others without confirming that there are no dangerous interactions. Check with your doctor or pharmacist before taking any other medication—including a nonprescription one—with digoxin.

Tips and other important things to know

- Keep all appointments for follow-up visits so your doctor can monitor your condition and response to this medication. He or she may order periodic blood tests while you take digoxin to determine, among other things, whether you are taking the proper dosage.

- Seniors may be particularly sensitive to the effects of digoxin.

Special precautions

- If you are pregnant or breast-feeding, discuss with your doctor the use of this medication *before* you start taking it.

- This medication has a great number of potentially hazardous interactions. Discuss with your doctor all the medications you take—including over-the-counter ones—before taking this one.

- Wearing a medical alert bracelet/necklace is advised.

Generic name Diltiazem

Brand names include
Cardizem, Dilacor

Principal uses

Diltiazem is prescribed to treat hypertension (high blood pressure) and to manage certain types of angina pectoris (chest pain). In injection form, it is used to control arrhythmias (irregular heartbeats). Diltiazem belongs to a class of medications known as calcium channel blockers.

Administration

Follow prescribing information from the doctor and pharmacist. Also:

- Never abruptly stop taking this medication if you have been taking it regularly. The dosage must be gradually reduced or your condition may worsen. Your doctor will guide you about tapering the dose.

- Take diltiazem tablets before meals and at bedtime or as otherwise prescribed. The dual-release capsules (Cardizem CD) may be taken without regard to meals. The extended-release capsules should be taken on an empty stomach (1 hour before or 2 hours after a meal). Preparations that need to be taken 3 times a day are rarely used.

- In addition to oral forms of diltiazem (tablets, extended-release capsules, sustained-release capsules), there is an injection form. The injection form of administration is not discussed here.

If you miss a dose: Take the missed dose immediately, unless it is within 8 hours of the next dose, in which case you should skip the missed dose and resume the regular schedule. Do not take two doses at once.

Warnings

- Of all the calcium channel blockers, diltiazem is the most likely to cause appetite loss and nausea. Other more serious adverse reactions include the development of heart block, slow heartbeat, fluid retention, and congestive heart failure.

- Never switch brands without discussing this with your doctor; the dosing schedule is different for the various brands currently available.

- Nitroglycerin or other nitrate medications may cause dizziness during diltiazem treatment. Discuss this reaction with your doctor; it is important to keep taking the diltiazem in most cases.

- Diltiazem passes into breast milk and in most cases should not be used while breast-feeding.

Tips and other important things to know

- The adverse reactions most commonly cited as reasons for stopping the medication include gastrointestinal upset, slow heartbeat, and skin eruptions.

- Your doctor will probably show you how to take your pulse and recommend taking it at certain times and calling if it drops to a certain level. A standard recommendation is to contact the doctor if the heartbeat drops below 50 beats per minute.

See the *amlodipine* entry on page 1506 for more information on how calcium channel blockers work, what to expect in terms of time of onset and side effects, and when to contact the doctor if problems develop. (Unless otherwise noted, the information for *amlodipine* applies to all calcium channel blockers.)

Generic name Doxazosin

Brand name Cardura

Principal uses

Doxazosin is prescribed to manage hypertension (high blood pressure). It is also used to treat benign prostatic hyperplasia, an enlargement of the gland surrounding the urinary canal in men, and associated complications, such as weak urine flow and frequent urination. Doxazosin belongs to a class of medications called alpha₁ blockers.

Administration

Follow prescribing information from the doctor and pharmacist. Also:

- The dosage must be increased gradually to avoid unwanted reactions.

- Doxazosin may be taken without regard to food.

- Take doxazosin at the same time every day; this will help you remember to take it.

Side effects and severe reactions

Side effects that are generally of no concern unless they are persistent or severe include:

- Nervousness, restlessness, unusual irritability, and runny nose. These reactions tend to dissipate as your body adjusts to the medication.

See the *terazosin* entry on page 1560 for more information on how alpha₁ blockers work, what to expect in terms of time of onset and side effects, and when to contact the doctor if problems develop. (Unless otherwise noted, the information for *terazosin* applies to all alpha₁ blockers.)

Generic name Enalapril

Brand name Vasotec

Principal uses

Enalapril is prescribed to manage hypertension (high blood pressure), to control the symptoms of congestive heart failure, and to treat a type of heart dysfunction. Some people with diabetes take it to help prevent worsening of kidney damage.

How does it work?

Enalapril is an angiotensin converting enzyme (ACE) inhibitor. This class of medications can significantly lower blood pressure by blocking the body's formation of angiotensin II, a chemical that leads to the constriction of blood vessels and increased blood pressure. ACE inhibitors also reduce the retention of salt and water. Other ACE inhibitors include *benazepril, lisinopril,* and *quinapril,* among others.

Administration

Follow prescribing information from the doctor and pharmacist. Also:

- Do not change the dosage on your own; your doctor has tailored it carefully to meet your body's response to this medication.

- Enalapril may be taken without regard to food.

- Take enalapril at the same time every day; this will help you remember to take it.

If you miss a dose: Take the missed dose as soon as possible, unless it is almost time for the next dose, in which case you should skip the missed dose and resume the regular schedule. Do not take two doses at once.

How quickly will it take effect?

Enalapril reduces blood pressure within 1 hour. The greatest lowering effect occurs at 4 to 6 hours. It may take several weeks of treatment for your blood pressure to reach an optimal level, however.

Side effects and severe reactions

Side effects that are generally of no concern unless they are persistent or severe include:

- A cough that is dry, tickling, and nonproductive

- Headache, diarrhea, nausea, and unusual tiredness; these are less common

Contact the doctor if any unusual, worrisome, or severe reactions occur or if you develop:

- Loss of taste, dizziness, lightheadedness, fainting, joint pain, skin rash, itching

- Symptoms of excessive potassium levels, including confusion, nervousness, difficulty breathing or shortness of breath, numbness or tingling in the hands, feet, or lips

- Symptoms of infection, such as fever, chills, and sore throat, all of which may indicate a lowered white blood cell count (white blood cells fight infection)

Seek emergency care if you develop:

- Symptoms of a serious allergic reaction, including sudden trouble in swallowing or breathing, hoarseness, or swelling of the face, tongue, lips, throat, mouth, or extremities

Warnings

- ACE inhibitors must be taken regularly and as prescribed to function as intended. Keep this in mind even if you feel well; high blood pressure causes few recognizable symptoms but can cause considerable harm.

- ACE inhibitors should not be taken during pregnancy, especially after the first 3 months of gestation, as they can cause serious harm or even death to the fetus. Report a pregnancy to your doctor immediately.

- Always report lightheadedness to your doctor. This common side effect, particularly notable in the first few days of starting the medication, can often be minimized with a dosage adjustment. Change the dosage only under your doctor's advice, however.

- Your blood pressure may drop too low while you are taking an ACE inhibitor if you start to perspire excessively, get dehydrated, or develop an illness with vomiting or diarrhea. Lightheadedness and fainting may occur. Similar symptoms can occur when a diuretic is added to an ACE inhibitor. Consult your doctor if you suspect your fluid volume has dropped significantly in these or any other ways.

- ACE inhibitors may worsen kidney function, especially if you already have kidney disease. If this is a concern, your doctor will check your kidney function with a blood test before starting the medication and while you are taking it.

- As with many medications, it is important to consult your doctor before taking others, including over-the-counter ones. This is particularly true with ACE inhibitors. Be sure to ask about preparations for treating colds.

- If you are taking an ACE inhibitor, avoid potassium supplements, sodium substitutes (many contain potassium), and low-salt milk unless your doctor recommends otherwise. These substances may lead to dangerously high levels of potassium in your blood.

Tips and other important things to know

- ACE inhibitors, such as enalapril, will help keep your blood pressure down but will not cure you of hypertension.

- Discuss with your doctor lifestyle measures you can take to lower your blood pressure, such as weight control, moderate exercise, and a healthy diet.

- Keep all appointments for follow-up visits so that your doctor can monitor you and check for unwanted reactions to the medication. He or she will likely perform periodic blood tests to ensure that your kidney functions and potassium levels are normal.

- To minimize dizziness or lightheadedness that you may experience, get up gradually from a sitting or lying position.

- When prescribed for high blood pressure, enalapril may be given alone or with a diuretic to counteract fluid retention.

- If you have been taking a diuretic, the doctor may advise you to stop taking that medication 2 to 3 days before starting the ACE inhibitor. This is to reduce the risk of very low blood pressure.

- If you have been prescribed other medications to take with an ACE inhibitor, be sure to get an overall picture from your doctor about what side effects to expect.

Special precautions

- If you are pregnant or breast-feeding, discuss with your doctor the use of this medication *before* you start taking it.

- This medication has a number of potentially hazardous interactions. Discuss with your doctor all the medications you take—including over-the-counter ones—*before* taking this one.

Generic name
Erythromycin

Brand names include E-Base, E-Mycin, Eryc, Ery-Tab, PCE, Robimycin

Principal uses

Erythromycin is prescribed for bacterial infections that affect the pelvis, genitals, urinary tract, intestines, respiratory tract, skin, and other parts of the body. It is used to treat syphilis, gonorrhea, and chlamydia and to prevent endocarditis (an inflammation of the heart lining) before dental procedures. The topical solution and ointment are prescribed for inflammatory acne. The eye ointment is instilled in the eyes of newborns to prevent infection. Erythromycin belongs to a class of medications known as macrolide antibiotics.

Administration

Follow prescribing information from the doctor and pharmacist. Also:

- Take the oral form of erythromycin with a full glass of water on an empty stomach (1 hour before or 2 hours after eating); food decreases the rate at which the medication is absorbed. The exception to this is the enteric-coated tablets, which are specially designed so that they can be taken with food.

- Be sure to chew the chewable tablets. Do not swallow them whole.

- When using the topical solutions, wash, rinse, and dry the affected area before applying the medication. Do not apply the solution near the eyes, nose, mouth, or other mucous membranes. Avoid sharing towels and washcloths.

- When using the eye ointment, first wash your hands well and clean away any excess pus or other material. Do not actually touch the eye or surrounding tissue with the applicator tube.

- Store the oral liquid form of erythromycin in the refrigerator to help preserve its taste.

- Erythromycin is taken orally as well as given by injection. The injection form of administration is not discussed here.

If you miss a dose: Take it as soon as possible, unless it is almost time for the next dose, in which case you should evenly space out the next two doses over the next 4 to 6 hours and then resume the regular schedule.

Side effects and severe reactions

Contact the doctor if any unusual, worrisome, or severe reactions occur or if you develop:

- When using the eye ointment: itchy eyelids, continuous burning sensations, or other indications of possible sensitivity to the ointment

- Hearing loss from the oral form. This hearing loss is reversible and mainly occurs in people with kidney problems.

Tips and other important things to know

- Erythromycin may alter the results of certain diagnostic tests. Make sure that all your doctors are aware that you are take this medication.

- Topical forms of erythromycin sometimes cause dryness and itching. Less commonly, they cause irritation, peeling, oily skin, burning, redness, hives, and other sensitivity reactions.

- If you are taking the topical form of erythromycin for acne, be aware that it may take up to 12 weeks to see the medication's fullest benefit.

Special precautions

- If you are pregnant or breast-feeding, discuss with your doctor the use of this medication *before* you start taking it.

See the *azithromycin* entry on page 1510 for more information on how macrolide antibiotics work, what to expect in terms of speed and side effects, and when to contact the doctor if problems develop. (Unless otherwise noted, the information for *azithromycin* applies to all macrolide antibiotics.)

Generic name Estrogen

Brand names include
Estraderm, Premarin

Principal uses

Estrogen is prescribed for such menopausal symptoms as dizziness, hot flashes, and vaginal dryness and to reduce the risk of heart disease because the medication has a beneficial effect on cholesterol levels. It is also used for ovarian failure and inadequate ovarian function, to prevent osteoporosis, to manage metastatic breast cancer in post-menopausal women, and, in men, to treat advanced prostate cancer. Estrogen creams for vaginal dryness and transdermal patches designed to deliver set amounts of estrogen are available.

How does it work?

Estrogens are naturally produced by a woman's ovaries. There are six naturally occurring estrogens. They are responsible for, among other things, producing female sexual characteristics and promoting the development of the female reproductive system and the growth of the vagina, uterus, and other organs. Estrogens also have numerous metabolic effects. Estrogen levels naturally drop after menopause.

Since the discovery of estrogen in human and animal urine in 1930, various synthetic versions have been created. Estrogens that are taken as supplements mimic the action of natural estrogen. When taken as directed, certain estrogens slow the progression of postmenopausal osteoporosis. They do this by enhancing the retention of critical minerals—calcium and phosphate—in the bones and by halting bone loss. Except for conjugated estrogen and estrogenic substances, which are usually obtained from the urine of pregnant mares, estrogens are manufactured in the laboratory. Estradiol (for example, Estraderm) is a commonly used estrogen. Estrogens given by injection are not discussed here. Estrogens are combined with other hormones for birth control; see *Estrogen and Progestin* on page 1526.

Administration

Follow prescribing information from the doctor and pharmacist. Also:

- Oral estrogens are typically administered in cycles.

- The doctor should describe how to apply the cream to the vagina. Look for package instructions as well.

- The transdermal patch is typically applied to the trunk of the body twice a week. Do not apply it to the

breasts. Wait for at least 1 week to reuse the same skin area.

- If you have not had a hysterectomy (surgical removal of the uterus), estrogen is usually given in combination with a progesterone combination.

If you miss a dose: Take the missed dose as soon as possible, unless it is almost time for the next dose, in which case you should skip the missed dose and resume the regular schedule. Do not take two doses at once.

How quickly will it take effect?

Although you may start to feel the effects of estrogen within 1 or 2 days, it may take 1 or more weeks for menopausal symptoms to respond fully. The time it takes to work varies widely among people.

Side effects and severe reactions

Side effects that are generally of no concern unless they are persistent or severe include:

- Nausea. This typically disappears with long-term therapy. Nausea may be reduced by taking the medication with meals or at bedtime (if only one dose a day is taken). Vomiting may also occur.

Contact the doctor if any unusual, worrisome, or severe reactions occur or if you develop:

- Bloated feeling, abdominal pain or swelling, breast swelling and tenderness, secretions from the breast, weight gain, loss of appetite, sun sensitivity, loss of libido, headache, changes in normal menstrual bleeding pattern, intolerance of contact lenses, increased problems with such long-term eyesight conditions as myopia, depression, fluid retention. A number of these reactions are not serious, but report any of them so that your doctor can make an individualized judgment.

- Abdominal pain, leg or buttock pain, numbness or stiffness in any part of the body, chest pain or pressure, pain in the calves or chest, sudden shortness of breath, coughing up of blood, severe headache, dizziness, faintness, unexpected vaginal

bleeding or discharge, flashing lights or other visual disturbances, yellowing of the skin or white of the eye, pale stools, dark urine, breast lumps, seizures

Seek emergency care if you develop:

- Signs or symptoms of a blood clot, a rare but very serious occurrence that requires immediate medical attention: coughing up blood; unexplained or sudden shortness of breath; severe headache; pain in the groin, chest, or leg (particularly the calf); loss of coordination; slurring of speech; sudden loss or change in vision; unexplained weakness or numbness or pain in an arm or leg; or abdominal or stomach pain that is sudden, severe, or persistent

Warnings

- Discuss with your doctor the risks of taking estrogen, especially of long-term use, which has been linked to increased rates of endometrial cancer, breast cancer (possibly), blood clotting disorders, and gallbladder disease. A complete personal and family medical history is important. Read the patient's package insert.

- If you become pregnant while taking birth control pills or estrogen therapy in any form, immediately stop taking the medication and contact your doctor for guidance.

- The risk of potentially fatal clots is markedly increased in women who smoke cigarettes, especially if they are over age 35.

- Estrogen poses particular risks to people with diabetes. If you have diabetes, discuss the effects of estrogen on your condition.

Tips and other important things to know

- Keep all appointments for follow-up visits so that your doctor can monitor your condition and reaction to this medication.

- Estrogen products are largely interchangeable, differing in the specific type of estrogen they contain, their source, the dose required, and in some cases the part of the body they affect.

- The hormone progestin is often added to estrogen replacement therapy to reduce the risk of abnormal changes in the uterine lining that can lead to cancer.

- Your doctor should show you how to perform a monthly breast self-examination (see Chapter 19).

- Men taking estrogens may develop breast enlargement or erectile dysfunction (impotence) that disappears when the medication is stopped.

- If you are taking estrogen for post-menopausal symptoms, remember that the bleeding you may experience during the week in which you take no estrogen does not mean you are ovulating. You cannot conceive.

- No data indicate that estrogen therapy reduces depression or nervousness associated with menopause.

- Estrogen may alter the results of certain diagnostic tests. Make sure that all doctors treating you are aware that you take this medication.

Special precautions

- If you are pregnant or breast-feeding, discuss with your doctor the use of this medication *before* you start taking it.

Generic name Estrogen and Medroxyprogesterone

Brand names include Premphase, Prempro

Principal uses

This estrogen replacement therapy is used to alleviate such menopausal symptoms as dizziness, hot flashes, and vaginal dryness; to reduce the risk of heart disease, because the medication has a beneficial effect on cholesterol levels; and to help prevent osteoporosis (bone thinning) and associated bone fractures.

How does it work?

This medication combines the hormones estrogen (conjugated) and medroxyprogesterone (a derivative of progesterone). When taken in supplement form, these hormones replace those that a woman's body produces less of due to menopause. Estrogen and medroxyprogesterone are also taken by women who have had their hormone-producing ovaries removed. This combination of medications is used for women who have their hormone producing ovaries but not their uterus removed.

Administration

Follow prescribing information from the doctor and pharmacist. Also:

- This medication may be taken without regard to food. Try taking it with food if it upsets your stomach, however.

If you miss a dose: Take the missed dose as soon as possible, unless it is almost time for the next dose, in which case you should skip the missed dose and resume the regular schedule. Do not take two doses at once.

How quickly will it take effect?

Although you may start to feel the effects of this medication within 1 or 2 days, it may take 1 or more weeks for menopausal symptoms to respond fully. The time it takes to work varies widely among people.

Side effects and severe reactions

Contact the doctor if any unusual, worrisome, or severe reactions occur or if you develop:

- Vaginal bleeding; this is common initially. You should report to your doctor the initial bleeding and any bleeding that persists for 2 months or more.

- Breast lump, yellowing of the skin or eyes, abdominal pain or tenderness, nausea, vomiting, enlargement of benign tumors ("fibroids") of the uterus, change in the amount of cervical secretions, fluid retention, changes in sex drive, spotty darkening of the skin, depression, hair loss, abnormal hairiness, unexpected weight changes

- Symptoms of a possible blood clot: sudden shortness of breath, pains in the calves or chest, coughing up of blood, severe headache or vomiting, faintness, dizziness, unexpected changes in speech or vision, weakness or numbness of an extremity.

Seek emergency care if you develop:

- Symptoms of pulmonary embolus or thrombophlebitis (shortness of breath, chest pain, coughing up blood, and persistent leg pain or swelling

Warnings

- Your doctor should carefully review with you the risks and benefits associated with taking this medication or any other estrogen replacement regimen.

- Certain groups of women are not typically prescribed this medication. These include women who have had cancer of the breast or uterus, women who have circulation problems, women who have had their uterus surgically removed (a hysterectomy), and women who have unusual vaginal bleeding that has not been medically evaluated. Your doctor will make a professional judgment about this medication's safety and potential for you on the basis of your personal and family medical history.

- One of the reasons that progestins are given along with estrogen is to minimize a risk associated with taking estrogen alone: the development of abnormal changes in the uterine lining, which can lead to cancer (endometrial cancer). Although progestin does not eliminate this risk, it does significantly reduce it. Your doctor should review these issues with you.

- If you become pregnant while taking this medication, immediately stop taking it and contact your doctor for guidance; it increases the risk of birth defects. The use of this hormone combination to test for pregnancy or prevent miscarriage is outdated and dangerous.

- The risk of potentially fatal clots is markedly increased in women who smoke cigarettes, especially if they are over age 35.

- The estrogen in this medication poses particular risks to people with diabetes. If you have diabetes, discuss with your doctor the effects of estrogen on your condition.

Tips and other important things to know

- Keep all appointments for follow-up visits so your doctor can monitor your condition and reaction to this medication.

- Your doctor should show you how to perform a monthly breast self-examination to check for the development of breast lumps while taking this medication (see Chapter 19).

- No data indicate that estrogen replacement therapy reduces depression or nervousness associated with menopause.

- This medication may alter the results of certain diagnostic tests. Make sure all your doctors are aware that you take it.

Special precautions

- If you are pregnant or breast-feeding, discuss with your doctor the use of this medication *before* you start taking it.

Generic name Estrogen and Progestin

Brand names include
Lo/Ovral, Ortho-Novum 7/7/7, Triphasil

Principal uses

The combination of estrogen and progestin is taken to prevent pregnancy.

How does it work?

This type of oral contraceptive contains two synthetic female hormones, estrogen and progestin. Estrogen inhibits the release of follicle stimulating hormone (FSH), the hormone active in the first half of the menstrual cycle and responsible for ovulation. Progestin functions as something of a backup mechanism, inhibiting ovulation by interfering with the release of luteinizing hormone (LH) in the second half of the menstrual cycle. Progestin also thickens the mucus in the cervix, making travel in the vagina more difficult for sperm, and causes alterations in the lining of the uterus that inhibit implantation of a fertilized egg.

The different types of oral contraceptives vary in the amount of estrogen and progestin they provide. So-called single-phase (or one-phase) products deliver a fixed amount of progestin and estrogen throughout the month (the cycle). Two-phase combinations deliver a varying amount of progestin (first an increase and then a decrease) with a low-level, steady amount of estrogen. Three-phase products deliver an even more varying pattern of progestin, whereas estrogen levels remain very low but steady. Oral contraceptives that contain only progestin are also available, but they are not discussed here.

Administration

Follow prescribing information from the doctor and pharmacist. Also:

- Keep the medication in its original container.

- Take the medication at the same time each day—at 24-hour intervals—to ensure constant medication levels in your system that protect you from pregnancy.

- If nausea is a problem, try taking the medication with food or directly after eating. Taking the medication at night may also reduce nausea or headaches.

If you miss a dose and you are normally on a 20-, 21-, or 24-day dosing schedule for one-phase or two-phase combination: Take the missed dose as soon as possible. If it is already the next day, take two tablets and continue the regular schedule. If you miss 2 days of the medication in a row, take two tablets a day for the next 2 days, then resume the regular schedule. If you miss taking this medication for 3 days in a row, stop taking the medication and use another form of contraception until your menstrual period starts or you confirm that you are not pregnant. Start a new cycle of tablets.

If you miss a dose and you are on a 28-day dosing schedule for one-phase or two-phase combination: Follow the above instructions. If the dose you miss is one of the last seven tablets of the cycle, however, take the first tablet of the next month's cycle on the regularly scheduled day.

If you miss a dose and you are normally on a 21-day dosing cycle for three-phase cycles: Take the missed dose as soon as possible. If you remember about the missed dose only the next day, take two tablets at the same time and continue on the regular schedule. Use an additional form of contraception until the end of the cycle, however. If you miss two doses in a row, take two tablets a day for 2 days and then continue the regular schedule while using an additional form of contraception until the end of the cycle. If you miss three doses, stop taking the medication and use another form of contraception until your menstrual period begins or you confirm that you are not pregnant. Start a new cycle of tablets.

If you miss a dose and you are on a 28-day dosing schedule for three-phase cycles: Follow the above instructions. If the dose you miss is one of the last seven tablets of the cycle, however, take the first tablet of the next month's cycle on the regularly scheduled day.

How quickly will it take effect?

This medication will not begin to protect you from pregnancy until you have taken it for at least 7 days.

Side effects and severe reactions

Side effects that are generally of no concern unless they are persistent or severe include:

- Acne, nausea, mild headache, stomach bloating, cramps in the lower stomach, appetite changes, breast tenderness and swelling, weight gain (not sudden), unusual tiredness or weakness, vaginal spotting and breakthrough bleeding. Many of these side effects should lessen after 3 to 6 months (or dosing cycles).

Contact the doctor if any unusual, worrisome, or severe reactions occur or if you develop:

- Unexpected changes in vaginal bleeding patterns; fainting; increased blood pressure; painful urination or frequent need to urinate; such skin irritations as rash or redness; vaginal itching or irritation; vaginal discharge that is thick, white, or curdlike; yellowing of eyes or skin; lumps in the breast or discharge from them; depression; stomach or abdominal pain or tenderness

Seek emergency care if you develop:

- Symptoms of a blood clot, a rare but very serious occurrence that requires immediate medical attention: coughing up blood; unexplained or sudden shortness of breath; severe headache; pain in the groin, chest or leg (particularly the calf); loss of coordination; slurring of speech; sudden loss of or change in vision; unexplained weakness, numbness, or pain in an arm or leg; or abdominal or stomach pain that is sudden, severe, or persistent

Warnings

- Use an additional form of birth control during the first week of treatment.

- If you suspect that you have become pregnant while taking this medication, stop taking it and contact the doctor right away. Progestin has been linked to birth defects when taken early in pregnancy.

- In rare cases, oral contraceptives cause serious conditions, such as blood clots, heart attack and stroke, noncancerous liver tumors, liver cancer, and uterine and gallbladder problems. Your doctor should discuss these risks with you.

- A number of medications may interfere with the pregnancy protection that estrogen and progestin provide. These include *ampicillin, phenylbutazone, rifampin, griseofulvin, oral neomycin, tetracycline,* and *valproic acid,* among others. Ask your doctor for guidance.

- Oral contraceptives do not protect you from venereal or sexually transmitted diseases, including acquired immunodeficiency syndrome (AIDS).

- Your doctor should discuss with you the risks of cigarette smoking while taking oral contraceptives, which include potential heart and circulation problems. The risks are particularly high among heavy smokers over age 35.

Tips and other important things to know

- Read the patient information sheet that comes with the medication. This will contain important information regarding the particular type of oral contraceptive you are taking.

- Keep all appointments for follow-up visits scheduled every 6 and 12 months so that your doctor can monitor your condition and reac-

tion to this medication. Annual gynecologic exams and Papanicolaou (Pap) tests are particularly important while taking estrogen and progestin.

- Ask your doctor about when it is safe to try to get pregnant after stopping an oral contraceptive and about potential delays that may occur. Waiting 2 months after stopping to try to get pregnant is standard.

- Weigh yourself twice a week and contact the doctor if your weight changes suddenly or if you notice swelling.

- Take extra care to keep the vaginal area clean; changes the medication causes in the texture of the cervical mucus increases susceptibility to infection.

- If you wear contact lenses and notice a change in their effectiveness or experience discomfort while wearing them, contact the doctor for guidance. Your prescription may need to be adjusted.

- Oral contraceptives may alter the results of a number of diagnostic tests. Make sure all the doctors and dentists who treat you, including those treating you in an emergency or performing surgery, are aware that you take contraceptive pills.

- Ask your dentist about the need to take particularly good care of your teeth while you are taking oral contraceptives. You may be more likely to develop tenderness, swelling, or bleeding of the gums.

- Keep an extra 1-month supply on hand.

Special precautions

- This medication may increase sensitivity to the sun; discuss with your doctor what precautions are appropriate.

- If you are pregnant or breast-feeding, discuss with your doctor the use of this medication *before* you start taking it.

- This medication has a number of potentially hazardous interactions. Discuss with your doctor all the medications you take—including over-the-counter ones—before taking this one.

Generic name Etodolac
Brand name Lodine

Principal uses

Etodolac is prescribed to control pain and to manage acute and chronic osteoarthritis and rheumatoid arthritis.

How does it work?

Etodolac belongs to a class of medications called nonsteroidal anti-inflammatory drugs (NSAIDs). Although much about how these medication work remains unclear, they are believed to help reduce pain, inflammation, and fever by interfering with the synthesis of chemicals in your system called prostaglandins.

Administration

Follow prescribing information from the doctor and pharmacist. Also:

- Etodolac may be taken without regard to food. If it causes stomach upset, try taking it with a meal or an antacid.

- Drink a full glass of water with the tablet or capsule and avoid lying down for the next 15 to 30 minutes.

- Follow prescription instructions exactly—do not take more or less than recommended—to ensure that it works for you and to avoid unwanted reactions.

If you miss a dose: If you normally take several doses a day, take the missed dose as soon as possible, unless it is within 4 hours of the next scheduled dose, in which case you should skip the missed dose and resume the regular schedule. If you normally only take one dose a day, take the missed dose as soon as possible if you remember it within 8 hours of when you should have taken it. Otherwise, skip the missed dose and resume the regular schedule. Do not take two doses at once.

How quickly will it take effect?

You will likely feel some relief from pain within 30 minutes, with a peak effect occurring in 1 to 2 hours and overall pain relief lasting 4 to 6 hours. Some arthritis symptoms may continue, depending on the type of joint problem being treated.

Side effects and severe reactions

Side effects that are generally of no concern unless they are persistent or severe include:

- Minor stomach upset, diarrhea, gas, nausea, constipation

Contact the doctor if any unusual, worrisome, or severe reactions occur or if you develop:

- Persistent stomach pain or upset or other worrisome gastrointestinal symptoms, as they may indicate bleeding, ulcers, or other serious problems. Minor stomach upset is common during the first few days of treatment, however.

- Malaise, weakness, dizziness, depression, nervousness, unusual weight gain or fluid retention (swelling), hallucinations, blurred vision or other visual disturbances, ringing in the ears, urination problems, persistent headache, chills or fever

Seek emergency care if you develop:

- Black or tarry stools or signs of bleeding

- Fever

- Signs of violent drug reaction

Warnings

- Toxic reactions in the gastrointestinal tract, from bleeding to ulcers and perforation, can occur at any time and without warning when you take an NSAID, especially for prolonged periods.

- Although toxic gastrointestinal reactions can occur in anyone, certain people are at greater risk: Older people who have had peptic ulcer disease or those prone to stomach ulcer problems because of smoking or alcohol use, for example.

Tips and other important things to know

- Stop the medication and call the doctor if severe side effects set in.

- If you take this medication regularly, keep all appointments for follow-up visits so that your doctor can properly monitor your condition and

check for unwanted reactions to the medication.

- Etodolac may alter the results of certain laboratory tests; be sure all doctors who treat you are aware that you take this medication.

Special precautions

- If you are pregnant or breast-feeding, discuss with your doctor the use of this medication *before* you start taking it.

- Until your reaction to this medication has been established, avoid activity that requires mental or physical alertness.

Generic name Famotidine

Brand names include Pepcid, Pepcid AC

Principal uses

Famotidine is prescribed for short periods of time to treat active duodenal (intestinal) and gastric (stomach) ulcers and for longer periods of time to help prevent duodenal ulcers. Famotidine is also prescribed for conditions involving excess stomach acid and to control gastroesophageal reflux disease (GERD; backflow of stomach contents). Many people take it to prevent and treat heartburn (Pepcid AC only). Famotidine belongs to a class of medications known as H_2 (gastric histamine) blockers.

Low-dose famotidine tablets are available without a prescription. Famotidine is also given by injection, but this form of administration is not discussed here.

Administration

Follow prescribing information from the doctor and pharmacist. Also:

- Famotidine may be taken without regard to food.

- Famotidine is commonly taken at bedtime.

- Before measuring out a dose of the oral suspension, shake it vigorously for 5 to 10 seconds. Discard any constituted (mixed with liquid) suspension after 30 days.

How quickly will it take effect?

You will likely start to feel some relief from heartburn and ulcer pain within a few hours.

Side effects and severe reactions

Contact the doctor if any unusual, worrisome, or severe reactions occur or if you develop:

- Headache, dizziness, constipation, diarrhea

Warnings

- Consult your doctor or pharmacist before taking famotidine with an enteric-coated medication, as the enteric-coated pills may dissolve more quickly than they were designed when taken with H_2-blockers.

See the *ranitidine* entry on page 1556 for more information on how H_2 blockers work, what to expect in terms of speed and side effects, and when to contact the doctor if problems develop. (Unless otherwise noted, the information for *ranitidine* applies to all H_2 blockers.)

Generic name Fluconazole

Brand name Diflucan

Principal uses

Fluconazole is used to treat serious fungal infections that affect the vagina, throat, urinary tract, and other parts of the body. Sometimes it is prescribed to prevent a fungal infection.

How does it work?

Fluconazole fights fungal infections by interfering with the normal functioning of certain elements within the fungal cell, causing the cell to stop growing and reproducing. Fluconazole has this effect on only certain fungi.

Administration

Follow prescribing information from the doctor and pharmacist. Also:

- Fluconazole works best when constant levels are present in your bloodstream. To ensure this, take it at the same time every day and do not miss any doses.

- Fluconazole is available in oral as well as injection form. The injection form is occasionally prescribed for home use, but it is not discussed here.

If you miss a dose: Take the missed dose as soon as possible, unless it almost time for the next dose, in which case you should skip the missed dose and resume the regular schedule. Do not take two doses at once.

How quickly will it take effect?

Fluconazole is prescribed for stubborn fungal infections. Although you may feel relief from symptoms relatively soon, it may take weeks or months for this medication to eradicate your infection.

Side effects and severe reactions

Side effects that are generally of no concern unless they are persistent or severe include:

- Diarrhea, constipation, indigestion, drowsiness, dizziness, headache, nausea, vomiting, loss of appetite, weight loss, abdominal pain, flushing or redness in the face or skin, change in taste

Contact the doctor if any unusual, worrisome, or severe reactions occur or if you develop:

- Dark or amber-colored urine; yellowish tint to the skin or eyes; reddening, peeling, blistering, or loosening of skin or mucous membranes; fever; chills; sore throat; unusual bleeding or bruising; notable weakness or tiredness

Seek emergency care if you develop:

- Peeling of skin
- Hallucinations
- Anaphylaxis
- Unusual bleeding

Warnings

- Take the full course of this medication exactly as prescribed to help clear up your infection, even if your symptoms seem to have lessened.
- Contact the doctor if your condition fails to improve—or if it worsens—over a few weeks or months. Ask your doctor what to expect given your particular condition.

- Fluconazole poses 1% risk of severe liver injury.
- If you are taking coumadin, your dose of fluconazole may need to be adjusted.

Tips and other important things to know

- Keep all appointments for follow-up visits so that the doctor can monitor your progress and check for side effects of the medication.
- Loss of hair may occur in patients taking the drug for more than 3 months, but this is reversible.

Special precautions

- If you are pregnant or breast-feeding, discuss with your doctor the use of this medication *before* you start taking it.

Generic name Fluoxetine
Brand names include Prozac, Prozac Pulvules

Principal uses

Fluoxetine is prescribed to treat major mental depression, obsessive-compulsive disorder, obesity, eating disorders, and alcohol dependence.

How does it work?

Fluoxetine belongs to a class of medications known as serotonin reuptake inhibitors. These medications readjust the brain's delicate balance of chemical messengers. Other commonly used serotonin reuptake inhibitors include *paroxetine* and *sertraline*.

Administration

Follow prescribing information from the doctor and pharmacist. Also:

- To ensure its effectiveness, take this medication regularly and exactly as prescribed. Try to take it at the same time every day to avoid missing doses.
- Fluoxetine may be taken without regard to food, but try taking it with a meal if it causes stomach upset.

If you miss a dose: Skip the missed dose and take the next dose at the regularly scheduled time. Do not take two doses at once.

How quickly will it take effect?

Depression may start to lift within 1 to 3 weeks, although it may take 4 weeks or longer for the medication's full benefits to be felt.

Side effects and severe reactions

Side effects that are generally of no concern unless they are persistent or severe include:

- Headache, nausea, diarrhea, insomnia, tremor, drowsiness or loss of alertness
- Dryness of the mouth. Contact your doctor or dentist if dryness persists for more than 2 weeks.

Contact the doctor if any unusual, worrisome, or severe reactions occur or if you develop:

- Anxiety, restlessness, nervousness, sweating, loss of appetite, weight loss, abnormal vision, decreased sex drive, apathy, fever, rapid speech, a feeling of being out of control, skin rash, hives or itching

Seek emergency care if you develop:

- Suicidal thoughts

Warnings

- Consult your doctor before starting any new medications, including over-the-counter ones, because fluoxetine interacts negatively with many.
- This drug may activate mania (or an unusually heightened and energetic state) in individuals with manic-depressive or other cyclic disorders.
- Discuss with your doctor the risks of drinking alcohol or ingesting any other substance that depresses (slows down) the central nervous system, as fluoxetine may increase their effects in potentially harmful ways.

Tips and other important things to know

- Keep all appointments for follow-up visits so that your doctor can monitor your condition and check for unwanted reactions to the medication.

- If you are bothered by mouth dryness, try sucking on a hard candy or ice chips, chewing sugarless gum, or taking a saliva substitute. Cavities and other mouth problems are more likely to develop if the mouth is constantly dry.

- Your doctor will decide which antidepressant is optimal for you. Fluoxetine has the benefit of causing fewer difficulties with dry mouth, dizziness, constipation, heart problems, weight gain, and drowsiness than do standard tricyclic antidepressants. But it is more likely to cause gastrointestinal reactions, such as nausea, as well as nervousness, anxiety, and insomnia.

- You will have mild to severe gastrointestinal symptoms–nausea, upset stomach, cramps, diarrhea–within the first days of taking this drug.

- Fluoxetine interacts with many other psychoactive drugs. It raises their blood levels and thereby causes toxicity. Discuss with your doctor any other medication that you take or plan to take.

Special precautions

- If you are pregnant or breast-feeding, discuss with your doctor the use of this medication *before* you start taking it.

- Ask your doctor about risks of taking this medication at the same time as alcohol or other central nervous system depressants (these slow down the nervous system).

- Until your reaction to this medication has been established, avoid activity that requires mental or physical alertness.

Generic name Fluticasone (Nasal Spray)

Brand name Flonase

Principal uses

Fluticasone is applied in the form of a nasal spray to relieve hay fever symptoms, such as sneezing, runny nose, and watery eyes.

How does it work?

Fluticasone is a corticosteroid ("steroid") medication. When inhaled through the nose, it helps to suppress many of the cellular reactions responsible for inflammation, thus reducing allergy symptoms, including nasal stuffiness. Fluticasone is also used in the forms of inhaled aerosols and topical creams or ointments, but these are not discussed here.

Administration

Follow prescribing information from the doctor and pharmacist. Also:

- Take this medication exactly as prescribed. Its effectiveness depends on regular and consistent use. To avoid the risk of potentially serious complications, do not take it in higher doses or more frequently than recommended.

- Carefully read the package insert. Do not advance the applicator past the opening of the nose.

- Remember to clear your nasal passages first by blowing your nose.

- Shake the container gently before use.

If you miss a dose: Take the missed dose right away if it is within 1 hour of when you should have taken it. Otherwise, skip the missed dose and resume the regular schedule. Do not take two doses at once.

How quickly will it take effect?

The nasal spray will start to relieve symptoms of allergic rhinitis within 12 hours or the first or second day of treatment, although it may take several days to experience the medication's full benefits.

Side effects and severe reactions

Side effects that are generally of no concern unless they are persistent or severe include:

- Mild and transient sensations of burning, dryness, or irritation in the nose; headache; cough; hoarseness; sneezing attacks; transient and mild nosebleeds; nausea; runny or stuffy nose; mild throat irritation; tearing of the eyes

Contact the doctor if any unusual, worrisome, or severe reactions occur or if you develop:

- Persistent or severe burning, irritation, or any other symptoms of an adverse reaction in the area where you applied the medication; joint pain; lassitude; depression; muscular pain

- Hives; itching; rash; dryness or bad taste in the mouth; sore throat; fever; notable fatigue or weakness; symptoms of a nose, sinus, throat, or other type of infection

Seek emergency care if you develop:

- Symptoms of a severe allergic reaction, such as swelling of the face, eyelids, or lips; difficulty breathing; increased shortness of breath

Warnings

- Contact the doctor if your condition fails to improve—or if it worsens—within a few days.

- Use this medication for only the condition for which your doctor has prescribed it; there are numerous nasal conditions for which it is not appropriate.

- Never increase the dose on your own; contact the doctor if you are concerned that your symptoms are not subsiding. Corticosteroid medications can cause unwanted and even serious complications if absorbed in large amounts into the body.

- If your doctor has recommended that you switch from an oral steroid medication to a nasal steroid such as this, he or she will watch you carefully for indications that the nasal steroid does not provide your system with enough steroid. This is dangerous and must quickly be rectified should it occur. Contact the doctor immediately for guidance if you experience a severe asthma attack or will undergo a period of physical stress, such as surgery, during this transition period or shortly thereafter. You may need supplementary steroids during this time because your body has not yet started to produce its own.

- Because steroids suppress the immune system, you may be more susceptible to infections than you would otherwise be. Such infections as chickenpox and measles can cause more serious complications in people on steroids, for example. Avoid exposure to these illnesses and contact the doctor immediately if you are exposed.

- This medication is not recommended for children under age 12 because its safety and effectiveness in this age group has not been established, although it is occasionally used in young children with severe allergic symptoms involving the nose.

Tips and other important things to know

- This medication does not have an immediate effect on allergy symptoms.

Special precautions

- If you are pregnant or breast-feeding, discuss with your doctor the use of this medication *before* you start taking it.

Generic name Fluvastatin

Brand name Lescol

Principal uses

Fluvastatin is prescribed to lower high levels of cholesterol fats in the blood. This is done in an attempt to prevent heart complications of coronary artery disease associated with cholesterol-clogged blood vessels.

Administration

Follow prescribing information from the doctor and pharmacist. Also:

- Take this medication exactly as prescribed. The dosage has been carefully tailored to your body's requirements and response. Do not take it in larger or smaller doses, more often, or for longer than recommended.
- Fluvastatin may be taken without regard to food. Taking it in the evening enhances its effectiveness.

If you miss a dose on one day: Skip the missed dose and resume the regular schedule the next day. Do not take two doses at once.

Contact the doctor if any unusual, worrisome, or severe reactions occur or if you develop:

- Severe muscle aches and pains

Tips and other important things to know

Fluvastatin belongs to a class of medications called hepatic hydroxymethylglutaryl coenzyme A (HMG CoA) reductase inhibitors (statins). Medications in this class may vary slightly with regard to when they are best taken, the side effects they produce, the research in which they have been used, and the amount of experience doctors have with them. Fluvastatin is the least expensive and least effective of the statins.

See the *simvastatin* entry on page 1559 for more information on how statins work, what to expect in terms of speed and side effects, and when to contact the doctor if problems develop. (Unless otherwise noted, the information for *simvastatin* applies to all statins.)

Generic name Furosemide

Brand name Lasix

Principal uses

Furosemide is used to reduce fluid retention caused by such conditions as congestive heart failure and kidney disease and to treat hypertension (high blood pressure).

How does it work?

Furosemide is a loop diuretic. It works primarily by increasing the amount of urine your body produces and eliminates—thus reducing fluid retention and lowering blood pressure—by inhibiting the resorption of sodium in the kidney's loop of Henle (hence the name *loop diuretic*). Furosemide is taken orally as well as given by injection, but the injection form is not discussed here.

Administration

Follow prescribing information from the doctor and pharmacist. Also:

- Take furosemide at the same time every day; this will help you remember to take it and avoid missing doses.
- Measure out the oral solution carefully.
- Furosemide will make you urinate more often and in greater volume. To avoid getting up to urinate during the night, try taking a single daily dose in the morning after breakfast. If you have been told to

take more than one dose a day, take the last one no later than 6 PM.

If you miss a dose: Take the missed dose right away, unless it is almost time for the next dose, in which case you should skip the missed dose and resume the regular schedule. Do not take two doses at once.

How quickly will it take effect?

Furosemide will start to increase urine production and output within 1 hour. The greatest effect will occur within 1 or 2 hours, and the overall effect will last 6 to 8 hours. Blood pressure takes time to fall; it may take several weeks to see the full benefits.

Side effects and severe reactions

Side effects that are generally of no concern unless they are persistent or severe include:

- Dizziness or lightheadedness when sitting up or lying down
- Tiredness, particularly when first starting furosemide

Contact the doctor if any unusual, worrisome, or severe reactions occur or if you develop:

- Dry mouth, increased thirst, muscle weakness or cramps, rapid or irregular heartbeat, mood or mental changes, nausea or vomiting, loss of appetite, unusual tiredness or weakness, rapid or excessive weight loss or gain (such as more than 2 lb per day), diarrhea
- Shortness of breath; difficult or labored breathing; pain in the chest, back, or legs

Seek emergency care if you develop:

- Constant dizziness or an inability to sit up

Warnings

- Take this medication as prescribed even if you feel well; hypertension is a largely symptom-free disease until organs become damaged.
- Do not make any drastic changes in your diet without discussing them with your doctor first.
- Contact the doctor for guidance if you perspire heavily, stand for long periods, drink alcohol, are exposed

to very hot weather, or develop an illness with severe nausea, vomiting, or diarrhea. Dizziness, lightheadedness, dehydration, and excessively low blood pressure are risks.

- If you have high blood pressure, avoid stimulant-containing over-the-counter medications, as some may increase blood pressure.

- Discuss with your doctor the considerable risks of sun sensitivity. Ultraviolet radiation alters the medication's structure such that certain people react to it in an allergic way. The reaction occurs 10 days to 2 weeks after the first exposure to the sun.

- As with all medications, it is important to tell all your doctors about the medications you take and your medical history. In the case of furosemide, it is particularly vital that you report liver disease and the use of a digitalis medication, such as digoxin.

Tips and other important things to know

- Furosemide will help keep your blood pressure down, but it will not cure you of hypertension.

- Keep all appointments for follow-up visits so that your doctor can monitor your condition and assess your reaction to this medication.

- Your doctor may recommend that you increase your consumption of potassium-rich foods or drinks or take a potassium supplement or other medication to help prevent potassium depletion. Potassium-rich foods include bananas, orange juice, whole and skim milk, and raisins. Salt restrictions may also be recommended.

- To minimize dizziness or lightheadedness that can occur especially with the first few doses, get up gradually from a sitting or lying position.

- If you have diabetes, be aware that furosemide may alter the results of urine glucose (sugar) tests.

Special precautions

- This medication may increase sensitivity to the sun; discuss with your doctor what precautions are appropriate.

- Ask your doctor about risks of taking this medication at the same time as alcohol or other central nervous system depressants (these slow down the nervous system).

- If you are pregnant or breast-feeding, discuss with your doctor the use of this medication *before* you start taking it.

Generic name Gemfibrozil

Brand name Lopid

Principal uses

Gemfibrozil is prescribed to reduce high serum levels of triglycerides (fatty substances in the blood) in people whose elevated triglycerides have not responded to dietary changes, weight loss, or other medications and who are at risk of coronary artery disease or pancreatitis.

How does it work?

This medication works by speeding the removal of triglycerides from the blood.

Administration

Follow prescribing information from the doctor and pharmacist. Also:

- Take gemfibrozil on an empty stomach 30 minutes before morning and evening meals. Try taking it with food if it causes stomach upset, however.

If you miss a dose: Take the missed dose as soon as possible, unless it is almost time for the next dose, in which case you should skip the missed dose and resume the regular schedule. Do not take two doses at once.

How quickly will it take effect?

The speed at which gemfibrozil starts to work varies widely among people. Your doctor will check your triglyceride levels in 4 to 6 weeks to determine if the medication is working.

Side effects and severe reactions

Side effects that are generally of no concern unless they are persistent or severe include:

- Mild stomach and abdominal pains, indigestion, gas, diarrhea, nausea, vomiting

Contact the doctor if any unusual, worrisome, or severe reactions occur or if you develop:

- Eczema, fatigue, headache, dizziness, blurred vision, depression, hives, itching, joint pain, muscle pain or weakness, yellowing of eyes or skin

Warnings

- Close medical supervision is important while taking this medication. Especially during the first year of treatment, your doctor will test your liver function and periodically check your blood cholesterol and triglyceride levels.

- For cases of mildly elevated triglyceride levels, HMG COA reductase inhibitors may be a better choice than gemfibrozil.

- Gemfibrozil can cause muscle inflammation, with aching and pain, and kidney failure when taken in combination with an HMG CoA reductase inhibitor.

- The dose of gemfibrozil must be reduced in people with kidney failure.

- Do not take gemfibrozil if you are pregnant or breast-feeding, unless you have had a bout of pancreatitis associated with severe triglyceride elevations during a prior pregnancy.

Tips and other important things to know

- Gemfibrozil should be used as a supplement to important lifestyle measures for reducing your risk for heart disease, such as restricting dietary fats and cholesterol, controlling weight, limiting or eliminating alcohol intake, and exercising regularly. Gemfibrozil should never be used as a substitute for these measures.

- Blood sugar (glucose) levels will be tested before you start taking this medication, because triglyceride levels are commonly elevated in people with diabetes and control of blood glucose levels in diabetics is essential to lower triglycerides.

- In some cases gemfibrozil can raise total and LDL cholesterol levels at the same time that it lowers triglycerides.

- In most cases, gemfibrozil has little effect on blood cholesterol levels.

Special precautions

- Until your reaction to this medication has been established, avoid activity that requires mental or physical alertness.
- If you are pregnant or breast-feeding, discuss with your doctor the use of this medication *before* you start taking it. See the *Warnings* section.

Generic name Glipizide

Brand names include
Glucotrol, Glucotrol XL

Principal uses

Glipizide is prescribed to lower blood glucose (sugar) levels in people with type 2 diabetes (formerly referred to as noninsulin dependent diabetes mellitus) whose condition cannot be controlled by diet alone.

How does it work?

Glipizide belongs to a class of antidiabetic medications called sulfonylureas which lower blood sugar levels by stimulating the release of insulin from the pancreas.

Administration

Follow prescribing information from the doctor and pharmacist. Also:

- Take glipizide at the same time every day.
- Glipizide is typically taken 30 minutes before a meal.

If you miss a dose: Take the missed dose right away, unless it is almost time for the next dose, in which case you should skip the missed dose and resume the regular schedule. Do not take two doses at once.

How quickly will it take effect?

Glipizide starts to work within 90 minutes; the most extensive blood sugar drop occurs within 2 to 3 hours. Glipizide's effects continue for 10 to 24 hours.

Side effects and severe reactions

Contact the doctor if any unusual, worrisome, or severe reactions occur or if you develop:

- Nausea, appetite loss, vomiting, heartburn, constipation, diarrhea, stomachache, mild dizziness, drowsiness, headache. These common reactions may respond to a doctor-recommended dosage adjustment.

Seek emergency care if you develop:

- A severe manifestation of any of the above
- Severe low blood sugar (hypoglycemia) (see page 1182 for more information).

Warnings

- Glipizide cannot be used in place of insulin; it is not an oral form of insulin.
- Your doctor will warn you about the symptoms of hyperglycemia (sugar levels too high) and hypoglycemia and what to do if they develop. Severe hypoglycemia is considered a medical emergency.
- The risk of hypoglycemia is increased by, among other things, missing meals, drinking a significant amount of alcohol, exercising much more than usual, and failing to take antidiabetic medications as prescribed.
- Limit alcohol while taking glipizide, as it may produce low blood sugar or cause other unwanted side effects.
- Certain heart problems tend to develop more frequently in people who take such oral hypoglycemia agents as glipizide. Be sure to discuss with your doctor any heart condition that you might have or that runs in your family.
- If you are pregnant or breast-feeding, do not take this medication.

Tips and other important things to know

- This medication is just one of several important tools for people with type 2 diabetes to lower blood sugar levels. A sound diet, exercise, and weight control are other critical measures. Your doctor should give you guidance on this.
- Check for sugar in your blood as recommended by your doctor. Be sure you understand what to do if these levels are abnormal.
- Symptoms of low blood sugar (hypoglycemia) possibly include an anxious feeling, abdominal or stomach pain, chills, cold sweats, dizziness, drowsiness, depressed mood, shakiness, fatigue, hunger, blurred vision, headache, irritability, continuous nausea or vomiting, confusion, poor concentration, loss of consciousness, or seizures. If you experience any of these symptoms, take a source of glucose; drink or eat a sugar-containing food. Tell your doctor at your next visit about the symptoms you have experienced, when and how often they occur.
- The effectiveness of such oral antidiabetic medications as glipizide tends to diminish over time, through either an increased resistance to the medication in your body or a worsening of the diabetes itself.
- Severe stress caused by injury, fever, acute infection, surgery, or other incidents may temporarily make it more difficult to properly control diabetes. Let your doctor know if you are (or will be) going through a period of great physical stress. Sometimes insulin is used instead of an oral medication during such times.

Special precautions

- This medication has a number of potentially hazardous interactions. Discuss with your doctor all the medications you take—including over-the-counter ones—before taking this one.
- Wearing a medical alert bracelet/necklace is advised.
- If you are pregnant or breast-feeding, discuss with your doctor the use of this medication *before* you start taking it. See *Warnings* section.

Generic name Glyburide
Brand names include
DiaBeta, Glynase, Glynase PresTab, Micronase

Principal uses

Glyburide is taken by people with type 2 diabetes mellitus (formerly referred to as non-insulin-dependent diabetes mellitus) whose blood glucose (sugar) levels cannot be controlled by diet alone.

How does it work?

Glyburide is one of the sulfonylurea antidiabetic medications. It helps to control diabetes by stimulating the pancreas to release insulin.

Administration

Follow prescribing information from the doctor and pharmacist. Also:

- Glyburide is taken once or twice a day with breakfast and dinner.
- To reduce the risk of stomach upset, take glyburide 30 minutes before eating.

If you miss a dose: Take the missed dose right away, unless it is almost time to take the next dose, in which case you should skip the missed dose and resume the regular schedule. Do not take two doses at once.

How quickly will it take effect?

Insulin concentrations generally begin to rise within 15 to 60 minutes, with a maximum effect in 1 to 2 hours and increased insulin concentrations persisting for up to 24 hours. A single morning dose of glyburide may help lower blood sugar levels for up to 24 hours.

Side effects and severe reactions

Contact the doctor if any unusual, worrisome, or severe reactions occur or if you develop:

- Nausea, unpleasant sensation of fullness in the stomach, heartburn, skin lesions, itching, redness, hives
- Symptoms of hyperglycemia (high blood sugar). These tend to develop more gradually than do those for low blood sugar. They may include excessive thirst or urination, drowsiness, dry or flushed skin, fruity odor to the breath, dryness in the mouth, loss of appetite, tiredness, trouble breathing (fast and deep), stomachache, nausea, or vomiting.
- Symptoms of a potentially severe allergic reaction, possibly including pale skin, unusual sweating, seizures, shortness of breath, and wheezing

Seek emergency care if you develop:

- Symptoms of severe low blood sugar, including disorientation, coma, pale skin, perspiration, body rash, seizures

Warnings

- Your doctor should discuss with you the risks of this medication—and describe alternatives to glyburide treatment.
- Take this medication exactly as prescribed. Potentially fatal low blood sugar concentrations can develop if too much is taken. Keep in mind the other common causes of low blood sugar as well: increased exercise, alcohol consumption, and missing meals.
- Watch for symptoms of high and low blood sugar and ask your doctor what to do should either occur.
- Limit alcohol while taking this medication.
- Glyburide should not be used during pregnancy.

Tips and other important things to know

- When properly used, glyburide will help manage your disease. It will not cure you of it, however.
- Antidiabetic medications, such as glyburide, constitute a critical—but only partial—element in an overall lifestyle approach for people with type 2 diabetes that includes a well-designed diet, exercise, weight control, and personal hygiene measures.
- Symptoms of low blood sugar (hypoglycemia) possibly include an anxious feeling, abdominal or stomach pain, chills, cold sweats, dizziness, drowsiness, depressed mood, shakiness, fatigue, hunger, blurred vision, headache, irritability, continuous nausea or vomiting, confusion, poor concentration, loss of consciousness, or seizures. If you experience any of these symptoms, take a source of glucose; drink or eat a sugar-containing food. Tell your doctor at your next visit about the symptoms you have experienced, when and how often they occur.
- Keep all appointments for follow-up visits so that your doctor can moni-

tor your condition and check for unwanted reactions to the medication.

- Your doctor will likely guide you about how to monitor your blood glucose (sugar) levels.
- Contact your doctor for guidance if you are going through (or anticipate) a period of physical stress, such as infection, trauma, surgery, or fever. In some cases, the doctor may want to stop glyburide and prescribe insulin for a short period of time.

Special precautions

- Ask your doctor about risks of taking this medication at the same time as alcohol or other central nervous system depressants (these slow down the nervous system).
- Wearing a medical alert bracelet/necklace is advised.
- This medication may increase sensitivity to the sun; discuss with your doctor what precautions are appropriate.

Generic name
Hydrochlorothiazide

Brand names include
Aquazide-H, Diaqua, Esidrix, Hydro-chlor, Hydro-D, HydroDIURIL, Mictrin, Oretic

Principal uses

Hydrochlorothiazide is prescribed for hypertension (high blood pressure). Its ability to increase the amount of salt excreted by the kidneys lowers blood pressure and benefits a number of other conditions.

How does it work?

Hydrochlorothiazide is a thiazide diuretic. It increases the production and output of urine and salt by blocking cells in the kidney that normally resorb salt and water. This lowers blood pressure. Diuretics are commonly referred to as "water pills."

Administration

Follow prescribing information from the doctor and pharmacist. Also:

- Take your medication at the same time every day to help avoid missing doses.
- To avoid getting up to urinate during the night, especially while first taking this medication, try taking a single daily dose in the morning after breakfast. Do not take the daily dose later than 6 PM if possible.
- Take hydrochlorothiazide with food if it upsets your stomach.

If you miss a dose: Take the missed dose as soon as possible, unless it is within 4 hours of the next dose, in which case you should skip the missed dose and resume the regular schedule. Do not take two doses at once.

How quickly will it take effect?

Hydrochlorothiazide will start to work within 2 hours and continue working for 6 to 12 hours overall. It may take several weeks for such a condition as high blood pressure to fully respond, however.

Side effects and severe reactions

Side effects that are generally of no concern unless they are persistent or severe include:

- Excessive urination, diarrhea, decreased sexual ability (impotence), loss of appetite, upset stomach, dizziness or lightheadedness when rising from a sitting or lying position, increased sun sensitivity

Contact the doctor if any unusual, worrisome, or severe reactions occur or if you develop:

- Severe stomach pain with nausea and vomiting, black or bloody stools, blood in the urine, cough, hoarseness, joint pain, fever or chills, difficult or painful urination, lower back or side pain, skin rash or hives, yellowing of eyes or skin, unusual bruising or bleeding
- Symptoms of excessive potassium loss: dry mouth, increased thirst, muscle cramps or pain, nausea or vomiting, mood changes, weak or irregular heartbeat, unusual tiredness, notable weakness
- Symptoms of excessive sodium loss: confusion, irritability, muscle cramps, convulsions, unusual tired-ness, notable weakness, mental slowness

Seek emergency care if you develop:

- Symptoms of a severe allergic reaction, such as sudden shortness of breath or swelling of the lips, tongue, or face

Warnings

- Take this medication as prescribed even if you feel well; hypertension is a largely symptom-free disease until organs become damaged.
- Do not make any drastic changes in your diet without discussing them with your doctor first.
- This medication can cause glucose (sugar) intolerance in some people. People with diabetes should have their blood sugar levels monitored and may, in some cases, need to have their insulin or blood sugar medication dosage adjusted.
- To prevent dehydration, contact the doctor for guidance if you develop an illness with severe nausea, vomiting, or diarrhea.
- If you have high blood pressure, you should generally avoid over-the-counter medications that can raise it, such as certain stimulant-containing cough and cold remedies. Ask your doctor or pharmacist for guidance.

Tips and other important things to know

- When taking hydrochlorothiazide for high blood pressure, keep in mind that it will help control your blood pressure but will not cure hypertension.
- Consult with your doctor about lifestyle measures you can take to help control hypertension, such as losing weight, exercising moderately, and following a healthy diet.
- Keep all appointments for follow-up visits so that your doctor can monitor your condition and assess your reaction to this medication.
- Hydrochlorothiazide for high blood pressure is commonly combined with medications that help prevent excessive potassium loss.
- Your doctor may recommend that you increase your consumption of potassium-rich foods or drinks or take a potassium supplement or other medications to help prevent the loss of this important mineral. Potassium-rich foods include bananas, orange juice, whole and skim milk, and raisins.
- Particularly when you start taking hydrochlorothiazide, you may feel unusually tired.
- To minimize dizziness or lightheadedness that sometimes occurs with this medication (especially the first few doses), get up gradually from a sitting or lying position.

Special precautions

- If you are pregnant or breast-feeding, discuss with your doctor the use of this medication *before* you start taking it.
- This medication may increase sensitivity to the sun; discuss with your doctor what precautions are appropriate.
- Ask your doctor about risks of taking this medication at the same time as alcohol or other central nervous system depressants (these slow down the nervous system).

Generic name
Hydrocodone and Acetaminophen

Brand names include
Bancap, Ceta Plus, Hydrocet, Hy-Ohen, Lorcet-HD, Lortab, Panacet, Vicodin, Zydone

Principal uses

The combination of hydrocodone and acetaminophen is prescribed to treat moderate to moderately severe pain.

How does it work?

This medication combines a painkiller (the narcotic analgesic hydrocodone) with a non-narcotic painkiller and fever reducer (acetaminophen). Hydrocodone, like other opiates, blocks certain pain receptors. Although its exact mechanism of action remains unclear, acetaminophen is believed to relieve pain by increasing the level at which you feel or experience pain. Other commonly used acetaminophen and narcotic combination pain relievers include *codeine with acetaminophen, propoxyphene with acetaminophen,* and *oxycodone with acetaminophen.*

Administration

Follow prescribing information from the doctor and pharmacist. Also:

- Take this medication exactly as prescribed. Do not take it in larger doses, more frequently, or for longer periods of time than recommended. There is a risk of physical and psychological dependence, liver damage, and overdose in such cases.

If you miss a dose and normally take this medication regularly: Take the missed dose as soon as possible, unless it is almost time for the next dose, in which case you should skip the missed dose and resume the regular schedule. Do not take two doses at once.

How quickly will it take effect?

This medication typically takes 30 to 60 minutes to start relieving pain.

Side effects and severe reactions

Side effects that are generally of no concern unless they are persistent or severe include:

- Drowsiness, dizziness, lightheadedness, faintness, nausea or vomiting, unexpected tiredness or weakness, dryness in the mouth, constipation

Contact the doctor if any unusual, worrisome, or severe reactions occur or if you develop:

- Bloody or cloudy urine, confusion, black or tarry stools, difficult or painful urination, hallucinations, severe constipation, worrisome visual disturbances, persistent pounding or fast heartbeat, irregular breathing, significant new skin rashes such as red spots on the skin, troubled breathing, yellowing of the skin or the whites of the eyes, uncontrolled muscle movements, sore throat and fever, unusual bleeding or bruising, skin rash or hives or itching, sudden reduction in urine output, frequent urge to urinate

- Nausea or vomiting, diarrhea, body aches, shivering or trembling, stomach cramps, notably fast heartbeat, weakness, restlessness, irritability, nervousness, sweating. These may occur days or weeks after stopping this medication after a period of prolonged use.

Seek emergency care if you develop:

- Symptoms of an overdose: seizures, confusion, notably slow or troubled breathing, severe drowsiness, severe dizziness, uncontrolled restlessness, weakness

Warnings

- Do not abruptly stop taking a narcotic analgesic and acetaminophen combination if you have been taking it regularly for several weeks. Contact your doctor for guidance. The dose may have to be gradually reduced to avoid unwanted reactions.

- If you find that the medication becomes less effective over time, contact the doctor. Do not increase the dose on your own.

- This medication may make you feel drowsy, lightheaded, or dizzy or give you a false sense of well-being. Lie down if you experience dizziness, lightheadedness, nausea, or vomiting; this may alleviate these sensations. Get up gradually from a sitting or lying position to avoid dizziness or lightheadedness. Make sure you know how you react to the medication before driving or engaging in any other potentially hazardous activity.

- Check the labels on all the medications you take, prescription or nonprescription, for the presence of a narcotic or acetaminophen. Do not take them without calling your doctor for guidance if any do, because taking them at the same time as a narcotic analgesic and acetaminophen combination could lead to an overdose.

- Drinking alcohol may increase the risk of liver damage with the acetaminophen in this medication.

Tips and other important things to know

- The risk of psychological or physi-

cal dependence is relatively low when the combination of a narcotic analgesic and acetaminophen is taken as prescribed for short periods. Significant physical dependence (with withdrawal symptoms when stopping the medication) emerges as a risk only after several weeks of continued use.

- If you are taking this medication regularly, be sure to keep all appointments for follow-up visits so that your doctor can monitor your condition and check for unwanted reactions.

- Check with your doctor or dentist before taking any other painkillers, including aspirin or other nonsteroidal anti-inflammatory drugs (NSAIDs), on a regular basis along with this one.

- Make sure all your doctors (including the dentist) are aware that you take this medication.

Special precautions

- Until your reaction to this medication has been established, avoid activity that requires mental or physical alertness.

- If you are pregnant or breast-feeding, discuss with your doctor the use of this medication *before* you start taking it.

- This medication has a number of potentially hazardous interactions. Discuss with your doctor all the medications you take—including over-the-counter ones—before taking this one.

- Ask your doctor about risks of taking this medication at the same time as alcohol or other central nervous system depressants (these slow down the nervous system).

Generic name Ibuprofen

Brand names include
Advil, Children's Advil, Medipren, Motrin, Nuprin, PediaProfen, Rufen, Trendar

Principal uses

Ibuprofen is prescribed to treat mild to moderate pain, stiffness, tenderness, and swelling associated with menstruation, arthritis, gout, dental extraction, and various other conditions. It also reduces fever. Ibuprofen belongs to a class of medications known as nonsteroidal anti-inflammatory drugs (NSAIDs).

Administration

Follow prescribing information from the doctor and pharmacist. Also:

- Take ibuprofen on an empty stomach (1 hour before or 2 hours after eating) to encourage full absorption. If it causes stomach upset, however, take it with food.

- Take the regular tablet with a full glass of water and avoid lying down for 15 to 30 minutes afterward.

- Do not mix the suspension with an antacid or other liquid.

How quickly will it take effect?

If you are taking this medication for arthritis, your symptoms may lessen within 7 days of regular ibuprofen use, although it may take 1 to 2 weeks before you experience the medication's full benefits.

Warnings

- Do not take more than six tablets (1.2 g) without a doctor's guidance.

- Do not take this medication for more than 10 days for pain relief or for a fever that lasts longer than 3 days, unless your doctor has recommended it. Contact the doctor if a painful area becomes red or swollen.

- Consult with your doctor before taking ibuprofen if you have peptic ulcer or kidney disease.

Tips and other important things to know

- Certain dosage forms of ibuprofen are available only by prescription.

- Adverse reactions to this medication are often related to the dose.

See the *nabumetone* entry on page 1546 for more information on how NSAIDs work, what to expect in terms of speed and side effects, and when to contact the doctor if problems develop. (Unless otherwise noted, the information for *nabumetone* applies to all NSAIDs.)

Generic name Insulin, Human

Brand names include

Humulin N, Humulin R

Principal uses

Insulin is used to treat all patients with type 1 diabetes mellitus. It is also prescribed for patients with type 2 diabetes whose illness is inadequately controlled by diet and oral glucose-lowering medications. It is administered in emergency settings to treat such serious complications as diabetic ketoacidosis (a dangerous accumulation of glucose and acids) and diabetic coma.

How does it work?

Under normal circumstances, the pancreas, a large gland near the stomach, produces insulin. This hormone helps remove glucose from the blood. When your body does not make enough insulin or the insulin it produces does not work properly, insulin is injected to replace the missing insulin or overcome the body's resistance to its action.

There are several types of insulin. They differ in terms of how quickly and for how long they work. Although animal insulins are still available, almost all diabetic patients are now treated with genetically engineered insulin (of recombinant DNA origin) that is structurally identical to the insulin normally produced by the human pancreas.

Administration

Follow prescribing information from the doctor and pharmacist. Also:

- The doctor or nurse will show you how to prepare the insulin and give yourself an injection. Also read the patient's instructions that come with the insulin package, which will give you detailed guidance about putting together the syringe and administering the injection.

- Careful instructions and follow-up are needed for those using an insulin pump.

- Insulin is typically injected before meals or at bedtime.

- Store unopened bottles of insulin in a dark, cool place such as the refrigerator. Do not let insulin freeze; also, avoid exposing it to very hot temperatures or sunlight.

- An opened insulin bottle may be kept at room temperature for a month. Discard insulin that has been at room temperature for longer than this. Also check the expiration date.

- The doctor should instruct you on selecting and rotating injection sites.

- Use disposable needles and syringes to avoid infection and dispose of them as directed by your doctor or pharmacist. A special container made for used needles is appropriate. If you choose to reuse your syringes or needles, ask the doctor or nurse to show you how to sterilize them properly.

If you miss a dose: Ask your doctor for general guidelines on what to do if you miss a scheduled insulin dose.

How quickly will it take effect?

Various types of insulin start to work at different speeds. Ask your doctor what to expect with the particular type that you use.

Side effects and severe reactions

Contact the doctor if any unusual, worrisome, or severe reactions occur or if you develop:

- Injection site itching, swelling, redness, stinging, hives, or warmth

- Symptoms of hyperglycemia (extremely high blood sugar). These tend to develop more gradually than those for hypoglycemia. They may include excessive thirst or urination, drowsiness, dry or flushed skin, fruity odor to the breath, dryness of the mouth, loss of appetite, tiredness, trouble breathing (fast and deep), stomachache, nausea, and vomiting.

- Symptoms of a potentially severe allergic reaction, possibly including perspiration, pale skin, seizures, rash, shortness of breath, wheezing, and shallow breathing

Seek emergency care if you develop:

- Symptoms of severe low blood sugar. These may include disorientation, coma, pale skin, perspiration, and seizures.

Warnings

- Take insulin exactly as prescribed. Doing otherwise puts you at risk for serious and even fatal complications.

- Never change your prescription in any way without consulting your doctor first: do not switch the type, brand, or strength of insulin you are using or the model or brand of syringe or needle. Do not alter the order of insulins you have been told to mix together. Find out from your doctor or pharmacist exactly what the insulin should look like—cloudy or clear—and examine it carefully before each use.

- Treat symptoms of both hypoglycemia and hyperglycemia quickly. Make sure you clearly know what to do before either occurs.

- Hypoglycemia may develop for various reasons, including taking too much insulin. If you develop symptoms of hypoglycemia, immediately eat sugar (glucose tablets and gel are available as well) or a sugar-based product, such as fruit juice, soft drink (nondiet), or honey. Make it a practice to keep hard candies or other sugar-containing products with you at all times. Contact your doctor at your next visit about symptoms of hypoglycemia, when and how often they occur.

- Hyperglycemia may develop for various reasons, including taking too little insulin or skipping a dose. Contact your doctor at your next visit about symptoms of hyperglycemia, when and how often they occur.

- Although insulin poses no risks to the mother or fetus, poorly controlled diabetes during a pregnancy may endanger the fetus. You should be monitored closely through a pregnancy.

Tips and other important things to know

- When properly used, insulin will help you manage your disease, but it will not cure diabetes.

- Get precise instructions on which kind of insulin to use, how often to give yourself an injection, when during the day to inject it, and how much

to use. Ask your doctor for guidance if you do not understand one of these aspects of your medication.

- Many aspects of daily living, from the food you eat, your exercise habits, the other medications you take, the common illnesses you get (especially with nausea or vomiting), and the traveling you do, may require temporary alterations in your insulin dosage. Work closely with your doctor to monitor your condition and readjust your insulin dosage as needed.

- Symptoms of low blood sugar (hypoglycemia) possibly include an anxious feeling, abdominal or stomach pain, chills, cold sweats, dizziness, drowsiness, depressed mood, shakiness, fatigue, hunger, blurred vision, headache, irritability, continuous nausea or vomiting, confusion, poor concentration, loss of consciousness, or seizures. If you experience any of these symptoms take a source of glucose; drink or eat a sugar-containing food (see *Warnings* section). Tell your doctor at your next visit about the symptoms you have experienced, when and how often they occur.

- The most important thing you can do to control your diabetes is to follow the special meal plan that your doctor has recommended. Eat regular meals. Ask your doctor what to do if you miss a meal. Other aspects of your lifestyle, from weight control to personal hygiene measures, are also extremely important.

- Keep a spare supply of insulin (and a syringe and needle) on hand at all times. This is particularly important when traveling. Stay alert to time zone changes that may alter you dosage schedule.

- Your doctor may prescribe a glucagon kit to use in certain emergency situations, such as unconsciousness due to extremely low blood glucose. Make sure that the people who spend the most time with you know where this kit is and how and when to use it.

- The medical alert bracelet or necklace that you wear should clearly state that you are taking insulin. This is important information for someone caring for you in an emergency.

- Regularly test for sugar in your blood. Blood glucose measurements are important guides to getting the most out of the insulin you take. Your doctor will instruct you on how frequently to carry out these tests and what to do with the results.

Special precautions

- Until your reaction to this medication has been established, avoid activity that requires mental or physical alertness.

- Wearing a medical alert bracelet/necklace is advised.

Generic name Ipratropium

Brand name Atrovent

Principal uses

Ipratropium is used long term to control bronchial spasms (wheezing) associated with such lung diseases as chronic bronchitis and emphysema. A nasal spray is also available, but it is not discussed here.

How does it work?

Ipratropium is an anticholinergic bronchodilator administered by means of a metered-dose inhaler or solution for nebulization (inhalation aerosol). Ipratropium makes breathing easier by opening up the air passages (bronchial tubes) of the lungs. Unlike most other bronchodilator medications, it targets the bronchial muscles, largely sparing the rest of the body from exposure to the medication.

Administration

Follow prescribing information from the doctor and pharmacist. Also:

- Proper use of metered-dose inhalers is the single most important factor in making sure that this medication works for you. See the patient's information sheet that comes with the medication and page 1464 for information on using inhalers.

- Taking more of this medication than recommended or taking it more frequently increases the risk that you will experience potentially serious side effects.

- To fully benefit from this medication, use it every day at regularly spaced intervals or as otherwise prescribed by the doctor.

- Shake the medication container well before using it.

- Avoid getting the inhalation aerosol solution into your eyes, where it may cause eye irritation or blurred vision for a short time. Keep your eyes closed when inhaling. If the medication does get into your eyes, rinse them out with cool water.

- When using the inhalation aerosol: Wait at least 5 minutes after using another bronchodilator inhalation aerosol if one has been prescribed for you. This is to avoid unwanted reactions. Get specific instructions from your doctor.

- Never mix the inhalation solution with cromolyn inhalation solution for use in a nebulizer. This could lessen the effect of the cromolyn.

- It is very important to store this medication away from heat and direct sunlight.

If you miss a dose: Take the missed dose as soon as possible, unless it is almost time for the next dose, in which case you should skip the missed dose and resume the regular schedule. If you use the medication regularly every day, take any remaining doses after the missed dose at regularly spaced intervals. Do not take two doses at once.

How quickly will it take effect?

You will likely feel some relief from symptoms in 5 to 15 minutes, with a maximum effect in 90 minutes to 2 hours. Ipratropium should work for 4 to 6 hours overall.

Side effects and severe reactions

Side effects that are generally of no concern unless they are persistent or severe include:

- Cough, dryness of the mouth or throat, nervousness, stomach upset, nausea, headache, dizziness, blurred vision or other vision changes, unpleasant taste in the mouth, unusual tiredness or weakness, sleeping problems, problems urinating

Contact the doctor if any unusual, worrisome, or severe reactions occur or if you develop:

- Skin rash or hives, mouth or lip sores

- Worsening of symptoms—or ones that do not lessen—within 30 minutes of taking this medication.

- Acute eye pain

Seek emergency care if you develop:

- Swelling of tongue or lips, difficulty swallowing

Warnings

- Do not use ipratropium for urgent situations requiring fast action. It takes time for the medication to open up the breathing tubes.

- Be sure to mention all your allergies to your doctor, including those to such foods as soybean or lecithin.

Tips and other important things to know

- If you develop bothersome dryness of your mouth or throat—ipratropium may inhibit salivation—try sucking on a sugarless hard candy or ice chips, chewing gum, or using a saliva substitute. Contact the doctor if the dryness persists for more than 2 weeks.

- See a dentist regularly when taking this medication; dryness of the mouth increases the risk of cavities and other types of dental disease.

Special precautions

- If you are pregnant or breast-feeding, discuss with your doctor the use of this medication *before* you start taking it.

Generic name Isosorbide Mononitrate

Brand names include Imdur, Ismo, Monoket

Principal uses

Isosorbide mononitrate is used to prevent angina pectoris (chest pain) caused by coronary artery disease.

Note: this medication is different from *sublingual nitroglycerine,* a medication placed under the tongue to relieve the pain of an angina attack that is underway. Isosorbide dinitrate is a similar medication but has a shorter duration of action. The information here applies only to the isosorbide mononitrate regular and extended-release tablets.

How does it work?

Isosorbide mononitrate belongs to a class of medications known as nitrates. These medications help reduce the frequency of angina attacks by increasing the supply of blood and oxygen to the heart. They accomplish this largely by dilating (opening up) blood arteries and veins. Nitrates do not dilate cholesterol plaque. This action is primarily to dilate less diseased or non-diseased vessels.

Administration

Follow prescribing information from the doctor and pharmacist. Also:

- To get the full protective effects of this medication, follow prescription instructions exactly. This is also important for helping to avoid increased resistance to the medication and significant withdrawal reactions and to prevent a recurrence of your condition.

- Typically, the first dose of the regular tablet is taken in the morning, followed by the second one 7 hours later. The extended-release tablet is typically taken once a day, in the morning.

- Isosorbide may be taken without regard to food.

- Never break, crush, or chew the extended-release tablet. Drink it with at least half a glass of water.

If you miss a dose: Take the missed dose as soon as possible, unless your next scheduled dose is within 2 hours, in which case you should skip the missed dose and resume the regular schedule. If you are taking the extended-release tablet, skip the missed dose, unless the next scheduled dose is within 6 hours, in which case you should skip the missed dose and resume the regular schedule. Do not take two doses at once.

How quickly will it take effect?

The regular tablets will start to demonstrate an effect in about 1 hour, with a peak effect in 1 to 4 hours. The extended-release tablets will provide benefit for approximately 12 hours.

Side effects and severe reactions

Side effects that are generally of no concern unless they are persistent or severe include:

- Headache (sometimes with throbbing), occasionally a decrease in blood pressure

Contact the doctor if any unusual, worrisome, or severe reactions occur or if you develop:

- Dizziness, lightheadedness, or fainting, particularly when rising from a sitting or lying position; dryness of the mouth, blurred vision, flushing of the face or neck, skin rash with redness and possible itching and peeling, fast pulse, weakness, sweating, nausea, vomiting

Warnings

- Isosorbide mononitrate will not relieve an angina attack that has already begun. It works too slowly to be able to do so.

- If you have been taking isosorbide regularly for several weeks or more and suddenly stop, you may develop angina attacks. Follow your doctor's instructions carefully regarding a gradual reduction in dosage.

- Do not switch brands without specific instructions from your doctor, as all brands are not equivalent.

- People with low blood pressure or who are taking blood pressure–lowering medications should use this medication with particular caution because it can cause severe low blood pressure. As with any medication, be sure to mention this and all other medical conditions to your doctor before starting the medication.

- Alcohol, hot weather, exercise, and long periods of standing may increase the risk of lightheadedness due to low blood pressure brought about by the medication. Ask your doctor for guidance. Remember that alcohol appears in some foods and medications; check labels.

Tips and other important things to know

- Headaches are a common side effect of this medication, particularly for the first few doses. Headaches are also an indication that the medication is working. Do not reduce the isosorbide dose in an attempt to get rid of the headache pain. Instead, treat the headache with an over-the-counter medication that your doctor recommends (typically aspirin or acetaminophen). The headaches will likely become less noticeable with time.

- Stand up slowly to avoid lightheadedness, dizziness, or faintness prompted by a drop in blood pressure.

Special precautions

- Ask your doctor about risks of taking this medication at the same time as alcohol or other central nervous system depressants (these slow down the nervous system).

- Until your reaction to this medication has been established, avoid activity that requires mental or physical alertness.

- If you are pregnant or breast-feeding, discuss with your doctor the use of this medication *before* you start taking it.

- This medication has a number of potentially hazardous interactions. Discuss with your doctor all the medications you take—including over-the-counter ones—before taking this one.

Generic name
Levothyroxine

Brand names include
Levoxyl, Synthroid

Principal uses

Levothyroxine is used to replace or supplement a deficiency in thyroxine, a condition called hypothyroidism. Thyroxine is a major hormone produced by the thyroid gland. This medication is also prescribed to treat thyroid cancer and to help shrink an enlarged thyroid gland (goiter). It is given by injection to newborns with congenital hypothyroidism (cretinism; an absence of normal thyroid

secretion), but this form of administration is not discussed here.

How does it work?

Levothyroxine is a synthetic thyroid hormone that is structurally related to and acts in the same way as the body's naturally produced thyroid hormone. It plays an important role in numerous metabolic functions, increasing the metabolism of body tissues and stimulating in protein synthesis and cell growth.

Administration

Follow prescribing information from the doctor and pharmacist. Also:

- Follow prescription instructions exactly to avoid symptoms of an overactive or underactive thyroid.

- To ensure a constant level in your body and to avoid missing doses, take levothyroxine at the same time every day. However, it can be taken at any time during the day if you forget to take it at your usual time.

If you miss a dose on one day: Resume your regular schedule the next day. Do not take two doses the next day.

How quickly will it take effect?

It may take days or even weeks for you to experience noticeable lessening of your symptoms.

Side effects and severe reactions

Contact the doctor if any unusual, worrisome, or severe reactions occur or if you develop:

- Hives, skin rash, severe headache in children

- Persistence of side effects of hypothyroidism—dry and puffy skin, clumsiness, listlessness, unusual weight gain, tiredness, weakness, sleepiness—despite taking the medication for some time (longer than a few weeks, for example)

- Chest pain

- Symptoms of hyperthyroidism (excessive thyroid hormone). The dosage may need adjustment. Look for increased appetite, diarrhea, fever, menstrual irregularities, leg cramps, sensitivity to heat, hand tremors, inability to sleep, weight loss, and increased sweating or vomiting.

Warnings

- Never stop taking levothyroxine without specific instructions from your doctor. It usually must be taken indefinitely if your condition involves a lack of thyroid hormone; ask your doctor what to expect.
- Do not switch brands without consulting your doctor. They may not be equivalent.
- Because of the risk of angina (chest pain) with heavy exercise or exertion, levothyroxine should be used with particular caution in people who already have angina problems, or who have hypertension (high blood pressure) or other heart disease.

Tips and other important things to know

- Keep all appointments for follow-up visits so your doctor can monitor your condition properly and check for your response to levothyroxine. Thyroid function tests are done periodically.
- Side effects are not common. They are most likely to occur when treatment is started or the dosage is being adjusted.
- Keep your prescription refills up to date.
- All doctors treating you, including dentists, should be told that you take this medication.
- Some brands of the tablets contain the dye tartrazine, an allergen for some people.

Generic name Lisinopril

Brand names include Prinivil, Zestril

Principal uses

Lisinopril is prescribed to treat hypertension (high blood pressure), to manage congestive heart failure, and to improve chances for survival for recent heart attack victims.

Administration

Follow prescribing information from the doctor and pharmacist. Also:

- Lisinopril may be taken without regard to food.

How quickly will it take effect?

It may take several weeks before you experience the full benefits of this medication.

Side effects and severe reactions

Contact the doctor if any unusual, worrisome, or severe reactions occur or if you develop:

- Symptoms of an infection, such as a sore throat or fever
- Lightheadedness; a change in the dosage may eliminate or significantly lessen this side effect
- A loss of taste perception

Seek emergency care if you develop:

- Symptoms of a severe allergic reaction, such as difficulty breathing or facial swelling

Warnings

- Avoid salt substitutes that contain potassium while taking lisinopril.

Tips and other important things to know

- Diuretics ("water pills") are sometimes taken along with lisinopril to help control blood pressure.
- The doctor will periodically check blood tests to monitor your kidney function and potassium levels while you take this medication.

See the *enalapril* entry on page 1522 for more information on how angiotensin converting enzyme (ACE) inhibitors work, what to expect in terms of time of onset and side effects, and when to contact the doctor if problems develop. (Unless otherwise noted, the information for *enalapril* applies to all ACE inhibitors.)

Generic name Loratadine

Brand name Claritin

Principal uses

Loratadine is prescribed to relieve hay fever symptoms, such as sneezing, stuffi-

ness, runny nose, tearing eyes, and itching. It has also been used to treat chronic allergy symptoms, such as rash, itching, and hives of unknown cause.

How does it work?

Loratadine is a tricyclic antihistamine. It relieves allergy symptoms by blocking the effects of histamine, a chemical that the body releases in response to irritants. It is considered "long acting" because it works for many hours. Loratadine is also available in combination with pseudoephedrine, a common decongestant; see *Loratadine with Pseudoephedrine* for more information.

Administration

Follow prescribing information from the doctor and pharmacist. Also:

- Take this medication on an empty stomach (1 hour before or 2 hours after a meal); food delays its action. If it causes an upset stomach, however, it may be beneficial to take with food.
- Loratadine is typically taken once a day. Follow your doctor's instructions, nonetheless.

If you miss a dose: Take the missed dose as soon as possible, unless it is almost time for the next dose, in which case you should skip the missed dose and resume the regular schedule. Do not take two doses at once.

How quickly will it take effect?

You will likely start to feel relief from allergy symptoms within 1 to 3 hours and feel the greatest effect in 8 to 12 hours. Loratadine generally works for 24 hours overall.

Side effects and severe reactions

Side effects that are generally of no concern unless they are persistent or severe include:

- Dry mouth, headache, drowsiness, mild fatigue

Contact the doctor if any unusual, worrisome, or severe reactions occur or if you develop:

- Sore throat and fever, notable tiredness or weakness, unusual bleeding or bruising

- Dizziness, fainting

Warnings

- Discuss with your doctor the risks of taking this medication while breast-feeding.

Tips and other important things to know

- Antihistamines, such as loratadine, do not cure you of hay fever or other allergic conditions, although they help control its symptoms.
- Loratadine tends to cause less sedation than do other antihistamines.
- Sleepiness, drowsiness, and other central nervous system reactions are usually a problem only when the medication is taken in higher than recommended doses or in seniors or in people who have liver or kidney disease.
- To avoid corrupting the results of an allergy skin test, stop taking loratadine at least 4 days beforehand.

Special precautions

- If you are pregnant or breast-feeding, discuss with your doctor the use of this medication *before* you start taking it.
- Until your reaction to this medication has been established, avoid activity that requires mental or physical alertness.

Generic name Loratadine with Pseudoephedrine

Brand name Claritin-D

Principal uses

This medication is prescribed to relieve hay fever symptoms, such as sneezing, stuffiness, runny nose, tearing eyes, and itching. It is especially useful for nasal stuffiness because it contains pseudoephedrine, a nasal decongestant.

Administration

Follow prescribing information from the doctor and pharmacist. Also:

- Although this medication may be taken without regard to food, it is best taken on an empty stomach (1 hour before or 2 hours after a meal) because food delays its action.

Side effects and severe reactions

Side effects that are generally of no concern unless they are persistent or severe include:

- Headache, insomnia, sleepiness, nervousness, dizziness, and fatigue

Contact the doctor if any unusual, worrisome, or severe reactions occur or if you develop:

- Restlessness, excitability, dizziness, weakness, insomnia, drowsiness, fast heartbeat, irregular heart rhythms

Warnings

- Certain people should avoid exposure to pseudoephedrine, including some who have successfully taken loratadine alone for hay fever symptoms in the past. The doctor will make a judgment on the basis of your medical history.
- Because of the presence of pseudoephedrine, a central nervous system stimulant, this medication has the potential for abuse. Higher than recommended doses may cause elevated mood, decreased appetite, irritability, and a sense of enhanced physical strength and mental capacity, among other reactions. Increasingly higher doses may subsequently be needed to produce these reactions, and unpleasant withdrawal reactions may develop when the medication is stopped under such circumstances.
- Check with your doctor before taking this medication with an over-the-counter antihistamine or decongestant, as excessive levels of certain ingredients may build up in your system.

See the *loratadine* entry on page 1522 for more information on how tricyclic antihistamines work, what to expect in terms of speed and side effects, and when to contact the doctor if problems develop. (Unless otherwise noted, the information for *loratadine* applies to all tricyclic antihistamines.)

Generic name Lorazepam

Brand names include Ativan

Principal uses

Lorazepam is used to treat anxiety, tension, agitation, irritability, and insomnia.

Administration

Follow prescribing information from the doctor and pharmacist. Also:

- Take this medication exactly as prescribed. Do not change the dosage without specific instructions from your doctor.
- Lorazepam may be taken without regard to food. Try taking it with food if it upsets your stomach, however.
- When taking the sublingual tablet (tablet placed under the tongue), let it dissolve slowly under your tongue. Avoid swallowing for at least 2 minutes to allow the medication to absorb sufficiently. Do not chew the tablet.
- Lorazepam is available in oral as well as injection forms, but the injection form is not discussed here.

Warnings

- When you are ending long-term therapy (3 months or more), the medication must be discontinued slowly over a period of weeks (in most cases) to avoid acute withdrawal reactions.
- Avoid consuming a lot of caffeine-containing products, as they may interfere with lorazepam's effectiveness.

See the *alprazolam* entry on page 1504 for more information on how benzodiazepines work, what to expect in terms of speed and side effects, and when to contact the doctor if problems develop. (Unless otherwise noted, the information for *alprazolam* applies to all benzodiazepines.)

Generic name Lovastatin

Brand name Mevacor

Principal uses

Lovastatin is prescribed to lower high levels of cholesterol in the blood. This is done in an attempt to prevent heart complications of coronary artery disease associated with cholesterol-clogged blood vessels.

Administration

Follow prescribing information from the doctor and pharmacist. Also:

- Take this medication exactly as prescribed. The dosage has been carefully tailored to you, based on your body's requirements and response. Do not take it in larger or smaller doses, more often, or for longer than recommended.
- Take lovastatin with food, as this enhances its effectiveness. Take a single daily dose with your evening meal.

If you miss a dose: Take the missed dose later the same night. If you do not take lovastatin on one day, resume the regular schedule the next day. Do not take two doses at once.

Side effects and severe reactions

Contact the doctor if any unusual, worrisome, or severe reactions occur or if you develop:

- Generalized muscle aches and pain

Warnings

Lovastatin belongs to a class of medications called HMG CoA reductase inhibitors (statins).

- In addition to side effects seen with other statins, lovastatin may cause trouble sleeping. This reaction may lessen and disappear as your body adjusts to the medication. If you have any concerns, discuss them with your doctor.

Tips and other important things to know:

- Statins vary slightly in when they are best taken, the research in which they have been used, the side effects they produce, and the amount of experience doctors have with them.

See the *simvastatin* entry on page 1559 for more information on how statins work, what to expect in terms of speed and side effects, and when to contact the doctor if problems develop. (Unless otherwise noted, the information for *simvastatin* applies to all statins.)

Generic name
Medroxyprogesterone

Brand names include
Amen, Curretab, Cycrin, Depo-Provera, Provera

Principal uses

Medroxyprogesterone is prescribed to restore absent menstrual cycles and to correct abnormal uterine bleeding due to female hormone imbalances. It is used in conjunction with estrogen replacement therapy to help prevent uterine cancer. Medroxyprogesterone is also used in injection form as a contraceptive for women, to treat advanced endometrial (uterine lining) and renal cancer, and to control sexually aggressive behavior in men.

How does it work?

Medroxyprogesterone is derived from progesterone, the female hormone critical to a woman's menstrual cycle rhythms and the development of milk-producing glands in the breast. When taken orally, medroxyprogesterone induces a change in endometrium (the cells that line the uterus). When injected, medroxyprogesterone reduces the likelihood of pregnancy by interrupting the hormonal messages that normally cause ovulation (a ripening of egg cells and their release from the ovaries) around the middle of the monthly menstrual cycle. It also initiates certain changes in the endometrium.

Administration

Follow prescribing information from the doctor and pharmacist. Also:

- Take the tablet on an empty stomach (1 hour before or 2 hours after eating). If it causes stomach upset, try taking it with food.
- The injection form of this medication is administered in the buttock or upper arm once every 3 months (13 weeks). This is done by a nurse or other health care professional.

If you miss a dose of the oral form: Take the missed dose as soon as possible, unless it is almost time for the next dose, in which case you should skip the missed dose and resume the regular schedule. Do not take two doses at once.

How quickly will it take effect?

For absent menstruation and abnormal uterine bleeding, ask your doctor what to expect on the basis of the regimen he or she has prescribed. In the standard scenario, bleeding typically begins within 3 to 7 days of stopping the medroxyprogesterone. If given at the proper time during a woman's menstrual cycle, the injection for contraception will start to protect against pregnancy right away.

Side effects and severe reactions

Side effects that are generally of no concern unless they are persistent or severe include:

- Changes in appetite, weight gain or loss, unusual tiredness or weakness, fluid retention in the ankles or feet, abdominal pain or discomfort (such as bloating), mild headache, dizziness, hair loss, acne, depression, hot flashes
- For the tablets (taken for any reason) especially: irregular menstrual bleeding, spotting, changes in menstrual flow, changes in cervical secretions, breast tenderness, weight gain or loss
- For the injection contraceptive especially: irregular and unpredictable menstrual periods or spotting for the first few months. An altogether absence of periods is more likely to occur over time with regular use of medroxyprogesterone. Weight gain is relatively common.

Contact the doctor if any unusual, worrisome, or severe reactions occur or if you develop:

- Unusually heavy or continuous vaginal bleeding
- Persistent pain, bleeding, or pus at the injection site, any of which may occur, in rare cases, with the contraceptive injection
- A delay in your menstrual period of 45 days from your last period
- Vaginal bleeding that persists much longer than normal

Seek emergency care if you develop:

- Symptoms of a rare yet serious and even potentially fatal blood clot, heart attack, stroke, or other complications: shortness of breath, chest pain, coughing up blood, loss of coordination, sudden or severe headache, jaundice (may be indicated by yellowing of the eyes or skin), sudden loss of vision (partial or complete) or double vision, slurred speech, calf or groin pain, unusual weakness, numbness, or persistent pain and swelling in an arm or leg

Warnings

- Discuss with your doctor the risks of taking medroxyprogesterone.

- Do not switch brands without talking to your doctor.

- Stop taking this medication and contact the doctor immediately if you suspect you have become pregnant. Especially during the delicate first 4 months of pregnancy, medroxyprogesterone increases the risk of birth defects in the baby's genitals.

- Medroxyprogesterone should never be taken as a test for pregnancy or to try to prevent miscarriage. Both uses are now outdated and recognized as potentially harmful to a growing fetus.

- The contraceptive injection should not be given to a pregnant woman. To ensure this, the first injection is given during the first 5 days of a normal menstrual period, or within the first 5 days after delivery of a baby if the mother is not breast-feeding, or at the sixth week after delivery if the mother is breast-feeding exclusively.

- The contraceptive injection does not protect you against human immunovirus (HIV) infection or acquired immunodeficiency syndrome (AIDS) or other sexually transmitted diseases.

Tips and other important things to know

- Keep all appointments for follow-up visits so that your doctor can monitor your progress and check for unwanted reactions to the medication. A physical examination, breast and pelvic exam, and cervical smear (Papanicolaou test, or Pap test) are standard features of these visits, which are scheduled for every 6 to 12 months.

- Medroxyprogesterone may mask the symptoms of menopause by causing regular menstrual periods despite the onset of menopause. Discuss this with your doctor if you are of menopausal age.

- Unless you are taking the tablet for birth control, the dosage you have been prescribed will most likely not result in a contraceptive effect. Ask your doctor if you have any questions.

- The use of medroxyprogesterone as a contraceptive injection is very effective, with fewer than 1 in every 100 women experiencing a pregnancy. Its reliability depends on your returning for a shot at the end of every 13-week period, however.

- The contraceptive effects of the birth control injection persist for some time after the final dose. Ask your doctor what to expect.

Special precautions

- If you are pregnant or breast-feeding, discuss with your doctor the use of this medication *before* you start taking it.

- This medication may increase sensitivity to the sun; discuss with your doctor what precautions are appropriate.

Generic name Metformin

Brand name Glucophage

Principal uses

Metformin is prescribed to lower blood glucose (sugar) levels in people with type 2 diabetes mellitus (formerly referred to as noninsulin dependent diabetes mellitus) whose condition is inadequately controlled by diet alone. It is sometimes prescribed to be taken along with other antidiabetic medications.

How does it work?

Metformin lowers blood glucose levels by reducing the liver's production of glucose and enhancing the body's uptake and use of glucose. A biguanide antihyperglycemia agent, it is unrelated to the sulfonylurea medications commonly used to control diabetes and offers the appeal of rarely producing hypoglycemia (low blood sugar) unless used in combination with other medications to lower blood glucose.

Administration

Follow prescribing information from the doctor and pharmacist. Also:

- Take metformin with meals to reduce the risk of stomach upset and diarrhea. If you have been prescribed one dose a day, take it with breakfast. If you have been prescribed two doses a day, take the first dose with breakfast and the second dose with dinner.

- If necessary, the dosage is increased gradually over time.

If you miss a dose: Take the missed dose as soon as possible, unless it is almost time for the next dose, in which case you should skip the missed dose and resume the regular schedule. Do not take two doses at once.

How quickly will it take effect?

Blood sugar levels may drop within a few days to 1 week, although it may take up to 2 weeks for metformin to exert its full effect.

Side effects and severe reactions

Side effects that are generally of no concern unless they are persistent or severe include:

- Diarrhea, nausea, vomiting, abdominal cramping or pain, abdominal bloating, loss of appetite, gas, unpleasant or metallic taste

Contact the doctor if any unusual, worrisome, or severe reactions occur or if you develop:

- Early symptoms of lactic acidosis, an uncommon but serious and potentially fatal metabolic disease in which lactic acid builds up in the blood. It can occur when too much metformin accumulates in the body. The symptoms include unexplained breathing problems, feeling very weak or sickly, unusual sleepiness, unusual or unexpected stomach trouble, feeling cold, and muscle pain. Stop taking metformin immediately if these symptoms occur.

Seek emergency care if you develop:

- Symptoms of severe hypoglycemia. These may include disorientation, coma, pale skin, perspiration, body rash, seizures, and breathing difficulties.

- Early symptoms of lactic acidosis. Full blown lactic acidosis produces a coma.

Warnings

- Do not change the dosage of this medication without specific instructions from your doctor.

- Because of the risk of lactic acidosis while taking metformin (a serious complication defined in the *Side effects and severe reactions* section above), tell your doctor right away if you develop an illness with severe vomiting, diarrhea, or fever or if you become dehydrated for some reason.

- Treat symptoms of hypoglycemia quickly because this condition can be fatal. Make sure you clearly know what to do *before* such a situation occurs.

- Lactic acidosis tends to occur when people with diabetes who have renal (kidney) insufficiency take metformin.

- Do not take metformin if you are pregnant or breast-feeding.

Tips and other important things to know

- Metformin should constitute just one component of a broader strategy to control your diabetes that features a well-designed diet, weight control, regular physical activity, personal hygiene measure, and attempts to avoid infection. Ask your doctor for guidance.

- Low blood sugar may develop if you delay or skip a meal, drink a large amount of alcohol, exercise more vigorously than usual, or get sick (especially if you vomit or develop diarrhea), among other things.

- Symptoms of low blood sugar (hypoglycemia) possibly include an anxious feeling, abdominal or stomach pain, chills, cold sweats, dizziness, drowsiness, depressed mood, blurred vision, shakiness, fatigue, hunger, headache, irritability, continuous nausea or vomiting, confusion, poor concentration, loss of consciousness, or seizures. If you experience any of these symptoms, take a source of glucose; drink or eat a sugar-containing food. Tell your doctor at your next visit about the symptoms you have experienced, when and how often they occur.

- Keep all appointments for follow-up visits so that your doctor can monitor your condition, conduct laboratory tests, and check your response to the medication.

- Stay in close contact with your doctor and let him or her know if you undergo a period of increased physical stress, such as an infection, trauma, fever, or surgery. The doctor may recommend that you take insulin during such periods (see *Insulin, Human*, page 1537).

- Make sure you can identify the symptoms of hypoglycemia and hyperglycemia (high blood sugar) and know what to do if it occurs.

- Because this medication is very dangerous to take if you have kidney impairment, the doctor should check your kidney function before prescribing this medication and annually thereafter.

- Follow your doctor's guidance about how and when to perform home blood sugar tests and what to do if the results are abnormal.

- Metformin should be temporarily stopped for a surgical procedure unless it is quite minor. The same is true for x-ray procedures with injectable contrast agents. Make sure all your doctors and your dentist are aware that you take metformin; follow their guidance on temporarily stopping it, if necessary.

Special precautions

- If you are pregnant or breast-feeding, discuss with your doctor the use of this medication *before* you start taking it.

Generic name
Methylphenidate

Brand name Ritalin

Principal uses

Methylphenidate is prescribed to treat the behavioral problem known as attention deficit hyperactivity disorder (ADHD) in children and adolescents. In adults, it is used to treat narcolepsy, a disorder involving uncontrolled sleeping or sudden periods of deep sleep.

How does it work?

Methylphenidate stimulates the central nervous system. This explains its use for narcolepsy. For unexplained reasons, however, it has the opposite effect on children, calming and stabilizing hyperactivity, decreasing distractibility and improving attention span.

Methylphenidate is available in the form of regular and sustained-release tablets. The sustained-release tablets deliver methylphenidate into the system more slowly and are occasionally recommended for children and adolescents who develop exaggerated symptoms when the regular medication wears off.

Administration

Follow prescribing information from the doctor and pharmacist. Also:

- Take methylphenidate exactly as prescribed. Do not alter the dosage in any way or stop taking the medication without the doctor's guidance.

- Take methylphenidate 30 to 45 minutes before eating. This enhances its effectiveness.

- If you are taking methylphenidate for narcolepsy, avoid sleeping problems by taking the first dose (of the regular tablet) when you wake up in the morning and the final one before 6 PM. If you are giving it to your child or adolescent for ADHD, give him or her the last dose (of the regular tablet) several hours before bedtime.

- Swallow the sustained-release tablets whole. Never crush or chew them.

If you miss a dose: Take the missed dose as soon as possible and take the rest of the day's doses at evenly spaced intervals throughout the day. Do not take two doses at once.

How quickly will it take effect?

The regular tablets will reach peak levels in your system within 2 hours and work for 3 to 6 hours overall. The sustained-release tablets will reach peak concentrations in 4 to 7 hours and work for up to 8 hours. A child or adolescent taking methylphenidate for ADHD may have to take the medication for at least a week or two before its full effects can be determined.

Side effects and severe reactions

Side effects that are generally of no concern unless they are persistent or severe include:

- Drowsiness, nausea, stomach aches, headache, such symptoms of overstimulation as nervousness and dizziness, insomnia

- Particularly in children: loss of appetite, stomach pain, sleeping difficulties, weight loss

Contact the doctor if any unusual, worrisome, or severe reactions occur or if you develop:

- Fast heartbeat, fever, chest pain, unusual bruising, joint pain, tics or other uncontrolled body movements, skin rash or hives, weight loss (in adults)

- After stopping the medication especially: severe depression, notable tiredness or weakness, unusual behavior

- Seizures, peeling or blistering skin

Seek emergency care if the child or adolescent develops:

- Depression, unusual behavior, hallucinations (especially at higher dosages)

Warnings

- Never abruptly stop taking this medication. This is particularly important if you have been taking it for a long time at high doses; suddenly stopping may unmask severe depression or cause other unwanted reactions. Follow your doctor's instructions.

- If you are concerned that this medication is losing its effectiveness, contact the doctor for guidance. Do not alter the dosage on your own.

- Methylphenidate may precipitate Gilles de la Tourette's syndrome (a movement disorder) and increase the risk of seizures in people predisposed to seizures.

- Methylphenidate may cause excessive blood pressure increases in the presence of tyramine, a substance found in such foods as chocolate, pepperoni, canned fish, and bologna. The doctor may recommend that you avoid these and other foods while taking this medication.

- Especially if you are taking methylphenidate for narcolepsy, avoid caffeine-containing drinks. This is important for avoiding excessive central nervous system stimulation.

- Methylphenidate is not generally recommended for women of childbearing age unless the potential benefits outweigh the risks. If you fall into this category, discuss your concerns with your doctor.

- Methylphenidate can become habit forming (especially in adults) if taken in larger amounts than recommended. Symptoms of mental or physical dependence include a strong desire to keep taking the medication, a need to increase the dose to experience the same effects, and the development of withdrawal side effects, such as notable tiredness or depression when stopping the medication.

Tips and other important things to know

- Rely on a trusted professional to determine whether your child needs this medication. It should be prescribed only after a careful evaluation. Psychological counseling and other measures to ensure that your child adapts well are also critical.

- Methylphenidate is considered the medication of choice for ADHD. Treatment is typically stopped once puberty sets in. It is not recommended for children under 6 years of age.

- If you are taking methylphenidate for narcolepsy, keep in mind that it is a potent medication that should not be used to treat normal fatigue.

- Contact the doctor if you detect no change in your child's condition after 1 month of treatment.

- Because the long-term use of methylphenidate has been associated with suppression of growth in hyperactive children, the doctor should monitor your child's growth and weight carefully. Most children will eventually grow to their natural height.

- Keep all appointments for follow-up visits so your doctor can monitor your condition and the development of reactions to the medication. He or she may check for altered blood counts, increased blood pressure, and other signs of excessive stimulation when the medication is taken for long periods.

- Sustained-release tablets (as opposed to regular tablets) enable a child to take one dose while still at home in the morning.

- Your doctor may discuss taking intermittent medication "holidays" on weekends and other less stressful times. This is done to avoid the need for increasingly higher doses, and for children and adolescents whose growth might be affected.

- Dependence and addiction to this medication are much more of a risk in adults than in children.

Special precautions

- Until your reaction to this medication has been established, avoid activity that requires mental or physical alertness.

- If you are pregnant or breast-feeding, discuss with your doctor the use of this medication *before* you start taking it.

Generic name
Nabumetone

Brand name Relafen

Principal uses

Nabumetone is prescribed to treat pain, stiffness, tenderness, and swelling associated with acute or chronic rheumatoid arthritis and osteoarthritis. It also reduces fever.

How does it work?

Nabumetone belongs to a class of medications called nonsteroidal anti-inflammatory drugs (NSAIDs). Other commonly used NSAIDs include *ibuprofen, naproxen,* and *oxaprozin*. Much remains to be learned about how NSAIDs exert their effect. They are believed to interfere with the synthesis of chemicals (prostaglandins) in the body that are active in inflammatory processes and pain.

Administration

Follow prescribing information from the doctor and pharmacist. Also:

- Take nabumetone with food, milk, or an antacid (preferably a magnesium- and aluminum-containing one) and a full glass (8 oz) of water to reduce the risk of stomach upset.

Taking it with food also boosts absorption.

- Sit or stand up for 15 to 30 minutes after taking the medication to help ensure that it does not get stuck in the esophagus.

If you miss a dose and take this medication regularly: Take the missed dose as soon as possible, unless it is almost time for the next dose, in which case you should skip the missed dose and resume the regular schedule. Do not take two doses at once.

How quickly will it take effect?

Pain is usually relieved within 1 hour or so, although arthritis-related inflammation and associated discomforts usually require a few days to 1 week (or several weeks in severe cases) of regular treatment to lessen. Maximum benefits may not be experienced for 2 to 4 weeks.

Side effects and severe reactions

Side effects that are generally of no concern unless they are persistent or severe include:

- Diarrhea, mild nausea, vomiting, mild stomach pain or cramps, lightheadedness, dizziness, drowsiness, fatigue, bloated feeling, excess gas, headache, indigestion, constipation, mild heartburn, ringing in the ears

Contact the doctor if any unusual, worrisome, or severe reactions occur or if you develop:

- Skin rash or itching
- Severe stomach or abdominal pain, burning, or cramping; black, bloody, or tarry stools; fainting; convulsions, chest pain; shortness of breath; troubled breathing; wheezing; chest tightness; hivelike swellings around the face or in the mouth; spitting up of blood; sudden decrease in urine volume; severe or persistent nausea or indigestion or heartburn; vomiting blood or material that looks like coffee grounds; weight gain; visual disturbances; unusual bleeding or bruising; or sore throat, fever, and chills

Seek emergency care if you develop:

- Signs of bleeding, violent drug reactions, loss of normal urination

Warnings

- NSAIDs are potent medications. Take them exactly as prescribed. Do not take them for longer or in larger amounts than recommended. People have died of overdoses.
- Unless your doctor specifically recommends it, do not regularly take other anti-inflammatory medications (including aspirin) while taking an NSAID.
- Drinking alcohol at the same time that you take an NSAID increases the risk of ulcers.
- Consult with your doctor *before* taking nabumetone if you have a history of peptic ulcer disease or kidney problems.

Tips and other important things to know

- NSAIDs are powerful tools for helping manage the pain and inflammation associated with rheumatoid conditions, but they do not reverse or cure the underlying ailment.
- To manage the pain of such a chronic condition as arthritis, NSAIDs may need to be taken regularly.
- If you are taking an NSAID long term, be sure to keep all appointments for follow-up visits so that your doctor can monitor your condition and check for unwanted reactions to the medication. Tests for blood counts and kidney and liver condition, and an examination for ulcers and gastrointestinal bleeding, are standard.
- Make sure any doctor or dentist who is to perform surgery on you is aware that you take an NSAID.

Special precautions

- Ask your doctor about risks of taking this medication at the same time as alcohol or other central nervous system depressants (these slow down the nervous system).
- If you are pregnant or breast-feeding, discuss with your doctor the use of this medication *before* you start taking it.
- Until your reaction to this medication has been established, avoid activity that requires mental or physical alertness.

Generic name

Naproxen

Brand names include

Aleve, Anaprox, Naprosyn

Principal uses

Naproxen is used to relieve mild to moderate pain and inflammation associated with menstruation, gout, osteoarthritis, rheumatoid arthritis, juvenile rheumatoid arthritis, sunburn, migraine headache (naproxen sodium only), and various other conditions. It also reduces fever. Naproxen belongs to a class of medications known as nonsteroidal anti-inflammatory drugs (NSAIDs).

Administration

Follow prescribing information from the doctor and pharmacist. Also:

- Take the regular tablet with a full glass of water and avoid lying down for 15 to 30 minutes afterward.
- Take the extended-release tablet with food or an antacid (a magnesium- or aluminum-containing one is preferable) to reduce stomach irritation.

If you miss a dose: Take the missed dose as soon as possible, unless the next scheduled dose is within 4 hours, in which case you should skip the missed dose and resume the regular schedule. If you normally take naproxen once a day and remember that you have missed a dose within 8 hours of your next scheduled dose, skip the missed dose and resume the regular schedule. Do not take two doses at once.

How quickly will it take effect?

Naproxen relieves pain within 1 hour and will continue to work for approximately 7 hours. Inflammation associated with arthritis may take several days to 2 weeks or so of regular treatment to decrease.

Side effects and severe reactions

Contact the doctor if any unusual, worrisome, or severe reactions occur or if you develop:

- Skin rash (in children especially)

Warnings

- This medication is available in two forms: naproxen (Naprosyn) and naproxen sodium (with salt; Aleve, Anaprox). Do not take both forms at the same time, as the body ultimately converts them into the same substance. A dose of 275 mg of naproxen sodium is equivalent to 250 mg of naproxen.

- Naproxen is available with or without a prescription. Follow recommended dosages carefully. People have died from taking excessive amounts of this medication.

- Naproxen has a number of potentially hazardous interactions. Discuss with your doctor all the medications you take—including such over-the-counter ones as aspirin and acetaminophen—before taking this one.

- Because of the risk of dizziness, drowsiness, tiredness, and headache with naproxen, avoid situations that demand physical or mental alertness until you know how you will react to it.

- Consult with your doctor *before* taking this medication if you have a history of peptic ulcer disease or kidney disease.

Tips and other important things to know

- Naproxen may alter the results of certain diagnostic tests. Make sure all your doctors and your dentist are aware that you take this medication.

- Naproxen may increase sensitivity to the sun; discuss with your doctor what precautions are appropriate.

See the *nabumetone* entry on page 1546 for more information on how NSAIDs work, what to expect in terms of speed and side effects, and when to contact the doctor if problems develop. (Unless otherwise noted, the information for *nabumetone* applies to all NSAIDs.)

Generic name Neomycin, Polymyxin B, and Hydrocortisone

Brand names include
Bacticort, Cortisporin, Drotic, Otocort

Principal uses

This combination medication is used to treat bacterial infections and inflammation of the skin or in the eyes or ears.

How does it work?

The two antibiotics (neomycin and polymyxin B) in this combination medication attack susceptible bacteria in different ways, and the corticosteroid ("steroid"; hydrocortisone) reduces inflammation.

Administration

Follow prescribing information from the doctor and pharmacist. Also:

- Wash your hands well before administering any form of this medication. Avoid spreading the infection by keeping the end of medication applicator from touching your fingers, the area you are treating, or any other surface other than the medication container.

- For the skin ointment: Clean the affected area gently with mild soap and water. Rub a very thin layer lightly into the skin. Let the area dry fully before covering it with loose clothing. Do not apply tight bandages or snug diapers (or plastic pants) that do not let air circulate. Do not apply the ointment to broken skin or to sensitive areas, such as the face, genitals, or rectal area, unless specifically told to do so.

- For the ear solution or suspension drops: Instill the prescribed number of drops into the ear and place the dropper directly back into the bottle.

- For the eye suspension drops: After instilling the prescribed number of drops, keep the eye closed for 1 to 2 minutes to allow for full absorption. Unless directed otherwise, wait at least 5 to 10 minutes before applying any other eye medication.

- For the eye ointment: See page 1462 for directions on administering an eye ointment.

If you miss a dose: Administer the missed dose right away, unless it is almost time for the next dose, in which case you should skip the missed dose and resume the regular schedule. Do not take two doses at once.

How quickly will it take effect?

Most conditions will start to clear up within a few days of regular treatment, although this will largely depend on the type and severity of your condition.

Side effects and severe reactions

Side effects that are generally of no concern unless they are persistent or severe include:

- For the eye medication: mild stinging, burning, or watering directly after application. The ointment may cause temporary blurred vision.

Contact the doctor if any unusual, worrisome, or severe reactions occur or if you develop:

- Failure to heal or increased irritation, itching, swelling, sensitivity, reddening, dryness, scaling, skin cracking, rash, or extra hair growth, acnelike eruptions, fine reddish lines, a new infection, discoloration in dark-skinned people (usually temporary)

- For the ear medication: persistent stinging or burning

Warnings

- Although it is important to complete the full course of medication to avoid a reappearance of the infection, you should also take care to limit your use of this medication to the amount and duration prescribed.

- Contact the doctor if your condition fails to improve—or if it worsens—within a few days.

- Ear or kidney damage may occur with extended use or systemic reactions to the steroid component of this combination medication can occur if it is used for very long periods or in high doses or is administered improperly. Ask your doctor for guidance if you have any questions about using this medication safely.

- Some forms of this medication contain sulfites. If you are allergic to sulfites, inform your doctor and pharmacist.

Generic name Nifedipine

Brand names include

Adalat, Procardia

Principal uses

Nifedipine is prescribed to manage hypertension (high blood pressure) and certain types of angina pectoris (chest pain). It belongs to a class of medications called calcium channel blockers.

Administration

Follow prescribing information from the doctor and pharmacist. Also:

- Nifedipine may be taken without regard to food.

- Never abruptly stop taking this medication if you have been taking it regularly. The dosage must be reduced gradually or your condition may worsen. Your doctor should give you guidance.

- Swallow the capsule whole unless otherwise directed by your doctor. Do not crush, break, or chew it unless specifically directed to do so.

- Nifedipine is available as short-acting (fast-acting; taken more than once a day) capsules and several types of long-acting (extended-release; taken once a day) tablets.

If you miss a dose: Take the missed dose immediately, unless it is almost time for the next one, in which case you should skip the missed dose and resume the regular schedule. Do not take two doses at once.

Warnings

- The first doses, or dosage increases, may temporarily exacerbate angina. Discuss this with your doctor if you have any questions.

- When altering the dosage, some people experience annoying symptoms of low blood pressure, such as dizziness, lightheadedness, flushing, headache, weakness, fainting, and nausea. If these reactions occur, discuss them with your doctor, because the dosage may need to be adjusted.

- Short-acting nifedipine is associated with more adverse reactions than other calcium channel blockers and should seldom be used. Discuss with your doctor any concerns you might have.

Tips and other important things to know

- If you take Procardia XL, you may notice the empty capsule shell in your stool. This is normal. The medication has been absorbed into your system.

- Nifedipine was once quite commonly used to reduce severely high blood pressure rapidly. Many experts now consider this use outdated because of associated risks.

- Short-acting nifedipine capsules may not be appropriate for treating angina, Raynaud's phenomenon (a vascular disorder), or preterm labor. Your doctor will make this judgment call.

- Nifedipine may alter the results of certain laboratory tests, so make sure all your doctors and your dentist are aware that you take it.

See the *amlodipine* entry on page 1506 for more information on how calcium channel blockers work, what to expect in terms of speed and side effects, and when to contact the doctor if problems develop. (Unless otherwise noted, the information for *amlodipine* applies to all calcium channel blockers.)

Generic name

Nitroglycerin

Brand names include

Nitro-Dur Transdermal, Nitrostat

Principal uses

Nitroglycerin is used to prevent and relieve the pain of angina pectoris (chest pain), including chronic angina attacks. It is also given by injection in certain emergency situations to treat heart attacks and critically high blood pressure.

How does it work?

Nitroglycerin helps relieve chest pain by improving the supply of blood and oxygen to the heart. Nitroglycerin is available in several forms. Orally, it is taken in the form of capsules, sprays, sublingual tablets (tablets placed under the tongue), and transmucosal tablets (tablets placed in the mouth where the medication can be absorbed through the mucous membranes). It is applied to the skin in the form of an ointment or a transdermal patch (patch that allows medication to be absorbed through the skin) that delivers a preset amount of medication gradually during the period of time that the patch is on, which is usually 24 hours. Nitroglycerin is also given by injection, but this form of administration is not discussed here.

Administration

Follow prescribing information from the doctor and pharmacist. Also:

- Make sure you understand how to use the form of nitroglycerin that the doctor has prescribed for you. Carefully read the patient's instructions that come with the medication.

- Do not drink, smoke, use chewing tobacco, or chew gum while a sublingual or transmucosal tablet is dissolving in your mouth.

Sublingual tablet:

- Take it at the first sign of an angina attack. Sit down. Wet the tablet with saliva, place it under your tongue, and wait for it to dissolve completely. Do not chew, crush, or swallow this tablet. Rest.

- Take another sublingual tablet in 5 minutes if the first one fails to relieve your pain. If 3 sublingual tablets (used consecutively with rest periods in between) fail to relieve the chest pain within 10 to 15 minutes, immediately contact your doctor or go to an emergency room.

- If the sublingual tablet causes an unpleasant tingling or burning sensation, try holding it between your cheek and tongue.

Transmucosal tablet:

- Place it under your upper lip and gum or between your tongue and cheek and let it dissolve gradually over 3 to 5 minutes. Do not chew or swallow this tablet. Avoid drinking hot liquids with it or touching it with your tongue, as this will make it dissolve more quickly.

Oral tablet:

- Swallow the tablet whole on an empty stomach (30 minutes before or 1 to 2 hours after eating).

Oral spray:

- Spray it on your tongue. Take care not to inhale it. Wait about 10 seconds before swallowing.

Ointment:

- Spread it onto hairless skin in a thin layer. Because absorption will not be as complete as for other forms, avoid applying it to the extremities of the arms or legs. Do not rub the ointment in. The doctor should show you how to apply a plastic film to enhance absorption and to protect your clothes. Ask the doctor about rotating application spots to avoid skin inflammation and rash.

Transdermal patch:

- Apply it as directed by the product insert or by your doctor. In general, avoid hairy spots or areas you move a lot. Avoid exposure to microwave ovens, as radiation that leaks from some ovens may heat up the metallic backing on the patch and burn the skin. Discard the patch properly, where children and pets cannot get access to it; There may still be medication in it.

If you miss a dose and are taking this medication regularly: Take the missed dose as soon as possible, unless the next scheduled dose is within 2 hours (or within 6 hours for sustained-release tablets or capsules), in which case you should skip the missed dose and resume the regular schedule. Do not take two doses at once.

How quickly will it take effect?

The speed at which nitroglycerin relieves chest pain depends on the form in which you take it. Sublingual tablets take 1 to 3 minutes to work and continue to have an effect for up to 30 minutes. The translingual spray (medication that is sprayed on the tongue, or oral spray) takes 2 minutes and continues to have an effect for 30 to 60 minutes. The transmucosal tablets take 3 minutes and continue to work for 5 hours. The ointment takes 20 to 60 minutes and continues to work for 3 to 6 hours. The oral (sustained-release) capsule takes 40 minutes and continues to work for 4 to 8 hours. The transdermal patch takes 40 to 60 minutes and continues to work for 18 to 24 hours.

Side effects and severe reactions

Side effects that are generally of no concern unless they are persistent or severe include:

- Headache, fast pulse, nausea or vomiting, restlessness, flushing
- Dizziness, lightheadedness, or flushing when getting up from a sitting or lying position

Contact the doctor if any unusual, worrisome, or severe reactions occur or if you develop:

- Blurred vision, persistent headache, dry mouth, skin rash

Seek emergency care if you develop:

- Persistent chest pain

Warnings

- For this medication to work as intended, you must take it exactly as directed.
- The sublingual tablet is used to relieve the pain of an angina attack that has already begun. The other forms of nitroglycerin are used to prevent angina; they generally work too slowly to relieve pain that has started.
- Do not suddenly stop taking this medication if you have been taking it regularly. Withdrawal should be gradual, as prescribed by the doctor, to reduce the risk of angina attacks.
- Because they may work differently, do not switch brands without consulting your doctor or pharmacist.

Tips and other important things to know

- Sublingual tablets are also occasionally prescribed to prevent angina during the night and before stressful situations.
- Headaches associated with the use of this medication are most common with the first doses and usually lessen as your body adjusts to the medication. They may be relieved by the use of standard headache medications. Talk to your doctor about reducing the dose.
- To reduce dizziness, flushing, or faintness when rising, get up gradu-

ally. Lie down if you start to feel dizzy. Descend stairs with care. Talk to your doctor about precautions you should take during hot weather and while exercising.

- If you have been prescribed the sublingual or translingual form of this medication, be sure to keep it nearby at all times.
- Take care in storing nitroglycerin; follow the label instructions carefully. Sublingual tablets, for example, should be tightly sealed away from heat and light. Take the cotton out of nitroglycerin containers; it absorbs the medication. Replace the supply every 3 months, or as otherwise directed, to keep the medication fresh.
- Nitroglycerin is not addictive.

Special precautions

- Ask your doctor about risks of taking this medication at the same time as alcohol or other central nervous system depressants (these slow down the nervous system).
- Until your reaction to this medication has been established, avoid activity that requires mental or physical alertness.
- If you are pregnant or breast-feeding, discuss with your doctor the use of this medication *before* you start taking it.

Generic name Nizatidine

Brand names include Axid, Axid AR

Principal uses

Nizatidine is prescribed to treat duodenal (intestinal) ulcers and associated symptoms. It is also prescribed to control gastroesophageal reflux disease (GERD; backflow of stomach contents). It is commonly taken for heartburn. Nizatidine belongs to a class of medications known as H_2 (gastric histamine) blockers.

Administration

Follow prescribing information from the doctor and pharmacist. Also:

- For heartburn, a capsule is taken 30 minutes before a meal. Do not take it more than twice a day.

Warnings

- The effects of long-term treatment (longer than 1 year) with nizatidine are not known.

Tips and other important things to know

- Low-dose nizatidine is available in nonprescription form for the treatment of heartburn.

See the *ranitidine* entry on page 1556 for more information on how H₂ blockers work, what to expect in terms of speed and side effects, and when to contact the doctor if problems develop. (Unless otherwise noted, the information for *ranitidine* applies to all H₂ blockers.)

Generic name Omeprazole

Brand name Prilosec

Principal uses

Omeprazole is used for short periods of time to treat active duodenal (intestinal) ulcers, severe inflammation of the esophagus, and gastroesophageal reflux disease (GERD; backflow of stomach contents). It has also been prescribed for long-term treatment of disorders involving excessive stomach acid secretion, such as Zollinger-Ellison syndrome, and erosion of the esophagus lining caused by acid from the stomach.

How does it work?

Omeprazole belongs to a class of medications called proton-pump inhibitors. It helps treat disorders involving excess stomach acid by interfering with the critical, final step of acid production within the stomach's mucous lining.

Administration

Follow prescribing information from the doctor and pharmacist. Also:

- Omeprazole is taken in the form of a delayed-release capsule. Swallow this capsule whole. Do not open, crush, or chew it.

- Take omeprazole immediately before meals for optimal effect.

- Omeprazole may be taken with an antacid to help relieve stomach pain, particularly before the omeprazole has had a chance to work. Discuss this option with your doctor.

If you miss a dose: Take the missed dose as soon as possible, unless it is almost time for the next dose, in which case you should skip that dose and resume the regular schedule. Do not take two doses at once.

How quickly will it take effect?

Omeprazole can halt the production of stomach acid within 1 hour. A single dose continues to inhibit acid production for up to 72 hours. Taken regularly, the medication builds up to an optimal level in your system. It may take several days to notice a decrease in stomach pain. Duodenal ulcers typically heal within 4 weeks.

Side effects and severe reactions

Side effects that are generally of no concern unless they are persistent or severe include:

- Abdominal or stomach pain, diarrhea or loose stools, gas, nausea, vomiting, headache, dizziness, heartburn

Contact the doctor if any unusual, worrisome, or severe reactions occur or if you develop:

- Persistent mouth sores or ulcers, difficult or painful urination, frequent urge to urinate, bloody or cloudy urine, sore throat and fever, notable tiredness or weakness

Warnings

- It is important to keep taking this medication even when you feel fine.

- Omeprazole may harm a fetus. Discuss with your doctor the risks and benefits of taking this medication while pregnant.

- The dosage may have to be specially adjusted in people of Asian descent because this group appears to process the medication differently than do other people.

Tips and other important things to know

- Keep all appointments for follow-up visits so that your doctor can monitor your condition properly and make an appropriate decision about when to stop treatment with omeprazole.

Special precautions

- If you are pregnant or breast-feeding, discuss with your doctor the use of this medication *before* you start taking it.

Generic name Oxaprozin

Brand name Daypro

Principal uses

Oxaprozin is prescribed to manage the pain of osteoarthritis and rheumatoid arthritis. It belongs to a class of medications known as nonsteroidal anti-inflammatory drugs (NSAIDs).

Administration

Follow prescribing information from the doctor and pharmacist. Also:

- Take oxaprozin with food or milk to reduce the risk of stomach upset.

- Drink a full glass (8 oz) of water with the caplet and avoid lying down for 15 to 30 minutes afterward.

Side effects and severe reactions

Contact the doctor if any unusual, worrisome, or severe reactions occur or if you develop:

- Symptoms of bleeding in your gastrointestinal tract, such as black or bloody stools, vomiting or coughing up of blood, or severe abdominal pain or tenderness

- Unexpected hearing or vision changes (blurred vision, ringing in the ears)

Tips and other important things to know

- This medication may increase sensitivity to the sun; discuss with your doctor what precautions are appropriate.

- If you take this medication long term, the doctor will likely check blood values periodically to confirm that no unwanted reactions are developing.

See the *nabumetone* entry for more information on how NSAIDs work, what to expect in terms of speed and side effects, and when to contact the doctor if problems develop. (Unless otherwise noted, the information for *nabumetone* applies to all NSAIDs.)

Generic name Oxycodone with Acetaminophen

Brand names include Percocet, Roxicet, Tylox

Principal uses

This medication combines a narcotic analgesic (oxycodone) with acetaminophen to treat moderate to moderately severe pain.

Administration

Follow prescribing information from the doctor and pharmacist. Also:

- Take this medication exactly as prescribed. Do not take it in larger doses, more frequently, or for longer periods of time than recommended. There is a risk of physical and psychological dependence, potentially fatal overdose, and liver damage in such cases.

Warnings

- There is a considerable risk of becoming psychologically and physically dependent on this medication when it is taken in higher doses or for long periods of time.

- This medication should be used with great care in combination with tranquilizers, muscle relaxants, antidepressants, antihistamines, or other substances that depress (slow down) the central nervous system and can make you sleepy, including alcohol. Consult your doctor about the risks of combining these types of substances with oxycodone and acetaminophen.

See the *hydrocodone and acetaminophen* entry on page 1535 for more information on how narcotic analgesic and acetaminophen combination medications work, what to expect in terms of speed and side effects, and when to contact the doctor if problems develop. (Unless otherwise noted, the information for *hydrocodone and acetaminophen* applies to all narcotic analgesic and acetaminophen combinations.)

Generic name Penicillin V Potassium

Brand names include Betapen-VK, Bopen-V-K, Ledercillin VK, V-Cillin K, Veetids

Principal uses

Penicillin V potassium is used to treat mild to moderate bacterial infections affecting the upper respiratory tract (such as "strep throat"), middle ear, urinary tract, skin, and other body tissues. It is commonly prescribed for severe gingivitis (gum disease) and to prevent rheumatic fever and endocarditis (an infection of the heart valves) in susceptible people undergoing dental surgery or minor procedures.

How does it work?

Penicillin V potassium is an antibiotic. It fights infection by adhering to the walls of susceptible invading organisms, ultimately killing them by interfering with their ability to make new cell walls. Penicillin V potassium is also used in injection form, but this form is not discussed here.

Administration

Follow prescribing information from the doctor and pharmacist. Also:

- Although it may be taken with meals, penicillin V potassium is most fully absorbed when taken on an empty stomach (1 hour before or 2 hours after eating).

- Keep the oral solution refrigerated and discard any unused portion after 14 days.

- Check the expiration date. Discard the solution if the date has passed.

If you miss a dose: Take the missed dose right away, unless it is almost time for the next dose, in which case you should skip the missed dose and resume the regular schedule. Do not take two doses at once.

How quickly will it take effect?

Penicillin V potassium will start to fight bacteria within 1 hour or less, but it will take 3 days or so for you to notice an improvement in your condition. How soon this happens depends on the type and severity of your infection, however.

Side effects and severe reactions

Contact the doctor if any unusual, worrisome, or severe reactions occur or if you develop:

- Severe stomach upset, nausea, vomiting, diarrhea, dizziness, mouth and tongue irritation (including soreness or a possible darkening or "hairiness" of the tongue)

- Symptoms of a mild allergic reaction, which may include skin rash, hives, itching

- Symptoms of a second (unrelated) infection

- Severe or bloody diarrhea. Do not take an antidiarrheal medication unless the doctor recommends it. In rare cases, diarrhea can signal the development of a serious bowel inflammation called pseudomembranous colitis.

Seek emergency care if you develop:

- Symptoms of a severe allergic reaction, which may include swelling of the mouth and tongue, fever, peeling skin, difficulty breathing, swollen or painful joints

- Seizures, unusual bleeding

Warnings

- Contact the doctor if your condition fails to improve—or if it worsens—within 3 to 5 days. A different medication may be needed.

- Take the full prescribed course of this medication, even if you are feeling well; otherwise, the infection may linger and resurface later. If you have a "strep" infection and fail to complete the medication regimen, you could put yourself at risk of developing serious heart problems later.

- Use this medication only for the infection—and the person—for which it has been prescribed.

- Severe allergic reactions are a particular risk in people who have had a reaction to penicillin or to cephalosporin antibiotics in any form.

- Certain types of the penicillin V potassium solution contain phenylalanine, a substance that certain people must avoid.

- If you take oral contraceptives (birth control pills) containing estrogen, beware that penicillin V potassium may make them less effective. Discuss with your doctor the risk of an unplanned pregnancy. He or she may recommend an additional (temporary) form of birth control.

Tips and other important things to know

- Penicillin V potassium was one of the first antibiotics introduced. Although it is powerful, it can fight only certain susceptible bacteria. It will have no impact on an infection caused by other organisms, such as viruses (as in the common cold), fungi, or parasites.

- If you have diabetes, be aware that penicillin V potassium may alter the results of certain urine glucose (sugar) tests. Discuss this with your doctor. The medication may alter the results of certain diagnostic tests as well.

Generic name Phenytoin

Brand names include Dilantin, Diphenylan

Principal uses

Phenytoin is an anticonvulsant medication prescribed to manage tonic-clonic (grand mal) and simple and complex partial seizures. Phenytoin is also used to control certain kinds of severe pain, such as migraine headache and trigeminal neuralgia, and rarely, to treat abnormal heart rhythms.

How does it work?

Phenytoin stabilizes many of the cellular mechanisms in nerve membranes that lead to seizure activity. It also stabilizes the conduction tissue of the heart that carries electrical signals.

Administration

Follow prescribing information from the doctor and pharmacist. Also:

- Take phenytoin at the same time every day to keep medication levels constant and seizures well controlled.
- Take phenytoin with food to reduce stomach upset.

If you miss a dose: Take the missed dose immediately, unless it is almost time for the next dose, in which case you should skip the missed dose. (If phenytoin is taken several times a day, take the missed dose only if it is within 4 hours of the next scheduled dose.) Do not take a two doses at once.

How quickly will it take effect?

Two to 3 weeks may be needed to determine how effective phenytoin is in reducing the severity and frequency of seizures.

Side effects and severe reactions

Side effects that are generally of no concern unless they are persistent or severe include:

- Fatigue and drowsiness, especially at first
- Slightly pink, red, or brownish urine

Contact the doctor if any unusual, worrisome, or severe reactions occur or if you develop:

- Fever, dizziness, headache, trouble sleeping, nervousness, nausea, vomiting, constipation, muscle twitching, overgrowth of the gums, extra body hair
- Symptoms of a new infection
- A severe skin reaction, yellowing of the skin or eyes, notable fatigue and weakness with fever, sore throat, abnormal bleeding or bruising, malaise, joint pain or swelling, mental confusion, double vision, unsteadiness, slurred speech, jerky eye movements, or enlarged lymph glands

Seek emergency care if you develop:

- Severe rash, fever, or pain

Warnings

- Never abruptly stop taking this medication or change the dose or brand without consulting your doctor; this can precipitate worse seizures. This includes switching from a brand-name to a generic version. The dosage should be increased gradually.

Tips and other important things to know

- Keep all appointments for follow-up visits; some adverse reactions can be detected only by laboratory tests or a physical examination.

- Discuss with your doctor the balance of sedation from the anti-seizure medication with your ability to function well.
- To minimize the potential for gum overgrowth, it is very important to brush and floss regularly.

Special precautions

- If you are pregnant or breast-feeding, discuss with your doctor the use of this medication *before* you start taking it. If you are at risk of pregnancy or on birth control pills, discuss with your doctor the use of this medication. Phenytoin can increase metabolism of birth control pills and make them ineffective, and has also been associated with birth defects.
- This medication increases your need for folic acid. Your doctor should monitor your blood levels of this vitamin and pregnant women should take folic acid supplements.
- Until your reaction to this medication has been established, avoid activity that requires mental or physical alertness.
- Ask your doctor about risks of taking this medication at the same time as alcohol or other central nervous system depressants (these slow down the nervous system).
- Wearing a medical alert bracelet/necklace is advised.

Generic name Potassium Supplements

Brand names include Apo-K, Cena-K, Kato, Klorvess, Klotrix, K-Tab, Potasalan, Rum-K, Slo-K, Ten-K

Principal uses

Potassium supplements are used to prevent or treat potassium depletion.

How does it work?

Your body needs potassium to function normally. Most people get the potassium they need through a balanced diet. For those who use diuretics ("water pills") that deplete potassium reserves or more rarely, the person who requires additional dietary potassium, potassium supplements are often recommended. Potassium salts, potassium acetate, potassium chloride, and potassium gluconate are discussed here, although the injection forms of these medications are not.

Administration

Follow prescribing information from the doctor and pharmacist. Also:

- Take potassium supplements immediately after eating.
- Slowly sip liquid forms of the medication or the water with which you take a pill—over 5 to 10 minutes—to reduce stomach irritation.
- For tablets and capsules: take with an 8-oz glass of water. Never crush or chew the sustained-release capsule.
- For powder, granules, or soluble tablets: mix the medication in at least 4 oz of water or juice. Allow the medication to dissolve completely and stop fizzing before drinking.
- For premixed liquid potassium products: dilute in at least 4 to 8 oz of water or as otherwise directed on the package or the prescription label.

If you miss a dose: Take the missed dose right away, unless it is more than 2 hours since when you should have taken the dose, in which case you should skip the missed dose and resume the regular schedule. Do not take two doses at once.

How quickly will it take effect?

The speed at which a potassium supplement starts to work depends on your condition and the reason for which you are taking it. Ask your doctor what to expect.

Side effects and severe reactions

Side effects that are generally of no concern unless they are persistent or severe include:

- Mild abdominal discomfort, nausea, vomiting, diarrhea, mild gas

Contact the doctor if any unusual, worrisome, or severe reactions occur or if you develop:

- Abdominal or stomach pain, cramping, or persistent soreness; chest or throat pain (possibly when swallowing)

Seek emergency care if you develop:

- Bloody or black stools; this may indicate stomach or intestinal bleeding
- Symptoms of hyperkalemia, a condition in which there is too much potassium in the blood: palpitations (irregular heartbeat), shortness of breath, notable tiredness or weakness in the legs, nausea and vomiting, abdominal pain, stomach pain, unexplained diarrhea, abnormal heart rhythms (to be determined by your doctor), numbness or tingling in the feet, fingers, or lips

Warnings

- Do not change the dose without your doctor's recommendation. Do not take more than recommended; potassium supplements are available only by prescription because excessive doses can cause severe reactions, including hyperkalemia. This condition can develop quickly and without warning, causing death if improperly treated.
- Avoid salt substitutes (including low-sodium milk) unless your doctor advises you to do otherwise; they tend to contain large amounts of potassium.
- Potassium supplements should not be taken when you are dehydrated and urinating small volumes. Extended sun exposure and sweating can cause dehydration; muscle cramps are a sign that they have indeed caused dehydration. Ask your doctor what to do should such a situation arise.
- Discuss with your doctor the risks of breast-feeding while taking potassium supplements. They appear to be safe to use during pregnancy, but you should discuss this with your doctor.

Tips and other important things to know

- Keep all appointments for follow-up visits so that your doctor can properly monitor your condition and reaction to this medication.
- Consuming foods rich in potassium may help you avoid the need for a potassium supplement. Potassium-rich foods include apricots, avocados, bananas, beans, broccoli, butternut squash, cantaloupe, dates, lentils, milk, orange juice, raisins, spinach, yogurt, watermelon, and zucchini.
- If you are on a sodium-restricted diet, do not use tomato juice to dilute the potassium supplement.
- The wax shell of the sustained-release tablet may appear in the stool a few hours later. This is normal and no cause for alarm; the potassium has been absorbed into your body.
- Liquid forms of potassium are often the best choices for people with certain heart, gastrointestinal, or esophageal disorders. Your doctor will make this judgment.

Generic name Pravastatin

Brand name Pravachol

Principal uses

Pravastatin is prescribed to lower high levels of cholesterol in the blood. This is done in an attempt to prevent heart complications of coronary artery disease associated with cholesterol-clogged blood vessels.

Administration

Follow prescribing information from the doctor and pharmacist. Also:

- Take this medication exactly as prescribed. The dosage has been carefully tailored to your body's requirements and response. Do not take it in larger or smaller doses, more often, or for longer than recommended.
- Pravastatin may be taken without regard to meals.
- Take pravastatin in the evening, preferably at bedtime, unless otherwise directed by your doctor.

Side effects and severe reactions

Contact the doctor if any unusual, worrisome, or severe reactions occur or if you develop:

- Severe muscle aches and pains

Tips and other important things to know

- Pravastatin belongs to a class of medications called hydroxymethyl-glutaryl coenzyme A (HMG CoA) reductase inhibitors (statins). Medications in this class may vary slightly in price, when they are best taken, the research in which they have been used, the side effects they produce, and the amount of experience doctors have with them.

- The dosage is typically readjusted every 4 to 6 weeks until the optimal dosage is determined.

See the *simvastatin* entry on page 1559 for more information on how statins work, what to expect in terms of speed and side effects, and when to contact the doctor if problems develop. (Unless otherwise noted, the information for *simvastatin* applies to all statins.

Generic name Prednisone

Brand names include
Meticorten, Orasone, Panasol, Deltasone

Principal uses

Prednisone is used to treat various allergic and inflammatory conditions, including severe asthma, nephritis (a kidney condition), inflammatory bowel disease, multiple sclerosis, and numerous rheumatic disorders, including systemic lupus erythematosus (SLE; lupus) and rheumatoid arthritis. Hydrocortisone (a similar substance to prednisone) has also been used to suppress rejection of transplanted organs and to treat severe skin reactions to medications, foods, plants, and other substances. Prednisone is sometimes taken if the body does not produce enough corticosteroids on its own.

How does it work?

Prednisone is a corticosteroid ("steroid"). It suppresses inflammation and immune system function in several ways. It limits the activity of certain disease-fighting white blood cells involved in causing inflammation, redness, and swelling. Our bodies naturally produce corticosteroids, therefore, when taken in pill or liquid form as medication, it can shut down the body's natural production.

Administration

Follow prescribing information from the doctor and pharmacist. Also:

If you miss a dose and you normally take one dose a day: Take the missed dose right away and resume the regular schedule. If you do not remember the missed dose until the next day, skip the missed dose.

If you normally take one dose every other day: Take the missed dose as soon as possible if it is still morning, and then resume the regular schedule. If it is later in the day, wait until the next morning to take the missed dose. If you normally take several doses a day, take the missed dose as soon as possible, and resume the regular schedule.

How quickly will it take effect?

Prednisone will reach peak concentrations in your bloodstream in 1 to 2 hours, but it may take several days for your condition to improve. This depends in part on the type and severity of your illness. Ask your doctor what to expect.

Side effects and severe reactions

Side effects that are generally of no concern unless they are persistent or severe include:

- Increased appetite, nervousness or restlessness, trouble sleeping, indigestion

Contact the doctor if any unusual, worrisome, or severe reactions occur or if you develop:

- Symptoms of an infection, increased thirst, decreased or blurred vision, frequent urination, confusion, mood swings or emotional instability, persistent depression, hallucinations, restlessness or worrisome changes in mental status

- With long-term use: acne, unusual rounding out of face ("moon face"), black or bloody stools, persistent abdominal or stomach pain, reddish purple lines on skin, thin and shiny skin, poorly healing wounds, rapid weight gain, muscle weakness and loss of muscle mass, black and blue marks on skin, excessive facial hair, mild dizziness, vision problems,

changes in fat distribution, thinning of bones

- Symptoms that your body is not adjusting well when you are stopping prednisone: stomach or abdominal pain, back pain, fever, dizziness, fainting, muscle or joint pain, nausea, persistent loss of appetite, shortness of breath, vomiting, unusual tiredness or weakness, weight loss, frequent or continuing headache, reappearance of disease being treated

Warnings

- Prednisone is a very powerful medication and extremely valuable in treating many conditions, but it must be used with care because of its potential to cause side effects.

- Never abruptly stop taking this medication. Doing this could cause very serious reactions, particularly if you have been taking prednisone for an extended period of time or in high doses. Contact your doctor if you become sick or are unable to take your medication for some other reason.

- Prednisone suppresses the immune system. For this reason, avoid exposure to serious infections, such as chickenpox or measles. This is particularly important for children who have not yet had these infections and have no immunity to them; the infection may have a much more severe course in them. Contact the doctor right away if you suspect you have been exposed to a such infections.

- Prednisone must be used with particular caution in children because of the risk of adverse reactions, including suppression of normal growth with large doses or long-term treatment. Ask your doctor what to expect.

- Do not get an immunization without your doctor's approval; the prednisone may limit your body's ability to mount an appropriate immune system response.

- Avoid using nonsteroidal anti-inflammatory drugs (NSAIDs) with prednisone. They may increase the risk of gastrointestinal upset and ulceration. As with any medication, it is important to discuss with your doctor all those you take before getting a prescription.

Tips and other important things to know

- Side effects associated with prednisone are largely related to the dose and the amount of time you take the medication. Ask the doctor what to expect, given your prescription.

- This medication may reduce your body's ability to properly handle stressful physical situations, such as surgery (including dental surgery) or emergency treatment. Make sure any doctor or dentist treating you in such circumstances is aware that you take prednisone. You may temporarily need extra doses.

- The doctor should recommend that you take calcium supplements or other medications to help prevent bone loss, a risk for bone fractures.

- Because prednisone may alter the results of certain diagnostic tests, tell the doctor performing the test that you take this medication.

Generic name
Propoxyphene with Acetaminophen

Brand names include
Darvocet, Wygesic

Principal uses

This medication is prescribed to treat mild to moderate pain and pain accompanied by fever. It combines a narcotic analgesic (propoxyphene) with acetaminophen.

Administration

Follow prescribing information from the doctor and pharmacist. Also:

- Take this medication exactly as prescribed. Do not take it in larger doses, take it more frequently, or take it for longer periods of time than recommended. There is a risk of physical and psychological dependence, potentially fatal overdose, and liver damage in such cases.

- Take this medication with food if it causes stomach upset.

Warnings

- There is a considerable risk of becoming psychologically and physically dependent on this medication when it is taken in higher doses or for longer than recommended.

- This medication should not be taken in people who have a history of addiction or who are suicidal. If either condition applies to you, contact your doctor immediately.

- This medication should be used with great care in combination with tranquilizers, muscle relaxants, antidepressants, antihistamines, or other substances that depress (slow down) the central nervous system and can make you sleepy, including alcohol. Consult your doctor about the risks of combining these types of medications with propoxyphene and acetaminophen.

See the *hydrocodone and acetaminophen* entry on page 1535 for more information on how narcotic (opioid) analgesic and acetaminophen combination medications work, what to expect in terms of speed and side effects, and when to contact the doctor if problems develop. (Unless otherwise noted, the information for *hydrocodone and acetaminophen* applies to all narcotic [opioid] analgesic and acetaminophen combinations.)

Generic name   Quinapril

Brand name   Accupril

Principal uses

Quinapril is prescribed to treat hypertension (high blood pressure) and to manage congestive heart failure. It belongs to a class of medications called angiotensin converting enzyme (ACE) inhibitors.

Administration

Follow prescribing information from the doctor and pharmacist. Also:

- Take this medication on an empty stomach (1 hour before or 2 hours after eating) because food, particularly if it is high in fat, can impair absorption of the medication.

How quickly will it take effect?

It may be several weeks before you experience the full benefits of this medication.

Side effects and severe reactions

Contact the doctor if any unusual, worrisome, or severe reactions occur or if you develop:

- Pronounced lightheadedness, fainting

- Unusual bruising or bleeding; symptoms of an infection, such as sore throat or fever

Seek emergency care if you develop:

- Symptoms of a severe allergic reaction, such as difficulty breathing or swelling of the eyes, lips, tongue, or face

Warnings

- Avoid salt substitutes that contain potassium while taking this medication.

Tips and other important things to know

- Diuretics ("water pills") are sometimes taken along with quinapril to help control blood pressure.

- Many people taking this medication feel lightheaded, especially during the first few days of treatment. Try getting up from a sitting or lying position slowly to minimize this sensation.

See the *enalapril* entry on page 1522 for more information on how ACE inhibitors work, what to expect in terms of time of onset and side effects, and when to contact the doctor if problems develop. (Unless otherwise noted, the information for *enalapril* applies to all ACE inhibitors.)

Generic name   Ranitidine

Brand name   Zantac

Principal uses

Ranitidine is used to manage gastric (stomach) and duodenal (intestinal) ulcers and to relieve associated symptoms. It is also prescribed to treat conditions involving excess stomach acid, to control gastroesophageal reflux disease (GERD; backflow of stomach contents), to prevent stress ulcers and damage from long-term use of nonsteroidal anti-inflammatory drugs (NSAIDs), and occasionally to treat heartburn, sour stomach, and various other disorders.

How does it work?

Ranitidine belongs to a class of medications known as H_2 (gastric histamine) blockers, also known as histamine$_2$—or H_2—antagonists. H_2 blockers inhibit the ability of the stomach to make acid. They do this by occupying the receptor sites on cells that histamine normally locks onto for this purpose. (These sites differ from histamine receptors involved in producing allergy symptoms, however.) Once acid levels drop, many ulcers heal on their own. Other commonly used medications in this class include *cimetidine, famotidine,* and *nizatidine.*

Ranitidine is available in both oral and injection forms, but the injection form is not discussed here.

Administration

Follow prescribing information from the doctor and pharmacist. Also:

- Swallow the tablet or capsule whole with plenty of water; do not chew it.

- Ranitidine may be taken without regard to food.

- Antacids may be taken along with the medication to relieve pain, but to avoid canceling out the H_2 blocker's effect, always take the antacid 2 to 3 hours before or after the H_2 blocker.

- If you have been prescribed one dose a day, take it at bedtime, unless otherwise advised by the doctor. If you have been prescribed two doses a day, take one in the morning and one at night. If you have been prescribed several doses a day, take them with meals and at bedtime.

If you miss a dose: Take the missed dose as soon as possible, unless it is almost time for the next dose, in which case you should skip the missed dose and resume the regular schedule. Do not take two doses at once.

How quickly will it take effect?

Heartburn should resolve in about 1 hour. It may take several days for ulcer-related stomach pain and other symptoms to dissipate with ranitidine, and possibly 4 to 8 weeks of regular use for the ulcer to heal.

Side effects and severe reactions

Contact the doctor if any unusual, worrisome, or severe reactions occur or if you develop:

- Headache, swelling of eyelids, tightness in chest, confusion, unusual bleeding or bruising, unusual tiredness or weakness, sore throat and/or fever, heartbeat that is fast, pounding, irregular, or slow

- Symptoms of a bleeding ulcer, such as vomiting of "coffee ground" material and the development of black or tarry stools

Warnings

- For proper healing, it is important to keep taking this medication as prescribed, even if you feel better.

- Contact the doctor if your ulcer pain persists or gets worse.

- Do not take an H_2 blocker for longer than prescribed; the long-term safety of most is not well established.

- Do not abruptly stop taking an H_2 blocker for peptic ulcer disease, as this increases the risk of a recurrence or perforation. Once you stop taking the medication, stay alert for symptoms of a recurrence.

- Do not take any over-the-counter medication for more than 2 weeks without checking with your doctor.

Tips and other important things to know

- The various H_2 blockers work the same way against ulcers and most gastrointestinal conditions and heal ulcers at about the same rate. They differ somewhat in potency, types of side effects associated with them, and interactions with other medications. The doctor will select the H_2 blocker most appropriate for you on the basis of your medical condition.

Because they work in the same way, it is unlikely that an ulcer that fails to heal with one H_2 blocker will respond to another.

- Keep all appointments for follow-up visits so that your doctor can properly monitor your condition and determine when the medication can safely be stopped.

- Just because symptoms have cleared with an H_2 blocker does not mean the illness has been eliminated; your doctor will have to make a professional judgment regarding your condition.

- H_2 blockers are typically prescribed after other strategies—eliminating the cause of the ulcer, taking antacids—have failed. Subsequent rounds of treatment with H_2 blockers may be necessary if the ulcer reappears.

- Most people experience few if any side effects with H_2 blockers.

- To encourage healing and lessen pain, avoid sodas, citrus products, alcohol, nonsteroidal anti-inflammatory drugs (NSAIDs; these include aspirin), and other foods and medications known to irritate the stomach. Eliminate other medications only under the advice of your doctor, however. Ask for guidance on limiting protein-rich foods known to increase stomach acid secretions.

- Smoking cigarettes tends to increase the amount of acid the stomach produces, especially at night. Stop smoking altogether or at least refrain from smoking after the last H_2 blocker dose of the day.

- Certain H_2 blockers may alter the results of laboratory tests for blood and platelet counts, skin allergies, sperm levels, and stomach acid production, among others. All your doctors and your dentist should be told that you take an H_2 blocker.

Special precautions

- If you are pregnant or breast-feeding, discuss with your doctor the use of this medication *before* you start taking it.

Generic name Salmeterol

Brand name Serevent

Principal uses

Salmeterol is taken regularly to help prevent bronchospasm (narrowing of the airways) and asthma symptoms. It has also been used to prevent exercise-induced bronchospasm.

How does it work?

This long-acting beta agonist opens up the airways in a process called bronchodilation. It promotes bronchodilation by acting on certain receptors in the muscles of the airways, relaxing them. This helps prevent bronchospasm and asthma attacks. *Albuterol* is a commonly used beta agonist that, although structurally and pharmacologically similar to salmeterol in many ways, is short acting (fast acting) rather than long acting and is therefore used differently.

Administration

Follow prescribing information from the doctor and pharmacist. Also:

- Take this medication exactly as prescribed. To avoid the risk of serious reactions, do not take more of it or take it more often than recommended.

- Salmeterol is administered by oral inhalation using a metered-dose inhaler. See the package insert for detailed instructions and ask your doctor or pharmacist for guidance if you are unclear on how to administer it. Also, see page 1464 for more information on inhalation medications.

- Clean the plastic case and cap for the metal canister in warm running water once a day and dry them well.

- Unless otherwise directed by your doctor, take this medication at 12-hour intervals to achieve the optimal effect.

- To prevent exercise-induced bronchospasm, salmeterol is typically taken 30 to 60 minutes before exercise.

- Spacer devices have been used successfully with the metered-dose inhaler. Ask your doctor for information about this if you have trouble administering the medication.

If you miss a dose: Take the missed dose right away and resume the regular dosing schedule.

How quickly will it take effect?

Studies indicate that in people with asthma or chronic bronchitis, a 42-microgram dose (2 puffs) of salmeterol produces effective bronchodilation in 10 to 25 minutes. Improvements in the condition of the airway continue for 12 hours or so.

Side effects and severe reactions

Side effects that are generally of no concern unless they are persistent or severe include:

- Headache (including sinus headache), tremor, cough, lower respiratory tract infection, sore throat, hay fever, stomach pain and other gastrointestinal upset, joint or back pain, muscle pains or cramps, dizziness, nervousness, malaise or fatigue, dental pain

Contact the doctor if any unusual, worrisome, or severe reactions occur or if you develop:

- Chest pain; rapid heartbeat; severe dizziness or faint feeling; bluish discoloration of skin; skin rash, hives, or itching; persistent flushing or redness of skin; swelling of face, lips, or eyelids

- Increased bronchospasm or other symptoms of worsening asthma

Warnings

- It is important to keep taking this medication, even when you feel fine.

- Ask your doctor for detailed guidance on which other asthma medications to continue using and which ones to stop.

- Never use salmeterol to treat acute asthma symptoms. Use an inhaled, short-acting (fast-acting) bronchodilator in such situations. Your doctor should give you information on handling these situations.

- If asthma symptoms become bothersome despite twice daily (recommended) doses of salmeterol, contact your doctor for guidance. Honestly discuss your use of asthma medications.

- Salmeterol is not a substitute for inhaled or oral corticosteroids ("steroids"). Do not reduce or stop the steroid dose your doctor may have prescribed for you, as your asthma may seriously worsen.

- Do not take extra doses of salmeterol for any condition, including to prevent exercise-induced asthma, unless the doctor specifically recommends it.

- If the salmeterol dose you take fails to control exercise-induced asthma, consult your doctor. Do not take more inhalations of salmeterol for at least 12 hours after taking the medication for exercise-induced asthma. Your doctor may give you a short-acting asthma medication to handle any acute symptoms not controlled by the salmeterol.

Tips and other important things to know

- Salmeterol is notable among asthma medications for its delayed onset and prolonged duration of action. This is why it is called *long acting.*

- Salmeterol is not usually started in people with rapidly deteriorating asthma whose condition can be managed by occasional doses of a short-acting (fast-acting) beta agonist, such as albuterol.

Special precautions

- If you are pregnant or breast-feeding, discuss with your doctor the use of this medication *before* you start taking it.

Generic name Sertraline

Brand name Zoloft

Principal uses

Sertraline is prescribed for mental depression. It belongs to a class of medications known as serotonin reuptake inhibitors.

Administration

Follow prescribing information from the doctor and pharmacist. Also:

- It is critical that you take this medication exactly as prescribed.

- Sertraline may be taken without regard to food, but try to take it consistently in relation to your meals.

This helps encourage even absorption.

If you miss a dose: Talk to your doctor about what to do.

How quickly will it take effect?

You may have to take sertraline for up to 4 weeks before noticing an improvement in your condition.

Side effects and severe reactions

Side effects that are generally of no concern unless they are persistent or severe include:

- Decreased appetite or weight loss, stomach cramps, lessened sexual drive, decreased sexual ability (impotence)

Contact the doctor if any unusual, worrisome, or severe reactions occur or if you develop:

- Fever; rapid speech; a feeling of being out of control; skin rash, hives, or itching

Warnings

- This medication may activate mania (or an unusually heightened and energized state) in people with manic-depressive or other cyclic disorders.

See the *fluoxetine* entry for more information on how serotonin reuptake inhibitors work, what to expect in terms of speed and side effects, and when to contact the doctor if problems develop. (Unless otherwise noted, the information for *fluoxetine* applies to all serotonin reuptake inhibitors.)

Generic name Simvastatin

Brand name Zocor

Principal uses

Simvastatin is prescribed to lower high levels of cholesterol in the blood. This is done in an attempt to prevent heart complications or coronary artery disease associated with cholesterol-clogged blood vessels.

How does it work?

Simvastatin belongs to a class of medications called hepatic hydroxymethylglu-

taryl coenzyme A (HMG CoA) reductase inhibitors (statins). Other common cholesterol-lowering medications in this class include *fluvastatin, lovastatin, pravastatin, atorvastatin,* and *cerivastatin.* These medications work by interfering with a critical step in the synthesis of cholesterol. They all reduce total cholesterol, low-density lipoprotein (LDL) cholesterol (so-called bad cholesterol), and triglyceride levels, but raise high-density lipoprotein (HDL) cholesterol (the so-called good cholesterol) levels.

Administration

Follow prescribing information from the doctor and pharmacist. Also:

- Take this medication exactly as prescribed. The dosage has been carefully tailored to your body's requirements and response.

- Simvastatin may be taken without regard to meals at any time during the day.

If you miss a dose on one day: Resume the regular schedule the next day. Do not take two doses the next day.

How quickly will it take effect?

Your doctor will likely schedule a follow-up visit for about 4 weeks after you started this medication to determine whether your cholesterol level has dropped.

Side effects and severe reactions

Side effects that are generally of no concern unless they are persistent or severe include:

- Diarrhea, constipation, gas

Contact the doctor if any unusual, worrisome, or severe reactions occur or if you develop:

- Unexplainable joint pain or muscle aches, pains, or tenderness; fever; malaise; unusual tiredness or weakness

- Abdominal pain, heartburn, headache, fatigue, vomiting, nausea, anorexia, skin rash, hair loss, itching, skin changes

Seek emergency care if you develop:

- Persistent muscle aches and pains

Warnings

- This medication must be taken regularly, as prescribed, for it to work. Do not stop taking it on your own; consult your doctor for guidance.

- As with all medications, it is important to discuss your medical history with your doctor before starting on one. With statins, this is particularly important in the case of recent major surgery and liver disease. Even if you do not have a liver disorder, your doctor will periodically check your liver function with a blood test.

- Statins should not be taken during pregnancy. Discuss with your doctor your plans for pregnancy before becoming pregnant, if possible. Contact the doctor right away if you unexpectedly become pregnant.

- These drugs may cause dangerous muscle inflammation, evidenced by muscle pain and kidney damage when taken in combination with certain drugs such as erythromycin, gemfibrozil, niacin, cyclosporin, and drugs used to treat fungus infections.

Tips and other important things to know

- No medication will eliminate the dangers associated with high cholesterol levels, but many help minimize the risks.

- Doctors typically prescribe such medications as simvastatin after attempting to lower cholesterol levels with dietary measures, weight reduction, exercise, and the treatment of an underlying disorder, should one exist. A typical cholesterol-lowering diet limits the intake of cholesterol and fats (total and saturated fat).

- It is critical that you continue intelligent dietary measures, weight control, and exercise once you start taking a cholesterol-lowering medication. No medication should be viewed as a substitute for these measures.

- If you have any questions about why controlling your cholesterol is important, talk to your doctor. Also, see Chapter 20 for a fuller discussion.

- The doctor may decide to reduce the medication dose if cholesterol levels fall below the target range.
- Keep all appointments for follow-up visits so that your doctor can monitor your cholesterol level and overall condition and check for unwanted reactions to the medication.
- Make sure all surgeons, dentists, and doctors who care for you are aware that you take this medication.
- Statins are less effective if you are notably overweight. Ask your doctor for guidance on dieting.

Special precautions

- Do not take this drug if you are pregnant or breast-feeding. Discuss with your doctor the use of this medication if you are planning to become pregnant.

Generic name Sumatriptan
Brand name Imitrex

Principal uses

Sumatriptan is used to treat severe migraine headaches and symptoms frequently associated with them, such as nausea, vomiting, and sensitivity to light and sound.

How does it work?

Sumatriptan apparently works by activating receptors in blood vessels in the brain that promote their constriction. This type of action has been associated with migraine pain relief.

Sumatriptan is available as an injection, tablets, and in nasal spray form for treatment of migraine and cluster headache. The injection form of administration is not discussed here.

Administration

Follow prescribing information from the doctor and pharmacist. Also:

- Take sumatriptan tablets with a full glass (8 oz) of water.
- Swallow the tablets whole. Do not break, chew, or crush them.
- Sumatriptan may be taken any time during the course of a migraine.
- If your migraine pain returns after initial relief with a first dose of suma-

triptan, take another dose of sumatriptan. Limit your doses to the number the doctor has recommended, however. Too much of this medication increases the risk of side effects.

- Ask the doctor what to do if you get no pain relief at all in 2 to 4 hours. In such situations, a second dose is unlikely to lessen the pain of that particular migraine, although it may help with future ones.

How quickly will it take effect?

Pain relief usually occurs within 30 minutes to 3 hours, with maximum relief between 3 to 6 hours.

Side effects and severe reactions

Side effects that are generally of no concern unless they are persistent or severe include:

- Dizziness; drowsiness; flushing, lightheadedness; nausea or vomiting; feeling cold or out of sorts; sensations of warmth, heat, burning, tightness, numbness, or tingling; muscle aches, cramps, or stiffness; discomfort in the mouth, jaw, tongue, sinuses, or nose

Contact the doctor if any unusual, worrisome, or severe reactions occur or if you develop:

- Difficulty swallowing, skin rash or bumps, pounding heartbeat
- Mild chest pain, chest or neck tightness or pressure; contact the doctor immediately if these symptoms persist for more than 1 hour.

Seek emergency care if you develop:

- Severe neck or chest pain; wheezing; swelling of the face, eyelids, or lips

Warnings

- Contact the doctor for guidance if your migraine headaches get worse or become more frequent or if sumatriptan fails to alleviate three migraine headaches in a row.
- Consult with your doctor about using sumatriptan if you have a history of poorly controlled hypertension or any history of coronary artery disease.

Tips and other important things to know

- Sumatriptan will relieve only that pain associated with migraine headaches (either with or without aura).
- Less potent medications should be tried before turning to this one.
- Sumatriptan does not prevent or reduce the frequency of migraine headaches. The doctor may recommend other medications for these purposes.
- Many migraine sufferers benefit from lying down in a dark, quiet room.
- Side effects with sumatriptan tend to appear within 1 hour of taking the medication and resolve within 1 hour.
- Many patients have a return of the headache in 12 hours.

Special precautions

- Until your reaction to this medication has been established, avoid activity that requires mental or physical alertness.
- If you are pregnant this medication is contraindindicated. If you are breast-feeding, discuss with your doctor the use of this medication *before* you start taking it.

Generic name Terazosin
Brand name Hytrin

Principal uses

Terazosin is prescribed to manage mild to moderate hypertension (high blood pressure). It is also used to treat benign prostatic hyperplasia (BPH; enlargement of the prostate gland surrounding the urinary canal) and associated complications, such as weak urine flow and frequent urination.

How does it work?

Terazosin is an alpha$_1$ blocker. Like other medications in its class, it helps lower blood pressure by blocking nerve endings called alpha$_1$ receptors, thus opening up blood vessels. In BPH, a type of muscle in the prostate and the bladder opening relaxes.

Administration

Follow prescribing information from the doctor and pharmacist. Also:

- Terazosin may be taken without regard to food.
- Take the first dose at bedtime unless otherwise directed.
- Take terazosin at the same time every day to avoid missing doses.

If you miss a dose and you normally take one dose a day: Take the missed dose right away, unless it is within 8 hours of the next dose, in which case you should skip the missed dose and resume the regular schedule. Do not take two doses at once.

How quickly will it take effect?

It will likely take several weeks for terazosin to maximally reduce your blood pressure.

Side effects and severe reactions

Side effects that are generally of no concern unless they are persistent, or severe include:

- Headache, weakness, fatigue, unusual tiredness, flu-like feeling, nausea, drowsiness, impotence
- Back or joint pain, nasal congestion, and blurred vision

Contact the doctor if any unusual, worrisome, or severe reactions occur or if you develop:

- Dizziness or lightheadedness (especially when standing up); sudden fainting; fluid retention with possible swelling of wrists, ankles, or lower legs; palpitations
- Irregular or pounding heartbeat, shortness of breath, difficult or labored breathing, chest pain

Warnings

- Take this medication as prescribed even if you feel well; hypertension is a largely symptom-free disease until organs become damaged.
- Avoid potentially hazardous activities, such as driving, for the first 12 hours after taking the first dose of this medication, increasing the dose or restarting the medication. Do this to avoid accidents caused by lack of alertness, dizziness, or lightheadedness. To avoid these side effects, this medication is usually started at a low dose which is then gradually increased.
- Avoid over-the-counter medications that contain stimulants, such as certain medications for colds; they can increase blood pressure. Ask your doctor or pharmacist for guidance.

Tips and other important things to know

- Alpha$_1$ blockers do not cure high blood pressure, but they do help to control it.
- Your doctor should give you guidance on other measures you can take to control high blood pressure, such as weight control, moderate exercise, and dietary measures.
- Alpha$_1$ blockers may help relieve the symptoms of BPH, but they will not alter the size of the prostate. In fact, the prostate may well continue to grow and require surgery.
- Lie or sit down if you get dizzy, faint, or feel in any other way out of sorts. These symptoms are due to a marked lowering of blood pressure. Until you know how this medication affects you, always get up gradually and carefully from a sitting or lying position. This is important to remember when getting up at night; turn on the light and take your time. These reactions are most likely to develop within 90 minutes of taking the medication, particularly during the first week of treatment.
- Because of the risk of dizziness or lightheadedness, take precautions in hot weather, during exercise, when drinking alcohol, or if standing for long periods.

Special precautions

- Until your reaction to this medication has been established, avoid activity that requires mental or physical alertness.
- If you are pregnant or breast-feeding, discuss with your doctor the use of this medication *before* you start taking it.
- Ask your doctor about risks of taking this medication at the same time as alcohol or other central nervous system depressants (these slow down the nervous system).

Generic name Tramadol
Brand name Ultram

Principal uses

Tramadol is prescribed to treat moderate to moderately severe pain. It is used for chronic back and cancer pain and during recovery from obstetric, orthopedic, and oral surgery.

How does it work?

It is not clear exactly how tramadol works, although its pain-relieving qualities have been attributed to its actions on the central nervous system.

Administration

Follow prescribing information from the doctor and pharmacist. Also:

- Take this medication exactly as prescribed. To avoid the risk of dependence and potentially serious reactions, do not take it in greater quantity or more frequently than recommended.
- Tramadol may be taken without regard to food.

If you miss a dose: Take the missed dose as soon as possible, unless it is almost time for the next dose, in which case you should skip the missed dose and resume the regular schedule. Do not take two doses at once.

How quickly will it take effect?

Pain relief should begin in 1 hour, with a peak effect within 2 to 4 hours and lasting for 3 to 6 hours overall.

Side effects and severe reactions

Side effects that are generally of no concern unless they are persistent or severe include:

- Indigestion, nausea, vomiting, constipation, dizziness

Contact the doctor if any unusual, worrisome, or severe reactions occur or if you develop:

- Nervousness or restlessness, tremor, emotional ability, sweating, headache,

- dry mouth, itching, sleepiness, weakness and fatigue
- Seizure, slowed or troubled breathing

Seek emergency care if you develop:

- Seizures, prolonged sedation, severe drug reaction

Warnings

- Tramadol can be habit forming, causing physical and emotional dependence. This is not a problem if it is taken as prescribed, however. Although it is not chemically related to opium, it is not recommended for people dependent on opiate painkillers or when drinking alcohol.
- Follow the doctor's guidance on when to stop this medication, as it can cause unpleasant withdrawal reactions under certain circumstances. It may also become less effective over time; ask your doctor for information.
- Because tramadol affects the central nervous system and may cause associated dizziness and other reactions, be careful when getting out of bed, walking, driving, or partaking in any other potentially dangerous activity until you know exactly how you react to the medication.
- Tramadol may increase the risk of seizures in people with a history of seizures or who are taking certain medications, such as monoamine oxidase (MAO) inhibitors, tricyclic antidepressants, selective serotonin reuptake inhibitor (SSRI) antidepressants, or antipsychotic medications.
- As with any medications, it is important to inform your doctor about allergic reactions to any other medications. In the case of tramadol, it is particularly important to report a previous allergic reaction to codeine or other opiates or to tramadol itself.
- Avoid consuming alcohol or ingesting any other central nervous system depressants, such as sedatives, tranquilizers, or opiates when taking tramadol. These substances may work together with tramadol to dangerously slow down the central nervous system.

Tips and other important things to know

- Tramadol may alter the results of certain laboratory tests. Make sure that any doctor who is performing tests is aware that you take it.

Special precautions

- Until your reaction to this medication has been established, avoid activity that requires mental or physical alertness.
- Ask your doctor about risks of taking this medication at the same time as alcohol or other central nervous system depressants (these slow down the nervous system). See the *Warnings* section.
- If you are pregnant or breast-feeding, discuss with your doctor the use of this medication *before* you start taking it.

Generic name
Triamcinolone

Brand names include
Aristocort, Azmacort, Kenacort

Principal uses

Triamcinolone is used in the form of an oral inhalant to treat severe, chronic bronchial asthma. It is used in the form of a nasal aerosol or spray to control hay fever symptoms, such as stuffiness and irritation, to control other allergic disorders and inflammatory conditions, and to prevent recurrent nasal polyps.

Triamcinolone is also available in tablet, syrup, injection, cream, lotion, ointment, paste, and solution forms for various ailments, but these are not discussed here. Triamcinolone is a corticosteroid ("steroid") medication.

Administration

Follow prescribing information from the doctor and pharmacist. Also:

- To function as intended, the oral and nasal forms of this medication must be used daily and at evenly spaced intervals as directed by your doctor.
- Carefully read the package insert. For extra guidance about administering the oral inhalation form of tri-

amcinolone, see page 1464. For the nasal inhalation or spray, see page 1464.

- To reduce the risk of serious reactions, do not use the oral inhalation medication more frequently, in larger doses, or for longer than recommended. Do not suddenly stop taking it; withdrawal should be gradual as directed by your doctor.
- After using the oral inhaler, rise out your mouth or drink a glass of water.
- Clean the inhaler regularly in warm water. Dry it thoroughly.

If you miss a dose of the oral inhalant: Take the missed dose as soon as possible, unless it is almost time for the next dose, in which case you should skip the missed dose and resume the regular schedule. Do not take two doses at once.

If you miss a dose of the nasal medication: Take the missed dose right away if it is within the hour of when you should have taken it. Otherwise, skip the missed dose and resume the regular schedule.

Tips and other important things to know

- The various oral and nasal steroids differ primarily, at least from the consumer's point of view, in the number and frequency of doses recommended for each.

See the *beclomethasone* entry on page 1511 for more information on how corticosteroid medications work, what to expect in terms of speed and side effects, and when to contact the doctor if problems develop. (Unless otherwise noted, the information for *beclomethasone* applies to all orally and nasally inhaled steroids.)

Generic name Triamterene with Hydrochlorothiazide

Brand names include
Dyazide, Maxzide

Principal uses

This medication is used to treat high blood pressure (hypertension) and fluid retention.

How does it work?

This medication combines two diuretics, one that increases loss of potassium in the urine (hydrochlorothiazide) and one that prevents potassium loss (triamterene).

Administration

Follow prescribing information from the doctor and pharmacist. Also:

- This medication may be taken without regard to food.

If you miss a dose: Take the missed dose as soon as possible, unless it is almost time for the next dose, in which case you should skip the missed dose and resume the regular schedule. Do not take two doses at once.

How quickly will it take effect?

This medication will start to work within 1 hour, with a peak effect in 2 to 3 hours. It may take several weeks of regular use for high blood pressure to respond fully, however.

Side effects and severe reactions

Side effects that are generally of no concern unless they are persistent or severe include:

- Tiredness, excessive urination, diarrhea, decreased sexual ability, loss of appetite, upset stomach, dizziness or lightheadedness when rising from a sitting or lying position, increased sun sensitivity

Contact the doctor if any unusual, worrisome, or severe reactions occur or if you develop:

- Symptoms of hyperkalemia, a condition in which there is too much potassium in the blood: shortness of breath, mental confusion, anxiety, notable tiredness or weakness in the legs, nausea and vomiting, abdominal pain, stomach pain, unexplained diarrhea, abnormal heart rhythms (to be determined by your doctor), numbness or tingling in the feet, fingers, or lips
- An illness with severe nausea, vomiting, or diarrhea

Seek emergency care if you develop:

- Symptoms of a severe allergic reaction, such as sudden shortness of breath or swelling of the lips, tongue, or face

Warnings

- Take this medication as prescribed even if you feel well; hypertension is a largely symptom-free disease until organs become damaged.
- Do not make any drastic changes in your diet without discussing them with your doctor first.
- This medication can cause glucose (sugar) intolerance in some people. People with diabetes should have their blood sugar levels monitored and may, in some cases, need to have their insulin or blood sugar medication dosage adjusted.
- If you have high blood pressure, you should generally avoid over-the-counter medications that can raise it, such as certain stimulant-containing cough and cold remedies. Ask your doctor or pharmacist for guidance.

Tips and other important things to know

- This combination medication is considered valuable because it reduces the tendency to lose excessive amounts of potassium, something that can occur when hydrochlorothiazide is taken alone.
- This medication will help control your blood pressure, but it will not cure you of the disease.
- Keep all appointments for follow-up visits so that your doctor can monitor your condition and assess your reaction to this medication.
- To minimize dizziness or lightheadedness that sometimes occurs with this medication (especially the first few doses), get up gradually from a sitting or down position.
- Your doctor should advise you on lifestyle measures to lower blood pressure, such as weight control, moderate exercise, and following a healthy diet.

Special precautions

- If you are pregnant or breast-feeding, discuss with your doctor the use of this medication *before* you start taking it.

Generic name

Trimethoprim/
Sulfamethoxazole

Brand names include

Bactrim, Septra

Principal uses

This medication is used to treat bacterial infections in the urinary tract, digestive tract (as in traveler's diarrhea), respiratory tract and bronchial tubes, middle ear, and other parts of the body. It is used to prevent and treat *Pneumocystis carinii* pneumonia. Trimethoprim/sulfamethoxazole is sometimes given by injection in the hospital for very serious infections, but this use is not discussed here.

How does it work?

The combination of these two antibiotics is so effective because each attacks the ability of susceptible bacteria to make folic acid—a nutrient the bacteria need to grow and reproduce—in different ways. The combination is particularly effective because bacteria are slow to develop resistance to both at the same time.

Administration

Follow prescribing information from the doctor and pharmacist. Also:

- Take this medication with a full glass (8 oz) of water and drink several extra glasses of water a day to help prevent side effects.
- Take this medication on an empty stomach (1 hour before or 2 hours after eating). If it upsets your stomach, however, try taking it with food or milk.

If you miss a dose: Take the missed dose as soon as possible, unless it is almost time for the next dose, in which case you should skip the missed dose and resume the regular schedule. Do not take two doses at once.

How quickly will it take effect?

A single dose of this medication will reach peak concentrations in your system within 1 to 4 hours. Depending on the type of infection you have and how severe it is, however, it may take several days or more of regular use for your condition to improve noticeably.

Side effects and severe reactions

Side effects that are generally of no concern unless they are persistent or severe include:

- Dizziness, headache, nausea or vomiting, loss of appetite

Contact the doctor if any unusual, worrisome, or severe reactions occur or if you develop:

- Increased skin sensitivity to the sun
- Pale skin; itching or skin rash; joint or muscle aches; swallowing difficulty; sore throat and fever; yellowing of skin or eyes; notable bleeding or bruising; seizures; skin redness, blistering, peeling, or looseness; loss of coordination
- Vaginal yeast infection

Seek emergency care if you develop:

- Shortness of breath, severe abdominal pain

Warnings

- Take all the prescribed medication, even if symptoms of the infection have cleared; otherwise, the infection may reappear or another kind of infection may develop.
- Contact the doctor if your condition does not improve—or if it worsens—within approximately 10 days.
- Do not share this medication. It should be used only by the person for whom it has been prescribed.
- Do not give this medication to children less than 2 months old.

Tips and other important things to know

- This medication is powerful, but it will have no impact on an infection caused by a virus, such as the common cold or flu, or by a number of other organisms.
- Keep all appointments for follow-up visits so that your doctor can monitor your progress and check for

unwanted reactions to the medication, especially if you are taking it for extended periods of time. It is particularly important to check for unwanted blood reactions.

- The sensitivity to the sun that this medication produces in some people may last for months after you stop taking it. Take precautions in the sun—discuss these with your doctor—and watch for your reaction to the sun. Contact the doctor if you have a severe reaction.
- Ask your doctor or dentist about precautions you should take in brushing your teeth, flossing, and other measures to avoid irritation or bleeding of the gums.

Special precautions

- If you are pregnant or breast-feeding, discuss with your doctor the use of this medication *before* you start taking it.
- This medication may increase sensitivity to the sun; discuss with your doctor what precautions are appropriate.
- Until your reaction to this medication has been established, avoid activity that requires mental or physical alertness.

Generic name Valproic Acid and derivatives

Brand names include Depakene, Depakote

Principal uses

Valproic acid is prescribed to manage various kinds of seizures, including simple and complex absence (petit mal) seizures, tonic-clonic (grand mal) seizures, mixed-type seizures, complex partial seizures, and psychomotor seizures. It is also used to control infantile spasms.

How does it work?

It is not exactly clear how valproic acid works. It appears to inhibit seizure signals from spreading through the brain, possibly by means of producing increased levels of brain chemicals involved in inhibiting nerve cell communication.

Administration

Follow prescribing information from the doctor and pharmacist. Also:

- Take this medication exactly as prescribed. Do not alter the dosage in any way without consulting your doctor, or you may increase the risk of seizures and side effects.
- Take this medication with food if it causes stomach upset.
- Swallow the regular capsules whole to avoid irritating your mouth or throat. Do not chew or break them. Take the pill with an noncarbonated liquid to prevent damaging its coating, which is designed to lessen stomach irritation. If the capsule dissolves too early, it may irritate your mouth or leave a bad taste.
- Swallow the delayed-release capsule or tablet whole. If you have trouble swallowing the delayed-release capsule, you may open it and sprinkle its contents over a small amount of soft food, such as pudding. Ingest this entire mixture immediately without chewing.
- If you dislike the taste of the syrup, you may mix it with a liquid or food, but make sure to consume the entire mixture right away.

If you miss a once-daily dose: Take the missed dose as soon as possible, unless it is already the next day, in which case you should skip the missed dose and resume the regular schedule.

If you miss a dose and normally take two or more doses a day: Take the missed dose if you remember within 6 hours of when you should have taken it, then space out the rest of the day's doses evenly through the rest of the day. Do not take two doses at once.

How quickly will it take effect?

You will likely have to take this medication for 2 weeks or more before its ability to control your seizure disorder can be determined.

Side effects and severe reactions

Side effects that are generally of no concern unless they are persistent or severe include:

- Drowsiness, dizziness, mild stomach

or abdominal cramps, diarrhea, nausea and vomiting, indigestion, hair loss, shifts in menstrual periods, hand or arm trembling, unusual weight gain or loss

Contact the doctor if any unusual, worrisome, or severe reactions occur or if you develop:

- Severe abdominal or stomach cramps, double vision, increase in seizures, loss of appetite, persistent nausea or vomiting, facial swelling, spots before the eyes, yellowing of the eyes or skin, continuous and uncontrolled rolling or back-and-forth movement of eyes, unusual bleeding or bruising

Warnings

- Never abruptly stop taking valproic acid. This may precipitate severe or prolonged seizures, particularly if you are taking the medication for a major seizure disorder.
- Valproic acid is often taken in combination with other anticonvulsant medications; ask your doctor about what side effects to look for with other medications you take.
- Check with your doctor before switching brands or switching to a generic version of this medication, as various brands may affect your seizure condition differently.
- Check with your doctor before drinking alcohol or using any other medication that depresses (slows down) the central nervous system, from sedatives to other anticonvulsants.
- Avoid use of this medication during pregnancy or if you are trying to conceive.

Tips and other important things to know

- Keep all appointments for follow-up visits so that your doctor can monitor your condition and check for side effects. This is particularly important during the first 6 months of treatment.
- Be sure that any doctor or dentist who is going to perform surgery on you is aware that you take this medication. This is important for several reasons, including the increased

likelihood of bleeding problems with valproic acid.

- Valproic acid may alter the results of certain laboratory tests. If you have diabetes, take note that this medication may produce a false positive result when you are testing for urine sugar.

Special precautions

- Ask your doctor about risks of taking this medication at the same time as alcohol or other central nervous system depressants (these slow down the nervous system).
- Until your reaction to this medication has been established, avoid activity that requires mental or physical alertness.
- Wearing a medical alert bracelet/necklace is advised.
- If you are pregnant or trying to conceive, discuss the use of this medication with your doctor *before* you start taking it. See the *Warnings* section.

Generic name Warfarin

Brand names include Coumadin, Panwarfin

Principal uses

Warfarin is prescribed to prevent and treat blood clots and pulmonary emboli (lung clots). It is also used to prevent clots from forming in the heart, which can lead to a stroke. Warfarin will not dissolve an existing clot, but it may stop it from increasing in size and causing serious and potentially fatal complications.

How does it work?

Warfarin is an anticoagulant. It decreases the clotting ability of the blood by slowing down the production of substances critical to making the blood clot. Warfarin is taken orally.

Administration

Follow prescribing information from the doctor and pharmacist. Also:

- For this medication to work properly and to reduce the risk of serious bleeding, it is extremely important that you take it exactly as prescribed. Do not take more of it, take

it more frequently, or take it for longer than recommended.

- Take warfarin on an empty stomach (1 hour before or 2 hours after a meal), unless it causes stomach upset, in which case you should try taking it with food.
- Protect the medication from light.

If you miss a dose: Take the missed dose as soon as possible, unless you do not remember until the next day, in which case you should skip the missed dose and take the regular scheduled dose alone. Do not take two doses at once. This could cause serious bleeding.

How quickly will it take effect?

A single dose of warfarin typically has an anticoagulant effect within 24 hours and works for 2 to 5 days overall. Daily doses may be required to reach and maintain a therapeutic amount of anticoagulation.

Side effects and severe reactions

Side effects that are generally of no concern unless they are persistent or severe include:

- Bloated stomach, gas, loss of appetite, unusual hair loss, cool fingers and toes

Contact the doctor if any unusual, worrisome, or severe reactions occur or if you develop:

- Heavy or persistent bleeding from superficial injuries, bleeding from gums when the teeth are brushed, unexplained nosebleeds, bruising or purplish spots on skin that appear to develop for no reason, noticeably heavy or unexpected menstrual bleeding, cloudy or dark urine, painful or difficult urination, pain and purplish color in toes, swelling, unexpected weight gain, yellow skin or eyes, sore throat, white spots or sores or ulcers in the mouth or throat, fever, chills, notable tiredness or weakness, sudden decrease in urine output
- Symptoms of internal bleeding: unusual bruising or bleeding, black or tarry stools, blood in the urine or stool, abdominal pain or swelling, back pain, constipation, coughing up blood, vomiting blood or mater-

ial that looks like coffee grounds, severe or continuing headache, joint pain, stiffness, or swelling

- An unrelated illness

Warnings

- Warfarin can be hazardous if not used properly. The dosage prescribed for you is carefully tailored to alter your body's blood-clotting function without causing severe bleeding. Blood clots are dangerous because they can cut off oxygen to critical organs and body tissue.

- There are a number of situations and conditions in which warfarin is not recommended. Make sure that your doctor knows about all your medical conditions.

- Avoid making drastic changes in your environment, diet, or physical state without discussing them first with your doctor, as some may alter your response to warfarin. For example, ingesting high concentrations of vitamin K, found in such foods as leafy green vegetables, counteracts the effects of warfarin. Also discuss with your doctor the risk of ingesting alcohol.

- Check with your doctor before starting or stopping any other medication (including aspirin), as many alter the way that warfarin (or the other medication) is processed. Some medications may also affect blood clotting. This could cause complications if you stop taking them without a readjustment of the warfarin dosage.

- Do not switch brands without checking with your doctor or pharmacist.

Tips and other important things to know

- It is extremely important to keep all appointments for follow-up visits so that your doctor can closely monitor your condition, observe your reaction to the medication (typically done by means of a weekly blood test to check for clotting time), and examine you for side effects.

- Tell all the doctors who treat you, including your dentist, that you take warfarin.

- Seniors must be followed particularly closely while taking an anticoagulant, such as warfarin, because they tend to be more sensitive to its effects.

- Your doctor may strongly advise you to stop partaking in contact sports or other activities that put you at risk for traumatic injury. Also avoid activities that put you at risk for getting cuts, scrapes, or bruises because of the risk of excessive bleeding. Discuss with your doctor what precautions are appropriate.

- When stopping warfarin therapy, be aware that the medication's effects may persist for about 2 to 5 days after the final dose.

Special precautions

- This medication has a number of potentially hazardous interactions. Discuss with your doctor all the medications you take—including over-the-counter ones—before taking this one.

- If you are pregnant or breast-feeding, discuss with your doctor the use of this medication *before* you start taking it.

- Wearing a medical alert bracelet or necklace is advised.

- Ask your doctor about risks of taking this medication at the same time as alcohol or other central nervous system depressants (these slow down the nervous system).

Generic name Zolpidem

Brand name Ambien

Principal uses

Zolpidem is prescribed for short periods to treat sleeping problems, such as difficulty falling asleep or staying asleep or awakening early.

How does it work?

Zolpidem is a sedative and tranquilizer. It interacts with central nervous system receptors responsible for alertness and the awake state, among other things. Zolpidem acts on the brain and exerts some of the same actions in the body that a class of traditional sedatives

known as benzodiazepines do, although it does not belong to this class.

Administration

Follow prescribing information from the doctor and pharmacist. Also:

- Zolpidem works quickly; take it just before you are ready to go to sleep for the night, preferably when you are already in bed as onset may be abrupt, or as otherwise prescribed by your doctor.

- Take this medication only when you have time for a full night's sleep (7 to 8 hours). If you wake up before this amount of time, the medication will not have worn off completely and may cause unwanted drowsiness and memory problems.

- Avoid taking zolpidem with a meal or immediately after one, as food delays absorption of the medication.

- When stopping this medication, follow your doctor's instructions carefully. If you take zolpidem for 1 or more weeks, stopping abruptly or rapidly reducing the dose may cause unpleasant withdrawal reactions, such as fatigue, nausea, vomiting, panic, or stomach cramps.

If you miss a dose: Take the missed dose if it is within 1 hour of when you should have taken the medication. Otherwise, skip the missed dose and resume the regular schedule. Do not take two doses at once.

How quickly will it take effect?

Zolpidem reaches peak concentrations in a little over 90 minutes. Because it works so quickly, be sure to take it directly before retiring for the night.

Side effects and severe reactions

Contact the doctor if any unusual, worrisome, or severe reactions occur or if you develop:

- Dizziness, diarrhea, mental depression, confusion, fainting, headache, constipation, indigestion, frequent falling, hallucinations, skin rash, facial swelling, difficulty breathing, dry mouth, medicated feeling, nausea, vomiting, heart palpitations, nervousness, unusual excitability, unusual thinking or behavior

Seek emergency care if you develop:

- Symptoms of an overdose: staggering, trouble breathing, or severe drowsiness, nausea, or vomiting

Warnings

- Follow prescription instructions exactly. Zolpidem can be habit forming, causing psychological or physical dependence, if taken for extended periods or at high doses.

- If the doctor specifically recommends that you take zolpidem for more than a few weeks, you should be aware that the medication may become less effective over time. Never increase the dose on your own in an attempt to boost its performance; contact the doctor for guidance.

- Some people experience dizziness, drowsiness, lightheadedness, unsteadiness, clumsiness, double vision or other visual disturbances, problems concentrating, or other lingering effects of zolpidem on arising the next morning and during that day. This is particularly a risk if you take the zolpidem in doses higher than recommended, drink alcohol, or are a senior. Make sure you know exactly how you react to this medication before driving, operating machinery, or do anything else that demands physical or mental alertness.

- Do not drink alcohol or take other substances that depress (slow down) your central nervous system; zolpidem may compound the effects of these depressants in potentially hazardous ways.

Tips and other important things to know

- Sleep problems are usually temporary and require medications for only brief periods of time, such as 1 or 2 days. It is uncommon for zolpidem to be needed for longer than 7 to 10 days, although your doctor may recommend that you use it for longer periods.

- Adverse reactions to zolpidem appear to be dose related.

- Seniors may be more sensitive to zolpidem's effects.

- Some people have trouble sleeping for the first few nights after stopping zolpidem. This is called rebound insomnia and is most likely to occur when the medication has been taken for 1 or more weeks.

- Do not take zolpidem on an overnight airplane flight that lasts less than 7 to 8 hours, as a special type of memory loss called "traveler's amnesia" may occur.

Special precautions

- Until your reaction to this medication has been established, avoid activity that requires mental or physical alertness.

- If you are pregnant or breast-feeding, discuss with your doctor the use of this medication *before* you start taking it.

- Ask your doctor about risks of taking this medication at the same time as alcohol or other central nervous system depressants (these slow down the nervous system).

Glossary

The *Johns Hopkins Family Health Book* Glossary provides clear definitions of commonly used medical terms. Rather than function as an encyclopedia of medical conditions, the glossary focuses on terms pertaining to human biology, signs and symptoms of disease, and the diagnostic and treatment techniques used to manage disease. Definitions of specific illnesses are located in the chapters and can be found quickly by using the index.

Abscess A localized, pus-filled cavity in an organ or tissue that is often accompanied by inflammation.

Acidosis A condition characterized by the presence of abnormally high levels of acid in the blood.

Acuity Sharpness.

Acupuncture A technique involving the insertion of thin needles into certain areas of the body to alleviate stress or pain or to treat disease.

Acute Occurring suddenly or lasting a short period of time.

Addiction A physical or emotional dependence on a substance (such as alcohol or drugs) or activity.

Adenoma A benign tumor that originates in a gland.

Adrenal cortex The outer portion of an adrenal gland in which the hormones aldosterone, cortisol, and dehydroepiandrosterone are produced. Hormones made in the adrenal cortex help to regulate blood pressure and fight infection and play a role in the production of sex hormones manufactured outside of the reproductive glands.

Adrenal gland One of a pair of small glands, 1 or 2 in. long, that sit atop each kidney and influence a variety of body functions through the production of certain hormones. See also Adrenal cortex and Adrenal medulla.

Adrenal medulla The inner region of an adrenal gland in which the hormones epinephrine and norepinephrine are produced. Hormones made in the adrenal medulla help to regulate blood pressure, heart rate, and carbohydrate and fat metabolism and play a role in the "fight-or-flight" response.

Aerobic exercise Prolonged activity that increases exercise tolerance by improving the way the body makes use of oxygen.

Aldosterone A hormone produced in the adrenal glands that helps to regulate the fluid volume of the body by signaling the kidney to exchange salt for potassium and acid.

Allergen An otherwise innocuous substance—such as animal dander, pollen, or food—that the body treats like an invading enemy and attacks with its immune defenses, resulting in physical reactions such as inflammation of the skin, eyes, or bronchial tubes.

Alveolus One of the millions of balloon-like structures located at the tips of bronchioles where oxygen is exchanged for carbon dioxide.

Ambulatory Having the ability to walk.

Amenorrhea A prolonged absence of menstrual periods.

Amino acid A nitrogen-containing building block of protein. Some amino acids essential to life are synthesized by the body, whereas others are found only in food.

Amnesia Memory loss.

Amniocentesis A procedure in which a thin, hollow needle inserted through the abdomen is used to draw amniotic fluid from the womb during pregnancy to determine the gender of the fetus or to identify an abnormality.

Amniotic fluid The liquid that surrounds and protects the fetus while the fetus is in the uterus.

Amniotic sac The thin, tough membrane that envelops the fetus while the fetus is in the uterus.

Amputation The surgical or traumatic removal of a part of the body, such as a limb or digit.

Analgesic A medication that relieves pain.

Anaphylaxis A severe allergic reaction characterized by flushing, itching, hives, lip and eyelid swelling, tightening of the throat, sudden hoarseness, nausea, vomiting, and abdominal pain. Anaphylaxis can begin within seconds of exposure to an allergen and can prove fatal in a matter of minutes if not immediately and appropriately treated.

Androgen A group of male reproductive hormones, including testosterone, made in the testes and adrenal glands and also found in small amounts in women.

Anemia A condition characterized by a deficiency in red blood cells, hemoglobin, or volume of blood.

Aneurysm A bulge or ballooned area in an artery resulting from pressure on a weak area of the artery wall.

Angina pectoris Chest discomfort due to inadequate blood supply to the heart.

Angioplasty A surgical procedure in which a long, slender catheter is inserted into a narrowed, plaque-filled artery where a balloon at the tip of the catheter is inflated to widen the artery and increase blood flow.

Anorexia nervosa A pathologic obsession with thinness and an abnormal need to control food, usually affecting young women, that often leads to emaciation, malnutrition, and related health problems. Can be fatal if not treated.

Anterior Forward.

Antibiotic A medication that kills disease-causing bacteria or prevents them from reproducing.

Antibody A molecule that attacks foreign substances, called antigens, in the body.

Anticoagulant A medication that delays or prevents blood clotting.

Antidiuretic hormone (ADH) A hormone produced in the pituitary gland that signals the kidneys to reabsorb water when the body becomes dehydrated and also causes constriction of certain blood vessels to increase blood pressure in response to a steep drop in blood pressure; also called vasopressin.

Antidote A medication or other substance that counteracts the toxic effects of a poison.

Antigen A protein, especially when appearing on the surface of cells, that if recognized as foreign triggers the manufacture of antibodies.

Antihistamine A medication that acts to block the action of histamine, the body chemical released during allergic reactions that is responsible for allergic symptoms.

Antipyretic Fever reducing.

Anus The canal, encircled by two rings of powerful muscles, that connects the rectum to the outside of the body. Muscle contractions in the colon force stool out of the body through the anus.

Aorta The main artery leading away from the heart that transports blood to the rest of the body.

Aphasia An inability to produce spoken language properly.

Aplasia The underdevelopment of an organ or tissue.

Apnea An involuntary cessation of breathing that is temporary.

Apocrine gland A gland located under the arms or in the genital region that is responsible for producing body odor.

Apoptosis The process by which cells are programmed to die.

Aqueous humor A clear, watery fluid that nourishes the lens of the eye.

Areola The light pink or brown tissue surrounding the nipple.

Arrhythmia An abnormality in heart rhythm.

Arteriole A small artery that connects a larger artery with a capillary.

Artery A type of blood vessel that transports blood away from the heart to other parts of the body.

Arthroplasty Replacement or repair of a joint by surgery.

Ascorbic acid Vitamin C.

Asphyxia Suffocation.

Aspiration A procedure in which a needle and syringe are used to withdraw fluid or gas from a body cavity.

Asthma A respiratory disorder characterized by frequent or occasional periods of breathlessness, wheezing, coughing, and chest tightness that can be mild or severe.

Asymptomatic Without symptoms.

Ataxia An inability to coordinate voluntary muscle movement.

Atherosclerosis A condition characterized by thickening and hardening of the arteries.

Atresia The abnormal closure or absence of an opening or passage in the body present at birth.

Atrium A chamber or cavity, such as either of the small filling chambers in the upper part of the heart, that receives blood from veins.

Atrophy The wasting away of an organ or tissue.

Augmentation mammoplasty The clinical name for the surgical technique of increasing breast size.

Aura One or more of a constellation of symptoms, such as seeing a halo of light, that sometimes precedes a migraine headache or convulsion.

Auricle See External ear.

Autoimmune response Misinterpretation of one's own tissue as foreign and the production of antibodies against it.

Autonomic nervous system The part of the nervous system that regulates involuntary functions such as breathing, heartbeat, and digestion.

Avulsion A cut or tear that removes flesh from underlying tissue or the knocking or tearing out of a tooth.

Axon One of the major parts of a nerve cell that conducts impulses away from the cell body.

Bacteria Single-celled microorganisms that can either aid in necessary biological processes or cause disease.

Basal cell A cell within the epidermal layer of the skin.

Benign When referring to tumors, noninvasive and not capable of distant spread (see Metastasis). Not cancerous.

Bile A powerful detergent-like substance, made in the liver and containing cholesterol, bile salts, and bilirubin, that works in the small intestine to render fats into digestible, microscopic fragments that are more easily absorbed by the body.

Bilirubin The pigment, derived from hemoglobin, that gives bile its distinctive yellow-brown color and makes stool brown.

Biochemical marker A substance found in blood or urine that helps doctors to better understand certain biological processes going on inside the body.

Biofeedback A technique that promotes the self-regulation of seemingly unconscious body functions, ranging from heart rate or blood pressure to the perception of pain, and can be used to manage associated discomfort and stress.

Biopsy The removal and microscopic analysis of a tissue sample.

Bladder A sac with muscular walls into which urine flows from the kidneys. As the bladder fills with urine, nerve fibers within its walls detect stretching and when full, signal the need to void.

Blepharoplasty A surgical procedure involving the removal of fat, muscle, and excess skin from the eyelids.

Boil A bacterial skin abscess that begins as a small, tender nodule and after several days spontaneously ruptures and drains pus; also called a furuncle.

Bone density The amount of mineral in any given volume of bone.

Bone density test A medical test used to measure the density of the bones.

Bone marrow A core of fatty tissue, lying deep within the cavities of certain bones, that houses the body's reservoir of blood stem cells—the cells that divide to produce a continuing supply of red and white blood cells throughout life.

Bone mass The total amount of bone in the skeleton.

Bowel See Small intestine.

Brachytherapy See Internal radiation therapy.

Bradycardia An abnormally slow heartbeat.

Brain stem The part of the brain, consisting of the medulla, pons, and midbrain, that connects the cerebral hemispheres to the spinal cord and helps to maintain vital functions such as breathing and heartbeat.

Bronchus One of the two breathing tubes connecting the windpipe to the lungs.

Bronchiole One of the many small airways of the lungs connecting the larger bronchi with the smaller alveoli.

Bronchodilator A medication used to temporarily open airways that have narrowed due to an asthma attack.

Bruise An injury resulting in broken blood vessels and pooled blood under the skin that causes temporary skin discoloration.

Bulimia An eating disorder characterized by episodes of binge eating followed by purging through self-induced vomiting or abuse of laxatives, enemas, suppositories, or diuretics. Bulimics often maintain a normal weight.

Bullous A blister-like skin rash.

Bursa One of the fluid-filled pouches that cushion and protect tendons as they cross joints or bones.

Calcitonin A hormone made in the thyroid gland that is necessary for maintenance of proper calcium levels in the blood and for preservation of bone density by preventing breakdown of bone.

Calculus Rocklike mineral deposits that form on teeth (as a result of plaque buildup) or in other parts of the body, such as kidney stones.

Callus A thickened area of skin.

Cancer An uncontrolled growth of abnormal cells.

Capillary The smallest type of blood vessel. Capillaries serve as the connection between small arteries and veins.

Carbohydrate A nutrient, found mainly in cereals, breads, fruits, and vegetables, that provides fuel for the body in the form of glucose—which is used to produce energy for every cell in the body—and assists in the metabolism of other nutrients.

Carbon monoxide A colorless and odorless gas that can be fatal if inhaled in high concentrations.

Carbuncle A cluster of interconnected, deep boils that occur most commonly on the back of the neck, armpits, shoulders, and buttocks.

Carcinogen A cancer-causing agent.

Carcinogenesis The process by which a normal cell becomes cancerous.

Carcinoma A tumor that originates in the skin or linings of internal organs that tends to spread to other parts of the body (see Metastasis).

Cardiac Relating to the heart.

Cardiac arrest The sudden cessation of heartbeat and blood circulation.

Cardiomyopathy Disease of the heart muscle.

Cardiopulmonary Relating to the heart and lungs.

Cardiopulmonary resuscitation (CPR) A technique designed to restore heartbeat and respiration in an unconscious victim whose heart has stopped and who is not breathing.

Cardiovascular Relating to the system consisting of the heart and blood vessels that is responsible for circulating blood in the body.

Carie A dental cavity.

Carotid artery One of the main arteries in the neck that transports blood to the head and brain.

Cartilage Specialized, dense connective tissue that provides support and protection in the nasal septum, ears, and the ends of bones where they face one another in a joint.

Catheter A small, flexible tube inserted into various parts of the body to inject or suction out fluids.

Cellulose A type of water-insoluble fiber found in wheat bran, whole grains, fruits, and vegetables.

Central nervous system The system, made up of the brain and spinal cord, that governs higher functions such as speech, thought, and memory; the movement of muscles; the perception of sensations such as touch, sound, and light; and involuntary functions such as breathing, heartbeat, and digestion.

Cerebellum The area of the brain that directs certain activities not under conscious control, such as the ability to maintain balance and coordinate movement.

Cerebral cortex The outer surface of the cerebrum.

Cerebrospinal fluid The thin, shock-absorbing layer of liquid that surrounds and protects the brain and spinal cord.

Cerebrovascular Relating to the blood vessels of the brain.

Cerebrum The largest part of the brain, containing the cerebral hemispheres and responsible for such higher functions as speech, vision, thought, reason, and memory.

Cerumen A protective wax, produced by glands in the skin of the outer portion of the ear, that lubricates the skin of the canal and traps foreign particles.

Cervix The lower end (neck) of the uterus.

Cesarean section A surgical procedure in which a baby is removed from the uterus via incisions made in the abdomen and uterine wall.

Chemotherapy The administration of medications to treat cancer and infections.

Cholesterol A soft, fatty substance, made in the liver and also found in foods that come from animals, necessary for the production of cell membranes and sex hormones.

Chorionic villi The fingerlike projections from the chorion, the membrane that forms the placenta.

Choroid The layer of tissue in the eye lying between the retina and the sclera that is rich with blood vessels that nourish the retina, and dissipate heat.

Chromosome One of the 46 structures, existing in pairs, in which genes are stored in the body.

Chronic Long term.

Chyme The mushy pulp that food is broken down into after being pushed through the esophagus and exposed to the gastric acids and churning action of the stomach, after which it reaches the small intestine via the pyloric valve.

Cilia Microscopic hairlike projections that move in a coordinated fashion to carry impurity-laden mucus from the bottom of the lungs toward the throat, where it can be coughed out or swallowed.

Cirrhosis Permanent scarring of the liver, usually due to severe liver damage or chronic liver disease, that obstructs blood flow and prevents the liver from operating effectively.

Claudication The pain felt in muscles, during exercise or exertion, due to insufficient blood flow.

Clavicle The collar bone.

Clitoris A small node of erectile tissue in women, situated where the folds of the labia meet in the front, that enlarges and stiffens during sexual arousal.

Cloning The sexless reproduction of life using genetic material of a single, already existing parent.

Coarctation A narrowing or constriction.

Coccyx The tailbone (tip end of the spine).

Cochlea The hearing portion of the inner ear in which sound vibrations are registered by hair cells and converted into nerve impulses. These impulses are then carried to the hearing centers of the brain.

Cognitive Relating to the thought process.

Coitus Sexual intercourse.

Colic Pain due to spasm of the intestine or other hollow organs; a condition in infants characterized by excessive crying or screaming presumably due to gastrointestinal discomfort.

Collagen A binding-like protein found primarily in ligaments, cartilage, skin, and bone.

Colon A tube about 6 feet long, connecting the small intestine with the rectum and anus, that converts what is left of digested food into stool by removing salts and water. The stool is then transported to the rectum for temporary storage; also called the large intestine or large bowel.

Colorectal Relating to the colon and rectum.

Colostrum A watery, yellowish fluid, produced in the female breast, which provides a newborn with protective antibodies that fight infection during the first few days of life.

Computed tomography (CT) scan A painless, noninvasive series of x-ray pictures taken by a machine that encircles the body like a giant tube. This series of separate pictures is integrated by a computer to create a comprehensive view of the body.

Conception The fertilization of an egg by a sperm.

Concussion A temporary disruption of brain function caused by head trauma.

Cone One of many nerve cells, located in the retina, that registers and converts light into electrical signals that are sent to the brain via the optic nerve. Cones help to provide sharp central vision and are integral to the brain's perception of color and details.

Congenital Present at birth.

Conjunctiva A mucous membrane, nourished by a dense network of tiny blood vessels, that covers the inner surface of the upper and lower eyelids and the sclera.

Contrast agent A dye, taken orally or injected or inserted into the body, that is sometimes used during x-ray examinations to accentuate areas of the body that otherwise cannot be adequately represented on x-ray images.

Cornea The curved surface in the center of the front of the eye, made up of layers of clear tissue, that bends or refracts the rays of light through the pupil. The cornea is responsible for approximately 65% of the focusing that the eye does.

Coronary Relating to the arteries that carry blood to the heart.

Cortical bone A type of bone that is hard and compact, making up 85% of all bone.

Corticosteroid A hormone made in the adrenal glands. Similar compounds are used in medications to treat inflammation and suppress autoimmune responses.

Cortisol A hormone produced in the adrenal cortex that is chiefly responsible for maintaining vital processes during periods of sustained stress and for containing inflammation.

Cranium The part of the skull that encloses the brain.

Creatinine A waste product, filtered from the blood by the kidneys and passed from the body through the urine, that is often measured to evaluate the functioning of the kidney.

Curettage The scraping away of growths or other material from a cavity wall or other part of the body, often with a curette (a medical instrument shaped like a spoon).

Cuticle The fold of the skin at the base of a nail that serves as a seal, keeping bacteria, yeast, and debris in the environment from entering the adjacent skin.

Cyanotic A state characterized by bluish skin due to lack of oxygen.

Cyst A fluid-filled cavity.

Dander Shed skin debris.

Dehydration Fluid deficiency.

Dementia A loss of cognitive function usually due to a brain disease.

Dendrite One of the short extensions of a nerve cell body through which the cell receives electrochemical impulses.

Dentin The main body of a tooth, underneath the layer of enamel, surrounding the chamber of soft, sensitive pulp.

Dermatitis Inflammation of the skin.

Dermis The middle layer of skin, made mostly of collagen and filled with blood vessels, nerve cells, muscle cells, lymph vessels, hair follicles, and sweat and sebaceous glands.

Dextrose See Glucose.

Dialysis The use of a filtering machine or filtering fluids to remove toxins from the body of a person with kidney failure.

Diaphragm The powerful fanlike muscle that separates the chest cavity from the abdominal cavity.

Differentiated cell A type of cell, such as that found in muscles and nerves, that cannot be replaced if damaged or lost because it cannot reproduce itself; also called a specialized cell.

Digit Any finger or toe.

Dilate Widen.

Dislocation The movement of a bone out of its joint.

Diuretic A medication or agent that increases the amount of urine excreted.

Dopamine A neurotransmitter, associated with feelings of pleasure and well-being, that helps to regulate important brain functions. Dopamine has been studied for its role in the development of diseases such as schizophrenia and Parkinson's disease and in the abuse of drugs such as cocaine and alcohol.

Duodenum A part of the small intestine, about a foot long, that secretes bicarbonate to buffer harsh stomach acids, absorbs iron and other minerals, and breaks down and absorbs fat with the aid of bile.

Dysarthria Impaired ability to articulate speech due to lack of muscular control.

Dysmenorrhea Painful menstrual periods.

Dysplasia Abnormal tissue development.

Eccrine gland One of the sweat glands located throughout the body (but primarily on the palms, soles, and forehead) that help to regulate body temperature.

Ectopic Tissue in an atypical location.

Eczema An acute or chronic inflammation of the skin, due to an allergy or with no apparent cause, that is often accompanied by itching, blistering, and scaling.

Edema Swelling, usually occurring in the legs and ankles but in other parts of the body as well, that results from excessive accumulation of fluid in the tissues.

Electrolyte A substance such as chloride, potassium, sodium, or bicarbonate that helps to regulate the proper balance of acid and base, and by moving across cell walls, alters electrical charge in nerve and muscle cells.

Embolism The obstruction of a blood vessel, as from a blood clot or air bubble.

Embryo The term used to describe a developing baby from the time of implantation in the uterus to the eighth week after conception, after which time the term fetus is used.

Emetic A vomit-inducing substance, such as ipecac syrup.

Endocardium The thin, interior membrane that lines the chambers of the heart.

Endocrine system The system of glands distributed throughout the body—including the pituitary gland in the brain, the thyroid and parathyroid glands in the neck, the adrenal glands that lie atop each kidney, and the specialized cells within the pancreas in the midabdominal region— that serve as a main regulation, control, and signaling network for many body functions.

Endocrinologist A doctor who specializes in the diagnosis and treatment of endocrine system disorders.

Endodontist A dentist who specializes in the diagnosis and treatment of diseases within the tooth cavity.

Endometrium The lining of the uterus.

Endorphin A neurotransmitter produced in the brain that is often referred to as the body's natural painkiller.

Enema The insertion of fluid into the rectum to stimulate a bowel movement.

Enzyme A protein found in cells and digestive juices that triggers chemical reactions.

Eosinophil A type of specialized white blood cell that responds in allergic reactions.

Epidermis The outermost layer of the skin, in which skin cells are made.

Epiglottis The flap-like cover that closes with swallowing to prevent food and liquid from entering the respiratory passages, but opens to admit air.

Epinephrine A hormone made in the adrenal glands that is released into the blood in response to fright, exercise, exposure to cold temperatures, and low blood sugar levels. It helps to raise blood sugar, blood pressure, and heart rate and to ready the body for emergency action (the fight-or-flight response). It is also a neurotransmitter for certain nerve cells.

Episiotomy A small incision made in the area between the vagina and the rectum to facilitate rapid childbirth and prevent tearing of the vulva or vagina during childbirth.

Erection The enlargement and stiffening of the penis due to sexual arousal.

Ergonomics The scientific discipline devoted to the study of human work, including the relationships between people at work, the tools they use, and the physical and psychological demands of the work environment.

Erythrocyte See Red blood cell.

Esophagus A muscular tube about 9 $\frac{1}{2}$ in. long connecting the throat to the stomach.

Estradiol The most abundant chemical form of estrogen—made in the ovaries, it operates from puberty to menopause, and is measured by doctors to determine estrogen levels.

Estrogen A group of female reproductive hormones made primarily in the ovaries. It is also present in men in small amounts.

Estrogen replacement therapy (ERT) Use of estrogen in menopausal and postmenopausal women to alleviate the symptoms of menopause and to prevent osteoporosis and heart disease.

Eustachian tube The tube that drains fluids and mucus from the ears down into the back of the throat and equalizes middle ear pressure with the air pressure on the outside.

External beam radiotherapy A type of radiation therapy involving the use of a machine that is positioned outside the body and that directs radiation to the affected tissue; also called teletherapy.

External ear The outer crescent-shaped portion of the ear that gathers sound waves like a radar scanner and funnels them to the eardrum; also called the auricle or pinna.

Fallopian tube One of a pair of slender hollow tubes that extend outward, draping their fringe-like ends near the ovaries to gather in the eggs released with each monthly reproductive cycle and transport them to the uterus.

Fat Compounds made of fatty acids and used by the cells of the body in the production of hormones, the conduction of nerve impulses, membrane formation, and many other functions. In medicine, the term lipid is often used.

Fatty acid A building block of fat.

Febrile Feverish.

Femur The thigh bone.

Fetus The term used to describe a developing baby starting at the ninth week after conception.

Fiber A type of carbohydrate found in the cell walls of plants. There are two types: water soluble and water insoluble. They have different actions in the body.

Fibroid A benign tumor of muscular and connective tissue.

Fibula The outer and smaller of the two main lower leg bones.

Fistula An abnormal connection between internal organs or between an organ and the outside of the body.

Flatulence Excessive gas in the stomach and colon.

Follicle A sac or thin tubular structure in the skin or other organ.

Follicle-stimulating hormone (FSH) A hormone produced by the pituitary gland that stimulates estrogen secretion and the growth of follicles in the ovary in women and the development and maturation of sperm in men.

Fontanel A soft area on the top of a newborn's head, covering openings in the skull that have not yet fused together.

Forceps A medical instrument resembling tongs that is used to grasp or compress.

Fovea A depression in the center of the macula of the retina, which is packed with cone cells and provides sharp vision.

Fracture The breaking of a bone.

Fungus A plant-derived organism, such as mold, that lacks chlorophyll and depends on a host organism for nourishment.

Furuncle See Boil.

Furunculosis A condition characterized by recurrent or multiple boils.

Gallbladder The organ, about the size and shape of a pear and located on the right side of the body just under the liver, that functions as a holding tank for bile.

Gamma globulin An infection-fighting protein in the blood.

Gastric Relating to the stomach.

Gastrin A hormone produced in the stomach and duodenum that stimulates the acid production necessary for proper digestion.

Gastroesophageal reflux disease (GERD) Inflammation of the esophagus due to acid from the stomach, usually manifested as chronic heartburn.

Gastrointestinal tract The esophagus, stomach, and small and large intestines.

Gene The basic unit of heredity, made of DNA, that instructs the body to make proteins and through which inheritable characteristics are transmitted from parent to offspring.

Genome The sum of a person's genetic material; the complete set of chromosomes.

Gland A hormone-producing organ or group of cells.

Globulin A group of plasma proteins, some of which work to destroy potentially disease-producing microorganisms, whereas others are active in the formation of blood clots.

Glomerulus One of a number of tiny blood vessels in the kidneys that help to filter out waste from the blood.

Glucagon Hormone produced by the pancreas, in response to low blood sugar levels, that raises levels of blood sugar and is integral to the retrieval and use of stored fuels.

Glucose Blood sugar; also called dextrose.

Goiter Enlargement of the thyroid gland.

Grand mal A major convulsion, or seizure, lasting as long as 5 minutes.

Granulocyte Granule-containing white blood cells that consume and destroy bacteria.

Groin The region of the body, located generally in the lower abdominal area, between the torso and the tops of the legs.

Growth hormone A hormone produced in the pituitary gland that stimulates the release from the liver of insulin-like growth factor 1 (IGF-1) and helps to maintain and repair the lean mass of the body.

Gum A type of water-soluble fiber found in legumes, oats, and other plants.

Halitosis Bad breath.

Hangnail A sometimes painful tear in the edge of the nail near the skin, or a projection or split of the skin that surrounds the nail.

Heart attack A sudden occlusion or blockage by clot of one of the arteries supplying blood to the heart muscle with resultant damage to the muscle.

Heartburn The discomfort associated with the backing up of gastric juices from the stomach into the esophagus.

Hemangioma A benign tumor composed of blood vessels.

Hemarthrosis Bleeding into a joint.

Hematemesis Vomiting of blood.

Hematoma An accumulation of blood under the skin (a bruise), often with swelling, or in an organ.

Hematuria Blood in the urine.

Hemicellulose A type of water-insoluble fiber found in wheat bran, whole grains, and vegetables.

Hemiplegia Paralysis affecting one side of the body.

Hemoglobin The protein-iron compound transported by red blood cells that plays a key role in carrying oxygen from the lungs to the tissues.

Hemolyze To break down red blood cells.

Hemorrhage Bleeding.

Hemorrhoid An abnormally swollen vein located beneath the lining of the anal canal, or in the area near the anus, that may cause pain, itching, or bleeding.

Hepatic Relating to the liver.

Hepatoma Liver cancer.

Hernia An outpouching or projection of an organ or a part of an organ through the wall that normally contains it.

High-density lipoprotein (HDL) A lipoprotein that transports cholesterol and other lipids away from the arteries to the liver, where it is made into other substances needed by the body or eliminated; also called good cholesterol.

Hirsutism Excessive facial or body hair growth.

Histamine The chemical released by the body during an allergic reaction that is responsible for allergic symptoms such as swelling in the nose and eyes, excess mucus, itching, sneezing, irritation, and constriction of the breathing passages in the lung.

Hives Red, raised, itchy areas of inflamed skin that result from an allergic reaction; also called urticaria.

Homocysteine An amino acid that at high levels may play a role in clogging arteries.

Hormone A chemical courier, produced by an organ or gland and sent via the bloodstream to deliver instructions to other organs and glands, that helps to maintain the healthy functioning of the body.

Hot flash A temporary sensation of heat in the neck, face, and chest that occurs during menopause.

Humerus The upper arm bone.

Hymen A thin membrane spanning the vaginal canal, fully or partially blocking the opening, that usually is stretched or broken either by athletic activities or first sexual intercourse.

Hypercalcemia Elevated blood calcium levels.

Hyperglycemia Elevated blood sugar levels.

Hyperplasia Abnormal overgrowth of organ tissue.

Hypertension High blood pressure.

Hyperthyroidism An overactive thyroid gland.

Hyperventilation Rapid breathing and breathlessness due to a medical condition such as asthma, or a syndrome brought on by anxiety or stress.

Hypoglycemia Low blood sugar levels.

Hypotension Low blood pressure.

Hypothalamus A portion of the brain that regulates body temperature, appetite, and blood pressure, among other functions, and is involved in stress reactions and the expression of emotion.

Hypothermia A dangerous loss of body heat due to the body's failure to maintain its core temperature.

Hypothyroidism An underactive thyroid gland.

Hypotonic Poor muscle tone.

Hypoxia Reduced oxygen in the blood or body tissues.

Hysterectomy A surgical procedure in which the entire uterus is removed.

Idiopathic A term used to describe a disease or disorder whose cause is unknown.

Ileum The third and last portion of the small intestine.

Ilium The upper part of the hipbone.

Impetigo A contagious bacterial skin infection most common in young children and characterized by tiny blisters or honey-colored crusts that appear on the face, scalp, arms, and legs.

Impotence The inability to have or maintain an erection.

Incontinence A failure to control the release of urine or stool.

Infarct Tissue death due to lack of oxygen.

Infection A disease due to a microorganism.

Inguinal nodes Lymph nodes located in the groin.

Inner ear The part of the ear that translates sound vibration and head movement into nerve impulses that the brain interprets as sound and position.

Inorganic A substance that does not contain carbon.

Insomnia Difficulty falling or staying asleep.

Insulin A hormone produced by the pancreas, in response to the rise in blood sugar that follows a meal, that primarily regulates the storage of nutrients within cells but which also stimulates the kidney to retain salt and fluid, the production and storage of glycogen in liver cells, and the storage of fat in fat cells.

Internal radiation therapy A type of radiation therapy involving the surgical implantation of a radioactive source directly into or near the tumor; also called brachytherapy.

Intracranial Inside the skull.

Intravenous Inside or into a vein.

Iris The round, colored part of the eye containing blood vessels and connective tissue that adjusts the size of the pupil and regulates the amount of light that reaches the retina in the back of the eye.

Ischemia Lack of adequate quantities of blood in an organ or part of an organ, usually due to the narrowing or blockage of an artery.

Jaundice Yellowing of the skin or whites of the eyes (sometimes accompanied by a brownish or orange tint in the urine) that results from an accumulation of bile pigment in the skin.

Jejunum The second part of the small intestine, about 8 feet long, that absorbs the most nutrients such as proteins, sugars, vitamins, and minerals.

Joint The movable juncture of two or more bones.

Jugular vein One of the large veins in the neck that transports blood from the head and neck to the heart.

Kidney One of a pair of bean-shaped organs, each about 11 centimeters long in adults, responsible for cleansing the blood of waste, regulating certain chemicals, and removing fluid from the body.

Kyphosis Abnormally increased curvature of the spine; also called hunchback.

Labia The visible external portion of a woman's genitals, consisting of two fleshy outer folds of skin, that help protect sensitive tissues such as the entrances to the urethra and vagina.

Laceration A tear.

Lactose intolerance A condition characterized by poor digestion of dairy products.

Lanugo The soft, downy hair often present on the shoulders, forehead, and cheeks of a newborn that generally disappears within the first weeks of life.

Large bowel See Colon.

Large intestine See Colon.

Larynx The speaking chamber or voicebox.

Lens The transparent structure in the eye that focuses light rays on the retina and changes the shape of its curvature, depending on the distance of the object being viewed.

Lesion A broad medical term describing an altered or injured area of tissue.

Leukemia Cancer of the blood-forming tissues.

Leukocyte See White blood cell.

Leukocytosis A very high white blood cell count.

Leukopenia A very low white blood cell count.

Leukoplakia A white, usually benign patch in the oral cavity that simple rubbing will not remove and which usually forms in response to chronic irritation such as poor-fitting dentures or smokeless tobacco.

Libido Sexual drive or desire.

Ligament A band or sheet of strong fibrous tissue that holds together the joints of bones and helps to control how much motion occurs between the bones.

Lignin A type of water-insoluble fiber found in wheat bran, whole grains, and vegetables.

Lipid Fats or fatlike substances.

Lipoprotein A protein that transports fats in the blood.

Liposuction A body-contouring surgical procedure in which a vacuum-like machine is used to suck out fat from under the skin through a tube that is inserted through one or more small incisions.

Liver A large, solid organ located in the upper right abdomen that filters and neutralizes toxins and wastes in the blood and makes substances such as protein, chemicals essential for blood clotting, and bile, among others.

Liver spot An evenly colored (tan to dark brown), dime-sized flat spot on the skin found most often on the face and back of the hands of people over age 40 and caused by exposure to ultraviolet rays.

Localized Limited to a specific area.

Low-density lipoprotein (LDL) A lipoprotein that carries cholesterol and other lipids from the liver to the walls of the arteries, where it may accumulate and form plaque; also called bad cholesterol.

Lumbar Relating to the lower back.

Lumpectomy The surgical removal of a cancerous portion of the breast.

Lunula The portion of a nail that looks like a whitish crescent.

Luteinizing hormone (LH) A hormone produced by the pituitary gland that stimulates estrogen and progesterone secretion, and the growth of follicles in the ovary in women. In men it stimulates the development and functioning of testicular cells.

Lymph The clear, watery fluid that acts as a conductor between blood and tissue cells by conveying oxygen and nutrients to cells from the blood and returning waste products such as carbon dioxide from cells to the blood.

Lymph gland See Lymph node.

Lymph node Rounded structures, ranging from the size of a pinhead to a grape, along lymphatic vessels, consisting of immune cells that function primarily to filter out bacteria and other toxic substances which are flushed out from the tissues by the lymph fluid.

Lymphatic system The system made up of lymphatic vessels and capillaries that circulate lymphatic fluid between the cells that make up different tissues.

Lymphoma A tumor that originates in the lymphatic system.

Macula The center of the retina, responsible for central vision.

Magnetic resonance imaging (MRI) A painless, noninvasive method of taking pictures of internal organs with a machine that encircles the body like a giant tube. A computer integrates the pictures to create a comprehensive view of the body.

Malignant Tumors having the ability to spread into neighboring tissues and migrate to distant places in the body. Cancerous.

Mammary gland The milk-producing part of the breasts.

Mammogram An x-ray of the breast used to help detect breast cancer.

Mandible Lower jawbone.

Mast cell One of the cells that release histamine and other chemicals in response to contact between an allergen and the lining of the nose or eyes of a susceptible person.

Mastectomy A surgical procedure in which part or all of the breast is removed.

Masticate Chew.

Maxilla Upper jawbone.

Meconium stool A tarry and greenish or black stool, produced by a newborn during the first 24 hours of life, that is composed of residual amniotic fluid and intestinal secretions.

Medulla The center of a bone, gland, or organ.

Melanin The darkly pigmented substance, produced by melanocyte cells in the skin, that gives skin its coloring and helps to protect it from the potentially harmful ultraviolet rays of the sun.

Melatonin A hormone produced in the brain and used in synthetic form by some people to treat insomnia.

Menarche The onset of menstruation.

Meninges The membranes covering the brain and spinal cord.

Meniscus A pad of cartilage, in the shape of a crescent, that reduces friction in the knee joints.

Menopause The day on which menstrual periods have ceased for 1 year due to loss of ovarian estrogen. The term menopause is also used to refer to the entire process by which the production of ovarian estrogen declines and finally stops, and to the sudden cessation of menstruation that occurs due to surgery or radiation.

Metastasis The spread of cancerous cells from one region of the body to another.

Methadone A synthetic opiate, as addictive but not as pleasurable as morphine or heroin, used with some success in the treatment of heroin, morphine, and other opiate addiction.

Microbe A one-celled organism such as a bacterium.

Middle ear The air chamber, lying behind the eardrum, containing three tiny bones (the malleus, stapes, and incus), that amplify sound vibration.

Mineral One of a group of inorganic substances that are necessary in certain amounts to maintain health and ensure proper development and functioning of the body.

Mitosis The process of orderly cell replication.

Mitral valve The valve that regulates blood flow between the left atrium and the left ventricle and keeps blood from flowing backward in the wrong direction.

Mole A spot on the skin, usually round and uniform in color (ranging from flesh tones to deep brown or black), that may be found anywhere on the body and that may be flat or raised.

Monounsaturated fat A type of unsaturated fat that may help to reduce blood cholesterol levels.

Morphine A powerful painkilling medication derived from opium.

Musculoskeletal Relating to the system consisting of the muscles, ligaments, tendons, and bones of the body.

Mutation An alteration in the DNA of a cell due to an accident or disruption in the process of cell division or due to the presence of a carcinogen.

Myalgia Muscle pain or tenderness.

Myelin An insulating material that coats axons.

Myocardial infarction A heart attack.

Myopathy A disease of the muscles.

Necrosis The death of cells surrounded by living tissue.

Neonatal Relating to an infant who is 4 weeks old or younger.

Nephron The functional unit of the kidney; tiny filtering units, about one million of which are contained in each kidney, that draw waste and fluid from the blood to make urine while allowing water and essential salts, minerals, and nutrients to be reabsorbed back into the bloodstream.

Neuron A nerve cell.

Neuropathy Any disease of the nerves.

Neurotransmitter A substance that sends messages between nerve cells.

Nicotine A poisonous, addictive central nervous system stimulant, found primarily in tobacco.

Node A small, round mass of tissue in the body.

Norepinephrine A hormone made in the adrenal glands that is released into the blood in response to fright, exercise, exposure to cold temperatures, and low blood sugar levels. It helps to raise blood sugar, blood pressure, and heart rate and to ready the body for emergency action (the fight-or-flight response). It is also a neurotransmitter for certain nerve cells. Also called noradrenaline.

Nucleus The structure within each cell containing the chromosomes and their genes.

Obesity The state of being 20% or more above ideal body weight.

Occlusion A blockage or obstruction in a passage or channel in the body, such as in a blood vessel.

Occult Difficult to detect.

Ocular Relating to the eye.

Ocularist A specialist who makes artificial eyes and prosthetic devices for people who have lost their eyes because of disease, injury, or congenital defect.

Olfactory Relating to the sense of smell.

Olfactory nerve A group of sensitive fibers in the upper portion of the nose that is responsible for detecting odors.

Oncologist A doctor who specializes in the prevention and treatment of cancer.

Ophthalmic Relating to the eye.

Ophthalmologist A doctor who specializes in diseases of the eye. An ophthalmologist can perform eye surgery and prescribe glasses or contact lenses.

Optic nerve The structure that connects the eye to the brain and transmits the electrical impulses created by the retina to the visual cortex of the brain, which translates the impulses into an image.

Organic Containing carbon.

Orthotic splint An arch-supporting shoe insert.

Osseous Relating to the bones.

Ossicle One of the three tiny bones in the middle ear—the malleus, the stapes, and the incus—that form a chain that conducts sound waves from the eardrum to the hearing portion of the inner ear, amplifying the sound.

Osteoblast A bone cell that creates new bone by removing calcium and other minerals from the bloodstream and depositing them in bone.

Osteoclast A bone cell that destroys old bone by removing calcium and other minerals from bone and sending them back into the bloodstream.

Osteopathy Any disease of the bones; more commonly, a philosophy of medicine that emphasizes a holistic approach.

Osteoporosis An age-related, gradual decrease in bone density (reduction in bone mass per unit of volume) that causes them to become vulnerable to fractures in response to minor trauma.

Ovary The female reproductive organ that produces eggs. The ovaries also produce estrogen (secreted by the follicles), and progesterone (secreted by the corpus luteum).

Palate The roof of the mouth.

Palpate To examine by touch.

Palsy Paralysis, numbness, or an inability to control movement.

Pancreas An oblong organ, located behind the stomach, that secretes enzymes and bicarbonate (used for digestion by the small intestine) and hormones such as insulin and glucagon.

Paralysis An inability to move a muscle.

Paranasal sinus One of a series of air-filled chambers in the bones of the skull on either side of the nose and in the forehead.

Parasite An organism that is attached to or lives inside another organism and feeds off its host.

Parathyroid gland One of a pair (occasionally more) of pea-sized collections of tissue, lying on either side of and behind the thyroid gland, that mainly regulate proper levels of calcium and phosphorus in the blood by the production of parathyroid hormone.

Parathyroid hormone (PTH) A hormone made in the parathyroid glands that helps to maintain proper amounts of calcium in the blood by stimulating the release of calcium from bone, increasing reabsorption of calcium by the kidney, and by enhancing absorption of calcium and phosphorus from the diet in response to low calcium levels. Also known as parathormone.

Parotid gland One of the salivary glands.

Patella The kneecap.

Patent Open.

Pathogen A microorganism or other substance capable of causing disease.

Peak bone density The maximum bone density attained by a person.

Pectin A type of water-soluble fiber found in apples, citrus fruits, legumes, and certain vegetables.

Pectoral Relating to the chest.

Pelvis The bone supporting the spine and connecting to the leg bones.

Peptic Relating to digestion.

Percutaneous Performed through the skin.

Perforation A small hole.

Pericarditis An inflammation of the pericardium, the covering of the heart.

Pericardium The two thin leaves of slick fibrous tissue (with a fine layer of fluid between them) that surround and cushion the heart and reduce the friction that would otherwise occur with continual beats.

Perimenopausal A term meaning around the time of menopause.

Perineum The strip of skin between the vulva and anus in women and between the scrotum and anus in men.

Peristalsis Process involving involuntary muscles of the digestive tract by which food is moved from the esophagus through the stomach and intestines to the rectum.

Peritoneum The membrane that lines the abdominal cavity.

Peritonitis An infection or inflammation of the peritoneum.

Petit mal A momentary blackout in which the victim stares blankly for a few moments or becomes unaware of surroundings.

Pharynx The throat.

Phenotype The expression of the genes present in an individual.

Phobia An intense, unreasonable fear of a specific activity, object, or situation.

Photosensitivity A sensitivity to light.

Pigment A substance that provides color.

Pinna External ear; auricle.

Pituitary gland The master endocrine gland, located at the base of the brain, that produces its own hormones—such as growth hormone and prolactin—and also hormones such as luteinizing hormone and follicle stimulating hormone that regulate the activity of other glands in the endocrine system.

Placebo A sugar pill or inactive agent used in clinical trials of medications.

Placenta The structure that develops in the uterus during pregnancy and functions as the means by which the fetus receives nourishment and oxygen, and eliminates waste.

Plaque A buildup of cholesterol and other substances on an artery wall, or an abnormal area on the skin or mucous membranes.

Plasma The faintly yellow liquid in which blood cells, platelets, and other substances such as protein, electrolytes, sugar, glucose, and fats are suspended. It also conveys a number of important hormones, is the medium for circulating minerals and vitamins, and is the means of chemical communication between different parts of the body.

Platelet One of many small, colorless, granular cells that originate in the bone marrow and clump together for blood clotting; also called thrombocytes.

Pleura The delicate membrane that encloses each lung and lines the inside of the chest wall.

Pleural effusion A buildup of excess fluid in the space between the two pleural, membranes that surround each lung.

Pleurisy A painful disorder in which the pleurae, the two-ply membranes that enclose each lung and line the chest cavity, become inflamed.

Polyunsaturated fat A type of unsaturated fat; diets high in unsaturated fat lower serum cholesterol levels.

Posterior Behind or in the back part of.

Postmenopausal A term referring to a woman who has completed menopause.

Postpartum After childbirth.

Priapism A prolonged, often painful erection that is not associated with sexual stimulation and which often results from the use of medications that affect the central nervous system or from diseases such as sickle cell disease or leukemia.

Progesterone A female sex hormone, made in the ovaries, that is chiefly responsible for preparing the uterus for the fertilized egg and for the growth and development of the fetus. It is sometimes added to estrogen replacement therapy to decrease the risk of cancer of the uterus.

Progestin A synthetic form of progesterone used in hormone replacement therapy.

Prognosis A forecast of the course that a disease or disorder will take and of the nature of recovery.

Prolactin A hormone made in the pituitary gland that directly stimulates the mammary glands to produce milk during and following pregnancy.

Prolapse A term used to describe an organ or other structure that has shifted out of its normal place in the body, especially sinking down through a natural opening.

Prostate gland A gland surrounding the neck of the bladder in men, that secretes a fluid that makes up one-third of the volume of semen.

Prostate specific antigen (PSA) test A blood test, measuring the level of a protein produced by the prostate cells, used to detect diseases of the prostate gland.

Prosthesis An artificial body part, such as that used to replace an arm.

Prosthodontist A dental specialist who creates artificial replacements for missing or defective teeth, such as crowns, bridgework, and dentures.

Protein A group of organic compounds composed of amino acids that are essential for growth and repair of internal organs, blood, muscles, bone, and skin and for the formation of antibodies, hormones, and enzymes.

Pruritus Itching.

Psychosis A mental condition characterized by being out of touch with reality.

Ptosis Drooping of upper eyelid or prolapse of a body part.

Pulmonary Relating to the lung.

Pulmonary function test A breathing test performed to assess how well the lungs function.

Pulmonary valve The valve that regulates blood flow between the right ventricle and the outflow to the lungs.

Pupil The dark area (actually an opening) in the middle of the iris that contracts to limit the amount of light entering the eye or expands to allow more light to enter.

Purulent Creating or containing pus.

Pus A thick, yellowish fluid usually found at the site of certain infections and containing white blood cells and bacteria.

Pustule An elevation of the skin containing pus, often with an inflamed base.

Pylorus A ring of muscle between the stomach and the duodenum that slowly releases tiny particles of food (smaller than 1 mm in diameter) into the small intestine.

Radiation A type of energy found in x-rays and ultraviolet light.

Radon A colorless and odorless radioactive gas—sometimes escaping from the ground and entering homes through basement foundations and floor drains—that may increase the risk of lung cancer after long-term exposure.

Rectum The storage chamber for stool located at the lowest part of the colon.

Red blood cell One of the cells, produced mainly in bone marrow, that shuttles oxygen from the lungs through the bloodstream to the tissues and returns carbon dioxide (a waste product of cell activity) to the lungs where it is breathed out; also called erythrocytes.

Reflex An involuntary response to a stimulus.

Relapse The reappearance of a disease that was thought to have abated.

Renal Relating to the kidneys.

Renewing cell A type of cell, such as that found in the skin, hair, and blood, that reproduces itself continually throughout life.

Retina The thin layer of transparent tissue, containing millions of light-sensing rods and cones, that lines the inside of the eye; the retina senses light and sends it for processing to the brain via the optic nerve. See also Cone, Rod.

Rhinoplasty A surgical procedure involving the removal of bone and cartilage from the nose in order to allow the nose to be reshaped and reconstructed to create a smaller or narrower nose or to improve breathing.

Rod One of many nerve cells, located in the retina, that senses light and converts it into electrical signals that are sent to the brain via the optic nerve.

Saccule A jelly-filled organ lined with sensitive, motion detector hair cells that forms part of the balancing mechanism of the ear.

Sacrum A triangle-shaped bone, composed of five vertebrae joined together, located at the base of the spine.

Sarcoma A tumor, usually malignant, that originates in the connective tissues, especially in muscles, bones, and cartilage.

Saturated fat One of two main types of fat, found chiefly in foods that come from animals and certain vegetable oils, that raises blood cholesterol levels, leading to heart disease and other chronic conditions.

Scapula The shoulder blade.

Sciatic nerve The largest nerve in the body. It exits the spine in the lower back, enters the soft tissues of the buttock through the sciatic notch, and then supplies the legs.

Sclera The white, opaque outer membrane that covers most of the surface of the eyeball, with the exception of the portion covered by the cornea.

Scrotum The sac in which the testicles are suspended.

Sebaceous gland One of a number of oil-producing glands found throughout the skin, except for the palms and the soles, that helps to keep skin soft and moist and gives hair its glossy appearance.

Sebum The skin-lubricating oil produced by sebaceous glands.

Semen A mixture of sperm and fluid secreted by the prostate gland and seminal vesicles.

Semicircular canals Fluid-filled chambers within the balance portion of the inner ear that help to maintain posture during head rotation.

Sensorineural hearing loss A loss of hearing due to a disorder of the sensory mechanism of the cochlea or the acoustic nerve.

Sepsis An infection of the blood by disease-causing microorganisms, usually resulting from an infected wound or tissue.

Septic shock An advanced state of infection, usually occurring in the presence of a wound, that may cause multiple organ failure and dangerously low blood pressure. Septic shock is the major cause of death in people who suffer severe burns.

Serotonin A neurotransmitter that helps to regulate mood and sleeping patterns. Serotonin also inhibits gastric juices and plays a role in the production of the hormone melatonin.

Sexual dysfunction The loss of sexual function or desire.

Shunt A channel designed to reroute the flow of fluid from one course to another.

Small intestine A loosely coiled, three-part tube, about an inch in diameter and stretching to more than 20 feet, that absorbs nutrients from food and drink through undulating fin-gerlike projections called villi that carpet the intestinal lining; also called the small bowel.

Specialized cell See Differentiated cell.

Speculum An instrument used to hold apart the walls of an organ, such as the vagina or the nose, during an examination.

Spinal column The collective name for the 33 vertebrae that surround and protect the spinal cord.

Spirometer A device used to measure the amount of air leaving the lungs and the speed with which it is exhaled.

Sprain The tearing of a ligament.

Squamous cell A flat, scale-like cell on the surface of the skin.

Stem cell See Renewing cell.

Stenosis An abnormal narrowing or constriction of an opening or channel in the body.

Sternum The breast bone (where the ribs meet in the center).

Strain Damage to a muscle or tendon due to overstretching.

Stroke Damage to part of the brain caused by lack of blood supply, usually due to a blockage in an artery or the rupturing of a blood vessel.

Subcutaneous Under the skin.

Subluxation The partial movement of a bone out of its joint.

Sunblock A cream, liquid, or ointment used to protect the skin from the potentially harmful effects of the sun's ultraviolet rays.

Synapse A specialized area at one end of a nerve cell, containing tiny sacs of neurotransmitters, that allows that cell to communicate with other nerve cells.

Syncope A sudden loss of consciousness.

Synovial fluid The transparent fluid within joints that keeps them lubricated.

Syrup of ipecac A medication used to induce vomiting.

Tachycardia An abnormally rapid heartbeat.

Tar The sticky, tar-like residue of the thousands of compounds found in tobacco smoke.

Teletherapy See External beam radiotherapy.

Tendon A tough, flexible fibrous tissue bundle that anchors muscle to bone, varying in size from the delicate strings of tissue in the minute muscles of the hands to the heavy tendons, thick as ropes, that anchor the thigh or calf muscles.

Testicle One of a pair of egg-shaped structures about 2 in. in size that hang suspended in the scrotal sac and are responsible for producing sperm cells and male reproductive hormones such as testosterone.

Testosterone A male reproductive sex hormone made in the testicles.

Thrombocytes See Platelets.

Thrombocytopenia An abnormally low level of circulating platelets.

Thrombocytosis An abnormally high level of circulating platelets.

Thrombus A blood clot.

Thrush A yeast infection in the mouth.

Thyroid gland A butterfly-shaped gland, lying across the base of the neck in front of the windpipe, that helps to regulate various processes in the body through its production of thyroid hormone and calcitonin.

Thyroid hormone A hormone made in the thyroid gland that helps to regulate growth and development, basal metabolic rate, body temperature, menstrual cycles, and the body's use of carbohydrate, protein, and cholesterol.

Tibia A lower leg bone.

Tinnitus Ringing in the ears.

Tonsils Immune defense tissues—the palatine tonsils are located at the back of the throat and the lingual tonsils at the base of the tongue—designed to identify and deactivate infectious bacteria.

Torsion Twist.

Toxin A poisonous substance.

Trabecular bone A type of bone that is spongelike, making up 15% of all bone.

Trachea The windpipe.

Transcutaneous electrical nerve stimulator (TENS) A device that transmits low-level electrical current through adhesive patches to reduce spasm and pain.

Transient ischemic attack A small stroke in which symptoms last less than 24 hours.

Transverse Lying or placed across.

Tricuspid valve The valve that controls blood flow between the right atrium and right ventricle.

Triglyceride The principal fat in the blood.

Tumor An abnormal growth of cells that may be benign or cancerous.

Tympanic membrane The eardrum.

Ulna The larger of the two main bones of the forearm.

Ulnar styloid The tip of the ulna.

Ultrasonography See Ultrasound.

Ultrasound A painless process that involves taking pictures of parts of the body using high-frequency sound waves.

Undifferentiated cell A type of cell, such as that found in the liver, kidneys, and glands, that has a limited ability to reproduce; also called a committed cell.

Unsaturated fat One of two main kinds of fat. Unsaturated fat may have a healthy effect on the heart (when used in moderation) by lowering cholesterol levels.

Urea A nitrogen-containing waste product, eliminated in the urinary tract, that is produced when protein is broken down.

Ureter The tube connecting the kidneys to the bladder.

Urethra The tube that conducts urine from the bladder to the outside of the body.

Urinary tract The structures in the body responsible for the production and release of urine. The urinary tract includes the kidneys, ureters, bladder, and urethra.

Urticaria See Hives.

Uterus A small (about 2.5 to 3 in. wide in the nonpregnant state), hollow organ shaped like an upside-down pear with thick muscular walls wherein the embryo and fetus develop during pregnancy; also called the womb.

Utricle A jelly-filled organ lined with sensitive, motion detector cells that forms part of the balancing mechanism of the ear.

Vaccine A medication, derived from killed or weakened microorganisms or manufactured materials, used to prompt the body to form infection-fighting antibodies to prevent disease.

Vagina The muscular canal, about 5 in. long, that connects the uterus to the outside of the body.

Varicose Abnormally swollen, usually in reference to veins.

Vas deferens The sperm passageway between the testicles and urethra.

Vascular Relating to the blood vessels, arteries, and veins.

Vasectomy Procedure in which the sperm passageway from the testicles to the urethra is cut in two and the ends sealed shut in order to prevent sperm from entering the ejaculate.

Vasopressin See Antidiuretic hormone (ADH).

Vein A blood vessel that transports blood back to the heart.

Vena cava The two large veins that collect oxygen-poor blood returning from the lower and upper parts of the body.

Venous Relating to the veins.

Ventricle Either of the major pumping chambers of the heart, located below the atria; also refers to any of the fluid-filled cavities of the brain.

Ventricular septum The wall separating the right and left ventricles.

Venule A small vein.

Vertebra One of the 33 bones of the spine.

Vertigo The sensation of spinning in the absence of head or body movement, sometimes accompanied by motion sickness.

Vesicle A small, fluid-containing sac in the body or a small blister on the skin.

Vestibule The portion of the inner ear behind the cochlea and in front of the semicircular canals.

Virus A package of genetic material (DNA or RNA) bundled in a protein packet that exists and replicates by invading and hijacking the machinery of living cells such as those of plants, humans, or animals.

Viscosity The resistance of a substance, usually a fluid, to flow.

Visual acuity The sharpness of a person's vision.

Visual cortex The area of the brain in which electrical impulses created by the retina are translated into mental images.

Visualization The use of consciously created mental images to control pain, relieve stress, increase blood flow to certain areas of the body, and slow heartbeat.

Vitamin One of a group of organic substances that are necessary in certain amounts to maintain health and ensure proper development and functioning of the body.

Vitreous humor A clear, gelatinous substance that nourishes the lens of the eye.

Vocal cord One of a pair of strong bands of elastic tissue, covered with a thin mucous membrane, that span the windpipe from front to back and produce sound when vibrated by air from the lungs.

Vulva The collective name for the mons pubis (the mound-shaped tissues covering the pubic bone), the labia, and the clitoris.

Wart A growth on the skin caused by a viral infection.

Weight-bearing exercise Exercise that puts stress on muscle and bone, increasing muscle mass and bone strength.

White blood cell One of the cells, produced in bone marrow and other parts of the body, that seeks out and destroys disease-causing microorganisms or other substances that have invaded the body; also called leukocytes.

Womb See Uterus.

Zygote A single, unique cell created from the union of sperm and egg from which the nearly 10 trillion cells that make up an adult are ultimately derived.

Growth Charts

Different children grow at different rates, but the rate of growth for any individual child should follow a steady course. The growth charts on the following pages are useful tools to chart a child's changes in height and weight as he or she grows.* These charts are based on growth rates published by the National Center for Health Statistics (NCHS) for children from birth to 36 months (boys on page 1584; girls on page 1585) and for children from 2 to 18 years (boys on page 1586; girls on page 1587). The 50 percent line represents the average rate of growth, but the natural rate of growth for many children is above or below this percentile. If a child consistently dips below his or her own percentile rate of growth and does not follow a steady upward course, you should speak to your pediatrician.

To find your child's position on a growth chart, first select the chart appropriate for your child's age and gender. Each chart shows the rate of growth for both height (length/stature, upper curves) and weight (lower curves), and these two indicators of growth are charted separately. Find your child's height (in. or cm) and age (months or years) on the chart; the point where these two values meet is your child's rate of growth for height (length/stature) for that age. To plot your child's rate of growth for weight, find the point where your child's weight (lb or kg) and age (months or years) intersect. Your child's growth rate for height may be different from his or her growth rate for weight.

Using the charts over a period of time will indicate whether your child's height and weight growth rates are keeping to the same percentiles or fluctuating from them.

---

*Growth charts courtesy of Ross Products Division, Abbott Laboratories, Columbus, OH; used with permission.

Length and Weight Percentiles for Boys—Birth to 36 Months

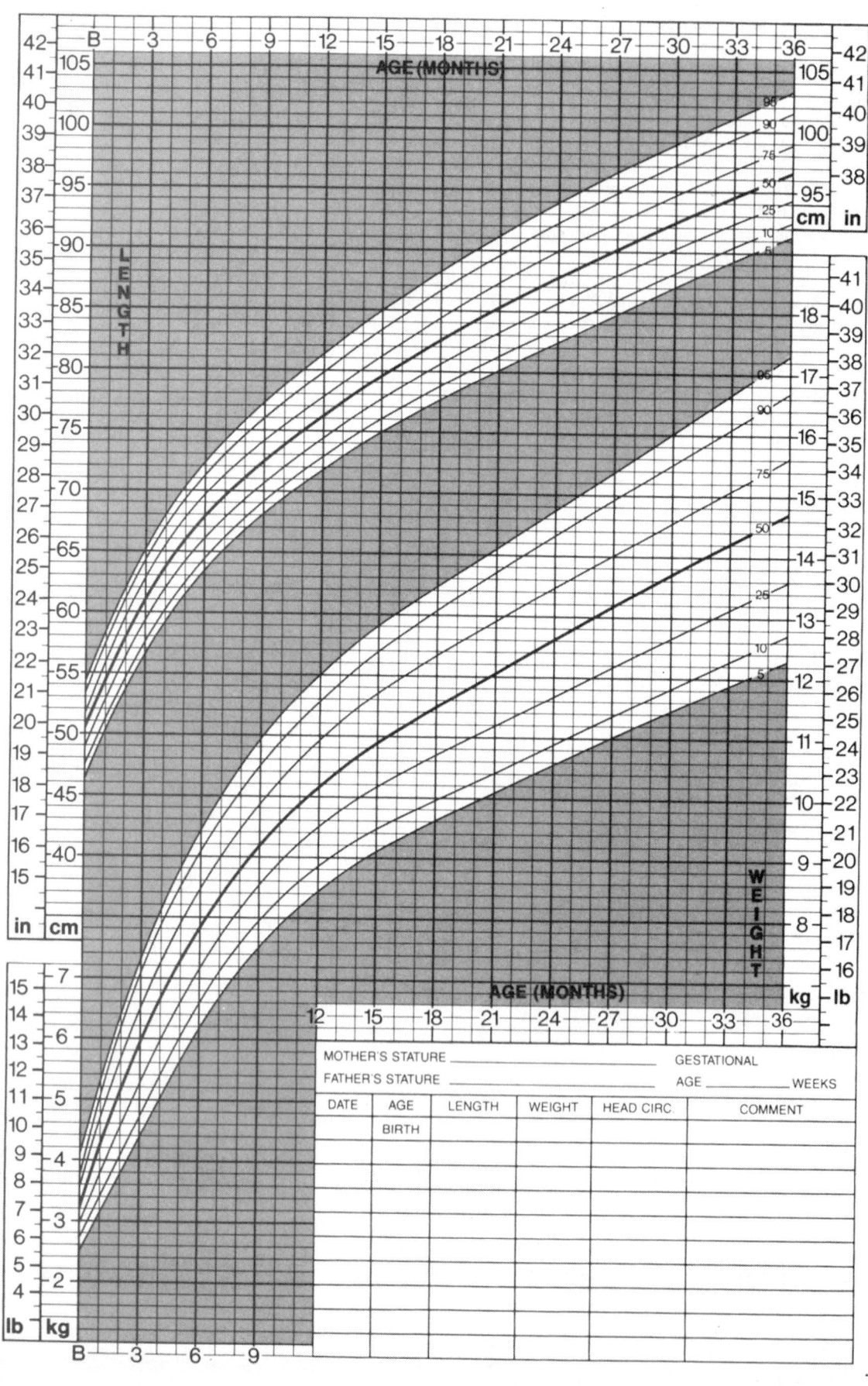

Length and Weight Percentiles for Girls—Birth to 36 Months

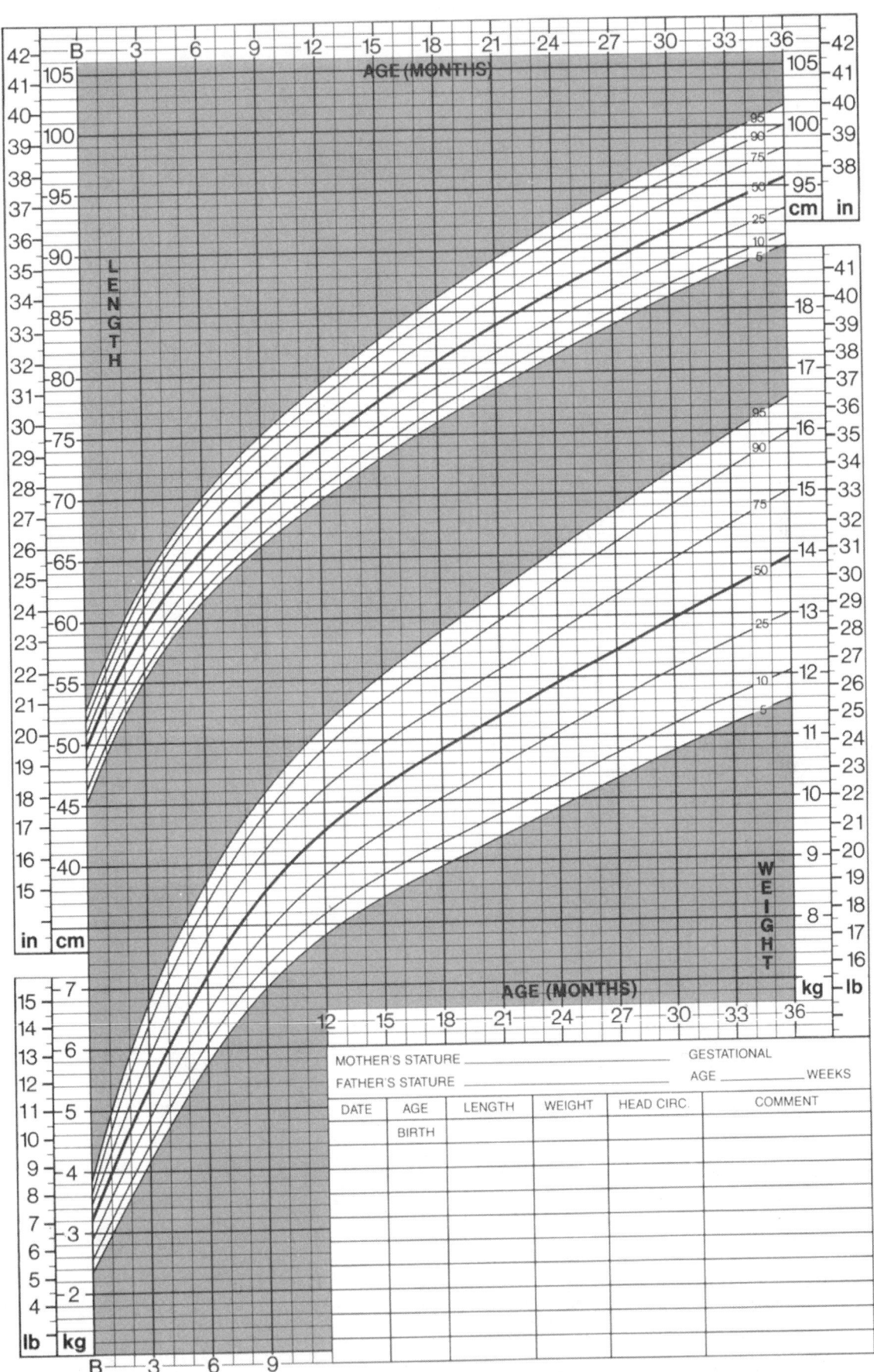

Stature and Weight Percentiles for Boys—2 to 18 Years

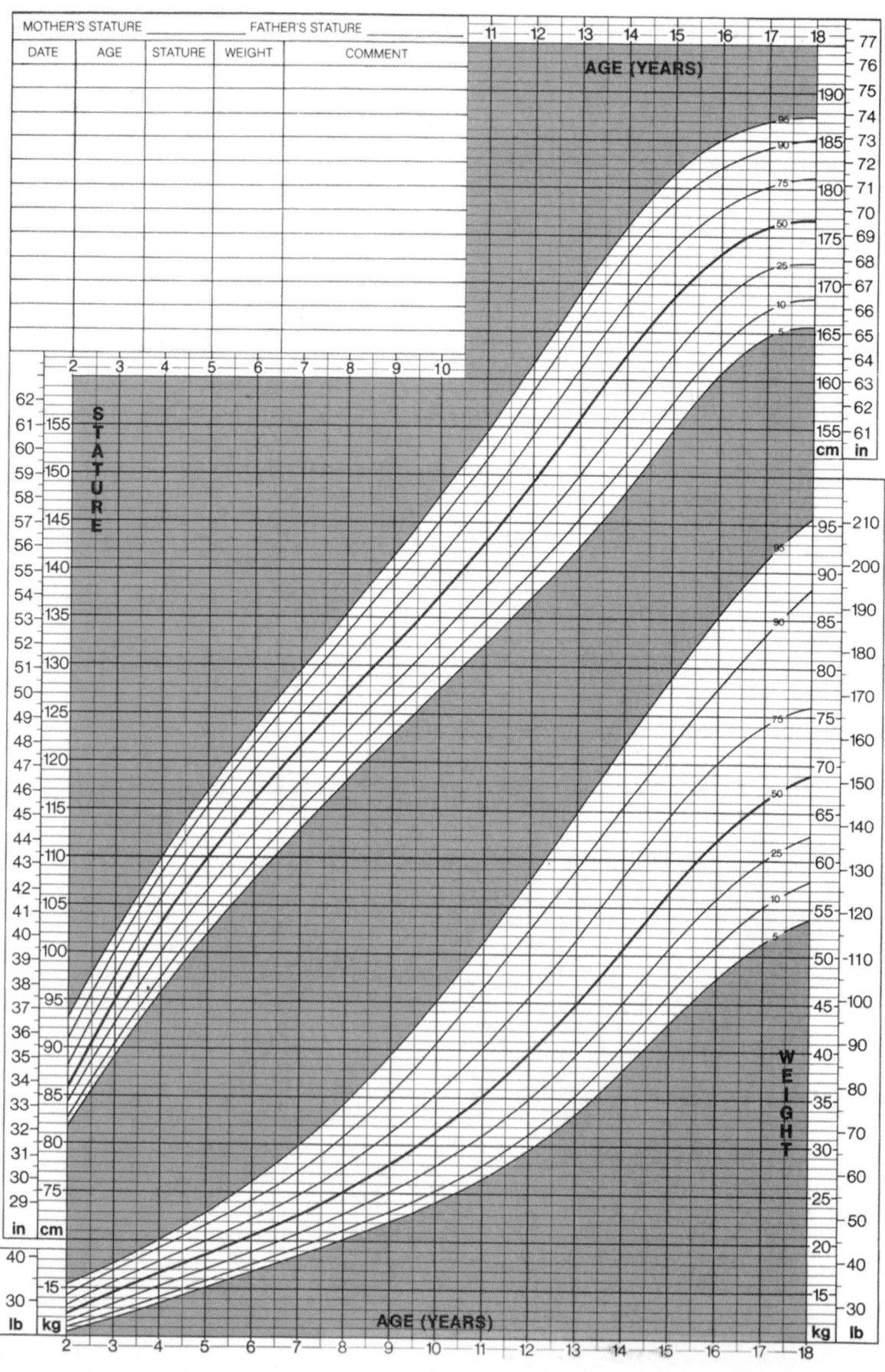

Stature and Weight Percentiles for Girls—2 to 18 Years

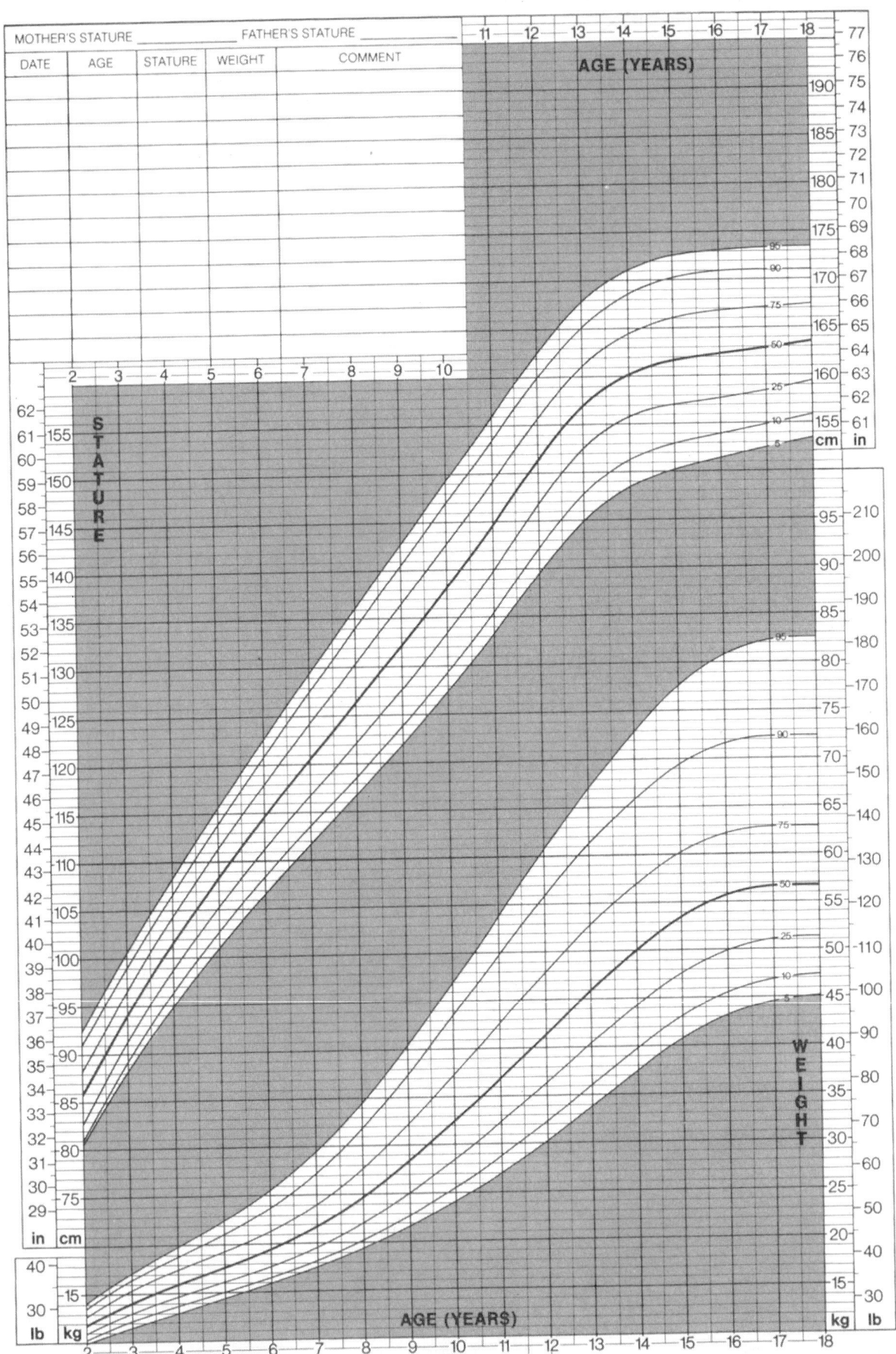

Living Wills and Advance Directives

Planning Your End-of-Life Care

Taking an active role in your health care also includes planning for the unthinkable. Every year, thousands of Americans are unable to make decisions about their health due to the effects of an accident or severe illness. These decisions often involve the use of life-sustaining machines or feeding tubes. You have an obligation to consider choices that may affect your end-of-life care. Planning for such a contingency ensures that your wishes will be carried out and that family or friends will not be forced to make difficult decisions about your treatment. You can make these decisions ahead of time through the use of health care agents, living wills, or advance directives. Examples of living will and advance directive forms appear on the next few pages (see also Chapter 35).

A Note on the Forms

The forms that appear on the next few pages are valid in the state of Maryland and are provided as examples only. These forms may or may not be valid in other states, depending on the laws there. While most states honor living wills and advance directives regardless of the origin of the forms, some require their own forms to be used. To obtain forms specific to your state, consult with your doctor or lawyer, local hospital, or senior citizen center.

When filling out your form, put your initials next to statements that you agree with and draw lines through the statements that you do not agree with. Do not use checkmarks or other symbols. While these forms do need to be signed by witnesses, most states do not require notarization, but check with your lawyer to see if your state requires notarization.

What is a Health Care Agent?

A health care agent is someone who makes decisions about your health when you are unable to do so. You can choose anyone age 18 or over to be your health care agent except someone who works for a health care facility in which you are receiving care. Your health care agent will be your voice during a health crisis and make sure that your treatment preferences are honored by a doctor or hospital. If you choose to designate a health care agent, you should give that person very clear instructions regarding your care in the event of a health crisis. The role of your health care agent is to carry out your wishes concerning end-of-life care. This person will not have any power over your financial or other affairs. In order to appoint a health care agent, fill out Part A of the advance directive form (see page 1591).

Living Will, Advance Directives, and Organ Donation Form

Whether or not you name a health care agent, you can use a living will or advance directive to notify a doctor or hospital of your treatment preferences in the event that you have an accident or severe illness that prevents you from making decisions about your care. You may fill out all or part

---

The forms on pages 1591 to 1597 are provided courtesy of the state of Maryland, Department of Legislative Reference, General Assembly of Maryland, and Office of the Attorney General.

of a living will or advance directive. You may also create your own versions of these forms, written the way you want. A living will or advance directive must always be signed by two witnesses. A doctor or hospital employee may be a witness but if you name a health care agent that person cannot be a witness. In addition, at least one of your witnesses may not be someone who may benefit financially from your death. These forms usually do not need to be notarized and you do not need a lawyer to fill them out. Your doctor may be able to explain some of the medical issues if they are not clear to you. Once you have created a living will or advance directive, you should give a copy to your doctor, health care agent, the hospital in which you are receiving care, and family members or close friends. Living wills and advance directives never expire, though you can change or revoke them at any time. It is a good idea to review your living will or advance directive periodically to make sure that it reflects your wishes. If you change or revoke it, you should notify all those who have a copy.

THE LIVING WILL

The living will is the shorter of the two forms (see page 1595). It allows you to select or reject life-sustaining procedures that may be used in the event that you have a terminal condition (a condition that ultimately results in death) or are in a persistent vegetative state. A persistent vegetative state is a state of permanent unconsciousness—what most people refer to as a coma. For example, a living will can be used to decide whether or not you wish to receive nutrition through an intravenous (IV) line. A living will cannot be used to name a health care agent or to make decisions regarding any health crisis beyond the two types mentioned above.

THE ADVANCE DIRECTIVE

An advance directive is more broad in scope. It has two parts, Part A (see page 1591) and Part B (see page 1593). Part A can be used to name a health care agent. Like a living will, Part B of an advance directive can be used to make decisions about your treatment in the event that you have a terminal condition or are in a coma. Part B can also be used to specify what life-sustaining procedures will be used if you have an end-stage condition. An end-stage condition is an advanced and progressive condition—such as advanced Alzheimer's disease—that cannot be cured and which makes you physically dependent on others. Unlike a living will, Part B of an advance directive can be used to make health care decisions that do not involve life-sustaining procedures. If you decide to make decisions about life-sustaining procedures in Part B of an advance directive, you do not need to fill out the living will form.

THE ORGAN DONATION FORM

The organ donation form (see page 1597) may be completed and attached to your living will or advance directive. This form allows you to make an anatomic gift to someone in need of an organ or tissue transplant. Many states also include such a form on their state driver's license. This form needs to be signed by two witnesses (see above). Speak to your doctor or lawyer for more information regarding organ donation (see also Chapter 35).

ADVANCE DIRECTIVE

PART A
APPOINTMENT OF HEALTH CARE AGENT

(Optional Form)

(Cross through this whole part of the form if you do not want to appoint a health care agent to make health care decisions for you. If you do want to appoint an agent, cross through any items in the form that you do not want to apply.)

1. I, _____ ,

   residing at _____

   _____

   appoint the following individual as my agent to make health care decisions for me:

   _____

   _____

   (Full Name, Address and Telephone Number of Agent)

   Optional: If this agent is unavailable or is unable or unwilling to act as my agent, then I appoint the following person to act in this capacity:

   _____

   _____

   (Full Name, Address and Telephone Number of Back-up Agent)

2. My agent has full power and authority to make health care decisions for me, including the power to:

A. Request, receive, and review any information, oral or written, regarding my physical or mental health, including, but not limited to, medical and hospital records, and consent to disclosure of this information;

B. Employ and discharge my health care providers;

C. Authorize my admission to or discharge from (including transfer to another facility) any hospital, hospice, nursing home, adult home, or other medical care facility; and

D. Consent to the provision, withholding, or withdrawal of health care, including, in appropriate circumstances, life-sustaining procedures.

Page 1 of 4

3. The authority of my agent is subject to the following provisions and limitations:

    _____

    _____

4. If I am pregnant, my agent shall follow these specific instructions:

    _____

    _____

5. My agent's authority becomes operative (*initial* only the one option that applies):

    _____   *When my attending physician and a second physician determine that I am incapable of making an informed decision regarding my health care; or*

    _____   *When this document is signed.*

6. My agent is to make health care decisions for me based on the health care instructions I give in this document and on my wishes as otherwise known to my agent. If my wishes are unknown or unclear, my agent is to make health care decisions for me in accordance with my best interest, to be determined by my agent after considering the benefits, burdens, and risks that might result from a given treatment or course of treatment, or from the withholding or withdrawal of a treatment or course of treatment.

7. My agent shall not be liable for the costs of care based solely on this authorization.

By signing below, I indicate that I am emotionally and mentally competent to make this appointment of a health care agent and that I understand its purpose and effect.

_____   _____
(Date)   (Signature of Declarant)

The declarant signed or acknowledged signing this appointment of a health care agent in my presence and, based upon my personal observation, appears to be a competent individual.

_____   _____
(Witness)   (Witness)

_____   _____

_____   _____

_____   _____

(Signatures and Addresses of Two Witnesses)

Page 2 of 4

ADVANCE DIRECTIVE

PART B
HEALTH CARE INSTRUCTIONS

(Optional Form)

*(Cross through this whole part of the form if you do not want to use it to give health care instructions. If you do want to complete this portion of the form, **initial** those statements you want to be included in the document and **cross through** those statements that do not apply.)*

If I am incapable of making an informed decision regarding my health care, I direct my health care providers to follow my instructions as set forth below. **(Initial** *all those that apply.)*

1. If my death from a terminal condition is imminent and even if life-sustaining procedures are used there is no reasonable expectation of my recovery:

   _____ *I direct that my life not be extended by life-sustaining procedures, including the administration of nutrition and hydration artificially.*

   _____ *I direct that my life not be extended by life-sustaining procedures, except that, if I am unable to take food by mouth, I wish to receive nutrition and hydration artificially.*

2. If I am in a persistent vegetative state, that is, if I am not conscious and am not aware of my environment nor able to interact with others, and there is no reasonable expectation of my recovery:

   _____ *I direct that my life not be extended by life-sustaining procedures, including the administration of nutrition and hydration artificially.*

   _____ *I direct that my life not be extended by life-sustaining procedures, except that, if I am unable to take food by mouth, I wish to receive nutrition and hydration artificially.*

3. If I have an end-stage condition, that is, a condition caused by injury, disease, or illness, as a result of which I have suffered severe and permanent deterioration indicated by incompetency and complete physical dependency and for which, to a reasonable degree of medical certainty, treatment of the irreversible condition would be medically ineffective:

   _____ *I direct that my life not be extended by life-sustaining procedures, including the administration of nutrition and hydration artificially.*

Page 3 of 4

_____   *I direct that my life not be extended by life-sustaining procedures, except that, if I am unable to take food and water by mouth, I wish to receive nutrition and hydration artificially.*

4. _____   I direct that, no matter what my condition, medication to relieve pain and suffering not be given to me if the medication would shorten my remaining life.

5. _____   I direct that, no matter what my condition, I be given all available medical treatment in accordance with accepted health care standards.

6. If I am pregnant, my decision concerning life-sustaining procedures shall be modified as follows:

_____

_____

_____

7. I direct (in the following space, indicate any other instructions regarding receipt or nonreceipt of any health care):

_____

_____

_____

By signing below, I indicate that I am emotionally and mentally competent to make this Advance Directive and that I understand the purpose and effect of this document.

_____   _____
(Date)   (Signature of Declarant)

The declarant signed or acknowledged signing these health care instructions in my presence and, based upon my personal observation, appears to be a competent individual.

_____   _____
(Witness)   (Witness)

_____   _____

_____   _____

_____   _____

(Signatures and Addresses of Two Witnesses)

Page 4 of 4

LIVING WILL

(Optional Form)

If I am not able to make an informed decision regarding my health care, I direct my health care providers to follow my instructions as set forth below. (***Initial*** *those statements you wish to be included in the document and **cross through** those statements which do not apply.)*

A. If my death from a terminal condition is imminent and even if life-sustaining procedures are used there is no reasonable expectation of my recovery:

_____   *I direct that my life not be extended by life-sustaining procedures, including the administration of nutrition and hydration artificially.*

_____   *I direct that my life not be extended by life-sustaining procedures, except that, if I am unable to take food by mouth, I wish to receive nutrition and hydration artificially.*

_____   *I direct that, even in a terminal condition, I be given all available medical treatment in accordance with accepted health care standards.*

B. If I am in a persistent vegetative state, that is, if I am not conscious and am not aware of my environment nor able to interact with others, and there is no reasonable expectation of my recovery within a medically appropriate period:

_____   *I direct that my life not be extended by life-sustaining procedures, including the administration of nutrition and hydration artificially.*

_____   *I direct that my life not be extended by life-sustaining procedures, except that, if I am unable to take in food by mouth, I wish to receive nutrition and hydration artificially.*

_____   *I direct that I be given all available medical treatment in accordance with accepted health care standards.*

C. If I am pregnant, my decision concerning life-sustaining procedures shall be modified as follows:

_____

_____

_____

By signing below, I indicate that I am emotionally and mentally competent to make this Living Will and that I understand its purpose and effect.

_____   _____
           (Date)   (Signature of Declarant)

The declarant signed or acknowledged signing this Living Will in my presence and, based upon my personal observation, the declarant appears to be a competent individual.

_____   _____
          (Witness)   (Witness)

_____   _____

_____   _____

_____   _____

(Signatures and Addresses of Two Witnesses)

ORGAN DONATION ADDENDUM

(Note: If you want to be an organ donor, you can attach this page to your living will or advance directive. Sign it and have it witnessed.)

I direct that if I am brain dead, an anatomical gift be offered on my behalf to a patient in need of an organ or tissue transplant. If a transplant occurs, I want artificial heart/lung support devices to be continued on my behalf only until organ or tissue suitability of the patient is confirmed and organ or tissue recovery has taken place.

By signing below, I indicate that I am emotionally and mentally competent to make this organ donation addendum and that I understand the purpose and effect of this document.

_____   _____
(Date)   (Signature of Declarant)

The declarant signed or acknowledged signing this organ donation addendum in my presence and based upon my personal observation appears to be a competent individual.

_____   _____
(Witness)   (Witness)

(Signatures of Two Witnesses)

Measurement Conversions

CUSTOMARY MEASURE	=	METRIC MEASURE

Length

1 inch	2.54 centimeters (cm)
1 foot	0.3 meters (m)
1 yard	0.9 m
1 mile	1.6 kilometer (km)

Area

1 square inch	6.5 square cm (cm^2)
1 square foot	0.09 square meters (m^2)
1 square yard	0.8 m^2
1 square mile	2.6 square kilometers (km^2)

Mass

1 ounce	28 grams (g)
1 pound	0.45 kilograms (kg)

Volume

1 teaspoon	5 milliliters (mL)
1 tablespoon	15 mL
1 fluid ounce	30 mL
1 cup	0.24 liters (L)
1 US pint	0.47 L
1 US quart	0.95 L
1 US gallon	3.8 L
1 cubic foot	0.03 cubic meters (m^3)
1 cubic yard	0.76 m^3

To convert metric units to customary measure, divide the metric unit by
its conversion from a single customary unit (right-hand column). For example:

5 centimeters = 5 ÷ 2.54 = 2 inches (rounded off) *and*

10 kilometers = 10 ÷ 1.6 = 6.25 miles.

CONVERTING TEMPERATURE

Fahrenheit to Centigrade (Celsius)   °F − 32 × 0.556 = °C

Centigrade (Celsius) to Fahrenheit   °C ÷ 0.556 + 32 = °F

To convert Fahrenheit degrees to Centigrade degrees, subtract 32 from the Fahrenheit value and multiply the result by 0.556. For example:

$$72°F − 32 = 40 × 0.556 = 22°C \text{ (rounded off)}.$$

To convert Centigrade degrees to Fahrenheit degrees, divide the Centigrade degrees by 0.556 and add 32 to the result. For example:

$$22°C ÷ 0.556 = 40 \text{ (rounded off)} + 32 = 72°F.$$

COOKING MEASUREMENTS

1 teaspoon	=	⅙ fluid ounce
3 teaspoons	=	1 tablespoon
1 tablespoon	=	½ fluid ounce
12 tablespoons (dry)	=	1 cup
16 tablespoons (wet)	=	1 cup
1 cup	=	8 fluid ounces
1 pint	=	2 cups or 16 fluid ounces
2 pints	=	1 quart
4 quarts	=	1 gallon

Laboratory Tests

Below are the normal values of commonly ordered laboratory tests. The range of normal values can vary depending on individual laboratories. If you have laboratory tests performed, check with that laboratory for the correct range of normal values.

COMMONLY ORDERED LABORATORY TESTS AND THEIR REFERENCE VALUES

LABORATORY TESTS	REFERENCE VALUES
Hematology	
White blood cell count	$5000-10,000$ mm^3
Differential	
Neutrophils	40–60%
Lymphocytes	20–40%
Monocytes	4–8%
Eosinophils	1–3%
Basophils	around 1%
Red blood cell count	
Male	$4.3-5.7$ m/mm^3
Female	$3.8-5.1$ m/mm^3
Reticulocyte count	$25-75 \times 10^3$ µL
Hemoglobin	$12.0-15.0$ g/dL
Hematocrit	36.0–46.0%
Platelet count	150,000–450,000
Erythrocyte sedimentation rate	0–20 mm/h
Prothrombin time (PT)	less than 2 sec deviation from control
Activated partial thromboplastin time (APTT)	25–35 sec
Diagnostic Immunology	
Antinuclear antibodies (ANA)	negative at a 1:8 dilution of serum
C3 complement level	$1200-1500$ µg/mL
C4 complement level	$350-600$ µg/mL
Rheumatoid factor	less than 1:80 dilution of serum (agglutination method) less than 60 (nephelometric method)
VDRL test for syphilis	negative
Chemistry*	
Acid phosphatase	$0.0-0.6$ U/L
Albumin	$3.5-5.0$ g/dL
Alkaline phosphatase	$50-120$ U/L
Amylase	$25-85$ U/L
alpha$_1$-Fetoprotein	less than 10 ng/mL
Vitamin B$_{12}$ level	$160-950$ pg/mL
Bicarbonate	$20-29$ mEq/L
Bilirubin direct	less than 0.2 mg/dL
Bilirubin total	$0.3-1.2$ mg/dL
Blood urea nitrogen (BUN)	$7-20$ mg/dL
Calcium (total)	$8.2-10.2$ mg/dL

*Serum, unless otherwise indicated.

LABORATORY TESTS	CONVENTIONAL UNITS
Chemistry (Continued)	
Chloride	96–106 mEq/L
Creatine kinase	
Male	38–174 U/L
Female	26–140 U/L
Creatine clearance (urine)	75–125 mL/min
Creatinine	0.8–1.4 mg/dL
Red blood cell folate level	166–640 ng/mL
Glucose	70–110 mg/dL
Glycosylated hemoglobin level	4–7%
Iron	60–150 µg/dL
Lactate dehydrogenase (LDH)	50–200 U/L
Lipase	14–280 mIU/mL
Lipid profile	
Total serum cholesterol	
Desirable	less than 200 mg/dL
Borderline	200–239 mg/dL
High	greater than or equal to 240 mg/dL
High-density lipoprotein cholesterol	
Male	35–65 mg/dL
Female	35–80 mg/dL
Low-density lipoprotein cholesterol	60–130 mg/dL
Triglycerides	10–190 mg/dL
Magnesium	
Serum	1.5–2.3 mg/dL
Phosphorus	
Serum	2.3–4.7 mg/dL
Urine	0.9–1.3 g/24 h
Potassium	3.5–5.0 mEq/L
Prostate-specific antigen (PSA)	less than 4.0 ng/mL
Parathyroid hormone (PTH)	10–50 pg/mL
Aspartate aminotransferase (SGOT)	10–30 U/L
Alanine aminotransferase (SGPT)	8–20 U/L
Sodium	136–142 mEq/L
Total protein	6.0–8.0 g/dL
Total triiodothyronine by radioimmunoassay (T3)	70–200 ng/dL
T3 resin uptake	25–35%
Total thyroxine by radioimmunoassay (T4)	5.5–12.5 µg/dL
Thyroid-stimulating hormone (TSH)	0.5–5.0 µIU/mL
Uric acid	4.0–8.5 mg/dL

Abbreviations key:

g/dL	grams per deciliter	mIU/mL	milli international units per milliliter
g/24 h	grams per 24 hours	mL/min	milliliters per minute
mEq/L	milliequivalents per liter	m/mm^3	millions of cells per cubic millimeter
µg/dL	micrograms per deciliter	mm/h	millimeters per hour
µg/mL	micrograms per milliliter	ng/dL	nanograms per deciliter
µIU/mL	micro international units per milliliter	ng/mL	nanograms per milliliter
µL	microliter	pg/mL	picograms per milliliter
mg/dL	milligrams per deciliter	U/L	units per liter

Index

Page numbers in boldface indicate primary discussion and those in italics indicate illustrations. Symptom main entries are printed in color, for quick access.

FAMILY HEALTH RECORD

Allergies

Family member   Allergy

_____

_____

_____

_____

_____

_____

_____

_____

_____

_____

_____

Medications taken

Family member   Medication

_____

_____

_____

_____

_____

_____

_____

_____

_____

_____

_____

_____

_____

FAMILY HEALTH RECORD

Illness record

Family member	Date	Remarks

Surgery record

Family member	Date	Remarks

FAMILY PHONE NUMBERS

Paramedics 911 or _____

Fire department _____

Police department _____

Poison control center _____

Pediatrician _____

Internist _____

Gynecologist _____

Dentist _____

Pharmacist _____

Electric company _____

Gas company _____

Insurance company _____

Mother at work _____

Father at work _____

Neighbor _____

Relative _____

_____

_____

_____

_____

_____

_____

_____

CONTROLLING SEVERE BLEEDING
(see page 380)

Using Direct Pressure (Wear latex gloves if you have them)

1. Place sterile gauze or the cleanest least fuzzy cloth available against the source of bleeding.

2. Apply firm pressure with your hands. This may be painful to the victim.

3. Apply a covering bandage over the gauze or cloth or have someone do this while you maintain pressure. Use the best available cloth you have and make sure that the cloth does not come into contact with the wound but only wraps around the wound to hold the dressing in place.

4. Maintain pressure on the wound until the bandage has been applied.

5. Knot the covering bandage directly over the wound and source of bleeding.

6. Do not remove the bandage. Leave this to EMS or other medical professionals.

7. If the wound bleeds through the dressing, enough pressure may not have been applied. Without removing the bandage, apply direct pressure again and put a second dressing and bandage over the first. This should control the bleeding.

8. If you have nothing to make into a bandage, maintain direct pressure with your hands until EMS arrives.

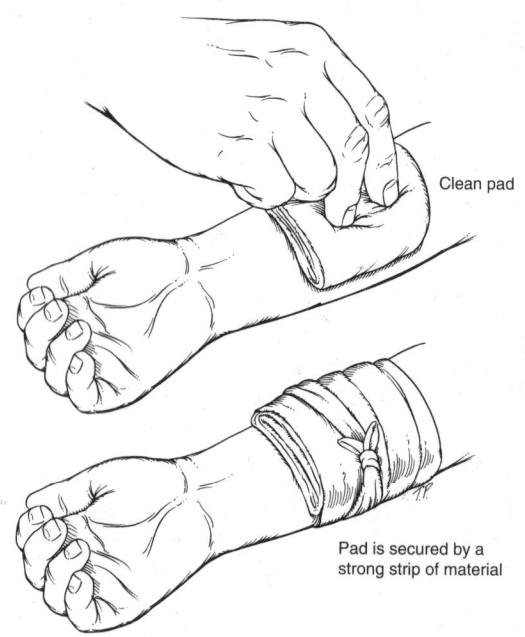

Clean pad

Pad is secured by a strong strip of material

Applying direct pressure and maintaining pressure.

Using Indirect Pressure

Use indirect pressure if direct pressure does not control the bleeding, you suspect a fracture, or there is an object embedded in the wound. Indirect pressure slows the blood flow to the wound with compression at locations other than the wound itself.

1. Use a finger to find the arterial pressure point closest to the wound (see illustration). If you are using indirect pressure in addition to direct pressure, maintain direct pressure throughout.

2. Apply pressure to the artery with your finger, gently pressing it toward the bone.

3. Maintain indirect pressure only long enough to control bleeding.

Using Tourniquets

Only use a tourniquet in cases of life-threatening bleeding, such as may accompany traumatic amputation (see page 390) or other uncontrollable arterial bleeding. *Improper use of a tourniquet may lead to further, serious injury including the destruction of tissue.*

1. Never use wire, rope, cable, or any other narrow cord, or anything that might cut into the skin. Tourniquets should ideally be at least 2 inches wide.

2. If you don't have an EMS tool kit containing a tourniquet, use your belt, shirt-sleeve, towel, or even duct tape. Be resourceful

3. Wrap the tourniquet tightly just above the wound.

4. If using cloth, try to knot it directly over the pressure point (see illustration), pressing the artery toward the bone.

5. Do *not* insert any sort of bar into the device to twist it tight.

6. Continue to apply direct pressure and indirect pressure if necessary.

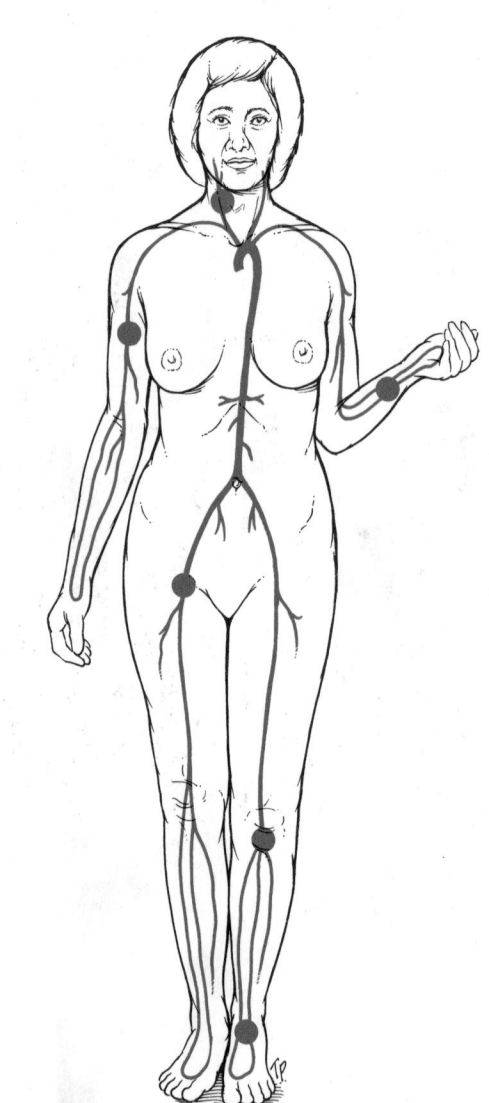

Circles show the arterial pressure points for applying indirect pressure.